New Oxford Textbook of

Psychiatry

VOLUME 1

New Oxford Textbook of Psychiatry

SECOND EDITION

Edited by

Michael G. Gelder

Emeritus Professor of Psychiatry, Warneford Hospital, University of Oxford, Oxford, UK

Nancy C. Andreasen

Director, Mental Health Clinical Research Centre, University of Iowa Hospital and Clinic, Iowa City, USA

Juan J. López-Ibor Jr.

Professor of Psychiatry, Complutense University, Madrid, Spain

and

John R. Geddes

Professor of Epidemiological Psychiatry University of Oxford, Warneford Hospital, Oxford, UK

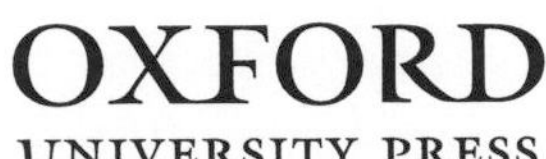

OXFORD
UNIVERSITY PRESS

Great Clarendon Street, Oxford OX2 6DP

Oxford University Press is a department of the University of Oxford.
It furthers the University's objective of excellence in research, scholarship,
and education by publishing worldwide in

Oxford New York

Auckland Cape Town Dar es Salaam Hong Kong Karachi
Kuala Lumpur Madrid Melbourne Mexico City Nairobi
New Delhi Shanghai Taipei Toronto

With offices in

Argentina Austria Brazil Chile Czech Republic France Greece
Guatemala Hungary Italy Japan Poland Portugal Singapore
South Korea Switzerland Thailand Turkey Ukraine Vietnam

Published in the United States
by Oxford University Press Inc., New York

First edition published 2000
Reprinted 2003

This edition published 2009

British Library Cataloguing in Publication Data
Data available

Library of Congress Cataloguing in Publication Data
Data available

Typeset in Cepha Imaging Pvt. Ltd., Bangalore, India
Printed in Italy on acid-free paper by Rotolito Lombarda SpA

ISBN 978-0-19-920669-8
ISBN 978-0-19-920669-8 (set)
ISBN 978-0-19-955992-3 (Volume 1)
ISBN 978-0-19-955993-0 (Volume 2)

10 9 8 7 6 5 4 3 2 1

Oxford University Press makes no representation, express or implied, that the drug dosages in this book are correct. Readers must therefore always check the product information and clinical procedures with the most up-to-date published product information and data sheets provided by the manufacturers and the most recent codes of conduct and safety regulations. The authors and the publishers do not accept responsibility or legal liability for any errors in the text or for the misuse or misapplication of material in this work. Except where otherwise stated, drug dosages and recommendations are for the non-pregnant adult who is not breast-feeding.

Preface to the second edition

This new edition, like the first, aims to present a comprehensive account of clinical psychiatry with reference to its scientific basis and to the ill person's perspective. As in the first edition, the authors are drawn from many countries, including the UK, the USA, 12 countries in continental Europe, and Australasia. The favourable reception of the first edition has led us to invite many of the original authors to revise their chapters for this second edition but 50 chapters are the work of new authors, many concerned with subjects that appeared in the first edition, while others are completely new. The forensic psychiatry section has the most new chapters, followed by the section on psychology as a scientific basis of psychiatry.

The overall plan of the book resembles that of the first edition (see preface to the 1st edition, reprinted on pages vii and viii). One important feature is that information about treatment appears in more than one place. The commonly used physical and psychological treatments are described in Section 6. Their use in the treatment of any particular disorder is considered in the chapter concerned with that disorder and the account is in two parts. The first part is a review of evidence about the effects of each of the treatments when used for that disorder. The second part, called Management, combines evidence from clinical trials with accumulated clinical experience to produce practical advice about the day to day care of people with the disorder.

Although much information can now be obtained from internet searches, textbooks are still needed to provide the comprehensive account of established knowledge into which new information can be fitted and against which recent findings can be evaluated. As well as seeking to provide an authoritative account of essential knowledge, each chapter in the new edition includes a brief list of sources of further information, including where appropriate, regularly updated web sites.

An essential component of good practice is the need to be aware of patients' perspectives, to respect their wishes, and to work with them, and often their families, as partners. The book opens with an important chapter on the experience of being a patient, and there are chapters on stigma, ethics, and the developing topic of values-based practice.

We are grateful to the following who advised us about parts of the book; Professor John Bancroft (Psychosexual Disorders), Professor Tom Burns (Social and Community Psychiatry), Professor William Fraser (Intellectual Disability), Professor Keith Hawton (Suicide and Deliberate Self Harm), Professor Susan Iversen (Psychology), Professor Robin Jacoby (Old Age Psychiatry), Professor Paul Mullen (Forensic Psychiatry), Sir Michael Rutter (Child and Adolescent Psychiatry), and Professor Gregory Stores (Sleep Disorders).

The editors

Preface to the first edition

Three themes can be discerned in contemporary psychiatry: the growing unity of the subject, the pace of scientific advance, and the growth of practice in the community. We have sought to reflect these themes in the *New Oxford Textbook of Psychiatry* and to present the state of psychiatry at the start of the new millennium. The book is written for psychiatrists engaged in continuous education and recertification; the previous, shorter, *Oxford Textbook of Psychiatry* remains available for psychiatrists in training. The book is intended to be suitable also as a work of reference for psychiatrists of all levels of experience, and for other professionals whose work involves them in the problems of psychiatry.

The growing unity of psychiatry

The growing unity in psychiatry is evident in several ways. Biological and psychosocial approaches have been largely reconciled with a general recognition that genetic and environmental factors interact, and that psychological processes are based in and can influence neurobiological mechanisms. At the same time, the common ground between the different psychodynamic theories has been recognized, and is widely accepted as more valuable than the differences between them.

The practice of psychiatry is increasingly similar in different countries, with the remaining variations related more to differences between national systems of health care and the resources available to clinicians, than to differences in the aims of the psychiatrists working in these countries. This unity of approach is reflected in this book whose authors practise in many different countries and yet present a common approach. In this respect this textbook differs importantly from others which present the views of authors drawn predominantly from a single country or region.

Greater agreement about diagnosis and nosology has led to a better understanding of how different treatment approaches are effective in different disorders. The relative specificity of psychopharmacological treatments is being matched increasingly by the specificity of some of the recently developed psychological treatments, so that psychological treatment should no longer be applied without reference to diagnosis, as was sometimes done in the past.

The pace of scientific advance

Advances in genetics and in the neurosciences have already increased knowledge of the basic mechanisms of the brain and are beginning to uncover the neurobiological mechanisms involved in psychiatric disorder. Striking progress has been achieved in the understanding of Alzheimer's disease, for example, and there are indications that similar progress will follow in uncovering the causes of mood disorder, schizophrenia, and autism. Knowledge of genetics and the neurosciences is so extensive and the pace of change is so rapid that it is difficult to present a complete account within the limited space available in a textbook of clinical psychiatry. We have selected aspects of these sciences that seem, to us and the authors, to have contributed significantly to psychiatry or to be likely to do so before long.

Psychological and social sciences and epidemiology are essential methods of investigation in psychiatry. Although the pace of advance in these sciences may not be as great as in the neurosciences, the findings generally have a more direct relation to clinical phenomena. Moreover, the mechanisms by which psychological and social factors interact with genetic, biochemical, and structural ones will continue to be important however great the progress in these other sciences. Among the advances in the psychological and social sciences that are relevant to clinical phenomena, we have included accounts of memory, psychological development, research on life events, and the effects of culture. Epidemiological studies continue to be crucial for defining psychiatric disorders, following their course, and identifying their causes.

Psychiatry in the community

In most countries, psychiatry is now practised in the community rather than in institutions, and where this change has yet be completed, it is generally recognized that it should take place. The change has done much more than transfer the locus of care; it has converted patients from passive recipients of care to active participants with individual needs and preferences. Psychiatrists are now involved in the planning, provision, and evaluation of services for whole communities, which may include members of ethnic minorities, homeless people, and refugees. Responsibility for a community has underlined the importance of the prevention as well as the treatment of mental disorder and of the role of agencies other than health services in both. Care in the community has also drawn attention to the many people with psychiatric disorder who are treated in primary care, and has led to new ways of working between psychiatrists and physicians. At the same time, psychiatrists have worked more in general hospitals, helping patients with both medical and psychiatric problems. Others have provided care for offenders.

The organization of the book

In most ways, the organization of this book is along conventional lines. However, some matters require explanation.

Part 1 contains a variety of diverse topics brought together under the general heading of the subject matter and approach to psychiatry. Phenomenology, assessment, classification, and ethical problems are included, together with the role of the psychiatrist as educator and as manager. Public health aspects of psychiatry are considered together with public attitudes to psychiatry and to psychiatric patients. Part 1 ends with a chapter on the links between science and practice. It begins with a topic that is central to good practice—the understanding of the experience of becoming a psychiatric patient.

Part 2 is concerned with the scientific foundations of psychiatry grouped under the headings neurosciences, genetics, psychological sciences, social sciences, and epidemiology. The chapters contain general information about these sciences; findings specific to a particular disorder are described in the chapter on that disorder. Brain imaging techniques are discussed here because they link basic sciences with clinical research. As explained above, the chapters are selective and, in some, readers who wish to study the subjects in greater detail will find suggestions for further reading.

Part 3 is concerned with dynamic approaches to psychiatry. The principal schools of thought are presented as alternative ways of understanding the influence of life experience on personality and on responses to stressful events and to illness. Some reference is made to dynamic psychotherapy in these accounts, but the main account of these treatments is in Part 6. This arrangement separates the chapters on the practice of dynamic psychotherapy from those on psychodynamic theory, but we consider that this disadvantage is outweighed by the benefit of considering together the commonly used forms of psychotherapy.

Part 4 is long, with chapters on the clinical syndromes of adult psychiatry, with the exception of somatoform disorders which appear in Part 5, Psychiatry and Medicine. This latter contains more than a traditional account of psychosomatic medicine. It also includes a review of psychiatric disorders that may cause medical symptoms unexplained by physical pathology, the medical, surgical, gynaecological, and obstetric conditions most often associated with psychiatric disorder, health psychology, and the treatment of psychiatric disorder in medically ill patients.

Information about treatment appears in more than one part of the book. Part 6 contains descriptions of the physical and psychological treatments in common use in psychiatry. Dynamic psychotherapy and psychoanalysis are described alongside counselling and cognitive behavioural techniques. This part of the book contains general descriptions of the treatments; their use for a particular disorder is considered in the chapter on that disorder. In the latter, the account is generally in two parts: a review of evidence about the efficacy of the treatment, followed by advice on management in which available evidence is supplemented, where necessary, with clinical experience. Treatment methods designed specially for children and adolescents, for people with mental retardation (learning disability), and for patients within the forensic services are considered in Parts 9, 10, and 11 respectively.

Social psychiatry and service provision are described in Part 7. Public policy issues, as well as the planning, delivery, and evaluation of services, are discussed here. Psychiatry in primary care is an important topic in this part of the book. There are chapters on the special problems of members of ethnic minorities, homeless people, and refugees, and the effects of culture on the provision and uptake of services.

Child and adolescent psychiatry, old age psychiatry, and mental retardation are described in Parts 8, 9, and 10. These accounts are less detailed than might be found in textbooks intended for specialists working exclusively in the relevant subspecialty. Rather, they are written for readers experienced in another branch of psychiatry who wish to improve their knowledge of the special subject. We are aware of the controversy surrounding our choice of the title of Part 10. We have selected the term 'mental retardation' because it is used in both ICD-10 and DSM-IV. In some countries this term has been replaced by another that is thought to be less stigmatizing and more acceptable to patients and families. For example, in the United Kingdom the preferred term is 'learning disability'. While we sympathize with the aims of those who adopt this and other alternative terms, the book is intended for an international readership and it seems best to use the term chosen by the World Health Organization as most generally understood. Thus the term mental retardation is used unless there is a special reason to use another.

In Part 11, Forensic Psychiatry, it has been especially difficult to present a general account of the subject that is not tied to practice in a single country. This is because systems of law differ between countries and the practice of forensic psychiatry has to conform with the local legal system. Although many of the examples in this part of the book may at first seem restricted in their relevance because they are described in the context of English law, we hope that readers will be able to transfer the principles described in these chapters to the legal tradition in which they work.

Finally, readers should note that the history of psychiatry is presented in more than one part of the book. The history of psychiatry as a medical specialty is described in Part 1. The history of ideas about the various psychiatric disorders appears, where relevant, in the chapters on these disorders, where they can be considered in relation to present-day concepts. The history of ideas about aetiology is considered in Part 2, which covers the scientific basis of psychiatric aetiology, while the historical development of dynamic psychiatry is described in Part 3.

Michael Gelder
Juan López-Ibor
Nancy Andreasen

Acknowledgements from the first edition

We are grateful to the many colleagues who have advised us about certain parts of the book.

The following helped us to plan specialized parts of the book: Dr Jeremy Holmes (Section 3, Psychodynamic Contributions to Psychiatry); Professor Richard Mayou (Section 5, Psychiatry and Medicine); Professor Robin Jacoby (Section 8, Psychiatry of Old Age); Sir Michael Rutter (Section 9, Child and Adolescent Psychiatry); Professor William Fraser (Section 10, Intellectual Disablity); Professor Robert Bluglass (Section 11, Forensic Psychiatry).

The following helped us to plan certain sections within Section 4, General Psychiatry: Professor Alwyn Lishman (delirium, dementia, amnestic syndrome, and other cognitive disorders); Professor Griffith Edwards (alcohol use disorders); Dr Philip Robson (other substance use disorders); Professor Guy Goodwin (mood disorders); Professor John Bancroft (sexuality, gender identity, and their disorders); Professor Gregory Stores (sleep–wake disorders); Professor Keith Hawton (suicide and attempted suicide). In Section 6, Professor Philip Cowen advised about somatic treatments, Dr Jeremy Holmes about psychodynamic treatments, and Professor David Clark about cognitive behavioural therapy. Dr Max Marshall provided helpful advice about forensic issues for Section 7. We also thank the many other colleagues whose helpful suggestions about specific problems aided the planning of the book.

Finally, we record our special gratitude to the authors and to the staff of Oxford University Press.

Contents
Volume 1

Preface to the second edition *v*

Preface to the first edition *vii*

Acknowledgements from the first edition *ix*

Contributors list *xxi*

Section 1 The Subject Matter of and Approach to Psychiatry

1.1 **The patient's perspective** *3*
Kay Redfield Jamison, Richard Jed Wyatt, and Adam Ian Kaplin

1.2 **Public attitudes and the challenge of stigma** *5*
Graham Thornicroft, Elaine Brohan, and Aliya Kassam

1.3 **Psychiatry as a worldwide public health problem** *10*

1.3.1 Mental disorders as a worldwide public health issue *10*
Benedetto Saraceno

1.3.2 Transcultural psychiatry *13*
Julian Leff

1.4 **The history of psychiatry as a medical specialty** *17*
Pierre Pichot

1.5 **Ethics and values** *28*

1.5.1 Psychiatric ethics *28*
Sidney Bloch and Stephen Green

1.5.2 Values and values-based practice in clinical psychiatry *32*
K. W. M. Fulford

1.6 **The psychiatrist as a manager** *39*
Juan J. López-Ibor Jr. and Costas Stefanis

1.7 **Descriptive phenomenology** *47*
Andrew Sims

1.8 **Assessment** *62*

1.8.1 The principles of clinical assessment in general psychiatry *62*
John E. Cooper and Margaret Oates

1.8.2 Assessment of personality *78*
C. Robert Cloninger

1.8.3 Cognitive assessment *85*
Graham E. Powell

1.8.4 Questionnaire, rating, and behavioural methods of assessment *94*
John N. Hall

1.9 **Diagnosis and classification** *99*
Michael B. First and Harold Alan Pincus

1.10 **From science to practice** *122*
John R. Geddes

Section 2 The Scientific Basis of Psychiatric Aetiology

2.1 **Brain and mind** *133*
Martin Davies

2.2 **Statistics and the design of experiments and surveys** *137*
Graham Dunn

2.3 **The contribution of neurosciences** *144*

2.3.1 Neuroanatomy *144*
R. C. A. Pearson

2.3.2 Neurodevelopment *156*
Karl Zilles

2.3.3 Neuroendocrinology *160*
Charles B. Nemeroff and Gretchen N. Neigh

2.3.4 Neurotransmitters and signalling *168*
Trevor Sharp

2.3.5 Neuropathology *177*
Peter Falkai and Bernhard Bogerts

2.3.6 Functional position emission tomography in psychiatry *185*
P. M. Grasby

2.3.7 Structural magnetic resonance imaging *191*
J. Suckling and E. T. Bullmore

2.3.8 Functional magnetic resonance imaging *196*
E. T. Bullmore and J. Suckling

2.3.9 Neuronal networks, epilepsy, and other brain dysfunctions *201*
John G. R. Jefferys

2.3.10 Psychoneuroimmunology *205*
Robert Dantzer and Keith W. Kelley

2.4 The contribution of genetics *212*

2.4.1 Quantitative genetics *212*
Anita Thapar and Peter McGuffin

2.4.2 Molecular genetics *222*
Jonathan Flint

2.5 The contribution of psychological science *234*

2.5.1 Development psychology through infancy, childhood, and adolescence *234*
William Yule and Matt Woolgar

2.5.2 Psychology of attention *245*
Elizabeth Coulthard and Masud Husain

2.5.3 Psychology and biology of memory *249*
Andreas Meyer-Lindenberg and Terry E. Goldberg

2.5.4 The anatomy of human emotion *257*
R. J. Dolan

2.5.5 Neuropsychological basis of neuropsychiatry *262*
L. Clark, B. J. Sahakian, and T. W. Robbins

2.6 The contribution of social sciences *268*

2.6.1 Medical sociology and issues of aetiology *268*
George W. Brown

2.6.2 Social and cultural anthropology: salience for psychiatry *275*
Arthur Kleinman

2.7 The contribution of epidemiology to psychiatric aetiology *280*
Scott Henderson

Section 3 Psychodynamic Contributions to Psychiatry

3.1 Psychoanalysis: Freud's theories and their contemporary development *293*
Otto F. Kernberg

3.2 Object relations, attachment theory, self-psychology, and interpersonal psychoanalysis *306*
Jeremy Holmes

3.3 Current psychodynamic approaches to psychiatry *313*
Glen O. Gabbard

Section 4 Clinical Syndromes of Adult Psychiatry

4.1 Delirium, dementia, amnesia, and other cognitive disorders *325*

4.1.1 Delirium *325*
David Meagher and Paula Trzepacz

4.1.2 Dementia: Alzheimer's disease *333*
Simon Lovestone

4.1.3 Frontotemporal dementias *344*
Lars Gustafson and Arne Brun

4.1.4 Prion disease *351*
John Collinge

4.1.5 Dementia with Lewy bodies *361*
I. G. McKeith

4.1.6 Dementia in Parkinson's disease *368*
R. H. S. Mindham and T. A. Hughes

4.1.7 Dementia due to Huntington's disease *371*
Susan Folstein and Russell L. Margolis

4.1.8 Vascular dementia *375*
Timo Erkinjuntti

4.1.9 Dementia due to HIV disease *384*
Mario Maj

4.1.10 The neuropsychiatry of head injury *387*
Simon Fleminger

4.1.11 Alcohol-related dementia (alcohol-induced dementia; alcohol-related brain damage) *399*
Jane Marshall

4.1.12 Amnesic syndromes *403*
Michael D. Kopelman

4.1.13 The management of dementia *411*
John-Paul Taylor and Simon Fleminger

4.1.14 Remediation of memory disorders *419*
Jonathan J. Evans

4.2 Substance use disorders *426*

4.2.1 Pharmacological and psychological aspects of drugs abuse *426*
David J. Nutt and Fergus D. Law

4.2.2 Alcohol use disorders *432*

4.2.2.1 Aetiology of alcohol problems *432*
Juan C. Negrete and Kathryn J. Gill

4.2.2.2 Alcohol dependence and alcohol problems *437*
Jane Marshall

4.2.2.3 Alcohol and psychiatric and physical disorders *442*
Karl F. Mann and Falk Kiefer

4.2.2.4 Treatment of alcohol dependence *447*
Jonathan Chick

4.2.2.5 Services for alcohol use disorders *459*
D. Colin Drummond

4.2.2.6 Prevention of alcohol-related problems *467*
Robin Room

4.2.3 Other substance use disorders *472*

4.2.3.1 Opioids: heroin, methadone, and buprenorphine *473*
Soraya Mayet, Adam R. Winstock, and John Strang

4.2.3.2 Disorders relating to the use of amphetamine and cocaine *482*
Nicholas Seivewright and Robert Fung

4.2.3.3 Disorders relating to use of PCP and hallucinogens *486*
Henry David Abraham

4.2.3.4 Misuse of benzodiazepines *490*
Sarah Welch and Michael Farrell

4.2.3.5 Disorders relating to the use of ecstasy and other 'party drugs' *494*
Adam R. Winstock and Fabrizio Schifano

4.2.3.6 Disorders relating to the use of volatile substances *502*
Richard Ives

4.2.3.7 The mental health effects of cannabis use *507*
Wayne Hall

4.2.3.8 Nicotine dependence and treatment *510*
Mª Inés López-Ibor

4.2.4 Assessing need and organizing services for drug misuse problems *515*
John Marsden, Colin Bradbury, and John Strang

4.3 Schizophrenia and acute transient psychotic disorders *521*

4.3.1 Schizophrenia: a conceptual history *521*
Nancy C. Andreasen

4.3.2 Descriptive clinical features of schizophrenia *526*
Peter F. Liddle

4.3.3 The clinical neuropsychology of schizophrenia *531*
Philip D. Harvey and Christopher R. Bowie

4.3.4 Diagnosis, classification, and differential diagnosis of schizophrenia *534*
Anthony S. David

4.3.5 Epidemiology of schizophrenia *540*
Assen Jablensky

4.3.6 Aetiology *553*

4.3.6.1 Genetic and environmental risk factors for schizophrenia *553*
R. M. Murray and D. J. Castle

4.3.6.2 The neurobiology of schizophrenia *561*
Paul J. Harrison

4.3.7 Course and outcome of schizophrenia and their prediction *568*
Assen Jablensky

4.3.8 Treatment and management of schizophrenia *578*
D. G. Cunningham Owens and E. C. Johnstone

4.3.9 Schizoaffective and schizotypal disorders *595*
Ming T. Tsuang, William S. Stone, and Stephen V. Faraone

4.3.10 Acute and transient psychotic disorders *602*
J. Garrabé and F.-R. Cousin

4.4 Persistent delusional symptoms and disorders *609*
Alistair Munro

4.5 Mood disorders *629*

4.5.1 Introduction to mood disorders *629*
John R. Geddes

4.5.2 Clinical features of mood disorders and mania *632*
Per Bech

4.5.3 Diagnosis, classification, and differential diagnosis of the mood disorders *637*
Gordon Parker

4.5.4 Epidemiology of mood disorders *645*
Peter R. Joyce

4.5.5 Genetic aetiology of mood disorders *650*
Pierre Oswald, Daniel Souery, and Julien Mendlewicz

4.5.6 Neurobiological aetiology of mood disorders *658*
Guy Goodwin

4.5.7 Course and prognosis of mood disorders *665*
Jules Angst

4.5.8 Treatment of mood disorders *669*
E. S. Paykel and J. Scott

4.5.9 Dysthymia, cyclothymia, and hyperthymia *680*
Hagop S. Akiskal

4.6 Stress-related and adjustment disorders *693*

4.6.1 Acute stress reactions *693*
Anke Ehlers, Allison G. Harvey and Richard A. Bryant

4.6.2 Post-traumatic stress disorder *700*
Anke Ehlers

4.6.3 **Recovered memories and false memories** *713*
Chris R. Brewin

4.6.4 **Adjustment disorders** *716*
James J. Strain, Kimberly Klipstein, and Jeffrey Newcorm

4.6.5 **Bereavement** *724*
Beverley Raphael, Sally Wooding, and Julie Dunsmore

4.7 Anxiety disorders *729*

4.7.1 **Generalized anxiety disorders** *729*
Stella Bitran, David H. Barlow, and David A. Spiegel

4.7.2 **Social anxiety disorder and specific phobias** *739*
Michelle A. Blackmore, Brigette A. Erwin, Richard G. Heimberg, Leanne Magee, and David M. Fresco

4.7.3 **Panic disorder and agoraphobia** *750*
James C. Ballenger

4.8 Obsessive–compulsive disorder *765*
Joseph Zohar, Leah Fostick, and Elizabeth Juven-Wetzler

4.9 Depersonalization disorder *774*
Nick Medford, Mauricio Sierra, and Anthony S. David

4.10 Disorders of eating *777*

4.10.1 **Anorexia nervosa** *777*
Gerald Russell

4.10.2 **Bulimia nervosa** *800*
Christopher G. Fairburn, Zafra Cooper, and Rebecca Murphy

4.11 Sexuality, gender identity, and their disorders *812*

4.11.1 **Normal sexual function** *812*
Roy J. Levin

4.11.2 **The sexual dysfunctions** *821*
Cynthia A. Graham and John Bancroft

4.11.3 **The paraphilias** *832*
J. Paul Fedoroff

4.11.4 **Gender identity disorder in adults** *842*
Richard Green

4.12 Personality disorders *847*

4.12.1 **Personality disorders: an introductory perspective** *847*
Juan J. López-Ibor Jr.

4.12.2 **Diagnosis and classification of personality disorders** *855*
James Reich and Giovanni de Girolamo

4.12.3 **Specific types of personality disorder** *861*
José Luis Carrasco and Dusica Lecic-Tosevski

4.12.4 **Epidemiology of personality disorders** *881*
Francesca Guzzetta and Giovanni de Girolamo

4.12.5 **Neuropsychological templates for abnormal personalities: from genes to biodevelopmental pathways** *886*
Adolf Tobeña

4.12.6 **Psychotherapy for personality disorder** *892*
Anthony W. Bateman and Peter Fonagy

4.12.7 **Management of personality disorder** *901*
Giles Newton-Howes and Kate Davidson

4.13 Habit and impulse control disorders *911*

4.13.1 **Impulse control disorders** *911*
Susan L. McElroy and Paul E. Keck Jr.

4.13.2 **Special psychiatric problems relating to gambling** *919*
Emanuel Moran

4.14 Sleep–wake disorders *924*

4.14.1 **Basic aspects of sleep–wake disorders** *924*
Gregory Stores

4.14.2 **Insomnias** *933*
Colin A. Espie and Delwyn J. Bartlett

4.14.3 **Excessive sleepiness** *938*
Michel Billiard

4.14.4 **Parasomnias** *943*
Carlos H. Schenck and Mark W. Mahowald

4.15 Suicide *951*

4.15.1 **Epidemiology and causes of suicide** *951*
Jouko K. Lonnqvist

4.15.2 **Deliberate self-harm: epidemiology and risk factors** *957*
Ella Arensman and Ad J. F. M. Kerkhof

4.15.3 **Biological aspects of suicidal behaviour** *963*
J. John Mann and Dianne Currier

4.15.4 **Treatment of suicide attempters and prevention of suicide and attempted suicide** *969*
Keith Hawton and Tatiana Taylor

4.16 Culture-related specific psychiatric syndromes *979*
Wen-Shing Tseng

Index

Contents
Volume 2

Preface to the second edition *v*

Preface to the first edition *vii*

Acknowledgements *ix*

Contributors list *xxi*

Section 5 Psychiatry and Medicine

5.1 Mind–body dualism, psychiatry, and medicine *989*
Michael Sharpe and Jane Walker

5.2 Somatoform disorders and other causes of medically unexplained symptoms *992*

5.2.1 Somatoform disorders and functional symptoms *992*
Richard Mayou

5.2.2 Epidemiology of somatoform disorders and other causes of unexplained medical symptoms *995*
Gregory Simon

5.2.3 Somatization disorder and related disorders *999*
Per Fink

5.2.4 Conversion and dissociation disorders *1011*
Christopher Bass

5.2.5 Hypochondriasis (health anxiety) *1021*
Russell Noyes Jr.

5.2.6 Pain disorder *1029*
Sidney Benjamin and Stella Morris

5.2.7 Chronic fatigue syndrome *1035*
Michael Sharpe and Simon Wessely

5.2.8 Body dysmorphic disorder *1043*
Katharine A. Phillips

5.2.9 Factitious disorder and malingering *1049*
Christopher Bass and David Gill

5.2.10 Neurasthenia *1059*
Felice Lieh Mak

5.3 Medical and surgical conditions and treatments associated with psychiatric disorders *1065*

5.3.1 Adjustment to illness and handicap *1065*
Allan House

5.3.2 Psychiatric aspects of neurological disease *1071*
Maria A. Ron

5.3.3 Epilepsy *1076*
Brian Toone

5.3.4 Medical conditions associated with psychiatric disorder *1081*
James R. Rundell

5.3.5 Psychiatric aspects of infections *1090*
José-Luis Ayuso-Mateos

5.3.6 Psychiatric aspects of surgery (including transplantation) *1096*
S. A. Hales, S. E. Abbey, and G. M. Rodin

5.3.7 Psychiatric aspects of cancer *1100*
Jimmie C. Holland and Jessica Stiles

5.3.8 Psychiatric aspects of accidents, burns, and other physical trauma *1105*
Ulrik Fredrik Malt

5.4 Obstetric and gynaecological conditions associated with psychiatric disorder *1114*
Ian Brockington

5.5 Management of psychiatric disorders in medically ill patients, including emergencies *1128*
Pier Maria Furlan and Luca Ostacoli

5.6 Health psychology *1135*
John Weinman and Keith J. Petrie

5.7 The organization of psychiatric services for general hospital departments *1144*
Frits J. Huyse, Roger G. Kathol, Wolfgang Söllner, and Lawson Wulsin

Section 6 Treatment Methods in Psychiatry

6.1 The evaluation of treatments *1151*

6.1.1 The evaluation of physical treatments *1151*
Clive E. Adams

6.1.2 The evaluation of psychological treatment *1158*
Paul Crits-Christoph and Mary Beth Connolly Gibbons

6.2 Somatic treatments *1168*

6.2.1 General principles of drug therapy in psychiatry *1168*
J. K. Aronson

6.2.2 Anxiolytics and hypnotics *1178*
Malcolm Lader

6.2.3 Antidepressants *1185*
Zubin Bhagwagar and George R. Heninger

6.2.4 Lithium and related mood stabilizers *1198*
Robert M. Post

6.2.5 Antipsychotic and anticholinergic drugs *1208*
Herbert Y. Meltzer and William V. Bobo

6.2.6 Antiepileptic drugs *1231*
Brian P. Brennan and Harrison G. Pope Jr.

6.2.7 Drugs for cognitive disorders *1240*
Leslie Iversen

6.2.8 Drugs used in the treatment of the addictions *1242*
Fergus D. Law and David J. Nutt

6.2.9 Complementary medicines *1247*
Ursula Werneke

6.2.10 Non-pharmacological somatic treatments *1251*

6.2.10.1 Electroconvulsive therapy *1251*
Max Fink

6.2.10.2 Phototherapy *1260*
Philip J. Cowen

6.2.10.3 Transcranial magnetic stimulation *1263*
Declan McLoughlin and Andrew Mogg

6.2.10.4 Neurosurgery for psychiatric disorders *1266*
Keith Matthews and David Christmas

6.3 Psychological treatments *1272*

6.3.1 Counselling *1272*
Diana Sanders

6.3.2 Cognitive behaviour therapy *1285*

6.3.2.1 Cognitive behaviour therapy for anxiety disorders *1285*
David M. Clark

6.3.2.2 Cognitive behaviour therapy for eating disorders *1298*
Zafra Cooper, Rebecca Murphy, and Christopher G. Fairburn

6.3.2.3 Cognitive behaviour therapy for depressive disorders *1304*
Melanie J. V. Fennell

6.3.2.4 Cognitive behaviour therapy for schizophrenia *1313*
Max Birchwood and Elizabeth Spencer

6.3.3 Interpersonal psychotherapy for depression and other disorders *1318*
Carlos Blanco, John C. Markowitz, and Myrna M. Weissman

6.3.4 Brief individual psychodynamic psychotherapy *1327*
Amy M. Ursano and Robert J. Ursano

6.3.5 Psychoanalysis and other long-term dynamic psychotherapies *1337*
Peter Fonagy and Horst Kächele

6.3.6 Group methods in adult psychiatry *1350*
John Schlapobersky and Malcolm Pines

6.3.7 Psychotherapy with couples *1369*
Michael Crowe

6.3.8 Family therapy in the adult psychiatric setting *1380*
Sidney Bloch and Edwin Harari

6.3.9 Therapeutic communities *1391*
David Kennard and Rex Haigh

6.4 Treatment by other professions *1399*

6.4.1 Rehabilitation techniques *1399*
W. Rössler

6.4.2 Psychiatric nursing techniques *1403*
Kevin Gournay

6.4.3 Social work approaches to mental health work: international trends *1408*
Shulamit Ramon

6.4.4 Art therapy *1413*
Diane Waller

6.5 Indigenous, folk healing practices *1418*
Wen-Shing Tseng

Section 7 Social Psychiatry and Service Provision

7.1 Public policy and mental health *1425*
Matt Muijen and Andrew McCulloch

7.2 Service needs of individuals and populations *1432*
Mike Slade, Michele Tansella, and Graham Thornicroft

7.3 Cultural differences care pathways, service use, and outcome *1438*
Jim van Os and Kwame McKenzie

7.4 Primary prevention of mental disorders *1446*
J. M. Bertolote

7.5 Planning and providing mental health services for a community *1452*
Tom Burns

7.6 Evaluation of mental health services *1463*
Michele Tansella and Graham Thornicroft

7.7 Economic analysis of mental health services *1473*
Martin Knapp and Dan Chisholm

7.8 Psychiatry in primary care *1480*
David Goldberg, André Tylee, and Paul Walters

7.9 The role of the voluntary sector *1490*
Vanessa Pinfold and Mary Teasdale

7.10 Special problems *1493*

7.10.1 The special psychiatric problems of refugees *1493*
Richard F. Mollica, Melissa A. Culhane, and Daniel H. Hovelson

7.10.2 Mental health services for homeless mentally ill people *1500*
Tom K. J. Craig

7.10.3 Mental health services for ethnic minorities *1502*
Tom K. J. Craig and Dinesh Bhugra

Section 8 The Psychiatry of Old Age

8.1 The biology of ageing *1507*
Alan H. Bittles

8.2 Sociology of normal ageing *1512*
Sarah Harper

8.3 The ageing population and the epidemiology of mental disorders among the elderly *1517*
Scott Henderson and Laura Fratiglioni

8.4 Assessment of mental disorder in older patients *1524*
Robin Jacoby

8.5 Special features of clinical syndromes in the elderly *1530*

8.5.1 Delirium in the elderly *1530*
James Lindesay

8.5.1.1 Mild cognitive impairment *1534*
Claudia Jacova and Howard H. Feldman

8.5.2 Substance use disorders in older people *1540*
Henry O'Connell and Brian Lawlor

8.5.3 Schizophrenia and paranoid disorders in late life *1546*
Barton W. Palmer, Gauri N. Savla, and Thomas W. Meeks

8.5.4 Mood disorders in the elderly *1550*
Robert Baldwin

8.5.5 Stress-related, anxiety, and obsessional disorders in elderly people *1558*
James Lindesay

8.5.6 Personality disorders in the elderly *1561*
Suzanne Holroyd

8.5.7 Suicide and deliberate self-harm in elderly people *1564*
Robin Jacoby

8.5.8 Sex in old age *1567*
John Kellett and Catherine Oppenheimer

8.6 Special features of psychiatric treatment for the elderly *1571*
Catherine Oppenheimer

8.7 The planning and organization of services for older adults *1579*
Pamela S. Melding

Section 9 Child and Adolescent Psychiatry

9.1 General issues *1589*

9.1.1 Developmental psychopathology and classification in childhood and adolescence *1589*
Stephen Scott

9.1.2 Epidemiology of psychiatric disorder in childhood and adolescence *1594*
E. Jane Costello and Adrian Angold

9.1.3 Assessment in child and adolescent psychiatry *1600*
Jeff Bostic and Andrés Martin

9.1.4 Prevention of mental disorder in childhood and other public health issues *1606*
Rhoshel Lenroot

9.2 Clinical syndromes *1612*

9.2.1 Neuropsychiatric disorders *1612*
James C. Harris

9.2.2 Specific developmental disorders in childhood and adolescence *1622*
Helmut Remschmidt and Gerd Schulte-Körne

9.2.3 Autism and the pervasive developmental disorders *1633*
Fred R. Volkmar and Ami Klin

9.2.4 Attention deficit and hyperkinetic disorders in childhood and adolescence *1643*
Eric Taylor

9.2.5 Conduct disorders in childhood and adolescence *1654*
Stephen Scott

9.2.6 Anxiety disorders in childhood and adolescence *1664*
Daniel S. Pine

9.2.7 Paediatric mood disorders *1669*
David Brent and Boris Birmaher

9.2.8 Obsessive–compulsive disorder and tics in children and adolescents *1680*
Martine F. Flament and Philippe Robaey

9.2.9 Sleep disorders in children and adolescents *1693*
Gregory Stores

9.2.10 Suicide and attempted suicide in children and adolescents *1702*
David Shaffer, Cynthia R. Pfeffer, and Jennifer Gutstein

9.2.11 Children's speech and language difficulties *1710*
Judy Clegg

9.2.12 Gender identity disorder in children and adolescents *1718*
Richard Green

9.3 Situations affecting child mental health *1724*

9.3.1 The influence of family, school, and the environment *1724*
Barbara Maughan

9.3.2 Child trauma *1728*
David Trickey and Dora Black

9.3.3 Child abuse and neglect *1731*
David P. H. Jones

9.3.4 The relationship between physical and mental health in children and adolescents *1740*
Julia Gledhill and M. Elena Garralda

9.3.5 The effects on child and adult mental health of adoption and foster care *1747*
June Thoburn

9.3.6 Effects of parental psychiatric and physcial illness on child development *1752*
Paul Ramchandani, Alan Stein, and Lynne Murray

9.3.7 The effects of bereavement in childhood *1758*
Dora Black and David Trickey

9.4 The child as witness *1761*
Anne E. Thompson and John B. Pearce

9.5 Treatment methods for children and adolescents *1764*

9.5.1 Counselling and psychotherapy for children *1764*
John B. Pearce

9.5.2 Psychodynamic child psychotherapy *1769*
Peter Fonagy and Mary Target

9.5.3 Cognitive behaviour therapies for children and families *1777*
Philip Graham

9.5.4 Caregiver-mediated interventions for children and families *1787*
Philip A. Fisher and Elizabeth A. Stormshak

9.5.5 Medication for children and adolescents: current issues *1793*
Paramala J. Santosh

9.5.6 Residential care for social reasons *1799*
Leslie Hicks and Ian Sinclair

9.5.7 Organization of services for children and adolescents with mental health problems *1802*
Miranda Wolpert

9.5.8 The management of child and adolescent psychiatric emergencies *1807*
Gillian Forrest

9.5.9 The child psychiatrist as consultant to schools and colleges *1811*
Simon G. Gowers and Sian Thomas

Section 10 Intellectual Disability (Mental Retardation)

10.1 Classification, diagnosis, psychiatric assessment, and needs assessment *1819*
A. J. Holland

10.2 Prevalence of intellectual disabilities and epidemiology of mental ill-health in adults with intellectual disabilities *1825*
Sally-Ann Cooper and Elita Smiley

10.3 Aetiology of intellectual disability: general issues and prevention *1830*
Markus Kaski

10.4 Syndromes causing intellectual disability *1838*
David M. Clarke and Shoumitro Deb

10.5 Psychiatric and behaviour disorders among mentally retarded people *1849*

10.5.1 Psychiatric and behaviour disorders among children and adolescents with intellectual disability *1849*
Bruce J. Tonge

10.5.2 Psychiatric and behaviour disorders among adult persons with intellectual disability *1854*
Anton Došen

10.5.3 Epilepsy and epilepsy-related behaviour disorders among people with intellectual disability *1860*
Matti Iivanainen

10.6 Methods of treatment *1871*
T. P. Berney

10.7 Special needs of adolescents and elderly people with intellectual disability *1878*
Jane Hubert and Sheila Hollins

10.8 Families with a member with intellectual disability and their needs *1883*
Ann Gath and Jane McCarthy

10.9 The planning and provision of psychiatric services for adults with intellectual disability *1887*
Nick Bouras and Geraldine Holt

Section 11 Forensic Psychiatry

11.1 General principles of law relating to people with mental disorder *1895*
Michael Gunn and Kay Wheat

11.2 Psychosocial causes of offending *1908*
David P. Farrington

11.3 Associations between psychiatric disorder and offending *1917*

11.3.1 Associations between psychiatric disorder and offending *1917*
Lindsay Thomson and Rajan Darjee

11.3.2 Offending, substance misuse, and mental disorder *1926*
Andrew Johns

11.3.3 Cognitive disorders, epilepsy, ADHD, and offending *1928*
Norbert Nedopil

11.4 Mental disorders among offenders in correctional settings *1933*
James R. P. Ogloff

11.5 Homicide offenders including mass murder and infanticide *1937*
Nicola Swinson and Jennifer Shaw

11.6 Fraud, deception, and thieves *1941*
David V. James

11.7 Juvenile delinquency and serious antisocial behaviour *1945*
Susan Bailey

11.8 Child molesters and other sex offenders *1960*
Stephen Hucker

11.9 Arson (fire-raising) *1965*
Herschel Prins

11.10 Stalking *1970*
Paul E. Mullen

11.11 Querulous behaviour: vexatious litigation, abnormally persistent complaining and petitioning *1977*
Paul E. Mullen

11.12 Domestic violence *1981*
Gillian C. Mezey

11.13 The impact of criminal victimization *1984*
Gillian C. Mezey and Ian Robbins

11.14 Assessing and managing the risks of violence towards others *1991*
Paul E. Mullen and James R. P. Ogloff

11.15 The expert witness in the Criminal Court: assessment, reports, and testimony *2003*
John O'Grady

11.16 Managing offenders with psychiatric disorders in general psychiatric sevices *2009*
James R. P. Ogloff

11.17 Management of offenders with mental disorder in specialist forensic mental health services *2015*
Pamela J. Taylor and Emma Dunn

Index

Contributors list

S.E. Abbey Associate Professor of Psychiatry, University of Toronto, Toronto, Canada
Chapter 5.3.6

Henry David Abraham Distinguished Life Fellow, American Psychiatric Association, USA
Chapter 4.2.3.3

Clive E. Adams Cochrane Schizophrenia Group, University of Oxford Department of Psychiatry, Warneford Hospital, Oxford, UK
Chapter 6.1.1

Hagop S. Akiskal Professor of Psychiatry and Director of the International Mood Center, University of California at San Diego, California, USA
Chapter 4.5.9

Nancy C. Andreasen Dept of Psychiatry, University of Iowa Hospitals & Clinics, Iowa City, USA
Chapter 4.3.1

Adrian Angold Associate Professor of Child and Adolescent Psychiatry, Duke University Medical Center, Durham, North Carolina, USA
Chapter 9.1.2

Jules Angst Emeritus Professor of Psychiatry, Zurich University, Switzerland
Chapter 4.5.7

Ella Arensman Director of Research, National Suicide Research Foundation, Ireland
Chapter 4.15.2

J.K. Aronson Reader in Clinical Pharmacology, University Department of Primary Health Care, Headington, Oxford, UK
Chapter 6.2.1

José-Luis Ayuso-Mateos Chairman, Department of Psychiatry, Universidad Autónoma de Madrid, Hospital Universitario de la Princesa, Spain
Chapter 5.3.5

Susan Bailey Consultant Child and Adolescent Forensic Psychiatrist, Salford NHS Trust and Maudsley NHS Trust; Senior Research Fellow, University of Manchester, UK
Chapter 11.7

Robert Baldwin Consultant, Old Age Psychiatrist, and Honorary Senior Lecturer, Manchester Royal Infirmary, UK
Chapter 8.5.4

James C. Ballenger Retired Professor and Chairman, Department of Psychiatry and Behavioral Sciences and Director, Institute of Psychiatry, Medical University of South Carolina, USA
Chapter 4.7.3

John Bancroft, The Kinsey Institute for Research in Sex, Gender, & Reproduction and Department of Psychiatry, University of Oxford, UK
Chapter 4.11.2

David H. Barlow Center for Anxiety and Related Disorders at Boston University, Massachusetts, USA
Chapter 4.7.1

Delwyn J. Bartlett Woolcock Institute of Medical Research, Sydney, Australia
Chapter 4.14.2

Christopher Bass Consultant in Liaison Psychiatry, John Radcliffe Hospital, Oxford, UK
Chapters 5.2.4 and 5.2.9

Antony W. Bateman Halliwick Psychotherapy Dept, St Ann's Hospital, London, UK
Chapter 4.12.6

Per Bech Professor of Psychiatry and Head of Psychiatric Research Unit, WHO Collaborating Centre, Frederiksborg General Hospital, Hillerød, Denmark
Chapter 4.5.2

Sidney Benjamin Senior Lecturer, University of Manchester, UK
Chapter 5.2.6

Thomas P. Berney Consultant Developmental Psychiatrist Honorary Research Associate, University of Newcastle upon Tyne, UK
Chapter 10.6

Jose M. Bertolote Chief, Mental Disorders Control Unit, World Health Organization, Geneva; Associate Professor, Department of Psychogeriatrics, University of Lausanne, Switzerland
Chapter 7.4

Zubin Bhagwagar CT Mental Health Center, Yale University, New Haven CT, USA
Chapter 6.2.3

Mary Beth Connolly Gibbons Assistant Professor of Psychology in Psychiatry Department of Psychiatry, University of Pennsylvania, Pennsylvania, USA
Chapter 6.1.2

Dinesh Bhugra Professor of Mental Health and Cultural Diversity, King's College London, Institute of Psychiatry, London, UK
Chapter 7.10.3

Michel Billiard Professor of Neurology, School of Medicine, Guide Chauliac Hospital, Montpellier, France
Chapter 4.14.3

Max Birchwood Director, Early Intervention Service, Northern Birmingham Mental Health Trust, and University of Birmingham, UK
Chapter 6.3.2.4

Boris Birmaher UPMC Western Psychiatric Institute, Pittsburgh, USA
Chapter 9.2.7

Stella Bitran, Center for Anxiety and Related Disorders, Boston University, Beacon, MA, USA
Chapter 4.7.1

Alan H. Bittles Centre for Comparative Genomics, Murdoch University, Perth, Australia
Chapter 8.1

Dora Black Honorary Consultant, Child and Adolescent Psychiatry, Traumatic Stress Clinic, London; Honorary Lecturer, University of London, UK
Chapters 9.3.2 and 9.3.7

Michelle A. Blackmore, Doctoral Student of Clinical Psychology Adult Anxiety Clinic at Temple University, Philadelphia, Pennsylvania, USA
Chapter 4.7.2

Carlos Blanco New York State Psychiatric Institute, New York, USA
Chapter 6.3.3

Sidney Bloch Professor of Psychiatry, University of Melbourne; Senior Psychiatrist, St Vincent's Hospital, Melbourne, Australia
Chapters 1.5 and 6.3.8

William V. Bobo Assistant Professor of Psychiatry, Vanderbilt University School of Medicine Nashville, Tennessee (USA)
Chapter 6.2.5

Bernhard Bogerts Department of Psychiatry, University of Magdeburg, Germany
Chapter 2.3.5

Jeff Bostic School of Psychiatry, Harvard Medical School, Cambridge MA, USA
Chapter 9.1.3

Nick Bouras Professor, Institute of Psychiatry - King's College London MHiLD - York Clinic, London, UK
Chapter 10.9

Christopher R. Bowie Department of Psychiatry, Mount Sinai School of Medicine, New York, USA
Chapter 4.3.3

Colin Bradbury Department of Psychological Medicine, Institute of Psychiatry, De Crespigny Park, London, UK
Chapter 4.2.4

Brian P. Brennan Instructor in Psychiatry, Harvard Medical School and Associate Director for Translational Neuroscience Research, Biological Psychiatry Laboratory, McLean Hospital, Belmont, MA, USA
Chapter 6.2.6

David Brent Dept of Psychiatry, University of Pittsburgh Medical School, Pittsburgh PA, USA
Chapter 9.2.7

Chris R. Brewin Research Dept of Clinical, Educational & Health Psychology, University College London, UK
Chapter 4.6.3

Elaine Brohan Institute of Psychiatry, David Goldberg Centre, De Crespigny Park, London, UK
Chapter 1.2

Ian Brockington Professor of Psychiatry, University of Birmingham, UK
Chapter 5.4

George W. Brown Professor of Sociology, Academic Department of Psychiatry, St Thomas's Hospital, London, UK
Chapter 2.6.1

Arne Brun Professor of Neuropathology. Department of Pathology, Lund University Hospital, Lund, Sweden
Chapter 4.1.3

Richard A. Bryant School of Psychology, University of New South Wales, Sydney NSW, Australia
Chapter 4.6.1

E.T. Bullmore Institute of Psychiatry, King's College London, UK
Chapters 2.3.7 and 2.3.8

Tom Burns Professor of social psychiatry, Dept of Psychiatry, University of Oxford, Warneford Hospital, Oxford, UK
Chapter 7.5

José Luis Carrasco Professor of Psychiatry, Hospital Fundacion Jimenez Diaz, Universidad Autonoma, Madrid, Spain
Chapter 4.12.3

D.J. Castle University of Western Australia, Fremantle, Australia
Chapter 4.3.6.1

Jonathan Chick Consultant Psychiatrist, NHS Lothian, and Senior Lecturer, Department of Psychiatry, University of Edinburgh, UK
Chapter 4.2.2.4

Daniel Chisholm Department of Health System Financing, Health Systems and Services, World Health Organization, Geneva, Switzerland
Chapter 7.7

David Christmas Dept of Psychiatry, University of Dundee, Dundee, UK
Chapter 6.2.10.4

David M. Clarke Consultant Psychiatrist, Lea Castle Centre, Kidderminster DY10 3PP, UK
Chapters 6.3.3.1 and 10.4

L. Clark Dept of Experimental Psychology, University of Cambridge, Cambridge, UK
Chapter 2.5.5

Judy Clegg Lecturer, Speech and language therapist, HPC, RCSLT Department of Human Communication Sciences University of Sheffield, UK
Chapter 9.2.11

C. Robert Cloninger Dept of Psychiatry, Washington University School of Medicine, St Louis MO, USA
Chapter 1.8.2

John Collinge Head of the Department of Neurodegenerative Disease at the Institute of Neurology, University College London and the Director of the UK Medical Research Council's Prion Unit, London, UK
Chapter 4.1.4

Henry O'Connell Consultant Psychiatrist, Co. Tipperary, Ireland
Chapter 8.5.2

Melissa A. Culhane Harvard Program in Refugee Trauma, Department of Psychiatry, Massachusetts General Hospital, Cambridge, USA
Chapter 7.10.1

John E. Cooper Emeritus Professor of Psychiatry, University of Nottingham, UK
Chapter 1.8.1

Sally-Ann Cooper Professor of Learning Disabilities, Division of Community Based Sciences, Faculty of Medicine, University of Glasgow, UK
Chapter 10.2

Zafra Cooper Principal Research Psychologist, Oxford University Department of Psychiatry, Warneford Hospital, Oxford, UK
Chapters 4.10.2 and 6.3.2.2

E. Jane Costello Department of Psychiatry and Behavioral Sciences, Duke University Medical Center, Brightleaf Square, Durham NC, USA
Chapter 9.1.2

Elizabeth Coulthard Institute of Neurology, University College London, UK
Chapter 2.5.2

F.-R. Cousin Psychiatrist, Centre Hospitalier Saint-Anne, Paris, France
Chapter 4.3.10

Philip J. Cowen Professor of Psychopharmacology, Department of Psychiatry, University of Oxford, UK
Chapter 6.2.10.2

Tom K.J. Craig Professor of Social Psychiatry, King's College London, Institute of Psychiatry, London, UK
Chapters 7.10.2 and 7.10.3

Paul Crits-Christoph Professor of Psychology in Psychiatry; Director, Center for Psychotherapy Research Department of Psychiatry, University of Pennsylvania. Pennsylvania, USA
Chapter 6.1.2

Michael Crowe Consultant Psychiatrist, South London and Maudsley NHS Trust; Honorary Senior Lecturer, Institute of Psychiatry, King's College London, UK
Chapter 6.3.7

D.G. Cunningham Owens Reader in Psychiatry, Department of Psychiatry, University of Edinburgh, UK
Chapter 4.3.8

Dianne Currier Division of Molecular Imaging & Neuropathology, Department of Psychiatry, Columbia University, USA
Chapter 4.15.3

Robert Dantzer Integrative Immunology and Behavior Program, University of Illinois at Urbana-Champaign, Edward R. Madigan Laboratory, West Gregory Drive, Urbana, IL, USA
Chapter 2.3.10

Rajan Darjee Division of Psychiatry, University of Edinburgh, Edinburgh, UK
Chapter 11.3.1

Anthony S. David Professor of Cognitive Neuropsychiatry, Institute of Psychiatry, King's College London, UK
Chapters 4.3.4 and 4.9

Kate Davidson Senior Research Psychologist, Department of Psychological Medicine, University of Glasgow, UK
Chapter 4.12.7

Martin Davies Dept of Experimental Psychology, University of Oxford, Oxford, UK
Chapter 2.1

Giovanni de Girolamo Health Care Research Agency, Emilia-Romagna Region, Bologna, Italy
Chapters 4.12.2 and 4.12.4

Shoumitro Deb Clinical Professor of Neuropsychiatry & Intellectual Disability, Division of Neuroscience, University of Birmingham, UK
Chapter 10.4

R.J. Dolan Institute of Neurology, University College London, UK
Chapter 2.5.4

Anton Došen Emeritus Professor of Psychiatric Aspects of Intellectual Disability at the Radboud University, Nijmegen, The Netherlands
Chapter 10.5.2

D. Colin Drummond Professor of Addiction Psychiatry, Section of Alcohol Research, National Addiction Centre, Division of Psychological Medicine and Psychiatry, Institute of Psychiatry, King's College London, UK
Chapter 4.2.2.5

Emma Dunn School of Medicine, Cardiff University, Cardiff, UK
Chapter 11.17

Graham Dunn Professor of Biomedical Statistics, Health Methodology Research Group, School of Community Based Medicine, University of Manchester, UK
Chapter 2.2

Julie Dunsmore Honorary Clinical Associate, SciMHA Unit, University of Western Sydney, Australia
Chapter 4.6.5

Anke Ehlers Department of Psychiatry, University of Oxford, UK
Chapters 4.6.1 and 4.6.2

Timo Erkinjuntti Professor of Neurology, Head of the University Department of Neurological Sciences, University of Helsinki and Head Physician, Department of Neurology and Memory Research Unit, Helsinki University Central Hospital, Finland
Chapter 4.1.8

Brigette A. Erwin Adult Anxiety Clinic of Temple University, Philadelphia, Pennsylvania, USA
Chapter 4.7.2

Colin A. Espie Professor of Clinical Psychology and Head of Department of Psychological Medicine, University of Glasgow, UK
Chapter 4.14.2

Jonathan J. Evans Section of Psychological Medicine, University of Glasgow, Glasgow, UK
Chapter 4.1.14

Christopher G. Fairburn Wellcome Principal Research Fellow and Professor of Psychiatry, University of Oxford, UK
Chapters 4.10.2 and 6.3.2.2

Peter Falkai Professor of Medical Psychology, Rheinische Friedrich-Wilhelms-Universität, Bonn, Germany
Chapter 2.3.5

Stephen V. Faraone Director, Medical Genetics Research, Professor of Psychiatry and of Neuroscience & Physiology, Director, Child and Adolescent Psychiatry Research, SUNY Upstate Medical University, New York, USA
Chapter 4.3.9

Michael Farrell Senior Lecturer and Consultant Psychiatrist, National Addiction Centre, South London and Maudsley NHS Trust, London, UK
Chapter 4.2.3.4

David P. Farrington Professor of Psychological Criminology, University of Cambridge, UK
Chapter 11.2

J. Paul Fedoroff Director, Sexual Behaviors Clinic Royal Ottawa Mental Health Centre and Director of Forensic Research University of Ottawa Institute of Mental Health Research, Canada
Chapter 4.11.3

Howard H. Feldman Professor and Head, Division of Neurology, Department of Medicine, University of British Columbia, Vancouver, BC, Canada
Chapter 8.5.1.1

Melanie J.V. Fennell Consultant Clinical Psychologist; Director, Oxford Diploma in Cognitive Therapy, University of Oxford Department of Psychiatry, Warneford Hospital, Oxford, UK
Chapter 6.3.2.3

Max Fink Emeritus Professor of Psychiatry and Neurology, State University of New York at Stony Brook; Professor of Psychiatry, Albert Einstein College of Medicine; Attending Psychiatrist, Long Island Jewish Medical Center, New York, USA
Chapter 6.2.10.1

Michael B. First Columbia University, New York, USA
Chapter 1.9

Per Fink Director, Research Unit for Functional Disorders, Aarhus University Hospital, Risskov, Denmark
Chapter 5.2.3

Philip A. Fisher Research Scientist, Oregon Social Learning Center, Eugene, Oregon, USA
Chapter 9.5.4

Martine F. Flament Chargée de Récherche INSERM, CNRS UMR 7593, Paris, France
Chapter 9.2.8

Simon Fleminger Consultant Neuropsychiatries, Lishman Brain Injury Unit, Maudsley Hospital, London, UK
Chapters 4.1.10 and 4.1.13

Jonathan Flint Wellcome Trust Centre for Human Genetics Roosevelt Drive, Oxford, UK
Chapter 2.4.2

Susan Folstein Professor of Psychiatry and Behavioral Sciences, Johns Hopkins School of Medicine, Baltimore, USA
Chapter 4.1.7

Peter Fonagy Freud Memorial Professor of Psychoanalysis, University College London; Director of Research, Anna Freud Centre, London, UK; Director, Child and Family Center and Clinical Protocols and Outcomes Center, Menninger Clinic, Topeka, Kansas, USA
Chapters 4.12.6, 6.3.5 and 9.5.2

Gillian C. Forrest Consultant Child and Adolescent Psychiatrist
Chapter 9.5.8

Leah Fostick Department of Psychiatry, Chaim Sheba Medical Centre, Tel Hashomer, Israel
Chapter 4.8

W. Fraser Division of Psychological Medicine, University of Wales College of Medicine, Cardiff, UK
Introduction to Section 10

Laura Fratiglioni Aging Research Centre, Karolinska Institute, Stockholm, Sweden
Chapter 8.3

David M. Fresco Adult Anxiety Clinic of Temple University, Philadelphia, Pennsylvania, USA
Chapter 4.7.2

K.W.M. Fulford Professor of Philosophy and Mental Health, University of Warwick; Honorary Consultant Psychiatrist, University of Oxford, UK
Chapter 1.5.2

Robert Fung, Specialist Registrar in Psychiatry, Sheffield Care NHS Trust, UK
Chapter 4.2.3.2

Pier Maria Furlan Director of Department of Mental Health San Luigi Gonzaga Hospital - University of Torino, Italy
Chapter 5.5

Glen O. Gabbard Bessie Walker Callaway Distinguished Professor of Psychoanalysis and Education in the Kansas School of Psychiatry, Menninger Clinic, Topeka; Clinical Professor of Psychiatry of Kansas School of Medicine, Wichita, Kansas, USA
Chapter 3.3

Jean Garrabé Honorary President of L'Evolution psychiatrique, Paris, France
Chapter 4.3.10

M. Elena Garralda Professor of Child and Adolescent Psychiatry, Imperial College of Medicine, London, UK
Chapter 9.3.4

Ann Gath Formerly of University College London, UK
Chapter 10.8

John R. Geddes Professor of Epidemiological Psychiatry, Department of Psychiatry, University of Oxford, Warneford Hospital, Oxford, UK
Chapters 1.10 and 4.5.1

David Gill Research Fellow, Department of Psychiatry, University of Oxford, UK
Chapters 5.2.9

Kathryn J. Gill MUHB Addictions Unit, McGill University, Montreal QC, Canada
Chapter 4.2.2.1

Julia Gledhill Clinical Research Fellow, Imperial College of Medicine, London, UK
Chapter 9.3.4

David Goldberg Director of Research and Development, Institute of Psychiatry, King's College London, UK
Chapter 7.8

Terry E. Goldberg The Zucker Hillside Hospital, Glen Oaks NY, USA
Chapter 2.5.3

Guy Goodwin Professor, University Department, Warneford Hospital, Oxford, UK
Chapter 4.5.6

Kevin Gournay Emeritus Professor, Institute of Psychiatry, King's College London, UK
Chapter 6.4.2

Simon G. Gowers Professor of Adolescent Psychiatry, University of Liverpool, UK
Chapter 9.5.9

Cynthia A. Graham, Oxford Doctoral Course in Clinical Psychology Warneford Hospital, Oxford and The Kinsey Institute for Research in Sex, Gender, & Reproduction, UK
Chapter 4.11.2

Philip Graham Emeritus Professor of Child Psychiatry, Institute of Child Health, London, UK
Chapter 9.5.3

P.M. Grasby Senior Lecturer, MRC Cyclotron Unit, Hammersmith Hospital, London, UK
Chapter 2.3.6

Richard Green Head, Gender Identity Clinic, and Visiting Professor of Psychiatry, Imperial College of Medicine at Charing Cross Hospital, London, UK; Emeritus Professor of Psychiatry, University of California, Los Angeles, California, USA
Chapters 4.11.4 and 9.2.12

Stephen Green Clinical Professor of Psychiatry, Georgetown University School of Medicine, Washington, D.C., USA
Chapter 1.5.1

Michael Gunn Professor of Law and Head of Department, Department of Academic Legal Studies, Nottingham Law School, Nottingham Trent University, UK
Chapter 11.1

Lars Gustafson Professor of Geriatric Psychiatry, Lund University Hospital, Lund, Sweden
Chapter 4.1.3

Francesca Guzzetta Bologna, Italy
Chapter 4.12.4

Jennifer Gutstein Department of Child Psychiatry, College of Physicians and Surgeons, Columbia University, New York, USA
Chapter 9.2.10

Sarah Harper Oxford Institute for Aging, University of Oxford, Oxford, UK
Chapter 8.2

Rex Haigh Project Lead, Community of Communities, Centre for Quality Improvement, Royal College of Psychiatrists, London; Consultant Psychiatrist, Berkshire Healthcare NHS Foundation Trust, UK
Chapter 6.3.9

S.A. Hales Psychiatry Fellow, Princess Margaret Hospital, University Health Network, Toronto, Canada
Chapter 5.3.6

John N. Hall Professor of Mental Health, School of Health and Social Care, Oxford Brookes University, Oxford, UK
Chapter 1.8.3

Wayne Hall Professor of Public Health Policy, University of Queensland, Herston, Australia
Chapter 4.2.3.7

Edwin Harari Consultant Psychiatrist, St Vincent's Hospital, Melbourne, Australia
Chapter 6.3.8

Sarah Harper Oxford Institute for Aging, University of Oxford, Oxford, UK
Chapter 8.2

James C. Harris Director Developmental Neuropsychiatry Clinic, Professor of Psychiatry and Behavioral Sciences, Pediatrics, and Mental Hygiene, The Johns Hopkins University School of Medicine, USA
Chapter 9.2.1

Paul J. Harrison Clinical Reader in Psychiatry, University of Oxford Department of Psychiatry, Warneford Hospital, Oxford, UK
Chapter 4.3.6.2

Allison G. Harvey Department of Experimental Psychology, University of Oxford, UK
Chapter 4.6.1

Philip D. Harvey Professor of Psychiatry and Behavioral Sciences, Emory University School of Medicine, Woodruff Memorial Building, Atlanta, GA, USA
Chapter 4.3.3

Keith Hawton Director, Centre for Suicide Research, University Department of Psychiatry, Warneford Hospital, Oxford, UK
Chapter 4.15.4

Richard G. Heimberg Adult Anxiety Clinic of Temple University, Philadelphia, Pennsylvania, USA
Chapter 4.7.2

Scott Henderson Emeritus Professor, The Australian National University, Canberra, Australia
Chapters 2.7 and 8.3

George R. Heninger Professor, Department of Psychiatry, Yale University School of Medicine, New Haven, Connecticut, USA
Chapter 6.2.3

Leslie Hicks, University of York, UK
Chapter 9.5.6

A.J. Holland Lecturer, Department of Psychiatry, University of Cambridge, UK
Chapter 10.1

Jimmie C. Holland Wayne E. Chapman Chair in Psychiatric Oncology, Department of Psychiatry and Behavioral Sciences, Memorial Sloan Kettering Cancer Center, New York, USA
Chapter 5.3.7

Sheila Hollins Professor of Psychiatry of Learning Disability, Department of Psychiatry and Disability, St George's Hospital Medical School, University of London, UK
Chapter 10.7

Jeremy Holmes Consultant Psychiatrist/Psychotherapist, North Devon District Hospital, Barnstaple; Senior Lecturer, University of Bristol, UK
Chapter 3.2

Suzanne Holroyd Professor, Director of Geriatric Psychiatry, Department of Psychiatry and Neurobehavioral Science, University of Virginia, Charlottesville VA, USA
Chapter 8.5.6

Geraldine Holt Honorary Senior Lecturer in Psychiatry at the Institute of Psychiatry, King's College London, UK
Chapter 10.9

Allan House Professor of Liaison Psychiatry, University of Leeds, UK
Chapter 5.3.1

Daniel H. Hovelson The Harvard program in refugee trauma, Massachusetts general hospital, Dept of psychiatry, USA
Chapter 7.10.1

Jane Hubert Senior Lecturer in Social Anthropology, Department of Psychiatry and Disability, St George's Hospital Medical School, University of London, UK
Chapter 10.7

Stephen Hucker University of Toronto, Toronto, Canada
Chapter 11.8

T. A. Hughes Consultant Psychiatrist, St Mary's Hospital, Leeds, UK
Chapter 4.1.6

Masud Husain Institute of Neurology & Institute of Cognitive Neuroscience, UCL, London and National Hospital for Neurology & Neurosurgery, London, UK
Chapter 2.5.2

Frits J. Huyse Psychiatrist, Consultant integrated care, Department of General Internal Medicine, University Medical Centre Groningen (UMCG), Groningen, The Netherlands
Chapter 5.7

Matti Iivanainen Professor, Department of Child Neurology, University of Helsinki, Finland
Chapter 10.5.3

Leslie Iversen Visting Professor, Department of Pharmacology, University of Oxford, UK
Chapter 6.2.7

Richard Ives National Children's Bureau, London, UK
Chapter 4.2.3.6

Assen Jablensky Professor of Psychiatry, University of Western Australia, Perth, Australia
Chapters 4.3.5 and 4.3.7

Robin Jacoby Clinical Reader in the Psychiatry of Old Age, University of Oxford, UK
Chapters 8.4 and 8.5.7

Claudia Jacova Assistant Professor, Division of Neurology, Department of Medicine, University of British Columbia, Vancouver, BC, Canada
Chapter 8.5.1.1

David V. James Consultant Forensic Psychiatrist, North London Forensic Service and Fixated Threat Assessment Centre, UK
Chapter 11.6

Kay Redfield Jamison Professor of Psychiatry, Johns Hopkins School of Medicine, Baltimore, Maryland, USA
Chapter 1.1

John G.R. Jefferys Department of Neurophysiology, Division of Neuroscience, University of Birmingham, UK
Chapter 2.3.9

Andrew Johns Consultant Forensic Psychiatry and Honorary Senior Lecturer, Maudsley Hospital, London, UK
Chapter 11.3.2.

E.C. Johnstone Professor of Psychiatry and Head, Department of Psychiatry, University of Edinburgh, UK
Chapter 4.3.8

David P.H. Jones Senior Clinical Lecturer in Child Psychiatry, Park Hospital for Children, University of Oxford, UK
Chapter 9.3.3

Peter R. Joyce Professor, Department of Psychological Medicine, Christchurch School of Medicine, Christchurch, New Zealand
Chapter 4.5.4

Elizabeth Juven-Wetzler Department of Psychiatry, Chaim Sheba Medical Centre, Tel Hashomer, Israel
Chapter 4.8

Horst Kachele Universitätsklinik Psychosomatische Medizin and Psychotherapie Universitätsklinik Ulm, Germany
Chapter 6.3.5

Adam Ian Kaplin Assistant Professor, Departments of Psychiatry and Neurology, Johns Hopkins University School of Medicine, Johns Hopkins Hospital, Baltimore, MD, USA
Chapter 1.1

Markus Kaski Director, Rinnekoti Research Foundation, Director and Chief Physician of Rinnekoti Foundation, Espoo, Finland
Chapter 10.3

Aliya Kassam Institute of Psychiatry, David Glodberg Centre, De Crespigny Park, London, UK
Chapter 1.2

Roger G. Kathol, Adjunct Professor of Internal Medicine and Psychiatry, University of Minnesota, President, Cartesian Solutions, Inc. Burnsville, MN, USA
Chapter 5.7

Paul E. Keck Jr. Lindner Center of HOPE, Mason, and Department of Psychiatry, University of Cincinnati College of Medicine, Cincinnati, OH, USA
Chapter 4.13.1

John Kellett St George's Hospital Medical School, London, UK
Chapter 8.5.8

Keith W. Kelley Department of Animal Sciences, University of Illinois, Urbana-Champaign, USA
Chapter 2.3.10

David Kennard Chair of the UK Network of the International Society for the Psychological Treatments of the Schizophrenias and other psychoses (ISPS UK); former Head of Psychology Services, The Retreat, York, UK
Chapter 6.3.9

Ad.J.F.M. Kerkhof Professor of Clinical Psychology, Vrije Universiteit, Amsterdam, The Netherlands
Chapter 4.15.2

Otto F. Kernberg Professor of Psychiatry, Cornell University Medical College, New York; Training and Supervising Analyst, Columbia University Center for Psychoanalytic Training and Research, New York, USA
Chapter 3.1

Falk Kiefer Professor of Addiction Research, Deputy Director, Department of Addictive Behaviour and Addiction Medicine, Central Institute of Mental Health CIMH, University of Heidelberg, Mannheim, Germany
Chapter 4.2.2.3

Arthur Kleinman Presley Professor of Anthropology and Psychiatry, Harvard University; Chair, Department of Social Medicine, Harvard Medical School, Cambridge, Massachusetts, USA
Chapter 2.6.2

Ami Klin Yale University, New Haven, Connecticut, USA
Chapter 9.2.3

Kimberly Klipstein Department of Psychiatry, Mount Sinai School of Medicine, New York, USA
Chapter 4.6.4

Martin Knapp Institute of Psychiatry, King's College London; London School of Economics and Political Science, University of London, UK
Chapter 7.7

Michael D. Kopelman Professor of Neuropsychiatry at King's College London, Institute of Psychiatry, UK
Chapter 4.1.12

Malcolm Lader Emeritus Professor of Clinical Psychopharmacology, King's College London, Institute of Psychiatry, Denmark Hill, London, UK
Chapter 6.2.2

Fergus D. Law Honorary Senior Registrar and Clinical Lecturer, Psychopharmacology Unit, University of Bristol, UK
Chapters 4.2.1 and 6.2.8

Brian Lawlor Conolly Norman Professor of Old Age Psychiatry, St. James's Hospital & Trinity College, Dublin, Ireland
Chapter 8.5.2

Dusica Lecic-Tosevski Professor of Psychiatry, Institute of Mental Health, School of Medicine, University of Belgrade, Belgrade, Serbia
Chapter 4.12.3

Julian Leff Emeritus Professor, Department of Psychological Medicine, Institute of Psychiatry, King's College London, UK
Chapter 1.3.2

R.J. Levin Department of Biomedical Science, University of Sheffield, UK
Chapter 4.11.1

Rhohel Lenroot Child Psychiatry Branch, NIMH, Bethesda MD, USA
Chapter 9.1.4

Peter F. Liddle Professor of Psychiatry, University of British Columbia, Vancouver, British Columbia, Canada
Chapter 4.3.2

Felice Lieh Mak Emeritus Professor, Department of Psychiatry, University of Hong Kong, Hong Kong
Chapter 5.2.10

James Lindesay Professor of Psychiatry for the Elderly, University of Leicester, UK
Chapters 8.5.1 and 8.5.5

Jouko K. Lonnqvist Professor, National Public Health Institute, Helsinki, Finland
Chapter 4.15.1

Juan J. López-Ibor Jr. Chairman, Department of Psychiatry, San Carlos University Hospital, Complutense University, Madrid, Spain
Chapters 1.6 and 4.12.1

Mª Inés López-Ibor San Carlos University Hospital, Complutense University, Madrid, Spain
Chapter 4.2.3.8

Simon Lovestone Professor of Old Age Psychiatry, NIHR Biomedical Research Centre for Mental Health, MRC Centre for Neurodegeneration Research, Departments of Psychological Medicine and Neuroscience, King's College London, Institute of Psychiatry, London, UK
Chapter 4.1.2

Leanne Magee Temple University, Philadelphia, Pennsylvania, USA
Chapter 4.7.2

Andrew McCulloch The Mental Health Foundation, London, UK
Chapter 7.1

Jane McCarthy Division of Mental Health, St George's Hospital, London, UK
Chapter 10.8

Susan L. McElroy Lindner Center of HOPE, Mason, and Department of Psychiatry, University of Cincinnati College of Medicine, Cincinnati, Ohio, USA
Chapter 4.13.1

Peter McGuffin Director and Professor of Psychiatric Genetics, Institute of Psychiatry, King's College London, UK
Chapter 2.4.1

I.G. McKeith Clinical Director, Institute for Ageing and Health, Newcastle University, Newcastle Upon Tyne, UK
Chapter 4.1.5

Kwame McKenzie Centre for Addictions and Mental Health, Toronto, Canada; University of Toronto, Canada; University of Central Lancashire, UK
Chapter 7.3

Declan McLoughlin Institute of Psychiatry, King's College London, UK
Chapter 6.2.10.3

Mark W. Mahowald Director, Minnesota Regional Sleep Disorders Center, Hennepin County Medical Center; Professor of Neurology, University of Minnesota Medical School, Minneapolis, Minnesota, USA
Chapter 4.14.4

Mario Maj Institute of Psychiatry, University of Naples, Italy
Chapter 4.1.9

Ulrik Fredrik Malt Professor of Psychiatry (Psychosomatic Medicine), National Hospital, University of Oslo, Norway
Chapter 5.3.8

J. John Mann Vice Chair for Research Scientific Director, Kreitchman PET Center, Columbia University and Chief, Division of Molecular Imaging & Neuropathology, New York State Psychiatric Institute, USA
Chapter 4.15.3

Karl F. Mann Professor and Chair in Addiction Research, Deputy Director Central Institute of Mental Health (CIMH), University of Heidelberg, Mannheim, Germany
Chapter 4.2.2.3

Russell L. Margolis Professor of Psychiatry and Neurology Director, Johns Hopkins Schizophrenia Program Director, Laboratory of Genetic Neurobiology Division of Neurobiology, Department of Psychiatry, Johns Hopkins University School of Medicine, Baltimore, USA
Chapter 4.1.7

John C. Markowitz Associate Professor of Psychiatry, Weill Medical College of Cornell University; Director, Psychotherapy Clinic, Payne Whitney Clinic, New York Presbyterian Hospital, New York, USA
Chapter 6.3.3

John Marsden Lecturer, Institute of Psychiatry, King's College London, UK
Chapter 4.2.4

Jane Marshall Senior Lecturer in the Addictions, National Addiction Centre, Institute of Psychiatry, King's College London, UK
Chapters 4.1.11 and 4.2.2.2

Andrés Martin Professor of Child Psychiatry, Child Study Center Yale University School of Medicine, New Haven, Connecticut, USA
Chapter 9.1.3

Keith Matthews Dept of Psychiatry, University of Dundee, Dundee, UK
Chapter 6.2.10.4

Barbara Maughan MRC Child Psychiatry Unit, Institute of Psychiatry, King's College London, UK
Chapter 9.3.1

Soraya Mayet National Addiction Centre, Institute of Psychiatry, King's College London, UK
Chapter 4.2.3.1

Richard Mayou Emeritus Professor of Psychiatry, University of Oxford, UK
Chapter 5.2.1

Nick Medford Institute of Psychiatry, King's College London, UK
Chapter 4.9

David Meagher Dept of Adult Psychiatry, Midwestern Regional Hospital, Limerick, Ireland
Chapter 4.1.1

Thomas W. Meeks Division of Geriatric Psychiatry, University of California San Diego, La Jolla CA, USA
Chapter 8.5.3

Pamela S. Melding Honorary Senior Lecturer, Department of Psychological Medicine, University of Auckland, New Zealand and Consultant in Psychiatry of Old Age, Mental Health Serviced, North Shore Hospital, Waitemata District Health Board, Takapuna, North Shore City, Auckland, New Zealand
Chapter 8.7

Herbert Y. Meltzer Bixler/May/Johnaon Professor of Psychiatry, Professor of Pharmacoloqy Vanderbilt University School of Medicine, Nashville, Tennessee, USA
Chapter 6.2.5

Julien Mendlewicz Department of Psychiatry, University Clinics of Brussels, Erasme Hospital, Brussels, Belgium
Chapter 4.5.5

Andreas Meyer-Lindenberg Dept of Psychiatry, Central Institute of Mental Health, Mannheim, Germany
Chapter 2.5.3

Gillian C. Mezey Consultant and Senior Lecturer in Forensic Psychiatry, Traumatic Stress Service, St George's Hospital Medical School, London, UK
Chapters 11.12 and 11.13

R.H.S. Mindham Emeritus Professor of Psychiatry, University of Leeds, UK
Chapter 4.1.6

Andrew Mogg Institute of Psychiatry, King's College London, UK
Chapter 6.2.10.3

Richard F. Mollica Director, Harvard Program in Refugee Trauma; Associate Professor of Psychiatry, Harvard Medical School and Harvard School of Public Health, Cambridge, Massachusetts, USA
Chapter 7.10.1

Emanuel Moran Consultant Psychiatrist, Grovelands Priory Hospital, London, UK
Chapter 4.13.2

Stella Morris Dept of Psychological Medicine, Hull Royal Infirmary, Hull, UK
Chapter 5.2.6

Matt Muijen WHO Regional Office for Europe, Copenhagen, Denmark
Chapter 7.1

Paul E. Mullen Professor of Forensic Psychiatry, Monash University; Clinical Director, Victorian Institute of Forensic Mental Health, Monash University, Melbourne, Australia
Chapters 11.10, 11.11 and 11.14

Alistair Munro Emeritus Professor of Psychiatry, Dalhousie University, Halifax, Nova Scotia, Canada
Chapter 4.4

Rebecca Murphy Research Psychologist, Oxford University Department of Psychiatry, Warneford Hospital, Oxford, UK
Chapters 4.10.2 and 6.3.2.2

Lynne Murray Winnicott Research Unit, University of Reading, Reading, UK
Chapter 9.3.6

R.M. Murray Institute of Psychiatry, King's College London, UK
Chapter 4.3.6.1

Norbert Nedopil Professor of Forensic Psychiatry, Head of the Department of Forensic Psychiatry at the Psychiatric Hospital of the University of Munich, Munich, Germany
Chapter 11.3.3

Juan C. Negrete Professor and Head, Addictions Psychiatry Program, University of Toronto, Canada
Chapter 4.2.2.1

Gretchen N. Neigh Dept of Psychiatry and Behavioral Sciences, Emory University, Atlanta GA, USA
Chapter 2.3.3

Charles B. Nemeroff Reunette W. Harris Professor and Chairman, Department of Psychiatry and Behavioral Sciences, Emory University School of Medicine, Atlanta, Georgia, USA
Chapter 2.3.3

Giles Newton-Howes Division of Neurosciences and Mental Health, Imperial College School of Medicine, London, UK
Chapter 4.12.7

Jeffrey Newcorm Mount Sinai School of Medicine, New York, USA
Chapter 4.6.4

Russell Noyes Jr. Department of Psychiatry, University of Iowa College of Medicine, Iowa City, Iowa, USA
Chapter 5.2.5

David J. Nutt Professor of Psychopharmacology and Head of Clinical Medicine, University of Bristol, UK
Chapters 4.2.1 and 6.2.8

Margaret Oates Senior Lecturer in Psychiatry, University of Nottingham, UK
Chapter 1.8.1

James R.P. Ogloff Victorian Institute of Forensic Mental Health, Thomas Embling Hospital, Fairfield VIC, Australia
Chapters 11.4 ,11.14, and 11.16

John O'Grady Knowle Hospital, Fareham, UK
Chapter 11.15

Catherine Oppenheimer Consultant Psychiatrist, Warneford Hospital, Oxford, UK
Chapter 8.5.8 and 8.6

Luca Ostacoli Liaison Psychiatry and Psychosomatic Unit, Department of Mental Health, San Luigi Gonzaga Hospital - University of Torino, Italy
Chapter 5.5

Pierre Oswald Dept of Psychiatry, ULB Erasme, Brussels, Belgium
Chapter 4.5.5

Barton W. Palmer Veterans Affairs Medical Center, University of California, San Diego CA, USA
Chapter 8.5.3

Gordon Parker Professor, University of New South Wales; and Executive Director, Black Dog Institute, Australia
Chapter 4.5.3

E.S. Paykel Emeritus Professor of Psychiatry, Department of Psychiatry, University of Cambridge, UK
Chapter 4.5.8

John B. Pearce Emeritus Professor of Child and Adolescent Psychiatry, University of Nottingham, UK
Chapters 9.4 and 9.5.1

†**R.C.A. Pearson** Department of Biomedical Science, University of Sheffield, UK
Chapter 2.3.1

Keith J. Petrie Associate Professor, School of Medicine,University of Auckland, New Zealand
Chapter 5.6

Cynthia R. Pfeffer Weill Medical College of Cornell University, New York Presbyterian Hospital-Westchester Division, White Plains, New York, USA
Chapter 9.2.10

Katharine A. Phillips Professor of Psychiatry and Human Behavior, The Warren Alpert Medical School of Brown University; Director, Body Dysmorphic Disorder Program, Butler Hospital, Providence, USA
Chapter 5.2.8

Pierre Pichot Académie Nationale de Médecine, Paris, France
Chapter 1.4

Harold Alan Pincus Columbia University, New York, USA
Chapter 1.9

Vanessa Pinfold 'Rethink', London, UK
Chapter 7.9

Daniel S. Pine Division of Intramural Research Programs, National Institutes of Health, Bethesda, USA
Chapter 9.2.6

Malcolm Pines Founding Member, Institute of Group Analysis, London, UK
Chapter 6.3.6

Harrison G. Pope Jr. Professor of Psychiatry, Harvard Medical School, Boston; Chief, Biological Psychiatry Laboratory, McClean Hospital, Belmont, Massachusetts, USA
Chapter 6.2.6

Robert M. Post Chief, Biological Psychiatry Branch, National Institute of Mental Health, Bethesda, Maryland, USA
Chapter 6.2.4

Graham E. Powell Psychology Services, Powell Campbell Edelmann, London, UK
Chapter 1.8.3

Herschel Prins Professor, Midlands Centre for Criminology and Criminal Justice, University of Loughborough, UK
Chapter 11.9

Paul Ramchandani Dept of Psychiatry, University of Oxford, Warneford Hospital, Oxford, UK
Chapter 9.3.6

Shulamit Ramon Professor of Interprofessional Health and Social Studies, Anglia Polytechnic University, Cambridge, UK
Chapter 6.4.3

Beverley Raphael University of Western Sydney Medical School, Sydney NSW, Australia
Chapter 4.6.5

James Reich Clinical Professor of Psychiatry, University of California, San Francisco Medical School and Adjunct Associate Professor of Psychiatry, Stanford School of Medicine, USA
Chapter 4.12.2

Helmut Remschmidt Director, Department of Child and Adolescent Psychiatry, Philipps Universität, Marburg, Germany
Chapter 9.2.2

Philippe Robaey Institute of Mental Health Research, Royal Ottawa Hospital, Ottawa, Canada
Chapter 9.2.8

Ian Robbins Consultant Clinical Psychologist, St George's Hospital, London, UK
Chapter 11.13

T.W. Robbins Section of Forensic Psychiatry, St George's Hospital Medical School, London, UK
Chapter 2.5.5

G.M. Rodin Professor of Psychiatry, University of Toronto, Toronto, Canada
Chapter 5.3.6

Maria A. Ron Professor of Neuropsychiatry, Institute of Neurology, University College London, UK
Chapter 5.3.2

Robin Room Professor, School of Population Health, University of Melbourne; and Director, AER Centre for Alcohol Policy Research, Turning Point Alcohol and Drug Centre, Fitzroy, Victoria, Australia
Chapter 4.2.2.6

W. Rössler Professor of Clinical Psychiatry and Psychology, University of Zürich, Switzerland
Chapter 6.4.1

James R. Rundell Department of Psychiatry and Psychology, Mayo Clinic Professor of Psychiatry, Mayo Clinic College of Medicine, USA
Chapter 5.3.4

Gerald Russell Emeritus Professor of Psychiatry, Director of the Eating Disorders Unit, Hayes Grove Priory Hospital, Hayes, Kent, UK
Chapter 4.10.1

B.J. Sahakian Dept of Psychiatry, University of Cambridge, Cambridge, UK
Chapter 2.5.5

Diana Sanders Chartered Counselling Psychologist, working in Psychological Medicine in Oxford, UK
Chapter 6.3.1

Paramala J. Santosh Great Ormond Street Hospital for Sick Children, London, UK
Chapter 9.5.5

Benedetto Saraceno Director of Department of Mental Health and Substance Abuse, World Health Organization WHO
Chapter 1.3.1

Gauri N. Savla, Veterans Affairs Medical Center, University of California, San Diego CA, USA
Chapter 8.5.3

Carlos H. Schenck Staff Psychiatrist, Minnesota Regional Sleep Disorders Center, Hennepin County Medical Center; Associate Professor of Psychiatry, University of Minnesota Medical School, Minneapolis, Minnesota, USA
Chapter 4.14.4

John Schlapobersky Consultant Psychotherapist, Trumatic Stress Clinic Middlesex/University College Hospital, formerly also of The Medical Foundation for the Care of Victims of Torture London, UK
Chapter 6.3.6

Fabrizio Schiffano, Chair in Clinical Pharmacology and Therapeutics Associate Dean, Postgraduate Medical School, Hon Consultant Psychiatrist Addictions, University of Hertfordshire, School of Pharmacy, College Lane Campus, Hatfield, UK
Chapter 4.2.3.5

Gerd Schulte-Körne Director of the Department of Child and Adolescent Psychiatry, Psychosomatics and Psychotherapy, University of Munich, Pettenkoferstr, München/Germany
Chapter 9.2.2

J. Scott Professor of Psychological Medicine, University of Newcastle & Honorary Professor, Psychological Treatments Research, Institute of Psychiatry, London and University Department of Psychiatry, Leazes Wing, Royal Victoria Infirmary, Newcastle upon Tyne, UK
Chapter 4.5.8

Stephen Scott Professor of Child Health & Behaviour, King's College London, Institute of Psychiatry, and Director of Research National Academy for Parenting Practitioners, London, UK
Chapters 9.1.1 and 9.2.5

Nicholas Seivewright Consultant Psychiatrist in Substance Misuse, Community Health Sheffield NHS Trust, Sheffield, UK
Chapter 4.2.3.2

David Shaffer Department of Child Psychiatry, College of Physicians and Surgeons, Columbia University, New York, USA
Chapter 9.2.10

Trevor Sharp Dept of Pharmacology, University of Oxford, Oxford, UK
Chapter 2.3.4

Michael Sharpe Professor of Psychological Medicine & Symptoms Research, University of Edinburgh, UK
Chapters 5.1 and 5.2.7

Jennifer Shaw Centre for Suicide Prevention, The School of Medicine, University of Manchester, UK
Chapter 11.5

Mauricio Sierra Institute of Psychiatry, King's College London, UK
Chapter 4.9

Gregory Simon Investigator, Center for Health Studies, Group Health Cooperative, Seattle, Washington, USA
Chapter 5.2.2

Andrew Sims Professor of Psychiatry, University of Leeds, UK
Chapter 1.7

Ian Sinclair Professor of Social Work, University of York, UK
Chapter 9.5.6

Mike Slade Health Service and Population Research Department and Institute of Psychiatry, King's College London, UK
Chapter 7.2

Elita Smiley Consultant Psychiatrist and Clinical Senior Lecturer, Division of Community Based Sciences, Faculty of Medicine, University of Glasgow, UK
Chapter 10.2

Wolfgang Söllner Department of Psychosomatic Medicine and Psychotherapy General Hospital Nuremberg, Prof.Ernst-Nathan-Str. 1, Nürnberg, Germany
Chapter 5.7

Daniel Souery Department of Psychiatry, University Clinics of Brussels, Erasme Hospital, Brussels, Belgium
Chapter 4.5.5

Elizabeth Spencer Senior Clinical Medical Officer, Early Intervention Service, Northern Birmingham Mental Health Trust, Birmingham, UK
Chapter 6.3.2.4

David A. Spiegel Center for Anxiety and Related Disorders at Boston University, Boston, Massachusetts, USA
Chapter 4.7.1

Costas Stefanis Honorary Professor of Psychiatry, University of Athens, Greece
Chapter 1.6

Alan Stein Royal Free and University College Medical School, University College London, and Tavistock Clinic, London, UK
Chapter 9.3.6

Jessica Stiles Department of Psychiatry and Behavioral Sciences, Memorial Sloan Kettering Cancer Center, New York, USA
Chapter 5.3.7

William S. Stone Assistant Professor of Psychology, Director of Neuropsychology Training and Clinical Services, Department of Psychiatry, Harvard Medical School, Massachusetts Mental Health Center Public Psychiatry, Division of the Beth Israel Deaconess Medical Center, Boston, USA
Chapter 4.3.9

Gregory Stores Emeritus Professor of Developmental Neuropsychiatry, University of Oxford, UK
Chapters 4.14.1 and 9.2.9

Elizabeth A. Stormshak Assistant Professor, University of Oregon, Eugene, Oregon, USA
Chapter 9.5.4

James J. Strain Professor/Director, Behavioral Medicine and Consultation Psychiatry, Mount Sinai School of Medicine, New York, USA
Chapter 4.6.4

John Strang National Addiction Centre, Institute of Psychiatry, King's College London, UK
Chapters 4.2.3.1 and 4.2.4

J. Suckling Brain Mapping Unit, Department of Psychiatry, University of Cambridge, Addenbrookes Hospital, Cambridge, UK
Chapters 2.3.7 and 2.3.8

Nicola Swinson Centre for Sucide Prevention, The School of Medicine, University of Manchester, UK
Chapter 11.5

Michele Tansella Professor of Psychiatry and Chairman, Department of Medicine and Public Health, Section of Psychiatry, University of Verona, Italy
Chapters 7.2 and 7.6

Mary Target Senior Lecturer in Psychoanalysis, Psychoanalysis Unit, University College London; Deputy Director of Research, Anna Freud Centre, London, UK
Chapter 9.5.2

Eric Taylor Head of Department, Child & Adolescent Psychiatry, King's College London, Institute of Psychiatry, UK
Chapter 9.2.4

John-Paul Taylor Academic Specialist Registrar, Institute for Ageing and Health Newcastle University, Campus for Ageing and Vitality, Newcastle upon Tyne, UK
Chapter 4.1.13

Pamela J. Taylor School of Medicine, Cardiff University, Cardiff, UK
Chapter 11.17

Tatiana Taylor Dept of Psychiatry, University of Oxford, Warneford Hospital, Oxford, UK
Chapter 4.15.4

Mary Teasdale 'Rethink', London, UK
Chapter 7.9

Anita Thapar Department of Psychological Medicine, School of Medicine, Cardiff University, UK
Chapter 2.4.1

June Thoburn Emeritus Professor of Social Work, University of East Anglia, Norwich, UK
Chapter 9.3.5

Sian Thomas Chester Young People's Centre, Chester, UK
Chapter 9.5.9

Lindsay Thomson Division of Psychiatry, University of Edinburgh, Edinburgh, UK
Chapter 11.3.1

Anne E. Thompson Emeritus Professor Child and Adolescent Psychiatry, University of Nottingham, UK
Chapter 9.4

Graham Thornicroft Professor of Community Psychiatry, Institute of Psychiatry, King's College London, UK
Chapters 1.2, 7.2 and 7.6

Adolf Tobeña Professor of Psychiatry, Director of the Dept. of Psychiatry and Forensic Medicine, Autonomous University of Barcelona, Bellaterra (Barcelona), Spain
Chapter 4.12.5

Bruce J. Tonge Head Monash University School of Psychology Psychiatry & Psychological Medicine, Monash Medical Centre, Clayton, Victoria, Australia
Chapter 10.5.1

Brian Toone Consultant, Maudsley Hospital; Honorary Senior Lecturer, Institute of Psychiatry, King's College London, UK
Chapter 5.3.3

David Trickey Leicester Royal Infirmary, Leicestershire Partnership NHS Trust, UK
Chapters 9.3.2 and 9.3.7

Paula Trzepacz Eli Lilly & Co, USA
Chapter 4.1.1

Wen-Shing Tseng Professor at Department of Psychiatry, University of Hawaii School of Medicine, USA
Chapters 4.16 and 6.5

Ming T. Tsuang Behavioral Genomics Endowed Chair and University Professor, University of California; Distinguished Professor of Psychiatry and Director, Center for Behavioral Genomics, Department of Psychiatry, University of California, San Diego, CA, USA
Chapter 4.3.9

André Tylee Director, Royal College of General Practitioners Unit for Mental Health Education in Primary Care, Institute of Psychiatry, King's College London, UK
Chapter 7.8

Amy M. Ursano Department of Psychiatry, University of North Carolina at Chapel Hill School of Medicine, Chapel Hill, North Carolina, USA
Chapter 6.3.4

Robert J. Ursano Professor and Chairman, Department of Psychiatry, Uniformed Services University of the Health Sciences, F. Edward Herbert School of Medicine, Bethesda, Maryland, USA
Chapter 6.3.4

Jim van Os Professor of Psychiatric Epidemiology, Maastricht University, Maastricht, The Netherlands and Visiting Professor of Psychiatric Epidemiology Institute of Psychiatry, London, UK
Chapter 7.3

Fred R. Volkmar Yale University, New Haven, Connecticut, USA
Chapter 9.2.3

Jane Walker Clinical Lecturer and Honorary Specialist Registrar in Liaison Psychiatry, Psychological Medicine & Symptoms Research Group, School of Molecular & Clinical Medicine, University of Edinburgh, UK
Chapter 5.1

Diane Waller Professor of Art Psychotherapy, Goldsmiths, University of London, UK
Chapter 6.4.4

Paul Walters MRC Fellow & Specialist Psychiatrist , Programme Leader MSc in Mental Health Services Research, Section of Primary Care Mental Health, Health Service and Population Research Department, David Goldberg Centre, Institute of Psychiatry, London, UK
Chapter 7.8

John Weinmann Professor of Psychology as applied to Medicine, Institute of Psychiatry, King's College London, UK
Chapter 5.6

Myrna M. Weissman Professor of Epidemiology in Psychiatry, College of Physicians and Surgeons of Columbia University; Chief, Division of Clinical and Genetic Epidemiology, New York State Psychiatric Institute, New York, USA
Chapter 6.3.3

Sarah Welch Gloucestershire Partnership NHS Foundation Trust, UK
Chapter 4.2.3.4

Ursula Werneke Consultant Psychiatrist, Norrkoping, Sweden
Chapter 6.2.9

Simon Wessely Professor of Epidemiological and Liaison Psychiatry, Institute of Psychiatry, King's College London, UK
Chapter 5.2.7

Kay Wheat Senior Lecturer in Law, Department of Academic Legal Studies, Nottingham Law School, Nottingham Trent University, UK
Chapter 11.1

Adam R. Winstock Senior Staff Specialist, Drug Health Services, Conjoint Senior Lecturer, National Drug and Alcohol Research Centre, UNSW, Australia
Chapters 4.2.3.1 and 4.2.3.5

Sally Wooding Senior Research Fellow, SciMHA Unit, University of Western Sydney, Australia
Chapter 4.6.5

Matt Woolgar Institute of Psychiatry, King's College London, UK
Chapter 2.5.1

Miranda Wolpert Director of Child and Adolescent Mental Health Services, Evidence Based Practice Unit, University College London and Anna Freud Centre, UK
Chapter 9.5.7

Lawson Wulsin Professor of Psychiatry and Family Medicine, University of Cincinnati, OH, USA
Chapter 5.7

Richard Jed Wyatt† National Institutes of Mental Health, Bethesda, Maryland, USA
Chapter 1.1

William Yule Professor of Applied Child Psychology, Institute of Psychiatry, King's College London, UK
Chapter 2.5.1

Karl Zilles Professor, Institute of Neuroscience and Biophysics, INB-3 Research Centre, Jülich and C.&O. Vogt Institute of Brain Research, University Düsseldorf, Germany
Chapter 2.3.2

Joseph Zohar Psychiatric Medical Center, Sheba Medical Center, Tel Hashomer and Sackler School of Medicine, Tel Aviv University, Israel
Chapter 4.8

SECTION 1

The Subject Matter of and Approach to Psychiatry

1.1 The patient's perspective *3*
Kay Redfield Jamison, Richard Jed Wyatt, and Adam Ian Kaplin

1.2 Public attitudes and the challenge of stigma *5*
Graham Thornicroft, Elaine Brohan, and Aliya Kassam

1.3 Psychiatry as a worldwide public health problem *10*

1.3.1 Mental disorders as a worldwide public health issue *10*
Benedetto Saraceno

1.3.2 Transcultural psychiatry *13*
Julian Leff

1.4 The history of psychiatry as a medical specialty *17*
Pierre Pichot

1.5 Ethics and values 28

1.5.1 Psychiatric ethics *28*
Sidney Bloch and Stephen Green

1.5.2 Values and values-based practice in clinical psychiatry *32*
K. W. M. Fulford

1.6 The psychiatrist as a manager *39*
Juan J. López-Ibor Jr. and Costas Stefanis

1.7 Descriptive phenomenology *47*
Andrew Sims

1.8 Assessment *62*

1.8.1 The principles of clinical assessment in general psychiatry *62*
John E. Cooper and Margaret Oates

1.8.2 Assessment of personality *78*
C. Robert Cloninger

1.8.3 Cognitive assessment *85*
Graham E. Powell

1.8.4 Questionnaire, rating, and behavioural methods of assessment *94*
John N. Hall

1.9 Diagnosis and classification *99*
Michael B. First and Harold Alan Pincus

1.10 From science to practice *122*
John R. Geddes

1.1

The patient's perspective

Kay Redfield Jamison, Richard Jed Wyatt,† and Adam Ian Kaplin

It is difficult to be a psychiatric patient, but a good doctor can make it less so. Confusion and fear can be overcome by knowledge and compassion, and resistance to treatment is often, although by no means always, amenable to change by intelligent persuasion. The devil, as the fiery melancholic Byron knew, is in the details.

Patients, when first given a psychiatric diagnosis, are commonly both relieved and frightened—relieved because often they have been in pain and anxiety for a considerable period of time, and frightened because they do not know what the diagnosis means or what the treatment will entail. They do not know if they will return to the way they once were, whether the treatment they have been prescribed will or will not work, and, even if it does work, at what cost it will be to them in terms of their notions of themselves, potentially unpleasant side-effects, and the reactions of their family members, friends, colleagues, and employers. Perhaps most disturbing, they do not know if their depression, psychosis, anxieties, or compulsions will return to become a permanent part of their lives. Caught in a state often characterized by personal anguish, social isolation and confusion, newly diagnosed patients find themselves on a quest to regain a sense of mastery of themselves and their surroundings. One of the main goals of therapies of all types is to empower the patient and give them some control back over their world.

The specifics of what the doctor says, and the manner in which he or she says it, are critically important. Most patients who complain about receiving poor psychiatric care do so on several grounds: their doctors, they feel, spend too little time explaining the nature of their illnesses and treatment; they are reluctant to consult with or actively involve family members; they are patronizing, and do not adequately listen to what the patient has to say; they do not encourage questions or sufficiently address the concerns of the patient; they do not discuss alternative treatments, the risks of treatment, and the risks of no treatment; and they do not thoroughly forewarn about side-effects of medications.

Most of these complaints are avoidable. Time, although difficult to come by, is well spent early on in the course of treatment when confusion and hopelessness are greatest, non-adherence is highest, and the possibility of suicide substantially increased. Hope can be realistically extended to patients and family members, and its explicit extension is vital to those whose illnesses have robbed them not only of hope, but of belief in themselves and their futures. The hope provided needs to be tempered, however, by an explication of possible difficulties yet to be encountered: unpleasant side-effects from medications, a rocky time course to meaningful recovery which will often consist of many discouraging cycles of feeling well, only to become ill again, and the probable personal, professional, and financial repercussions that come in the wake of having a psychiatric illness.

It is terrifying to lose one's sanity or to be seized by a paralysing depression. No medication alone can substitute for a good doctor's clinical expertise and the kindness of a doctor who understands both the medical and psychological sides of mental illness. Nor can any medication alone substitute for a good doctor's capacity to listen to the fears and despair of patients trying to come to terms with what has happened to them. A good doctor is a therapeutic optimist who is able to instill hope and confidence to combat confusion and despair. Great doctors are able to provide the unwavering care to their patients that they would want a member of their own family to receive, blending empathy, and compassion with expertise.

Doctors need to be direct in answering questions, to acknowledge the limits of their understanding, and to encourage specialist consultations when the clinical situation warrants it. They also need to create a therapeutic climate in which patients and their families feel free, when necessary, to express their concerns about treatment or to request a second opinion. Treatment non-adherence, one of the major causes of unnecessary suffering, relapse, hospitalization, and suicide, must be addressed head-on. Young males, early in the course of their illness, are particularly likely to stop medication against medical advice, and the results can be lethal.[1,2] Unfortunately, doctors are notoriously variable in their ability to assess and predict adherence in their patients.[3]

Asking directly and often about medication concerns and side-effects, scheduling frequent follow-up visits after the initial diagnostic evaluation and treatment recommendation, and encouraging adjunctive psychotherapy, or involvement in patient support groups, can make a crucial difference in whether or not a patient takes medication in a way that is most effective. Aggressive treatment of unpleasant or intolerable side-effects, minimizing the dosage and number of doses, and providing ongoing, frequently repetitive

†Deceased.

education about the illness and its treatment are likewise essential, if common-sense, ways to avert or minimize non-adherence.

Education is, of course, integral to the good treatment of any illness, but this is especially true when the illnesses are chronic. The term 'doctor' derives originally from the Latin word for teacher, and it is in their roles as teachers that doctors provide patients with the knowledge and understanding to combat the confusion and unpredictability that surrounds mental illness. Patients and their family members should be encouraged to write down any questions they may have, as many individuals are intimidated once they find themselves in a doctor's office. Any information that is given orally to patients should be repeated as often as necessary (due to the cognitive difficulties experienced by many psychiatric patients, especially when acutely ill or recovering from an acute episode) and, whenever feasible, provided in written form as well. Additional information is available to patients and family members in books and pamphlets obtainable from libraries, bookstores, and patient support groups, as well as from audiotapes, videotapes, and the Internet.(2,4) Visual aids, such as charts portraying the natural course of the treated and untreated illness, or the causes and results of sleep deprivation and medication cessation, are also helpful to many.(5–7) Finally, providing the patients with self-report scales to monitor their daily progress, such as mood charts in affective disorder, not only provides invaluable clinical data, but also teaches patients to better understand their own illness and its response to therapeutic interventions as well as exacerbating stressors. Patients, when they are well, often benefit from a meeting with their family members and their doctor, which focuses upon drawing up contingency plans in case their illness should recur. These meetings also provide an opportunity to shore up the support system the patient has by educating their caregivers about the nature, cause, manifestations, and treatment of their loved one's mental illness. Such meetings may also include what is to be done in the event that hospitalization is required and the patient refuses voluntary admission, a discussion of early warning signs of impending psychotic or depressive episodes, methods for regularizing sleep and activity patterns, techniques to protect patients financially, and ways to manage suicidal behaviour should it occur. Suicide is the major cause of premature death in the severe psychiatric illnesses,(8,9) and its prevention is of first concern. Those illnesses most likely to result in suicide (the mood disorders, comorbid alcohol and drug abuse, and schizophrenia) need to be treated early, aggressively, and often for an indefinite period of time.(2,10) The increasing evidence that treatment early in psychiatric illness may improve the long-term course needs to be considered in light of the reluctance of many patients to stay in treatment.(10,11)

No one who has treated or suffered from mental illness would minimize the difficulties involved in successful treatment. Modern medicine gives options that did not exist even 10 years ago, and there is every reason to expect that improvements in psychopharmacology, psychotherapy, and diagnostic techniques will continue to develop at a galloping pace. Still, the relationship between the patient and doctor will remain central to the treatment, as Morag Coate wrote 35 years ago in *Beyond All Reason*:(12)

> Because the doctors cared, and because one of them still believed in me when I believed in nothing, I have survived to tell the tale. It is not only the doctors who perform hazardous operations or give life-saving drugs in obvious emergencies who hold the scales at times between life and death. To sit quietly in a consulting room and talk to someone would not appear to the general public as a heroic or dramatic thing to do. In medicine there are many different ways of saving lives. This is one of them.

Further information

Non-Governmental Mental Health Websites: US

http://www.nami.org/

http://www.dbsalliance.org/site/PageServer?pagename=home

Governmental Mental Health Websites: US

http://www.nimh.nih.gov/

http://www.hhs.gov/samhsa/mentalhealth/

Non-Governmental Mental Health Websites: UK

http://www.mentalhealth.org.uk/

http://www.depressionalliance.org/index.html

Governmental Mental Health Websites: US

http://www.dh.gov.uk/en/Healthcare/NationalServiceFrameworks/Mentalhealth/index.html

http://www.mentalhealthcare.org.uk/

References

1. Jamison, K.R., Gerner, R.H., and Goodwin, F.K. (1979). Patient and physician attitudes toward lithium: relationship to compliance. *Archives of General Psychiatry*, **36**, 866–9.
2. Goodwin, F.K. and Jamison, K.R. (2007). *Manic-depressive illness* (2nd edn.). Oxford University Press, New York.
3. Osterberg, L. and Blaschke, T. (2005). Adherence to medication. *The New England Journal of Medicine*, **353**, 487–97.
4. Wyatt, R.J. and Chew, R.H. (2005). *Practical psychiatric practice. Forms and protocols for clinical use* (3rd edn). American Psychiatric Association, Washington, DC.
5. Post, R.M., Rubinow, D.R., and Ballenger, J.C. (1986). Conditioning and sensitisation in the longitudinal course of affective illness. *The British Journal of Psychiatry*, **149**, 191–201.
6. Wehr, T.A., Sack, D.A., and Rosenthal, N.E. (1987). Sleep reduction as a final common pathway in the genesis of mania. *The American Journal of Psychiatry*, **144**, 201–4.
7. Baldessarini, R.J., Tondo, L., and Hennen, J. (2003). Lithium treatment and suicide risk in major affective disorders: update and new findings. *The Journal of Clinical Psychiatry*, **64**(Suppl. 5), 44–52.
8. Harris, E.C. and Barraclough, B. (1997). Suicide as an outcome for mental disorders. A meta-analysis. *The British Journal of Psychiatry*, **170**, 205–28.
9. Institute of Medicine (IoM). (2002). *Reducing suicide: a national imperative*. National Academy Press, Washington, DC.
10. Wyatt, R.J. (1995). Early intervention for schizophrenia: can the course of the illness be altered? *Biological Psychiatry*, **38**, 1–3.
11. Berger, G., Dell'Olio, M., Amminger, P., *et al.* (2007). Neuroprotection in emerging psychotic disorders. *Early Intervention in Psychiatry*, **1**, 114–27.
12. Coate, M. (1964). *Beyond all reason*. Constable, London.

1.2

Public attitudes and the challenge of stigma

Graham Thornicroft, Elaine Brohan, and Aliya Kassam

Introduction

The starting point for this discussion is the idea of stigma. This term (plural stigmata) was originally used to refer to an indelible dot left on the skin after stinging with a sharp instrument, sometimes used to identify vagabonds or slaves.[1–4] In modern times stigma has come to mean 'any attribute, trait or disorder that marks an individual as being unacceptably different from the 'normal' people with whom he or she routinely interacts, and that elicits some form of community sanction.'[5–7]

Understanding stigma

There is now a voluminous literature on stigma.[5,8] [9–13,13–19] The most complete model of the component processes of stigmatization has four key components:[20]

i) Labelling, in which personal characteristics, which are signalled or noticed as conveying an important difference.

ii) Stereotyping, which is the linkage of these differences to undesirable characteristics.

iii) Separating, the categorical distinction between the mainstream/normal group and the labelled group as in some respects fundamentally different.

iv) Status loss and discrimination: devaluing, rejecting, and excluding the labelled group. Interestingly, more recently the authors of this model have added a revision to include the emotional reactions which may accompany each of these stages.[21,22]

Shortcomings of work on stigma

Five key features have limited the usefulness of stigma theories. First, while these processes are undoubtedly complex, academic writings on stigma (which in the field of mental health have almost entirely focused upon schizophrenia) have made relatively few connections with legislation concerning disability rights policy[23] or clinical practice. Second, most work on mental illness and stigma has been descriptive, overwhelmingly describing attitude surveys or the portrayal of mental illness by the media. Very little is known about effective interventions to reduce stigma. Third, there have been notably few direct contributions to this literature by service users.[24] Fourth, there has been an underlying pessimism that stigma is deeply historically rooted and difficult to change. This has been one of the reasons for the reluctance to use the results of research in designing and implementing action plans. Fifth, stigma theories have de-emphasized cultural factors and paid little attention to the issues related to human rights and social structures.

Recently there have been early signs of a developing focus upon discrimination. This can be seen as the behavioural consequences of stigma, which act to the disadvantage of people who are stigmatized.[23,25–27] The importance of discriminatory behaviour has been clear for many years in terms of the personal experiences of service users, in terms of devastating effects upon personal relationships, parenting and childcare, education, training, work, and housing.[28] Indeed, these voices have said that the rejecting behaviour of others may bring greater disadvantage than the primary condition itself.

Stigma can therefore be seen as an overarching term that contains three important elements: [29]

- problems of knowledge ignorance
- problems of attitudes prejudice
- problems of behaviour discrimination

Ignorance: the problem of knowledge

At a time when there is an unprecedented volume of information in the public domain, the level of accurate knowledge about mental illnesses (sometime called 'mental health literacy') is meagre.[30] In a population survey in England, for example, most people (55 per cent) believe that the statement 'someone who cannot be held responsible for his or her own actions' describes a person who is mentally ill.[31] Most (63 per cent) thought that fewer than 10 per cent of the population would experience a mental illness at some time in their lives.

There is evidence that deliberate interventions to improve public knowledge about depression can be successful, and can reduce the effects of stigmatization. At the national level, social marketing campaigns have produced positive changes in public attitudes towards people with mental illness, as shown recently in New Zealand and Scotland.[32,33] In a campaign in Australia to increase knowledge about depression and its treatment, some states and territories received this intensive, co-ordinated programme, while others did not. In the former, people more often recognized the features of depression, were more likely to support help seeking for depression, or to accept treatment with counselling and medication.[34]

Prejudice: the problem of negative attitudes

Although the term prejudice is used to refer to many social groups, which experience disadvantage, for example minority ethnic groups, it is employed rarely in relation to people with mental illness. The reactions of a host majority to act with prejudice in rejecting a minority group usually involve not just negative thoughts but also emotion such as anxiety, anger, resentment, hostility, distaste, or disgust. In fact prejudice may more strongly predict discrimination than do stereotypes. Interestingly, there is almost nothing published about emotional reactions to people with mental illness apart from that which describes a fear of violence.[35]

Discrimination: the problem of rejecting and avoidant behaviour

Surveys of attitude and social distance (unwillingness to have social contact) usually ask either students or members of the general public what they would do in imaginary situations or what they think 'most people' who do, for example, when faced with a neighbour or work colleague with mental illness. Important lessons have flowed from these findings. This work has emphasized what 'normal' people say without exploring the actual experiences of people with mental illness themselves about the behaviour of normal people towards them. Further it has been assumed that such statements (usually on knowledge, attitudes, or behavioural intentions) are congruent with actual behaviour, without assessing such behaviour directly. Such research has usually focussed on hypothetical rather than real situations, neglecting emotions, and the social context, thus producing very little guidance about interventions that could reduce social rejection. In short, most work on stigma has been beside the point.

Global patterns

Do we know if discrimination varies between countries and cultures? The evidence here is stronger, but still frustratingly patchy.[36] Although studies on stigma and mental illness have been carried out in many countries, few have been comparison of two or more places, or have included non-Western nations.[37]

In Africa one study described attitudes to mentally ill people in rural sites in Ethiopia. Among almost 200 relatives of people with diagnoses of schizophrenia or mood disorders, 75 per cent said that they had experienced stigma due to the presence of mental illness in the family, and a third (37 per cent) wanted to conceal the fact that a relative was ill. Most family members (65 per cent) said that praying was their preferred of treating the condition.[38] Among the general population in Ethiopia schizophrenia was judged to be the most severe problem, and talkativeness, aggression, and strange behaviour were rated as the most common symptoms of mental illness.[39] The authors concluded that it was important to work closely with traditional healers.

In South Africa,[40,41] a survey was conducted of over 600 members of the public on their knowledge and attitudes towards people with mental illness.[42] Different vignettes, portraying depression, schizophrenia, panic disorder, or substance misuse were presented to each person. Most thought that these conditions were either related to stress or to a lack of willpower, rather than seeing them as medical disorders.[43] Similar work in Turkey,[44] and in Siberia and Mongolia[45] suggests that people in such countries may be more ready to make the individual responsible for his or her mental illness and less willing to grant the benefits of the sick role.

Most of the published work on stigma is by authors in the USA and Canada,[11,27,46,47] but there are also a few reports from elsewhere in the Americas and in the Caribbean.[48] In a review of studies from Argentina, Brazil, Dominica, Mexico, and Nicaragua, mainly from urban sites, a number of common themes emerged. The conditions most often rated as 'mental illnesses' were the psychotic disorders, especially schizophrenia. People with higher levels of education tended to have more favourable attitudes to people with mental illness. Alcoholism was considered to be the most common type of mental disorder. Most people thought that a health professional needs to be consulted by people with mental illnesses.[49]

A great deal of work has studied the question of stigma towards mentally ill people in Asian countries and cultures.[50–52] Within China,[53] a large scale survey was undertaken of over 600 people with a diagnosis of schizophrenia and over 900 family members.[54] Over half of the family members said that stigma had an important effect on them and their family, and levels of stigma were higher in urban areas and for people who were more highly educated.

In the field of stigma research we find that schizophrenia is the primary focus of interest. It is remarkable that there are almost no studies, for example, on bipolar disorder and stigma. A comparison of attitudes to schizophrenia was undertaken in England and Hong Kong. As predicted, the Chinese respondents expressed more negative attitudes and beliefs about schizophrenia, and preferred a more social model to explain its causation. In both countries most participants, whatever their educational level, showed great ignorance about this condition.[55] This may be why most of population in Hong Kong are very concerned about their mental health and hold rather negative views about mentally ill people.[56] Less favourable attitudes were common in those with less direct personal contact with people with mental illness (as in most Western studies), and by women (the opposite of what has been found in many Western reports).[57]

Little research on stigma has been conducted in India. Among relatives of people with schizophrenia in Chennai (Madras) in Southern India, their main concerns were: effects on marital prospects, fear of rejection by neighbours, and the need to hide the condition from others. Higher levels of stigma were reported by women and by younger people with the condition. [58] Women who have mental illness appear to be at a particular disadvantage in India. If they are divorced, sometimes related to concerns about heredity,[59] then they often receive no financial support from their former husbands, and they and their families experience intense distress from the additional stigma of being separated or divorced.[60]

In Japan mental illnesses are seen to reflect a loss of control, and so are not subject to the force of will power, both of which lead to a sense of shame.[61–63] Although, it is tempting to generalize about the degree of stigma in different countries, reality may not allow such simplifications. A comparison of attitudes to mentally ill people in Japan and Bali, for example showed that views towards people with schizophrenia were less favourable in Japan, but that people with depression and obsessive-compulsive disorder were seen to be less acceptable in Bali.[64]

What different countries do often share is a high level of ignorance and misinformation about mental illnesses. A survey of teachers' opinions in Japan and Taiwan showed that relatively few could describe the main features of schizophrenia with any accuracy. The general profile of knowledge, beliefs, and attitudes was similar to that found in most Western countries, although the degree of social rejection was somewhat greater in Japan.[65]

In a unique move aimed to reduce social rejection, the name for schizophrenia has been changed in Japan. Following a decade of pressure from family member groups, including Zenkaren, the name for this condition was changed from *seishi buntetsu byo* (split-mind disorder) to *togo shiccho sho* (loss of co-ordination disorder).[66,67] The previous term went against the grain of traditional, culturally-valued concepts of personal autonomy, as a result of which only 20 per cent of people with this condition were told the diagnosis by their doctors.[68–70] There are indications from service users and family members that the new term is seen as less stigmatizing and is more often discussed openly.

Little is written in the English language literature on stigma in Islamic communities, but despite earlier indications that the intensity of stigma may be relatively low,[52] detailed studies indicate that on balance, it is no less than we have seen described elsewhere.[71–74] A study of family members in Morocco found that 76 per cent had no knowledge about the condition, and many considered it chronic (80 per cent), handicapping (48 per cent), incurable (39 per cent), or linked with sorcery (25 per cent). Most said that they had 'hard lives' because of the diagnosis.[75] Turning to religious authority figures is reported to be common in some Moslem countries.[76,77] Some studies have found that direct personal contact was not associated with more favourable attitudes to people with mental illness,[78,79] especially where behaviour is seen to threaten the social fabric of the community.[80,44]

What sense can we make of all these fragments of information? Several points are clear. First there is no known country, society, or culture in which people with mental illness are considered to have the same value and to be as acceptable as people who do not have mental illness. Second, the quality of information that we have is relatively poor, with very few comparative studies between countries or over time. Third, there do seem to be clear links between popular understandings of mental illness, if people in mental distress want to seek help, and whether they feel able to disclose their problems.[81] The core experiences of shame (to oneself and for others) and blame (from others) are common everywhere stigma has been studied, but to differing extents. Where comparisons with other conditions have been made, then mental illnesses are more, or far more, stigmatized,[82,83] and have been referred to as the 'ultimate stigma' [9]. Finally, rejection and avoidance of people with mental illness appear to be universal phenomena.

Conclusions

If we deliberately shift focus from stigma to discrimination, there are a number of distinct advantages. First attention moves from attitudes to actual behaviour, not if an employer *would* hire a person with mental illness, but if he or she *does*. Second, interventions can be tried and tested to see if they change behaviour towards people with mental illness, without *necessarily* changing knowledge or feelings. The key candidates as active ingredients to reduce stigma are: (i) at the local level, direct social contact with people with mental illness;[84–86] and (ii) social marketing techniques at the national level. Third, people who have a diagnosis of mental illness can expect to benefit from all the relevant anti-discrimination policies and laws in their country or jurisdiction, on a basis of parity with people with physical disabilities. Fourth, a discrimination perspective requires us to focus not upon the 'stigmatized' but upon the 'stigmatizer'. In sum, this means sharpening our sights upon human rights, upon injustice, and upon discrimination as actually experienced by people with mental illness.[7,24,87,88]

Further information

Thornicroft, G. (2006). *Shunned: Discrimination against people with mental illness*. Oxford University Press, Oxford.

Hinshaw, S. (2007). *The mark of shame: stigma of mental illness and an agenda for change*. Oxford University Press, Oxford.

Corrigan, P. (2005). *On the stigma of mental illness*. American Psychological Association, Washington, DC.

Sartorius, N. and Schulze, H. (2005). *Reducing the stigma of mental illness*. A report from a global programme of the World Psychiatric Association. Cambridge University Press, Cambridge.

References

1. Cannan, E. (1895). The stigma of pauperism. *Economic Review*, 380–91.
2. Thomas Hobbes of Malmesbury. (1657). *Markes of the absurd geometry, rural language, Scottish church politics, and barbarisms of John Wallis professor of geometry and doctor of divinity*. Printed for Andrew Cooke, London.
3. Gilman, S.L. (1982). *Seeing the insane*. Wiley, New York.
4. Gilman, S.L. (1985). *Difference and pathology: stereotypes of sexuality, race and madness*. Cornell University Press, Ithaca.
5. Goffman, I. (1963). *Stigma: notes on the management of spoiled identity*. Penguin Books, Harmondsworth, Middlesex.
6. Scambler, G. (1998). *Stigma and disease: changing paradigms*. Lancet, **352**, 1054–5.
7. Hinshaw, S.P. and Cicchetti, D. (2000). Stigma and mental disorder: conceptions of illness, public attitudes, personal disclosure, and social policy. *Development and Psychopathology*, **12**(4), 555–98.
8. Mason, T. (2001). *Stigma and social exclusion in healthcare*. Routledge, London.
9. Falk, G. (2001). *Stigma: how we treat outsiders*. Prometheus Books, New York.
10. Heatherton, T.F., Kleck, R.E., Hebl, M.R., *et al.* (2003). *The social psychology of stigma*. Guilford Press, New York.
11. Corrigan, P. (2005). *On the stigma of mental illness*. American Psychological Association, Washington, DC.
12. Wahl, O.F. (1999). *Telling is a risky business: mental health consumers confront stigma*. Rutgers University Press, New Jersey.
13. Pickenhagen, A. and Sartorius, N. (2002). *The WPA global programme to reduce stigma and discrimination because of schizophrenia*. World Psychiatric Association, Geneva.

14. Sartorius, N. and Schulze, H. (2005). *Reducing the stigma of mental illness: a report from a global association*. Cambridge University Press, Cambridge.
15. Hayward, P. and Bright, J.A. (1997). Stigma and mental illness: a review and critique. *Journal of Mental Health*, **6**(4), 345–54.
16. Link, B.G., Cullen, F.T., Struening, E.L., *et al.* (1989). A modified labeling theory approach in the area of mental disorders: an empirical assessment. *American Sociological Review*, **54**, 100–23.
17. Link, B.G., Struening, E.L., Rahav, M., *et al.* (1997). On stigma and its consequences: evidence from a longitudinal study of men with dual diagnoses of mental illness and substance abuse. *Journal of Health and Social Behaviour*, **38**(2), 177–90.
18. Link, B.G., Phelan, J.C., Bresnahan, M., *et al.* (1999). Public conceptions of mental illness: labels, causes, dangerousness, and social distance. *American Journal of Public Health*, **89**(9), 1328–33.
19. Smith, M. (2002). Stigma. *Advances in Psychiatric Treatment* **8,** 317–25.
20. Link, B.G. and Phelan, J.C. (2001). Conceptualizing stigma. *Annual Review of Sociology*, **27,** 363–85.
21. Link, B.G., Yang, L.H., Phelan, J.C., *et al.* (2004). Measuring mental illness stigma. *Schizophrenia Bulletin*, **30**(3), 511–41.
22. Jones, E., Farina, A., Hastorf, A., *et al.*(1984). *Social stigma: the psychology of marked to relationships*. W.H. Freeman & Co., New York.
23. Sayce, L. (2000). *From psychiatric patient to citizen. Overcoming discrimination and social exclusion*. Palgrave, Basingstoke.
24. Chamberlin, J. (2005). User/consumer involvement in mental health service delivery. *Epidemiologia e Psichiatria Sociale*, **14**, 10–14.
25. Corrigan, P.W., Larson, J.E., Watson, A.C., *et al.* (2006). Solutions to discrimination in work and housing identified by people with mental illness. *Journal of Nervous and Mental Disease*, **194**(9), 716–18.
26. Angermeyer, M.C. and Matschinger, H. (2005). Labeling—stereotype—discrimination. An investigation of the stigma process. *Social Psychiatry and Psychiatric Epidemiology*, **40**(5), 391–5.
27. Estroff, S.E., Penn, D.L., and Toporek, J.R. (2004). From stigma to discrimination: an analysis of community efforts to reduce the negative consequences of having a psychiatric disorder and label. *Schizophrenia Bulletin*, **30**(3), 493–509.
28. Thornicroft, G. (2006). *Shunned: discrimination against people with mental illness*. Oxford University Press, Oxford.
29. Thornicroft, G., Rose, D., Kassam, A., *et al.* (2007). Stigma: ignorance, prejudice or discrimination? *British Journal of Psychiatry*, **190,** 192–3.
30. Crisp, A., Gelder, M.G., Goddard, E., *et al.* (2005). Stigmatization of people with mental illnesses: a follow-up study within the changing minds campaign of the Royal College of Psychiatrists. *World Psychiatry*, **4,** 106–13.
31. Department of Health. (2003). *Attitudes to mental illness 2003 report*. Department of Health, London.
32. Vaughn, G. (2004). Like minds, like mine. In *Mental health promotion: case studies from countries* (eds. S. Saxena and P. Garrison), pp. 62–6. World Health Organization, Geneva.
33. Dunion, L. and Gordon L. (2005). Tackling the attitude problem. The achievements to date of Scotland's 'see me' anti-stigma campaign. *Mental Health Today*, **4**, 22–5.
34. Jorm, A.F., Christensen, H., and Griffiths, K.M. (2005). The impact of beyondblue: the national depression initiative on the Australian public's recognition of depression and beliefs about treatments. *Australian and New Zealand Journal of Psychiatry*, **39**(4), 248–54.
35. Graves, R.E., Cassisi, J.E., and Penn, D.L. (2005). Psychophysiological evaluation of stigma towards schizophrenia. *Schizophrenia Research*, **76**(2–3), 317–27.
36. Littlewood, R. (2004). Cultural and national aspects of stigmatisation. In *Every family in the land* (ed. A.H. Crisp), pp. 14–17. Royal Society of Medicine, London.
37. Fabrega, H., Jr. (1991). The culture and history of psychiatric stigma in early modern and modern western societies: a review of recent literature. *Comprehensive Psychiatry*, **32**(2), 97–119.
38. Shibre, T., Negash, A., Kullgren, G. *et al.* (2001). Perception of stigma among family members of individuals with schizophrenia and major affective disorders in rural Ethiopia. *Social Psychiatry and Psychiatric Epidemiology*, **36**(6), 299–303.
39. Alem, A., Jacobsson, L., Araya, M., *et al.* (1999). How are mental disorders seen and where is help sought in a rural Ethiopian community? A key informant study in Butajira, Ethiopia. *Acta Psychiatrica Scandinavica*, **397**(Suppl.), 40–7.
40. Stein, D.J., Wessels, C., Van Kradenberg, J., *et al.* (1997). The mental health information centre of South Africa: a report of the first 500 calls. *Central African Journal of Medicine*, **43**(9), 244–6.
41. Minde, M. (1976). History of mental health services in South Africa. Part XIII. The national council for mental health. *South African Medical Journal*, **50**(3F), 1452–6.
42. Hugo, C.J., Boshoff, D.E., Traut, A., *et al.* (2003). Community attitudes toward and knowledge of mental illness in South Africa. *Social Psychiatry and Psychiatric Epidemiology*, **38**(12), 715–19.
43. Cheetham, W.S. and Cheetham, R.J. (1976). Concepts of mental illness amongst the rural Xhosa people in South Africa. *Australian and New Zealand Journal of Psychiatry*, **10**(1), 39–45.
44. Ozmen, E., Ogel, K., Aker, T., *et al.* (2004). Public attitudes to depression in urban Turkey—the influence of perceptions and causal attributions on social distance towards individuals suffering from depression. *Social Psychiatry and Psychiatric Epidemiology*, **39**(12), 1010–16.
45. Dietrich, S., Beck, M., Bujantugs, B., *et al.* (2004). The relationship between public causal beliefs and social distance toward mentally ill people. *Australian and New Zealand Journal of Psychiatry*, **38**(5), 348–54.
46. Link, B.G., Yang, L.H., Phelan, J.C., *et al.* (2004). Measuring mental illness stigma. *Schizophrenia Bulletin*, **30**(3), 511–41.
47. Corrigan, P., Thompson, V., Lambert, D., *et al.* (2003). Perceptions of discrimination among persons with serious mental illness. *Psychiatric Services*, **54**(8), 1105–10.
48. Villares, C. and Sartorius, N. (2003). Challenging the stigma of schizophrenia. *Revista Brasasileira de Psiquiatria*, **25,** 1–2.
49. de Toledo Piza, P.E. and Blay, S.L. (2004). Community perception of mental disorders—a systematic review of Latin American and Caribbean studies. *Social Psychiatry and Psychiatric Epidemiology*, **39**(12), 955–61.
50. Ng, C.H. (1997). The stigma of mental illness in Asian cultures. *Australian New Zealand Journal of Psychiatry*, **31**(3), 382–90.
51. Leong, F.T. and Lau, A.S. (2001). Barriers to providing effective mental health services to Asian Americans. *Mental Health Services Research*, **3**(4), 201–14.
52. Fabrega, H. Jr. (1991). Psychiatric stigma in non-western societies. *Comprehensive Psychiatry*, **32**(6), 534–51.
53. Kleinman, A. and Mechanic, D. (1979). Some observations of mental illness and its treatment in the people's republic of China. *Journal of Nervous and Mental Disease*, **167**(5), 267–74.
54. Phillips, M.R., Pearson, V., Li, F., *et al.* (2002). Stigma and expressed emotion: a study of people with schizophrenia and their family members in China. *British Journal of Psychiatry*, **181,** 488–93.
55. Furnham, A. and Chan, E. (2004). Lay theories of schizophrenia. A cross-cultural comparison of British and Hong Kong Chinese attitudes, attributions and beliefs. *Social Psychiatry and Psychiatric Epidemiology*, **39**(7), 543–52.
56. Chou, K.L., Mak, K.Y., Chung, P.K., *et al.* (1996). Attitudes towards mental patients in Hong Kong. *International Journal of Social Psychiatry*, **42**(3), 213–9.
57. Chung, K.F., Chen, E.Y., and Liu, C.S. (2001). University students' attitudes towards mental patients and psychiatric treatment. *International Journal of Social Psychiatry*, **47**(2), 63–72.

58. Thara, R. and Srinivasan, T.N. (2000). How stigmatising is schizophrenia in India? *International Journal of Social Psychiatry*, **46**(2), 135–41.
59. Raguram, R., Raghu, T.M., Vounatsou, P., *et al.* (2004). Schizophrenia and the cultural epidemiology of stigma in Bangalore, India. *Journal of Nervous and Mental Disease*, **192**(11), 734–44.
60. Thara, R., Kamath, S., and Kumar, S. (2003). Women with schizophrenia and broken marriages—doubly disadvantaged? Part II: family perspective. *International Journal of Social Psychiatry*, **49**(3), 233–40.
61. Desapriya, E.B. and Nobutada, I. (2002). Stigma of mental illness in Japan. *Lancet*, **359**(9320), 1866.
62. Hasui, C., Sakamoto, S., Suguira, B., *et al.* (2000). Stigmatization of mental illness in Japan: images and frequency of encounters with diagnostic categories of mental illness among medical and non-medical university students. *Journal of Psychiatry & Law*, **28**(Summer), 253–66.
63. Sugiura, T., Sakamoto, S., Kijima, N., *et al.* (2000). Stigmatizing perception of mental illness by Japanese students: comparison of different psychiatric disorders. *Journal of Nervous and Mental Disease*, **188**(4), 239–42.
64. Kurihara, T., Kato, M., Sakamoto, S., *et al.* (2000). Public attitudes towards the mentally ill: a cross-cultural study between Bali and Tokyo. *Psychiatry and Clinical Neuroscience*, **54**(5), 547–52.
65. Kurumatani, T., Ukawa, K., Kawaguchi, Y. *et al.* (2004). Teachers' knowledge, beliefs and attitudes concerning schizophrenia—a cross-cultural approach in Japan and Taiwan. *Social Psychiatry and Psychiatric Epidemiology*, **39**(5), 402–9.
66. Desapriya, E.B. and Nobutada, I. (2002). Stigma of mental illness in Japan. *Lancet*, **359**(9320), 1866.
67. Takizawa, T. (1993). Patients and their families in Japanese mental health. *New Directions for Mental Health Service*, (**60**), 25–34.
68. Goto, M. (2003). Family psychoeducation in Japan. *Seishin Shinkeigaku Zasshi*, **105**(2), 243–7.
69. Kim, Y. and Berrios, G.E. (2001). Impact of the term schizophrenia on the culture of ideograph: the Japanese experience. *Schizophrenia Bulletin*, **27**(2), 181–5.
70. Mino, Y., Yasuda, N., Tsuda, T., *et al.* (2001). Effects of a one-hour educational program on medical students' attitudes to mental illness. *Psychiatry and Clinical Neuroscience*, **55**(5), 501–7.
71. Karim, S., Saeed, K., Rana, M.H., *et al.* (2004). Pakistan mental health country profile. *International Review of Psychiatry*, **16**(1–2), 83–92.
72. Al-Krenawi, A., Graham, J.R., and Kandah, J. (2000). Gendered utilization differences of mental health services in Jordan. *Community Mental Health Journal*, **36**(5), 501–11.
73. Al-Krenawi, A., Graham, J.R., Ophir, M., *et al.* (2001). Ethnic and gender differences in mental health utilization: the case of Muslim Jordanian and Moroccan Jewish Israeli out-patient psychiatric patients. *International Journal of Social Psychiatry*, **47**(3), 42–54.
74. Cinnirella, M. and Loewenthal, K.M. (1999). Religious and ethnic group influences on beliefs about mental illness: a qualitative interview study. *British Journal of Medical Psychology*, **72**(Pt 4), 505–24.
75. Kadri, N., Manoudi, F., Berrada, S., *et al.* (2004). Stigma impact on Moroccan families of patients with schizophrenia. *Canadian Journal of Psychiatry*, **49**(9), 625–9.
76. Al-Krenawi, A., Graham, J.R., Dean, Y.Z., *et al.* (2004). Cross-national study of attitudes towards seeking professional help: Jordan, United Arab Emirates (UAE) and Arabs in Israel. *International Journal of Social Psychiatry*, **50**(2), 102–14.
77. Loewenthal, K.M., Cinnirella, M., Evdoka, G., *et al.* (2001). Faith conquers all? Beliefs about the role of religious factors in coping with depression among different cultural-religious groups in the UK. *British Journal of Medical Psychology*, **74**(Pt 3), 293–303.
78. Arkar, H. and Eker, D. (1992). Influence of having a hospitalized mentally ill member in the family on attitudes toward mental patients in Turkey. *Social Psychiatry and Psychiatric Epidemiology*, **27**(3), 151–5.
79. Arkar, H. and Eker, D. (1994). Effect of psychiatric labels on attitudes toward mental illness in a Turkish sample. *International Journal of Social Psychiatry*, **40**(3), 205–13.
80. Coker, E.M. (2005). Selfhood and social distance: toward a cultural understanding of psychiatric stigma in Egypt. *Social Science & Medicine*, **61**(5), 920–30.
81. Littlewood, R. (1998). Cultural variation in the stigmatisation of mental illness. *Lancet*, **352**(9133), 1056–7.
82. Lai, Y.M., Hong, C.P., and Chee C.Y. (2001). Stigma of mental illness. *Singapore Medical Journal*, **42**(3), 111–14.
83. Lee, S., Lee, M.T., Chiu, M.Y., *et al.* (2005). Experience of social stigma by people with schizophrenia in Hong Kong. *British Journal of Psychiatry*, **186**, 153–7.
84. Link, B.G. and Cullen, F.T. (1986). Contact with the mentally ill and perceptions of how dangerous they are. *Journal of Health and Social Behaviour*, **27**(4), 289–302.
85. Pinfold, V., Toulmin, H., Thornicroft, G., *et al.* (2003). Reducing psychiatric stigma and discrimination: evaluation of educational interventions in UK secondary schools. *British Journal of Psychiatry*, **182**, 342–6.
86. Pinfold, V., Huxley, P., Thornicroft, G., *et al.* (2003). Reducing psychiatric stigma and discrimination—evaluating an educational intervention with the police force in England. *Social Psychiatry and Psychiatric Epidemiology*, **38**(6), 337–44.
87. Rose, D. (2001). *Users' voices, the perspectives of mental health service users on community and hospital care.* The Sainsbury Centre, London.
88. Kingdon, D., Jones, R., and Lonnqvist, J. (2004). Protecting the human rights of people with mental disorder: new recommendations emerging from the council of Europe. *British Journal of Psychiatry*, **185**, 277–9.

1.3

Psychiatry as a worldwide public health problem

Contents

1.3.1 Mental disorders as a worldwide public health issue
Benedetto Saraceno

1.3.2 Transcultural psychiatry
Julian Leff

1.3.1 Mental disorders as a worldwide public health issue

Benedetto Saraceno

Magnitude and burden of mental disorders

The twentieth century has witnessed significant improvements in somatic health in most countries. A number of key public health threats have been eradicated or brought under control under the leadership of WHO. Priority was given to communicable diseases in view of their inherent potential to spreading.

At the present time, a focus on non-communicable diseases and mental health would now appear as the next natural step in public health priorities. In the case of mental health, this is due to the capacity of mental disorders to proliferate not only as a result of complex and multiple biological, psychological but also social determinants. WHO estimates that at any given time 450 million people suffer from some form of mental or brain disorder, including alcohol and substance use disorders. In other words, one in four of the world's population suffer from different forms of mental, behavioural, and neurological disorders.(1)

The World Development Report: investing in health(2) and the development of the disability-adjusted life-year for estimating the global burden of disease, including years lost because of disability(3,4) and the World Health Report 2001, have all raised the awareness of the global burden of mental disorders. Mental disorders already account for more than 13.46 per cent of the GBD. Furthermore, it is estimated that by the year 2015, the GBD from all neuropsychiatric illnesses will reach 14.14 per cent and by 2030, 14.42 per cent. According to WHO, mental disorders accounted for 6 of the 20 leading causes of disability worldwide for the 15–44 age group, the most productive section of the population.(1) While a greater proportion of the burden is found in high-income countries (21.4 per cent) including those with formerly socialist economies (16.4 per cent), low- and middle-income countries are greatly affected and are likely to see a disproportionately large increase in the burden attributable to mental disorders in the coming decades as infectious diseases are brought under better control and as the population ages. The growing burden of mental, neurological, and substance use disorders is exacerbated in low and middle-income countries due to a projected increase in the number of young people entering the age of risk for the onset of certain mental disorders. An estimated 849 000 people commit suicide every year. This figure represents 1.4 per cent of the global burden of disease as estimated using Disability Adjusted Life Years (DALY) methodology. The proportion of the global disease burden due to suicide varies from 0.2 per cent in Africa up to 2.5 per cent in the Western Pacific region. In the European, South East Asian, and Western Pacific regions, this proportion exceeds the world average. Suicide among young people is of significant concern; in some regions, suicide is the third leading cause of death in the age group of 15–35 years. Suicide is the leading cause of death for this age group in China and the second in the European region. Alcohol consumption alone is responsible for 4 per cent of the global disease burden.(5) In 2000, the global use of alcohol was estimated to have caused 1.8 million deaths or 3.2 per cent of the total deaths from all causes that year. It is estimated that 2.2 million people died from alcohol-related causes in 2005 and increase of 22 per cent from 2000. The population of injecting drug users comprises approximately 10 million people worldwide. Globally, 4–12 per cent of all HIV cases are due to injection drug use, a driving force behind the HIV/AIDS epidemic in many parts of the world.

Economic and social costs of mental disorders

The economic and social costs of mental disorders fall on societies, governments, people with mental disorders, and their carers and families. Given the long-term nature of mental disorders, the most evident economic burden is that of direct treatment costs. For example, the most important contributor to direct costs of depression is hospitalization, accounting for around half of the total in the United Kingdom and three-quarters in the United States.[6] However a common finding from studies of the economic burden of mental disorders in high-income countries is that the 'indirect' costs of lost productivity and premature mortality outweigh the 'direct' costs of treatment and care.[7] Three recent mental health economic studies carried out in India have likewise shown that lost production and other time costs greatly exceed the costs of targeted clinical intervention.[8–10]

In most countries, families bear a significant proportion of these economic costs because of the absence of publicly funded comprehensive mental health service networks. However, ultimately governments and societies pay a price in terms of reduced national income and increased expenditure on social welfare programmes. Thus, the economic logic for societies and countries is simple: treating mental disorders is expensive but leaving them untreated can be more expensive.

In addition to the obvious suffering caused by mental disorders there is a hidden burden of stigma and discrimination and human rights violations. Rejection, unfair denial of employment opportunities and discrimination in access to services, health insurance, and housing are common as are violations of basic human rights and freedoms, as well as denials of civil, political, economic, and social rights, in both institutions and communities. Much of this goes unreported and therefore the burden remains unquantified. Families and primary care providers also incur social costs, such as the emotional burden of looking after disabled family members, diminished quality of life, social exclusion, stigmatization, and loss of future opportunities for self-improvement.

Global resources for mental health

The WHO survey of mental health resources (Project Atlas) highlighted the huge existent gap between the burden of mental disorders and available resources.[11,12]

Mental health policy and legislation

Mental health services and strategies must be well coordinated with other services, such as social security, education, and public interventions in employment and housing through an adequate mental health policy. In spite of this, only 62 per cent of countries have a

Table 1.3.1.1 Policy and legislation on mental health in WHO regions and the world—countries (%)

WHO regions	Policy (N: 190)	Legislation (N: 173)
Africa	50%	80%
Americas	73%	75%
Eastern Mediterranean	73%	57%
Europe	71%	92%
South-East Asia	55%	64%
Western Pacific	48%	76%
World	62%	78%

Source: The World health report 2001–Mental Health: New Understanding, New Hope, © 2001, World Health Organization, www.who.int

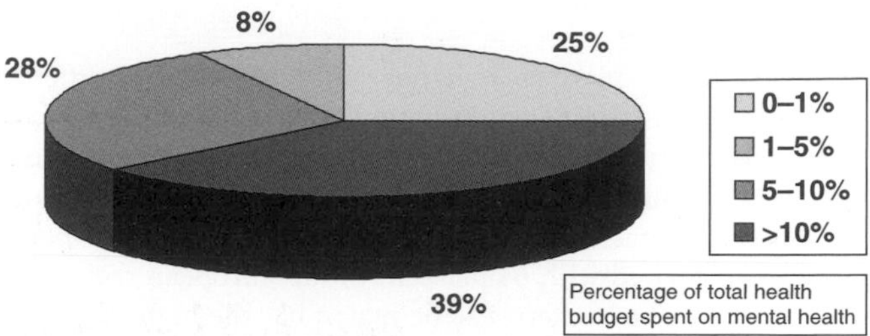

Fig. 1.3.1.1 Percentage of total health budget spent on mental health—countries (%) (*N* = 101). Taken from The World health report 2001–Mental Health: New Understanding, New Hope © 2001, World Health Organization, www.who.int

policy in the mental health field (see Table 1.3.1.1). Mental health legislation is essential to guarantee the dignity of patients and protect their fundamental human rights, though 22 per cent of countries do not have legislation in the field of mental health.

Mental health budget

In spite of the importance of mental health burden in the world (representing more than 13.46 per cent of global burden of diseases), out of only 101 countries that reported having a specific budget, 25 per cent spend less than 1 per cent of the total health budget on mental health (Fig. 1.3.1.1).

Methods of financing mental health care

The tax-based method is the preferred method for financing mental health care present in 63 per cent of countries (Fig. 1.3.1.2), while all the countries with out-of-pocket financing as the primary method are low- or middle-income countries. However, families of people with severe chronic mental disorders are often among the poorer and, in addition to the family burden, can access to basic mental health care.

Community care for mental health

Community care has a better effect than institutional treatment on the outcome and quality of life of individuals with chronic mental disorders. Globally, 68 per cent of countries reported to have at least some community care facilities for mental health. Community care facilities in mental health are only present in 52 per cent of the low-income countries versus 97 per cent of high-income countries.

Though community-based services are recognized to be most effective, 65 per cent of all psychiatric beds are still in mental hospitals—eating away the already meagre budgets while providing largely custodial care in an environment that violates basic human rights of inmates.[10]

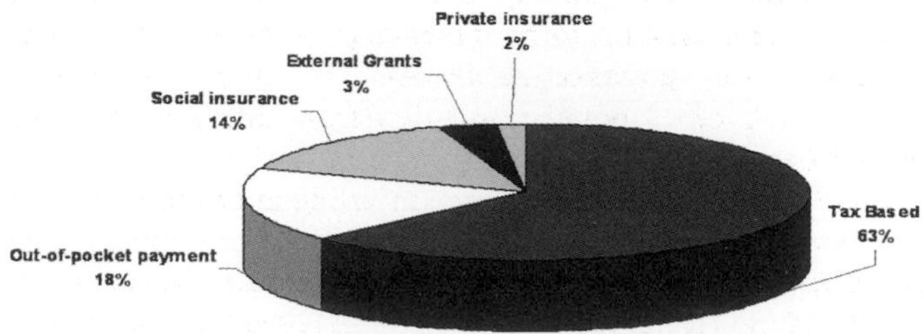

Fig. 1.3.1.2 Methods of financing mental health care in the world—countries (%) (*N* = 180). Taken from The World health report 2001–Mental Health: New Understanding, New Hope, © 2001, World Health Organization, www.who.int

Psychiatric beds

The distribution of psychiatric beds by setting across different income countries also varies. In low-income countries 74 per cent of the psychiatric beds are located in mental hospitals, while in high-income countries only 55 per cent. Across different regions, south-east Asia has 83 per cent of its psychiatric beds in mental hospitals compared with 64 per cent in the European region (see Table 1.3.1.2). The Western Pacific region has the highest proportion of psychiatric beds in general hospitals (35 per cent), followed by Europe with 22 per cent of their total psychiatric beds. In approximately 41 per cent of countries there is less than one psychiatric bed per 10 000 of the population. The proportion of beds which are not located in mental hospitals or in general hospitals includes those in private and military hospitals, hospitals for special groups of population or long-term rehabilitation centres.

Professionals working in mental health

All the countries in the south-east Asia region and most of countries in the African region have less than one psychiatrist per 100 000 population compared to 10 psychiatrist per 100 000 populations in the European region (see Table 1.3.1.3).

The median number of psychiatric nurses per 100 000 population varies from 0.10 in the south-east Asia region to 25 in the European region.

The median number of psychologists in mental health per 100 000 population varies from 0.03 in the south-east Asia and Western Pacific region to 3.10 in the European region and 2.80 in the American region.

In the world there is less than one psychologist per 100 000 population in 61.6 per cent of countries and in low-income countries almost all the population has access to less than one psychologist per 100 000.

The median number of social workers working in mental health per 100 000 population varies from 0.04 in the south-east Asian region to 1.50 in the European region. In about 64 per cent of countries there is less than one social worker per 100 000 population. In the African and Eastern Mediterranean regions more than 85 per cent of the population has access to less than one social worker per 100 000 population.

Table 1.3.1.2 Psychiatric beds per 10 000 population and proportion of psychiatric beds in mental hospitals in WHO regions and the world (*N* = 185)

WHO regions	Median per 10,000 population	Mental hospitals (%)
Africa	0.34	73.0
Americas	2.60	80.6
Eastern Mediterranean	1.07	83.0
Europe	8.00	63.5
South-East Asia	0.33	82.7
Western Pacific	1.06	60.1
World	1.69	68.6

Source: Taken from The World health report 2001–Mental Health: New Understanding, New Hope, © 2001, World Health Organization, www.who.int

Treatment gap for mental disorders

A large proportion of the individuals who suffer from mental disorders do not receive any health care for their condition. The treatment gap for most mental disorders is high. According to a recent review done by WHO from published sources, originating from the United States, Europe, Brazil, Chile, China, India, Zimbabwe, and others,[13] the percentages of people in need for treatment not receiving it are as follows (see Table 1.3.1.4).

Improving mental health care

The mental health infrastructure and services in most countries is grossly insufficient for the large and growing needs. In order to deliver a high standard of mental health treatment and care, WHO emphasizes the adoption of an integrated system of service delivery which attempts to comprehensively address the full range of psychosocial needs of people with mental disorders. A number of policy recommendations for service organizations have been highlighted in the World Health Report 2001.[1] They include (i) shifting care away from large psychiatric hospitals, (ii) developing community mental health services, and (iii) integrating mental health care into general health services.

Table 1.3.1.3 Median number of psychiatrists, psychiatric nurses, psychologists and social workers working in mental health per 100 000 population in WHO regions and the world

WHO regions	Psychiatrists (N=176)	Psychiatric nurses (N=187)	Psychologists in mental health (N=177)	Social workers in mental health (N=161)
Africa	0.04	0.2	0.05	0.05
Americas	2	2.6	2.80	1.00
Eastern Mediterranean	0.95	1.25	0.60	0.40
Europe	9.8	24.8	3.10	1.50
South-East Asia	0.2	0.1	0.03	0.04
Western Pacific	0.32	0.5	0.03	0.05
World	1.2	2	0.60	0.40

Source: Taken from The World health report 2001–Mental Health: New Understanding, New Hope, © 2001, World Health Organization, www.who.int

Table 1.3.1.4 Treatment gap for some mental and substance use disorders

Schizophrenia	32.2%
Depression	56.3%
Bipolar disorder	50.2%
Panic disorder	55.9%
Obsessive compulsive disorder	57.3%
Alcohol abuse and dependence	78.1%

Source: Taken from The World health report 2001–Mental Health: New Understanding, New Hope, © 2001, World Health Organization, www.who.int

Essentially, ethical and scientific considerations have given impetus to the movement to transfer mental health care from mental hospitals to primary health care, general hospitals, and a range of community services in the expectation of enhancing accessibility and acceptability of services, achieving better 'mental' and 'physical' health outcomes, and also a better rationalization of resources.

A large part of mental health care can be self-managed and/or managed by informal community mental health services and low-cost resources can be made available in the community to this effect. Where additional expertise and support is needed a more formalized network of services is required. In ascending order these include primary care services, followed by psychiatric services based in general hospitals and formal community mental health services and lastly by specialist and long stay mental health services.

The mental health field is developing rapidly. There is an evolving information base to guide policy, legislation, service development, and clinical practice. However, there remains a gap between what we know in terms of what works and what is actually occurring in practice in countries around the world. This gap needs to be closed by continued advocacy efforts to raise mental health on the agenda of governments, by continued dissemination of information on effective policies, service development and clinical practice, and the dissemination of international human right standards.

Acknowledgements

M. Garrido Cumbrera has contributed to this publication providing significant comments and technical assistance during the preparation of this manuscript.

Disclaimer

B. Saraceno is a staff member of the World Health Organization. The author alone is responsible for the views expressed in this publication and they do not necessarily represent the decisions, policy or views of the World Health Organization.

Further information

WHO Mental Health website: http://www.who.int/mental_health/en/

References

1. World Health Organization (2001). *The World Health Report 2001: mental health: new understanding, new hope.* World Health Organization, Geneva.
2. World Bank (1993). *World Development Report: investing in health.* Oxford University Press, New York.
3. Murray, C.J.L. and Lopez, A.D. (1996). *The global burden of diseases: a comprehensive assessment of mortality and disability from diseases, injuries and risk factors in 1990 and projected to 2020.* Harvard School of Public Health, World Health Organization and World Bank, Boston.
4. Murray, C.J.L. and Lopez, A.D. (2000). Progress and directions in refining the global burden of disease approach: a response to Williams. *Health Economics*, **9**, 69–82.
5. World Health Organization (2004). *Global status report on alcohol.* World Health Organization, Geneva.
6. Berto, P., D'Ilario, D., Ruffo, P., *et al.* (2000). Depression: cost-of-illness studies in the international literature, a review. *The Journal of Mental Health Policy and Economics*, **3**, 3–10.
7. Hu, T-W. (2004). An International Review of the Economic Costs of Mental Illness. Disease Control Priorities Project. Working Paper No. 31. University of California, Berkeley. Available at: http://www.dcp2.org/file/45/wp31.pdf
8. Chisholm, D., Sekar, K., Kumar, K.K., *et al.* (2000). Integration of mental health care into primary care. Demonstration cost-outcome study in India and Pakistan. *The British Journal of Psychiatry*, **176**, 581–8.
9. Patel, V., Chisholm, D., Rabe-Hesketh, S., *et al.* (2003). Efficacy and cost-effectiveness of drug and psychological treatments for common mental disorders in general health care in Goa, India: a randomised, controlled trial. *Lancet*, **361**(9351), 33–9.
10. Srinivasa Murthy, R., Kishore Kumar, K.V., Chisholm, D., *et al.* (2005). Community outreach for untreated schizophrenia in rural India: a follow-up study of symptoms, disability, family burden and costs. *Psychological Medicine*, **35**(3), 341–51.
11. World Health Organization (2005). *Mental health atlas 2005.* World Health Organization, Geneva.
12. Saxena, S., Sharan, P., Garrido Cumbrera, M., *et al.* (2006). World Health Organization's mental health atlas 2005: implications for policy development. *World Psychiatry*, **5**(3): 179–84.
13. Kohn, R., Saxena, S., Levav, I., *et al.* (2004). The treatment gap in mental health care. *Bulletin of the World Health Organization*, **82**(11): 856–66.

1.3.2 Transcultural psychiatry

Julian Leff

Clinical relevance of transcultural psychiatry

With the mass movements of populations that have characterized the second half of the twentieth century, there can be few psychiatrists who do not encounter members of an ethnic minority group in their practice. The principles of transcultural psychiatry are obviously of relevance to this type of psychiatrist–patient interaction, but they are also of central importance even when the psychiatrist and patient share the same ethnic background. This is because within a particular ethnic group there are invariably many subcultures, for example based on religious affiliation, which encompass a diversity of beliefs. It is essential that the psychiatrist be aware of the common belief systems likely to be encountered, not simply to enhance rapport with patients and relatives, but in order to avoid serious mistakes in ascribing pathology to experiences that are accepted as normal by the subculture. For example, it is important to be aware that between 10 and 17.5 per cent of the general population report experiencing psychotic symptoms.[1,2] The political repercussions of ignorance of such subcultural phenomena are illustrated by the accusations of misdiagnosis of Black patients by White psychiatrists which have come from both outside and within the profession. It is somewhat reassuring that the only published scientific study of this contention fails to support it.[3]

There are two main streams of thought and enquiry that have shaped the development of transcultural psychiatry: social anthropology and psychiatric epidemiology. In a number of ways these disciplines are opposed; the former is concerned with qualitative data and emphasizes cultural relativity (see Chapter 2.6.2.), while the latter relies on quantitative data and prioritizes a search for universal disease categories (see Chapter 2.7). The tools of the epidemiologist are standardized interview schedules which are linked with definitions of symptoms and signs, and rules for reaching a diagnosis. These have been introduced in an attempt to reduce the subjectivity of the psychiatrist's judgement to a minimum. By contrast, it is the person's subjective experience of illness that is the prime focus of the anthropologist. Consequently the use of standardized psychiatric interviews has been criticized by anthropologists as imposing a western biomedical model of disease on the rich variety of experience of illness and distress. The two approaches are not mutually exclusive and are best viewed as contributing complementary material to our understanding of psychiatric morbidity.[4]

The contribution of psychiatric epidemiology

Cultural influences on the psychoses

Epidemiologists have been keen to discover whether psychiatric conditions are universal and appear with the same incidence across human populations. Universality would minimize the role of culture in shaping the form of a condition, while a uniform incidence would indicate that biological factors played a major role in aetiology. Schizophrenia has been the focus of many epidemiological surveys, especially the cross-national studies conducted by the World Health Organization (WHO). The International Pilot Study of Schizophrenia[5] showed that it was possible to conduct a psychiatric epidemiological study across a wide variety of cultures and languages.[6] The use of standardized assessment and diagnostic techniques revealed that the core symptoms of schizophrenia were subject to few cultural variations. The most striking difference in the form of the illness was that catatonic symptoms were relatively frequent in patients from developing countries, but rare in the other centres.

The success of this study led to an even more ambitious project—the Determinants of the Outcome of Severe Mental Disorders. The main aim was to collect epidemiologically based samples of psychotic patients making a first contact with health services in centres around the world. It was found that the incidence of narrowly defined schizophrenia was remarkably uniform across a diversity of countries.[7] However, when patients with a broad diagnosis of schizophrenia but lacking the core Schneiderian symptoms were considered, the incidence rates across centres showed a threefold difference which was highly significant. This suggests that socio-cultural factors are likely to play a much greater role in the aetiology of non-Schneiderian schizophrenia than in the narrowly defined form, although the nature of these factors remains to be determined.

Dramatic differences in outcome at a 2-year follow-up were found, patients with schizophrenia in developing centres faring considerably better than those in developed centres despite a paucity of psychiatric personnel and facilities. This was not explained by a higher proportion of cases with an acute onset in the developing centres, raising intriguing questions about the beneficial aspects of traditional cultures. Explanations that have been proposed include beliefs that the causes of illness are external to the patient, the low demands for productivity and punctuality in an agrarian economy enabling the employment of disabled patients, and the quality of traditional family life. Only the latter has been investigated and appears to make an important contribution, since family carers in India are far less critical and more tolerant of patients with schizophrenia than their counterparts in Britain.[8]

The existence of relatively large populations of people of ethnic minority status in developed countries has facilitated the study of cultural influences on psychoses. Such research has revealed a remarkably elevated incidence of both schizophrenia and mania in some of these groups.[9,10] Of a number of possible explanations, the most likely lie in the social environment.[11]

Mania has been the focus of much less transcultural research than schizophrenia, but what little there is suggests that psychotic experiences are more common in Nigerian and African–Caribbean patients than in patients from European countries.[12,13]

Cultural influences on the neuroses

(a) Variations in frequency across cultures

Whereas neither the form nor the incidence of psychoses vary much across cultures, neuroses show dramatic variations in both respects. So-called culture-bound syndromes are an extreme example of variation in frequency since it is claimed that they are confined to specific cultural groups (see Chapter 4.16.). It is an error to think of these as exotic manifestations in traditional societies, since eating disorders, while increasingly common in developed countries are infrequent elsewhere.[14] Even with common conditions such as depression, the range of prevalence rates from studies across cultures is extremely wide.[15] This is partly attributable to a greater focus on bodily symptoms in patients in developing countries. The significance of somatic symptoms may well be missed by standardized interviews designed to detect the cognitive experiences of depression.

The emphasis on the measurement of prevalence of neuroses as opposed to incidence is due to the small proportion of new cases of neurosis that present to psychiatric services. In order to detect the majority of new cases of neuroses it is necessary to conduct population surveys, which are costly in terms of time and trained personnel. The few population surveys that have been conducted in both developed and developing countries using the same methods of interviewing and case ascertainment have shown either no difference in the prevalence of neuroses[16,17] or a higher rate in the developing country.[18,19]

(b) Variations in form across cultures

One of the most striking transcultural aspects of the neuroses is the great variation in the frequency of classical conversion hysteria. Whereas this condition is rarely seen in psychiatric and neurological services in developed countries today, it is still a common form of presentation in developing countries.[20] This is another manifestation of the tendency to present emotional distress in bodily terms that prevails in those cultures. Somatization is by no means uncommon in patients in developed countries, particularly in individuals of lower socio-economic status, but somatic symptoms are more likely to dominate the picture in patients in a developing country. This is determined partly by beliefs about illness (see Chapter 2.6.2.) and partly by mutual expectations of patients and doctors and of traditional healers, who treat the majority of people with neuroses in developing countries.

Contributions of anthropology

Help-seeking behaviour

In general people seek help from healers who hold the same beliefs as they do (see Chapter 7.3). Traditional healers in developing countries have the advantage of sharing the same belief system about illness with their clients, so that they can take for granted a great deal of common ground and do not need to embark on long explanations. Clients of traditional healers often present their distress in terms of somatic symptoms. Skilled healers are adept at understanding the relationship problems that underlie the client's bodily complaints, and their prescription of rituals is aimed at involving the client's social network and regularizing relationships.[21] Problems in communication arise when the patient brings somatic symptoms to the western trained doctor, who may fail to detect the emotional distress generating the symptoms[22] and is unable to recognize the relationship difficulties that have prompted the comlaints.

Traditional healers are by no means confined to developing countries or to ethnic minority groups in developed countries. Alternative medicine flourishes where western biomedicine is perceived by the public to be ineffective, and psychiatry is one of those areas. Patients with psychiatric conditions are very likely to seek help from acupuncture, spiritual healing, homeopathy, or herbal remedies, in addition to consulting the general practitioner or psychiatrist. Sympathetic questioning of psychiatric patients will elicit their use of a number of sources of alternative medicine in their neighbourhood.

The concept of depression

At the same time as the evidence for a biological basis for depression appears to be strengthening, the western concept of depression has been criticized by transcultural researchers. Obeyesekere[23] considers that each culture has developed its own methods for dealing with painful emotions, for example, the Buddhists of Sri Lanka cope with the loss of a loved person by meditating on the illusory nature of the world of sense, pleasure, and domesticity. Obeyesekere[23] refers to these coping measures as 'the work of culture' and views the construction of a disease known as depression as a western cultural resource. Its incorporation into international classifications of diseases could be viewed as 'the imposition of western cultural standards that are presented as universal and inseparable parts of an emerging new world order'.[24] If a biological basis for the neuroses was firmly established such a formulation could be readily dismissed, but the efficacy of non-biological treatments for depression and anxiety, such as cognitive therapy, couple therapy, and behaviour therapy, indicates that Obeyesekere's view deserves serious consideration. It represents a specific example of the general premise that western biomedicine is itself a cultural construction and needs to be seen as one of many different ways of dealing with the experience of illness and distress.[24] The achievement of biomedicine in ridding the world of smallpox and other fatal diseases is undeniable, but in the field of psychiatry in particular we need to remain open to the ways other cultures have developed for helping people with what we would term psychiatric illness.

Further information

Kleinman, A. (1988). *Patients and healers in the context of culture: an exploration of the borderland between anthropology, medicine and psychiatry*. University of California Press, Berkeley.

Swartz, L. (2000). *Culture and mental health: a Southern African view*. Oxford University Press, Oxford.

References

1. Van Os, J., Hanssen, M., Bijl, R.V., *et al.* (2001). Prevalence of psychotic disorder and community level of psychotic symptoms: an urban-rural comparison. *Archives of General Psychiatry*, **58**, 663–8.
2. Wiles, N.J., Zammit, S., Bebbington, P., *et al.* (2006). Self-reported psychotic symptoms in the general population. Results from the longitudinal study of the British National Psychiatric Morbidity Survey. *British Journal of Psychiatry*, **188**, 519–26.
3. Hickling, F.W., McKenzie, K., Mullen, R., *et al.* (1999). A Jamaican psychiatrist evaluates diagnoses at a London psychiatric hospital. *British Journal of Psychiatry*, **175**, 283–5.
4. Morgan, C., Mallett, R., Hutchinson, G., *et al.* (2004). Negative pathways to psychiatric care and ethnicity: the bridge between social science and psychiatry. *Social Science and Medicine*, **58**(4), 739–52.
5. World Health Organization (1973). *The international pilot study of schizophrenia*, Vol. 1. WHO, Geneva.
6. Westermeyer, J. and Janca, A. (1997). Language, culture and psychopathology: conceptual and methodological issues. *Transcultural Psychiatry*, **34**, 291–311.
7. Jablensky, A., Sartorius, N., Ernberg, G., *et al.* (1992). Schizophrenia: manifestations, incidence and course in different cultures: a World Health Organization ten-country study. *Psychological Medicine*, **20**, 1–97.
8. Wig, N., Menon, D.K., Bedi, H., *et al.* (1987). Expressed emotion and schizophrenia in North India. II. Distribution of expressed emotion components among relatives of schizophrenic patients in Aarhus and Chandigarh. *British Journal of Psychiatry*, **151**, 160–5.
9. Cantor-Graae, E., Pedersen, C.B., McNeil, T.F., *et al.* (2003). Migration as a risk factor for schizophrenia: a Danish population-based cohort study. *British Journal of Psychiatry*, **182**, 117–22.
10. Fearon, P., Kirkbride, J. B., Morgan, C., *et al.* (2006) Incidence of schizophrenia and other psychoses in ethnic minority groups: results from the MRC AESOP study. *Psychological Medicine*, **36**, 1541–50.
11. Mallett, R., Leff, J., Bhugra, D., *et al.* (2002). Social environment, ethnicity and schizophrenia: a case control study. *Social Psychiatry and Psychiatric Epidemiology*, **37**, 329–35.
12. Leff, J.P., Fischer, M., and Bertelsen, A. (1976). A cross-national epidemiological study of mania. *British Journal of Psychiatry*, **129**, 428–37.
13. Makanjuola, R.O. (1982). Manic disorder in Nigerians. *British Journal of Psychiatry*, **141**, 459–63.
14. Greenberg, L., Cwikel, J., and Mirsky, J. (2007). Cultural correlates of eating attitudes: a comparison between native-born and immigrant university students in Israel. *International Journal of Eating Disorders*, **40**, 51–8.

15. Üstün, T.B. and Sartorius, N. (eds.) (1995). *Mental illness in general health care.* Wiley, New York.
16. Leighton, A.H., Lambo, T.A., Hughes, C.C., *et al.* (1963). *Psychiatric disorder among the Yoruba.* Cornell University Press, Ithaca, New York.
17. Stanley, D. and Wand, R.R. (1995). Obsessive-compulsive disorder: a review of the cross-cultural epidemiological literature. *Transcultural Psychiatric Research Review*, **32**, 103–36.
18. Orley, J. and Wing, J.K. (1979). Psychiatric disorders in two African villages. *Archives of General Psychiatry*, **36**, 513–20.
19. Hollifield, M., Katon, W., Spain, D., *et al.* (1990). Anxiety and depression in a village in Lesotho, Africa: a comparison with the United States. *British Journal of Psychiatry*, **156**, 343–50.
20. Wig, N.N. and Pershad, D. (1975–1977). *Triennial statistical report.* Department of Psychiatry, Postgraduate Institute of Medical Education and Research, Chandigarh, India.
21. Nichter, M. (1981). Negotiation of the illness experience: ayurvedic therapy and the psychosocial dimension of illness. *Culture, Medicine and Psychiatry*, **5**, 5–24.
22. Jacob, K.S., Bhugra, D., Lloyd, K.R., *et al.* (1998). Common mental disorders, explanatory models and consultation behaviour among Indian women living in the UK. *Journal of the Royal Society of Medicine*, **91**, 66–71.
23. Obeyesekere, G. (1985). Depression, buddhism and the work of culture in Sri Lanka. In *Culture and depression: studies in the anthropology and cross-cultural psychiatry of affect and disorder* (eds. A. Kleinman and B. Good), pp. 134–52. University of California Press, Berkeley, CA.
24. Bibeau, G. (1997). Cultural psychiatry in a creolizing world: questions for a new research agenda. *Transcultural Psychiatry*, **34**, 9–41.
25. Kakar, S. (1995). Clinical work and cultural imagination. *Psychoanalytic Quarterly*, **64**, 265–81.

1.4

The history of psychiatry as a medical specialty

Pierre Pichot

Introduction

In 1918, Emil Kraepelin wrote:[1]

> A hundred years ago, they were practically no alienists. The care of the mental patients was nearly everywhere in the hands of head supervisors, attendants and administrators of the houses for the mentally ill and the role of the physicians was limited to the treatment of the physical illnesses of the patients.

He pointed out that, in the first decades of the 19th century, many of the books dealing with psychiatric themes were still written by medical doctors, such as Reil (who coined the word psychiatry), who had few contacts with mental patients or even by philosophers and theologians, and that only in the great scientific centres had specialists appeared 'who had decided to spend their life in the study and treatment of mental diseases'.

The history of psychiatry as a medical specialty has to be distinguished from the history of psychiatric medical knowledge which began in ancient Greece with the birth of medicine as a science. For more than 2000 years, only physicians observed and treated mental illnesses, and institutions were created in which the 'lunatics' and the 'insane' were received. But, as rightly pointed out by Kraepelin, the truth is that psychiatry was not really a medical specialty. One can argue about the precise date of the appearance of psychiatry as a specific field of medicine and of the psychiatrist as a specialist, devoting his professional competence exclusively to the care of the mentally ill. Denis Leigh recognizes that 'some degree of specialization occurred [in England] among respectable physicians' in the middle of the eighteenth century when the monopoly of Bethlem was broken and new 'lunatic hospitals', such as St Luke's were opened.[2] On the other hand, the American historian Jan Goldstein stresses that in France the language, as an exact reflection of the underlying reality, began to use expressions such as *homme spécial* to describe a physician specializing in a branch of medicine such as psychiatry only around 1830.[3]

Pinel and the birth of psychiatry as a branch of medicine

Despite those divergences, it is generally accepted that the work of Philippe Pinel constitutes a turning point. His role has several aspects. He is known worldwide as the physician who 'liberated the insane from their chains' in a dramatic initiative he started in 1793, at the height of the French revolution, at the Bicêtre asylum, and completed 3 years later at the Salpêtrière asylum. However, the reality is more complex.

Pinel, who was born in 1745, had studied medicine, translated Cullen's books into French, and published scientific papers on various subjects. He acted as a physician in a small Parisian 'madhouse', the Pension Belhomme, in which wealthy lunatics were confined at the request of their families. At that time most of the Parisian insanes were confined for a few weeks in the general hospital—the Hôtel Dieu. If their state did not rapidly improve, they were considered as incurable and send to Bicêtre or the Salpêtrière, built a century before, which also received other social deviants like beggars and prostitutes. Pinel, who was known by his politically influential friends for his progressive scientific ideas, was appointed physician to Bicêtre. The division for the insane was under the direction of an overseer (*surveillant*), Pussin, who had already introduced humanitarian reforms in the care of the patients. Pinel's merit was to approve and systematically develop Pussin's empirical measures and to propose an explicit scientific theory for their mode of action. Inspired by Crichton's views about the nature of the 'passions' by Condillac's psychology, and by the ideas of Jean-Jacques Rousseau, he created the *traitement moral* which he claimed to be effective with patients previously considered as incurably ill.

The improvement of the conditions in which the insane were cared for, supported and expanded by Pinel, was not an isolated French phenomenon. In Tuscany, Chiarugi in 1789 had already asserted that the basis of the extensive reforms he had introduced in the local asylum for the insane was that 'it is a supreme moral duty and a medical obligation to respect the mental patient as a person'. In England, where public had been shocked by the inhuman treatment to which King George III had been submitted during his mental illness; and where, a pious Quaker, William Tuke, deeply affected by the conditions in which the wife of a member of the Society of Friends had died in York lunatic asylum, decided to set up a special institution under the government of the Friends 'for the care and accommodation of their own members'. At the Retreat, opened in 1796 near York, physical restraints were largely abolished, and religious and moral values were emphasized in relations with the patients.

Chiarurgi's reforms did not survive the upheavals caused by subsequent wars and the political divisions of Italy, and Tuke's creation of the Retreat had not been prompted by medical considerations but was the expression of religious humanitarian purposes. The role played by Pinel was decisive, not so much because of the changes he promoted in the conditions of the patients, although they had a profound influence, but because he made the study and treatment of mental disorders a branch of medicine.

In 1801, Pinel published the *Medico-philosophical Treatise on Mental Alienation*. In it, he presented the various clinical manifestations he had observed; proposed a simple nosological system largely borrowed from older authors; examined possible aetiological factors; and described his 'moral treatment' in detail. The book has remained a landmark in the history of psychiatry, even being considered by the philosopher Hegel as a 'moment of capital importance in the history of humanity'. For Pinel, insanity was a disease and the patient affected by it remained, despite the loss of his reason, a human being. Its study, like the rest of medicine, had to be 'a science which consists of carefully observed facts'. Goldstein[(3)] has shown that Pinel's main preoccupation was to prove this scientific nature of the new medical specialty by repudiating the previous practices of the 'empirics' and 'charlatans'—the two terms being practically synonymous. He had accepted the method Pussin had developed empirically and transformed it in his moral treatment by providing a scientific theory of its mode of action. A curiously premonitory aspect of his emphasis on the necessity of a scientific methodology is to be found in his *Tables to Determine How Probable is the Curability of Alienation*, published in 1808. He provided statistical data on the efficacy of his therapeutic method according to the types of mental disorders and in comparison with spontaneous evolution, and concluded that medicine can only be a true science through the use of the calculus of probability!

Psychiatry as a profession: Esquirol and the clinical approach

If, because of the international influence of the ideas expressed in his book, Pinel is the founder of psychiatry as a medical discipline, he was not a psychiatric specialist in the strict meaning of the term. Although he retained his position at the Salpêtrière until his death in 1826 and is known today for his contributions to mental medicine, he had many other medical interests which gave him, in his time, a leading position among the Paris physicians; his *Philosophical Nosology*, published in 1796 and a classical reference for several decades, deals with general pathology. The case of his pupil and successor, Esquirol, who became the prototype of the psychiatric specialist was very different. At the Salpêtrière he was only in charge of the 'section of the insane'. He was later appointed medical director of the Charenton psychiatric asylum near Paris and owned in addition a small clinic, in which he treated his private patients. All his activities were exclusively dedicated to the study and treatment of mental disorders and the teaching of psychiatry. His book, *On Mental Diseases* published in 1838, in which he collected his previous publications, acquired a fame as great as Pinel's *Treatise*. In 1913, Karl Jaspers recognized that the later great representatives of German psychiatry, such as Griesinger and Kraepelin, were strongly indebted to Esquirol. He, and the school he founded, effectively developed one of the basic tenets of the new medical specialty. For Esquirol, careful objective observation and analysis of the symptoms and the behaviour of the patients were fundamental. He originated the descriptive clinical approach expanded by his pupils. Even more than Pinel, he was suspicious of unproved theories and when he eventually suggested relations between pathogenic factors and syndromes, he remained extremely cautious in his interpretations. Zilboorg, the psychoanalytically oriented historian of psychiatry, has accused this predominantly descriptive approach of creating a 'psychiatry without psychology' because, lacking psychodynamic concepts, its attempted objectivity remained at an allegedly superficial level.[(4)] The truth is that it laid the foundations of the present description of the mental disorders. The 'atheoretical' descriptive approach adopted in the present nosological systems—both the American *Diagnostic and Statistical Manual* and the *International Classification of Diseases*—whose proclaimed purpose is to emphasize the medical character of psychiatry is, in this respect, a return to Esquirol's principles.

The social aspects of psychiatry and the asylum system

By the end of the eighteenth century it was recognized that the study of mental alienation was part of medicine. However, mental diseases were of such a nature that it was not possible to treat the insane in the same conditions as patients affected by other diseases. Their most obvious manifestations had social consequences. According to the prevailing philosophical view, the mentally ill were deprived of free-will by their illness. In practice, they were unable to participate in the normal life of the society and were often considered as potentially dangerous. Because of this, they had generally been confined in madhouses of various kinds. One of the aspects of the reforms initiated by Pinel had been to make more explicit the difference in nature between the socially deviant behaviour of the insane, which, being the consequence of an illness, belonged exclusively to medicine, and the other deviations which society had to control and eventually to repress. The implementation of this fundamental distinction during the first half of the 19th century helped to give psychiatry its specific shape as a profession by being at the origin of forensic psychiatry and by leading to the formulation of precise rules concerning the commitment of the insane to institutions of a strictly medical character.

The legal code promulgated by Napoleon in 1810 stipulated that 'no crime or delict exists if commited in a state of dementia', with the old term dementia being used as a synonym of Pinel's mental alienation. This legal provision, introduced in similar forms in other countries, opened an important domain of activity to the medical profession of psychiatrist. Because of their now recognized specialized knowledge, the alienists were to help the judges in determining whether the mental state of an individual convicted of a 'crime or delict' was normal or pathological, with decisive consequences on the subsequent decision. The title of Esquirol's *Treatise* mentions explicitly that it describes mental diseases 'in their medical, hygienic and medico-legal aspects'. The conflict (which still exists) between the judges, usually supported by public opinion, who took a restrictive view of the concept of mental disease; and the psychiatrists, who tended to expand it to include new types of deviant behaviour, is illustrated by the violent controversies provoked by Esquirol's description of 'homicidal monomania'. They had an even more famous counterpart in England. J.C. Pritchard, an admirer of

Esquirol, had isolated 'moral insanity' as a specific mental disorder in two books published in 1837 and 1842; in the second, he examined its 'relations to jurisprudence'. Half a century later, in 1897, Henry Maudsley, who was in favour of the use of this diagnosis, recognized that this category, although internationally accepted by the psychiatrists, corresponded to

> . . . a form of mental alienation which has so much the look of vice and crime that may persons regard it as an unfounded medical invention'. Judges have repeatedly denounced it from the bench as a 'most dangerous medical doctrine', 'a dangerous innovation' which, in the interest of society, should be reprobated.

The general acceptance of the new medical concept of mental alienation implied the existence of adequate facilities for the treatment of the patients. The creation of new asylums—the term was retained—and the reorganization of the old ones were the answers. The French law of 1838 that fixed the detailed rules for the expansion of the new system to the whole country and for its functioning and financial support had a model character. Similar results were obtained in, for example, England with the Asylum Act 1828 and the Lunacy Act 1845. Outwardly, the new system was the extension, under more humane conditions, of the previous institutional practices. However, it had radically original features. While recognizing the necessity of protecting society, it stressed the fact that the insane had a fundamental right to be protected and medically treated in a competent way. The deprivation of liberty for the patients which it still implied, was strictly controlled to prevent possible misuse and was anyway justified, according to Esquirol and most contemporary psychiatrists, not only by the loss of free will, which was a consequence of the illness, but also by the therapeutic value of separation from a pathogenic milieu.

The asylum system became the central element of psychiatric care and was both the consequence and determining factor of the emergence of psychiatry as a medical specialty to which it gave, until the end of the 19th century and even beyond, an original character. The asylums acquired a quasi-monopoly in the care of the mentally ill. The few private institutions reserved for the wealthier members of the population, which often belonged to alienists in charge of the asylum, were generally submitted to the same legal rules. Private practice with ambulatory patients, as existing today, was exceptional or dealt with cases which were not then considered to belong to mental alienation. As a result, the study of mental illness was predominantly restricted to the more severe forms of disorder. Another consequence was that the alienists in charge of patients committed to the asylums had a dual function, a fact that differentiated them from other hospital physicians. In addition to their medical duties, they were involved in legal procedures which determined the conditions of admission, stay, and eventually release of the mentally ill. As superintendents, they also often had economic and financial responsibilities, being in charge of the material as well as the medical aspects of the functioning of their institutions.

Despite the fact that the laws now strictly differentiated the nature of the limitations of liberty in asylums and in prisons, the participation of the alienist in a form of social control was eventually perceived negatively by the public, and often by other physicians, and contributed to accentuating the specificity of psychiatry inside medicine. During the third and the fourth decades of the 19th century, which saw the birth of the asylum system, the psychiatrists became really conscious of their identity as a professional group. In England, France, Germany, and the United States they founded societies and began to publish journals with specialized scientific goals. Such a description oversimplifies an evolution which was progressive and in some cases took different directions. The creation and the extension of the asylum system took many years; it did not reach its classical form until the last part of the century, as testified by the famous campaign conducted in the United States during the 1840s by Dorothea Dix who complained that many of the mentally ill were still incarcerated in almshouses and prisons. The moral treatment practized in the institutions was eventually used to justify brutal measures, alleged to be therapeutic, and the behaviour of the attendants, who were not usually medically trained (significantly, they were known as *surveillants* in France), was too often of a purely repressive character. It was a long time before the proposals made in 1856 by the British psychiatrist John Conolly in his book, *The Treatment of the Insane without Mechanical Restraints* were put into practice everywhere.

The biological and the psychological model

The clinical orientation of Pinel, Esquirol, and their followers was basically empirical. By concentrating on describing observable symptoms and abnormal behaviours, it avoided theoretical controversies. However, many believed that if psychiatry was to become a branch of the medical sciences and to progress, it had to adopt models similar to those accepted by the rest of medicine. According to the anatomoclinical perspective, which was now dominant, diseases were distinct entities. Each disease was defined by a characteristic pattern of symptoms provoked by a lesion or eventually, a dysfunction of an organ to be discovered at autopsy. In 1821, Bayle, following this scheme, described the typical clinical symptoms and lesions of the brain in the general paralysis of the insane. Despite the disappointing results of the further anatomopathological studies (brain lesions were observed in only a small proportion of cases), there was increasing conviction that, with better investigation methods, mental disorders, like other diseases, could be explained by somatic causes. The degeneration theory, proposed in 1857 by Morel, which attributed many forms of insanity to the hereditary transmission of dysfunction of the nervous system produced by the noxious effects of environmental factors, and whose influence lasted until Kraepelin, is another expression of this biological orientation whose aim was to give psychiatry an undisputed medical status.

The biological and the purely clinical approaches were concerned with different conceptual levels—the discovery of the causes of insanity and the description of its manifestations respectively. Therefore, they could easily coexist. Even when the followers of Pinel and Esquirol expressed reservations about the applicability of the biological model to every type of mental disorder, they still believed in the medical nature of psychiatry. The situation created in the German-speaking countries by the school of the 'mentalists' (the term *Psychiker* by which they were known means 'psychologically oriented'), who were predominant during the first half of the 19th century, was very different. Influenced by philosophical, religious, and romantic trends, these psychiatrists took a radical dualistic position, postulating the absolute difference between the physical body and the spiritual soul. The soul was the source of the whole psychic life and hence eventually of its abnormal aspect—insanity. A term such as disease, appropriate for the somatic illness, could only be used metaphorically in psychiatry. The sins of the patients were the origin of the mental disorders, and psychiatry belonged more to moral philosophy than to medicine. These ideas were developed in various related forms by the majority of the German psychiatrists of the period (Heinroth, Ideler, Langerman, and many others). Their ideological position had two consequences: scientific relations with other schools, such as the French and the English who saw in the publications of the mentalists obscure philosophical theories devoid of medical character, were largely cut off, and they provoked a violent reaction in Germany itself. The most extreme representatives of the contending group of 'somatists' (*Somatiker*), such as Jakobi and Friedreich, saw the mental disorders as symptoms of somatic diseases, not necessarily of the brain. In fact for them mental diseases as such did not exist. They defended aggressively their biological and sometimes bizarre hypotheses, such as the aetiological role of intestinal worms, against the mentalists. Finally, around 1850, they gained the upper hand. The publication in 1845 of *Pathology and Therapy of the Nervous Diseases* by Wilhelm Griesinger, an heir to their school who was also influenced by the French alienists, is a landmark in the history of the German psychiatry. With his appointment in 1865 as professor of psychiatry in Berlin, where he succeeded the mentalist Ideler, medical psychiatry was definitely established in Germany as a branch of the natural sciences.

The rise of neuropsychiatry

Romberg's *Lehrbuch der Nervenkrankheiten* symbolizes the birth of neurology as an autonomous medical specialty studying and treating the diseases of the nervous system. It was published 5 years after Griesinger's *Textbook* in which, adopting and expanding Bayle's anatomoclinical model he had affirmed: 'Mental diseases are diseases of the brain'. If both psychiatric and neurological symptoms originated in the nervous system, some form of association between the two specialties was a logical step, at least at the conceptual level. One aspect of their complex relationship was the creation of neuropsychiatry which developed its most characteristic aspects in the German-speaking countries.

The universities acquired considerable power and influence in the second half of the 19th century. From the 1850s on, chairs were created for the teaching of the new common discipline and special institutions, the university clinics, were built with hospital beds for psychiatric patients (if their disorders became chronic they were sent to the nearest asylum), laboratories for research on neurophysiology and neuroanatomy, and special wards for the neurological cases were developed. Griesinger's first move when he took over the chair of psychiatry at Berlin was the creation of neurological wards at the Charité. The leading neuropsychiatrists in charge of these institutions often performed research in both fields with equal competence, as shown by the work of Wernicke and Westphal, and later of Kleist and Bonhöffer, in Germany and of Meynert in Austria.

The concept of neuropsychiatry, appearing at a period during which the German school was progressively gaining influence, had a deep impact on psychiatric thought and on the psychiatric profession, even if its institutional driving force, the university clinic system, was not developed everywhere to the same extent as in Germany. For example, it was conspicuously absent in England, despite the fact that the theoretical position taken by the most important psychiatrist of the time, Henry Maudsley, was very close to that of Griesinger. The National Hospital in Queen's Square, London, founded in 1860, retained a virtual monopoly on the teaching of neurology for many decades, and psychiatry, taught essentially in hospitals, was not represented at university level until the 1930s. However, in most countries, neuropsychiatric institutions coexisted with the asylums where the alienists had the unenviable task of caring for chronic mental patients, often with inadequate means. The concept of neuropsychiatry reflected a basically biological perspective on the aetiology of the mental illnesses, expressed in the creation of a new specialty associating competence in the two previously separated domains of medicine. However, it provoked ideological and professional tension between the 'pure' psychiatrists, mainly those in charge of asylums, and the neuropsychiatrists, predominantly involved in teaching and research. In the long term, this conflict was one of the factors which finally led, in the 1960s, to the almost complete administrative and institutional separation of the two specialties in countries such as France where they had been, at least formally, associated. But many traces of the old situation remain. The most influential scientific journal published in German, *Nervenarzt*, still deals equally with neurology and psychiatry, and the term 'neuropsychiatric' survives in the titles of many teaching and research institutions.

The neuroses and the birth of the psychotherapies

The study of the neuroses, in which the relation between psychiatry and neurology was also involved, resulted in completely different, but equally important changes to psychiatry as a medical specialty. The term neurosis had been coined in 1769 by Cullen to describe a class of diseases he attributed to a dysfunction of the nervous system. In this very heterogenous group, two entities of very ancient origin, hysteria and hypochondriasis, had predominantly psychological manifestations. Since the affected patients were not usually commited to asylums, they were not normally studied by alienists, but by specialists in internal medicine such as Briquet, who in 1859, wrote the classical *Treatise on Hysteria*. Because of the assumed nature of the neuroses, the new discipline of neurology rapidly took an interest in them.

Charcot, the founder of the French neurological school, was responsible for the internal medicine wards at the Salpêtrière—they were not associated with the 'divisions of the insane' at the same hospital, the domain of the alienists. In about 1880, he became interested in hysterical patients who, because of their seizures, were admitted to the same ward as the epileptics. He developed a purely neurological theory of the disease which he described and studied using hypnosis. This was the former 'animal magnetism', long fallen into disrepute, but to which he gave a new scientific status. Charcot's descriptions of the *grande hystérie*, which he demonstrated on selected patients in his famous public lectures, were justly criticized later, but his international fame attracted students from all over the world. One of them, was a young lecturer in neuropathology at the University of Vienna, Sigmund Freud, who, impressed by Charcot's lectures, decided to devote all his energies to the study and the treatment of the neuroses. Another was a French professor of philosophy (psychology was then a branch of philosophy), Pierre Janet, who had become interested in the psychological aspects of the neuroses. He was later to develop, in parallel with Freud, a psychopathological theory which, despite the traces it has left (the concepts of psychasthenia and the dissociative processes in hysteria) was not to be as internationally successful as Freud's psychoanalysis. Charcot's ideas were opposed by Bernheim, the professor of internal medicine at the Nancy Medical School and also an adept of hypnosis. He attacked the neurological interpretations of the Salpêtrière and claimed that suggestion played a central role in the phenomena described by Charcot.

The general interest in the neuroses, which extended beyond medicine to *fin de siècle* literature, was an international phenomenon. In 1880, Beard, an American neurologist, described a new neurosis, neurasthenia, which soon aroused even more interest than Charcot's hysteria. Psychiatry had played almost no part in this evolution, but this was to change under the influence of three related developments: the changes which took place within the concept of neurosis, the birth of the psychotherapies, and the incorporation in the field of psychiatry of psychopathological manifestations, even if they were of minor intensity.

The transformation of the concept of neurosis is apparent in the position taken by Kraepelin in the 1904 edition of his *Textbook*. He introduced a chapter,'The psychogenic neuroses', on the grounds that 'among the neuroses, to which belong epilepsy and chorea, one must isolate a sub-group characterized by the purely psychological cause of the apparition of the symptoms'. The disintegration of the old concept left to neurology, which from now on abandoned the generic term, diseases (such as epilepsy and chorea) whose somatic manifestations could be shown to express a dysfunction of a precise part of the nervous system. Psychiatry took charge of hysteria, hypochondriasis, neurasthenia, and the related phobic, obsessional, and anxious disorders, which constituted the new neuroses. This concept was justified by the psychological nature of the symptoms and the causes recognized even by a biologically oriented psychiatrist such as Kraepelin. This redrawing of the frontier between the neurological and psychiatric specialties also testified to the extension of the limits of psychiatry. Pinel's insanity, until then defined by the necessity of commitment to special institutions, was replaced by a broader concept. A new class corresponding to our present personality disorders had already appeared in the 1894 edition of Kraepelin's *Textbook*. It had been isolated for the first time in 1872–1874 by the psychiatrist Koch. Like the neuroses, the cases were rarely observed in asylums but, nevertheless, they were now considered as belonging to the psychiatric field of study.

This field was further modified by the birth of the psychotherapies. In fact, they had a long history. In 1803, one of the first German mentalists, Reil, had described under the name of 'psychic therapy' (*psychische Curmethode*) a number of procedures, including very violent somatic ones, which could influence the 'perturbed passions of the soul', and Pinel's moral therapy contained psychotherapeutic elements. However, psychotherapies as techniques whose formal rules were based on an explicit theory about their psychological mechanisms of action, derived mainly from Mesmer's animal magnetism as rehabilitated by Charcot. The emergence of the psychotherapies, characteristic of the last decades of the 19th century, was intimately related to the renewed study of the neuroses. After he had abandoned hypnosis, Freud developed psychoanalysis, but many other techniques evolved during the same period, which were as well or even better known at the time, although they were to have a less lasting success. One of these was the method of Janet, who still occasionally used hypnosis. In 1904, Dubois, a Swiss neuropathologist from Bern, introduced a technique influenced by Bernheim's theory of suggestion in *The Psychoneuroses and their Moral Treatment*, and claimed to produce a 'psychological re-education' by a combination of rational and persuasive elements. His international reputation brought him patients from all over the world. The 'rest cure', proposed in 1877 by the American neurologist S. Weir Mitchell for the treatment of hysteria and later of neurasthenia, was combined with Dubois' method by Dejerine, Charcot's successor as the professor of neurology in Paris.

This very incomplete summary illustrates the striking fact that, because of their intimate connections with the neuroses, the psychotherapies originated inside neurology. When the study and treatment of the neuroses were incorporated into psychiatry, the psychiatrists considered that they were an integral part of their activity and tried to retain the monopoly of their practice. They never completely succeeded. Already Freud had, according to his biographer Jones, 'warmly welcomed the incursion in the therapeutic field of suitable people from another walk of life than medicine'. The problem of the 'lay analysts', a source of conflict within the psychoanalytic movement, is only an aspect of a broader question which was later to involve the relations of the medical specialty of psychiatry with the new professional group of clinical psychologists.

From the beginning of the 20th century to the Second World War

During the first half of the 20th century, psychiatry developed in many directions. Kraepelin's monumental synthesis[5] established around 1900, a nosological system which, in its broad outlines, has remained valid until today. Without being radically altered it was completed, to mention only a few contributions, in 1911, by Bleuler's description of schizophrenia and in 1913, by Jaspers' psychopathological perspective, developed by the Heidelberg school and Kurt Schneider, and by other psychiatrists working in academic institutions. However, the old conflict between the 'mentalists' and the 'somatists' reappeared in a modified form. The mainstream of psychiatry had abandoned the extreme positions of the 'brain pathologists' of the Meynert-Wernicke type but, while recognizing a limited influence of psychological factors, admitted in a general way the biological origin of the more severe mental disorders—the psychoses. The empirical discoveries of biological treatments—of general paralysis by malaria therapy (Wagner von Jauregg in 1917), of schizophrenia by insulin coma (Sakel in 1933) or by chemically induced seizures (von Meduna in 1935), and of depression by electroconvulsive therapy (Cerletti in 1938)—not only helped to dispel the prevailing therapeutic pessimism, but provided supporting arguments. However, an opposing ideological current represented by psychoanalysis had arisen from the study of the neuroses. Its attention was concentrated on the study of complex psychopathological mechanisms postulated to be at the origin of the neurotic, and later also of the psychotic symptoms, favoured psychogenetic aetiological theories, and advocated psychotherapy as the fundamental form of treatment. Psychoanalysis expanded steadily during this period and gained enthusiastic adherents in many countries. However, partly because of the suspicion and even hostility of many members of the psychiatric establishment, they remained isolated in close-knit groups with their own teaching system independent of the official medical curriculum, and the use of their therapeutic technique was restricted to a small number of mostly neurotic patients seen in outpatient clinics or, more often, in private practice.

The great majority of patients suffering from mental disorders were still confined in asylums, and the enormous increase in their number, mainly related to the social changes accompanying industrialization and urbanization, although other factors have been invoked, was striking. In Great Britain it grew from 16 000 in 1860 to 98 000 in 1910, three times more rapidly than the population. A similar phenomenon was observed in all countries and persisted until the end of the 1940s despite the introduction of the first biological therapies. In the United States, there were already 188 000 patients in mental hospitals in 1910, and by the end of the Second World War, 850 000 were lodged in huge institutions which were overpopulated, understaffed, and could only provide custodial care. This obvious degeneracy of the asylum system, contrasting with the progresses in the scientific field, stimulated efforts to improve the practice of psychiatry and its institutional framework. Most of these improvements took place after 1920 and, although their results remained relatively limited, they were the forerunners of later more drastic changes.

The education of psychiatric specialists, which had varied widely from country to country, was improved and systematized. A convergence of evolution is apparent during this period which can be said, to some extent, to have seen the formal administrative recognition of psychiatry as a medical specialty. Educational programmes and controls of the level of competence were introduced which extended beyond psychiatrists in academic positions. A limited teaching of psychiatry became compulsory even in the general medical curriculum. In France, psychiatrists for public asylums and, in some cases, residents in psychiatry were selected by a competitive examination system. In England, the Board of Control recommended in 1918, that a leading position in a psychiatric institution could only be occupied by a physician who had obtained a Diploma in Psychological Medicine awarded by the Royal College of Physicians and by five universities. In the United States, the moving force behind the reforms was Adolf Meyer, the Director of the Henry Phipps Clinic at Johns Hopkins University from 1913 to 1939, who organized a systematic residency system and promoted the creation of the Board of Neurology and Psychiatry. This Board was established in 1936 and awarded a diploma which it became necessary to hold, to be recognized as a specialist.

The changes were reflected in the vocabulary. The term psychiatry, originating in the German-speaking countries and mostly used there, was adopted everywhere at the beginning of the century. In France, the health authorities officially substituted '*hôpital psychiatrique*' for '*asile d'aliénés*' and '*psychiatre*' for '*aliéniste*' in the 1930s. In England, a Royal Commission used the words 'hospital', 'nurse', and 'patient' instead of 'asylum', 'attendant', and 'lunatic' for the first time between 1924 and 1926. However, efforts were also made to dissociate, when possible, the social protection function of the institutions from their medical role by allowing them to admit patients under the same conditions as the general hospitals. In 1923, a special section was created in the Paris Sainte-Anne asylum which provided treatment to voluntary patients and had both hospital beds and a large outpatient department. In England, the Mental Health Act of 1930 made voluntary admissions to psychiatric hospitals possible; by 1938, they already constituted 35 per cent of all admissions.

Social considerations had always been evident in psychiatry, but their traditional expressions had mainly been of a negative nature, i.e., the confinement of patients in asylums. The new possibility of free admissions reflected an increase in tolerance towards the disturbing character of mental illness. At the same time, a differently oriented and broader social perspective appeared. The concept of mental hygiene originated in the United States in 1919 with the creation by a former patient, Clifford Beers, of an organization whose internationally growing influence was manifested by well-attended congresses held in Washington in 1930 and in Paris in 1937. From its beginning, the movement was not purely medical and was influenced by various humanitarian philosophical trends. It emphasized the role of social factors, such as living conditions or educational practices, in the origin of mental disturbances and promoted their prevention and treatment by the close co-operation of psychiatrists and nurses with non-medical groups in the community. One of the institutional consequences of these ideas was the creation of the profession of social worker. They began their activity in Adolf Meyer's clinic (Adolf Meyer had been an early supporter of the mental hygiene movement whose principles converged with his own ideas) at the Sainte-Anne Hospital in Paris, in England where the London School of Economics opened a special training course in 1929, and elsewhere.

Contemporary with the emergence of psychiatric social work was the expansion of clinical psychology. The Binet-Simon scale for the measurement of intelligence, developed in 1905, was the first application to psychiatry of the new discipline of experimental psychology which had originated at the end of the previous century. This initial contribution led to the creation of a professional class of clinical psychologists who were initially concerned with the development and use of psychological assessment instruments and with theoretical research in a few psychiatric centres. Their number initially remained low; in 1945 the United States, where they were most numerous, had about 4 000 psychiatrists but only 200 clinical psychologists.

The expansion of psychiatry after 1945

The Second World War coincided with a major transformation of the psychiatric specialty. The war had vividly demonstrated the frequency of mental disorders in the United States; they had proved to be the leading cause of medical discharges from the military service and the primary cause of almost 40 per cent of selective service rejections. The previously prevailing view that psychiatry was a minor and often somewhat despised medical discipline, concerned primarily with the custodial care of psychologically deviant and potentially troublesome individuals, was progressively dispelled. The preservation and the restoration of mental health—an expression from now on often used by national and international institutions—began to be considered by governments as an important task. The fundamental changes which took place after 1945 and shaped psychiatry as we know it today were the result of this new atmosphere and of the emergence of new perspectives in the three traditional domains— the psychological, the social, and the biological. Some appeared in slightly different forms at different times, their relative influence was submitted to variations, and eventually they came into conflict. The result has been an impressive expansion and increase of the efficacy of psychiatry, profound institutional transformations, and successive ideological waves which have had a major impact on the professional position of the psychiatrist.

The demographic data reflect the new importance of psychiatry in medicine. In the United States, the proportion of psychiatrists in the medical profession was 0.7 per cent in 1920, 1.4 per cent in 1940, and 5.5 per cent in 1970, the rate of growth having doubled after the Second World War. In France, at present there are 18 psychiatrists for 100 000 habitants; they constitute 6 per cent of all physicians. Similar levels were reached during the postwar decades in the developed countries and remain relatively stable today. Even before this spectacular increase in numbers, psychiatrists had been becoming conscious of the necessity to affirm the identity of their discipline. The First World Congress of Psychiatry, held in Paris in 1950, has been followed by periodic meetings and by the creation of the World Psychiatric Association to which almost every national society of psychiatry belongs. The health authorities of various countries have become conscious of the necessity to provide adequate financial means to support research and training in the discipline. In 1946, the United States government created the National Institutes of Mental Health for such a purpose, and similar efforts were made in many countries although the structures of the organizations formed were different. To promote the same goals at the international level, the World Health Organization, created immediately after the Second World War, had a Section (later Division) of Mental Health which, among other co-ordinating activities, tried to overcome the difficulties of communication between the national schools by establishing a common nosological language.

While the changes affected almost all countries, they were most spectacular in the United States. From the end of the 19th century until the 1930s, the concepts developed in the German-speaking countries had been the most influential. This disappeared with the advent of the National Socialist regime which, under cover of racist theories, expelled many of the leading psychiatrists from Germany and Austria, introduced compulsory sterilization for several varieties of mental illnesses, and promoted the voluntary killing in psychiatric hospitals of mentally-retarded children and chronic patients. The United States, which had emerged from the Second World War as the most powerful country in the world, began to exert a widespread influence in psychiatry as in the rest of medicine. Because of the prestige of its research and teaching institutions and the worldwide influence of its scientific publications, reinforced by the progressive adoption of English as the language of international scientific communication, American psychiatry became a model in many countries, even though many of the theoretical trends and technical advances it adopted and developed had originated in Europe. However, in the United States, with a local colouring, they took on a special intensity.

The psychodynamic wave

An important factor in the spread of the doctrine of psychoanalysis was the emigration of a relatively large number of German and Austrian psychoanalysts to the United States from 1933 onwards. They had been compelled to leave their home countries for racial reasons—psychoanalysis had been condemned by the National Socialist regime as Jewish and Freud's books had been publicly burned. Many of the young psychiatrists trained in large numbers to answer the demands of the armed forces adopted psychoanalysis under the influence of some of those in charge of the programmes. For a generation, until the end of the 1960s, psychoanalysis became the dominant ideology in American psychiatry.

The American form of psychodynamism often deviated from Freudian orthodoxy, but it emphasized the role of psychogenetic factors, the value of the study of intrapsychic mechanisms, and the basic importance of psychotherapy, while giving little consideration to the traditional clinical approach and to nosology. The domination of this essentially psychological orientation, sometimes compared with the success of the German mentalist school during the first half of the 19th century, had important consequences. Although the disorders of hospitalized psychotics were eventually interpreted according to psychoanalytic theory, psychotherapy was mostly used, as it has been since its beginning, on ambulatory neurotic patients. As early as 1951–1952, 3 000 of the 7 500 American psychiatrists identified private practice as their main activity, and in 1954, the number of private psychiatrists exceeded that of their salaried colleagues for the first time, with a quarter of the former devoted exclusively to psychotherapy. However, with the initial encouragement of official institutions such as the Veterans Administration, the clinical psychologists began to engage in psychotherapeutic activities. The number of members of the Clinical Psychology Section of the American Psychological Association reached 20 000 in 1980, at a time when they were 26 000 psychiatrists in the United States. In public opinion, and to a certain extent in general medical opinion also, psychiatry was assumed to consist only of psychotherapy and psychology.

In most other countries the developments that occurred in the United States were not as intense, generally appeared later, and were modified by local traditions and influences. In the German-speaking countries they were delayed by the still powerful neuropsychiatric perspective and the temporary vogue for existential phenomenology. In the United Kingdom, the eclectic current fostered by the influential London Institute of Psychiatry during the decades following the war restricted the advance of psychodynamism; in 1956, *Time Magazine* could affirm, as a conclusion of a survey, that 'all of Great Britain [had] half as many analysts as New York City'. In France, the psychoanalyst Jacques Lacan gave the doctrine a special colouring. On the whole, however, the rise of psychodynamism was a general phenomenon, except in the communist countries where Freud's doctrine had been condemned on ideological grounds.

A reaction began in the 1960s with the successes of the new pharmacotherapies. Clinical psychologists had developed alternative radically different psychotherapeutic methods based on learning theories, especially the behaviour therapy introduced in 1958 by Wolpe, supported in the United Kingdom by Eysenck, and the cognitive therapy often associated with it. These methods competed successfully with the psychodynamic techniques and conquered a large part of the field. Psychodynamism did not disappear; many of its concepts retained their place in psychiatry and psychotherapeutic methods continued to be practized, but it lost its predominant ideological position. In addition to its theoretical contributions, when its influence on the professional aspect of psychiatry is considered from a historical perspective, it has been an important factor in the further expansion of the activity of psychiatrists in the treatment of relatively minor disorders and has also encouraged clinical psychologists to play an active and independent role in this field.

The social wave

At the end of the Second World War there was a great desire for social change; one of its aspects was the belief that everyone had a 'right to health' or at least the right to receive adequate medical care regardless of the ability to pay. This resulted in the creation of the National Health Service in the United Kingdom in 1948 and the Social Security system in France, together with similar developments in other countries. The social perspective, which was one of the basic principles underlying these developments, initiated major institutional changes in psychiatry. They were the result of a number of factors—the necessity to give to the whole population an easy access to psychiatric care, and also the belief that social elements played an important role in the aetiology of the mental disorders and that they could greatly contribute to the healing process, with the aim of progressively reintegrating the patient in the community.

The most spectacular aspect of the new policy was the decline of the asylum system, still in a dominant position in psychiatry; in fact, the number of patients in psychiatric hospitals in the developed countries reached its peak in 1955. The criticisms of the 'degeneration' of the functioning of psychiatric hospitals and the segregation of patients in institutions, often located far from their homes and families, were not new. However, the previous partial improvements, such as the decrease in the number of compulsory commitments or the creation of outpatient departments, were replaced by the creation of completely new structures. Ideally, the country would be divided into geographical zones or sectors with a population of about 100 000, and each zone would have a multidisciplinary team of psychiatrists, nurses, clinical psychologists, social workers, and occupational therapists responsible for mental health. Visits and therapeutic interventions in the patient's home and easily accessible outpatient departments were to play an increasingly important role. If hospitalization was necessary, it should be as far as possible in small units located in a general hospital where the time of stay was to be reduced to the absolute minimum. Special institutions such as day hospitals, night hospitals, and specially adapted workshops would contribute to the progressive readaptation of the patient to the life in the community. The introduction of this 'community care', which was expected to work in close co-operation with general practitioners and various public and private institutions, would result in the disappearance of the traditional psychiatric hospital and to 'deinstitutionalize' psychiatry. The new system was introduced in various forms in most countries after 1969. In the United States, the Community Mental Health Center Act was promulgated in 1967. In the United Kingdom, which had strong traditions of social psychiatry, plans for the implementation of community care were discussed in the 1960s, and in 1975, the Government White Paper *Better Services for the Mentally Ill* encouraged the formation of multidisciplinary 'primary care teams' which also included general practitioners. In France, an official directive in 1960 created the *psychiatrie de secteur* which was expected to result in the progressive elimination of *hospitalocentrisme*. The World Health Organization (WHO) encouraged all its member countries to adopt similar practices.

Although, in the last 40 years community care has become the official doctrine everywhere, except in Japan where the rate of hospitalization in mostly private hospitals has grown continuously, its implementation has not been easy despite the major therapeutic improvements brought about by pharmacotherapy. In some parts of the United States, the sudden closure of public psychiatric hospitals combined with the inadequacies of the Community Mental Health Centers were for a time at the origin of an appalling lack of care for a number of mentally ill people. The expected 'fading out' of hospitalization has been slow. According to the WHO, in 1976 the number of mental health beds (including beds for the mentally retarded) per 1 000 population was 6.5 in Sweden, 5.5 in the United Kingdom, 3 in France, and 2 in Germany. These figures have since decreased and the types of hospitalization have changed. In 1955, 77 per cent of the 'psychiatric care episodes' in the United States occurred in public psychiatric hospitals, compared with 20 per cent in 1990. In 1994, 1.4 million mental patients were hospitalized, but only 35 per cent in public psychiatric hospitals compared with 43 per cent in general hospitals and 11 per cent in private psychiatric hospitals, which increased in number from 150 in 1970 to 444 in 1988. In France, where the total number of psychiatric patients treated in public institutions (including children) is now about a million, 60 per cent are seen exclusively on an ambulatory basis, but the number of hospital beds has only been reduced by half.

Reflecting the increasing influence of social perspectives, the organizational changes modified psychiatry as a profession. The increase in the number of psychiatrists in private practice was paralleled, in general to a lesser extent, by an increase in the public sector where their role was modified. In the traditional asylum, the authority of the psychiatrist was unchallenged and limited only by the legal provisions related to the procedures of commitment. The nurses, and later the clinical psychologists, social workers, and occupational therapists, were 'paramedical auxiliaries' in a subordinate position. The creation of multidisciplinary teams, working in various settings, gave the psychiatrist a function of co-ordination made increasingly complex by the claims of professional autonomy made by the former auxiliaries. In some cases, such as in the American Mental Health Centers, the psychiatrists who were a small minority in the team and had less and less control over its functioning, resented what they considered to be the loss of their medical status.

The importance given to social factors was not limited to the system by which care was delivered. Sometimes, combined with radical ideological and political attitudes, it took more extreme forms. The criticisms, which first centred on the inadequacies of the existing institutions, extended to the concept of mental disease itself. The antipsychiatric movement claimed that mental diseases were artificial constructs which were not related to diseases in the medical meaning of the term. The allegedly pathological behaviours, such as those conceptualized as schizophrenia, were in fact normal reactions to an inadequate social system. The so-called treatments were techniques used by the ruling classes to preserve the social order of which they were the beneficiaries. The only solution was a drastic reform of society. Such theses varied in their content and in the arguments used. They were developed by authors such as Szasz, Laing, and Cooper in the English-speaking world, the philosopher Foucault in France, and the psychiatrist Basaglia in Italy. They reached their greatest influence in the 1960s and a few attempts were made to put their ideological principles into practice. Although they attracted much attention at the time, they were very limited and short lived. One of the few countries where this movement had a practical impact was Italy. Basaglia's strongly politically oriented theories were influential in the later legal reform of the antiquated asylum system, but, despite the apparently revolutionary character of some of the new administrative provisions, the changes made were very similar to those taking place in other countries.

The biological wave

Psychotropic drugs, such as opium, had been used since the origin of the medical treatment of psychiatric patients. During the 19th and the first half of the 20th century, synthetic drugs such as the bromides, the barbiturates, and the amphetamines were developed. Some of them, especially the sedatives and hypnotics, had a real but in practice, marginal value in alleviating some symptoms. They had never constituted an effective treatment of mental disorders. Modern psychopharmacology not only initiated what has been rightly called a therapeutic revolution in psychiatry but also gave a powerful new impulse to the biological perspective. Its date of birth is usually considered to be 1952, when the remarkable activity of chlorpromazine on the symptoms of schizophrenia and mania was discovered. This had been preceded in 1949 by the demonstration of the value of lithium salts in manic states. A few years later, it was shown that the continuous administration of lithium salts prevented the recurrence of manic and depressive phases in the mood disorders. This was followed by the introduction of drugs acting on the depressive manifestations (imipramine and the monoamine oxidase inhibitors in 1957) and on anxiety (including chlorediazepoxide, the prototype of the benzodiazepines, in 1960). In one decade, clinicians had empirically discovered the fields of application of the main classes of psychoactive drugs—the neuroleptics, the antidepressants, the anxiolytics, and the mood stabilizers—which had been synthesized by biochemists and previously tested by pharmacologists on animal models. The scale and rapidity of the spread of their use had major repercussions.

The first was a modification of the image of psychiatry. The layman generally expected a physician to prescribe drugs to treat the disease from which he suffered. In part, because it did not conform to the expected therapeutic behaviour, psychiatry had been seen as an atypical and almost non-medical specialty. In addition to the specificity of the institutions in which it was generally practized, psychological techniques were unknown in the rest of medicine, and even the recently introduced biological techniques (the shock therapies and the lobotomy) had a somewhat strange and frightening character. The establishment of pharmacotherapy contributed strongly to modifying this perception, even if it did not completely remove the traditional prejudices.

The second consequence was even more important. There were, at least initially, controversies about the roles of pharmacotherapy and of the new social perspectives in the restructuring of the mental health care system. In fact, the number of inpatients in psychiatric hospitals began to decrease from 1955 on, and it seems obvious that the main cause was the therapeutic efficacy of the drugs. They reduced the mean length of hospitalization and eventually even made it unnecessary. Although some types of patients did not benefit from them and the mental state of others was only improved, many who had previously been condemned to long stays in the hospital were able to return to the community, with their treatment eventually being continued in rehabilitation settings and often on an ambulatory basis. Pharmacotherapy had made possible the practical implementation of social trends. In addition to this basic contribution to the 'deinstitutionalization' movement, pharmacotherapy was an essential factor in the growth of private practice. The success of psychotherapy had been one contribution to this, but the complexity of its techniques, the length of the treatment, its applicability to only a few types of disorders, and the uncertainty of the results limited its use to a relatively small number of selected patients, even in the United States during the period of the greatest popularity of psychodynamism. Pharmacotherapy could be used much more easily, on a much larger number of patients, and did not require a long and complex training. Some of the drugs, such as the anxiolytics, had an immediate symptomatic effect, and others (the antidepressants and the neuroleptics) could attenuate or suppress the pathological manifestations in a few weeks and, outside the acute phase requiring hospitalization, could be used on an ambulatory basis. It was not only private psychiatrists who were able to treat many of their patients successfully; general practitioners also began to prescribe psychotropic drugs on a large scale.

The third consequence was the explosive development of biological research in psychiatry. The first therapeutic discoveries were largely empirical, but new biochemical techniques allowed some of the modes of action of the drugs to be elucidated. From 1960 on, studies of the influence of these drugs on various aspects of neurotransmission in the brain stimulated hypotheses about the abnormal biochemical mechanisms considered to be the physical substrate of the mental disorders. Meanwhile new methods had been introduced for examination of morphological modifications of the living brain and even of the nature and localization of the biochemical processes taking place in its different parts. The discovery by Watson and Crick in 1953, of the chemical basis of heredity and the subsequent spectacular advances in molecular biology gave a fresh impulse to psychiatric genetics, which had been partly discredited by their misuse by the National Socialist regime. Under the name of neurosciences, these new fields of enquiry progressively acquired a dominant role in psychiatric research at the same time as the introduction of an ever-increasing number of drugs, eventually more potent, usually with less inconvenient side-effects, and sometimes with new therapeutic indications.

'Remedicalization' of psychiatry

In 1983, Melvin Sabshin, the Director of the American Psychiatric Association, summarized the overlapping chronologies of the psychodynamic, biological, and social waves as follows:[6]

> Psychoanalysis surged through the United States during the 1940s and the 1950s. During the 1950s, a new psychopharmacological approach emerged which had great impact on psychiatric practice generally . . . The 1960s saw the dawning of a community psychiatric approach which attempted to accomplish a massive desinstitutionalization of patients from public psychiatric hospitals.

Although less radical and not strictly identical, the general picture was similar in other countries. The 1960s saw an often uneasy coexistence of three schools. 'During that decade', wrote Sabshin, 'American psychiatry enlarged its boundaries and its practices so broadly that many critics grew increasingly concerned with the 'bottomless pit' of the field'. The extension of the practice of psychotherapy, frequently to cases with no clear pathological character, tended to blur the limits of the mental disease concept and to neglect the traditional diagnostic approach. Social work was also tempted to concern itself with problems with no obvious medical nature, such as those still described in 1978 in the United States by the President's Commission of Mental Health, which asserted that 'American mental health cannot be defined only in terms of disabling mental illness and identified mental disorders' and identified as a domain of concern for workers in the field 'unrelenting poverty and unemployment and the institutionalized discrimination that occurs on the basis of race, sex, class, age . . .'. In sharp contrast, the new biological psychiatry recognized only a strictly medical model, stressing the necessity of an accurate diagnosis for the prescription of the drugs and for the testing of their efficacy, and advocated restrictive limits in the definition of the mental diseases.

Around 1970, a profound change took place. Although the institutional modifications of the care system favoured by the generalization of drug therapy continued and expanded under its various forms everywhere, the influence of psychodynamism began to decline within the psychiatric profession. According to the Director of the National Institutes for Mental Health 'it was nearly impossible in 1945 for a non-psychoanalyst to become Chairman of a Department of Psychiatry (in the United States)' but by the mid-1970s the situation was reversed. The publication by the American Psychiatric Association of the Third Revision of the Diagnostic and Statistical Manual of Mental Disorders (DSM-III) is often considered as the symbolic expression of the change. This took place in 1980, but its origins were more than a decade previously, and it was significantly presented by its apologists, such as Klerman, as 'a decisive turning point in the history of American psychiatry . . . an affirmation of its medical identity'. The new nosology, which was categorical in nature and which introduced diagnostic criteria borrowed from experimental psychology in the delimitation of the categories, did not allow any reference to 'unproven' aetiological factors or pathogenic mechanisms, unless 'scientifically demonstrated'. It claimed to be purely descriptive and therefore acceptable as a means of communication by all psychiatrists, whatever their individual orientation may be. It was in fact perceived, not only in its country of origin, as a reaction against the extreme socio-psychological positions—the deletion of the term neurosis because of its usual association with the psychoanalytic theory of intra-psychic conflicts raised violent controversies—and, despite its proclaimed 'a-theorism', as favouring the biological medical model. Although initially exclusively devised for the use of the American psychiatrists, to the surprise of its authors it was rapidly accepted in all countries and the WHO adopted finally its principles in its own nosological system, the International Classification of Diseases. Originally the result of a brutal reversal of trends in the American psychiatry, it expressed a general change of direction in the psychiatric way of thinking towards the affirmation, against the forces believed to threaten it of the medical character of psychiatry.

Crisis in psychiatry?

At first glance, the new status of psychiatry seems to have taken firm root in the last three decades. It rests on the general acceptance of the medical definition of the concept of mental disease and of the progressive realization of a diversified but co-ordinated institutional system of mental health care. The biological perspective, even if it has taken a prominent place in research and therapy, is now combined with psychological and social approaches in the bio-psychosocial model. The psychiatrist, in accordance with his medical professional responsibilities, occupies a central position in a multidisciplinary team whose members contribute their special competences to the common goal.

This idyllic picture is far from a reflection of reality, even in the developed countries, and the existence of a crisis in psychiatry is evoked with increasing frequency. An indication of the loss of prestige of psychiatry in the medical profession is the alarming decrease of the proportion of American medical students choosing a psychiatric residency; it fell to 2 per cent in 1990, a level much too low to ensure the maintenance of the present demography. Under the pressure of economic constraints, efforts are made everywhere to control the rising burden of medical care. They have taken different forms according to the country—from the managed care system in the United States to the *numerus clausus* system in France, in which the number of internships available is determined by the government—but their common aim is to limit the number of psychiatrists and the cost of their activities. Paradoxically, the recognition of the frequency of the mental disorders and the growing demand for psychiatric treatments has been associated with a reduction in the domain of action of psychiatrists, who are now often vastly outnumbered by clinical psychologists and social workers. In the United States, by 1990, 80 000 'clinical' social workers were active in the psychiatric socio-psychological domain, a quarter of them in part- or full-time private practice. The claims of these powerful professional groups are not limited to a completely autonomous status but, in the case of the clinical psychologists, extend to the demand for a legal recognition of such typical 'medical privileges' as the right to hospitalize patients and to prescribe drugs. Even within medicine, psychiatry is under attack. In Germany, a medical psychotherapeutic specialty distinct from psychiatry has been created. The most impressive change has been in the proportion of mental disorders being now treated by general practitioners as a result of the availability of psychotropic drugs with fewer side-effects; in France, 60 per cent of antidepressants are now prescribed by general practitioners. These examples may not be a fair representation of the global picture, but there is undoubtedly a movement towards a limitation of the psychiatric specialty to the care of the most severe cases—in practice, the psychotic cases. However, some neuroscientists raise doubts about the usefulness of maintaining psychiatry as a specialty even in this field. Influential biologically oriented psychiatrists have recently proposed on theoretical and practical grounds, that psychiatry should be absorbed into a new medical discipline, akin to the former neuropsychiatry, and all or most of its socio-psychological aspects should be left to non-medical professions.

Since psychiatry has emerged as a specialty, it has been submitted to conflicting forces. The demands of society, changes in the concept of mental disorder and of its limits, variations in the role played by different theoretical perspectives, and successive scientific discoveries have been responsible for an evolution reflected in the professional status and role of the psychiatrist. Displacements of the centre of gravity of a complex structure in which biological, psychological, and social factors interact have modified the image of psychiatry. The threat of being incorporated in other medical specialties or being deprived of its medical character is but another transitory episode in its history.

Further information

Hunter, R. and Macalpine, I. (1963). *Three hundred years of psychiatry 1535–1860*. Oxford University Press, London.

Pichot, P. (1996). *Un siècle de psychiatrie*. Synthelabo, Le Plessis-Robinson.

Postel, J. and Questel, U. (ed.) (1994). *Nouvelle histoire de la psychiatrie.* Dunod, Paris.

Shorter, E.A. (1997). *History of psychiatry: from the era of the asylum to the age of Prozac.* Wiley, New York.

References

1. Kraepelin, E. (1918). Hundert Jahre Psychiatrie. *Zeitschrift für die gesamte Neurologie und Psychiatrie*, **38**, 161–275.
2. Leigh, D. (1961). *The historical development of British psychiatry.* Vol. I, *Eighteenth and nineteenth centuries.* Pergamon Press, Oxford.
3. Goldstein, J. (1987). *Console and classify: the French psychiatric profession in the nineteenth century.* Cambridge University Press.
4. Zilboorg, G. (1941). *A history of medical psychology.* Norton, New York.
5. Kraepelin, E. (1904). *Psychiatrie* (7th edn). Barth, Leipzig.
6. Sabshin, M. (1983). Preface. In *International perspectives on DSM-III* (ed. R.L. Spitzer, J.B.W. Williams, and A.E. Skodol). American Psychiatric Press, Washington, DC.

1.5

Ethics and values

Contents

1.5.1 Psychiatric ethics
Sidney Bloch and Stephen Green

1.5.2 Values and values-based practice in clinical psychiatry
K. W. M. Fulford

1.5.1 Psychiatric ethics

Sidney Bloch and Stephen Green

A myriad of ethical problems pervade clinical practice and research in psychiatry. Yet with few exceptions,[1–3] psychiatric ethics has generally been regarded as an addendum to mainstream bioethics. An assumption has been made that 'tools' developed to deal with issues like assisted reproduction or transplant surgery can be used essentially unmodified in psychiatry. These tools certainly help the psychiatrist but the hand-me-down approach has meant that salient features of psychiatric ethics have been prone to misunderstanding. Psychiatric ethics is concerned with the application of moral rules to situations and relationships specific to the field of mental health practice. We will focus on ethical aspects of diagnosis and treatment that challenge psychiatrists, and on codes of ethics. Resolution of ethical dilemmas requires deliberation grounded in a moral theoretical framework that serves clinical decision-making, and we conclude with our preferred theoretical perspective.

Diagnostic issues

Conferring a diagnosis of mental illness on a person has profound ethical sequelae since the process may embody substantive adverse effects, notably stigma, prejudice, and discrimination (e.g. limited job prospects, inequitable insurance coverage). Furthermore, those deemed at risk to harm themselves or others may have their civil rights abridged. These consequences justify Reich's[4] call for the most thorough ethical examination of what he terms the clinician's 'prerogative to diagnose'.

Psychiatrists strive to diagnose by using as objective criteria as possible and information gained from previous clinical encounters. The process is relatively straightforward when findings such as gross memory impairment and life-threatening social withdrawal strongly suggest severe depression. Other situations are not so obvious. For instance, the distress felt by a bereaved person may incline one clinician towards diagnosing clinical depression whereas another may construe the picture as normal grief. Expertise, peer review, and benevolence combine to protect against arbitrariness and idiosyncrasy. Notwithstanding, psychiatrists must, to some extent, apply what might be termed as 'reasoned subjectivism'. Thus, specified criteria in the American Psychiatric Association's (APA) DSM-IV[5] and the World Health Organization's ICD-10[6] do not preclude debate about the preciseness or legitimacy of syndromes like Attention Deficit Hyperactivity Disorder (ADHD) and sexual orientation disturbance. Concern about the intrusion of value judgements into contemporary classification has led to the contention that some diagnoses reflect pejorative labelling rather than scientific decisions. For example, charges of sexism were leveled against DSM-III[7] on the grounds that masculine-based assumptions shaped criteria, resulting in women receiving unwarranted diagnoses like premenstrual dysphoria.[8]

The issue central to this debate is whether certain mental states are grounded in fact or value judgements. Szasz[9] takes a radical position, arguing that disordered thinking and behaviour are due to objective abnormalities of the brain whereas mental illness *per se* is a 'myth', created by society in tandem with the medical profession in order to exert social control. The 'anti-psychiatrist movement'[10,11] posits that mental illnesses are social constructs, reflecting deviations from societal norms. This argument is supported by the role of values in both defining homosexuality in the past as a psychiatric disorder, then reversing that position, in the case of American psychiatry through a ballot among members of the APA in 1973.[12] Legitimate diagnoses necessarily combine aspects of fact and value, as Wakefield[13] avows in his conception of 'harmful dysfunction'. He views 'dysfunction' as a scientific and factual term, based in biology, which refers to the failure of an internal evolutionary mechanism to perform a natural function for which it is designed and 'harmful' as a value-oriented term which covers the consequences of the dysfunction deemed detrimental in socio-cultural terms. Applying this notion to mental functioning, Wakefield describes beneficial effects of natural mechanisms like those mediating cognition and emotional regulation, and judges their dysfunction harmful when it yields effects disvalued by society (e.g. self-destructive acts). Diagnosable conditions occur when the inability of an internal mechanism to perform its natural function causes harm to the person. DSM-IV[5] rightly emphasizes that mental disorders should not be diagnosed solely by reference to social norms. The deterioration of functioning by which schizophrenia is (partly) defined under Criterion B, or the norm violations of antisocial personality disorder, must therefore be, in DSM-IVs phrase, 'clinically significant'. What this amounts to, then, is that a negative value judgement is insufficient to diagnose. The repercussions of these issues can be considerable, (e.g. exposing children erroneously labelled as ADHD to long-term medication with its attendant risks).[14] A related matter, so-called 'cosmetic psychopharmacology', involves the use of medication to enhance psychological functioning. As Kramer[15] notes, fluoxetine may modulate emotions like anxiety, guilt, and shame, raising ethical questions regarding a person's capacity to possess 'two senses of self'. Psychiatric diagnosis may also mitigate legal and personal results of one's actions (e.g. interpreting excessive sexual activity as a variant of obsessive-compulsive disorder rather than as wilful).

Some of the worst perversions of psychiatry, in which it has been deployed as a form of social control, have been driven by misuse of its diagnostic concepts. In the former Soviet Union, for example, thousands of political, religious, and other dissidents were committed to psychiatric hospitals on the basis of 'delusions of reformism' and other similar tainted concepts.[16]

Treatment issues

Assessing and treating patients require a working alliance in conjunction with informed consent. Many psychiatric patients are in a position to understand and appreciate the nuances of treatment options, to express an informed preference, and to feel allied with a therapist in the task. When the process of informed consent is responsibly handled, particularly with reference to benefits and risks of therapeutic options, mentally ill people are in a comparable position to their counterparts in general medicine. This comparability is grounded in two concepts—competence[17] and voluntarism. [18] The former satisfies the required criterion that the person facing choices in treatment has the 'critical faculties' to appreciate the implications of each course of action. Voluntarism refers to a state in which the process of consent is devoid of any form of coercion. Obviously, given that the organ of decision-making is the same one that is impaired in many psychiatric conditions, profound ethical complications may ensue when seeking informed consent.

Other issues also present themselves in this context; these have been conveniently examined as a series of rights—to treatment, effective treatment, and refusal of treatment—and involuntary treatment.

The right to treatment

The asylum revealed tragically how this right was never actualized; the overcrowded institution became little more than a warehouse.[19] Its custodial nature persisted even after the advent of psychotropics and psychosocial therapies. It took a plaintiff[20] to determine that a person committed involuntarily had the 'right to receive treatment that would offer him a reasonable opportunity to be cured or to improve his mental condition'. Diagnosed with schizophrenia in 1957, Kenneth Donaldson received minimal treatment for the next decade and a half. The US Supreme Court concluded in 1975 that a patient who does not pose a danger to himself or to others and who is not receiving treatment should be released into the community.

The right to effective treatment

The right to treatment has been revisited in subsequent judgements, predominantly in the United States.[21] However, the right has lacked a guarantee that patients will receive effective treatment, reflected vividly in Osheroff v Chestnut Lodge (a private psychiatric hospital in the United States). In this case, the plaintiff sued the staff for their failure to provide antidepressant treatment in the face of his deteriorating depression. Klerman[22] subsequently argued that the clinician is duty-bound to use only' 'treatments for which there is substantial evidence' 'or seek a second opinion in the absence of a clinical response. Stone[23] countered this position which he averred was tantamount to '. . . promulgating more uniformed scientific standards of treatment in psychiatry, based on . . . opinion about science and clinical practice'. Moreover, he posited that legal standards of care should not be established by one 'school' for the whole profession, even if enveloped in science. Instead, we should depend on 'the collective sense' of psychiatry, as well as apply the 'respectable minority rule', namely that a relatively small group within psychiatry can legitimately devise novel therapies.

The right to refuse treatment

As a voluntary patient, Osheroff could have refused treatment of any type as part of informed consent. He pinpointed the institution's alleged failure to offer him an alternative treatment in the face of his worsening state with the therapy that was administered. If principles of informed consent had been applied correctly, his freedom to choose one treatment over others, and to withdraw consent at any stage thereafter, would have prevailed.

The situation differs radically when the patient is committed involuntarily to hospital or community treatment. The right to refuse treatment then looms large.[24] A key event in this context was another US legal judgement when a court ruled that detained patients have a right to refuse treatment.[25] This coincided with changing commitment laws in many jurisdictions from criteria linked to need for treatment to those highlighting the danger posed to oneself and/or others. The ethical repercussions are profound. If psychiatrists are empowered to detain a patient, is it not a contradiction if they are then powerless to provide treatment should the person refuse? The argument rests on the premise that someone disturbed enough to warrant involuntary admission is axiomatically entitled to treatment, and the psychiatrist well placed to give it. Without this arrangement, the psychiatrist's functions are reduced to the custodial.

A countervailing argument is grounded in constitutional rights. Merely because people are committed does not mean they are incapable of participating in the process of informed consent. In the event they cannot appreciate the rationale for a course of action, a form of substituted judgement should be employed thereby ensuring that their rights remain prominent.

An assortment of legal remedies has emerged in response to this ethical quandary, ranging from a full adversarial process to reliance on a guardian. Appelbaum[24] has contributed a lucid account of available options and a predilection for a treatment-driven model in which patients are committed because their capacity to decide about their medical care is lacking as part of their disturbed mental functioning. His own research demonstrates that most 'refusing' patients voluntarily accept treatment within 24 h.[26]

In another pragmatically oriented account Stone[27] proposes that presumption of competence should be dealt with before admission to hospital. Dealing with commitment and competence together obviates the problem of compulsory admission without the powers to treat. The snag is the fluidity of the mental state. What patients think about treatment during the maelstrom of being detained may well change once they settle in and are suitably cared for.

Involuntary treatment

A consensus has prevailed universally that a proportion of psychiatric patients lack the capacity for self-determination. They are prone to harming themselves and/or others, acting in ways they will later regret (e.g. a manic patient's sexual indiscretions); and suffer from self-neglect (e.g. malnourished and physically ill schizophrenic patients). What is not universally agreed is how best to deal with such vulnerable people. Society has, generally, devised laws as the vehicle to respond to the thorny issue of how to protect this group. However, variations in legislation and its application are legion, reflecting, in part, the ethical underpinnings of the process. Psychiatrists and society need to establish coherent arguments concerning relevant moral principles. A good start is Mill's[28] contention that the 'only purpose for which power can be rightfully exercised over any member of a civilized community, against his will, is to prevent harm to others. His own good, either physical or moral, is not a sufficient warrant'. Mill's caveat that an exception must be made in the case of children and mentally disturbed people (i.e. 'delirious' or in a 'state of excitement or absorption incompatible with the full use of the reflecting faculty') suggests they can legitimately be assisted.

Chodoff[29] has addressed the awesome question of compulsorily treating a person on the grounds of mental illness. He finds classical moral theory wanting and therefore proposes a 'chastened and self-critical' paternalism, one 'willing to commit to strong safeguards against abuse'. This humanism is epitomized in a concluding sentiment: involuntary treatment is not a conflict of right versus wrong but one over the right to remain at liberty against the right 'to be free from dehumanizing disease'.

Our account hitherto has referred to patients as a homogeneous group. Loss of critical faculties may be a unifying feature but ethical factors will vary according to particulars of the clinical state. One noteworthy example is suicidal behaviour. Szasz[30] sees suicide as the act of a moral agent. The State should therefore not assume power to prevent self-killing although it may opt to advise for or against. This argument is a libertarian one, with the corollary that everyone should have the right to end their life. Szasz has, however, neglected Mill's[28] point that when respecting a person's right to liberty, a possible exception is loss of critical faculties. This is not to aver that all suicidal behaviour is the product of a disordered mind. Suicide in the wake of debilitating illness and a long-standing commitment to euthanasia, seems rational—for example, the British author, Arthur Koestler, left a suicide note demonstrating that he arrived at his decision authentically and competently in terms of psychological function.[31]

The suicidal patient epitomizes the psychiatrist's dilemma in having no choice but to impose treatment in various circumstances and having to declare a person's incapacity, by dint of mental illness, to make rational judgements about what is in their best interests.[32] Van Staden and Kruger[33] cover this topic by highlighting its dimensions, namely the failure to understand relevant information, choose decisively between options, and accept that the need for treatment prevails. They refer to the utility of a 'functional approach' in determining capacity, especially the temporal factor, so that a patient incapable of consenting at one point in their illness may become able at another. Ethical arguments to justify detention in a hospital can be extrapolated into the community setting. Similar restrictions on liberty lie at the heart of the moral dilemma and the psychiatrist again has to consider patients' competence. Munetz and his colleagues[34] apply three ethical arguments in a compelling fashion—utilitarian, communitarian, and beneficence—concluding that all three support the use of compulsory treatment in the community setting. Advance directives are a means to obviate some of the ethical complications of compulsory treatment. In summary, patients prone to recurrence of their illness during which they may be too disturbed to provide informed consent reach an agreement with their psychiatrist about what constitutes the best course of action should they suffer an episode in the future and be unable to decide appropriately what treatment is in their best interest. Given that several mental illnesses have a recurring course and are associated with incapacity, advanced directives would appear, on the face of it, to have a useful role. Empirical studies to examine this potential are a clear option; promising results have been achieved in work carried out hitherto.[35]

Codes of ethics

The development of codes of ethics in the history of medicine reflects their possible role in promoting sound clinical practice (and research). Some codes have been a direct response to the collapse of professional standards—the Nuremberg Statement, for instance, was formulated in the aftermath of the Nazi medical crimes—but they obviously also have positive functions.

Promoting professional cohesion is one such function. Despite George Bernard Shaw's depiction of professions as 'conspiracies against the laity' and the risk that professional codes may indeed be self-serving—a charter for restrictive practices, protectionist rather than protective—a profession can only function effectively if it is cohesive and acts in a collegial way. Thus, a code which sets out its members' obligations to one another can contribute substantially to achieving this goal. Most codes have emphasized medicine's tradition of commitment and dedication to society; some even call for 'whistle blowing' in appropriate circumstances.

A second function of codes is to enhance high standards of practice. Professions are characterized, in part, by a corpus of specialized knowledge and skills, not readily available to others, and offered to a dependent, often vulnerable clientele.[36] To the extent, therefore, that it takes an expert to judge relevant expertise, a degree of self-regulation is essential. But this must be balanced by external monitoring. Where bad practice becomes the norm, self-regulation may reinforce it: the abuse of psychiatry to suppress dissent in the former Soviet Union was, in effect, promoted by leaders of the profession.[16] It can be argued that a prescriptive ethical code is unnecessary, since implicit discipline and a shared ethos suffice to maintain standards. As we have noted, history contradicts this, with codes often appearing as a response to compromised care. What kind of codes best promote sound practice will vary with circumstances. They have therefore differed widely in form and content, ranging from aspirational principles to practice guidelines which are set out in considerable detail. The latter are pertinent, especially for education and training. The code of the Royal Australian and New Zealand College of Psychiatrists[37] and the American Psychiatric Association[38] combine general principles with a series of annotations on specific areas such as confidentiality, respect for professional boundaries, and informed consent. Codes also vary in ethical focus, some are virtue-driven, emphasizing character traits which support best possible practice whereas others are duty-based in that they lay out specific responsibilities and obligations.

Codes thus have several meritorious purposes. Furthermore, these support one other. For instance, their inherent educational quality serves to enhance sound ethical clinical practice and their stipulation of potential hazards in ethical decision-making may prevent compromised care, even misuse of expert knowledge.

Conclusion

We have readily noted how the psychiatrist faces ethical quandaries at several levels, both diagnostically and therapeutically, and the potential role of codes of ethics to grapple with them. Diverse moral theories have also been promulgated to aid the practitioner[1,2] and we conclude with our own preferred approach, a combination of principlism[39] and care ethics.[40] Principlism (or principle-based ethics) relies on a set of well-recognized moral principles to identify and analyse ethical problems: respect for autonomy (literally self-government), non-maleficence (first of all, do no harm), beneficence (acting in peoples' best interests), and justice (treating people fairly). The essence of care ethics revolves around the 'natural' propensity of health professionals to extend care to dependent, vulnerable people and to react with such 'moral' feelings as compassion, sensitivity, and trustworthiness.[40] The approach fits well with psychiatry since its practitioners depend day in, day out, on empathy in order to understand the interests and needs of patients and their families. A synthesis of care ethics and principlism permits sound moral reflection within an emotionally based environment in which connectedness between patient and therapist is paramount. We believe this approach, a complementarity between feeling and reason, acknowledges and best exploits the role of 'moral emotions'[41] when clinicians are presented with the many, nuanced ethical conundrums of psychiatric practice.

Further information

Bloch, S. and Green, S. (eds.) (1999). *Psychiatric ethics* (3rd edn). Oxford University Press, Oxford.

Green, S. and Bloch, S. (2006). *An anthology of psychiatric ethics*. Oxford University Press, Oxford.

Post, S. (ed.) (2004). *Encyclopedia of bioethics* (3rd edn). Macmillan, New York.

References

1. Green, S. and Bloch, S. (2006). *An anthology of psychiatric ethics*. Oxford University Press, Oxford.
2. Bloch, S., Chodoff, P., and Green, S. (1999). *Psychiatric ethics* (3rd edn). Oxford University Press, Oxford.
3. Dickenson, D. and Fulford, W. (2001). *In two minds: a casebook of psychiatric ethics*. Oxford University Press, Oxford.
4. Reich, W. (1999). Psychiatric diagnosis as an ethical problem. In *Psychiatric ethics* (ed. S. Bloch, P. Chodoff, and S. Green) (3rd edn). Oxford University Press, Oxford, pp. 193–224.
5. American Psychiatric Association. (1994). *Diagnostic and statistical manual of mental disorders* (4th edn). APA, Washington, DC.
6. World Health Organization. (1992). *International statistical classification of diseases and related health problems*, 1989 revision. WHO, Geneva.
7. Kaplan, M. (1983). A woman's view of DSM-III. *American Psychologist* **38**, 786–92.
8. Chesler, P. (1972). *Women and madness*. Avon, New York.
9. Szasz, T. (1960). The myth of mental illness. *American Psychologist*, **15**, 113-8.
10. Scheff, T. (1966). *Being mentally ill: a sociological theory*. Aldine, Chicago.
11. Laing, R. (1969).*The divided self*. Pantheon, New York.
12. Stoller, R., Marmor, J., Bieber, I., *et al.* (1973). A symposium: should homosexuality be in the APA nomenclature. *American Journal of Psychiatry*, **130**,1207–16.
13. Wakefield, J. (1992). The concept of mental disorder: on the boundary between biological facts and social values. *American Psychologist*, **47**, 373–88.
14. Halasz, G. (2002). A symposium of attention deficit hyperactivity disorder (ADHD): an ethical perspective. *Australian and New Zealand Journal of Psychiatry*, **36**, 472–5.
15. Kramer, P. (1993). *Listening to Prozac*. Viking, New York.
16. Bloch, S. and Reddaway, P. (1977). *Russia's political hospitals*. Gollancz, London (Published in the US as *Psychiatric Terror*, New York: Basic Books).
17. Lidz, C.W., Meisel, A., Zerubavel, E., *et al.* (1984). *Informed consent: a study of decision making in psychiatry*. Guilford, New York.
18. Roberts, L. (2002). Informed consent and the capacity for voluntarism. *American Journal of Psychiatry*, **159**, 705–12.
19. Bloch, S. and Pargiter, R. (2002). A history of psychiatric ethics. *Psychiatric Clinics of North America*, **25**, 509–24.
20. Donaldson v O'Connor, F. 2d 5th Cir, decided Apr. 26, 1974; O'Connor v Donaldson 422US. **563**, 1975.
21. Wyatt v Stickney 325F Supp 781 (1971); Wyatt v Stickney 344F Supp 373, 376, 379–85 (1972).
22. Klerman, G. (1990). The psychiatric patient's right to effective treatment: implications of Osheroff v Chestnut Lodge. *American Journal of Psychiatry*, **147**, 419–27.
23. Stone, A. (1990). Law, science, and psychiatric malpractice: a response to Klerman's indictment on psychoanalytic psychiatry. *American Journal of Psychiatry*, **147**, 419–27.
24. Appelbaum, P. (1988). The right to refuse treatment with antipsychotic medications: retrospect and prospect. *American Journal of Psychiatry*, **145**, 413–9.
25. Rogers v Okin, 478F Supp 1342 (D Mass, 1979); Rogers v Commissioner of the Department of Mental Health, 458NE 2d 308 (Mass Sup Jud Ct, 1983).
26. Appelbaum, P. and Gutheil, T. (1979). 'Rotting with their rights on': constitutional theory and clinical reality in drug refusal by psychiatric patients. *Bulletin of the American Academy of Psychiatry and the Law*, **7**, 308–17.
27. Stone, A. (1981). The right to refuse treatment: why psychiatrists should and can make it work. *Archives of General Psychiatry*, **38**, 358–62.
28. Mill, J.S. (1976). On liberty. In *Three essays*. Oxford University Press, Oxford.

29. Chodoff, P. (1984). Involuntary hospitalisation of the mentally ill as a moral issue. *American Journal of Psychiatry*, **141**, 384–9.
30. Szasz, T. (1986). The case against suicide prevention. *American Psychologist*, **41**, 806–12.
31. Cesarani, D. (1998). *Arthur Koestler: the homeless mind*. Heinemann, London.
32. Heyd, D. and Bloch, S. (1998). The ethics of suicide. In: *Psychiatric ethics* (ed. S. Bloch, P. Chodoff, and S. Green) (3rd edn). Oxford University Press, Oxford, pp. 441–60.
33. Van Staden, C. and Kruger, C. (2003). Incapacity to give informed consent owing to mental disorder. *Journal of Medical Ethics*, **29**, 41–3.
34. Munetz, M., Galon, P., and Frese, F. (2003). The ethics of mandatory community treatment. *Journal of the American Academy of Psychiatry and the Law*, **31**,173–83.
35. Green, S. and Bloch, S. (2006). *An anthology of psychiatric ethics*. Oxford University Press, Oxford. pp. 183–84.
36. Fullinwinder, R. (1994). *Codes of ethics and the professions* (ed. M. Coady, S. Bloch). Melbourne University Press, Melbourne, pp. 72–87.
37. Royal Australian and New Zealand College of Psychiatrists. (2001). *Code of ethics* (3rd edn). Melbourne.
38. American Psychiatric Association. (2001). *Principles of medical ethics with annotations especially applicable to psychiatry* (5th edn). APA, Washington, DC.
39. Beauchamp, T. and Childress, J. (2001). *Principles of biomedical ethics* (5th edn). Oxford University Press, New York.
40. Baier, A. (2004). Demoralization, trust and the virtues. In: *Setting the moral compass* (ed. C. Calhoun). Oxford University Press, New York, pp. 176–88.
41. Hume, D. (1969). *A treatise of human nature*. Penguin, Harmondsworth.

1.5.2 Values and values-based practice in clinical psychiatry

K. W. M. Fulford

Introduction

Values-based practice is a new skills-based approach to working more effectively with complex and conflicting values in health and social care. This chapter illustrates some of the ways in which combining values-based with evidence-based approaches supports the day-to-day practice of the clinical psychiatrist, particularly in the context of multidisciplinary teamwork.

What are values?

Perhaps one of the most familiar ways in which values impact medicine is by way of ethics. But values are wider than ethics. Ethical values are indeed one kind of value. But there are many other kinds of values, such as aesthetic and prudential values. Values also extend to needs, wishes, preferences, indeed to any and all of the many different ways in which we express negative or positive evaluations and value judgments. Within each and all of these areas, moreover, there are wide differences in the particular values held by different individuals, by different cultures, and at different historical periods.

Given the breadth and complexity of values, it is small wonder that the term 'values' means different things to different people. This is illustrated by Table 1.5.2.1 which lists the responses of a group of trainee psychiatrists when asked, at the start of a training session on values-based practice, to write down three words or short phrases that they associate with 'values'. As the table shows, although there is some overlap, every member of the group came up with a different set of associations.

If our values are diverse, however, they are not completely idiosyncratic. To the contrary, there are many values that are widely shared, at least within a given group at a particular period. The values of patient autonomy (freedom of choice) and of acting in the patient's best interests, for example, are shared values that underpin contemporary medical ethics, and these two values are indeed among the values evident in Table 1.5.2.1.

It is the diversity of human values, and how this can be linked with the shared ethical values underpinning clinical practice, that is the starting point for values-based practice. There is a sense in which medicine has always been values-based just as there is a sense in which it has always been evidence-based.[1] The need for values-based practice in contemporary practice, again like the need for evidence-based practice, arises from the growing complexity of medicine; the growing complexity of the evidence underpinning medicine has led to the need for the new tools of evidence-based medicine; the growing complexity of the values underpinning medicine has led to the need for the new tools of values-based medicine.

The growing complexity of values, as well as evidence, is particularly evident in psychiatry. 'Autonomy' and 'best interests', for example, although both shared ethical values, are often in tension. In the past, most people were content to allow doctors to decide what is in their best interests and this is still the case in many parts of the world.[2] Increasingly though, at least in Europe and North

Table 1.5.2.1 What are values?

Faith Internalization Acting in best interests	How we treat people Attitudes Principles Autonomy
Integrity Conscience Best interests Autonomy	Love Relationships
Respect Personal Difference . . . diversity	Non-violence Compassion Dialogue
Beliefs Right/wrong to me What I am	Responsibility Accountability Best interests
Belief Principles Things held dear	What I *believe* What makes me tick What I won't compromise
Subjective merits Meanings Person-centred care	'Objective' core Confidentiality Autonomy
A *standard* for the way I conduct *myself* Belief about how things *should* be Things you would not want to change	Significant Standards Truth

America, a growing emphasis on patient autonomy has led to complex interactions between these two values in clinical care. In particular, autonomy and best interests come into direct conflict in relation to issues of compulsory treatment (Chapter 1.5.1). Then again, even considered in isolation, 'best interests' have highly complex applications in practice, in the sense that what is 'best' for one person may be very different from what is 'best' for another, according to differences in their personal values and the values of others concerned. Establishing 'best interests' thus presents particular challenges in areas such as old age psychiatry, for example, where patients may lack the decision-making capacity to exercise genuine autonomy on their own behalf.

One response to the growing complexity of the values bearing on clinical practice is to write ever more detailed rules aimed at fixing in advance the 'right outcomes' for any given clinical situation. It is this response that is driving the growing volume of ethical codes and regulatory bodies concerned with medicine. Values-based practice offers quite a different albeit complementary response. It switches the focus from pre-set *right outcomes* to a reliance on *good process*. Values-based practice, that is to say, focuses not so much on *what* is done but on *how* it is done. Starting from the 'democratic' ethical premise of respect for differences of values, values-based practice relies on good process (in particular good clinical skills, see below) to support balanced decision-making within the framework of shared values defined by codes of ethical practice.[3]

Values-based and evidence-based medicine

As a process-based approach to clinical decision-making, values-based practice is complementary not only to regulatory ethics but also to evidence-based practice. The processes of values-based practice and of evidence-based practice are of course very different. Evidence-based practice, as John Geddes describes (Chapter 1.10), relies on statistical and other methods for combining evidence from methodologically sound research. Values-based practice, by contrast, relies primarily on learnable clinical skills. There are other components of the process of values-based practice, including a number of specific links between values-based and evidence-based practice.[3] But at the heart of values-based practice are four areas of clinical skill. As set out more fully in Table 1.5.2.2, these are, raised awareness of values and of differences of values, reasoning about values, knowledge of values, and communication skills.

The close interdependence of values-based and evidence-based approaches has been well recognized by many of those involved in the development of evidence-based medicine. Indeed, there is perhaps no clearer statement of this inter-dependence than the very definition of evidence-based medicine given by David Sackett and his colleagues in their book, *Evidence-Based Medicine: How to Practice and Teach EBM*.[1] Evidence-based medicine is standardly thought to be concerned only with research evidence, as outlined above. To the contrary, Sackett *et al.* say (p. 1), evidence-based medicine combines three distinct elements. The first element is, certainly, best research evidence. In clinical practice, however, best research evidence has to be combined with the experience and skills of practitioners, and, crucially, with patients' values. 'By patients' values', Sackett *et al.* continue, 'we mean the unique preferences, concerns and expectations each patient brings to a clinical encounter and which must be integrated into clinical decisions if they are to serve the patient'. Furthermore, they conclude, it is only 'when these three elements (best research 'evidence, clinicians' experience and patients' values) are integrated, (that) clinicians and patients form a diagnostic and therapeutic alliance which optimizes clinical outcomes and quality of life.'

Table 1.5.2.2 The four key skills areas underpinning values-based practice

Skills area	Applications in values-based practice
1. Raising Awareness of Values	Values, our own and those of others, are often implicit: thus a first step towards balanced decision-making is to raise awareness, 1) of values as such, 2) of differences of values, (See text)
2. Reasoning about Values	In ethics and law, various methods of reasoning are used to derive ethical conclusions. In values-based practice, the same range of methods is used but primarily to explore and open up the range of values bearing on a given situation. These include principles, casuistry (case-based reasoning), utilitarianism (balancing utilities, used especially in health economics), and deontology (rule-based reasoning, used especially in law). (See Further information)
3. Knowledge of Values	Values-based practice draws on evidence about values derived from, 1) the full range of empirical methods (including qualitative social science methods), 2) a range of philosophical methods, 3) combined methods (see text, also Further Reading).
4. Communication Skills	In values-based practice, communication skills are central to, 1) eliciting and understanding individual values, 2) resolving conflicts of values, for example by negotiation and conflict resolution (see text).

Values in the multidisciplinary team

In many parts of the world, psychiatric services are increasingly delivered through multidisciplinary and multi agency teams (Chapter 1.8.1). The move to multidisciplinary team-working reflects a broadly evidence-based recognition that different professional groups offer different but complementary resources of knowledge and skills. It was realized early on, however, that differences of perspective (which include different value perspectives) between different professional groups may lead to communication and other problems of effective team-working.[4,5] This is where values-based practice can help to support the leadership role of the clinical psychiatrist in the multidisciplinary team. To anticipate a little, values-based practice, as we will see in this section and the next, 1) helps to make differences of perspective between team members more transparent, thus improving communication and shared decision-making; and 2) converts these differences of perspective between team members from a barrier into a positive resource for decision-making that is sensitive to the particular and often very different values—the needs, wishes, preferences, etc.—of individual patients and their families.

First, then, what are the differences of perspective between different team members? The perhaps surprising extent of these differences is illustrated by Table 1.5.2.3. This is based on a study, led by the British social scientist, Anthony Colombo, of multidisciplinary teams in the UK concerned with the community care of people with long-term schizophrenia.(6) To understand the significance of Table 1.5.2.3, we need to look briefly at the background to Colombo's study and how it was carried out.

Colombo was interested in implicit models of disorder and how such models might influence the processes of decision-making in day-to-day clinical care within multidisciplinary teams. Asked directly, most team members, from whatever professional background, will indicate that they share much the same broadly biopsychosocial model of schizophrenia. This is their shared *explicit* model, then. The hypothesis guiding Colombo's study, however, was that, notwithstanding their explicit commitment to a shared biopsychosocial model, in actual practice different team members would be guided by different *implicit* models. These different implicit models reflected different weightings or priorities (hence values), in turn reflecting differences of professional background and training, that different team members might attach to the different aspects of a given case. Their different implicit models, furthermore, just in being implicit rather than explicit, could help explain the difficulties of communication and other problems of shared decision-making within multidisciplinary teams that had been identified in the literature (as above).

The aim of Colombo's study, therefore, was to access the *implicit* models (including values) guiding different professional groups in their responses to patients with schizophrenia. Colombo's method, correspondingly, was indirect rather than direct. He presented subjects with a standardized case vignette, of a man called 'Tom', with features of schizophrenia (though without using that term as such), and then explored their responses using a semi-structured interview and carefully validated scoring system. In previous work, Colombo had shown how different models of disorder (six of which are represented by the columns in Table 1.5.2.3) could be analysed

Table 1.5.2.3 Comparison of models grids for psychiatrists and social workers (shared elements of models shown highlighted)

	Models - Psychiatrists					
Elements	**Medical (Organic)**	**Social stress**	**Cognitive behaviour**	**Psychotherapeutic**	**Family (interaction)**	**Political**
1. Diagnosis/Description	P					
2. Interpretation of Behaviour	P					
3. Labels	P					
4. Aetiology	P					
5. Treatment	P					
6. Function of the Hospital	**P**	**P**				**P**
7. Hospitality & Community	P					
8. Prognosis	P					
9. Rights of the Patient	**P**					
10. Rights of Society	**P**					
11. Duties of the Patient	P		**P**			
12. Duties of Society	P					
	Models - Social Workers					
1. Diagnosis/Description				S		
2. Interpretation of Behaviour				S		
3. Labels				S		
4. Etiology				S		
5. Treatment		S			S	
6. Function of the hospital	**S**	**S**				**S**
7. Hospitality & Community		S		S		
8. Prognosis				S		
9. Rights of the Patient	**S**	S				S
10. Rights of Society	**S**					
11. Duties of the Patient			**S**			
12. Duties of Society		S				

and compared along 12 key dimensions (diagnosis, causal factors, etc.) as represented by the lines in Table 1.5.2.3. Responses to the semi-structured interview thus allowed a profile to be developed for each subject, and cumulatively for each professional group, of their implicit models. These profiles, or 'models grids', gave an overall picture of the implicit model on which an individual or group was drawing in their responses to Tom.

It is the 'models grids' for psychiatrists and psychiatric social workers respectively that are compared in Table 1.5.2.3. As this shows, notwithstanding their shared explicit commitment to a biopsychosocial model, psychiatrists and social workers, working in similar teams in the same area of the UK, had widely different *implicit* models. Direct comparison of the two models grids shows that psychiatrists and approved social workers coincided on only six out of a total possible of 72 elements! Small wonder, then, given that team members were unaware of these differences of implicit models, that difficulties of communication and of shared decision-making often arose. They all accepted an explicitly biopsychosocial approach. But their different professional perspectives, including value perspectives, led them to attach very different priorities to different aspects of 'Tom', and, by extension, to the real patients with whom they were concerned in the real world of day-to-day multidisciplinary care.

Values-based practice in the multidisciplinary team

Colombo's study illustrates how careful research may improve our knowledge of values (skills area 3, Table 1.5.2.2 above) and his research has subsequently been adapted and developed as part of a training manual for values-based practice.[7] Research is as important in values-based practice as in any other aspect of medicine. There is a widespread assumption that understanding each other's values is a matter of relatively transparent intuition. But in addition to empirical studies, surveys,[8] patient narratives,[9] and other sources all point to the extent to which our perceptions of each other's values are often *mis*perceptions. Colombo's study also illustrates the inter-dependence of the four skills areas. As a contribution to skills area 3 (knowledge), the study also contributes to raising awareness of values and of differences of values (skills area 1) in the specific context of multidisciplinary team working.

Merely raising awareness of differences of implicit models may itself be enough to improve communication between team members and hence, shared decision-making as the basis of effective multidisciplinary care. There are circumstances, however, in which raising awareness may not be sufficient. Where team values are directly conflicting, for example, raising awareness may even have the effect of accentuating rather than reducing difficulties of shared decision-making. So, how should differences of values be managed? Different responses are possible here. One approach is to try to create a homogenized composite model. At a relatively abstract level, this is what the biopsychosocial model offers. A different response is to seek to establish a 'top' model that takes priority over all other models. It is a natural enough assumption of any given professional group that their own particular model should be the 'top' model.

Rather than either a composite model or a 'top' model, values-based practice suggests that differences of value perspective, as incorporated into implicit models of disorder, far from being suppressed should be acknowledged and built on as a positive resource for effective multidisciplinary teamwork. This is essentially because, as the models grids in Table 1.5.2.4 show, differences in implicit models between different team members reflect corresponding differences among *patients themselves*.

The models grids in Table 1.5.2.4 were derived in Colombo's study using precisely the same methods as the models grids for the professional groups (i.e., using the same standardized case vignette, interview schedule, etc.). The patients involved in Colombo's study, however, were not recruited through multidisciplinary teams. Rather, they were recruited as volunteers from local MIND, a mental health NGO in the UK that 'advocates for patients' rights. To volunteer for the study, a patient had to have had a diagnosis of schizophrenia for at least three years. There was no requirement that they should agree with the diagnosis. Rather, the aim was to explore the implicit models of a group of subjects who had had this diagnosis 'willing or no' for an extended period. The expectation in the study was that this group of patients, recruited in this way, would include a significant number with a 'political', or 'anti-psychiatric', model of disorder, represented by the right-hand column of the models grids. In fact, as Table 1.5.2.4 shows, the patient group divided naturally into two sub-groups, one with implicit models very close to those of the psychiatrists in the study, the other with implicit models very close to those of the social workers.

The correlation in Colombo's study between different professional models and different patient models, gives a whole new values-based rationale for multidisciplinary teamwork. From an evidence-based perspective, multidisciplinary team working offers a diversity of knowledge and skills in meeting patients' needs. From a values-based perspective, multidisciplinary team working brings, in addition to different knowledge and skills, different value perspectives. In a well-functioning multidisciplinary team, these different value perspectives can help to ensure that professionals' knowledge and skills are matched appropriately to the different values—the needs, wishes, preferences, etc.—of individual patients and their families.

In helping to bring together the different perspectives of team members in a positive and well-balanced way, values-based practice thus, directly supports the leadership role of the consultant psychiatrist in the multidisciplinary team. Again, all four skills areas of values-based practice are closely interdependent here. In addition to knowledge of values, the reasoning skills noted in Table 1.5.2.2 may be helpful. Good communication skills are also crucial. As Table 1.5.2.2 indicates, these include in particular, skills for eliciting and understanding values, and where values conflict, skills of negotiation and conflict resolution.

Conclusions

This chapter has introduced a number of key points about values-based practice (summarized in Table 1.5.2.5) as a new skills-based approach to working more effectively with complex and conflicting values. The importance of values-based as well as evidence-based approaches has been illustrated particularly by reference to the leadership role of the consultant psychiatrist in the multidisciplinary team. Multidisciplinary team-working is of course not unique in its requirement for values-based as well as evidence-based approaches. As Sackett *et al.*[1] reminded us at the start of this chapter, it is only by combining best research evidence with practitioners' knowledge and skills and with patients' values, that we can

Table 1.5.2.4 Comparison of models grids for two groups of Patients—Group 1 similar to Medical Psychiatrists (Pt-Med), Group 2 similar to Social Workers (Pt-SW) (See also Table 1.5.2.3)

	Models - Group 1 (similar to psychiatrists)					
Elements	**Medical (Organic)**	**Social stress**	**Cognitive behaviour**	**Psycho-therapeutic**	**Family (interaction)**	**Political**
1. Diagnosis/Description	Pt-Med					
2. Interpretation of Behaviour			Pt-Med	Pt-Med		
3. Labels	Pt-Med					
4. Aetiology	Pt-Med					
5. Treatment	Pt-Med					
6. Function of the hospital	Pt-Med	Pt-Med				Pt-Med
7. Hospitality & Community		Pt-Med		Pt-Med		
8. Prognosis	Pt-Med					
9. Rights of the Patient	Pt-Med					Pt-Med
10. Rights of Society		Pt-Med				
11. Duties of the Patient		Pt-Med	Pt-Med			
12. Duties of Society	Pt-Med		Pt-Med			Pt-Med
	Models - Group 2 (similar to social workers)					
1. Diagnosis/Description				Pt-SW		
2. Interpretation of Behaviour				Pt-SW		
3. Labels			Pt-SW	Pt-SW		
4. Aetiology				Pt-SW		
5. Treatment		Pt-SW		Pt-SW		
6. Function of the hospital	Pt-SW					Pt-SW
7. Hospitality & Community		Pt-SW		Pt-SW		
8. Prognosis				Pt-SW		
9. Rights of the Patient	Pt-SW	Pt-SW				Pt-SW
10. Rights of Society		Pt-SW				
11. Duties of the Patient		Pt-SW	Pt-SW			
12. Duties of Society			Pt-SW			Pt-SW

build the 'diagnostic and therapeutic alliance' on which in any area of medicine, good clinical care crucially depends.

Two further points are worth adding in conclusion. The first is that values-based practice as introduced here, as being based primarily on learnable clinical skills, is only one among a number of new disciplinary resources supporting more effective ways of working with complex and conflicting values in healthcare. Further and quite different resources are provided by such empirical disciplines as decision theory,[(10)] for example, and health economics, an innovative use of which has recently been developed by a group at the Centre for Value-Based Medicine in the States.[(11)] Values-based practice itself is so underpinned by a branch of analytic philosophy, called philosophical value theory (see Further Reading, below) that, as an analytic discipline, it is a natural partner both of empirical research, as in Colombo's study,[(12)] and of other philosophical disciplines more familiar in psychiatry, notably phenomenology.[(13)] As Andreasen[(14)] has argued, these and other philosophical disciplines, have a growing practical importance not only in clinical psychiatry, as illustrated in this chapter, but also in the new neurosciences.

The second concluding point has to do with the place of psychiatry as a science-led medical discipline in the 21st century. As the most value-laden area of medicine, psychiatry was widely stigmatized in the 20th century as being, at best, scientifically underdeveloped,[(15)] at worst outwith medicine altogether;[(16)] and debates about eliminate values from psychiatric diagnostic concepts continue in the context of current revisions of the ICD and DSM classifications.[(17, 18)] Philosophical value theory, as the discipline underpinning values-based practice, shows to the contrary that the value-ladenness of psychiatry, far from reflecting any deficiency in its science, is a direct consequence of the fact that psychiatry, in being concerned with the higher functions of emotion, desire, volition, sexuality, and so forth, is by the same token concerned with areas of experience and behaviour where human value themselves are highly diverse ([(19)], especially chapters 4 and 5, building on[(20)]).

Table 1.5.2.5 Key points about values-based practice for clinical psychiatry

1. Values are wider than ethics and include all the many ways in which we express positive and negative evaluations, i.e., preferences, needs, wishes, etc. as well as ethical values
2. Values-Based Practice is a new skills-based approach to working with complex and conflicting values in medicine
3. Ethical principles provide a framework of shared values – such as 'best interests' and 'autonomy of patient choice' - that guide the *outcomes* of clinical decision-making supported by codes of practice and regulatory bodies
4. Values-based practice is complementary to regulatory ethics in focusing on the *process* of clinical decision-making: ethics focuses on 'right outcomes' (reflecting shared values); values-based practice focuses on 'good process' (reflecting complex/conflicting values)
5. In focusing on process rather than outcomes, values-based practice (concerned with complex and conflicting values) is fully complementary to evidence-based practice (concerned with complex and conflicting evidence) in clinical decision-making
6. At the heart of the 'good process' on which values-based practice depends are four key areas of clinical skills: 1) awareness of values and of diversity of values, 2) reasoning about values, 3) knowledge of values, and 4) communication skills (including skills in such areas as negotiation and conflict resolution)
7. Among other applications, values-based practice supports the role of the consultant psychiatrist in multidisciplinary teams by, 1) improving understanding of differences of values between different team members (thus improving communication and shared decision-making), and 2) improving understanding of the particular and often very different values of individual patients and carers (thus improving the extent to which care and treatment are appropriately matched to the particular needs, preferences and wishes of each individual patient and their families)
8. Values-based practice is research-based, drawing in particular on the resources of philosophical value theory and a number of other areas of the philosophy of psychiatry, such as phenomenology, in addition to empirical social science methods, patient narratives and other sources
9. In clinical work, values-based practice is supported by a wide range of training materials and is the basis of a number of both national and international developments in psychiatry aimed at building a strong diagnostic and therapeutic alliance between professionals and patients in mental health and social care
10. The skills-based approach of values-based practice is one of a number of disciplinary resources for working with complex and conflicting values in medicine: in addition to ethics, other important disciplines include health economics and decision theory

Psychiatry, therefore, in addition to being *scientifically* complex, is shown by philosophical value theory to be *evaluatively* complex. This is why it has been appropriate that values-based practice, as a skills-based approach to working with complex and conflicting values, should have developed first in psychiatry. But with the growing complexity of the values bearing on all areas of medicine, it seems likely that, as Sackett *et al.* anticipated (as above), values-based as well as evidence-based approaches will become increasingly crucial in the 21st century not only in psychiatry but across the board. The effect of this will be to reverse the 20th century stigmatization of psychiatry. Instead of being perceived as a scientific also-ran, psychiatry, by being first in the field with values-based practice as an essential partner to evidence-based practice, will be seen to have led the way with a 21st century model of medicine that is not only fully science-based but also genuinely patient-centred.

Acknowledgments

The information on which Tables 1.5.2.3 and 1.5.2.4 are based is derived from the study of models of disorder described in the text and first published in Colombo *et al.* 2003. [6]

Further information

1) Skills training for values-based practice

Woodbridge, K., and Fulford, K.W.M. (2004). *Whose Values? A workbook for values-based practice in mental health care.* London: Sainsbury Centre for Mental Health. (see website www.scmh.org.uk); also by mail from The Sainsbury Centre for Mental Health, 134–8, Borough High Street, London SE1 1LB

2) The theory of values-based practice

Fulford, K.W.M. (1989, reprinted 1995 and 1999). *Moral Theory and Medical Practice.* Cambridge: Cambridge University Press.

Fulford, K.W.M. (2004). Ten Principles of Values-Based Medicine. Ch 14 In *The Philosophy of Psychiatry: A Companion* (ed. J. Radden), pp. 205–34. New York: Oxford University Press. (Describes the links between values-based and evidence-based approaches in clinical decision-making).

3) Values-based practice and the new philosophy of psychiatry

Fulford, K.W.M., Thornton, T., and Graham, G. (2006). *The Oxford Textbook of Philosophy and Psychiatry.* Oxford: Oxford University Press. (see especially chapter 18, setting values-based practice in context with more familiar approaches to ethics; and chapter 21, showing how values-based alongside evidence-based approaches are important in diagnostic assessment as well as in treatment and care planning).

References

1. Sackett, D.L., Straus, S.E., Scott Richardson, W., *et al.* (2000). *Evidence-Based Medicine: How to Practice and Teach EBM* (2nd edn.). Edinburgh and London: Churchill Livingstone.
2. Okasha, A. (2000). Ethics of Psychiatric Practice: Consent, Compulsion and Confidentiality. *Curr Op in Psychiatry*, **13**, 693–8.
3. Fulford, K.W.M. (2004). Ten Principles of Values-Based Medicine. Ch 14 In *The Philosophy of Psychiatry: A Companion* (ed. J. Radden), pp. 205–34. New York: Oxford University Press.
4. Clunis Report: North East Thames and South East Thames Regional Health Authorities. (1994). *The Report of The Enquiry into the Care tnd Treatment of Christopher Clunis.* London: HMSO.
5. Department of Health. (1999). *Still Building Bridges: The Report of a National Inspection of Arrangements for the Integration of Care Programme Approach with Care Management.* London: Department of Health.
6. Colombo, A., Bendelow, G., Fulford, K.W.M., *et al.* (2003). Evaluating the influence of implicit models of mental disorder on processes of shared decision making within community-based multi-disciplinary teams. *Social Science and Medicine*, **56**, 1557–70.
7. Woodbridge, K., and Fulford, K.W.M. (2004). *Whose Values? A workbook for values-based practice in mental health care.* London: Sainsbury Centre for Mental Health.
8. Rogers, A., Pilgrim, D. and Lacey, R., (1993). *Experiencing Psychiatry: Users' Views of Services.* London: The Macmillan Press.

9. Fulford, K.W.M., Dickenson, D. and Murray, T.H. (eds.) (2002) *Healthcare Ethics and Human Values: An Introductory Text with Readings and Case Studies.* Malden, USA, and Oxford, UK: Blackwell Publishers.
10. Hunink, M., Glasziou, P., Siegel, J., *et al.* (2001). *Decision Making in Health and Medicine: Integrating Evidence and Values.* Cambridge: Cambridge University Press.
11. Brown, M. M., Brown, G.C. and Sharma, S. (2005). *Evidence-Based to Value-Based Medicine.* Chicago: American Medical Association Press.
12. Fulford, K.W.M. and Colombo, A. (2004). *Six Models of Mental Disorder: A Study Combining Linguistic-Analytic and Empirical Methods.* Philosophy, Psychiatry, & Psychology, **11/2**, 129–44.
13. Stanghellini, G. (2004). Deanimated bodies and disembodied spirits. In *Essays on the Psychopathology of Common Sense.* Oxford: Oxford University Press.
14. Andreasen, N.C. (2001). *Brave New Brain: Conquering Mental Illness in the Era of the Genome.* Oxford: Oxford University Press.
15. Kendell, R.E. (1975). The concept of disease and its implications for psychiatry. *British Journal of Psychiatry*, **127**, 305–15.
16. Szasz, T.S. (1961; revised 1974). *The Myth of Mental Illness.* Foundations of a Theory of Personal Conduct. New York, USA: Harper and Row.
17. Sadler, J.Z. (2004). *Values and Psychiatric Diagnosis.* Oxford: Oxford University Press.
18. Wakefield, J.C. (2000). Aristotle as Sociobiologist: The 'Function of a Human Being' Argument, Black Box Essentialism, and the Concept of Mental Disorder. *Philosophy, Psychiatry, & Psychology,* **7/1**, 17–44.
19. Fulford, K.W.M. (1989, reprinted 1995 and 1999). *Moral Theory and Medical Practice.* Cambridge: Cambridge University Press.
20. Hare, R.M. (1952). *The Language of Morals.* Oxford: Oxford University Press.
21. Fulford, K.W.M., Thornton, T., and Graham, G. (2006). *The Oxford Textbook of Philosophy and Psychiatry.* Oxford: Oxford University Press.

1.6

The psychiatrist as a manager

Juan J. López-Ibor Jr. and Costas Stefanis

Introduction: integrating two perspectives

The past years have witnessed the introduction and implementation of strict macro and micro economical principles in the planning and delivery of health care. The change is a consequence of the limitation of resources and the obligation to optimize their utilization in the delivery of health care to those in need. This has led to the birth of a new domain of management science dealing with hard choices and with the selection of priorities in the delivery of health care.[1] Even Western European countries, where a tradition of equity presides over health care and developing countries, with a tradition of care based on welfare system are adopting strategies built upon managed care principles. Of course, the private health care present in many forms in the different countries has been a driving force in this movement.

The new management perspective is based on the standards of management discipline but has to adapt to the main ethical concerns of delivery of care to suffering human beings. Because management has oftentimes been imposed as an 'external' mandate to the clinical community, clinicians, lacking understanding for the basics behind management, are reluctant to accept it; they often feel degraded by managers and develop negative attitudes towards them.

The objective of the present chapter is to provide clinicians with some input on how to manage the resources at hand and how to understand and communicate with managers in order to reach priorities closer to the needs of patients.

Health professionals and managers differ in many aspects. They belong to two different cultures which are summarized in Table 1.6.1.

However, many managerial skills are extremely useful to deal with psychiatric diseases, because they are chronic, they are accompanied by high degrees of disability, they require an interdisciplinary perspective, and they have important interactions with the social environment. Nowadays, most psychiatrists work as members of a multidisciplinary team, need to develop collaborative working relationships with other professionals, should have an understanding of the roles and the limits and extent of involvement of other agencies, and lastly, of the lines of accountability. Furthermore, the concerns about the competence of psychiatrists that is the framework for training programmes include some such as: the psychiatrist is a medical expert, a communicator, a collaborator, a manager, a health promoter, a professional and somebody able to tolerate ambiguity and uncertainty. In most of those, managerial skills are essential. Unfortunately, those skills are not taught in most medical schools.

There are three levels at which there is a parallel between a manager and a psychiatrist: a) the psychiatrist as a manager of the interventions needed to implement an individualized treatment plan for his patient, b) the psychiatrist as a manager of the involvement of other professionals in clinical settings, and c) the psychiatrist as a manager of health care resources available to his practice.

The psychiatrist as a manager of his patient's needs is a consequence of the introduction of processes of disease and patient management by most health care organizations. These play an increasing emphasis on prioritizing health care provision on the basis of limited resources and increased sensitivity to specialized patient needs. Therefore, the clinician has to keep a delicate balance between cost containment principles and quality in care provided. It is crucial for the psychiatrist to be able to identify and implement practices that assure quality of care without sacrificing this to any external pressures for containment of cost within his clinical practice. The *Madrid Declaration* of the World Psychiatric Association (WPA)[2] has one item on the rights of psychiatrists that in essence

Table 1.6.1 Two different cultures

	Health professionals	Managers
Values	Health and fighting diseases	Economy and administration
Main interest	1. Patients 2. The profession	1. Organization 2. Management
Principal loyalty	The profession	The institution
Main concern	Patients	Health policy
Persons are	Patients	Clients, stakeholders
Terminology	Medical	Business-like
Training in management	No	Yes
Clinical training	Yes	No
Worries about costs	No	Yes
Stability in working places	Long	Short

declares that the first right of the psychiatrist is to be able to practice the profession without external constraints of any kind.

The psychiatrist as a manager of other professionals in clinical settings is consequently working as an element of a multidisciplinary team. Everybody in a team should at least possess an understanding of the essence, the extent and the limitations of cooperation and accountability. Managing other professional also largely refers to managing other psychiatrists within the same clinical settings. Management goes beyond the simple 'coordination' of various roles and steps in the process of providing health care, in the professional education of colleagues, the training of young professionals and the sharing of experience.

The psychiatrist as a manager of health care services has to struggle to reach a satisfactory degree of equity and in order to do so, the clinician has to become familiar with issues such as human resource management, customer satisfaction and change, crisis and conflict management.

What is management?

The word management derives from the Italian *maneggiare* 'to handle' (i.e., a horse), from *mano* 'hand', from Latin *manus*. Management is 'the art of getting things done through people';[3] it is the act (sometimes the art) of conducting or supervizing something (initially a business) and the thoughtful use of means to accomplish an end. Management needs to direct and to control a group of people or entities for the purpose of coordinating and harmonizing that group towards accomplishing a goal and it often encompasses the deployment and handling of human, financial, technological, and other resources.

Management in health care is not new. Physicians have a long tradition of being supervisors or conductors of a team. The simplest form of management is the partnership, an essential model for the doctor–patient relationship.

Management can also refer to the person or people who perform the acts of management; in this sense management has to do with power by position, whereas leadership involves power by influence.

From a functional perspective, management consists of measuring a quantity on a regular basis and of adjusting some initial plan in order to reach an intended goal. This applies even in situations where planning does not take place.

Functions of management

Management has several functions, which are summarized as following:

Planning: deciding what needs to happen in the future and generating plans for action.

Organizing: making optimum use of the resources required to enable the successful carrying out of plans.

Leading and motivating: exhibiting skills in these areas for getting others to play an effective part in achieving plans.

Coordinating: making different people or equipments work together for a goal or effect.

Controlling (monitoring): checking progress against plans, which may need modification based on feedback.

Basic managerial concepts

Although in the following paragraphs we will, as often as possible, replace managerial jargon by one more pleasant to clinicians, there some basic concepts which need a definition.

Efficacy is the ability to produce a desired effect and it is measured by the closeness to an achievable goal.

In clinical settings, efficacy is the degree of the benefit for patients, induced by an intervention (treatment, procedure or service) in ideal research conditions (i.e., in a controlled trial). It indicates that the therapeutic effect is acceptable. 'Acceptable' refers to a consensus that it is at least as good as other available interventions to which it will have ideally been compared to in a clinical trial.

Effectiveness, on the contrary, refers to the impact in real world situations.

Efficiency is the achieved results or effects related to the effort invested in terms of money, time and other resources. It is the maximization of some desired output or effect for the least amount of input, means or effort. Usually, the larger the ratio, the greater the efficiency.

Efficiency is not a pure scientific concept as it carries a value judgement. Efficiency is achieved through design, the process by which intelligence is substituted for matter and energy in technological systems.

Productivity is a measure of efficiency; it is the amount of output created (in terms of goods produced or services rendered) per unit input used. For instance, labour productivity is measured as output per worker or output per labour-hour.

Equity is social justice, the way of providing services according to the needs of each individual in a defined population. It is not an equalitarian principle because each individual should not get the same, but what he or she would need in a specific situation.

The light bulb example: the efficacy is the amount of visible light measured in lumens; the efficiency is the ratio of lumens to the amount of energy consumed to produce them, measured in Watts. Equity will measure the reach of the lumens to the needs of, let's say, the passers by on a street.

Ethical aspects of management in clinical settings

Health care and economic management are two different cultures. Cultures are defined by their values and peculiarities, among them ethics. Specific values are part of the property of a culture and belong to the identity of every social group.

There are three stages in the development of medical ethics,[4] each one adding value to the previous one without replacing it totally. In each one of them particular managerial skills are helpful.

The **ethics of welfare** is the traditional medical ethics, first appeared in Hippocratic writings. According to it, the doctor's primary goal and duty are the well-being of the patient and as much as possible, harm avoidance. The doctor is perceived and behaves as a good father, to be fully trusted, convinced that the physician will act adequately to the benefit of the patient. To meet this obligation, the doctor has to increase to the maximum his own medical knowledge and to assume a series of obligations. The scientific advances increase the paternalism of the professional who has to learn how to manage information. The ***Madrid Declaration*** of the WPA expressed this notion in the following way: *Psychiatry is a medical discipline concerned with the provision of the best treatment for mental disorders. Psychiatrists serve patients by providing the best therapy available consistent with accepted scientific knowledge and ethical principles. It is the duty of psychiatrists to keep abreast scientific developments of the specialty.*

The USA influence, with its strong emphasis on autonomy and individualism, has lead to the **ethics of autonomy**. The ethics of autonomy considers the patient as an autonomous human being, adult and free and consequently, able to take his/her own decisions. The values and beliefs of the patient are the background for the moral responsibilities of the doctor. As a consequence, doctors have to truly inform patients about all possible diagnoses and treatments so that patients are able to decide. The basic element of this new way of establishing the doctor-patient relationship is the informed consent.(5) From this perspective, patient-doctor relationship is defined in new terms: *The patient should be accepted as a partner by right in therapeutic process. The therapist-patient relationship must be based on mutual trust and respect to allow the patient to make free and informed decisions. It is the duty of psychiatrists to provide the patient with relevant information so as to empower the patient to come to a rational decision according to his or her personal values and preferences* (WPA *Madrid Declaration*).

The **ethics of equity** is a consequence of the impact of economic factors in medicine. The need of equal access to health care resources for all patients, including those suffering from mental illnesses and the principle of equity in a period of intrinsic and extrinsic limitations to health care cost, is leading to a third stage of bioethics which has also been called the **ethics of management**. The main reasons for the increase or imbalance of the costs are partially due to the successful developments of modern medicine: health care by itself is increasingly expensive (implementation of new and expensive technologies, incorporation of new professions into medicine, financing research in biomedical sciences, and applying resources for the training of physicians and specialists); the better control of acute diseases which increases the proportion of chronic illness requiring care; the increased demand due to ageing of the population and in social security systems, the change in the population pyramid, decreases the population of those paying compared to those making the expenses.

Resources to be invested in health care are limited. The first one to ask for limits was President Carter in the USA, during his first public speech after assuming the presidency, when he claimed for a ceiling of the 7 per cent of the GNP to be devoted to health care. This was in 1977. But, why such a limit? Why could it not be possible for an enlightened society to decide to devote 10, 20 or even 50 per cent of its GNP to health care and less, for instance, to defence? President Carter expressed it very well: too much spending in this area would decrease investments in education and care of the environment, which would lead to a deterioration of health.(8) In Europe, the cost of brain disorders (to be precise brain diseases and mental disorders) is more than the double of the cost of all cancers and diabetes together.(7)

The fact that more is not better is evident when comparing health indexes, and among them the bottom line, which is life expectancy. This is much lower in the US which dedicate over twice the percentage of their GNP to health care, than countries such as Japan, France, Italy, or Spain.

Economic factors can limit the access to health care, either because individuals lack sufficient insurance coverage or because of waiting lists. In the last few years, limitations have been imposed by governments which through different approaches try to control the access of patients to interventions which are not considered economically worthy. Again the WPA has addressed these issues in several documents such as the *Hawaii Declaration* (rev.), the *WPA Statement and Viewpoints on the Rights and Legal Safeguards of the Mentally Ill*, the first official document on the rights of mentally ill, and the *Madrid Declaration* of the WPA. This last code of ethics states '*As members of society, psychiatrists must advocate for fair and equal treatment of the mentally ill, for social justice and equity for all. While doing so, psychiatrists should be aware of and concerned with the equitable allocation of health resources*'.

Therefore, the goal of cost control should not be considered in isolation from other goals, such as quality assurance and equity. Here a managerial approach is useful, when based on three pillars: Information (to know what we physicians do, how patients behave on long-term outcome of medical interventions and on the impact on quality of life), consensus (on the right approaches to decide interventions), and a new social contract on sustainable health care. This approach is not limited to health care, it has a great influence on the culture of modern enterprises and in post-modern perspectives.(9,10)

Nature of managerial activity

Workplace democracy has become more common and advocated. Management is based on classical military type of command-and-control but it should not throw itself to the other extreme here all management functions are distributed among all workers, each of whom takes on a portion of the work, and the institution is run by assemblies of staff and of patients as was common in some anti-psychiatry experiences. Management relies increasingly more on facilitating, promoting and supporting collaborative activity, which is essential in health care. Modern management embraces democratic principles, in that, in the long term, workers must give majority support to management; otherwise they leave to find other work, or go on strike.

In for-profit organizations, the primary function of management is the satisfaction of a range of stakeholders. This typically means making profit (for the shareholders), creating valued products at a reasonable cost (for customers), and providing rewarding employment opportunities (for employees). In non-profit management, other functions are added, such as keeping the faith of donors, attaining social and political goals such as increasing health and fighting diseases.

In most models of management, shareholders vote for the board of directors, and the board then appoints senior management. This model is rarely applied in health care (or in Academic life).

Management also has the task of innovating and improving the functioning of organizations.

Categories of management

There are many categories of management. The most important are: human resource management, production (operations) management, strategic management, marketing management, financial management, and information technology management.

Nevertheless, as more and more processes simultaneously involve several categories, it is better to think in terms of the various processes, tasks, and objects subject to management.

Management science and organizational psychology

Whether management is rightly claiming a scientific status is debatable. It is more appropriate to classify it as a branch of economic sciences often confounded with its practical arm, operations research. Management science is the discipline of using analytical methods, to help make better decisions. Among others methods are decision-making analysis, optimization, simulation, forecasting, game theory[(11)] (which had a strong impact in psychotherapy[(12)]), network (transportation) forecasting models, mathematical modelling, data mining, probability and statistics, morphological analysis, resources allocation, and project management.

Industrial and organizational psychology consists of the application of psychological theories, research methods, and intervention strategies to workplace issues in order to hire suitable employees for the job, to reduce absenteeism, to improve communication and to increase job satisfaction.

Information systems

An information system is the array of persons, data records and activities that process the data and information in a given organization, including manual processes or automated processes. Information systems are also social systems whose behaviour is heavily influenced by the goals, values and beliefs of individuals and groups, as well as the performance of the technology. An information system consists of three components: human, technology, and organization.[(13)]

The systems rely on data from the unit as well as data acquired outside it (such as literature research, scientific meetings, consensus documents and others) and data provided by others (i.e. the Health Care System, partners, suppliers, and customers).

A computer based information system is a technologically implemented medium for recording, storing, and disseminating linguistic expressions, as well as for drawing conclusions from such expressions.[(14)]

Managerial levels and styles

The management of a large organization usually has three self-evident levels: senior management, middle management, and low-level management.

There are several management styles that can be applied depending on the nature of the activity, the type of the task, the characteristics of the workforce, and the personality and skills of the leaders. As the style of leadership is dependent upon the prevailing circumstance, leaders should exercise a range of leadership styles and should deploy them as appropriate.[(15)]

An **autocratic** or authoritarian manager makes all the decisions and keeps the information and decision-making among the senior management. Objectives and tasks are set and the workforce is expected to do exactly as required. The communication involved with this method is mainly downward, from the leader to the subordinate. The main advantage of this style is that the direction of the business is stable and the decisions are similar and comparable. This in turn projects the image of a trustworthy and well managed business. However, this method can lead to a decrease in motivation of employees and subordinates who may become highly dependant on the leaders and close supervision may be unavoidable.

A **paternalistic** approach is also dictatorial; however, the decisions tend to be in the best interests of the employees rather than the business. This can help balance out the lack of worker motivation caused by an autocratic management style. Feedback is again generally downward; however, feedback to the management will occur in order for the employees to be kept happy. This style can be highly advantageous, and can engender loyalty from the employees, leading to a lower labour turnover, thanks to the emphasis on social needs. It shares the same disadvantages of the authoritarian style; employees becoming highly dependant on the leader, and if wrong decisions are made, then employees may become dissatisfied with the leader.

In a **democratic** style, the manager allows the employees to take part in decision-making; therefore everything is agreed by the majority. The communication is extensive in both directions (from subordinates to leaders and vice-versa). This style can be particularly useful when complex decisions that require a range of specialized skills need to be made. From the overall business point of view, job satisfaction and quality of work will improve. However, the decision-making process is severely slowed down, and the need of a consensus may avoid taking the 'best' decision for the business. It can go against a better choice of action.

In a **laissez-faire** leadership style, the leader's role is peripheral and the staffs manage their own areas of the business; the leader therefore evades the duties of management leading to an uncoordinated delegation. The communication in this style is horizontal, meaning that it is equal in both directions; however, very little communication occurs in comparison with other styles. The style brings out the best in highly professional and creative groups of employees; however, in many cases it is not deliberate and is simply a result of poor management. This leads to a lack of staff focus and sense of direction, which in turn leads to much dissatisfaction, and a poor company image.

Roles and responsibilities of heads of clinical units and leaders

The head of a clinical unit is a managing director. In business, the principal leader is the Managing Director, who is in charge of the definition, the development and implementation of the strategic plan of their unit or service in the most cost-effective and time-efficient manner.

The managing director is responsible for both the day-to-day running of the company and developing business plans for the long-term future of the organization. In business, the managing director is accountable to the board and the shareholders of the company. It is the board that grants the managing director the authority to run the company. In clinical settings, the head of a unit is accountable to and gets the power from the health authorities.

A head of a unit may or may not have direct clinical responsibilities and is usually burdened by much office-based work, but he or she is the leader of the organization, chairing different sorts of meetings, motivating the workforce and developing the culture and style of the organization.

As the title suggests, the managing director needs to manage everything. This includes the staff, the patients, the budget and the resources to make the best use of them and increase the company's profitability.

Strategic planning

Strategic planning is the process of defining the goal of an organization and of making decisions on allocating resources to pursue the goal. In order to determine where it is going, the organization needs to know exactly where it stands, then determine where it wants to go (over the next years, typically 3 to 5) and how it will get there.[16] The resulting document is called the 'strategic plan'.

Strategic planning deals with at least one of three key questions: 1 'What do we do?' 2. 'For whom do we do it?' and 3. 'How do we excel?'

There are many approaches to strategic planning. Typically it is done in a stepwise manner:

1 Vision (define the vision and set a mission statement with a hierarchy of goals);
2 SWOT analysis (strengths, weaknesses, opportunities and threats);
3 Formulation (of the actions and processes to be taken to attain these goals);
4 Implementation (of the agreed upon processes);
5 Controlling (to get full control of the operation); and
6 Monitoring (to get feedback from implemented processes).[17]

Situational analysis. When developing strategies it is important to analyze the organization and its environment in the present moment and how it may develop in the future. The analysis has to be executed both at internal as well as at external levels to identify all opportunities and threats of the new strategy. Analysis of the external environment normally focuses on the customer (the needs of patients).

Goals, objectives and targets: Vision, mission and values. These are essential components of strategic planning. They are specific, time-bound statements of intended future results, and general and continuing statements of intended future results.

A **Vision statement** outlines what a clinical unit wants to be in the future; it is a source of inspiration and provides clear decision-making criteria. It reflects the optimistic, perhaps utopic view of the organization's future.

A **Mission statement** describes what the unit or service is at present. It defines the customers (kinds of patients), critical processes and it informs about the desired level of performance.

A vision statement is different from a mission statement. The Vision describes a future identity and the Mission describes why it will be achieved.

A **Values statement** describes the main values protected by the organization during the progression, reflecting the organization's culture and priorities.

Management by objectives

Management by Objectives (MBO)[18] is a method of agreeing on objectives within an organization. The management and the head of clinical units reach a consensus on the objectives to attain in a certain time period (typically one year). The objectives have to comply with some criteria, usually described by the acronym SMART (Specific, Measurable, Achievable, Realistic, and Time-Specific). They usually represent an increased level of performance than the one attained during the previous period of time. The objectives of each clinical unit are part of the global objectives of the hospital or the higher level organization (i.e., the health care area) which are the result of the consensus between the organization and the health care authorities. Some objectives are collective, while others can be individualized. Ideally, the responsible of a clinical unit shares and divides the objectives among the responsible staff under his authority.[19]

The achievement (or non-achievement) of the objectives should lead to incentives (or penalties). In health care, significant pay incentives (bonuses) are not common, and this is an advantage because high bonuses trigger unethical behaviour such as distorting financial figures to achieve short term individual targets. This is the main criticism of management by objectives.

Quality management

Quality management is an exceptionally useful tool for the running of clinical services. It is based on scientific excellence which includes research on efficacy and efficiency. In can include systems to control costs but accompanied by methods to sustain and increase quality. The basic assumption is that cost control and quality of care can run in parallel. Of the several approaches, we have chosen for this chapter, the European Foundation for Quality Management (EFQM)[20] model, because it is increasingly been used by health care administration in many countries and not only by Europeans, and although developed for the management of very large companies it soon became evidence of their advantages for the public sector.

The EFQM model relies on the strive over Excellence, which is defined as the *outstanding practice in managing the organization and achieving results*. Truly Excellent organizations are those that strive to satisfy their stakeholders by what they achieve, how they achieve it, what they are likely to achieve, and the confidence they have that the results will be sustained in the future. Being excellent requires total leadership commitment and acceptance of the fundamental concepts, a set of principles on which the organization bases its behaviours, activities, and initiatives.

Excellence relies on a few fundamental concepts (Fig. 1.6.1):

1 Results Orientation: Excellence is achieving results that delight all the organization's stakeholders.
2 Customer Focus: Excellence is creating sustainable customer (patient) value.
3 Leadership and Constancy of Purpose: Excellence is visionary and inspirational leadership, coupled with constancy of purpose.
4 Management by Processes and Facts: Excellence is managing the organization through a set of interdependant and interrelated systems, processes and facts.
5 People Development and Involvement: Excellence is maximizing the contribution of employees through their development and involvement.
6 Continuous Learning, Innovation and Improvement: Excellence is challenging the status quo and effecting change by utilizing learning to create innovation and improvement opportunities.
7 Partnership Development: Excellence is developing and maintaining value-adding partnerships.

Results orientation
Public responsibility
Customer focus
Partnership development
Leadership and constancy of purpose
Continuous learning, improvement and innovation
Management by processes and facts
People development and involvement

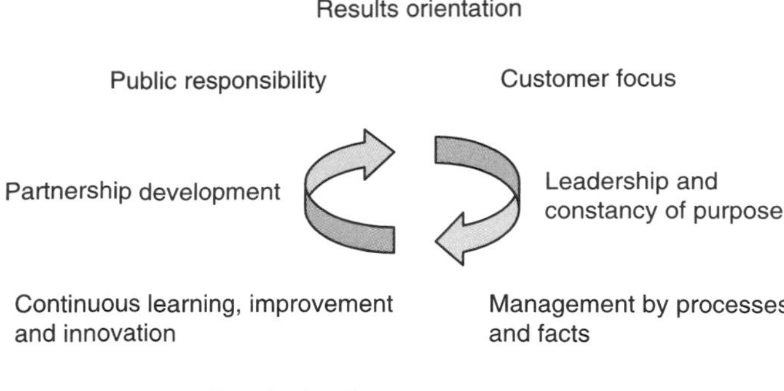

Fig. 1.6.1 Concepts of excellence.

8 Corporate Social Responsibility: Excellence is exceeding the minimum regulatory framework in which the organization operates and strives to understand and respond to the expectations of their stakeholders in society.

The EFQM Excellence Model is a practical tool that can be used in a number of different ways: as a tool for self-assessment; as a way to benchmark with other organizations; as a guide to identify areas for improvement; as the basis for a common vocabulary and a way of thinking; as a structure for the organization's management system.

The EFQM Excellence Model is a non-prescriptive framework based on nine criteria (Fig. 1.6.2). Five of these are 'Enablers' and four are 'Results'. The 'Enabler' criteria covers what an organization does. The 'Results' criteria covers what an organization achieves. 'Results' are caused by 'Enablers' and 'Enablers' are improved using feedback from 'Results'.

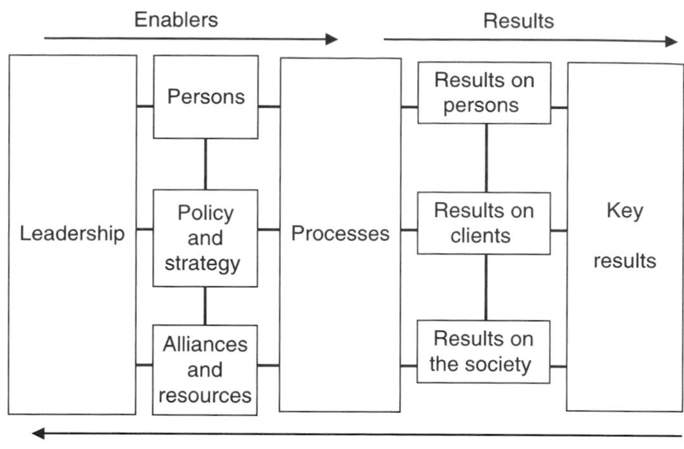

Fig. 1.6.2 European Foundation for Quality Management.

Risk management

Risk management is a discipline for living with the possibility that future events may cause adverse effects. The term is increasingly been used in the health sector.

Risk analysis includes risk assessment (identifying sources of potential harm, assessing the likelihood that harm will occur and the consequences if harm does occur), risk management (evaluation of the risks identified that require action and selection and implementation of the procedures to control those risks), and risk communication (interactive dialogue between all parties involved in the risk).

There are seven principles in the management of risk:

1 Global perspective (recognizing both the potential value of opportunities and the potential impact of adverse effects);

2 Forward-looking view (identifying uncertainties, anticipating potential outcomes);

3 Open communication (encouraging free-flowing information at and between all levels);

4 Integrated management (risk management is an integral part of management);

5 Continuity (maintaining constant vigilance);

6 Shared vision (common purpose, collective communication, and focusing on results); and

7 Teamwork (pooling talents, skills, and knowledge).

The experience of psychiatrists in disaster and traumatic events has made them highly valuable experts in risk management.

Types of health care and management systems

Health Systems throughout the world share the same, although sometime distant, goals: accessibility, equity, and extensive range of coverage. But there is also a wide array of organizational and financing types (taxation, employer-employee based private insurance, mixed), which have a strong impact on their efficiency, effectiveness, equity, and productivity. On the basis of financial policy, the following three main health care systems can be distinguished:

1 The social insurance system: It is also known as Bismarck model. It is based on obligatory insurance funded by both the employer and the employees. It guarantees collectivity, bilateral consent, and social solidarity. There is only marginal interference by the state, which however, is the main provider of health care facilities. Patients are free to choose their primary care physician, who is either a free professional or salaried to an insurance agency. In some countries, this system has evolved into the next one.

2 Government-state controlled through taxation system: Introduced by Beveridge in the U.K., it guarantees free of charge access of all citizens to health care services. Planning, programming, financing, and administration of services, as well as prevention and public health policy are centrally controlled. The system is financed through taxes as health care is considered a right of the citizens. Interestingly enough, it often co-exists with a non-negligible private insurance sector, which offers reduced waiting lists, better accommodation facilities, a more free election of the doctors and other privileges. In both cases, there are some limitations to access such as, having the primary care physician as the first contact and gate-keeper.

3 The private health system: The system is financed either through private insurance or by direct (out of the pocket) payment by the patient. Population insurance is not obligatory. Both, the patients and the physicians preserve the right of choice and payment is based on fee per service. The private system flourishes in the USA where about 2/3 of Health Services belong

to private or to managed care for profit or non-profit organizations. Governmental contribution to health care free of charge for patients is limited to the uninsured, very poor, and elderly as well as to patients in emergency through the Medicare and Medicaid Federal Government programs.

The more recent trend is towards adopting a mixed system of financing of health services, with an increasing collaboration of the private sector both in financing the services and in providing medical care.

Managed care

Managed care is the use of business managerial principles, strategies and techniques in health care. As it started in the USA during the presidency of Ronald Reagan, in a restricted sense is only applied to this country as a way to control Medicare and Health Maintenance Organizations' (HMO's) payouts. However, nowadays every system including those more controlled by governments use the same approach to control costs. Governmental run systems are just big nationwide HMO's and confront clinicians with the same restrictions to their work, patients with limitations of access, be it only waiting lists, conflicts of interests and confrontation of cultures. Essentially, it is a reform of health care from its longstanding not-for-profit business principles into a for-profit model that would be driven by the insurance industry or governmental bodies ruled by the same principles.

The reason for the beginning of managed care is the need to control cost and to reduce the so-called medical inflation which in the 1980s and 90s, was running at twice or thrice the general inflation rate. Nevertheless, managed care has not been so successful at this role, but has brought rationality in the use of public resources in health care, and often into attracting private resources to a successful for-profit business model.

There are several forms of managed care. Plans range from more restrictive to less restrictive, and include:

Health Maintenance Organization (HMO)

An HMO is an insurance plan under which an insurance company gears most aspects of the health care of the insured person. Each insured person is assigned a 'gatekeeper', usually a primary care physician who is responsible for the overall care of members assigned to him/her. Specialty services require a specific referral from the primary care physician to the specialist. Non-emergency hospital admissions also require specific pre-authorization by the PCP. Typically, services are not covered if performed by a provider not an employee of or specifically approved by the HMO, unless it is an emergency as defined by the HMO. The HMO concept was introduced in 1960 by Dr. Paul Elwood[(21)] and was adopted by the Nixon Administration.

Preferred Provider Organization (PPO)

PPO is a coinsurance system, which provides patients a co payment (generally around 80 per cent) of the costs of care, for an insurance fee. The deductible is the first part of the coverage and is paid by the patient. After the deductible is met, the coinsurance portion applies. Because the patient is picking up a substantial portion of the 'first dollars' of coverage, PPO is the least expensive type of coverage.

Point of Service (POS)

A POS plan utilizes some of the features of each of the above plans. Members of a POS plan do not make a choice about which system to use until the point at which the service is being used. For example, if the patient stays in a network of providers and seeks a referral to use a specialist, they may have a co payment only. However, if they use a network provider, but do not seek a referral, they will pay more.

Conclusions

It is clear that the modern role of both the physicians, in general, and psychiatrists, in particular, requires intensive decision-making which is helped by management principles.

Psychiatrists, in addition to their clinical qualifications and skills are asked to occupy positions and undertake responsibilities as clinical executives, directors of health care facilities, administrators of Academic units and even Mental Health Commissioners, all of them requiring managerial knowledge and leadership qualities.

Increased pressure by patients for improved quality of services and access to new and innovative treatments needs to be balanced against the expectation of the health care system of the physician to act 'economically', following cost containment guidelines and staying within expenditure ceilings.

Such decisions require specialized knowledge and a deep understanding of the principles and the functions of management and health economics. Such knowledge is only gained through specialized training by introducing management teaching, either at the undergraduate level or preferably at the residency level, as part of the core curriculum or as an elective which may include items such as administration principles, quality assurance, budgeting, resource allocation, accreditation procedures and what is close to the psychiatrist's clinical background the personnel management. This may be extended to ongoing professional education programmes for psychiatrists who are already active in the field.

Further information

Harvard Business Review http://harvardbusinessonline.hbsp.harvard.edu

World Psychiatric Association Section on Mental Health Economics Prof. Katarzyna Prot, Chair Institute of Psychiatry & Neurology. IV Dept. of Psychiatry Ceglowska 80. Warsaw, Poland 01-809 T: (40-21) 230-0653; F: (40-21) 230-7832 prot@bukareszt.ro; http://www.wpanet.org

References

1. Porter, M.E. and Teisberg, E.O. (2006). *Redefining Health Care: Creating Value-Based Competition on Results*. Harvard Business School Press, Boston.
2. World Psychiatric Association (1998). The Madrid Declaration. *Current Opinion in Psychiatry*, **11**, 1.
3. Follett, M. P. (1951). *Creative Experience*. Peter Smith, New York.
4. López-Ibor, J.J. and Crespo Hervás, M.D. (2000). A West Mediterranean Perspective. In *Ethics, Culture and Psychiatry. International Perspectives*. (eds. A. Okasha, J. Arboleda-Florez, and N. Sartorius). American Psychiatric Press, Inc. Washington, DC.
5. López-Ibor, J.J. and Crespo Hervás, M.D. (1996). Informed Consent in Spain. In *Informed Consent in Psychiatry. European Perspectives of Ethics, Law and Clinical Practice*. (eds. H.G. Koch, S. Reiter-Theil, and H. Helmchen), pp. 233–7. Medizin in Recht und Ethik, Band 33, Nomos, Baden-Baden.

6. López-Ibor, J.J. (1997). Psychiatric Care under the Present Economic Era. An International Perspective. *European Psychiatry*, **12** (suppl 2), 88–91.
7. Andlin-Sobocki, P., Jonsson, B., Wittchen, H.U., *et al.* (2005). Cost of disorders of the Brain in Europe. *European Journal of Neurology*, *Jun.* **12** (suppl 1), 1–27.
8. World Psychiatric Association (1990). *The WPA Bulletin* VI N.2–3.
9. Naisbitt, J. (1982). *Megatrends: Ten New Directions Transforming our Lives*. Macdonald.
10. Callahan, P. (1991). *What kind of Life*. Simon & Schuster, New York.
11. Morgenstern, O. and von Neumann, J. (1947). *The Theory of Games and Economic Behavior*. Princeton University Press
12. Berne, E. (1964). *Games People Play – The Basic Hand Book of Transactional Analysis*. New York: Ballantine Books.
13. Angell, I.O. and Smithson, S. (1991). *Information Systems Management: Opportunities and Risks*. Macmillan, London.
14. Langefors B. (1973). *Theoretical Analysis of Information Systems*. Philadelphia, Auerbach Publishers.
15. Tannenbaum, R.and Schmidt, W.H. (1985). How to Choose a Leadership Pattern. *Harvard Bussines Review*, March–April, 95–101.
16. Bradford, R.W., Duncan, P. and Tarcy, B. (2000). *Simplified Strategic Planning*. Chandler House Press, Worcester, MA.
17. Fahe, L. and Narayanan, V.K. (1986). *Macroenvironmental Analysis for Strategic Management*. West Publishing Company, New York.
18. Drucker, P. (1964). *Managemet for Results*. Harper & Row, New York.
19. Goldratt, E.M. and Cox, J. (2004). *The Goal: A Process of Ongoing Improvement*. North River Press, Great Barrington, MA.
20. http:// www.efqm.org
21. Ellwood, P.M. Jr., Anderson, N.N., Billings, J.E., *et al.* (1971). Health maintenance strategy. *Medical Care*, **9**(3), 291–8.

1.7

Descriptive phenomenology

Andrew Sims

Principles of descriptive phenomenology

Definitions and explanations

Psychopathology is the systematic study of abnormal experience, cognition, and behaviour. It includes the **explanatory psychopathologies**, where there are assumed causative factors according to theoretical constructs, and **descriptive psychopathology**, which precisely describes and categorizes abnormal experiences as recounted by the patient and observed in his behaviour.[1] Therefore the two components of descriptive psychopathology are the observation of behaviour and the empathic assessment of subjective experience. The latter is referred to by Jaspers as **phenomenology**,[2] and implies that the patient is able to introspect and describe what these internal experiences are, and the doctor responds by recognizing and understanding this description. Descriptive phenomenology, as described here, is synonymous with phenomenological psychopathology, and involves the observation and categorization of abnormal psychological events, the internal experiences of the patient, and consequent behaviour. The attempt is made to observe and understand this psychological event or **phenomenon** so that the observer can, as far as possible, know what the patient's experience must feel like.

Mental phenomena in health and cultural variation

It is not surprising that the identification and classification of the phenomena of mental illness is a difficult task as there is no consensus concerning what would be acceptable as normal healthy experiences. Mental illness has variously been considered as the products of a diseased brain, the symptoms that doctors treat, or a statistical variation from the norm carrying biological disadvantage, and mental illness often has legal implications. It is best to retain the use of the word 'normal' in a statistical sense; thus a phenomenon, such as hypnagogic hallucination, may be statistically abnormal but not an indicator of ill health or mental disease. Similarly, it is unwise to extrapolate from a population of mentally ill people and make assertions about the origins of behaviour in those who are not mentally ill.

It is important to recognize the effect of **culture** on subjective experience, the expression of psychological symptoms, and their manifestation in behaviour. In some cultures the very expression of subjective experience and emotion is discouraged and censored, in others feelings tend to be somatized, and in yet others the subjective experience of the individual tends to be subjugated to the sense of well being of the immediate social group. There are specific culture-bound expressions of subjective distress concerning body image in those who suffer from anxiety disorders. For delusions of passivity, although the psychopathological form remains relatively constant, the description of content will vary according to culture; for example, 'the djinn made me do it', 'my thoughts are controlled by the television'. Similarly, for possession state, although the psychopathological description remains similar, the actual cultural expression is very different between a member of a fundamentalist sect in the American Appalachian Mountains and a Buddhist girl in Sri Lanka.

Understanding the patient's symptoms

Although in internal medicine a clear distinction is made between **symptom** (the complaint which the patient makes) and **sign** (the indicator of specific disease observed or elicited on examination), in psychiatry both are contained within the speech of the patient. He complains about his unpleasant mood state, therefore identifying the *symptom*; he ascribes the cause of the pain in his knee to alien forces outside himself, thus revealing a *sign* of psychotic illness. Because both symptoms and signs emanate from the patient's conversation, in psychiatric practice the term symptom is often used to include both. For a symptom to be used diagnostically, its occurrence must be typical of that condition and it must occur relatively frequently.

Fundamental to psychiatric examination is the use of **empathic understanding** to explore and clarify the patient's subjective experiences. The method of empathy implies using the ability to 'feel oneself into' the situation of the other by proceeding through an organized series of questions, rephrasing, and reiterating where necessary until one is quite sure of what is being described by the patient. The final stage is recounting back to the patient what you, the psychiatrist, believe the patient's experience to be, and the patient recognizing that as indeed an accurate representation of their own internal state. Empathy uses the psychiatrist's capacity, as a fellow human being, to experience what the patient's subjective state must feel like as it arises from a combination of external environmental and internal personal circumstances.

Identifying phenomena as specific indicators of defined psychopathology may be difficult. It may require hearing much conversation from the patient for significant words and sentences to be revealed. The psychiatrist, when in the role of psychopathologist, has to assume that all speech of the patient, all behaviour of the patient, and every nuance has meaning, at least to the patient at the time the speech or behaviour takes place; it is not just an epiphenomenon of brain functioning.

Jaspers has contrasted **understanding** with **explaining**; descriptive phenomenology is concerned with the former. Understanding is the perception of personal meaning of the patient's subjective experience and involves the human capacity for empathy. That is, I understand because I am able to put myself into my patient's situation and know for myself how he is feeling, I feel those feelings of misery myself. Explanation is concerned with observation from outside and working out causal connections as in scientific method. In psychopathology, the terms *primary* and *secondary* are based upon this important distinction between meaningful and causal connections. That which is primary can be reduced no further by understanding, i.e. by empathy. What is secondary emerges from the primary in a way which can be understood by putting oneself into the patient's situation at the time; that is, if I were as profoundly depressed as my patient, I could have such a bleak feeling that I believed the world had come to an end—a nihilistic secondary delusion.

Subjective experience and its categorization

Within certain limits subjective experience is both predictive and quantifiable. When an individual loses a close relative it can be predicted that he or she will experience misery and loss. It is possible to quantify depressive symptoms and compare the degree of depression at different times in the same individual or differences between individuals at the same time. An important distinction for psychopathology is that between form and content. The **form** of psychological experience is the description of its structure in phenomenological terms (e.g. a delusion). Its **content** is the psychosocial environmental context within which the patient describes this abnormal form: 'Nurses are coming into the house and stealing my money'. The form is dependent upon the nature of the mental illness, and ultimately upon whatever are the aetiological factors of that condition. Content is dependent upon the life situation, culture, and society within which the patient exists. The distinction is important for diagnosis and treatment; determining the psychopathological form is necessary for accurate diagnosis, whereas demonstrating the patient's current significant concerns from the content of symptoms will be helpful in constructing a well-directed treatment regime.

Whereas most science is concerned with objectivity and with trying to eliminate the observer as far as possible from being a variable within the experiment, descriptive phenomenology tries to make evaluation of the subjective both quantifiable and scientific. It is a mistake to discredit subjectivity in our clinical practice. Inevitably we use it all the time and we should learn to use it skilfully and reliably. When I make an assessment that my patient is depressed, I am, at least to some extent, making a subjective judgement based upon the experienced and disciplined use of empathy: 'If I felt as my patient looks and describes himself to be, I would be feeling sad'. In psychopathology the distinction is also made between **development**, where a change of thinking or behaviour can be seen as emerging from previous patterns by understanding what the individual's subjective experience is, and **process**, where an event is imposed from outside and this cannot be understood in terms of a natural progression from the previous state. Anxiety symptoms could be seen as a development in a person with anankastic personality confronted with entirely new external circumstances; epilepsy and its psychiatric symptoms would be a process imposed upon the individual and not understandable in terms of previous life history.

Theoretical bases of descriptive phenomenology

There are important theoretical differences from dynamic psychopathology. Descriptive psychopathology does not propose explanations accounting for subjective experience or behaviour, but simply observes and describes them. Psychoanalytic psychopathology studies the roots of current behaviour and conscious experience through postulated unconscious conflicts and understands abnormalities in terms of previously described theoretical processes. The distinction between form and content and between process and development is not seen as important in psychoanalysis, but symptoms are considered to have an unconscious psychological basis. Descriptive phenomenology makes no comment upon the unconscious mind. It depends upon the subject being able to describe internal experiences, i.e. conscious material. Descriptive psychopathology is not dependent upon brain localization but on clarifying the nature of the subjective phenomena in discussion with the patient; if links can then be shown between certain phenomena and specific brain lesions, that is, of course, highly advantageous in furthering psychiatric knowledge. Descriptive phenomenology can be a unifying factor between concepts of brain and mind; it does not depend on philosophical stance on the nature of mind or brain.

Disorders of perception

Perception is not restricted to the screening of physical signals by sense organs but implies the processing of these data to represent reality. Ideas from the philosophy of mind have influenced psychiatric concepts of perception and the constitution of reality. Recently the distinction between sensory screening and interpretation has been confirmed by neurocognitive research.

Hundert[(3)] used the philosophical idea contained in the Kantian distinction between *a priori* categories and *a posteriori* experiences as a framework for differentiating perception by the sense organs from the secondary evaluation process. Kant's emphasis on the interplay between 'distal' perception and 'proximal' conceptualization can be exemplified by the perception and recognition of faces, disturbed in the Capgras syndrome and to a lesser degree in schizophrenia. The processing of visual perception is organized on at least four levels of complexity: the retina, the lateral geniculate body, the occipital visual cortex, and the hippocampus. The occipital cortex, where we actually 'see', does not contain an image any more than do the preceding levels; rather, it holds a database composed of signals from specific neurones for edges, angles, curves, sudden movements, and so on. Compared with the perceptual screen of the retina, these signals are 'scrambled' but even so they form a notion of what we perceive as reality. Recognition of faces needs further processing, probably in the hippocampal area where associations from other cortical fields are integrated with the visual information (e.g. the voice belonging to the face). In psychiatry we deal with heterogeneous aetiologies, and perceptual disturbances may originate from different levels of processing, usually from a more integrated level than in neurological disease, and further from the immediate screening of physical stimuli by the sense organs. Thus, psychiatric disorders of perception affect different stages of information processing—from disturbances in the sense organs to complex phenomena involving feelings and ideas.

Here we shall mainly focus on hallucinations and some related phenomena, which are relevant for psychiatric illnesses.

Definitions of perceptual disturbances

Cutting[4] defines **hallucination** as 'perception without an object or as the appearance of an individual thing in the world without any corresponding material event'. The problem with this definition is that although some hallucinating patients mistake a hallucinatory perception for a real one, others can differentiate them: as demonstrated experimentally by Zucker,[5] there is an 'as if' quality even when patients assert that they perceive real objects or events. Voices described in detail by hallucinating patients were imitated and presented to the patients without warning. They had no difficulty in discriminating these external voices from their hallucinations. For this reason Janzarik[6] defined hallucinations, without associating them with perception at all, as 'free running psychic contents' (using a concept similar to Jackson's disinhibition). In keeping with this idea, lack of perception may facilitate hallucinations as in sensory deprivation or in the oneiroid states of paraplegic patients.[7]

The perceptual quality of hallucinations differs from similarity to sensory experiences, as in delirium, to the bizarre apprehensions of some with schizophrenia. Also, the extent to which the person is affected varies from descriptions of hallucinations as film-like in amphetamine psychoses to the affectively overwhelming experiences of hallucinations associated with delusional mood.

The term **pseudohallucination**, sometimes, is used to describe a perception recognized as *unreal*. Jaspers[8] defined hallucination as corporeal and tangible; pseudohallucination lacks this quality. According to Jaspers, pseudohallucinations are not tangible and real as hallucinatory perceptions; they appear spontaneously; they are discernible from real perception; and, they are difficult, but not impossible, to overcome voluntarily. Kandinsky illustrated Jaspers' definition of pseudohallucination: spontaneously arising images of acquaintances arose when a patient kept his eyes closed. He was fully aware of the unrealistic character of this experience and could abandon it by opening his eyes. Thus, to Jaspers, pseudohallucinations are close to imagined images except that they arise spontaneously and are more vivid. Jaspers' definition is not used consistently; in some Anglo–American literature it has been sufficient for the definition of pseudohallucination that there be subjective awareness that the percept lacks a real external equivalent and arises from the subject.

Imagery describes vivid visual experiences, which can be produced and manipulated voluntarily. It occurs in trance states when the perceptions are produced voluntarily, but are more real and last longer than in a normal state.

Illusions differ from hallucinations in being based on a misinterpretation of a real object or event, often associated with a mood. Illusions have to be distinguished from delusional perceptions which are percepts based on real objects to which an incorrect meaning has been attached. In delusional perceptions this 'error' cannot be corrected by the patient; in illusions the patient can recognize the true meaning.

Kurt Schneider described *Gedankenlautwerden* (*écho de la pensée*, or thoughts heard aloud) as a transitional phenomenon between vivid imagination and auditory hallucination. The patient recognizes that the words he hears are his own thoughts, but he cannot voluntarily control them. *Gedankenlautwerden* can disturb concentration when talking to other people. It can be differentiated from thought insertion and from auditory hallucinations in that there is a lesser degree of alienation.

Klosterkötter[9] has described transitions from elementary unformed hallucinatory sensations, like a crack, bump, or hiss, through more meaningful perceptions which still can be localized 'inside' the head, to complex hallucinations which become part of a delusional cognitive structure. These transitions were related to increasingly affective involvement in the themes of the hallucination. Klosterkötter's observations support Janzarik's interpretation of hallucinations as 'free running psychic contents', as do experimental studies of model psychoses which show a regular sequence of three psychopathological states: vegetative arousal, affective change, and 'productive' phenomena-like hallucinations and delusions.

Some misperceptions, found mainly in schizophrenic patients, are less complex than hallucinations, appear to be more closely related to neuropsychological disturbances, and include less systematization. They include **optical distortions** of size, colour, distance, and perspective, which can resemble experiences reported by people taking cannabis or other psychoactive drugs. These fluctuating, circumscribed misperceptions exemplify the way in which a more complex phenomenon of psychopathology can be built upon something more basic. Krause *et al.*[10] videotaped the non-verbal behaviour of schizophrenic patients and their healthy partners in a conversation. Brief non-verbal cues play an important part in dialogue. Schizophrenic patients miss these non-verbal brief cues and are poor at judging the intentions of others; their own non-verbal communication is poorly co-ordinated. The ensuing dysfunction diminishes social competence. Schizophrenic painters, trained before the onset of their illness, have been shown to misperceive perspective.[11]

Sensory modalities

Hallucinations can affect every sense modality. The most common, in the idiopathic psychoses, are **auditory hallucinations**, usually in the form of voices, although other kinds of sound may be associated with delusional contents. Voices talking to each other about the patient, and voices commenting about the patient's ongoing acting or thinking, are considered to be typical of, but not specific to, schizophrenia.[12] Voices calling the patient's name or talking without comments to the patient are diagnostically non-specific.

Visual hallucinations are most frequently found in organic psychosis, particularly delirium, in which they may occur for only a couple of hours during the night if the syndrome is not full blown. Visual hallucinations, more often than those in other sensory modalities, depict animals and scenes with several persons. In alcoholic delirium in particular, optical hallucinations of fine structures (such as hairs, threads, or spider webs) occur, and are especially likely to appear if the patient stares at a white wall. A typical, although not specific, combination of hallucination and delusion in organic psychosis is the 'siege experience', in which patients believe they are besieged by enemies and have to bar their doors and windows.

Bodily, tactile, or coenaesthetic hallucinations are associated more often with schizophrenia than with affective or organic psychoses. The phenomenology includes simple tactile sensations of the skin, sexual sensations, sensations of the contraction, expansion, or rotation of inner organs, or atypical pain. Usually these sensations are associated with delusional explanations. Tactile hallucinations localized in the skin can underlie the **delusion of parasitosis**. Elderly patients in the early stages of organic cerebral alterations are at highest risk.

Coenaesthesia is a bodily misperception, which may last for minutes to days. It fluctuates (sometimes in relation to stress), and is usually not attributed to external agents or explained by delusional ideas. Patients seldom report them spontaneously. Klosterkötter[9] suggests that when coenaesthesia is attributed strongly to external influences, it is likely to be followed by schizophrenia.

Hallucinations may be **gustatory** or **olfactory**, for example, a smell of gas (perhaps thought to emanate from neighbours trying to kill the patient). Blunting of gustatory sensations or misperception of food as oversalted or overspiced is occasionally reported by melancholic patients.

Aetiological theories of hallucination

Aetiological theories are of three kinds:

1. overstimulation affecting different levels of information processing;
2. failure of inhibition of mental functions;
3. distortion of the processing of sensory information at the interpretive level.

The work of Penfield and Perot[13] has suggested that **overstimulation** may be a pathogenic mechanism. They stimulated the temporal regions of 500 patients, of whom 8 per cent reported scenic hallucinations, some in several modalities. Stimulation of the visual occipital cortex led to simple hallucinations-like flashes, circles, stars, or lines. This phenomenon has been observed in drug-induced experimental psychosis. It is interesting that schizophrenic patients can usually distinguish drug-induced hallucinations from those arising from their disorder. Using neural network theories, Emrich[14] simulated hallucinations by using Hopfield networks; overloading the storage capacity of the network generated what appeared to be the equivalent of hallucinations.

Disinhibition theory originated with Hughlings Jackson, who considered that productive symptoms were caused by the disinhibition of controlling neural activities, while negative symptoms resulted from damage to the systems, which generate the productive symptoms. More recently, sensory deprivation research has yielded inconsistent results; hallucinations, narrowly defined, seldom occur after deprivation, which may be of greater relevance to vivid, usually visual, imaginative experiences. Disinhibition may also underlie the 'hypnagogic hallucinations' which can occur in healthy subjects shortly before they fall asleep.

The role in the production of hallucinations of post-sensory interpretation and evaluation of stimuli is uncertain. In these terms, hallucinations are a sort of deception, but this is not a sufficient description of their nature. Recent neurophysiological hypotheses and findings from neuroimaging studies have suggested that there is an 'inner censorship' involved in clarifying ambiguities of perception.[14]

Disorders of thinking

Types of thinking

Three types of thinking can be distinguished which represent a continuum, without sharp boundaries, and intertwined in everyday life, from low to high regard for external reality and goal-directness: fantasy thinking, imaginative thinking, and rational thinking.[15] Since each of these types can predominate under some conditions, this distinction is useful to understand certain abnormal phenomena.

Fantasy thinking (also called dereistic or autistic thinking) produces ideas, which have no external reality. This process can be completely non-goal-directed, even if the subject is to some extent aware of the mood, affect, or drive, which motivates it. In other cases fantasy serves to exclude reality, which may require material with which the subject does not want to engage. This type of fantasy thinking is directed. Its goal is not to solve a problem but to avoid it via neglect, denial, or distortion of reality. Normal subjects use fantasy thinking deliberately and sporadically. However, if its content becomes subjectively accepted as fact, it becomes abnormal. This pathological exclusion of reality can remain limited in extent (e.g. in hysterical conversion and dissociation, pseudologia phantastica, and some delusions) or it may be manifested as withdrawal from the real world.

Rational (conceptual) thinking attempts to resolve a problem through the use of logic, excluding fantasy. The accuracy of this endeavour depends on the person's intelligence, which can be affected by various disturbances of the different components involved in understanding and reasoning.

Imaginative thinking comes between fantasy thinking and rational thinking. It is a process of forming a representation of an object or a situation using fantasy but without going beyond the rational and possible. This thinking is goal-directed but frequently leads to more general plans than the solution of immediate problems. Imaginative thinking becomes pathological if the person attaches more weight to his representation of events than to other objectively equally possible interpretations. In overvalued ideas, the imagined interpretation surpasses other interpretations in strength; in delusions, all other possibilities are excluded.

Delusions

The term 'delusion' signifies a complex edifice of thinking in which 'delusional ideas' are linked with other ('normal') thoughts. Delusions are communicated to others in the form of judgement. In this context, the term 'delusional idea' customarily refers to pathologically false judgement for which three criteria have been proposed: the unrivalled conviction with which they are held, their lack of amenability to experiences or compelling counter-arguments, and the impossibility of their content.[16] The last criterion must be discarded for two reasons. Firstly, collective beliefs derived from the socio-cultural setting of a person can be considered, in other surroundings, as false or impossible. Taking this into account, delusion is often defined as a 'false unshakable belief, which is out of keeping with the patient's social and cultural background'.[15] Secondly, in certain delusions (e.g. delusional jealousy) the content does not go beyond the possible. Thus delusions are best defined as overriding, rigid, convictions which create a self-evident, private, and isolating reality requiring no proof.[17]

(a) The genesis of delusions

Jaspers[18] introduced a distinction between primary and secondary delusions. He supposed that the first, called true *delusional ideas*, are characterized by their 'psychological irreducibility', whereas the second, called *delusion-like ideas*, emerge understandably from disturbing life experiences or from other morbid phenomena, such as pathological mood state or misperception. This led to the assumption that primary delusions are the direct expression of the underlying condition considered to be the basis of schizophrenia. Four types of primary delusion have been distinguished in this perspective.

1 **Delusional intuition** (autochthonous delusion), occurring spontaneously, 'out of the blue'.

2 **Delusional percept**, in which a normal perception acquires a delusional significance. Schneider[19] assumed that 'psychological irreducibility' was clearly evident in this process, and included *delusional percept* among his 'first-rank symptoms' of schizophrenia.

3 **Delusional memory** can be distorted or false memory coming spontaneously into the mind, like delusional intuition. In other cases they occur, like delusional percept, in two stages, which means that normal memories are interpreted with delusional meaning.

4 **Delusional atmosphere** refers to an ensemble of minuscule and almost unnoticed experiences, which impart a new and bewildering aspect to a situation. The world seems to have been subtly altered; something uncanny seems to be going on in which the subject feels personally involved, but without knowing how. From this uncertainty evolves first certainty of self-reference, and then the formation of fully structured and specific delusional meaning. The apparent change in the surrounding situation is accompanied by tension, depression, or suspicion, and by anxious or even exciting expectations, so that it is often called 'delusional mood'.

The primary–secondary distinction assumes that the delusional atmosphere is part of the process underlying all primary delusional phenomena. If this preliminary disturbance is not perceived clearly or is not communicated by the patient as a general change in the situation, delusion may be manifested only as delusional percept, intuition, or memory. When the initial change in atmosphere is experienced clearly, a subsequent alteration in the environment, or a fully formed delusional idea, can lead to release from the preceding perplexity. The origin of primary delusions is commonly attributed to a basic cognitive anomaly disturbing information-processing, which reduces the influence of past experience on current perception. This is considered to entail a heightened awareness of irrelevant stimuli and an ambiguous unstructured sensory input allowing the intrusion of unexpected and unintended material from long-term memory.[20]

(b) The content of delusions

The content of delusions is determined by the mood in which they emerge and evolve, by the patient's personality and socio-cultural background, and by previous life experiences. In principle, the content can embrace all kinds of presumptions in separate categories. The following six delusional themes are usually distinguished:

- **delusion of persecution** based on the assumption that the patient is pursued, spied upon, or harassed
- **delusional jealousy**
- **delusion of love** characterized by the patient's conviction that another person is in love with him or her
- **delusion of guilt**, unworthiness, and poverty which may sometimes reach the degree of 'nihilistic delusion', in which the patient believes the real world has disappeared completely
- **grandiose delusion** in which patients are convinced that they have great talents, are prominent in society, or possess supernatural powers
- **hypochondriacal delusion** founded on the conviction of having a serious disease.

The mood state when delusional ideas emerge favours certain themes. Delusion of guilt, or unworthiness, and hypochondriacal delusion are strongly linked with depression. Grandiose and erotic delusion generally occurs in excited or manic states. Delusions of persecution and jealousy emerge most frequently from suspicious mood states or a delusional atmosphere, but may occur in depressed subjects.

Some further specific contents of delusions are:

- **religious delusion**, which may occur with grandiose delusion or delusion of guilt
- **delusion of infestation**, a subtype of hypochondriacal delusion, and characterized by the conviction of infestation by small organisms
- **delusional misidentification** in which the patient believes, on the basis of a delusional percept, that a perceived person has been replaced by an imposter, or in which he is convinced that another person has been physically transformed into his own self
- **delusion of control** in which the patient experiences sensations, feelings, drives, volition, or thoughts as *made* or influenced by others (this schizophrenic delusion is believed to result from cognitive dysfunction consisting of a failure of the system which monitors willed intentions).[21]

(c) The structure of delusions

1 The alternatives, 'logical' or 'paralogical', indicate whether or not the connection of ideas is consistent with logical thinking.

2 The notions, 'organized' or 'unorganized', indicate whether or not the delusional idea is integrated into a formed concept. Highly organized, logical delusions are described as *systematized*.

3 The relationship between delusion and reality varies:
   - in **polarized delusion**, delusional reality is inextricably intermingled with actual fact
   - if the delusional belief and reality exist side by side without influencing each other, we speak of **juxtaposition**
   - in **autistic delusion** the patient takes no account of reality and lives in a delusional world.

Overvalued idea

An overvalued idea is an acceptable, comprehensible idea pursued beyond the bounds of reason.[22] Overvalued idea causes disturbed functioning or suffering to the person himself or others.

Overvalued ideas of prejudice (overvalued paranoid ideas) are characterized by an underlying self-referent interpretation of the behaviour or sayings of others; patients assume themselves to be overlooked, slighted, unfairly treated, provoked, or loved. Overvalued apprehension may become apparent as morbid jealousy, hypochondriacal phobia (e.g. parasitophobia), or dysmorphophobia, in which patients assume that they attract attention because of a real or presumed bodily defect. In anorexia nervosa subjects are preoccupied by the endeavour to remain thin, and in transsexualism by the desire to change gender because they feel that they belong to the opposite sex.

Overvalued ideas generally occur with abnormal personality under stressful situations. Those with paranoid personality traits may develop, on the basis of a presumed injustice, querulous, or litiginous overvalued idea. Sometimes ideas become overvalued only during abnormal mood states (of various origins) which set aside counterbalancing influences.

Thinking in mood disorders

The content of thought in mood disorders is coloured by affect. Negative thinking about self, the future, and the world prevails.[23] Mishaps and failures are attributed to personal faults; success is attributed to the action of other people. This depressive thinking spreads from the starting point of negative life events to more general events, and it tends to become long lasting. The fixed viewpoint that emerges is called 'cognitive schema'. After recovery from an acute episode this schema may become latent, but it can be reactivated by distressing life events. It can also prolong symptoms. Negative thinking started by minor misfortunes can become autonomous, driving down mood—which in turn intensifies negative thinking. The negative schema can prolong a depressive episode or precipitate a new one. It is probable that such schemas are activated by both cognitions and emotions. Guilty thoughts are closely connected with this type of thinking, and may reach the intensity of a delusion. To a degree, guilty thinking in depression is dependent on culture. In mania, the content of thought is related to the mood of elation, with diminished self-criticism and excessive self-importance. In phobic and other anxiety states, thinking centres on situations leading to anxiety. Typical contents of delusional thinking in depression concern guilt, religious failure, condemnation, personal insufficiency, impoverishment, hypochondriasis, and nihilistic ideas. In mania, delusional ideas may be feelings of spiritual or economic power. In contrast with schizophrenic delusions, affective delusions grow out of the underlying, excessive mood and do not appear as something new and alien to the personality.

Phobic and anankastic phenomena

Phobic and anankastic (obsessional) phenomena have in common that the patient experiences them as unwanted, but cannot suppress them. They often occur together.

(a) Phobia

Phobias are inappropriate, exaggerated fears which are not under voluntary control, cannot be reasoned away, and entail avoidance behaviour.[24] The fears are kindled by particular stimuli. These may either be perceived objects, such as animals (animal phobia) or pustules (in some illness phobias), or situations such as open places (agoraphobia) or confined rooms (claustrophobia).

Phobias initially triggered by a very specific stimulus can eventually generalize. Thus, an elevator phobia may become extended to all kinds of closed rooms. Some phobias are linked with broader circumstances from the beginning. In social phobia, for instance, patients avoid meeting people because they fear that they will be noticed. Identical types of fears can be triggered by different stimuli in different subjects. Thus, illness phobia is activated in some patients by observed body changes, but in others by situations involving the risk of infection.

Phobias are characterized by avoidance behaviour: patients avoid anxiety-provoking objects or situations. Because of stimulus generalization, this can lead to severe impairment; for instance, they cannot leave home.

(b) Anankastic symptoms

Anankastic phenomena occur as obsessions or compulsions:

1 Obsessions occur as repeated thoughts, memories, images, ruminations, or impulses that patients know to be their own but are unable to prevent. The content of these ideas is often unpleasant, terrifying, obscure, or aggressive.

2 Compulsions are actions, rituals, or behaviours that the patient recognizes as part of his own behaviour, but cannot resist.

(c) Combined syndromes

In phobic–anankastic syndromes patients attempt to reduce their phobic fears by certain actions, such as hand washing in the case of an infection phobia. If obsessional thoughts or impulses induce anxiety (e.g. obscene ideas during worship, or the impulse to lean too far over a balustrade) and entail the avoidance of the situations that provoke them, the term anankastic–phobic syndrome is used.

Phobias, obsessions, and compulsions result most frequently from neurotic conflicts, but they also occur with functional or organic mental disorders. Anankastic personalities, characterized by perfectionism, rigidity, sensitivity, and indecisiveness, are especially prone to develop obsessions and compulsions.

Disorder of the thinking process

Disturbance of thinking may be recognized by the patient himself or deduced by an observer from the subject's speech.

Impairments of thought production are conventionally named 'formal thought disorder' and contrast with abnormalities of the 'content of thought' observed in delusions. In the deviant reality-testing of deluded patients there is always a disturbance of the form of thinking.

(a) Disorders of the flow of thinking

Each remembered idea is linked with a number of other notions, related closely as well as distantly. In rational thinking, a 'determining tendency'[25] guides the flow of ideas in the chosen direction and excludes associations which do not conform with this goal. This procedure can be disturbed in various ways which are commonly grouped together under the heading of 'formal thought disorder'.

(i) *Disturbances of the speed of thinking*

In **acceleration** of thinking, associations are still formed normally but at grossly accelerated speed. The goal is not maintained for long and the intervention of new thoughts produces 'flight of ideas'.

Retardation refers to a slowing down of the thinking process, which hampers formation of associations and may prevent reaching the original goal of thoughts. This results in difficulties in concentration and decision-making.

Acceleration and retardation of thinking are due to a change of affect, and are characteristic of mood disorders.

(ii) *Circumstantiality*

In circumstantiality the determining tendency is maintained but the patient can reach the goal only after having exhaustively explored unnecessary associations arising in his mind. When answering a question, he relates many irrelevant details before returning to the point. This inability to exclude unimportant associations occurs in organic mental disorders and in mental retardation.

(iii) *Perseveration*

Perseveration is found in organic mental disorders and is defined as an inability to shift from one theme to another; a thought is retained long after it has become inappropriate in the given context. For example, a patient may give a correct answer to the first question, but repeats the same response to a subsequent, completely different inquiry.

(iv) *Interruptions in the flow of thinking*

Thought blocking is a sudden unintended cessation in the train of thought, experienced by the patient as 'snapping off'. After this break, which may occur in the middle of a sentence, the previous thought may be taken up again or replaced by another. Thought blocking occurs in organic states, in depression, and frequently in schizophrenia where it is described as part of negative thought disorder.

In **loosening of association** the flow of thinking is interrupted by deviation towards distant or unrelated thought, in contrast with flight of ideas in which there is only a speeding up of access to nearby associations. Loosening of association is a type of formal thought disorder. In **tangentiality** the ideas deviate towards an obliquely related theme. In **fusion**, different kinds of association evoked by an original thought are blended to produce a word or sentence. **Derailment** is characterized by the interpolation of ideas which neither the patient nor the observer can link with the previous stream of thought. **Muddling** designates an extreme degree of derailment and fusion.

In organic states, incoherent thinking, which is clinically similar to derailment, may be attributable to a primary intellectual impairment and not to an increased spread of associations.

(b) Overinclusive thinking

This kind of thought disorder is not based on an interruption of the flow of thought but on an inability to preserve conceptual boundaries; ideas only distantly related to the concept under consideration become incorporated within it,[26] for example, when asked to indicate the essential components of a *room*, *table* might be included as well as *ceiling*, *wall*, and *floor*.

(c) Concrete and abstract thinking

In organic mental disorders and mental retardation, inability to think abstractly may be attributed to a diminished capacity to structure a concept. There have been various theories used to explain the **concrete thinking** of schizophrenia, involving memory, conceptualization, and intrusion of delusions. The process may be enhanced by loosening of associations. The fact that schizophrenia sometimes manifests excessively **abstract thinking** may also be explained by a disturbance of working memory such that the concrete meaning of the initial thought is not retained.

(d) Disorder of control of thinking

In **obsessions** and **compulsions** the subject recognizes his thoughts as being produced by himself but is unable to control them.

In **passivity of thought**, the patient experiences his thoughts as manipulated by outside influences. The interpretation resulting from this feeling is described as 'thought withdrawal', 'thought insertion', or 'thought broadcasting' (which denotes the patient's conviction that his thoughts are diffused to other people). These 'delusions of the control of thought' were included by Schneider[27] among his 'first-rank symptoms' of schizophrenia.

A particular variation of thought insertion occurring in schizophrenia is **crowding of thoughts**. In this condition, the patient experiences an excessive increase in the amount of thoughts imposed from the outside and compressed in his mind.

Language and speech disorder

'Speech disorder' refers to defects in the ability to generate and articulate verbal statements, whereas 'language disorder' designates deficits in the use of language. The terms 'aphasia' and 'dysphasia' are often used interchangeably for speech disorders.

(a) Disturbed generation and articulation of words

Aphonia designates the inability to vocalize. Thus, whispering occurs in somatic illnesses (paralysis of cranial nerve IX or disease of the vocal cords) and hysteria. **Dysphonia** is a somatic impairment with hoarseness.

Dysarthria refers to disorders of articulation occurring in various malformations or diseases, which impair the mechanisms of phonation, in lesions of the brain stem, in schizophrenia, and in psychogenic disorders.

The causes of **stuttering and stammering** are unclear, but are sometimes considered to be of neurotic origin. **Logoclonia** (the spastic repetition of syllables) occurs in Parkinsonism.

(b) Disturbance in talking

'Disturbances in talking' was proposed by Scharfetter[28] as a generic term for disorders of speech or language not belonging to the preceding group of disturbances.

Changes in volume of sound and in intonation occur in affective and schizophrenic states, and refer to loud excited and quiet monotonous speech.

Bradyphasia (decelerated talking) and **tachyphasia** (accelerated talking) occur in mood disorders, schizophrenia, and organic dysphasias.

Logorrhea (verbosity) is observed in various disorders, especially in manic states.

Alogia (poverty of speech) is a decrease in spontaneous talking; it occurs in depression and schizophrenia.

In **poverty of content of speech**, the amount of speech is adequate but conveys little information. This is often related to schizophrenic disorganization of thinking.

Verbigeration is the monotonous repetition of syllables and words observed in organic language disorders, schizophrenia, and agitated depression.

Echolalia is the repetition of words or parts of sentences that are spoken by others. It can be observed in schizophrenia, organic states, and subnormality.

Sometimes patients give **approximate answers**: i.e. they avoid giving the correct answer to a question that they have understood, just missing being correct. This occurs in organic disorders, schizophrenia, and hysteria.

Paraphasia denotes the enunciation of an inappropriate sound instead of a word or phrase. This happens in organic speech disorders but may also have psychogenic causes.

Speech may be unintelligible for various reasons. **Paragrammatism** and **parasyntax** (loss of grammatical and syntactical coherence) occur in organic mental disorders and excited manic states, and in schizophrenia, when severe thought derailments become manifest as 'word salad'. **Private symbolism** can be observed in schizophrenia in three forms: use of existing words with a particular symbolic meaning, creation of 'neologisms' (new words with an idiosyncratic meaning), and production of a private incomprehensible language, which may be spoken (cryptolalia) or written (cryptographia).

Mutism (refraining from speech) may be found in various kinds of psychiatric disorder. It is a cardinal feature of stupor and also occurs as an 'hysterical' reaction to stress.

Pseudologia fantastica is characterized by fluent lying, which is developed into a fantastic construct. This 'mythomania' occurs in histrionic and asocial personality disorders.

(c) Organic language disorders

This refers to impairments of spontaneous language, naming, writing, and reading, occurring as a result of brain dysfunction. These disorders can be divided into 'sensory' (receptive), 'motor' (expressive) defects, or both combined, containing the following principal subcategories:

(i) Sensory language disorders

In **primary sensory dysphasia** the patient cannot understand the speech of others. His own speech remains fluent, but contains errors in the use of words, syntax, and grammar. Writing and reading are also impaired. If, in this condition, the patient's speech becomes unintelligible, the disturbance is called 'jargon aphasia'. If only the repetition of a message is disturbed, the disorder is named 'conduction dysphasia'.

In **pure word-deafness** speech, reading, and writing are fluent and correct. The patient hears words as sounds, but cannot recognize their meaning. In **pure word-blindness** (alexia) speech and writing are normal but the patient cannot read with understanding.

(ii) Motor language disorders

In **primary motor dysphasia** the verbal or written expression of words and the construction of sentences is disturbed, but the understanding of speech and writing are preserved.

In **pure word-dumbness** the disturbance is limited to an inability to produce and repeat words at will. **Pure agraphia** is an isolated inability to write. **Nominal dysphasia** is an inability to produce names and nouns.

Disorders of intellectual performance

(a) Conceptualization of intelligence

'Intelligence' refers to the capacity to solve problems, to cope with new situations, to acquire skills through learning and experience, to establish logical deductions, and to form abstract concepts. There has been a classical debate amongst psychologists as to whether intelligence represents different and specific abilities or a unitary, general factor of intelligence.

(b) Measurements of intelligence

Individual intellectual capacity is graded by reference to the intelligence quotient (**IQ**), which is defined as the ratio of a subject's intelligence to the average intelligence for his or her age. The assessment of intelligence is considered in Chapter 1.8.3.

In addition to the global assessment of intelligence, numerous tests have been developed to assess organic impairment, scholastic achievement, and aptitude.

(c) Mental retardation (learning disability)

If the development of intellectual performance does not reach an IQ level of 70, the condition is designated 'mental retardation'. This is subdivided according to severity, with four levels recognized in ICD-10:

- mild (IQ 50–69)
- moderate (IQ 35–49)
- severe (IQ 20–34)
- profound (IQ below 20).

The causes of mental retardation are considered in Section 10.

Disorders of later onset

In these disorders normally developed intellectual performance declines. This can occur as a result of organic brain disorders, and in psychotic and affective disorders.

Organic disorders may have toxic, traumatic, inflammatory, or hypoxic causes. If these conditions are treated successfully, the disturbance can be arrested or even reversed.

In dementia there is a progressive disintegration of intellectual function, which usually begins insidiously and is often first recognized through an impairment of memory.

In psychotic states the distorted testing and evaluation of reality can impair intellectual performance. In schizophrenia, formal thought disorder may contribute to this effect.

Severe affective disorder can impair perception, attention, and motivation, leading to poor intellectual performance. These disturbances are observed more often in depression, but can occur in manic mood.

Disorders of mood

This section outlines the psychopathological elements comprising mood disorders, in particular the different varieties of depression, mania, anxiety state, and depersonalization.

Mood is a state of mind, which is longer lasting than affect or feeling. Mood encompasses all mental processes; it is not influenced by will, and is strongly related to values. Heidegger(29) has considered mood as the fundamental expression of an individual's being. Kierkegaard(30) emphasized the role of existential orientation in determining mood, especially general anxiety.

The extent and type of deviation of mood is important in affective disorders. Although there are no sharp boundaries between the normal variations and pathological states of mood, severe states are clearly abnormal and difficult to understand. Mood can be abnormal in several ways: sad or anxious in depressive disorders; euphoric in mania; irritated in mania or agitated depression; dysphoric in depression or in mixed manic—depressive disorders; morose in chronic-depressed states, often with a component of resentment; blunted (the feeling of 'having no feelings' or 'petrified' feelings) in prolonged, severe depressive disorder. Stanghellini(31) analysed depressed patients and described how morose affect may emerge when the patient struggles against declining abilities and experiences resistance. In such cases feelings of timidity and despair may contrast with an outward appearance of hostility.

Two types of **euphoria** should be differentiated: one shows elation and feelings of increased spiritual, intellectual, or physical power, and the other results from disinhibition in organic states and dementia. This second type, rather than elation, may show lack of interest and an attitude of negligence towards the patient's actual situation.

These abnormal moods are related to altered **bodily feelings** and thinking.

Abnormal **somatic** symptoms can be divided into physical symptoms, such as cardiovascular dysregulation, increased sweating, and feeling cold, and hypochondriacal symptoms, such as headache and feeling of tightness in the chest, heavy limbs, being choked, or difficulty in swallowing. These latter symptoms are related to feeling of loss of energy.

Lopez-Ibor(32) suggested the term 'depression-equivalent' for conditions in which somatic symptoms (e.g. headaches which vary on a diurnal pattern) dominate the clinical picture. Cross-cultural research has found higher rates of such somatic symptoms in depression in Africa(33) and South America,(34) and a lower rate of guilt compared with Western industrialized countries. However, the results are not wholly consistent and variation may reflect cultural differences or differing patterns of consultation with doctors, and what patients expect doctors to treat.

A feedback loop may develop between anxiety and physical **arousal**, e.g. palpitations, which accompanies it.(35,36) The prevalence of mitral valve prolapse is higher in anxiety disorder (37 per cent) than in the general population (5 per cent).(37) This finding is consistent with the idea that palpitation may lead to a conditioned anxiety response. The behaviour therapy technique of exposure aims to decondition this reflex. In social phobia and panic disorder anxiety is often complicated by anxiety-provoking situations which may lead to severe social disablement. Somatic symptoms of anxiety may be so prominent in some depressive states that patients are misdiagnosed as medically ill, with loss of weight, atypical pain, or sensory or motor disturbances. This type of depression has been called 'depressio sine depressione', or 'somatoform depression'.

Disturbances of diurnal rhythm can influence all the other symptoms of mood disorder.(38) There are changes associated with sleep in the electroencephalogram, with shorter REM latency (phase advance), and also changes in endocrine and cardiovascular circadian rhythms. In depression, sleep disturbance is characterized by early awakening, whereas falling asleep in the evening is often undisturbed. About 70 per cent of melancholic patients show diurnal distribution of mood, psychomotor activity, somatic symptoms, and slowed and impoverished thinking.

Psychomotor retardation or acceleration is one of the most prominent symptoms of mood disorder. Often the patient's appearance and expressive movements reveal more than words. The retarded patient's movements are slow, the limbs are rigid, the body is bent, and the expression is sad or anxious, and does not respond to the situation. The subjective feeling may be of emptiness, weakness, and tension. If the condition is severe, it can be difficult to discriminate between depressive and catatonic stupor; patients with depressive stupor seldom have increased muscular tension or rigidity. Increased psychomotor activity can appear in depression as agitation, i.e. restlessness without the ability to attain goals or organize behaviour. In mania, increased psychomotor activity is also seen in sexual excesses and extravagant spending.

Psychomotor retardation, and probably also acceleration, may be accompanied by a changed experience of time.(39) Depressed patients overemphasize the past, remembering guilt-connected events; manic patients feel that the future is immanent. Inability to distinguish wishes from reality results in poor decision-making in both depression and mania. Some depressives are unable even to decide how to dress in the morning. A manic patient's workroom can reflect the dissolution of his ability to give priority to important things, for example tools for immediate and frequent use and those seldom used. Extreme retardation is seen in depressive stupor when patients do not move, speak, eat, or drink. Extreme acceleration occurs in mania ('boiling over') and may be accompanied by a sense of confusion.

Retardation and acceleration are closely related to depressive and manic **thought disorder**. In depression the flow of associations is reduced and slowed, and short-term memory can appear impaired (pseudodementia). Depressed patients often ruminate about negative topics and have difficulty in terminating these thoughts. In mania, acceleration of thinking leads to a plethora of associations, 'flight of ideas', and pressure of speech. Unlike patients with schizophrenic thought disorder, depressed patients retain logical connections.

Depersonalization (see later) can occur alone or as part of a depressive state. In the latter, part of the body, the self, the mind, actions, or thinking are sensed as being alienated—not belonging to the self. In mood disorders, depersonalization does not usually reach the intensity of delusion, as it can in schizophrenia.

Although anxiety disorders and major depression have been defined by operational criteria in the diagnostic manuals, the clinical symptoms of mood states vary considerably. Attempts have been made to define a core syndrome by using factor analysis to identify latent trait symptom profiles derived from several assessment scales and from different samples of depressed patients. Cross-cultural comparisons of symptom profiles can also help to identify core symptoms. Among the latent traits, retardation was found most often, together with loss of interest and alteration of diurnal rhythm. Guilt, death wish, and affective reactivity occurred inconsistently.(40)

Disorders of self and body image

Disorders of self

These describe the abnormal inner experiences of I-ness and my-ness which occur in psychiatric disorders. Scharfetter has added the characteristic of awareness of being or ego vitality to the four formal characteristics previously described by Jaspers: feeling of awareness of activity, awareness of unity, awareness of identity, and awareness of the boundaries of self.[41,42]

(a) Disorder of the awareness of being

This is demonstrated by **nihilistic delusions**, which frequently occur in severe depressive illness and are a feature of the eponymous Cotard's syndrome.[43] Non-psychotic abnormality is exemplified by **depersonalization** in which the sufferer experiences his mental activity, body, or surroundings as changed in quality to become unreal, remote, or automatized.

(b) Disorder of awareness of activity

Disorder of the awareness of activity occurs with neurological lesions, such as some dyspraxias, and also in psychotic conditions in which the individual believes that no action has occurred when it has, or vice versa. This does not include action that the patient knows he has executed but with a belief it was under the influence of another. Non-psychotic disorder of activity occurs when an individual believes that he has no freedom of action and that his range of choice is limited by external circumstances, for instance a person with depressive symptoms who believes that he is inevitably incompetent.

(c) Disorder of awareness of singleness

In health, one assumes that 'I am one person'. Disorder occurs in the rare visual perceptual experience of **autoscopy**.[44] Non-psychotic examples of disorder of singleness include the double phenomenon, described by Jaspers,[45] and **multiple personality disorder,** which is the apparent existence of two or more distinct personalities within an individual, only one of them being evident at any time. The **double phenomenon** is much more frequent, and describes the self-experience of those who feel that there are two different parts of themselves in conflict with each other; they are fully aware of both at the same time.

(d) Disorder of awareness of identity

Disorder of identity occurs in **delusion of control** or **passivity experience**, in which the sufferer believes that he has been taken over by an alien, with the belief that there is a break in continuity from 'myself' who was there before. Non-psychotic disorder of awareness of identity is exemplified by **possession disorder**, in which there is a temporary loss of the sense of personal identity and the individual may act *as if* they have been taken over by another personality, spirit, or force.

(e) Disorder of the awareness of boundaries of self

Disorder of boundaries of self occurs in first-rank symptoms of schizophrenia such as thought withdrawal, control, and diffusion.[46] The patient believes that thoughts 'are being taken out of me, influenced by an outside source'. Non-psychotic disorder of the boundaries of self occurs in ecstasy states, characteristically described as an 'as if' experience. There is disturbance of boundaries of self in that the individual may feel that there is no limit between self and the outside world.

Depersonalization and derealization

Depersonalization is the experience of one's own feelings and experiences being detached, distant, not one's own, lost or altered. Derealization is the same range of subjectivity describing awareness of the outside world. The sufferer recognizes that this is a subjective change and is not imposed by outside forces. Because the sufferer finds it difficult to describe, this experience tends to be underdiagnosed, but the misery it causes and the disturbance in functioning is considerable; it is experienced as being so subjectively unpleasant that not uncommonly deliberate self-harm results.

Insight

The clinical assessment of a patient's capacity to understand the nature, significance, and severity of his or her own illness has been called insight. There is current interest in describing its characteristics and establishing how it correlates with other measures of illness.[47] The attitude of patients towards their illness has clear clinical implications, and the assessment of insight tries to investigate the patient's awareness concerning the impact their illness has, and their capacity to adapt to the changes brought about by illness. The patient's awareness of illness and the extent to which it is interfering with function affects compliance for prescribed treatment. David has proposed that insight implies the ability to relabel unusual mental events as *pathological*, the recognition that one has mental illness, and compliance with treatment. Some parallels have been drawn between the loss of insight in psychiatric patients and the denial of disease or loss of function that occurs in certain neurological conditions.

Because of its importance for clinical management, there have been many attempts over recent years to measure insight, all of which depend upon a precise operational definition of the concept. McEvoy *et al.*[48] developed a questionnaire to measure the patients' awareness of the pathological nature of their experiences and also their acceptance of the need for treatment. The measure constructed by David *et al.*[49] added the ability to relabel unusual mental events as 'pathological' to the recognition of mental illness and compliance with treatment.

The relationship between impairment of insight and the presence of other aspects of psychopathology is complicated; there is no clear association between impairment of insight and intellectual or neuropsychological deficit.[50] Not surprisingly, patients with unimpaired insight are found to be significantly less likely to require readmission to hospital, tend to be more compliant with treatment, and show an improved prognosis.[51] Surprisingly, and this shows how little is known about this subject, many patients are prepared to comply with treatment, even though they do not believe themselves to be ill, if the social milieu is conducive to receiving treatment.[48]

Insight is a multifaceted phenomenon with considerable clinical significance as it predicts the likelihood of patients complying with treatment. Most studies of insight have been concerned with patients suffering from schizophrenia, and it is important to extend work to other serious mental illnesses.

Disorders of awareness of the body

(a) Bodily complaint without organic cause

Such conditions create difficulties for psychopathological understanding.

1 Aetiology is often obscure, sometimes with doubt that there may be an unrevealed physical cause.

2 The descriptive terms used come from different theoretical backgrounds and have changed their meaning over the years.

3 There is often discrepancy between the meanings attached to the symptoms by the patient and by the doctor.

'Somatoform disorders', which include both somatization and hypochondriacal disorders[52] are, characteristically, repeated presentation of physical symptoms with persistent requests for medical investigation, despite negative findings, and reassurance by doctors that the symptoms have no physical basis. The patient with **somatization** as the prominent disorder complains of multiple recurrent, and often changing, physical symptoms in different bodily systems over a prolonged time. The patient with **hypochondriasis** has a persistent preoccupation with bodily function, the possibility of illness, and the seriousness with which symptoms should be treated. Not infrequently these two groups of symptoms overlap. Co-morbid anxiety and depression is quite frequent with both somatization and hypochondriasis. The content of hypochondriasis may take the form of delusion, overvalued ideas, hallucination, anxious or depressive rumination, or anxious preoccupation.

The term 'Dissociative (conversion) disorder' has replaced the confusing, but graphic, hysteria. **Conversion symptoms** can be categorized as motor, sensory (including pain), or psychological. Motor symptoms include weakness or paralysis of limbs or part of a limb and abnormality of gait; sensory symptoms include glove, and stocking anaesthesia. Amongst the psychological symptoms is a narrowing of the field of consciousness with selective amnesia such as may occur in fugue states. For conversion disorder, or hysteria, to be diagnosed, symptoms should appear to be psychogenic in nature, causation should be considered unconscious, symptoms may carry some sort of advantage to the patient, and they occur by the mediation of the processes of conversion or dissociation.

Artefactual illness includes two categories: *elaboration* of physical symptoms for psychological reasons, and intentional production or *feigning* of symptoms or disabilities, either physical or psychological. Conversion symptoms are believed to arise without the patient's conscious involvement, but artefactual illness implies that the illness, lesion, or complaint is ultimately the individual's own conscious production. **Malingering** implies feigning or producing symptoms expressly for the social advantages of being regarded as ill, while the broader category of artefactual illness includes other motivations and simply describes the behaviour.

Narcissism is an exaggerated concern with one's self-image, especially with personal appearance. This absorption with self is usually associated with feelings of insecurity and ambivalence concerning the self and feelings of threat to one's integrity.

Dislike of the body and distortion of body image are subjectively different experiences but often occur together, for example in anorexia nervosa or with gross obesity. In **dysmorphophobia** the primary symptom is the patient's belief that he or she is unattractive. Sufferers believe themselves to have a physical defect, such as the size of their nose or breasts, that is noticeable to other people, but objectively their appearance may lie within normal limits. The content disorder of dysmorphophobia is an overvalued idea in which the degree of concern and consequent distress is clearly out of proportion and comes to dominate the whole of life. The overvalued idea of dysmorphophobia may be associated with an underlying personality disorder of anankastic or dependent type, or with other psychiatric disorders.

Awareness of body size and **disturbance of eating** frequently occur together; alteration of body image is associated with eating disorder. Obesity in adolescence, in diet-conscious Western societies, frequently results in self-loathing, more frequently in girls than boys, with overestimation of body fatness. Disturbance of body image occurs in sufferers from anorexia nervosa, characteristically an overestimate of width with an accurate estimation of height or the width of inanimate objects. The more 'over-fat' an individual considers herself to be, the more dissatisfaction with herself she will experience.[53] Such disorders of self-image, with significant overestimation of size and discrepancy between perceived and desired size, also occur in bulimia nervosa, and may be associated with depression of mood and feelings of guilt and unworthiness.

(b) Organic changes in body image

Organic change may result from either damage to the conceptualized object (e.g. following amputation, with a phantom limb) or damage to the process of conceptualization (e.g. section of the corpus callosum). Hyperschemazia, pathological accentuation of body image, occurs when physical illness or neurological lesion causes enhancement of perception of an organ. Diminished or absent body image (hyposchemazia, aschemazia) may occur with loss of innervation, or with parietal lobe lesions. The diminution of body image may be simple (e.g. loss or neglect of a limb) or complex. There may also be distortions of the body image (paraschemazia), in which enhancement or diminution of parts of the body may occur.

(c) Disorder of gender and sexuality

Core gender identity is established very early in life and then retained; it is biologically influenced and socially reinforced. **Transsexualism** is a disorder of gender identity, much more common in biological males, in which there is discrepancy between anatomical sex and the gender that the person assigns to himself. The subjective belief is an overvalued idea. Other disorders of sexuality are considered elsewhere. (See Chapter 4.11.3)

(d) Pain as a psychopathological entity

Pain is a subjective experience, which is hard to describe and categorize; it is not well-charted phenomenologically. It appears to have more in common with mood than perception. Pain associated with psychiatric illness tends to be more diffuse and less well localized and to spread with non-anatomical distribution. It also tends to be complained of constantly, becoming even more severe at times but persisting without remission. It may clearly be seen to be associated with underlying disturbance of mood, which appears to be primary in time and causation. Psychogenic pain tends to progress in severity and extent over time. Persistent, severe, and distressing pain, which cannot be explained fully by a physiological process or physical disorder has been designated **persistent somatoform pain disorder**. (See Chapter 5.2.6.)

Motor symptoms and signs

Motor symptoms and signs may be due to a neurological disorder causing organic brain syndrome, such as rigidity in Parkinson's disease, or may be related to emotional states such as restlessness or tremor in anxiety. However, there is a further group of symptoms, which affect voluntary movements and often occur in functional psychoses. These symptoms are neither unequivocally neurological nor clearly psychogenic in origin and are termed **motility disorder** by some authors. Table 1.7.1 gives a glossary of disordered motility. Whether patients are unable or unwilling to move normally is still a matter of debate. The origin of motility symptoms may well be a functional (rather than a morphological) abnormality of basal ganglia.

A further classification of motility disorder distinguishes psychomotor hyperphenomena (e.g. tic disorder), hypophenomena (e.g. stupor), and paraphenomena (e.g. mannerism). **Tics** are rapid, irregular movements involving groups of facial or limb muscles. **Stupor** is a state in which a patient does not communicate, i.e. does not speak (mutism) or move (akinesia), although he or she is alert. **Mannerisms** are uncommon; they are conspicuous expressions by gesture, speech, or objects (e.g. dress) that seem to have a particular meaning, often delusional.

Catatonia is a psychopathological syndrome of disturbed motor behaviour. It is generally reversible, and it occurs with mood disorders, general medical conditions, toxic and psychotic states, and neurological disorders. Brain tumour, encephalitis, endocrine, and metabolic disorders may elicit catatonic symptoms. In Western countries catatonia is considered, nowadays, to be uncommon in general psychiatric practice, however, some catatonic symptoms have been found to occur in 5–10 per cent of acute psychiatric in-patients.[54]

Table 1.7.1 Symptoms and signs of motility disorder

Catalepsy (synonym; waxy flexibility, flexibilitas cerea)	Maintaining uncomfortable positions against resistance
Posturing	Maintaining uncomfortable positions that may have a delusional meaning
Stupor	Inability to communicate despite being awake
Akinesia	Inability to move
Mutism	Inability to speak
Echolatia	Repetition of another person's speech
Echopraxia	Repetition of another person's acts
Mannerism	Uncommon conspicuous expression by gestures, speech, or objects
Grimacing	Uncommon conspicuous facial expression
Stereotypy	Repetition of actions
Verbigeration	Repetition of speech
Tic	Rapid movements of facial or limb muscles
Akathisia	Inability to remain seated or standing
Psychomotor retardation	Slowing of mental and motor activity
Psychomotor agitation	Arousal of mental and motor activity (typically by anxiety)

Stupor, *mutism*, and *negativism* are the classical triad of symptoms demarcating the catatonia syndrome, and automatic obedience and stimulus-bound behaviour, stereotypy, and catalepsy contribute to the syndrome in manic patients.[55] Lesser symptoms may occur, and catatonia may take the form of hypomobility, with stupor only in extreme cases. Patients in stupor remain persistently unresponsive for hours, days, or even longer. They appear to be unaware of events around them and are mute.

Catatonic excitement presents as excessive motor activity. Such patients may talk incessantly, especially when in an 'exalted stage'.[56] There may be outbursts of talking, singing, dancing, and removing their clothes. Such states carry the risk of exhaustion, dehydration, and injury; it may be harmful and dangerous to the patient and to others.

In **negativism** the patient resists the examiner's manipulations with force equal to that applied by the examiner. In **catalepsy** (posturing), the patient maintains posture for long periods. These include facial postures, such as grimacing or *schnauzkrampf* (lips in a pucker); body postures, such as *psychological pillow* (lying on his back with head elevated as if on a pillow); lying in a 'jack-knife' position; and many other uncomfortable and bizarre postures maintained against gravity or attempts to rectify them. An examiner trying to move a cataleptic limb passively will notice **waxy flexibility**, in which initial resistance to an induced movement changes to gradually allowing the imposition of a posture, like bending a candle.

Stereotypy is non-goal directed, repetitive behaviour, the verbal form of which is called *verbigeration*, endless repetition of phrases and sentences. **Automatic obedience** occurs when, despite instructions to the contrary, the patient permits the examiner to move his limbs into a new posture. This may then be maintained against instructions to the contrary. In **ambitendency** the patient appears stuck in indecisiveness, resisting the examiner's non-verbal signals, but showing hesitancy in doing so.

Echo phenomena may occur when the patient is interacting with another person and present as *echolalia* (imitation of the speech of others) or *echopraxia* (imitation of the actions of others). **Mannerisms** are strange but purposeful movements characteristic of that person. They may be exaggerated caricatures of ordinary movements.

Disordered speech may also be regarded as a sign of disordered motility, as in mutism or verbigeration.

In **delirium**, tremor often occurs. Anxiety is accompanied by restlessness. In a particular motor pattern in delirium tremens (alcohol withdrawal delirium) the patient appears to be collecting objects or brushing away dust. Typically, the movements never seem to achieve what they are meant to and, of necessity therefore, are repetitive. Suggestibility in delirium may lead to movements, which are based on erroneous assumptions, such as trying to take hold of a proffered, but non-existent, thread. Patients may develop panic and try to flee. Speech may be hurried and indistinct. In some cases of delirium, such as that due to hepatic failure, patients may be hypoactive before becoming drowsy and comatose. Hepatic failure may also result in catatonic disorder.

Many conditions, such as brain tumour, encephalitis, and endocrine and metabolic disorders, may elicit catatonic symptoms. Patients with a variety of mental disorders may show abnormal movements that are of histrionic nature. They may throw themselves to the ground, seek and maintain bodily contact, or show psychomotor agitation. Alternatively, there may be psychogenic paresis.

In dementia there may be general disturbance of psychomotor functions leading to disturbed co-ordination and clumsiness. During the further progress of dementia, lethargy, and akinesia may occur.

Sequelae of encephalitis are known to include a number of motor symptoms apart from parkinsonism, as seen in the epidemic of encephalitis lethargica that occurred around 1920. **Tardive dyskinesia** is a side-effect of neuroleptic therapy. However, since signs of tardive dyskinesia such as perioral hyperkinesia and dystonias were described before the introduction of neuroleptics,[57] it is also a motor symptom of mental disorder in its own right.

Disorders of memory

The psychology of memory is discussed in Chapter 2.5.3.

Memory may be differentiated into short-term or recent memory and long-term or remote memory. Furthermore, ultra-short-term memory may be distinguished from short-term memory. Ultra-short-term memory encompasses immediate registration within the span of attention. Short-term memory reflects new learning. Long-term memory is usually associated with earlier data or other information that has been stored for months or years.

Additional terms describing memory functions are *declarative* and *procedural* memory. Declarative memory contains facts, which may be consciously recalled, whereas procedural memory contains skills and automatic activities. In dementia—both degenerative (Alzheimer type) and vascular (multi-infarct dementia)—recent memory is usually impaired earlier than remote memory.

Biographical memory is the recall of events in a person's past, which have an emotional loading, and therefore an impact on understanding depression.

Amnesia is a period of time, which cannot be recalled, and it may be global or partial. With regard to time it may be retrograde—an expression derived from the idea that one is looking backwards from an event (such as brain trauma or electroconvulsive therapy) to find the period that is deleted before the event. Correspondingly, anterograde amnesia means a period of deleted memory after an event. Although it is difficult to distinguish between types of amnesia, focal lesions in the hippocampus seem to affect remote memory less than recent memory, whereas diffuse brain disease often affects both. In psychogenic amnesia it is sometimes possible to recognize specific personal meaning in the events which cannot be recalled.[58] Amnestic disorders should strongly alert the examiner to the possibility of cerebral pathology.

Disorders of memory are closely connected with other disorders, such as disorders of consciousness; there is often amnesia for episodes of disturbed consciousness.

Some patients are aware of memory disorder and complain about it; others tend to neglect their memory deficits and manifest secondary signs such as confabulation. Confabulations are inventions, which substitute for missing contents in gaps of memory; the patient is not aware that they are not true memories.

A disorder of short-term memory, as in Korsakoff's syndrome or transient global amnesia, is often neglected by the patient. Behaviour appears normal, and it often seems that the personality is intact. Such a patient may be engaged in lively conversation or seemingly purposeful actions, and only after further investigation does it become obvious that these activities are not based on facts. This memory disorder can be assessed directly by examining the patient. Other forms become apparent retrospectively on taking the patient's history. In these cases the patient complains about periods of global or partial amnesia. Memory for certain events may have faded or become obscured by layers of other events (palimpsest); this is typical of repeated amnestic periods following bouts of drinking. In mood disorder there may be complaints about impaired memory, although no memory deficit is found in objective tests. Examples of false memory (paramnesia) are *déjà vu*, an erroneous feeling of familiarity with, for example, a person or a room, and jamais vu, a feeling of unfamiliarity for a well-known object. *Déjà vu* may occur in temporal lobe epilepsy, although it is not specific for that disorder. Delusional memories are also examples of paramnesia.

Disorders of consciousness

Consciousness is the sum of various mental functions—in the words of Jaspers[59] 'the whole of present mental life'. Lipowski,[60] who regards the concept of consciousness to be 'completely redundant', describes what is commonly meant by clouding of consciousness on the basis of a number of behavioural features (Table 1.7.2). In contrast with Lipowski, the concept of consciousness has recently elicited fresh interest in philosophy and clinical neurology. (See Chapter 2.1)

Consciousness is a mode of relatedness between mind and world. Disordered consciousness may occur on a dimension of severity, which ranges from lucidity via clouding and then towards unconsciousness. The latter represents a state of coma. In addition, consciousness may be assessed on a dimension of vigilance.[61] Ey[62] regards consciousness as an attribute of wakefulness. Indeed, sleepiness implies a reduction in consciousness; but consciousness may also be reduced despite normal vigilance. Likewise, consciousness is impaired by a disorder of memory, orientation, or coherence, as in the clouded consciousness of delirium.

When consciousness is impaired there is clouding of perception, ideas, and images. The intensity of perception is diminished and there is a disintegration of order in the perceptive field. Accordingly, patients become disoriented.

The term 'confusional state' is a synonym for delirium that emphasizes thought disorder and disorientation. **Disorientation** may concern time, place, or person. Temporal and geographical disorientation are common. Remote contents are better remembered than recent ones; name or date of birth is usually more available than age, or name of the hospital. It is useful, after a polite excuse, to ask direct questions concerning orientation, even if they sound trivial, since some patients are skilful in avoiding topics that show the degree of their disorientation.

Table 1.7.2 Behavioural features indicating clouding of consciousness

The person is awake but may be drowsy
Awareness of the self and the environment is reduced
Both immediate and recent memory are impaired
Thinking is disorganized, and may be dreamlike; for instance perception is faulty and misperceptions may occur
The ability to (learn new material is reduced) learn
The person is unable to overcome this state by deliberate effort

Another abnormality is described by the term **narrowing of consciousness**, which means that awareness of a person's environment is restricted, for example, owing to an abnormal affective or delusional state.

In epileptic aura or after taking certain drugs, consciousness may be experienced as heightened with increased intensity of awareness.

Twilight state is a well-defined interruption of the continuity of consciousness. Consciousness is clouded and sometimes narrowed. Despite the disorder of consciousness, the patient is able to perform certain actions, such as dressing, driving, or walking around. Subsequently, there is amnesia for this state. Twilight states may occur in epilepsy, alcoholism (*mania à potu* is a twilight state), brain trauma, general paresis, and dissociative disorder. *Mania à potu* describes the situation where a person reacts excessively by developing twilight state with small amounts of alcohol. Often these patients have an increased vulnerability due to pre-existing organic brain pathology. Twilight state occasionally leads to violent behaviour.

In an **oneiroid state** the patient experiences narrowing of consciousness together with multiple scenic hallucinations. Oneiroid states may occur in schizophrenia, but are also observed in patients who have to be totally passive and dependent on others. The atmosphere is perceived as strange and dreamlike. Accordingly patients may be aloof and behave like dreamers.[(63)] Unlike twilight states, the contents of oneiroid states are often remembered.

Disorders of attention and concentration

Attention and concentration imply the directing of mental activities towards a particular object. Attention is associated with present alertness, and concentration with longer lasting achievement and performance; there is a distinction between *selective* and *shared* attention. Attention and concentration may be impaired by clouded consciousness or individual aspects, such as sleepiness, incoherence, or memory deficit. However, there may be other reasons for inattention such as hallucination or mood disturbances. Attention deficit is a permanent feature in the childhood disorder, attention-deficit hyperactivity disorder.

Assessment of attention and concentration may consist of simple arithmetical tasks and include psychometric performance test in addition to the clinical examination. Psychometric performance tests are also valuable tools in assessing disorder of memory and consciousness.

Disorders of sleep are described in Chapter 4.14.

Disorder of personality

It is the expression of disordered personality which is the consideration of descriptive phenomenology, the observation of characteristic behaviour and the subject's self description. Schneider has defined personality as 'the unique quality of the individual, his feelings and personal goals'[(64)] *Abnormality of personality* is present when a characteristic or trait of clinical relevance is developed in the patient to a statistically abnormal extent, that is either deficient or excessive. *Personality disorder* is present when that abnormality causes suffering to the patient or to other people. A person with antisocial personality disorder not uncommonly causes discomfort to other people; with obsessive-compulsive personality disorder the abnormal characteristics may frequently cause distress to the individual himself.

Both ICD 10 and DSM-IV are derived from Schneider's description of personality types. The advantage of such a typological approach is that it does not imply any specific theory of causation. The accurate description of personality characteristics and type is valuable in clinical practice for diagnosis, prognosis and the rational planning of treatment. The skills of psychopathology are ideally suited to the observation of consistent personality traits, and forming an opinion unprejudiced by preconceived theoretical considerations. Descriptions of different personality types and disorders are developed elsewhere.

Acknowledgements

This revised chapter, prepared by Andrew Sims, is based on that in the first edition by Andrew Sims, Christoph Mundt, Peter Berner, and Arnd Barocka. The contributions of these authors to the original text is gratefully acknowledged.

Further information

Sims, A. (2003). *Symptoms in the mind* (3rd edn). W.B. Saunders, London.

Jaspers, K. (1963). *General psychopathology* (7th edn) (trans. J. Hoenig and M.W. Hamilton). Manchester University Press.

Cutting, J. (1997). *Principles of psychopathology*. Oxford University Press.

References

1. Sims, A. (2003). *Symptoms in the mind* (3rd edn). W.B. Saunders, London.
2. Jaspers, K. (1963). *General psychopathology* (7th edn) (trans. J. Hoenig and M.W. Hamilton). Manchester University Press.
3. Hundert, E.M. (1995). *Lessons from an optical illusion*. Harvard University Press, Cambridge, MA.
4. Cutting, J. (1997). *Principles of psychopathology*. Oxford University Press.
5. Zucker, K. (1928). Experimentelles über Sinnestäuschungen. *Archiv für Psychiatrie und Nervenkrankheiten*, **83**, 706–54.
6. Janzarik, W. (1988). *Strukturdynamische Grundlagen der Psychiatrie*. Enke, Stuttgart.
7. Schmidt-Degenhard, M. (1992). *Die oneiroide Erlebnisform*. Springer, Berlin.
8. Jaspers, K. (1965). *Allgemeine psychopathologie*. Springer, Berlin.
9. Klosterkötter, J. (1992). The meaning of basic symptoms for the development of schizophrenic psychoses. *Neurology, Psychiatry, and Brain Research*, **1**, 30–41.
10. Krause, R., Steimer, E., Sänger-Alt, C., *et al.* (1989). Facial expression of schizophrenic patients and their interactionpartners. *Psychiatry: Interpersonal and Biological Processes*, **52**, 1–12.
11. Allderidge, P. (1974). *The late Richard Dadd*, pp. 1817–86. Tate Gallery, London.
12. Huber, G. and Gross, G. (1989). The concept of basic symptoms in schizophrenia and schizoaffective psychoses. *Recenti Progressi in Medicina*, **80**, 646–52.
13. Penfield, W. and Perot, P. (1963). The brain's record of auditory and visual experience. *Brain*, **86**, 595–696.
14. Emrich, H.M. (1989). A three-component-system hypothesis of psychosis. Impairment of binocular depth inversion as an indicator of a functional dysequilibrium. *British Journal of Psychiatry*, **155** (Suppl. 5), 37–8.

15. Hamilton, M. (1974). *Fish's clinical psychopathology. Signs and symptoms in psychiatry* (revised reprint). John Wright, Bristol.
16 Jaspers, K. (1975). *Allgemeine psychopathologie* (8th edn). Springer, Berlin.
17. Scharfetter, C. (1980). *General psychopathology*. Cambridge University Press.
18. Jaspers, K. (1963). *General psychopathology* (7th edn) (trans. J. Hoenig and M.W. Hamilton), p. 98. Manchester University Press.
19. Schneider, K. (1962). *Klinische psychopathologie* (6th edn). Thieme, Stuttgart.
20. Hemsley, D.R. (1994). An experimental psychological model for schizophrenia. In *Search for the causes of schizophrenia* (ed. H. Häfner, W.F. Gattaz, and W. Janzarik), pp. 179–88. Springer, Berlin.
21. Frith, C.D. and Done, D.J. (1989). Experiences of alien control in schizophrenia reflect a disorder in the central monitoring of action. *Psychological Medicine*, **19**, 359–63.
22. McKenna, P.J. (1984). Disorders with overvalued ideas. *British Journal of Psychiatry*, **145**, 579–85.
23. Beck, A.T., Rush, A.J., Shaw, B.F., *et al.* (1979). *Cognitive therapy of depression*. Guilford Press, New York.
24. Marks, J.M. (1969). *Fears and phobias*. Heinemann, London.
25. Jaspers, K. (1963). *General psychopathology* (7th edn) (trans. J. Hoenig and M.W. Hamilton), p. 162. Manchester University Press.
26. Payne, R.W. (1996). The measurement and significance of overinclusive thinking and retardation in schizophrenic patients. In *Psychopathology of schizophrenia* (ed. P.H. Hoch and J. Zubin), pp. 77–97. Grune and Stratton, New York.
27. Schneider, K. (1962). *Klinische psychopathologie* (6th edn). Thieme, Stuttgart.
28. Scharfetter, C. (1980). *General psychopathology*, p. 114. Cambridge University Press.
29. Heidegger, M. (1963). *Sein und Zeit*. Niemeyer, Tübingen.
30. Kierkegaard, S. (1849). *Die Krankheit zum Tode*, Vol. 8. Diederichs, Jena.
31. Stanghellini, G. (1995). The interplay between personality and affective vulnerability: the case of dysphoria. Presented at World Psychiatry Association Regional Symposium, Prague.
32. Lopez-Ibor, J.J. (1969). Depressive Äquivalente. In *Das depressive syndrom* (ed. H. Hippius and H. Selbach), pp. 403–7. Urban und Schwarzbenberg, Munich.
33. Mundt, C. (1991). Endogenität von Psychosen—Anachronismus oder aktueller Wegweiser für die Pathogeneseforschung? *Nervenarzt*, **62**, 3–15.
34. Escobar, J.I., Gomez, J., and Tuason, V.B. (1983). Depressive phenomenology in North and South American patients. *American Journal of Psychiatry*, **140**, 47–51.
35. Lader, M. (1983). The psychophysiology of anxiety. *Encephale*, **9**, 205B–10B.
36. Kellner, R. (1988). Anxiety, somatic sensations, and bodily complaints. In *Handbook of anxiety* (ed. R. Noyes Jr, M. Roth, and G.D. Burrows), Vol. 2, pp. 213–37. Elsevier, Amsterdam.
37. Albus, M. (1990). Psychophysiologie der Angsterkrankungen. *Nervenarzt*, **61**, 639–46.
38. Stallone, F., Huba, G.J., Lawlor, W.G., *et al.* (1973). Longitudical studies of diurnal variations in depression: a sample of 643 patient days. *British Journal of Psychiatry*, **123**, 311–8.
39. Mundt, C., Richter, P., van Hees, H., *et al.* (1998). Zeiterleben und Zeitschätzung depressiver Patienten. *Nervenarzt*, **69**, 38–45.
40. Philipp, M., Maier, W., and Benkert, O. (1985). Operational diagnosis of endogenous depression. II. Comparison of 8 different operational diagnoses. *Psychopathology*, **18**, 218–25.
41. Jaspers, K. (1963). *General psychopathology* (7th edn) (trans. J. Hoenig and M.W. Hamilton), pp. 121–7. Manchester University Press.
42. Scharfetter, C. (1981). Ego-psychopathology: the concept and its empirical evolution. *Psychological Medicine*, **11**, 273–90.
43. Cotard, M. (1882). Nihilistic delusions. Reprinted in *Themes and variations in European psychiatry* (ed. S.R. Hirsch and M. Shepherd). John Wright, Bristol.
44. Lukianowicz, N. (1958). Autonoscopic phenomena. *Archives of Neurology and Psychiatry*, **80**, 199–220.
45. Jaspers, K. (1963). *General psychopathology* (7th edn) (trans. J. Hoenig and M.W. Hamilton), pp. 92–3. Manchester University Press.
46. Sims, A.C.P. (1993). Schizophrenia and permeability of self. *Neurology, Psychiatry and Brain Research*, **1**, 133–5.
47. David, A.S. (1990). Insight and psychosis. *British Journal of Psychiatry*, **156**, 798–808.
48. McEvoy, J.P., Apperson, L.J., and Appelbaum, P.S. (1989). Insight in schizophrenia: its relationship to acute psychopathology. *Journal of Nervous and Mental Disease*, **177**, 43–7.
49. David, A.S., Buchanan, A., and Reed, A. (1992). The assessment of insight in psychosis. *British Journal of Psychiatry*, **161**, 599–602.
50. Kemp, R. and David, A. (1996). Insight and psychosis: a social perspective. *Psychological Medicine*, **25**, 515–20.
51. McEvoy, J.P., Freter, S., and Everett, C. (1989). Insight and the clinical outcome in schizophrenia. *Journal of Nervous and Mental Diseases*, **177**, 48–51.
52. World Health Organization (1992). International statistical classification of diseases and related health problems, 10th revision. WHO, Geneva.
53. Slade, P.D. (1988). Body image in anorexia nervosa. *British Journal of Psychiatry*, **153** (Suppl. 2), 20–2.
54. Rosebush, P.I., Hildebrand, A.M., Furlong, B.G., *et al.* (1990). Catatonic syndrome in a general psychiatric population: frequency, clinical presentation and response to lorazepam. *Journal of Clinical Psychiatry*, **51**, 357–62.
55. Fink, M. and Taylor, M.A. (2003). *Catatonia: a clinician's guide to diagnosis and treatment*. Cambridge University Press.
56. Kahlbaum, K.L. (1874). *Die Katatonie oder das Spannungsirresein*. (trans. Y. Levis and T. Pridon 1973) Verlag August Hirshwald, Berlin. Johns Hopkins University Press, Baltimore.
57. Berrios, G. (1996). *The history of mental symptoms*. Cambridge University Press.
58. Lishman, W.A. (1997). *Organic psychiatry*. Blackwell Science, Oxford.
59. Jaspers, K. (1963). *General psychopathology* (7th edn) (trans. J. Hoenig and M.W. Hamilton), p. 138. Manchester University Press.
60. Lipowski, Z. (1990). *Delirium*. Oxford University Press, New York.
61. Sims, A. (2003). *Symptoms in the mind* (3rd edn), p. 41. W.B. Saunders, Edinburgh.
62. Ey, H. (1963). *La conscience*. Presse Universitaire de France, Paris.
63. Mayer-Gross, W., Slater, E., and Roth, M. (1955). *Clinical psychiatry*. Cassell, London.
64. Schneider, K. (1950). *Psychopathic personalities* (9th edn) (trans. M.W. Hamilton, 1958). Cassell, London.

1.8

Assessment

Contents

1.8.1. The principles of clinical assessment in general psychiatry
John E. Cooper and Margaret Oates

1.8.2 Assessment of personality
C. Robert Cloninger

1.8.3 Cognitive assessment
Graham E. Powell

1.8.4 Questionnaire, rating, and behavioural methods of assessment
John N. Hall

1.8.1. The principles of clinical assessment in general psychiatry

John E. Cooper and Margaret Oates

Introduction

This chapter is focused on the needs of the clinician in a service for general adult psychiatry, who has to carry-out the initial assessment of the patient and family, working either in the context of a multi-disciplinary team or independently. Within this quite wide remit, the discussion is limited to general principles that guide the practice of all types of psychiatry. The chapter does not include the special procedures and techniques also needed for assessment of children and adolescents, the elderly, persons with mental retardation, persons with forensic problems, and persons requiring assessment for suitability for special types of psychotherapy.

It is assumed that the reader has already had significant experience of clinical psychiatry and has completed the first stages of a postgraduate psychiatric training programme. Therefore details of the basic methods recommended in commonly used textbooks or manuals of instruction for obtaining and recording information on essentials such as the history, personal development, mental state, and behaviour of the patient are not included in this chapter.[1]

Three topics have been given special attention. These are assessment by means of a multi-disciplinary **team**, the trio of concepts **diseases, illness, and sickness**, and the development of **structured interviewing and rating schedules**. The first two have a special connection that justifies emphasis in view of the recent increase in multi-disciplinary styles of assessment. For instance, when different members of the team appear to be in disagreement about what should be done, it is usually a good idea to ask the question: 'What is being discussed—is it the patient's possible physical disease, the patient's personal experience of symptoms and distress, or the interference of these with social activities?' It will then often become apparent that the issues in question are legitimate differences in emphasis and priority of interest, rather than disagreements. The third topic is given prominence in order to illustrate some aspects of the background of the large number of such schedules (or 'instruments') that are now available. They are usually given the shortest possible mention in research reports, but since most advances in clinical methods and service developments come from studies in which an assessment instrument has been used, clinicians should know something about them.

The aim of the initial clinical assessment is to allow the clinician and team to arrive at a comprehensive plan for treatment and management that has both short-term and longer-term components. The achievement of this will be discussed under the following headings.

- Concepts underlying the procedures of assessment
- Contextual influences on assessment procedures
- Assessment as a multi-disciplinary activity
- Instruments for assessment
- The condensation and recording of information
- Making a prognosis
- Reviews
- Writing reports

Concepts underlying the procedures of assessment

The separation of form from content, and from effects on activities

In psychiatric practice more than in other medical disciplines, the key items of information that allow the identification of signs and symptoms of psychiatric disorders are often embedded in a mixture of complaints about disturbed personal and social relationships, together with descriptions of problems to do with work, housing, and money. These complaints and problems may be a contributing cause or a result of the symptoms of psychiatric disorders, or they may simply exist in parallel with the symptoms. A preliminary sorting out into overall categories of information is therefore essential.

The distinction between the form and the content of the symptoms is particularly important, together with the differentiation of both of these from their effects upon the functioning of the patient (function is used here in a general sense as applying to all activities, in contrast to the specific meaning given to it in the classification of disablements). This differentiation is discussed in Chapter 1.7, so only a brief mention is needed here.

The presenting complaint of the patient is often the interference with functions, but enquiry about the reasons for this should then reveal the contents of the patient's thoughts and feelings. The form of the symptoms (i.e. the technical term, such as phobia or delusion used to identify a recurring pattern of experience or behaviour known to be important) allows the identification of the psychiatric disorder. Knowledge of the effects on functions is essential for decisions about the management of patient and family, and is an important aspect of the severity of the disorder.

This sorting into different types of information often implies a conflict of priorities during the interview. The clinician must be seen to acknowledge the concerns and distress of the patient, but also must ask questions that will allow the identification of symptoms. Learning to balance this conflict of interest is an essential part of clinical training, and has been well recognized by previous generations of descriptive psychiatrists, including Jaspers. The separation of the social effects of a symptom from the symptom itself is also a necessary part of the assessment process. Further comments on this and related issues have been made by Post(2) and by McHugh and Slavney.(3)

Categories of information: subjective, objective, and scientific

Is there such a thing as a truly objective account of events? If 'objective' is intended to mean absolutely true and independent of all observers, the answer must be negative. Students and trainee psychiatrists often come to psychiatric clinical work from medical and surgical disciplines where they have been encouraged to 'search for the facts' with the implication that 'true' facts exist. They may need to be reminded that the supposed facts of all medical histories, even those of clearly physical illnesses, depend upon the perceptions, opinions, and memories of individuals who may give different versions of the same events at different times.

'Objective' has several shades of meaning in ordinary usage, but in clinical assessment it's most useful meaning is that an account of an event or behaviour is based on agreement between two or more persons or sources. In contrast, 'subjective' can be used to indicate that the account comes from only one person. Objective information is likely to be safer to act upon than subjective, so efforts should always be put into raising as much as possible of the information about a patient into the objective category. Nevertheless, many of the most important symptoms in psychiatry can only be subjective, since they refer to the inner experience of the one person who can describe them.

When assessing the reliability and usefulness of other types of information, such as the results of treatment or possible explanations of causes, a further useful distinction can be made between objective defined as above and 'scientific', taking this to mean that systematic efforts have been made to obtain evidence based upon comparisons (or 'controls') which demonstrate that one explanation can be preferred out of several possibilities that have been considered.

Simple definitions such as these are useful in clinical discussions, but it must be remembered that in the background are many complicated and unsolved problems of philosophy and semantics. Some of these suggestions on the status of information in clinical work are based upon the writings and clinical teaching of Kraupl Taylor.(4)

Disease, illness, and sickness

These concepts have existed in the medical and sociological literature for many years, and are best regarded as useful but inexact concepts that refer to different but related aspects of the person affected, namely pathology (disease), personal experience (illness), and social consequences (sickness), respectively.(5) They are useful as a trio because they serve as a reminder that all three levels should be considered in a clinical assessment, even though for different patients they will vary greatly in relative importance. There are no simple answers to questions about how they are best defined and how exactly they are related to each other, but time spent on these issues is not wasted because they reflect quite naturally some of the different interests and priorities of the different health professions (and are therefore often the basis of different viewpoints put forward by various members of a multi-disciplinary team).

Another reason for being familiar with these concepts is that in legal and administrative settings, simple and categorical pronouncements about the presence of mental illness or mental disease and their causes and effects may be required whatever the medical viewpoint might be about the complexity of these concepts.

Clinicians of any medical discipline know from everyday experience that the complete sequence of disease—illness—sickness does not apply to many patients. Although disease usually causes the patient to feel ill and the state of illness then usually interferes with many personal and social activities, in practice there are many exceptions. Potentially serious physical, biochemical, or physiological abnormalities (disease) may be discovered in surveys of apparently healthy persons before any symptoms, distress, or interference with personal activities (illness) have developed, and some patients may have either or both of illness and sickness (interference with social activities) without any detectable disease.

A number of sociologists, anthropologists, and philosophers have joined psychiatrists in trying to define mental illness and mental health, but without achieving much clarification. Aubrey

Lewis[6] and Barbara Wootton,[7] although writing from the different contexts of clinical psychiatry and sociology, both arrived at the conclusion that neither mental illness nor mental health could be given precise definitions, although they are useful terms in everyday language (and the same applies equally to physical health and physical illness).

More positive conclusions have resulted from attempts to define disease, in that Scadding (a general physician) has suggested that it should be defined as an abnormality of structure or function that results in 'a biological disadvantage'.[8,9] This seems reasonable if one is dealing only with conditions that have a clear physical basis, but if applied in psychiatry it implies that, for instance, behaviours such as homosexuality that reduce the likelihood of reproduction would have to be regarded as diseases alongside infections, carcinoma, and suchlike. This seems to be stretching a traditional concept too far, and different approaches clearly need to be explored.

One way forward is to accept that simple definitions and concepts encompassed by one word cannot cope with complicated ideas such as disease or health, and to take care to differentiate between definitions of these as concepts in their own right, and attempts to develop **models of medical practice**. The debate noted above refers to concepts of health, disease, and disorder, and it has been continued more recently with respect to psychiatry in two quite extensive reviews, in terms of the types of concepts,[10] and of their possible contents.[11] What follows below is better regarded as about *models of medical practice*, and two points are suggested as a basis for the discussion. First, more than one dimension or aspect of the person affected always needs to be included in descriptions of health status. Second, models of medical practice and thinking do not necessarily have to start with the assumption that physical abnormalities (diseases) are the basic concept from which all others are derived.

Regarding the first point (of more than one aspect or dimension), soon after the contribution of Susser and Watson[5] noted above, Eisenberg, a psychiatrist with social and anthropological interests,[12] made a plea for all doctors, but particularly psychiatrists, to recognize the importance of appropriate illness behaviours in addition to giving the necessary attention to the diagnoses and treatment of serious and dangerous disorders.[13] He gave special emphasis to the need to minimize problems that may arise from discrepancies between disease as it is conceptualized by the physician and illness as it is experienced by the patient: 'when physicians dismiss illness because ascertainable disease is absent, they fail to meet their socially assigned responsibilities'. A similar model with a more overtly three-dimensional structure usually referred to as 'bio-psychosocial' has also been described by Engel.[14] and also by Susser.[15] Historically, all these can be regarded as variations on and explicit developments of a theme that has been accepted implicitly by generations of psychiatrists influenced by the 'psychobiology' of Adolf Meyer and his many distinguished pupils, manifest in the importance given to the construction of the traditional clinical formulation.

The second point, to do with the disease level not being the best starting point for conceptual models of medical practice, is of more recent and specifically psychiatric origin. Both Kraupl Taylor[16] and, more recently, Fulford[17] give detailed arguments for the conclusion that the illness experience of the patient is the most satisfactory starting point from which to develop a model of medical practice. Taylor presents his case as a matter of logic, and Fulford works through lengthy philosophical and ethical justifications. This new viewpoint has the virtue of starting with the encounter between patient and doctor, which has the strength of being one of the few things that is common to all types of clinical practice. In Taylor's terms, by describing symptoms and distress the patient arouses 'therapeutic concern' in the doctor and so first establishes 'patienthood'. Whether or not a diagnosis is reached or a disease is later found to be present, and whether or not the social activities of the patient are also interfered with, are other issues of great importance, but they do not diminish the primary importance of the first interaction; in this, both patient and doctor play their appropriate roles according to their personal, social, cultural, and scientific backgrounds.

If medical training and practice are guided by this model, there is no interference with the essential obligation of the doctor to identify and treat any serious disease that may be present. However, a parallel obligation to satisfy the patient and family that the illness (comprising complaints and distress) and the sickness (interference with activities) have also been recognized and will be given attention, is equally clear.

How to answer questions by the patient and family about whether the patient has a mental illness or not, and what this implies, needs careful discussion. Within a multi-disciplinary team it is usually best for the team to reach early agreement on a particular way of describing the patient's illness so that conflicting statements will not be made inadvertently by different members if asked about it. This is because the patient or family may expect this type of statement, and not because distinctions between, for instance, mental illness and physical illness, or between nervous illness and emotional upset, are regarded as fundamental from a psychiatric viewpoint. This difficult issue will be made easier if something about the patient's ideas about the nature and implications of terms such as 'mental illness' and 'nervous breakdown' is always included as part of the initial assessment information. Similarly, all members of the team need to be familiar with the concept of illness behaviour and the way this is determined by cultural influences[18] (see Chapter 2.6.2).

The diagnostic process: disorders and diagnoses

Psychiatrists learn during their general medical training that the search for a diagnosis underlying the presenting symptoms is one of the central purposes of medical assessment. This is because if an underlying cause can be found, powerful and logically based treatments may be available. But even in general medicine, as Scadding pointed out 'the diagnostic process and the meaning of the diagnosis which emerges are subject to great variation . . . the diagnosis which is the end-point of the process may state no more than the resemblance of the symptoms and signs to a previously recognized pattern'.[8,9] In psychiatry, 'may' becomes 'usually', and this has been recognized by the compilers of both ICD-10 and DSM-IV, in that these are presented not as classifications of diagnoses, but of disorders. These classifications use similar definitions of a disorder; the key phrases in ICD-10 are 'the existence of a clinically recognizable set of symptoms or behaviour associated in most cases with distress and with interference with personal functions', and in DSM-IV 'a clinically significant behavioural or psychological syndrome or pattern that occurs in an individual and that is associated with present distress or disability . . . '.

The use of such broad definitions is necessary because of the present limited knowledge of the causes of most psychiatric disorders, and a similarly limited understanding of processes that underlie their constituent symptoms. To avoid overoptimistic assumptions, there is much to be said for psychiatrists avoiding the use of the term 'diagnosis' except for the comparatively small minority of instances in which it can be used in the strict sense of indicating knowledge of something underlying the symptoms. A consequence of this viewpoint is that the currently used 'diagnostic criteria' in both these classifications should be relabelled as 'criteria for the identification of disorders'.

In spite of this, it must be accepted that the patient and family are likely to expect statements to be made about the cause of their distress and symptoms. The members of all human groups expect their healers to discover the causes of their misfortunes (i.e. to make a diagnosis), and to provide remedies. This is so whether the group is a sophisticated and scientifically oriented modern society, or a non-industrialized society that relies on ethnic healers and folk remedies. The obvious relief of a patient or family on the pronouncement of an 'official' diagnosis is often evident in any type of healing activity, even though the diagnostic terms themselves mean very little. The pronouncement of an official diagnosis is taken to show that the doctor knows what is wrong, and therefore will be able to provide successful treatment or advice. If the diagnosis is expressed in terms that the patient can understand, it will have additional power as an explanatory force.

The readiness of ethnic healers and practitioners of complementary (or alternative) medicine to provide a diagnosis and treatment in terms that have a meaning and therefore a powerful appeal to their customers is probably one of the main reasons for their continued survival and popularity alongside scientifically based medicine. This is a separate issue from the question of whether or not the treatments of complementary practitioners are successful in the sense of having effects that could be demonstrated by means of a controlled clinical trial.

Within psychiatry and clinical psychology, the medical habit of searching for a diagnosis has at times been misunderstood as an unjustified preoccupation with the presence of physical disease as a cause of mental disorders. This was most marked in the United States during the 1950s and 1960s, expressed particularly in the writings of Menninger in which the diagnostic process and attempts to classify patients were dismissed as a waste of time.[19] This viewpoint ignores two points made here and by many others; first, the choice of a diagnostic term is only one part of the overall process of assessment that leads also to a personal formulation. Second, any assessment of a person, whether made as statements about psychodynamic processes, as statements about structural and biochemical abnormalities, or as statements about interference with activities, is unavoidably an act of classification of some sort.

More detailed discussions about the importance of diagnosis have been provided by Scadding[8] as a general physician, and by Kendell[20] and Cooper.[21] as psychiatrists.

Concepts of disablement

Disablement will be used here as an overall term to cover any type of interference with activities by illness. This is often of more concern to the patient than the symptoms of the illness itself, since the fear of long-term dependence upon others is usually present, even though not voiced in the early stages. The question arises whether to leave the description and assessment of disablement to different members of the team as it arises in various forms, or whether in addition to encourage reference to one of the systematic descriptive schemes that are now available. Even if not used as fully as their authors intend, these have the merit of serving as checklists or reminders for the whole team, to ensure that the many different effects of the illness have been considered.

Two widely used descriptive schema are the *International Classification of Functioning, Disability and Health* (*ICF*),[22] and a broadly similar framework described by Nagi[23] that is often used in the United States, particularly by neurologists. These are best regarded as descriptive conceptual frameworks rather than classifications, sharing a basic structure of several levels of concepts. For the ICIDH, these are **functioning**, **disability**, and the **contextual factors (both environmental and personal)** relevant to what is being assessed. These terms and concepts are defined in the manuals published by WHO Geneva. The ICF is published as both a short and a long version, and it is probably wise for interested users to start by examining the short version. As noted in Fig. 1.8.1.1, these three concepts can be put alongside the sequence of ideas that leads from complaints, through symptoms to the identification of disorders or diagnoses. This may represent a causal sequence in some individuals, and this is clearest in acute physically based illnesses. But for many patients encountered in psychiatric practice, whose illnesses often have prominent social components, causal relationships may be absent or even in the opposite direction. For instance, sudden bereavement, i.e. loss of a social relationship, may be the clear cause of interference with the ability to perform daily activities (disability), and also of uncontrolled weeping (an impairment of the normal control of emotions). Social handicaps can also be imposed unjustifiably by other persons, as when a patient who is partly or fully recovered from long-standing psychiatric illness and quite able to work is refused employment due to the prejudice of a potential employer.

Many mental health workers find that to use a scheme such as Fig. 1.8.1.1 or the ICF helps to clarify how different aspects of a patient's problems fit together. Similarly, the different members of the team may be able to see more clearly how their activities with the patient and family complement one another, since the different concepts in the framework correspond approximately with the interests of different health disciplines. Social workers will focus on assessment of work and social relationships, occupational therapists will have a special expertise in the assessment of daily activities, and clinical psychologists are skilled in the assessment of cognitive and other psychological functions. Researchers in the various health disciplines have naturally devised rating scales that reflect their own interests and ideas, independently of the ICF or other overall schema, but it is usually found that such scales correspond quite closely with one or other of the concepts just discussed. The reluctance of both researchers and clinicians to adopt a standard set of terms to cover the various levels or concepts continues to be a problem; the reader needs to be aware that the terms impairment, disability, and handicap are often used synonymously by different authors.

The description of social and interpersonal relationships is in principle included in comprehensive schemas such as the ICF and that of Nagi, but many separate instruments that cover relationships in great detail have been devised over the years by psychotherapists, family therapists, and others.[24–26]

The sequence of assessment: collection, analysis, synthesis, and review

As information accumulates and is discussed, several different but related aspects of the patient and the illness have to be kept in mind. Good psychiatric practice is a part of what is sometimes referred to as 'whole-person medicine' in which at different times the contrasting but complementary processes of both analysis and synthesis of the information available will be needed. The patient must be seen both as an individual with a variety of attributes, abilities, problems, and experiences, and as a member of a group that is subject to family, social, and cultural influences; at different stages in the process of assessment each of these aspects will need separate consideration.

Analysis is needed to identify those attributes, experiences, and problems of the patient and the family that might require specific interventions by different members of the team. This must then be followed by several types of synthesis (or bringing together of information) to enable attempts to understand both subjective and objective relationships between the patient and the illness. First, possible interventions must be placed in order of priority for action. Second, the whole programme needs to be reviewed at intervals so as to assess progress and decide about any additional interventions that are required. At these times of review, and particularly towards the end of the whole episode of illness, global statements about 'overall improvement', or changes in 'quality of life' may be additional useful ways of summarizing and evaluating what has been happening from the viewpoint of the patient.

From complaints to formulation

Figure 1.8.1.1 demonstrates how the information contained in the complaints presented by the patient needs to be sorted out into different conceptual categories so that it can form the basis of actions by the various members of the multi-disciplinary team.

The top box represents the complaints. Unpleasant symptoms are likely to head the list, but inability to do everyday activities or a description of problems with relationships may well come first. Symptoms that give a clue to disorders, diagnoses, and possible treatments may not be identified without close questioning by someone who knows what to ask about.

The second box indicates that the complaints need to be sorted out into symptoms and impairments (an impairment in this sense is interference with a normal physiological or psychological function, as explained below). Some complaints are both symptoms and impairments: symptoms because it is known that they can contribute towards the recognition of an underlying diagnosis or towards the identification of a disorder, and impairments because they indicate measurable interference with the function of a part of the body or of a particular organ. For instance, inability to remember the time of the day is a symptom (disorientation in time) that may contribute towards a diagnosis of some kind of dementia. It is also an impairment of cognitive functioning that is likely to interfere with the performance of everyday activities such as getting up and going to bed at the correct time, and organizing housework.

The left-hand side of Fig. 1.8.1.1 represents the progress towards the identification of a disorder and perhaps even an underlying diagnosis. These are important concepts because they may indicate useful treatments and likely eventual outcomes. The right-hand side shows the progression from impairment of functions of parts of the body or organs, through interference with personal and daily activities to interference with participation in social activities.

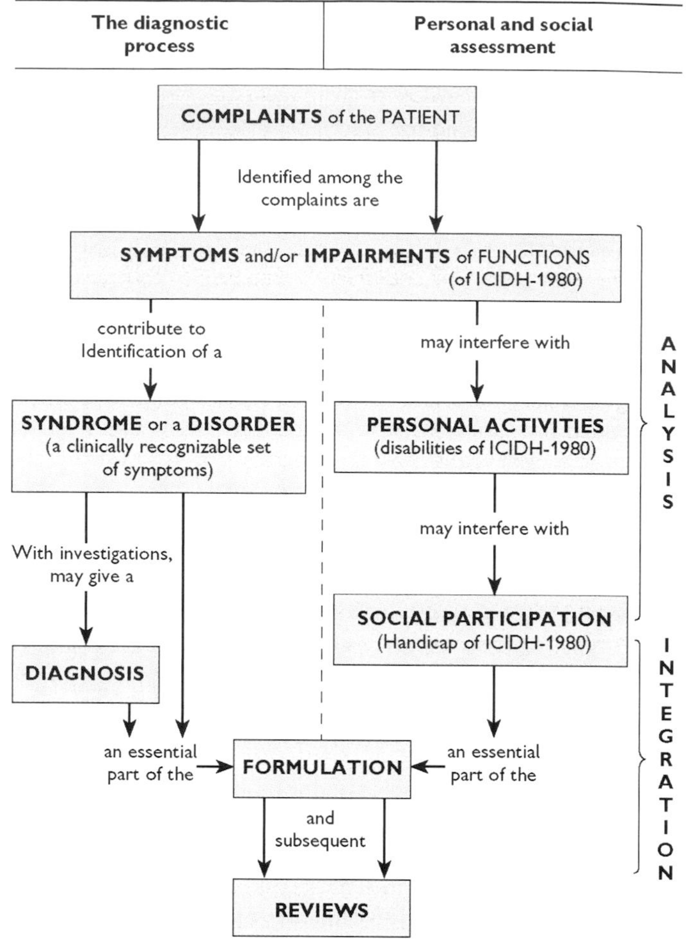

Fig. 1.8.1.1 Analysis and integration of information.

A clinical assessment is not complete until all the components of both sides of Fig. 1.8.1.1 have been considered. In doing this, the different components and the two pathways of concepts will need to be given widely varying emphasis for different patients, and also for the same patient at different times. For instance, if there is a physical cause for a disturbance of behaviour, an accurate diagnosis of this will lead to the best possible chance of rapid and successful treatment. In contrast, if a disturbance of social behaviour has its origin in personal relationships or has been imposed upon the patient by the social prejudices of others, the correct diagnostic category is unlikely to add much. An assessment of social networks and supportive relationships will be more relevant to deciding upon useful actions.

Life events and illness

For clarity, the right-hand side of Fig. 1.8.1.1 is given in a very compressed form, but in practice it is likely to need dividing into several components. The possibility of discovering relationships in time between life events and the onset of symptoms or interference with activities, particularly if repeated, should always be kept in mind, since this may be relevant to management plans and the assessment of prognosis. The best guide to this will be a lifechart. The opinions of patients and families about the causes of illness must be listened to with respect, while bearing in mind that the attribution of illness to the effects of unpleasant experiences is a more or less universal human assumption that often has no logical justification. Clinicians have to arrive at their own conclusions about such relationships by means of experience, common sense, and some acquaintance with research findings. Researchers seeking robust evidence on this topic are faced with a very difficult task, since the assessment of vulnerability to life events is a surprisingly complicated and controversial issue. The leading method in this field is the Life Events and Difficulties Schedule developed by Brown and Harris; a bulky training manual has to be mastered during a special course, and this then serves as a guide to an interview which may last for several hours. The length and detail of these procedures illustrate well the technical and conceptual problems that have to be faced.[27–29]

Psychodynamics and the life story

'Psychodynamics' refers in a general sense to the interactions between discrete life events, personal relationships, and personality attributes, in addition to its use to cover internal psychological processes (such as defence mechanisms and coping strategies). All of these need to be examined when trying to understand which of several possible causes of an illness at a particular time is the most likely.

A mixture of knowledge about local social and cultural influences and more technical psychological issues is needed for this appraisal of the patient's life story, and suggestions about different components of the overall pattern may well come from different members of the team.

The internal psychodynamics of the patient often need to be considered in detail, and one way to do this would be to construct a subdivision of the right-hand side of Fig. 1.8.1.1 to show interpersonal relationships and psychodynamic processes. In some patients a major conclusion of the initial assessment will be that these aspects are paramount, indicating the need for referral to a specialist psychotherapy service. The assessment of suitability for specific forms of psychotherapy and cognitive behavioural approaches are dealt with in section 6.

Contextual influences on assessment procedures

The place of assessment should not be regarded as automatically fixed in the outpatient or other clinical premises. One or more assessment interviews at home should be considered,[30] since the patient and family may feel much more at ease and therefore likely to express themselves more freely in familiar surroundings, but with the proviso that privacy may be more difficult to achieve. The assessor will often be surprised how much useful information about the home and family circumstances is gained from an interview at home, even when there appeared to be no special reason for this at first. In addition, the behaviour of both the patient and family members in the clinic or hospital is often different from that observed in familiar home surroundings. There are also obvious advantages to both assessment and care at home for mothers who have psychiatric disorders in the puerperium.[31]

Interviews on primary care premises are also often appreciated by patients who dislike going to hospitals of any sort, and the ease of consultation with the general practitioner is an additional advantage. The adoption of regular visits by a consultant psychiatrist to primary care premises as a major element in cooperation between psychiatrists and general practitioners is a style of work that seems to be spreading, with advantages to all concerned.[32]

Privacy of interviewing and **confidentiality** of what is discussed needs careful consideration; there are few absolute rules, but the following points of procedure should be explained clearly to both patient and relatives from the start. First, the patient and any member of the family should know that if they wish they are entitled to speak to the doctor in private, and they must be able to feel that what they say will not be conveyed to any other member of the family unless they request this. Second, in addition to the usual rules of professional secrecy, the patient must agree not to question other family members about what they said to the doctor, and vice versa. These may seem to be elementary points to trained professionals, but they are often not appreciated by patients or relatives who may be in fear of each other, or at least apprehensive about the reaction of the other on learning that statements they might construe as critical have been made about them. These are all points by which trust is established and maintained between patient and doctor, and for the same reason any attempts by relatives to seek interviews on condition that the occasion is kept secret from the patient should be firmly resisted.

An interpreter should always be sought if the patient cannot speak fluently in the language of the interviewer. Mental health professionals who can also act as interpreters are increasingly available nowadays due to the presence of almost all communities of sizeable ethnic minorities. Because of the issues of confidentiality noted above, a professional of the same sex as the patient should always be preferred to family members when interpretation is needed.

Language barriers are usually, but not always, accompanied by a cultural difference. The interviewer must remember that the concept of a private interview between two strangers in which personal and often unpleasant events and experiences are discussed freely comes from 'middle-class western' culture, and is not necessarily shared by persons from other cultures. A discussion of this point before the interview with a mental health professional familiar with the patient's background will help the interviewer to determine what to aim at in terms of intimate or possibly distressing information.

Multiple sources of information are always an advantage for those topics (mainly events) for which objective accounts are possible. Clinical experience is the best guide as to which account to use when conflicts of information arise. Serious conflicts of information arising during the initial assessment that involve the patient's account of events are best resolved by trying to obtain more information. Confrontation of the patient with important conflicts of information should be avoided since it easily leads to misunderstandings. If done at all, confrontation should be reserved for later stages in the overall management when it forms part of a planned intervention with a special purpose.

Assessment as a multi-disciplinary activity

Multi-disciplinary teams can take many forms, varying from the tightly organized and necessarily hierarchical surgical theatre team in which the role of each member is clearly defined and unchanging, to loosely knit groups in other types of health service in which only some of those attending meetings about patients regard what is taking place as a team event. For the purposes of discussion of the types of multi-disciplinary teamwork increasingly to be found in the mental health services, it is useful to differentiate between multi-disciplinary practice, familiar to many generations of mental health workers, and the more recently evolved multi-disciplinary teamwork. Both of these styles of work have many variations, but they both have some key features that need to be recognized by those involved.

In **multi-disciplinary practice** the consultant or most senior doctor present at clinical meetings or 'ward rounds' is accepted by all as the leader of the group, and listens to (and usually depends upon) the views of the senior nurses and other health professionals who may or may not be present. But the decisions about treatment and management are clearly acknowledged to be the responsibility of the doctors present. In most settings the only essential attendees at these meetings are the doctors and nurses; attendance of other health professionals is usually welcomed and valued, but they are not regarded as necessary members of the group.

Multi-disciplinary teamwork has probably developed in response to a marked increase in the number of social workers, occupational therapists, clinical psychologists, and others, in those medical services in which patients and families with multiple needs are the rule rather than the exception. Clinical skills and techniques that were not previously available are now available, and the health professionals offering these expect quite naturally to be given increased personal and professional recognition; this can usually be found as a member of a multi-disciplinary team of the sort described here. The most fully developed style of multi-disciplinary teamwork involves a very significant commitment of professional time by each member so that all the team meetings can be attended, in addition to the time spent directly with the patient and family.

Some sharing of responsibilities and blurring of roles is needed, but each member also must be seen as retaining the professional skills of their parent discipline. Role blurring is most obvious in the information-gathering and information-sharing phases of assessment, and in the team discussions that lead to agreement about the content of a programme of activities.

Leadership

The concept of a team implies that a team leader is recognized, but a leader does not have to be an obviously dominant speaker and decision maker. Many successful team leaders 'lead from behind' to great effect and to everyone's satisfaction. The main reasons for having an agreed leader are, first, to keep discussions acceptably brief and to a practical timetable; second, to facilitate decisions between reasonable alternatives; and third, to arbitrate when insoluble disagreements arise between team members.

There are a number of settings within the mental health services in which there may be no need for the leader for everyday purposes to be a doctor. This occurs most frequently in special crisis intervention and emergency units, in rehabilitation units, and in services for those with mental retardation. However, members of such teams have to acknowledge that decisions about the presence of physical illness, and the need for medication or laboratory investigations, can only be made by a medically qualified person. The team then has to accept the authority of the doctor on these occasions because of the unique ethical and legal responsibilities that accompany a medical qualification.

In teams running an inpatient unit such as an acute admission ward, there is a clear need for the whole team to accept that medical and nursing members have free access to all the patients for purposes of physical examination, laboratory investigations, the administration of medication, and a variety of nursing procedures.

Key workers and the planning of care

The allocation of a team member as key worker (or case manager) for each patient being assessed is the usual method of work in teams of this sort. Which member becomes key worker for which patient depends upon the ability of the team to match the needs of each patient with the skills available amongst the team members, according to their training. Although all patients are discussed in detail at team meetings, and any team member can contribute suggestions and viewpoints, it is usually accepted that once a programme of activities is identified and agreed upon, most if not all of the contacts with the patient and family will be made by the key worker. The key worker also has the responsibility of reporting back to the team about progress, and about problems encountered which might require new major decisions or changes in the programme.

In the United Kingdom, due to yet another recent reorganization of primary care and hospital services, the situation with respect to urgent assessments and psychiatric emergencies has recently become complicated. Fundamental structural changes are taking place as a result of administrative and financial pressures rather than because of evidence from studies of the previous pattern of services. There is, however, now an element common to all areas in that the provision of a written plan for the care proposed is now a statutory responsibility for all patients. Further changes seem likely, and it is beyond the remit of the general principles of assessment described here to try to describe the present situation in the United Kingdom in detail. Reviews by Burns[(33)] and others[(34)] are very helpful guides through the complexities and terms used to cover some of these developments in the United Kingdom.

In addition to the specific medical responsibilities noted above, psychiatrists as members of a multi-disciplinary team have other important areas of expertise that should be recognized by the other members. Experienced psychiatrists are likely to have special skills in the assessment of dangerousness and risks of various sorts, and psychiatrists at any stage in their training should be able to show that they are specially trained to summarize information by the production of an overall *formulation* that reflects the agreed policies of the team.

To be an efficient and accepted long-term member of a multi-disciplinary team of this type requires personal characteristics not necessarily possessed by all mental health professionals. Tolerance of the different viewpoints of other team members is essential, in addition to the professional skills needed to carry-out the work required.

The frequency of team meetings is determined by the size and nature of the workload. Special meetings to discuss topics not directly related to the patients are also usually found to be necessary, so as to deal with issues such as team policies, recruitment and appointments, relationships with outside agencies (for instance about too few, too many, or inappropriate referrals), interpersonal problems between team members, and work-related stress in the team members. This last problem is particularly important in teams dealing with crisis intervention and psychiatric emergencies because of the need to maintain a rapid turnover of patients and families who are seen over only a limited period of time.

A different type of problem that may need sensitive handling by the team leader and others in authority outside the team itself is the relationship between the team members and their immediate superiors (or 'line managers') in the hierarchy of their own discipline. Each team member has to strike a balance between personal needs for professional supervision and training, and the ability to make decisions within the team because of special skills not possessed by other team members. This type of problem will be minimized if team members are comparatively senior and experienced within their parent discipline. Student health workers are not appropriate as team members, but they can benefit greatly if attached to the team as observers. They will have the opportunity to learn something about how other disciplines operate, which is an aspect of training usually absent from the rest of their training.

Disagreements often arise within a team about the best time for patients to be discharged from care, or about the precise time for referral when it is in the patient's interests to be assessed by another service. In countries where outpatient services and inpatient services are staffed by different teams under different organizations, there will be many such breaks in care, and multi-disciplinary teamwork can become frustrating. But where continuity of care between different parts of the general psychiatric services is the norm, the most frequent changes of care result from the need for the patient to be assessed for more specialized treatment such as rehabilitation, cognitive behavioural therapy, or intensive psychotherapy. The team needs to develop agreed policies for these occasions, and these will depend largely upon the structure of the local services available.

Although no systematic information is available, there is little doubt that the style of multi-disciplinary teamwork just described has become accepted in the mental health services in many countries. Its popularity and success are probably due to the recognition of multiple rather than single needs in a large proportion of psychiatric patients and families, plus an increased job satisfaction experienced by the non-medical team members. Multi-disciplinary styles of working are especially important in emergency psychiatric services and crisis intervention units.[35,36]

Instruments for assessment

Reasons for the development of structured interviewing and rating instruments

The training of all mental health professionals includes instruction in some system of information-gathering and recording based upon a conceptual structure that helps them to organize the large amount of information they usually need to collect. With training, the list of headings under which this information is collected becomes incorporated in the professional's mind as an automatically available guide to the conduct of assessment interviews. For research purposes, however, it is necessary to demonstrate overtly that the essential topics have been covered in a comprehensive and systematic manner. In many types of research not only the headings covered but the detailed items also need to be recorded so that others studying the results of the research can be confident that nothing was missed, and that the information obtained was not a biased selection of the total that might have been available. It has also been generally recognized since the 1950s that for purposes of communication between researchers in different centres, conclusions must be based upon information that has been shown to have a satisfactory inter-rater reliability.

With these aims in mind, detailed and comprehensive structured interviewing and rating schedules for recording many varieties of information have been developed (nowadays these are usually called 'instruments'; for brevity this term will be used to cover any sort of published interviewing and rating schedule). The most common types cover the present mental state and behaviour. Most of these instruments are not appropriate for use in everyday clinical work because they have been designed for research studies, but nevertheless it is useful for clinicians to know something about how they originated.[37]

Since the first appearance of partly or fully structured psychiatric rating instruments in the 1950s, there has been a steady increase in their number, type, and complexity. In the discussion that follows, some of the most widely used instruments are commented upon as examples but many others are available that are not mentioned. Comprehensive lists of such instruments can be found in catalogues of instruments and reviews by the WHO and others.[38–42]

A word of warning is needed about the use of these instruments in ordinary clinical work. Any of them can be used as useful checklists by clinicians to improve the range of information collected. But this does not mean that the quality of information recorded will necessarily be high. Most instruments were originally designed for use in research studies in which they were used by researchers specially trained in their use, and occasional use by untrained staff will not produce information of the same quality and usefulness.

Instruments for the assessment of mental state and behaviour

The instruments now available can be grouped according to the main purposes for which they were designed.

Screening instruments such as the General Health Questionnaire[43] are needed for the identification of likely cases or high-risk individuals amongst large populations. These tend to be short and economical in use, since they have to be administered to large numbers of subjects. They are designed to generate a simple score that indicates the status of the subject in relation to the populations upon which the instrument was developed and validated. This is essential for screening and for epidemiological studies, but this single score does not convey much about the details of the subject's feelings or behaviour, and so is of limited interest to the clinician.

Screening instruments are often questionnaires, defining this to mean that they are simply a means of recording the answers to a set of questions, without any further questions or enquiry about the extent to which the subject understands the question or wishes to qualify answers given. Questionnaires are usually filled in by the subject as a 'paper-and-pencil' exercise, as in the General Health Questionnaire, but one widely used questionnaire that has a very detailed content (the *Composite International Diagnostic Interview*[44,45]) is completed by an interviewer.

Detailed instruments may contain the following:

1 Symptoms of only one type, as in Hamilton's rating scale for depression,[46] or the Scale for Assessment of Negative Symptoms.[47]

2 A selection of symptoms for the study of the relationships between two closely related types, such as depressive and schizophrenic symptoms in the Schedule for Affective Disorders and Schizophrenia.[48]

3 A limited number of items covering different symptoms and behaviour selected as being of special importance, as in the recently developed Health of the Nation Scales of the United Kingdom.[49]

4 A more or less comprehensive array of symptoms that allows the study of the relative distribution of symptoms of many different types, such as Schedules for Clinical Assessment in Neuropsychiatry[50] and the Composite International Diagnostic Interview.[44,45] Other widely used but less tightly structured instruments with a comprehensive content are the Brief Psychiatric Rating Scale[51] and the Comprehensive Psychopathological Rating Scale,[52] aimed at measuring change.

The source and method for collection of information is usually specified by the designers of an instrument. These can include interviews with patients, relatives, and carers, observation of the patient, extracts from other documents, and any combination of these.

The more detailed instruments usually depend upon an interview, and the style of interviewing recommended and the training needed to achieve this depend upon both the quality of the information required and the type of research interviewer for whom the instrument is designed. These vary widely; for instance, Schedules for Clinical Assessment in Neuropsychiatry require a clinical professional training plus a special course for the instrument itself; the Comprehensive Psychopathological Rating scale, the Brief Psychiatric Rating scale, and the *Structured Clinical Interview for DSM*[53] assume a clinical professional training only. The Composite International Diagnostic Interview requires experience in interviewing such as market research plus a special course for the instrument itself, but no clinical professional training.

The time period covered varies from a cross-sectional picture of the present mental state and behaviour ('present' usually being taken to mean the immediately recent period of 2 or 4 weeks), to longer periods of follow-up, personal history, and development, and lifetime histories of psychiatric disorders. The more complicated and lengthy instruments that cover these longer periods are usually designed for particular studies, so are rarely suitable for general use.

Developments since the 1950s

A historical approach is helpful in trying to understand how and why the many instruments now available have developed. Hamilton's Rating Scale for Depression, published in 1959, is a good example of the first generation of instruments, most of which are comparatively short and simple.[46] Its contents can easily be printed on one page, and comprise the following:

1 the names of the symptoms to be rated

2 a rating scale, the same for all the symptoms, by which the presence or absence and the severity of each symptom is recorded

3 a box in which the rating of each symptom is placed

No special recommendations about length and style of interview are given, and no explanations or definitions of the symptoms are given other than what is provided on the rating sheet itself. In other words, the interpretation of the ratings is based on the assumption that the raters have sufficient experience and training to know what most of their contemporaries also mean by the named symptoms. Data analysis is left to the user, other than recommendations about the likely meaning of the sum of the ratings with respect to severity of illness and 'caseness'. This and other early instruments were not tied to the use of any particular set of diagnostic categories, probably because the diagnostic classifications that were available in the 1950s and 1960s were not widely used.

The first generation of instruments made it much easier for researchers to communicate the detailed results of their clinical studies to others, mainly by facilitating the study of changes in symptoms over comparatively short periods of time. The need for this was no doubt connected with the increasing numbers of psychotropic medicines that became available around that time. Measurement of change in symptoms is more immediately useful for the study of response to treatment than reliance upon statements about overall improvement or waiting for a change in diagnosis. But in the absence of guidance about how the symptoms are defined, problems still remain in the interpretation of the results.

Improvements in more recent instruments leading to better quality and meaning of the data they collect have been of two main types, in that the structure and the associated procedures of the instruments have become more elaborate as time has passed. First, the input has been improved by the provision of written descriptions and definitions of symptoms, and by recommending particular styles of interviewing. This implies that researchers using the instrument should carry-out preliminary training work so that satisfactory levels of inter-rater reliability are achieved before starting the main study. Second, the output has been improved by the use of computers to organize and summarize the symptom ratings, allied with the development of widely used psychiatric classifications.

Computer programs based upon decision trees (algorithms) first appeared in the 1970s, and are now commonplace. They allow the specification of sets of symptoms that identify disorders or indicate diagnoses, so that the resulting statements about symptom profiles or the presence of disorders or diagnoses are free from errors of human judgement such as carelessness, simple forgetting, and personal variations from one occasion to the next. But the biases and assumptions built into the programs by their authors still remain, and these may be a problem to others with different opinions.

Programs can also be written to assign disorders and diagnoses according to a selected classification, such as ICD-10 or DSM-IV, and some of the most recently developed instruments such as Schedules for Clinical Assessment in Neuropsychiatry and the Comprehensive International Diagnostic Interview are of this type. When used as intended, the data output from these more recent structured instruments is versatile and of high reliability, but to obtain these benefits the researcher has to pay the penalty of working hard to achieve and to maintain inter-rater reliability.

There are, of course, still plenty of uses for the simpler types of instruments; it is up to those designing and carrying out a study to decide what type of information they need and why, and to select their instruments accordingly. For the sake of those who will be interested in trying to interpret the results, a justification of the quality of the information obtained should always be included in the description of the findings.

Once an instrument (or often a related group of instruments) has demonstrated its usefulness it is likely to stay in use for many years, while at the same time being subject to extensions and improvements. Families of instruments and traditions of interviewing style therefore develop and persist in the major research centres and groups, and it is possible to identify some of these and follow them over the years.

Three such traditions of instrument development are selected for mention so as to illustrate the continuity and close relationships that sometimes exist between different instruments; these relationships may not be apparent from reports of studies in which they have been used. Three research centres that have produced particularly prominent sets of instruments are the Medical Research Council Social Psychiatry Unit at the Institute of Psychiatry in London, Biometrics Research at the New York State Psychiatric Institute at Columbia University, New York, and the Department of Psychiatry at Washington University, St Louis, Missouri. The instruments mentioned below are only a small proportion of the many in the literature, but they are well known because of their association with some large collaborative international research studies and with widely used classifications of psychiatric disorders such as ICD-8, ICD-9, and ICD-10, and DSM-III, DSM-IIIR, and DSM-IV.

At approximately the same time in the early 1960s, but independently, research groups headed by John Wing, at the Institute of Psychiatry of the University of London (at the Maudsley Hospital), and by Robert Spitzer, at the Biometrics Research Unit at the New York State Psychiatric Institute at Columbia University, began to produce structured interviewing and rating schedules that provided extensive coverage of symptoms and were accompanied by recommendations for training procedures.

The present state examination

The present state examination (**PSE**)[54] is a semi-structured procedure, based upon an interview schedule containing items that are rated as the interview proceeds. The content of the PSE has always been more or less comprehensive and it contains a number of symptoms, such as worry, muscular tension, restlessness, etc. that are not associated with particular diagnoses. These symptoms are included because they are often clinically obvious and also important to the patient (see comments below on 'bottom-up' and 'top-down' organization of interview schedules).

The ratings made by the interviewer do not depend entirely upon the immediate reply of the subject, but represent the interviewer's clinical judgement as to whether or not the subject has the symptoms as described in the glossary of definitions learned during the interview training. Questions are provided for all the symptoms and items and are used whenever possible in the order provided, but the order may be varied if the interviewer thinks fit. The interviewer is also encouraged to ask any other questions that seem relevant to determine the timing, frequency, and severity of the symptoms, as in an ordinary clinical interview. In other words, the interviewer aims to conduct a clinical interview that has been structured as much as possible so as to allow symptoms to be rated with high inter-rater reliability, but without seeming to be unpleasantly rigid to either the subject or the interviewer. Much practice and training are required before these aims can be achieved, but there is no doubt that it is possible.

The PSE was not developed with any particular diagnostic classification in mind. It was intended from the start simply to be a means of arriving at a comprehensive and defined set of symptoms described in a reliable manner, with the user being left to decide whether and how to condense the symptoms into groups and what to do with the results. This is sometimes referred to as a 'bottom-up' style of instrument organization. Versions 7 and 8 of the PSE were first used on a large scale in two studies that involved international collaboration and comparisons, namely the United States–United Kingdom Diagnostic Project between London and New York,[55,56] and the International Pilot Study of Schizophrenia coordinated by the WHO, Geneva.[57] Since then its content has been revised and extended as versions 9 and 10, but the techniques of interviewing and rating remain the same. PSE-10 is one of the main components of Schedules for Clinical Assessment in Neuropsychiatry.

Schedule for affective disorders and schizophrenia, and the structured clinical interview for DSM

The series of instruments developed by Spitzer and his colleagues at Biometrics of the New York State Psychiatric Institute have been of several different kinds and, in the early years at least, had a much more rigid structure than the PSE. Users of the Mental Status Schedule and the longer Psychiatric Status Schedule were instructed to follow the order of the questions as printed in the schedule, the only deviation from this being a repetition of the same questions if thought necessary by the interviewer. However, later instruments such as the Schedule for Affective Disorders and Schizophrenia[48] and, more recently, the Structured Clinical Interview for DSM-III and DSM-IV[53] allow more flexibility for the interviewer in both interview style and the choice of a little or a lot of training (despite its length, the Structured Clinical Interview for DSM is recommended for clinical use as well as for research). There has also been an increasing tendency for instruments from the New York group to be dedicated to a particular purpose. For instance, the content of the Schedule for Affective Disorders and Schizophrenia is keyed towards the study of relationships between schizophrenia and affective disorders, and the Structured Clinical Interview for DSM contains only those items that are necessary for identifying disorders present in the corresponding DSM. Like the Diagnostic Interview Schedule mentioned in the next section, the Schedule for Affective Disorders and Schizophrenia and the Structured Clinical Interview for DSM have a 'top-down' structure, meaning that their content is determined from the start by an already existing set of criteria or symptoms.

The instruments produced by these two centres in the 1960s and 1970s have been used widely in many countries, and their success led to the production of many similar instruments by other researchers. The adoption of the PSE for use by the WHO in a number of international collaborative studies also led to its being translated into more than 25 languages, with varying but never extensive degrees of adaptation to fit the different cultures and social settings involved.

The diagnostic interview schedule

The third major research group is based at Washington University, St Louis, Missouri, and is well known as the originator of the first widely used sets of *Diagnostic Criteria for Research*.[58] Following the publication of DSM-III in 1980, there was considerable interest in discovering how the disorders it contained were distributed in the American population. Supported by the National Institute of Mental Health, Lee Robins and her colleagues designed the Diagnostic Interview Schedule (**DIS**)[59] for this purpose. This is composed of questions covering the symptoms required to identify what were considered to be the 15 most important disorders in DSM-III. The Epidemiological Catchment Area study of the National Institute of Mental Health, the very large study in which the DIS was first used, included a population sample of more than 18 000 subjects in five largely urban areas.[60]

So as to avoid the costs and other problems involved in employing trained psychiatrists or psychologists as interviewers, the DIS was designed as a highly structured questionnaire administered as an interview by lay interviewers. The interviewers, usually already experienced in interviewing for market research, had to undergo a week-long intensive training course on the DIS. The DIS questions must be given in the order printed in the schedule. Possible symptoms are not rated as present if in the opinion of the subject they may be due to physical disorders, but there is no free questioning about timing, severity, and other details of the symptoms. Questions may be repeated, but only questions provided in the schedule may be asked of the subject. This is a very different concept from that of the PSE technique, and it is based upon the assumption made by the designers of the DIS that by controlling the interviewer in this way, the DIS would 'enable the interviewer to obtain psychiatric diagnoses comparable to those a psychiatrist would obtain'.[60] Put in another way, this is an assumption that expressed complaints can be used as near equivalents of inferred symptoms for the purposes of identifying psychiatric disorders.

Schedules of clinical assessment for neuropsychiatry and the composite international diagnostic interview

Although originating from different groups with different traditions and purposes, the PSE and the DIS have now given rise to direct descendants, namely the Schedules of Clinical Assessment for Neuropsychiatry (**SCAN**) and the Composite International Diagnostic Interview (**CIDI**), that are closely connected. During the early 1980s, a collaborative programme of work between WHO and the National Institute of Mental Health of the United States (known as the Joint Project) resulted in the transformation of DIS into CIDI[61] by increasing its contents by adding large parts of first DSM-IIIR and then of the drafts of ICD-10 and DSM-IV. This was matched by the evolution of PSE-9 into PSE-10, the centrepiece of SCAN,[50] whose content similarly covers almost all of both ICD-10 and DSM-IV. The only sections of ICD-10 and DSM-IV not now covered by SCAN and CIDI are those dealing with disorders of adult personality, disorders of childhood and adolescence, and mental retardation.

The coordination by WHO of the development of the final stages of SCAN and CIDI has been aimed at the production of two instruments with different but complementary uses in epidemiological studies. CIDI can be administered to comparatively large numbers of subjects in the community since the use of lay interviewers keeps costs to a minimum. SCAN is more suitable for the professional (and therefore more expensive) assessment of subjects with obvious or severe disorders, whether these have been selected from a larger population by means of CIDI or other screening instruments, or whether they are being studied clinically for other reasons. The latest development in this long-term programme has been the establishment of WHO-sponsored training centres in a number of countries. Psychiatrists and other mental health professionals can now obtain the necessary training for both SCAN and CIDI in English, French, German, Spanish, Chinese, Japanese, and Arabic.[61]

These and other instruments will no doubt be developed further, but every new instrument and every change to an existing one carries with it problems of data interpretation. Even though the content of changed or new instruments may seem to be the same as their predecessors, quite small changes in the method or the sequence of questions may have important effects, particularly for highly structured instruments in which the ratings are not filtered through the clinical judgement of a trained mental health professional. For instance, a recent report from the United States[62] discusses the possibility that the differences in prevalence rates for some disorders found between the Epidemiological Catchment Area study[60] and the more recent Co-morbidity Study[63] are due at least in part to changes in the 'stem questions' that introduce other specific questions rather than being due to real differences in the community subjects.

There are also unsolved problems in the study of individuals in the community, who have not sought professional help, by means of instruments originally designed for the study of psychiatric patients already in contact with services. To fulfil the criteria for a psychiatric disorder does not necessarily indicate a need for treatment, since the assessment of 'caseness' requires more than a simple count of symptoms. The debate about this problem has now stretched over 20 years, but needs to continue,[64,65] together with further examination of the closely related topic of clinical validity.[66]

Other selected issues

The importance of **negative symptoms** in the assessment of individuals with schizophrenic syndromes has led to the development of instruments devoted to these symptoms; the Scale for the Assessment of Negative Symptoms[47] is one of the most widely used, particularly in the United States. The Psychological Impairments Rating Scale (WHO/PIRS)[67] has been found to be acceptable in a variety of cultural settings, and has been used in several large international collaborative studies coordinated by the WHO. Both these instruments and a variety of others are useful as checklists for ordinary clinical purposes.[68] However, because of the nature of the symptoms being assessed, most of them are still beset with significant problems about inter-rater reliability and the exact meaning of their constituent items.

The **assessment of personality** poses special problems because to obtain a satisfactory account of a individual's personality, however the concept is defined, requires much more than the views of that individual; additional accounts of personal development and relationships from relatives or close friends are needed for comparison. Current concepts of personality disorders as listed in ICD-10 and DSM-IV also have serious limitations; the problems are well illustrated by a recent large international collaborative study coordinated by the WHO, using the International Personality Disorder Examination (IPDE).[61] Several hours of skilled interviewing are required, with at least two informants, to cover the content of the items that are needed to identify the disorders of adult personality contained in both the above classifications.

This study and others with similar aims have found that if an individual fulfils the criteria for one disorder of personality, they are quite likely to fulfil the criteria for at least one more. This implies that the present categories reflect only parts of the overall personality; this may be quite useful, but a fairly drastic overhaul of the currently used categories is clearly needed.

Clinically, it is useful to assess three aspects of personality, according to the salience of personal characteristics and problems arising from them. First, one or more of the personality disorders described in ICD-10 or DSM-IV should be used only if there are quite clear accounts of repeated problems and behaviours as specified, and they are not due to symptoms of any other disorders that may be present. Second, for less severe but repeated problems and behaviours, the concept of 'accentuated personality type' is often useful, described simply by a short list of ordinary adjectives. These indicate recurring behaviours and attitudes likely to cause a variety of mild interpersonal or social problems, again not attributable to symptoms of other disorders. Finally, even though neither of these first two types of personality disturbance is present, it is always worthwhile describing the usual characteristics of the patient by means of a few adjectives (such as 'a worrier', somewhat shy and socially inhibited, definitely gregarious, etc.). Vaguely optimistic terms commonly offered by friends and relatives, such as 'happy-go-lucky', should be avoided.

Multiaxial descriptive systems (often optimistically called classifications) have been available for many years,[69] and now apply to both ICD-10 and DSM-IV. Multiaxial systems describe several aspects of the person in addition to the disorder, and can be regarded as providing a systematized formulation that facilitates the coded recording of several aspects of the person concerned. Most of them have been designed more for research than for everyday clinical use, but they can all serve as very useful checklists when preparing for clinical reviews. DSM-IV, like DSM-III, is presented as a multiaxial scheme covering five aspects of the subject (Axis I, clinical disorders; Axis II, personality disorders and mental retardation; Axis III, General Medical Conditions; Axis IV, Psychosocial and Environmental Problems; Axis V, Global Assessment of Functioning). Similar instruments are now available for ICD-10,[70] covering general adult psychiatry and the psychiatry of childhood and adolescence (see Chapter 1.9 and 9.1.1).

Quality of life has come to the fore in recent years, but in the same way as for multiaxial assessment, to use this term does no more than make explicit something that has always been implicit in a good clinical assessment. Examination of the content of the many assessment instruments that are now available with this title shows that they contain various mixtures of almost every possible attribute of the person, the illness, and the environment. There is no point in using a new term when the information collected refers only to already familiar problems such as symptoms, disablements, how the patient's time is occupied, and contacts with medical services. There is even a considerable literature on the 'quality of life' of whole communities and countries, in which indices are calculated from national or regional statistics about, for instance, standards of housing, education, transport, and consumption of material resources. Such indices are of value to economists and demographers, but are far removed from clinical assessments. There is much to be said for using the term in clinical work only when it indicates 'higher-level' value-judgements and concepts such as personal satisfaction, self-fulfilment, and freedom from distress. Most of these are subjective and difficult to measure, but in many ways they reflect the ultimate aims of all medical care. An excellent recent review of this topic from the viewpoint of psychiatry is available,[71] which illustrates well the wide range of subjects now covered by the term.

Service research into the closely related **needs assessment** has resulted in the production of some detailed instruments that, again, are of interest to clinicians largely as potential checklists. A good example from the United Kingdom is the MRC Needs for Care Assessment.[72]

Administrative pressure to provide some sort of **quantification of clinical outcome** has resulted in several comparatively brief instruments designed for clinical use. Two widely used examples are the Global Assessment of Functioning (**GAF**) scale (Axis V of DSM-IV) and, in the United Kingdom, the recently developed Health of the Nation Outcome Scale (**HONOS**).[49]

In both of these, the assessor uses whatever information is available about the patient to make judgements about the presence and severity of symptoms and troublesome behaviour, and the extent to which these interfere with activities, relationships, and social performance. In the GAF scale this is expressed as a single overall score. In HONOS, 12 separate ratings are made which can be used independently, or added together to give an overall score if required. This type of instrument is likely to become increasingly important as the demand for 'evidence-based medicine' spreads, since they are designed for use by virtually any health professional in almost any setting. So long as precautions are always taken to ensure that the ratings made are as reliable and as valid as the setting permits, and likely sources of bias and error are kept in mind, their use can be a valuable aid to many forms of clinical assessment.

One further example of a **comprehensive assessment instrument** should be mentioned because it was designed for both research and clinical purposes, and it has been at times widely used in a number of European countries. The ADMP (an acronym in both German and English for the Association of Methodology and Documentation in Psychiatry) exists in English, German, French, Spanish, and Japanese versions, covering virtually all the information needed for a comprehensive assessment by means of lists of items to be coded as present or absent. It is up to the user to decide the meaning of each item, and how much to train with fellow raters (or not) so as to improve inter-rater reliability.[73]

The condensation and recording of information

Summary and formulation

The skills required to produce summaries and formulations should be acquired early on in professional training, since they are central to the process of getting the information about the patient into a form which facilitates the making of decisions and the allocation of priorities for actions. Useful preliminaries to the writing of both summary and formulation are the preparation of a problem list and a lifechart; how to prepare these should also be covered in the early stages of training. The summary for an individual patient should be more or less the same whoever prepares it, since it should be a simple record of what is known, arranged under conventional headings. A 'telegram' style of writing is acceptable for the sake of brevity. In contrast, a formulation should be written as a grammatically correct narrative, and there is no necessary expectation that two different clinicians using the same summary about a patient would arrive at exactly the same conclusions in their formulations. This is because a formulation is an attempt by the writer to understand, and therefore to some extent to interpret, what has been influencing (and perhaps causing) the feelings and behaviour of the patient, and what relationships might exist between life events, illness, and contact with medical services.

Like the rest of the written medical records, the summary, formulation, and problem lists should be regarded as being as much for future readers as for the present carers. A clearly written summary and a well-argued formulation recorded in the case records will ensure that the reasons for treatments and decisions to do with the present illness are clear, and will be of great help to others if the patient has to be assessed in subsequent episodes of illness.

Summaries and formulations written by psychiatric members of a multi-disciplinary team should be freely available to all the team, so that they can be discussed before the meetings at which a diagnosis is agreed and care programmes are set-up. But it is not usually appropriate to send summaries and formulations made for hospital and team purposes to general practitioners or to consultants in other specialties. Specially written and shorter letters are best for this, taking into account the possibility that the patient or family may gain sight of, or even be shown, documents about them sent to other medical professionals.

Differential, main, subsidiary, and alternative diagnoses

A differential diagnosis should be placed in the case records in a prominent place, with a clear indication of who made it ('diagnosis' will be used in this section because of current conventions, but the difference between identifying a disorder and inferring an underlying diagnosis already noted must be kept in mind). When the patient suffers from more than one disorder it is usually possible to select one as the main diagnosis and specify the other(s) as additional or subsidiary diagnoses. The main diagnosis will usually be the one that is leading to immediate action, but the choice may depend upon the purposes for which the diagnoses are being recorded. Usually it reflects the reason for the current contact with services or admission but there are patients and occasions when, for instance, it makes more sense to record a lifetime diagnosis (such as schizophrenia or bipolar disorder) as the main diagnosis, even though something else such as anxiety or a phobic disorder is the reason for the current episode of care.

When one main diagnosis clearly applies yet does not account for some symptoms which, although a significant part of the clinical picture, still fall short of fulfilling the criteria for another disorder, it is useful to record these simply as 'additional symptoms' (for instance, depressive disorder with some obsessional symptoms; agoraphobia with some depressive symptoms, etc.). Neither ICD-10 nor DSM-IV mention this way of recording symptoms 'leftover' after the main disorder has been accounted for, even though it is a useful clinical custom familiar to many generations of clinicians in a variety of countries. However, omission from formal classifications should not be allowed to inhibit clinicians from following clinical habits they find useful.

When there is reasonable debate about what is the best diagnosis out of two or more possibilities, one must be chosen provisionally as the main diagnosis as a basis for action but the other should be recorded as an alternative diagnosis. It is also good practice in quite early stages of the assessment process to record provisional diagnoses, which can then be changed as more information becomes available. About a third of psychiatric patients fulfil the criteria for more than one disorder as defined in current classifications, but as already noted, this does not carry the same implications about underlying morbid physiological, psychological, or anatomical processes as would a statement about the presence of the same number of medical or surgical diagnoses.

Making a prognosis

The final statement in the formulation should be the prognosis. This attempt to predict what will happen to the patient in the future should be expressed as clear statements about likely outcomes, avoiding vague comments such as 'the prognosis is guarded' (found all too often in case records). The patient and family usually hope to be told about the prospects for recovery and the likelihood of relapse. Efforts should be made to do this, but with due care to emphasize that a prognosis is only an estimate that may be proved wrong by events. A prognostic statement should contain predictions of such things as:

1 immediate response to treatment, assuming compliance
2 duration of this episode of illness and/or stay in hospital
3 degree of recovery from this illness (i.e. partial or complete) in terms of both symptoms and return to previous activities
4 risk of recurrence, stated as the likely position at specific points in time, depending upon the circumstances of the case (6 months, 1 year, and 2 years from the present are often appropriate)

However difficult it may seem, attempts should be made to record a prognosis in these terms, and to sign it. To do this will fulfil the legitimate expectations of the patient and family, and the clinician will make possible a uniquely valuable learning experience when faced in the future with such statements about those patients seen in further episodes of care.

Reviews

The initial assessment should produce a list of agreed actions to be carried out in a stated order of priority by the various members of the team. Division into immediate and medium-term actions will help the whole process, and also indicate the timescale of reviews to assess progress. One of the main functions of the acknowledged team leader is to keep an eye on the progress of all the patients in the care of the team, discussing with each key worker both outside and within team meetings the best timing of the next review. Review meetings should be recorded as such in the case documents, with conclusions about progress made and any changes in plans or objectives. It is particularly important, again for future readers of the records, to write down clearly whether there was any response treatment (it is very frustrating to read in a case record of treatments given in the past, and then to find no indication of the result.)

Writing reports

Consultant psychiatrists are often asked by external agencies to provide written reports on patients for whom they have a current clinical responsibility, and requests may also be received for a report on a patient they have not seen previously. The purpose of these external reports is usually different to that of the usual clinical communications undertaken in the ordinary clinical care of the patient, in that the request is usually for an opinion about one specific issue. These requests frequently involve an opinion on the risk posed to others by the patient's inability to perform certain skills, or by the positive adverse effect of the patient's problems on others. An opinion on the capacity of the patient to understand and competently agree about important issues is also frequently requested.

The purposes of reports

Reports requested by individuals or agencies (both judicial and non-judicial) will usually fall into one of four broad groups:

1 Protection of the public or an institution:

   (a) life assurance and mortgage companies who are interested in the risk of suicide, or loss of earnings due to future illnesses;

   (b) licensing authorities and transport companies who are concerned with fitness to drive or risks due to the public, due to impairment of skills and judgement consequent upon psychiatric illness;

   (c) employment and benefit agencies who are concerned with fitness to work;

   (d) employers or occupational health physicians who are concerned about the risk posed by the patient's psychiatric disorder to an institution's clients, or about the likelihood of periods of absence because of sick leave.

2 Protection of the patient:

   (a) solicitors or courts may require reports on the competence of individual patients to conduct their financial affairs, to protect themselves from exploitation, and to engage in civil contracts;

   (b) bodies concerned with the Mental Health Act (in the United Kingdom the Mental Health Act Commission and Mental Health Review Tribunals) may require reports on the competence of individuals to give informed consent to non-voluntary psychiatric treatment or inpatient care, and the risk to the safety and well-being of the individual patient posed by such treatment.

3 Child protection:

   (a) Social Services Child Care Departments and others involved in the welfare of children may request reports of the supervising psychiatrist for Child Protection Case Conferences on the contribution of a psychiatric disorder to the childcare problem, and on the likely impact of the psychiatric disorder on the future parenting of the patient;

   (b) solicitors acting for all parties in childcare proceedings (the child, the Social Services Department, and the patient) may ask for a psychiatric report on a mentally ill parent about the likely risk to the child of suffering significant physical, developmental, or emotional harm from the patient in question.

4 Medico-legal and compensation proceedings: lawyers acting for either the patient or an agency being sued may ask for a report on the impact of the event on the mental health of the patient, together with the nature of the psychiatric disorder and its prognosis. Such reports may be requested of the supervising consultant, or of another psychiatrist as an independent expert.

Reports for forensic or criminal proceedings are dealt with in Chapter 11.15.

Guiding principles

The general principles noted below apply to all reports, whether the psychiatrist knows the patient because of current or previous clinical responsibility, or whether the report is on a patient whom the psychiatrist has not seen before (this latter is known as providing an 'expert opinion').

(a) Confidentiality

In most situations written consent must be obtained from the patient before personal information can be given to an outside agency. In almost all situations involving the writing of a report on an individual to an outside agency, that individual will gain sight of the report or will be entitled to do so. It is therefore good clinical practice for the patient to be aware of the content of the report, and particularly of any opinions or recommendations it may contain. Nevertheless, there are certain situations where the duty of care to the public or to a child overrides the duty of confidentiality, and in such circumstances the psychiatrist may write the report even without the patient's consent.

(b) Partiality

The opinion of the psychiatrist is being sought as an expert professional. The report should not be biased in favour of one side or another and should not be influenced unduly by the interests of the commissioning agency or the psychiatrist's view of the best interests of their patient. This may cause difficulties if the patient is in the personal care of the psychiatrist because in most clinical situations psychiatrists try to be non-critical, non-judgemental, and supportive, tending to encourage rather than to prevent. But the best interests of the patient will not be served by being put in a situation where the likely outcomes are failure to do what is expected or to function at a suboptimal level.

Structure of reports

All reports should have three main sections. First, the report should begin with the patient's personal details and the reasons for which the report has been requested, together with the identity of the commissioning agency. It should also specify the relationship between the writer and the patient. If the patient is or was in the clinical care of the writer the duration of the care should be noted, and the date of the last occasion the patient was seen should be given. If a special interview had to be arranged with a patient not previously known, the duration and date of the interview should be stated. The sources of information other than the patient used to prepare the report should then be detailed, plus any other documents that have been read. Reports for civil, judicial, and child protection proceedings will also require a short paragraph on the current employment and status of the author of the report, and a note of any special experience of relevance.

The second section should describe in appropriate detail the patient's personal, social, medical, and psychiatric history, the mental state and behaviour at examination, the diagnosis and differential diagnosis, and comments upon aetiology, management, and prognosis. In almost all reports, the prognosis is the primary concern, so this should be given special attention. It is important to remember that one of the most reliable predictors of the recurrence of behaviours or episodes of illness in the future is the frequency of their occurrence in the past. Similarly, the vulnerability of the patient in the past (that is, any enduring predisposing factors and patterns of past precipitants) will tend to predict future vulnerability and the likelihood of further episodes of illness. Some mention of the past will therefore always be necessary, but in many instances this can be brief and reduced to a commentary of a few lines. But in other situations, particularly those involving civil court actions or childcare proceedings, a more detailed account of the past will be necessary.

Certain aspects of the patient's past history and previous levels of functioning will need to be highlighted depending upon the purposes of the report and the nature of the questions asked of the psychiatrist. For example, if the report has been requested by an occupational physician about the fitness of a patient to return to work, then attention will need to be paid in the report to the duration of illnesses in the past and the amount of sick leave that has been taken. Detail will need to be given about the impact, if any, that the patient's ill health has had on the past to his or her capacity to work. If the report has been requested in relation to the safety of the patient to care for a child, then information will need to be given in the past history of the patient about the previous impact of the patient's illness on his or her capacity to care for children or any risks that the patient posed to a child in the past. Life assurance and mortgage companies are likely to be particularly interested in suicidal behaviour.

The last section should contain the opinion of the psychiatrist about the specific questions posed by the commissioning agent. These questions may be unrealistically simple or there may be requests for categorical assertions of outcome that are simply not possible. The writer must avoid falling into the trap of complying with unreasonable requests about certainties. One way of avoiding this is to give opinions about risks or outcomes by stating criteria that would indicate different outcomes with different likelihoods, expressed by words such as possible, probable, and definite.

In situations where one of the variables involved in the patient's prognosis is the response of helping agencies and the availability of resources, great care must be exercised on the part of the report writer to ensure that this contingency is made clear. If possible, suggestions should be made as to how the availability of the required resources can be assured. When considering the likely impact of a future breakdown in the mental health of a patient on some other person, such as a child, consideration should be given not only to the direct impact of the illness but also to the indirect consequences and the presence or absence of other protective factors. For example, if a woman with schizophrenia lives with her parents who can safely take over the care of her child, then the impact of a further episode on that child may be much less than if she is living alone and the child needs to be removed into the care of the local authority.

An opinion is often requested on whether an accident or an act of omission such as medical negligence caused the current psychiatric disorder or disabilities of the patient. If the psychiatrist concludes that the accident or omission was definitely a contributing cause but not in itself sufficient to cause all aspects of the existing disorder and disability, then further comments will be expected on other possible contributing influences, such as predisposing personal traits, or special vulnerability to current adversities. In such circumstances, there should be an attempt to weigh the contributing factors in order of their aetiological importance.

The last section of the report is usually the best place to list the sources of information used for the report, making clear distinctions between personal observations and information obtained by the writer, opinions and observations made by other team members, and written information obtained from other documents. There should always be a clear distinction between opinions based upon objective information and direct examination, and suppositions based upon interpretations, speculation, and past clinical experience. If opinions based upon research conducted by others are given, then the sources of this information should be acknowledged and referenced in the usual manner.

The language of the report should be appropriate to the commissioning agency. If the report has been requested by an occupational physician or medical officer working for a company, then it is appropriate to use accepted medical and psychiatric terminology. If the report has been requested by a civil or judicial authority, non-technical language should be used wherever possible and any medical or psychiatric terms used should be defined. At all times when writing psychiatric reports it is important to use psychiatric terms in an appropriate fashion according to a stated international classification, and to avoid idiosyncrasies.

Further information

Moller, H.J., Engel, R.R., and Helmsley, D.R. (2001). Standardised measurement instruments in psychiatry. In *Contemporary psychiatry. Foundations of psychiatry*, Vol. 1 (eds. H. Henn, N. Sartorius, H. Helmchen, and H. Lauter), pp. 113–35. Springer-Verlag, Berlin.

Grounds, A. (1993). Psychiatric reports for legal purposes in forensic psychiatry. In *Clinical, legal and ethical issues* (eds. J. Gunn and P.J. Taylor), Chap. 22, p. 826–55. Butterworth—Heineman Ltd, Oxford.

References

1. Gelder, M., Gath, D., Mayou, R., *et al.* (1996). *Oxford textbook of psychiatry* (3rd edn). Oxford University Press, Oxford.
2. Post, F. (1983). The clinical assessment of mental disorders. In *Handbook of psychiatry*, Vol. 1 (eds. M. Shepherd and O.L. Zangwill), pp. 210–20. Cambridge University Press, Cambridge.
3. McHugh, P.R. and Slavney, P.R. (1986). *The perspectives of psychiatry*. Johns Hopkins University Press, Baltimore, MD.
4. Taylor, F.K. (1971). A logical analysis of the medico-psychological concept of disease: Part 1. *Psychological Medicine*, **1**, 356–64.
5. Susser, M.W. and Watson, W.B. (1971). *Sociology in medicine* (2nd edn), pp. 16–17, 216–18, 295ff. Oxford University Press Oxford.
6. Lewis, A.L. (1953). Health as a social concept. *The British Journal of Sociology*, **4**, 109–204.
7. Wootton, B. (1959). Social pathology and the concepts of mental health and mental illness. *Social science and social pathology*. Allen and Unwin, London.
8. Scadding, J.G. (1967). Diagnosis, the clinician and the computer. *Lancet*, **2**, 877–82.
9. Scadding, J.G. (1996). Essentialism and nominalism in medicine: the logic of diagnosis in disease terminology. *Lancet*, **348**, 594–6.
10. Kerr, A. and McClelland, H. (1991). *Concepts of mental disorder: a continuing debate*. Gaskell Press, London.

11. Tyrer, P. and Steinberg, D. (1993). *Models for mental disorders: conceptual models in psychiatry*. Wiley, Chichester.
12. Eisenberg, L. (1998). The social construction of mental illness (editorial). *Psychological Medicine*, **18**, 1–9.
13. Eisenberg, L. (1977). Disease and illness. Distinctions between professional and popular ideas of sickness. *Culture, Medicine and Psychiatry*, **1**, 9–24.
14. Engel, G.L. (1978). The biopsychosocial model and the education of health professionals. *Annals of the New York Academy of Sciences*, **310**, 169–81.
15. Susser, M. (1990). Disease, illness, sickness; impairment, disability and handicap (editorial). *Psychological Medicine*, **20**, 471–4.
16. Taylor, F.K. (1979). *Psychopathology: its causes and symptoms*. Quartermaine House, Sunbury on Thames.
17. Fulford, K.W.M. (1989). *Moral theory and medical practice*. Cambridge University Press, Cambridge.
18. Mechanic, D. (1986). The concept of illness behaviour; culture, situation and personal predisposition. *Psychological Medicine*, **16**, 1–8.
19. Menninger, K. (1948). Changing concepts of disease. *Annals of Internal Medicine*, **29**, 318–25.
20. Kendell, R.E. (1975). *The role of diagnosis in psychiatry*. Blackwell Science, Oxford.
21. Cooper, J.E. (1983). Diagnosis and the diagnostic process. In *Handbook of psychiatry. General psychopathology*, Vol. 1, Part III (eds. M. Shepherd and O.L. Zangwill), pp. 199–209. Cambridge University Press, Cambridge.
22. World Health Organization. (2001). *International Classification of Functioning, disability and health (ICF) short version*. WHO, Geneva.
23. Nagi, S.Z. (1965). Some conceptual issues in disability and rehabilitation. In *Sociology and rehabilitation* (ed. M.B. Sussman), pp. 110–13. American Sociological Association, Washington, DC.
24. Weissman, M.M. (1975). The assessment of social adjustment: a review of techniques. *Archives of General Psychiatry*, **32**, 357–65.
25. Gurland, B.J., Yorkston, N.J., Stone, A.R., *et al.* (1972). The Structured and Scaled Interview to Assess Maladjustment (SSIAM). I. Description, rationale and development. *Archives of General Psychiatry*, **27**, 259–64.
26. Claire, A.W. and Cairns, V.E. (1978). Design, development and use of a standardised interview to assess social maladjustment and dysfunction in community studies. *Psychological Medicine*, **8**, 589–604.
27. Brown, G.W. and Harris, T.O. (1986). *Social origins of depression; a study of psychiatric disorder in women*. Tavistock Publications, London.
28. Brown, G.W. and Harris, T.O. (1986). Stressor, vulnerability and depression; a question of replication (editorial). *Psychological Medicine*, **16**, 739–44.
29. Andrews, G. and Tennant, C. (1978). Life events and psychiatric illness (editorial). *Psychological Medicine*, **8**, 545–9.
30. Jones, S.J., Turner, R.J., and Grant, J. (1987). Assessing patients in their homes. *Bulletin of the Royal College of Psychiatrists*, **11**, 117–19.
31. Oates, M.R. (1988). The development of an integrated community-oriented service for severe post-natal mental illness. In *Motherhood and mental illness*, Vol. 3 (eds. R. Kumar and I. Brockington), pp. 133–58. John Wright, London.
32. Tyrer, P. (1984). Psychiatric clinics in general practice: an extension of community care. *The British Journal of Psychiatry*, **145**, 9–14.
33. Burns, T. (1997). Case management, care management and care programming (editorial). *The British Journal of Psychiatry*, **170**, 393–5.
34. Holloway, F., Oliver, N., Collins, E., *et al.* (1995). Case management: a critical review of the literature. *European Psychiatry*, **10**, 113–28.
35. Katschnig, H. and Cooper, J.E. (1991). Psychiatric emergency and crisis intervention services. In *Community psychiatry: the principle* (eds. D.H. Bennet and H.L. Freeman), pp. 517–42. Churchill Livingstone, Edinburgh.
36. Cooper, J.E. (1990). Professional obstacles to implementation and diffusion of innovative approaches to mental health care. In *Mental health care delivery: innovations, impediments and implementation* (eds. I. Marks and R. Scott), pp. 233–53. Cambridge University Press, Cambridge.
37. Henderson, A.S. (1988). The tools of social psychiatry. In *An introduction to social psychiatry*, pp. 6–29. Oxford University Press, Oxford.
38. Thompson, C. (ed.) (1989). *The instruments of psychiatric research*. Wiley, Chichester.
39. World Health Organization. (1993). *Catalogue of assessment instruments used in the studies coordinated by the WHO mental health programme*. WHO/MNH/92.5. Division of Mental Health, World Health Organization, Geneva.
40. Sartorius, N. and Janca, A. (1996). Psychiatric assessment instruments developed by the World Health Organization. *Social Psychiatry and Epidemiology*, **31**, 55–69.
41. Janca, A. (1997). Current trends in the development of psychiatric assessment instruments. *Current Opinion in Psychiatry*, **10**, 457–61.
42. Thornicroft, G. and Tansella, M. (eds.) (1997). *Mental health outcome measures*. Springer-Verlag, Berlin.
43. Goldberg, D.P. and Hillier, V.F. (1979). A scaled version of the general health questionnaire. *Psychological Medicine*, **9**, 139–45.
44. Wittchen, H.-U., Robins, L.N., Cottler, L.B., *et al.* (1991). Cross-cultural feasibility, reliability and sources of variance of the Composite International Diagnostic Interview (CIDI)—results of the multi-centre WHO/ADAMHA field trials (wave 1). *The British Journal of Psychiatry*, **159**, 645–53.
45. World Health Organization. (1993). *The Composite Diagnostic Interview, core version 1.1*. American Psychiatric Press, Washington, DC.
46. Hamilton, M. (1960). Rating scale for depression. *Journal of Neurology, Neurosurgery, and Psychiatry*, **23**, 56–62.
47. Andreason, N.C. (1989). The Scale for Assessment of Negative Symptoms (SANS): conceptual and theoretical foundations. *The British Journal of Psychiatry*, **155**(Suppl. 7), 49–52.
48. Endicott, J. and Spitzer, R.L. (1978). A diagnostic interview: the schedule for affective disorders and schizophrenia. *Archives of General Psychiatry*, **35**, 837–44.
49. Wing, J.K., Curtis, R., and Beevor, A. (1994). 'Health of the Nation': measuring mental health outcomes. *Psychiatric Bulletin: Journal of Trends in Psychiatric Practice*, **18**, 690–1.
50. Wing, J.K., Babor, T., Brugha, T., *et al.* (1990). SCAN: Schedules for Clinical Assessment in Neuropsychiatry. *Archives of General Psychiatry*, **47**, 589–93.
51. Overall, J.E. and Gorham, D.R. (1962). The Brief Psychiatric Rating Scale (BPRS). *Psychological Reports*, **10**, 799–812.
52. Asberg, M., Montgomery, S.A., Perris, C., *et al.* (1978). A Comprehensive Psychopathological Rating Scale (CPRS). *Acta Psychiatrica Scandinavica. Supplementum*, **271**, 5–28.
53. Spitzer, R.L., Williams, J.B.W., and Gibbon, M. (1987). *Structured clinical interview for DSM-IV (SCID)*. Biometrics Research, New York State Psychiatric Institute, New York.
54. Wing, J.K., Cooper, J.E., and Sartorius, N. (1974). Measurement and classification of psychiatric symptoms: an instruction manual for the PSE and the CATEGO program. Cambridge University Press, London.
55. Cooper, J.E., Kendell, R.E., Gurland, B.J., *et al.* (1969). Cross-national study of diagnosis of mental disorders; some results from the first comparative investigation. *The American Journal of Psychiatry*, **125**(Suppl.), 21–9.
56. Cooper, J.E., Kendell, R.E., Gurland, B.J., *et al.*(1972). *Psychiatric diagnosis in New York and London: a comparative study of mental hospital admissions*. Maudsley Monograph No. 20. Oxford University Press, Oxford.
57. Sartorius, N., Jablensky, A., and Shapiro, R. (1977). Two year follow–up of the patients included in the WHO international pilot study of schizophrenia: preliminary communication. *Psychological Medicine*, **7**, 529–41.

58. Feighner, J.P., Robins, E., Guze, S.B., *et al.* (1972). Diagnostic criteria for use in psychiatric research. *Archives of General Psychiatry*, **26**, 57–63.
59. Robins, L.N., Helzer, J.E., Croughan, J., *et al.* (1981). National Institute of Mental Health Diagnostic Interview Schedule. Its history, characteristics and validity. *Archives of General Psychiatry*, **38**, 381–8.
60. Regier, D.A., Boyd, J.H., Burke, J.D., *et al.* (1988). One month prevalence of mental disorders in the United States: based on the five epidemiological catchment area sites. *Archives of General Psychiatry*, **45**, 977–86.
61. Pull, C. and Wittchen, H.-U. (1991). CIDI, SCAN and IPDE: structured diagnostic interviews for ICD–10 and DSMIII–R. *European Journal of Psychiatry*, **6**, 277–85.
62. Regier, D.A., Kaelber, C.T., Rae, D.S., *et al.* (1998). Limitations of diagnostic criteria and assessment instruments for mental disorders. *Archives of General Psychiatry*, **55**, 9–115.
63. Kessler, R.C., McGonagle, K.A., Zhao, S., *et al.* (1994). Lifetime and 12 month prevalence of DSM–III–R psychiatric disorders in the United States; results from the National Co-morbidity Study. *Archives of General Psychiatry*, **51**, 8–19.
64. Wing, J.K., Bebbington, P., and Robins, L.N. (1981). *What is a case? The problem of definition in psychiatric community surveys*. Grant McIntyre, London.
65. Spitzer, R.L. (1998). Diagnosis and need for treatment are not the same (commentary). *Archives of General Psychiatry*, **55**, 120.
66. Kendell, R.E. (1989). Clinical validity. *Psychological Medicine*, **19**, 45–56.
67. Biehl, H., Maurer, K., Jablensky, A., *et al.* (1989). The WHO/PIRS: introducing a new instrument for rating observed behaviour, and the rationale of the psychological impairment concept. *The British Journal of Psychiatry*, **155**(Suppl. 7), 68–81.
68. Barnes, T.R.E. (ed.) (1989). Negative symptoms in schizophrenia. *The British Journal of Psychiatry*, **155**(Suppl. 7).
69. Mezzich, J.E. (1979). Patterns and issues in multiaxial psychiatric diagnosis. *Psychological Medicine*, **9**, 125–37.
70. World Health Organization. (1997). *Multiaxial presentation of ICD–10 for use in adult psychiatry*. Cambridge University Press, Cambridge.
71. Katschnig, H., Freeman, H., and Sartorius, N. (1997). *Quality of life in mental disorders*. Wiley, Chichester.
72. Bebbington, P., Brewin, C.R., Marsden, L., *et al.* (1996). Measuring the need for psychiatric treatment in the general population: the community version of the MRC Needs for Care Assessment. *Psychological Medicine*, **26**, 229–36.
73. Woggon, B. (1986). The AMDP-III: a comprehensive instrument for recording psychiatric information. In *Assessment in depression* (eds. N. Sartorius and T. Baan), pp. 112–20. Springer–Verlag, Berlin.

1.8.2 Assessment of personality

C. Robert Cloninger

Introduction

The assessment of personality provides the context needed to understand someone as a whole person with particular goals and values that they pursue with a unique emotional style. A person's way of adapting to life experience can tell an experienced clinician much about his level of well-being and his vulnerability to various forms of psychopathology. Knowing a person's personality well can allow a psychiatrist to predict what other mental and physical disorders are likely to occur in the same person or in the same family. For example, individuals with antisocial personality are more likely to have substance abuse and less likely to have Parkinson's disease than others.[1] On the other hand, if you learn someone has substance abuse, then you can reasonably suspect that they may be impulsive or novelty seeking. Recognition of the many associations between personality and psychopathology can greatly enhance clinical assessment and differential diagnosis in general.

Assessment of personality also helps to establish a therapeutic alliance and mutual respect, because it involves the sharing of unique personal and social information that distinguishes one person's style of life from others. Patients feel understood and appreciated when their psychiatrist understands their motivation and can predict their reactions to different situations and people. On the other hand, no one likes to be reduced to a 'case' or a 'label'. Everyone is unique, and yet it is possible to explore the mystery of each person's uniqueness in a systematic way. Consequently, effective clinical assessment of personality is designed to understand a person's emotions, goals and values, strengths and weaknesses in the context of the narrative of his life.

Understanding personality also helps in treatment planning because people differ markedly in the types of treatments to which they respond and with which they will comply. For example, personality traits predict much of the variability in response to antidepressants, whereas the symptoms of depression or other psychopathology do not.[2,3]

Fortunately, personality can be well assessed clinically without psychometric testing in ways that are simple and brief as part of routine history taking and mental status examination. The clinical assessment of personality requires little extra time if the clinician is alert to non-verbal cues in a person's general appearance, expressions, and behavior, as well as to the significance of what is said and how it is said. Only brief questions to clarify complaints and their context may be needed.

Personality develops over time in response to a changing internal and external environment. As a result, the longitudinal course of a person's development of personality and psychopathology is a key element in the clinical assessment of personality. Specifically, it is highly informative to know what a patient's personality was like as a child when assessing him in the presence of additional psychopathology, like a depression or anxiety state that modifies his emotions, thoughts, and behaviour. However, personality traits are not fixed and completely stable. Rather, each of us has a range of thoughts, feelings, and behaviours at any given point in time. As a result, our personality traits frequently vary within that range and occasionally change by moving beyond the previous range in response to particular internal and external events. Understanding the course of a person's development during his life is what allows the psychiatrist to understand him as a unique person.

In this chapter, I will try to explain the basic constructs and methods of personality assessment, so that a clinician can apply this knowledge in a flexible and practical manner. If you have to ask standardized questions that are not tailored to opportunities that arise in the course of an interview, then you don't understand the basic constructs adequately. On the other hand, some clinical features about personality traits are sufficiently high in yield and diagnostic value, that they should be assessed in a final review if they haven't been come up more spontaneously during the interview.

What is personality?

In order to assess something it is crucial to have a good understanding of what it is and what it is not. People differ markedly from one another in their outlook on life, in the way they interpret their experiences, and in their emotional and behavioral responses to those experiences. These differences in outlook, thoughts, emotions, and are what actions characterize an individual's personality. More generally, personality can be defined as the dynamic organization within the individual of the psychobiological systems that modulate his or her unique adaptations to a changing internal and external environment.[4] Each part of this definition is important for a clinician to appreciate. Personality is 'dynamic', meaning, it is constantly changing and adapting in response to experience, rather than being a set of fixed traits. Inflexibility of personality is actually an indicator of personality disorder. Personality is regulated by 'psychobiological' systems, meaning, personality is influenced by both biological and psychological variables. Consequently, treatment of personality disorders requires growth in psychological self-understanding and not just treatment with medications, although these can be helpful adjuncts to therapy.[5,6] These systems involve interactions among many internal processes, so that each person's pattern of adjustment is 'unique' to them, even though they follow general rules and principles of development as complex adaptive systems.[7] Finally, to understand personality and its development, we must pay attention to both the 'internal' and 'external' processes by which an individual interacts with and adapts to his own internal milieu and external situation. For example, when a person is under stress, he is likely to think and feel differently about himself and other people. On the other hand, when he is calm and encouraged, he may act more maturely and happily. Everyone has personal sensitivities or 'rough spots' that surface when they are under stress. Everyone has 'good days' and 'bad days', and this pattern of variability over time is what characterizes a person's unique personality configuration.

An individual's personality can only be adequately characterized in terms of interactions among different internal and external forces that influence a person's emotions, thoughts, and behaviour. A person may feel and act differently on a date, at work, with trusted friends, at school, or in church. His personality doesn't change, rather his personality can only be adequately assessed when the psychosocial context is specified. Some traits are strong and pervasive regardless of the situation, but other aspects of personality may be markedly affected by the situation. Furthermore, the internal processes may modify a person's outlook, as when his outlook is influenced by prior or anticipated events, or when his goals and values allow him to change his outlook in ways that are not predictable by what he has previously done. Human beings have an amazing ability to change their outlook for the better or the worse in ways that are unpredicted by their past or present circumstances. Personality traits can be described in ways that are moderately stable over time and situations, but a prudent clinician must never mistake average probabilities with predictive certainty.

Five major types of situations are useful to distinguish for human beings: Sexual situations involving reproduction and sexuality; Material situations involving the quest for material possessions and power; Emotional situations involving emotions and social attachments; Intellectual situations involving communication and culture; Spiritual situations involving the quest for what is beyond individual human existence. The average person is concerned with material situations most of the time—obtaining food, clothing, shelter, transportation, and striving for power and wealth. However, to understand a person fully it is essential to recognize his feelings, thoughts, and intuitions in other types of situations ranging from the sexual to the spiritual. The way a person adapts to these five different types of situations correspond to layers of an individual's personality. The treatment of psychopathology can be viewed as a working-through of problems and blind spots in these five layers of everyone's personality, enabling the development of self-awareness in the full range of life situations.[8]

Personality involves much more than the description of a fixed set of traits that allow the prediction of a person's behavior. Personality involves the interaction of internal and external forces that influence the development of a person's behavior, but nevertheless allow for the potential of a person to grow in self-awareness and thereby change in ways that cannot be predicted from his past behavior.[9]

How can personality be described quantitatively?

Personality refers to the motivational systems *within* a person, not between individuals. In other words, to understand what motivates a person we need to recognize empathically what he is thinking and feeling within his own being. We need a model of the dynamic psychobiological processes within a human being. Unfortunately, the people who have developed most personality tests often treat each person as a black box that emits self-reports. As a result, most personality psychologists have failed to understand the internal dynamics underlying the thoughts and feelings of the people they assess. However, it is possible to describe a person's internal processes, which interact with his or her external situations. In order to account for both the internal and the external influences on personality, it is essential to distinguish the dimensions of a person's temperament and those of his character.[4]

The temperament traits are biases in emotional responses that are fully developed early in life and relatively stable thereafter. On the other hand, character involves higher cognitive processes that develop in a stepwise manner over the life course to enable a person to regulate his emotions, achieve certain goals, and maintain particular values and virtues. Initially, it was thought that character was less heritable than temperament, but empirical studies have shown that both are moderately heritable. The key difference is the difference in the pattern of learning and memory: the procedural learning of habits and skills influences the conditioning of temperament, whereas propositional learning of goals and values influences the development of character. Both procedural and propositional learning interact with one another in self-aware consciousness so that a person can maintain a personal sense of continuity throughout many episodes of experience as the story of his life unfolds.

Temperament can be assessed in terms of four quantifiable dimensions, as measured by the Temperament and Character Inventory.[4] These are described in Table 1.8.2.1, which shows that each trait is manifested in slightly different ways depending on the situation. A situation necessarily depends on both the person's outlook and the external circumstances themselves. For example, a person is described as high in Harm Avoidance if he is easily fatigued, fearful, shy, pessimistic, and inhibited. On the other hand, a person is described as low in Harm Avoidance if he is vigorous, risk-taking, beguiling, optimistic, and uninhibited.

Table 1.8.2.1 Descriptions of temperaments according to emotional responses elicited by particular external situations and internal outlooks

Temperament	Sexual situations	Material situations	Emotional situations	Intellectual situations	Spiritual situations
Harm Avoidance	Fatigable vs Vigorous	Fearful vs Risk-taking	Shy vs Beguiling	Pessimistic vs Optimistic	Inhibited vs Uninhibited
Novelty Seeking	Craving vs Reserved	Extravagant vs Frugal	Irritable vs Stoical	Impulsive vs Rigid	Exploratory vs Immobile
Reward Dependence	Insecure vs Independent	Sympathetic vs Aloof	Sociable vs Distant	Sentimental vs Indifferent	Attached vs Detached
Persistence	Ambitious vs Apathetic	Overachieving vs Underachieving	Loyal vs Fickle	Determined vs Ambivalent	Perfectionistic vs Pragmatic

However, the level of Harm Avoidance varies moderately between situations. For example, some people who are shy are not easily fatigued, and some people who are shy meeting strangers are risk-takers when driving an automobile. The components of Harm Avoidance that are manifested in different situations are moderately correlated, and so it is useful to consider all these as part of a higher order trait that is moderately heritable and moderately stable across time and situations. Likewise, Novelty Seeking, Reward Dependence, Persistence are also moderately heritable and stable dimensions of temperament.

Likewise, there are three dimensions of character, which quantify the nature of a person's goals and values (Table 1.8.2.2). Each of these character traits is comprised of components that are expressed in different situations. The character dimensions also correspond to key functions of a person's mental self-government. As a result, character traits provide a rich description of key features of the mental status examination, including insight and judgment.

Insight refers to the depth of a person's ability to recognize and understand the inner nature of things, rather than basing opinions on superficial appearances. Insight is quantifiable as the character trait of Self-transcendence. A person with deep insight is respectful, mindful, and holistic in perspective, whereas one with little insight is unrealistic, shallow, and fragmented in perspective.

Judgment refers to a person's legislative ability to cooperate and get along with others in ways that are appropriate and flexible, and can be quantified as the character trait of Cooperativeness. A person with good judgment is cooperative and principled, whereas a person who has poor judgment is uncooperative and opportunistic.

Foresight refers to a person's executive ability to anticipate what will be satisfying in the long-term or in the future. This executive function allows a person to follow a life path that maintains well-being. A person who is far-sighted is responsible, purposeful, resilient, and resourceful, whereas one who learns from hindsight only is irresponsible, aimless, fragile, and inadequate. In addition, foresight leads to cheerfulness and spontaneity, whereas reliance on hindsight is associated with moodiness and conventionality. Accordingly, the degree of a person's foresight provides important clinical information about a person's ability to appreciate what is real, meaningful, and satisfying. As a result, a person's self-directedness is an important indicator of reality testing, maturity, and vulnerability to mood disturbance. Self-directedness is high

Table 1.8.2.2 Descriptions of the three dimensions of character according to the five layers of everyone's personality, which are defined by the predominant focus of the person's internal perspective on the external situation. Within each layer of personality, maturation and integration involves increasing each of the three character dimensions, which describe the functions of insight, judgment, and foresight. Integration of the whole person requires working through these functions in each of the layers of personality

Cognitive function (Character dimension)	Characteristics of the sexual layer	Characteristics of the material layer	Characteristics of the emotional layer	Characteristics of the intellectual layer	Characteristics of the spiritual layer
Insight (Self-Transcendence)	Trustful vs Alienated (prelogical categorizing)	Free-Flowing vs Compulsive (concrete-vivid logic)	Identifying vs Avoiding (emotive imagery)	Creative vs Imitative (abstract symbols)	Intuitive vs Conventional (preverbal schemas)
Judgment (Cooperativeness)	Tolerant vs Prejudiced	Forgiving vs Revengeful	Empathic vs Inconsiderate	Helpful vs Unhelpful	Principled vs Opportunistic
Foresight (Self-Directedness)	Responsible vs Irresponsible	Purposeful vs Aimless	Resilient vs Moody	Resourceful vs Inadequate	Spontaneous vs Predetermined

in people who are mature and happy, whereas it is low in people with personality disorders and in those vulnerable to psychoses and mood disorders.

Psychometric testing of personality traits

A wide variety of psychometric tests can be used to describe personality traits, so it is useful for a clinician to understand the relationships among alternative measures. The number and content of traits describing personality vary but there is actually extensive overlap among the traits measured. Hans Eysenck popularized tests that measured three factors called Neuroticism, Extraversion, and Psychoticism.(10) The Eysenck Personality Questionnaire also includes validity measure called 'Lie'. Nearly all tests subsequently developed include factors corresponding closely to Neuroticism and Extraversion at least. Later, Jeffrey Gray showed that individual differences in rates of learning corresponded to weighted combinations of Neuroticism and Extraversion.(11) In other words, people who are most prone to anxiety and respond most sensitively to punishment are neurotic introverts (that is, they are high in Neuroticism and low in Extraversion). On the other hand, people who are most impulsive and respond most sensitively to rewards are stable extraverts (that is, they are low in Neuroticism and high in Extraversion). As a result, both Zuckerman and Cloninger developed tests that correspond to these individual differences in learning and vulnerability to psychopathology, as summarized in Table 1.8.2.3. Essentially, people who are most prone to anxiety are those who are described as neurotic introverts by Eysenck, neurotic or anxiety-prone by Zuckerman and Gray, and harm-avoidant by Cloninger. On the other hand, people who are most prone to impulsivity, anger, and substance abuse are called stable extraverts by Eysenck, impulsive sensation-seekers by Zuckerman and Gray, and Novelty seekers by Cloninger.

Later, Cloninger and others showed that all seven of the dimensions of his Temperament and Character Inventory had unique genetic determinants and unique brain processes, suggesting that a seven dimensional model is needed to account for the dynamic processes within each individual that regulates his personality. Nevertheless, five factor models like Zuckerman and Kuhlman's Personality Qeustionnaire or Costa and McCrae's NEO personality inventory can capture most of the information about personality in a statistical sense, even though they ignore the non-linear structure of personality resulting from its complex evolutionary history. Tables 1.8.2.3 and 1.8.2.4 and 4 show the correlations between measures of Cloninger's seven factor model and alternative five factor models (Zuckerman's ZKPQ in Table 1.8.2.3, Costa's NEO-PI in Table 1.8.2.4). As in Eysenck's Neuroticism factor, Neuroticism in five factor models is a composite of anxiety-proneness (as measured by high Harm Avoidance) and personality disorder (as measured by low Self-directedness). Extraversion is a composite of intrapsychic processes involving risk-taking (as measured by low Harm Avoidance), impulsivity (as measured by high Novelty Seeking), and sociability (as measured by high Reward Dependence), and personality maturity (as measured by high Self-directedness).(12) Essentially, Neuroticism and Extraversion are composites of traits leading to maladaptive and adaptive emotional styles. Five factor models now also distinguish traits related to agreeability and sociability (as measured by TCI Reward Dependence and Cooperativeness, low ZKPQ hostility, and high NEO agreeability). There is also consistent recognition of a trait variously identified as conscientiousness, persistence, and vigorous activity, which has been identified by a specific resistance to extinction of intermittently reinforced behaviour regulated by specific brain circuitry in rodents and humans.(13)

Beyond these four personality traits (anxiety-proneness, impulsive anger-proneness, social attachment, and persistence), alternative models of personality vary according to how the remaining features of personality are measured. Five factor models like the ZKPQ and NEO do not measure the personality trait underlying self-awareness, which leads to insight, creativity, and spirituality; however, this trait is measured as Self-transcendence in the TCI. Individual differences in serotonergic receptor function has been found to be strongly related to Self-transcendence.(14)

No consensus is possible to choose among alternative structures derived from factor analysis because an infinity of alternative rotations are statistically equivalent. Information beyond statistics is needed to choose among alternative models, as has been done by Gray, Zuckerman, and Cloninger. Such information includes brain imaging, genetics, development, or utility for developing insight

Table 1.8.2.3 Correlations (r x 100) between the Temperament and Character Inventory (TCI) scales and those of the Eysenck Personality Questionnaire (EPQ-revised) and the Zuckerman-Kuhlman Personality Questionnaire (correlations over 0.4 in bold, significant correlations only shown, n = 207. Reprinted from Personality and Individual Differences, 21, Zuckerman, M. and Cloninger, C.R. Relationship between Coninger's, Zuckerman's, and Eysenck's dimensions of personality, 283–5. Copyright 1996, with permission from Elsevier.

	Harm avoidance	Novelty seeking	Reward dependence	Persistence	Self-directed	Cooperative	Self-transcendent
EPQ Neuroticism	**59**				**– 45**		
EPQ Extraversion	**–53**	**44**	23		18		
EPQ Psychoticism		**41**	**–45**	–29	–31	**–42**	
EPQ Lie		–21			25	34	
ZKPQ Neuroticism	**66**				**–49**		
ZKPQ Impulsive Sensation	–39	**68**	–20				28
ZKPQ Hostility			–27		–32	**–60**	
ZKPQ Sociability	–38	37	31				
ZKPQ Activity	–29			**46**	36		

Table 1.8.2.4 Correlations between the scales of Temperament and Character Inventory-Revised (TCI-R) and the NEO-PI-Revised (correlations over 0.4 in bold, significant correlations only shown, multiple correlation also shown, n = 662, adults in the USA)

	Harm avoidance	Novelty seeking	Reward dependence	Persistence	Self-directed	Cooperative	Self-transcendent	mR
NEO Neuroticism	**63**			−20	**−62**	−28		75
NEO Extraversion	**−55**	40	**52**	40	25		22	77
NEO Openness	−25	**43**	25				37	54
NEO Conscience	−26	−34		**51**	**41**			70
NEO Agreeability		−23	40		31	**61**	20	66
mR	76	65	68	60	67	65	45	

into intrapsychic processes, as described in more detail elsewhere.[7] Fortunately, familiarity with the strong relationships among alternative measures will allow the clinician to interpret flexibly whatever information is available.

The assessment of personality can also be based upon abnormal traits indicative of personality disorder, as has been done by Livesley and others.[15] Whether the starting point is normal or abnormal personality traits, the same structure of personality is observed.[11,16] This shows that personality disorders are particular configurations of traits that vary quantitatively in the general population, not qualitatively in discrete disorders.

Clinical assessment of personality

Personality can be well assessed by allowing the patient to tell his life story and conducting a standard mental status examination. A checklist of signs and symptoms is not adequate for the assessment of personality because narratives only provide an account of a person's continuity of self-awareness over his lifespan. Within the life story, the key elements on which temperament ratings are made are the narrative account of emotional style, particularly in childhood, and general appearance and behaviour on mental status examination. The key elements on which character ratings are based are the range of a person's thoughts, the nature of his interpersonal relationships, and his insight and judgment. The clinician must consider not only the words of the patient, which may involve little or no cognitive insight or self-awareness, but also recognize the significance of non-verbal signs from body posture, facial expression, and gestures to understand his way of perceiving and relating to others.

The level of a person's foresight reflects all of these other sources of information. Lack of foresight is the cardinal feature of personality disorder. Other consistent features of personality disorders are summarized in Table 1.8.2.5.

Temperament involves emotional biases that can be directly observed and felt by an experienced clinician. The tendency of a person to elicit strong emotions from others or 'to get under the skin' of another is a sign of extreme temperament traits or personality disorder. For example, the person with extreme temperament may elicit an urge to be rescued or hostility in the examiner. His general appearance and behavior may be ingratiating or negativistic. Specific features of temperament that distinguish subtypes of personality disorders are summarized in Table 1.8.2.6.

Character traits are assessed partly on intuitive recognition and partly on history. A person who frequently blames others or elicits strong emotional responses in the examiner should be suspected of having a personality disorder. The ratings of character are more precisely based on observations of key functions of self-awareness obtained in the life narrative and the mental status examination. The most informative finding concerns the level of a person's self-awareness, as described in Table 1.8.2.7. The presence of personality disorder means essentially that a person is usually not self-aware (stage 0 in Table 1.8.2.7). Most adults are in the first stage of self-awareness most of the time: they are responsible, have initiative, and are able to delay gratification if they want, but are egocentric. As previously mentioned, they are preoccupied with material concerns. Such individuals may have problems with jealousy or pride, but are sufficiently self-aware so that they are not considered personality disordered. Elsewhere, a simple exercise to evaluate level of self-awareness is described as the Silence of the Mind meditation.[7] It can also be used to help a person improve his level of self-awareness, so it is useful for both assessment and treatment. The ability to reach the second or third stage of self-awareness is the key to improvement in psychotherapy, as described in detail elsewhere.[3] Such growth in self-awareness or

Table 1.8.2.5 Qualitative description of personality disorders

Discriminating features
A maladaptive pattern of responses to personal and social stress that is
stable and enduring since teens
inflexible and pervasive
causing subjective distress
and/or impaired work and/or social relations
Consistent features
lack of foresight (that is, the ability to anticipate what will be satisfying in the long run)
strong emotional reactions elicited from others
(like anger or urge to rescue)
efforts to blame and change others, rather than oneself
Variable features
odd, eccentric
erratic, impulsive
anxious, fearful

Table 1.8.2.6 Qualitative clusters and subtypes of personality disorders according to the American Psychiatric Association (DSM-IV, 1994)

Cluster	Subtype	Discriminating features
Odd/Eccentric	(Low Reward Dependence)	
	Schizoid	socially indifferent
	Paranoid	suspicious
	Schizotypal	eccentric
Erratic/Impulsive	(High Novelty Seeking)	
	Antisocial	disagreeable
	Borderline	unstable
	Histrionic	attention-seeking
	Narcissistic	self-centered
Anxious/Fearful	(High Harm Avoidance)	
	Avoidant	inhibited
	Dependent	submissive
	Obsessive	perfectionistic
Not otherwise specified		
	Passive-Aggressive	negativistic
	Depressive	pessimistic

character traits corresponds closely to the stages of cognitive and character development as described by Piaget, Freud, and Erikson (Table 1.8.2.8). For example, the first stage of self-awareness corresponds to the presence of initiative in Erikson's terms. The second stage involves the presence of generativity. More fine-grained ways to quantify the range of a person's thoughts and human relationships are also described elsewhere.[3] Such refined ratings are important for treatment but not for initial diagnosis.

Table 1.8.2.7 Three stages of self-awareness on the path to well-being (Reproduced from Cloniger, C.R. (2004). *Feeling Good: The Science of Well Being*, with permission of Oxford University Press, New York)

Stage	Description	Psychological characteristics
0	unaware	irresponsible, seeking immediate gratification ('child-like' ego-state)
1	average adult cognition	purposeful but egocentric able to delay gratification, but has frequent negative emotions (anxiety, anger, disgust) ('adult' ego-state)
2	meta-cognition	resourceful and allocentric aware of own subconscious thinking calm and patient, so able to supervise conflicts and relationships ('parental' ego-state, 'mindfulness')
3	contemplation	creative and holistic perspective wise, spontaneous, and loving able to access what was previously unconscious as needed without effort or distress able to anticipate what will be satisfying in future ('state of well-being', 'foresight')

Insight and judgment are also important for assessing character because they are really simply alternative terms for describing the character traits of Self-transcendence and Cooperativeness, as previously discussed. The person's history about his family of rearing, education, marriage, and work history provide the key information for evaluating character. It is important to inquire about a person's goals and his hobbies and recreational activities, whether someone has secure friends, particularly anyone they fully trust and can confide in now or in the past, is important to know as a measure of capacity for intimacy and as a predictor of capacity for forming a therapeutic alliance. Relationships with prior counselors, as well as history of disability claims and law-suits provide important information about personality.

Remember that it is often important with psychiatric patients to assess their personality when they were children or adolescents. In other words, it is as important to evaluate their personality retrospectively as well as in practical, particularly at an age before the onset of other psychopathology, like substance abuse or depression. Current anxiety or depression is expected to inflate Harm Avoidance ratings. Stress or intoxication tends to release temperaments from higher cortical control by character. Likewise, chronic substance abuse, depression, or psychosis arrest character development while active, so early onset of mental disorders is often associated with character deficits. It is usually easy for a patient to provide meaningful information about his childhood personality if the clinician simply asks about the child's early relationships with parents, siblings, schoolmates, and other childhood friends.

Remember also that the single most important dimension of personality to assess in rating a person's level of maturity is his degree of foresight, measured as his Self-directedness. Is the person responsible, or does he tend to blame his problems on other people on unfortunate circumstances? Is the person purposeful, or does he lack clear goals in his life? Is he resourceful, or does he feel inadequate himself and depends on others to solve his problems for him? Assessment of Self-directedness alone is sufficient to determine if a person has a personality disorder of at least moderate severity.[2,4] In contrast, the finding of high Neuroticism is not the same as finding of low Self-directedness, even though they are strongly correlated: a person with anxiety or mood disorder and no personality disorder may be high in Neuroticism but not low in Self-directedness.

Some mild personality disorders also require consideration of the person's capacity to get along with others, as measured by his Cooperativeness. In addition, high functioning individuals who do not merit a diagnosis of personality disorder may nevertheless have specific blind spots in their insight and judgment that leads to severe problems. For example, a competent physician may usually be self-aware but lacks a capacity for intimacy or a sense of fairness in business. Such specific deficits may have severe impairment, even if a person is self-aware in other situations. As a result, it is important to consider the overall profile of a person's life in all five types of situations mentioned earlier. Simply deciding whether or not a person has a personality disorder is insufficient for an assessment of his personality and risk for psychopathology. An adequate initial assessment of a person's personality should allow ratings of all four dimensions of temperament and three dimensions of character, which in turn provide a basis for understanding a person's capacity for well-being and vulnerability to psychopathology.

Table 1.8.2.8 Comparison of different descriptions of character development

Stage of character development	Stage of Piaget	Stage of Freud	Stage of Erikson	Judgment (Cooperative)	Insight (Self-Transcendent)	Foresight (Self-directed)
0	Reflexive					
1	Enactive			Tolerance		
2		Oral	Trust		Trust	
3						Responsible
4	Intuitive	Anal	Autonomy	Forgiving		
5		Phallic	Initiative		Free-Flowing Productivity	
6	Concrete Operations	Latency	Industry			Purposeful
7		Early Genital		Empathic		
8					Transpersonal Identification	
9	Abstract Operations		Identity			Resilient
10		Later Genital	Intimacy	Helpful		
11			Keeper of Meaning		Creativity	
12						Resourceful
13			Integrity	Principled		
14					Holistic Intuition	
15						Spontaneous

Clinical value of psychometric testing

Most experienced clinicians should be able to make valid personality assessments without psychometric testing. However, psychometric testing may still be useful for at least three reasons. First, it helps the clinician to refine his or her clinical assessments by asking more questions with comparisons to normative data than is usually practical during a clinical session. Second, it provides the patient written feedback that can be studied and reflected upon, which does not depend on the clinicians' subjective biases—it reflects back to the patient what was said and provides a language that can be used for accurate communication between the patient and the doctor. Third, it provides a standard for comparison to later assessments as a means of measuring growth. As a result, it is often useful to supplement clinical impression with documentation that allows the patient to describe himself or herself without reliance on the judgment of anyone else. The patient's effort to describe himself or herself often has the therapeutic value of stimulating the patient to begin to understand the motives underlying the pattern of his behaviour. In addition, comparison of psychometric test scores with clinical impression is a helpful way for the clinicians to train themselves in the art of personality assessment.

Further information

The Washington University Center for Well-Being: psychobiology.wustl.edu
The Anthropaideia Foundation: aidwellbeing.org

References

1. Kaasinen, V., and Aalto, S. *et al.* (2004). Insular dopamine D2 receptors and novelty seeking personality in Parkinson's disease. *Movement Disorders*, **19**(11), 1348–51.
2. Cloninger, C. R. (2000). A practical way to diagnose personality disorder: A proposal. *Journal of Personality Disorders*, **14**(2), 99–108.
3. Joyce, P. R., Mulder, R. T. *et al.* (1994). Temperament predicts clomipramine and desipramine response in major depression. *Journal of Affective Disorders*, **30**, 35–46.
4. Cloninger, C. R., Svrakic, D. M. *et al.* (1993). A psychobiological model of temperament and character. *Archives of General Psychiatry*, **50**, 975–90.
5. Joyce, P. R., Mulder, R. T. *et al.* (2003). Borderline personality disorder in major depression: differential drug response, and 6-month outcome. *Comprehensive Psychiatry*, **44**(1), 35–43.
6. Oldham, J. M., Gabbard, G. O. *et al.* (2001). *Practice guidelines for the treatment of patients with borderline personality disorder*. Washington, DC., American Psychiatric Press.
7. Cloninger, C. R. (2004). *Feeling Good: The Science of Well Being*. New York, Oxford University Press.
8. Perls, F. S. (1969). *Gestalt Therapy Verbatim*. Lafayette, California, Real People Press.
9. Lowen, A. (2003). *The language of the body: Physical dynamics of character structure*. Alchua, Florida, Bioenergetics Press.
10. Eysenck, H. J., (ed.) (1981). *A Model of Personality*. New York, Springer-Verlag.
11. Gray, J. A. (1981). A critique of Eysenck's Theory of Personality. *A Model of Personality*. H. J. Eysenck. New York, Springer-Verlag: 246–76.
12. Zuckerman, M. and Cloninger, C. R. (1996). Relationships between Cloninger's, Zuckerman's, and Eysenck's dimensions of personality. *Personality & Individual Differences*, **21**, 283–5.
13. Gusnard, D. A., Ollinger, J. M. *et al.* (2003). Persistence and brain circuitry. *Proceedings of the National Academy of Sciences USA*, **100**(6), 3479–84.
14. Borg, J., Andree, B. *et al.* (2003). The serotonin system and spiritual experiences. *American Journal of Psychiatry*, **160**(11), 1965–1969.

15. Livesley, W. J., Jang, K. L. *et al.* (1998). Phenotypic and genetic structure of traits delineating personality disorder. *Archives of General Psychiatry* **55**, 941–48.
16. Strack, S., (ed.) (2006). *Differentiating normal and abnormal personality*. Springer Publishing, New York.

1.8.3 Cognitive assessment

Graham E. Powell

Principles of assessment

Assessment, testing, or measurement is the evaluation of the individual in numerical or categorical terms, adhering to a range of statistical and psychometric principles. Examples of measurement are, assigning people or behaviour to categories, using scales to obtain self-ratings or self-reports, using tests of ability and performance, or collecting psychophysiological readings. Even diagnosis is a form of measurement and should have various psychometric properties such as satisfactory reliability and validity. In this chapter we concentrate on cognitive or neuropsychological assessment, which typically employs standardized psychometric tests, but it is axiomatic that the basic principles are applicable to all forms of measurement without exception. For example, stating that a patient does or does not have a symptom is potentially just as much of a measurement as stating his or her IQ. It should be noted that this account is of English language tests, and readers elsewhere should note the principles but ask local psychologists what tests they use.

Psychometric tests aim to measure a real quantity—the degree to which an individual possesses or does not possess some feature or trait, such as social anxiety or spelling ability or spatial memory. This real quantity is known in classical test theory as the **true score** *t*, and the score that is actually obtained on the given test is the **observed score** *x*. It is assumed that the observed score is a function of two values, the true score plus a certain amount of **error** *e*, because no test is perfect. Therefore we have the most basic equation in psychometrics: $x = t + e$. The statistical aim of psychometric measurement is to keep the error term to an absolute minimum so that the observed score is equal to the true score, which happens when the error term is reduced to zero. Of course, this is never achieved, but the error term can be reduced to the minimum by making the test as reliable as possible, where reliability is simply the notion that the test gives the same answer twice.

In practice, of course, if a test were repeated many times, each occasion would give a slightly different result, depending on how the person felt, the precise way questions were asked, the details of how answers were scored, or whether there has been any lucky guessing. In other words, observed scores would cluster around the true score. Like the distribution of any variable, the distribution of observed scores would have a mean and a standard deviation. The mean is obviously the true score, and this standard deviation is called the **standard error of measurement (SEM)**. The aim of a good test is to keep the SEM as near as possible to zero, and test manuals should state the actual SEM.

There is a relationship between SEM and the reliability of the test:

$$\text{SEM} = \text{SD}\sqrt{(1 - r_{11})}$$

where SD is the standard deviation of the test and r_{11} is the test–retest reliability of the test (expressed as a correlation coefficient ranging from −1 to +1). If the reliability of the test is perfect (+1), as can be seen the SEM will be zero:

$$\text{SEM} = \text{SD}\sqrt{(1-1)} = \text{SD}\sqrt{0} = 0.$$

Thus a test should be as reliable as possible because then the observed score will be the true score and the standard error of measurement will be zero.

An unreliable test is always useless, but if reliability can be achieved then it is worth considering the test score and, more specifically, what it measures. The degree to which a test measures what it is supposed to measure is known as **validity**. There may be various threats to validity. For example, a test of numeracy may be so stressful that scores are highly dependent upon the patient's anxiety level rather than on his or her ability, or a test of social comprehension may have questions which are culturally biased and so scores may depend in part upon the person's ethnic background.

In practice, there are various types of reliability and validity, and these are summarized in Tables 1.8.3.1 and 1.8.3.2. Further discussion can be found in Kline.[1]

Having used a reliable and valid test, the next issue is how the numbers are analysed and expressed. It has to be noted first that there are three types of scale of measurement. A **nominal** scale is when numbers are assigned to various categories simply to label the categories in a manner suitable for entry onto a computer database—the categories actually bear no logical numerical relationship to each other. Examples would be marital test status or ethnic background or whether one's parents were divorced or not. Nominal scales are used to split people into groups and all statistics

Table 1.8.3.1 Types of reliability

Scorer or rater reliability	The probability that two judges will (i) give the same score to a given answer, (ii) rate a given behaviour in the same way, or (iii) add up the score properly. Scorer reliability should be near perfect.
Test–retest reliability	The degree to which a test will give the same result on two different occasions separated in time, normally expressed as a correlation coefficient. A reliability of less than 0.8 is dubious.
Parallel-form reliability	The degree to which two equivalent versions of a test give the same result (usually used when a test cannot be exactly repeated because, say, of large practice effects).
Split-half reliability	If a test cannot be repeated and there are no parallel forms, a test can be notionally split in two and the two halves correlated with each other (e.g. odd items versus even items). There is also a mathematical formula for computing the mean of all possible split halves (the Kuder–Richardson method).
Internal consistency	The degree to which one test item correlates with all other test items, i.e. an 'intraclass correlation' such as the a coefficient, which should not drop below 0.7.

Table 1.8.3.2 Types of validity

Face validity	Whether a test seems sensible to the person completing it; i.e. does it appear to measure what it is meant to be measuring? This is in fact not a statistical concept, but without reasonable face validity, a patient may see little point in co-operating with a test that seems stupid.
Content validity	The degree to which the test measures all the aspects of the quality that is being assessed. Again, this is not a statistical concept but more a question of expert judgement.
Concurrent validity	Whether scores on a test discriminate between people who are differentiated on some criterion (e.g. are scores on a test of neuroticism higher in those people with a neurotic disorder than in those without such a disorder!). Also, whether scores on a test correlate with scores on a test known to measure the same or similar quality.
Predictive validity	The degree to which a test predicts whether some criterion is achieved in the future (e.g. whether a child's IQ test predicts adult occupational success; whether a test of psychological coping predicts later psychiatric breakdown). For obvious reasons, these last two types of validity are often jointly referred to as *criterion-related validity*.
Construct validity	Whether a test measures some specified hypothetical construct, i.e. the 'meaning' of test scores. For example, if a test is measuring one construct, there should not be clusters of items that seem to measure different things; the test should correlate with other measures of the construct (*convergent validity*); it should not correlate with measures that are irrelevant to the construct (*divergent validity*).
Factorial validity	If a test breaks down into various subfactors, then the number and nature of these factors should remain stable across time and different subject populations.
Incremental validity	Whether the test result improves decision-making (e.g. whether knowledge of neuropsychological test results improves the detection of brain injury).

are based on the frequency of people in each group. The relationship or association between groups can be examined using χ^2 statistics, for example to test whether there is a relationship between being divorced and having parents who divorced. Next there is an **ordinal** scale, in which larger numbers indicate greater possession of the property in question. Rather like the order of winning a race, no assumptions are made about the magnitude of the difference between any two scale points; it does not matter whether the race is won by an inch or a mile. Ordinal scales allow people to be rank ordered and numerical scales can be subjected to non-parametric statistical analysis (which is that branch of statistics which makes minimal assumptions about intervals and distributions), including the comparison of means and distributions and the computation of certain correlation coefficients. Finally comes the **interval** scale in which each scale point is a fixed interval from the previous one, like height or speed. The types of test described in this chapter for the most part aspire to be interval scales, allowing use of the full range of parametric statistics (which assume equal intervals and normally distributed variables).

Having obtained a test score for someone, that score then has to be interpreted in the light of how the general population or various patient groups generally perform on that test. There are two general characteristics of a scale that have to be remembered. The first is the measure of central tendency. Typically one would consider the mean (the arithmetic average), but it is also sometimes useful to consider the median (the middle score) and the mode (the most frequently obtained score). This will be the first hint as to whether the score is normal or whether it is more typical of one group than another. However, in order to gauge precisely how typical a given score is, it is necessary to take into account the **standard deviation (SD)** of the test (other measures relating to the dispersion of test scores, such as the range or skew, can be considered but are not of such immediate relevance).

As long as the mean and SD of the test are known, it is possible to work out exactly what percentage of people obtain up to the observed score x. This is done by converting the observed score into a **standard score** z and converting the z-score to a **percentile**. A standard score is simply the number of SDs away from the mean m, and it will have both negative and positive values (because an observed score can be either below or above the mean, respectively). In other words, $z = (x - m)/\text{SD}$. For reference, Table 1.8.3.3 gives some of the main values of z and what percentage of people score up to those values. It is this percentage that is known as the percentile and it is obtained from statistical tables. For example, a score at the 25th percentile means that 25 per cent of people score lower than that specific score. Obviously, the 50th percentile is the mean of the test. For illustration, the equivalent IQ scores (IQ scores have a mean of 100 and SD of 15) and broad verbal descriptors are also given in Table 1.8.3.3.

A knowledge of percentile scores can help to decide to which category a patient may belong. For example, if a patient completes a token test of dysphasia and scores at the 5th percentile for normal controls and the 63rd percentile for a group of dysphasics, the score is clearly more typical of the dysphasic group.

However, in clinical practice it is often not just a comparison with others that is needed, but a comparison between two of the patient's own scores. For example, verbal IQ might seem depressed

Table 1.8.3.3 *z*-scores, percentiles, IQ scores, and descriptions

z-score	Percentile	IQ	Description
−2.00	2.5th	70	Scores below the 2.5th percentile are *deficient* or in the *mentally retarded* range
−1.67	5th	75	
−1.33	10th	80	Scores between the 2.5th and 10th percentile are *borderline*
−1.00	16th	85	
−0.67	25th	90	Scores between the 10th and 25th percentile are low average
−0.33	37th	95	
0.00	50th	100	The mean score
+0.33	63rd	105	
+0.67	75th	110	Scores between the 25th and 75th percentile are in the *average* range
+1.00	84th	115	
1.33	90th	120	Scores between the 75th and 90th percentile are high average
		120+	Scores over the 90th percentile are *superior*

in comparison with spatial IQ, or the patient's memory quotient might seem too low for his or her IQ. These are known as **difference scores**, and their analysis is a crucial part of the statistical analysis of a patient's profile. There are two key concepts: the **reliability of difference scores** and the **abnormality of difference scores**. Failure to distinguish between these two leads to all manner of erroneous conclusions. In brief, a reliable difference is one that is unlikely to be due to chance factors, so that if the person were to be retested then the difference would again be found. If the test is very reliable (see the previous discussion of reliability), even a small difference score, may be reliable. As a concrete example, the manual of the Wechsler Adult Intelligence Scale—Third Edition (**WAIS-III**)[1] indicates that a difference of about nine points between verbal IQ and performance IQ is statistically reliable at the 95 per cent level of certainty.

However, although a difference of this size would be reliable, this does not necessarily mean that it is abnormal and therefore indicative of pathology. The abnormality of a difference score is the percentage of the general population that has a difference score of this size or greater. Published tables,[2] show that 18 per cent of adults have a discrepancy of at least 10 points between verbal and performance IQ, so a difference of 10 points is not at all unusual. In fact, to obtain an abnormal difference between verbal and performance IQ the discrepancy has to be of the order of 22 points for adults and 26 points for children (i.e. less than 5 per cent of adults or children have discrepancy scores of this size).

Having introduced the basic concepts of psychometric assessment, this is an appropriate point, prior to the description of specific tests, at which to summarize the information that can (or should) be found in a typical test manual, and this is set out in Table 1.8.3.4.

Table 1.8.3.4 What to expect in a good test manual

Theory	The history of the development of the concept and earlier versions of the test The nature of the construct and the purpose of measuring it
Standardization	Characteristics of the standardization sample, how the sampling was carried out. and how well these characteristics match those of the general population Similar data on any criterion groups Similar data for each age range if the test is for children
Administration	How to administer the test in a standard fashion so as to minimize variability of administration as a factor in the error term
Scoring	How to score the test, and criteria for awarding different scores, so as to minimize scorer error
Statistical properties	Means and standard deviations of all groups Reliability coefficients and how they were obtained Validity measures and how they were derived Standard error of measurement Reliability of difference scores Abnormality of difference scores Other data on the scatter of subtest scores Scores of criterion groups
Special considerations	Groups for whom the test is not suitable or less suitable, i.e. the range of convenience of the tests Ceiling effects: at what point does the test begin to fail to discriminate between high scorers? Floor effects: at what point does the test begin to fail to discriminate between low scorers?

Tests of cognitive and neuropsychological functioning

General ability and intelligence

A very useful broad screening test, especially when it is suspected that mental functions are severely compromised, is the Mini-Mental State Examination.[3,4] It is brief, to the point, and can be repeated over time to gauge change. It measures general orientation in time and place, basic naming, language and memory functions, and basic non-verbal skills, and has good norms for a middle age range, especially the elderly, with appropriate adjustment for age. The maximum score is 30, and a score of 24 or less raises the possibility of dementia in older persons, especially if they have had nine or more years of education (a score of 24 is at about the 10th percentile for people aged 65 and older).

However, the Mini-Mental State Examination is only a screening test and the presence or nature of cognitive impairment cannot be diagnosed on the basis of this test alone. A detailed cognitive assessment is provided by the Wechsler scales, i.e. the Wechsler Adult Intelligence Scale—Third Edition UK Version (**WAIS-III^{UK}**),[1] the Wechsler Intelligence Scale for Children—IV UK Version (**WISC-IV^{UK}**),[5] or the Wechsler Preschool and Primary Scale of Intelligence—Revised (**WPPSI-III**).[6] Outlines of the WAIS-III^{UK} and WISC-IV^{UK} are given in Table 1.8.3.5.

IQ scores themselves are very broad measures, drawing upon a wide range of functions. This does not only mean that the scores are very stable (reliable), but also that the IQ score is relatively insensitive to anything except quite gross brain damage. Rather, a careful analysis of subtest scores is needed, always bearing in mind the concepts of reliability and abnormality of difference scores. For example, it takes a subtest range of 11 to 12 points to be considered abnormal (i.e. found in less than 5 per cent of people) on the WAIS-III^{UK} and the WISC-IV^{UK}.

Sometimes the patient may have a language disorder or English may not be his or her first language. In such circumstances Raven's Progressive Matrices Test,[7] which is a non-verbal test of inductive reasoning (non-verbal in the sense that it requires no verbal instructions and no verbal or written answers), can be used. The present author avoids the new norms because they were not collected in the normal fashion (i.e. not in a formal test session under the direct supervision of a psychologist), but the old norms are good. The Matrices Test has the additional advantage of having an advanced version for people in the highest range of ability.[8] No non-English versions of the WAIS-III^{UK} or the WISC-IV^{UK} are available, but the non-verbal scores can be used with caution as there may be unexpected cross-cultural effects.

Speed of processing

Reasoning is not just about solving difficult problems, but also about solving them quickly; the difference between power and speed. IQ tests as above do have timed subtests sensitive to speed, but it can be useful to administer specific tests that are not quite so confounded with intellectual ability.

One example, particularly sensitive to even quite mild concussion, is the Paced Auditory Serial Addition Test (**PASAT**).[9,10] Here, the

Table 1.8.3.5 Outline of the WAIS-III^{UK} and WISC-IV^{UK}

	WAIS-III^{UK}	WISC-IV^{UK}
Age range	16–89 years	6.0–16.11 years
Verbal subtests	Vocabulary Similarities Arithmetic Digit span Information Comprehension Letter-number sequencing	Similarities Digit span Vocabulary Letter-number sequencing Comprehension Information Arithmetic Word reasoning
Non-verbal or spatial subtests	Picture completion Digit symbol Block design Matrix reasoning Picture arrangement Symbol search Object assembly	Block design Picture concepts Coding Matrix reasoning Symbol search Picture completion Cancellation
IQ score	Verbal IQ (VIQ) Performance IQ (PIQ) Full scale IQ (FSIQ)	Full scale IQ (FSIQ)
Index scores	Verbal comprehension Perceptual organization Working memory Processing speed	Verbal comprehension Perceptual reasoning Freedom from distractibility Processing speed
Mean IQ or index scores	100 (SD of 15)	100 (SD of 15)
Mean subtest scores	10 (SD of 3)	10 (SD of 3)
Test–retest reliability of IQ	0.98 for Full scale IQ	0.97 for Full scale IQ
Standard error of measurement of FSIQ	About 2.5, so all scores are about ±5 points[a]	About 2.68, so all scores are about ±5 points
Reliable differences (p <.05)	About 9 points between VIQ and PIQ	About 11 points between VCI and PRI
Abnormal differences (p <.05)	About 22 points between VIQ and PIQ	About 26 points between VCI and PRI
Validity	Highly related to other tests of ability and to criteria related to ability	Highly related to other tests of ability and to criterion groups

[a]95% of the time, true scores are the observed score ±1.96 SEM. In other words, the likely true score is within the range defined by about 2 SEMs either side of the score obtained.

client is read a list of numbers, and as each one is read out so it has to be added to the previous number and the answer spoken aloud (Table 1.8.3.6). This has to be done quickly or the next number will come along. There are several trials in which the numbers are delivered at a faster and faster pace, from one number every 2.4 s down to every 1.2 s. It sounds easy but in actuality is very demanding; even at the slowest speed the average score is only about 70 per cent correct, and this falls away to only about 40 per cent at the fastest speed. Indeed, if a patient has any significant mental slowing, they often cannot do the test at all. Obviously the test cannot be used if the patient has a stammer, or is dysarthric or innumerate.

A less stressful test of mental speed is the Speed of Comprehension Test,(11) in which the person indicates as fast as possible whether simple sentences are true or false (e.g. tomato soup is a liquid, grapes are people). The test can be given orally for patients who cannot read.

Two visual tests of mental speed are Map Search (looking for target symbols on a map as fast as possible) and Telephone Search (looking for various symbols on a page from a telephone directory).(12)

One test that tries to disentangle the relative contribution of slowed motor speed versus slowed mental speed, often a crucial issue in patients with motor deficits, is the Adult Memory and Information Processing Battery,(13) which has two useful timed tests of cancelling target digits.

Attention and concentration

There are various aspects of attention and concentration: the ability to focus resources, the ability to focus on the right aspect, the ability to sustain this attention, the ability to ignore extraneous

Table 1.8.3.6 Sample from PASAT

Number on tape	(Mental process)	Patient says
7		
5	(5+7)	12
1	(1+5)	6
4	(4+1)	5
9	(9+4)	13

information or distracting events, and the ability to divide attention between different tasks. The tests on speed listed above are of course also measures of attention, because highly focused and selective attention has to be sustained for the duration of a pressured task. Digit span on the WAIS-III^{UK} is also a test of attention, as any lapse in attending to the incoming digits will necessarily result in a wrong answer.

However, in addition to these tests, a battery may be used, such as the Test of Everyday Attention(12) which has eight different subtests. Test–retest reliability is quite good, over 0.83 for Map Search and Telephone Search, for example. In terms of validity, the tests are very sensitive to the effects of head injury and stroke.

Memory

Memory is a complex set of processes whereby the person registers, stores, and retrieves information within different modalities (e.g. verbal memory versus spatial memory) and across different time periods (e.g. primary or shorter-term memory versus secondary or longer-term memory or learning). Therefore, as with intelligence, various batteries have evolved with subtests that tap these various aspects. Two examples of batteries are the Wechsler Memory Scale—Third Edition(14) for adults and the Children's Memory Scale,(15) which are both summarized in Table 1.8.3.7. Another battery, which makes a special effort to reflect real-life tasks, is the Rivermead Behavioural Memory Test,(16) which also has a child's version.(17)

Sometimes time constraints make it difficult to give complete memory batteries. Often, just a few key subtests are selected, or other individual tests may be given. For example, to gauge verbal learning the Rey Auditory-Verbal Learning Test is well researched,(18) a test of visual memory is the Rey–Osterrieth Complex Figure Test(19); and a forced choice recognition tests for words and faces is the Recognition Memory Test.(20) If the ability of the patient to recall details of his or her past life is an issue, the Autobiographical Memory Interview can be used.(21)

Language

Commonly used batteries for the assessment of language deficits are the Boston Diagnostic Aphasia Examination(22) and the closely related Western Aphasia Battery.(23) The Boston Examination covers auditory comprehension, oral expression, understanding written language, and writing. These tests can take a long time to give and so brief screening tests are often used, such as the Boston Naming Test(24) or the Graded Naming Test,(25) which both assess word finding, or the Token Test,(26) which assesses verbal comprehension. Finally, a good test to gauge reading and spelling ability is the Wechsler Objective Reading Dimensions Test(27) which will produce reading and spelling ages, and give the abnormality of difference scores between IQ and reading or spelling scores.

Frontal and executive functions

The term executive function derives from the theory that there is a supervisory system exerting executive control of attention. Deficits of this system cause broad patterns of cognitive and behavioural change called the dysexecutive syndrome,(28) which includes changes in volition, poor planning, a disruption of purposive action, and reduced efficacy of performance. One of the most frequent causes of this syndrome is damage to the frontal lobes (frontal-lobe syndrome is a dysexecutive syndrome) but it may also be caused by other patterns of lesion. Table 1.8.3.8 lists some of the features of the dysexecutive syndrome, and examples of tests that are sensitive to them.

Table 1.8.3.7 Summary of two memory batteries

	Wechsler memory Scale-III	Children's memory scale
Age range	16–89 years	5–16 years
Subtests	Information and orientation Logical memory[a] Faces[a] Verbal paired associates[a] Family pictures[a] Word lists[a] Visual reproduction[a] Letter—number sequencing Spatial span Mental control Digit span (Means typically 10, SDs typically 3)	Dot locations[a] Stories[a] Faces[a] Word pairs[a] Family pictures[a] Word lists[a] Numbers Sequences Picture locations (Means of 10, SDs of 3)
Index Scores	Auditory immediate Visual immediate Immediate memory Auditory delayed Visual delayed Auditory recognition delayed General memory Working memory (Means of 100, SDs of 15)	Verbal immediate Verbal delayed Verbal delayed recognition Learning Visual immediate Visual delayed Attention/concentration General memory (Means of 100, SDs of 15)
Reliability	0.60–0.87 for the index scores (i.e. rather low, and note a practice effect of up to 15 points across 5 weeks)	0.76–0.91 for the index scores (note a large practice effect of about 10–15 points across a 2-month interval)
Standard error of measurement	3.88–7.40 (so true scores are at best ±8 points from the observed score)	4.5–7.4 (so true scores are at best ±9 points from the observed score)
Validity	See manual for content, criterion-related, construct, and other types of validity	See manual for content, construct, and criterion-related validity

[a]Also delayed trial.

Some clinical issues

Sources of tests and test data

A good summary of the principles of test theory is given by Halligan *et al.*(36) Information about tests and where to order them from can be found in Lezak's *Neuropsychological Assessment*,(37) Strauss's *Compendium of Neuropsychological Tests*(2) and Mitrushina's(38) *Handbook of Normative Data.*

Understanding tests

The onus is upon the test user to be sufficiently knowledgeable about test theory to gauge the strengths and limitations of tests. Common problems with tests are small standardization sample sizes, unknown or unstable factor structure, poor or no theoretical adequacy, poor or no use of criterion groups, vague scoring

Table 1.8.3.8 Features and tests of the dysexecutive syndrome

Features	Tests
Behavioural change	The Dysexecutive Questionnaire (DEX), both self-report and other report[29]
Planning and impulsivity	Mazes subtest of the WISC-IV^{UK}[7]
Fluency	Of generating words and designs, the DKEFS[30]
Concept formations and ability to shift mental set	Modified Card Sorting Test[31] Rule Shift Cards Test[33]
Estimation	Of various amounts, the Cognitive Estimates Test[32,33] Temporal Judgement Test of time estimation[29]
Alternating plans	Switching between plans based on numbers or letters, the Trail Making Test, see DKEFS[30]
Screening out distracting information	The Stroop Test,[34] e.g. reading the word 'BLUE' when it is printed in red ink
Suppression of competing responses	The Hayling Test[35] which requires patients to choose connected or unconnected words to finish a sentence
Rule attainment	Brixton Test, requiring the patient to learn the rule whereby a pattern changes[35]
Planning	Action Program Test, to use given materials to achieve a given end[29] Zoo Map Test of organizing a route[29] Modified Six Elements Test of planning the order of tasks according to rules[29]

criteria, and poor or no information on difference scores within or between tests.

Even a well-normed and proven test may not actually be applicable to the particular patient at hand; tests only have a certain range of convenience. Tests have to be very carefully chosen when confounding factors are present, such as when English is not the patient's first language or when there is a sensory or motor deficit.

Indeed, there are a range of potentially confounding variables even in those patients who are within the range of convenience of the test. These include effects of medication, fatigue as the testing progresses, motivation, mental state, disturbed behaviour, cultural background and beliefs, and educational background. Test manuals may provide information on such potentially confounding variables, but often it is necessary to know the primary research on the test and its sensitivity to such factors.

Assessing children

Special issues arise in the assessment of children because the neuropsychology theory and conceptual framework are different, the effects of specified lesions change with age, the pattern of recovery of function varies with age, extensive developmental norms, covering the age range, are needed, and children may be more stressed by tests or may find it harder to cooperate with test procedures. These and other issues are fully discussed in texts on developmental neuropsychology,[39] paediatric neuropsychology,[40] and head injury in children.[41] Several children's tests have already been cited by name in preceding sections, and many of the adult tests cited have also been standardized on children, often in subsequent research studies not necessarily carried out by the original test author. Examples of tests with children's norms are word fluency, design fluency, auditory verbal learning, the original Wechsler Memory Scale, the Stroop Test, the Token Test, the Trail-making Test, Wisconsin Card Sorting, the Paced Serial Addition Test, and the Progressive Matrices Test.

Assessing premorbid ability

In order to understand the effects of a brain injury, to gauge intellectual loss, to plan rehabilitation, and to advise on issues relating to personal injury compensation, it is necessary to estimate premorbid intelligence. A summary of strategies for estimating premorbid IQ is given in Table 1.8.3.9.

Capacity

Within the context of intellectual and cognitive functioning, a person is incapable of managing his or her own affairs if two

Table 1.8.3.9 Strategies for estimating premorbid IQ

Strategy	Test and/or comment
Assume highest subtest score on the WAIS-III represents original level	Normal individuals have a profile of abilities and show quite a wide range of subtest scores. It makes no sense at all to say that a person's best score is his or her 'real' potential. Anyone using this method will grossly over-estimate IQ loss
Consider scores on subtests thought to be relatively insensitive to the effects of brain injury	Vocabulary is highly correlated with IQ and is also such a deeply ingrained ability that it is relatively insensitive to the affects of brain injury. Therefore, scores on the Vocabulary subtest can indeed be a guide to premorbid IQ
Gauge IQ from educational record	This is reasonable as long as the person had (i) full access to education, and (ii) the motivation to take and pass exams. Gauging ability band is made easier now that national statistics on examination pass rates are published annually in the UK
Gauge IQ from occupational record	Again this is reasonable as a broad approximation, but cultural and sociological constraints on choice of work or progress in work have to be taken into account
Tests of overlearned skills such as reading	Reading ability is highly correlated with IQ, and is a very overlearned skill, not easily affected by brain injury. This is the best and safest method, as long as the patient had no history of dyslexia and is not currently dysphasic. Tests include the Wechsler Test of Adult Reading[42] and the Spot the Word Test[11]
Genetic endowment	If the patient was damaged at birth, or if the damage caused gross physical deficits adversely affecting educational and occupational potential, then the ability and educational and occupational record of natural parents and siblings may be considered

criteria are met. First, they must have an objective deficit likely to impair problem-solving and decision-making. Second, they must be incapable of sensibly delegating or of appropriately seeking advice. Cognitive assessment obviously bears upon both of these issues. In the first instance assessment can help gauge whether there is a deficit at all, and if so its severity and precise nature. For example, most people would be able to manage their own lives despite some mild reduction in intellectual efficiency or some mild memory problem—after all, this is in any case the course of natural ageing but it is much more difficult to cope with a severe memory deficit. In the second instance, cognitive assessment can point to deficits which make it unlikely that the person can appropriately delegate certain responsibilities. For example, those with dysexecutive syndrome may be gullible or impulsive over whom to approach for advice, or may be reluctant to accept advice, may delegate only inconsistently, or may say they accept certain advice but then do the opposite. In short, they cannot plan to delegate, or if they do make such plans, the plans are poorly monitored and inconsistently implemented.

Malingering

There is no single test of malingering (i.e. consciously motivated deliberate underperformance on tests). Rather, a pattern builds up which gradually raises the suspicion of malingering.[2] Features of test performance which raise the issue are as follows:

1. a degree of deficit that is disproportionate to the severity of the injury;
2. bizarre errors not typically seen in patients with genuine deficits;
3. patterns of test performance that do not make sense;
4. not showing expected patterns;
5. inconsistencies between test performance and behaviour in real life;
6. inexplicable claims of remote memory loss even for important life events like weddings;
7. random responding on forced-choice tests;
8. below random responding on forced-driven tests;
9. poor performance on effort tests that look hard but are in fact easy;
10. the absence of severe anxiety or profoundly low mood such as might cause a collapse in performance;
11. after head injury, the absence of any improvement or indeed a worsening of performance over time;
12. failure to report deficits following a brain injury when in retrospect those deficits are claimed to have been severe;
13. relative absence of a history of somatization or related disorders.

Typical clinical neuropsychological assessment

Having set out the theory, tests, and issues, we can build up a picture of a typical clinical neuropsychological assessment, as given in Table 1.8.3.10.

Table 1.8.3.10 Typical protocol for a clinical neuropsychological assessment and report

Aims	The purpose of the assessment, e.g. to describe deficits. monitor improvement, inform rehabilitation planning, address certain specific issues
Background of patient	Information relevant to the interpretation of test findings, e.g. language, handedness, age, educational history, occupational history, medical and psychiatric history
Nature of the brain injury	For example, time since injury, age at injury, mechanisms of injury, retrograde amnesia, loss of consciousness, post-traumatic amnesia, results of neurological examination, results of scans
Behaviour and mental state	Motivation, co-operation with procedures, anxiety, mood, any aspect that threatens reliability or validity, a clear statement as to whether or not reliability has been compromised
Intelligence	Verbal, non-verbal, skills profile
Speed	Verbal, non-verbal, motor
Attention and concentration	Verbal/spatial tasks General behaviour and lapses on tests
Memory	Verbal/non-verbal Immediate/delayed recall Learning
Language	Reading Screening tests for dysphasia Aphasia battery if needed
Construction skills	Refer to performance subtests Copying a complex figure
Sensory deficits	Note gross deficits and subjective account Record problems noted on tests Refer to neurological examination Tests of spatial neglect Tests of visual agnosia
Motor deficits	Note gross problems and subjective accounts Record problems noted on tests Refer to neurological examination Tests of apraxia
Executive functions	Fluency Planning Estimation Personality/behaviour Record dysexecutive problems noted on other tests
Life situation	Way of life, typical day, leisure activities Nature and amount of any support Impact of deficits upon everyday living
Interview with other informant	An observer's account of deficits, changes, coping, etc.
Formulation	A coherent account of the injury and its repercussions, taking all information into account, focusing on the aims of the assessment

Generalizability theory and ecological validity

There is a broad issue how to generalize from an observation made in one context to what might be observed in other contexts. Traditional divisions between reliability and validity become blurred because they are both expressions of the degree to which a score can be generalized. This sweeps away the notion of a true score, to be replaced by the notion of a universe score, which is the mean of all possible observations under all possible conditions. Classical test theory is replaced by generalizability theory, in which variance in a test score is apportioned to various factors. However, in practice generalizability theory informs test construction rather than replacing classical test theory.(15)

There is one very important aspect of generalizability, and this is ecological validity or the degree to which a test score predicts real-life functioning. Some of the various threats to ecological validity are listed in Table 1.8.3.11 (see Long(43) for a fuller discussion), but the recent trend is to make neuropsychological tests increasingly a distillation of real-life tasks so as to lessen this generalizability problem.(12,16,29)

Table 1.8.3.11 Threats to the ecological validity of test results

The assessment session	Data are collected in a quiet sterile focused environment, whereas real life is noisy and full of distractions
Type of test	Cognitive tests are often constructed to measure a single pure aspect of processing, whereas real-life tasks are multidimensional
Type of interaction	The behaviour of the patient is constrained by the nature of the examiner-patient relationship, and is unlike spontaneous behaviour
Content of tests	The limited number and content of tests that can be given may not tap the real-life problems that are complained of (e.g. reduced sense of humour)
Confounding factors	Test anxiety Motivation to co-operate with the assessment or to perform in a certain way Short test sessions to avoid fatigue whereas most problems are reported when the patient *is* fatigued
Over-reliance on test data	Blinkered adherence to numbers to the exclusion of background information, general observation, information from others, and common sense
Failure to consider ecological validity	Lack of understanding of the issue Failure to follow up patients in such a way as to obtain feedback on the ecological validity of the original assessment, which is necessary to shape ecologically valid assessment procedures
Solutions	Use tests of concentration and distraction Develop new tests or new versions of tests reflecting real-life tasks Find sources of information about real-life behaviour Continue to widen the range of tests available, focusing test development on clinical need Estimate effects of confounding factors Treat numbers as only one form of data Specifically address ecological issues in the final report

Cognitive assessment of psychiatric disorders

It is possible to give only a summary of findings from the cognitive assessment of psychiatric and neuropsychiatric disorders. A fuller account is given by Grant and Adams(44) and McCaffrey.(45)

Epilepsy

There is no single cognitive profile of people with epilepsy. The relationship between epilepsy and the presence of mental retardation (learning disability) will mainly be mediated by the original brain damage causing both the epilepsy and the mental retardation. However, some patients do deteriorate intellectually if seizures are frequent or uncontrolled or if there are lapses into status epilepticus. In terms of partial seizures, the most common pattern is disturbance of verbal memory if there is a left temporal (dominant) focus and of non-verbal memory if there is a right focus. Anticonvulsants themselves may mildly impair performance on a wide variety of intellectual, cognitive, and speeded tasks.

Parkinsonism

The pattern of deficits in patients without overt dementia is memory disturbance and dysexecutive syndrome (e.g. reduced fluency, concept formation, ability to shift set). If there is an overt (subcortical) dementia, aphasia, agnosia, and severe amnesia are relatively uncommon, but mood change is frequent.

Dementia

The most common early sign of Alzheimer's disease is poor performance on delayed verbal memory, possibly with dysexecutive signs, eventually joined by a deterioration in the meaningfulness of speech with a breakdown in semantic relationships and understanding; speech becomes empty of content and frontal dysexecutive deficits emerge.

Depression

In younger neurologically intact persons, depression affects attention and memory. After head injury, the presence of anxiety or depression can make a significant to test scores, including IQ, mental speed, and verbal and spatial memory.

Alcohol

There is a typical neurocognitive profile found in chronic detoxified alcoholics after 2 to 4 weeks abstinence: intact IQ and verbal skills, but impairment of novel problem-solving, abstract reasoning, learning and memory, visual spatial analysis, and complex perceptual–motor integration. If severe thiamine deficiency arises, Wernicke–Korsakoff syndrome may ensue, with profound anterograde amnesia.

Other drugs(37)

Findings regarding the long-term neuropsychological effects of marijuana are equivocal, but if there are long-term changes they probably involve attention. Long-term cocaine use may also affect attention and memory. There are conflicting reports about the long-term use of opiates, but there may be a diffuse effect upon visuospatial and visuomotor activities. Chronic solvent abuse leads to cerebellar ataxia and also some impairment of IQ and memory.

Schizophrenia

There is a growing awareness of dysexecutive deficits in the aetiology of schizophrenic symptoms, relating to disorders of willed action for example. Patients with schizophrenia score poorly on the Behavioural Assessment of the Dysexecutive Syndrome and show other dysexecutive features.

Summary, conclusion, and future directions

Psychometric methods based on classical test theory have permitted the development of reliable and valid tests assessing a wide range of intellectual and cognitive functions. Test results assist in formulation and diagnosis, guide rehabilitation and management, provide baseline measures to detect change, and generally assist clinical decision-making regarding such issues as capacity. Tests and assessment procedures are being further developed so as to improve their ecological validity, enabling better prediction of real-life behaviour and functioning.

Further information

Appleton, R. and Baldwin, T. (ed.) (2006). *Management of brain-injured children*. Oxford University Press, New York. AssessmentPsychology.com

Halligan, P.W. and Wade, D.T. (ed.) (2005). *Effectiveness of rehabilitation for cognitive deficits*. Oxford University Press, London.

Stern, Y. (ed.) (2007). *Cognitive reserve: theory and applications*. Taylor & Francis, New York.

References

1. Wechsler, D. (1997). *Wechsler Adult Intelligence Scale* (3rd edn). Psychological Corporation, Cleveland, OH.
2. Strauss, E., Sherman, E.M.S., and Spreen, O. (2006). *A compendium of neuropsychological tests: administration, norms, and commentary* (3rd edn). Oxford University Press, New York.
3. Folstein, M.F., Folstein, S.E., and McHugh, P.R. (1975). 'Mini-Mental State'. A practical method for grading the cognitive state of patients for the clinician. *Journal of Psychiatric Research*, **12**, 189–98.
4. Tombaugh, T.N., McDowell, I., Krisjansson, B., *et al.* (1966). Mini-Mental State Examination (MMSE) and the modified MMSE (3MS): a psychometric comparison and normative data. *Psychological Assessment*, **8**, 48–59.
5. Wechsler, D. (2004). *Wechsler Intelligence Scale for Children* (4th edn) *UK: manual*. Harcourt Assessment, London.
6. Wechsler, D. (1989). *Manual for the Wechsler Preschool and Primary Scale of Intelligence* (revised). Psychological Corporation, San Antonio, CA.
7. Raven, J.C. (1996). *Progressive matrices*. Oxford Psychologists Press, Oxford.
8. Raven, J.C. (1994). *Advanced progressive matrices, sets I and II*. Oxford Psychologists Press, Oxford.
9. Gronwall, D.M.A. (1977). Paced auditory serial addition task: a measure of recovery from concussion. *Perceptual and Motor Skills*, **44**, 367–73.
10. Stuss, D.T., Stethem, L.L., and Pelchat, G. (1988). Three tests of attention and rapid information processing: an extension. *Clinical Neuropsychologist*, **2**, 246–50.
11. Baddeley, A.D., Emslie, H., and Nimmo-Smith, I.N. (1992). *The speed and capacity of language-processing tests*. Thames Valley Test Company, Bury St Edmunds.
12. Robertson, I.H., Ward, T., Ridgeway, V., *et al.* (1994). *The test of everyday attention*. Thames Valley Test Company, Bury St Edmunds.
13. Coughlan, A.K. and Hollows, S.E. (1985). *The Adult Memory and Information Processing Battery (AMIPB): test manual*. Psychology Department, St James's University Hospital, Leeds.
14. Wechsler, D. (1997). *Wechsler Memory Scale* (3rd edn). Psychological Corporation, San Antonio, CA.
15. Cohen, M.J. (1997). *Children's Memory Scale*. Psychological Corporation, San Antonio, CA.
16. Wilson, B., Cockburn, J., and Baddeley, A. (1985). *The Rivermead Behavioural Memory Test*. Thames Valley Test Company, Bury St Edmunds.
17. Wilson, B.A., Ivani-Chalian, R., and Aldrich, F. (1991). *The Rivermead Behavioural Memory Test for Children Aged 5–10 Years*. Thames Valley Test Company, Bury St Edmunds.
18. Schmidt, M. (1996). *Rey Auditory–Verbal Learning Test*. Western Psychological Services, Los Angeles, CA.
19. Meyers, J. and Meyers, K. (1995). *The Meyers scoring system for the Rey Complex Figure and the Recognition Trial: professional manual*. Psychological Assessment Resources, Odessa, TX.
20. Warrington, E.K. (1984). *Recognition Memory Test manual*. NFER–Nelson, Windsor.
21. Kopelman, M., Wilson, B., and Baddeley, A. (1990). *The autobiographical memory interview*. Thames Valley Test Company, Bury St Edmunds.
22. Goodglass, H. and Kaplan, E. (1983). *The assessment of aphasia and related disorders* (2nd edn). Lea and Febiger, Philadelphia, PA.
23. Kertesz, A. (1982). *Western aphasia battery*. Psychological Corporation, San Antonio, CA.
24. Kaplan, E.F., Goodglass, H., and Weintraub, S. (1983). *The Boston Naming Test* (2nd edn). Lea and Febiger, Philadelphia, PA.
25. McKenna, P. and Warrington, E.K. (1983). *Graded Naming Test*. NFER–Nelson, Windsor. (New norms in 1997.)
26. McNeil, M.M. and Prescott, T.E. (1978). *Revised Token Test*. Pro-ed, Austin, TX.
27. Wechsler, D. (1993). *Wechsler objective reading dimensions: manual*. Psychological Corporation, London.
28. Baddeley, A.D. and Wilson, B.A. (1988). Frontal amnesia and the dysexecutive syndrome. *Brain and Cognition*, **7**, 212–30.
29. Wilson, B.A., Alderman, N., Burgess, P.W., *et al. Behavioural assessment of the dysexecutive syndrome*. Thames Valley Test Company, Bury St Edmunds.
30. Delis, D.C., Kaplan, E., and Kramer, J.H. (2001). *Delis Kaplan Executive Function System (DKEFS): manual*. The Psychological Corporation, San Antonio, TX.
31. Nelson, H.E. (1976). A modified card sorting test sensitive to frontal lobe defects. *Cortex*, **12**, 313–24.
32. Shallice, T. and Evans, M.E. (1978). The involvement of the frontal lobes in cognitive estimation. *Cortex*, **14**, 292–303.
33. O'Carroll, R., Egan, V., and Mackenzie, D.M. (1994). Assessing cognitive estimation. *British Journal of Clinical Psychology*, **33**, 193–7.
34. Sachs, T.L., Clark, C.R., Pols, R.G., *et al.* (1991). Comparability and stability of performance of six alternate forms of the Dodrill–Stroop Color–Word Tests. *Clinical Neuropsychologist*, **5**, 220–5.
35. Burgess, P.W. and Shallice, T. (1997). *The Hayling and Brixton tests*. Thames Valley Test Company, Bury St Edmunds.
36. Halligan, P.W., Kischka, U., and Marshall, J.C. (2003). *Handbook of clinical neuropsychology*. Oxford University Press, New York.

37. Lezak, M.D., Howieson, D.B., Loring, D.W., *et al.* (2004). *Neuropsychological assessment* (4th edn). Oxford University Press, New York.
38. Mitrushina, M., Boone, K.B., Razani, J., *et al.* (2005). *Handbook of normative data for neuropsychological assessment* (3rd edn). Oxford University Press, New York.
39. Spreen, O., Risser, A.H., and Edgell, D. (1995). *Developmental neuropsychology*. Oxford University Press, New York.
40. Baron, I.S, Fennell, E.B., and Voeller, K.K.S. (1995). *Paediatric neuropsychology in the medical setting*. Oxford University Press, New York.
41. Broman, S.H. and Michel, M.E. (ed.) (1995). *Traumatic head injury in children*. Oxford University Press, New York.
42. The Psychological Corporation. (2001). *Wechsler Test of Adult Reading (WTAR): manual*. The Psychological Corporation, San Antonio, TX.
43. Long, C.J. (1996). Neuropsychological tests: a look at our past and the impact that ecological issues may have on our future. In *Ecological validity of neuropsychological testing* (ed. R.J. Sbordone and C.J. Long), pp. 1–41. GR Press–St Lucie Press, Delray Beach, FL.
44. Grant, I. and Adams, K.M. (ed.) (1996). *Neuropsychological assessment of neuropsychiatric disorders* (2nd edn). Oxford University Press, New York.
45. McCaffry, R.J., Palav, A.A., O'Bryant, S.E., *et al.* (ed) (2003). *Practitioner's guide to symptom base rates in clinical neuropsychology*. Kluwer Academic/Plenum Publishers, New York.

1.8.4 Questionnaire, rating, and behavioural methods of assessment

John N. Hall

The earliest forms of psychiatric assessment were based on direct interviews with patients, on reported observations by those who knew the patient, and on direct observations by attendants—later nurses—in the care setting. Attempts to codify these forms of assessment had begun over 90 years ago, as illustrated by the 'Behavior Chart' of Kempf.[1] The present range of structured psychiatric assessment methods grew from the 1950s in association with the introduction of neuroleptic medication and the development of psychiatric rehabilitation programmes. The two most frequently used types of systematic and structured assessment used in both clinical practice and research continue to be questionnaires and ratings. Their value lies in the systematic coverage of relevant content, and the potential for comparing scores across individuals and groups and over time.

This section covers assessment methods that are appropriate for both self-report by patients and others—questionnaires—and observations and judgements made by others about the patient and their immediate circumstances—rating methods. This section will also briefly describe behavioural approaches to assessment of clinical relevance.

Questionnaires offer the respondent a preset range of written questions covering the area of clinical interest, such as depression. The questions are usually completed by marking one of a set of provided response categories (**forced-choice** questions), but may be completed by the patient writing their own response in free text. **Self-report** and 'self-monitoring' methods are similar to the latter form of questionnaire, in that the patient completes a diary or pre-marked sheets. These are more open-ended, and any associated thoughts of the patient may be included. Self-report measures are used widely in cognitive behavioural interventions.

Ratings are judgements about the quality or characteristics of a defined attribute or behaviour, completed subjectively, or on the basis of direct observation of the behaviour in question. While questionnaires are usually self-completed, ratings may be completed by one person with respect to another person. In psychiatric practice, ratings include those made by professional staff, often a nurse or care worker, or by a family member or informal carer, about a patient.

Ratings and behavioural measures have a special use in the assessment of disturbed or bizarre behaviour, where the patient may have little insight or knowledge of the nature or degree of their disturbance, which may pose a major ongoing management problem, or a barrier to their placement in the community. An example of such a measure is the Aberrant Behavior Checklist.[2] This is a 58-item behavioural rating scale completed by an informant, with the content covering five subscales: irritability, agitation, and crying; social withdrawal and lethargy; stereotyped behaviour; hyperactivity and non-compliance; and inappropriate speech.

The purpose of questionnaire, rating, and behavioural assessments

Scales may be used for a number of purposes:

- for the initial assessment of a patient as part of a clinical formulation
- for ongoing monitoring during the course of treatment
- as outcome measures
- for assigning patients from a larger population to a particular therapeutic regime
- for service planning

Normally an assessment will focus on the presented or referred patient. However, it may be helpful to either focus on a family member or on a formal or informal direct carer of the patient. Another potential focus is the patient's environment. The range of behaviour a patient can display is limited by the physical nature of their environment, by the range of equipment or materials available to the patient, and by the social rules of the setting (such as rules against smoking). A rating of environmental restrictiveness would then survey both environmental constraints and the range of formal institutional regulations and informal rules followed by care staff.

Most measures simply describe the current functioning of the patient, without offering a framework for translating the obtained scores into clinical priorities for treatment. An important development in rating methodology has been the 'needs assessment' approach that incorporates the views of patients and carers when taking into account the extent to which their needs have been met, or remain unmet. The Camberwell Assessment of Need (CAN) family of measures[3] has adopted a consistent set of content domains, which has been applied to separate need assessment schedules which can now be applied to adults, older adults, people with learning disabilities, and in forensic settings.

Scale content

A questionnaire or rating is defined by both **overall content** and **item format**. The content of a measure should logically be determined by its purpose. One model of assessment[4] suggests that there are four main content areas for assessment, including cognition, affect (including verbal-subjective components of behaviour), physiological activity, and overt behaviour. The content should cover all the domains of clinical relevance, including current and past behaviour, and psychopathology. While most rating scales cover a relatively limited number of functional areas, and are often designed for use with a specific client group or clinical population, some measures are designed for wider use.

The format of each item typically consists of an **item stem**, or question, followed by a set of **response options**. The item stem and responses should be grammatically complementary, and the total set of response options for each item should together cover all logically possible response options. Responses should use exact frequencies (such as 'twice a day' or 'at least every hour') rather than vague terms such as 'often' or 'frequently'. Response options may be set out verbally, or may have a numerical value attached. Usually the responses for each item will be laid out in sequence to form a graded series of increasing or decreasing severity or quality of response. These items may be set out in **unipolar** (where one end is 'zero' or nil occurrence) or **bipolar** (with the mid-point being neutral or 'normal') form. In general, if an item has more than five response options there is a risk of poor reliability. Figure 1.8.4.1 illustrates the most common individual item formats.

Most items in questionnaires and rating scales are designed to produce ordinal scores—that is, the score simply gives the relative order of items, without implying any mathematical equality of the differences between scores. This limits the statistical methods that can be used with the scores arising from these measures.

Criteria for evaluating questionnaires and rating scales

There are a number of technical and practical factors to bear in mind in appraising and selecting a measure. Anyone using a published questionnaire or rating scale should examine the technical qualities of the measure, which should be included in the original publication or on a scale manual. This is both to critically assess whether or not a specific measure is suitable for the intended purpose, and also to understand how best to use the scale in practice—including any training requirements.

Direct frequency count

How many cigarettes a day do you smoke? ....

Dichotomous or binary item (used in checklists)

Have you ever smoked a cigarette? Yes ☐ No ☐

Three or more response options

a. Nominal scaling: please describe your marital status

Single ☐ Married ☐ Separated/divorced ☐ Widowed ☐

b. Ordinal Unipolar: how often do you feel constipated?

Never ☐ Between 1 and 3 times a week ☐ 4 or more times a week ☐

c. Ordinal Bipolar: how good are you as a car driver?

Above average ☐ average ☐ below average ☐

Linear or **Visual analogue** scale (the line is usually 10 cm long)

What quality of care have you received?

Very poor ________________________ Very good

Fig. 1.8.4.1 Examples of item formats.

Psychometric adequacy

Psychometric criteria are the most important technical ways to evaluate the quality of a measure. Chapter 1.8.3 outlines those minimum psychometric principles and properties that are applicable to all psychological measures, including the classical approaches to scaling, reliability, validity, and sensitivity to change, as well as generalizability approaches. The most widely known psychometric requirements of any scale are validity and reliability: neither of these are inherent properties of a scale. Scales are valid for specific purposes, which should be clearly described in the original published article about a scale.

The form of reliability most characteristic of rating scales, and of other behavioural measures, is inter-rater or inter-observer reliability, which examines the similarity of scores when two or more different raters administer a scale. Ideally the manual for a scale should describe a rater training procedure. If not, it is always sensible to carry out some basic rater training, carrying out some assessments prior to the main study, analyzing score discrepancies, and ensuring that raters have discussed these differences and why they arose.

Typically, ratings may be completed after an observation period varying from a few minutes or hours, to a few days. For those ratings based on observation periods of more than a day, there is then a variable delay between the relevant observations and the completion of the rating, and also any one observer will only have been present or on duty for a proportion of the observation period. Unless the observer against whom reliability is being assessed is observing for exactly the same period, the periods of observation will not be coincident. Under these circumstances a double rating may not be strictly a reliability check, but more of a check of the stability of the behaviour. Patel *et al.*[5] discuss how the use of a simple checklist of the occurrence of key events can substantially improve the reliability of this type of scale.

A further technical issue for observer-based scales is that of reactivity, which is the change in behaviour due to the patient's awareness of the presence of an observer. *Any* live observer will induce some reactivity effects, and this issue is often ignored. Reactivity factors may be reduced by making the observation procedure as minimally intrusive as possible by, for example, careful siting of the observer.

Practical factors and an example

Because of their apparent simplicity, the limitations of questionnaires are not always considered. Bowling[6] has reviewed the main sources of variation in data quality between four modes of administering questionnaires, comparing face-to-face interviews, telephone interviews, self-administration, and electronic procedures. The quality of data was defined in terms of overall response rates, item response rates, response accuracy, and social desirability response bias. These different ways of administering questionnaires have differing cognitive demands on respondents, so that face-to-face interviews tend to yield higher quality data. Regier *et al.*[7] point out the need to standardize measures for both clinical and epidemiological work, given the 'drift' or 'mutations' that can occur with repeated use of even the most carefully designed measures, with major consequences, for example, for public health and policy if prevalence estimates cannot be made reliably.

Practically, scales should be written at the level of vocabulary simple enough for the lowest level of educational attainment likely to be found among scale users. Usually one type of item format is used throughout the scale: sometimes the wish to have one format means that some items are then not easy to understand because that one format is not suited to the content of every item. Shorter scales are usually preferred to longer ones. Some scales are in the public domain. Others are copyright and payments should then be made each time a copy of the scale is used.

There are several steps involved in creating a questionnaire or rating scale. The creation of the original item pool is the first step in designing a new measure, and often existing measures provide some of the items, as well as those identified from any other surveys or studies. Individual items must be selected from this pool, implying, making judgements about the most important topics to cover, and about the bandwidth of the possible range of response options from 'normal' to the most extreme likely to be found.

McGuire *et al.*[8] give a very clear description of the construction of a new rating scale to assess the quality of the clinician–patient therapeutic relationship in community care. They describe the four stages in the creation of the scale:

- generating an item pool
  - conducting semi-structured interviews with clinicians and patients
  - reviewing the content of existing scales covering the same phenomena
- identifying factors and items in the new scale
  - original pool of items rated by clinicians and patients
  - rating scores subjected to principal components factor analysis
- conducting a test–retest reliability study of the new scale
- testing the factorial structure of the revised new scale in a new sample of clinicians and patients

Multiple measures

In both clinical practice and research, the concurrent use of several different measures may be helpful, addressing different categories of functioning and behaviour, with care taken to consider the overall assessment load on any one staff member in the light of their other clinical commitments. Rutter,[9] in reviewing changes in child psychiatry, pays particular attention to the importance of sound measurement by contrasting standardized interviews and checklists, and points out that multiple measures involving different informants, which are repeated over time, are necessary to reduce error and minimize rater bias. Self-completed questionnaires may supplement observer-completed ratings or checklists in the assessment of specific behavioural problems. Deale *et al.*[10] in evaluating the outcome of a treatment trial for chronic fatigue, used 10 outcome measures, namely: three functional impairment measures; two fatigue measures; two psychological distress questionnaires or inventories; and three other variables, including a global self-rating and a self-written statement of illness attributions.

Behavioural and observational assessment methods

A number of existing simple observational methods were refined alongside the clinical introduction of behaviour therapy procedures in the 1960s, and these continue to be associated with contemporary cognitive behavioural interventions (see Fig. 1.8.4.2).

These methods focus on current overt behaviour, and are used for the immediate recording of events, for example counting the number of times an event occurs (leading to frequency counts), or coding observed event by using a set of prescribed behavioural categories that exhaustively and mutually exclusively cover all anticipated possibilities. Direct observation methods can be used in a standardized manner for a group of patients. But they also lend themselves to flexible modification, so that the frequency and the duration of observation periods, and coding systems, can be chosen to suit the requirements of the behavioural difficulties of an individual.

Functional analysis

The term 'functional analysis' generally refers to attempts to discern the variables controlling or maintaining a phenomenon. It usually describes the observation of an individual's behaviour of clinical significance, linked to the observation of those events in the immediate environment that directly preceded, were concurrently associated with, and followed, the target behaviour. This sequence of **antecedent** environmental events, target **behaviour** and concurrent events, and **consequent** environmental events, is often called an **ABC** analysis. For example, incidents of aggression by a particular client in a day-setting may be a function of who is near them or talking to them, so that a record of their presence or absence would be important.

Sampling

A key issue with both rating and direct observational methods is the spread of observation periods over the waking day. Since many behaviours vary in their natural frequency during the waking day, many events should, theoretically, be observed continuously throughout the day. However, since the time needed for continual observation is usually unavailable, a representative sample of the whole day should be observed. Ideally, a random sample of time

Functional analysis Event sampling Time sampling Response coding Self-report and self-monitoring methods Psychophysiological methods

Fig. 1.8.4.2. Categories of behavioural and observational assessment methods.

periods throughout the day should be observed. When events of clinical interest are very complex, it may take too long to code each event fully, so then only, say, every fifth or tenth event is coded in detail—this is termed as **event sampling**. When events are happening very rapidly, or if they tend to happen at about the same rate during the day, it is time-wasting to observe all the time, so observations may then be made only every 15 or 30 min—this is termed as **time sampling**.

Response coding

A set of qualitative coding categories should cover all the most likely events, using clear and unambiguous language, coding categories should be simple enough to be entered quickly. When continuous observation is used, especially for high rates of behaviour, the observer must be allowed regular rest periods.

Psychophysiological methods

These methods typically involve the use of surface sensors to measure changes in, for example, skin electrical conductivity (as in measuring changes in sweating), in light transmission (as in measuring changes in finger blood flow), and in volume (as in plethysmography). These sensors are now always electronic, so the electrical signals from them are calibrated with the associated physical change, which is taken as a proxy measure for the assumed underlying change in physiological arousal. The small size, low weight, and the sophistication and reliability of electronic recording equipment, including hand-held electronic event recorders, now allows the immediate and unobtrusive recording of events, with concurrent data analysis.

Standard or individualized measures?

There are many standard ratings and questionnaires already in existence covering most areas of clinical interest. However, the fact that a scale is well used does not necessarily mean that it is psychometrically sound, or that the content covered is appropriate for a given clinical or research purpose. Rating scales may continue to be used widely when they are no longer the best scales technically, but because the volume of published research in which they have been used permits comparisons with other studies.

Solutions to this dilemma are either to create a totally new measure, making sure it *is* better than its predecessor, or to improve systematically the properties of an existing measure. Parker *et al.*[11] describe a modification of the well-established parental bonding instrument to include abusive parenting, which was omitted in the original version. Their article demonstrates both how to modify an original measure to improve item wording, and at the same time incorporate additional material to increase the value of the measure. An unsound solution is to change the measure in an *ad hoc* way—scale vandalization!—with no awareness of the principles of sound scale and item construction. This only results in an instrument that will then be of poor or unknown reliability or validity.

Conclusions

The value of rating and questionnaire methods is that they can be used by a variety of assessors who do not need to be qualified mental health professionals—although the need for at least some training in rating methods should not be overlooked. They can be presented in very short versions therefore making minimal demands on both assessors and patients, and so can lead to high levels of compliance. Since they can be used by patients, they can themselves be tools to increase engagement and to give patients direct feedback about their own current state. Behavioural and observational assessment measures constitute a clinically useful subgroup of methods, which potentially have high validity with respect to day-to-day functioning. However, the apparent simplicity of all of these methods masks the need for care in their construction, the importance of training in their use, and caution in over-sophisticated interpretation of data arising from their use.

Further information

There are a number of helpful core texts, describing general technical issues in questionnaire and rating scale design (see Streiner & Norman[a] and McDowell[b]). Similarly Haynes & O'Brien[c] and Hersen[d] cover the general principles of behavioural assessment. Andrews *et al.*[e] give an excellent review of outcome measures in mental health, covering many of the most commonly used rating scales. McDowell[b] and Bowling[f] include extensive lists of the most commonly used scales in health and social care, including those covering mental health issues.

(a) Streiner, D.L. and Norman, G.R. (2003). *Health measurement scales*. Oxford University Press, Oxford.
(b) McDowell, I. (2006). *Measuring health: a guide to rating scales and questionnaires*. Oxford University Press, Oxford.
(c) Haynes, S.N. & O'Brien, W.H. (2000). *Principles and practice of behavioural assessment*. Springer, New York.
(d) Hersen, M. (2005). *Clinician's handbook of adult behavioral assessment*. Academic Press, New York.
(e) Andrews, G., Peters, L., and Teesson, M. (1994). *The measurement of consumer outcome in mental health: a report to the National Mental Health Information Strategy Committee*. Clinical Research Unit for Anxiety Disorder, Sydney, Australia.
(f) Bowling, A. (2004). *Measuring health*. Open University Press, Maidenhead.

References

1. Kempf, E.J. (1915). The behavior chart in mental diseases. *American Journal of Insanity*, **71**, 761–72.
2. Aman, M.G., Singh, N.N., and Stewart, A.W. (1985). The aberrant behavior checklist: a behavior rating scale for the assessment of treatment effects. *American Journal of Mental Deficiency*, **89**, 485–91.
3. See www.iop.kcl.ac.uk/hsr/prism/can
4. Eifert, G.H. and Wilson, P.H. (1991). The triple response approach to assessment: a conceptual and methodological reappraisal. *Behaviour Research and Therapy*, **29**, 283–92.
5. Patel, V., Hope, T., Hall, J.N., *et al.* (1995). Three methodological issues in the development of observer-rated behaviour rating scales: experience from the development of the rating scale for aggressive behaviour in the elderly. *International Journal of Methods in Psychiatric Research*, **5**, 21–7.
6. Bowling, A. (2005). Mode of questionnaire administration can have serious effects on data quality. *Journal of Public Health*, **27**, 281–91.

7. Regier, D.A., Kaelber, C.T., Rae, D.S., *et al.* (1998). Limitations of diagnostic criteria and assessment instruments for mental disorders. *Archives of General Psychiatry*, **55**, 109–15.
8. McGuire-Snieckus, R., McCabe, R., Catty, R., *et al.* (2007). A new scale to assess the therapeutic relationship in community mental health care: STAR. *Psychological Medicine*, **37**, 85–95.
9. Rutter, M. (1997). Child psychiatric disorder: measures, causal mechanisms, and interventions. *Archives of General Psychiatry*, **54**, 785–9.
10. Deale, A., Chalder, T., Marks, I., *et al.* (1997). Cognitive behaviour therapy for chronic fatigue syndrome: a randomized controlled trial. *American Journal of Psychiatry*, **154**, 408–14.
11. Parker, G., Roussos, J., Hadzi-Pavlovic, D., *et al.* (1997). The development of a refined measure of dysfunctional parenting and assessment of its relevance in patients with affective disorders. *Psychological Medicine*, **27**, 1193–203.

1.9

Diagnosis and classification

Michael B. First, and Harold Alan Pincus

In Psychiatry, as in all of medicine, diagnosis is a key function and central to developing a plan of treatment for patients. Psychiatry, however, faces special challenges. The etiopathogenesis of most psychiatric disorders is not known. For the most part, a clinician must rely on reports from, and direct observation of patients to gather the necessary information to determine a diagnosis. Until very recently, laboratory tests had little relevance. Even diagnostic information found in medical records may not be useful, since the clinician cannot ascertain whether the historically recorded diagnoses of previous clinicians were based on reliable observations, the application of similar diagnostic approaches, or even the same system of classification. These special challenges faced by the field have ensured that diagnosis and classification in psychiatry has a long and rich history.

Definitions

The term 'diagnosis' can mean both the name of a particular disease as well as the process of determining or 'making' a diagnosis. In medicine, generally, various terms are used to describe a pathological entity. When there is the presence of objective pathology or the presumed understanding of aetiology, the term 'disease' is generally used, e.g., pancreatic cancer, strep throat, Alzheimer's disease. In instances of unknown aetiology or when the disease process is not apparent, the term 'disorder' is usually applied with a syndromic characterization, i.e., definition based on symptom presentation, history, and sometimes, associated laboratory findings. Other terms are also used in common parlance, such as 'illness' for an individual's subjective awareness of distress and 'sickness' for the inability to perform usual social roles. For the most part, in psychiatry, the term 'disorder' is used.

Classification represents the process of placing diagnostic entities into various groupings in a systematic way, based on a set of principles with regard to the similarities and differences among these categories. Depending upon the principles and conceptual framework underlying the categorization process, classifications can be very different.

Goals of the classification

In some ways, the most important question may be 'whose needs is the classification primarily intended to address?' Clinicians want a classification that can categorize as many people that come in for help as possible. They want the classification to facilitate the identification and treatment of patients and provide guidance on prognosis and cause. Researchers want to have groupings that are highly homogeneous in order to test the efficacy of specific treatments and to better understand the aetiology of specific disorders. Educators want a classification system to offer a structure for teaching about psychopathology and differential diagnosis. Public health administrators want to track epidemiology, health utilization, and costs over time. Some argue that psychiatric diagnosis is a reductionistic labelling of individual differences or social deviance and exposes individuals to potential stigma. At a minimum, they would like a psychiatric diagnostic system to be less prone to misuse. Ultimately, most classifications attempt to balance among those competing priorities, not always successfully. In some cases, e.g., the ICD-10, different products are developed for different target groups, i.e., research diagnostic criteria for investigators, a simpler, more aggregated classification for primary care providers, etc.

Conceptual issues

A range of conceptual issues and their resolution determines the principles and rules governing a system of classification. It is important to note, however, that classification systems do not necessarily apply these rules in a consistent manner. Some of the issues noted below may not be resolved in an absolute manner, but in a way that employs compromises among multiple priorities, e.g. balancing the needs of clinicians, researchers, educators, and public health administrators or having some diagnostic groupings based on a descriptive approach and others on a theory-based approach.

Descriptive v. theory-based: Do the classification principles emanate from a theory regarding the aetiology or mechanisms of psychopathology (e.g. psychodynamics, behavioural, neurobiological) or does the classification attempt to provide a theoretical heuristic framework for describing syndromic entities?

Pathology v. normalcy: What assumptions underlie distinguishing what constitutes a 'mental disorder' or 'caseness' from normative behavior?

Categorical v. dimensional: Does the classification assume discrete categories with sharp boundaries or does it assume that psychopathology lies on a continuum across a range of dimensions (and if so, what dimensions and how were they chosen?)

Lumping v. splitting: Does the classifications system establish a smaller number of broad, relatively heterogeneous categories or numerous homogeneous categories?

Multiple v. single diagnosis: Is there a hierarchy where certain diagnoses have priority and 'trump' other diagnoses if an individual fits into more than one category or are multiple simultaneous diagnoses (i.e. comorbidity) encouraged to communicate more complete diagnostic information?

The development of modern classifications

The first international classification of diseases in 1855 was concerned with a nomenclature of causes of death.[1] After many revisions this list was adopted by the World Health Organization (WHO) in 1948 and the so-called *Sixth Revision of the International Statistical Classification of Diseases, Injuries and Causes of Death* (ICD-6) was produced.[2] The sixth edition of the ICD included for the first time a classification of mental disorders, containing 10 categories of psychoses, nine categories of psychoneurosis, and seven categories of character, behaviour, and intelligence. A number of problems with this classification (e.g., many important categories such as the dementias, many personality disorders, and adjustment disorders were not included) rendered it unsatisfactory for use in most countries; only five countries, including the United Kingdom, adopted it officially. The first edition of the American Psychiatric Association's Diagnostic and Statistical Manual of Mental Disorders (DSM-I)[3] was published in the United States as an alternative to ICD-6. For the first time in an official classification, glossary definitions of the various disorders were included in addition to the names of the disorders.

Work on ICD-8 began in 1959 with the goal of developing a classification system that would be acceptable to all of its member nations. The resulting system, ICD-8, went into effect in 1968, and in 1974 added a glossary which was largely based on British views about diagnostic concepts.[4] Coincident with the development of ICD-8, the American Psychiatric Association prepared a second edition of its DSM based on ICD-8, defining each disorder for use in the United States.[5]

The early 1970s saw the introduction of explicit operationalized diagnostic criteria that were developed for research purposes. Although the glossary definitions of disorders in DSM-II and ICD-8 were an improvement over just having a list of diagnostic categories, these brief descriptions were too vague to be useful in identifying diagnostically homogeneous populations for study. Researchers responded to this need by developing their own operationalized criteria. The first set of diagnostic criteria that covered a wide range of disorders was developed by Robins and Guze at Washington University in St. Louis[6] with the stated purpose of 'provid[ing] common ground for different research groups so that diagnostic definitions can be emended constructively as further studies are completed'. (p. 57). They were known as the 'Feighner criteria' after the first author of the paper that presented them. Criteria sets for 16 disorders were presented and listed those features required for each diagnosis (known as 'inclusion criteria') as well as features whose presence would rule out the disorder (known as 'exclusion criteria'). The Feighner criteria proved to be enormously useful to the research community as illustrated by the large number of times they were cited in other papers (i.e. 1650 citations from 1972 to 1982 as compared to the typical average of 2.1 citations per paper). Several years later, an expanded set of research criteria based on the Feighner criteria was developed to meet the needs of a National Institute of Mental Health-sponsored collaborative project on the psychobiology of depression.[7] These criteria, known as the Research Diagnostic Criteria (RDC) subsequently became very popular among researchers and were heavily used, especially in research on mood and psychotic disorders.

To develop the mental disorders section for ICD-9, WHO initiated an intensive program to identify problems encountered by psychiatrists in different countries in the use of the mental disorders section of ICD-8 and to formulate recommendations for their solution. A series of eight international seminars were held annually from 1965 to 1972, each of which focussed on a recognized problem in psychiatric diagnosis. The outcome of the seminars formed the basis for the recommendations made for ICD-9,[8] which was ultimately published in 1978.

As work progressed on the development of ICD-9, the American Psychiatric Association decided to develop a third edition of its diagnostic manual, DSM-III.[9] This decision was made both because of identified inadequacies of the ICD-9 for research and clinical use, and because the ICD-9 did not include important innovations that had already been demonstrated by researchers to be both technically feasible and useful, like operationalized diagnostic criteria. Under the leadership of Robert L. Spitzer, successive drafts of DSM-III were prepared by 14 advisory committees, with the drafts being distributed among both American and international psychiatrists for comments and review. Many of the DSM-III criteria sets were based on the RDC criteria, with the rest developed based on expert consensus.

The improvement in reliability over DSM-II (which provided only glossary definitions) was demonstrated by a large NIMH-supported field trial in which clinicians were asked to independently evaluate patients using drafts of the DSM-III criteria.[10] The explicit diagnostic criteria provided for each of the disorders in the classification were based on the symptomatic presentation of the disorder rather than on theories about the underlying cause. Even though the DSM-III was a product of the American Psychiatric Association, its adoption of this 'descriptive approach' resulted in its widespread acceptance by all mental health professionals in the United States, regardless of their theoretical orientation. For example, clinicians from different orientations might have very different understandings of what causes panic attacks; a cognitively-oriented clinician might attribute a panic attack to the person's tendency to catastrophize in response to normal physical sensations like increased heart rate; a neurobiologically-oriented clinician might consider panic attacks to be due to overactivity of brain circuitry involved in fight-or-flight responses, and a psychodynamically-oriented clinician might see panic as a consequence of the breakdown of the defense organization at various levels. Despite these divergent hypotheses, however, all of these clinicians can agree on how a panic attack presents (i.e. a discrete period of apprehension or fear with at least four symptoms such as shortness of breath, palpitations, chest pain, choking, dizziness, etc), thus facilitating communication among them.

DSM-III also introduced the use of a multiaxial system for recording the diagnostic evaluation. The multiaxial system facilitated the use of a biopsychosocial model of evaluation by separating (and thereby calling attention to) developmental and personality disorders (Axis II), physical conditions (Axis III), stressors (Axis IV), and degree of adaptive functioning (Axis V) from the usually more florid presenting diagnoses (Axis I).

Despite initial opposition among some psychiatrists (most especially those with a psychoanalytic orientation), DSM-III proved to be a great success, becoming the common language of mental health clinicians and researchers for communicating about mental disorders. Although it was intended primarily for use in the United States, it was translated into 13 languages and was widely used by the international research community.

Experience with DSM-III in the few years after its publication in 1980, revealed a number of inconsistencies and lack of clarity in the diagnostic criteria sets. Furthermore, research conducted in the early 1980's demonstrated errors in some of the assumptions that went into the construction of the DSM-III criteria sets. For example, the DSM-III prohibition against giving an additional diagnosis of Panic Disorder to individuals with both Major Depressive Disorder and panic attacks was shown to be incorrect based on data demonstrating that relatives of individuals with both Major Depressive Disorder and Panic Attacks can have either Major Depressive or Panic Disorder.[11] For these reasons, work began on a revision of the DSM-III, which was published as DSM-III-R in 1987.[12]

Initial work began on the development of the psychiatric section of the *10th Revision of the International Classification of Diseases* (ICD-10), in 1982 under the chairmanship of Norman Sartorius. After a meeting of WHO representatives and consultants together with representatives of the American Drug and Mental Health Administration in Copenhagen in 1982, several further meetings took place (e.g. in Djakarta and in Geneva in 1984) in which a provisional psychiatric classification was designed. It was decided that the ICD-10 classification of mental disorders would be produced in several versions. The first of these is to be used, as are other parts of the International Classification of Diseases, mainly for statistical purposes, and included a short glossary definition for each category.[13] This is the version that was officially approved by the World Health Assembly and thus, is the version for which international compatibility is mandated by treaty agreements. The second version, Clinical Descriptions and Diagnostic Guidelines is for the use of the practicing clinician.[14] Each category in this version has a detailed definition specifying the main features of the disorder followed by diagnostic guidelines. The third version, the Diagnostic Criteria for Research is primarily intended for research and contains diagnostic criteria which are stricter in form than those in the clinical diagnostic guidelines from which they were derived.[15] For example, while the guidelines may indicate that a particular disorder 'usually starts in early childhood', the diagnostic criteria for research would specify that the diagnosis 'should not be made if the onset is after the age of 30', The decision to separate the criteria for research from the clinical guidelines was made because clinicians in their daily work do not observe overly strict rules when making diagnoses, which are of cardinal importance for research.[16] Finally, a version of the mental disorders section was produced for use in primary care settings.[17] It contains a much smaller number of categories (i.e. those that are frequently encountered in every day general practice) as well as treatment guidelines corresponding to these categories.

By 1986, a first draft of the psychiatric chapter, including details of the categories, code numbers, diagnostic guidelines, and precise diagnostic criteria for research had been written, and by June 1987, the clinical diagnostic guidelines were being circulated by WHO's division of mental health for field trials in 194 different centers in 55 different countries.[18] In 1989, the International Revision Conference, attended by representatives of the health ministries of a majority of WHO member states gave formal approval to the basic categories and text. A draft of the diagnostic criteria for research was produced in 1990 and field trials to evaluate inter-rater agreement, confidence in diagnosis, and ease of use began later in the year.[19] Finally, in 1990, the World Health Assembly formally approved its introduction in member states starting in January 1, 1993.

The American Psychiatric Association started work on the development of DSM-IV in 1988, shortly after the publication of DSM-III-R, spurred on by the need to coordinate its development with the already ongoing development of ICD-10. DSM-IV continued the descriptive atheoretical approach advanced by both DSM-III and DSM-III-R, but this time also incorporated a meta-analytic data-based revision process to guide changes.[20,21] This was in contrast to both DSM-III and DSM-III-R which by necessity, given the paucity of available empirical data, relied almost exclusively on expert consensus. The DSM-IV workgroups began their deliberations by identifying a series of diagnostic questions to be considered and problems to be addressed and employed a three-stage empirical review process to address, these questions. The first stage involved a systematic comprehensive review of the published literature guided by literature searches using rules established at a DSM-IV methods conference. The second stage involved supplementing the literature reviews with a data reanalysis project funded by the MacArthur foundation in which existing data sets collected for other studies were combined and analyzed using meta-analytic methods. These data reanalyses were useful in answering a number of diagnostic questions (e.g. determining the minimum number of panic attacks required in order to justify a diagnosis of panic disorder) but were unfortunately limited by incompatibilities in the data sets and the fact that the data needed to answer specific diagnostic questions often had not been collected. Proposed criteria sets formulated based on the literature reviews and data reanalyses were then tested in 15 NIMH-funded multi-site field trials. The entire empirical review process and the reasons underlying the decisions made by the DSM-IV workgroups have been documented in the four volume DSM-IV Sourcebook.[22–25]

In order to increase compatibility between ICD-10 and DSM-IV, a collaborative relationship was established between the DSM-IV workgroups and the developers of ICD-10. Two meetings were convened in which the respective workgroups joined forces with the goal of minimizing the differences between diagnostic definitions in the two systems. Unfortunately, the potential to make the two systems identical was seriously constrained by differences in the timelines between the two revision processes. By the time the DSM-IV workgroups were first convened in 1989, the categories and basic text of the ICD-10 had already been settled by the International Revision Conference.[26] Thus, although final DSM-IV and ICD-10 systems were much more similar than were DSM-III and ICD-9, a number of mostly small differences in criteria sets persist. While some of the discrepancies are the result of genuine differences in diagnostic outlook (e.g., the one month duration of ICD-10 schizophrenia vs. 6 month duration of DSM-IV schizophrenia), the overwhelming majority appear not to have any justification.[27]

One of the most important uses of the DSM-IV has been as an educational tool. This is especially true of the descriptive text that accompanies the criteria sets for the DSM-IV disorders. Given that the interval between DSM-IV and DSM-V was being extended from seven years between DSM-III and DSM-III-R, and between DSM-III-R and DSM-IV to at least 12 years, concerns were raised that the information in the text would become increasingly out-of-date over time. Therefore, in order to bridge the span between DSM-IV and DSM-V, a revision of the DSM-IV text was undertaken.[28] The primary goal of the DSM-IV-TR was to maintain the currency of the DSM-IV text, which reflected the empirical literature up to 1992. Thus, most of the major changes in DSM-IV-TR were confined to the descriptive text. Changes were made to a handful of criteria sets in order to correct errors identified in DSM-IV. In addition, some of the diagnostic codes were changed to reflect updates to the ICD-9-CM coding system adopted by the U.S. Government.

Differences between DSM-IV and ICD-10

A fundamental difference between the ICD-10 and the DSM-IV reflects the different purposes of the two systems, i.e., that ICD-10 is set up as a classification system whereas DSM-IV is a diagnostic nomenclature. The primary goal of the ICD is to facilitate the collection of statistics about those individuals who present themselves to a health care professional. Thus, the ICD has been designed to provide the coder with an unambiguous choice of diagnostic category given a particular case. The main rule for deciding whether to include a diagnostic category in the ICD is its common international usage. Inclusion of a category in the ICD carries with it no implication of diagnostic validity—in fact, a number of categories included in ICD-10 were considered for inclusion in DSM-IV—but were not added because of concerns about their validity (e.g., mixed anxiety depression). In contrast, inclusion of a category in the DSM implies that the category has been officially sanctioned by the American Psychiatric Association as appropriate for clinical and research usage, i.e., the category has both clinical utility and is backed up by an empirical data base. It should be noted, however, that the empirical data base is not equivalent for all of the categories—to minimize disruption, diagnostic categories, that were included in earlier editions of the DSM have been 'grandfathered' in. Starting with DSM-IV, new categories were only added if they met these higher standards.

Another important difference between the DSM and ICD approach is the role of impairment in the definition of a disorder. With only a few exceptions (e.g., dementia, phobias), mental disorders in ICD-10 are defined exclusively by the symptomatic presentations—there is no requirement that the symptoms cause any impairment in the individual's level of functioning. Impairment in functioning caused by the symptoms is indicated in ICD-10 by using an orthogonal scale, the International Classification of Functioning.[29] In contrast, most of the DSM-IV criteria sets include a criterion (known as the 'clinical significance criterion') requiring that the disturbance causes clinically significant distress or impairment in social, occupational, or other important areas of functioning. According to the introduction of the DSM-IV, this criterion has been included to help establish 'the threshold for the diagnosis of a disorder in those situations in which the symptomatic presentation by itself (particularly in its milder forms) is not inherently pathological and may be encountered in individuals for whom a diagnosis of 'mental disorder' would be inappropriate'. (p. 8). Accordingly, the only diagnoses that do not include this criterion are those whose symptomatic presentations are considered to be inherently indicative of psychopathology (e.g., the psychotic disorders).

The diagnostic implications of this difference can be illustrated in the different ways that specific phobia is defined in DSM-IV and ICD-10. In DSM-IV, a phobia is diagnosed only if 'the avoidance, anxious anticipation, or distress in the feared situation interferes significantly with the person's normal routine, occupational (or academic) functioning or social activities or relationships, or there is marked distress about having the phobia'. (p. 449, DSM-IV-TR). ICD-10 has no such requirement; the phobia is diagnosed so long as there is a marked fear or avoidance of a specific object or situation. Thus, an individual residing in New York City who has a snake phobia but who never has any occasion to encounter a snake would not be diagnosed as having a mental disorder in DSM-IV-TR because the phobia does not have any impact on the person's functioning whereas in ICD-10 such an individual would be diagnosed as having a snake phobia because the person would react with fear or avoidance if he or she had the occasion to be confronted with a snake.

Separating symptoms from the functional impairment that results from them certainly makes conceptual sense. In other areas of medicine, the diagnosis of a disorder is based solely on the presence of pathology and not on the effect that the pathology exerts on a person's life (e.g., a patient is diagnosed with pneumococcal pneumonia if the patient's lungs are infected with the pneumococcus bacillus regardless of the impact of the pneumonia on the patient's level of functioning). The problem with diagnosing mental disorders in this way is that it is not currently possible to define the presence of a mental disorder based on the identification of its underlying pathology. The descriptive symptoms that make up the definitions of mental disorders in the DSM-IV and ICD-10 are not specific to mental disorders but can and do occur in individuals without any mental disorder. Thus, defining disorders exclusively in terms of presenting symptomatology, much of which can occur in normal individuals, can lead to false positive diagnoses. For this reason, in order to avoid false positive diagnoses in the absence of objective evidence of disease, DSM relies on functional impairment or distress to help set the diagnostic threshold between normality and disorder.

The structure of ICD-10, (Chapter V)

The psychiatric classification is part of the general medical classification. There are 21 chapters, each designated by a Roman numeral. The psychiatric disorders are included in Chapter V which is also identified by the letter F. The letter F is followed by Arabic numbers, the so-called second digit for the larger diagnostic groups and the third digit for more special groups. Thus the use of three digits allows a choice of 100 diagnostic possibilities. Proceeding further with a fourth digit, 1000 possible diagnoses are available, of which about one-third are used at present. This system is thus designed to allow the addition of new diagnoses in future without having to change substantial parts of the classification.

Furthermore, it is possible to code the course over time or characteristic features of a disorder by using a fifth or sixth digit. By using codes from other chapters of ICD-10, such as X, Y, and Z, additional circumstances (e.g. suicide) or special symptoms (e.g. nausea) as well as psychosocial factors can be coded. Somatic comorbidity is coded from the related chapters, for example diseases of ear, nose, and throat from Chapter VIII headed by the letter H (e.g. tinnitus H93.1) or diseases of the gastrointestinal system from Chapter XI headed by the letter K (e.g. alcohol gastritis K29.2). The specific challenges encountered in diagnosing psychiatric disorders reliably over the years has led WHO to include short definitions plus inclusion and exclusion terms for all psychiatric disorders in Chapter V (F). In all other chapters, diagnoses are named without further explanation.

As described earlier in this chapter, Chapter V of ICD-10 is not just a catalogue of disorders for statistical purposes, but is also a clinical manual, a textbook of diagnoses, and an instrument for research for different users. Therefore, a group of texts had to be produced to serve the various purposes—the so-called 'ICD-10 family of documents'

The *Short Glossary of ICD-10, Chapter V (F)* is part of the basic work known as the *International Statistical Classification of Diseases and Related Health Problems* The Short Glossary is part of the first of three volumes, the general systematic classification, and gives short definitions which are useful not only for medical personnel but also for statisticians, health insurance clerks, and others who are not in medical or related professions.

The *Clinical Descriptions and Diagnostic Guidelines (CDDG Version)*, known as the Blue Book because of the colour of its cover, was developed first and can be regarded as the central part of the psychiatric classification[14] intended for use by psychiatric clinicians in their daily practice. The *Diagnostic Criteria for Research* (DCR), known as the Green Book, has been developed for scientific use[15] and is intended to be used together with the diagnostic guidelines. Compared with the Blue Book, the symptom criteria are more clearly defined, the time criteria are stricter, and the inclusion and exclusion criteria are more precise in the Green Book. Thus, many unclear cases which are unsuitable for research are excluded. However, despite its title, this book is also useful for diagnosticians in clinical practice.

The *multiaxial version* of the ICD-10 classification of mental disorders allows different aspects of the patient's health and social situation to be assessed. Introduced by Rutter and colleagues,[30] multiaxial diagnosis has been employed for many years in child and adolescent psychiatry. It contains clinical syndromes, problems of development, intelligence, somatic disorders, and psychosocial problems. To a considerable degree, the multiaxial version of ICD-10 is comparable with that of DSM-IV. However, in DSM-IV, axis I is for psychiatric clinical disorders, axis II is for personality disorders and intellectual disability, and axis III is for general medical conditions. In ICD-10, axis I includes all disorders. Thus, psychiatric disorders (F1–F5), personality disorders (F6) and intellectual disability (F7), and the chapters on somatic comorbidity all use one axis.

Axis II of ICD-10 is for disability. To facilitate its use, WHO developed an instrument, the short disability assessment schedule (WHO DAS-S), which helps to describe and assess the consequences of axis I disorders.[31] Axis II corresponds to the widely used DSM-IV axis V, Global Assessment of Functioning (GAF). In connection with the disability axis, the International Classification of Functioning created by WHO for the whole of rehabilitative medicine, of which psychiatry is only a part, should be mentioned.[29] Axis III of ICD-10 covers psychosocial and other problems, and corresponds to DSM-IV axis IV (psychosocial and environmental problems).

The *primary health care* (PHC) version of the ICD-10 classification of mental disorders was developed because of the great importance of psychiatric disorders in general practice, for example the high prevalence of depressions, anxiety disorders, and dependence on alcohol and psychotropic drugs.[17] There are 24 syndromes, including dementia, delirium, depression, etc. Each disorder is understood in a rather broad sense, and not subdivided, and the descriptions are simpler than those in the main classification. A flipcard containing symptoms, diagnostic criteria, differential diagnoses, and counselling and treatment of the patient and the family is provided for every syndrome.

At first glance, the structure of ICD-10, Chapter V (F), follows that of ICD-8 or ICD-9 (See Appendix 1). The classification begins with the 'organic disorders', followed by disorders due to the abuse of psychoactive substances. The next section of the classification contains schizophrenia and other psychotic disorders. This is followed by affective disorders and then neurotic and personality disorders. The chapter ends with intellectual disability and disorders of childhood and adolescence. Closer examination of the classification reveals that the traditional dualistic principle—psychoses on the one hand (in ICD-9: codes 290–299) and neuroses on the other (in ICD-9: codes 300–310)—has been abandoned. The diagnostic terms now used take a more phenomenological descriptive approach. According to the authors of ICD-10, the same psychiatric disorder may show both psychotic and non-psychotic symptoms. 'Psychotic' is defined as the manifestation of productive symptoms. The term 'neurosis' did not appear in the first drafts of ICD-10 because it is used in different and contradictory ways and is supposedly based on theories of intrapsychic processes which many of the WHO experts regarded as not generally accepted. However, after protests and objections by many clinicians worldwide, it was concluded that 'psychotic' and 'neurotic' should be used, although only as descriptive terms and not as diagnostic rubrics. Thus the term 'neurotic disorders' follows the traditional use of the word but does not imply an etiological theory.

(a) Organic, including symptomatic, mental disorders

Disorders of organic aetiology are grouped in this subchapter, independent of whether they contain psychotic or non-psychotic symptoms. However, the use of the term 'organic' does not imply that conditions elsewhere in the classification are non-organic in the sense of having no cerebral substrate.

(b) Mental and behavioural disorders due to psychoactive substance use

An improvement over ICD-9 is the compilation of all mental and behavioural disorders due to psychoactive substances within a single subchapter. The third digit indicates which substance or class of substances (e.g. F10 Alcohol) is responsible for the disorder, which is coded as a fourth digit (e.g. F10.3 Alcohol withdrawal state) or a fifth digit (e.g. F10.31 Alcohol withdrawal state with convulsions). It is possible to differentiate acute intoxication, harmful use, dependence syndrome, withdrawal state with or without delirium, different psychotic disorders, amnesic syndrome, and a number of other disorders. Thus, the psychopathological syndrome can be described and related to the dominant substance class.

(c) Schizophrenia, schizotypal, and delusional disorders

This subchapter covers schizophrenia, acute psychotic disorders, schizoaffective disorders, delusional disorders, and schizotypal disorders. Before schizophrenia can be diagnosed the symptoms have to be observed for at least one month, unlike DSM-IV where symptoms should be observed for six months before using this diagnosis. Special care is taken with the description of short-lasting psychoses, since acute and transient psychotic disorders are of particular interest to psychiatrists from developing countries where short-lasting acute psychoses with a good prognosis are observed quite frequently.

(d) Mood (affective) disorders

All mood disorders are combined in this subchapter, which represents a considerable change compared with ICD-9. The disorders previously known as endogenous and neurotic depressions are coded in this subchapter; the differentiation between these categories has been abandoned. The ICD-9 category of neurotic depression (300.4) is no longer found in ICD-10; most of these cases are now coded as dysthymia (F34.1). Single manic episodes are coded as F30, while recurrent manic episodes are now coded as bipolar affective disorder (F31), regardless of whether or not there has been a previous depressive episode.

(e) Neurotic, stress-related, and somatoform disorders

The disorders in this subchapter are divided into a large number of categories. For instance, dissociative disorders are divided into seven subcategories, some of which represent rather rare disorders. The term hysteria is no longer used. In this subchapter, reactions to severe stress and adjustment disorders are enumerated according to time criteria and severity. Here, aetiology is generally accepted to mean exceptional mental stress or special life events. A new group of disorders in this classification are the somatoform disorders, which are of particular importance in developing countries. The traditional term neurasthenia is still maintained for a special category, in contrast with DSM-IV.

(f) Behavioural syndromes associated with physiological disturbances and physical factors

This subchapter brings together eating disorders, non-organic sleep disorders, sexual dysfunction, mental and behavioural disorders associated with the puerperium, and abuse of non-dependence-producing substances. In ICD-9, all sexual disorders were contained in one subchapter. In ICD-10, only disorders of sexual dysfunction are in F5; disorders of gender identity and sexual preference have been assigned to two different sections in subchapter F6 on personality disorders. The special code F54, psychological and behavioural factors associated with disorders or diseases classified elsewhere, allows classification of psychosomatic disorders by coding an additional somatic diagnosis.

(g) Disorders of adult personality and behaviour

Specific personality disorders are coded in this subchapter. Cyclothymic personality is not included, but an equivalent appears in F3 as cyclothymia. Also, schizotypal disorders could have been assigned to this subchapter but appear instead in F2 (as F21). The emotionally unstable personality disorder is found in this subchapter, where it is subdivided into an impulsive type (F60.30) and a borderline type (F60.31). A new entity is the factitious disorder, i.e. the intentional production or feigning of symptoms or disabilities, either physical or psychological (F68.1). If desired, narcissistic personality disorder and passive–aggressive personality disorder may be coded by using the criteria in Annex 1 of the Diagnostic Criteria for Research.

An important aspect of this subchapter is the inclusion of enduring personality changes after catastrophic experience (F62.0) or after psychiatric illness (F62.1). Personality changes after surviving a concentration camp or torture are coded under the first of these.

(h) Remaining subchapters

F7 intellectual disability, F8 Disorders of psychological development, and F9 Behavioural and emotional disorders with onset during childhood and adolescence are

The structure of DSM-IV-TR

The 'DSM-IV-TR Classification of Mental Disorders' refers to the comprehensive listing of the official diagnostic codes, categories, subtypes, and specifiers (see Appendix 2). It is divided into various 'diagnostic classes' which group disorders together based on common presenting symptoms (e.g., mood disorders, anxiety disorders), typical age-at-onset (e.g., disorders usually first diagnosed in infancy, childhood, and adolescence), and aetiology (e.g., substance-related disorders, mental disorders due to a general medical condition).

Disorders usually first diagnosed in infancy, childhood, or adolescence

The DSM-IV-TR classification begins with disorders usually first diagnosed in infancy, childhood, or adolescence. The inclusion of a separate 'childhood disorders' section in DSM-IV-TR is only for convenience—some of these conditions are sometimes diagnosed for the first time in adulthood (e.g., attention-deficit/hyperactivity disorder) and many disorders included in the rest of DSM-IV-TR can start in childhood (e.g., major depressive disorder, schizophrenia). Thus, a psychiatrist doing a diagnostic assessment of a child or adolescent should not only focus on those disorders listed in this section but also consider disorders from throughout the DSM-IV-TR. Similarly, when evaluating an adult, the psychiatrist should also consider the disorders in this section since many of them persist into adulthood (e.g., stuttering, learning disorders, tic disorders).

While the first set of disorders included in this section (i.e., intellectual disability learning and motor skills disorders, and communication disorders) are not, strictly speaking, regarded as mental disorders they are included in the DSM-IV-TR to facilitate differential diagnosis. Autism and other pervasive developmental disorders are characterized by gross qualitative impairment in social relatedness, in language, and in repertoire of interests and activities and include autistic disorder, Asperger's disorder, Rett's disorder, and childhood disintegrative disorder. The Disruptive Behaviour Disorders (i.e. Attention-deficit/hyperactivity disorder, conduct disorder, and oppositional-defiant disorder) are grouped together because they are all characterized (at least in their childhood presentations) by disruptive behavior. The Feeding Disorders of Infancy and Early Childhood include the DSM-IV-TR categories of pica, rumination disorder, and feeding disorder of infancy and early childhood (also known as failure to thrive). Tic disorders, elimination disorders, and other disorders of infancy and early childhood (which include separation anxiety disorder, selective mutism, reactive attachment disorder, and stereotypic movement disorder) round out the childhood section.

Delirium, dementia, amnestic disorder, and other cognitive disorders

In DSM-III-R, delirium, dementia, amnestic disorder, and other cognitive disorders, along with substance-induced mental disorders and mental disorder due to a general medical condition, were included in a section called 'organic mental disorders', which contained all disorders that were due to either a general medical condition or substance use. In DSM-IV, the term 'organic' was completely eliminated from the classification because of the misleading implication that disorders not included in that section (e.g., schizophrenia, bipolar disorder) did not have an organic component[32]. In fact, virtually all mental disorders have both psychological and biological components, and to designate some disorders as 'organic' and the remaining disorders in the DSM-IV as 'non-organic' reflected a reductionistic mind-body dualism.

As a result of the elimination of the Organic Mental Disorder diagnostic grouping, those disorders originally included in that section had to be redistributed throughout DSM-IV into other diagnostic classes. Delirium, dementia, and amnestic disorder were thus grouped together into a major diagnostic class because of their central roles in the differential diagnosis of cognitive impairment. Although both delirium and dementia are characterized by multiple cognitive impairments, delirium is distinguished by the presence of clouding of consciousness which is manifested by an inability to appropriately maintain or shift attention. Three types of delirium are included in DSM-IV based on causative factors: delirium due to a general medical condition, substance-induced delirium, and delirium due to multiple etiologies.

Dementia is defined by clinically significant memory impairment accompanied by impairment in one or more other areas of cognitive functioning (e.g. language, executive functioning). DSM-IV-TR includes several types of dementia based on aetiology, including dementia of the Alzheimer's type, vascular dementia, a variety of dementia due to general medical and neurological conditions (e.g., HIV, Parkinson's disease), substance-induced persisting dementia, and dementia due to multiple etiologies. In contrast to dementia, amnestic disorder is characterized by memory impairment occurring in the absence of other cognitive impairments. Two types are included in DSM-IV: amnestic disorder due to a general medical condition and substance-induced persisting amnestic disorder.

Mental disorders due to a general medical condition not elsewhere classified

In DSM-IV-TR, most of the mental disorders due to a general medical condition have been distributed alongside their 'non-organic' counterparts in the classification (e.g. mood disorder due to a general medical condition and substance-induced mood disorder was included in the mood disorders section). Two specific types of mental disorders due to a general medical condition (i.e. catatonic disorder due to a general medical condition and personality change due to a general medical condition) do not fit into any of the other diagnostic classes and therefore, are included here in this diagnostic class.

Substance-related disorders

In DSM-IV, substance-related disorders include psychiatric disturbances that result from medication side effects and the consequences of toxin exposure, in addition to those that arise due to drug and alcohol abuse. Two types of substance-related disorders are included in DSM-IV: substance use disorders (dependence and abuse), which focus on the maladaptive nature of the pattern of substance use; and substance-induced disorders, which cover psychopathological processes caused by the direct effects of substances (including toxins and medications) on the central nervous system.

Schizophrenia and other psychotic disorders

Included in this grouping are those disorders in which psychosis is the primary characteristic symptom (i.e. schizophrenia, schizophreniform disorder, schizoaffective disorder, delusional disorder, shared psychotic disorder and brief psychotic disorder). It should be noted that other disorders that may have psychotic features are not included in this grouping (e.g. mood disorders with psychotic features, delirium).

Mood disorders

This diagnostic class includes disorders in which the predominant disturbance is in the individual's mood. Although the term 'mood' is generally considered to include emotions such as depression, euphoria, anger, and anxiety, DSM-IV includes in this section only disorders characterized by depressed, elevated, or irritable mood. This diagnostic class is further divided into depressive and bipolar disorders. The term 'bipolar' is misleading because the name implies the presence of both 'down' and 'up' moods. In fact, bipolar disorder is defined by the presence of one or more manic or hypomanic episodes. Thus, patients with multiple manic episodes (i.e. unipolar mania) are considered to be bipolar despite the lack of the second 'pole'.

Anxiety disorders

The common thread tying together disorders in this section is the fact that the clinical presentation of these disorders is typically characterized by significant anxiety. The rationale for this grouping has been criticized because of evidence suggesting that at least some of the disorders are likely to be etiologically distinct from the others. For example, it has been argued that obsessive-compulsive disorder is most likely part of an obsessive-compulsive spectrum that might include tic disorders, hypochondriasis, body dysmorphic disorder, and perhaps trichotillomania.[33]

Somatoform disorders

Somatoform disorders are characterized by their presentation in general medical settings by individuals who do not consider themselves to be suffering from a mental disorder. Individuals with somatoform disorders present with somatic complaints or bodily concerns that are not adequately explained by an underlying general medical condition. Conceptually, the somatoform disorders can be divided into three general types: 1) those in which the individual's focus is on the physical symptoms themselves (somatization disorder, undifferentiated somatoform disorder, pain disorder, and conversion disorder); 2) those who are preoccupied by the belief that one has a serious physical illness despite medical reassurance (hypochondriasis); and 3) those who are preoccupied by the belief that a part or parts of their body are physically defective (body dysmorphic disorder).

Factitious disorders

Individuals with a factitious disorder intentionally produce or feign a physical or psychological symptom, motivated by the psychological need to assume the sick role and be taken care of. This is in contrast to malingering (which is not considered to be a mental disorder) in which the person is motivated by secondary gain (e.g. to evade criminal responsibility, to receive disability benefits).

Dissociative disorders

Dissociation is the core element of this group of disorders, which is defined as a disruption in the usually integrated functions of consciousness, memory, identity, and perception. Four specific disorders are included (dissociative amnesia, dissociative fugue, dissociative identity disorder, and depersonalization disorder).

Sexual and gender identity disorders

This diagnostic class groups together disorders involving three relatively distinct aspects of human sexuality: sexual dysfunctions, which involve disturbances in sexual desire or functioning, paraphilias which involve unusual sexual preferences that interfere with functioning (or in the case of preferences that involve harm to others like paedophilia, merely acting on those preferences), and gender identity disorder that entail one's internal identity of maleness and femaleness (gender identity) being at odds with one's anatomical sexual characteristics.

Eating disorders

Disorders in this section involve abnormal eating behavior; either the refusal to maintain adequate body weight (anorexia nervosa) or discrete episodes of uncontrolled eating accompanied by excessive effects to counteract the effects of these binges (bulimia nervosa).

Sleep disorders

Sleep disorders are subdivided into four groups based on presumed aetiology (primary, related to another mental disorder, due to a general medical condition, and substance induced). Two types of primary sleep disorders have been included: dyssomnias (problems in regulation of amount and quality of sleep) and parasomnias (events that occur during sleep). The dyssomnias include primary insomnia, primary hypersomnia, circadian rhythm sleep disorder, narcolepsy, and breathing-related sleep disorder, whereas the parasomnias include nightmare disorder, sleep terror disorder, and sleepwalking disorder.

Impulse control disorders not elsewhere classified

Many disorders in the DSM-IV-TR are characterized by problems with impulse control (e.g. borderline personality disorder, substance dependence, attention-deficit/hyperactivity disorder). This diagnostic grouping is for those impulse-control disorders not included in other sections of the DSM-IV-TR. Included are problems controlling angry impulses (intermittent explosive disorder), problems controlling impulses to steal (kleptomania) or set fires (pyromania), problems controlling impulses to pull out one's hair (trichotillomania) and problems controlling impulses to gamble (pathological gambling).

Adjustment disorders

This diagnostic class is for presentations that do not meet criteria for specific disorders (i.e. subthreshold presentations) that represent a maladaptive response to a stressor. For example, if depression occurring after a job loss is severe enough to meet full symptomatic criteria for a major depressive episode, then major depressive disorder would be diagnosed. If the job-loss-related depression falls symptomatically short of this diagnostic threshold, then adjustment disorder with depressed mood is diagnosed.

Personality disorders

Each of us has a personality, that is our characteristic way of experiencing and processing the world and ourselves. When an individual's characteristic patterns of relating, feeling, and thinking are so inflexible and maladaptive that they interfere with his or her functioning, then that person is considered to have a personality disorder. 10 specific personality disorders are included in DSM-IV-TR: paranoid personality disorder (pervasive distrust and suspiciousness of others), schizoid personality disorder (lack of desire for social relationships and a restricted expression of emotions), schizotypal personality disorder (acute discomfort with close relationships, odd beliefs, perceptual distortions, and eccentricities of behaviour), antisocial personality disorder (disregard for the rights of others), borderline personality disorder (instability of personal relationships and self-image, fears of abandonment, and marked impulsivity), histrionic personality disorder (extensive emotionality and attention seeking), narcissistic personality disorder (grandiosity, need for admiration, and lack of empathy), avoidant personality disorder (social inhibition, and hypersensitivity to negative evaluation), dependent personality disorder (excessive need to be taken care of), and obsessive-compulsive personality disorder (preoccupation with orderliness, perfectionism, stubbornness).

Research planning for DSM-V and ICD-11

It is currently anticipated that the DSM-V will be published in 2012 and that the ICD-11, although likely to be in a final draft form around the same time, will be officially published a few years later after approval by the WHO Assembly. When the last major revision of the DSM, DSM-IV, was published in 1994, the American Psychiatric Association decided to hold off on starting work on the next revision of the DSM until at least 2010, at least partly in response to the criticism that the seven year interval between prior versions of the DSM was too short.[34] Similarly, resistance to the implementation of ICD-10 by many countries (including the United States) ensured that the next revision of the ICD would also be put off for a number of years. The American Psychiatric Association decided to take advantage of this delay in the diagnostic revision process by partnering with the National Institute of Mental Health and the World Health Organization in order to initiate a research planning process with the aim of stimulating potentially informative research prior to the formal beginning of the DSM-V and ICD-11 revision processes.

Part of the impetus for encouraging research in advance of the next diagnostic revision is the general frustration felt by both researchers and clinicians with the superficially descriptive approach taken by DSM-IV and ICD-10. Although the operationalized criteria in DSM-III were developed based largely on expert consensus, there was a general understanding that the categories would continually be revised and improved in future editions of the DSM, ultimately culminating in the identification of the underlying disease processes.

Unfortunately, in the more than 25 years since the publication of DSM-III, the goal of validating these syndromes and discovering the underlying pathophysiology has remained elusive. Despite many proposed candidates, not one laboratory marker has been found to be diagnostically useful for any DSM category.[35] Epidemiological and clinical studies have shown extremely high rates of comorbidities among the disorders, undermining the hypotheses that these syndromes represent distinct etiologies. Regarding treatment, lack of treatment specificity is the rule: SSRI's effective for treating disorders across the diagnostic spectrum (e.g. depression, panic, generalized anxiety disorder, posttraumatic stress disorder, social anxiety, body dysmorphic disorder, obsessive-compulsive disorder, pathological gambling, trichotillomania, borderline personality disorder, etc.). Results of twin studies have also contradicted DSM-IV's assumptions that separate syndromes have a distinct underlying genetic basis (e.g. major depressive disorder and generalized anxiety disorder have the same genetic risk factors).

The considerable limitations of the DSM paradigm have fueled the desire that DSM-V and ICD-11 would be etiologically-based rather just descriptive. The main barrier to making DSM-V and ICD-11 more etiological is, of course, the enormous gaps in our understanding of the pathophysiology of mental disorders. Therefore, in order to help move the field forward towards the goal of a primarily etiological classification, a series of 'white papers' was commissioned under joint sponsorship of the American Psychiatric Association, the National Institute of Mental Health (NIMH), National Institute for Alcoholism and Alcohol Abuse (NIAAA), and the National Institute for Drug Abuse (NIDA). Research planning workgroups responsible for the development of these white papers were constituted for two primary reasons: 1) to stimulate research that will enrich the empirical data base prior to the start of the DSM-V revision process; and 2) to devise a research and analytic agenda that would facilitate the integration of findings from animal studies, genetics, neuroscience, epidemiology, clinical research, cross-cultural research, and clinical services research, which will lead to the eventual development of an etiologically-based, scientifically-sound classification system. In order to encourage thinking beyond the current DSM-IV framework, most of the workgroup members had not been closely involved in the DSM-IV development process. Furthermore, rather than organizing the white paper workgroups around the traditional diagnostic categories, the workgroups focused instead on cross-cutting issues, which included 1) a basic nomenclature workgroup, focusing on a variety of issues that had to do with the way disorders are classified in the DSM; 2) a neuroscience and genetics workgroup whose focus was to develop a basic and clinical neuroscience and genetics research agenda to guide the development of a future pathophysiologically-based classification; 3) a developmental science workgroup which outlined a research agenda to inform developmental aspects of the diagnostic classification; 4) a workgroup focusing on two major gaps in the DSM-IV, namely inadequacies in the classification of personality disorders and of relational disorders; 5) a mental disorders and disability workgroup which focused on disentangling the concepts of symptom severity and disability; and 6) a culture and psychiatric diagnosis workgroup which considered cross-cultural issues in diagnosis and classification. It should be noted that given the breakthrough nature of the suggested research and the relatively short time frame leading up to the anticipated publication of DSM-V and ICD-11, it was understood that most of the proposed research agenda was unlikely to bear fruit until DSM-VI/ICD-12 or later.

The six white papers were published by American Psychiatric Publishing, Inc. in 2002 in a monograph entitled 'A Research Agenda for DSM-V'.[36] Three additional white papers, one focusing on gender issues, one focusing on diagnostic issues in the geriatric population, and one focusing on mental disorders in infants and young children were commissioned subsequently and appear in a second volume of the research agenda.[37]

The second phase of the DSM-V Research Planning Process consisted of 11 research planning conferences (plus a methods conference) that occurred from 2004 to 2007. These conferences were being organized with the assistance and support of the World Health Organization and are co-funded by APA, NIMH, NIAAA, and NIDA. Unlike the white papers in the first phase which focused on general cross-cutting issues, these conferences for the most part focussed on specific diagnostic topics. The primary goals of these conferences were to stimulate the empirical research necessary to allow informed decision-making regarding crucial diagnostic deficiencies identified in DSM-IV and ICD-10, and to promote international collaboration in order to increase the likelihood of developing a future unified DSM/ICD (i.e. each conference had two co-chairs, one from the United States and the other outside the US, each conference included an equal number of the US and international participants, and half the conferences took place outside the US). Conference topics were selected after consultation with the US and international experts. Finite resources necessitated that the number of conferences be limited to a total of 11 (and the number of participants to 25); thus a number of potentially important topics could not be included. The 11 diagnostic-topic focused conferences covered Dimensional Approaches Personality Disorders (December 2004, Arlington, VA);[38] Substance-Related Disorders (February 2005, Rockville, MD);[39] Stress-Induced and Fear Circuitry Disorders (June 2005, Arlington, VA); Dementia (September 2005, Geneva, Switzerland),[40] Deconstructing Psychosis (February 2006, Arlington, VA);[41] Obsessive-Compulsive Spectrum Disorders (June 2006, Arlington, VA);[33] Dimensional Approaches to Diagnosis (July 2006, Bethesda, MD);[42] Somatic Presentations (September 2006, Beijing, China); Externalizing Disorders of Childhood (February 2007, Mexico City); Comorbidity of Anxiety and Depression (June 2007, London, UK), and Public Health Implications (September 2007, Geneva, Switzerland). An additional conference on Autism spectrum disorders was also convened in Sacramento, CA in February 2008. Summaries of the conferences are available on the DSM-V website: www.dsm5.org.

The future

Despite the ubiquitous desire to move from a descriptive classification system to an etiologically-based classification system defined by objective laboratory findings, results of the research planning process indicate that disorders in DSM-V and ICD-11 will continue to be defined based on descriptive symptomatology. Despite the advances in neuroimaging, genetics, and biological markers over the past 10 years, it is unlikely that any objective laboratory findings will be part of the definition of any DSM-V or ICD-11 disorder, with the one exception being polysomnography findings to define sleep disorders given that such findings are already part of the diagnostic definitions of sleep disorders in the International Classification of Sleep Disorders – 2nd Edition (ICSD-2).(43) Although research studies have reliably demonstrated differences in a wide variety of objective measures between groups of affected individuals and controls (for example, brain ventricular size in individuals with schizophrenia as compared to unaffected controls),(44) when it comes down to applying the findings to a particular individual for the purpose of making a diagnosis, none of these findings have been shown to be sufficiently sensitive or specific.

A central question being raised as part of the DSM-V/ICD-11 revision process is whether psychiatric diagnosis would be better served by a dimensional approach rather than the current categorical approach. This topic was the exclusive focus of one of the 11 research planning conferences being held in advance of the DSM-V/ICD-11 revision (i.e. 'Dimensional Approaches in Diagnostic Classification: A Critical Appraisal', held in Arlington VA, July 27–28, 2006)(42), was the main focus of the Personality Disorders Research Planning conference which proposed a research agenda for adopting a dimensional approach to personality disorders(45) and was a important component of the other diagnostic-related conferences (e.g. 'Should there be both categorical and dimensional criteria for the substance use disorders in DSM-V'.(46)) Much of the impetus for moving toward a dimensional approach comes from dissatisfaction with categorical diagnoses expressed by the research community.(47–58) There are a number of persuasive arguments for the superiority of a dimensional approach over a categorical one, including, 1) the lack of evidence for discrete breaks or demarcations in distributions of symptoms; 2) evidence of a superior fit of empirical data to latent structuring models that correspond to dimensional vs. categorical approaches; 3) higher levels of diagnostic reliability and stability over time; and 4) elimination of the problematic artifacts of the categorical system, like excessive diagnostic comorbidity and arbitrary diagnostic thresholds.(59) On the other hand, a categorical approach to diagnosis remains critically important because of its clinical and administrative utility. Clinicians typically must make dichotomous decisions in everyday practice (i.e. whether to treat or not treat, to hospitalize or not hospitalize, to refer or not refer, etc.) and need to assign diagnostic categories to their patients for the purposes of reimbursement.(60) Categorical labels also facilitate clinical communication by providing a convenient shorthand when discussing a patient's diagnosis (e.g. it is more efficient for a clinician to use a single diagnostic term when talking about a patient who has a borderline personality disorder rather than having to describe all the dimensions that went into that summary judgment). Given the relative advantages of each approach, DSM-V and ICD-11 will most likely adopt some sort of hybrid approach, retaining the categorical diagnoses for communication and decision-making purposes but also providing accompanying dimensions.

Finally, there is a strong push for DSM-V and ICD-11 to become more developmentally focused. ICD-10 and DSM-IV provide definitions of mental disorders that, as far as possible, are applicable across age groups. Given that most disorders can occur at any time during an individual's lifespan, for the most part, the definitions of disorder ignore developmental variations in presentation. It should be noted that DSM-IV does include some age-appropriate modifications in the diagnostic definitions (e.g. in PTSD, criterion B(1), 'recurrent and intrusive distressing recollections of the event, including images, thoughts, or perceptions' is supplemented by 'in young children, repetitive play may occur in which themes or aspects of the trauma are expressed'), these modifications are the exceptions. It is anticipated that DSM-IV and ICD-11 will pay considerably more attention to these issues, reviewing longitudinal studies that track the evolution of disorders across the lifespan and also consider whether definitions should be modified to take into account developmental context.

Appendix 1

International classification of diseases, 10th revision

F00–F09 Organic, including symptomatic, mental disorders

F00 Dementia in Alzheimer's disease

F00.0 Dementia in Alzheimer's disease with early onset
F00.1 Dementia in Alzheimer's disease with late onset
F00.2 Dementia in Alzheimer's disease, atypical or mixed type
F00.9 Dementia in Alzheimer's disease, unspecified

F01 Vascular dementia

F01.0 Vascular dementia of acute onset
F01.1 Multi-infarct dementia
F01.2 Subcortical vascular dementia
F01.3 Mixed cortical and subcortical vascular dementia
F01.8 Other vascular dementia
F01.9 Vascular dementia, unspecified

F02 Dementia in other diseases classified elsewhere

F02.0 Dementia in Pick's disease
F02.1 Dementia in Creutzfeldt–Jakob disease
F02.2 Dementia in Huntington's disease
F02.3 Dementia in Parkinson's disease
F02.4 Dementia in human immunodeficiency virus (HIV) disease
F02.8 Dementia in other specified diseases classified elsewhere

F03 Unspecified dementia

A fifth character may be added to specify dementia in F00–F03, as follows:

.x0 Without additional symptoms
.xl Other symptoms, predominantly delusional
.x2 Other symptoms, predominantly hallucinatory
.x3 Other symptoms, predominantly depressive
.x4 Other mixed symptoms

F04 Organic amnesic syndrome, not induced by alcohol and other psychoactive substances

F05 Delirium, not induced by alcohol and other psychoactive substances

F05.0 Delirium, not superimposed on dementia, so described
F05.1 Delirium, superimposed on dementia
F05.8 Other delirium
F05.9 Delirium, unspecified

F06 Other mental disorders due to brain damage and dysfunction and to physical disease

F06.0 Organic hallucinosis
F06.1 Organic catatonic disorder
F06.2 Organic delusional (schizophrenia-like) disorder
F06.3 Organic mood (affective) disorders
.30 Organic manic disorder
.31 Organic bipolar disorder
.32 Organic depressive disorder
.33 Organic mixed affective disorder
F06.4 Organic anxiety disorder
F06.5 Organic dissociative disorder
F06.6 Organic emotionally labile (asthenic) disorder
F06.7 Mild cognitive disorder
F06.8 Other specified mental disorders due to brain damage and dysfunction and to physical disease
F06.9 Unspecified mental disorder due to brain damage and dysfunction and to physical disease

F09 Unspecified organic or symptomatic mental disorder

F07 Personality and behavioural disorders due to brain disease, damage and dysfunction

F07.0 Organic personality disorder
F07.1 Postencephalitic syndrome
F07.2 Postconcussional syndrome
F07.8 Other organic personality and behavioural disorders due to brain disease, damage, and dysfunction
F07.9 Unspecified organic personality and behavioural disorder due to brain disease, damage, and dysfunction

F10–F19 Mental and behavioural disorders due to psychoactive substance use

F10 Mental and behavioural disorders due to use of alcohol
F11 Mental and behavioural disorders due to use of opioids
F12 Mental and behavioural disorders due to use of cannabinoids
F13 Mental and behavioural disorders due to use of sedatives or hypnotics
F14 Mental and behavioural disorders due to use of cocaine
F15 Mental and behavioural disorders due to use of other stimulants, including caffeine
F16 Mental and behavioural disorders due to use of hallucinogens
F17 Mental and behavioural disorders due to use of tobacco
F18 Mental and behavioural disorders due to use of volatile solvents
F19 Mental and behavioural disorders due to multiple drug use and use of other psychoactive substances

Four- and five-character categories may be used to specify the clinical conditions, as follows

F1*x*.0 Acute intoxication
.00 Uncomplicated
.01 With trauma or other bodily injury
.02 With other medical complications
.03 With delirium
.04 With perceptual distortions
.05 With coma
.06 With convulsions
.07 Pathological intoxication
F1*x*.1 Harmful use
F1*x*.2 Dependence syndrome
.20 Currently abstinent
.21 Currently abstinent, but in a protected environment
.22 Currently on a clinically supervised maintenance or replacement regime (controlled dependence)
.23 Currently abstinent, but receiving treatment with aversive or blocking drugs
.24 Currently using the substance (active dependence)
.25 Continuous use
.26 Episodic use (dipsomania)
F1*x*.3 Withdrawal state
.30 Uncomplicated
.31 Convulsions
F1*x*.4 Withdrawal state with delirium
.40 Without convulsions
.41 With convulsions
F1*x*.5 Psychotic disorder
.50 Schizophrenia-like
.51 Predominantly delusional
.52 Predominantly hallucinatory
.53 Predominantly polymorphic
.54 Predominantly depressive symptoms
.55 Predominantly manic symptoms
.56 Mixed
F1*x*.6 Amnesic syndrome
F1*x*.7 Residual and late-onset psychotic disorder
.70 Flashbacks
.71 Personality or behaviour disorder
.72 Residual affective disorder
.73 Dementia
.74 Other persisting cognitive impairment
.75 Late-onset psychotic disorder
F1*x*.8 Other mental and behavioural disorders
F1*x*.9 Unspecified mental and behavioural disorder

F20–F29 Schizophrenia, schizotypal, and delusional disorders

F20 Schizophrenia

F20.0 Paranoid schizophrenia
F20.1 Hebephrenic schizophrenia
F20.2 Catatonic schizophrenia
F20.3 Undifferentiated schizophrenia
F20.4 Post-schizophrenic depression
F20.5 Residual schizophrenia
F20.6 Simple schizophrenia
F20.8 Other schizophrenia
F20.9 Schizophrenia, unspecified

A fifth character may be used to classify course
*x*0 Continuous
.*x*1 Episodic with progressive deficit
.*x*2 Episodic with stable deficit
.*x*3 Episodic remittent
.*x*4 Incomplete remission
.*x*5 Complete remission
.*x*8 Other
.*x*9 Period of observation less than one year

F21 Schizotypal disorder

F22 Persistent delusional disorders

F22.0 Delusional disorder
F22.8 Other persistent delusional disorders
F22.9 Persistent delusional disorder, unspecified

F23 Acute and transient psychotic disorders

F23.0 Acute polymorphic psychotic disorder without symptoms of schizophrenia
F23.1 Acute polymorphic psychotic disorder with symptoms of schizophrenia
F23.2 Acute schizophrenia-like psychotic disorder
F23.3 Other acute predominantly delusional psychotic disorders
F23.8 Other acute and transient psychotic disorders
F23.9 Acute and transient psychotic disorders unspecified

A fifth character may be used to identify the presence or absence of associated acute stress

.*x*0 Without associated acute stress
.*x*1 With associated acute stress

F24 Induced delusional disorder

F25 Schizoaffective disorders

F25.0 Schizoaffective disorder, manic type
F25.1 Schizoaffective disorder, depressive type
F25.2 Schizoaffective disorder, mixed type
F25.8 Other schizoaffective disorders
F25.9 Schizoaffective disorder, unspecified

F28 Other non-organic psychotic disorders

F29 Unspecified non-organic psychosis

F30–F39 Mood (affective) disorders

F30 Manic episode
F30.0 Hypomania
F30.1 Mania without psychotic symptoms
F30.2 Mania with psychotic symptoms
F30.8 Other manic episodes
F30.9 Manic episode, unspecified

F31 Bipolar affective disorder

F31.0 Bipolar affective disorder, current episode hypomanic
F31.1 Bipolar affective disorder, current episode manic without psychotic symptoms
F31.2 Bipolar affective disorder, current episode manic with psychotic symptoms
F31.3 Bipolar affective disorder, current episode mild or moderate depression

.30 Without somatic symptoms
.31 With somatic symptoms

F31.4 Bipolar affective disorder, current episode severe depression without psychotic symptoms
F31.5 Bipolar affective disorder, current episode severe depression with psychotic symptoms
F31.6 Bipolar affective disorder, current episode mixed
F31.7 Bipolar affective disorder, currently in remission
F31.8 Other bipolar affective disorders
F31.9 Bipolar affective disorder, unspecified

F32 Depressive episode

F32.0 Mild depressive episode

.00 Without somatic symptoms
.01 With somatic symptoms

F32.1 Moderate depressive episode

.10 Without somatic symptoms
.11 With somatic symptoms

F32.2 Severe depressive episode without psychotic symptoms
F32.3 Severe depressive episode with psychotic symptoms
F32.8 Other depressive episodes
F32.9 Depressive episode, unspecified

F33 Recurrent depressive disorder

F33.0 Recurrent depressive disorder, current episode mild

.00 Without somatic symptoms
.01 With somatic symptoms

F33.1 Recurrent depressive disorder, current episode moderate

.10 Without somatic symptoms
.11 With somatic symptoms

F33.2 Recurrent depressive disorder, current episode severe without psychotic symptoms
F33.3 Recurrent depressive disorder, current episode severe with psychotic symptoms
F33.4 Recurrent depressive disorder, currently in remission
F33.8 Other recurrent depressive disorders
F33.9 Recurrent depressive disorder, unspecified

F34 Persistent mood (affective) disorders

F34.0 Cyclothymia
F34.1 Dysthymia
F34.8 Other persistent mood (affective) disorders
F34.9 Persistent mood (affective) disorder, unspecified

F38 Other mood (affective) disorders

F38.0 Other single mood (affective) disorders

.00 Mixed affective episode

F38.1 Other recurrent mood (affective) disorders

.10 Recurrent brief depressive disorder

F38.8 Other specified mood (affective) disorders

F39 Unspecified mood (affective) disorder

F40–F48 Neurotic, stress-related, and somatoform disorders

F40 Phobic anxiety disorders
F40.0 Agoraphobia

.00 Without panic disorder
.01 With panic disorder

F40.1 Social phobias
F40.2 Specific (isolated) phobias
F40.8 Other phobic anxiety disorders
F40.9 Phobic anxiety disorder, unspecified

F41 Other anxiety disorders

F41.0 Panic disorder (episodic paroxysmal anxiety)
F41.1 Generalized anxiety disorder
F41.2 Mixed anxiety and depressive disorder
F41.3 Other mixed anxiety disorders
F41.8 Other specified anxiety disorders
F41.9 Anxiety disorder, unspecified

F42 Obsessive-compulsive disorder

F42.0 Predominantly obsessional thoughts or ruminations
F42.1 Predominantly compulsive acts (obsessional rituals)
F42.2 Mixed obsessional thoughts and acts
F42.8 Other obsessive-compulsive disorders
F42.9 Obsessive-compulsive disorder, unspecified

F43 Reaction to severe stress, and adjustment disorders

F43.0 Acute stress reaction
F43.1 Post-traumatic stress disorder
F43.2 Adjustment disorders

.20 Brief depressive reaction

.21 Prolonged depressive reaction
.22 Mixed anxiety and depressive reaction
.23 With predominant disturbance of other emotions
.24 With predominant disturbance of conduct
.25 With mixed disturbance of emotions and conduct
.28 With other specified predominant symptoms
F43.8 Other reactions to severe stress
F43.9 Reaction to severe stress, unspecified

F44 Dissociative (conversion) disorders

F44.0 Dissociative amnesia
F44.1 Dissociative fugue
F44.2 Dissociative stupor
F44.3 Trance and possession disorders
F44.4 Dissociative motor disorders
F44.5 Dissociative convulsions
F44.6 Dissociative anaesthesia and sensory loss
F44.7 Mixed dissociative (conversion) disorders
F44.8 Other dissociative (conversion) disorders
.80 Ganser's syndrome
.81 Multiple personality disorder
.82 Transient dissociate (conversion) disorders occurring in childhood and adolescence
.88 Other specified dissociative (conversion) disorders
F44.9 Dissociative (conversion) disorder, unspecified

F45 Somatoform disorders

F45.0 Somatization disorder
F45.1 Undifferentiated somatoform disorder
F45.2 Hypochondriacal disorder
F45.3 Somatoform autonomic dysfunction
.30 Heart and cardiovascular system
.31 Upper gastrointestinal tract
.32 Lower gastrointestinal tract
.33 Respiratory system
.34 Genitourinary system
.38 Other organ or system
F45.4 Persistent somatoform pain disorder
F45.8 Other somatoform disorders
F45.9 Somatoform disorder, unspecified

F48 Other neurotic disorders

F48.0 Neurasthenia
F48.1 Depersonalization-derealization syndrome
F48.8 Other specified neurotic disorders
F48.9 Neurotic disorder, unspecified

F50–F59 Behavioural syndromes associated with physiological disturbances and physical factors

F50 Eating disorders

F50.0 Anorexia nervosa
F50.1 Atypical anorexia nervosa
F50.2 Bulimia nervosa
F50.3 Atypical bulimia nervosa
F50.4 Overeating associated with other psychological disturbances
F50.5 Vomiting associated with other psychological disturbances
F50.8 Other eating disorders
F50.9 Eating disorder, unspecified

F51 Non-organic sleep disorders

F51.0 Non-organic insomnia
F51.1 Non-organic hypersomnia
F51.2 Non-organic disorder of the sleep-wake schedule
F51.3 Sleepwalking (somnambulism)
F51.4 Sleep terrors (night terrors)
F51.5 Nightmares
F51.8 Other non-organic sleep disorders
F51.9 Non-organic sleep disorder, unspecified

F52 Sexual dysfunction, not caused by organic disorder or disease

F52.0 Lack or loss of sexual desire
F52.1 Sexual aversion and lack of sexual enjoyment
.10 Sexual aversion
.11 Lack of sexual enjoyment
F52.2 Failure of genital response
F52.3 Orgasmic dysfunction
F52.4 Premature ejaculation
F52.5 Non-organic vaginismus
F52.6 Non-organic dyspareunia
F52.7 Excessive sexual drive
F52.8 Other sexual dysfunction, not caused by organic disorders or disease
F52.9 Unspecified sexual dysfunction, not caused by organic disorder or disease

F53 Mental and behavioural disorders associated with the puerperium, not elsewhere classified

F53.0 Mild mental and behavioural disorders associated with the puerperium, not elsewhere classified
F53.1 Severe mental and behavioural disorders associated with the puerperium, not elsewhere classified
F53.8 Other mental and behavioural disorders associated with the puerperium, not elsewhere classified
F53.9 Puerperal mental disorder, unspecified

F54 Psychological and behavioural factors associated with disorders or diseases classified elsewhere

F55 Abuse of non-dependence-producing substances

F55.0 Antidepressants
F55.1 Laxatives
F55.2 Analgesics
F55.3 Antacids
F55.4 Vitamins
F55.5 Steroids or hormones
F55.6 Specific herbal or folk remedies
F55.8 Other substances that do not produce dependence
F55.9 Unspecified

F59 Unspecified behavioural syndromes associated with physiological disturbances and physical factors

F60–F69 Disorders of adult personality and behaviour

F60 Specific personality disorders
F60.0 Paranoid personality disorder
F60.1 Schizoid personality disorder
F60.2 Dissocial personality disorder
F60.3 Emotionally unstable personality disorder
.30 Impulsive type
.31 Borderline type
F60.4 Histrionic personality disorder
F60.5 Anankastic personality disorder

F60.6 Anxious (avoidant) personality disorder
F60.7 Dependent personality disorder
F60.8 Other specific personality disorders
F60.9 Personality disorder, unspecified

F61 Mixed and other personality disorders

F61.0 Mixed personality disorders
F61.1 Troublesome personality changes

F62 Enduring personality changes, not attributable to brain damage and disease

F62.0 Enduring personality change after catastrophic experience
F62.1 Enduring personality change after psychiatric illness
F62.8 Other enduring personality changes
F62.9 Enduring personality change, unspecified

F63 Habit and impulse disorders

F63.0 Pathological gambling
F63.1 Pathological fire-setting (pyromania)
F63.2 Pathological stealing (kleptomania)
F63.3 Trichotillomania
F63.8 Other habit and impulse disorders
F63.9 Habit and impulse disorder, unspecified

F64 Gender identity disorders

F64.0 Transsexualism
F64.1 Dual-role transvestism
F64.2 Gender identity disorder of childhood
F64.8 Other gender identity disorders
F64.9 Gender identity disorder, unspecified

F65 Disorders of sexual preference

F65.0 Fetishism
F65.1 Fetishistic transvestism
F65.2 Exhibitionism
F65.3 Voyeurism
F65.4 Paedophilia
F65.5 Sadomasochism
F65.6 Multiple disorders of sexual preference
F65.8 Other disorders of sexual preference
F65.9 Disorder of sexual preference, unspecified

F66 Psychological and behavioural disorders associated with sexual development and orientation

F66.0 Sexual maturation disorder
F66.1 Egodystonic sexual orientation
F66.2 Sexual relationship disorder
F66.8 Other psychosexual development disorders
F66.9 Psychosexual development disorder, unspecified

A fifth character may be used to indicate association with:

.*x*0 Heterosexuality
.*x*l Homosexuality
.*x*2 Bisexuality
.*x*8 Other, including prepubertal

F68 Other disorders of adult personality and behaviour

F68.0 Elaboration of physical symptoms for psychological reasons
F68.1 Intentional production or feigning of symptoms or disabilities, either physical or psychological (factitious disorder)
F68.8 Other specified disorders of adult personality and behaviour
F69 Unspecified disorder of adult personality and behaviour

F70–F79 Mental retardation (intellectual disability)

F70 Mild mental retardation (intellectual disability)

F71 Moderate mental retardation (intellectual disability)

F72 Severe mental retardation (intellectual disability)

F73 Profound mental retardation (intellectual disability)

F78 Other mental retardation (intellectual disability)

F79 Unspecified mental retardation (intellectual disability)

A fourth character may be used to specify the extent of associated behavioural impairment:

F7x.0 No, or minimal, impairment of behaviour
F7x.1 Significant impairment of behaviour requiring attention or treatment
F7x.8 Other impairments of behaviour
F7x.9 Without mention of impairment of behaviour

F80–F89 Disorders of psychological development

F80 specific developmental disorders of speech and language

F80.0 Specific speech articulation disorder
F80.1 Expressive language disorder
F80.2 Receptive language disorder
F80.3 Acquired aphasia with epilepsy (Landau-Kleffner syndrome)
F80.8 Other developmental disorders of speech and language
F80.9 Developmental disorder of speech and language, unspecified

F81 Specific developmental disorders of scholastic skills

F81.0 Specific reading disorder
F81.1 Specific spelling disorder
F81.2 Specific disorder of arithmetical skills
F81.3 Mixed disorder of scholastic skills
F81.8 Other developmental disorders of scholastic skills
F81.9 Developmental disorder of scholastic skills, unspecified

F82 Specific developmental disorder of motor function

F83 Mixed specific developmental disorders

F84 Pervasive developmental disorders

F84.0 Childhood autism
F84.1 Atypical autism
F84.2 Rett's syndrome
F84.3 Other childhood disintegrative disorder
F84.4 Overactive disorder associated with mental retardation and stereotyped movements
F84.5 Asperger's syndrome
F84.8 Other pervasive developmental disorders
F84.9 Pervasive developmental disorder, unspecified

F88 Other disorders of psychological development

F89 Unspecified disorder of psychological development

F90–F98 Behavioural and emotional disorders with onset usually occurring in childhood and adolescence

F90 Hyperkinetic disorders

F90.0 Disturbance of activity and attention
F90.1 Hyperkinetic conduct disorder
F90.8 Other hyperkinetic disorders
F90.9 Hyperkinetic disorder, unspecified

F91 Conduct disorders

F91.0 Conduct disorder confined to the family context
F91.1 Unsocialized conduct disorder

F91.2 Socialized conduct disorder
F91.3 Oppositional defiant disorder
F91.8 Other conduct disorders
F91.9 Conduct disorder, unspecified

F92 Mixed disorders of conduct and emotions

F92.0 Depressive conduct disorder
F92.8 Other mixed disorders of conduct and emotions
F92.9 Mixed disorder of conduct and emotions, unspecified

F93 Emotional disorders with onset specific to childhood

F93.0 Separation anxiety disorder of childhood
F93.1 Phobic anxiety disorder of childhood
F93.2 Social anxiety disorder of childhood
F93.3 Sibling rivalry disorder
F93.8 Other childhood emotional disorders
F93.9 Childhood emotional disorder, unspecified

F94 Disorders of social functioning with onset specific to childhood and adolescence

F94.0 Elective mutism
F94.1 Reactive attachment disorder of childhood
F94.2 Disinhibited attachment disorder of childhood
F94.8 Other childhood disorders of social functioning
F94.9 Childhood disorders of social functioning, unspecified

F95 Tic disorders

F95.0 Transient tic disorder
F95.1 Chronic motor or vocal tic disorder
F95.2 Combined vocal and multiple motor tic disorder (de la Tourette's syndrome)
F95.8 Other tic disorders
F95.9 Tic disorder, unspecified

F98 Other behavioural and emotional disorders with onset usually occurring in childhood and adolescence

F98.0 Non-organic enuresis
F98.1 Non-organic encopresis
F98.2 Feeding disorder of infancy and childhood
F98.3 Pica of infancy and childhood
F98.4 Stereotyped movement disorders
F98.5 Stuttering (stammering)
F98.6 Cluttering
F98.8 Other specified behavioural and emotional disorders with onset usually occurring in childhood and adolescence
F98.9 Unspecified behavioural and emotional disorders with onset usually occurring in childhood and adolescence

F99 Unspecified mental disorder

F99 Mental disorder, not otherwise specified

Appendix 2

Diagnostic and Statistical Manual of Mental Disorders (4th edition)

NOS = Not Otherwise Specified.

An x appearing in a diagnostic code indicates that a specific code number is required.

An ellipsis (. . .) is used in the names of certain disorders to indicate that the name of a specific mental disorder or general medical condition should be inserted when recording the name (e.g., 293.0 Delirium Due to Hypothyroidism).

If criteria are currently met, one of the following severity specifiers may be noted after the diagnosis

Mild
Moderate
Severe

If criteria are no longer met, one of the following specifiers may be noted

In Partial Remission
In Full Remission
Prior History

Disorders usually first diagnosed in infancy, childhood, or adolescence

Mental retardation

Note: *These are coded on Axis II.*

317 Mild Mental Retardation
318.0 Moderate Mental Retardation
318.1 Severe Mental Retardation
318.2 Profound Mental Retardation
319 Mental Retardation, Severity Unspecified

Learning disorders

315.00 Reading Disorder
315.1 Mathematics Disorder
315.2 Disorder of Written Expression
315.9 Learning Disorder NOS

Motor skills disorder

315.4 Developmental Coordination Disorder

Communication disorders

315.31 Expressive Language Disorder
315.32 Mixed Receptive–Expressive Language Disorder
315.39 Phonological Disorder
307.0 Stuttering
307.9 Communication Disorder NOS

Pervasive Developmental disorders

299.00 Autistic Disorder
299.80 Rett's Disorder
299.10 Childhood Disintegrative Disorder
299.80 Asperger's Disorder
299.80 Pervasive Developmental Disorder NOS

Attention-deficit and disruptive behaviour disorders

314.xx Attention-Deficit/Hyperactivity Disorder
 .01 Combined Type
 .00 Predominantly Inattentive Type
 .01 Predominantly Hyperactive-Impulsive Type
314.9 Attention-Deficit/Hyperactivity Disorder NOS
312.xx Conduct Disorder
 .81 Childhood-Onset Type
 .82 Adolescent-Onset Type
 .89 Unspecified Onset

313.81 Oppositional-Defiant Disorder
312.9 Disruptive Behaviour Disorder NOS

Feeding and eating disorders of infancy or early childhood

307.52 Pica
307.53 Rumination Disorder
307.59 Feeding Disorder of Infancy or Early Childhood

Tic disorders

307.23 Tourette's Disorder
307.22 Chronic Motor or Vocal Tic Disorder
307.21 Transient Tic Disorder
Specify if: Single Episode/Recurrent
307.20 Tic Disorder NOS

Elimination disorders

—.— Encopresis
787.6 With Constipation and Overflow Incontinence
307.7 Without Constipation and Overflow Incontinence
307.6 Enuresis (Not Due to a General Medical Condition)
Specify type: Nocturnal Only/Diurnal Only/Nocturnal and Diurnal

Other disorders of infancy, childhood, or adolescence

309.21 Separation Anxiety Disorder
Specify if: Early Onset
313.23 Selective Mutism
313.89 Reactive Attachment Disorder of Infancy or Early Childhood
Specify type: Inhibited Type/Disinhibited Type
307.3 Stereotypic Movement Disorder
Specify if: With Self-Injurious Behaviuor
313.9 Disorder of Infancy, Childhood, or Adolescence NOS

Delirium, dementia and amnestic and other cognitive disorders

Delirium

293.0 Delirium Due to . . . [Indicate the General Medical Condition]
—.— Substance Intoxication Delirium (refer to Substance-Related Disorders for substance-specific codes)
—.— Substance Withdrawal Delirium (refer to Substance-Related Disorders for substance-specific codes)
—.— Delirium Due to Multiple Etiologies (code each of the specific etiologies)
780.09 Delirium NOS

Dementia

294.xx Dementia of the Alzheimer's Type, With Early Onset (also code 331.0 Alzheimer's disease on Axis III)
.10 Without Behavioural Disturbance
.11 With Behavioural Disturbance
294.xx Dementia of the Alzheimer's Type, With Late Onset (also code 331.0 Alzheimer's disease on Axis III)
.10 Without Behavioural Disturbance
.11 With Behavioural Disturbance
290.xx Vascular Dementia
.40 Uncomplicated
.41 With Delirium
.42 With Delusions
.43 With Depressed Mood
Specify if: With Behavioural Disturbance

Code presence or absence of a behavioural disturbance in the fifth digit for Dementia Due to a General Medical Condition:
294.10 = Without Behavioural Disturbance
294.11 = With Behavioural Disturbance
294.1x Dementia Due to HIV Disease (*also code 042 HIV on Axis III*)
294.1x Dementia Due to Head Trauma (*also code 854.00 head injury on Axis III*)
294.1x Dementia Due to Parkinson's Disease (*also code 331.82 Dementia with Lewy Bodies on Axis III*)
294.1x Dementia Due to Huntington's Disease (*also code 333.4 Huntington's disease on Axis III*)
294.1x Dementia Due to Pick's Disease (*also code 331.11 Pick's disease on Axis III*)
294.1x Dementia Due to Creutzfeldt–Jakob Disease (*also code 046.1 Creutzfeldt–Jakob disease on Axis III*)
294.1x Dementia Due to . . . [*Indicate the General Medical Condition not listed above*] (*also code the general medical condition on Axis III*)
—.— Substance-Induced Persisting Dementia (*refer to Substance-Related Disorders for substance-specific codes*)
—.— Dementia Due to Multiple Etiologies (*code each of the specific etiologies*)
294.8 Dementia NOS

Amnestic disorders

294.0 Amnestic Disorder Due to . . . [*Indicate the General Medical Condition*]
Specify if: Transient/Chronic
—.— Substance-Induced Persisting Amnestic Disorder (*refer to Substance-Related Disorders for substance-specific codes*)
294.8 Amnestic Disorder NOS

Other cognitive disorder

294.9 Cognitive Disorder NOS

Mental disorders due to a general medical condition not elsewhere classified

293.89 Catatonic Disorder Due to . . . [*Indicate the General Medical Condition*]
310.1 Personality Change Due to . . . [*Indicate the General Medical Condition*]
Specify type: Labile Type/Disinhibited Type/Aggressive Type/Apathetic Type/Paranoid Type/Other Type/Combined Type/Unspecified Type
293.9 Mental Disorder NOS Due to . . . [*Indicate the General Medical Condition*]

Substance-related disorders

The following specifiers apply to Substance Dependence as noted:
[a]With Physiological Dependence/Without Physiological Dependence

[b]Early Full Remission/Early Partial Remission Sustained Full Remission/Sustained Partial Remission

[c]In a Controlled Environment

[d]On Agonist Therapy/

The following specifiers apply to Substance-Induced Disorders as noted:

[I]With Onset During Intoxication/[W]With Onset During Withdrawal

Alcohol-related disorders

Alcohol use disorders

303.90 Alcohol Dependencea,b,c
305.00 Alcohol Abuse

Alcohol-induced disorders

303.00 Alcohol Intoxication
291.81 Alcohol Withdrawal
Specify if: With Perceptual Disturbances
291.0 Alcohol Intoxication Delirium
291.0 Alcohol Withdrawal Delirium
291.2 Alcohol-Induced Persisting Dementia
291.1 Alcohol-Induced Persisting Amnestic Disorder
291.x Alcohol-Induced Psychotic Disorder
.5 With Delusions[I,W]
.3 With Hallucinations[I,W]
291.89 Alcohol-Induced Mood Disorder[I,W]
291.89 Alcohol-Induced Anxiety Disorder[I,W]
291.89 Alcohol-Induced Sexual Dysfunction[I]
291.82 Alcohol-Induced Sleep Disorder[I,W]
291.9 Alcohol-Related Disorder NOS

Amphetamine (or Amphetamine-like)-related disorders

Amphetamine use disorders

304.40 Amphetamine Dependence[a,b,c]
305.70 Amphetamine Abuse

Amphetamine-Induced Disorders

292.89 Amphetamine Intoxication
Specify if: With Perceptual Disturbances
292.0 Amphetamine Withdrawal
292.81 Amphetamine Intoxication Delirium
292.xx Amphetamine-Induced Psychotic Disorder
.11 With Delusions[I]
.12 With Hallucinations[I]
292.84 Amphetamine-Induced Mood Disorder[I,W]
292.89 Amphetamine-Induced Anxiety Disorder[I]
292.89 Amphetamine-Induced Sexual Dysfunction[I]
292.85 Amphetamine-Induced Sleep Disorder[I,W]
292.9 Amphetamine-Related Disorder NOS

Caffeine-related disorders

Caffeine-induced disorders

305.90 Caffeine Intoxication
292.89 Caffeine-Induced Anxiety Disorder[I]
292.85 Caffeine-Induced Sleep Disorder[I]
292.9 Caffeine-Related Disorder NOS

Cannabis-related disorders

Cannabis use disorders

304.30 Cannabis Dependence[a,b,c]
305.20 Cannabis Abuse

Cannabis-induced disorders

292.89 Cannabis Intoxication
Specify if: With Perceptual Disturbances
292.81 Cannabis Intoxication Delirium
292.xx Cannabis-Induced Psychotic Disorder
.11 With Delusions[I]
.12 With Hallucinations[I]
292.89 Cannabis-Induced Anxiety Disorder[I]
292.9 Cannabis-Related Disorder NOS

Cocaine-related disorders

Cocaine use disorders

304.20 Cocaine Dependencea,b,c
305.60 Cocaine Abuse

Cocaine-induced disorders

292.89 Cocaine Intoxication
Specify if: With Perceptual Disturbances
292.0 Cocaine Withdrawal
292.81 Cocaine Intoxication Delirium
292.xx Cocaine-Induced Psychotic Disorder
.11 With Delusions[I]
.12 With Hallucinations[I]
292.84 Cocaine-Induced Mood Disorder[I,W]
292.89 Cocaine-Induced Anxiety Disorder[I,W]
292.89 Cocaine-Induced Sexual Dysfunction[I]
292.85 Cocaine-Induced Sleep Disorder[I,W]
292.9 Cocaine-Related Disorder NOS

Hallucinogen-related disorders

Hallucinogen use disorders

304.50 Hallucinogen Dependence[b,c]
305.30 Hallucinogen Abuse

Hallucinogen-induced disorders

292.89 Hallucinogen Intoxication
292.89 Hallucinogen Persisting Perception Disorder (Flashbacks)
292.81 Hallucinogen Intoxication Delirium
292.xx Hallucinogen-Induced Psychotic Disorder
.11 With Delusions[I]
.12 With Hallucinations[I]
292.84 Hallucinogen-Induced Mood Disorder[I]
292.89 Hallucinogen-Induced Anxiety Disorder[I]
292.9 Hallucinogen-Related Disorder NOS

Inhalant-related disorders

Inhalant use disorders

304.60 Inhalant Dependence[b,c]
305.90 Inhalant Abuse

Inhalant-induced disorders

292.89 Inhalant Intoxication
292.81 Inhalant Intoxication Delirium
292.82 Inhalant-Induced Persisting Dementia

292.xx Inhalant-Induced Psychotic Disorder
.11 With Delusions[I]
.12 With Hallucinations[I]
292.84 Inhalant-Induced Mood Disorder[I]
292.89 Inhalant-Induced Anxiety Disorder[I]
292.9 Inhalant-Related Disorder NOS

Nicotine-related disorders

Nicotine use disorder

305.1 Nicotine Dependence[a,b]

Nicotine-induced disorders

292.0 Nicotine Withdrawal
292.9 Nicotine-Related Disorder NOS

Opioid-related disorders

Opioid use disorders

304.00 Opioid Dependence[a,b,c,d]
305.50 Opioid Abuse

Opioid-induced disorders

292.89 Opioid Intoxication
Specify if: With Perceptual Disturbances
292.0 Opioid Withdrawal
292.81 Opioid Intoxication Delirium
292.xx Opioid-Induced Psychotic Disorder
.11 With Delusions[I]
.12 With Hallucinations[I]
292.84 Opioid-Induced Mood Disorder[I]
292.89 Opioid-Induced Sexual Dysfunction[I]
292.85 Opioid-Induced Sleep Disorder[I,W]
292.9 Opioid-Related Disorder NOS

Phencyclidine (or Phencyclidine-like)-related disorders

Phencyclidine use disorders

304.60 Phencyclidine Dependence[b,c]
305.90 Phencyclidine Abuse

Phencyclidine-induced disorders

292.89 Phencyclidine Intoxication
Specify if: With Perceptual Disturbances
292.81 Phencyclidine Intoxication Delirium
292.xx Phencyclidine-Induced Psychotic Disorder
.11 With Delusions[I]
.12 With Hallucinations[I]
292.84 Phencyclidine-Induced Mood Disorder[I]
292.89 Phencyclidine-Induced Anxiety Disorder[I]
292.9 Phencyclidine-Related Disorder NOS

Sedative-, Hypnotic-, Oranxiolytic-related disorders

Sedative, Hypnotic, or Anxiolytic use disorders

304.10 Sedative, Hypnotic, or Anxiolytic Dependence[a,b,c]
305.40 Sedative, Hypnotic, or Anxiolytic Abuse

Sedative-, Hypnotic-, or Anxiolytic-induced disorders

292.89 Sedative, Hypnotic, or Anxiolytic Intoxication
292.0 Sedative, Hypnotic, or Anxiolytic Withdrawal
Specify it: With Perceptual Disturbances
292.81 Sedative, Hypnotic, or Anxiolytic Intoxication Delirium
292.81 Sedative, Hypnotic, or Anxiolytic Withdrawal Delirium
292.82 Sedative-, Hypnotic-, or Anxiolytic-Induced Persisting Dementia
292.83 Sedative-, Hypnotic-, or Anxiolytic-Induced Persisting Amnestic Disorder
292.xx Sedative-, Hypnotic-, or Anxiolytic-Induced Psychotic Disorder
.11 With Delusions[I,W]
.12 With Hallucinations[I,W]
292.84 Sedative-, Hypnotic-, or Anxiolytic-Induced Mood Disorder[I,W]
292.89 Sedative-, Hypnotic-, or Anxiolytic-Induced Anxiety Disorder[W]
292.89 Sedative-, Hypnotic-, or Anxiolytic-Induced Sexual Dysfunction[1]
292.85 Sedative-, Hypnotic-, or Anxiolytic-Induced Sleep Disorder[I,W]
292.9 Sedative-, Hypnotic-, or Anxiolytic-Related Disorder NOS

Polysubstance-related disorder

304.80 Polysubstance Dependence[a,b,c,d]

Other (or Unknown) substance-related disorders

Other (or Unknown) substance use disorders

304.90 Other (or Unknown) Substance Dependence[a,b,c,d]
305.90 Other (or Unknown) Substance Abuse

Other (or Unknown) substance-induced disorders

292.89 Other (or Unknown) Substance Intoxication
Specify it: With Perceptual Disturbances
292.0 Other (or Unknown) Substance Withdrawal
Specify it: With Perceptual Disturbances
292.81 Other (or Unknown) Substance-Induced Delirium
292.82 Other (or Unknown) Substance-Induced Persisting Dementia
292.83 Other (or Unknown) Substance-Induced Persisting Amnestic Disorder
292.xx Other (or Unknown) Substance-Induced Psychotic Disorder
.11 With Delusions[I,W]
.12 With Hallucinations[I,W]
292.84 Other (or Unknown) Substance-Induced Mood Disorder[I,W]
292.89 Other (or Unknown) Substance-Induced Anxiety Disorder[I,W]
292.89 Other (or Unknown) Substance-Induced Sexual Dysfunction[1]
292.85 Other (or Unknown) Substance-Induced Sleep Disorder[I,W]
292.9 Other (or Unknown) Substance-Related Disorder NOS

Schizophrenia and other psychotic disorders

295.xx Schizophrenia

The following Classification of Longitudinal Course applies to all subtypes of Schizophrenia.

Episodic With Interepisode Residual Symptoms (*specify if*: With Prominent Negative Symptoms)/Episodic With No Interepisode Residual Symptoms/Continuous (*specify if*: With Prominent Negative Symptoms)

Single Episode In Partial Remission (*specify if*: With Prominent Negative Symptoms)/Single Episode In Full Remission
Other or Unspecified Pattern
.30 Paranoid Type
.10 Disorganized Type
.20 Catatonic Type
.90 Undifferentiated Type
.60 Residual Type
295.40 Schizophreniform Disorder
Specify it: Without Good Prognostic Features/With Good Prognostic Features
295.70 Schizoaffective Disorder
Specify type: Bipolar Type/Depressive Type
297.1 Delusional Disorder
Specify type: Erotomanic Type/Grandiose Type/Jealous Type/ Persecutory Type/Somatic Type/Mixed Type/Unspecified Type
298.8 Brief Psychotic Disorder
Specify it: With Marked Stressor(s)/Without Marked Stressor(s)/ With Postpartum Onset
297.3 Shared Psychotic Disorder
293.xx Psychotic Disorder Due to . . . [Indicate the General Medical Condition]
.81 With Delusions
.82 With Hallucinations
—.— Substance-Induced Psychotic Disorder (refer to Substance-Related Disorders for substance-specific codes)
Specify it: With Onset During Intoxication/With Onset During Withdrawal
298.9 Psychotic Disorder NOS

Mood disorders

Code current state of Major Depressive Disorder or Bipolar I Disorder in fifth digit:
1 = Mild
2 = Moderate
3 = Severe Without Psychotic Features
4 = Severe With Psychotic Features
Specify: Mood-Congruent Psychotic Features/Mood-Incongruent Psychotic Features
5 = In Partial Remission
6 = In Full Remission
0 = Unspecified
The following specifiers apply (for current or most recent episode) to Mood Disorders as noted
[a]Severity/Psychotic/Remission Specifiers/[b]Chronic/[c]With Catatonic Features/[d]With Melancholic Features/[e]With Atypical Features/[f]With Postpartum Onset
The following specifiers apply to Mood Disorders as noted:
[g]With or Without Full Interepisode Recovery/[h]With Seasonal Pattern/[i]With Rapid Cycling

Depressive disorders

296.xx Major Depressive Disorder,
.2x Single Episodea,b,c,d,e,f
.3x Recurrenta,b,c,d,e,f,g,h
300.4 Dysthymic Disorder
Specify it: Early Onset/Late Onset
Specify: With Atypical Features
311 Depressive Disorder NOS

Bipolar disorders

296.xx Bipolar I Disorder,
.0x Single Manic Episode[a,c,f]
Specify if: Mixed
.40 Most Recent Episode Hypomanic[g,h,i]
.4x Most Recent Episode Manic[a,c,f,g,h,i]
.6x Most Recent Episode Mixed[a,c,f,g,h,i]
.5x Most Recent Episode Depressed[a,b,c,d,e,f,g,h,i]
.7 Most Recent Episode Unspecified[g,h,i]
296.89 Bipolar II Disorder[a,b,c,d,e,f,g,h,i]
Specify (current or most recent episode): Hypomanic/Depressed
301.13 Cyclothymic Disorder
296.80 Bipolar Disorder NOS
293.83 Mood Disorder Due to . . . [*Indicate the General Medical Condition*]
Specify type: With Depressive Features/With Major Depressive-like Episode/With Manic Features/With Mixed Features
—.— Substance-Induced Mood Disorder (*refer to Substance-Related Disorders for substance-specific codes*)
Specify type: With Depressive Features/With Manic Features/ With Mixed Features
Specify if: With Onset During Intoxication/With Onset During Withdrawal
296.90 Mood Disorder NOS

Anxiety Disorders

300.01 Panic Disorder Without Agoraphobia
300.21 Panic Disorder With Agoraphobia
300.22 Agoraphobia Without History of Panic Disorder
300.29 Specific Phobia
Specify type: Animal Type/Natural Environment Type/Blood-Injection-Injury Type/Situational Type/Other Type
300.23 Social Phobia
Specify if: Generalized
300.3 Obsessive–Compulsive Disorder
Specify if: With Poor Insight
309.81 Posttraumatic Stress Disorder
Specify if: Acute/Chronic
Specify if: With Delayed Onset
308.3 Acute Stress Disorder
300.02 Generalized Anxiety Disorder
293.89 Anxiety Disorder Due to . . . [*Indicate the General Medical Condition*]
Specify if: With Generalized Anxiety/ With Panic Attacks/With Obsessive–Compulsive Symptoms
—.— Substance-Induced Anxiety Disorder (*refer to Substance-Related Disorders for substance-specific codes*)
Specify if: With Generalized Anxiety/ With Panic Attacks/With Obsessive–Compulsive Symptoms/With Phobic Symptoms
Specify if: With Onset During Intoxication/With Onset During Withdrawal
300.00 Anxiety Disorder NOS

Somatoform disorders

300.81 Somatization Disorder

300.82 Undifferentiated Somatoform Disorder
300.11 Conversion Disorder
Specify type: With Motor Symptom or Deficit/With Sensory Symptom or Deficit/With Seizures or Convulsions/With Mixed Presentation
307.xx Pain Disorder
.80 Associated With Psychological Factors
.89 Associated With Both Psychological Factors and a General
Medical Condition
Specify if: Acute/Chronic
300.7 Hypochondriasis
Specify if: With Poor Insight
300.7 Body Dysmorphic Disorder
300.82 Somatoform Disorder NOS

Factitious disorders

300.xx Factitious Disorder
.16 With Predominantly Psychological signs and Symptoms
.19 With Predominantly Physical Signs and Symptoms
.19 With Combined Psychological and Physical Signs and Symptoms
300.19 Factitious Disorder NOS

Dissociative disorders

300.12 Dissociative Amnesia
300.13 Dissociative Fugue
300.14 Dissociative Identity Disorder
300.6 Depersonalization Disorder
300.15 Dissociative Disorder NOS

Sexual and gender identity disorders

Sexual dysfunctions

The following specifiers apply to all primary Sexual Dysfunctions:
Lifelong Type/Acquired Type Generalized Type/Situational Type Due to Psychological Factors/Due to Combined Factors

Sexual desire disorders

302.71 Hypoactive Sexual Desire Disorder
302.79 Sexual Aversion Disorder

Sexual arousal disorders

302.72 Female Sexual Arousal Disorder
302.72 Male Erectile Disorder

Orgasmic disorders

302.73 Female Orgasmic Disorder
302.74 Male Orgasmic Disorder
302.75 Premature Ejaculation

Sexual pain disorders

302.76 Dyspareunia (Not Due to a General Medical Condition)
306.51 Vaginismus (Not Due to a General Medical Condition)

Sexual dysfunction due to a general medical condition

625.8 Female Hypoactive Sexual Desire Disorder Due to . . . [*Indicate the General Medical Condition*]
608.89 Male Hypoactive Sexual Desire Disorder Due to . . . [*Indicate the General Medical Condition*]
607.84 Male Erectile Disorder Due to . . . [*Indicate the General Medical Condition*]
625.0 Female Dyspareunia Due to . . . [*Indicate the General Medical Condition*]
608.89 Male Dyspareunia Due to . . . [*Indicate the General Medical Condition*]
625.8 Other Female Sexual Dysfunction Due to . . . [*Indicate the General Medical Condition*]
608.89 Other Male Sexual Dysfunction Due to . . . *Indicate the General Medical Condition*]
—.— Substance-Induced Sexual Dysfunction (*refer to Substance-Related Disorders for substance-specific codes*)
Specify if: With Impaired Desire/With Impaired Arousal/With Impaired Orgasm/With Sexual Pain
Specify if: With Onset During Intoxication
302.70 Sexual Dysfunction NOS

Paraphilias

302.4 Exhibitionism
302.81 Fetishism
302.89 Frotteurism
302.2 Pedophilia
Specify if: Sexually Attracted to Males/Sexually Attracted to Females/Sexually Attracted to Both
Specify if: Limited to Incest
Specify type: Exclusive Type/Nonexclusive Type
302.83 Sexual Masochism
302.84 Sexual Sadism
302.3 Transvestic Fetishism
Specify if: With Gender Dysphoria
302.82 Voyeurism
302.9 Paraphilia NOS

Gender identity disorders

302.xx Gender Identity Disorder
.6 in Children
.85 in Adolescents or Adults
Specify if: Sexually Attracted to Males/Sexually Attracted to Females/Sexually Attracted to Both/Sexually Attracted to Neither
302.6 Gender Identity Disorder NOS
302.9 Sexual Disorder NOS

Eating disorders

307.1 Anorexia Nervosa
Specify type: Restricting Type; Binge-Eating/Purging Type
307.51 Bulimia Nervosa
Specify type: Purging Type/Nonpurging Type
307.50 Eating Disorder NOS

Sleep disorders

Primary sleep disorders

Dyssomnias

307.42 Primary Insomnia
307.44 Primary Hypersomnia
Specify if: Recurrent

347.00 Narcolepsy
780.57 Breathing-Related Sleep Disorder
327.3X Circadian Rhythm Sleep Disorders
.31 Delayed Sleep Phase Type
.35 Jet Lag Type
.36 Shift Work Type
.30 Unspecified Type
Type/Unspecified Type
307.47 Dyssomnia NOS

Parasomnias

307.47 Nightmare Disorder
307.46 Sleep Terror Disorder
307.46 Sleepwalking Disorder
307.47 Parasomnia NOS

Sleep disorders related to another mental disorder

327.02 Insomnia Related to . . . *[Indicate the Axis I or Axis II Disorder]*
327.15 Hypersomnia Related to . . . *[Indicate the Axis I or Axis II Disorder]*

Other sleep disorders

780.xx Sleep Disorder Due to . . . *[Indicate the General Medical Condition]*
.52 Insomnia Type
.54 Hypersomnia Type
.59 Parasomnia Type
.59 Mixed Type
—.— Substance-Induced Sleep Disorder (*refer to Substance-Related Disorders for substance-specific codes*)
Specify type: Insomnia Type/Hypersomnia Type/Parasomnia Type/ Mixed Type
Specify if: With Onset During Intoxication/With Onset During Withdrawal

Impulse control disorders not elsewhere classified

312.34 Intermittent Explosive Disorder
312.32 Kleptomania
312.33 Pyromania
312.31 Pathological Gambling
312.39 Trichotillomania
312.30 Impulse-Control Disorder NOS

Adjustment disorders

309.xx Adjustment Disorder
.0 With Depressed Mood
.24 With Anxiety
.28 With Mixed Anxiety and Depressed Mood
.3 With Disturbance of Conduct
.4 With Mixed Disturbance of Emotions and Conduct
.9 Unspecified
Specify if: Acute/Chronic

Personality disorders

Note: *These are coded on Axis II*

301.0 Paranoid Personality Disorder
301.20 Schizoid Personality Disorder
301.22 Schizotypal Personality Disorder
301.7 Antisocial Personality Disorder
301.83 Borderline Personality Disorder
301.50 Histrionic Personality Disorder
301.81 Narcissistic Personality Disorder
301.82 Avoidant Personality Disorder
301.6 Dependent Personality Disorder
301.4 Obsessive–Compulsive Personality Disorder
301.9 Personality Disorder NOS

Other conditions that may be a focus of clinical attention

Psychological factors affecting medical condition

316 . . . *[Specified Psychological Factor]*
Affecting . . . *[Indicate the General Medical Condition]*
Choose name based on nature of factors:
Mental Disorder Affecting Medical Condition
Psychological Symptoms Affecting Medical Condition
Personality Traits or Coping Style Affecting Medical Condition
Maladaptive Health Behaviours Affecting Medical Condition
Stress-Related Physiological Response Affecting Medical Condition
Other or Unspecified Psychological Factors Affecting Medical Condition

Medication-induced movement disorders

332.1 Neuroleptic-Induced Parkinsonism
333.92 Neuroleptic Malignant Syndrome
333.7 Neuroleptic-Induced Acute Dystonia
333.99 Neuroleptic-Induced Acute Akathisia
333.82 Neuroleptic-Induced Tardive Dyskinesia
333.1 Medication-Induced Postural Tremor
333.90 Medication-Induced Movement Disorder NOS

Other medication-induced disorder

995.2 Adverse Effects of Medication NOS

Relational problems

V61.9 Relational Problem Related to a Mental Disorder or General Medical Condition
V61.20 Parent–Child Relational Problem
V61.10 Partner Relational Problem
V61.8 Sibling Relational Problem
V62.81 Relational Problem NOS

Problems related to abuse or neglect

V61.21 Physical Abuse of Child (*code 995.54 if focus of attention is on victim*)
V61.21 Sexual Abuse of Child (*code 995.53 if focus of attention is on victim*)
V61.21 Neglect of Child (*code 995.52 if focus of attention is on victim*)
—.— Physical Abuse of Adult
V61.12 (if by partner)
V62.83 (if by person other than partner) (*code 995.83 if focus of attention is on victim*)

—.— Sexual Abuse of Adult
V61.12 (if by partner)
V62.83 (if by person other than partner) (*code 995.83 if focus of attention is on victim*)

Additional conditions that may be a focus of clinical attention

V15.81 Noncompliance With Treatment
V65.2 Malingering
V71.01 Adult Antisocial Behaviour
V71.02 Child or Adolescent Antisocial Behaviour
V62.89 Borderline Intellectual Functioning

Note: *This is coded on Axis II*

780.93 Age-Related Cognitive Decline
V62.82 Bereavement
V62.3 Academic Problem
V62.2 Occupational Problem
313.82 Identity Problem
V62.89 Religious or Spiritual Problem
V62.4 Acculturation Problem
V62.89 Phase of Life Problem

Additional codes

300.9 Unspecified Mental Disorder (nonpsychotic)
V71.09 No Diagnosis or Condition on Axis I
799.9 Diagnosis or Condition Deferred on Axis I
V71.09 No Diagnosis on Axis II
799.9 Diagnosis Deferred on Axis II

Acknowledgement

ICD-10 section of the chapter prepared by Michael B. First and Harold Alan Pincus is adapted from Delling's original text. The contribution of the author to the original text is gratefully acknowledged.

References

1. Kramer, M. (1988). Historical roots and structural basis of the International Classification of Diseases. In *International classif cation in psychiatry* (eds. Mezzich, J. and von Cranach, M.), pp. 3–29. Cambridge University Press, Cambridge.
2. World Health Organization. (1949). *Manual of the International Statistical Classification of Diseases, Injuries and Causes of Death (ICD-6).* World Health Organization, Geneva, Switzerland.
3. American Psychiatric Association. (1952). *Diagnostic and Statistical Manual of Mental Disorders.* American Psychiatric Association, Washington, DC.
4. World Health Organization. (1967). *Glossary of mental disorders and guide to their classification, for use in conjunction with the International Classification of Diseases* (8th revision). World Health Organization, Geneva, Switzerland.
5. American Psychiatric Association. (1968). *Diagnostic and Statistical Manual of Mental Disorders,* (2nd edn.). Psychiatric Association, Washington, DC.
6. Feighner, J., Robins, E., Guze, S.B., *et al.* (1972). Diagnostic criteria for use in psychiatric research. *Archive of General Psychiatry,* **26**(1), 57–63.
7. Spitzer, R.L., Endicott, J. and Robins, E. (1978). Research diagnostic criteria: rationale and reliability. *Archives of General Psychiatry,* **35**(6), 773–82.
8. World Health Organization. *(1978) Mental disorders: glossary and guide to their classification, for use in conjunction with the Ninth Revision of the International Classification of Diseases.* World Health Organization, Geneva, Switzerland
9. American Psychiatric Association. (1980). *Diagnostic and Statistical Manual of Mental Disorders,* (3rd edn.) Psychiatric Association, Washington, DC.
10. Spitzer, R., Forman, J. and Nee, J. (1979) DSM-III field trials: I. initial interrator diagnostic reliabiltiy. *American Journal of Psychiatry,* **136,** 815–7.
11. Leckman, J., Weissman, M., Merikangas, K., *et al.* (1983). Panic disorder and major depression. Increased risk of depression, alcoholism, panic, and phobic disorders in families of depressed probands with panic disorder. *Archives of General Psychiatry,* **40**(10), 1055–60.
12. American Psychiatric Association. (1987). *Diagnostic and Statistical Manual of Mental Disorders* (3rd edn. – Revised) *(DSM-III-R).* American Psychiatric Association, Washington, DC.
13. World Health Organization. (1992). *International Statistical Classification of Diseases and Related Health Problems,* (10th Revision) *(ICD-10).* World Health Organization, Geneva
14. World Health Organization. (1992). *The ICD-10 Classification of Mental and Behavioural Disorders: Clinical Descriptions and Diagnostic Guidelines.* World Health Organization, Geneva
15. World Health Organization. (1993). *The ICD-10 Classification of Mental and Behavioural Disorders: Diagnostic Criteria for Research.* World Health Organization, Geneva.
16. Sartorius, N. (1990). Classifications in the field of mental health. World Health. *Statistics Quarterly,* **43**(4), 269–72.
17. World Health Organization. (1996). *Diagnostic and management guidelines for mental disorders in primary care: ICD-10* Chapter V Primary Care Version. Göttingen.: WHO-Hogrefe and Huber.
18. Sartorius, N., Kaelber, C., Cooper, J., *et al.* (1993). Progress toward achieving a common language in psychiatry. Results from the field trial of the clinical guidelines accompanying the WHO classification of mental and behavioural disorders in ICD-10. *Archives of General Psychiatry,* **50**(2), 115–24.
19. Sartorius, N., Ustun, T., Korten, A., *et al.* (1995). Progress toward achieving a common language in psychiatry, II: Results from the international field trials of the ICD-10 diagnostic criteria for research for mental and behavioural disorders. *American Journal of Psychiatry,* **152**(10), 1427–37.
20. Frances, A., Widiger, T. and Pincus, H. (1989). The development of DSM-IV. *Archive of General Psychiatry,* **46**, 373–5.
21. Widiger, T., Frances, A., Pincus, H., *et al.* (1991). Toward an empirical classification for the DSM-IV. *Journal of Abnormal Psychology,* **100**(3), 280–8.
22. Widiger, T., Frances, A., Pincus, H. *et al.* (eds.) (1994). *DSM-IV Sourcebook Vol. 1.* American Psychiatric Association, Washington, DC.
23. Widiger, T., Frances, A., Pincus, H., *et al.* (eds.) (1996). *DSM-IV Sourcebook Vol. 2.* American Psychiatric Association, Washington DC.
24. Widiger, T., Frances, A., Pincus, H., *et al.* (eds.) (1997). *DSM-IV Sourcebook Vol. 3.* American Psychiatric Association, Washington, DC.
25. Widiger, T., Frances, A., Pincus, H., *et al.* (eds.) (1998). *DSM-IV Sourcebook Vol. 4.* American Psychiatric Association, Washington, DC.
26. Kendell, R. (1991). The relationship between DSM-IV and ICD-10. *Journal of Abnormal Psychology,* **100**(3), 297–301.
27. First, M. and Pincus, H. (1999). Classification in psychiatry: ICD-10 vs. DSM-IV. A response. *British Journal of Psychiatry,* **175**, 205–9.
28. First, M. and Pincus, H. (2002) The DSM-IV Text Revision: rationale and potential impact on clinical practice. *Psychiatric Services,* **53**(3), 288–92.
29. World Health Organization. (2001). *International Classification of Functioning, Disability, and Health (ICF).* World Health Organization, Geneva.
30. Rutter, M., Shaffer, D. and Sturge, C. (1975). *A multi-axial classification of child psychiatric disorders.* World Health Organization, Geneva.

31. Janca, A., Kastrup, M., Katschnig, H., *et al.* (1996). The World Health Organization Short Disability Assessment Schedule (WHO DAS-S): a tool for the assessment of difficulties in selected areas of functioning of patients with mental disorders. *Social Psychiatry and Psychiatric Epidemiology,* **31**(6), 349–54.
32. Spitzer, R., First, M., Williams, J., *et al.* (1992). Now is the time to retire the term 'organic mental disorders'. *American Journal of Psychiatry,* **149**(2), 240–4.
33. Hollander, E., Kim, S. and Zohar, J. (2007). OCSDs in the forthcoming DSM-V. *CNS Spectrums,* **12**(5), 320–3.
34. Zimmerman, M. (1988). Why are we rushing to publish DSM-IV? *Archive of General Psychiatry,* **45**(12), 1135–8.
35. Charney, D., Barlow, D., Botteron, K., *et al.* (2002). Neuroscience research agenda to guide development of a pathophysiologically based classification system. In *A research agenda for DSM-V* (ed. Regier D.), pp. 31–84. American Psychiatric Association, Washington, DC.
36. Kupfer, D., First, M. and Regier, D. (eds.) (2002). *A Research Agenda for DSM-V.* American Psychiatric Publishing, Washington, DC.
37. Narrow, W., First, M., Sirovatka, P., *et al.* (2007). *Age and Gender Considerations in Psychiatric Diagnosis: A Research Agenda for DSM-V.* Arlington, American Psychiatric Association, VA
38. Widiger, T. and Simonsen, E. (2005). Alternative Dimensional Models of Personality Disorder: finding a common ground. *Journal of Personality Disorders,* **19**(2), 110–30.
39. Saunders, J., Schuckit, M., Sirovatka, P., *et al.* (eds.) (2007). *Diagnostic Issues in Substance Use Disorders Refining the Research Agenda for DSM-V.* Amerincan Psychiatric Association, Arlington, VA.
40. Sunderland, T., Jeste, D., Baiyewu, O., *et al.* (eds.) (2007). *Diagnostic Issues in Dementia Advancing the Research Agenda for DSM-V.* American Psychiatric Association, Arlington, VA
41. Allardycce, J., Gaebel, W., Zielasek, J., *et al.* (2007). Deconstructing Psychosis Conference February 2006: the validity of schizophrenia and alternatiuve approaches to the classification of psychosis. *Schizophrenia Bulletin,* **33**(4), 863–7.
42. Helzer, J., Kraemer, H., Krueger, R., *et al.* (eds.) (2008). *Dimensional Approaches in Diagnostic Classification: Refining the Research Agenda for DSM-V.* American Psychiatric Association, Arlington, VA.
43. American Sleep Disorders Association. (2005). *Diagnostic Classification Steering Committee. International Classification of Sleep Disorders: Diagnostic and Coding Manual.* American Academy of Sleep Medicine, Westchester, IL.
44. Andreasen, N., Olsen, S., Dennert, J., *et al.* (1982). Ventricular enlargement in schizophrenia: relationship to positive and negative symptoms. *American Journal of Psychiatry,* **139**, 297–302.
45. Widiger, T., Simonsen, E., Krueger, R., *et al.* (2005). Personality disorder research agenda for the DSM-V. *Journal of Personality Disorder,* **19**(3), 315–38.
46. Helzer, J., Van den Brink, W. and Guth, S. (2006). Should there be both categorical and dimensional criteria for the substance use disorders in DSM-V. *Addiction,* **101**(suppl. 1), 17–22.
47. Krueger, R., Watson, D. and Barlow, D. (2005). Introduction to the Special Section: toward a dimensionally-based taxonomy of psychopathology. *Journal of Abnormal Psychology,* **114**, 491–3.
48. Cloninger, C. (1998). A new conceptual paradigm from genetics and psychobiology for the science of mental health. *Australian and New Zealand Journal of Psychiatry,* **33,** 174–86.
49. Lenzenweger, M. (1999). Schizophrenia: refining the phenotype, resolving the endophenotype. *Behaviour and Research Therapy,* **37**(3), 281–95.
50. Livesley, W. and Jang, K. (2000). Toward an empirically-based classification of personality disorder. *Journal of Personality Disorder,* **14,** 137–51.
51. Meyer, R. (2001). Finding paradigms for the future of alcoholism research: an interdisciplinary perspective. *Alcohol, Clinical and Experimental Research,* **25**(9), 1393–406.
52. Peralta, V., Cuesta, M., Giraldo, C., *et al.* (2002). Classifying psychotic disorder: issues regarding categorical vs. dimensional approaches and time frame to assess symptoms. *European Archives of Psychiatry and Clinical Neuroscience,* **252**, 12–18.
53. Serreti, A., Macciardi, F. and Smeraldi, E. (1996). Identification of symptomatologic patterns concern in major psychoses: proposal for a phenotype definition. *American Journal of Medical Genetics,* **67**(4), 393–400.
54. Van Os, J., Gilvarry, C., Bale, E., *et al.* (1999). A comparison of the utility of dimensional and categorical representations of psychosis. *Psychological Medicine,* **29**, 595–606.
55. Clark, L. (2005). Temperament as a Unifying Concept in the Study of Personality and Psychopathology. *Journal of Abnormal Psychology,* **114**(4), 505–21.
56. Goldberg, D. (1996). A dimensional model for common mental disorders. *British Journal of Psychiatry,* **168**(suppl. 30), 44–9.
57. Krueger, R. and Piasecki, T. (2002). Toward a dimensional and psychometricallyinformed approach to conceptualizing psychopathology. *Behaviour and Research Therapy,* **40**(5), 485–99.
58. Widiger, T. and Samuel, D. (2005). Diagnostic categories or dimensions: a question for the diagnostic and statistical manual of mental disorders (5th edn.). *Journal of Abnormal Psychiatry,* **114**(4), 494–504.
59. First, M. (2005). Clinical Utility: A Prerequisite for the Adoption of a Dimensional Approach in DSM. *Journal of Abnormal Psychiatry,* **114**(4), 560–4.
60. Kraemer, H., Noda, A. and O'Hara, R. (2004). Categorical versus dimensional approaches to diagnosis: methodological challenges. *Journal of Psychiatric Research,* **38,** 17–25.

1.10

From science to practice

John R. Geddes

The difficulties in keeping up to date

Clinicians need accurate and up-to-date information about emerging knowledge on assessment and treatment as well as other developments in practice. The presentation of this knowledge needs to be timely, accurate, and unbiased. In an ideal world, every psychiatrist would have instantaneous access to the original scientific articles. As this is not feasible because clinicians are busy and the skills needed for an adequate systematic search, critical appraisal, and interpretation of research articles are not routinely available. Further, the volume of research articles is staggering: about 2 million papers are published in 20 000 biomedical journals every year,[1] and even if a psychiatrist restricted her reading to those clinical psychiatry journals it would be necessary to read about 5500 papers each year—equivalent to 15 papers every day.[2] Clearly, a strategy is required for efficient and timely identification of research that is both methodologically sound and clinically relevant.

Traditionally, clinicians have used a number of methods of keeping up to date with research, including consulting colleagues and reading textbooks and journals. Smith[3] reviewed the research on the information needs of doctors and rated sources of information on several dimensions: their relevance to clinical practice, their scientific validity, how easy they were to use, and an overall estimate of their usefulness. Most of the sources that scored highly on all dimensions (such as regularly updated evidence-based textbooks) were of limited availability. Traditional methods of obtaining information (such as conventional textbooks and lecture-based continuing medical education) were more widely available, but of limited validity.

The difficulty in accessing reliable information means that many clinical decisions are made with a greater degree of uncertainty than is necessary. The gap between research and clinical practice is often filled by an unsystematic combination of beliefs, opinions, and clinical experience, which inevitably leads to unnecessary variations in clinical practice. These have been widely documented in psychiatry and include variations in the use of electroconvulsive therapy,[4,5] the use of antipsychotics,[6,7] and the treatment of depression.[8–10] The existence of these variations can only mean that some patients are not receiving the optimum treatment.

Methods of improving use of best available evidence

A coherent set of strategies designed as a clinical tool to link the best available evidence directly to the care of individual patients was first formulated at McMaster University in Canada—an approach called **evidence-based medicine.**[11] Evidence-based medicine is problem-based and splits the process of linking research to practice into five stages (Fig. 1.10.1) plus the identification of clinical questions in need of more research.

To make evidence-based practice feasible in real-life clinical practice, a number of problems need to be solved at each stage of the process.

Formulating a structured clinical question

When uncertainty arises in clinical practice, the clinician needs to formulate a structured clinical question. This step is fundamental to the process of evidence-based medicine because it allows the

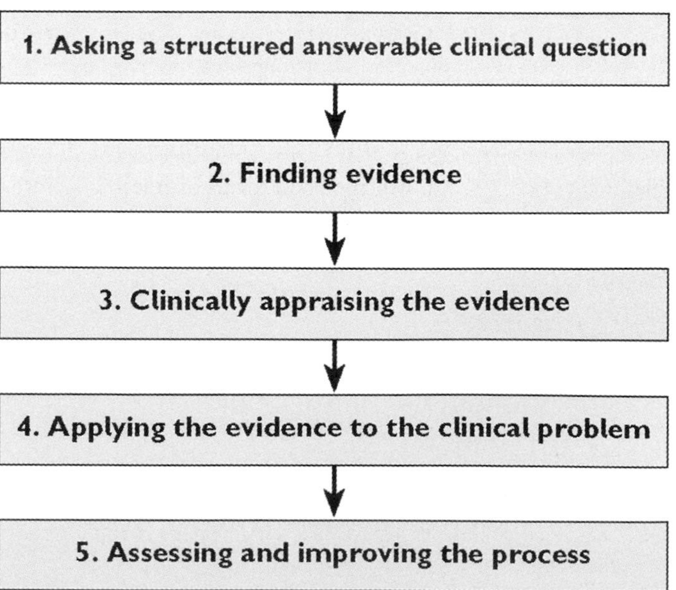

Fig. 1.10.1 The five stages of evidence-based medicine.

clinician first to classify the question, second to identify the research architecture that is most likely to yield a reliable result, and finally to determine the most efficient way of looking for the most reliable research.

(a) Example

Consider a patient who has suffered from two episodes of major depressive disorder both of which have caused substantial functional impairment. On each occasion his symptoms have responded to treatment with a selective serotonin reuptake inhibitor. Following remission of symptoms, the patient has been advised to continue treatment for 6 months before gradually discontinuing the drugs. His psychiatrist is now considering whether or not to advise long-term treatment with antidepressant medication to reduce the risk of relapse. The patient wants to know the risk of relapse without treatment and how much this would be reduced by continuing the drugs. The process of rapidly finding the best answer begins by formulating a clinical question:

1 in patients with major depressive disorder who have responded to drug treatment (the **problem**)

2 how effective are antidepressants (the **intervention**)

3 compared with alternative treatments (including none) (the **comparison intervention**)

4 in preventing relapse (the **outcome**)?

The next step is to classify the question. This example clearly concerns a question about therapy. Most of the questions that arise in clinical practice concern therapy, diagnosis, prognosis, or aetiology. Once the question has been formulated and classified, this suggests the most reliable research architecture (Table 1.10.1)

Table 1.10.1 Types of clinical question and most reliable study architecture

Type of question	Form of the question	Most reliable study architecture
Diagnosis	How likely is a patient who has a particular symptom, sign, or diagnostic test result to have a specific disorder?	A cross-sectional study of patients suspected of having the disorder comparing the proportion of the patients who really have the disorder who have a positive test result with the proportion of patients who do not have the disorder who have a positive test result.
Treatment	Is the treatment of interest more effective in producing a desired outcome than an alternative treatment (including no treatment)?	Randomized evidence in which the patients are randomly allocated to receive either the treatment of interest or the alternative: this is usually a systematic review of RCTs or a single high-quality RCT.
Prognosis	What is the probability of a specific outcome in this patient?	A study in which an inception cohort (patients at a common stage in the development of the illness—especially first onset) are followed up for an adequate length of time.
Aetiology	What has caused the disorder?	A study comparing the frequency of an exposure in a group of persons with the disease (cases) of interest with a group of persons without the disease (controls)—this may be an RCT, a case-control study. or a cohort study.

RCT, randomized controlled trial.

Finding evidence and advances in the organization of clinical knowledge

Identification of the nature of the clinical question and the most reliable study design enables the clinician to do a focused and efficient literature search. One of the main advances of evidence-based medicine has been the development of methods of research synthesis, or the process of identifying, appraising, and summarizing primary research studies into clinically usable knowledge. There are two main approaches to research synthesis—systematic reviews and clinical practice guidelines. Both these approaches are based on an explicit methodology that begins with the construction of a hierarchy of evidence in which certain forms of research architecture are considered to be reliable than others. The methodology is most clearly developed for questions about therapy and these will be the focus here.

(b) Levels of evidence

A commonly used hierarchy of evidence for studies of treatments is as follows:

Ia Evidence from a systematic review of randomized controlled trials,

Ib Evidence from at least one randomized controlled trial,

IIa Evidence from at least one controlled study without randomization,

IIb Evidence from at least one other type of quasi-experimental study,

III Evidence from non-experimental descriptive studies, such as comparative studies, correlation studies, and case-control studies,

IV Evidence from expert committee reports or opinions and/or clinical experience of respected authorities.

In this hierarchy, randomized evidence is considered, on average, to be more reliable thsan non-randomized evidence, and a systematic review of randomized evidence is considered to be the best defence against systematic bias.

Hierarchies of evidence have also been formulated for non-therapeutic studies, such as studies of aetiology, diagnosis, and prognosis. Again, the fundamental feature of these hierarchies is that the study architectures with the least susceptibility to bias are considered most reliable. The study design considered most reliable for each type of clinical question is shown in Table 1.10.1.

(c) Systematic reviews

The need for systematic reviews and the methodology used are described in Chapter 6.1.1.2. The recognition of the need for systematic reviews of randomized controlled trials, and the development of the scientific methodology of reviews, has been one of the most striking advances in health services research over the last decade. One key development was the founding of the Cochrane Collaboration, an international organization with the objective of producing regularly updated systematic reviews of the effectiveness of all health care interventions.[12]

(d) Clinical practice guidelines

In some areas of health care there is sufficient evidence, coexisting with substantial clinical uncertainty, that it is worth developing clinical practice guidelines. Clinical practice guidelines have been defined as 'systematically developed statements to assist practitioner decisions about appropriate health care for specific clinical circumstances'.[13] Guidelines have been developed for several years, but there have been recent advances in the methodology of producing explicitly evidence-based guidelines. Evidence-based clinical practice guidelines are developed by a guideline development group consisting of key stakeholders who decide on the precise clinical questions to be answered. The evidence is then systematically reviewed and classified according to a hierarchy of evidence (see above) and presented to the guideline development group. The group then makes recommendations as appropriate. The degree to which the recommendations are directly based on the evidence is described using a second level of classification[14]:

1 directly based on category I evidence;

2 directly based on category II evidence or extrapolated recommendation from category I evidence;

3 directly based on category III evidence or extrapolated recommendation from category I or II evidence;

4 directly based on category IV evidence or extrapolated recommendation from category I, II, or III evidence.

Clinical practice guidelines are usually developed at a national level and need tailoring to suit local circumstances. Professional and scientific bodies such as the American Psychiatric Association and the British Association for Psychopharmacology often take the lead in developing national guidelines. Increasingly, health care providing organizations are developing clinical practice guidelines as a way of assuring quality, increasing standardization of care and controlling costs. For example, in the United Kingdom, the National Institute for Health and Clinical Excellence (NICE) is now the main body producing guidelines across all disease areas. These guidelines are extremely rigorous in terms of methodology and also routinely include economic analyses of the cost-effectiveness of health care technologies. At their best, these guidelines produce the most accurate syntheses of current knowledge available. NICE also produces Health Technology Appraisals (HTAs) of single interventions to determine the cost-effectiveness of new technologies (mainly medicines) prior to their introduction into the taxpayer-funded National Health Service. Cost-effectiveness analysis requires the translation of disease-specific estimates of clinical effectiveness into the common metric of Quality Adjusted Life Years (QALYs) using sophisticated modelling techniques. Decisions about whether to allow reimbursement of the treatment depends on the cost per QALY (incremental cost-effectiveness ratio, ICER): a treatment with an ICER of more than £30 000 is unlikely to be approved. NICEs HTA decisions are particularly likely to be controversial when there is some evidence that the treatment works, but that the ICER is found to be too high—for example, in the case of acetylcholinesterase inhibitors in Alzheimer's disease.

There are several limitations to clinical practice guidelines. Firstly, evidence-based clinical practice guidelines are expensive and time consuming to produce and rapidly become out of date. Secondly, to influence practice, evidence-based clinical practice guidelines need to be actively disseminated and implemented. Guidelines that are developed nationally and passively sent out to doctors are often not used.[15] A number of active approaches are effective in helping change clinicians' behaviour:[16]

- outreach visits (also known as academic detailing)
- local opinion leaders
- patient-mediated interventions (including patient education)
- multifaceted interventions involving a range of techniques.

There is some evidence that guidelines can improve patient outcomes by their effect on clinical practice, especially when they are made relevant to local circumstances.[15] In one study in the United States, 217 patients with depressive disorders were randomly assigned to usual care or a multifaceted intervention designed to achieve the Agency for Health Care Policy and Research guidelines on management of depression.[17] Patients in the intervention group were much more likely to be treated in accordance with the guidelines, and this led to improved outcomes in patients with major depressive disorder (more than 50 per cent reduction on the Symptom Checklist-90 Depressive Symptom Scale at 4 months in 74 per cent of experimental patients compared with 44 per cent of control patients).

Understandably, clinicians also seek guidance in important clinical questions that are poorly served by high-quality, especially randomized, evidence. To assist in these clinical decisions, Frances and his colleagues have developed an innovative method of guideline development based on a systematic survey of the views of clinical experts.[18,19]

(e) Use of electronic communication and the Internet

The development of the Internet—or World Wide Web—during the 1990s facilitated the development of evidence-based practice. The Internet has now become a vast information resource for doctors and patients. Improved access to information afforded to patients means that they are often very well informed about their condition. This is one of the factors contributing to the need for doctors to improve their own access to information. The Internet has several drawbacks including the disorganization of the information and the lack of quality control.[20,21] Web portals have been developed that provide organized and indexed access to critically appraised websites (e.g. www.nelh.nhs.uk). The Web has now become the main medium for transmitting and storing knowledge.

(f) Improving current awareness

Another area of improvement has been the development of tools to assist doctors to maintain their current awareness of advances in research. The idea of review and abstracting journals is not new, but there has been a recognition that such journals also need a methodology to allow them to identify the most reliable and clinically important research studies.

A number of new journals have been produced with the aim of improving the availability of high-quality evidence to clinicians. The first of these was *ACP Journal Club* (targeted primarily at general physicians), followed by *Evidence-Based Medicine* (targeted primarily at family doctors) and, more recently, Evidence-Based Mental Health (aimed at mental health clinicians of all disciplines).

Evidence-Based Mental Health scans over 200 journals regularly and selects only those articles that both meet explicit methodological criteria (see Box 1.10.1) and are clinically important. The articles are then summarized in structured abstracts and published on one page with an accompanying commentary by a clinical expert.

A systematic approach to searching for the best available evidence

The developments in the organization of clinical knowledge make it possible for a clinician to search rapidly and efficiently for current best evidence using a standard approach (Fig. 1.10.2). This approach will change as new methods of organizing knowledge are developed.

(a) Example (continued)

Although a recent clinical guideline has been produced by NICE, it does not include sufficient quantitative information to answer the patient's question.

Box 1.10.1 Examples of the criteria for selection and review of articles for abstracting in Evidence-Based Mental Health

Articles are considered for abstracting if they meet the following criteria

Basic criteria

- Original or review articles
- In English
- About humans
- About topics that are important to the practice of clinicians in the broad field of mental health

Studies of prevention or treatment must meet these additional criteria

- Random allocation of participants to comparison groups
- Follow-up (endpoint assessment) of at least 80% of those entering the investigation
- Outcome measure of known or probable clinical importance
- Analysis consistent with study design

Studies of diagnosis must meet these additional criteria

- Clearly identified comparison groups, at least one of which is free of the disorder or derangement of interest
- Interpretation of diagnostic standard without knowledge of test results
- Interpretation of test without knowledge of diagnostic standard result
- Diagnostic(gold) standard(e.g. diagnosis according to DSM-IV or ICD-10 criteria after assessment by clinically qualified interviewer) preferably with documentation of reproducible criteria for subjectively interpreted diagnostic standard(e.g. report of statistically significant measure of agreement among observers)
- Analysis consistent with study design.

Studies of prognosis must meet additional criteria

- Inception cohort (first onset or assembled at a uniform point in the development of the disease) of individuals, all initially free of the outcome of the interest
- Follow-up of at least 80% of patients until the occurrence of a major study endpoint
- Or to the end of the study
- Analysis consistent with study design.

Studies of causation must meet these additional criteria

- Clearly identified comparison group for those at risk of, or having, the outcome of interest (i.e. randomized controlled trial quasi-randomized controlled trial, non-randomized controlled trial, cohort analytical study with case by-case matching, or statistical adjustment to create comparable groups, case-control study)
- Masking of observers of outcomes to exposures (this criterion is assumed to be met if the outcome is objective), observers of exposures masked to outcomes for case-control studies, or masking of subjects to exposure for all other study designs
- Analysis consistent with study design.

Geddes, J.R., Carney, S.M., Davies, C., Furukawa, T.A., Kupfer, D.J., Frank, E., Goodwin. G.M. Relapse prevention with antidepressant drug treatment in depressive disorders. *Lancet* 2003, **361:** 653–61.[22]

This is a systematic review of randomized controlled trials comparing a number of antidepressants (including tricyclics, selective serotonin reuptake inhibitors, monoamine oxidase inhibitors, and low-dose antipsychotics) with placebo in the prevention of relapse in depressive disorder.

1. Search for an evidence-based clinical practice guideline

↓

2. Search for a good-quality systematic review of randomized controlled trials of the intervention
Cochrane Database of Systematic Reviews
Database of Abstracts of Reviews of Effectiveness
Evidence-Based Mental Health
Electronic bibliographic database (Medline, EMBASE, or PsycLIT)

↓

3. Search for a single randomized controlled trial
Cochrane Controlled Trials Register
Evidence-Based Mental Health
Electronic bibliographic database (Medline, EMBASE, or PsycLIT)

↓

4. Search for the next level of evidence
Electronic bibliographic database (Medline, EMBASE, or PsycLIT)

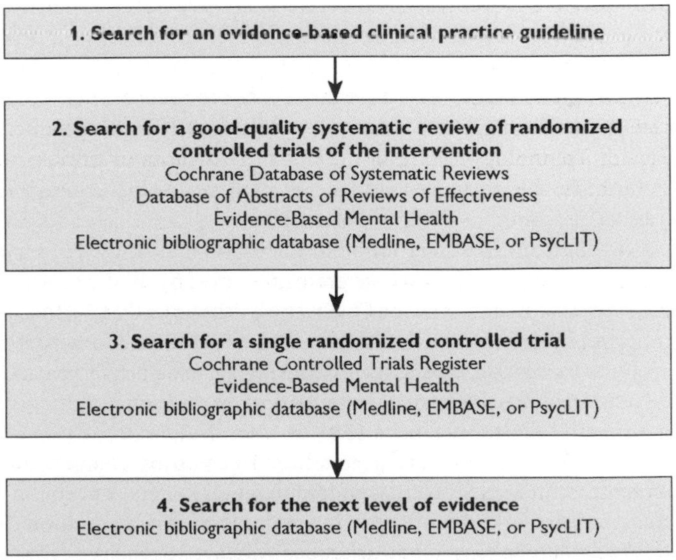

Fig. 1.10.2 A systematic approach to identifying the best evidence about a therapy.

Critical appraisal of research articles

Once the evidence has been found, it needs to be critically appraised for its reliability and usefulness. Psychiatrists need to be able to assess the scientific value and clinical importance of a study. This requires a range of epidemiological and biostatistical skills that have not traditionally been considered to be key skills for psychiatrists. In the United Kingdom, the Royal College of Psychiatrists introduced in 1999 a new part of the main professional examination that is designed to test these skills, recognizing their fundamental importance for clinical psychiatrists.[23]

Structured critical appraisal is an active process that involves a systematic assessment of the key methodological aspects of the paper. In particular, critical appraisal focuses systematically on those aspects of the study methodology that are most likely to lead to unreliability of results. A number of checklists, designed to make the appraisal quicker and more systematic, have been produced for different research study designs.[24] For example, the critical appraisal of a systematic review involves an assessment of those aspects of methodology described in Chapter 6.1.1.2. A commonly used checklist for systematic reviews is shown in Table 1.10.2.

(a) Example (continued)

Using the checklist, the review can be quickly critically appraised. It is a review of the efficacy of antidepressant drugs in preventing recurrence of depression in patients who responded to acute phase therapy with antidepressants and so appears relevant to the clinical question. The authors have only included randomized controlled trials, and this will make systematic error less likely and improve the reliability of the review. The literature search strategy is clearly documented and included electronic databases (Medline, Psyclit, Embase, Lilacs, and the Cochrane Library), hand searching of journals, and correspondence with researchers active in the field and drug companies. The quality of the randomized controlled trials was rated both from the description of the allocation of treatment and by assessing other methodological issues such as whether the primary analysis was done as an intention-to-treat analysis and the degree of blinding of the clinician and patient. It can be concluded that the reviewers have made a reasonable effort to identify the primary studies, although it is possible that other studies, perhaps with negative results, have not been published (publication bias, see Chapter 6.1.1.2).

The results of the primary studies are shown graphically as odds ratios (see Glossary) in Fig. 1.10.3. Odds ratios falling to the left of the vertical line indicate that the outcome (relapse of depressive symptoms) occurred less frequently in patients who continued treatment with an antidepressant. The smaller the odd ratio, the larger the treatment effect found in that particular study. For each study, the central diamond represents the most likely value of the relative risk and the box around the relative risk shows the 95 per cent confidence interval (**CI**). The larger studies (e.g. **Rouillon *et al.*[25]) have narrower confidence intervals because they are larger and therefore have less random error and greater precision.

From the figure, it can be seen that, the odds ratio of the all the studies included fall on the left-hand side of the line and therefore found the same direction of treatment effect. There is considerable overlap in the confidence intervals from study to study and, although there is some statistically significant heterogeneity between them (see Chapter 6.1.1.2), this appears to be in the size—rather than the nature—of the positive treatment effect. At the bottom of the figure is the estimate of the combined treatment effect of the trials. This is expressed as a pooled odds ratio. Combining the study results produces a more precise estimate of the drug's relative effectiveness, with tighter confidence intervals. The overall pooled odds ratio of relapse for patients taking antidepressants compared with placebo is 0.30 (95 per cent CI (see Glossary), 0.22–0.38).

Table 1.10.2 Checklist to assist the critical appraisal of a systematic review

Validity
1. Did the review address a clearly focused clinical question? Did the review describe: the population studied? the intervention given? the outcomes considered?
2. Did the authors select the right sort of studies for the review? The right studies would: address the review's question have an adequate study design (e.g. for a question re therapy, an RCT)
3. Were the important relevant studies included in the review? Which bibliographic databases were used? Personal contact with experts Search for unpublished as well as published studies Search for non-English language studies
4. Did the review's authors assess the quality of the included studies? Did they use: description of randomization? a rating scale?
Results
5. Were the results similar from study to study? Are the results of all the included studies clearly displayed? Are the results from different studies similar? If not, are the reasons for variations between studies discussed?
6. What is the overall result of the review? Is there a clear clinical conclusion (a clinical bottom-line)? What is it? What is the numerical result?
7. How precise are the results? Is there a confidence interval?
Clinical relevance of the results
8. Can I apply the results to my patient? Is this patient so different from those in the trial that the results do not apply?
9. Should I apply the results to my patient? How great would the benefit of therapy be for this particular patient? Is the intervention consistent with my patient's values and preferences? Were all the clinically important outcomes considered? Are the benefits worth the harms and costs?

RCT, randomized controlled trial.

Methods of using research findings at the level of individual patients

After the study has been critically appraised for its validity, the clinician needs to determine what the results are, and their importance for the patient. Patients in research studies are always different from those in real-life clinical practice in ways that may be difficult to determine even only if because they–or at least the

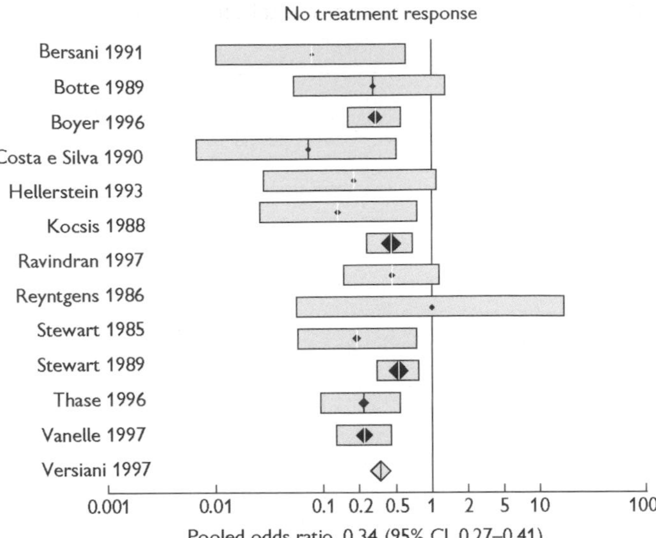

Fig. 1.10.3 Antidepressant versus placebo for the prevention of relapse in depressive disorder. (Reprinted from the *Lancet*, **361**, Geddes, J.R., Carney, S.M., Davies, C., *et al.* (2003), Relapse prevention with antidepressant drug treatment in depressive disorders, 653–61 Copyright 2003, with permission from Elsevier).[22]

episode of illness–was in the past rather than the present. Therefore, the use of results from research studies in clinical practice should be cautious and always requires a degree of extrapolation. The contribution of clinical epidemiology is in developing methods of applying research results to individual patients that are biologically and statistically robust and are explicit about any assumptions made. One of the most useful questions to ask when applying the results of a research study is: 'Is my patient so different from those in the study that the results cannot be used'? The next step is to try to interpret the study results for a particular patient, in terms of his or her clinical characteristics and treatment preferences.

An alternative measure of treatment effect which many find more clinically useful than the relative risk or odds ratio is the number needed to treat (**NNT**).[26,27] The NNT is an estimate of the number of patients that would need to be treated with the intervention of interest, compared with the alternative, in order to achieve one good outcome or to avoid one harmful outcome. The NNT is calculated by taking the reciprocal of the difference between the rates of the outcome of interest in the experimental and control groups.

(a) Example (continued)

Although the review supports the general conclusion that continued therapy with the same antidepressant that was effective in acute phase therapy is very much likely to decrease the risk of relapse, a clinician may wish to check the evidence for a specific drug. For example, how strong is the evidence for reboxetine? The systematic review identifies one trial that directly answers this question[28]. This was a multicentre trial performed in centres in Europe and South America. The trial recruited 358 outpatients who met DSM-IIIR criteria for an acute recurrence of major depressive disorder to open-label reboxetine and randomized the 285 patients who achieved >50 per cent reduction in baseline depressive symptoms on the Hamilton Depression Rating Scale to either continued reboxetine or placebo (mean age reboxetine 43.4 years, placebo 42.3 years, women 79.3 per cent reboxetine: 67.4 per cent men). One group of 145 patients were allocated to reboxetine, 4 mg b.d. and 141 patients were allocated to placebo. Treatment was continued for a further 46 weeks and the primary outcome was relapse (increase in the Hamilton Depression Rating Scale of 50 per cent or more and/or a total score of ≥18 points).

(i) Appraising the validity of a randomized controlled trial

The appraisal of an individual randomized controlled trial also addresses issues of internal and external validity. The main difference compared with the appraisal of a systematic review is that the reader can appraise the trial directly, rather than relying on the author of the review to have made an adequate assessment of the quality of the studies included. The most important questions to answer during the appraisal of the article are those relating to methodological issues that have been randomly shown to affect the reliability of the results (Table 1.10.3).

This study[28] was a **randomized controlled trial**. The method of randomization is not stated and no details are provided about the **concealment of treatment allocation**. Concealment of allocation is one of the most important features to appraise in a randomized controlled trial, and refers to how well the treatment allocation of the next patient was concealed from the participating clinician.[29] If a clinician has definite knowledge of, or can reasonably predict, the next allocation, he may decide not to enter a patient if he favours either treatment in that specific case. This would obviously lead to a subversion of randomization and biased results. This is why methods of quasi-randomization, such as alternate allocation, are often unsatisfactory. The most satisfactory methods of random allocation are when allocation is performed by a third party following entry of the patient into the study, for example using a centralized telephone service. Concealment of allocation should be distinguished from **blinding** of treatment allocation. Blinding refers to whether the patient (**single blind**), or both the patient and the clinician (**double blind**), are kept unaware of which arm of the study the patient has been allocated to *following* randomization. Blinding protects against bias in the treatment during the trial and in the assessment of subjective outcomes, but can be difficult to maintain when the experimental treatment has characteristic side-effects (e.g. antidepressants). This study was reported to be double blind; however, it is difficult to tell how effective the blinding was and whether this affected the treatment that the patients received or the ratings of outcome.

Of the patients who were randomized, 79/145 (54 per cent) of those allocated to reboxetine and 65/141 (46 per cent) of those allocated to placebo completed the trial. The reasons for drop-out are clearly stated and all the patients who entered the study are accounted for. Patients who drop out of a study may be different from those who complete it—this is a particular problem if there

Table 1.10.3 Questions that must be answered during the appraisal of an article

1. Was the assignment of the patients randomized?
2. Was the randomization list concealed?
3. Were all the subjects who entered the trial accounted for at its conclusion?
4. Were they analysed in the groups to which they were randomized?
5. Were subjects and clinicians 'blind' to which treatment was being received?
6. Other than the experimental treatment, were the groups treated equally?
7. Were the groups similar at the start of the trial?

is **differential drop-out** between the arms of the study. For this reason, the most statistically reliable and clinically useful method of analysis is to include all patients who were randomized in the analysis. This is called an **intention-to-treat analysis (ITT)**. In the reboxetine trial(28) the primary analysis was done on an ITT basis (although three patients who dropped out before the first follow-up assessment were excluded from the primary analysis—these were included in the systematic review), and the patients were analysed in the groups to which they were randomized. Lastly, although randomization will avoid bias in treatment allocation, it is possible that, by chance, the groups will be unbalanced on some key prognostic factors such as age, sex, duration, and severity of illness. Therefore it is important to assess the baseline characteristics of the patients to identify any obvious differences. In Versiani *et al.*(28) the patients were reasonably similar on baseline characteristics at entry into the trial, although the proportion of females was a little higher in the reboxetine group.

(ii) Are the results relevant for your patient?

To determine the relevance of the study to real-life patients, it is important to examine the inclusion and exclusion criteria of the trial. The main inclusion criteria are discussed above. Patients excluded from the trial were those with coexisting psychotic features or chronic depression, those with a first episode at the time of screening and patients with a history of seizures, serious brain injury, clinically significant haemopoietic or cardiovascular disease, urinary retention, or glaucoma. The user of the study results will have to take these inclusion and exclusion criteria into account, and the clinician needs to judge the relevance of the results for the individual patient.

(iii) What are the results?

Of the 145 patients treated with reboxetine, 29 relapsed, giving an experimental event rate (**EER**), of 20 per cent or a probability of relapse of 0.2. In the placebo-treated group 73 of 141 patients relapsed giving a control event rate (**CER**) of 52 per cent. Therefore the absolute difference between the rates was

$$\text{EER} - \text{CER} = 32 \text{ per cent}$$

and the difference between the probabilities is 0.32. This means that for every 100 patients treated with reboxetine, compared with placebo, 32 fewer relapsed. Therefore, to prevent one relapse over 46 weeks, 100/32, or about three patients, would need to be treated (NNT) with reboxetine.

(b) Interpretation of numbers needed to treat

The clinical interpretation of NNT depends on the seriousness of the outcome and the nature (and cost) of the intervention.

For example, if the number needed to treat with aspirin following acute stroke to avoid one death in the short-term is 100, this seems a very useful intervention because death is such a serious outcome that it is worth treating a lot of patients to save a few from dying—especially as aspirin is very cheap. Some examples of NNTs are given in Table 1.10.4.

Table 1.10.4 Examples of numbers needed to treat for interventions in psychiatry assessment and report

Intervention	Outcome	NNT	95% CI	Reference
Cognitive therapy in bulimia nervosa	Long-term remission	2		30
Antidepressants in dysthymic disorder	Clinical response	5	3–10	31
Family therapy in schizophrenia	Relapse at 1 year	**7**	4–14	32
SSRIs compared with TCAs in depressive disorder	Remain in treatment at 6 weeks	39	20–426	28

SSRI, selective serotonin reuptake inhibitor, TCA tricyclic antidepressant.

Critical appraisal of other research designs

The approach taken to the appraisal of research designs applied to other clinical questions is similar to that outlined above. Rather than passively reading the article or abstract, the clinician actively searches out the most important methodological features to determine the reliability of the study. By applying the methods developed by clinical epidemiologists, the results presented in the paper can be used to calculate more clinically meaningful measures. These can, in turn, be tailored to suit the characteristics of the individual patient. The clinician needs to develop a practical knowledge of the tools to allow him to use them routinely and quickly in clinical practice and also to develop sufficient familiarity to be able describe the results of studies to colleagues and patients.

Glossary

- **Absolute risk reduction (risk difference)** is the absolute arithmetic difference in the risk of the adverse outcome between control group (CER) and experimental group (EER). When an intervention increases the probability of a beneficial outcome it is known as the absolute benefit increase (ABI).
- **Confidence interval (CI)** is the range within which the true value of a statistical measure can be expected to lie. The CI is usually accompanied by a percentage value (usually 95 per cent) which shows the level of confidence that the true value lies within this range.
- **Event rate** is the proportion of patients in a group in whom the event is observed. In control patients, this is called the control event rate (CER) and in experimental patients it is called the experimental event rate (EER). The patient expected event rate (PEER) refers to the rate of events that would be expected in a patient who received no treatment or conventional treatment.
- **Number needed to treat (NNT)** is the reciprocal of the absolute risk reduction and is the number of patients that need to be treated to prevent one bad outcome or to achieve one beneficial outcome.
- **Odds ratio** is the odds of the outcome in the experimental group divided by the odds of the outcome in the control group. The odds ratio is often reported in meta-analyses because of its useful statistical properties.
- **Relative risk** is the risk of the outcome in the experimental group divide by the risk of the outcome in the control group. The risk ratio is increasingly reported in meta-analyses because it is easier to interpret clinically than the odds ratio.

Further information

Straus S.E., Richardson, S., Rosenberg, W., *et al.* (2001). *Evidence-based medicine: how to practise and teach EBM* (2nd edn). Churchill Livingstone, London.

Geddes, J.R. and Harrison, P.J. (1997). Evidence-based psychiatry: closing the gap between research and practice. *British Journal of Psychiatry*, **176**, 220–5.

References

1. Mulrow, C.D. (1994). Rationale for systematic reviews. *British Medical Journal*, **309**, 597–9.
2. Geddes, J.R., Wilczynski, N., Reynolds, S., *et al.* (1999). Evidence-based mental health—the first year. *Evidence-Based Mental Health*, **2**, 3–5.
3. Smith, R. (1996). What clinical information do doctors need? *British Medical Journal*, **313**, 1062–8.
4. Pippard, J. (1992). Audit of electroconvulsive treatment in two national health service regions. *The British Journal of Psychiatry*, **160**, 621–37.
5. Hermann, R.C., Dorwart, R.A., Hoover, C.W., *et al.* (1995). Variation in ECT use in the United States. *The American Journal of Psychiatry*, **152**, 869–75.
6. Meise, U., Kurz, M., and Fleischhacker, W.W. (1994). Antipsychotic maintenance treatment of schizophrenia patients: is there a consensus? *Schizophrenia Bulletin*, **20**, 215–25.
7. Lehman, A.F. and Steinwachs, D.M. (1998). Patterns of usual care for schizophrenia: initial results from the Schizophrenia Patient Outcomes Research Team (PORT) Client Survey. *Schizophrenia Bulletin*, **24**, 11–20.
8. Wells, K.B., Katon, W., Rogers, B., *et al.* (1994). Use of minor tranquilizers and antidepressant medications by depressed outpatients: results from the medical outcomes study. *The American Journal of Psychiatry*, **151**, 694–700.
9. Hirschfeld, R.M., Keller, M.B., Panico, S., *et al.* (1997). The National Depressive and Manic-Depressive Association consensus statement on the undertreatment of depression. *Journal of the American Medical Association*, **277**, 333–40.
10. Munizza, C., Tibaldi, G., Bollini, P., *et al.* (1995). Prescription pattern of antidepressants in out-patient psychiatric practice. *Psychological Medicine*, **25**, 771–8.
11. Evidence-Based Medicine Working Group (1992). Evidence-based medicine. A new approach to teaching the practice of medicine. *Journal of the American Medical Association*, **268**, 2420–5.
12. Chalmers, I., Dickersin, K., and Chalmers, T.C. (1992). Getting to grips with Archie Cochrane's agenda. *British Medical Journal*, **305**, 786–8.
13. Field, M.J. and Lohr, K.N. (1990). *Clinical practice guidelines: direction of a new agency*. Institute of Medicine, Washington, DC.
14. Eccles, M., Freemantle, N., and Mason, J. (1988). North of England evidence based guidelines development project: methods of developing guidelines for efficient drug use in primary care. *British Medical Journal*, **316**, 1232–5.
15. Grimshaw, J.M. and Russell, I.T. (1993). Effect of clinical guidelines on medical practice: a systematic review of rigorous evaluations. *Lancet*, **342**, 1317–22.
16. Oxman, A.D., Thomson, M.A., Davis, D.A., *et al.* (1995). No magic bullets: a systematic review of 102 trials of interventions to improve professional practice. *Canadian Medical Association Journal*, **153**, 1423–31.
17. Katon, W., Von Korff, M., Lin, E., *et al.* (1995). Collaborative management to achieve treatment guidelines. Impact on depression in primary care. *Journal of the American Medical Association*, **273**, 1026–31.
18. Kahn, D.A., Docherty, J.P., Carpenter, D., *et al.* (1997). Consensus methods in practice guideline development: a review and description of a new method. *Psychopharmacology Bulletin*, **33**, 631–9.
19. Frances, A.J., Docherty, J.P., and Kahn, D.A. (1998). The Expert Consensus Guideline Series: treatment of bipolar disorder. *The Journal of Clinical Psychiatry*, **57**, 1–88.
20. Jadad, A.R. and Gagliardi, A. (1998). Rating health information on the Internet: navigating to knowledge or to Babel? *Journal of the American Medical Association*, **279**, 611–14.
21. Silberg, W.M., Lundberg, G.D., and Musacchio, R.A. (1997). Assessing, controlling, and assuring the quality of medical information on the Internet: caveant lector et viewor–let the reader and viewer beware. *Journal of the American Medical Association*, **277**, 1244–5.
22. Geddes, J.R., Carney, S.M., Davies, C., *et al.* (2003). Relapse prevention with antidepressant drug treatment in depressive disorders. *Lancet*, **361**, 653–61.
23. Critical Review Paper Working Party (1997). MRCPsych Part II examination: proposed critical review paper. *Psychiatric Bulletin*, **21**, 381–2.
24. Sackett, D.L., Richardson, S., Rosenberg, W., *et al. Evidence-based medicine: how to practise and teach EBM*. Churchill Livingstone, London.
25. Rouillon, F., Berdeaux, G., Bisserbe, J.C., *et al.* (2000). Prevention of recurrent depressive episodes with milnacipran: consequences on quality of life. *Journal of Affective Disorders*, **58**, 171–80.
26. Sackett, D.L., Deeks, J.J., and Altman, D.G. (1996). Down with odds ratios! *Evidence-Based Medicine*, **1**, 164–6.
27. Cook, R.J. and Sackett, D.L. (1995). The number needed to treat: a clinically useful measure of treatment effect. *British Medical Journal*, **310**, 452–4.
28. Versiani, M., Mehilane, P., Gaszner, P., *et al.* (1999) Reboxetine, a unique selective NRI, prevents relapse and recurrence in long-term treatment of major depressive disorder. *The Journal of Clinical Psychiatry*, **60**, 400–406.
29. Shulz, K. (2000). Assessing allocation concealment and blinding in randomised controlled trials: why bother? *Evidence-Based Mental Health*, **3**, in press.
30. Fairburn, C.G., Norman, P.A., Welch, S.L., *et al.* A prospective study of outcome in bulimia nervosa and the long-term effects of three psychological treatments. *Archives of General Psychiatry*, **52**, 304–12.
31. Vanelle, J.M., Attar, L.D., Poirier, M.F., Bouhassira, M., Blin, P., and Olie, J.P. (1997). Controlled efficacy study of fluoxetine in dysthymia. *The British Journal of Psychiatry*, **170**, 345–50.
32. Mari, J.J. and Streiner, D. (1998). Family intervention for schizophrenia. In *Cochrane database of systematic reviews* (ed. M. Oakley-Brown), Update Software.
33. Anderson, I.M. and Tomenson, B.M. (1995). Treatment discontinuation with selective serotonin reuptake inhibitors compared with tricyclic antidepressants: a meta-analysis. *British Medical Journal*, **310**, 1433–8.

SECTION 2

The Scientific Basis of Psychiatric Aetiology

2.1 **Brain and mind** *133*
Martin Davies

2.2 **Statistics and the design of experiments and surveys** *137*
Graham Dunn

2.3 **The contribution of neurosciences** *144*

2.3.1 **Neuroanatomy** *144*
†R. C. A. Pearson

2.3.2 **Neurodevelopment** *156*
Karl Zilles

2.3.3 **Neuroendocrinology** *160*
Charles B. Nemeroff and Gretchen N. Neigh

2.3.4 **Neurotransmitters and signalling** *168*
Trevor Sharp

2.3.5 **Neuropathology** *177*
Peter Falkai and Bernhard Bogerts

2.3.6 **Functional position emission tomography in psychiatry** *185*
P. M. Grasby

2.3.7 **Structural magnetic resonance imaging** *191*
J. Suckling and E. T. Bullmore

2.3.8 **Functional magnetic resonance imaging** *196*
E. T. Bullmore and J. Suckling

2.3.9 **Neuronal networks, epilepsy, and other brain dysfunctions** *201*
John G. R. Jefferys

2.3.10 **Psychoneuroimmunology** *205*
Robert Dantzer and Keith W. Kelley

2.4 **The contribution of genetics** *212*

2.4.1 **Quantitative genetics** *212*
Anita Thapar and Peter McGuffin

2.4.2 **Molecular genetics** *222*
Jonathan Flint

2.5 **The contribution of psychological science** *234*

2.5.1 Development psychology through infancy, childhood, and adolescence *234*
William Yule and Matt Woolgar

2.5.2 **Psychology of attention** *245*
Elizabeth Coulthard and Masud Husain

2.5.3 **Psychology and biology of memory** *249*
Andreas Meyer-Lindenberg and Terry E. Goldberg

2.5.4 **The anatomy of human emotion** *257*
R. J. Dolan

2.5.5 **Neuropsychological basis of neuropsychiatry** *262*
L. Clark, B. J. Sahakian, and T. W. Robbins

2.6 **The contribution of social sciences** *268*

2.6.1 **Medical sociology and issues of aetiology** *268*
George W. Brown

2.6.2 **Social and cultural anthropology: salience for psychiatry** *275*
Arthur Kleinman

2.7 **The contribution of epidemiology to psychiatric aetiology** *280*
Scott Henderson

2.1

Brain and mind

Martin Davies

History of the mind–brain relation

The thesis that the brain, rather than the heart, is the seat of the mind was already widely accepted by the ancient Greeks; but it was not universally accepted—Aristotle was an exception. Many issues in psychiatry resonate with the ancient debates over the roles of the heart and the brain. But a brief review of modern thinking about the mind–brain relation can begin two millennia later with René Descartes, who held that minds are real things of a fundamentally different kind from material bodies.[(1)]

Dualism: Descartes

Descartes's world-view included bodies or material things, whose essence is to be extended in space, and minds, which are immaterial things whose essence is thinking. According to **Cartesian dualism**, the mind is not literally housed within the body, because spatial properties belong to matter and not to mind. But, when he talked about the way we experience the states of our own body, Descartes sometimes spoke of the mind being 'mixed up with' the body.

Early theories of the brain as the seat of the mind assigned an important role to the ventricles. On Descartes's view, mechanical operations involving the release of animal spirits in the ventricles were adequate to explain animal behaviour but intelligent human action required something more. He postulated that the immaterial mind could modulate processes in the material brain by way of a causal interaction operating through the pineal gland.

The motion of bodies and the completeness of physics

Dualist interactionism is challenged by theories about the motion of bodies. According to Descartes's own theory, quantity of motion (defined as mass times speed) is conserved. Because motion is not a directional notion, this conservation law allowed that the immaterial mind could bend the trajectory of a physical particle in the pineal gland. But Gottfried Leibniz's superior theory, with conservation laws for momentum (a directional notion) and kinetic energy, had the consequence that only impacts with other bodies could cause changes in the direction or speed of physical particles. This left no room for immaterial causes of material changes and, while Leibniz was a dualist, he was not an interactionist dualist but believed, instead, in a **pre-established harmony** between the material and immaterial worlds.

By departing from the idea that impact was the only force on bodies, and allowing action at a distance, Isaac Newton reopened the possibility of distinctively mental forces affecting the trajectory of bodies. These forces were not even ruled out by the law of conservation of energy, which was widely accepted by the middle of the nineteenth century, but advances in biochemistry and neurophysiology during the first half of the twentieth century made appeal to vital and mental forces seem increasingly unmotivated. Since around 1950, the dominant theories of the mind–brain relation have been compatible with a broadly physicalist world-view and with the completeness of physics: physical effects have wholly physical causes.[(2)]

Behaviourism: Ryle

From the 1920s to the 1950s, particularly in the United States, behaviourism was a dominant approach within psychology. This was not just methodological behaviourism, which is a restriction on the kinds of evidence that can be used, but a radical reconception of psychology as the science of behaviour rather than the science of the mind. In philosophy, **analytical behaviourism** was a doctrine about the meaning of our mental discourse. The idea was to analyse or translate our mental talk into talk about patterns of behaviour.

Gilbert Ryle promoted behaviourism as a response to what he called 'Descartes's myth' of 'the ghost in the machine'.[(3)] A dualist would regard talk about being in love, or wanting to visit Paris, as talk about an immaterial mind whose states lie hidden behind observable bodily behaviour. Ryle proposed to analyse this mental talk as being about the observable behaviour itself. He did not, however, aim to replace all mental terms by terms appropriate to the science of material bodies moving through space. He analysed believing that the ice is thin as, in part, being 'prone to skate warily' and it was enough, for his purposes, that skating warily is an observable and recognizable kind of behaviour, even if it is not readily defined in terms of the trajectories of body parts.

Because action is explained in terms of what the agent believes and what the agent wants, analytical behaviourism faces a major objection of principle. There is no pattern of behaviour associated with a belief, by itself. Someone who believes that the ice is thin but has an unusual desire to be immersed in ice-cold water may not skate warily. So there is no prospect of analysing any belief in terms of behaviour. We might elevate this point into a general requirement on the description of any creature as having beliefs. Attributions of beliefs are not warranted if they merely summarize the creature's dispositions to exhibit patterns of behaviour. A belief is a mental state that can figure in the explanation of indefinitely many different actions in pursuit of different goals.

The identity theory: Place and Smart

Ryle's behaviourism involved a clear rejection of Descartes's duality of material and immaterial substances, but **central state materialism** (also known as the **identity theory**) encapsulated a more thoroughgoing commitment to the physicalist world-view. If the physical effects of our experiences, thoughts, and volitions have wholly physical causes then there is no causal work left for distinct mental items to do. To avoid epiphenomenalism, mental states, processes and events were to be identified with physical states, processes and events, and mental properties with physical properties. Place advanced a precursor of the identity theory, restricted to the case of conscious experiences,[(4)] and this was generalized by Smart, who identified beliefs and desires, intentions and hopes, as well as sensations and experiences, with brain states or processes.[(5)]

The identity theory defends the idea of **mental causation** by identifying each mental state with a physical state that is a locus of causal powers. But, taken literally, the identity theory is bound to seem chauvinistic. No being with a physical constitution radically different from ours could be described as feeling anything, or thinking anything, or wanting anything.

Functionalism: Putnam and Lewis

The functionalist response to the identity theory is that what a system does is more important than what it is made from. Physically different computing machines can run the same software and one version of the functionalist theory of the mind–brain relation is that the mind is the software of the brain.[(6)]

In an early version of **functionalism**, Hilary Putnam proposed that mental states are functional states like the states of an abstractly defined Turing machine rather than physical states like the states of a human brain.[(7)] This **machine functionalism** had the advantage of not tying mental states to a particular physical substrate but also a disadvantage. Since a Turing machine is in only one state at a time, machine states are not analogous to mental states like being in love or wanting to visit Paris.

The dominant version of contemporary functionalism, attributable to David Lewis, is **analytical functionalism**.[(8)] The leading idea is that commonsense specifications of the interconnected causal roles of mental states can be taken as interlocking analyses of mental state terms. For any physical being with a mind, there will be physical states playing each of the mental state causal roles but different physical states may play the same causal role in physically different minded beings—in human beings and Martians, for example.

Functionalism thus avoids the apparent chauvinism of the identity theory by allowing that a human being may be in the same mental state as a being with a very different physical constitution. But functionalism faces the opposite problem of apparently being too liberal. It seems to be possible to make up examples in which physical states play the causal roles that are supposed to define mental states, yet where, intuitively, there is no intelligence and no mental life.[(9)]

Challenges to functionalism

The dominant contemporary theories of the mind–brain relation are compatible with a broadly physicalist world-view and analytical functionalism, in particular, is consistent with a version of physicalism, **a priori physicalism**, that is both ontologically and conceptually **reductionist**.[(10)]

Ontologically, analytical functionalism is like the identity theory in its commitment to types of physical state that *realize* mental states. Functionalism does not quite say that being in pain is to be identified with having C-fibres firing (the standard example for the identity theory); but it does say that the causal role of the mental state of being in pain is played, in human beings, by the physical state of having C-fibres firing.

Despite this ontological similarity to the identity theory, analytical functionalism is *conceptually* more like analytical behaviourism in being a thesis about the meanings of our mental terms. According to behaviourism, it is a matter of meaning, or **conceptual analysis**, that being in a mental state is being disposed to produce particular patterns of behaviour. According to functionalism, it is equally a matter of meaning that being in a mental state is being in a state that plays a particular causal role. Consequently, analytical functionalism is *conceptually reductionist*. The mental facts, as conceived by the functionalist, are *entailed a priori* by the physical facts.

As we shall now see, both the ontological and the conceptual commitments of analytical functionalism face challenges.

Rylean behaviourism revisited

A theorist of the mind–brain relation who was sympathetic to Rylean behaviourism might challenge the *ontological* commitments that are shared by functionalism and the identity theory. The neo-behaviourist might accept the idea that if a system has a disposition to exhibit a particular pattern of behaviour then there must be a basis for this disposition in the system's inner constitution. But he might argue that identifying individual mental states with physical states, or insisting that mental states are individually realized by physical states, goes beyond what is required by this idea.

Dispositions do not float free of inner constitution and the behavioural dispositions of human beings are, presumably, underpinned by states and processes of the brain. But it is not obviously required that there must be a single brain state that underpins precisely the dispositions that are associated with the attribution of a single mental state. This neo-behaviourism may draw support from remarks made by Wittgenstein.[(11)]

Neo-behaviourism will be open to objection so long as it retains the unattainable commitment to an analysis of belief attributions in behavioural terms. But there is an alternative view that abandons those analytical ambitions. The **interpretationist** says that mentalistic interpretation is answerable to a creature's behaviour in various actual and hypothetical circumstances, but that this answerability is a matter of 'making sense' of the creature and cannot be codified mental state by mental state.[(12)] Rather, the interpreter casts a net of psychological description—'X is in pain; X is in love; X wants to visit Paris; X believes that the ice is thin; ...'—over a writhing mass of behaviour. Tracts of human behaviour normally support this interpretive project and, presumably, the behaviour is susceptible of causal explanation. But we should not assume that the physical causes of behaviour must have an articulation that matches the structure of the interpreter's description.[(13)]

Interpretationism is compatible with a broadly physicalist worldview but it involves some departure from apparently plausible claims about mental reality and mental causation. The interpretationist is not committed to the claim that there are individual mental states—for example, individual beliefs such as my belief that there is a bottle of white wine in the refrigerator, or that I have an appointment at 9 a.m.—that are bearers of causal powers.

Consciousness and the explanatory gap

The *conceptual* commitments of analytical functionalism are challenged by our conception of **conscious mental states**.

According to functionalism, all mental states are realized by physical, specifically neural, states and the phenomenal properties of conscious mental states are physical properties of those neural states. We can ask what makes the difference between conscious mental states and unconscious mental states. Is there, for example, something distinctive about the neural underpinnings of conscious mental states? If we had a plausible answer to that question, there would be the further question *why* mental states with that distinctive neural nature are *conscious* mental states. This question is apt to seem puzzling and even unanswerable. But, according to analytical functionalism, there would be no puzzling 'why?' question about consciousness. All the mental facts, including the facts about consciousness and phenomenology, are entailed a priori by the physical facts.

A powerful intuition thus speaks against the conceptual commitments of analytical functionalism. For it seems that even the full physical story about the world would not settle a priori the question whether a creature was in a conscious mental state. It seems to be conceivable (not ruled out a priori) that there could be a creature physically just like one of us yet lacking consciousness—a *zombie*—or even a complete physical duplicate of our world from which consciousness was totally absent—a *zombie world*.(14) Between the physical sciences and the facts of consciousness there seems to be an **explanatory gap**.(15)

Thomas Nagel has drawn attention to a difference between two kinds of conception. Conceptions of conscious mental states are **subjective**; they are accessible from some, but not all, points of view. The conscious mental states that we can *conceive* are limited to relatively modest imaginative extensions from the conscious mental states that we ourselves *undergo*. In contrast, the conceptions deployed in grasping theories in the physical sciences are **objective**; they are accessible from many different points of view. The physical theories that we can grasp are limited, not by our sensory experience, but by our intellectual powers.(16) Many contemporary philosophers of consciousness argue that the explanatory gap is a product of this duality of conceptions. There is no a priori entailment from the physical and functional facts *objectively conceived* to the phenomenal facts *subjectively conceived*.

The majority of these philosophers maintain that a duality of conceptions does not require an ontological dualism of substances, states, or properties and that the explanatory gap is consistent with physicalism as an ontological doctrine. But there is an important minority view that acceptance of an explanatory gap must lead to a rejection of physicalism. David Chalmers, beginning from the intuition of an explanatory gap, recommends a return to some form of dualism.(17) Others argue in the opposite direction, embracing physicalism, denying that there is an explanatory gap, and accepting the counterintuitive conceptual reductionism of analytical functionalism.

Personal and subpersonal levels of description and explanation

The mind–brain relation is an aspect of a more encompassing relationship between persons and the physical systems of which they are constituted, including systems of neural information processing.

Our conception of persons as such is a conception of subjects and agents. At the personal level of description and explanation, we describe what people feel, think, want and do, and we explain what people do in terms of their sensations, beliefs, and desires. As the case of conscious mental states illustrates, our personal-level *descriptions* are not always entailed a priori by physical and functional descriptions of the systems that constitute us. Personal-level descriptions involve subjective and normative concepts that are different from the objective and descriptive concepts that figure in the physical sciences.

Our personal-level *explanatory practices* seem to be different in kind from our scientific practices of explaining the operation of mechanical systems. McDowell describes personal-level explanations as 'explanations in which things are made intelligible by being revealed to be, or to approximate to being, as they rationally ought to be'.(18) In a similar spirit, Dennett describes them as 'non-mechanistic'. A mechanistic account of what happens when a person feels, thinks, wants, and acts would belong at a quite different level of description and explanation, not the 'level of people and their sensations and activities', but 'the *subpersonal* level of brains and events in the nervous system'.(19)

One extreme view of the relationship between the personal and subpersonal levels highlights what is distinctive about the personal level and regards it as substantially independent from the subpersonal level. This view might encourage the interpretationist account of personal-level psychological descriptions, minimizing the ontological and causal commitments of personal-level discourse to avoid constraints on that discourse from the subpersonal level of neuroscience.

The opposite extreme view is the conceptually reductionist view of analytical functionalism. The personal level is the level of mental states whose causal roles are revealed by conceptual analysis while the subpersonal level is the level of neural states that play those roles. There are no explanatory gaps. All that is true at the personal level is entailed a priori by physical truths at the subpersonal level.

According to an attractive view that is intermediate between these two extremes, the relationship between the personal and subpersonal levels is one of *interaction without reduction*.(20) As against the first extreme view, the personal level is not independent of the subpersonal level but constrained by it, because our personal-level descriptions—cast in terms of experience, thought, planning, and agency—carry commitments about causal structure in the brain. But, as against the second extreme view, there are also explanatory gaps that reveal themselves when we try to construct illuminating accounts of those personal-level notions using only the subpersonal-level resources of neuroscience.

Conclusion

Descartes's ontological dualism of mind and body made it difficult for him to describe the phenomenology of embodiment, the way we experience our own body. Contemporary theories of the mind–brain relation are predominantly physicalist, rather than dualist, in their ontology. But the duality of objective and subjective conceptions still presents a challenge for the sciences of the mind. Persons understood as such, partly from the first-person perspective—persons conceived as subjects and agents, with their experiences, thoughts, plans and actions—will not be visible in a purely objective, scientific story of the physical world.

Further information

Anthology

Chalmers, D.J. (ed.) (2002). *Philosophy of mind: classical and contemporary readings*. Oxford University Press, Oxford.

Textbook

Braddon-Mitchell, D. and Jackson, F.C. (2007). *Philosophy of mind and cognition: an introduction* (2nd edn). Blackwell Publishing, Oxford.

References

1. Descartes, R. (1641). *Meditations on first philosophy* In Descartes, R. (1988). *Selected philosophical writings* (trans. eds. J. Cottingham, R. Stoothoff, and D. Murdoch). Cambridge University Press, Cambridge, UK.
2. Papineau, D. (2002). *Thinking about consciousness*, Appendix. Oxford University Press, Oxford.
3. Ryle, G. (1949). Descartes' myth. In *The concept of mind*, Chap. 1. Penguin Books, Harmondsworth.
4. Place, U.T. (1956). Is consciousness a brain process? *The British Journal of Psychology*, **47**, 44–50.
5. Smart, J.C.C. (1959). Sensations and brain processes. *Philosophical Review*, **68**, 141–56.
6. Block, N. (1995). The mind as the software of the brain. In *An invitation to cognitive science* (2nd edn), Vol. 3 (eds. E.E. Smith and D.N. Osherson), pp. 377–425. MIT Press, Cambridge, MA.
7. Putnam, H. (1967). The nature of mental states. Originally titled 'Psychological predicates'. In *Art, mind, and religion* (eds. W.H. Capitan and D.D. Merrill), pp. 37–48. University of Pittsburgh Press, Pittsburgh, PA.
8. Lewis, D. (1972). Psychophysical and theoretical identifications. *Australasian Journal of Philosophy*, **50**, 249–58.
9. Block, N. (1978). Troubles with functionalism. In *Minnesota studies in the philosophy of science*, Vol. 9 (ed. C. Wade Savage), pp. 261–325. University of Minnesota Press, Minneapolis, MN.
10. Jackson, F.C. (2005). The case for a priori physicalism. In *Philosophy—science—scientific philosophy: main lectures and colloquia of GAP.5* (eds. C. Nimtz and A. Beckermann), pp. 251–65. Fifth International Congress of the Society for Analytical Philosophy, Bielefeld, 22–26 September 2003. Mentis, Paderborn.
11. Wittgenstein, L. (1981). *Zettel*, (eds. G.E.M. Anscombe and G.H. von Wright, trans. G.E.M. Anscombe), Sections 608–9. Basil Blackwell, Oxford.
12. Davidson, D. (1973). Radical interpretation. *Dialectica*, **27**, 313–28. Reprinted in Davidson, D. (1984). *Inquiries into truth and interpretation*, pp. 125–39. Oxford University Press, Oxford.
13. Dennett, D.C. (1987). True believers: the intentional strategy and why it works. In *The intentional stance*, pp. 13–35. MIT Press, Cambridge, MA.
14. Chalmers, D.J. (1996). *The conscious mind: in search of a fundamental theory.* Oxford University Press, Oxford.
15. Levine, J. (1983). Materialism and qualia: the explanatory gap. *Pacific Philosophical Quarterly*, **64**, 354–61.
16. Nagel, T. (1974). What is it like to be a bat? *Philosophical Review*, **83**, 435–50. Reprinted in Nagel, T. (1979). *Mortal questions*, pp. 165–80. Cambridge University Press, Cambridge, UK.
17. Chalmers, D.J. (2007). Naturalistic dualism. In *The Blackwell companion to consciousness* (eds. M. Velmans and S. Schneider), pp. 359–68. Blackwell Publishing, Oxford.
18. McDowell, J. (1985). Functionalism and anomalous monism. In *Actions and events: perspectives on the philosophy of Donald Davidson* (eds. E. LePore and B.P. McLaughlin), pp. 387–98. Basil Blackwell, Oxford.
19. Dennett, D.C. (1969). *Content and consciousness*, pp. 91–4. Routledge and Kegan Paul, London.
20. Davies, M. (2000). Interaction without reduction: the relationship between personal and sub-personal levels of description. *Mind and Society*, **1**, 87–105.

2.2

Statistics and the design of experiments and surveys

Graham Dunn

Introduction

Research into mental illness uses a much wider variety of statistical methods than those familiar to a typical medical statistician. In many ways there is more similarity to the statistical toolbox of the sociologist or educationalist. It would be a pointless exercise to try to describe this variety here but, instead, we shall cover a few areas that are especially characteristic of psychiatry. The first and perhaps the most obvious is the problem of measurement. Measurement reliability and its estimation are discussed in the next section. Misclassification errors are a concern of the third section, a major part of which is concerned with the estimation of prevalence through the use of fallible screening questionnaires. This is followed by a discussion of both measurement error and misclassification error in the context of modelling patterns of risk.

Another major concern is the presence of missing data. Although this is common to all areas of medical research, it is of particular interest to the psychiatric epidemiologist because there is a long tradition (since the early 1970s) of introducing missing data by design. Here we are thinking of two-phase or double sampling (often confusingly called two-stage sampling by psychiatrists and other clinical research workers). In this design a first-phase sample are all given a screen questionnaire. They are then stratified on the basis of the results of the screen (usually, but not necessarily, using two strata—likely cases and likely non-cases) and subsampled for a second-phase diagnostic interview. This is the major topic of the third section.

If we are interested in modelling patterns of risk, however, we are not usually merely interested in describing patterns of association. Typically we want to know if genetic or environmental exposures have a causal effect on the development of illness. Similarly, a clinician is concerned with answers to the question 'What is the causal effect of treatment on outcome?' How do we define a causal effect? How do we measure or estimate it? How do we design studies in order that we can get a valid estimate of a causal effect of treatment? Here we are concerned with the design and analysis of randomized controlled trials (RCTs). This is the focus of the fourth section of the present chapter.

Finally, at the end of this chapter pointers are given to where the interested reader might find other relevant and useful material on psychiatric statistics.

Reliability of instruments

In this section we consider two questions:

- What is meant by 'reliability'?
- How do we estimate reliabilities?

Models and definitions

Most clinicians have an intuitive idea of what the concept of reliability means, and that being able to demonstrate that one's measuring instruments have high reliability is a good thing. Reliability concerns the consistency of repeated measurements, where the repetitions might be repeated interviews by the same interviewer, alternative ratings of the same interview (as a video recording) by different raters, alternative forms or repeated administration of a questionnaire, or even different subscales of a single questionnaire, and so on. One learns from elementary texts that reliability is estimated by a correlation coefficient (in the case of a quantitative rating) or a kappa (κ) or weighted κ statistic (in the case of a qualitative judgement such as a diagnosis). Rarely are clinicians aware of either the formal definition of reliability or of its estimation through the use of various forms of intraclass correlation coefficient rho (ρ).

First consider a quantitative measurement X. We start with the assumption that it is fallible and that it is the sum of two components: the 'truth' T and 'error' E. If T and E are statistically independent (uncorrelated), then it can be shown that

$$\text{Var}(X) = \text{Var}(T) + \text{Var}(E) \tag{2.2.1}$$

where Var(X) is the variance of X (i.e. the square of its standard deviation), and so on. The reliability ρ_x of X is defined as the proportion of the total variability of X (i.e. Var(X)) that is explained by the variability of the true scores (i.e. Var(T)):

$$\rho_x = \frac{\text{Var}(T)}{\text{Var}(X)} = \frac{\text{Var}(T)}{\text{Var}(T) + \text{Var}(E)} \tag{2.2.2}$$

This ratio will approach zero as the variability of the measurement errors increases compared with that of the truth. Alternatively, it will approach one as the variability of the errors decreases. The standard deviation of the measurement errors (i.e. the square root of Var(E)) is usually known as the instrument's standard error of measurement. Note that reliability is not a fixed characteristic of an instrument, even when its standard error of measurement (i.e. its precision) is fixed. When the instrument is used on a population that is relatively homogeneous (low values of Var(T)), it will have a relatively low reliability. However, as Var(T) increases then so does the instrument's reliability. In many ways the standard error of measurement is a much more useful summary of an instrument's performance, but one should always bear in mind that it too might vary from one population to another—a possibility that must be carefully checked by both the developers and users of the instrument.

Now let us complicate matters slightly. Suppose that a rating depends not only on the subject's so-called true score T and random measurement error E, but also on the identity R, say, of the interviewer or rater R. That is, each rater has his or her own characteristic bias (constant from assessment to another) and the biases can be thought of as varying randomly from one rater to another. Again, assuming statistical independence, we can show that, if $X = T + R + E$, then

$$\mathrm{Var}(X) = \mathrm{Var}(T) + \mathrm{Var}(R) + \mathrm{Var}(E) \qquad (2.2.3)$$

But what is the instrument's reliability? It depends. If subjects in a survey or experiment, for example, are each going to be assessed by a rater randomly selected from a large pool of possible raters, then

$$\rho_{xa} = \frac{\mathrm{Var}(T)}{\mathrm{Var}(X)} = \frac{\mathrm{Var}(T)}{\mathrm{Var}(T) + \mathrm{Var}(R) + \mathrm{Var}(E)} \qquad (2.2.4)$$

However, if only a single rater is to be used for all subjects in the proposed study, there will be no variation due to the rater and the reliability now becomes

$$\rho_{xb} = \frac{\mathrm{Var}(T)}{\mathrm{Var}(T) + \mathrm{Var}(E)} \qquad (2.2.5)$$

Of course, $\rho_{xb} > \rho_{xa}$. Again, the value of the instrument's reliability depends on the context of its use. This is the essence of generalizability theory.(1) The three versions of ρ given above are all intraclass correlation coefficients and are also examples of what generalizability theorists refer to as generalizability coefficients.

Designs

Now consider two simple designs for reliability (generalizability) studies. The first involves each subject of the study being independently assessed by two (or more) raters but that the raters for any given subject have been randomly selected from a very large pool of potential raters. The second design again involves each subject of the study being independently assessed by two (or more) raters, but in this case the raters are the same for all subjects. Equations (2.2.1) and (2.2.2) are relevant to the analysis of data arising from the first design, whilst eqns (2.2.3–2.2.5) are relevant to the analysis of data from the second design.

Estimation of ρ and κ from ANOVA tables

When we come to analyse the data it is usually appropriate to carry out an analysis of variance (ANOVA). For the first design we carry out a one-way ANOVA (X by subject) and for the second we perform a two-way ANOVA (X by rater and subject). In the latter case we assume that there is no subject by rater interaction and accordingly constrain the corresponding sum of squares to be zero. We assume that readers are reasonably familiar with an analysis of variance table. Each subject has been assessed by, say, k raters. The one-way ANOVA yields a mean square for between-subjects variation (**BMS**) and a mean square for within-subjects variation (**WMS**). WMS is an estimate of Var(E) in eqn. (2.2.1). Therefore, the square root of WMS provides an estimate of the instrument's standard error of measurement. The corresponding estimate of ρ_x is given by

$$r_x = \frac{\mathrm{BMS} - \mathrm{WMS}}{\mathrm{BMS} + (k-1)\mathrm{WMS}} \qquad (2.2.6)$$

where r_x is used to represent the estimate of ρ_x rather than the true, but unknown, value. In the case of $k = 2$, r_x becomes

$$r_x = \frac{\mathrm{BMS} - \mathrm{WMS}}{\mathrm{BMS} + \mathrm{WMS}} \qquad (2.2.7)$$

In the slightly more complex two-way ANOVA, the ANOVA table provides values of mean squares for subjects or patients (**PMS**), raters (**RMS**), and error (**EMS**). We shall not concentrate on the details of estimation of the components of eqn. (2.2.3) (see Fleiss(2) or Streiner and Norman(3)) but simply note that ρ_{xa} is estimated by

$$r_{xa} = \frac{n(\mathrm{PMS} - \mathrm{EMS})}{n \times \mathrm{PMS} + k \times \mathrm{RMS} + (nk - n - k)\mathrm{EMS}} \qquad (2.2.8)$$

where n is the number of subjects (patients) in the study.

In reporting the results of a reliability study, it is important that investigators give some idea of the precision of their estimates of reliability, for example by giving an appropriate standard error or, even better, an appropriate confidence interval. The subject is beyond the scope of this chapter, however, and the interested reader is referred to Fleiss(2) or Dunn(4) for further illumination.

Finally, what about qualitative measures? We shall not discuss the estimation and interpretation of κ in any detail here but simply point out that for a binary (yes/no) measure one can also carry out a two-way analysis of variance (but ignore any significance tests since they are not valid for binary data) and estimate r_{xa} as above. In large samples r_{xa} is equivalent to κ.(3) A corollary of this is that κ is another form of reliability coefficient and, like any of the reliability coefficients described above, will vary from one population to another (i.e. it is dependent on the prevalence of the symptom or characteristic being assessed).

Prevalence estimation

Following Dunn and Everitt,(5) we ask the following questions of a survey report.

- Do the authors clearly define the sampled population?
- Do the authors discuss similarities and possible differences between their sampled population and the stated target population?
- Do the authors report what sampling mechanism has been used?
- Is the sampling mechanism random? If not, why not?
- Exactly what sort of random sampling mechanism has been used?
- Do the methods of data analysis make allowances for the sampling mechanism used?

Of course, it is vital that what counts as a case should be explained in absolute detail, including the method of eliciting symptoms (e.g. structured interview schedule), screening items, additional impairment criteria, and so on, as well as operational criteria or algorithms used in making a diagnosis. In the following we concentrate on the statistical issues. First, we consider survey design (and the associated sampling mechanisms), and then we move on to discuss the implications of design for the subsequent analysis of the results.

Survey design

Here we are concerned with the estimation of a simple proportion (or percentage). We calculate this proportion using data from the sample and use it to infer the corresponding proportion in the underlying population. One vital component of this process is to ensure that the sampled population from which we have drawn our subjects is as close as possible to that of the target population about which we want to draw conclusions. We also require the sample to be drawn from the sample population in an objective and unbiased way. The best way of achieving this is through some sort of random sampling mechanism. Random sampling implies that whether or not a subject finishes up in the sample is determined by chance. Shuffling and dealing a hand of playing cards is an example of a random selection process called simple random sampling. Here every possible hand of, say, five cards has the same probability of occurring as any other. If we can list all possible samples of a fixed size, then simple random sampling implies that they all have the same probability of finishing up in our survey. It also implies that each possible subject has the same probability of being selected. But note that the latter condition is not sufficient to define a simple random sample. In a systematic random sample, for example, we have a list of possible people to select (the sampling frame) and we simply select one of the first 10 (say) subjects at random and then systematically select every tenth subject from then on. All subjects have the same probability of selection, but there are many samples which are impossible to draw using this mechanism. For example, we can select either subject 2 or subject 3 with the same probability (1/10), but it is impossible to draw a sample which contains both.

What other forms of random sampling mechanisms might be used? Perhaps the most common is a stratified random sample. Here we divide our sampled population into mutually exclusive groups or strata (e.g. men and women, or five separate age groups). Having chosen the strata, we proceed, for example, to take a separate simple random sample from each. The proportion of subjects sampled from each of the strata (i.e. the sampling fraction) might be constant across all strata (ensuring that the overall sample has the same composition as the original population), or we might decide that one or more strata (e.g. the elderly) might have a higher representation. Another commonly used sampling mechanism is multistage cluster sampling. For example, in a national prevalence survey we might chose first to sample health regions or districts, then to sample post codes within the districts, and finally to select patients randomly from each selected post code. (See Kessler[6] and Jenkins *et al.*[7] for discussions of complex multistage surveys of psychiatric morbidity.)

One particular design that has been used quite often in surveys designed to estimate the prevalence of psychiatric disorders is called two-phase or double sampling. Psychiatrists frequently refer to this as two-stage sampling. This is unfortunate, since it confuses the two-phase design with simple forms of cluster sampling in which the first-stage involves drawing a random sample of clusters and the second-stage a random sample of subjects from within each of the clusters. In two-phase sampling, however, we first draw a preliminary sample (which may be simple, stratified, and/or clustered) and then administer a first-phase screening questionnaire such as the General Health Questionnaire (see Chapter 1.8.1). On the basis of the screen results we then stratify the first-phase sample. Note that we are not restricted to two strata (likely cases versus the rest), although this is perhaps the most common form of the design. We then draw a second-phase sample from each of the first-phase strata and proceed to give these subjects a definitive psychiatric assessment. The point of this design is that we do not waste expensive resources interviewing large numbers of subjects who not appear (on the basis of the first-phase screen) to have any problems. Accordingly, the sampling fractions usually differ across the first-phase strata. However, it is vital that each of the first-phase strata have a reasonable representation in the second-phase, and it is particularly important that all of the first-phase strata provide some second-phase subjects. The reader is referred to Pickles and Dunn[8] for further discussion of design issues in two-phase sampling (including discussion of whether it is worth the bother).

Analysis of the results

Here we are particularly concerned with the last of the questions posed at the beginning of the section. In fact, it is a question that should be asked not only of prevalence surveys but of all investigations whether they are epidemiological surveys, intervention studies, or laboratory experiments. How was the design incorporated in the analysis? Frequently the required information is missing. Either the authors are ignorant of the implications of the design, or the journal editor has insisted that technical details are stripped from the report, or both.

Consider a hypothetical sample of 100 participants who have contributed to an estimate of prevalence of, say, depression using a definitive psychiatric interview.

Seventy of the participants have been given a diagnosis of depression. What is a valid estimate of prevalence? What is the standard error of the estimate? Assuming that the data have arisen through simple random sampling, the prevalence p is estimated by 0.70 and its variance is given by

$$\mathrm{Var}(p) = \frac{1}{np(1-p)} \qquad (2.2.9)$$

where n is the sample size. The standard error is then given by the square root of this expression.

Suppose that we are now told that the results were obtained from a two-phase survey. The size of the first-phase sample was 300. Of these, 100 were screen positive and 200 were screen negative. The second-phase sample consisted of 70 screen positives, of whom 65 were found to be depressed on interview, together with 30 screen negatives, of whom 5 were found to be depressed on interview. The estimate of prevalence is given by

$$\begin{aligned} p &= P(\text{screen +ve}) \times P(\text{interview +ve}|\text{screen +ve}) + P(\text{screen} - \text{ve}) \\ &\quad \times P(\text{interview +ve}|\text{screen}-\text{ve}) \\ &= (100/300) \times (65/70) + (200/300) \times (5/30) \\ &= 0.42 \qquad (2.2.10) \end{aligned}$$

where $P(A)$ should be read as 'probability of A' and $P(A|B)$ should be read as 'probability of A given B' or 'probability of A conditional on B having occurred'. The vertical '|' should not be confused with division, represented by '/'.

The prevalence estimate from the two-phase survey is considerably lower than if simple random sampling had been assumed. How has this arisen? Obviously the second-phase sample has been enriched for people who are likely to be depressed. The sampling fraction for the screen positives is 70/100, that is each second-phase participant can be thought of as representing 100/70 of screen positives from the original sample. Similarly, the sampling fraction for the screen negatives is 30/200, and each second-phase participant represents 200/30 screen-negative participants from the first-phase sample. The reciprocal of the sampling fraction is called the sampling weight. The total weighted second-phase sample size is $70 \times (100/70) + 30 \times (200/30) = 300$, the first-phase sample. Similarly, the total weighted number of cases of depression is $65 \times (100/70) + 5 \times (200/30) \approx 126$. The latter is the estimate of the number of cases in the first-phase sample. Hence the estimate of prevalence is $126/300 = 0.42$, as before. To recapitulate in a slightly more technical way, if the ith individual in the second-phase sample is assigned a sampling weight w_i, and if the interview outcome y_i has a value of 1 if the ith subject is a case and is 0 otherwise, then the weighted prevalence estimate is given by

$$p = \Sigma w_i y_i / \Sigma w_i \qquad (2.2.11)$$

where Σ means 'sum over all observations in the second-phase sample' and x_i is simply an indicator that the observation is, indeed, a second-phase observation ($x_i = 1$ for everyone). This estimator is an example of the well-known Horwitz–Thompson estimator from the sampling survey literature[9] but it is not particular familiar to psychiatrists or medical statisticians. We shall discuss the use of weighting adjustments again below.

Returning to our original two-phase calculations, let $A = P$(screen +ve) and $B = 1–A = P$(screen –ve). Also, let $p = P$(interview +ve|screen +ve) and $q = P$(interview +ve|screen –ve), so that eqn. (2.2.10) becomes

$$p = Ap + Bq \qquad (2.2.12)$$

The variance of the estimate of prevalence from the two-phase design is given by[10]

$$\mathrm{Var}(p) = \frac{A^2 p(1-p)}{n_1} + \frac{B^2 q(1-q)}{n_2} + \frac{(p-q)^2 AB}{n_3} \qquad (2.2.13)$$

where n_1 is the number of first-phase screen positives and n_2 is the number of first-phase screen negatives (and $n = n_1 + n_2$ is the total (first phase) sample size).

Validation of screening questionnaires

It is frequently the case that data from a two-phase survey which has been designed to estimate prevalence are also used to examine the characteristics of the screen questionnaire (in particular, sensitivity and specificity). Readers who are unfamiliar with these concepts are referred to Chapter 2.7 or to Goldberg and Williams.[11] Sensitivity is the proportion of true cases who are screen positive. Specificity is the proportion of true non-cases who are screen negative. The trouble is caused because we used the screen first and then differentially subsampled to carry out the definitive diagnostic interview. Readers familiar with the use of Bayes' theorem will realize how to solve the problem, but here we use another version of the Horwitz–Thompson estimator:

$$\text{Sensitivity} = \Sigma w_i y_i z_i / w_i y_i \qquad (2.2.14)$$

and

$$1\text{–specificity} = \Sigma w_i (1-y_i) z_i / \Sigma w_i (1-y_i) \qquad (2.2.15)$$

where, as before, y_i indicates whether the ith subject was a true case of depression (1 = yes, 0 = no). This ensures that the calculations in eqn (2.2.14) are only being carried out on the true cases and, similarly, that the calculations in (2.2.15) are only being carried out on the non-cases. Again, w_i is the second-phase sampling weight. The new variable z_i indicates whether the screen result was positive (1 = yes, 0 = no). An alternative, and perhaps easier, approach is to split the second-phase sample into two: cases and non-cases. Estimation of sensitivity and specificity in these two subfiles (assuming that they are being stored on a computer) is then computationally exactly the same as the weighted estimation of prevalence discussed in the previous section. In the first file, sensitivity is simply the weighted sum of the screen positives divided by the weighted sum of the cases. Similarly, in the second file, specificity is the weighted sum of the screen negatives divided by the weighted sum of the non-cases.

Many readers will be familiar with the idea of choosing a range of cut-points for the screen questionnaire and then estimating sensitivity and specificity at each of the choices. A plot of sensitivity against 1—specificity is called a receiver operating characteristic (**ROC**) curve. If the screen is of no use, then the plot will be a straight line through the origin with unit slope. A good screen will produce a convex curve (the greater the area between the observed curve and that indicated by a straight line with unit slope, the better the screen is at discriminating between cases and non-cases). It is sometimes said that one cannot investigate ROC curves using two-phase data. This view is, in fact, mistaken. One can think of the two-phase sampling design as a mechanism by which one can deliberately introduce the analogues of verification bias.[12] Note that there is no necessity to restrict the first-phase stratification to just two strata (potential cases versus non-cases) to define the sampling fractions for the second-phase of the survey. We start by calculating observed sampling fractions for each discrete outcome of the screening questionnaire. These define the corresponding sampling weights. We then consider all the possibilities for defining z_i in eqns (2.2.14) and (2.2.15)—there is no need for the z_i to correspond to the way that the second-phase sampling fractions were determined. We then repeatedly use eqns (2.2.14) and (2.2.15), keeping the weights constant as we change the definition of the z_i. One important point to bear in mind is that if the characteristics of the screen are not fairly well known beforehand and if one of the major aims of the survey is to carry out an ROC analysis, then this is not a particularly efficient design to use. It would be better to go back to the simple random sample—all subjects assessed by both screen and interview.

If one needs, say, confidence intervals for estimates of sensitivity and specificity, it is relatively straightforward to do this via a weighted logistic regression (see next section). The file can be split into cases and non-cases and then, using appropriate software (see below), one fits a logistic model containing a predictor variable which has the value of 1 for all subjects (i.e. just fitting a constant). One then obtains the confidence interval for the intercept term in the output. Finally, the inverse of the logistic transformation of the lower and upper confidence limits will yield the corresponding limits for the sensitivity (specificity) itself. Note that the interval will be asymmetric and will be within the permitted bounds of zero and unity.

Modelling patterns of risk

Henderson (see Chapter 2.7) has introduced the idea of an odds ratio to measure the association between a suspected risk factor and disease. In a linear logistic model the response variable is the natural logarithm of the odds (of disease). Therefore the difference between two groups on this logistic scale (i.e. $\log(a/b)-\log(c/d)$ using Henderson's notation) is equivalent to the logarithm of the odds ratio (i.e. $\log(ad/bc)$). This provides us with an easy way to calculate confidence intervals for odds ratio: log(odds ratio) or $\log(ad/bc)$ is normally distributed with variance $1/a + 1/b + 1/c + 1/d$ (the corresponding standard error is the square root of this variance). The 95 per cent confidence interval for the log(odds ratio), for example, is then the point estimate plus or minus 1.96 standard errors. Taking exponents (antilogarithms) of these limits provides the corresponding limits for the odds ratio itself. The exponent of the parameter estimate in the output of the logistic regression run provides the point estimate for the corresponding odds ratio.

The great advantage of logistic regression is that it enables us to model the potential effects of several risk factors simultaneously. It allows us to adjust for the effects of suspected confounder(s) in assessing the effects of a risk factor of interest. Logistic regression can also be generalized to cope with the use of sampling weights, either to cope with data missing by design (as in a two-phase survey) or to allow for non-response and/or attrition.(13) However, one must be very wary of using weights in software packages that do not explicitly deal with sampling weights. Many packages have weighting functions but these are interpreted as frequency weights—the number of times the observation has been made instead of the number of times it might have been made (as in the case of a sampling weight). The use of frequency weights, as opposed to sampling weights, produces standard errors, and confidence intervals that are far too small. This is not a subtle effect; it can make an enormous difference to a P value, giving the impression of a highly significant effect when, in reality, there is little or nothing there.(14) We illustrate this point by reference to a two-phase survey of psychiatric morbidity in Cantabria in Northern Spain.(15,16) The weighted prevalence estimate from these data is 31 per cent. The appropriate 95 per cent confidence interval (**CI**), obtained using sampling weights is (26 per cent, 40 per cent). The naive use of frequency weights produces a 95 per cent CI of (28 per cent, 35 per cent), which is much too narrow. The odds ratio indicating how much higher the prevalence of disorder is in women compared with men is 2.02 with a 95 per cent CI of (0.86, 4.74). The naive use of frequency weights gives the same point estimate (2.02), but here the 95 per cent CI is (1.45, 2.77); again, this is much too narrow. In the analysis of a similar study from Verona in Northern Italy, Dunn *et al.*(14) found a corresponding odds ratio of 2.85 with a 95 per cent CI of (1.31, 6.19). The P value for this odds ratio is about 0.008. The incorrect use of frequency weights gives us a 95 per cent CI of (2.31, 3.53) and a corresponding P value of less than 0.00001—at least an 800-fold difference!

Evaluating treatment effects

Readers will be familiar with the challenges posed by confounding in trying to validly infer an effect of an exposure on the development of illness from data arising from an observational study (or epidemiological survey). We can model patterns of risk (as in the above section) but we can never be sure that we have allowed for all possible sources of confounding (i.e. the effects of unmeasured variables that are associated with the exposure of interest and also influence outcome) in assessing the effect of a particular risk factor. The same challenges apply to the use of observational data to the evaluation of the effect of a treatment or other intervention. Although it may be possible to obtain valid treatment effect estimates from observational data,(17,18) the ideal is to use a randomized experiment. Allocation of treatments by randomization ensures that there are no systematic selection effects (i.e. no biases arising from hidden confounding) and enables the investigator to obtain valid measurements of uncertainty (i.e. valid p-values, standard errors, and confidence intervals).

How do we define a causal effect of treatment? Following Rubin(19) we define it as the comparison between potential outcomes or counterfactuals. For a patient who has received treatment we define the treatment effect as a comparison between the outcome that we have observed after the receipt of treatment (Y_t, say) with that we would have observed if, contrary to fact, the same patient had not received the treatment (Y_c, say the subscript c indicating a control condition). For a patient who has not received treatment we compared the observed outcome (Y_c, in this case) with the unobserved counterfactual (Y_t). Typically, we might be interested in the difference (Y_t-Y_c) but ratios might also be of interest. We define the Average Causal Effect (ACE) of treatment as the average (*Ave*—over the whole of the population of interest) of the individual treatment effects, that is

$$\text{ACE} = \text{Ave}(Y_t-Y_c) \tag{2.2.16}$$

But, of course we can only ever observe either Y_t or Y_c, not both. We can never observe an individual treatment effect and therefore cannot obtain a direct estimate of the average. But we note that

$$\text{ACE} = \text{Ave}(Y_t) - \text{Ave}(Y_c) \tag{2.2.17}$$

and if we could obtain valid estimates of Ave(Y_t) and Ave(Y_c) then the problem would be solved. The only sure way of knowing that we have a valid estimate of these two averages (i.e. no selection biases) is to make sure that the allocation of treatment is completely random. Hence the Randomized Controlled Trial (RCT). Of course, we have to ensure that we have eliminated or reduced all other potential sources of bias (e.g. by masking treatment allocation from the people assessing outcomes) and one must not automatically assume that randomization has led to a perfect trial. In the critical appraisal of a clinical trial report, one might ask:

- What is the target population for the evaluation of the treatment, and were the trial participants representative of this population?
- Were the treatment and control conditions clearly defined and operationalized? In particular, was the control condition convincing?

- Were outcomes clearly defined and reliably measured?
- Was the trial adequately powered (i.e. was the number of randomized participants adequate for the job at hand)?
- Was randomization used to allocate treatment and how was the randomization actually implemented?
- Was it possible to blind mask treatment allocation from all those concerned with the assessment of outcomes? What evidence has been provided to indicate that masking has been effective?
- What methods were used to estimate the treatment effects and their precision? Were they fully compatible with the trial design (the randomization procedure)? Did the analysis take account of everyone randomized? In particular, did the analysis deal adequately with missing outcome data?
- If the trial used a non-standard design (randomization of groups of participants rather than of individuals; use of group-based therapies; and so on) were the power calculations and methods of statistical analysis appropriate for this design?

Estimation of treatment efficacy in the presence of non-compliance

What if the trial participants, despite giving their consent to be randomized, do not receive the treatment to which they were allocated? In a drug trial the participants may not take the tablets, or take less than the prescribed amount. They may even receive the active medication despite being allocated to the placebo (control) condition. In a psychotherapy trial they may not turn up to all or even any of the planned sessions of therapy. The standard method of analysis (and justifiably so) is based on the so-called Intention-to-Treat (ITT) principle: we analyse as randomized. We evaluate the effect of the offer of treatment as opposed to its receipt. But what do we do if we wish to evaluate (estimate) the effect of the treatment actually received? Two commonly used methods of analysis are called per Protocol and As Treated estimators. In the first method the effect of randomization is evaluated after first discarding the people who did not adhere to (or comply with) their allocated treatment. In the second, we compare the outcomes of all those who receive the treatment with all of those who received the control condition, regardless of their random allocation. Both methods are potentially flawed—they take no account of possible selection effects (confounding). A much better approach is to estimate the effect of randomization in that subgroup of participants who would always have complied with their treatment allocation whatever the outcome of the randomization. We call this subgroup the Compliers (the rest being non-compliers), and we aim to estimate the Complier-Average Causal Effect of Treatment (CACE).[20,21] In effect we are obtaining an ITT effect for the Compliers. Randomization ensures that, on average, the proportion (P) of Compliers is the same in each arm of the trial. The overall ITT effect is a weighted average of the ITT effect in the Compliers and the ITT effect in the non-compliers (the weights being P and 1-P, respectively). If we are prepared to assume that there is no direct effect of randomization on outcome (in particular, there is no effect of randomization on outcome in the non-compliers) then

$$\begin{aligned} \text{ITT}_{\text{All}} &= P.\text{ITT}_{\text{Compliers}} + (1-P).\text{ITT}_{\text{non-compliers}} \\ &= P.\text{ITT}_{\text{Compliers}} \end{aligned} \tag{2.2.18}$$

It follows that

$$\text{CACE} = \text{ITT}_{\text{compliers}} = \frac{\text{ITT}_{\text{All}}}{P} \tag{2.2.19}$$

It is easy to show that in a trial in which no-one allocated to the control condition gets access to the (potentially) active treatment the proportion of Compliers (P) is estimated by the proportion of Compliers in the treatment group (this follows directly from randomization). In the situation in which participants allocated to the control condition can get access to treatment P is estimated by the difference between the two randomized groups with respect to the proportion of participants receiving treatment. Considering everyone randomized, eqn (2.2.19) is the ratio of the ITT effect on outcome to the ITT effect on receipt of treatment. Note that ITT_{All} and CACE ($\text{ITT}_{\text{Compliers}}$) share the same null hypothesis (when one is zero, so is the other) and a significance test for one of them is equivalent to the corresponding significance test for the other. The estimation of the CACE is simply a way of adjusting the overall ITT estimate to allow to attenuation in the presence of non-compliance. It will not reveal a significant treatment effect when we already have a non-significant ITT estimate.

We do not advocate the replacement of ITT estimates by CACE estimation, but we do recommend that investigators supplement their primary ITT analyses with more detailed explanatory methods, particularly when there are situations in which non-compliance is strongly associated with subsequent loss to follow-up (i.e. missing outcome data). Valid ITT (and any other) estimates are particularly difficult to obtain in the presence of missing data. This is an active area of theoretical development in medical statistics, but the more easily understood methods are now beginning to make the transition to the more easily accessible clinical journals. For example, a relatively non-technical discussion of the potential application to mental health trials is provided by Dunn *et al.*[22,23]

We refer readers to Everitt and Wessely[24] and Dunn[25] for a much more detailed discussion of the methodological pitfalls for RCTs in psychiatry. One important point needs stressing again, however. It is vital that RCTs involve the randomization of sufficient numbers of subjects to be confident that the trial has sufficient power to detect the *minimum* treatment effect that still has *clinical* (as opposed to statistical) significance. This minimum effect should be defined in terms of its importance and *not* by naively observing the results of previous trials or pilot investigations.

Conclusions

The recently published *Encyclopedia of Biostatistics*[26] comprises of six large volumes of chapters such as this one, covering every area of conceivable interest to the statistically interested clinical research worker. Therefore it is inevitable that this chapter should be very restricted. Inevitably, the choice of topics might be thought to be rather idiosyncratic. Areas which might have been covered, but have been ignored, include survival modelling (particularly recent developments in so-called frailty modelling), longitudinal data analysis (with special reference to modelling patterns of attrition), genetics, and a whole range of classical multivariate methods such as principal components and factor analysis, discriminant analysis (although logistic modelling is one of the better methods of discriminant analysis), multidimensional scaling, and cluster analysis.

Henderson (see Chapter 2.7) has also mentioned exciting possibilities for the development of latent trait (item response theory) and latent class models. Several years ago I was often asked to teach trainee psychiatrists all they needed to know about statistics in two 2-h sessions. The first was to cover univariate methods, and the second, multivariate analysis. It cannot be done!

Further information

So, where should the reader go from here? Which are the most useful textbooks? In terms of general medical statistics, the obvious choice is Armitage, Berry, and Matthews. Everitt and Dunn and Everitt provide general introductions to multivariate methodology. Measurement error problems, including structural equation modelling, are covered by Dunn. The role of statistics in genetics is well covered by Sham. Although there are many texts on the use of statistics in psychology and education (e.g. Plewis which includes an introduction to multilevel modelling), the only specialist reference for psychiatrists appears to be that by Dunn.

Armitage, P., Berry, G., and Matthews, J.N.S. (2002). *Statistical methods in medical research* (4th edn). Blackwell Science, Oxford.

Everitt, B.S. and Dunn, G. (2001). *Applied multivariate data analysis* (2nd edn). Arnold, London.

Everitt, B.S. (1996). *Making sense of statistics in psychology*. Oxford University Press, Oxford.

Sham, P. (1998). *Statistics in human genetics*. Arnold, London.

Dunn, G. (1999). *Statistics in psychiatry*. Arnold, London.

Plewis, I. (1997). *Statistics in education*. Arnold, London.

References

1. Shavelson, R.J. and Webb, N.M. (1991). *Generalizability theory: a primer*. Sage, Thousand Oaks, CA.
2. Fleiss, J.L. (1987). *The design and analysis of clinical experiments*. Wiley, New York.
3. Streiner, D.L. and Norman, G.R. (2003). *Health measurement scales: a practical guide to their development and use* (3rd edn). Oxford University Press, Oxford.
4. Dunn, G. (2004). *Statistical evaluation of measurement errors: design and analysis of reliability studies* (2nd edn). Arnold, London.
5. Dunn, G. and Everitt, B.S. (1995). *Clinical biostatistics: an introduction to evidence based medicine*, Chap. 4. Arnold, London.
6. Kessler, R.C. (1994). The National Comorbidity Survey of the United States. *International Review of Psychiatry*, **6**, 365–76.
7. Jenkins, R., Bebbington, P., Brugha, T., *et al.* (1997). The National Psychiatric Morbidity Surveys of Great Britain—strategy and methods. *Psychological Medicine*, **27**, 765–74.
8. Pickles, A. and Dunn, G. (1998). Prevalence of disease, estimation from screening data. In *Encyclopedia of biostatistics*, Vol. 5 (eds. P. Armitage and T. Colton), pp. 3484–90. Wiley, Chichester.
9. Lehtonen, R. and Pahkinen, E.J. (1995). *Practical methods for design and analysis of complex surveys*. Wiley, Chichester.
10. Cochran, W.G. (1977). *Sampling techniques* (3rd edn). Wiley, New York.
11. Goldberg, D.P. and Williams, P. (1988). *A user's guide to the General Health Questionnaire*. NFER-Nelson, Windsor.
12. Begg, C.B. and Greenes, R.A. (1983). Assessment of diagnostic tests when disease verification is subject to selection bias. *Biometrics*, **39**, 207–15.
13. Dunn, G. (1998). Compensating for missing data in psychiatric surveys. *Epidemiologia e Psichiatria Sociale*, **6**, 159–62.
14. Dunn, G., Pickles, A., Tansella, M., *et al.* (1999). The role of two-phase epidemiological surveys in psychiatric research. *The British Journal of Psychiatry*, **174**, 95–100.
15. Pickles, A., Dunn, G., and Vázquez-Barquero, J.L. (1995). Screening for stratification in two-phase ('two-stage') epidemiological surveys. *Statistical Methods in Medical Research*, **4**, 75–91.
16. Vázquez-Barquero, J.L., Garcia, J., Artal Simón, J., *et al.* (1997). Mental health in primary care: an epidemiological study of morbidity and use of health resources. *The British Journal of Psychiatry*, **170**, 529–35.
17. Rubin, D.B. (2007). The design versus the analysis of observational studies for causal effects: parallels with the design of randomized trials. *Statistics in Medicine*, **26**, 20–36.
18.. Luellin, J.K., Shadish, W.R., and Clark, M.H. (2005). Propensity scores: an introduction and experimental test. *Evaluation Review*, **29**, 530–58.
19. Rubin, D.B. (1974). Estimating causal effects of treatments in randomized and non-randomized studies. *Journal of Educational Psychology*, **66**, 688–701.
20. Bloom, H.S. (1984). Accounting for no-shows in experimental evaluation designs. *Evaluation Review*, **8**, 225–46.
21. Angrist, J.D., Imbens, G.W., and Rubin, D.B. (1996). Identification of causal effects using instrumental variables (with discussion). *Journal of the American Statistical Association*, **91**, 444–72.
22. Dunn, G. Maracy, M., Dowrick, C., *et al.* Estimating psychological treatment effects from an RCT with both non-compliance and loss to follow-up. *The British Journal of Psychiatry*, **183**, 323–31.
23. Dunn, G., Maracy, M., and Tomenson, B. (2005). Estimating treatment effects from randomized clinical trials with non-compliance and loss to follow-up: the role of instrumental variable methods. *Statistical Methods in Medical Research*, **14**, 369–95.
24. Everitt, B.S. and Wessely, S. (2004). *Clinical trials in psychiatry*. Oxford University Press, Oxford.
25. Dunn, G. (2006). Psychotherapy for depression. In *Textbook of clinical trials* (2nd edn) (eds. D. Machin, S. Day, and S. Green), pp. 377–93. John Wiley & Sons, Chichester.
26. Armitage, P. and Colton, T. (eds.) (1998, 2nd edn 2005). *Encyclopedia of biostatistics*. Wiley, Chichester.

2.3

The contribution of neurosciences

Contents

2.3.1 Neuroanatomy
†R. C. A. Pearson

2.3.2 Neurodevelopment
Karl Zilles

2.3.3 Neuroendocrinology
Charles B. Nemeroff and Gretchen N. Neigh

2.3.4 Neurotransmitters and signalling
Trevor Sharp

2.3.5 Neuropathology
Peter Falkai and Bernhard Bogerts

2.3.6 Functional positron emission tomography in psychiatry
P. M. Grasby

2.3.7 Structural magnetic resonance imaging
J. Suckling and E. T. Bullmore

2.3.8 Functional magnetic resonance imaging
E. T. Bullmore and J. Suckling

2.3.9 Neuronal networks, epilepsy, and other brain dysfunctions
John G. R. Jefferys

2.3.10 Psychoneuroimmunology
Robert Dantzer and Keith W. Kelley

2.3.1 Neuroanatomy

†R. C. A. Pearson

Introduction

The symptoms, signs, and syndromes of psychiatry, whether organic or biological psychiatric disease or not, in the main reflect alterations in functions which reside in the cerebral cortex, including the limbic lobe, and those structures and pathways closely related to the cortex. These cortical manifestations of psychiatric disease include alterations in thought, language, perception, mood, memory, motivation, personality, behaviour, and intellect. Therefore, this brief account of brain structures and pathways that are important in psychiatry will concentrate on the cerebral cortex and related structures and pathways. Readers who require a fuller account of central nervous system anatomy are referred to the many standard texts, which give a more complete coverage of the subject.

Broadly speaking, neuroanatomy can be subdivided into two parts—the topographical organization of the brain and spinal cord, and the anatomical connections forming functional pathways in the central nervous system. The former is of vital importance clinically, since pathologies rarely respect the boundaries of functional systems, and knowledge of the spatial relationships of different brain structures is increasingly useful as modern imaging methods more accurately visualize detailed brain structure *in vivo*. However, it is the second subdivision of the subject which makes the greater contribution to understanding the biological basis of psychiatric disease, and it is this that will be at the centre of the present account.

The structure and organization of the cerebral cortex

The lobes of the cerebral cortex

A variable pattern of fissures (sulci) and folds (gyri), many of which have specific names, extensively groove the surface of the cerebral hemisphere. A few are relatively constant and are used to subdivide the cerebral hemisphere into lobes, named for the bones of the skull which they underlie (Fig. 2.3.1.1).

The deep lateral sulcus, also called the Sylvian fissure, extends from the uncus, anteriorly and medially, to the parietal lobe, posteriorly and medially. It has a short stem, and anterior, ascending, and posterior rami. The anterior and ascending rami embrace the pars triangularis of the frontal lobe, which houses Broca's motor speech area. The much longer posterior ramus is used in defining the lobes of the hemisphere. The central sulcus is prominent approximately midway along the anteroposterior extent of the

† Dr. Pearson died while this new edition was being prepared. The editors pay tribute to his scientific achievements and to his contributions to this book.

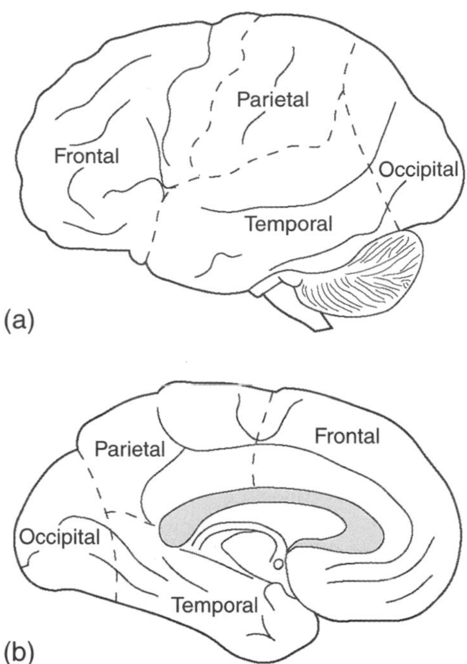

Fig. 2.3.1.1 The lobes of the cerebral cortex.

lateral surface of the hemisphere and, most commonly, extends over the medial margin, where its inferomedial tip is embraced by the U-shaped paracentral lobule. On the lateral surface, it passes from the medial margin, forwards and laterally, to reach the lateral sulcus. The line of the central sulcus closely approximates the line of the coronal suture of the adult skull, i.e. the junction between the frontal and parietal bones; consequently, the sulcus separates the frontal and parietal lobes. The demarcation of the occipital lobe is the parieto-occipital sulcus dorsally and medially, and the pre-occipital sulcus ventrally and laterally, with an imaginary line connecting the two and intersecting the posterior tip of the lateral sulcus. The temporal lobe lies anterior to this line and inferior (ventral) to the lateral sulcus. The deep lateral sulcus broadens out at its fundus, with an area of cortex forming the extensive floor of the sulcus, particularly in its anterior two-thirds. This cortex is the insula, which does not form part of any of the lobes mentioned above. The insula is surrounded by the circular sulcus, and is overhung by the frontal and parietal opercula superiorly, and the temporal operculum inferiorly (ventrally). The anatomical borders of the lobes of the cerebral cortex, and other sulcal and gyral landmarks, are only loosely paralleled by functional boundaries. However, lobar terminology is so firmly embedded in clinical and non-clinical neuroscience that consideration of their anatomical features is essential.

(a) The frontal lobe (Fig. 2.3.1.2)

The precentral gyrus, immediately in front of the central sulcus and continuing onto the medial surface, contains the primary motor cortex. The precentral sulcus usually defines the anterior boundary, and in front of this lies the premotor cortex. The inferior

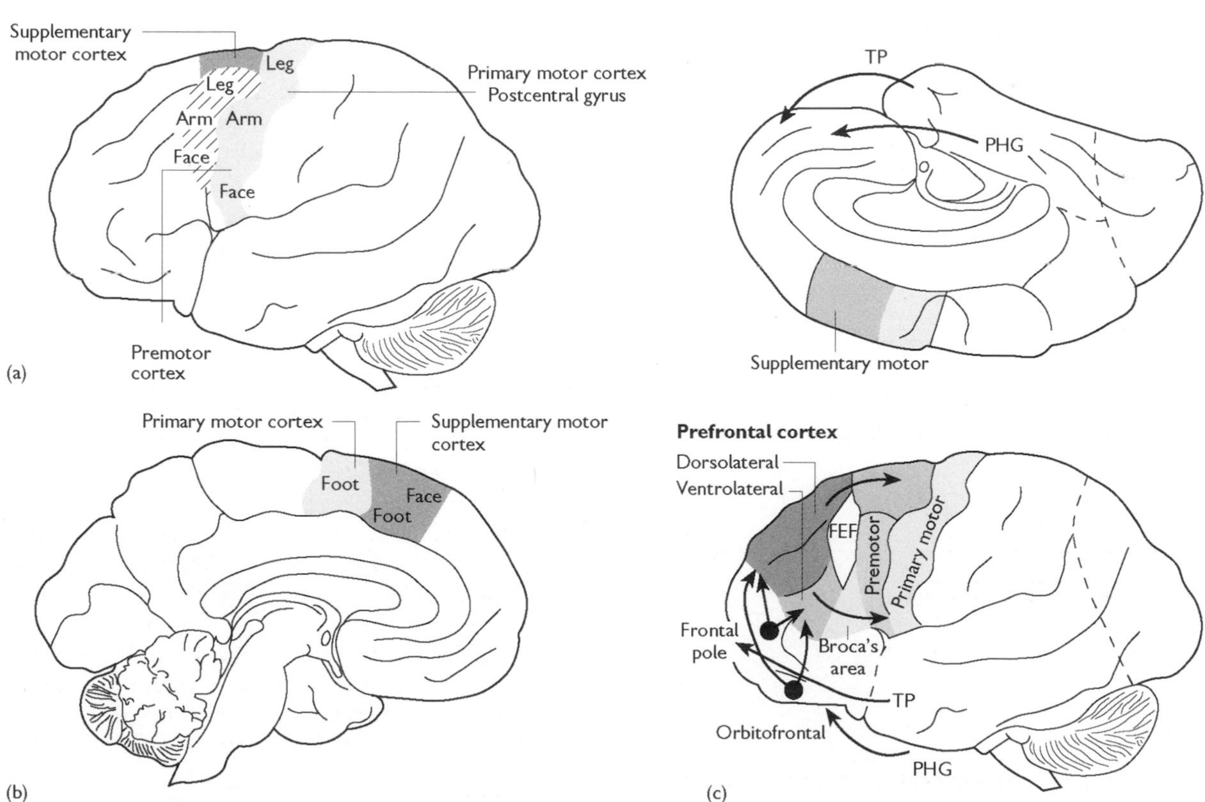

Fig. 2.3.1.2 Motor areas of the frontal lobe: TP, temporal pole; PHG, parahippocampal gyrus; FEF, frontal eyefields.

margin of the sulcus runs into the pars triangularis, which includes Broca's motor speech area. On the medial margin and surface, the cortex includes the supplementary motor area. The lateral prefrontal cortex, in front of these motor and associated areas, is usually grooved by two major horizontal sulci, defining the superior, middle, and inferior frontal gyri. The cortex on the medial surface of the frontal lobe anterior to the prefrontal gyrus forms the medial prefrontal cortex. The concave inferior surface of the frontal lobe, overlying the bony orbit *in vivo*, is the orbitofrontal cortex.

(b) The parietal lobe (Fig. 2.3.1.3)

Behind the central sulcus, the primary somatic sensory cortex (SI), extending onto the medial surface to occupy the posterior part of the paracentral lobule, where the sacral spinal segments are represented, occupies the postcentral gyrus. The postcentral sulcus limits the postcentral gyrus posteriorly. Behind this, the sulcal pattern is variable, but one or more horizontal intraparietal sulci divide the lobe into superior and inferior parts. The second somatic sensory cortex (SII) is located in the parietal operculum, close behind the inferolateral tip of the central sulcus. Specific sulcal patterns in the transition region between the parietal lobe and the occipital and temporal lobes (the supramarginal and angular gyri) are important landmarks for the detailed localization of language functions.

(c) The occipital lobe (Fig. 2.3.1.4)

The occipital lobe is predominantly involved in vision and visual perception. The medial surface is grooved by the deep horizontal calcarine sulcus, which typically reaches the posterior pole of the hemisphere. Within its walls is the primary visual cortex. This area (area 17 of Brodmann) is often called the striate cortex; in the freshly sliced brain, a thin band of white matter, the stria of Gennari, is clearly visible running in the centre of the cortical grey ribbon. The extent of this stria precisely demarcates the primary visual cortex. Surrounding areas of the medial and lateral surface, the prestriate and peristriate cortex, contain some of the numerous separate visual association areas.

(d) The temporal lobe (Figs 2.3.1.5 and 2.3.1.6)

Two horizontal sulci, the superior and inferior temporal sulci, divide the lateral surface of the temporal lobe into the superior, middle, and inferior gyri. The latter, extending onto the inferior surface, is also known as the inferotemporal cortex. On the medial surface, the collateral sulcus runs from close to the temporal pole to the calcarine sulcus posteriorly. Medial to this is the parahippocampal gyrus. Anteriorly, this curves dorsally and caudally to form the hook-shaped uncus. The entorhinal cortex occupies approximately the anterior third of the parahippocampal gyrus. Lateral to this, in the walls of the rhinal sulcus, lies the perirhinal cortex. The uncus closely overlies the amygdala; the primary olfactory cortex, the piriform cortex, lies immediately in front. The choroid fissure limits the parahippocampal gyrus medially. Passing into the floor of the lateral ventricle, the subicular areas of cortex lead to the hippocampus proper. A detailed consideration of the anatomy of the hippocampus is given below.

The cortex of the temporal operculum contains Heschl's gyri, within which lies the primary auditory cortex. Diverse auditory

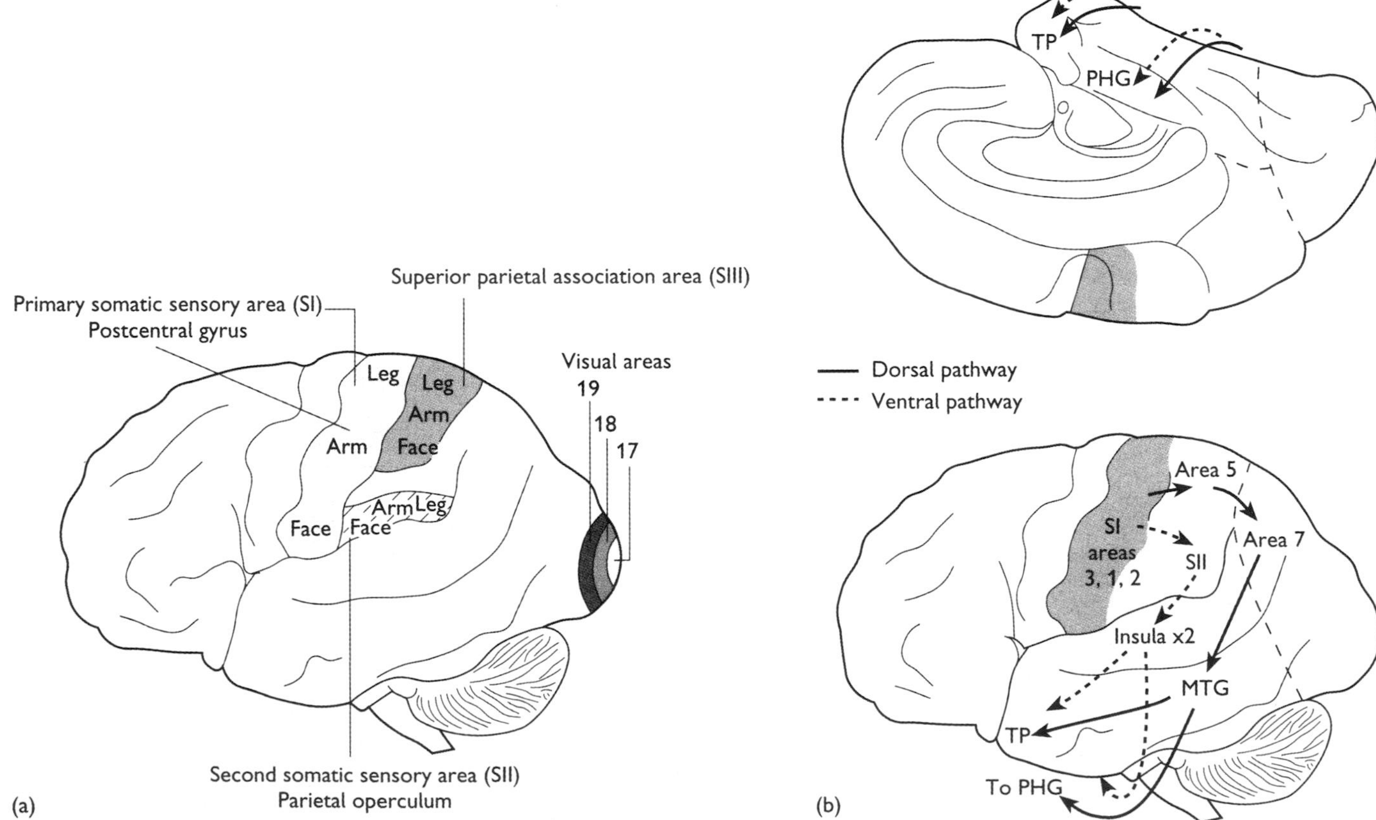

Fig. 2.3.1.3 (a) Areas of the parietal lobe; (b) somatic sensory association pathways. TP, temporal pole; PHG, parahippocampal gyrus; MTG, middle temporal gyrus.

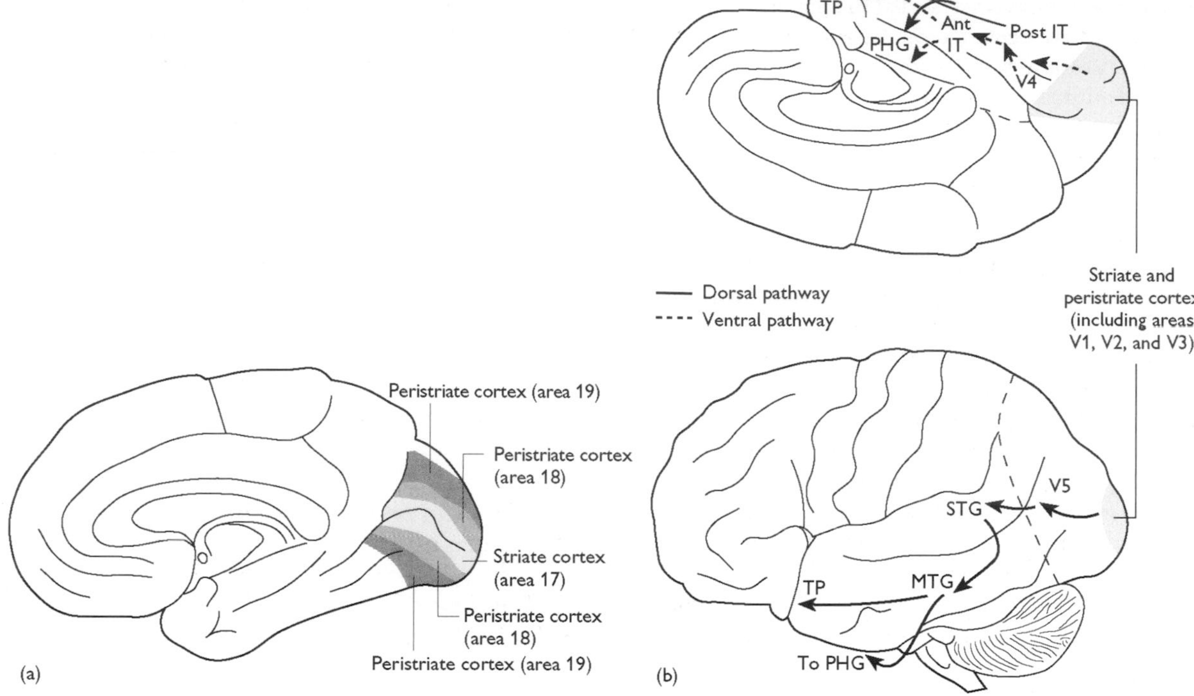

Fig. 2.3.1.4 The occipital lobe: (a) visual areas; (b) visual association pathways. TP, temporal pole; IT, inferotemporal cortex; PHG, parahippocampal gyrus; STG, superior temporal gyrus; MTG, middle temporal gyrus; Ant, anterior; Post, posterior.

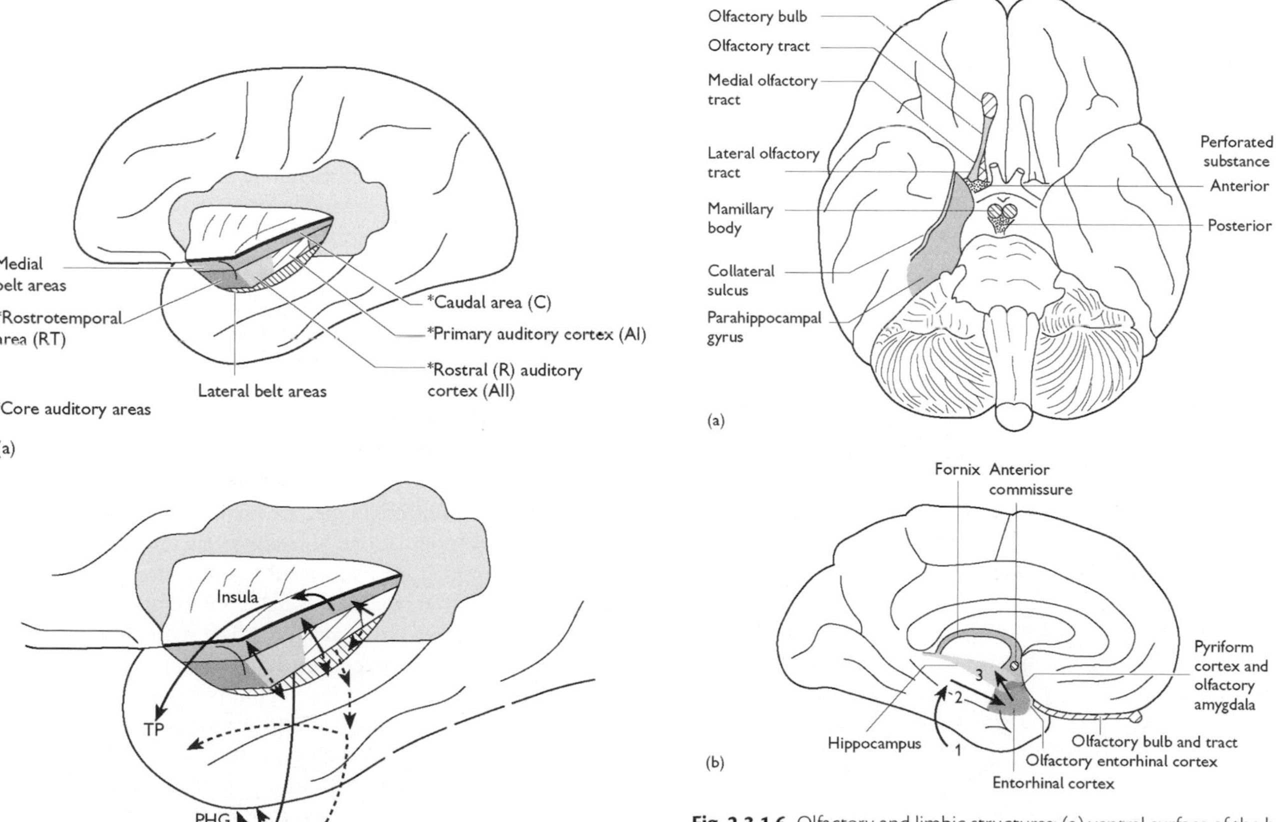

Fig. 2.3.1.5 Auditory association connections. TP, temporal pole; PHG, parahippocampal gyrus.

Fig. 2.3.1.6 Olfactory and limbic structures: (a) ventral surface of the brain; (b) medial temporal lobe. 1, Association cortex to parahippocampal gyrus; 2, parahippocampal gyrus to entorhinal cortex; 3, entorhinal cortex to hippocampus (perforant path).

association areas surround this, extending into the superior temporal gyrus. The functions of the cortex of the middle temporal gyrus are uncertain, but include complex visual, auditory, and somatic sensory association areas. The inferotemporal cortex is largely concerned with visual perception and cognition. The anatomical pathways that underlie these functions are considered below.

(e) The insula

The anterior margin of the insula, where the cortex becomes continuous with the anterior perforated substance, is known as the limen insulae. Above and below, where the insular cortex rolls round onto the opercula, lies the circular sulcus, the superior and inferior rami of which fuse posterosuperiorly to form the apex of the insula. Several variable sulci mark the insula, but little is known of the functional subdivisions of this cortex; gustatory, somatic sensory, and auditory areas have been described.

The structure of the neocortex

The neocortical grey matter is usually described as having six layers (Plate 1(a)). Wide variation in the nature of this microscopic lamination underlies the subdivision of neocortex into a multiplicity of (usually numbered) areas. At its simplest, two types of neurones make up the grey matter—pyramidal and non-pyramidal (or granular) cells. An apparent predominance of one or other type gives the extremes of granular and agranular cortex, equating with sensory areas (granular) and the motor cortex (agranular). In fact, the proportion of different cell types is constant in all areas. Indeed, with the single exception of the primary visual cortex, the numbers of neurones under a fixed surface area is also constant in all cortical areas. Variations in the size of pyramidal cells in particular lead to an apparent change in proportions. These variations probably reflect differences in the axonal volume of individual pyramidal cells, reflecting the distance and volume of projection fibres from a cortical area.

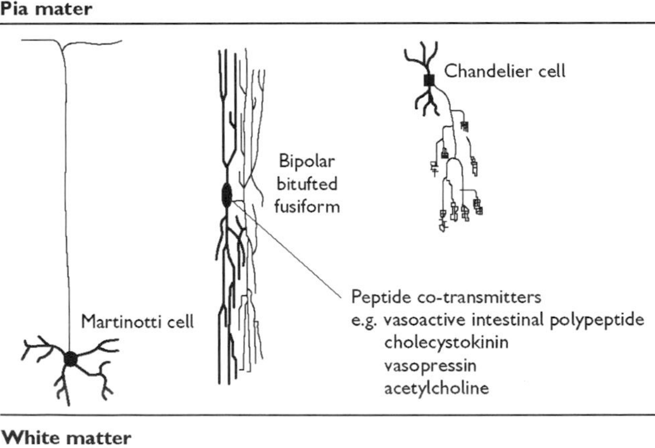

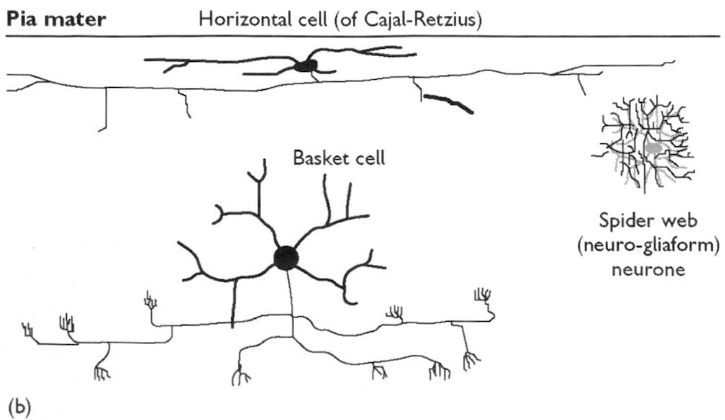

Fig. 2.3.1.7 Inhibitory (GABA-ergic) neurones of the neocortex: (a) vertical; (b) horizontal.

Pyramidal cells have a single main apical dendrite ascending towards the pial surface, and several horizontally spreading basal dendrites. All dendrites bear dendritic spines, which receive synapses (Plate 1(b)). All pyramidal cells use excitatory amino acids as neurotransmitters and have axons which enter the subcortical white matter; hence they are all projection neurones. They constitute approximately 60 per cent of all the neurones in the cortex. A second spiny neuronal type, the spiny stellate cells, is the next most numerous. These also use an excitatory amino acid, most probably glutamate, as their neurotransmitter. Unlike pyramidal cells, however, their axons remain confined to the cortical grey matter; they are interneurones, accounting for a further 25 per cent of cortical neurones. All the other neurones are inhibitory interneurones, using γ-aminobutyric acid (GABA) as their major neurotransmitter. Many also contain one or more neuropeptides, and their content of specific calcium-binding proteins varies. They have a wide range of axonal and dendritic forms, and have been multiply classified in the past. Broadly speaking, they can be grouped into those with horizontal axonal arborizations, those whose axons ramify at right angles to the pial surface, i.e. through the depth of the cortex, and those with radial axons (Fig. 2.3.1.7).

The structure of the allocortex

The allocortex comprises a number of different areas, all with very different structures. They are either limbic or olfactory (or both) and are found predominantly in the medial temporal lobe. The largest of these regions is the hippocampus. Essentially, this includes the three-layered cortex of the hippocampus, together with the transitional areas between it and neocortex, which are variably said to have three, four, five, or six laminae. The hippocampal formation comprises the dentate gyrus, Ammon's horn (CA fields), and the subiculum. Both the dentate gyrus and the CA fields have a prominent single layer of neurones, with an overlying molecular layer and a subjacent polymorphic layer. In the dentate gyrus, the cells are granule cells, whereas in the CA fields they are predominantly large pyramidal cells—the stratum pyramidale. Both cell types are excitatory and are projection neurones. Scattered populations of GABA-ergic inhibitory interneurones are found immediately subjacent to the main cellular laminae and in the molecular layers. The CA fields are numbered 1, 2, and 3, from the subiculum to the dentate gyrus. The subiculum is the zone of transition between the three-layered hippocampus proper, and the entorhinal cortex and cortex of the parahippocampal gyrus laterally. It is sometimes further subdivided into subzones including the presubiculum, between the lateral cortex and the subiculum, and the prosubiculum, between the subiculum proper and CA1 of the hippocampus. The histological appearance of the hippocampus and adjacent areas are shown in Fig. 2.3.1.8, and their connections are considered in detail below.

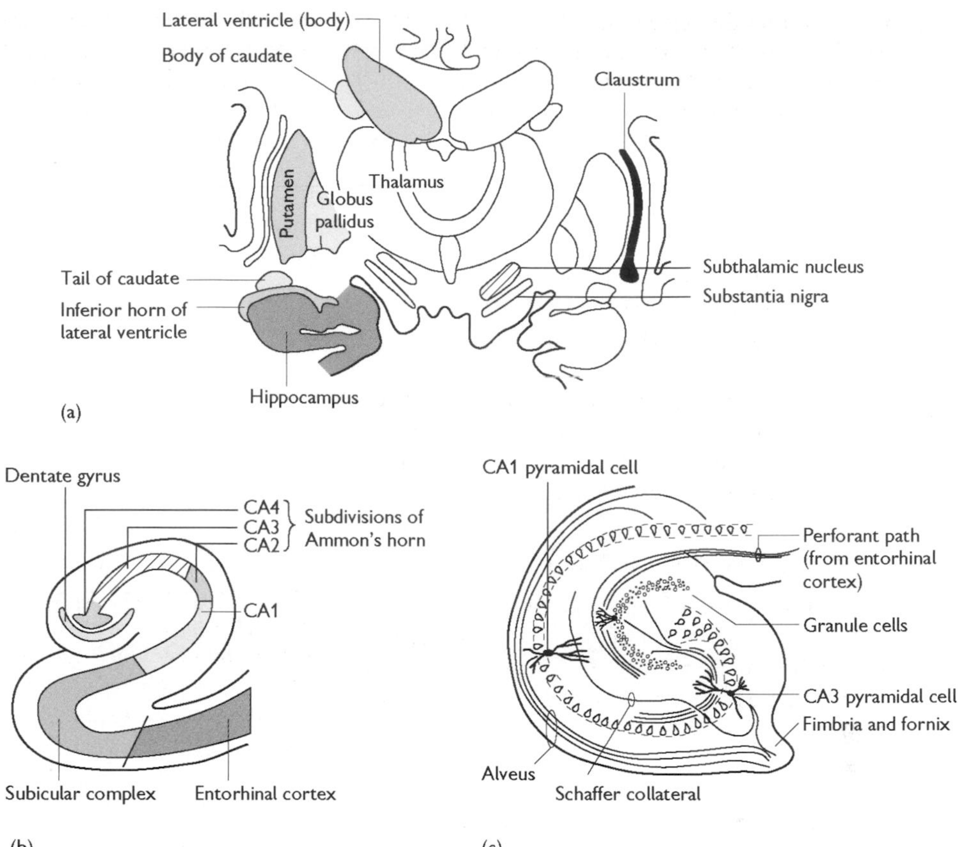

Fig. 2.3.1.8 (a) Hippocampal formation in the temporal lobe; (b) subdivisions of the hippocampal formation; (c) organization of the hippocampus.

Table 2.3.1.1 General connections of the cerebral cortex

Nucleus/area	Afferents	Efferents
Subcortical		
Thalamus		
Principal	+	+
Intralaminar	+	+
Locus coeruleus (NA)	+	–
Raphe (serotonin)	+	–
Basal nucleus (ACh)	+	–
Hypothalamus (histamine)	+	–
SN and VTA (dopamine)	+	–
Claustrum	+	+
Striatum	–	+
Pons	–	+
Superior colliculus and reticular formation	–	+
Specific (e.g. corticospinal)	–	(+/–)
Cortical		
Contra lateral		
Homotopic	+	+
Heterotopic	+	+
Ipsilateral		
Short	+	+
Long	+	+

NA, noradrenaline; ACh, acetylcholine; SN, substantia nigra; VTA, ventral tegmental area.

The general pattern of connectivity of the cortex

All cortical areas share a broadly similar pattern of connections. What differs is the relative quantity of connections in each category, as well as the precise detail of origin and termination. The broad categories of connections which all cortical areas share are most easily seen in a table (Table 2.3.1.1). These will be dealt in detail in subsequent sections.

A central feature of the connections of the neocortex is their organization relative to the cortical laminae (Plate 1(a)). For simplicity, it can generally be assumed that the forward-flowing stream of connections for perception and action use the central laminae, descending projections originate in deeper layers, and feedback and non-specific afferents terminate in both superficial and deep laminae. Thus, in primary sensory areas the thalamic input from the principal nuclei (e.g. the lateral geniculate nucleus in the visual cortex) terminates in layer IV. Projections to higher association areas originate from pyramidal cells immediately adjacent, in layer III. As the ipsilateral association pathway progresses from area to area, the association fibres terminate in this central region, and the thalamic afferents end in superficial and deep laminae. Projections to subcortical nuclei, such as the striatum, arise in layer V, and corticothalamic axons come from layer VI. It is as if the input of major importance, requiring detailed, focused, and faithful transmission, arrives in layer IV and is passed on from the deeper part of layer III. Inputs which moderate or modulate this pass to either side of the central layers, and outputs which are not directly part of this progression arise from deeper layers.

There is a general principle in the organization of connectivity with the cerebral cortex of overlapping connectivity of functionally related areas throughout the range of connections made. In other words, functionally related cortical areas, which are connected with each other, also tend to have overlapping or interdigitating connections with other structures. This is seen on the striatum, the thalamus, the claustrum, the cholinergic basal forebrain, and the pontine nuclei.

Subcortical afferents to the cerebral cortex

The thalamus (Plate 2)

Thalamic nuclei can be classified as specific (principal) or non-specific. In general, the specific nuclei degenerate completely when the cortex is removed, whereas the non-specific nuclei do not. This is because the sole major projection of the specific nuclei is to the cerebral cortex. The non-specific nuclei are the intralaminar and midline nuclei, which project to the basal ganglia as well as to cortex, and the reticular nucleus, which projects only to other thalamic nuclei.

All cortical areas receive afferents from at least one specific thalamic nucleus, and an additional input from the intralaminar/midline nuclei. Corticothalamic fibres reciprocate all thalamocortical projections, probably without exception.

(a) Specific nuclei

The cortical projections of the specific nuclei are shown in Plate 2. Subclassification of the specific thalamic nuclei depends upon their afferent subcortical connections. The primary relay nuclei receive the major sensory pathways—the lateral and medial geniculate nuclei for the optic tract and auditory pathway respectively, and the ventral posterior nucleus for the somatic sensory pathways. The secondary relay nuclei are those which receive a known major subcortical pathway which is not sensory. These are usually taken to include the caudal subdivision of the ventral lateral nucleus, which receives the cerebellar pathway, the anterior division of the ventral lateral nucleus and the ventral anterior nucleus, which both receive fibres from the internal segment of the globus pallidus, and the anterior nuclei, which receive the mammillothalamic tract. The association nuclei are those which were not previously understood to receive a major subcortical pathway, predominantly the medial nucleus and the pulvinar. This view is no longer really tenable, since the pulvinar is now known to receive a major input from the superior colliculus, and the various subdivisions of the medial nucleus receive fibres from the ventral pallidum and the olfactory pathway, amongst others. The subcortical afferents to the principal thalamic nuclei are shown in Plate 2(a).

(b) The non-specific nuclei

The reticular nucleus lies lateral to the main body of the thalamus, separated from it by the external medullary lamina. Cells in the nucleus are inhibitory, using GABA as their neurotransmitter. Excitatory thalamocortical and corticothalamic fibres, passing to and from the main nuclei, traverse the reticular nucleus and give axon collaterals to the reticular nucleus cells. There is a very tight arrangement, whereby the branches of axons from the thalamus to a particular cortical area terminate in the reticular nucleus in close proximity to the corticothalamic axons from the same cortical area. The reticular nucleus cells in turn send their inhibitory axons into the thalamus, to terminate precisely in the nuclei from which they receive a collateral input.

The intralaminar and midline nuclei receive afferents from the major pathways to their adjacent principal nuclei and project to the striatum (caudate, putamen, and ventral striatum) as well as to the cortex. There is a broad topographic relationship in their projection to both areas. The midline nuclei innervate the ventral striatum (nucleus accumbens) and the limbic cortex, including the hippocampal formation. The anterior intralaminar nuclei connect with the prefrontal, parietal, occipital, and temporal cortex, and project to all parts of the caudate. The posterior intralaminar nuclei, of which the centromedian nucleus is the largest, project to the putamen and are reciprocally related to the motor, premotor, and supplementary motor areas of cortex in the frontal lobe. Many axons to the cortex from the intralaminar nuclei are collateral branches of thalamostriate axons. The cortical and striatal areas to which they each project are precisely those parts of the cortex and striatum which are themselves directly connected by corticostriate fibres.

Non-thalamic subcortical afferents to the cerebral cortex

A variety of nuclei send afferents to the cerebral cortex. These fall into two categories: fibres from the so-called isodendritic core of the brainstem and basal forebrain, which are non-reciprocal and aminergic, and the two-way interconnections with the claustrum.

Acetylcholine and the basal forebrain

A system of cholinergic nuclei extend from the septum verum anteriorly, through the nuclei of the diagonal band of Broca to the basal nucleus of Meynert in the substantia innominata, ventral to the globus pallidus, most posteriorly. From these, cholinergic fibres pass to the entire cerebral cortex. Alternative nomenclature for these nuclei uses a numeric system, (Ch1 to Ch4). The anterior cell groups project to the hippocampus and entorhinal cortex, and to the olfactory bulb and cortex. There is an approximate topographic relationship in the projection of the basal nucleus to the neocortex, but with considerable overlap; adjacent or overlapping regions of the nucleus project to widely separated but functionally related and interconnected areas of neocortex. Degeneration of this system is associated with the dementias of Alzheimer's disease and Lewy body disease.

Cholinergic cells in the pedunculopontine nucleus of the midbrain project to the thalamus, particularly to the midline and intralaminar nuclei.

(a) Serotonin, noradrenaline (norepinephrine) and adrenaline (epinephrine): the raphe and associated nuclei

The median group of nuclei of the brainstem reticular formation is made up largely of the various raphe nuclei, all of which use serotonin (5-hydroxytryptamine) as their neurotransmitter. Their projections are very widespread throughout the central nervous system. Broadly speaking, there is a rostrocaudal topography to the efferent projections of these nuclei. The most rostral, notably the dorsal median raphe nucleus in the midbrain tegmentum, send projections to the entire cerebral cortex and striatum. There is a prominent projection to the thalamus, notably to the midline nuclei which in turn project in part to the hippocampal formation.

The serotoninergic raphe-spinal tract, which has important functions in the gating of pain, arises from the most rostral nuclei, the raphe obscurus and the raphe magnus.

The locus coeruleus lies in the dorsolateral pons, immediately deep to the ventricular ependyma. Together with the subceruleus immediately deep to it, this nucleus supplies noradrenergic fibres to most of the central nervous system. Ascending fibres pass to the thalamus and hypothalamus, the entire cerebral cortex (neo- and allocortex), the amygdala, the septal nuclei, and the olfactory bulb. Adrenergic cells in the brainstem do not appear to send ascending projections to the cortex.

(b) Dopamine: the substantia nigra and adjacent nuclei

The major dopaminergic cell group of the midbrain is the pars compacta of the substantia nigra, which projects to the striatum (caudate, putamen, nucleus accumbens, and olfactory tubercle). Two other adjacent nuclei, the ventral tegmental area of Tsai and the pigmented parabrachial nucleus, are also dopaminergic. Together, these three cell groups project rostrally in the medial forebrain bundle to innervate the thalamus and hypothalamus, the hippocampal formation, the entorhinal cortex and amygdala, and widespread areas of the neocortex, especially the prefrontal, orbitofrontal, and cingulate cortex.

(c) Histamine and the posterior hypothalamus

The entire cerebral cortex, including the limbic lobe, receives a histaminergic projection from the tuberomamillary nucleus of the posterior hypothalamus. Postsynaptic receptors appear to be of two types, H1 and H2, with broadly opposing effects.

(d) The cortex and the claustrum

The claustrum is a thin plate of grey matter lying immediately deep to the cortex of the insula, and separated from it by the white matter of the extreme capsule. Medially, the external capsule (Fig. 2.3.1.8(a)) separates it from the putamen. The nucleus receives fibres from and projects to the whole cortex, including the allocortex. The reciprocal connection is topographically organized, but with overlapping zones projecting to widely separated but functionally related and interconnected cortical areas. Many of the neurones of the claustrum have branching axons with collaterals going to two or more such interconnected areas. For example, the superior parietal cortex (area 5) is widely separated from the premotor cortex (area 6) but is connected to it by ipsilateral association fibres, and the two areas are functionally closely related. Both these areas project to and receive from an overlapping zone of the claustrum, and many axons of claustral cells in this zone may branch to both areas.

(e) Modulation of cortical activation and the anatomy of the reticular activating system

Specific information to the cerebral cortex, for example relating to sensory stimuli in the periphery, is relayed via the main thalamic nuclei. The other, diffusely projecting, systems are most likely to be involved in the regulation of cortical responsivity. Such a role has been demonstrated electrophysiologically for the claustrum, and the pharmacology of the antihistamines indicates a role for this transmitter system in the regulation of cortical arousal. The cholinergic input from the basal forebrain is necessary for the proper functioning of the cortex, and its degeneration is associated with cognitive decline and memory impairment. The possible relationship of mesolimbic dopamine pathways to schizophrenia is well known. Similarly, the psychopharmacology of serotonin also implies a major role for this transmitter system in the proper functioning of the cortex. There are two routes by which these 'non-specific' pathways affect the cortex: direct projections, and an indirect pathway through the thalamus. Brainstem nuclei send fibres to the intralaminar and midline nuclei, which in turn send fibres to the entire cortex including the hippocampus. The cholinergic input from the interpeduncular nucleus to the intralaminar nuclei is prominent. Serotonin is particularly concentrated in the midline nuclei. There are other reticular formation projections to these nuclei, but the transmitters remain uncertain. This latter indirect route by which the reticular formation of the brainstem impinges on the cerebral cortex via the thalamus constitutes the reticular activating system. The role of this system in cortical arousal is well documented.

Corticocortical connections

(a) The corpus callosum and the commissural connections of the cerebral cortex

All cortical areas, both send fibres to and receive fibres from the opposite hemisphere, although the connections are not necessarily throughout the whole area. In most of the cortex, commissural fibres pass to the contralateral side in the corpus callosum. The anterior commissure carries fibres that interconnect the anterior third or so of the temporal lobe with its partner, as well as fibres that interconnect the olfactory bulbs on each side. Some fibres in the fornix cross the midline, the so-called commissure of the fornix, to interconnect the two hippocampal formations. Commissural fibres are of two types, homotopic and heterotopic. Homotopic fibres pass from one area of cortex to the same area on the other side. Heterotopic fibres pass from one area to a different, although, often functionally related, area on the other side. As a generalization, the functions of the commissures can be subdivided into two categories. First, they serve to interconnect representations of the contralateral sensory surround across the midline, for example, the representations of the two halves of the body, the two visual hemifields, and so on. In areas containing a lateralized sensory representation, of either the body or the visual field, the callosal fibres are confined, in both origin and termination, to the parts of the area containing a representation of midline and adjacent regions. Thus the representation of the trunk in somatic sensory areas sends and receives commissural fibres, whereas the hand and foot representations are not connected across the midline. Similarly, the vertical meridians in visuotopic representations are interconnected by callosal fibres, whereas the periphery is not. In contrast, the second function of the commissures is to connect areas in one hemisphere with areas on the other side, where the functions of each are represented on only one side, i.e. they are lateralized. Of course, this is most apparent for language areas; for example, objects held in the non-dominant hand cannot be named following callosal section because the sensory cortex of the non-dominant hemisphere cannot communicate across the midline with the language and speech areas in the dominant hemisphere.

(b) Ipsilateral corticocortical association connections

All cortical areas interconnect with other areas in the same hemisphere. The primary sensory areas are in the parietal, occipital, and temporal lobes. From these, parallel pathways emanate in an approximately hierarchical sequence through multiple areas in the adjacent association cortex, passing towards the medial temporal lobe where all pathways converge on the parahippocampal gyrus and the cortex of the temporal pole. In general, three 'tiers' of association areas can be recognized in this sequence; the first tier receives from the core sensory areas, and the third projects into the temporal pole and the parahippocampal gyrus. Connections passing in the direction of the medial temporal cortex from the primary sensory areas have a feedforward pattern of termination, whereas the reciprocal connections have a feedback character. Although the interconnections of the multiple areas along this sequence of connections are complex, a broad pattern common to all the sensory pathways can be discerned. Essentially, each sensory modality has a core zone in the cortex, comprising three areas. Each of these is linked to the relevant main thalamic nuclei and contains a complete representation of the sensory surround. They are linked together by short association connections passing forwards from the first thalamo-recipient zone in a stepwise fashion to the other two. Two streams of connections, dealing with different aspects of sensory perception, emanate from these into the surrounding association areas. One of these, the ventral stream (the 'stimulus-relevant' or 'what' system), is primarily concerned with a detailed perception and characterization of the stimulus. The second, the dorsal stream (the 'self-relevant' or 'where' system), is concerned mainly with spatial location, particularly in extrapersonal space. Each area in this sensory hierarchy is reciprocally connected to a part of the frontal lobe, where the dual-pathway streams are represented by a dorsal and a ventral prefrontal subdivision, feeding onto the supplementary and premotor cortex, and so to the motor cortex.

(c) Cortical association pathways for vision (Fig. 2.3.1.4)

The three core visual areas are V1 (the primary visual cortex, striate cortex), V2 which surrounds V1 and is contained within Brodmann's area 18, and outside this the V3 complex which is probably still within area 18. From these, feedforward projections pass to areas in the inferior parietal and superior temporal cortices, as the dorsal stream, and to V4, within Brodmann's area 19, at the junction of the occipital association cortex with the inferior temporal gyrus on the medial surface, forming the ventral pathway. Areas in the superior temporal sulcus and middle temporal gyrus form the next two tiers of association cortex for the dorsal pathway. The ventral route progresses via the posterior inferotemporal cortex on to the anterior inferotemporal cortex. Both the anterior inferotemporal and middle temporal cortical areas at the distal end of these two visual association pathways project to the cortex of the temporal pole, and to the parahippocampal gyrus. The parahippocampal gyrus projects to the entorhinal cortex more anteriorly, and the temporal pole connects with the amygdala. The entorhinal cortex provides a major input to the dentate gyrus of the hippocampus via the perforant path as seen in the figure. Similarly, the amygdala projects into the hippocampal formation.

(d) Cortical association pathways for somatic sensation (Fig. 2.3.1.3)

The three core areas for the somatic sensory cortex are Brodmann's areas 3, 1, and 2 on the postcentral gyrus, together constituting the classical primary somatic sensory cortex. Each receives a major input from the ventral posterior nucleus of the thalamus and contains a complete representation of the body. Area 3 projects forwards to areas 1 and 2, and area 1 projects similarly to area 2. All three areas project in a feedforward fashion to the second somatic sensory area in the parietal operculum. This represents the first step on the ventral association pathway. The dorsal pathway begins with the projection of all subdivisions of the primary somatic sensory cortex to Brodmann's area 5 in the superior parietal cortex. Further steps along the ventral pathway are areas in the insula. In the ventral pathway, information flows from the superior to the inferior parietal cortex, and so to the middle temporal gyrus. Areas at the ends of both these paths project onto the parahippocampal gyrus and the temporal pole.

(e) Cortical association pathways for hearing (Fig. 2.3.1.5)

The association pathways from the auditory cortex are less well understood. The three core areas lie along Heschl's gyrus in the temporal operculum, with the classical primary auditory area (AI) most posterior, the rostral auditory area (AII) more anterior, and the rostrotemporal auditory area in front of that. Each of these contains a complete representation of the auditory surround, organized tonotopically, and connects with the medial geniculate nucleus. On either side of these lie multiple auditory association areas, termed the medial and lateral belt areas, representing the first steps along the two association streams of connections, although it is unclear which is 'dorsal' and which is 'ventral' in a functional sense. The medial belt areas have connections with parts of the insula, whereas the lateral belt areas project into the association cortex of the superior temporal gyrus. The first association pathway probably continues through areas of the anterior part of the superior temporal gyrus, and so to the parahippocampal gyrus and the temporal pole. The second continues from the superior to the middle temporal gyrus, and thence to the parahippocampal cortex and the temporal pole.

(f) The olfactory pathway to the cerebral cortex (Fig. 2.3.1.6)

The olfactory pathway is unique among the sensory modalities in having direct access to the cerebral cortex without passing through the thalamus. The primary olfactory receptor neurones of the olfactory mucosa send their axons (the fila olfactaria) through the cribriform plate of the ethmoid bone directly into the overlying olfactory bulb, where they contact the mitral cells in synaptic glomeruli. Axons of the mitral cells pass caudally in the olfactory tract to the anterior perforated substance. Here the olfactory tract splits into medial and lateral olfactory striae. All the mitral cell axons pass in the lateral stria. The medial stria contains axons mainly from the anterior olfactory nucleus, which are destined for the contralateral olfactory bulb by way of the anterior commissure. The lateral olfactory stria passes to the medial temporal lobe, where the axons terminate in the anterior margin of the entorhinal cortex, the pyriform cortex, and the corticomedial subdivision of the amygdala. All three termination zones interconnect. The olfactory entorhinal cortex and the olfactory amygdala both have connections with their non-olfactory partners, i.e. with the more posterior entorhinal subdivisions and the basolateral part of the amygdala respectively.

(g) The limbic cortex and the amygdala (Figs 2.3.1.6 and 2.3.1.8)

The latter stages of the sensory association pathways all converge on the entorhinal cortex, the perirhinal cortex, and the amygdala, which are themselves interconnected. These in turn project to the hippocampus. The perirhinal cortex lies lateral to the entorhinal cortex in the banks of the rhinal fissure. It appears to receive afferents from the later stages of the sensory association pathways, notably from the temporal pole, and is extensively interconnected with the amygdala, the entorhinal cortex, and the hippocampus. The amygdala projects to the CA pyramidal cells, notably to CA1. The entorhinal input to the hippocampus arises from cell clusters in layer II and forms the perforant pathway, with axons terminating on the dendrites of granule cells of the dentate gyrus. Additional entorhinal fibres pass to the CA pyramidal cells. Axons of the dentate gyrus granule cells pass out into the molecular layer of the CA fields, notably CA3, where they synapse on the apical dendrites of pyramidal neurones. CA3 pyramidal cells project out via the fimbria, but also send collateral axons to synapse with the pyramidal cells of CA1 in particular. The activity of pyramidal neurones in the CA fields is regulated by inhibitory GABA-ergic interneurones in the molecular layer and by the basket cells, which are also GABA-ergic, sited immediately subjacent to the pyramidal layer. The latter inhibitory neurones have axons that branch around the pyramidal cell bodies, forming the baskets of terminal fibres from which they are named. CA1 sends some fibres into the fornix, but projects heavily to the subicular complex. The major output of the hippocampal formation comes from the subicular complex, and passes out into the fornix via the alveus and fimbria. The projection of fibres in the fornix to the hypothalamus, including the mamillary nuclei, is considered below. However, some hippocampal efferent fibres bypass these nuclei and enter the mamillothalamic tract without synapsing. Rather they pass directly to the anterior thalamic nuclei, where they terminate. From the anterior thalamic nuclei, of which there are several subdivisions, axons project to the cortex of the cingulate gyrus along the whole of its length, extending into the parahippocampal gyrus inferiorly. Fibres forming the cingulum bundle interconnect these medial cortical areas, running predominantly from anterior to posterior and ending in the parahippocampal gyrus, so that they reach the entorhinal cortex. This completes Papez's circuit and defines the structures of the limbic lobe—hippocampal formation, mamillary nuclei and anterior thalamus, cingulate cortex, parahippocampal gyrus and cingulate cortex. The term 'limbic system' is often extended to include structures, such as the amygdala, which have strong connections with these components.

(h) Association connections of the frontal lobe (Fig. 2.3.1.2)

The hierarchical sequence of connections in the sensory association pathways outlined above is reflected in a similar sequence passing from association areas of the prefrontal cortex back towards the primary motor cortex of the precentral gyrus. The two streams of connections are tightly linked together by long association pathways, with each tier of connections in the sensory association pathways interconnected with an area of the frontal lobe. The medial temporal areas, including the entorhinal cortex, the perirhinal cortex and the parahippocampal gyrus are closely interconnected with areas in the orbitofrontal cortex. The temporal pole is reciprocally connected with the frontal pole (Brodmann's area 10). The tiers of sensory association areas in the parietal, occipital, and temporal cortex are interconnected with the dorsolateral and ventrolateral prefrontal association cortex, occupying Brodmann's areas 9, 46, and 45. Broadly speaking, the association areas on the dorsal stream of connections for each modality interconnect with the dorsolateral prefrontal areas 9 and 46. In contrast, the ventral stream areas interconnect with the ventrolateral prefrontal cortex in areas 45 and 46. Like the sensory association areas, these regions seem to separate functionally into a dorsal hierarchy, dealing with internally generated actions, and a ventral hierarchy related to externally guided behaviours. Connections from the dorsolateral prefrontal cortex pass preferentially to the supplementary motor cortex, whereas the more ventrally placed prefrontal cortex feeds into the premotor cortex. Both the supplementary and the premotor cortex feed into the primary motor cortex of the precentral gyrus. The frontal eye-field (Brodmann's area 8), which has major ipsilateral association connections with the visual areas in the occipital lobe, is strategically placed between the prefrontal and premotor areas. It also receives ipsilateral association connections from the dorsolateral and ventrolateral prefrontal association areas.

(i) Speech areas of the cerebral cortex

Because speech and language are not present in the subhuman primate species commonly used for neuroanatomical investigation of cortical connections, little is known about the connections of these in the human. The posterior speech area (Wernicke's area) occupies a large extent of the posterior temporal and inferior parietal cortex at the posterior limits of the superior temporal and lateral sulci, and is often taken as extending anteriorly along the superior temporal gyrus. It includes the angular and supramarginal gyri (Fig. 2.3.1.9). This would represent a region where the association pathways of all three modalities—somatic sensation, vision, and hearing—lie close together. It would include many auditory association areas along the superior temporal gyrus. Within the frontal lobe, Broca's area occupies the pars triangularis between the anterior and ascending rami of the lateral sulcus. It is closely adjacent to the face area in the lateral premotor cortex. Similarly, the medial speech area lies on the medial surface immediately in front of the face representation in the supplementary motor cortex. It is, perhaps, not unreasonable to suppose that these two areas function to some extent as the premotor and supplementary motor speech areas.

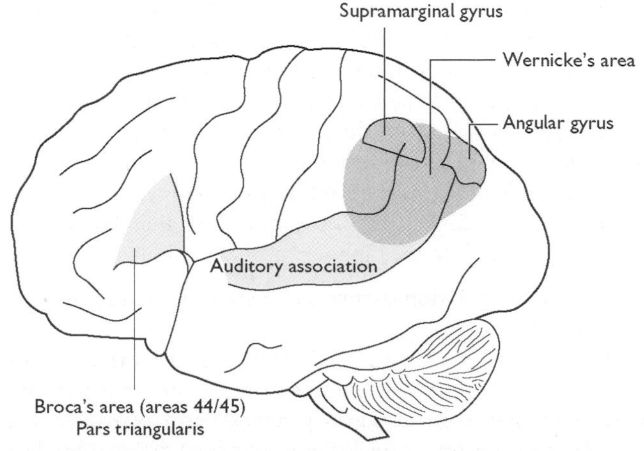

Fig. 2.3.1.9 Auditory association cortex and Wernicke's sensory speech area.

Subcortical efferent pathways of the cerebral cortex

The corticostriate pathway and the basal ganglia (Fig. 2.3.1.10)

The anatomical definition of the basal ganglia comprises those deep grey matter nuclei that develop from the telencephalic (cerebral) vesicle. Strictly, this would include the components of the striatum, the globus pallidus, the amygdala, and the claustrum. Because these latter two are better considered with the cortex and limbic system respectively, they are usually excluded from the term basal ganglia. Similarly, because of their close anatomical and functional relationship with the striatum and globus pallidus, the substantia nigra and subthalamic nucleus are usually included with the basal ganglia. The caudate and putamen are developmentally, anatomically, pharmacologically, and functionally a single structure, secondarily subdivided by the development of the internal capsule. The two fuse below the inferior margin of the anterior limb of the internal capsule to form the nucleus accumbens. This fusion comes to the surface of the hemisphere at the anterior perforated substance, an area sometimes called the olfactory tubercle. Together, the caudate, putamen, nucleus accumbens, and olfactory tubercle make up the striatum. The globus pallidus consists of two parts, an external segment (GPe) and an internal segment (GPi), separated by a thin white-matter lamina. Both segments extend ventrally in the region of the substantia innominata, below the anterior commissure, to form the ventral pallidum. The pars reticulata of the substantia nigra (SNpr) is developmentally, anatomically, pharmacologically and functionally a part of the internal segment of the globus pallidus, which has been separated off by the development of the fibres of the internal capsule passing into the crus cerebri of the midbrain. Therefore, in this account the basal ganglia and related nuclei will comprise the striatum, GPe, GPi-SNpr, and the subthalamic nucleus (see Fig. 2.3.1.10).

The entire cerebral cortex projects to the striatum. The putamen receives predominantly from the sensorimotor cortex around the central sulcus. The caudate receives the input from most of the parietal, occipital, temporal, and frontal lobes. The limbic areas, including the entorhinal and perirhinal cortex, the hippocampus, and the amygdala, project to the ventral striatum (nucleus accumbens and olfactory tubercle) and the adjacent ventral portion of the head of the caudate. The corticostriate pathway arises from pyramidal cells predominantly in layer V of the cortex and is excitatory, using glutamate as its neurotransmitter. The termination of the pathway is broadly topographically organized, but with considerable interdigitation or overlap of the projections from different cortical areas. Individual cortical areas project to a longitudinal strip of striatum orientated anteroposteriorly. The strips receiving from the frontal lobe extend more rostrally, whereas those receiving from the parietal, occipital, and temporal lobes extend more caudally. Anteriorly, zones receiving projections from interconnected areas in the frontal lobe interdigitate or overlap; centrally, zones receiving from frontal areas overlap with zones connected to areas within the parietal, temporal, or occipital cortex with which the frontal areas are connected by ipsilateral association fibres. More posteriorly, interconnected sensory association areas

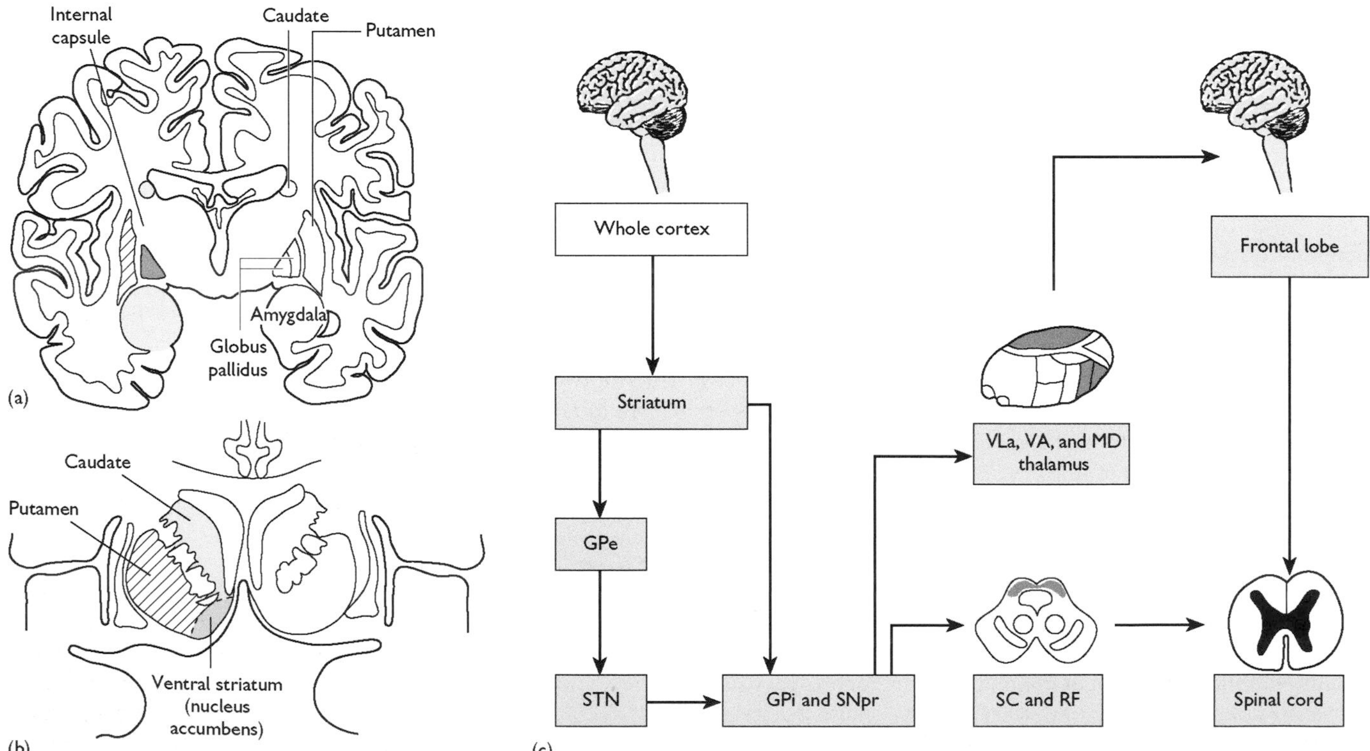

Fig. 2.3.1.10 The corticostriate pathway and the basal ganglia: (a) component nuclei of the basal ganglia; (b) striatum; (c) major pathways through the basal ganglia. GPe, external segment of the globus pallidus; STN, subthalamic nucleus; GPi, internal segment of the globus pallidus; SNpr, pars reticula of the substantia nigra.

project to overlapping zones in the striatum. The striatum itself is compartmentalized, on the basis of acetylcholinesterase (AChE) histochemistry, into AChE-poor patches (striosomes) and AChE-rich matrix. The cortex projects into both compartments, but with a slightly different laminar origin. Pyramidal neurones in the deeper part of lamina V project to the patches, whereas more superficial lamina V cells and some lamina III cells project to the matrix. It is possible that apparently overlapping corticostriate projections from different cortical areas are segregated into the different compartments. The projection from a single cortical area may switch between compartments along the anteroposterior length of its zone of termination. The intralaminar nuclei of the thalamus sends excitatory (glutamatergic) axons to the entire striatum. The nuclei project to those parts of the caudate or putamen which receive from the cortical areas and to which the particular intralaminar nucleus projects. Many, if not all, interconnected areas in the frontal, parietal, occipital, and temporal lobes also receive a shared projection from a single intralaminar nucleus. Thus, there is a tightly organized but complex topographical relationship between the connections of functionally related cortical areas with each other, with the striatum, and with the intralaminar nuclei of the thalamus. A closely similar relationship is seen in the cortical connections of the claustrum and the basal forebrain, and possibly even in the cortical projection to the pontine nuclei. Another major projection to the striatum is dopaminergic and comes from the pars compacta of the substantia nigra and adjacent nuclei. There is some topography in this projection, with the lateral and central parts of pars compacta of the substantia nigra projecting to the caudate and putamen. The medial part and the adjacent nuclei, such as the ventral tegmental area, project to the ventral striatum. The effect of dopamine on striatal neurones appears to be different in the two compartments. Additional striatal afferents come from the brainstem raphe nuclei (serotonin) and the amygdala (to the ventral striatum and the head of the caudate).

The output of the striatum passes to all parts of the globus pallidus (the ventral pallidum, GPe, and GPi-SNpr). These fibres are inhibitory, using GABA as their neurotransmitter. Here, the pathway through the basal ganglia separates into a direct and an indirect route, ultimately passing to the thalamus. Fibres from the striosomes (patches) of the striatum are rich in substance P (as well as being GABA-ergic) and project to GPi. Axons from GPi go directly to the anterior part of the ventral lateral nucleus and the adjacent ventral anterior nucleus of the thalamus, forming the direct route. Neurones in the striatal matrix compartment contain enkephalin as a cotransmitter with GABA and project to GPe. Axons from GPe go to the subthalamic nucleus, which in turn projects to GPi (the indirect pathway). The ventral pallidum has equivalent pathways, but the final destination of the pallidal output is the mediodorsal nucleus of the thalamus. All efferents from the globus pallidus are GABA-ergic and inhibitory. The neurones of the subthalamic nucleus are glutamatergic and excitatory. Activation of the striatal output through the direct pathway leads to a reduced tonic inhibition of the thalamus. In contrast, activation via the indirect pathway leads to increased activation of GPi, and hence increased inhibition of the thalamus. The balance between these opposite effects is crucial in the normal functioning of the basal ganglia. Disruption of this balance is used to explain much of the pathophysiology of the extrapyramidal disorders. The ventral anterior and rostral ventral lateral nuclei of the thalamus project mainly to the premotor and supplementary motor areas of the frontal lobe. The ventral pallidal pathway through the mediodorsal thalamus feeds onto the prefrontal association areas. The major pathways through the basal ganglia are summarized in Fig. 2.3.1.10(c)).

The corticopontine pathway and the cerebellum

There is a major projection from the cortex to the pontine nuclei. The extent to which individual cortical areas contribute to this pathway varies. The greatest projection comes from the regions around the central sulcus, which also contribute to the pyramidal tract (see below). However, there is a substantial projection from the prefrontal cortex and a significant number of fibres from the occipital lobe. Many fewer corticopontine axons arise from temporal neocortex, although some areas send some and it is possible that most areas send at least a few.

The pontine nuclei send their axons to the cerebellar cortex of the lateral parts of the posterior lobe. They terminate as mossy fibres, contacting granule cells. Axon collaterals pass, in addition, to the lateral dentate deep cerebellar nucleus. The anterior lobe and the midline and paramedian region of the posterior lobe are related to the spinocerebellar inputs. The flocculonodular lobe is connected to the vestibular pathway. The Purkinje cells of the cerebellar cortex send inhibitory fibres to the deep cerebellar nuclei, and it is from these that the output of the cerebellum arises. The intermediate (globose and emboliform) and medial (fastigial) deep nuclei project to the red nucleus and the vestibular nuclei and reticular formation. The dentate nucleus projects to the posterior part of the ventral lateral nucleus of the thalamus. This in turn provides the major thalamic input to the primary motor cortex of the precentral gyrus. In this way, the neocortical input to the cerebellum is transmitted via the pontine nuclei,and to the motor cortex via the thalamus.

The fornix and the cortical projection to the hypothalamus

Fibres leaving and entering the hippocampus form a thin white-matter covering on the ventricular surface, deep to the ependyma, called the alveus. These fibres pass into the fornix via the fimbria. The fornix passes initially posteriorly and superiorly, then anteriorly, curving around the outer curve of the lateral ventricle and angling towards the midline in its course. The fornices of the two sides come together at about the junction of the posterior third and anterior two-thirds of the corpus callosum. Many fibres pass across the midline, the commissure of the fornix, and turn caudally to enter the contralateral hippocampus. The two fornices, united in the midline, are suspended from the corpus callosum by the septum pellucidum as they arch over the roof of the third ventricle and the choroid fissure of the body of the lateral ventricle. They turn ventrally, immediately in front of the interventricular foramen of Monroe. The two fornices separate, and each divides into an anterior and a posterior column, passing in front of and behind the anterior commissure. The anterior column carries axons to and from the septal nuclei CA3, CA1, and the subiculum project to the lateral septal nucleus. This has diverse efferent projections to the hypothalamus, the epithalamus, and the midline thalamus, but also projects to the adjacent medial septal nucleus. The medial septal nucleus is the major source of cholinergic fibres to the hippocampus via the fornix. The posterior column of the fornix curves posteriorly through the hypothalamus, giving off many fibres to medial and lateral hypothalamic nuclei. It ends in the mamillary nuclei, which in turn project via the mamillothalamic tract to the anterior thalamus. This projection is partially bilateral.

There is a major input to the hypothalamus from the amygdala, via the stria terminalis, a white-matter tract that follows the curve of the caudate nucleus around the lateral ventricle, lying between the caudate and the thalamus. The connections between the hypothalamus and amygdala are reciprocal.

Direct projections to the cortex from the hypothalamus have been discussed earlier. Direct projections from neocortex to the hypothalamus have been described, but their extent and distribution are disputed. If they exist in the human, they probably arise from the prefrontal/orbitofrontal and insular cortex.

The corticobulbar and corticospinal pathways

The direct projection of the cortex to the brainstem and spinal cord, the pyramidal tract, arises from the cortex in front of and behind the central sulcus. About 40 per cent of fibres arise from the primary somatic sensory cortex and the adjacent superior parietal lobe. In the frontal lobe, axons arise from the primary motor, premotor, and supplementary motor areas. Apart from the direct innervation of the spinal cord and motor nuclei of the cranial nerves, direct cortical fibres innervate the red nucleus, the vestibular nuclei, the reticular formation, and the superior colliculus. In the case of the first two of these, the origin of the fibres is probably very similar to the areas of origin of the pyramidal tract. In contrast, the cortical projections to the reticular formation and superior colliculus have a much wider origin, and may include most neocortical areas to a greater or lesser degree.

The contribution of neuroanatomy to psychiatry

The above is a necessarily abbreviated account of the anatomy of the central nervous system, centring on the organization and connections of the cortex including the limbic lobe. Topographical neuroanatomy has been ignored, despite its importance in the reading of modern images of the brain in living patients. For psychiatry, the importance of the connectionist view of the brain lies in the contribution it can make to the understanding of the normal and pathological functioning of the central nervous system. Present-day neuropsychology and cognitive neuroscience are aimed towards understanding the highest levels of central nervous system processing and function. It is these areas or systems that are commonly involved in the signs and symptoms of major psychiatric disease. It is to the pathways underlying cognition, perception, memory, mood, and attention that the psychiatrist interested in the pathophysiology of mental illness must turn his or her attention, and it is this area that the above account has attempted to review.

Further information

Gloor, P. (1977). *The temporal lobe and limbic system*. Oxford University Press.

Pearson, R.C.A. (1995). Dorsal thalamus. In *Gray's anatomy* (38th edn) (ed. P.L. Williams, L.H. Bannister, M.M. Berry, *et al.*), pp. 1080–91. Churchill Livingstone, Edinburgh.

Pearson, R.C.A. (1995). Cerebral cortex. In *Gray's anatomy* (38th edn) (ed. P.L. Williams, L.H. Bannister, M.M. Berry, *et al.*), pp. 1141–71. Churchill Livingstone, Edinburgh.

Passingham, R. (1993). *The frontal lobes and voluntary action*. Oxford University Press.

Paxinos, G. (ed.) (1990). *The human nervous system*. Academic Press, San Diego, CA.

Tovée, M.J. (1996). *An introduction to the visual system*. Cambridge University Press.

Zeki, S. (1993). *A vision of the brain*. Blackwell Science, Oxford.

2.3.2 Neurodevelopment

Karl Zilles

Neural induction

The central nervous system originates from the midline region of the embryo as a specialized area of ectoderm, the neuroectoderm, or neural plate. FGF (fibroblast growth factor) signalling and BMP (bone morphogenetic protein) as well as Wnt (wingless gene) inhibition are required as steps for neural induction.(1) However, the complete set of factors and their respective interactions are presently not sufficiently understood in the mammalian embryo. As the neuroectodermal cells proliferate the neural plate is transformed into an indentation, the neural groove. The lateral parts of this groove approach each other and join in the midline, forming the neural tube. The folds begin to fuse in the central part of the groove but the most rostral and caudal parts close only later, leaving initially rostral and caudal neuropores. A small transitional zone between the neural plate and the surrounding ectoderm provides the cells of the neural crest, which develop into the postganglionic cells of the sympathetic and parasympathetic nervous system, the sensory neurons of the spinal ganglia and ganglia of cranial nerves, Schwann cells, and chromaffine cells of the suprarenal glands.

Neural tube formation requires a controlled expression of cell adhesion molecules in the lateral folds of the neural groove. If the rostral neuropore fails to close, the development of the forebrain is impaired leading to anencephaly. If the caudal neuropore fails to close, the most severe result is rachischisis, a malformation with a dorsally exposed neural groove. The mildest result is spina bifida occulta which is a cleft of a vertebral arch covered by epidermis.

As development continues, the neural tube and crest move to a position between the ectoderm and the notochord. The rostral part of the neural tube differentiates into the brain; the caudal part (behind the fifth somite) differentiates into the spinal cord.

Organogenesis of the central nervous system

The embryonic brain has three vesicular enlargements: the forebrain, telencephalon and diencephalon, the midbrain, mesencephalon, and the hindbrain, rhombencephalon. Because the brain grows much faster than the rest of the embryo, it becomes deflected ventrally. A dorsally convex cephalic flexure marks the border between hindbrain and midbrain, and a cervical flexure marks the border between spinal cord and hindbrain (Fig. 2.3.2.1). The ventrally convex pontine flexure forms the hindbrain. During week 5, the forebrain differentiates further into the rostral telencephalon and the more caudal diencephalon. The telencephalon consists of two hemispheric vesicles connected by a thin lamina terminalis, the most dorsal part of which develops into the commissural plate, the *Anlage* of the corpus callosum. The ventral part of the lamina terminalis differentiates into the anterior commissure. The central cavity of the diencephalon (the third ventricle) is connected with the cavities of the hemispheric vesicles (the lateral ventricles) by the interventricular foramen. The diencephalon develops bilateral evaginations, the eye vesicles, which differentiate into the retina and the optic nerve. Meanwhile the hindbrain becomes subdivided into a rostral metencephalon and a caudal myelencephalon.

The cerebellum starts to develop from the metencephalon during week 6 (Fig. 2.3.2.1). At first, the enlarged central cavity of the neural tube (the future fourth ventricle) has a thin roof plate bordered by two thickenings of the neural tube, the rhomboid lips, which merge in the midline. These thickenings develop into the cerebellar hemispheres, while the midline part develops into the vermis of the cerebellum. Fissures appear in the cerebellar hemispheres, forming the anterior and posterior lobes and the uvula.

The rhombencephalon is temporarily divided into eight rhombomeres,[2] whose borders are specified by specific combinations of transcription factors (e.g. Hox, Krox, Wnt genes) disappear during further development. Local expression of homeobox genes leads to the formation of the pallium and the ganglionic hill in the forebrain.

The hindbrain develops in close association with the visceral arches, which appear during week 4. It innervates these arches and the organs derived from them by a group of branchial nerves, which later become the trigeminal (V), facial (VII), glossopharyngeal (IX), vagal (X), and accessory (XI) cranial nerves. Other cranial nerves develop connections between the hindbrain and peripheral organs not derived from the visceral archs. They are the oculomotor (III), trochlear (IV), abducens (VI), vestibulocochlear (VIII), and hypoglossal (XII) nerves. The olfactory (I) and optic (II) nerves arise separately as evaginations of the forebrain.

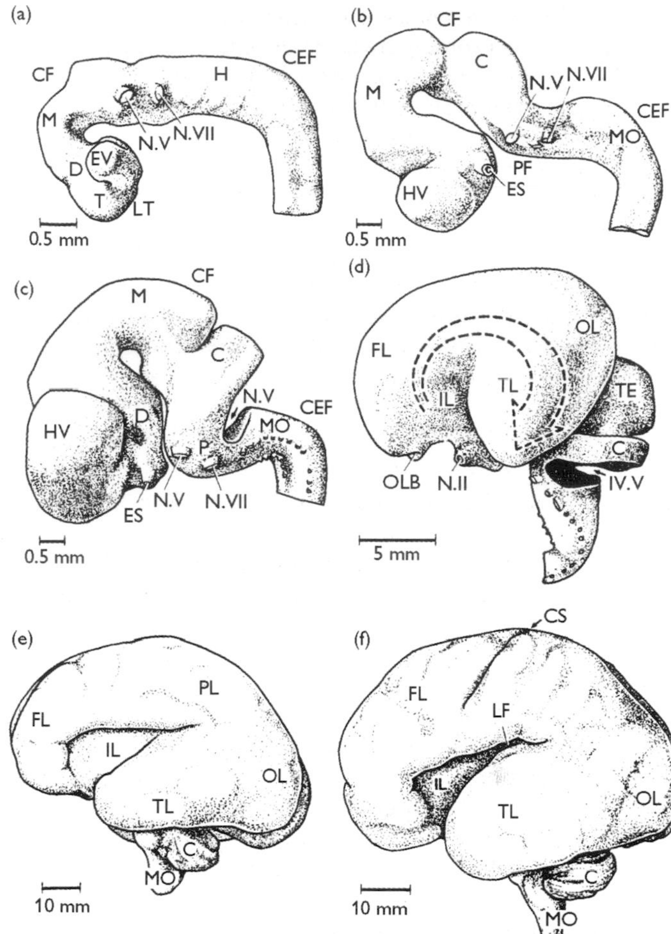

Fig. 2.3.2.1 Development of the human brain. Brains of (a) 4 mm, (b) 10.4 mm (c), 13.8 mm, and (d) 53 mm human embryos, and (e) 21 week and (f) 24 week fetuses. C, cerebellum or cerebellar *Anlage*; CEF, cervical flexure; CF, cephalic flexure; CS, central sulcus; D, diencephalon; ES, eye stalk; EV, eye vesicle; FL, frontal lobe; H, hindbrain; HV, hemispheric vesicle; IL, insular lobe; LF, lateral fissure; LT, lamina terminalis; M, mesencephalon; MO, medulla oblongata; N.II, optic nerve; N.V, trigeminal nerve; N. VII, facial nerve; OL, occipital lobe; OLB, olfactory bulb; P, pons; PF, pontine flexure; PL, parietal lobe; T, telencephalon; TE, tectum; TL, temporal lobe; IV.V, fourth ventricle.

Histogenesis of the spinal cord

The neural tube initially consists of a single layer of neuroepithelial cells surrounding a central canal filled with the cerebrospinal fluid. The outer surface of the future spinal cord has an external limiting membrane, and the inner surface bordering the central canal has an inner limiting membrane. The entire wall of the early neural tube is called the ventricular zone.[3]

The cells of the ventricular zone proliferate, and the surface of the spinal cord enlarges. The cord then thickens as cells divide further to produce a multilayered epithelium. The daughter cells have different potentialities: one type of cell (the neuroblast) retains the capability for mitosis, whereas another type (the proneurone) is postmitotic and represents an immature neurone. The proliferation of neurones is almost complete around birth.

Some neuroepithelial cells develop into precursors of glial cells, glioblasts, which differentiate into astroglial, oligodendroglial, and microglial cells. The first glioblasts differentiate into radially extended cells spanning the entire width of the wall of the spinal cord (the same occurs in the cerebral hemispheres and the cerebellar cortex as described below). During later development these cells are transformed into ependymal cells and astroglia.

The histogenesis of the spinal cord starts at the cervical level and progresses in a caudal direction. After week 3, a longitudinal sulcus limitans is recognizable on the inner surface of the neural tube, dividing the wall into dorsal (alar) and ventral (basal) plates. The dorsal plates of both sides are connected by a thin roof plate, and the ventral plates by a thin floor plate. The dorsal plate differentiates into a sensory zone, the dorsal horn of the adult spinal cord, and the ventral plate differentiates into a motor zone, the ventral horn. The sympathetic preganglionic neurones form the lateral horn, which is present only at thoracic levels. The subdivision into dorsal and ventral plates is functionally important not only in the spinal cord, but also in the brainstem (see below).

During week 5, three concentrically organized zones—a cell-dense ventricular zone, a less-dense intermediate or mantle zone, and a superficially located marginal zone free of neuronal cells—develop in the wall of the spinal cord. Proneurones leave the ventricular zone and migrate along radial glial cells into the intermediate zone where they become organized into cell groups, nuclei. The motor neurones develop the axons of the ventral root, and the processes from spinal ganglionic cells grow into the spinal cord to form the dorsal roots. Synapses develop first in the motor zone, and later in the sensory zone, during the weeks 10 to 13.

During the third month, the ventricular zone is reduced to a small rim surrounding the central canal and is finally transformed into the ependymal cell layer. The intermediate zone becomes organized into dorsal, ventral, and (at thoracic levels) lateral horns. The ascending and descending fibre tracts of the spinal cord are increased in size in the marginal zone. During weeks 14 and 15, oligodendrocytes begin to myelinate these fibre tracts. The corticospinal, or pyramidal, tract is visible for the first time during week 14 and reaches its target neurones, mainly motor neurones of the ventral horn, between weeks 17 and 29. The myelination of the pyramidal tract is completed between the first and second postnatal years. This late myelination explains the presence of the Babinski reflex in newborns and its disappearance during the first 2 years.

Histogenesis of the brainstem and cerebellum

At the level of the fourth ventricle the various zones of the hindbrain are arranged in a lateral-to-medial sequence (somatosensory-viscerosensory-visceromotor-somatomotor). In the hindbrain, proneurones not only migrate radially, as in the spinal cord, but also tangentially and longitudinally. This complex migration and the growth of fibre tracts lead to changes of the lateral-to-medial sequence of cranial nerve nuclei (e.g. the facial nucleus) in the adult.

In the cerebellum, between weeks 10 and 11, neuroblasts migrate from the ventricular zone through the intermediate zone into an area (the external granular layer) at the surface of the marginal zone. During weeks 12 and 13, proneurones from the ventricular zone begin to migrate along radially extended glial cells, Bergmann glia, into a region below this external granular layer, where they form the Purkinje cells of the ganglionic layer of the cerebellar cortex. Other proneurones from the ventricular zone develop into the cerebellar nuclei. Proneurones from the external granular layer then migrate inwards to form the internal granular layer and the basket and star cells of the molecular layer. The migration of cerebellar proneurones is not completed until the first postnatal year. During weeks 16 and 26, synapses develop and afferent fibre systems begin to form. The external granular layer finally disappears during the first 2 years of life, leaving the three-layered organization (molecular, ganglionic, and internal granular layers) of the adult cerebellar cortex.

Histogenesis of the cerebral cortex

Initially, the entire wall of the hemispheric vesicle consists of very densely packed mitotic cells. These cells undergo more than 28 mitotic rounds in the human brain.[4] In week 5, this develops into an inner cell-dense periventricular zone and an outer cell-poor marginal zone. In week 6, postmitotic proneurones leave the inner periventricular zone and form an intermediate (mantle) zone between the marginal and periventricular zones. By the end of week 6, the periventricular zone is further subdivided into a cell-dense ventricular zone and a less cell-dense subventricular zone.

During week 8, the cortical plate between the marginal and intermediate zones is formed by proneurones which have migrated along radial glial cells from the ventricular and subventricular zones through the intermediate zone.[3–7] A single radial glial cell can span the entire distance between the ventricular and pial surfaces. As the proneurones 'climb' to the cortical plate along the processes of the radial glial cell, they produce a vertically oriented cortical cell column. This radially guided migration is responsible for the architectonic organization of cortical layers II–VI. It is a prototype of the cortical map of the adult brain.[8] A further feature of cortical migration is the inside-to-outside layering, with the earliest proneurones being found in the deepest layers of the cortical plate and the latest in the most superficial layers. Thus layers V and VI of the adult cortex are generated before layer IV, and layer IV is generated before layers III and II. When cortical proneurones are migrating radially, their 'stop signal' is Reelin, produced by specialized cells (Cajal–Retzius cells) in the marginal layer. In this way, Reelin organizes the inside-to-outside layering of the cortex.[4] In addition to Reelin, the microtubule-associated protein (LIS1), Doublecortin (DCX), and the tumour-suppressor p73 are crucial for the normal migration of the proneurones. These radially migrating cells develop into the glutamatergic projection neurones (pyramidal neurones) of the cortex. At the same time there is much tangential migration of cells born in the ganglionic eminence, migrating into the cortical *Anlage*, and developing into γ-aminobutyric acid producing (GABAergic) cortical interneurones.[4,9]

Regional differences in the development of the cortical plate subdivide the hemisphere into segments. The lateral segment, with a well-developed cortical plate and presubplate, develops into the neocortex. The mediodorsal segment, with a wide marginal zone and a thin-folded cortical plate, develops into the archicortex, including the hippocampus. The mediobasal segment, with its inconspiciously developed cortical plate, is the precursor of the palaeocortex. The basolateral segment, ganglionic eminence, generates cortical interneurones (see above) and develops into the corpus striatum, the amygdala, and the septum.

During weeks 10 and 12, the axons of the serotoninergic and noradrenergic neurones contribute to the first synapses in the marginal and presubplate zones, where neurotrophin receptors (see below) are expressed. During the following 3 weeks, the subplate zone develops as axons grow in from the basal forebrain and thalamus, dendrites enlarge, and synapses form. From weeks 16 to 24, the cortical *Anlage* has a small marginal zone, a wide cell-dense cortical plate, and a very wide and less cell-dense subplate.

The transformation into the adult neocortical pattern starts between weeks 25 and 34 as the migration and proliferation of proneurones diminishes. Dendrites begin to differentiate and synapses begin to develop in the deepest cortical layers, progressing to the most superficial layer. Before birth, six cortical layers can be recognized in all regions of the neocortex. In the postnatal period, layer IV (inner granular layer) disappears as part of the differentiation of the motor cortex, leaving the five-layered agranular neocortex of the motor region.[10] Shortly before birth, the subplate, the subventricular zone, and most of the ventricular zone disappear, neuronal proliferation ceases, and the intermediate zone is transformed into the white matter of the pallium. The remaining ventricular zone contributes to the ependymal layer of the ventricular surface.

Dendritic and axonal differentiation continues after birth and into adult life. Synaptogenesis reaches a maximum during the first postnatal year, but continues at a lower rate during childhood. The myelination of the vestibular system is finished shortly before birth, that of the somatosensory, visual, auditory, pyramidal, and extrapyramidal fibre tracts is nearly complete by the end of the third postnatal year, and that of the associative fibre tracts in the cerebral hemispheres is continued until the second decade.[11] The key change in synapses after birth is pruning; the density of synapses in the adult brain is half that in neonates.

The development of the neocortex is summarized in Fig. 2.3.2.2.

Hemispheric shape and the formation of gyri

The spherical shape of the early foetal hemisphere is transformed into the adult shape by differing rates of growth in the various regions of the telencephalon (Fig. 2.3.2.1). The future insular lobe grows less than other telencephalic regions, so that by the eighth month it is covered by the frontal, parietal, and temporal lobes. In the adult brain the insula is completely buried in the depth of the lateral fissure.

The extensive growth of the parieto-occipito-temporal association cortex leads to a bend in the temporal lobe around the lateral fissure. At the same time the temporal pole is pushed rostrally. This direction of growth (Fig. 2.3.2.1(d)) also affects the structures situated dorsomedially, i.e. the archicortex with the hippocampus, the corpus striatum, and the lateral ventricles. The corpus striatum is split by the ingrowing fibres of the internal capsule into the caudate nucleus and the putamen. The head of the caudate is situated ventrolaterally to the corpus callosum in the frontal lobe, and the tail of the caudate is located in the temporal lobe dorsal to the inferior horn of the lateral ventricle. The hippocampus forms its largest extension (the retrocommisssural part) in the temporal lobe, bends around the posterior end (splenium) of the corpus callosum, and reaches a position on top of the corpus callosum (the supracommissural part). The precommissural part of the hippocampus ends in front of the genu of the corpus callosum.

After the appearance of the lateral fissure, the neocortical surface develops many sulci and gyri. The central, collateral, cingulate, parieto-occipital, superior temporal, and calcarine sulci appear between weeks 16 and 21, followed by the pre- and postcentral, frontal, temporal, and intraparietal sulci. Highly variable secondary and tertiary sulci develop between week 29 and birth, when all sulci have been formed.[12,13]

The reasons for the formation of gyri in many mammalian brains, including the human brain, are not completely understood. Since the basic organization of the cerebral cortex is vertically oriented, with cell columns positioned side by side, growth of the cortex inevitably leads to a considerable enlargement of the cortical surface. A large unfolded cortical surface would have two disadvantages: the volume of the skull would increase to such a degree during foetal development that a normal delivery would be impossible; the distance between cortical regions interconnected by intrahemispheric projection fibres would increase and with it the information transmission time. Gyri allow the maximal cortical surface in the minimal volume, and they increase the speed of neural transmission between neighbouring cortical areas. Recent measurements show that gyrification is greatest in the association cortices. Although all gyri and sulci are present at birth, the depth of the sulci increases until two-thirds of the cortical surface is hidden in them.[12]

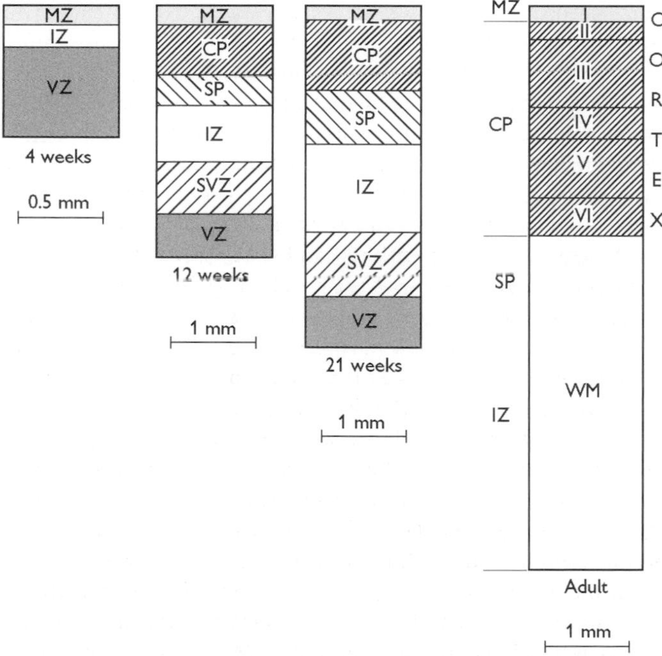

Fig. 2.3.2.2 Development of the neocortex between 4 weeks of gestation and adulthood. Roman numerals indicate the six cytoarchitectonically defined layers of the neocortex, which originate from the marginal zone (layer I) and the cortical plate. CP, cortical plate; IZ, intermediate zone; MZ, marginal zone; SP, subplate; SVZ, subventricular zone; VZ, ventricular zone; WM, white matter.

Genetic factors during development

The co-ordinated expression, in space and time, of many genes underlies neurodevelopment. Mutations in these 'neurodevelopmental genes' are increasingly being recognized as causes of developmental neurological disorders such as cortical dysplasia and epilepsy; they may also be relevant to learning disability and schizophrenia. Different gene families are involved in the major component processes of neurodevelopment, such as organogenesis, neurogenesis, neuronal migration, synaptogenesis, and programmed cell death (apoptosis).[14,15] The details are beyond the scope of this book, but a few examples are given here.

Neurotrophins (growth factors) are genes which, as their name suggests, are critical for neuronal growth and survival, especially via their influence on apoptosis which is promoted by insuffiency of neurotrophins such as nerve growth factor and inhibited by enhanced nerve growth factor functioning. The effects of neurotrophins are mediated by specific tyrosine kinase (Trk) receptors (Table 2.3.2.1). Classical neurotransmitters and their receptors are also involved in neurodevelopment, both directly in the formation of synaptic connections and indirectly through regulation of neurotrophins and Trk receptors; particular roles have been shown for glutamate, acting via *N*-methyl-D-aspartate receptors, as well as for γ-aminobutyric acid (GABA) and acetylcholine.

Table 2.3.2.1 Important neurotrophins, their sites of synthesis in the central nervous system, receptors, and target structures

Neurotrophin	Site of synthesis	Receptors	Target structures
NGF	Hippocampus Neocortex	TrkA, p76^{NTR}	Cholinergic neurones in the basal forebrain
BDNF	Hippocampus Neocortex	TrkB. p75^{NTR}	Dopaminergic neurones in the midbrain; retinal ganglionic cells; cholinergic neurones in the basal forebrain
NT-3	Hippocampus Cerebellum	TrkC, p75^{NTR}	Dopaminergic neurones in the midbrain; neurones of the nucleus mesencephalicus nervi trigemini; neurones of origin of the pyramidal tract

NGF, nerve growth factor; BDNF, brain-derived neurotrophic factor; NT-3, neurotrophin 3.

Further information

Rao, M.S. and Jacobson, M. (eds.) (2005). *Developmental neurobiology*. Kluwer Academic/Plenum Publishers, New York.

Sanes, D.H., Reh, T.H. and Harris, W.A. (2006). *Development of the nervous system* (2nd edn). Academic Press, Amsterdam.

Squire, L.R., Bloom, F.E., McConnell, S.K., *et al.* (eds.) (2005). *Fundamental neuroscience* (2nd edn), chapters 14–21. Academic Press, Amsterdam.

References

1. Ladher, R. and Schoenwolf, G.C. (2005). Making a neural tube: neural induction and neurulation. In *Developmental neurobiology* (eds. M.S. Rao and M. Jacobson), pp. 1–20. Kluwer Academic/Plenum Publishers, New York.
2. Lumsden, A. and Krumlauf, R. (1996). Patterning the vertebrate neuraxis. *Science*, **274**, 1109–15.
3. Kostovic, I. (1990). Zentralnervensystem. In *Humanembryologie* (ed. K.V. Hinrichsen), pp. 381–448. Springer-Verlag, Berlin.
4. Meyer, G. (2007). Genetic control of neuronal migrations in human cortical development. *Advances in Anatomy Embryology and Cell Biology*, **189**, 1–114.
5. Levitt, P. and Rakic, P. (1980). Immunoperoxidase localization of glial fibrillary acid protein in radial glial cells and astrocytes of the developing rhesus monkey brain. *Journal of Comparative Neurology*, **193**, 815–40.
6. Rakic, P. (1985). Limits of neurogenesis in primates. *Science*, **227**, 154–6.
7. Supèr, H., Soriano, E., and Uylings, H.B.M. (1998). The functions of the preplate in development and evolution of the neocortex and hippocampus. *Brain Research Reviews*, **26**, 40–64.
8. Rakic, P. (1988). Specification of cerebral cortical areas. *Science*, **241**, 170–6.
9. Rakic, P. (1995). Radial versus tangential migration of neuronal clones in the developing cerebral cortex. *Proceedings of the National Academy of Sciences of the United States of America*, **92**, 11323–7.
10. Brodmann, K. (1909). *Vergleichende Lokalisationslehre der Großhirnrinde in ihren Prinzipien dargestellt auf Grund des Zellenbaues*. Barth, Leipzig.
11. Yakovlev, P.I. and Lecours, A.-R. (1967). The myelogenetic cycles of regional maturation of the brain. In *Regional development of the brain in early life* (ed. A. Minkowski), pp. 3–70. Blackwell Science, Oxford.
12. Zilles, K., Armstrong, E., Schleicher, A., *et al.* (1988). The human pattern of gyrification in the cerebral cortex. *Anatomy and Embryology*, **179**, 173–9.
13. Armstrong, E., Zilles, K., Omran, H., *et al.* (1995). The ontogeny of human gyrification. *Cerebral Cortex*, **5**, 56–63.
14. Levitt, P., Barbe, M.F., and Eagleson, K.L. (1997). Patterning and specification of the cerebral cortex. *Annual Review of Neuroscience*, **20**, 1–24.
15. Lambert de Rouvroit, C. and Goffinet, A.M. (1998). A new view of early cortical development. *Biochemical Pharmacology*, **56**, 1403–9.

2.3.3 Neuroendocrinology

Charles B. Nemeroff and Gretchen N. Neigh

Definitions and principles

In the late 1950s, a controversy arose in endocrinology and neuroscience concerning whether neurones are capable of manufacturing and secreting hormones; that is to say, is it possible that certain neurones subserve endocrine functions? Much of the ensuing debate, which persisted for approximately two decades, was centred on two major findings. First, led by a husband and wife team, the Scharrers, a number of neurohistologists working with mammalian as well as with lower vertebrate and invertebrate species documented the presence—by both light and electron microscopy—of neurones that had all the characteristics of previously studied endocrine cells. They stained positive with the Gomori stain, which is claimed to be specific to endocrine tissues, and they incorporated granules or vesicles containing the endocrine substance purportedly released by these cells. The second major avenue of investigation centred around the brain's control of the secretion of the pituitary trophic hormones, which in turn were long known to control the secretion of the peripheral target endocrine hormones such as thyroid hormones, gonadal steroids, adrenal steroids, etc. A critical observation by several investigators had earlier demonstrated the existence of a vital neuroendocrine system, namely the magnocellular cells of the paraventricular nucleus of the hypothalamus that synthesized vasopressin and oxytocin, the nonapeptides that are transported down the axon to the nerve terminals of these neurones in the posterior pituitary (neurohypophysis) and released in response to physiological stimuli. For example, the release of vasopressin, or the antidiuretic hormone, as it is commonly named, acts as a critical regulator of fluid balance, and oxytocin is known to regulate the milk-letdown reflex during breast feeding.

It is now firmly established that neurones are indeed capable of functioning as true endocrine tissues, synthesizing and releasing substances, known as (neuro)hormones, which are released directly into the circulatory system and transported to distant sites of action. The release of vasopressin from the posterior pituitary gland and its action on the kidney is one often cited example; the action of the hypothalamic release and release-inhibiting factors on the anterior pituitary trophic hormone-producing cells is another.

Pleiotropic roles—endocrine factors and neurotransmitters

Although, it was clearly important to document the ability of neurones to function as neuroendocrine cells, particularly those in the central nervous system (CNS), the focus on an artificial classification system with clear demarcations of endocrine versus neuronal versus neuroendocrine, quickly lost its heuristic value. Indeed, we now recognize that the very same substance, often function at one site as an endocrine substance and at another as a neurotransmitter. Thus, adrenaline (epinephrine) functions as a hormone in the adrenal medulla and as a conventional neurotransmitter substance in the mammalian CNS. Similarly corticotrophin-releasing factor (CRF) functions as a true hormone in its role as a hypothalamic hypophysiotrophic factor in the hypothalamic anterior pituitary complex, yet it is apparently a 'conventional' neurotransmitter in cortical and limbic brain areas. It may act as a paracrine substance in the adrenal medulla (see Fig. 2.3.3.1). Thus, the field has progressed to the stage where we now strive to characterize the role of a particular chemical messenger in a particular region or endocrine axis. The traditional endocrine and neurotransmitter roles for several peptides alluded to above are firmly established, but the equally important paracrine roles for such substances, namely the secretion of a substance from one cell where it acts upon nearby cells, remain largely unexplored. This is, perhaps, best illustrated in the gastrointestinal tract where several peptides that function as hormones or neurotransmitter substances in other sites, including the CNS, act to influence local cellular function. Examples would include vasoactive intestinal peptide, cholecystokinin, and somatostatin.

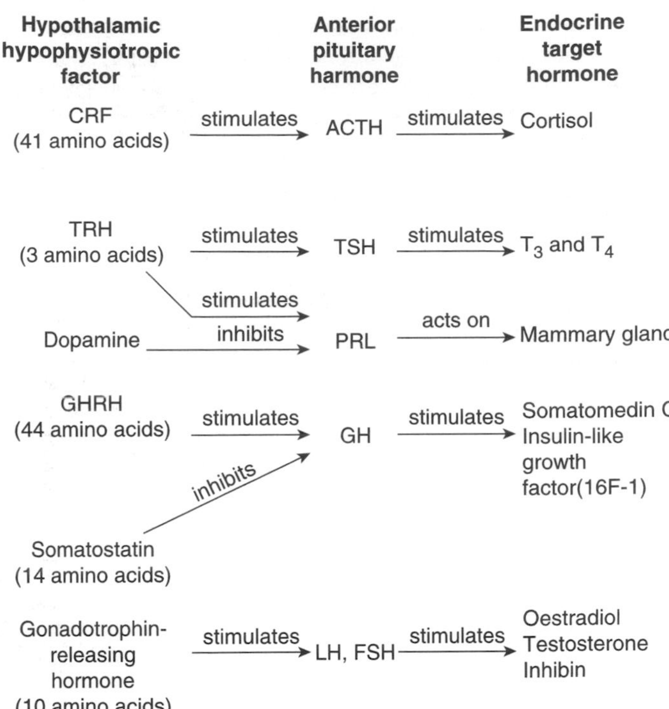

Fig. 2.3.3.1 Hormones of the hypothalamic-pituitary-end-organ axes: CRF, corticotrophin-releasing factor; TRH, thyrotrophin-releasing hormone; TSH, thyroid-stimulating hormone; T_3, tri-iodothyronine; T_4, thyroxine; PRL, prolactin; GHRH, growth-hormone releasing hormone; GH, growth hormone; LH, luteinizing hormone; FSH, follicle-stimulating hormone.

Neuroendocrinology

Neuroendocrinology thus, comprises the study of the endocrine role of neuronal or glial cells as well as the neural regulation of endocrine secretion, with a major portion of the latter consisting of the biology of the various hypothalamic-pituitary-end-organ axes and the major neurohypophyseal hormones, vasopressin and oxytocin. Because of the elegant and precise regulation of peripheral endocrine hormone secretion, afforded in part by the feedback of peripherally secreted hormones at pituitary and a variety of CNS sites, the actions of such hormones on the brain has become an integral part of this discipline. The related discipline of **psychoneuroendocrinology** arose with the realization that there are binding sites (receptors) for peripheral hormones within the CNS that have little to do with the feedback regulation of the hypothalamic-pituitary-end-organ axes, and the further recognition of the seminal role of the CNS in regulating endocrine function, for example in the effect of stress on several such measures. Often cited as beginning with the pioneering observations of Berthold, who reported that removing roosters' testosterone-secreting gonads abolished their sexual behaviour, psychoneuroendocrinology has been expanded to include the effects of hormones on behaviour, as well as the study of endocrine alterations in psychiatric disorders and, the converse, psychiatric symptomatology in endocrine disorders. Indeed, this stepchild of neuroendocrinology and psychosomatic medicine has been one of the most rapidly growing areas of research in psychiatry, now boasting an international society (International Society of Psychoneuroendocrinology), an annual meeting, and its own journal (Psychoneuroendocrinology).

Neuroendocrine window

One of the most commonly used strategies in the 1970s and 1980s, still in occasional use today, is the so-called neuroendocrine 'window' strategy. Until the relatively recent development and availability of functional brain-imaging techniques, the brain remained relatively inaccessible for study, with the exception of cerebrospinal fluid (CSF) and postmortem tissue studies. With the emergence of the monoamine theories of mood disorders and schizophrenia, many investigators attempted to draw conclusions about the activity of noradrenergic, serotonergic, and dopaminergic circuits in patients with various psychiatric disorders by measuring the basal and stimulated secretion of pituitary and end-organ hormones in plasma. There is little doubt that such an approach has severe limitations, but the results, now coupled with more modern approaches, have contributed to the substantial progress made in elucidating the pathophysiology of mood and anxiety disorders and, to a considerably lesser extent, schizophrenia. One assumption of the neuroendocrine window strategy is that the monoamine-containing neurones that regulate endocrine secretion are disordered (or not disordered) to the same extent as those monoamine circuits posited to be involved in the pathophysiology of the disorder under study. Such an assumption may well be true in neural circuits in which the cells of origin are found in a circumscribed area and project to widely diffused areas of the CNS (for example, the serotonergic and noradrenergic projections to the forebrain from the raphe and locus coeruleus cells in the brainstem, respectively). In contrast are the various dopaminergic circuits in the CNS, with their well-known topographic point-to-point distribution. Thus, there is little reason to believe that the activity of the major dopamine-containing hypothalamic projection, the tuberoinfundibular system, with perikarya in the arcuate and periventricular hypothalamic nuclei and projections to the median eminence, is in any way related to the activity of the mesolimbicocortical dopamine pathway, with cell bodies in the ventral tegmentum of the midbrain and projections to the nucleus accumbens, amygdala, and cortical regions. This latter pathway has been implicated in the pathophysiology of schizophrenia. Thus, the study of the dopamine modulation of prolactin secretion in schizophrenia is unlikely to inform about the nature of limbic and cortical dopamine neuronal alterations in this devastating disorder.

Hypothalamic-pituitary-end-organ axes

Because a large portion of neuroendocrinology relevant to psychiatry is concerned with the hypothalamic-pituitary-end-organ axes, alterations in each of these systems in patients with a major psychiatric disorder are described later in this chapter. To avoid repetition, a generic description of the hierarchical organization of the various components of these systems is briefly outlined here. More comprehensive reviews of this subject are available.[1] In general, the hypothalamus contains neurones that synthesize release and release-inhibiting factors. These peptide hormones, summarized in Fig. 2.3.3.1, are synthesized by a process beginning with transcription of the DNA sequence for the peptide prohormone. After translation in the endoplasmic reticulum and processing during axonal transport and packaging in the vesicles in the nerve terminals, the now biologically active peptide is released from nerve terminals in the median eminence and secreted into the primary plexus of the hypothalamohypophyseal portal vessels. They are transported humorally to the sinusoids of the adenohypophysis where they act on specific membrane receptors on their specific target: the pituitary trophic hormone-producing cells. Activation of their receptors results in the release or inhibition of release of the pituitary trophic hormone. The increase or decrease in pituitary trophic hormone secretion produces a corresponding increase or decrease in end-organ hormone secretion. Thus **gonadotrophin-releasing hormone** (**GnRH**), a decapeptide, induces the release of the gonadotrophins, luteinizing hormone, and follicle-stimulating hormone from the anterior pituitary gland, which in turn stimulate the secretion of oestrogen and progesterone in women, and testosterone in men. The exogenous, intravenous administration of GnRH, comprises the GnRH stimulation test, a very sensitive test of hypothalamic-pituitary-gonadal (**HPG**) axis activity. Such stimulation tests are thought to be a sensitive measure of the activity of the axis because it is influenced by GnRH secretion, gonadotrophin secretion, and feedback at the pituitary and brain by gonadal steroids. The organization of, and major feedback mechanisms thus far demonstrated in the hypothalamic–anterior pituitary–end-organ axes are illustrated in Fig. 2.3.3.2.

In summary, neuroendocrinology (and the related discipline psychoneuroendocrinology) broadly encompasses the study of the following:

- the neural regulation of peripheral, target-organ hormone secretions, pituitary trophic hormone secretions, and secretions of the hypothalamic-hypophysiotrophic hormones;
- the role of neurotransmitter systems in the regulation of the above;

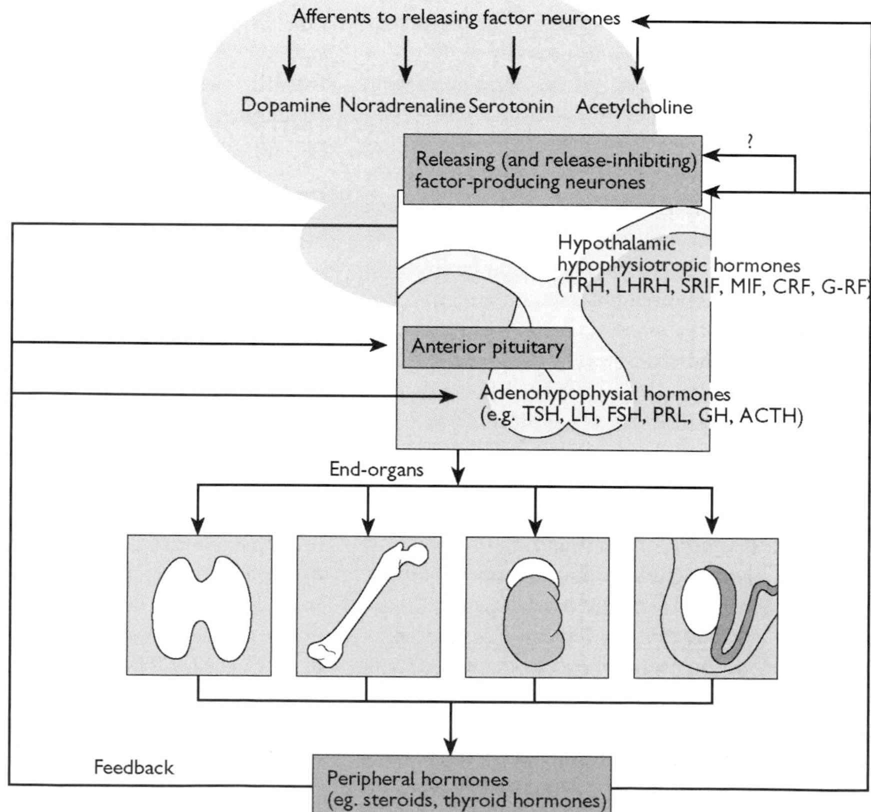

Fig. 2.3.3.2 Relationships between brain neurotransmitter systems, hypothalamic peptidergic (releasing-factor) neurones, anterior pituitary, and peripheral endocrine organs, illustrating established feedback loops: LHRH, luteinizing-hormone releasing hormone; SRIF, somatostatin; MIF, melanotrophin release-inhibiting factor; GHRF, growth-hormone releasing factor. Other abbreviations as in Fig. 2.3.3.1.

- the hormone effects of each of the endocrine axes on the CNS, alterations in the activity of the various endocrine axes in major psychiatric disorders, and conversely the behavioural consequences of endocrinopathies;
- the effects of target gland hormones on the CNS in normal individuals—for instance, the effects of synthetic glucocorticoids on memory processes.

The hypothalamic-pituitary-thyroid axis

It has been recognized for more than a century that adult patients with hypothyroidism exhibit profound disturbances in CNS function, including cognitive impairment and depression. In more recent years, attention has focused on more subtle alterations of the hypothalamic-pituitary-thyroid (**HPT**) axis in depressed patients. **Hypothyroidism** is most frequently subclassified as in four grades as follows:

- Grade 1 hypothyroidism is classic primary hypothyroidism (increased **thyroid-stimulating hormone** (**TSH**), decreased peripheral thyroid hormone concentrations, and an increased TSH response to **thyrotrophin-releasing hormone** (**TRH**)).
- Grade 2 hypothyroidism is characterized by normal, basal thyroid-hormone concentrations, but an increase in basal TSH concentrations and an exaggerated TSH response to TRH.
- Grade 3 hypothyroidism can only be detected by a TRH-stimulation test; patients have a normal basal thyroid hormone and TSH concentrations, but an exaggerated TSH response to TRH.
- Grade 4 hypothyroidism is defined as normal findings on the three thyroid axis function tests noted above, but the patients have antithyroid antibodies.

Left untreated, most, if not all, patients' progress from grade 4 to grade 1 hypothyroidism. Several studies have revealed an inordinately high rate of HPT axis dysfunction, largely hypothyroidism, in patients with major depression. In our pilot study, patients with comorbid depression and anxiety were especially likely to exhibit HPT axis abnormalities, especially the presence of grade 4 hypothyroidism, i.e. symptomless autoimmune thyroiditis. Patients with other major psychiatric diagnoses including schizophrenia and anxiety disorders appear to exhibit normal HPT axis function. For patients who require thyroid hormone replacement secondary to thyroid ablation, Bunevicius *et al.*[2] recently reported that treatment with a combination of **tri-iodothyronine** (**T3**) and **thyroxine** (**T4**) is optimal for mood and cognitive function, rather than the standard medication of T_4 alone.

In addition, a blunted TSH response to TRH is observed in approximately 25 per cent of patients with major depression. This observation, first reported by Prange *et al.*[3] and Kastin *et al.*,[4] more than 25 years ago, has been replicated in many studies. Unfortunately, the pathophysiological underpinnings of this observation remain obscure, though there is considerable evidence that it may be due, at least in part, to chronic hypersecretion of TRH and subsequent TRH-receptor downregulation in the anterior pituitary gland. Indeed, our group[5] and others have reported elevated TRH concentrations in the CSF of drug-free depressed patients.

TRH was the first of the hypothalamic-releasing factors to be chemically characterized. Immunohistochemical and radio-immunoassay methods revealed a heterogeneous brain distribution of TRH. This was the first in a series of experimental results that led to the inexorable conclusion that this peptide, and, as discussed below, other release and release-inhibiting hormones, function in extrahypothalamic brain regions as neurotransmitter substances. Thus, TRH has been shown to produce direct brain effects, independent of its action on the pituitary thyrotrophs. Antidepressant effects of intravenously and intrathecally applied TRH have been reported,[3] but the results have not been confirmed in large, controlled clinical trials.[6] In contrast, several reports over the last 30 years have documented the efficacy of T_3 (25–50 mg daily) in both accelerating the rate of onset of antidepressant response,[7] and in converting antidepressant non responders to responders,[8] the later confirmed in the recent NIMH-funded STAR-D trial.[9] Studies also suggest that T_4 (100–300 μg daily) supplementation is a viable strategy for increasing the response to antidepressants.[10] These studies were initiated when it became apparent that patients (and laboratory animals) with hypothyroidism do not respond to antidepressant agents. This led to the hypothesis that patients with subtle forms of hypothyroidism (grades 2–4) may not respond optimally to antidepressants unless they are adequately treated with exogenous thyroid hormone. With the cloning of the thyroid hormone receptor and its localization within the CNS, studies of its regulation in depression, as well as the regulation of TRH biosynthesis, can now be conducted in postmortem brain tissue.

The hypothalamic-pituitary-adrenal axis

Although, first identified in crude form in 1955 by Saffran *et al.*,[11] **corticotrophin-releasing factor** (**CRF**) was not chemically identified until 1981 by Vale and colleagues.[12] This discovery finally permitted the comprehensive assessment of hypothalamic-pituitary-adrenal (**HPA**) axis activity, and also led to scrutiny of the role of this peptide, which is now known to co-ordinate the endocrine, immune, autonomic, and behavioural effects of stress in a variety of psychiatric disorders.

CRF hypothesis of depression

Most investigators would agree that the most important finding in all of biological psychiatry is the hyperactivity of the HPA axis observed in a significant subgroup of patients with major depression. The magnitude of HPA axis hyperactivity has been reported to be correlated to the severity of the depression.[13] Literally thousands of reports on this subject have appeared since the original and independent observations of research groups led by Board, Bunney, and Hamburg, as well as by Carroll, Sachar, Stokes, and Besser. These studies, conducted from the late 1950s to the 1980s, applied the tests largely developed for the diagnosis of Cushing's syndrome to patients with major depression and other psychiatric disorders. A panoply of such tests, ranging from urinary free-cortisol, to CSF levels of cortisol, to the dexamethasone suppression test led to the inexorable conclusion that a sizeable percentage of depressed patients exhibited HPA axis hyperactivity. Our group and others, focusing on the mechanism(s) responsible for these findings, documented adrenocortical enlargement[14] and pituitary gland enlargement[15] in depressed patients, using CT and magnetic resonance imaging (**MRI**) respectively. The hypersecretion of cortisol is associated with hypersecretion of ACTH (and its co-secreted product of the precursor pro-opiomelanocortin), which due to its trophic properties also causes adrenocortical gland enlargement. Both direct measurements of CRF in CSF,[16] and of CRF and gene expression for CRF (CRF mRNA expression) in postmortem tissue confirmed the hypothesized hypersecretion of CRF in depressed patients.[17] In addition, CRF hypersecretion results in CRF1 receptor downregulation observed in both receptor binding studies[18] and CRF mRNA expression studies conducted on post-mortem tissue from suicide victims.[19] Like the hypersecretion of cortisol, CRF hypersecretion normalizes upon recovery from depression. Indeed, there is now considerable evidence, derived from both preclinical and clinical studies, that CRF neuronal hyperactivity is reduced by treatment with several antidepressants including paroxetine and fluoxetine, the selective serotonin-reuptake inhibitors (**SSRIs**), reboxetine (the noradrenaline-reuptake inhibitor), venlafaxine (the dual noradrenaline/serotonin-reuptake inhibitor), desipramine (the tricyclic antidepressant), and tranylcypromine (the monoamine oxidase inhibitor), as well as by electroconvulsive therapy.[20]

When patients who are drug free but depressed are given CRF intravenously, they exhibit, as a group, a blunted ACTH response compared with normal control subjects. This is believed to be secondary to either the downregulation of CRF receptors on the corticotrophs after long-standing CRF hypersecretion and/or intact negative feedback of the hypersecreted cortisol at anterior pituitary and higher CNS centres. As with the other measures of HPA axis function, this endocrine abnormality normalizes upon recovery from depression. Indeed, persistent alterations in HPA axis function, whether due to dexamethasone non-suppression or CSF-CRF hypersecretion, is the harbinger of a poor response to antidepressant treatment. In recent years, Holsboer *et al.*[21] have pioneered the use of the combined **dexamethasone-CRF test**, in which patients are given the synthetic glucocorticoid and the following day receive a standardized CRF stimulation test. The results reveal that this test has a much greater sensitivity in detecting increases in HPA axis activity; it has now been used to detect axis alterations in the first-degree relatives of depressed patients who have never been symptomatic, raising for the first time the question of a trait (vulnerability) component to this measure.[22]

Space constraints preclude a more comprehensive discussion of this rich literature, but a few additional points are certainly worth interjecting. First, a robust preclinical literature has documented the depressogenic and anxiogenic effects of exogenously administered CRF in laboratory animals. When CRF was directly injected into the central nervous system it produced effects reminiscent of the cardinal symptoms of depression in patients, including decreased libido, reduced appetite and weight loss, sleep disturbances, and neophobia. Indeed, newly developed CRF1-receptor antagonists represent a novel putative class of antidepressants. Such compounds exhibit activity in virtually every preclinical screen for antidepressants and anxiolytics currently employed, and in an open study a CRF1 receptor antagonist was shown to possess antidepressant properties.[23] A second CRF receptor, the CRF2 receptor, exhibits genetic polymorphism (i.e. it occurs in more than one naturally occurring isoform or splice variant), and it is believed to utilize the urocortins as endogenous ligands. The long-term consequences of cortisol hypersecretion in depression are just now being scrutinized. One such sequela appears to be neuronal loss in the hippocampus, one of the major feedback sites for glucocorticoids in the CNS. This has now been documented by structural brain-imaging studies that utilized MRI techniques.[24] If the degeneration of neurones that represent glucocorticoid feedback sites indeed occur in depressed patients, then this should further increase HPA axis hyperactivity, which would explain the many reports of increasing adrenocortical hyperactivity of elderly depressed patients when compared with matched younger depressed patients.

Future studies will focus on the development of positron emission tomography (**PET**) ligands for both the glucocorticoid receptor and the CRF receptor, the role of the CRF binding protein—a unique protein which binds CRF in extracellular fluid and in plasma, preventing its availability to act on its receptor—and the role of the CRF peptidase, which degrades the peptide, in normal and pathological states. Finally, are the studies from our group and others, which have documented the long-term persistent increases in the HPA axis and extrahypothalamic CRF neuronal activity after exposure to early untoward life events—for example, child abuse and neglect in both laboratory animals (rats and non-human primates) as well as in both male and female patients.[20,25,26] This phenomenon has been posited to underlie the now well-documented association between early abuse and neglect and increased vulnerability to mood disorders.[27–29] Indeed, we have recently demonstrated single nucleotide polymorphisms (SNPs) of the CRF1 receptor that confer vulnerability or resistance to the development of depression after exposure to child abuse.[30] An early intervention strategy using CRF receptor antagonists may prevent such long-term alterations in the central nervous system.

HPA axis and other psychiatric disorders

HPA axis alterations have also been investigated in other psychiatric disorders. When depression is comorbid with a variety of other disorders such as multiple sclerosis, Alzheimer's disease, multi-infarct dementia, Huntington's disease, and others, both CRF hypersecretion and HPA axis hyperactivity are common. There is little evidence for HPA axis dysfunction in schizophrenia. In contrast, at least one anxiety disorder, post-traumatic stress disorder, is associated with extrahypothalamic CRF hypersecretion, as evidenced by elevated CSF concentrations of CRF,[31] but normal or reduced measures of adrenocortical activity. Finally, CRF neuronal degeneration is now well known to occur in the cerebral cortex of patients with Alzheimer's disease,[32, 33] an effect which temporally occurs prior to the better-studied cholinergic neuronal involvement. With the reduction in CRF concentrations in the cerebral cortex there is a reciprocal increase in CRF receptor density. Whether modification of the disease-associated effects on the CRF neuronal system in the cortex and hippocampus represents a novel strategy for the treatment of this common dementing disorder remains unclear at the present time.

The hypothalamic-growth hormone axis

Although the HPA and HPT axes have been more closely scrutinized in patients with psychiatric disorders, there is virtually universal agreement that the blunted growth-hormone response to a variety of provocative stimuli (particularly clonidine, an α2-adrenergic agonist) in depressed patients is the most consistent finding in affective disorders research.[34] The mechanism underlying this phenomenon remains obscure, but it is of particular interest that, at least in some studies, it appears to persist upon recovery from depression, suggesting that it is a trait marker for depression vulnerability. There are reports of similar findings with other growth hormone-provocative stimuli, such as the use of apomorphine, desipramine, or levodopa. In addition, the blunted growth-hormone response to clonidine in depressed patients is particularly robust in those who have recently attempted suicide. Clearly, further work in this area is warranted, especially in the context of several reports of alterations in basal growth-hormone secretion in this disorder. The nature of this alteration is a reduction in the normal nocturnal rise in growth-hormone secretion, though this is not a universally agreed-upon finding. Alterations in growth-hormone secretion in other psychiatric disorders (particularly schizophrenia) have also been reported, though the results may have largely been due to long-term treatment of such patients with dopamine-receptor antagonists, antipsychotic drugs.

The secretion of growth hormone and the regulation of this axis are distinct from that of the other endocrine axes for several reasons. First, this is the one axis in which two hypothalamic-hypophysiotrophic hormones have unequivocally been shown to play a physiological role. The first discovered was **somatostatin** or **growth hormone-inhibiting hormone**. It is distributed in the CNS not only in cells of the periventricular nucleus of the hypothalamus, which projects to the median eminence, but in a variety of extrahypothalamic areas as well. Indeed, somatostatin is known to function as a CNS neurotransmitter and is of particular interest to psychiatrists because of its early involvement in the Alzheimer's disease process. Our group and others have documented the marked reduction in somatostatin concentrations in this dementing disorder.(33) In addition, somatostatin concentrations are markedly elevated in the basal ganglia of patients with Huntington's disease;(35) the pathological implications of this finding remain obscure. In contrast to the other peptide receptors described above in which one or at most two receptor subtypes have been identified, several distinct somatostatin receptor subtypes have now been structurally identified. Such diversity suggests the possibility of specific receptor-subtype agonists and antagonists as putative therapeutic agents.

Several years after the elucidation of the structure of somatostatin, the long-postulated **growth hormone-releasing factor (GHRF)** was found. This peptide has the most limited CNS distribution of all the hypothalamic-releasing hormones thus far studied. The vast majority of the peptide is found in the arcuate nucleus of the hypothalamus from where it projects nerve terminals to the median eminence. Unlike the other axes, the growth-hormone axis is also unique in not having a single target endocrine gland. Indeed, growth hormone does stimulate the release of **somatomedin C** from the liver and it also exerts direct effects on a variety of targets including bone and muscle. Most, but not all, investigators have reported a blunted growth-hormone response to GHRF in depressed patients, but the total number of patients studied pales in comparison to the TRH- and CRF-stimulation test data. There are no data published on somatomedin C responses to GHRF in depressed patients. No published studies are available in which GHRF concentrations or GHRF-mRNA expression have been studied in postmortem tissue of depressed patients and matched controls, an obvious study in view of the data reviewed above.

The hypothalamic-pituitary-gonadal axis

In view of the remarkable gender differences in the prevalence rate of depression, the relatively high rates of postpartum depression, as well as the reduction in libido that is so characteristic of depression, it is plausible to posit a reduction in HPG axis activity in depressed patients. Therefore, it is somewhat surprising that so little research has been conducted on HPG axis activity in depression and other psychiatric disorders. Indeed, a comprehensive database on this extraordinarily important area is simply not available, but the field has been reviewed.(36) A series of older studies documented no differences in basal gonadotrophin levels in depressed patients when compared to controls. The **gonadotrophin-releasing hormone (GnRH)** stimulation test has only been administered to a relatively small number of depressed patients; although the results revealed a blunted or normal response, no firm conclusions can be drawn from this limited data set. Indeed, such studies require control for menopausal status, menstrual-cycle phase, use of oral contraceptives, as well as the measurement of baseline progesterone, oestrogen, and gonadotrophin plasma concentrations. One remarkable finding relevant to these questions is the remarkable effectiveness of the GnRH agonist, leuprolide, in the treatment of the premenstrual syndrome. It is believed to act by producing a chemical ovariectomy through a marked downregulation of adenohypophyseal GnRH receptors and the expected resultant reduction in gonadotrophin and gonadal steroid secretion. Long-term treatment with this compound could theoretically result in bone-density reductions and a risk of cardiovascular disease. Therefore, supplementation with oestrogen and progesterone has been suggested in combination with leuprolide, though there are reports that such a strategy reduces the effectiveness of the treatment.

GnRH was the second of the hypothalamic-hypophysiotrophic hormones to be chemically characterized. It is relatively limited in distribution to hypothalamic regions and to the preoptic area and septum. It stimulates the secretion of both luteinizing hormone and follicle-stimulating hormone in both men and women. GnRH is known to act by stimulating GnRH receptors in the anterior pituitary gland, which results in the increased synthesis and release of the pituitary gonadotrophins, in turn causing the release of oestrogen and progesterone in women and testosterone in men. There is some evidence that oestrogens, which have receptors localized extensively throughout the CNS, may possess some antidepressant activity, in perimenopausal and postpartum depression, though the data is far from clear.(37) There are hints from the clinical trial literature that postmenopausal women on oestrogen replacement may respond better to treatment with fluoxetine than women who are not receiving such treatment,(38) though the database is small and fraught with many confounds. Further, emphasizing the potential role of sex steroids in affective disorders is the clinical study that demonstrates that in hypogonadal depressed men, testosterone treatment possessed antidepressant properties.(39)

The hypothalamic-prolactin axis

Prolactin, a pituitary hormone which acts on the mammary gland, plays a critical role in lactation. Unlike the other axes described, this axis is unique in having a non-peptide release-inhibiting factor, dopamine. In addition, although there is relatively strong evidence for the existence of a prolactin-releasing factor, its isolation and characterization has not yet been realized. One of the difficulties in completing this task is the presence of TRH, which is a potent prolactin-releasing factor, and may in fact function physiologically in this regard. Interestingly, although the TSH response to TRH in depressed patients is often blunted, the prolactin response is not. Although the results are not unequivocal, most studies have not observed alterations of prolactin secretion in depressed patients.[40] In contrast to this small database is a remarkably large database on the use of provocative tests of prolactin secretion in patients with psychiatric disorders. To summarize briefly, the prolactin response to agents that increase serotonergic neurotransmission such as l-tryptophan, 5-hydroxytryptophan (5-HTP), l-(+)- and d-(+)-fenfluramine, clomipramine, and also to direct serotonin-receptor agonists, is blunted in depressed patients, as well as in patients with cluster-B personality disorder and borderline personality disorder. The available data would suggest that this blunted prolactin response is mediated by alterations in 5-HT1A-receptor responsiveness.

Discussion and summary

Although, the hypothesis that the neuroendocrine window strategy would ultimately provide the long searched for information concerning the nature of monoamine circuit alterations in patients with psychiatric disorders has never been realized, the approach has led to major advances in biological psychiatry. It has led to the **CRF hypothesis of depression**, which is supported by a considerable multidisciplinary database, and this in turn has directed the field towards the development of novel therapeutic approaches, namely CRF receptor antagonists. It also apparently explains the neurobiological mechanisms responsible for the increase in depression (first postulated by Freud in the early part of the 20th century) in patients exposed to trauma during their early life. If CRF is indeed the 'black bile' of depression, responsible for the endocrinopathy of depression, as well as several of the other cardinal features of this disorder, then CRF-receptor antagonists should represent a novel class of antidepressants that will be a welcome addition to the armamentarium. Indeed, a number of pharmaceutical companies are now testing CRF-receptor antagonists as novel anxiolytics and antidepressants in preclinical studies and clinical trials.

In addition to the now widely replicated HPA axis and CRF alterations in depression, are the HPT axis abnormalities. Most depressed patients, in fact, exhibit alterations in one of these two axes. Furthermore, there is the widely replicated blunting of the growth-hormone response to clonidine and other provocative stimuli and the blunted prolactin response to serotonergic stimuli in depressed patients. The vast majority of studies have focused on patients with mood disorders, particularly unipolar depression. Clearly other disorders, including eating disorders, anxiety disorders, schizophrenia, and axis II diagnoses should also be critically evaluated and compared to the literature on depression. The original neuroendocrine window strategy may well have failed in terms of gleaning information about monoamine-circuit activity, but the mechanistic studies that followed have been remarkably fruitful. As repeatedly noted above, the availability of ligands that can be utilized with positron-emission tomography to determine peptide-receptor alterations in the brain and pituitary of patients with psychiatric disorders will advance the field, as will the long-elusive ability to measure receptors for the endocrine target hormones (glucocorticoids, oestrogens, thyroid hormones, etc.) in the brains of patients with these severe mental illnesses.

Finally, it is important to note the increasing database suggesting that depression is a systemic disease with major implications for vulnerability to other disorders. Thus, depressed patients are much more likely to develop coronary artery disease and stroke, and perhaps cancer. They have been shown to have reduced bone density, rendering them more at risk for hip fracture and increasing a variety of measures of inflammation. Such findings may well be mediated by the described endocrine alterations in depression. This should provide a further impetus for investigating the neuroendocrinology of psychiatric disorders.

Further information

Psychoneuroendocrinology http://www.elsevier.com/wps/find/journaldescription.cws_home/473/description#description

Hormones and Behavior http://www.elsevier.com/wps/find/journaldescription.cws_home/622842/description#description

Neuroendocrinology http://content.karger.com/ProdukteDB/produkte.asp?Aktion=JournalHome&ProduktNr=223855

References

1. Campeau, S., Day, H.E.W., Helmreich, D.L., *et al.* (1998). Principles of psychoneuroendocrinology. *Psychiatric Clinics of North America*, **21**, 259–76.
2. Bunevicius, R., Kazanavicius, G., Zalinkevicius, R., *et al.* (1999). Effects of thyroxine as compared with thyroxine plus triiodothyronine in patients with hypothyroidism. *New England Journal of Medicine*, **340**, 424–9.
3. Prange, A.J., Wilson, I.C., Lara, P.P., *et al.* (1972). Effects of thyrotropin-releasing hormone in depression. *Lancet*, **2**, 999–1002.
4. Kastin, A.J., Ehrensing, R.H., Schlach, D.S., *et al.* (1972). Improvement in mental depression with decreased thyrotropin response after administration of thyrotropin-releasing hormone. *Lancet*, **ii**, 740–2.
5. Banki, C.M., Bissette, G., Arato, M., *et al.* (1988). Elevation of immunoreactive CSF TRH in depressed patients. *American Journal of Psychiatry*, **145**, 1526–31.
6. Nemeroff, C.B. and Evans, D.L. (1989). Thyrotropin-releasing hormone (TRH), the thyroid axis and affective disorder. *Annals of the New York Academy of Sciences*, **553**, 304–10.
7. Prange, A.J., Wilson, I.C., Rabon, A.M., *et al.* (1969). Enhancement of imipramine antidepressant activity by thyroid hormone. *American Journal of Psychiatry*, **126**, 457–69.
8. Joffe, R.T., Singer, W., Levitt, A.J., *et al.* (1993). A placebo-controlled comparison of lithium and triiodothyronine augmentation of tricyclic antidepressants in unipolar refractory depression. *Archives of General Psychiatry*, **50**, 387–94.
9. Nierenberg, A.A., Fava, M., Trivedi, M.H., *et al.* (2006). A comparison of lithium and T(3) augmentation following two failed medication treatments for depression: a STAR*D report. *American Journal of Psychiatry*, **163**, 1519–30.
10. Baumgartner, A. (2000). Thyroxine and the treatment of affective disorders: an overview of the results of basic and clinical research. *International Journal of Neuropsychopharmacology*, **3**, 149–65.
11. Saffran, M., Schally, A.V., and Benfey, B.G. (1955). Stimulation of the release of corticotropin from the adenohypophysis by a neurohypophysial factor. *Endocrinology*, **57**, 439–44.
12. Vale, W., Spiess, J., Riveir, C., *et al.* (1981). Characterization of a 41 residue ovine hypothalamic peptide that stimulates secretion of corticotropin and β-endorphin. *Science*, **213**, 1394–7.

13. Evans, D.L. and Nemeroff, C.B. (1987). The clinical use of the dexamethasone suppression test in DSM-III affective disorders: correlation with the severe depressive subtypes of melancholia and psychosis. *Journal of Psychiatric Research*, **21**, 185–94.
14. Nemeroff, C.B., Krishnan, K.R.R., Reed, D., *et al.* (1992). Adrenal gland enlargement in major depression: a computed tomography study. *Archives of General Psychiatry*, **49**, 384–7.
15. Krishnan, K.R.R., Doraiswamy, P.M., Lurie, S.N., *et al.* (1991). Pituitary size in depression. *Journal of Clinical Endocrinology and Metabolism*, **72**, 256–9.
16. Heit, S., Owens, M.J., Plotsky, P., *et al.* (1997). Corticotropin-releasing factor, stress and depression. *Neuroscientist*, **3**, 186–94.
17. Raadsheer, F.C., Hoogendijk, W.J.G., Stam, F.C., *et al.* (1994). Increased number of corticotropin-releasing hormone neurones in the hypothalamic paraventricular nuclei of depressed patients. *Neuroendocrinology*, **60**, 436–44.
18. Nemeroff, C.B., Owens, M.J., Bissette, G., *et al.* (1988). Reduced corticotropin releasing factor binding sites in the frontal cortex of suicide victims. *Archives of General Psychiatry*, **45**, 577–9.
19. Merali, Z., Du, L., Hrdina, P., *et al.* (2004). Dysregulation in the suicide brain: mRNA expression of corticotropin-releasing hormone receptors and GABA(A) receptor subunits in frontal cortical brain regions. *Journal of Neuroscience*, **24**, 1478–85.
20. Nemeroff, C.B. (1999). The preeminent role of early untoward experience on vulnerability to major psychiatric disorders: the nature-nurture controversy revisited and soon to be resolved. *Molecular Psychiatry*, **4**, 106–8.
21. Holsboer, F., Von Bardeleben, U., Weidemann, K., *et al.* (1987). Serial assessment of corticotropin-releasing hormone response after dexamethasone in depression-implications for pathophysiology of DST nonsuppression. *Biological Psychiatry*, **22**, 228–34.
22. Holsboer, F., Lauer, C.J., Schreiber, W., *et al.* (1995). Altered hypothalamic-pituitary-adrenocortical regulations in healthy subjects at high familial risk for effective disorders. *Neuroendocrinology*, **62**, 340–7.
23. Zobel, A.W., Nickel, T., Kunzel, H.E., *et al.* (2000). Effects of the high-affinity corticotropin-releasing hormone receptor 1 antagonist R121919 in major depression: the first 20 patients treated. *Journal of Psychiatric Research*, **34**, 171–81.
24. Sheline, Y.I., Wang, P.W., Gado, M.H., *et al.* (1996). Hippocampal atrophy in recurrent major depression. *Proceedings of the National Academy of Sciences of the United States of America*, **93**, 3908–13.
25. Coplan, J.D., Andrews, M.W., Rosenblum, L.A., *et al.* (1996). Persistent elevations of cerebrospinal fluid concentrations of corticotropin-releasing factor in adult non-human primates exposed to early life stressors: implications for the pathophysiology of mood and anxiety disorders. *Proceedings of the National Academy of Sciences of the United States of America*, **93**, 1619–23.
26. Heim, C., Newport, D.J., Bonsall, R., *et al.* (2001). Altered pituitary-adrenal axis responses to provocative challenge tests in adult survivors of childhood abuse. *American Journal of Psychiatry*, **158**, 575–81.
27. Kendler, K.S., Neale, M.C., Kessler, R.C., *et al.* (1992). Childhood parental loss and adult psychopathology in women. A twin-study perspective. *Archives of General Psychiatry*, **49**, 109–16.
28. McCauley, J., Kern, D., Kolodner, K., *et al.* (1997). Clinical characteristics of women with an history of childhood abuse. *Journal of the American Medical Association*, **277**, 1362–8.
29. Agid, O., Shapira, B., Zislin, J., *et al.* (1999). Environment and vulnerability to major psychiatric illness: a case control study of early parental loss in major depression, bipolar depression and schizophrenia. *Molecular Psychiatry*, **4**, 163–72.
30. Bradley, R.G., Binder, E.B., Epstein, M.P., *et al.* (2007). Influence of child abuse and trauma on adult depression is moderated by the corticotrophin releasing hormone receptor gene. *In review*.
31. Bremner, J.D., Licinio, J., Darnell, A., *et al.* (1997). Elevated CSF corticotropin-releasing factor concentrations in posttraumatic stress disorder. *American Journal of Psychiatry*, **154**, 624–9.
32. Bissette, G., Reynolds, G.P., Kilts, C.D., *et al.* (1985). Corticotropin-releasing factor-like immunoreactivity in senile dementia of the Alzheimer type: reduced cortical and striatal concentrations. *Journal of the American Medical Association*, **254**, 3067–9.
33. Bissette, G., Cook, L., Smith, W., *et al.* (1998). Regional neuropeptide pathology in Alzheimer's disease: corticotropin-releasing factor and somatostatin. *Journal of Alzheimer's Disease*, **1**, 1–15.
34. Checkley, S.A., Slade, A.P., and Shur, P. (1981). Growth hormone and other responses to clonidine in patients with endogenous depression. *British Journal of Psychiatry*, **138**, 51–5.
35. Nemeroff, C.B., Youngblood, W.W., Manberg, P.J., *et al.* (1983). Regional brain concentrations of neuropeptides in Huntington's chorea and schizophrenia. *Science*, **221**, 972–5.
36. Young, E. and Korszun, A. (2002). The hypothalamic-pituitary-gonadal axis in mood disorders. *Endocrinology and Metabolism Clinics of North America*, **31**, 63–78.
37. Schmidt, P., Rubinow, D., Neuman, L., *et al.* (2000). Estrogen replacement in perimenopause-related depression: a preliminary report. *American Journal of Obstetrics and Gynecology*, **183**, 414–20.
38. Schneider, L.S., Small, G.W., Hamilton, S.H., *et al.* and the fluoxetine collaborative study group (1997). Estrogen replacement and response to fluoxetine in a multicenter geriatric depression trial. *American Journal of Geriatric Psychiatry*, **5**, 97–106.
39. Pope, H.G., Cohane, G.H., Kanayama, G., *et al.* (2003). Testosterone gel supplementation for men with refractory depression: a randomized, placebo-controlled trial. *American Journal of Psychiatry*, **160**, 105–11.
40. Nicholas, L., Dawkins, K., and Golden, R. (1998). Psychoneuroendocrinology of depression-prolactin. *Psychiatric Clinics of North America*, **21**, 341–58.

Nemeroff, Charles B (3-27-08)

Research Grants

NIH

Scientific Advisory Board

AFSP; AstraZeneca; Forest Laboratories; NARSAD; Quintiles; Janssen/Ortho-McNeil, PharmaNeuroboost, Mt. Cook Pharma, Inc

Stockholder or Equity

Corcept; Revaax; NovaDel Pharma; CeNeRx, PharmaNeuroboost

Board of Directors

American Foundation for Suicide Prevention (AFSP); George West Mental Health Foundation; NovaDel Pharma, Mt. Cook Pharma, Inc

Patents

Method and devices for transdermal delivery of lithium (US 6,375,990 B1)

Method to estimate serotonin and norepinephrine transporter occupancy after drug treatment using patient or animal serum (provisional filing April, 2001)

Neigh, Gretchen N. (7-11-08)

Research Grants

NIH, NARSAD, AHA

2.3.4 Neurotransmitters and signalling

Trevor Sharp

By the end of the 19th century it was recognized that signalling from one neurone to the next occurs at specialized contacts – Sherrington coined the term 'synapse'. It took another 50 years for scientists to accept that information passes between neurones principally through the movement across synapses of chemicals and not electrical current. Today changes in chemical transmission at brain synapses are accepted as being key to the successful drug treatment, and cause, of many forms of psychiatric illness. This article focuses on general aspects of chemical transmission and describes some recent advances relevant to psychiatry that point the direction of future research.

Otto Loewi identified the first chemical neurotransmitter, acetylcholine, in 1921. Today evidence suggests that there are many tens if not hundreds of molecules in the brain that have neurotransmitter properties. These molecules include not only the three major classes of neurotransmitters—amines, amino acids and neuropeptides—but also specific purines, trophic factors, inflammatory mediators (chemokines and cytokines), lipids, and even gases. Examples of molecules that serve neurotransmitter functions in the brain are listed in Table 2.3.4.1. This list is not exhaustive and more are likely to be discovered.

Table 2.3.4.1 Examples of neurotransmitters in the brain

Chemical class	Example
Amines	Dopamine Noradrenaline 5-hydroxytryptamine Histamine Melatonin Acetylcholine
Amino acids	γ-aminobutyric acid (GABA) Glutamate Glycine
Neuropeptides	Substance P Leu- and Met-enkephalin Galanin
Purines	Adenosine Adenosine triphosphate (ATP)
Neurotrophic factors#	Neurotrophins (e.g. BDNF, NGF) Insulin-like growth factor (IGF) Vascular endothelial growth factor (VEGF)
Cytokines*	Interleukin-1 (IL-1) Tumor necrosis factor-α (TNF-α)
Chemokines*	CC Chemokines (e.g. Interleukin-8 [IL-8]) CXC Chemokines
Endocannabinoids#	Anandamide 2-Arachidonyl-glycerol (2-AG)
Gases#	Nitric oxide (NO) Carbon monoxide (CO)

*Putative class of neurotransmitters.

#Retrograde messengers.

Basic principles of chemical transmission

Typically a molecule is classified as a neurotransmitter if it is localized in neurones, released from nerve terminals (and often soma and dendrites) on membrane depolarization, and exerts physiological and molecular effects through acting on postsynaptic receptors. However, the degree to which a particular molecule satisfies these criteria may vary. For example, the term 'neurotransmitter' was once used to cover only those molecules that exert fast synaptic effects, whereas molecules that exerted slow synaptic effects were termed 'neuromodulators'. These distinctions are less useful today (and will not be used herein) as it is recognized that many molecules are capable of exerting both fast and slow synaptic effects, depending on the receptor activated. Moreover, it is now recognized that certain molecules transfer information at a synapse in a 'retrograde' direction. In this case the molecules are located in the postsynaptic neurone and, when their synthesis is activated, the molecule diffuses across the synapse to act presynaptically.

The general principles of the chemical transmission at central synapses are similar across all neurotransmitter molecules but there are often important differences between molecules especially across molecules of different size, in particular small molecule transmitters such as amines and amino acids, and peptides (Fig. 2.3.4.1).(1)

Small molecule neurotransmitters

Typically small neurotransmitter molecules such as amines and amino acids are synthesized at the nerve terminal by one or a few enzymatic steps and packaged in small vesicles via proton-coupled vesicular transporters, prior to release into the synapse on arrival of a depolarizing action potential. After release, the neurotransmitter diffuses across the synapse to interact with receptors on the postsynaptic neurone to trigger electrical and/or biochemical changes in the postsynaptic cell. Small molecule neurotransmitters are also released from the soma and dendrites of neurones, one purpose being to interact with presynaptic receptors that signal negative feedback to the neurone.

Once released the small neurotransmitters are selectively taken up by sodium-coupled transporters that are located in the plasma membrane of the nerve terminal or neighbouring cells (neurones or glial cells). This transport terminates transmission at the postsynaptic receptor, maintains low extracellular levels of transmitter, and allows reuse of the neurotransmitter by the neurone. Transport into the nerve terminal also presents the transmitter to catabolic enzymes to generate biologically inactive metabolites, for instance, monoamine oxidase in the case of the amine transmitters.

Neurotransmitter transporters

Advances in cloning technology has lead to new discoveries regarding the structural and pharmacological identity of transporters located on the plasma membrane, as well as vesicular transporters

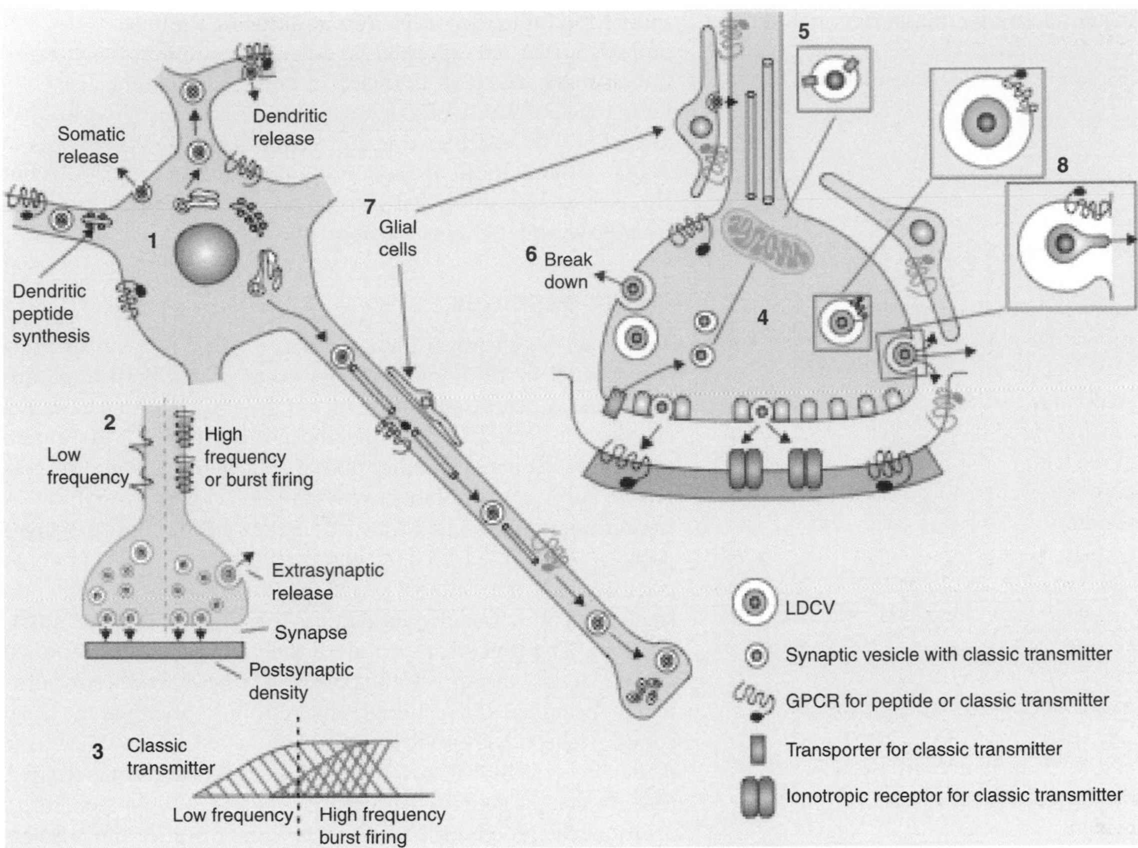

Fig. 2.3.4.1 Summary of the principal steps involved in chemical neurotransmission in the brain. Neuropeptides are synthesized in the cell body and then packaged in large dense core vesicles (LDCVs) that are transported into axons and dendrites (1). Small 'classic' neurotransmitters (e.g. amines and amino acids), are synthesized at the nerve terminal and stored in synaptic vesicles, and released into the synaptic cleft (2). LDCVs contain proteolytic enzymes (convertases) that generate the active neuropeptide from the precursor. Neurotransmitter receptors are either of the G-protein-coupled (metabotropic) or ligand-gated ion channel (ionotropic) type and are present on cell soma, dendrites, axons, and nerve endings (1,4). The small neurotransmitters are released during low and high frequency firing, whereas neuropeptides are preferentially released under burst or high frequency firing (2–4). Small transmitters have reuptake mechanisms (transporters) at both the plasma membrane and the vesicle membrane (5), which terminate neurotransmitter action and allow recycling (4). In contrast, neuropeptides are broken down by extracellular peptidases (6), and replacement occurs via axonal transport. Glial cells can express neurotransmitter receptors and transporters (7). Receptors are trafficked to and from the cell membrane by G-protein interacting proteins (8). Reprinted from The Lancet Neurology, 2, Hokfelt T, Bratfai T, Bloom F, Neuropeptides: opportunities for drug discovery, 465, copyright 2003, with permission from Elsevier.

located inside the nerve terminal.[2] The latter transporters concentrate transmitters in synaptic vesicles prior to release and play a key role in determining the neurotransmitter phenotype of a neurone.[3] A summary of plasma membrane and vesicular transporters is given in Table 2.3.4.2.

Plasma membrane transporters

Specific plasma membrane transporters for the amine neurotransmitters, dopamine (DAT), noradrenaline (NET), 5-HT (SERT), have been identified, sequenced and, investigated in detail at the molecular level because they are the site of action of stimulants such as amphetamines and cocaine, as well as many antidepressant drugs.[2] Indeed, the drug-binding site and the precise molecular mechanism of transporter inhibition by tricyclic antidepressant drugs have recently been revealed.[4]

Molecular cloning techniques have uncovered the genes for four transporters for the inhibitory neurotransmitter GABA; GAT-1, GAT-2, GAT-3 and BTG-1, the latter being localized primarily in the kidney. These transporters are highly homologous but pharmacologically distinct, with GAT-1 and GAT-3 being the most abundant subtypes and present on both neurones and glial cells. Although the significance of these transporters is yet to be fully understood, they display overlapping but different expression patterns in the CNS, suggesting distinct functional roles. The anticonvulsant effect of tiagabine is likely mediated by blockade of GAT-1, and there is much scope for new GABA uptake inhibitors of as yet unclear utility.

Glycine, another inhibitory amino acid transmitter, also has specific transporters located preferentially on the plasma membranes of glial cells in the forebrain (GLYT1) and neurones of the hindbrain and spinal cord (GLYT2). Interestingly, glycine is a positive allosteric co-modulator of glutamate NMDA receptors, and glycine

Table 2.3.4.2 Example of neurotransmitter transporters in the brain

Neurotransmitter	Transporter name
Plasma membrane transporters	
Dopamine	DAT
Noradrenaline	NET
5-Hydroxytryptamine	SERT
GABA	GAT-1
	GAT-2
	GAT-3
	BGT-1 (primarily in kidney)
Glutamate	EAAT-1 (GLAST1)
	EAAT-2 (GLT-1)
	EAAT-3 (EAAC1)
	EAAT-4
	EAAT-5
Glycine	GLYT-1
	GLYT-2
Acetylcholine (choline)	CHT
Vesicular transporters	
Monoamines (dopamine, noradrenaline, 5-HT,	VMAT1
histamine)	VMAT2
GABA	
Glutamate	VGAT
	VGLUT1
	VGLUT2
Acetylcholine	VGLUT3
	VAchT

transport blockade may offer a means to facilitate the functioning of this receptor without incurring excitotoxic effects. The antipsychotic potential of glycine transport blockers is currently under investigation because of consistent evidence of a link between the symptoms of schizophrenia and low glutamate function.[2]

Four transporters for the excitatory amino acid neurotransmitter, glutamate, have been cloned; EAAT1 (excitatory amino acid transporter1; synonym GLAST), EAAT2 (synonym GLT1), EAAT3, EAAT4, and EAAT5.[5] These transporters are located on both neurones (EAAT3) and glial cells (predominantly EAAT1/2) and serve to maintain low extracellular concentrations of glutamate, as well as providing a source of intracellular glutamate for metabolism. Whilst pharmacological blockade of glutamate transport increases excitotoxicity, pharmacologically enhanced EAAT expression appears to be neuroprotective.[6]

Vesicular transporters

Vesicular monoamine transporter 2 (VMAT2) has been identified and shown to be present in neurones of dopamine, noradrenaline and 5-HT (and histamine). In addition, vesicular monoamine transporter 1 (VMAT1) is an integral protein in the membrane of secretory vesicles of neuroendocrine and endocrine cells. Reserpine is a blocker of VMAT and causes depletion of amines, and the drug's tranquillizer effects are directly linked to this action. Acetylcholine is loaded into synaptic vesicles by a distinct transporter, VAchT.

Three homologous vesicular transporters for glutamate, VGLUT1, VGLUT2, and VGLUT3, have been cloned and characterized at the molecular level. Whilst all possess similar molecular properties, they are expressed on different neurone populations.[3] Interestingly, VGLUT3 is found in amine-containing neurones, raising the possibility of glutamate being a co-transmitter in these neurones. The vesicular transporter for GABA is VGAT. Loss of VGAT causes a drastic reduction in release of not only GABA but also glycine, indicating that glycinergic neurones do not express a separate vesicular glycine transporter.

Neuropeptides

Following the chemical identification of the first neuropeptide Substance P in 1971, evidence has accumulated that numerous peptides play neurotransmitter roles in the brain.[1] Some examples are shown in Table 2.3.4.3. The neuropeptides comprise 3–100 amino acids and together with other putative signalling peptides such as growth factors and cytokines, are synthesized in the nucleus by DNA transcription followed by translation from mRNA into precursor polypeptides (Fig. 2.3.4.1). These precursors typically undergo extensive post-translational processing that includes cleavage into smaller peptides by endopeptidases as well as other enzymic modifications. The precursor peptide usually contain an N-terminal signal sequence that directs the transport of newly synthesized protein to the lumen of the endoplasmic reticulum, and then the Golgi complex where the peptide is packaged into vesicles (so called large dense core vesicles) that are transported along the axon to the synapse. This obviates the need for neuropeptide vesicular transporters.

Proteolytic processing of a single precursor peptide often generates not one but a family of biologically active peptides, although the proteolytic steps may be tissue-specific. The opioid peptides provide one of the best worked out examples of this form of processing. Proopiomelanocortin (POMC) is a hypothalamic precursor opioid peptide whose structure contains sequences for adrenocorticotropic hormone (ACTH), α-melanocyte stimulating hormone (α-MSH) and β-endorphin. In the anterior lobe of the pituitary gland POMC is processed to form ACTH, whilst in the intermediate lobe POMC is processed to form α-MSH and β-endorphin. On the other hand, post-translational processing of the opioid precursor peptide, proenkephalin, gives rise to multiple copies of the pentapeptide met-enkephalin as well as a copy of leu-enkephalin, whilst a third opioid precursor, prodynorphin, gives rise to dynorphin. In total, the 3 separate opioid peptide genes give rise to at least 18 endogenous peptides with opiate-like activity.

Multiple proteolytic enzymes have been cloned and extensively characterized, including prohormone convertases that produce striking phenotypic effects when genetically manipulated in mutant mouse models.[7] The therapeutic utility of pharmacological manipulation of neuropeptide synthesis and degradation in the brain has yet to be realized. However, the success of inhibitors of the prohormone convertase that synthesizes angiotensin in the periphery (ACE inhibitors), for the treatment of hypertension, sets an important precedent.

Another mechanism to generate neuropeptide diversity is through alternative RNA splicing of a single gene. For example, in the case of the tachykinins alternative splicing of preprotachykinin gene A mRNA results in 3 splice variants which, after translation and post-translational processing, collectively generate the five biologically active peptides of the tachykinin family (including Substance P).

Table 2.3.4.3 Examples of families of neuropeptides

Opioid peptides	Leu-enkephalin Met-enkephalin Dynorphin β-endorphin Nociceptin
Tachykinins	Substance P Neurokinin A Neurokinin B
Hypothalamic releasing factors	Thyrotrophin releasing factor (TRH) Corticotrophin releasing factor (CRF) Growth hormone releasing hormone (GHRH) Somatostatin
Gut-brain peptides	Cholecystokinin (CCK) Galanin Insulin Neurotensin Neuropeptide Y (NPY) Vasointestinal polypeptide (VIP)
Other peptides	Bradykinin Calcitonin gene-related peptide Melanin concentrating hormone (MCH) Melanocortin Orexin Oxytocin Vasopressin

To date, there is little evidence that neuropeptides are cleared from the synapse by transporters in the plasma membrane, indicating that these particular transmitters are not recycled after release. Rather, evidence suggests that their action is terminated by peptidases that are thought to be located on extracellular membranes. Thus, replenishment of neuropeptides during high levels of synaptic activity is dependent on the proteolytic enzymes that generate the active peptides in the neurones.

A feature of most if not all neuropeptides is their co-localization with classic neurotransmitters. Some of the best examples include co-localization between GABA/dynorphin in movement control pathways (striatonigral neurones), CCK/dopamine in reward pathways (mesoaccumbens neurones), and glutamate/Substance P in pain pathways (dorsal root ganglion neurones). The functional significance of this co-localization is not fully clear but evidence suggests that peptide release requires higher frequencies of neuronal discharge than classic transmitters, and once released the neuropeptide either facilitates or opposes the function of the co-localized transmitter.[1] In a recent example, co-localization between 5-HT and galanin in midbrain raphe neurones was investigated to reveal an action of the peptide on 5-HT feedback mechanisms. This knowledge has been exploited to develop galanin ligands that are under development as novel antidepressant strategies.[8]

Neurotrophic factors

Neurotrophic factors are brain peptides that were originally recognized for their role in supporting growth, differentiation and survival of neurones but today are thought to possess many of the properties of neurotransmitters including neuronal localization and release, and an ability to modulate synaptic function. Moreover, there is evidence that trophic factors signal in a retrograde fashion (see later). Neurotrophic factors are currently named according to the action with which they were originally characterized (brain-derived neurotrophic factor — BDNF, nerve growth factor — NGF) and they comprise many families.[9]

Certain features distinguish neurotrophic factors from neuropeptides (see above). In particular, neurotrophic factors are larger molecules; for example, BDNF has a molecular size of 14 kDa whereas neuropeptides are typically much smaller peptides. Also whilst neuropeptides signal via G-protein coupled receptors (see below), neurotrophic factors signal via direct activation of a class of transmembrane spanning protein kinases called protein tyrosine kinases (Trk receptors) of which four types have been identified so far (TrkA, TrkB, TrkC and p75), and that phosphorylate proteins on tyrosine residues.[10] In some cases, the neurotrophic factor receptor and protein tyrosine kinase reside in the same protein, while in other cases, the receptor recruits an intracellular protein tyrosine kinase. Specific neurotrophic factors signal via specific protein kinases (e.g. NGF – via TrkA, BDNF – via TrkB). Activation of the protein tyrosine kinase triggers cascades of further protein phosphorylation that produce not only trophic effects but also changes in synaptic transmission.

Much recent interest in neurotrophic factors derives from findings that they regulate synaptic transmission in the adult brain, and that neurotrophic factor expression can be modulated through interactions with amine and amino acid neurotransmitters. For example, evidence suggests that repeated administration with amine-targeted antidepressants increases BDNF expression in animal models and depressed patients, whereas decreases in BDNF have been linked to depression. These data contribute to a currently popular hypothesis that changes in BDNF are important to the symptoms of depression as well as the relief of these symptoms by antidepressant drug treatment.[11, 12]

Chemokines and cytokines

Chemokines and cytokines comprise large families of homologous small proteins (6–10 kDa) and differ from neuropeptides and neurotrophic factors in that they are key signalling molecules of the immune system. However, recent findings suggest that these molecules and some of their receptors are also present in the brain in both glial cells and neurones, raising the possibility that they might also have neurotransmitter-like functions. Although the evidence is incomplete, data show that chemokine and cytokine molecules have several of the characteristics that define neurotransmitters including modulation of release of other neurotransmitters or neuropeptides.[13] The pharmacological development of agonists and antagonists that are selective for chemokine and cytokine receptors and can cross the blood-brain barrier, would open an intriguing new era of research in neuroscience.

Retrograde messengers

It is now recognized that in contrast to classical neurotransmitters and neuropeptides, a small number of brain molecules signal information at a synapse in a 'retrograde' direction that is released from the postsynaptic neurone to act on the presynaptic neurone. Molecules falling into this category include certain neurotrophic factors (see above), gaseous molecules and lipid messengers.

Nitric oxide

One putative retrograde gaseous messenger is nitric oxide (NO) that is produced in neurones from the amino acid L-arginine by a neurone-specific isoform of NO synthase (NOS), which has a widespread abundance in the brain. The first evidence of a role for NO as a neurotransmitter came from findings that stimulation of glutamate NMDA receptors by glutamate caused the release of a diffusible messenger, which was subsequently identified as NO.[14] The current thinking is that increased glutamatergic activity triggers in postsynaptic neurones an NMDA-mediated activation of NOS, and then increased synthesis of NO that diffuses across the synapse to enhance presynaptic transmission. The latter occurs at least in part through NO acting on guanylate cyclase to increase production of the second messenger cGMP. In postsynaptic neurones, NO regulates certain protein kinase pathways and gene transcription factors, and also changes cell signalling events by S-nitrosylation.

On the basis of studies on the effects of NO donors, and pharmacological and genetic modulation of NOS, increased NO production is associated with a range of CNS functions including cognition, induction and maintenance of synaptic plasticity, and NO may be neuroprotective under some conditions.[15] However, because excess NO has neurotoxic potential, and because of the difficulty of delivering NO to the CNS without inducing side effects through the many actions of NO on peripheral tissues, the development of NO-based therapies for the treatment of CNS disorders will be very challenging.

Endocannabinoids

Examples of lipid retrograde messengers are the endocannabinoids, which are a recently discovered family of naturally occurring lipids (including anandamide) that interact with cell surface receptors that are targeted by Δ^9-tetrahydrocannabinol (THC). The latter is the principle biologically active constituent of marijuana, the dried leaves of the cannabis plant.[16] In essence, endocannabinoids appear to be to THC what opiate peptides are to morphine.

It is now apparent that endocannabinoids are synthesized enzymically on demand within the postsynaptic neurone and once produced, diffuse across the synapse in a retrograde direction. Endocannabinoids then suppress neurotransmitter release through activation of presynaptic cannabinoid receptors, the main type in the brain being classified CB_1 (analogous in terms of structure and function to opiate receptors but quite distinct pharmacologically).

Many of the central effects of THC, including analgesia, increased appetite and euphoria, are thought to be mediated by CB_1 receptors. Since CB_1 receptors have a powerful influence on synaptic transmission in the brain and have limited distribution in the periphery (although CB_2 receptors are abundant in the immune system), drugs targeting these receptors and/or the enzymes involved in endocannabinoid synthesis and metabolism may have interesting therapeutic possibilities. Such drugs are currently under investigation as analgesic and anorectic agents, amongst many others.

Neurotransmitter receptors

Neurotransmitter receptors are located on the cell surface of both pre- and postsynaptic neurones, and as a general rule can be divided into two main types; one type activates an ion channel that is intrinsic to the receptor (ligand-gated ion channel, sometimes called ionotropic receptor), the other type activates a GTP binding protein which acts as a transducer between the receptor and effector system (G-protein coupled receptor [GPCR], sometimes called metabotropic receptor). An exceptions to this general rule are certain trophic factors and cytokines which signal via direct activation of a unique class of protein kinases, protein tyrosine kinases. In addition, steroid hormones signal in the brain by crossing the plasma membrane and activating receptors in the neuronal cytoplasm that translocate to the nucleus where they bind DNA and function as transcription factors.

Ligand-gated ion channels typically comprise a multimeric plasma membrane receptor complex (4–5 subunits each with 4 transmembrane spanning domains) that gate the influx of ions to evoke fast changes in synaptic signalling. GPCRs comprise a superfamily of single proteins (7 transmembrane spanning domains) that evoke slower changes in synaptic signalling through the generation of second messengers and interactions with intracellular signalling pathways.

One of the most remarkable advances in molecular neuropharmacology in the last 20 years, which has been made possible through advances in molecular cloning technology and the virtual completion of the human genome project, has been the discovery of huge diversity in neurotransmitter receptors. This complexity takes the form of not only several hundred GPCRs[17] but also considerable heterogeneity in ligand-gated ion channels produced through the assembly of multiple receptor subunits.[18, 19]

Most, and probably all, neurotransmitters have more than one receptor type, which were once classified solely according to their pharmacological properties, but today are grouped more precisely in terms of their pharmacological, functional, and structural properties. Many neurotransmitter receptor subtypes have been cloned and their distribution within the brain is known; the challenge is to turn these advances at the molecular level into a better understanding of synaptic function, and novel therapies. Neurotransmitter receptors are too numerous to describe individually but examples are shown in Table 2.3.4.4 and recent detailed reviews are available elsewhere.[10]

Ligand-gated ion channels

The amino acids glutamate and GABA are, respectively, the principal fast excitatory and inhibitory transmitters in the brain and exert their effects via ligand-gated ion channels. However, other transmitters are also capable of fast transmission via ligand-gated ion channels and these include acetylcholine (nicotinic receptors), 5-HT (5-HT_3) and ATP (P_{2X}). However, to date there is no known neuropeptide with a ligand-gated ion channel.

Ligand-gated ion channels for glutamate

Glutamate elicits fast excitatory effects by activating ligand-gated ion channels on postsynaptic membranes of which there are three types; α-amino-3-hydroxy-5-methyl-4-isoxazolepropionic acid (AMPA) receptors, N-methyl-d-aspartate (NMDA) receptors and less abundant kainate receptors, all of which were originally named according to their preferred synthetic agonist and gate cations (Na^+, K^+, and Ca^{2+}) with varying degrees of selectivity. There is likely to be additional heterogeneity because each receptor can be assembled as a tetramer of one or more of multiple subunits. For instance, AMPA receptors can be formed from tetramers of combinations of

Table 2.3.4.4 Examples of neurotransmitter receptors

Transmitter	Receptor	Signal transduction
Dopamine	D_1 family (Dopamine D_1, D_5)	Adenylate cyclase (G_s)
	D_2 family (Dopamine D_2, D_3, D_4)	Adenylate cyclase ($G_{i/o}$)
Noradrenaline	α_1 family ($\alpha_{1A,B,D}$)	Phospholipase C (G_q)
	α_2 family ($\alpha_{2A,B,C}$)	Adenylate cyclase ($G_{i/o}$)
	β family ($\beta_{1,2,3}$)	Adenylate cyclase (G_s)
5-hydroxytryptamine	5-HT_1 family (5-$HT_{1A, B, D,E, F}$)	Adenylate cyclase ($G_{i/o}$)
	5-HT_2 family (5-$HT_{2A, B, C}$)	Phospholipase C (G_q)
	5-HT_3	Cation channel
	5-HT_4	Adenylate cyclase (G_s)
	5-HT_5 family (5-$HT_{5A, B}$)	Not certain
	5-HT_6	Adenylate cyclase (G_s)
	5-HT_7	Adenylate cyclase (G_s)
Acetylcholine	M_1 (muscarinic)	Phospholipase C (G_q)
	M_2	Adenylate cyclase ($G_{i/o}$)
	M_3	Phospholipase C (G_q)
	M_4	Adenylate cyclase ($G_{i/o}$)
	M_5	Phospholipase C (G_q)
	Nicotinic (α1–10, β1–4, δ, ε, γ)	Cation channel
GABA	$GABA_A$ (α1–6, β1–3, γ1–3, σ1–3, δ, ε, π, o)	Chloride channel
	$GABA_B$	Adenylate cyclase ($G_{i/o}$)
Glutamate	AMPA ($GluR_{1-4}$)	Cation channel
	NMDA (NR_1, NR_{2A-D}, NR_{3A-B})	Cation channel
	Kainate ($GluR_{5-7}$, KA_1, KA_2)	Cation channel
	Group I family ($mGluR_{1/5}$)	Phospholipase C (G_q)
	Group II family ($mGluR_{2-3}$)	Adenylate cyclase ($G_{i/o}$)
	Group III family ($mGluR_{4/6,7,8}$)	Adenylate cyclase ($G_{i/o}$)
Tachykinin (including substance P)	NK_1	Phospholipase C (G_q)
	NK_2	Phospholipase C (G_q)
	NK_3	Phospholipase C (G_q)
Opioid	δ	Adenylate cyclase ($G_{i/o}$)
	κ	Adenylate cyclase ($G_{i/o}$)
	μ	Adenylate cyclase ($G_{i/o}$)
Galanin	GAL1	Adenylate cyclase ($G_{i/o}$)
	GAL2	Adenylate cyclase ($G_{i/o}$)
	GAL3	Adenylate cyclase ($G_{i/o}$)
Adenosine	A_1	Adenylate cyclase ($G_{i/o}$)
	A_2 family ($A_{2A, B}$)	Adenylate cyclase (G_s)
	A_3	Adenylate cyclase ($G_{i/o}$)
ATP	P2X family ($P2X_{1-7}$)	Cation channel
	$P2Y_1$	Phospholipase C (G_q)
	$P2Y_2$	Phospholipase C (G_q)
	$P2Y_4$	Phospholipase C (G_q)
	$P2Y_6$	Phospholipase C (G_q)
	$P2Y_{11}$	Phospholipase C (G_q)
	$P2Y_{12}$	Adenylate cyclase ($G_{i/o}$)
	$P2Y_{13}$	Adenylate cyclase ($G_{i/o}$)
	$P2Y_{14}$	Phospholipase C (G_q)
Cannabinoid	CB1	Adenylate cyclase ($G_{i/o}$)
	CB2	Adenylate cyclase ($G_{i/o}$)

four subunits (GluR1–GluR4) and NMDA receptors from two subunits (NR1, NR2). There are a large number of naturally occurring variants of both AMPA and NMDA subunits generated through RNA editing and alternative splicing.

The pharmacological and functional significance of this complexity is not yet clear although evidence suggests that certain agents are able to distinguish between different receptor assemblies.[10] Interestingly, recent data suggest that changes in AMPA receptor subunit composition at the postsynaptic membrane cause differences in ion (Ca^{2+}) permeability that change synaptic efficacy, the best-characterized form of which is long-term potentiation (LTP), a widely accepted neurophysiological correlate of learning and memory.[19]

An interesting feature of many ligand-gated ion channels is the presence of multiple chemically-sensitive sites (allosteric modulatory sites), in addition to the site(s) which bind the natural transmitter ligand. This is the case for both the AMPA and NMDA receptors. Thus, in addition to the glutamate binding site AMPA receptors are sensitive to 'AMPAkines' which comprise a chemically diverse group of agents that potentiate the function of the receptor in *in vitro* models, and elicit associated procognitive effects *in vivo*.[20] Non-glutamate sites on the NMDA receptor include a site for Mg^{2+} that is the source of a voltage-dependent NMDA receptor block which requires membrane depolarization to open, as well as positive modulatory sites for glycine and polyamines. Whilst glutamate is released from presynaptic terminals in an activity-dependent fashion and acts as a neurotransmitter, glycine and the polyamines act as extracellular modulators that are present at more constant levels. The latter binding sites are under investigation as a possible source of NMDA receptor enhancing agents that do not suffer the potential excitotoxic effects of agonists at the glutamate site.[21]

Ligand-gated ion channels for GABA

GABA elicits fast inhibitory effects by activating the $GABA_A$ receptor ion channel complex. $GABA_A$ receptors are heteropentameric membrane proteins that form a GABA-gated chloride channel. There are at least 18 types of $GABA_A$ receptor subunits (α1–6, β1–3, γ1–3, Π, δ, θ and p1–3). Although studies co-expressing different $GABA_A$ receptor subunits indicate the potential for several hundreds if not thousands of $GABA_A$ receptor subunit combinations, studies on $GABA_A$ receptor subunit distribution and abundance in native brain tissue indicate that the number of naturally occurring types of $GABA_A$ receptors may be of the order of 10 or fewer.[22]

As with the glutamate ionotropic receptors, $GABA_A$ receptors have a number of allosteric modulatory sites including those sensitive to certain endogenous steroids, anaesthetic agents (for example alfaxalone) and alcohol (ethanol). However, the vast majority of $GABA_A$ receptors are characterized by their sensitivity to benzodiazepines. Both genetic and medicinal chemistry approaches have been used to identify the pharmacological significance of $GABA_A$ receptor subtypes, and specifically to determine whether the multiple behavioural effects of benzodiazepines such as diazepam (sedation, anxiolysis, amnesia, motor in-coordination etc.) can be attributed to specific $GABA_A$ receptor subunit combinations.[18]

In particular, studies with point-mutated mice have revealed that the sedative effect of diazepam is mediated by α1-containing $GABA_A$ receptors, whereas the anxiolytic action is mediated by α2/α3-containing $GABA_A$ receptors. Moreover, findings that ligands with selective actions at α2- and/or α3-containing $GABA_A$ receptors display anxiolytic activity, raise the possibility of future benzodiazepines with behaviourally selective actions. Interestingly, α5-containing $GABA_A$ receptors may be an important site of action of alcohol. The $GABA_A$ receptor subunit(s) targeted by steroids and anaesthetics to produce the CNS inhibitory effects of these agents are currently under investigation.

G-protein coupled receptors

Almost all neurotransmitters signal effects via GPCRs and most neurotransmitters signal via more than one type of GPCR. For example, the amine 5-HT possesses 14 receptor subtypes (comprising seven receptor families, 5-HT_{1-7}), 13 of which are GPCRs and one is a ligand-gated ion channel. Each 5-HT GPCR has high affinity and selectivity for 5-HT but individually the receptors demonstrate different selectivity for other ligands, arise from different (but homologous) genes, and are formed from different protein sequences with different distributions and signalling effects.[23] Since several 5-HT GPCRs can co-localize at a single synapse, the signal received by a postsynaptic neurone may be quite complicated. This complexity for 5-HT can be seen in many other transmitters including dopamine (D_{1-5}), glutamate ($mGluR_{1-8}$), noradrenaline ($\alpha_{1A,B,D}$, $\alpha_{2A,B,C}$, β_{1-3}), endocannabinoids (CB_{1-2}) and neuropeptides (Table 2.3.4.4).

Typically GPCRs comprise a single membrane protein with seven transmembrane spanning domains, an N-terminus facing the extracellular space, a C-terminus facing the cytoplasm, and several intracellular transmembrane domain linking loops. The N-terminus of some GPCRs ($mGluR_{1-8}$, $GABA_B$) contains the ligand binding site, while for most GPCRs the predicted ligand binding site lies within the transmembrane domains. Both the C-terminus and the third transmembrane intracellular loops are targets for phosphorylation by protein kinases; the third intracellular loop is the main site of G-protein interaction.

G-proteins

Each G-protein is a heterotrimer comprised of α, β and γ subunits that dissociate on binding of ligand to the GPCR. On dissociation, the α subunit binds GTP and through intrinsic GTPase activity directly regulates a number of specific downstream effector enzymes and ion channels. The β/γ subunits are also biologically active and regulate some of the same effector proteins.

There are four major types of G-proteins, Gs, Gi, Gq and G_0 that produce the following signalling effects; activation of adenylate cyclase, inhibition of adenylate cyclase, activation of phospholipase C and interaction with Ca^{2+} and K^+ channels, respectively. Changes in the activity of adenylate cyclase results in altered intracellular levels of the 'second messenger' cyclic adenosine monophosphate (cAMP). Similarly, phospholipase C (PLC) alters intracellular levels of inositol triphosphate (IP_3) and diacyl glycerol (DAG). Altered levels of these second messengers trigger changes in activity of specific signalling cascades and ultimately changes in physiological responses (see below).

The opening of ion channels in response to neurotransmitter-induced GPCR activation leads to direct effects (excitatory or inhibitory) on the electrical properties of neurones, albeit on a slightly slower timescale than effects produced by ligand-gated ion channels. Almost all neurotransmitter classes are able to evoke changes in ion channel opening via GPCRs, and some may be clinically important. For example, the α_2-adrenoceptor-induced opening of K^+ channels on noradrenaline neurones that causes a fall in noradrenergic activity and release, may contribute to the anxiolytic and sedative properties of α_2-adrenoceptor agonists such as clonidine. On the other hand, the 5-HT_{2A} receptor-induced closing of K^+ channels on cortical neurones that causes an increase in cortical neurone activity, may underlie the psychotic effects of LSD and related hallucinogens.(23)

GPCR regulation

Recent discoveries of interactions between GPCRs and other intracellular proteins have lead to a new understanding of how the receptors are regulated and trafficked to and from the plasma membrane. Studies commencing on the β-adrenceptor, have identified two families of regulatory proteins called β-arrestins and GPCR kinases (GRKs). Within seconds of being activated by an agonist the GPCR is phosphorylated by a GRK on the C-terminal cytoplasmic tail and other intracellular domains. This phosphorylation promotes the interaction of β-arrestins with the GPCR, which limits the signal duration, and causes loss of sensitivity to agonist activation, and then receptor internalization from the cell surface.(24)

In addition to β-arrestins the C-termini of GPCRs associate with a large variety of transmembrane or soluble proteins, termed 'GPCR-interacting proteins' (GIPs). Some GIPs are themselves GPCRs that form homo- or heterodimers, while other GIPs are ionic channels, ionotropic receptors and proteins that control GPCR trafficking(25). One interesting example of a GIP is the molecule p11, which reportedly functions to traffic a 5-HT GPCR (5-HT_{1B}) to the plasma membrane. Evidence suggests that p11 expression is reduced in postmortem brain of patients committing suicide, and that mice with genetic deletion of p11 have a depressive-like phenotype.(26)

Small G proteins

In addition to the G-proteins associated with GPCRs, there is a super family of 'small G-proteins' which also bind GTP and possess intrinsic GTPase activity but these are not modulated by agonist binding. Rather, small G-proteins function as molecular switches that control several cellular processes ranging from vesicle trafficking and exocytosis (e.g. Rab) to assembly of cytoskeletal structures (e.g. Rho). Among the best characterized small G-proteins are those that comprise the Ras family. Numerous types of cell signals including those of most neurotrophic factors converge on Ras and related proteins to regulate MAP-kinase pathways.

Second messengers

The generation of the second messengers cAMP and DAG by adenylate cyclase and phospholipase C, respectively, leads to activation of protein kinases that add phosphate groups to specific protein targets to change their activity and ultimately trigger diverse physiological responses (Fig. 2.3.4.2). Enzymes called phosphatases,

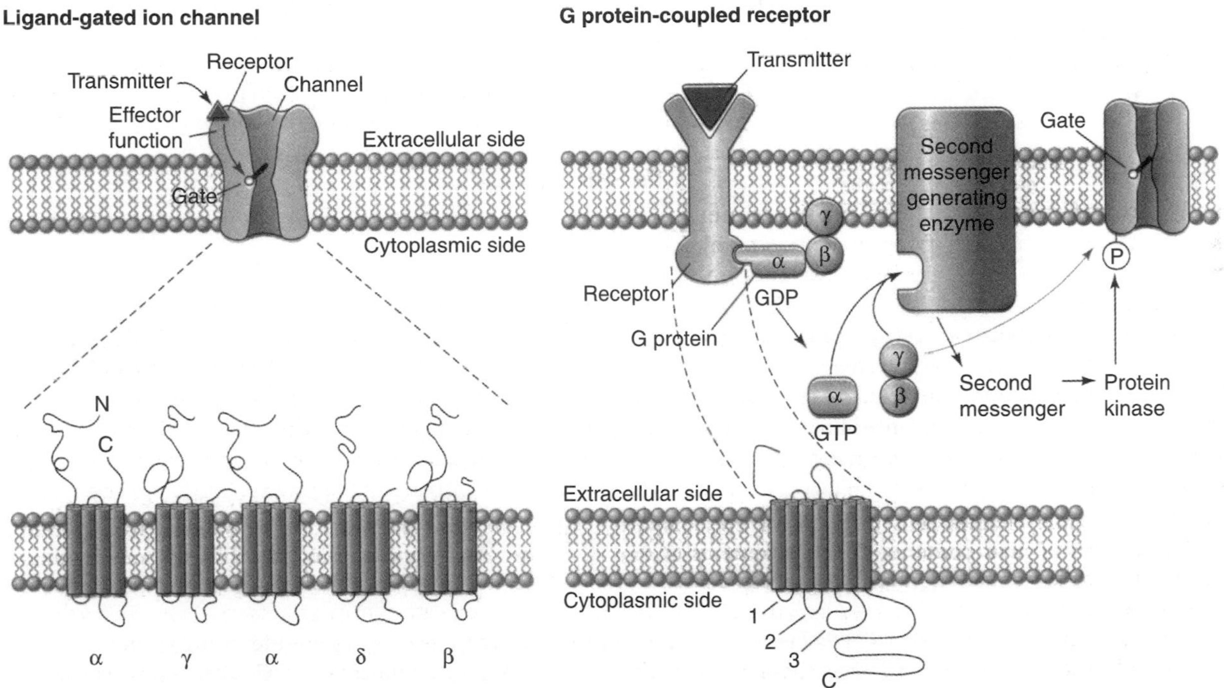

Fig. 2.3.4.2 Diagrammatic representation of ligand-gated ion channel and G-protein coupled receptors. Ligand-gated ion channels comprise multiple protein subunits that form a central pore in the plasma membrane. On binding of the neurotransmitter, this receptor mediates fast excitatory or inhibitory transmission depending on whether the pore gates cations or chloride ions, respectively. G-protein coupled receptors comprise a single membrane spanning protein. On binding of the neurotransmitter, this receptor mediates slow transmission by enabling the dissociation of the G-protein into α subunit monomer and β/γ subunit dimer, both of which may activate an effector enzyme to generate a second messenger. Also, the β/γ subunit dimer may directly interact with ion channels. Second messengers may also indirectly modulate ion channels through phosphorylation by activating protein kinases. Reproduced from Nestler EJ, Hyman SE and Malenka RC (2001) *Molecular Neuropharmacology*, p. 64, Copyright 2001, McGraw-Hill, New York.

which remove the phosphate groups, oppose these signalling effects. Guanylate cyclase is a cytosolic enzyme which also generates a second messenger, cGMP. As noted above, guanylate cyclase is activated by NO to produce effects on presynaptic function.

Based on molecular cloning studies, nine forms of adenylate cyclase have been identified (I–IX) and each exhibits a distinct distribution in brain and peripheral tissues.(27) The full implication of this complexity is not yet understood but it suggests that regulation of cAMP formation varies depending on the form of adenylyl cyclase expressed in neuronal cells.

Both cAMP and cGMP are degraded by phosphodiesterases (PDEs) which are expressed in numerous forms (types 1–11) in brain and periperal tissues.(10) At high concentrations, caffeine and related methylxanthines inhibit PDE and this action contributes to the pharmacological effects of these drugs. Much effort is being made to develop inhibitors that are selective for brain-specific forms of PDE. Rolipram inhibits all isoforms of PDE4; this drug showed promise as an antidepressant, but its clinical utility was limited by peripheral side effects. However, because the PDE4 enzymes comprise a number of isoforms, an inhibitor of one isoform may lead to the development of an effective antidepressant without the side effects of rolipram.

GPCR-induced activation of PLC causes the breakdown of phosphatidylinositol, resulting in the generation and recycling of the second messengers, IP_3 and DAG (phosphoinositide cycle). Both IP_3 and DAG produce downstream signalling effects, IP_3 through the mobilization of intracellular calcium stores and DAG through activating a protein kinase. There are two major isoforms of PLC in brain, β and γ, the β isoform being predominantly responsible for mediating the effects of GPCRs linked to Gq.

After its formation, IP_3 is recycled via a series of dephosphorylations to form inositol which is used in the regeneration of phosphatidylinositol. Interestingly, lithium, which is an important drug in the treatment of manic depressive illness, inhibits one of the enyzymes involved in the recycling of IP_3 (inositol-1-monophosphatase) and causes inositol depletion. Because inositol does not easily enter the blood-brain-barrier, brain inositol levels are thought to fall and production of the second messengers diminishes. It is a popular hypothesis that inositol depletion is responsible for lithium's clinical effects but this remains unproven. Indeed, lithium is known to interact with a range of signalling systems including various ion channels, adenlyate cyclases and protein kinases. Recent interest has focussed on the inhibition by lithium and mood stabilizing anticonvulsants such as valproate, of glycogen synthase kinase 3β that has a range of targets and effects ranging from formation of inositol to trophic mechanisms.(28)

Downstream signalling cascades

The activation or inhibition of second messenger signalling cascades by GPCRs can profoundly change the intracellular environment of a neurone by regulating the activity of protein kinases and other proteins, including gene transcription factors and even enzymes involved in regulation of chromatin structure. Consequently, these cascades may regulate gene transcription and protein synthesis and activate multiple downstream effectors, including those that form the cytoskeleton or contribute to mechanisms underlying synaptic plasticity. Such effects can have long-lasting effects on neuronal function. Increasing evidence suggests that the neuroadaptive responses to repeated psychotropic drug administration are underpinned by changes in gene expression that result in the remodelling of synaptic function and structure. This thinking has been applied to explain a range of processes including compulsive recreational drug use as well as the therapeutic action of antipsychotic drugs.

As an example, the past decade has seen the evolution of a fascinating theory to explain the delayed onset of antidepressant effect of drugs like fluoxetine and imipramine that act to inhibit plasma membrane amine transporters (see above). This theory posits that elevated amine levels trigger GPCR signalling cascades that activate gene programmes to enhance neuronal survival and connectivity, the latter having failed because of the adverse effects of stress and other environmental factors.(11, 29, 30) Some of the key genes involved in this process include trophic factors such as BDNF, which may be a trigger for the production of newly formed neurones (Fig. 2.3.4.3). Although this line of thought is driving promising pharmacological strategies for improved antidepressant therapies, our knowledge of the key molecules that are changed by antidepressants to bring about the relief of the symptoms of depression is far from complete.

Concluding remarks

Until recently, studies on the chemistry of synaptic neurotransmission have focused on a small number of neurotransmitters and a narrow group of proteins involved in neurotransmitter function,

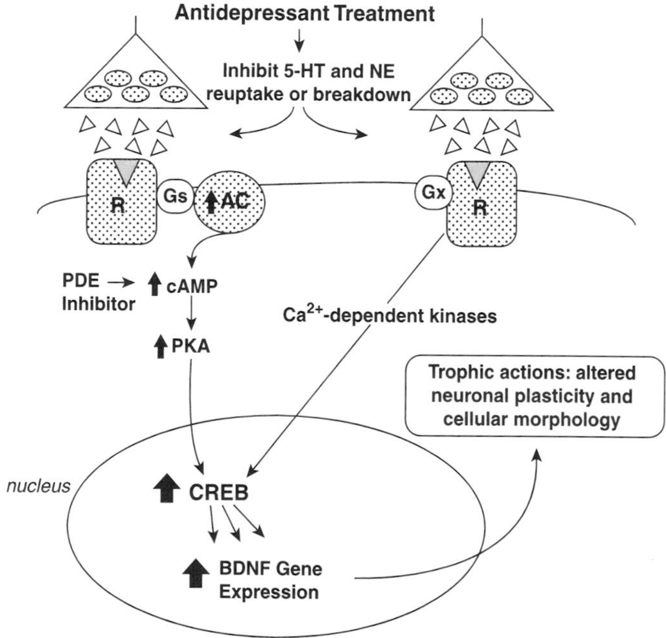

Fig. 2.3.4.3 Hypothetical signal transduction pathways regulated by antidepressant drugs leading to increased neurotrophic factor expression and neurogenesis. Antidepressant treatment increases synaptic amine levels that stimulate GPCRs (Gs) linked to adenylyl cyclase (AC). The subsequent increase in cAMP levels activates cAMP-dependent protein kinase (PKA) which, possibly together with Ca^{2+}-dependent protein kinases, increases the function and expression of the gene transcription factor, cAMP response element binding protein (CREB). CREB enhances the expression of brain derived neurotrophic factor (BDNF) that may underpin trophic effects of antidepressant treatment, including synaptic remodeling and increased neurogenesis. Reprinted by permission from Macmillan Publishers Ltd: Molecular Psychiatry, DOI: 10.1038/sj/mp/4001016.

specifically neurotransmitter receptors, transporters and enzymes which bring about neurotransmitter synthesis or degradation. Today, powerful molecular and genetic approaches are being used to identify and understand new proteins and mechanisms involved in neurotransmitter function and control. So far, just a few tens of perhaps thousands of neurotransmitter-related proteins, have been successfully targeted by pharmacological agents that have translated into important treatments of psychiatric disorder but there is promise of many more such treatments to come. Moreover, this huge diversity of neurotransmitter-related proteins is now emerging as a large resource for studies of genetic risk factors of psychiatric disorder and investigations of biological markers of illness diagnosis and progression, and treatment outcome.

Further information

International Union of Basic and Clinical Pharmacology (IUPHAR) committee official database on receptor nomenclature and drug classification, http://www.iuphar-db.org/index.jsp.

Kandel, E.R., Schwartz, J., Jessell, T. (2000) *Principles of Neural Science*, (4th edn.), McGraw-Hill, New York. Further details are available at http://en.wikipedia.org/wiki/Principles_of_Neural_Science.

Nestler, E.J., Hyman, S.E., and Malenka, R.C. (2008). *Molecular Neuropharmacology*, 2nd edn. McGraw-Hill, New York.

References

1. Hökfelt, T., Bartfai, T. and Bloom, F. (2003). Neuropeptides: opportunities fordrug discovery. *Lancet Neurology,* **2**, 463–72.
2. Iversen, L. (2006). Neurotransmitter transporters and their impacton the development of psychopharmacology. *British Journal of Pharmacology,* **147**, Suppl 1, S82-8.
3. Fremeau ,R.T., Voglmaier, S., Seal, R.P., *et al.* (2004). VGLUTs define subsets of excitatory neurones and suggest novel roles for glutamate. *Trends in Neurosciences,* **27**, 98–103.
4. Zhou, Z., Zhen, J., Karpowich, N.K., *et al.* (2007). LeuT-desipramine structure reveals how antidepressants block neurotransmitter reuptake. *Science,* **317**, 1390–3.
5. Shigeri, Y., Seal, R.P. and Shimamoto, K. (2004). Molecular pharmacology of glutamate transporters, EAATs and VGLUTs. *Brain Research,* **45**, 250–65.
6. Rothstein, J.D., Patel, S., Regan, M.R., *et al.* (2005). Beta-lactam antibiotics offer neuroprotection by increasing glutamate transporter expression. *Nature,* **433**, 73–7.
7. Scamuffa, N., Calvo, F., Chretien, M., *et al.* (2006). Proprotein convertases: lessons from knockouts. *Faseb Journal,* **20**, 1954–63.
8. Ögren, S.O., Kuteeva, E., Hökfelt, T, *et al.* (2006). Galanin receptor antagonists: a potential novel pharmacological treatment for mood disorders. *CNS Drugs,* **20**, 633–54.
9. Chao, M.V. (2003). Neurotrophins and their receptors: a convergence point for many signalling pathways. *Nature Reviews* **4**, 299–309.
10. Alexander, S.P., Mathie, A. and Peters, J.A. (2007). Guide to Receptors and Channels (GRAC), 2nd edition (2007 Revision). *British Journal of Pharmacology,* **150**, Suppl 1, S1–S168.
11. Castren, E. (2005). Is mood chemistry? *Nature Reviews,* **6**, 241–6.
12. Martinowich, K., Manji, H. and Lu, B. (2007). New insights into BDNF function in depression and anxiety. *Nature Neuroscience,* **10**, 1089–93.
13. Rostene, W., Kitabgi, P. and Parsadaniantz, S.M. (2007). Chemokines: a new class of neuromodulator? *Nature Reviews,* **8**, 895–903.
14. Garthwaite, J. and Boulton, C.L. (1995). Nitric oxide signaling in the central nervous system. *Annual Review of Physiology,* **57**, 683–706.
15. Calabrese, V., Mancuso, C., Calvani, M., *et al.* (2007). Nitric oxide in the central nervous system: neuroprotection versus neurotoxicity. *Nature Reviews,* **8**, 766–75.
16. Piomelli, D. (2003). The molecular logic of endocannabinoid signalling. *Nature Reviews,* **4**, 873–84.
17. Fredholm, B.B., Hokfelt, T. and Milligan, G. (2007). G-protein-coupled receptors: an update. *Acta physiologica,* **190**, 3–7.
18. Rudolph, U. and Mohler, H. (2006). GABA-based therapeutic approaches: GABAA receptor subtype functions. *Current Opinion in Pharmacology,* **6**, 18–23.
19. Schuman, E.M. and Seeburg, P.H. (2006). Signalling mechanisms. *Current Opinion in Neurobiology,* **16**, 247–50.
20. Lynch, G. and Gall, C.M. (2006). Ampakines and the threefold path to cognitive enhancement. *Trends in Neurosciences,* **29**, 554–62.
21. Kemp, J.A. and McKernan, R.M. (2002). NMDA receptor pathways as drug targets. *Nature Neuroscience,* **5** Suppl,1039–42.
22. McKernan, R.M. and Whiting, P.J. (1996). Which GABAA-receptor subtypes really occur in the brain? *Trends in Neurosciences,* **19**,139–43.
23. Barnes, N.M. and Sharp, T. (1999). A review of central 5-HT receptors and their function. *Neuropharmacology,* **38**,1083–152.
24. Lefkowitz, R.J. (2007). Seven transmembrane receptors: something old, something new. *Acta physiologica,* **190**, 9–19.
25. Bockaert, J., Roussignol, G., Becamel, C., *et al.* (2004). GPCR-interacting proteins (GIPs): nature and functions. *Biochemical Society Transactions,* **32**, 851–5.
26. Svenningsson, P., Chergui, K., Rachleff, I., *et al.* (2006). Alterations in 5-HT1B receptor function by p11 in depression-like states. *Science,* **311**, 77–80.
27. Cooper, D.M. (2003). Regulation and organization of adenylyl cyclases and cAMP. *Biochemical Journal,* **375**, 517–29.
28. Gould, T.D. and Manji, H.K. (2005). Glycogen synthase kinase-3: a putative molecular target for lithium mimetic drugs. *Neuropsychopharmacology,* **30**, 1223–37.
29. Pittenger, C. and Duman, R.S. (2008). Stress, depression, and neuroplasticity: a convergence of mechanisms. *Neuropsychopharmacology,* **33**, 88–109.
30. Duman, R.S. (2002). Synaptic plasticity and mood disorders. *Molecular Psychiatry,* **7**, Suppl 1, S29–34.

2.3.5 Neuropathology

Peter Falkai and Bernhard Bogerts

Introduction

The traditional domains of neuropathology are well-defined organic brain diseases with an obvious pathology, such as tumours, infections, vascular diseases, trauma, or toxic and hypoxemic changes, as well as degenerative brain diseases (e.g. Alzheimer's disease, Parkinson's disease, and Huntington's chorea). Neuropathological investigations of these brain disorders have been rewarding, because patients with any of these conditions can be expected to have gross morphological or more or less specific neurohistological anomalies related to the clinical symptoms of the disorders. Moreover, the type of brain pathology of these well-defined disease entities is quite homogenous. For example, it is highly unlikely that a patient with Parkinson's disease would not exhibit morphological changes and Lewy bodies in the nigrostriatal system, just as much a person with Huntington's chorea would have a normal striatum, or a patient with Pick's or Alzheimer's disease would have no changes in the cerebral cortex.

In contrast, the history of the neuropathology of psychiatric disorders outside primary degenerative diseases is much more controversial, because no such obvious and homogenous types of brain pathology (as seen in neurological disorders) have yet been detected for the major psychiatric illnesses such as schizophrenia, affective disorders, substance-related disorders, or personality disorders.

The scope of this chapter is to summarize the neuropathological findings in schizophrenia, affective disorders, and alcoholism. Tables 2.3.5.1, 2.3.5.2, 2.3.5.3, and 2.3.5.4 highlight the significant findings. It goes beyond the scope of this chapter to review the large body of literature on the dementias, including specifically Alzheimer's disease. Concerning this matter, the reader is referred to several comprehensive reviews (e.g. Jellinger and Bancher 1998).[1]

Schizophrenia and other psychotic disorders

Studies between 1898 and 1975

In 1898, Alois Alzheimer (1898)[2] described subtle changes in the neocortex of patients with schizophrenia. Subsequently to Alzheimer, Southard reported cortical atrophy in schizophrenia and mentioned association areas of the cerebral cortex to be most affected in this disorder.[4] Vogt and Vogt and their coworkers reported cellular alterations in the cortex, thalamus, and basal ganglia of schizophrenics.[5] These considerable efforts on the part of many well-known neuroanatomists and neuropathologists to prove schizophrenia to be a primary brain disorder ended in inconsistent and unsubstantiated findings.[6] To a large extent, these inconsistencies can be attributed to a variety of methodological inadequacies including diagnostic uncertainties, inadequate control samples, flawed tissue-handling procedures, variable choice of brain regions for neuropathological studies, limitations in the sensitivity and specificity of classical histological stains, as well as lack of quantitative methods to delineate and analyse subtle brain abnormalities.[7]

Table 2.3.5.1 Gross morphometric findings in schizophrenia

Region/parameter	Finding
General	
Brain length	(↓)
Brain weight	↓
Ventricular area/volume	↑
Cortex thickness	↓
Temporal lobe	
Lobar area/volume	—
Hippocampal area/volume	↓
Parahippocampal area/volume	↓
Parahippocampal cortical thickness	↓
Amygdala area/volume	—
Sylvian fissure length, planum temporal volume	↓
Sulcogyral pattern	Abnormal
Frontal, parietal, and occipital lobes	
Cingulate cortical thickness	—
Insula area/volume	—
Corpus callosum thickness	(↑)
Internal capsula area/volume	—
Basal ganglia	
Globus pallidum area/volume	(↓)
Nucleus accumbens area/volume	↓
Cautdate-putamen area/volume	↑
Thalamus	
Mediodorsal nucleus area/volume	(↓)
Whole and various nuclei area/volume	—
Cerebellum	
Anterior vermis area	↓
Brainstem	
Substantia nigra volume	↓
Locus coeruleus volume	—
Periventricular grey volume	↓

In comparison with controls: ↓, reduced; ↑, increased; —, no difference; ( ), finding not or only partially replicated.

Adapted from Arnold and Trojanowski.[3]

Table 2.3.5.2 Neuronal morphometric findings in schizophrenia

Region/parameter	Finding
Temporal lobe	
Superior temporal gyrus (Tpt) neurone density	↓
Hippocampal neurone density	(↓)
Hippocampal neurone size	(↓)
Entorhinal cortex neurone density	(↓)
Entorhinal cortex neurone size	↓
Amygdala neurone density (basolateral n.)	—
Frontal lobe	
Prefrontal cortex pyramidal neurone density	↑
Prefrontal cortex interneurone density	(↓)
Prefrontal cortex neurone size	↓
Cingulate (anterior) pyramidal neurone density	↓
Cingulate interneurone density	↓
Cingulate neurone size	↓
Motor cortex neurone density	(↓)
Motor cortex neurone size	—
Basal ganglia	
Globus pallidus neurone counts	—
Nucleus accumbens neurone counts	↓
Nucleus basalis of Meynert neurone counts	—
Thalamus	
Mediodorsal nucleus neurone counts	(↓)
Cerebellum	
Purkinje cell density	↓
Brainstem	
Substantia nigra neurone density	↓
Substantia nigra neurone size	—
Locus coeruleus neurone density	
Locus coeruleus neurone size	
Pedunculopontine nucleus neurone density	↓

In comparison with controls: ↓, reduced; ↑, increased; —, no difference; ( ), finding not or only partially replicated.

Adapted from Arnold and Trojanowski.[3]

Neuropathological findings in schizophrenia since 1975

Advances in the last 30 years have produced more reliable psychiatric diagnostic criteria, improved structural and functional neuroimaging techniques, a large array of highly sensitive and specific molecular probes and labeling procedures, suitable for use in neuropathological studies, and computer-assisted image analysis methodologies. For these and other reasons, there has been a resurgence of interest in the neurobiological substrates of schizophrenia, and contemporary neuropathological studies have enumerated many findings in the brains of patients with schizophrenia (for reviews see[7, 8, 9]). Finally, the recent description of the first risk genes like Neuregulin-1 or Dysbindin has provided this field with reliable research targets.[8, 9] To identify the role of these genes for the pathophysiology of schizophrenia their expression pattern in human brain tissue has to be established in the near future.

(a) Diagnostic neuropathology

Stevens (1982)[10] surveyed the brains of 28 schizophrenic patients for gross and microscopic abnormalities using standard diagnostic stains. She discovered no abnormalities in temporal (including the amygdalohippocampal region), frontal, or parietal lobes or in the thalamus, but detected assorted abnormalities in other regions, including neuronal loss or infarction in the globus pallidus in five patients, increased cerebellar white matter gliosis in five patients, excessive Purkinje cell loss in 13 cases, and, most notably, increased fibrillary gliosis in periventricular, periaqueductal, and basal forebrain regions bilaterally.

In another prospectively accrued series,[10] she found that of 56 schizophrenics five were afflicted with other distinct neurological illnesses (multiple sclerosis, Friedreich's ataxia, epilepsy, stroke) and three had been treated with prefrontal leukotomies. The remaining 48 showed no differences to controls in the frequency of large- or small-vessel cerebrovascular disease, senile plaques, or neurofibrillary degeneration. However, there was an 'increased incidence of unexpected pathology in the schizophrenic group compared with the control group'. Of these 48 schizophrenics, 21 exhibited some degree of focal pathology compared to 12 of 56 controls, but these abnormalities were diverse in nature and location. Holzer staining suggested a significant increase in fibrous gliosis in the cortex, white matter, and periventricular structures, but generally for those brains showing other focal pathology. After removal of these cases, the 'adjusted' group showed no evidence of increased gliosis.

In a series of 101 elderly schizophrenics,[12] Golier *et al.* found only 10 with definite or probable Alzheimer's disease by modern neuropathological diagnostic criteria, 29 with senile plaques, 15 with vascular lesions, two with Parkinson's disease, three with unspecified tumour, and five with 'other' findings.

Another review concluded extensive neuropathological investigations due to lack of any evidence of neurodegeneration or neural injury beyond what typically is observed in brains of individuals without neuropsychiatric illness.[8]

(b) Morphometric studies

Macroscopic findings (Table 2.3.5.1)

Several planimetric postmortem studies of the entire cortex have been performed, some reporting significant reduction of cortical volume (12 per cent) and central grey matter (6 per cent), and others reporting no difference in volumes of cortex, white matter and whole hemispheres between schizophrenics and controls. Others that measured general brain parameters have shown reduced brain length, brain weight, and increased ventricular area/volume.

Since the publication of the first report of reduced tissue volume in temporolimbic structures of schizophrenics,[13, 14] numerous quantitative or qualitative anatomical postmortem studies on limbic structures of schizophrenics have been conducted. The majority of these studies substantiated subtle structural changes (15–20 per cent mean volume reduction) in at least one of the investigated areas, whereas only a few yielded entirely negative results. The findings comprise reduced volumes or cross-sectional areas of the hippocampus, amygdala, parahippocampal gyrus, which were later corroborated by morphometric magnetic resonance imaging (MRI) studies. Figure 2.3.5.1 demonstrates the subtle bilateral volume reduction of the hippocampus in schizophrenics and furthermore visualizes the kind of hypoplastic appearance of the anterior hippocampus, which can be seen in about one third of the patients

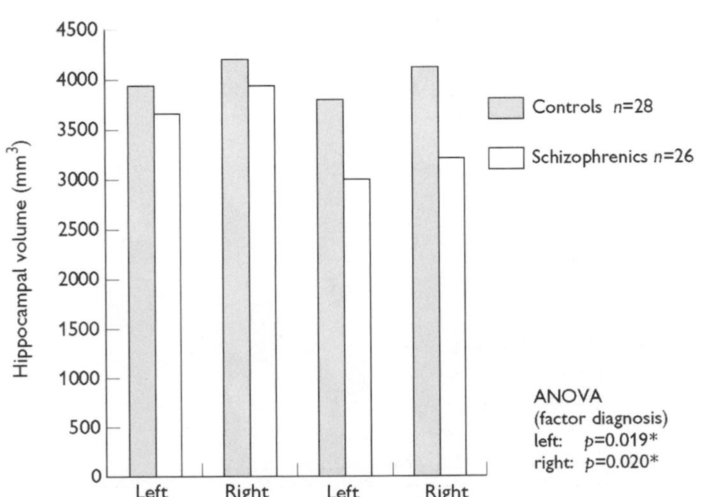

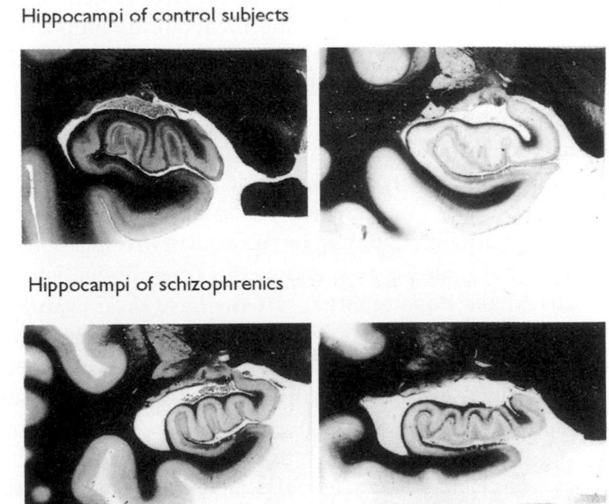

Fig. 2.3.5.1 Left side: hippocampal volumes in schizophrenic patients and controls; Right side: lippocampal atrophy macroscopically seen in about one-third of patients with schizophrenia (upper row) compared to control subjects (lower row) (from Bogerts 1990).

(lower row of the photographs). Other findings in limbic brain regions are left temporal horn enlargement, white-matter reductions in parahippocampal gyrus or hippocampus, and an increased incidence of a cavum septi pellucidi.

Unchanged volumes of the striatum and external pallidum but a subtle volume decrease in the internal pallidal segment were found in brains from the preneuroleptic era. Pallidal volume reduction was due to a reduction in the catatonic subgroup.(15) These initial findings have to be pursued, as longitudinal MRI studies suggest that enlargement of basal ganglia can be seen in schizophrenia as a consequence of treatment with classical neuroleptics, which can be reversed by the use of atypical substances.(16)

After initially finding no volumetric changes in the thalamic nuclei, subsequently the area/volume of the mediodorsal nucleus and anteroventral thalamic nucleus were found to be decreased.(17)

Changes in area measurements of the corpus callosum were described in some studies. The findings, however, are inconsistent; there are reports of increased as well as of decreased midline areas. More consistent are reports of shape abnormalities, in that the sex difference in anterior and posterior callosal thickness in normal controls seems to be reversed in schizophrenics and the mean curvature in the corpus callosum is bent upwards.(18)

Findings of decreased volume of the substantia nigra and the periventricular grey matter as well as no volumetric change in the locus coeruleus await replication.

Microscopic findings (Table 2.3.5.2)

There are a number of studies of neurone number, density, and size in schizophrenia. As summarized in Table 2.3.5.2, the majority of these have focused on the ventromedial temporal and frontal lobes.

In the lateral prefrontal cortex, an increase in neurone density has been reported inconsistently, which may relate to the observed decrease in neurone size (with decreased dendritic arborization and a decreased neuropil compartment).(20) In the anterior cingulate could be observed decreased pyramidal and local circuit neurone density accompanied by increased vertical axon density and altered dopaminergic innervation. These findings have been interpreted as representing disturbed connections in the anterior cingulate.

Within the ventromedial temporal lobe, reduced cell numbers or cell size and abnormal cell arrangements in the hippocampus or entorhinal cortex were described. However, some groups could not confirm cellular disarray in the hippocampus(21) just as little find significant volume and cell number reductions in the hippocampus and entorhinal cortex.(22)

Original studies demonstrating decreased neuronal counts in the mediodorsal and anteriorventral nucleus of the thalamus have been partially supported by subsequent investigations.(17)

The lateral (nigrostriatal) and medial (mesolimbic) parts of the mesencephalic dopaminergic systems have been evaluated and the size of the nerve cell bodies found to be significantly reduced in the medial part by 16 per cent, while the cell numbers were unchanged. The reduced cell size of the medial, mesolimbic neurones were taken to indicate dopaminergic underactivity. Two qualitative reports on degenerative changes in cholinergic cells in the basal nucleus of Meynert of schizophrenics have been published; more recent quantitative studies found normal cell numbers in the basal nucleus of schizophrenics. Volume measurements and cell counts in the noradrenergic locus coeruleus revealed a trend for decreased locus coeruleus volume without loss of neurones, indicating a reduction of neuropil in schizophrenics. These results appear comparable to those described in the substantia nigra, as mentioned above. Investigating the brainstem reticular formation revealed a twofold increased number of the cholinergic neurones of the pedunculopontine nucleus and the dorsal tegmental nucleus as well as a reduced cell size in the locus coeruleus.(23,24) However, these results are not undisputed as newer studies using state of the art stereology demonstrate opposite findings.(25)

Schizophrenia as a disorder of brain maturation

There is evidence from clinical research implicating aberrant neurodevelopmental processes in the pathophysiology of schizophrenia,(26) but there is also a growing literature suggestive of progressive deterioration in the disease for a substantial proportion of patients.(27) It should be noted that abnormal neurodevelopmental processes are not mutually exclusive of neurodegenerative mechanisms in the pathogenesis of complex neuropsychiatric disorders. Indeed, while some genetic disorders are mainly developmental (e.g. fragile X syndrome) and others mainly neurodegenerative (e.g. Huntington's disease), some have both developmental and degenerative pathologies (e.g. Down syndrome). Based on the neuropathological literature of the last 30 years some suggestions can be made concerning the pathophysiology of schizophrenia.

(c) Gliosis

Glial cells, mainly astrocytes (Figs. 2.3.5.2 and 2.3.5.3), show changes in response to almost every type of injury or disease in the central nervous system. Therefore, in typical degenerative brain disorders such as Alzheimer's disease or Huntington's chorea increased glial cell densities are found. Most studies using glial cell counts, neuron-to-glial ratios and glial cell nuclear volumes found no difference between schizophrenics and controls in temporolimbic structures, the thalamus, and cingulate cortex. In our own large-scale study we counted the number of astrocytes in several key regions such as the area surrounding the temporal horn and found no evidence for astrogliosis in schizophrenia (Fig. 2.3.5.3).(28) Although the question of fibrous gliosis (i.e. increase in glial cell fibres) remains more controversial, the well-controlled study by Bruton *et al.* (1990)(11) also rejects fibrous gliosis in schizophrenia.

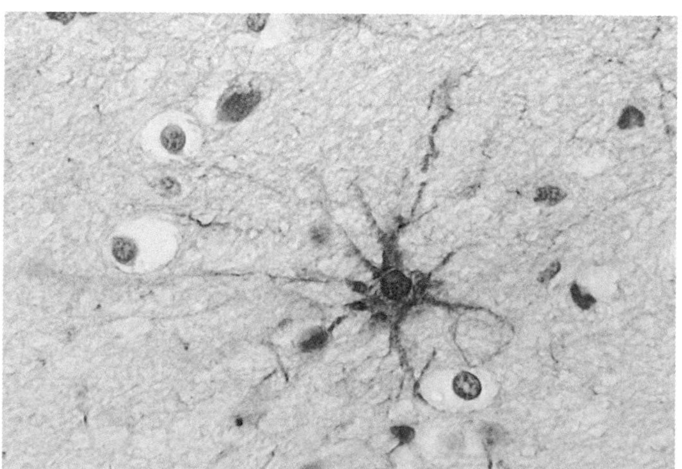

Fig. 2.3.5.2 Macroglia in a control subject: Glial fibrillary acid protein (GFAP) positive astrocyte in the human cortex.

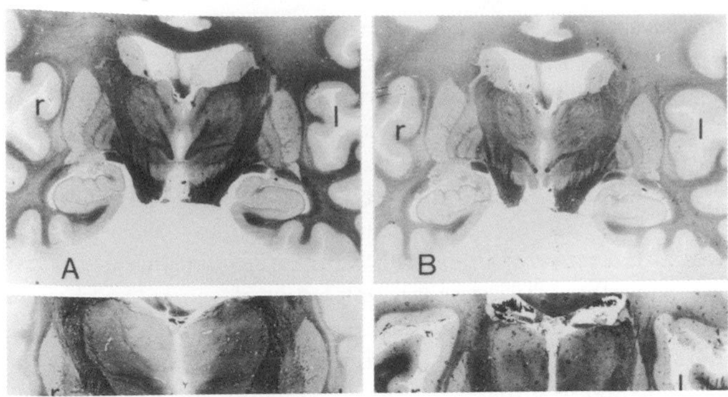

Fig. 2.3.5.3 No significant increase of GFAP positive cells around the left temporal horn in schizophrenia.

Therefore, it seems unlikely that the majority of schizophrenic patients show a considerable degree of astrogliosis. There is, on the contrary, some evidence demonstrating reduced macroglial densities in major depression and schizophrenia.(29) In this respect, specifically the oligodendroglia demonstrates qualitative and quantitative changes in schizophrenia(30) which is an interesting view of the riskgene Neuregulin-1 regulating myelin thickness via these cells. Some recent studies found evidence for the activation of microglia in the cortex of patients with schizophrenia.(31, 32, 33) As microglia respond to neuronal injury within 24 to 48 hours, studies are needed to link psychopathology with these markers. The examination of apoptic processes constitutes another interesting line of research supporting atypical degeneration with schizophrenia. Some recent studies demonstrate low-grade apoptotic processes in circumscribed brain regions in schizophrenia(34, 35) which is in line with other degenerative disorders showing similar features.(36)

(d) Neurohistological indications of disturbed brain development

Subtle cytoarchitectural anomalies were described in the hippocampal formation, frontal cortex, cingulate gyrus, and entorhinal cortex in patients suffering from schizophrenia compared with control subjects. For example, significant cellular disarray in the CA3-CA4 interface was described in the left and replicated in the right hippocampus.(37) This was interpreted as a bilateral migrational abnormality and broadly correlated with the degree of disease severity. One subsequent study was not able to fully replicate these findings, but did confirm a within-case correlation with severity; whereas another examination did not find any significant disarray distinguishing schizophrenics from controls. Another prominent finding was of an abnormal sulcogyral pattern or abnormal gross configuration of the temporal lobe and cytoarchitectonic abnormalities of the rostral entorhinal region as well as of the ventral insular cortex of schizophrenics.(38, 39) The cytoarchitectonic abnormalities of the rostral entorhinal region consisted of heterotopic pre-α-cells in the pre-β-layer (layer III), which would normally belong to the pre-α-layer (layer II). This observation stimulated considerable research, with some studies supporting these findings,(40, 41) while others did not.(42)

In conclusion, cytoarchitectonic abnormalities recently described in different limbic structures in schizophrenia are very subtle and can easily be missed using classical neuropathological methods. Quantifying them often needs sophisticated staining methods, for example, immunohistochemistry, serial sections and a matched control group and even then replicating original findings seems difficult, as outlined above. These findings can be interpreted as a sign for disturbed late neuronal migration or could mirror disturbed programmed cell death as heterotopias are frequently found in the temporal cortex of autopsied children, which seem to disappear in adults.

(e) Summary and pathophysiological conclusions

There is growing evidence for pathomorphological abnormalities in the postmortem brains of patients suffering from schizophrenia. The changes are focused on the frontal lobe and temporolimbic regions. They are subtle, lacking the typical signs of degeneration, and point to problems in prenatal (cell migration) and postnatal (connectivity) periods of brain development. Currently, underlying causes remain ambiguous, but the interaction between genetic and non-genetic factors (e.g. birth complications) is presently discussed on the basis of the recently found risk genes like Neuregulin-1 or Dysbindin.

Mood disorders (Table 2.3.5.3)

The number of published pathoanatomical studies in schizophrenia contrasts with the scant number of neuropathological examinations in affective disorders. In reviewing the world literature up to 1988, Jeste *et al.* (1988)(43) counted 15 neuropathological studies on affective disorders. Seven of them were published between 1949 and 1969, attended to less than four cases, and utilized qualitative tissue evaluation. Searching for 'unipolar depression and neuropathology' and 'bipolar depression', resulted in 56 and 77 hits in pubmed up to 2007, proving this field of research to speed up lately. Comprehensive reviews(44, 45, 46) highlight several aspects in more detail and are suggested for further reading. Table 2.3.5.3 summarizes the most relevant findings from morphometric post-mortem studies.

Macroscopic findings

Four studies examined macroscopic measures such as the gross brain morphology,(47) brain weight and ventricular volume,(48) and the area or volume of specific regions such as the hippocampus, parahippocampal gyrus (Altshuler *et al.* 1990), striatum, globus pallidus, and corpus callosum.(48, 49) In comparison to schizophrenic patients and/or non-psychiatric control subjects, patients with affective disorders revealed caudate lesions,(47) reduced area of the right parahippocampal gyrus,(50) increased brain and reduced ventricular volume.(48)

Microscopic findings

Several studies examined the cytoarchitecture and nerve cell, interneuronal or glial numbers of the pre- and orbitofrontal cortex,(51, 52, 53) entorhinal and insular cortex,(54, 55) anterior cingulated(56, 57) cerebellum,(58) brainstem(49, 59) and the peripheral nervous system.(60) Findings in patients with affective disorders included overall reduced neuronal numbers, together with disurbed cytoarchitecture of entorhinal cortex, reduced neuronal and glial numbers in the prefrontal cortex, the rostroventral insula and dorsal raphe, reduced Purkinje cells in anterior and posterior vermis and hemispheres of the cerebellum, reduced interneuronal numbers in layer II of the cingulate, but increased neuronal numbers of the locus coeruleus and peripheral motor neurone branching. In a series of studies focusing on the hypothalamus in affective disorders, the number of nitric oxide synthase (NOS) positive cells was reduced in the nucleus suprachiasmaticus[61] and the paraventricular nucleus[62] in patients with affective disorder stressing the importance of this anatomical region for these illnesses.

Summary and pathophysiological conclusions

In summary, the number of postmortem studies on mood disorders is still limited but growing. There is some evidence for changes in key cortical regions, the basalganglia, the hypothalamus and brainstem. Structural brain imaging studies support the notion of mood disorders being associated with regional structural brain abnormalities, in particular regions involved in mood regulation. Because small numbers of subjects were studied, only some post-mortem studies distinguished between unipolar and bipolar depression.[49] Nevertheless, recent structural imaging studies regarded this distinction worthwhile. The main abnormalities found in unipolar depression are smaller basal ganglia, cerebellum, frontal lobe and hippocampus, which may reflect disease-course-related atrophy. Bipolar disorder appears to be associated with larger third ventricle, smaller cerebellum, possibly smaller temporal lobe, and perhaps increased amygdala volume on the right side. In both groups, there seems to be an increased rate of subcortical white-matter lesions and periventricular hyperintensities. Whether the rate of subcortical white-matter lesions and periventricular hyperintensities are predictive of a later development of Alzheimer´s disease is yet unclear. Hippocampal plaques and tangles are increased in patients with Alzheimer´s disease with a lifetime history of major depression.[63] Further studies are needed, combining endocrine/biochemical parameters with structural parameters to identify the key regions involved in processes central to mood disorders such as changes in the regulation of the hypothalamic-pituitary-adrenal axis.

Alcoholism (Table 2.3.5.4)

The best known neuropathological feature of alcoholism is Wernicke's encephalopathy, which is characterized by degenerative changes including gliosis and small hemorrhages in structures surrounding the third ventricle and aqueduct (i.e. the mamillary bodies, hypothalamus, mediodorsal thalamic nucleus, colliculi, and midbrain tegmentum), as well as cerebellar atrophy. Most of the clinical features associated with the Wernicke-Korsakoff syndrome including ophthalmoplegia, nystagmus, ataxia, and mental symptoms such as confusion, disorientation, and even coma can be related to damaged functional systems in the hypothalamus, midbrain, and cerebellum.[64] Other important neuropathological manifestations of chronic alcoholism are central pontine myelinolysis, Marchiafava syndrome, and foetal alcohol syndrome (see Chapter 4.2.2.3).

Studies on alcohol-specific brain damage

Most of the changes mentioned above occur in association with thiamin deficiency, which is frequently, but not always, correlated with the long-term use of excessive amounts of alcohol. One major challenge is to identify those lesions caused by alcohol itself (uncomplicated alcoholism)[65] and those caused by other common

Table 2.3.5.3 Morphometric post-mortem studies in affective disorders

Study	Number of patients/controls	Region/parameter	Finding
General			
Jellinger (1977)[46]	4/15	Entire brain	Caudate lesions
Temporal lobe			
Altshuler *et al.* (1990)[49]	12/27	Hippocampal area	—
		Parahippocampal area	↓
Beckmann and Jakob (1991)[53]	4/0	Cytoarchitecture of entorhinal cortex	Disturbed
		Rostroventral insula nerve cell number	↓
Casanova *et al.* (1991)[54]	5/10	Entorhinal cortex neuronal numbers	↓
Other cortical and subcortical regions			
Brown *et al.* (1986)[47]	70/32	Lobar structures	—
		Callosal thickness	—
		Corpus striatum	—
		Brain weight	↑
		Lateral ventricles	↓
Diekmann *et al.* (1998)[55]	12/12	Cingulate cortex (interneurones in layer II)	↓
Baumann *et al.* (1999)[48]	8/8	Accumbens, putamen, caudate, external pallidal volumes	↓
Bernstein *et al.* (1998)[62]		NOS positive cells in the nucleus paraventricularis	↓
Bernstein *et al.* (2002)[61]		NOS positive cells in the nucleus suprachiasmaticus	↓
Cerebellum			
Lohr and Jeste (1986)[57]	12/23	Cerebellum: Purkinje cells in anterior and posterior vermis and hemispheres	—
Brainstem			
Hankoff and Peress (1981)[58]	4/26	Brainstem	—
Baumann *et al.* (1999)[48]	12/12	Locus coeruleus neuronal number	↑
Peripheral nervous system			
Ross-Stanton and Meltzer (1981)[60]		Motor neurone branching (peripheral)	↑

In comparison with controls: ↓, reduced; ↑, increased; —, no difference; ( ), finding not or only partially replicated.

Table 2.3.5.4 Morphometric post-mortem studies in alcoholism

Region/parameter	Finding
General	
Brain weight	↓
Intracranial volume	↓
Ventricular volume	↑
White > grey matter volume	↓
Temporal lobe	
Hippocampal neuronal numbers	(↓)
Amygdala neuronal numbers	↓
Frontal, parietal, and occipital lobes	
Superior frontal cortex, neuronal numbers (BA 8)	↓
Primary motor cortex, neuronal numbers (BA 4)	—
Frontal cingulated cortex, neuronal numbers (BA 32)	—
Inferior temporal cortex, neuronal numbers (BA 20 + 36)	—
Superior frontal cortex, GABAergic pyramidal neurones	—
Thalamus	
Medial dorsal and anterior nuclei of the thalamus, volumes	(↓)
Supraoptic and paraventricular nuclei of the hypothalamus, neuronal numbers	↓
Arginine-vasopressin immunoreactive neurones	↓
Basal ganglia	
Caudate, putamen, or globus pallidus volumes	—
Cerebellum	
Cerebellar volume in general	↓
Vernal, intermediate, and lateral zone volumes	↓
Purkinje cell densities	↓
Brainstem	
Locus coeruleus noradrenergic, neuronal numbers	(↓)
Median and dorsal raphe nuclei, neuronal numbers	—
Other brain structures	
Basal nucleus, neuronal structures	—

In comparison with controls: ↓, reduced; ↑, increased; —, no difference; ( ), finding not or only partially replicated.

alcohol-related factors, principally thiamin deficiency. The following paragraph summarizes recent results in this field, which has been reviewed in detail by others.[65, 66] Brain shrinkage can be found in uncomplicated alcoholism, which can largely be accounted for by loss of white matter. Some of this damage appears to be reversible. However, alcohol-related neuronal loss has been documented in specific regions of the cerebral cortex (superior frontal association cortex), hypothalamus (supraoptic and paraventricular nuclei), and cerebellum. The data are conflicting for the hippocampus, amygdala, and locus coeruleus. No changes are found in the basal ganglia, nucleus basalis, or serotonergic raphe nuclei. Concerning the prefrontal lobe it is interesting to note that although alcohol related pathology affects both neuronal and glial cells, the effects on glia are more dramatic than on neurones.[52] The cellular changes are more prominent and spread across cortical layers in alcohol dependent subjects compared to subjects with mood disorders.[52] As pointed out above, many of the regions being normal in uncomplicated alcoholics are damaged in those with Wernicke-Korsakoff syndrome. Dendritic and synaptic changes have been documented in uncomplicated alcoholics, and these, together with receptor and transmitter changes, may explain functional changes and cognitive deficits that precede the more severe structural neuronal changes.

Summary and pathophysiological considerations

In summary, there is neuropathological evidence showing that alcohol *per se* causes damage to both grey and white matter. White-matter damage is predominant and results in a reduction in brain volume. A component of the white-matter loss appears to be reversible in some cases, given a significant period of abstinence. The grey-matter damage appears to be regionally selective, but many areas of the brain appear to be resistant to damage.

Thiamin deficiency accounts for a major component of the brain damage in alcoholics. Animal models suggest the distribution and extent of neuronal loss to be dependent on the duration of alcohol exposure, the magnitude and mode of exposure (ingestion, inhalation, etc.), the genetic susceptibility of the species, and the strain of animals studied.[65] It has been suggested that alcohol withdrawal may play a role in brain damage, evidenced by the fact that a number of workers have shown loss of granule cells in the dentate gyrus of the hippocampus continuing even after alcohol exposure stops.[67] It was furthermore suggested that up-regulation of *N*-methyl-d-aspartate receptors may lead to withdrawal seizures and enhanced susceptibility to excitotoxicity, which may explain the continuing damage described.[68]

Further information

http://www.psychiatrie.med.uni-goettingen.de/falkai_publikationen.html
http://www.med.uni-magdeburg.de/fme/znh/kpsy/cv/bogerts%20de.htm

References

1. Jellinger, K.A. and Bancher, C. (1998). Neuropathology of Alzheimer's disease: a critical update. *Journal of Neural Transmission Supplementum*, **54**, 77–95.
2. Alzheimer, A. (1898). Beiträge zur pathologischen Anatomie der Hirnrinde und zur anatomischen Grundlage der Psychosen. *Monatsschrift Psychiatrie und Neurologie*, **2**, 82–120.
4. Southard, E.E. (1915). On the topographic distribution of cortex lesions and anomalies in dementia praecox with some account of their functional significance. *American Journal of Insanity*, **71**, 603–71.
5. Vogt, C. and Vogt, O. (1952). Resultats de l'etude anatomique de la schizophrenie et d'autres psychoses dites fontionelles faite a l'institut du cerveau de Neustadt, Schwarzwald. In *First International Congress of Neuropathology*, Vol. 1, pp. 515–32. Rosenberg and Sellier, Turin.
7. Harrison, P.J. (1999). The neuropathology of schizophrenia. A critical review of the data and their interpretation. *Brain*, **122**, 593–624.
8. Arnold, S.E., Talbot, K. and Hahn, C.G. (2005) Neurodevelopment, neuroplasticity, and new genes for schizophrenia. *Progress Brain Research*, **147**, 319–45.
9. Harrison, P.J. and Weinberger, D.R. (2005). Schizophrenia genes, gene expression, and neuropathology: on the matter of their convergence. *Molecular Psychiatry*, **10**, 40–68.
10. Stevens, J.R. (1982). Neuropathology of schizophrenia. *Archives of General Psychiatry*, **39**, 1131–9.
11. Bruton, C.J., Crow, T.J., Frith, C.D., *et al.* (1990). Schizophrenia and the brain: a prospective clinico-neuropathological study. *Psychological Medicine*, **20**, 285–304.
12. Golier, J.A., Davidson, M., Haroutunian, V., *et al.* (1995). Neuropathological study of 101 elderly schizophrenics: preliminary findings. *Schizophrenia Research*, **15**, 120.
13. Bogerts, B., Meertz, E., and Schönfeldt-Bausch, R. (1983). Limbic system pathology in schizophrenia: a controlled post mortem study. *7th World Congress of Psychiatry*, Vienna, 1983, Vortrag, Abstract F6.

14. Bogerts, B., Meertz, E. and Schonfeldt-Bausch, R. (1985). Basal ganglia and limbic system pathology in schizophrenia. A morphometric study of brain volume and shrinkage. *Archives of General Psychiatry*, **42**(8), 784–91.
15. Stevens, J.R. (1997). Anatomy of schizophrenia revisited. *Schizophr Bull*, **23**(3), 373–83.

    Bogerts, B. and Lieberman, J. (1993). Neuropathology in the study of psychiatric disease. In *International review of psychiatry* (ed. N.C. Andreasen and M. Sato), Vol. 1 pp. 515–55. American Psychiatric Press, Washington, DC.
16. Chakos, M.H., Lieberman, J.A., Alvir, J., *et al.* (1995). Caudate nuclei volumes in schizophrenic patients treated with typical antipsychotics or clozapine. *Lancet*, **345**(8947): 456–57.

    Broca, P. (1865). Sur la faculté du langage articulé. *Bulletins de la Societé d'Anthropologie*, **6**, 377–93.
17. Danos, P., Schmidt, A., Baumann, B., *et al.* (2005). Volume and neuron number of the mediodorsal thalamic nucleus in schizophrenia: a replication study. *Psychiatry Research* 140(3), 281–9.
18. Innocenti, G.M., Ansermet, F., and Parnas, J. (2003). Schizophrenia, neurodevelopment and corpus callosum. *Molecular Psychiatry*, **8**(3), 261–74.
19. Bogerts, B. (1990). *Die Hirnstruktur Schizophrener und ihre Bedeutung für die Pathophysiologie und Psychopathologie der Erkrankung.* Thieme, Stuttgart
20. Lewis, D.A., Cruz, D., Eggan, S., *et al.* (2004). Postnatal development of prefrontal inhibitory circuits and the pathophysiology of cognitive dysfunction in schizophrenia. *Annuals of the New York Academy of Scienes*, **1021**, 64–76.
21. Christison, G.W., Casanova, M.F., Weinberger, D.R., *et al.* (1989). A quantitative investigation of hippocampal pyramidal cell size, shape and variability of orientation in schizophrenia. *Archives of General Psychiatry*, **46**, 1027–32.
22. Heckers, S., Heinsen, H., Heinsen, Y.C., *et al.* (1990). Limbic structures and lateral ventricle in schizophrenia. *Archives of General Psychiatry*, **47**, 1016–22.
23. Karson, C.N., García-Rill, E., Biedermann, J., *et al.* (1991). The brain stem reticular formation in schizophrenia. *Psychiatry Research*, **40(1)**, 31–48.
24. Lohr, J.B. and Jeste, D.V. (1988) Locus ceruleus morphometry in aging and schizophrenia. *Acta Psychiatr Scand*, **77**(6), 689–97.
25. Marner, L., Soborg, C., and Pakkenberg, B. (2005). Increased volume of the pigmented neurons in the locus coeruleus of schizophrenic subjects: a stereological study. *Journal of Psychiatric Research*, **39**(4), 337–45.
26. Weinberger, D.R. (1996). On the plausibility of 'the neurodevelopmental hypothesis' of schizophrenia. *Neuropsychopharmacology*, **14**, 1S-11S.
27. Woods, B.T., Yurgelun-Todd, D., Goldstein, J.M., *et al.* (1996). MRI brain abnormalities in chronic schizophrenia: one process or more? *Biological Psychiatry*, **40**, 585–96.
28. Falkai, P., Honer, W.G., David, S., *et al.* (1999). No evidence for astrogliosis in brains of schizophrenic patients. A post-mortem study. *Neuropathology and Applied Neurobiology*, **25**, 48–53.
29. Cotter, D.R., Pariante, C.M. and Everall, I.P. (2001). Glial cell abnormalities in major psychiatric disorders: the evidence and implications. *Brain Research Bulletin*, **55**, 585–95.
30. Uranova, N.A., Vostrikov, V.M., Vikhreva, O.V., *et al.* the role of oligodendrocyte pathology in schizophrenia. *International Journal of Neuropsychopharmacology*, **Feb 21**, 1–9 (Epub ahead of print).
31. Bayer, T.A., Buslei, R., Havas, L., *et al.* (1999). Evidence for activation of microglia in patients with psychiatric illnesses. *Neuroscience Letters*, **271**, 126–8.
32. Radewicz, K., Garey, L.J., Gentleman, S.M. *et al.* (2000). Increase in HLA-DR immunoreactive microglia in frontal and temporal cortex of chronic schizophrenics. *Journal of Neuropathology and Experimental Neurology*, **59**, 137–50.
33. Foster, R., Kandanearatchi, A., Beasley, C., *et al.* (2006). Calprotectin in microglia from frontal cortex is up-regulated in schizophrenia: evidence for an inflammatory process? *European Journal of Neuroscience*, **24**, 3561–6.
34. Jarskog, L.F., Miyamoto, S. and Lieberman, J.A. (2007). Schizophrenia: new pathological insights and therapies. *Annu Rev Med*, **58**, 49–61.
35. Benes, F.M., Matzilevich, D., Burke, R.E., *et al.* (2006). The expression of proapoptosis genes is increased in bipolar disorder, but not in schizophrenia. *Molecular Psychiatry*, **11**, 241–51.
36. Glantz, L.A., Gilmore, J.H., Lieberman, J.A. *et al.* (2006). Apoptotic mechanisms and the synaptic pathology of schizophrenia. *Schizophrenia Research*, **18**, 47–63.
37. Kovelman, J.A. and Scheibel, A.B. (1984). A neurohistological correlate of schizophrenia. *Biological Psychiatry*, **19**, 1601–21.
38. Jakob, J. and Beckmann, H. (1986). Prenatal developmental disturbances in the limbic allocortex in schizophrenics. *Journal of Neural Transmission*, **65**, 303–26.
39. Jakob, H. and Beckmann, H. (1989). Gross and histological criteria for developmental disorders in brains of schizophrenics. *Journal of the Royal Society of Medicine*, **82**, 466–9.
40. Falkai, P. Schneider-Axmann, T. and Honer, W.G. (2000). Entorhinal cortex pre-alpha cell clusters in schizophrenia: quantitative evidence of a developmental abnormality. *Biological Psychiatry*, **47**, 937–43.
41. Kovalenko, S., Bergmann, A., Schneider-Axmann, T.,*et al.* (2003). Regio entorhinalis in schizophrenia: more evidence for migrational disturbances and suggestions for a new biological hypothesis. *Pharmacopsychiatry*, **36**, **Suppl 3**: S158–61.
42. Krimer, L.S., Herman, M.M., Saunders, R.C., *et al.* (1997). A qualitative and quantitative analysis of the entorhinal cortex in schizophrenia. *Cereb Cortex*, **7**, 732–9.
43. Jeste, D.V., Lohr, J.B., and Goodwin, F.K. (1988). Neuroanatomical studies of major affective disorders. A review and suggestions for further research. *British Journal of Psychiatry*, **153**, 444–59.
44. Harrison, P.J. (2002). The neuropathology of primary mood disorder. *Brain*, **125**, 1428–49.
45. Baumann, B. and Bogerts, B. (2001). Neuroanatomical studies on bipolar disorder. *British Journal of Psychiatry Supplemental*, **41**, S142–7.
46. Haldane, M. and Frangou, S. (2004) New insights help define the pathophysiology of bipolar affective disorder: neuroimaging and neuropathology findings. *Progress neuropsychopharmacol Biological Psychiatry*, **28**, 943–60.
47. Jellinger, K.A. (1977). Neuropathologic findings after neuroleptic long term therapy. In *Neurotoxicology* (eds. L. Roizin, H. Shiraki, and N. Grcevic), pp. 25–42. Raven Press, New York.
48. Brown, R., Colter, N., Corsellis, J.A.N., *et al.* (1986). Postmortem evidence of structural brain changes in schizophrenia. Differences in brain weight, temporal horn area and parahippocampal gyrus compared with affective disorder. *Archives of General Psychiatry*, **43**, 36–42.
49. Baumann, B., Danos, P., Krell, D., *et al.* (1999). Unipolar-bipolar dichotomy of mood disorders is supported by noradrenergic brainstem system morphology. *Journal of Affective Disorders*, **54**, 217–24.
50. Altshuler, L.L., Casanova, M.F., Goldberg, T.E., *et al.* (1990). The hippocampus and parahippocampus in schizophrenic, suicide, and control brains. *Archives of General Psychiatry*, **47**, 1029–34.
51. Rajkowska, G., Halaris, A. and Selemon, L.D. (2001). Reductions in neuronal and glial density characterize the dorsolateral prefrontal cortex in bipolar disorder. *Biological Psychiatry*, **49**, 741–52.
52. Miguel-Hidalgo, J.J. and Rajkowska, G. (2003) Comparison of prefrontal cell pathology between depression and alcohol dependence. *Journal of Psychiatric Research*, **37**, 411–20.

53. Bielau, H., Steiner, J., Mawrin, C., *et al.* (2007) Dysregulatin of GABAergic neurotransmission in mood disorders: a postmortem study. *Annals of New York Academy of Sciences*, **1096**, 157–69.
54. Beckmannn, H. and Jakob, H. (1991). Prenatal disturbances of nerve cell migration in the entorhinal region: a common vulnerability factor in functional psychoses? *Journal of Neural Transmission. General Section*, **84**, (1–2), 155–64.
55. Casanova, M.F., Saunder, R., Altshuler, L., *et al.* (1991). Entorhinal cortex pathology in schizophrenia and affective disorders. In *Biological Psychiatry* (ed. G. Racagni *et al.*), pp. 504–6. Elsevier, Amsterdam.
56. Diekmann, S., Baumann, B., Schmidt, U., *et al.* (1998). Significant decrease in calretinin immunoreactive neurons in layer II in the cingulate cortex in schizophrenics. *Pharmacopsychiatry*, **31**, 12.
57. Chana, G., Landau, S., Beasley, C., *et al.* (2003) Two-dimensional assessment of cytoarchitecture in the anterior cingulate cortex in major depressive disorder, bipolar disorder, and schizophrenia: evidence for decreased neuronal somal size and increased neuronal density. *Bioliological Psychiatry*, **53**, 1086–98.
58. Lohr, J.B. and Jeste, D.V. (1986). Studies of cerebellum and hippocampus in major psychiatric disorders. In *Biological psychiatry* (ed. C. Shagass *et al.*), pp. 1024–6. Elsevier, New York.
59. Hankoff, L.D. and Peress, N.S. (1981). Neuropathology of the brain stem in psychiatric disorders. *Biological Psychiatry*, **16**, 945–52.
60. Ross-Stanton, J. and Meltzer, F.A. (1981). Motor neuron branching patterns in psychotic patients. *Archives of General Psychiatry*, **38**, 1097–103.
61. Soares, J.C. and Mann, J.J. (1997). The anatomy of mood disorders-review of structural neuroimaging studies. *Biological Psychiatry*, **41**, 86–106.
61. Bernstein, H.G., Heinemann, A., Krell, D., *et al.* (2002) Further immunohistochemical evidence for impaired NO signaling in the hypothalamus of depressed patients. *Annals of New York Academy of Sciences*, **973**, 91–3.
62. Bernstein, H.G., Stanarius, A., Baumann, B., *et al.* (1998). Nitric oxide synthase-containing neurons in the human hypothalamus: reduced number of immunoreactive cells in the paraventricular nucleus of depressive patients and schizophrenics. *Neuroscience*, **83**, 867–75.
63. Rapp, M.A., Schnaider-Beeri, M., Grossman, H.T., *et al.* (2006). Increased hippocampal plaques and tangles in patients with Alzheimer disease with a lifetime history of major depression. *Archive of General Psychiatry*, **63**, 161–7.
64. Victor, M., Adams, R.D., and Collins, G. (1989). *The Wernicke-Korsakow syndrome and related neurologic disorders due to alcoholism and malnutrition.* Davis, Philadelphia, PA.
65. Harper, C.G. and Kril, J.J. (1990). Neuropathology of alcoholism. *Alcohol and Alcoholism*, **25**, 207–16.
66. Harper, C.G. (1998). The neuropathology of alcohol-specific brain damage, or does alcohol damage the brain? *Journal of Neuropathology and Experimental Neurology*, **57**, 101–10.
67. Vogt, C. and Vogt, O. (1948). Über anatomische Substrate. Bemerkungen zu pathoanatomischen Befunden bei Schizophrenie. *Ärztliche Forschritte*, **3**, 1–7.
67. Cavazos, J.E., Das, I., and Sutula, T.P. (1994). Neuronal loss induced in limbic pathways by kindling: evidence for induction of hippocampal sclerosis by repeated brief seizures. *Journal of Neuroscience*, **14**, 3106–21.
68. Hoffmann, P.L., Iorio, K.R., Snell, L.D., *et al.* (1995). Attenuation of glutamate-induced neurotoxicity in chronically ethanol-exposed cerebellar granule cells by NMDA receptor antagonists and ganglioside GM1. *Alcoholism, Clinical and Experimental Research*, **19**, 721–6.

2.3.6 Functional positron emission tomography in psychiatry

P. M. Grasby

Introduction

Positron emission tomography (**PET**) and single-photon emission tomography (**SPET**) are powerful tools for investigating the pathophysiology of psychiatric illnesses and the action of psychotropic drugs. With these techniques monoaminergic, cholinergic, opioid and benzodiazepine receptors, regional cerebral blood flow, glucose and oxygen metabolism can be measured in the living brain (Table 2.3.6.1). Thus, neural function of direct relevance to neurochemical and anatomical theories of psychiatric illnesses can be sampled.

Methodology of PET and SPET[(1)]

In brief, PET and SPET comprise the following:

- The production and incorporation of a positron or gamma-emitting radio-isotope into a molecule of biological interest to form a radiotracer administered to humans (Plate 3).
- The use of PET or SPET cameras to detect the emitted gamma radiation from the decaying radio-isotope and hence the 3D distribution of the radiotracer, over minutes to hours, in living human brain (Plate 4).
- Quantification of a physiological parameter of interest, such as number of available receptors or regional cerebral blood flow, from the mathematical modeling of the measured radio-activity in the brain over time (Plates 5 and 6).

Production of isotopes

Common PET radio-isotopes, produced by a cyclotron, are oxygen-15 ($(^{15})O$), carbon-11 ($(^{11})C$), and fluorine-18 ($(^{18})F$) (with half-lives of 2.03 min, 20.4 min, and 109.8 min respectively) whilst SPET radio-isotopes include technetium ($(^{99m})Tc$) and iodine-123 ($(^{123})I$) (with half-lives of 6.02 h and 13.2 h respectively). With appropriate radiochemistry, isotopes can be incorporated into specific molecules to make radiotracers. Following quality control procedures, to estimate specific activity and radiochemical purity, the radiotracer is injected intravenously into subjects lying in the PET camera (Plate 3). Importantly, the total mass of radiotracer injected is very small (typically less than 5 μg) and therefore the radiotracer has no pharmacological effect itself.

PET versus SPET

SPET radiotracers are less diverse than PET tracers. However, SPET is cheaper than PET and less technically demanding, making it more readily available in hospitals and research centres. PET radiochemical procedures require in-house automated rapid synthetic chemistry facilities in dedicated hot cells, whereas SPET chemistry is more straight-forward and does not require such extensive facilities. For research and quantitation purposes, PET is far superior to SPET, although any widespread commercial/clinical application is

Table 2.3.6.1 Established and novel radiotracers for psychiatry

Radiotracer	Application	Comments
PET radiotracers		
$H_2{}^{15}O$	Blood flow	Used to map dysfunctional brain areas involved in psychiatric illnesses. Effectively replaced by functional MRI techniques such as BOLD.
^{18}F-FDG	Glucose metabolism	Used for many resting state studies and nowadays to define psychotropic drug effects.
^{11}C-SCH 23390 ^{11}C-NNC 112	Dopamine D_1 receptor	Receptor occupancy studies with neuroleptics. Reports of altered cortical D_1 receptors in drug naive schizophrenics.
^{11}C-Raclopride	Dopamine D_2 receptor	Robust demonstration of no elevation of striatal D2 receptors in drug naive schizophrenics. Striatal D_2 receptor occupancy studies with many neuroleptics. Frequently used to index dopamine release.
^{11}C-FLB-457	Dopamine D_2 receptor	High affinity ligand; enabling extrastriatal D_2 populations to be measured. Studies in schizophrenia in progress. Binding may be sensitive to endogenous dopamine release.
^{18}F-Fallypride	Dopamine D_2 receptor	High affinity ligand; enabling striatal and extrastriatal D_2 populations to be measured. Binding may be sensitive to endogenous dopamine release.
^{18}F-Fluorodopa	Dopamine synthesis capacity	Radiotracer predominantly imageable in basal ganglia, cortical signal weak. Consistent reports of raised ^{18}FDOPA in schizophrenia.
^{11}C-Flumazenil	Central benzodiazepine receptors	Labels all subtypes of central receptor.
^{11}C-MDL-100907	5-HT_{2A} receptors	Most suitable ligand for imaging 5-HT_2 receptors.
^{11}C-WAY 100635 ^{11}C-desmethyl WAY ^{11}C – FCWAY ^{18}F - MPPF	5-HT_{1A} receptors	Reports of reduced 5-HT1A availability in depressive and anxiety disorders
^{11}C-DASB ^{11}C-McN 5652	5-HT transporter	Studies in depressive illness. Occupancy studies of SSRIs. Used to examine effects of ecstasy
SPECT radiotracers		
^{99m}TcHMPAO	Blood flow	Many resting state and two scan activation studies in psychosis.
^{123}I-Iodobenzamide	Dopamine D2 receptors	Occupancy and dopamine release studies in schizophrenia
^{123}I-Epidepride	Dopamine D2 receptors	Striatal and Extrastriatal D2 receptors. Used to show 'limbic selectivity' of certain neuroleptics
^{123}I-QNB	Muscarinic acetycholine receptors	
^{123}I-CIT	Dopamine and 5-HT reuptake sites	Studies in depressive illness

likely to be SPET based because of the technology restraints and costs associated with PET scanning.

Imaging of radiotracer, data collection, and analysis

PET utilizes the disintegration of positrons emitted from unstable nuclei such as$^{(11)}$C (Plate 4). Emitted positrons travel a short distance in tissue before annihilation by collision with an electron.(1) On annihilation, two high-energy gamma rays are generated with a separation angle of 180° (Plate 4). Radiation detectors (e.g. bismuth germanate), 180° apart and linked in electronic coincidence circuits, detect the resulting gamma radiation and therefore localize the source of radiation to a volume between any two detectors (Plate 3). By arranging rings of detectors around the subject's head and using computer-based back-projection techniques, the distribution of radiotracer within tomographic slices of the brain can be obtained.(1) SPET radioisotopes, in contrast, decay by emitting a single gamma ray and therefore the radiation detectors are not linked in coincidence circuits. State-of-the-art PET and SPET cameras have transaxial spatial resolutions of the order of 4 to 5 mm and can detect subnanomolar concentrations of receptors.(1)

Positron-emitting isotopes can be incorporated into molecules associated with diverse biochemical processes in the brain. For example, the positron emitter$^{(11)}$C can be incorporated into a molecule WAY 100635, which selectively binds to 5-HT_{1A} receptors, and injected intravenously in tracer amounts. Brain regions will show different profiles of radio-activity accumulation over time as the radiotracer binds in areas with a high density of 5-HT_{1A} receptors (medial temporal cortex) whilst in regions with no or sparse receptors (cerebellum), it will be washed out (Plate 5). By this means, specific and non-specific binding can be distinguished. With an appropriate model of the radiotracer's history in tissue over time, a quantitative measurement of 5-HT_{1A} receptor number in tomographic slices of the human brain can be obtained.(1) With some radiotracers (e.g. [11C]diprenorphine to label opiate receptors) it may be necessary to undertake radial artery cannulation to obtain an 'input function'(1) that describes the time course of presentation of radiotracer to the brain (Plate 6), whereas others tracers can be modeled with a 'pseudo' input function from a reference region.

Technical and practical limitations of PET and SPET compared with other imaging modalities

PET and SPET excel in the measurement of neurochemical parameters *in vivo* at very low (subnanomolar) concentration. Such sensitivity cannot be matched by other *in vivo* methods such as proton magnetic resonance spectroscopy (millimolar range). However, radiation dosimetry limits the number of scans that subjects may receive. Full quantitation can often be achieved with PET, unlike

SPET. However, for imaging blood flow change, or its correlates such as BOLD arterial spin labeling (ASL) and functional magnetic resonance imaging (fMRI), now offer the possibility of repeated measures (without radiation exposure) that far exceed that possible with PET- and SPET-based methods of flow mapping. Full quantitation of blood flow is not yet readily achievable with functional MRI without injection of contrast agents. In contrast, MRI based ASL can achieve full quantification. One disadvantage of functional MRI over PET, for some subjects, is the noisy claustrophobic environment of the scanner, but generally subjects and paradigms studied with PET flow mapping can be readily investigated with functional MRI (see Chapter 2.3.8), although all test materials in the vicinity of the scanner have to be non-magnetic.

Structural MRI scanning is often used in conjunction with PET activation and ligand binding techniques. The high-resolution anatomical information contained in MRI images can be used to precisely define areas of activation or radiotracer binding observed in PET studies from single subjects.

PET and SPET, and even functional MRI, have relatively poor temporal resolution (seconds) compared with electrophysiological methods such as EEG, event-related potentials, and magnetoencephalography (milliseconds), but these methods in turn suffer from poor spatial resolution. Attempts to integrate information from these different modalities are a major focus of methodological research in many imaging centres.

PET and SPET imaging strategies in psychiatry

These techniques (see Table 2.3.6.2) are used to either measure brain receptors and neurochemistry, or map functional brain activity via the indices of regional blood flow and glucose utilization.

Table 2.3.6.2 Summary of PET functional brain imaging approaches

Functional brain mapping: rCBF or metabolism is measured as an index of local neural activity
(a) Studies in normal volunteers in which 'activation' paradigms are used to identify functional anatomy that is relevant to psychiatric disorders
(b) Activation studies in patients who are compared with matched control subjects
(c) Studies in which the biological variable (e.g. rCBF) is correlated with a relevant clinical variable (e.g. hallucinations) within the patient group
(d) The longitudinal comparison of patients before and after various treatments and into clinical recovery
(e) Cross-sectional studies of resting-state brain activity in patient groups in comparison with appropriate controls
Radioligand imaging: the specific uptake and binding of radiolabelled tracer compounds is measured
(a) To estimate baseline radioligand uptake at rest in patient groups in comparison with controls
(b) Within-patient group correlations between radioligand uptake and particular symptoms/signs
(c) Longitudinal comparison of radioligand uptake in patients before and after various treatments and into clinical recovery
(d) 'Displacement' or radioligand activation studies designed to detect changes in the levels of intrasynapcic neurotransmitters in response to a pharmacological or cognitive challenge
(e) Investigation of the receptor binding and occupancy characteristics of psychotropic drugs

rCBF, regional cerebral blood flow.

Each approach attempts to define trait and state abnormalities of psychiatric illnesses or the effect of psychotropic drug action.

Because of the technical complexities, it is important to bear in mind the following questions when judging experimental results.

- What assumptions are made about the behaviour of the radiotracer *in vivo*?
- Has the radiotracer been well validated for the apparent physiological parameter measured ?
- Does the mathematical model of the radiotracer's behaviour give a good fit to the raw data?
- Is the spatial resolution of the PET camera sufficient for the regions measured?
- What is the test-test reliability for the PET radiotracer measure?
- How have the raw PET images been modified/treated in the data analysis?
- How have regions of interest been defined?
- Is there a possibility of observer bias in the measurements made?
- What statistical techniques have been used, and are the statistical thresholds appropriate?
- Do the statistics reflect fixed or random effects and the multiple comparisons made?

Measuring brain receptors and neurochemisty

Many neurochemical hypotheses, generated by post-mortem and animal data, can be rigorously tested with PET and SPET in the living brain whilst avoiding many of the confounding variables inherent in *in vitro* techniques. Many receptor systems can be studied (Table 2.3.6.1). For receptor mapping, particular successes in this area are the range of tracers available to image select components of dopaminergic and serotoninergic neurotransmission. For example, with presently available radiotracers it is possible to measure Dopamine D_1, striatal D_2, extrastriatal D_2, Dopamine reuptake sites, index Dopamine synthesis and endogenous dopamine release. For the serotonin system, 5-HT_{1A}, 5-HT_{2A} and 5-HT transporters can be readily measured. However, the rate of discovery of new radiotracers, suitable for use in humans, is relatively slow. Many conditions have to be satisfied to produce a suitable radiotracer for human use including blood-brain barrier permeability, high specific binding, receptor selectivity, absence of radioactive metabolites in brain, and adequate modelling of tracer kinetics (Plate 6). Practically, the increasing use of PET neuroreceptor mapping in the pharmaceutical sector should lead to a greater range of tracer availability due to the large chemical libraries within the industry.

Mapping brain activity by imaging blood flow and glucose metabolism

Regional cerebral blood flow and glucose metabolism are indicators of regional neuronal synaptic activity.[(2)] Radiotracers for these processes, such as $H_2{}^{(15)}O$ to index blood flow, are used to image brain activity in psychiatric illness. Glucose metabolic mapping using $[^{(18)}F]$deoxyglucose has some disadvantages over flow mapping. Radiation dosimetry limits for $[^{(18)}F]$deoxyglucose and the long half-life of the tracer restrict repeated measurement in a subject over a short time-scale. In contrast, $^{(15)}O$-based methods allow, for example, 12 measurements of regional blood flow over a 3 h period in a single subject.

The rapid development of PET cameras and automated data analysis techniques in the last few decades has established flow-based functional imaging as a large and active research activity.(2)

As the techniques of regional cerebral blood flow mapping have advanced there has been an equivalent sophistication of experimental design with rest state studies being overshadowed by activation paradigms.(2) In an activation design, subjects are engaged in a specific cognitive task whilst being scanned, for instance generating words, and the blood flow pattern is compared with flow present in a baseline condition such as repeating words. PET activation experiments may involve categorical, correlational, and factorial designs.(2) Although, the more recent advent of fMRI-based methods is now surpassing PET-based methods for functional brain activation mapping, there are certain situations where PET-based methods may be preferred. These include functional measurements in brain areas prone to susceptabilty artifacts in fMRI such as the temporal poles/basal frontal areas. In addition, PET [^{18}F]deoxyglucose remains a more direct measure of neural activation than all flow-related methods including fMRI and ASL, a potentially important consideration when investigating the central functional effects of CNS drugs that might also alter blood flow directly.

Novel designs and data analysis for PET studies

Developments in this area have been very rapid.(2) Examples would include the use of principal components technique to analyze PET activation data sets and attempts to determine measures of functional and effective connectivity between brain regions activated by a given task. For PET receptor studies, the use of cluster analysis, parametric approaches and simplified reference region models are of considerable interest and are now in common use.(3) Furthermore, attempts are being made to relate PET neurochemical measures to other imaging modalities and genetic factors. Examples of studies in these areas would include explorations of the relationship between densities of 5-HT$_{1A}$ receptors and amygdala reactivity during emotional processing,(4) and influence of genetic polymorphisms on 5-HT$_{1A}$ receptor expression.(5)

Imaging pathophysiology: examples from schizophrenia research

Imaging dopamine receptors

Much research effort has focused on *in vivo* PET/SPET measurement of striatal dopamine D$_2$-receptor number in schizophrenia following the initial post-mortem reports of increased striatal dopamine receptor number. Initially, using [^{11}C]N-methylspiperone as a radiotracer, a two- to threefold raised striatal D$_2$-receptor number in drug-naive schizophrenics was reported.(6) However, subsequently other investigators using [^{11}C]raclopride, [^{11}C]N-methylspiperone, [^{123}I]iodobenzamide, [^{76}Br]bromolisuride failed to detect such elevations of striatal dopamine D$_2$-receptor number.(7,8) The different radiotracer methodologies used, the selectivity of radiotracers for dopamine D$_2$, D$_3$, and D$_4$ receptor subtypes, and the clinical characteristics of the patients studied have been advanced as possible explanations for the failure to replicate raised striatal dopamine D$_2$-receptor number. However, given these conflicting but essentially negative results, attention has shifted in recent years to reports of increased presynaptic dopaminergic function measured with [^{18}F]dopa(9) and cortical dopamine D$_1$ receptors measured with [^{11}C]SCH 23390 and [^{11}C]NNC 112(10) in schizophrenia. Most recently low density extrastriatal D$_2$ receptors are being imaged with [^{11}C]FLB-457 and [^{18}F]Fallypride. However, the newer patient studies reporting changes of cortical D$_1$ and extrastriatal D$_2$ receptors await further replication.

A novel extension to studies utilizing PET/SPET radiotracers for imaging dopamine D$_2$ receptors has been to index dopamine release during a pharmacological challenge in schizophrenia. Theoretically, PET/SPET has the potential to detect neurotransmitter release associated with behavioural and pharmacological challenges if sufficient endogenous neurotransmitter is released to cause appreciable change (via receptor occupancy) in the number of 'available' receptors that can be 'seen' by a radioligand. For example, pre-dosing animals and human subjects with d-amphetamine, which releases dopamine, results in decreased [^{11}C]raclopride and [^{123}I]iodobenzamide binding to dopamine D$_2$ receptors.(11) Enhanced release of striatal dopamine in acutely symptomatic patients with schizophrenia following pharmacological challenge has been reported in a large cohort.(10,12) In these studies, the displacement of radiotracer (presumably reflecting increased release of dopamine) correlated with worsening of positive symptoms. This important finding of increased dopaminergic responsivity, together with the consistent reports of raised [^{18}F] FDOPA uptake, provide some of the most convincing *in vivo* evidence to support the hypothesis of subcortical dopamine overactivity in schizophrenia.

Imaging blood flow change, hypofrontality and cortical inefficiency

From the outset of the functional neuroimaging of schizophrenia there has been discussion as to whether the frontal lobes of patients are 'less active' than those of normal subjects.(13) However, hypofrontality, whether at rest or during cognitive challenge, has not been a universal finding in all studies, making it a somewhat unreliable trait marker of schizophrenia. It has been found in about 50 per cent of resting-state studies but more often in activation paradigms.(14) Discrepant results might be attributable to the nature and demands of the task used, task performance, and the symptom profiles of patients studied. For example, Frith *et al.*(15) and Fletcher *et al.* used PET to study paced verbal fluency activations in chronic and acute schizophrenic patients, on and off neuroleptic medication, respectively, and failed to find hypofrontality. But pacing tasks could be criticized on the grounds that slowing the task so that patients and normal subjects perform equally, fails to address a dysfunction that may be expressed when patients are required to produce 'normal' levels of performance. This is a difficult issue to resolve. Pacing patients and controls means that performance levels may be matched, and therefore differences of brain activation are not confounded by the patients' failure to do the task. Yet it may be instructive to image patients attempting to perform a task that stresses (dysfunctional) cognitive processes, produces altered brain activity and hence impaired performance.

Many authors have suggested hypofrontality may be most pronounced in schizophrenic patients who have predominantly 'negative' symptoms. This view has received support from a large cross-sectional study of chronically symptomatic patients where resting blood flow was measured in 30 patients.(16) Within this group of schizophrenic patients, greater hypofrontality was seen among those with the most pronounced negative symptoms as assessed by factor analysis. That symptoms and not the diagnosis of schizophrenia *per se* may be an important factor in hypofrontality is apparent in one study where poverty of speech (a sign of psychomotor retardation or poverty) was associated with reduced regional cerebral blood flow in the left dorsolateral prefrontal cortex, irrespective of diagnosis of depression or schizophrenia.[17] Some SPET and PET studies also suggest a relationship between hypofrontality and the presence of positive symptoms,[18,19] and hypofrontality (at rest or on activation) may resolve when symptoms improve.[20] Finally, contrary to the earlier notions of hypofrontality an alternative view of 'cortical inefficiency' has been advocated whereby patients with schizophrenia are suggested to have over activation (i.e. hyperfrontality) of frontal areas. In these studies it has been suggested that when patients and controls are performing at similar levels, patients show enhanced cortical activation reflecting the inefficient signal processing within the frontal cortex.[21]

Imaging pathophysiology: examples from depressive disorders

Imaging 5-hydroxytryptamine receptors

Impressive progress has seen the development of new radiotracers for the 5-hydroxytryptamine (**5-HT**) system; hypothesized to be dysfunctional in affective illness and to be the prime target for many antidepressant treatments. In particular, radioligands for 5-HT_{1A},5-HT_{2A} receptors, and the 5-HT transporter, are now established (Table 2.3.6.1).

One notable success is the radioligand [^{11}C]WAY 100635 for imaging 5-HT_{1A} receptors in the human brain.[22] As many antidepressant treatments alter 5-HT_{1A} receptor function in rodents, and 5-HT_{1A} knock out mice are anxious this ligand is proving useful investigating 5-HT_{1A} receptor populations in depressed or anxious patients before and after treatment. Studies in anxiety and depression are now being reported with suggestions of reductions of 5-HT_{1A} availability in these conditions.[23]

[^{11}C]N-methylspiperone, [^{18}F]altanserin, [^{18}F]ethylspiperone, [^{18}F]setoperone or [^{18}F]altanserin, and the SPET tracer [^{123}I]ketanserin have been used to measure 5-HT_2 receptor number; a receptor implicated in depressive illness, suicidal behaviour, and psychosis. Many of these 5-HT_2 ligands have been hampered by either the lack of selectivity, or the relatively low ratio of specific to non-specific signal obtained in the human brain,[24] although a few studies have appeared, reporting reduced 5-HT_2 receptor number in drug-free depressed patients. Further studies are needed using more selective ligands with higher signal-to-noise ratios, such as [^{11}C]MDL 100907, a promising selective ligand for 5-HT_{2A} receptors (Table 2.3.6.1). For the serotonin transporter, of the available tracers, [^{11}C]DASB gives a reasonable signal to noise ratio and studies have convincingly shown that standard efficacious doses of SSRI antidepressants are associated with substantial occupancy at this site.[25] Occupancy at the 5-HTT site occurs after first dosing, and responders and non responders do not differ in terms of SSRI occupancy levels, suggesting 5-HTT occupancy is perhaps a necessary but not sufficient explanation for the antidepressant effect.

Imaging blood-flow change in depressive disorder

Similarly to brain-mapping studies of patients with schizophrenia, regional deficits of neural activity (indexed by cerebral blood flow or glucose utilization) can be detected in the 'resting' brains of depressed patients.[26,27] Many resting-state studies have shown a reduction of regional brain functional activity, most frequently reported in the prefrontal cortex, compared with normal controls. However, the exact location of prefrontal change (dorsolateral, ventrolateral, orbitofrontal, and medial frontal areas) has been variably emphasized by different authors.[26–28]

As demonstrated in schizophrenia, significant associations between cortical activity and cognitive function, symptom clusters, including mood, and response to treatments are apparent.[27,28] Similar to schizophrenia, the resting-state functional brain abnormalities may represent the physiological correlates of aspects of the depressed state such as depressed mood, retardation, or cognitive impairment rather than trait markers of the illness itself.

Psychological challenge paradigms have been applied in studies in depressed cohorts to test whether specific brain regions, subserving select cognitive processes, are impaired in depressed patients. Currently, however, the majority of challenge paradigms in depressed subjects are undertaken with fMRI methods.

Imaging psychotropic drug action

Of direct clinical relevance are imaging studies of antipsychotic drug action where clinical efficacy and side-effects are related to receptor occupancy.[29,30]

Many studies have investigated the occupancy of striatal dopamine D_1 and D_2 and cortical serotonin 5-HT_2 receptors by neuroleptic drugs. Farde's group first demonstrated that clinically efficacious doses of a variety of classical antipsychotics cause between 65 per cent and 89 per cent occupancy of central dopamine D_2 receptors.[29] Higher receptor occupancy [(gt)85 per cent] is associated with an increased incidence of extrapyramidal side effects. Thus, there may be a therapeutic window for occupancy of between 65 per cent and 85 per cent, which is antipsychotic and yet less likely to cause extrapyramidal side effects. In contrast, treatment with classical antipsychotics produces variable levels of occupancy of striatal D_1 receptors. Interestingly, efficacious doses of the atypical antipsychotic clozapine are associated with a relatively low D_2 receptor occupancy (38–63 per cent) and a D_1 occupancy of 38 to 52 per cent.[29] This unexpected finding of low D_2 receptor occupancy, reproduced in different patient groups with both PET and SPET techniques, has challenged theories of a simple relationship between D_2 occupancy *per se* and clinical efficacy. Further evidence for this view comes from studies showing that schizophrenic antipsychotic non-responders have the same levels of dopamine D_2 occupancy as responders and that occupancy occurs as rapidly as 2 h after acute administration of the antipsychotic yet efficacy takes weeks to appear.

PET/SPET is also proving useful in the characterization of atypical antipsychotics. The binding of antipsychotic drugs to central 5-HT_2 receptors is a possible candidate for the mechanism of 'atypicality' and studies suggest high cortical 5-HT_2 occupancy with many atypicals including risperidone (80 per cent) and clozapine (84–90 per cent).[29,30] Other targets for some atypical neuroleptics include the 5-HT_{1A} receptor[31] and in addition, limbic selectivity (i.e. neuroleptic limbic occupancy > striatal occupancy) is an actively researched explanation for atypicality.[32]

Conclusions

So far, the PET and SPET radiotracer techniques have been immediately valuable in assessing the receptor occupancy effects of antipsychotic drugs and of mapping the neural correlates of dysfunctional cognitive processes and psychiatric symptoms. Although the applications described have not yielded a diagnostic test, the techniques are undoubtedly providing unique information about the pathophysiology of psychiatric illnesses. Such information is likely to be key for the development of truly novel treatments.

Further information

www.crump.ucla.edu/lpp/lpphome.html A website that gives more detailed information on the methodology of PET scanning and clinical applications.

Journals publishing regular research articles on PET neuroscience include *Biological Psychiatry, Neuroimage, Synapse, Brain, Human Brain Mapping, Journal of Nuclear Medicine, Molecular Psychiatry and Neuropsychopharmacology* amongst others. Annual and biannual meetings of the Society of Nuclear Medicine, Organization for Human Brain Mapping and the Society of Cerebral Blood Flow and Metabolism include many 'cutting edge' PET neuroscience reports.

References

1. Myers, R., Cunningham, V., Bailey, D., *et al.* (1996). *Quantification of brain function using PET*. Academic Press, London.
2. Frackowiak, R.S.J., Friston, K.J., Frith, C.D., *et al.* (1997). *Human brain function.* Academic Press, San Diego, CA.
3. Gunn, R.N., Gunn S.R. and Cunningham, V.J. (2001). Positron emission tomography compartmental models. *Journal of Cerebral Blood Flow and Metabolism,* **6**, 635–52.
4. Fischer, P.M., Meltzer, C.C., Ziolko, S.K., *et al.* (2006). Capacity for 5-HT1A-mediated autoregulation predicts amygdala reactivity. *Nature Neuroscience,* **11**, 1362–3.
5. David, S.P., Murthy, V.M., Rabiner, E.N., *et al.* (2005). A functional genetic variation of the serotonin (5-HT) transporter affects 5-HT1A receptor binding in humans. *Journal of Neuroscience,* **10**, 2586–90.
6. Wong, D.F., Wagner, H.N., Tune, L.E., *et al.* (1986). Positron emission tomography reveals elevated D2-dopamine receptors in drug-naïve schizophrenia. *Science,* **234**, 1558–63.
7. Farde, L., Wiesel, F.-A., Stone-Elander, S., *et al.* (1990). D2 dopamine receptors in neuroleptic naive schizophrenic patients. *Archives of General Psychiatry,* **47**, 213–19.
8. Sedvall, G. and Farde, L. (1995). Chemical brain anatomy in schizophrenia. *Lancet,* **346**, 743–9.
9. Hietala, J., Syvalahti, E., Vuorio, K., *et al.* (1995). Presynaptic dopamine function in striatum of neuroleptic naive schizophrenic patients. *Lancet,* **346**, 1130–1.
10. Guillin, O., Abi-Dargham, A. and Laruelle, M. (2007). Neurobiology of Dopamine in Schizophrenia. *International Review of Neurobiology,* **78**, 1–39.
11. Volkow, N.D., Wang, G.-J., Fowler, J.S., *et al.* (1994). Imaging endogenous dopamine competition with 11C-raclopride in the human brain. *Synapse,* **16**, 255–62
12. Laruelle, M., Abi-Dargham, A., van Dyck, C.H., *et al.* (1996). Single photon emission computerized tomography imaging of amphetamineinduced dopamine release in drug-free schizophrenia subjects. *Proceedings of the National Academy of Sciences of the United States of America,* **93**, 9235–40.
13. Weinberger, D.R. and Berman, K.F. (1996). Prefrontal function in schizophrenia: confounds and controversies. *Philosophical Transactions of the Royal Society of London. Series B: Biological Sciences,* **351**, 1495–503.
14. Chuam, S.E. and McKenna, P.J. (1996). Schizophrenia—a brain disease? A critical review of structural and functional cerebral abnormality in the disorder. *British Journal of Psychiatry,* **166**, 563–82.
15. Frith, C.D., Friston, K.J., Herold, S., *et al.* (1995). Regional brain activity in chronic schizophrenic patients during the performance of a verbal fluency task. *British Journal of Psychiatry,* **167**, 343–9.
16. Liddle, P.F., Friston, K.J., Frith, C.D., *et al.* (1992). Patterns of cerebral blood flow in schizophrenia. *British Journal of Psychiatry,* **160**, 179–86.
17. Dolan, R.J., Bench, C.J., Liddle, P.F., *et al.* (1993). Dorsolateral prefrontal cortex dysfunction in the major psychoses; symptom or disease specificity? *Journal of Neurology, Neurosurgery and Psychiatry,* **56**, 1290–4.
18. Andreasen, N.C., O'Leary, D.S., Flaum, M., *et al.* (1997). Hypofrontality in schizophrenia: distributed dysfunctional circuits in neurolepticnaive patients. *Lancet,* **349**, 1730–4.
19. Sabri, O., Erkwoh, R., Schreckenberger, M., *et al.* (1997). Correlation of positive symptoms exclusively to hyperperfusion or hypoperfusion of cerebral cortex in never-treated schizophrenics. *Lancet,* **349**, 1735–9.
20. Spence, S.A., Hirsch, S.R., Brooks, D.J., *et al.* (1998). Prefrontal cortex activity in people with schizophrenia and control subjects. Evidence from positron emission tomography for remission of 'hypofrontality' with recovery from acute schizophrenia. *British Journal of Psychiatry,* **172**, 316–23.
21. Callicott, J.H., Mattay, V.S., Verchinchi, B.A., *et al.* (2003). Complexity of prefrontal cortical dysfunction in schizophrenia: more than up or down. *American Journal of Psychiatry,* **12**, 2209–15.
22. Pike, V., McCarron, J.A., Lammerstma, A.A., *et al.* (1995). First delineation of 5-HT1A receptors in the living human brain using (11)CWAY-100635. *European Journal of Pharmacology,* **283**, R1–R3.
23. Sargent, P.A., Kjaer, K.H., Bench, C.J., *et al.* (2000). Brain serotonin1A receptor binding measured by positron emission tomography with [11C]WAY-100635: effects of depression and antidepressant treatment. *Archives of General Psychiatry,* **2**, 174–80.
24. Pike, V. (1993). Positron emitting radioligands for studies *in vivo*—probes for human psychopharmacology. *Journal of Psychopharmacology,* **7**, 139–58.
25. Meyer, J. (2007). Imaging the serotonin transporter during major depressive disorder and antidepressant treatment. *Journal Psychiatry and Neuroscience,* **2**, 86–102.
26. Goodwin, G. (1996). Functional imaging, affective disorder and dementia. *British Medical Bulletin,* **52**.
27. Drevets, W.C., Price, J.L., Simpson, J.R., *et al.* (1997). Subgenual prefrontal cortex abnormalities in mood disorders. *Nature,* **386**, 824–7.
28. Grasby, P.M. and Bench, C.J. (1997). Neuroimaging of mood disorders. *Current Opinion in Psychiatry,* **10**, 73–8.
29. Farde, L., Nordstrom, A.-L., Wiesel, F.A., *et al.* (1992). Positron emission tomographic analysis of central D1 and D2 dopamine receptor occupancy in patients treated with classical neuroleptics and clozapine. Relation to extrapyramidal side effects. *Archives of General Psychiatry,* **49**, 538–54.
30. Nyberg, S., Farde, L., and Erikson, L. (1993). 5-HT2 and D2 dopamine receptor occupancy in the living human brain: a PET study with risperidone. *Psychopharmacology,* **110**, 265–72.

31. Bantick, R.A., Deacon, J.F., and Grasby, P.M. (2001) The 5-HT1A receptor in schizophrenia: a promising target for novel atypical neuroleptics? *Journal of Psychopharmacology*, 1, 37–46.
32. Bressan, R.A., Erlandsson, K., Jones, H.M. *et al.* (2003) Optimizing limbic selective D2/D3 receptor occupancy by risperidone: a [123I]-epidepride SPET study. *Journal of Clinical Psychopharmacology*, 1, 5–14.

2.3.7 Structural magnetic resonance imaging

J. Suckling and E. T. Bullmore

Introduction

Magnetic resonance imaging (**MRI**) is a versatile and evolving technology for visualizing the structure, function, and metabolism of the living human brain. All kinds of MRI data can be acquired without exposing subjects to ionizing radiation or radioactive isotopes. Installing the hardware for MRI represents a major capital investment, of approximately £1.5 million. For these three reasons of versatility, safety, and (relative) affordability, MRI continues to be the dominant brain-imaging technique in psychiatric practice and research.

In this chapter, we introduce the principles and practicalities of MRI and describe common methods of structural MRI data acquisition and analysis. Chapter 2.3.8 on functional MRI provides greater detail on statistical issues arising in image analysis.

Magnetization

If iron filings are scattered on a piece of paper they will be oriented at random. If a bar magnet is then placed under the paper, the iron filings will align themselves so that each filing lies parallel to the magnetic field produced by the magnet. More technically, we can say that iron filings have a susceptibility to be magnetized by a static magnetic field.

Susceptibility refers both to the effect of a magnetic field on an object, and the effect of that object on the field. Paramagnetic materials, like some metals, tend to be attracted by magnets and cause a local increase in the magnetic field strength. Diamagnetic materials, like carbon and many organic compounds, tend to be repulsed by magnets and cause a local decrease in field strength.

The brain also has a susceptibility to be magnetized. It is largely composed of water and each molecule of water comprises, of course, two hydrogen atoms and one oxygen atom. The hydrogen nucleus is a single positively charged proton, which has a dynamic property called spin. Like all moving charged particles, spinning protons generate a magnetic field. The axis of the magnetic dipole generated by a spinning proton is sometimes called its magnetic moment, and is drawn as a vector.

When the brain is placed in a strong magnetic field, the spinning protons align themselves with the external field, just as iron filings align themselves to the field of a bar magnet. The angle of alignment between each proton's moment and the (longitudinal) axis of the external magnetic field is α. Protons obey the laws of quantum mechanics, and so two modes of alignment or spin states are possible, one with the magnetic moment in the direction of the field ($\alpha = 0°$) and one with the moment in the opposite direction ($\alpha = 180°$). Depending on the strength of the applied field, the spin states have slightly different probabilities, with those protons aligned in the direction of the field in excess by about 5 ppm at an external field strength of 1.5 T. (Magnetic field strength is measured in units of gauss (**G**) or tesla (**T**): 1 T = 10 000 G. The earth's magnetic field is approximately 0.5 G; a child's toy magnet has a field of around 10 G.)

Thus, if the magnetic moments for all spinning protons are averaged, the net, or bulk, magnetization vector for the brain as a whole will have $\alpha = 0°$. The length of the net magnetization vector then represents the strength of longitudinal magnetization (Fig. 2.3.7.1).

Protons aligned with a static magnetic field are not static themselves, they rotate or precess at very high frequency around the axis of the external field. The precession frequency, or Larmor frequency, is constant for a given type of atomic nucleus and external field strength. For protons, the Larmor frequency at 1.5 T is 63.9 MHz. However, although all hydrogen nuclei in the brain precess at the same frequency in the same field, they will not all precess with the same phase. At any given time, different nuclei have reached a different point in their rotation around the external field axis.

Nuclear magnetic resonance

When a wineglass is tapped by a knife, it produces a high-pitched sound of characteristic frequency. If a singer can exactly match that frequency with her voice then the glass will resonate and may break. The basic idea is that if an object has a characteristic frequency of oscillation, exposing it to energy precisely at that frequency will cause a change in physical state.

Analogously, if we supply a pulse of radio-frequency energy at (and only at) the Larmor frequency to a brain located in a magnetic field, the protons within the brain will absorb the energy and resonate—this is nuclear magnetic resonance (**NMR**)—and their angle of alignment α with the external field will increase. If sufficient energy is supplied to cause $\alpha = 90°$, the radio-frequency pulse is called a '90° pulse'. If the net magnetization vector is flipped to an angle $\alpha = 180°$, the radio-frequency pulse is called a '180° pulse'. At the same time as the angle of alignment is increased by radio-frequency irradiation, the phase of precession becomes coherent over all protons. In other words, in place of the random variation in the phase of precession that existed before the radio-frequency pulse, protons are now 'marching in step' with each other around the axis of the external field.

After the radio-frequency pulse has ceased, the resonating nuclei gradually relax back to the equilibrium state of random precession in alignment with the external field. The two components of this relaxation process are characterized by relaxation times. The first relaxation time (T_1), also called the spin-lattice relaxation time, describes the time taken for the strength of longitudinal magnetization to return to 63 per cent of its value before radio-frequency irradiation. This is a measure of the time taken for α to return to zero having been flipped to 90° or 180°. T_1 is determined by interactions between protons and their long-range (molecular) environment

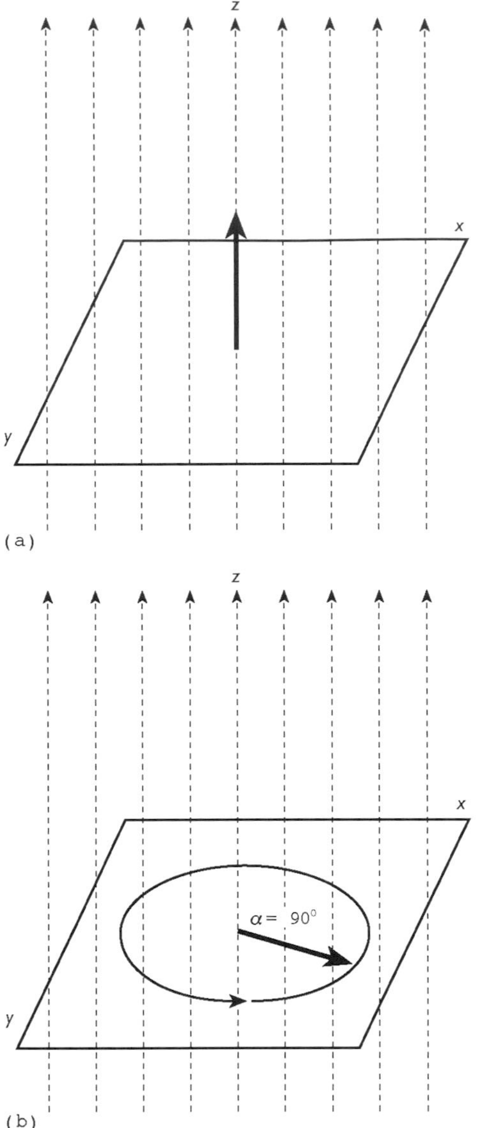

Fig. 2.3.7.1 Net magnetization vector.
(a) In a static magnetic field, the vector is aligned parallel to the longitudinal **z** axis of the field and **α** = 0.
(b) Immediately after a 90° excitation pulse of radio-frequency energy at Larmor frequency, the angle of alignment **α** is increased (transverse magnetization) and the phase of precession in the **x–y** plane is coherent over all protons in the brain. As protons relax following excitation, the angle of the net vector becomes smaller (return of longitudinal magnetization) and the phase of precession becomes more variable from one proton to another (dephasing).

or lattice. The second relaxation time (T_2), also called the spin–spin relaxation time, describes the time taken for the flipped nuclei to stop 'marching in step' around the axis of the field. This process of dephasing begins as soon as the radio-frequency pulse stops, but its rate is determined by the immediate (atomic) environment of the protons. Small variations in the applied magnetic field accentuate spin–spin relaxation, resulting in an observed relaxation time T_2* which is somewhat faster than the 'true' relaxation time T_2 that would have been observed in an ideally homogeneous field.

As protons relax, they release the energy absorbed from the radio-frequency pulse in the form of a weak radio-frequency signal, which decays at a rate normally determined by T_2*. This process is called free induction decay, and the emitted signal forms the data from which magnetic resonance images are ultimately constructed.

Magnetic resonance imaging

Spin echo sequence

A widely used MRI technique is the spin echo sequence. A 90° radio-frequency pulse is repetitively applied to the brain with a constant repetition time (TR ms) between consecutive pulses. Following each 90° pulse, protons are excited and then relax. The dephasing component of relaxation can be reversed by applying a second 180° pulse some time (TE/2 ms) after the 90° pulse. Following the first 90° pulse, protons immediately begin to precess idiosyncratically and the emitted signal decays. By reversing this process, the 180° pulse causes rephasing and an increase in emitted signal which has a maximum or echo at TE ms (time to echo) after the initial 90° pulse (Fig. 2.3.7.2).

The spatial location of the radio-frequency signal emitted by free induction decay in a given volume of the brain is encoded in three spatial dimensions by slice-selective radio-frequency irradiation combined with frequency- and phase-encoding gradients. To improve scan time, multiple slices can be excited in an interleaved fashion (multislice acquisition). This means that after the output signal is detected from one slice, and while the net magnetization vector is relaxing back to its equilibrium state, other slices can be excited. The in-plane resolution (voxel size) of the image is determined by the field of view and the number of voxels in the image. Typically, in-plane resolution at 1.5 T is in the order of 0.5 to 2 mm, and slice thickness is 2 mm or more.

Tissue contrast

The outstanding advantage of MRI for the anatomical examination of the brain is the easily visible contrast in the images between grey matter, white matter, and cerebrospinal fluid. In particular, contrast between parenchymal tissues (grey and white matter) has made MRI the imaging research tool of choice for identifying subtle cortical abnormalities in a wide variety of psychiatric disorders.

Tissue contrast in magnetic resonance images is determined by differences in the density of protons, and their physical and chemical environment. A tissue such as the cerebrospinal fluid, that is

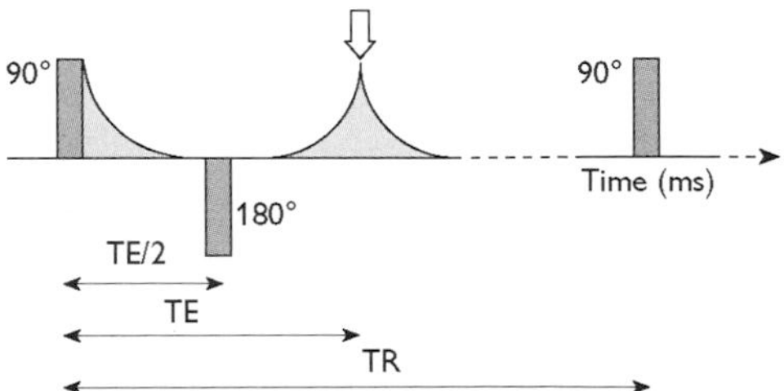

Fig. 2.3.7.2 Spin echo pulse sequence. A 90° excitation pulse of radio-frequency energy is immediately followed by exponential decay of the T_2-weighted signal. A 180° pulse TE/2 ms later causes rephasing of proton spins and an exponential increase in T_2-weighted signal with maximum (echo) TE ms after the 90° pulse. Images are acquired at TE (thick arrow). The protons are allowed to relax completely before the next 90° pulse, TR ms after the previous excitation.

composed largely of water, will have a lower proton density than parenchymal brain tissues. The physicochemical environment of protons has a marked effect on spin-lattice relaxation. If protons are mainly in freely diffusing water molecules, as they are in cerebrospinal fluid, T_1 will be prolonged, whereas if they are mainly bound to large macromolecules, as they are in fat, T_1 will be short (Table 2.3.7.1). Since grey matter contains proportionally less fat than myelinated white matter, T_1 is longer for grey matter. Spin–spin relaxation is likewise determined, in part, by the immediate physical environment of protons in the tissue; liquid tissues will have prolonged T_2 times compared with solid tissues. Other effects on apparent relaxation times (T_2*) include minute fluctuations or inhomogeneities in the strength of the external magnetic field, which may be due to the local paramagnetic effects of iron-containing compounds such as haemoglobin.

The parameters of the spin echo pulse sequence, repetition time (TR), and time to echo (TE), can be judiciously adjusted to acquire images that are sensitive to or weighted by one or other of these possible sources of tissue contrast.

If TR is long (>1000 ms) and TE is short (<20 ms), contrast in the images will be weighted by differences between tissues in proton density. Proton-density-weighted images show good contrast between relatively hyperintense parenchymal tissue and hypointense cerebrospinal fluid (Plate 7).

If TR is short (<1000 ms) and TE is also short (<20 ms), contrast in the images will be weighted by tissue differences in spin-lattice relaxation. T_1-weighted images show excellent contrast between hyperintense white matter and relatively hypointense grey matter (Plate 7). For this reason, T_1-weighted images are widely used to measure quantitative abnormalities in size or shape of the cerebral cortex.

If TR is long (>1000 ms) and TE is also long (>20 ms), contrast in the images will be weighted by tissue differences in spin–spin relaxation. T_2-weighted images show strong contrast between hyperintense cerebrospinal fluid and parenchymal tissues (Plate 7), unless there is congestion or oedema of the parenchyma, in which case the T_2-weighted signal will be increased. For this reason, T_2-weighted images are widely used to identify acute, inflammatory, and ischaemic lesions.

Structural imaging sequences

An enormous range of sequences are available for brain imaging. For example, fast spin echo imaging provides a pair of dual-echo images with complementary tissue contrasts (proton density and T_2-weighted) for no increase in scan time over the spin-echo sequence. Spins can also be manipulated through changes in the applied magnetic field gradients. These sequences yield images of high-spatial resolution and a range of contrasts. Additionally, there are methods for suppressing signals due to blood flow or fat, improving signals from pathology.

Table 2.3.7.1 Relaxation times at 1.5 T for different tissue types

Tissue type	T_1 (ms)	T_2 (ms)
Grey matter	980–1040	64–71
White matter	740–770	64–70
CSF	>2000	>300
Fat (at 1 T)	180	90

CSF, cerebrospinal fluid.

Diffusion-weighted imaging

Diffusion-weighted imaging can provide information about the organization of white matter tracts in the brain that cannot be obtained by other MRI methods.

The basic idea is that protons move within and between cells by random motion. Typically, a proton may travel around 20 μm in 100 ms by this Brownian motion or diffusion. The rate of proton diffusion is related to how constrained they are by physical barriers such as myelinated cell membranes. The rate of diffusion affects the spin–spin relaxation time, with rapidly diffusing protons tending to relax more quickly. To acquire images that are weighted by differences in diffusion, two extra gradients are briefly applied during a spin echo sequence.(1)

White matter is generally hyperintense in diffusion-weighted imaging because closely packed axonal tracts provide the greatest barrier to the free diffusion of water in the brain. Furthermore, it is possible to deduce from diffusion-weighted imaging data how compactly organized the white matter is, and even to estimate in what direction the fibre tracts are oriented (Plate 8). This information is of considerable interest to psychiatry, since the pathology of many psychiatric disorders may involve the axonal connections between multiple cortical areas.(2)

Safety

MRI is absolutely contraindicated in patients who have any strongly magnetized metal object in their heads. This includes aneurysm clips, reconstructive metal plates, traumatically embedded metal fragments, or implanted electronic devices such as cardiac pacemakers. It is advisable to screen all subjects undergoing MRI by questionnaire for possible contraindications. A skull radiograph is a useful preliminary examination if there is any doubt about the presence of intracranial metal. All subjects need to provide informed consent in writing.

Static magnetic fields used in MRI cause no harmful effects to biological tissue. Rapid switching of field gradients can induce electrical currents in tissue, but at the switching speeds used in MRI these induced currents are several times less than needed for muscle contraction. Since radio-frequency energy can cause heating, limits to the amounts of energy absorbed are set by national standards.

Artefacts

Quality assurance protocols and diligent hardware servicing are necessary to maintain high standards in MRI. Image artefacts refer to loss of image quality (i.e. spatial resolution or tissue contrast) owing to a specific cause. It is often possible to effect a remedy and an awareness of their causes can often pre-empt the problem.

Movement

Subject motion is the most common artefact and has two components: voluntary and involuntary (physiological). The result of voluntary motion during acquisition may be an obvious blurring (Plate 7). The cooperation of subjects is vital and special regard is required for children, the elderly, and those with neurological or psychiatric disorders who may find the MRI environment disconcerting. The subject's head may be physically restrained by additional padding and by Velcro straps placed across the forehead. Involuntary motion arises primarily from the cardiorespiratory cycle causing pulsation of the blood vessels and cerebrospinal fluid. This is most apparent in structural images showing major arteries.

Susceptibility

Where two materials with very different susceptibilities are closely adjacent, there may be severe distortion of the magnetic field, causing artefactual loss or exaggeration of the magnetic resonance signal. This is clearly seen in an image acquired with a metallic clip placed close to the scalp (Plate 7). Ferromagnetic (highly paramagnetic) materials that may cause artefacts include metallic dental fillings and plates, hairgrips, ear or nose rings, and even some cosmetics. A less obvious form of susceptibility artefact arises if more (diamagnetic) tissue is situated at one end of the image field of view than the other. A field gradient is set-up across the image resulting in signal loss. This is termed bulk susceptibility artefact and is often seen in images of both the head and neck (Plate 7).

Partial volume

Voxel sizes are larger than some scales of anatomical organization in the brain. A voxel may represent a heterogeneous mixture of tissue classes, or be only partially occupied by tissue of a single type. This partial volume artefact is particularly evident at the interface between cortical grey matter and sulcal cerebrospinal fluid, and at the interface between cortical grey matter and central white matter. It causes error in the estimation of tissue class volumes.

MRI hardware

Superconducting magnet

The superconducting magnets used for MRI require liquid helium cooling equipment to keep the temperature low enough (4 K) for superconduction. Cooling consumes the majority of the supplied power. Only a small current is initially required to generate the field, which is then self-sustaining.

Small variations in the homogeneity of the magnetic field give rise to distortions and artefacts. The field is minutely adjusted to improve homogeneity using additional magnets in an automated procedure known as shimming.

Magnetic field gradients are essential to MRI. Rapid switching of gradient coils produces the loud 'knocking' sound associated with magnetic resonance scanners. Three orthogonal gradients are available which are coupled to generate gradients in any direction.

Radio-frequency coil

The function of the radio-frequency coil is two-fold—to transmit the radio-frequency pulses of the imaging sequences and to receive the emitted signal. Head coils used for neuroimaging fit snugly over the subject's head, and are often of a three-dimensional design with good sensitivity throughout the volume they enclose. Surface coil designs are used to image small regions with high-spatial resolution, and phased-array coils combine several surface coils for more extensive coverage.

Computers

MRI produces large quantities of data, which require rapid processing and storage so that images may be viewed and other sequences prescribed during the same session. The computer system is integral to the machine and contains specialized hardware and software for data acquisition and image reconstruction, as well as control of the scanner.

The scanner suite

The room housing the scanner must be specially designed. It must have a reinforced floor and be environmentally controlled to maintain a constant temperature and humidity. The walls and ceiling contain a magnetic shield, which both prevents leakage of the field outside the room and stops FM radio broadcasts from being picked up by the radio-frequency coil.

MRI studies

Case-control design

Structural MRI studies in psychiatry have commonly adopted a cross-sectional or case-control design. This involves scanning two groups of subjects, patients, and matched controls, on a single occasion. The objective is generally to identify anatomical differences in brain structure between cases and controls. In evaluating or planning such a study, it is important to pay attention to several design issues, some of which are summarized below.

Power

What is the power of the study to refute the null hypothesis (zero anatomical difference between the case and control populations) when it is not true? In general, the power of a study is proportional to the sample size (the number of subjects scanned), the effect size (the anatomical difference between populations), and the probability threshold or p value adopted for hypothesis testing. The p value will often be decided in relation to the number of tests conducted—the greater the number of tests, the smaller is the appropriate p value. Therefore, the risk of low power and associated type 2 error is likely to be greatest when differences between two small groups have been multiply tested on the basis of many anatomical variables.

Representativeness

What population is represented by the sample of patients studied, and is this the population of interest? If the ambition of the study is to make inferences about the population of patients with, say, manic-depressive disorder, then it is important that the diagnosis is made according to standard and reliable criteria and that the sampling procedure is such that any patient in that population has an equal chance of being included in the study. This means that the authors of the study will need to sample cases from general practice and the community as well as from hospital clinics and wards. Sampling hospital patients is generally much easier; the patients are already well characterized and hospital treatment facilities are likely to be relatively few in number and close to the scanning unit. However, if only hospital patients are sampled, it follows that inference can only be made about the population of hospital patients, rather than the larger and more general population of individuals with the disorder.

Heterogeneity

Diagnostic categories in psychiatry may subsume considerable heterogeneity in terms of phenomenology and aetiology. For example, patients with a diagnosis of schizophrenia may differ profoundly in terms of positive or negative symptom profiles, cognitive deficit, and genetic or environmental risk factors. These natural sources of heterogeneity may be compounded by differences in treatment. Any or all of these factors may affect brain structure. Studies that simply ignore heterogeneity, or attempt to deal with it by *post hoc* statistical correction, may have less power to detect a group difference than studies which define cases according to refined or subdiagnostic criteria. Thus, studying a sample of schizophrenic patients with high negative symptom scores and marked working memory deficits may be more likely to reveal anatomical abnormalities of frontal cortex than studying an unrefined sample of patients with schizophrenia.

Matching

Ideally, the control or comparison subjects should be indistinguishable from the patients in every characteristic apart from features of the disorder. For example, it is important that cases and controls should be matched for age, handedness, and sex, since all of these factors may affect brain structure. Unfortunately, there are a number of other possible confounding factors that are not so obviously unrelated to presence of the disorder. For example, an unrefined sample of patients with schizophrenia will generally have lower IQ and smaller head size than an age- and sex-matched group of comparison subjects. Should we try to correct these differences as if they were spurious (by either refined sampling or *post hoc* statistical modelling), or should we accept that they represent real features of the disorder? In practice, most published studies tend to correct group differences on global variables by statistical modelling in order to focus attention on regional differences that may be more interesting. A comparable problem arises in relation to medication.

Other designs

A probable future trend in psychiatric MRI research over the next few years is that the hypotheses under investigation will become more concerned with aetiological mechanisms and pathogenetic models and less concerned with the basic question of whether a given group of patients has abnormal brain structure. This shift in hypothetical interest will dictate a shift in design away from case-control or cross-sectional studies.

Longitudinal designs, in which a cohort of volunteers or patients are scanned repeatedly over a period of months or years, are a powerful way of demonstrating normal and abnormal developmental changes in brain structure.[(3)] They have the obvious disadvantage that they are time consuming to complete and subjects may not attend for multiply repeated examination.

Genetic designs involve subjects that are defined genotypically, rather than phenotypically. Imaging studies of monozygotic twins discordant for a disorder,[(4)] and of families multiply affected by a disorder, are examples of genetic designs in which there may be complete knowledge about the proportion of genetic information that is shared between subjects but incomplete knowledge about the genetic constitution of each subject.

Overall, there is no single perfect design for an imaging study. Often designing a study will entail finding pragmatic and arguably justifiable solutions to problems. Furthermore, the 'goodness' of a design can really only be judged in relation to the hypothesis under investigation and the methods of analysis applied to the data. The best imaging studies will convey a sense that the design is both ingenious and inevitable, given the hypothesis and available methods, and will also include a frank discussion of the limitations or implications of the particular design adopted.

Data analysis

Clinical analysis

Structural MRI is most often used in clinical practice to exclude non-psychiatric causes for psychopathology. Clinical examination of these cases may also sometimes reveal abnormalities such as hippocampal sclerosis or callosal agenesis which suggest that psychopathology has been determined by birth injury or abnormal development. In assessment of a patient with dementia, MRI may usefully demonstrate signs of vascular disease (such as infarcts or periventricular white matter changes), or a focal pattern of grey matter atrophy suggestive of Pick's disease (frontal cortex) or Huntington's disease (caudate nucleus and frontal cortex). All of these abnormalities may be detected simply by skilled visual examination of the data. However, clinical diagnosis of the subtler abnormalities associated with, say, schizophrenia, obsessive–compulsive disorder, or autism require quantitative analysis of the patient's data and access to normative MRI measurements on appropriately matched samples of the general population. Neither quantitative analysis nor normative databases are widely used in current radiological practice, thus limiting the value of MRI to clinical psychiatry, but this may be expected to change in the future.

Quantitative analysis

There are broadly two requirements for quantitative analysis of structural MRI data. The first is to measure the anatomical structure of the brain (this is often called morphometry). The second is to test hypotheses of interest on the basis of these morphometric variables.[(5)] Here we shall focus on morphometry.

(a) Morphometry

A widely used method of measuring brain structure from magnetic resonance images is based on the hypothetical expectation that one or more anatomically defined regions of the brain are particularly relevant to the disorder.[(6)] The area or volume of each of these regions of interest (**ROIs**) can then be measured directly by drawing a line around the region on a computerized display of the data and counting the number of voxels enclosed by the line. Measurements of several ROIs may be combined to produce summary measures of asymmetry[(7)] or of spatially distributed anatomical systems. The advantages of ROI morphometry are that it is conceptually simple and that it allows measurement of structures (e.g. the hippocampus) or parts of structures (e.g. segments of the corpus callosum) that may be difficult to measure otherwise. Some familiar disadvantages are that it is time consuming and imperfectly reliable. More fundamentally, ROI morphometry is of limited use if it is not obvious in advance what the region of interest is, or there are several possible regions of abnormality (as is likely if the disorder is determined by an insult early in the course of brain development).

Computerized techniques are varied, but commonly adopt an approach summarized in Plate 9. In this scheme, the first step in image processing is removal of extracerebral tissues like skull and scalp leaving an image of the brain alone. The brain image is then segmented into the three main tissue classes. There are a variety of techniques for segmentation or brain tissue classification,[8] but generally the quality of segmentation is improved if multiple images of different contrasts (e.g. proton density, T_2-weighted) are available.

Once the brain image has been divided into its component classes, or even prior to segmentation, it can be automatically registered in a standard anatomical space. The value of making this transformation is potentially two-fold. First, it then becomes possible to compare brain structure between individuals at the spatial resolution of the image, that is in terms of the percentage occupancy of each voxel by each tissue class. This means that one is able ultimately to test anatomical differences between groups over the whole brain in detail, without having to assume a priori that pathological change is located in a particular region.[9,10] The second major advantage of image registration is that the parameters of the transformation used to align the image with the template may themselves be used as measures of brain structure. Thus, if an image represents a brain that is structurally abnormal in some way, the mathematical deformation which must be applied to align it with a standard template may be abnormally great.[11]

(b) Statistical testing

Morphometric variables can be used to test hypotheses by a variety of statistical analyses. For example, the null hypothesis of zero difference in brain structure between two groups can be addressed by a t-test of a single ROI or by many thousands of t-tests of, say, grey matter occupancy measured at each and every voxel. Similarly hypotheses concerning the relationship between brain structure and psychological function can be addressed by testing the correlation between a morphometric variable and the subjects' scores on a psychometric instrument. Alternatively, the relationships between several morphometric variables may be explored by multivariate methods such as partial least squares.[12]

Further information

MRI theory and practice—McRobbie, D.W., Moore, E.A., Graves, M.J., *et al.* (2007). *MRI from picture to proton* (2nd edn). Cambridge University Press, Cambridge.

Reviews of structural imaging in psychiatry—Symms, M., Jager, H.R., Schmierer, K., *et al.* (2004). A review of structural magnetic resonance neuroimaging. *Journal of Neurology, Neurosurgery, and Psychiatry*, **75**, 1235–44.

Hyman, S.E. (2007). Can neuroscience be integrated into the DSM-V? *Nature Reviews Neuroscience*, **8**, 725–32.

Online repository of methods and data—The Internet Brain Segmentation Repository (http://www.cma.mgh.harvard.edu/ibsr/) provides manually guided expert segmentation results along with magnetic resonance brain image data.

References

1. Basser, P.J. and Jones, D.K. (2002). Diffusion tensor MRI: theory, experimental design and data analysis—a technical review. *NMR in Biomedicine*, **15**, 456–67.
2. Taylor, W.D., Hsu, E., Krishnan, K.R.R., *et al.* (2004). Diffusion tensor imaging: background, potential and utility in psychiatric research. *Biological Psychiatry*, **55**, 201–7.
3. Giedd, J.N., Blumenthal, J., Jeffries, N.O., *et al.* (1999). Brain development during childhood and adolescence: a longitudinal MRI study. *Nature Neuroscience*, **2**, 861–3.
4. McDonald, C., Bullmore, E.T., Sham, P.C., *et al.* (2004). Association of genetic risks for schizophrenia and bipolar disorder with specific and generic brain structural endophenotypes. *Archives of General Psychiatry*, **61**, 974–84.
5. Bullmore, E.T., Suckling, J., Overmeyer, S., *et al.* (1999). Global, voxel and cluster tests, by theory and permutation, for a difference between two groups of structural MR images. *IEEE Transactions on Medical Imaging*, **18**, 32–42.
6. Wright, I.C., Rabe-Hesketh, S., Woodruff, P.W.R., *et al.* (2000). *The American Journal of Psychiatry*, **157**, 16–25.
7. Shenton, M.E., Dickey, C.C., Frumin, M., *et al.* (2001). A review of MRI findings in schizophrenia. *Schizophrenia Research*, **49**, 1–52.
8. Zhang, Y., Brady, M., and Smith, S. (2001). Segmentation of brain MR images through a hidden Markov random field model and the expectation-maximisation algorithm. *IEEE Transactions on Medical Imaging*, **20**, 45–57.
9. Ashburner, J. and Friston, K.J. (2000). Voxel-based morphometry—the methods. *NeuroImage*, **11**, 805–21.
10. Ananth, H., Popescu, I., Critchley, H.D., *et al.* (2002). Cortical and subcortical gray matter abnormalities in schizophrenia determined through structural magnetic resonance imaging with optimized voxel-based morphometry. *The American Journal of Psychiatry*, **159**, 1497–505.
11. Chung, M.K., Worsley, K.J., Robbins, S., *et al.* (2003). Deformation-based surface morphometry applied to gray matter deformation. *NeuroImage*, **18**, 198–213.
12. Nestor, P.G., O'Donnell, B.F., McCarley, R.W., *et al.* (2002). A new statistical method for testing hypotheses of neuropsychological/MRI relationships in schizophrenia: partial least squares analysis. *Schizophrenia Research*, **53**, 57–66.

2.3.8 Functional magnetic resonance imaging

E. T. Bullmore and J. Suckling

Introduction

Functional magnetic resonance imaging (**fMRI**) is a relatively new technique for measuring changes in cerebral blood flow. The first fMRI studies, showing functional activation of the occipital cortex by visual stimulation and activation of the motor cortex by finger movement, were published in the early 1990s.[1–3] In the years since then, fMRI has been used to investigate the physiological response to a wide variety of experimental procedures in both normal human subjects and diverse patient groups. In the next 10 years, fMRI will probably establish a role for itself in radiological and psychiatric practice; currently the clinical role of fMRI is limited to specialized applications such as assessment of hemispheric dominance prior to neurosurgery.[4]

The outstanding advantage of fMRI over alternative methods of imaging cerebral blood flow, such as positron emission tomography (**PET**) and single-photon emission computed tomography (**SPECT**), is that it does not involve exposure to radioactivity. This means that a single subject can safely be examined by fMRI on many occasions, and that the ethical problems of examining patients are minimized. Functional MRI also has superior spatial resolution (in the order of millimetres) and temporal resolution (in the order of seconds) compared with PET and SPECT.

In this chapter, we provide an introduction to technical issues relevant to fMRI data acquisition, study design, and analysis. An introduction to the basic physical principles of magnetization and nuclear magnetic resonance, and the technology, is given in Chapter 2.3.7.

Many excellent specialist texts covering all aspects of functional magnetic resonance imaging are available for the reader seeking more detailed treatment of the issues.[5–7]

Cerebral activation and blood-flow changes

Try closing your eyes and then opening them again. At the moment that you open your eyes, neurones in the occipital cortex that are specialized for the perception of visual stimuli will show a sudden and dramatic increase in their rate of discharge. There is a short delay (approximately 100 ms) between the stimulus and neural response owing to the propagation of electrical activity from the retina via the optic nerves and tracts to the visual cortex. Later, some 3 to 8 s after stimulus onset, there will be an accompanying change in the local blood supply to the stimulated area of cortex. Blood flow increases without a commensurate increase in oxygen uptake by the visual cortex, leading to a local increase in the ratio of oxygenated to deoxygenated forms of haemoglobin.

The linkage between neural activity and regional cerebral blood flow, sometimes called neurovascular coupling, has been known since Roy and Sherrington first reported 'changes in blood supply in accordance with local variations of functional activity' in 1894. However, the biophysical and biochemical mechanisms for neurovascular coupling are complex and not yet completely defined in detail.[7]

Endogenous contrast agents

The fact that neural activity is linked to local blood flow provides the opportunity for functional MRI. The most common, and non-invasive, approach exploits the paramagnetic properties of iron in deoxygenated haemoglobin as an endogenous contrast agent. Neural activity causes a local reduction in the ratio of deoxygenated to oxygenated haemoglobin, so that the paramagnetic effects of deoxyhaemoglobin are 'diluted'. Since apparent spin–spin relaxation or dephasing is accelerated by microscopic inhomogeneities in the magnetic field due to the presence of paramagnetic contrast agents, the net effect of diluting deoxyhaemoglobin will be to prolong T_2^* times in areas of the brain that receive an increased blood flow as a consequence of neural activity. The haemodynamic effect on spin–spin relaxation can be measured by a T_2^*-weighted signal change (of 3 per cent or less) which is blood oxygen level dependent (**BOLD**).

Imaging sequences for fMRI

Several different pulse sequences can be used to collect MRI data that are sensitive to functionally determined changes in signal strength. Here we will concentrate on gradient echo sequences which, combined with special techniques for very rapid data acquisition, are most widely used to date for fMRI. However, spin echo sequences can also be used for functional MRI data acquisition, and gradient echo sequences can be used for structural MRI.

Gradient echo sequence

The basic principle is similar to spin echo imaging. An initial excitation pulse of radiofrequency energy is supplied at the Larmor frequency to the brain in the presence of a powerful static magnetic field. Protons are excited to a state characterized by increased transverse magnetization and a coherent phase of precession around the axis of the external field. Immediately the radiofrequency pulse has ceased, protons begin to relax back to their equilibrium state of maximum longitudinal magnetization and random phase of precession, emitting a radiofrequency signal by free induction decay.

In gradient echo imaging, the process of spin–spin relaxation (dephasing) is first accelerated by briefly applying a gradient to the magnetic field shortly after the excitation pulse. Then, at some time (TE/2) after the excitation pulse, a second gradient is applied to reverse the process of dephasing, causing rephasing and a signal maximum or echo some time (TE) after excitation. The sequence is repetitively applied with a constant time interval between consecutive excitations (TR).

The objective is to manipulate spin–spin relaxation by brief perturbations of the external magnetic field rather than by supplying additional pulses of radiofrequency energy as in spin echo imaging. Frequency- and phase-encoding gradients are applied to locate the sources of signal in three-dimensional space (see Chapter 2.3.7).

One advantage of gradient echo imaging is that TE and TR can both be shorter than in spin echo imaging, allowing an overall reduction in scanning time. However, if TR is short, spoiler gradients or radiofrequency pulses may be needed to ensure that the protons have returned to equilibrium before the next excitation pulse is supplied. The flip angle α induced by radiofrequency excitation can be adjusted to generate images weighted by different sources of tissue contrast. T_1-weighted images are generated by radiofrequency pulses causing flip angles of the order of $10°$ to $20°$. For functionally sensitive T_2-weighted images, more radiofrequency energy must be supplied in the excitation pulse to give a flip angle approaching $90°$.

Echoplanar imaging

The gradient echo sequence equivalent to a fast spin echo sequence is obtained by rapidly applying, or blipping, a series of rephasing gradients following the excitation pulse and dephasing gradient. Gradient blipping is done extremely rapidly (<1 ms), and up to 128 echoes can be generated from a single excitation. Clearly, the advantage of such echoplanar imaging is the speed of acquisition. Multislice images of the entire cortex, with slice thickness of only a few millimetres, can be acquired in 2 s or less. Such high-speed imaging is highly desirable for functional MRI, where we wish to detect physiologically determined changes in magnetic resonance signal with the best possible temporal resolution. However, the hardware required for rapid gradient blipping has only become widely available in the last few years.

Artefacts

The main sources of artefact in functional MRI are the same as for structural MRI (see Chapter 2.3.7).

Movement

Movement of the subject's head during fMRI data acquisition is inevitable, and attempts to eliminate it by fixing the head in the scanner may paradoxically exacerbate the problem. The best approach of minimizing movement is to ensure that the subjects are not unduly anxious about the scanning procedure, that they understand clearly what they are being asked to do, and that they are comfortable in the scanner before data acquisition begins. Experiments should be designed so that they do not require the subject to move extensively; small finger movements required for button pressing do not generally cause severe head movement. However, even very small movements of the head (less than 1 mm) can cause significant artefacts in fMRI data.

Involuntary or physiological movements are mostly due to the cardiorespiratory cycle causing pulsation of the cerebrospinal fluid and vascular spaces. Therefore, these movements often occur at a higher frequency than the frequency of image volume acquisition, and are aliased into the signal as a low frequency confound.

Susceptibility

The susceptibility artefact is exaggerated by gradient echoplanar imaging, typically causing signal loss in inferior temporal and orbitofrontal brain regions close to bone or sinuses. The problem is further compounded if subjects are asked to speak during scanning, since slight deformations of the sinuses associated with overt articulation can cause changes in susceptibility artefact, which can mimic signal changes due to speech-related neural activity. If overt articulation is necessary to monitor the subject's performance on the experimental task, then it is advisable to design the sequence so that images are not acquired while the subject is speaking.

Hardware

The hardware requirements for functional MRI include a superconducting magnet, a radiofrequency coil, computers, and a purpose-built room, as described in Chapter 2.3.7.

Gradient coils

The essential extra prerequisite is gradient coils capable of very rapidly blipping the external magnetic field for echoplanar imaging. The gradients required are small compared with the external field (1 to 10 mT/m) but may need to be applied for less than 1 ms. The speed with which the gradient is switched on, the slew rate, is necessarily fast (up to 200 mT/m/s). Such rapidly changing gradients can cause eddy currents in the gradient coils, adversely affecting the homogeneity of the field. This problem is minimized by actively shielding the coils, which requires yet another set of coils.

Audiovisual equipment

It must be possible to present visual and auditory stimuli to subjects while they are lying with their heads in the bore of the magnet. Headphones are required to clearly present auditory stimuli in the presence of the loud background noise of gradient switching. Visual stimuli can be projected on to a screen, viewed through a periscope. The subject should have access to an alert button. In addition, it is generally useful for subjects to use a button-press device to indicate their response to cognitively demanding experimental tasks. These behavioural data will need to be monitored during scanning.

Experimental design

The basic principle of experimental design in fMRI is to manipulate the subject's experience or behaviour in some way that is likely to produce a functionally specific neurovascular response. It is usually important that the experiment should be designed to allow some other measure of response, for instance a button press, to be monitored simultaneously. We shall illustrate these and other principles by considering how one might design an experiment to identify the regions of the brain that are important in making a (semantic) decision about the meaning of words. As will become clear, no single design is ideal; each has its strengths and weaknesses, and the choice between them should also be considered carefully in the light of the particular hypothesis one is using fMRI to test.

Blocked periodic design

This experimental design, in its simplest form, involves alternately presenting the subject with two conditions: an activation (A) condition and a baseline (B) condition. Each condition is presented for an identical epoch of time. During each epoch, several stimuli are sequentially presented with an interstimulus interval (**ISI**) that is less than the epoch length. The cycle of alternation between A and B conditions is repeated a number of times over the course of each experiment.

For example, during each 30-s epoch of the A condition, we could visually present subjects with a series of 12 common concrete nouns (ISI = 2.5 s) and ask them to decide for each word whether it refers to an animate object (e.g. 'goat') or an inanimate object (e.g. 'bucket'). The subjects could be asked to indicate their decision by pressing one of two buttons: left for living objects and right for non-living objects. During each 30-s epoch of the B condition, we could present words at the same rate, but ask subjects to decide whether they are written in upper- or lowercase letters. This decision could be monitored by button press as in the A condition. The two epochs could be presented alternately, beginning with the B condition, in five cycles for a total experimental time of 5 min. Functional MRI data would be acquired continuously throughout the experiment (Fig. 2.3.8.1).

The rationale for this design is that the two conditions are matched in all respects apart from semantic analysis; words are visually presented at an identical rate, and subjects are asked to signal their decision by an identical device. But while condition A demands semantic analysis of the words (what do they mean?), condition B demands only orthographic analysis (what do they look like?). We assume that only those regions of the brain that are specifically responsible for semantic analysis will show an increased magnetic resonance signal during condition A; those regions responsible for visual perception and motor output will be activated identically under both conditions, and so will not demonstrate a periodic signal change at the frequency of AB alternation. This set of assumptions is sometimes referred to as cognitive subtraction.

Blocked periodic designs can generate robust signal changes in fMRI, as long as the two conditions are not too closely matched. The drawbacks are that it is impossible to assess the response to a single stimulus and the critical assumption of cognitive subtraction may not always be valid. Sometimes two experimental tasks that appear to differ only in terms of one component process may actually invoke entirely different cognitive strategies and so cause activation of entirely different neurocognitive networks.

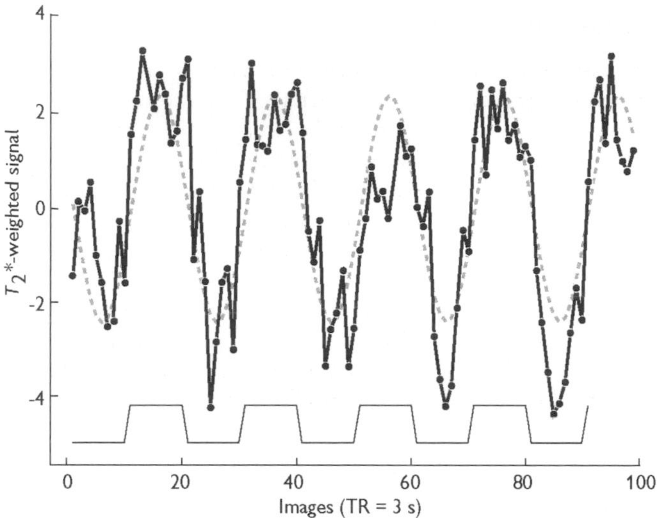

Fig. 2.3.8.1 Design, response, and modelled response for a blocked periodic experiment. The experimental design or input function is represented by a square wave (solid line), which alternates periodically between a baseline (B) and an activation (A) condition. The B condition is presented first, and the BA cycle is repeated five times in the course of the experiment. Images are acquired every 3 s during the experiment, and the T_2^*-weighted signal observed at an activated voxel is shown by points joined by a solid line. There is clearly a signal increase during the A condition. The modelled response is shown by the broken line.

Parametric design

Parametric designs are so called because the same task is presented throughout the experiment but some continuously variable parameter of the task is experimentally manipulated. For example, we could ask subjects to perform the semantic analysis task for 5 min, but continuously vary the interval between consecutive stimuli (words) from 10 s at the start of the experiment to 1 s at the end. Here we are assuming that as the task becomes more difficult, i.e. the interstimulus interval becomes shorter, blood flow to the regions specialized for semantic analysis will increase. The main advantage of this design is that it avoids the assumption of cognitive subtraction; the main disadvantage is that it may lack specificity. Motor and visual cortex, as well as brain regions specialized for semantic analysis, will probably show an increased blood flow as the rate of stimulus presentation is increased.

Event-related design

Event-related designs are composed of a series of individual stimuli. They may be coupled with sequences for very rapid image acquisition so that the temporal pattern of response to a single event can be resolved in detail. An event-related design would be advantageous for our semantic analysis experiment if we were particularly interested in correlating some aspect of the behavioural response to each stimulus, for instance accuracy of decision or reaction time, with the neurovascular response measured using fMRI. A disadvantage of such designs is that signal changes induced by a single trial are generally weak compared with the 2 to 5 per cent signal changes that are typical in blocked periodic experiments.

Beyond a single experiment

Generally, the hypothesis in question demands the investigation of more than a few subjects and/or more than one experimental condition. When designing the studies it is important that randomization should be used appropriately to eliminate confounding effects of the order in which experiments are conducted, and of the order in which different subjects are scanned. Practice on a task may substantially alter the neurovascular response, and so all subjects should receive preliminary training on the task according to a standard protocol. If there is considerable variability between subjects in their ability to perform a task, consider adjusting the difficulty of the task presented in the scanner so that each subject is performing at the same level in terms of accuracy or reaction time. The use of functional MRI to study longitudinal changes by repeated examination of the same subject(s), for instance before and after the administration of a drug, will generally improve the statistical power to detect the effect of interest by controlling for idiosyncratic variability of functional response between subjects.

Data analysis

General principles of data analysis are reviewed here; for more detailed coverage of the issues and the methods implemented in a variety of software packages, see.[(5–7)]

Movement estimation and correction

The first step in fMRI data analysis is to estimate the extent of head motion during data acquisition and to correct it. Due to the multislice acquisition protocols generally used for fMRI, the magnetic field to which the brain is exposed will change dramatically within the space of a few micrometres at the superior and inferior edges of a selectively irradiated slice. This means that minute head movements (<1 mm) can have disproportionately large effect on magnetic resonance signal.

Head movement occurring at the same time as time as experimental stimuli are present, namely stimulus correlated motion, can artefactually exaggerate the neurovascular response. Head movement occurring randomly with respect to the experimental design is more likely to cause the opposite problem of artefactually attenuating the measured response. Therefore it is essential to use a computerized method for movement estimation and correction.

Statistical models for the neurovascular response

The next step in analysis is to estimate the strength of the experimentally determined signal change in the time series of magnetic resonance signal measurements at each voxel in the image. This requires some sort of model for the response. The simplest model, for a blocked periodic design, is a square wave at the same frequency as the experimental input function. This model assumes that a brain region activated specifically by condition A will show an immediate increase in signal intensity, which is sustained throughout the epoch until the onset of condition B. The problem with this model is that the increase in magnetic resonance signal during condition A is due to changes in blood flow and oxygenation, which are dispersed and delayed by several seconds relative to the onset of condition A. Furthermore, this haemodynamic delay between stimulus onset and measurable response will be variable from one voxel to another. Therefore it is important that the experimental effect should be modelled as an increase in signal intensity that is arbitrarily delayed relative to the onset of the activating stimulus. The most general way of achieving this is to convolve the experimental input function (the vector coding changes in experimental conditions) with a model of the haemodynamic response. The haemodynamically convolved input function can then be regressed on the fMRI time series at each voxel to estimate the neurovascular response to changing experimental conditions.

In fitting linear regression models to fMRI time series, one important technical issue is that the residuals of the regression will generally not be white noise or serially independent. Rather the residuals will typically have long-range dependency or long memory in time and this will need to be addressed for proper estimation of linear model parameters.[8] There are probably several possible artefactual sources of autocorrelation in fMRI time series residuals—including imperfectly modelled experimental activation, uncorrected head movement, and aliased cardiorespiratory pulsation. However, recently attention has focused on the role of low frequency, spatially coherent, endogenous oscillations of large neuronal ensembles as a source of long memory in fMRI time series.[9] This hypothesis has encouraged studies of the univariate and multivariate properties of fMRI data recorded at rest, i.e. in the absence of experimentally controlled task processing.[10,11]

Activation mapping

The next step in analysis is often to decide which of the several thousand voxels in the image have demonstrated such a strong response to the experiment that it is unlikely to be due to chance. In other words, we want to identify the significantly activated voxels. Let us assume that we have estimated the neurovascular response by the magnitude of a linear model coefficient at each and every voxel, and refer to this as our test statistic. The problem is then to assign a probability to each test statistic under the null hypothesis that the experiment had no effect on the brain. To do this we need to know the probability distribution of our test statistic under the null hypothesis. There are broadly two ways we can know this distribution: we can work it out from mathematical theory, or we can sample it by randomly permuting the data. Theoretical distributions are quicker to evaluate than permutation distributions, but permutation entails many fewer assumptions and is the gold standard against which the validity of theoretical approximations should be checked.

Once we have a probability distribution for the test statistic, we still have to decide what p-value we wish to adopt as our threshold for activation. If we choose a small (conservative) p-value (e.g. <0.00001), only those voxels that demonstrate a very powerful response will be identified as activated. There will be few false-positive or type 1 errors, i.e. almost all the voxels we identify as activated will truly be activated. But there will probably be a large number of false-negative or type 2 errors, i.e. many voxels that are truly activated will not be identified as such. Conversely, if we choose a large (lenient) p-value (e.g. <0.01), there will be a larger number of false-positive errors but a smaller number of false-negative errors. The choice of p-value should be informed by the search volume, or the number of voxels tested for significance. The larger the search volume, the smaller the p-value will need to be for an acceptable degree of type 1 error control. A rule of thumb is that the p-value should be approximately the reciprocal of the search volume. More elaborate methods have been advocated for correcting p-values for large numbers of tests on imaging data.

An alternative approach to testing tens of thousands of voxels against a suitably small probability threshold, with an associated risk of major type 2 error, is to combine information about the experimental response over several voxels. For example, we can initially apply a lenient threshold ($p = 0.05$) to the test statistics estimated at each voxel, and set to zero any voxel that does not have a test statistic greater than the corresponding critical value. The result will be a map of several spatially contiguous clusters, ranging in size from a single voxel to several hundred voxels (Plate 10). We can ascertain the probability distribution for cluster size under the null hypothesis either by theory or permutation. Then we can proceed to identify significantly activated clusters instead of voxels. The advantage of hypothesis testing at cluster level is a greater power to detect significant foci of activation, partly because there will be many fewer clusters than voxels to test, so the p-value can be legitimately increased. The disadvantage is the loss of spatial resolution of activation.

Multivariate approaches

Many of the 'higher-order' cognitive tasks that are likely to be of greatest interest to psychiatric research do not activate a single modular region of the brain. Instead, they typically activate several spatially distinct or distributed regions that together comprise a large-scale neurocognitive network for performance of the task. It may then be of interest to investigate functional integration between different regions or nodes of the network. The simplest way to do this is by estimating the correlation between a pair of fMRI time series observed at different voxels or regions. Large correlations, whether negative or positive, may be described as evidence for functional connectivity. Psychiatric disorders may be characterized by abnormal functional relationships between coactivated regions, or functional dysconnectivity.

More sophisticated techniques for investigating functional relationships between large numbers of voxels or regions include multivariate methods such as principal component analysis, discriminant analysis, and path analysis. These methods are equally applicable to structural MRI data, where they may provide indirect evidence for anatomical connectivity between regions.

Within- and between-group analysis

Once a measure or parameter of experimental response has been estimated in each fMRI time series, the resulting parameter maps can be registered in standard space. There are many possible computational algorithms for spatial registration. The most commonly used at present is an affine transformation, which applies a global and linear rescaling in three dimensions to each individual image. A commonly adopted standard space is that represented in a stereotactic atlas of the brain originally written by Talairach and Tournoux to assist neurosurgeons in locating subcortical structures.[12] In these systems, each voxel is assigned a set of $\{x, y, z\}$ coordinates which define its position. In Talairach–Tournoux space, the coordinates are defined relative to the cerebral midline and a line is drawn between the anterior and posterior commissures (intercommissural or AC–PC line). After registration, parameter maps are usually smoothed by applying a two- or three-dimensional Gaussian filter to accommodate variability in sulcogyral anatomy between subjects and error in spatial registration.

It is then possible to test a wide variety of hypotheses about the response parameters measured over several subjects at each voxel in standard space. For example, one can test the null hypothesis that there is zero mean or median power of experimental response within a group, or the null hypothesis that there is zero difference in the power of response between two groups. It is also possible to test for correlations between the power of functional response and some behavioural or symptom measure within a group.

Visualization

The final result of fMRI data analysis will often be visualized as a map in standard space. The background for the map will generally be a grey-scale image of cerebral anatomy, such as a structural MRI dataset with fine spatial resolution and good tissue contrast between grey and white matter. In this case, one should beware of the potential discrepancy in geometric distortion between images of the same brain acquired using different sequences.

The background image will often be combined with, or substituted by, a rectangular grid allowing any feature of interest to be referred directly to the appropriate atlas of standard anatomical space. If the image is displayed as a series of two-dimensional slices, the z coordinate for each slice in standard space should also be displayed and the left and right sides of the right clearly indicated.

Voxels or clusters that demonstrate a significant effect are generally coloured against the grey-scale background image (Plate 11). A range of colours can be used to encode additional information. For example, the haemodynamic delay of response at each generically activated voxel may be colour coded by a continuous spectrum. Other strategies for visualization include use of three-dimensional rendering to show foci of activation in the context of the sulcogyral anatomy of a whole hemisphere, and 'flat mapping' whereby the template image is deformed to a smooth sphere and then mapped to a plane before activation foci are superimposed on it.

Further information

Comprehensive background information on fMRI physiology, experimental design, and data analysis:

Jezzard, P., Matthews, P.M., and Smith, S.M. (eds) (2003). *Functional magnetic resonance imaging: an introduction to methods.* (2nd edn) Oxford University Press, Oxford.

The physiological origins of the BOLD effect:

Logothetis, N.K., Pauls, J., Augath, M.A., *et al.* (2001). Neurophysiological investigation of the basis of the fMRI signal. *Nature*, **412**, 150–7.

Current perspectives of fMRI applications:

Matthews, P.M., Honey, G.D., and Bullmore, E.T. (2006). Applications of fMRI in translational medicine and clinical practice. *Nature Reviews. Neuroscience*, **7**, 732–44.

Community web site for information about Brain Mapping and methods: www.brainmapping.org

References

1. Kwong, K.K., Belliveau, J.W., Chesler, D.A., *et al.* (1992). Dynamic magnetic resonance imaging of human brain activity during primary sensory stimulation. *Proceedings of the National Academy of Sciences of the United States of America*, **89**, 5675–9.
2. Stehling, M.K., Turner, R., and Mansfield, P. (1991). Echo-planar imaging: magnetic resonance imaging in a fraction of a second. *Science*, **254**, 43–50.
3. Le Bihan, D. and Karni, A. (1995). Applications of magnetic resonance imaging to the study of human brain function. *Current Biology*, **5**, 231–7.
4. Matthews, P.M., Honey, G.D., and Bullmore, E.T. (2006). Applications of fMRI in translational medicine and clinical practice. *Nature Reviews Neuroscience*, **7**, 732–44.
5. Jezzard, P., Matthews, P.M., and Smith S. (2001). *Functional magnetic resonance imaging: an introduction to methods.* Oxford University Press, Oxford.
6. Frackowiak, R.S.J., Ashburner, J.T., Penny, W.D., *et al.* (2002). *Human brain function.* Academic Press, San Diego.
7. Buxton, R.B. (2002). *An introduction to functional magnetic resonance imaging: principles and techniques.* Cambridge University Press, Cambridge.
8. Maxim, V., Sendur, L., Fadili, J., *et al.* (2005). Fractional Gaussian noise, functional MRI and Alzheimer's disease. *NeuroImage*, **25**, 141–58.
9. Leopold, D.A., Murayama, Y., and Logothetis, N.K. (2003). Very slow activity fluctuations in monkey visual cortex: implications for functional brain imaging. *Cerebral Cortex*, **13**, 422–33.
10. Greicius, M.D., Krasnow, B., Reiss, A.L., *et al.* (2003). Functional connectivity in the resting brain: a network analysis of the default mode hypothesis. *Proceedings of the National Academy of Sciences of the United States of America*, **101**, 4637–42.
11. Achard, S., Salvador, R., Whitcher, B., *et al.* (2006). A resilient, low-frequency, small-world human brain functional network with highly connected association cortical hubs. *The Journal of Neuroscience*, **26**, 63–72.
12. Talairach, J. and Tournoux, P. (1988). *Co-planar stereotaxic atlas of the human brain.* Thieme, Stuttgart.

2.3.9 Neuronal networks, epilepsy, and other brain dysfunctions

John G. R. Jefferys

Introduction

The dynamics of highly interconnected networks of neurones are fundamental to both normal and pathological functioning of the brain.[1,2] Epilepsy is perhaps the most dramatic example of a dysfunctional neuronal network,[3] characterized by intense and highly synchronous neuronal activity, but more subtle dysfunction is associated with other conditions, such as schizophrenia.[4]

This chapter will largely focus on the hippocampus, and to a lesser degree on the neocortex. The hippocampal formation is implicated in several important psychiatric and neurological problems. The hippocampus and amygdala are often the site of epileptic foci, which can lead to problems in learning and memory, emotion, anxiety, and other problems. This kind of epilepsy is variously known as temporal lobe epilepsy, complex partial seizures, or limbic epilepsy. The hippocampus and associated limbic areas have been linked both to affective disorders and to psychoses. This chapter will consider the cellular organization of the hippocampus and then outline aspects of the emergent properties of neuronal networks in the hippocampus and speculative role in psychiatric disorders. Cellular and network mechanisms of focal epilepsy, and learning impairments associated with limbic epilepsy will be reviewed.

Hippocampal organization

Anatomy

The hippocampus resembles the neocortex in containing a majority of excitatory neurones, the pyramidal cells, and granule cells, which use glutamate as their neurotransmitter (E in Fig. 2.3.9.1).[1,2] Most of the remaining 10–20 per cent of neurones in the hippocampus are inhibitory, and use γ-aminobutyric acid (GABA) as their neurotransmitter (I in Fig. 2.3.9.1). The inhibitory neurones fall into several distinct subtypes according to where their axons go (and hence which cells they inhibit), where their cell bodies are, the shapes of their dendrites, whether they contain more than one transmitter, and whether they contain particular calcium-binding proteins. This chapter will ignore most of the diversity of interneurones.[5]

There are many more excitatory pyramidal cells (E and triangles) than inhibitory interneurones (I and circles). As with most neurones, they receive inputs onto their dendrites and somata (the latter contain the nucleus and are represented by a triangle or circle). The level of simplification is clear from the observation that each pyramidal cell receives tens of thousands of synapses. Axons from other regions, known as afferents, make excitatory synapses (e) with both pyramidal cells and interneurones. Most of the interneurones make inhibitory synapses (i) onto pyramidal cells. The inhibition of the pyramidal cell is called 'feed-forward' (f.f.) when the interneurones were excited by afferent axons and 'feed-back' (f.b.) when they were excited by pyramidal cells. Interneurones also inhibit each other forming a mutually inhibitory network (m.i.); this network is important in some kinds of physiological network oscillation (see text). Finally, pyramidal cells make excitatory synapses onto each other (r.e.), which can lead to epileptic discharges if not held in check by inhibitory mechanisms.

Evoked responses

Each hippocampal (or neocortical) area receives 'afferent' synaptic inputs from other areas. Most afferents are excitatory; stimulating them provides a convenient tool to study the operation of the neuronal circuits involved. The responses evoked in hippocampal neurones typically start with an excitatory postsynaptic potential. If the excitatory postsynaptic potential is strong enough, it will result in an action potential triggered at a low-threshold zone near the cell body, probably a short distance down the axon. The excitatory postsynaptic potential is followed by a fast and a slow inhibitory postsynaptic potential. Both the fast inhibitory and excitatory postsynaptic potentials are due to ligand-gated channels where the transmitter receptor is part of the same molecular structure as the ion channel. In the case of inhibition this is the $GABA_A$ receptor, which allows chloride ions to pass. In the case of excitation it is a variety of glutamate receptors, which are permeable to sodium, potassium, and in some cases calcium ions, and which are further subdivided into α-amino-3-hydroxy-5-methyl-4-isoxazolepropionic acid (AMPA)/kainic acid, *N*-methyl-D-aspartate (NMDA) and other classes. The slow inhibitory postsynaptic potential is due to $GABA_B$ receptors, which are G protein coupled and use second messengers to open separate potassium channels. Many other kinds of G-protein couple receptors exist, and often are involved in modulating neuronal excitability or synaptic function.

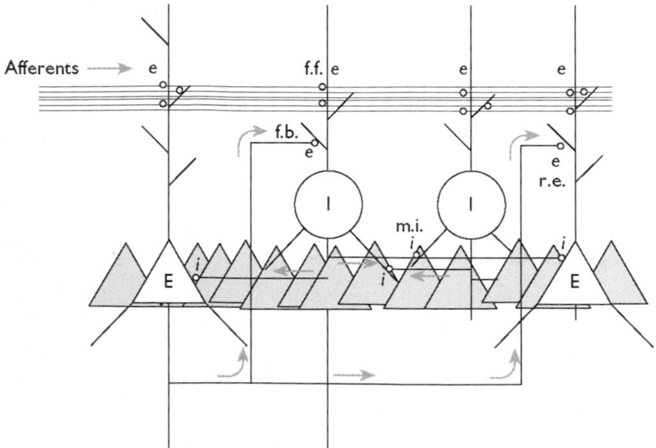

Fig. 2.3.9.1 Schematic illustration of hippocampal neuronal network.

Inhibitory neurones can be triggered both by activity in the principal cells (pyramidal or granule), resulting in recurrent or feedback inhibition, and directly by the incoming afferents, resulting in feed-forward inhibition. Experimentally, the synchrony of the stimulation of the afferent input imposes synchrony on the response with the useful consequence that the extracellular currents generated by the activity of individual pyramidal or granule cells can summate (because the cells are located in tight layers) and produce large 'field potentials' comprising a population excitatory postsynaptic potential, followed by a population spike.

Field potentials evoked by local stimulation are over in 10 to 20 ms and the slowest intracellular components end within a few 100 ms to 1 s. However, stimulation can have much more prolonged effects. The best known of these is long-term potentiation, in which a brief train of stimuli can result in an increase, lasting hours or days, in the response to a fixed test stimulus. The modest conditioning event and the enduring consequence make long-term potentiation an attractive model of learning and memory, although the evidence that it really is the direct cellular substrate for learning remains circumstantial.[6] It is perhaps more likely that long-term potentiation provides an artificial experimental tool that depends on cellular and molecular mechanisms that may also be involved in learning and/or other plastic changes in synaptic strength.

Local circuits

Hippocampal neurones are not just arranged as a simple synaptic relay where afferents excite target cells to produce an output depending on the size of the input and the state of inhibition at that time. Instead there exists a complex synaptic network, or local circuit, interlinking neurones of all kinds (Fig. 2.3.9.1 gives a very much simplified illustration of some of the salient features of hippocampal local circuits). This chapter considers two kinds of emergent network activity that arise from this organization: focal epilepsy and gamma rhythms.

Experimental approaches

Unravelling the cellular and network mechanisms of emergent network phenomena depends on a combination of electrophysiology, pharmacology, anatomy, and realistic computer simulations.[2,7] Two practical issues may need a brief introduction.

Brain slices have played a pivotal role in developing theories on the operation of neuronal networks. Slices about 0.4 mm thick are cut from the brains of deeply anaesthetized or recently killed experimental animals, or sometimes from humans undergoing neurosurgery. Brain slices can survive many hours *in vitro* in an artificial cerebrospinal fluid, usually equilibrated with 95 per cent oxygen and 5 per cent carbon dioxide (with bicarbonate providing a pH buffer). If the slices are prepared under sterile conditions, they can survive for weeks as 'organotypic slice cultures'. In both cases the visualization of the anatomy of the living slice helps locate electrodes, the mechanical stability greatly simplifies recordings from inside neurones, and the lack of a blood–brain barrier facilitates drug applications and changes in ion concentrations. Brain slices have proved immensely popular and successful, but it is important to remember that they are only one tool in the armoury needed to study brain function, and that ultimately results from them must be put in the context of the whole organism.

Realistic computer simulations provide the means to determine whether what we know at one level, for instance of the properties of individual neurones and their interconnections, are necessary and sufficient to explain the emergent properties at the next level, here of circuits of a few thousand neurones. The most useful models for this purpose are tightly constrained by experimental data, and ideally are used to make experimentally testable predictions. Mostly they consist of several 'compartments' to represent the anatomy of the neurone's dendrites and soma. Each compartment consists of several differential equations representing specific ion channels, which may be gated by membrane potential, extracellular neurotransmitters, or intracellular calcium. Large number of neurones can then be wired together in larger-scale simulations, using biologically realistic anatomical connectivity and synaptic properties.[2,7]

Emergent properties of hippocampal networks

Hippocampal rhythms

The organization of hippocampal networks (Fig. 2.3.9.1) leads to several distinct kinds of oscillation, which can be considered as 'emergent' properties of the network. Perhaps the most prominent rhythm in the hippocampus is theta (3–7 Hz), which, at least in rats, is associated with spatial navigation,[8] and may play a role in memory.[9] Theta results from interactions of the hippocampus with two other limbic structures, the septum and the entorhinal cortex. Often superimposed on theta is a faster rhythm known as gamma (30–100 Hz). The best evidence we have now is that gamma is generated by local circuits in the hippocampus and that inhibitory neurones play a crucial role.[2] The role of gamma in the hippocampus remains unclear; in the neocortex it has been implicated in higher cognitive processes such as the 'binding' of individual sensory features into coherent perceived objects.[10]

Networks for gamma rhythms

The first strong clue that inhibitory neurones played a central role in gamma rhythms came from hippocampal and neocortical slices in which fast excitatory postsynaptic potentials had been blocked by drugs. Excitation by pulses of glutamate or agonist drugs acting at metabotropic (i.e. G-protein-coupled) glutamate receptors resulted in rhythmic inhibitory postsynaptic potentials in the gamma frequency band. A series of experimental tests of predictions from realistic computer simulations showed that this gamma rhythm was generated by the mutual inhibition of inhibitory neurones, which produced a synchronous interruption of the fast discharge the metabotropic glutamate receptor activation would otherwise have evoked. These interruptions lasted for a time, of the order of 25 ms, that depended on the time course of the inhibitory postsynaptic potentials in interneurones. We named this phenomenon 'interneuronal network gamma'.

During interneuronal network gamma pyramidal cells generate rhythmic inhibitory postsynaptic potentials, but do not reach threshold unless they are driven by some other input. Another kind of gamma rhythm occurs when slices are exposed to cholinergic drugs such as carbachol, and/or to non-desensitizing glutamate agonist drugs such as kainic acid. Here each pyramidal cell fires on some cycles of the rhythm,[11,12] so that on average some fluctuating fraction of pyramidal cells fires on each cycle. This is closer to the situation *in vivo*.[13]

Significance of fast coherent cortical oscillations

Rhythms such as gamma have been linked with sensory processing and with perception and other cognitive functions. They may be disrupted in people with some degree of cognitive impairment, for instance normal age-related cognitive decline,[14] or there may be a more general disruption of cortical rhythms in more severe conditions such as schizophrenia.[4] The complexity of the circuits responsible for cortical oscillations means that individuals with apparently normal number of neurones and neuronal organization may still have rather subtle changes on their synaptic networks that can have profound effects on collective oscillations and behaviour.

Gamma rhythms are intimately linked with epilepsy. Coherent neural activity at gamma frequencies is associated with some kinds of epileptic activity. Gamma rhythms are disrupted in at least one chronic model of epilepsy associated with learning impairments. Finally, the ideas behind the synaptic network mechanisms of the two kinds of phenomena have much in common.

Epilepsy—an emergent property of neuronal networks

Epileptic discharges typically involve excessively synchronous activity in principal neurones. In experimental focal epilepsy this excessive synchronization is due to the mutual excitation of pyramidal cells in the hippocampus, neocortex, or related areas. The essential idea is of a chain reaction. Areas that are especially prone to epileptic discharges have strong synaptic interconnections between their principal cells (e.g. the pyramidal cells of the CA3 region of the hippocampus or layers 3 and 5 of the neocortex). Activity in a few pyramidal cells can propagate through the synaptic network to recruit the whole population of neurones. Normally this propagation is held in check by inhibitory neurones; if the control mechanism is ineffective then epileptic discharges result. In experimental models the balance of synchronization versus control is compromised by treatments that weaken inhibition (usually by drugs such as bicuculline or picrotoxin), strengthen excitation (incubating brain slices in solutions lacking magnesium ions) or strengthen synaptic potentials in general (4-aminopyridine). Combined experimental and theoretical studies of such models have led to some general principles.[7] Synchronous epileptic discharges will result under the following conditions.

1 Connections between excitatory neurones are divergent, that is each connects to more than one postsynaptic excitatory neurone.

2 Connections between excitatory neurones are powerful enough to make their postsynaptic cells fire with a high probability. Precisely how high a probability can be depends on factors such as the connectivity and size of the network. The 'intrinsic' electrical properties of the neurones are important. Many epilepsy-prone areas have cells with prominent voltage-sensitive calcium currents, which are more prolonged than the classical voltage-sensitive sodium currents of the axonal action potential, and which cause neurones to fire bursts of fast sodium action potentials. Such intrinsic bursts greatly amplify transmission between pyramidal cells.

3 The network is large enough to allow all the neurones to link together. The critical mass for a network where the probability of any two cells being directly connected is 1 per cent, and the probability of one cell exciting its target cells is approximately 50 per cent, works out at about 1000 to 2000 neurones.

These features explain experimental brief epileptic discharges very effectively. The brain contains inhibitory mechanisms, both synaptic (inhibitory postsynaptic potentials, presynaptic inhibition) and intrinsic (voltage- and calcium-sensitive potassium channels), to terminate hypersynchronous discharges. Other mechanisms are needed to overcome the burst-termination mechanisms for the crucial transition to full-blown seizures lasting tens of seconds to minutes. These include slower synaptic mechanisms (both *N*-methyl-D-aspartate and metabotropic glutamate receptors, GABA, which paradoxically can become depolarizing if present in excess), non-synaptic mechanisms (potassium accumulation, electric fields), and abnormal activity arising in axons (ectopic spikes, gap junctions).

Convulsant drugs can trigger seizures in normal brains. People with epilepsy have a reduced seizure threshold that means they have seizures without an obvious triggering chemical or event. The reasons are far from clear, but may include abnormalities in intrinsic properties of neurones or in the connectivity of the neurones. Improvements in non-invasive imaging and in neuropathology increasingly reveal misplaced neurones and other more or less subtle anatomical malformations in many focal epilepsies, which suggests that the local circuitry is disturbed.

Other kinds of epilepsy have very different mechanisms. Absence epilepsy is the other major class where cellular mechanisms are relatively well understood. They involve the interaction of the thalamus and neocortex, although the received wisdom on the underlying mechanism has recently been challenged by experiments on one of the key animal models of absence epilepsy.[15]

Epilepsy—learning and memory

Patients with temporal lobe epilepsy can have problems with learning and memory. Antiepileptic drugs can have marked side effects, but the observation that chronic animal models of temporal lobe epilepsy also have impairments in learning and memory suggests that this is not the only cause. Memory impairments could result from gross damage, such as hippocampal sclerosis. Gross hippocampal pathology will have effects similar to experimental lesions of the hippocampus, but the observation that at least some of the chronic animal models lack gross hippocampal pathology does not support neuronal death as being the sole cause of impaired learning and memory.

At least two chronic experimental epilepsies have either limited or no cell loss during their induction. These are kindling and stereotaxic injection of a minute dose of tetanus toxin. The tetanus toxin model results in a well-characterized and enduring impairment of learning and memory, which outlasts the active epileptic syndrome in all except a few rats that show relapse. The absence of medication and of gross cell loss suggest that the psychological impairments in this model have some functional cause. Long-term potentiation remains intact, at least over a period of up to an hour. There is an association of learning impairment with the size of population spikes recorded from the same rats *in vivo* and under anaesthesia. Inhibition remains impaired in rats at a stage (>3 months after injection) when they had gained remission from epileptic seizures, but retained learning impairments.[16,17] Abnormalities of the cellular electrophysiology of the postepileptic phase can lead to disruption of network properties, including gamma rhythms, which may, in time, provide a link to the behavioural problem.

Humans with limbic epilepsy often do have substantial hippocampal damage, and this will contribute to learning impairments. The experimental evidence suggests that even in the absence of gross hippocampal damage learning impairments can arise as a result of functional disruption of the hippocampal network.

Conclusions

Understanding the operation of networks of neurones provides valuable insight into a range of neurological and psychiatric diseases. The role of synaptic networks of excitatory neurones in focal epilepsies is now well established. The ways in which brief epileptic discharges transform into events lasting as long as full seizures are starting to be clarified, and may offer new avenues for developing rational therapies. New ideas on the generation of physiological rhythms suggest novel models of psychiatric and neurological problems ranging from impairments in learning and memory in limbic epilepsies to (more speculatively) the disruption of sensory perception in psychoses. Real clinical cases will inevitably be much more complex, but the ideas and models outlined above will aid the understanding of the underlying mechanisms.

Further information

Traub, R.D., Jefferys, J.G.R., and Whittington, M.A. (1999). *Fast oscillations in cortical circuits*. The MIT Press, Cambridge, MA (ISBN 0-262-20118-6).

Jefferys, J.G.R. (2007). Epilepsy *in vitro*: electrophysiology and computer modeling. In *Epilepsy: a comprehensive textbook* (eds. J. Engel Jr., T.A. Pedley, J. Aicardi, *et al.*). Lippincott, Williams & Wilkins, Philadelphia (ISBN 978-0781757775).

Winterer, G. and Weinberger, D.R. (2003). Cortical signal-to-noise ratio: insight into the pathophysiology and genetics of schizophrenia. *Clinical Neuroscience Research*, **3**, 55–66.

http://www.neuroscience.bham.ac.uk/neurophysiology/

References

1. Traub, R.D., Jefferys, J.G.R., and Whittington, M.A. (1999). Functionally relevant and functionally disruptive (epileptic) synchronized oscillations in brain slices. *Advances in Neurology*, **79**, 709–24.

2. Traub, R.D., Jefferys, J.G.R., and Whittington, M.A. (1999). *Fast oscillations in cortical circuits.* The MIT Press, Cambridge, MA.
3. Jefferys, J.G.R. (2003). Models and mechanisms of experimental epilepsies. *Epilepsia*, **44** (Suppl. 12), 44–50.
4. Winterer, G. and Weinberger, D.R. (2004). Genes, dopamine and cortical signal-to-noise ratio in schizophrenia. *Trends in Neurosciences*, **27**, 683–90.
5. Somogyi, P. and Klausberger, T. (2005). Defined types of cortical interneurone structure space and spike timing in the hippocampus. *The Journal of Physiology*, **562**, 9–26.
6. Bliss, T.V.P. and Collingridge, G.L. (1993). A synaptic model of memory: long-term potentiation in the hippocampus. *Nature*, **361**, 31–9.
7. Jefferys, J.G.R. (2007). Epilepsy *in vitro*: electrophysiology and computer modeling. In *Epilepsy: a comprehensive textbook* (eds. J. Engel Jr and T.A. Pedley). Lippincott, Williams & Wilkins, Philadelphia.
8. O'Keefe, J. and Burgess, N. (2005). Dual phase and rate coding in hippocampal place cells: theoretical significance and relationship to entorhinal grid cells. *Hippocampus*, **15**, 853–66.
9. Axmacher, N., Mormann, F., Fernandez, G., *et al.* (2006). Memory formation by neuronal synchronization. *Brain Research Reviews*, **52**, 170–82.
10. Usrey, W.M. and Reid, R.C. (1999). Synchronous activity in the visual system. *Annual Review of Neuroscience*, **61**, 435–56.
11. Fisahn, A., Pike, F.G., Buhl, E.H., *et al.* (1998). Cholinergic induction of network oscillations at 40 Hz in the hippocampus *in vitro*. *Nature*, **394**, 186–9.
12. Mann, E.O., Suckling, J.M., Hajos, N., *et al.* (2005). Perisomatic feedback inhibition underlies cholinergically induced fast network oscillations in the rat hippocampus *in vitro*. *Neuron*, **45**, 105–17.
13. Csicsvari, J., Jamieson, B., Wise, K.D., *et al.* (2003). Mechanisms of gamma oscillations in the hippocampus of the behaving rat. *Neuron*, **37**, 311–22.
14. Vreugdenhil, M. and Toescu, E.C. (2005). Age-dependent reduction of gamma oscillations in the mouse hippocampus *in vitro*. *Neuroscience*, **132**, 1151–7.
15. Manning, J.P., Richards, D.A., Leresche, N., *et al.* (2004). Cortical-area specific block of genetically determined absence seizures by ethosuximide. *Neuroscience*, **123**, 5–9.
16. Vreugdenhil, M., Hack, S.P., Draguhn, A., *et al.* (2002). Tetanus toxin induces long-term changes in excitation and inhibition in the rat hippocampal CA1 area. *Neuroscience*, **114**, 983–94.
17. Jefferys, J.G.R. and Mellanby, J. (1998). Behaviour in chronic experimental epilepsies. In *Disorders of brain and mind* (eds. M.A. Ron and A.S. David), pp. 213–32. Cambridge University Press, Cambridge.

2.3.10 Psychoneuroimmunology

Robert Dantzer and Keith W. Kelley

Introduction

Mind-body literature, in the form of magazines and self-help books on stress and healing, is full of definitive claims for the existence of powerful influences of emotions and psychosocial stressors on the immune system, leading to onset or progression of cancers or infectious diseases. This literature often makes explicit reference to research in psychoneuroimmunology to support these claims. Psychoneuroimmunology is a multi-disciplinary field that has grown rapidly during the last three decades at the crossroads of immunology, behavioural neurosciences, neuroendocrinology, and psychology. It studies mechanisms and functional aspects of bidirectional relationships between the brain and the immune system. Although still controversial, there is evidence that psychological events including emotions can and do influence the outcome of infectious, autoimmune, and neoplastic diseases via modulation of cells of the immune system. A surprising finding has been that immune events occurring in the periphery also affect mood, behaviour, and metabolism by modulating brain functions, thereby providing a biologically important link between the immune system and brain. The original discovery that activation of the innate immune system in the periphery causes clinical signs of sickness that are processed in the brain is now being extended to the involvement of the immune system in depressive disorders. This new information has solidified the idea that neurotransmitters, neuropeptides, neural pathways, and immune-derived signals such as cytokines are the minimal essential elements that permit the immune system and brain to communicate with one another. These new data offer the unexpected conclusion that the immune system is likely to be involved in not only how emotions affect health but also how immune events regulate the development and expression of emotions.

Brain influences on immunity

Early investigations

The concept that stressors can have a negative impact on immunity and ultimately induce a reduction in host resistance to infectious pathogens and even to tumour progression is not new. As a follow-up of the early studies of Hans Selye on stress, several scientists demonstrated in the 1950s and 1960s that laboratory rodents exposed to various stressors, including inescapable painful electric shocks, displayed an altered resistance to viral, bacterial, and parasitic infections. These effects of stressors were accompanied by decreases in antibody responses to the specific microbial pathogen under study. In view of the already demonstrated immunosuppressive effects of glucocorticoids and the pivotal role of glucocorticoids in the stress response, pathophysiological mechanisms of the immunosuppressive effects of stressors were easy to determine. However, it was already clear at that time that mechanisms of the effects of stressors on immunity were not that simple since decreases as well as increases in immunity could be observed, depending on the immune response under study, the type of stressor and the time point at which the stressor took place during the mounting of the immune response. Furthermore, administration of glucocorticoids at physiological instead of pharmacological doses had little effect on some aspects of immunity and evolution of the disease process.

There was little innovation in this field until the 1980s when a few pioneer immunologists and neuroscientists decided to work together in order to understand how the central nervous system communicates with the immune system. One impetus for this was the demonstration that immune responses can be submitted to Pavlovian conditioning in apparently the same way as the salivary response, as discovered by Robert Ader at the University of Rochester.[(1)] Mice exposed to a new taste paired with an immunosuppressive agent such as cyclophosphamide during the development of an antibody response were found to display further decreases in antibody titres when re-exposed to the taste alone in the absence of any immunomodulating agent. For this to occur, there must be pathways of communication from the brain to the immune system that are activated by the taste paired with cyclophosphamide. The search for these pathways of communication resulted in the demonstration of innervation of the primary (thymus) and secondary (spleen and lymphoid nodes) lymphoid organs by the sympathetic nervous system.[2] Sympathetic efferent nerves enter lymphoid organs with the vasculature but ultimately separate from blood vessels to innervate the parenchyma, where both B and T lymphocytes reside and can proliferate. Sympathetic fibres innervating lymphoid organs contain all the neurotransmitter machinery of other sympathetic neurones, including noradrenaline and neuropeptides such as substance P, neuropeptide Y (NPY), and calcitonin gene-related peptide (CGRP). This implies that the chemical composition of the microenvironment in which lymphocytes are present ultimately depends on activity of the autonomic nervous system. These findings gained in prominence when it was discovered that specific subsets of leukocytes have receptors for these neuronal communication signals.

Receptors within the immune system

In addition to cytoplasmic receptors that bind steroid hormones including glucocorticoids and sex hormones, lymphocytes, and other cells of the immune system have been found to have membrane receptors that bind and respond to most neurotransmitters and neuropeptides and are quasi-identical to brain neurotransmitter and neuropeptide receptors. As supported by an important body of literature, activation of these receptors in leukocytes has functional consequences on immune responses whether immunity is measured in vivo or in vitro.[3] As an typical example, growth hormone (GH), a pituitary hormone known for its growth-promoting activity and with no known immune function, was shown to restore the resistance of hypophysectomized rats to an infection with *Salmonella typhimurium*, with an efficacy comparable to that of a tetracycline antibiotic or the macrophage-stimulating factor interferon-gamma (IFN-γ).[4,5] These results obtained in vivo were replicated in vitro.[6] GH activated highly purified populations of pulmonary macrophages in the same way as IFN-γ. Both factors were able to prime macrophages triggered with opsonized zymosan to secrete superoxide anion O_2^-, an index of macrophage activation, even if GH was less active in this system than IFN-γ. Antibody blocking studies demonstrated that the priming activity of GH was independent of IFN-γ, and vice versa the activity of IFN-γ was distinct from that of GH. This priming had functional consequences since both IFN-γ and GH increased the capability of macrophages to kill *Pasteurella multocida*. Since most of the effects of GH on its target cells are mediated by the local production of insulin-growth factors (IGF), the capability of IGF-I to prime alveolar macrophages in vitro was also tested and found to be similar to that of GH, although the priming effects of GH were independent of the local production of IGF-I.[7] Other studies were showing at the same time that non-stimulated as well as immune-activated leukocytes were able to produce a GH-like peptide that was identical to pituitary GH,[8] conferring credibility to the important hypothesis that communication signals originally identified in the neuroendocrine system can actually be used by immune cells. In the same vein, corticotropin-releasing hormone (CRH), the main regulator of the hypothalamic–pituitary–adrenal axis, has been identified in the immune system in which it functions as an autocrine/paracrine mediator of inflammation.[9] In particular, CRH causes degranulation of mast cells and the release of histamine and several proinflammatory mediators.

The neuropeptides that are contained in sympathetic nerve endings that innervate lymphoid organs can play an important role in the modulation of the fine balance between the different populations of T helper (Th) cells that regulate cellular and humoral immunity. Th1 cells normally produce IFN-γ and interleukin-2 (IL-2), and both promote cellular immunity. In contrast, Th2 cells normally produce IL-4 and IL-10 that down-regulate cellular immunity and promote humoral immunity. CGRP and NPY drive Th1 cells towards the production of IL-4 whereas Th2 cells are driven by somatostatin and CGRP to produce IL-2 and IFN-γ.[10] If these effects that were observed in vitro are also true under in vivo conditions, they provide a possible mechanism by which stress can polarize immune responses in the direction of either Th1 or Th2 cells.

A recent potentially important discovery is that of the inhibition exerted by the parasympathetic nervous system on the production of proinflammatory cytokines by macrophages. Direct electrical stimulation of the peripheral vagus nerve that innervates the liver inhibited the production of proinflammatory cytokines by Kupffer cells in response to a lethal dose of endotoxin and prevented development of septic shock.[11] This vagal function was termed the cholinergic anti-inflammatory pathway[12] and it is mediated by nicotinic acetylcholine receptors containing an alpha-7 subunit.

Neural influences on the immune system

Since the immune system makes use of communication signals and receptors that are identical to those used by the central nervous system, the immune system should be very sensitive to neural influences. Besides the cholinergic anti-inflammatory pathway already mentioned, many data attest to the fact that brain events have an impact on immune responses. For instance, lesions in the neuroendocrine brain have profound influences on immunity. As an example, destruction of the tubero-infandibular region of the hypothalamus in mice persistently abrogates natural killer cell cytotoxic activity without altering T and B cell populations, but cortical and sham lesions had only a short-lived effect.[13] In other studies, ablation of the left sensori-motor cortex decreased cellular immunity whereas ablation of the right sensory-motor cortex increased it, showing that brain influences on immunity are lateralized.[14] This lateralization phenomenon was later demonstrated to exist in the absence of any lesion since left-handed mice, labelled as such based on their predominant use of the left paw to reach a food pellet in a tube that only enabled them to use one paw, displayed higher cellular immune responses than right-handed mice.[15] The mechanisms for this lateralized influence of the brain on immunity are still elusive.

The impact of stressors on immune responses represents another example of the influence of brain events on immunity. At the time these studies were carried out it was already well known that the influence of psychosocial stressors on the hypothalamic–pituitary–adrenal axis are not simply a function of the intensity and duration of the stressors but also depend upon their psychological features. Novelty, predictability, and controllability are the key factors that ultimately determine the neuroendocrine impact of stressors. It was therefore not surprising that the same psychological features were pivotal in the influence of stress on immunity. For instance, rats exposed to inescapable electric shocks 24 h after injection of syngenic tumour cells displayed more rapid tumour growth and a higher mortality rate than rats exposed to controllable electric shocks, despite the fact that the intensity and duration of electric shocks were exactly the same in both groups.[16] Lack of control had the same influence on the rejection of non-syngenic tumours[17] and cellular immunity as measured by the proliferative response of lymphocytes to T-cell mitogens.[18] It cannot be inferred that uncontrollability is always immunosuppressive. Lack of control over the occurrence of electric shocks was later found to increase rather than decrease humoral immunity, as measured by antibody titres against sheep red blood cells injected into rats that were submitted chronically to controllable or uncontrollable electric shocks.[19] The same difference in the way the immune system responds to an uncontrollable stressor was confirmed in an experiment in which mice were exposed to the odour of a stressed congener. A 24 h exposure to this stressor decreased the cellular immune response, as measured by proliferation of T cells to mitogens and natural killer cell cytotoxicity, but increased antibody titres against keyhole limpet haemocyanin.[20]

Stress and the immune system

Studies of the influence of stress on the immune system have also been carried out in human subjects in experimental settings or in real-life conditions. In these studies, the immune end points are either measured on blood lymphocytes or deduced from the result of an already existing pathological process. The group of Janice Kiecolt-Glaser at Ohio State University in Columbus is certainly the pioneer in this field. For instance, first year medical students were shown to display a reduction in the production of IFN-γ by circulating leukocytes and a reduced cytotoxicity of natural killer cells during the end of the year examination period, and these changes were independent on lifestyles.[21] As a result of extensive studies on different populations at risk, such as spouses experiencing marital conflict, caregivers of patients with Alzheimer's disease, and aged subjects, Kiecolt-Glaser's group proposed that negative emotions and stressful experiences can contribute to prolonged infection and delayed wound healing. In addition, negative emotions were proposed to directly produce the production of proinflammatory cytokines and therefore increase the risk for a spectrum of conditions associated with ageing, including cardiovascular disease, osteoporosis, arthritis, type 2 diabetes, certain cancers, frailty and functional decline, and periodontal disease.[22]

The influence of stressful life events on immune responses also appear to be modulated by coping strategies, as exemplified by a study carried out on susceptibility to upper respiratory tract illness in an adult population sample.[23] In a little less than 30 per cent of a population sample of adults between 18 and 65 years of age, the occurrence of clinical episodes of upper respiratory tract illness over a 15-week period was more frequent in those individuals who experienced high life event stress both before and during the study period. The impact of life events was buffered by an avoidance coping style.

In accordance with the hypothesis that negative emotions negatively impact the immune system, major depressive disorders were initially thought to be associated with depressed immune responses. This association has been confirmed for the number of circulating lymphocytes, proliferative response of lymphocytes to non-specific mitogens, and natural killer cell cytotoxicity.[24,25] However, more recent studies have revealed signs of activation of the innate immune system in at least some forms of depression.[25,26]

Although most of the literature deals with the influence of stressors and negative emotions, positive emotions have also been studied in their relation to immune events. In graduate students vaccinated against hepatitis B, dispositional positive affect was associated with a greater antibody response to vaccination.[27] The same trait was associated with decreased vulnerability to upper respiratory infections. Dispositional optimism, as defined by generalized positive expectations for the future, is positively related to measures of cellular immunity in cancer and HIV patients only when stressors are brief, relatively straightforward and controllable whereas the reverse relationship is observed when stressors are complex, persistent, and uncontrollable.[28]

Mechanisms of the relationship between stressful life events, emotions, and immunity are rarely investigated because of the many biobehavioural pathways that can be implicated in mediating relationship. In view of the postulated immunosuppressive effects of glucocorticoids, it has been important to demonstrate that not all effects of stress on immunity are mediated by activation of the hypothalamic–pituitary–adrenal axis. As an example, implantation of a corticosterone pellet after adrenalectomy in rats that were submitted to inescapable electric shocks so as to prevent the stress-induced increases in plasma corticosterone did not alter the decreased proliferative response of blood lymphocytes observed in stressed rats.[29] Evidence for a role of the sympathetic nervous system was provided by experiments using beta-adrenergic receptor antagonists or sectioning of the sympathetic nerve innervating the spleen. For instance, administration of propranolol prevented the decreased lymphoproliferative response in rats re-exposed to the cage in which they had been previously exposed to inescapable electric shocks.[30] Other possible biological mediators are CRH and endogenous opioids. In the clinic, the search for possible biological mediators of the relationship between stress and immunity is not easily found, and often confounded by the impact of stress and negative emotions on illness behaviour, via for instance deterioration in health-promoting behaviour and alterations in symptom perception.[31]

Susan Lutgendorf at the University of Iowa recently summarized the current view of interactions between health behaviours and psychosocial and biological factors that can combine to affect a multitude of disease outcomes in a biopsychosocial model (Fig. 2.3.10.1).[32]

The immune system as a true sensory organ

In a recent longitudinal study on the relationship between positive affect and clinical signs during a bout of influenza in volunteers inoculated with rhinovirus or influenza virus, production of inflammatory mediators by cells of the innate immune system in the nasal secretions was associated with reduced positive affect.[33] Since 1-day lagged analyses showed that daily production of inflammatory mediators predicted lower positive affect on the next day, it was difficult to interpret these findings in terms of the previously described relationship between emotions and immunity, negative emotions, or decreased positive affect increasing innate immunity. On the contrary, the authors interpreted their findings as supporting a causal association between pathogen-induced local cytokine production and changes in positive affect.

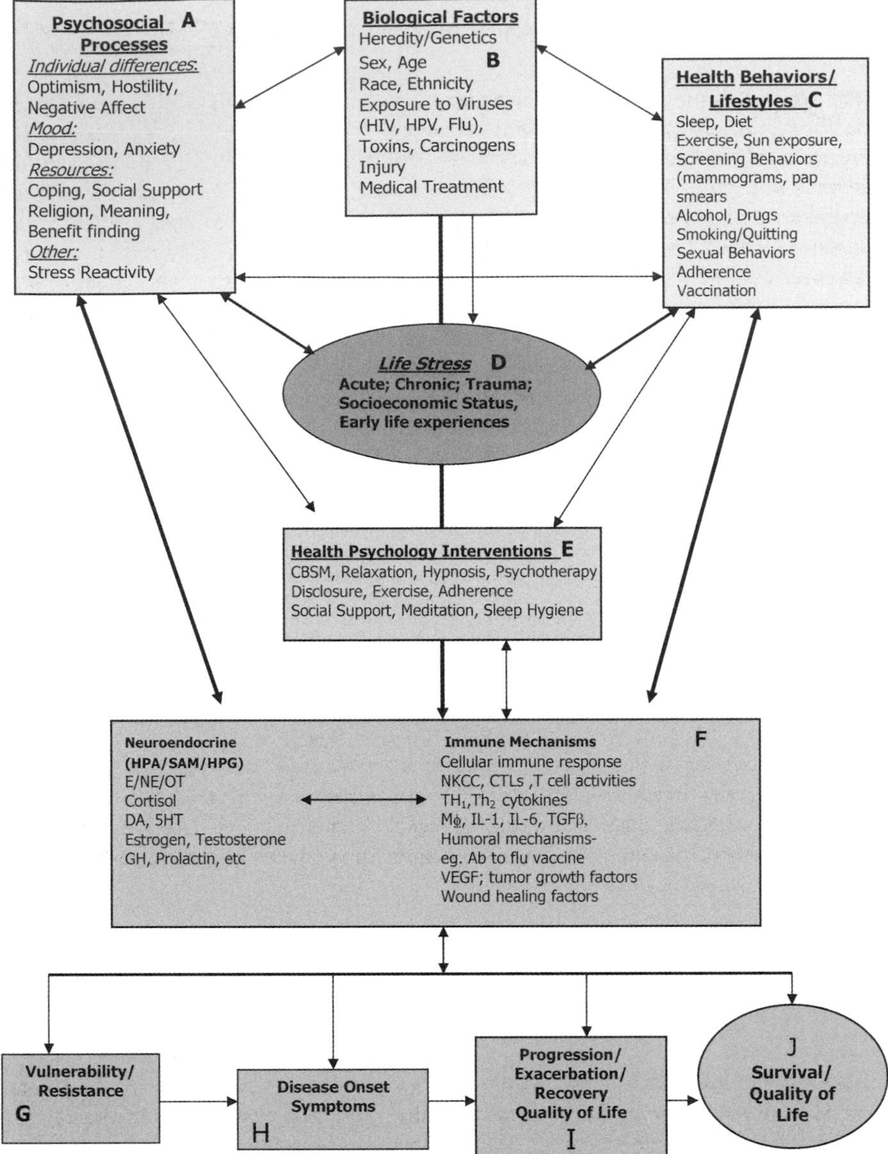

Fig. 2.3.10.1 The figure illustrates the biopsychosocial model in health psychology. The interaction between psychosocial processes (Box A), biological factors (Box B), and health behaviours (Box C) leads to a vulnerability (or resistance) to illness (Box G), disease onset and symptoms (Box H), progression, exacerbation, recovery, with concomitant quality of life (Box I), and survival with concomitant quality of life (Box J) via processes involving neuroendocrine and immune mechanisms (Box F). Effects of life stress (Box D) are filtered through psychosocial processes (Box A) and health behaviours (Box C) in their resultant effects on downstream mechanisms. Health psychology interventions (Box E) can modulate effects of psychosocial processes and health behaviours on neuroendocrine and immune mechanisms and on resultant health outcomes. There are also pathways between biobehavioural factors and disease outcomes not involving neuroendocrine or immune mechanisms, but other pathways are not included in this figure. Psychosocial processes (A) encompass psychological and social factors, particularly those that involve interpretation of and response to life stressors. These include personality variables (e.g., optimism, hostility, and negative affect), mental health and mood variables (e.g., depression and anxiety), coping, social support, spirituality, and sense of meaning. Health behaviours (C) include drug and alcohol use, smoking, sleep, nutrition, exercise, adherence to medical regimens, physical examinations, risk screenings, and risky sexual behaviours, among others. Health psychology interventions (E) can be used to alter psychosocial processes (A: e.g., decrease depression, increase coping) or improve health behaviours (C: e.g,. smoking cessation) to provide a more positive influence on neuroendocrine and immune factors and perhaps slow disease progression/exacerbation. Interventions include cognitive behavioural stress management (CBSM), relaxation, hypnosis, meditation, emotional disclosure, adherence-based interventions, sleep hygiene, exercise, social support groups, psychotherapy, imagery, distraction, behavioural pain management, yoga, massage, biofeedback, drug/alcohol prevention/rehabilitation, psychotherapy, and behavioural conditioning. These interventions can be used at all points of the trajectory of the disease or condition. Box F shows selected mechanisms involved in the bidirectional interactions between neuroendocrine and immune axes that mediate the relationships between biobehavioural factors (A–D) and disease outcomes (G–J). This by no means is an all-inclusive list of mechanisms, but it represents some of the commonly studied factors in this literature. Once vulnerability (G) has been established, continued interaction with positive or negative psychosocial factors (A: e.g., depression/social support), disease factors (B), adaptive/maladaptive health behaviours (C) and stress (D) will contribute to expression (or lack thereof) of disease symptoms (H), disease-free intervals/progression/exacerbation, and quality of life (e.g., functional, physical, emotional, and social well-being) (I), and survival (J). HPA, hypothalamic–pituitary–adrenocortical axis; SAM, sympathoadrenomedullary axis; HPG, hypophyseal pituitary gonadal axis; OT, oxytocin; DA, dopamine; 5HT, seratonin; GH, growth hormone; NKCC, natural killer cell cytotoxicity; CTLs, cytotoxic lymphocytes; $M_Ð$, macrophage; IL-1, interleukin 1; IL-6, interleukin 6; TGFÐ, transforming growth factor beta; Ab, antibody; and VEGF, vascular endothelial growth factor. (Reprinted from Brain Behaviour and Immunity, 17(4), ASK Lutgendorf and Es Costanzo, Psychoneuroimmunology and health psychology: an integrative model, 225–32, Copyright 2003, with permission from Elsevier.)

Plates for Chapter 2.3.1

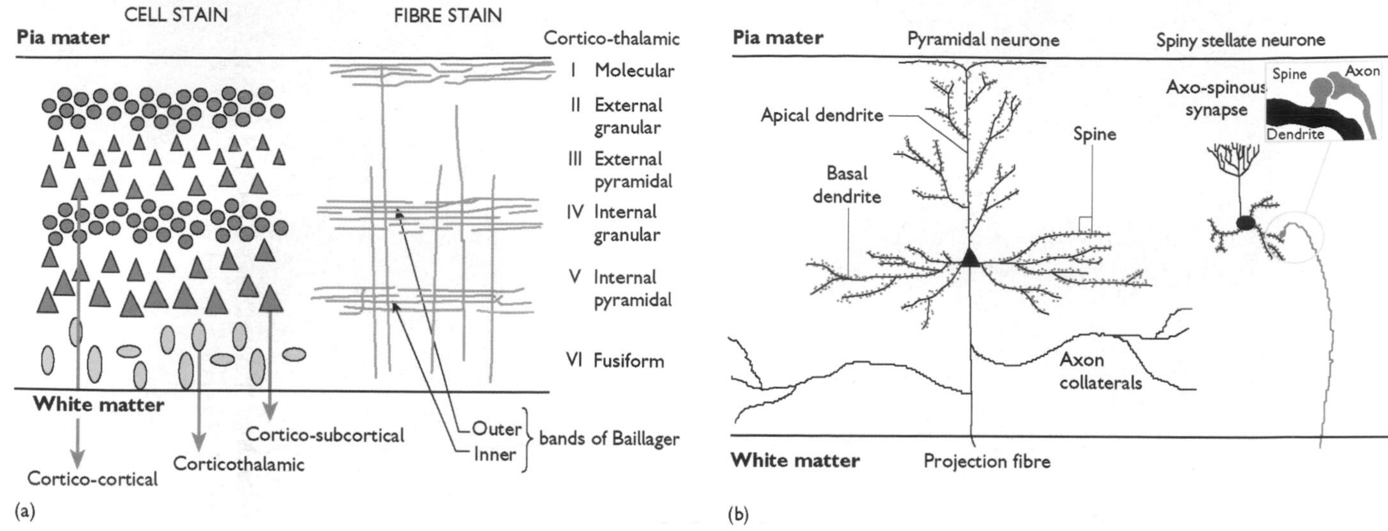

Plate 1 (a) Laminar structure of the cerebral neocortex; (b) excitatory amino acid using spiny neurones of the neocortex.

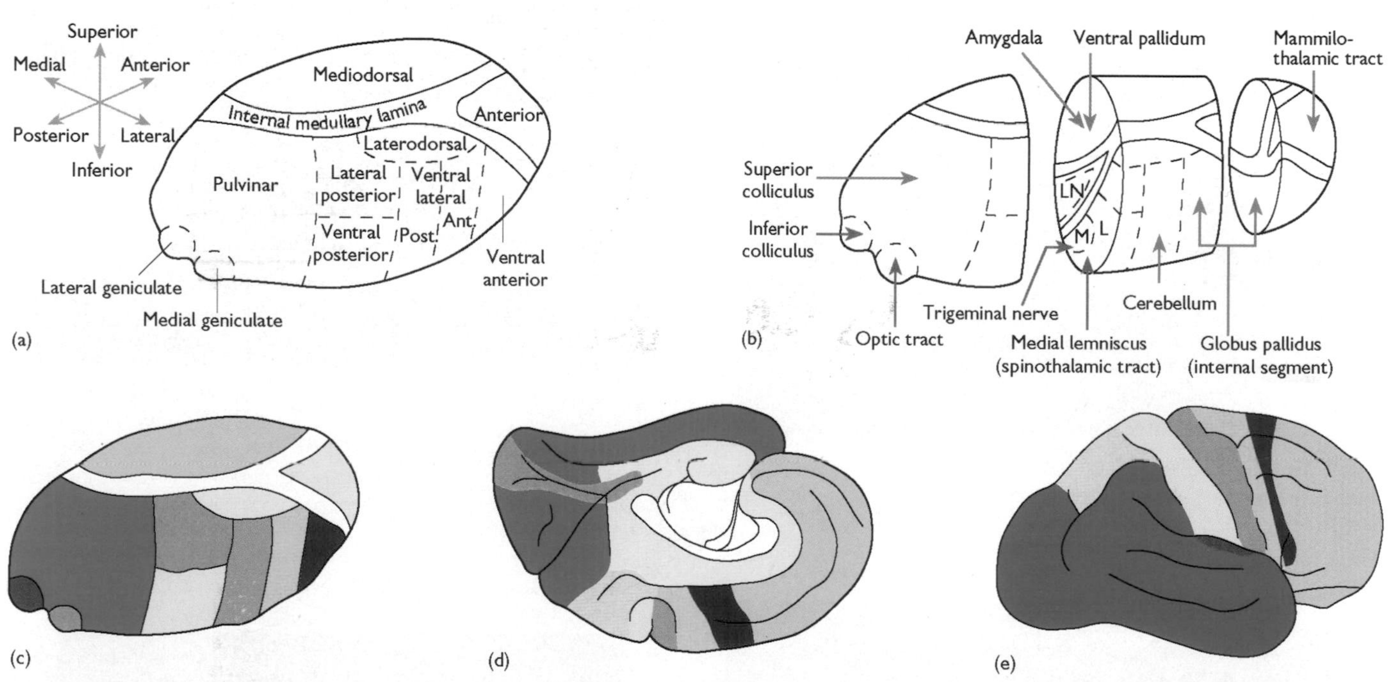

Plate 2 (a) The thalamus is shown as if removed from the brain at the top, with the individual major nuclei indicated. (b) Schematic diagram showing the isolated thalamus divided approximately at the middle of its anteroposterior extent; the arrows indicate known sources of major subcortical afferents to the individual named nuclei. (c) The diagram of the isolated thalamus shown in (a) with the individual main nuclei colour coded. (d), (e) Schematic diagrams of the cerebral surfaces (medial and lateral) showing the regions of cortex colour coded to correspond to the main thalamic nuclei with which they have major connections.

Plates for Chapter 2.3.6

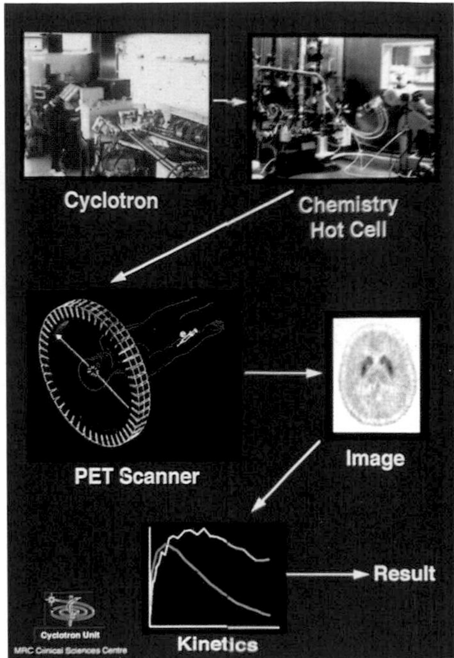

Plate 3 Steps in the production and use of PET radio-isotopes.

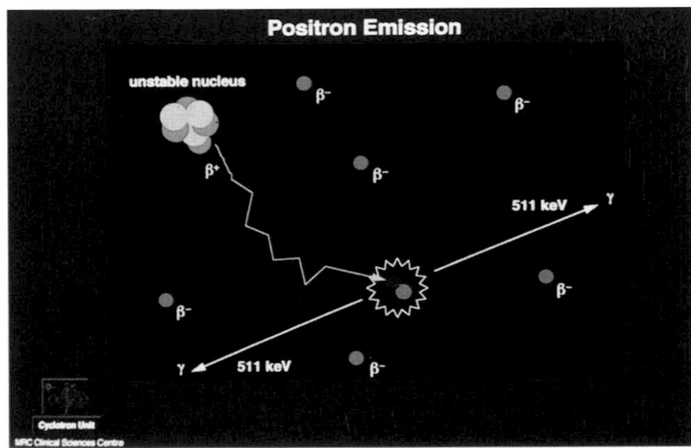

Plate 4 Principles of positron emission: β^- is an electron and β^+ is a positron. Two high-energy gamma rays (γ) are produced on annihilation of a positron by an electron

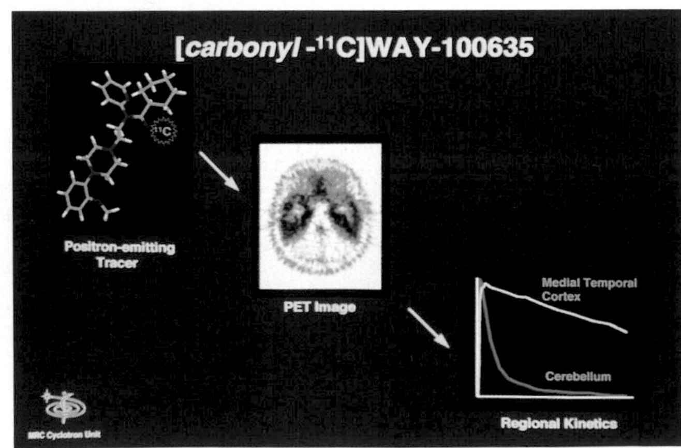

Plate 5 Use of a PET radiotracer to image 5-HT$_{1A}$ receptors in the human brain.

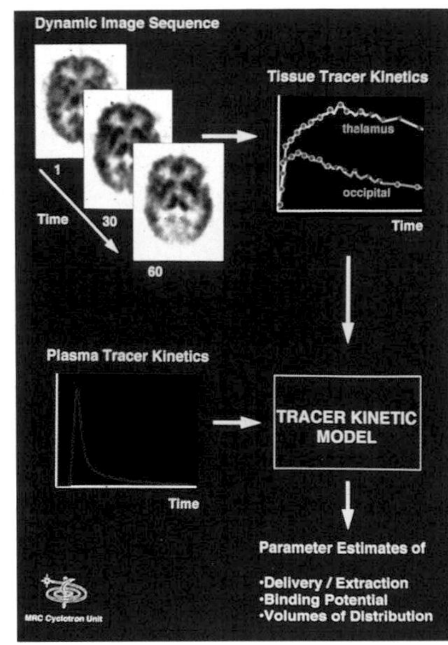

Plate 6 Steps in the data analysis of a PET radiotracer.

Plates for Chapter 2.3.7

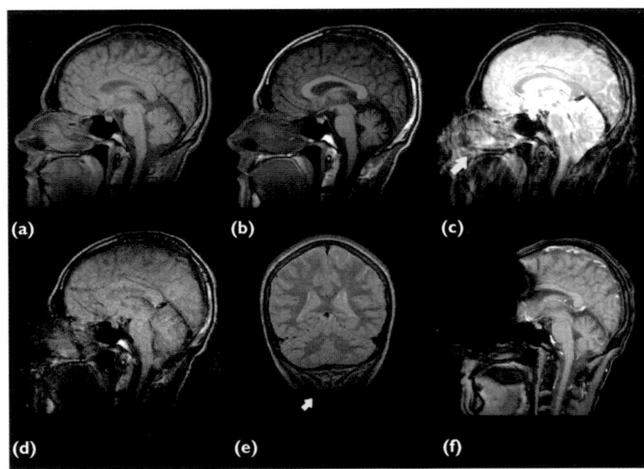

Plate 7 Spin echo MR images and artefacts. Top row, spin echo images: left, proton density image (TR = 2000 ms, TE = 20 ms); middle, T_1-weighted image (TR = 350 ms, TE = 20 ms); right, T_2-weighted image (TR = 2000 ms, TE = 90 ms). The arrow on the T_2-weighted image indicates blurring caused by movement (swallowing) during acquisition. Bottom row, examples of poor tissue contrast and susceptibility artefact: left, spin echo image showing poor contrast due to injudicious prescription of pulse sequence (TR = 350 ms, TE = 90 ms); middle, bulk susceptibility artefact; right, ferromagnetic susceptibility artefact caused by a metallic hairgrip.

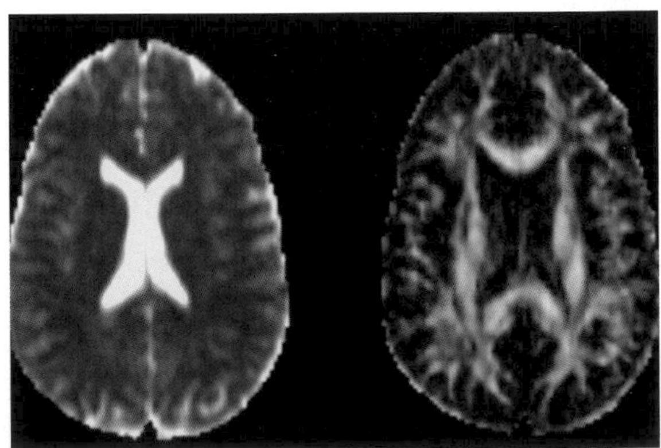

Plate 8 Diffusion-weighted MRI data can be used to generate maps of (left) the apparent diffusion coefficient (**ADC**) and (right) the anisotropy of diffusion. Diffusion of protons is most rapid and isotropic in cerebrospinal fluid, and least rapid and most anisotropic in white matter. White matter is clearly defined by relative hyperintensity in the anisotropy map.

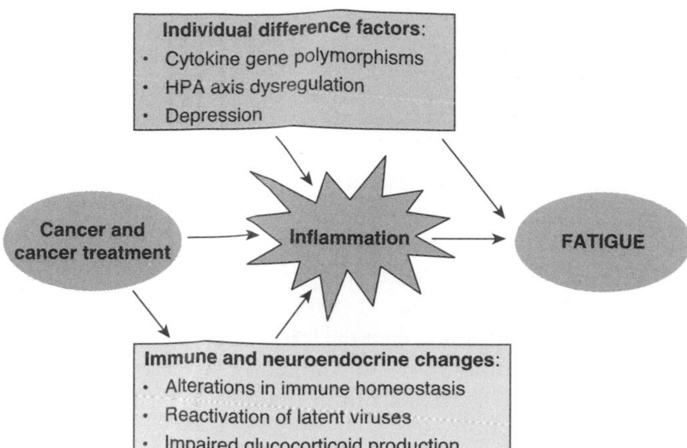

Fig. 2.3.10.2 Potential mechanisms for cancer-related fatigue. Cancer and its treatment can activate the proinflammatory cytokine network, leading to symptoms of fatigue through cytokine effects on the central nervous system. Chronic inflammation may develop when cancer and cancer treatments induce long-term changes in immune homeostasis, including alterations in immune cell subsets, alterations in expression and signaling of Toll-like receptors, and latent virus reactivation. Cancer-related changes in neuroendocrine function may also contribute to chronic inflammation, particularly impairments in glucocorticoid production that result in ineffective control of inflammatory processes. In addition, individual difference factors may increase the risk for chronic inflammation following cancer diagnosis and treatment. Potential risk factors include single nucleotide polymorphisms in cytokine genes, alterations in HPA axis function, and depressive symptoms. Of note, HPA dysregulation and depression may also have direct effects on fatigue. (Reprinted from Brain Behaviour and Immunity, 21(7), JE Bower, Cancer related fatigue, 863–871, Copyright 2007, with permission from Elsevier.)

is really a sixth sensory system.(45) Humans cannot see, smell, touch, hear, or taste pathogenic micro-organisms. However, cells of the immune system, whether they be T cells, B cells, macrophages, microglial cells, or dendritic cells are uniquely endowed with the molecular machinery to detect an endless array of pathogens. One way that the immune system informs the brain that a pathogen has entered the body is by immune cells recognizing these invaders. These leukocytes respond by releasing proinflammatory cytokines, which act as messenger systems to alert the brain that something is amiss in the periphery. The foundation for this conceptual system has strengthened during the last 20 years. It forms the intellectual basis for the notion that emotions are regulated by the immune system, and the immune system affects expression of emotions.

Further information

Ader, R. (2007). *Psychoneuroimmunology*, 2 volumes (4th edn). Elsevier, Amsterdam.

Psychoneuroimmunology Research Society: http://www.pnirs.org

References

1. Ader, R. (2003). Conditioned immunomodulation: research needs and directions. *Brain, Behavior, and Immunity*, **17**(Suppl. 1), S51–7.
2. Felten, D.L. and Felten, S.Y. (1988). Sympathetic noradrenergic innervation of immune organs. *Brain, Behavior, and Immunity*, **2**(4), 293–300.
3. Sanders, V.M. (2006). Interdisciplinary research: noradrenergic regulation of adaptive immunity. *Brain, Behavior, and Immunity*, **20**(1), 1–8.
4. Edwards, C.K. III, Yunger, L.M., Lorence, R.M., *et al.* (1991). The pituitary gland is required for protection against lethal effects of Salmonella typhimurium. *Proceedings of the National Academy of Sciences of the United States of America*, **88**(6), 2274–7.
5. Kelley, K.W., Weigent, D.A., and Kooijman, R. (2007). Protein hormones and immunity. *Brain, Behavior, and Immunity*, **21**(4), 384–92.
6. Edwards, C.K. III, Arkins, S., Yunger, L.M., *et al.* (1992).The macrophage-activating properties of growth hormone. *Cellular and Molecular Neurobiology*, **12**(5), 499–510.
7. Fu, Y.K., Arkins, S., Fuh, G., *et al.* (1992). Growth hormone augments superoxide anion secretion of human neutrophils by binding to the prolactin receptor. *The Journal of Clinical Investigation*, **89**(2), 451–7.
8. Baxter, J.B., Blalock, J.E., and Weigent, D.A. (1991). Expression of immunoreactive growth hormone in leukocytes in vivo. *Journal of Neuroimmunology*, **33**(1), 43–54.
9. Kalantaridou, S., Makrigiannakis, A., Zoumakis, E., *et al.* (2007). Peripheral corticotropin-releasing hormone is produced in the immune and reproductive systems: actions, potential roles and clinical implications. *Frontiers in Bioscience*, **12**, 572–80.
10. Levite, M. (1998). Neuropeptides, by direct interaction with T cells, induce cytokine secretion and break the commitment to a distinct T helper phenotype. *Proceedings of the National Academy of Sciences of the United States of America*, **95**(21), 12544–9.
11. Borovikova, L.V., Ivanova, S., Zhang, M., *et al.* (2000). Vagus nerve stimulation attenuates the systemic inflammatory response to endotoxin. *Nature*, **405**(6785), 458–62.
12. Pavlov, V.A. and Tracey, K.J. (2005). The cholinergic anti-inflammatory pathway. *Brain, Behavior, and Immunity*, **19**(6), 493–9.
13. Forni, G., Bindoni, M., Santoni, A., *et al.* (1983). Radiofrequency destruction of the tuberoinfundibular region of hypothalamus permanently abrogates NK cell activity in mice. *Nature*, **306**(5939), 181–4.
14. Renoux, G., Biziere, K., Renoux, M., *et al.* (1983). A balanced brain asymmetry modulates T cell-mediated events. *Journal of Neuroimmunology*, **5**(3), 227–38.
15. Neveu, P.J., Barneoud, P., Vitiello, S., *et al.* (1988). Brain modulation of the immune system: association between lymphocyte responsiveness and paw preference in mice. *Brain Research*, **457**(2), 392–4.
16. Sklar, L.S. and Anisman, H. (1979). Stress and coping factors influence tumor growth. *Science*, **205**(4405), 513–5.
17. Visintainer, M.A., Volpicelli, J.R., and Seligman, M.E. (1982). Tumor rejection in rats after inescapable or escapable shock. *Science*, **216**(4544), 437–9.
18. Laudenslager, M.L., Ryan, S.M., Drugan, R.C., *et al.* (1983). Coping and immunosuppression: inescapable but not escapable shock suppresses lymphocyte proliferation. *Science*, **221**(4610), 568–70.
19. Mormede, P., Dantzer, R., Michaud, B., *et al.* (1988). Influence of stressor predictability and behavioral control on lymphocyte reactivity, antibody responses and neuroendocrine activation in rats. *Physiology & Behavior*, **43**(5), 577–83.
20. Cocke, R., Moynihan, J.A., Cohen, N., *et al.* (1993). Exposure to conspecific alarm chemosignals alters immune responses in BALB/c mice. *Brain, Behavior, and Immunity*, **7**(1), 36–46.
21. Kiecolt-Glaser, J.K., Glaser, R., Strain, E.C., *et al.* (1986). Modulation of cellular immunity in medical students. *Journal of Behavioral Medicine*, **9**(1), 5–21.
22. Kiecolt-Glaser, J.K., McGuire, L., Robles, T.F., *et al.* (2002). Psychoneuroimmunology and psychosomatic medicine: back to the future. *Psychosomatic Medicine*, **64**(1), 15–28.
23. Cobb, J.M. and Steptoe, A. (1996). Psychosocial stress and susceptibility to upper respiratory tract illness in an adult population sample. *Psychosomatic Medicine*, **58**(5), 404–12.
24. Herbert, T.B. and Cohen, S. (1993). Depression and immunity: a meta-analytic review. *Psychological Bulletin*, **113**(3), 472–86.

To understand this interpretation, it is necessary to replace the relationship between the immune system and the brain in the context of regulatory immunophysiology. If the brain communicates with the immune system via neuroendocrine factors and autonomic neuronal pathways, it is probably because the immune system needs the brain to regulate its function and do what it cannot do by itself, (i.e., engage the whole organism in the fight against microbial pathogens). If this is the case, then it ensues that the immune system needs to inform the brain of its state of activity. In other words, brain-to-immune communication pathways need to be activated by immune-to-brain communication pathways. This interpretation makes the immune system a true sensory organ, specialized in the detection of the non-self and able to transmit this information to the brain.

Looking through the mirror: immune modulation of emotions and mood

The isolation, cloning, and expression of proinflammatory cytokines and their receptors in the late 1980s, coupled with the discovery of pathogen-associated molecular patterns (PAMPs) and their pathogen recognition receptors (PRRs), are two of the major advances in immunology that set the stage for defining immune-to-brain communication pathways. Interleukin-1 (IL-1) is a prototypical proinflammatory cytokine that is released from activated macrophages following activation of some PRRs. Other proinflammatory cytokines include tumour necrosis factor (TNF-α), IL-6, and IL-8. Injection of IL-1 or TNF-í, either systemically in the form of intraperitoneal administration or centrally via an intracerebroventricular route, induces the classical signs of illness, including fever, activation of the hypothalamic–pituitary–adrenal axis, and sickness behaviour, as evidenced by decreased interaction with the physical and social environment, reduced appetite, disappearance of body care activities, fatigue, malaise, and mild cognitive impairments.[34–37] These actions take place in the brain since pretreatment of rats with the specific antagonist of IL-1 receptors into the lateral ventricles of the brain significantly impairs the ability of systemic IL-1 to cause behavioural deficits.

At the molecular and cellular levels, it is now clear that IL-1 and other proinflammatory cytokines produced by activated innate immune cells in the periphery during the inflammatory response induce expression of the same cytokines in innate immune cells of the brain, including meningeal and perivascular macrophages, microglial cells in the brain parenchyma and mast cells. Peripheral cytokines are relayed to the brain via a humoral pathway involving the action of PAMPs on PRRs located in circumventricular organs at the interface of the brain and periphery and a neural pathway involving activation of the afferent nerves that innervate the body region in which the inflammatory response takes place. At the organism level, this central representation of the peripheral inflammatory response imposes a new mode of functioning on the brain so as to allow the organism to better cope with infection. The elevated body temperature actively maintained by the increased thermogenesis and decreased thermolysis that characterizes the fever response promotes a number of immune events and reduces microbial proliferation. At the same time, zinc and iron that are normally essential for cellular multiplication are sequestered and acute phase proteins including complement proteins are synthesized by hepatocytes to help killing microbial pathogens. The increased glucocorticoid levels that occur as a consequence of the hypothalamic effect of cytokines negatively feed back on activated innate immune cells and significantly limit the intensity and duration of the inflammatory response. Sickness behaviour itself helps to reduce physical activities detrimental to thermogenesis and facilitates the reduction of thermolysis. It also limits the spread of infection within the social group by reducing social activities and reduces pain that is enhanced by proinflammatory cytokines.

Once an infection, and therefore cytokine synthesis, resolves over the time course of a few days, behavioural symptoms of sickness normally disappear. However, if the infection does not resolve, or if there is ongoing autoimmune inflammatory processes of a chronic nature, such as rheumatoid arthritis, multiple sclerosis, inflammatory bowel disease, the synthesis of cytokines and their downstream products continues to be elevated. The chronic action of proinflammatory cytokines acting in the brain has now led to the hypothesis that these very same proteins are somehow involved in development of affective disorders such as depression. In the clinic, this hypothesis is supported by the high prevalence of major depressive disorders that is observed in patients with a chronic inflammatory condition[38] and the observation that chronic administration of recombinant IL-2 and/or IFN-α to cancer or hepatitis C patients induces alterations in mood that are characteristic of depression. In the laboratory, acute or chronic activation of the peripheral immune system induces depression-like behaviour that is apparent even when sickness behaviour has dissipated.[39] A leading candidate protein for this effect is a cytokine-activated enzyme known as indoleamine 2,3 dioxygenase (IDO)[40] which has an ubiquitous cellular localization and is also present in the brain. This enzyme degrades tryptophan, an essential amino acid that is required for the synthesis of the mood-regulating neurotransmitter serotonin. Increased degradation of tryptophan associated with inflammation results in a relative deficit in brain serotonin neurotransmission that can precipitate depression and an increased production of tryptophan neuroactive derivatives, including kynurenine, 3-hydroxy kynurenine, and quinolinic acid. These molecules act as agonists or antagonists of the NMDA receptor. Since brain IDO enzymatic activity is increased during activation of the peripheral immune system, these molecules gain access to the brain because they freely cross the blood–brain barrier. In addition, these metabolites are also produced in the brain.

There is accumulating evidence that activation of immune-to-brain communication pathways is responsible not only for the adaptive sickness behavioural response and the maladaptive syndrome of depression that develops in vulnerable individuals but also for the symptom burden that is experienced by physically ill patients, including fatigue[41] (see Fig. 2.3.10.2), pain[42], sleep disorders,[43] and impaired learning and memory.[44]

Concluding comments

A few years ago, scientists who proffered the idea that mood disorders could be induced by an infective process were considered heretic. That view has changed considerably with the discovery that cytokines from the immune system act as elements that permit active communication between the brain and the rest of the body. Indeed, it was in 1984 when a pioneering scientist in psychoneuroimmunology, J. Edwin Blalock, proposed that the immune system

Plate for Chapter 4.2.1

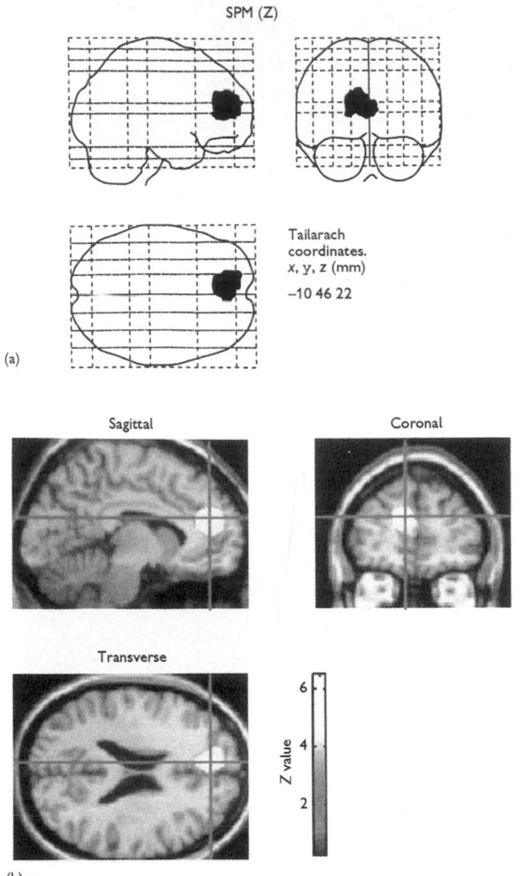

Plate 13 Area of activation during opiate craving: (a) [^{15}O]H_2O PET SPM image; (b) area of activation superimposed on magnetic resonance image.

Plate for Chapter 4.5.6

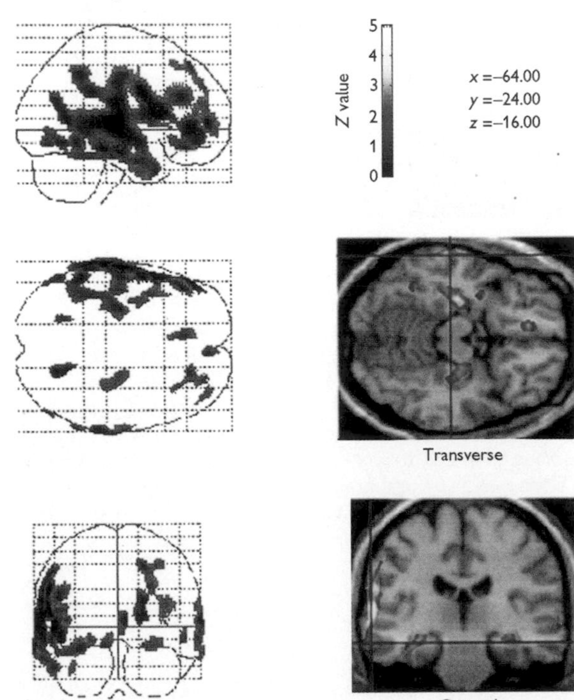

Plate 14 Statistical parametric maps ($p < 0.001$) for reductions in grey matter densities in subjects with chronic refractory depression compared with controls. Effects are controlled for age. (Reproduced with permission from P.J. Shah *et al.* (1998). Cortical grey matter reductions associated with treatment-resistant chronic unipolar depression: controlled MRI study. *British Journal of Psychiatry*, **72**, 527–32.)

Plates for Chapter 6.2.10.4

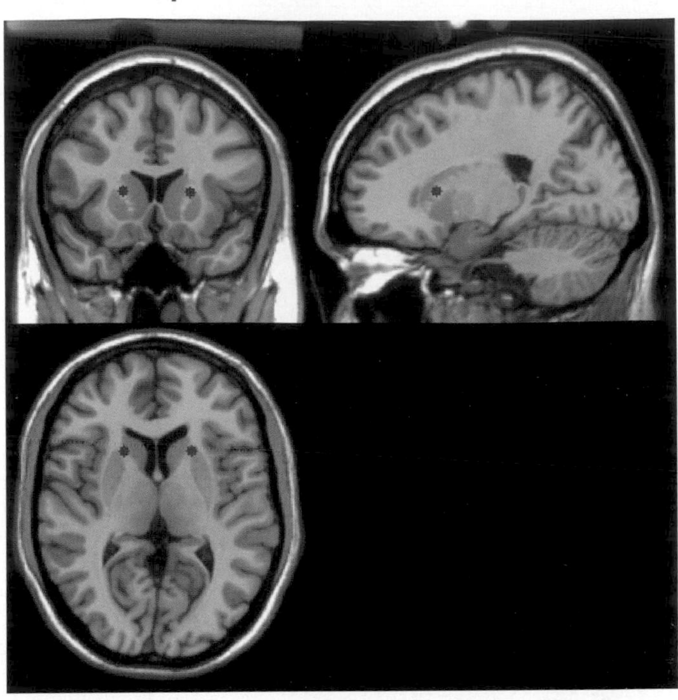

Plate 15 Typical locations of anterior capsulotomy lesions superimposed upon normalized T1 MRI scan. Lesions not to scale.

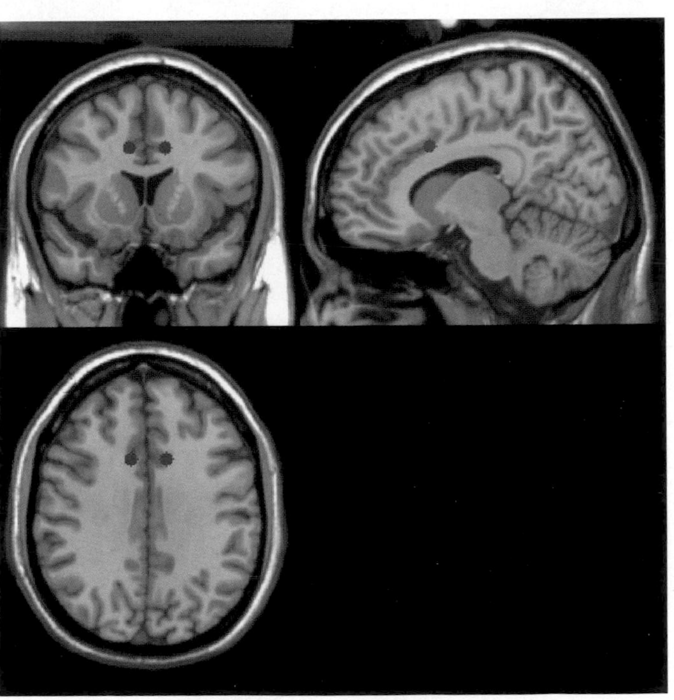

Plate 16 Typical locations of anterior cingulotomy lesions superimposed upon normalized T1 MRI scan. Lesions not to scale.

Plates for Chapter 2.3.7 *(continued)*

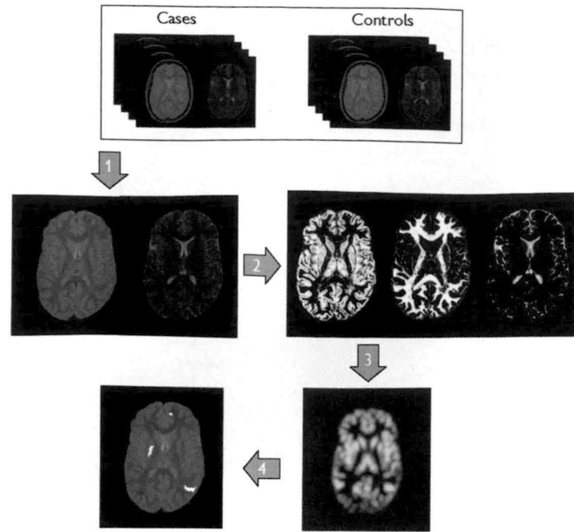

Plate 9 Steps in computerized image analysis. Dual-echo (fast spin echo) data are acquired from several cases and controls in a cross-sectionally designed study. Extracerebral tissue is removed (1) from each image before segmentation or tissue classification (2). Tissue-calssified images are registered with a template image in standard space (3) before hypothesis testing (4). Voxels or clusters, which demonstrate a significant difference in tissue class volume between groups, are colour coded.

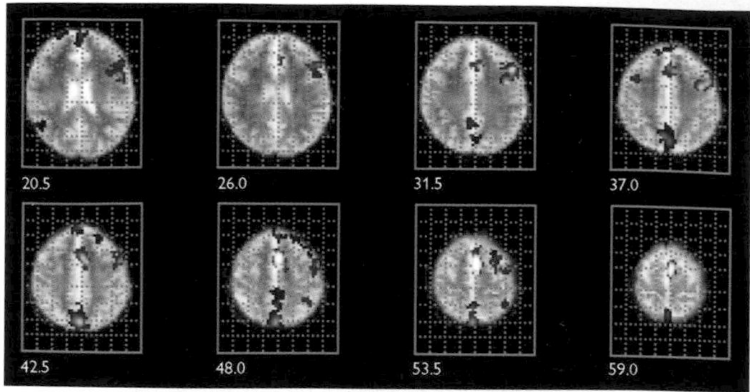

Plate 11 Activation map. Generically activated voxels are colour coded against a grey-scale background of gradient echoplanar imaging data. The grid respresents the standard Talairach-Tournoux Space;[12] z-coordinates for each slice are shown at the bottom left. Colour codes the timing and power of a periodic response to a covert verbal-fluency experiment. Blue voxels show increased magnetic responance signal during condition B (repeat a word covertly); light blue represents a greater power of response than dark blue. Red voxels show increased magnetic resonance signal during condition. A (generate a word beginning with a cue letter); yellow and orange represent a greater power of response than dark red. The voxel-wise probability of a false-positive error is $p = 0.0001$. The main areas activated during conditioin A are the dorsolateral prefrontal cortex, inferior frontal gyrus, and supplementary motor area; the main areas activated during condition B are the medial parietal cortex and posterior cingulate gyrus.

Plates for Chapter 2.3.8

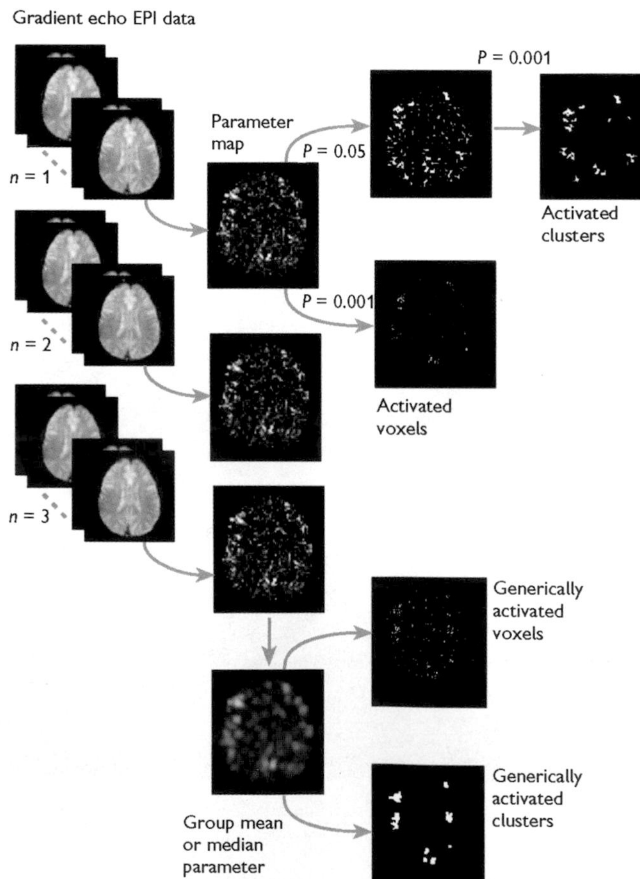

Plate 10 Steps in computerized data analysis. Gradient echoplanar imaging data have been acquired from three subjects under identical conditions. The time series at each voxel is analysed to estimate a measure or parameter of the experimental effect, which is represented as a parameter map. Significantly activated voxels or clusters can be identified in each individual image. Parameter maps can be averaged over individuals and generically activated voxels or clusters identified over the group of subjects. The power to detect activation is enhanced by cluster-level analysis and by combining data from several subjects.

Plate for Chapter 4.1.3

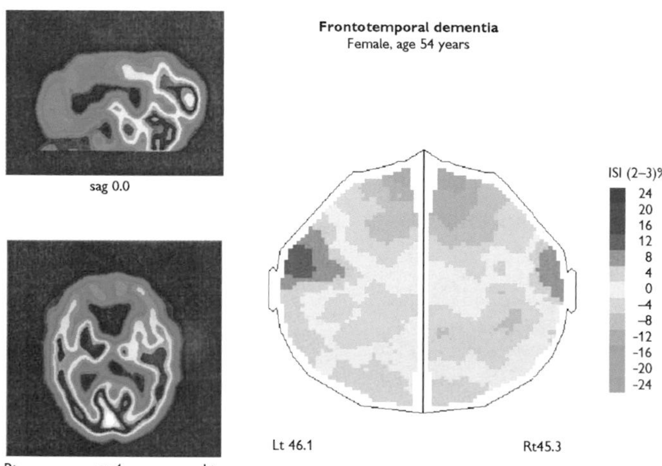

Plate 12 Regional cerebral blood flow (rCBF) measured using SPECT with exametazine (left) and the Xenon-133 inhalation method (right) in a 54-year-old female with clinical signs of FTD. The variation of regional cerebral blood flow is measured with xenon-133, above (red) or below (green) the average flow level, as indicated by the colour code. The patient showed the first signs of personality change, and stereotypy of speech and behaviour at the age of 48 years. EEG was normal, and CT and MRI showed slight frontal cortical atrophy. The regional cerebral blood flow measurement with xenon-133 showed a normal average flow level and marked bilateral, frontal flow decreases. The SPECT scan showed a severe perfusion deficit in the frontal and anterior cingulate cortex. (Courtesy of Department of Neurophysiology, University Hopital, Lund, Sweden.)

25. Zorrilla, E.P., Luborsky, L., McKay, J.R., *et al.* (2001). The relationship of depression and stressors to immunological assays: a meta-analytic review. *Brain, Behavior, and Immunity*, **15**(3), 199–226.
26. Maes, M., Smith, R., and Scharpe, S. (1995). The monocyte-T-lymphocyte hypothesis of major depression. *Psychoneuroendocrinology*, **20**(2), 111–16.
27. Marsland, A.L., Cohen, S., Rabin, B.S., *et al.* (2006). Trait positive affect and antibody response to hepatitis B vaccination. *Brain, Behavior, and Immunity*, **20**(3), 261–9.
28. Segerstrom, S.C. (2005). Optimism and immunity: do positive thoughts always lead to positive effects? *Brain, Behavior, and Immunity*, **19**(3), 195–200.
29. Keller, S.E., Weiss, J.M., Schleifer, S.J., *et al.* (1983). Stress-induced suppression of immunity in adrenalectomized rats. *Science*, **221**(4617), 1301–4.
30. Lysle, D.T., Cunnick, J.E., and Maslonek, K.A. (1991). Pharmacological manipulation of immune alterations induced by an aversive conditioned stimulus: evidence for a beta-adrenergic receptor-mediated Pavlovian conditioning process. *Behavioral Neuroscience*, **105**(3), 443–9.
31. Cohen, S. and Williamson, G.M. (1991). Stress and infectious disease in humans. *Psychological Bulletin*, **109**(1), 5–24.
32. Lutgendorf, S.K. and Costanzo, E.S. (2003). Psychoneuroimmunology and health psychology: an integrative model. *Brain, Behavior, and Immunity*, **17**(4), 225–32.
33. Janicki-Deverts, D., Cohen, S., Doyle, W.J., *et al.* (2007). Infection-induced proinflammatory cytokines are associated with decreases in positive affect, but not increases in negative affect. *Brain, Behavior, and Immunity*, **21**(3), 301–7.
34. Kent, S., Bluthe, R.M., Kelley, K.W., *et al.* (1992). Sickness behavior as a new target for drug development. *Trends in Pharmacological Sciences*, **13**(1), 24–8.
35. Konsman, J.P., Parnet, P., and Dantzer, R. (2002). Cytokine-induced sickness behaviour: mechanisms and implications. *Trends in Neurosciences*, **25**(3), 154–9.
36. Dantzer, R. (2001). Cytokine-induced sickness behavior: mechanisms and implications. *Annals of the New York Academy of Sciences*, **933**, 222–34.
37. Dantzer, R. and Kelley, K.W. (2007). Twenty years of research on cytokine-induced sickness behavior. *Brain, Behavior, and Immunity*, **21**(2), 153–60.
38. Steptoe, A. (ed.) (2007). *Depression and physical illness.* Cambridge University Press, Cambridge.
39. Frenois, F., Moreau, M., O'Connor, J., *et al.* (2007). Lipopolysaccharide induces delayed FosB/DeltaFosB immunostaining within the mouse extended amygdala, hippocampus and hypothalamus, that parallel the expression of depressive-like behavior. *Psychoneuroendocrinology*, **32**(5), 516–31.
40. Capuron, L. and Dantzer, R. (2003).Cytokines and depression: the need for a new paradigm. *Brain, Behavior, and Immunity*, **17**(Suppl. 1), S119–24.
41. Bower, J.E. (2007). Cancer-related fatigue: links with inflammation in cancer patients and survivors. *Brain, Behavior, and Immunity*, **21**(7), 863–71.
42. Wieseler-Frank, J., Maier, S.F., and Watkins, L.R. (2005). Immune-to-brain communication dynamically modulates pain: physiological and pathological consequences. *Brain, Behavior, and Immunity*, **19**(2), 104–11.
43. Irwin, M. (2002). Effects of sleep and sleep loss on immunity and cytokines. *Brain, Behavior, and Immunity*, **16**(5), 503–12.
44. Krabbe, K.S., Reichenberg, A., Yirmiya, R., *et al.* (2005). Low-dose endotoxemia and human neuropsychological functions. *Brain, Behavior, and Immunity*, **19**(5), 453–60.
45. Blalock, J.E. (1984).The immune system as a sensory organ. *Journal of Immunology*, **132**(3), 1067–70.

2.4

The contribution of genetics

Contents

2.4.1 Quantitative genetics
Anita Thapar and Peter McGuffin

2.4.2 Molecular genetics
Jonathan Flint

2.4.1 Quantitative genetics

Anita Thapar and Peter McGuffin

Patterns of inheritance

Our understanding of how traits and disorders are passed from one generation to the next began with the work carried out by an Augustinian monk, Gregor Mendel. Although Mendel's published work in 1866 was initially ignored, its rediscovery at the beginning of the twentieth century heralded the beginning of modern genetics. Mendel's experiments on pea plants and his observations of the patterns of inheritance of certain characteristics led to the development of his particulate theory of inheritance. It was only later in 1909 that the units of inheritance that he had described were named genes and alternative forms of a gene were termed alleles. It was also at this time that the terms phenotype, used to describe the observed characteristic, and genotype, used to refer to the genetic endowment, were introduced.

Mendel's laws

Mendel examined clear-cut dichotomous characteristics such as smooth versus wrinkled coats in peas. He first noted that when parents of different types were crossed, the first generation (F1) offspring displayed **uniformity** of that characteristic. He inferred that this uniformity was due to one phenotype being dominant and the other being recessive. Thus, when homozygous parents AA and aa produced heterozygote Aa offspring, these offspring displayed the phenotype of the AA parent rather than manifesting a phenotype intermediate to those of both parents.

Mendel then demonstrated that when the F1 heterozygotes (Aa) were intercrossed (Aa × Aa), **segregation** resulted in the second F2 generation showing recessive and dominant phenotypes in the ratio of 1 to 3. He then inferred that this F2 generation consisted of three types (AA, Aa, and aA, aa) occurring with a probability of 1:2:1.

Finally, Mendel showed that when the transmission of two different phenotypic traits was studied, they showed **independent assortment**. We now know that independent assortment occurs when the genes coding for these traits are either located far apart on the same chromosome or are on different chromosomes (see linkage).

Single-gene disorders

Although disorders showing a simple Mendelian pattern of inheritance are rare, they tend to be clinically severe and collectively impose a significant burden.

For **autosomal dominant** disorders to manifest themselves, only one disease allele is necessary, i.e. both heterozygotes as well as homozygotes (those who carry both disease genes) will be affected. In most instances, where there is one affected parent who is a heterozygote for the disease, approximately 50 per cent of the offspring will show the disorder. Autosomal disorders tend to be severe and manifest themselves in every generation. Huntington's disease and acute intermittent porphyria are examples of autosomal dominant conditions that are often present with psychiatric symptoms.

Autosomal recessive conditions such as phenylketonuria require the presence of two disease alleles to show clinical manifestations of the disorder. Thus, they often appear to skip generations. These disorders usually occur in the offspring of two 'carrier' heterozygote parents and are more common where there is a high rate of consanguinity (e.g. marriages between cousins) as these inbred populations will show greater homozygosity at all loci.

The other group of single-gene disorders consists of **sex-linked** conditions such as fragile X syndrome. Normal females have two X chromosomes whereas normal males have one X chromosome and one Y chromosome. Thus, for recessive disorders on the X chromosome, if the mother is a carrier (X^*X) and assuming that the father is unaffected (XY), half of her sons will manifest the disorder (X^*Y) and half of her daughters will be carriers (X^*X). Where the father is affected by an X-linked recessive condition, all the daughters will be carriers. As sons have to inherit their

X chromosome from their mother, there will be an absence of father to son transmission. X-linked dominant conditions are extremely rare.

Continuous traits

Mendel's laws are based on the transmission of dichotomous characteristics, yet many important human phenotypes such as height, weight, and blood pressure are continuously distributed. However, we are able to show that Mendelian principles can also be applied for these types of quantitative traits.

Let us first consider a phenotype measured on a continuous scale which results from the influence of a single gene with two alleles A_1 and A_2 (see Fig. 2.4.1.1). We can now describe the phenotypes of the three possible genotypes in terms of a quantitative value on the continuous scale. A_1A_1 has a value of $-a$; A_2A_2 has a value of $+a$; and A_1A_2, the heterozygote, has a value of d. When $d = 0$, A_1A_2 lies exactly half way between A_1A_1 and A_2A_2, that is the genetic contribution is entirely additive. When $d = -a$, A_2 is recessive to $A_1$and when $d = +a$, A_2 is dominant to A_1.

At the simplest level, we assume that there are no dominance effects and that there is no mutation, selection, migration, or inbreeding in the population. If p is the frequency of allele $A_1$and q is the frequency of A_2 in the population where $p + q = 1$ then the frequency of genotypes can be expressed as follows:

$$\begin{array}{ccc} A_1A_1 & A_1A_2 & A_2A_2 \\ p^2 & 2pq & q^2 \end{array}$$

This is known as the Hardy–Weinberg equilibrium. If we now simplify further and state allelic frequencies where $p = q = 0.5$, then the phenotypic values of A_1A_1, A_1A_2, and A_2A_2 would be distributed in the population with relative frequencies of 1:2:1.

Now if we consider a trait which results from two genes each of which has two alleles of equal frequency and additive effect, there would be five possible phenotypic values with relative frequencies of 1:4:6:4:1. Overall as the number of genetic loci (n) increases, the number of phenotypic values increases ($2n + 1$) and the distribution of phenotypic values more closely approximates a normal distribution. It is thought that most quantitative or continuous traits result from the additive action of genes at many loci which is otherwise known as **polygenic** inheritance. Where familial transmission is explained by environmental factors as well as by multiple genes, we then call this a **multifactorial** mode of inheritance.

Complex disorders and irregular phenotypes

(a) Polygenic/multifactorial threshold models

Most common human psychiatric and medical disorders such as schizophrenia, diabetes, and heart disease do not show a Mendelian pattern of inheritance. Neither can they be considered as continuous traits in that people are described as being affected or unaffected.

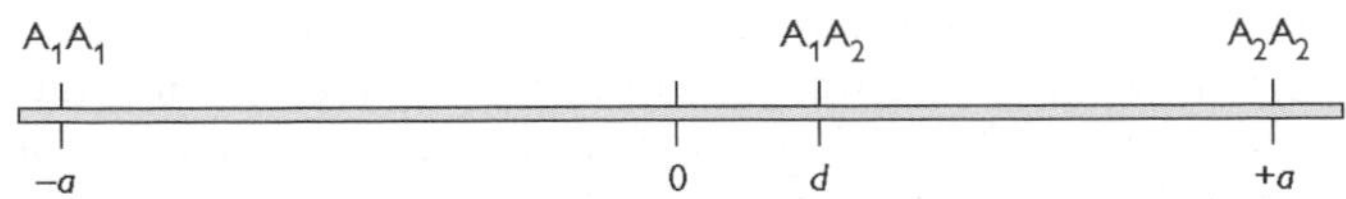

Fig. 2.4.1.1 A phenotype, measured on a continuous scale, resulting from a single gene with two alleles A_1 and A_2.

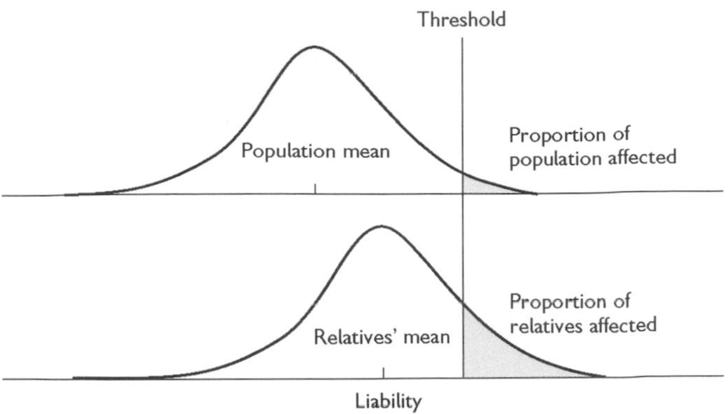

Fig. 2.4.1.2 A polygenic or multifactorial threshold model of disease transmission.

However, these conditions could be regarded as quasi-continuous in that those who are affected can be graded along a continuum of severity. It is possible to extend this to assume that there is an underlying liability to develop the disorder which is continuously distributed in the population. Those who pass a certain threshold manifest the condition. If the underlying liability to develop the disorder is inherited in a polygenic or multifactorial fashion, then we can assume that the distribution will be approximately normally distributed (Fig. 2.4.1.2). The genetic liability of relatives of affected individuals will be increased and their liability distribution will be shifted to the right (Fig. 2.4.1.2). Thus, the proportion of relatives above the disease threshold will be greater compared with the general population. If we know the proportion of affected relatives of probands and the proportion of those affected in the general population, it is possible to calculate the correlation in liability between pairs of relatives using this type of model.

(b) Single major locus model and atypical patterns of Mendelian inheritance

An alternative to a polygenic model of complex disease is a single major locus model. Single-gene disorders do not always show typical Mendelian patterns of inheritance. For example familial transmission can be modified by variable **expression** and **penetrance**. Some conditions can show great variability in terms of clinical expression. For example neurofibromatosis, an autosomal dominant disorder can express itself as the full blown disorder or merely as a few café-au-lait spots. Penetrance is defined as the probability of manifesting the disorder given a particular genotype. For Mendelian disorders this is always 1 or 0, but irregular patterns of inheritance may occur because of incomplete penetrance where the probability of manifesting the disorder is greater than 0 but less than 1.

Finally, there are now molecular explanations for other types of unusual patterns of inheritance for single genes. Anticipation where disorders show a progressively earlier onset and greater severity with subsequent generations is now known to be explained by heritable unstable nucleotide repeat sequences (see later). Huntington's chorea and fragile X syndrome are examples of disorders caused by heritable unstable repeats. For some conditions such as the Angelman syndrome and the Prader–Willi syndrome, manifestation of the disorder depends on the parental origin of the gene. This is known as imprinting.

(c) Other models

Alternative explanations of how complex conditions such as psychiatric disorders are inherited include mixed and oligogenic patterns of transmission. A mixed model includes a major gene and a polygenic/multifactorial contribution. However, for many of these disorders, genes of major effect may not exist. It may be that these irregular phenotypes are best explained by oligogenic models where the co-action or interaction of a small number of genes contributes to the disorder. These issues remain to be resolved by molecular genetic studies (see later).

Components of phenotypic variation

We will now consider the different influences that contribute to phenotypic variation in a population. The total variation in an observed trait (phenotype v_p) at the simplest level (ignoring non-additive effects) can be partitioned into a proportion due to genetic influences (v_g), a component explained by shared environmental factors (v_c), and a remainder accounted by non-shared environmental factors which includes error (v_e):

$$v_p = v_g + v_c + v_e$$

Shared or common environmental influences are aspects of the environment that result in greater similarity of family members for a given phenotype. Non-shared environmental factors refer to environmental influences that have effects which are specific to individuals and that contribute to phenotypic differences between family members.

Although we have so far only considered one type of genetic contribution, the genetic variance v_g can be further subdivided into variance due to additive genetic influences (v_a) and dominance effects (v_d).

The relative influence of genetic factors is expressed as **heritability** and when defined as the proportion of the total phenotypic variance attributable to additive genetic variance, is known as **narrow-sense heritability**:

$$h_n^2 = v_a / v_p.$$

Heritability is also sometimes used to describe the proportion of variance explained by the *total* genetic variance (additive and non-additive genetic variance) and it is then known as **broad-sense heritability**:

$$h_b^2 = v_a / v_g.$$

Similarly we can estimate the proportion of the total phenotypic variance explained by shared environment where $c^2 = v_c/v_p$ and the remaining proportion attributable to non-shared environmental factors and error (e^2).

It is important to remember that the estimate of heritability and the contribution of shared environment and non-shared environment are proportions of total variation within a given population, i.e. these parameters tell us about sources of difference between individuals in a population and have no meaning at an individual level. For example, if an individual was selected from a population where IQ had been shown to have a heritability of 50 per cent, it could not be said that 50 per cent of that individual's IQ was determined by genes. Another important point is that these estimates are specific to the population studied and may differ for other populations. Finally, the contribution of genetic and environmental influences to a phenotype does not allow any inferences about the extent to which that phenotype is modifiable by environmental factors. For example, phenylketonuria is a Mendelian condition that is determined by the presence of a single-gene mutation. Yet the clinical manifestations of the syndrome are prevented by dietary intervention.

Non-additive genetic effects

So far we have simplistically assumed that phenotypic variation is influenced in an additive fashion. However, the contribution of genes and environment is more complex than this. We have already referred to genetic **dominance** effects where there is non-additive interaction of alleles within a locus. Another potential source of influence is the non-additive interaction between alleles at different loci which is known as gene–gene interaction or **epistasis**.

Gene–environment interaction

Gene–environment interplay represents another important form of non-additive genetic contribution to complex phenotypes.[1] The term gene–environment interaction (G × E) is used here to refer to individual genetic differences in response to specific environmental factors. In the presence of gene–environment interaction, individuals who are at genetic risk of a disorder do not manifest the condition unless they are exposed to a specific environmental risk factor. Gene–environment interaction also means that not all those exposed to an environmental risk factor will show disorder. Later, we consider direct investigation of gene–environment interaction through molecular genetic studies. Twin and adoption study designs have also been used to examine G × E, in an indirect way. Here, genetic liability is inferred by virtue of having affected relatives rather than through possession of a specific genetic risk variant.

Gene–environment correlation

Gene–environment correlation further adds to the complexity of interplay between genes and environment. Gene–environment correlation arises when a person's genotype is correlated with the environment that they are exposed to. For example, sociable parents not only endow their children with genes but also provide an environment that encourages greater sociability in their children (passive gene–environment correlation). Moreover, positive gene–environment correlation would result where a sociable child actively seeks out more situations where socializing occurs (active gene–environment correlation) or where he or she evokes friendly responses in others (evocative gene–environment correlation). There is evidence that many important environmental risk factors in psychiatry (for example, life events) do correlate with genetic risk for specific disorders (for example, depression). Where that is the case, genetically sensitive designs are needed to investigate whether environmental risk factors have true environmentally mediated risk effects on disorder or whether the association has arisen because of genetic factors contributing to both the environmental risk exposure and disorder.

The presence of gene–environment interaction and gene–environment correlation highlights that the action of genes and environment must be considered together. Another important point is that in traditional twin study designs, G × E and G – E correlation effects are subsumed within the heritability estimate or in some circumstances the environmental variance component (see twin studies).

Research methods

Family, twin, and adoption studies

So far we have considered the theoretical basis of inheritance and possible sources of phenotypic variation and familial resemblance. Clearly, the investigation of the genetic basis of psychiatric disorders first requires us to examine to what extent genes and environment contribute to a given disorder or trait. Secondly, we need to know how genes and environmental influences exert their risk effects and finally we have to investigate the genetic basis of disorders at a molecular level.

Traditional methods in psychiatric genetics research include family, twin, and adoption studies. Family studies enable us to examine to what extent a disorder or trait aggregates in families. Familiality of a disorder can of course by explained by shared environmental influences as well as by shared genes. Twin and adoption studies allow us to disentangle the effects of genes and shared environment.

Family studies

(a) Methods

Family studies allow us to determine whether a disorder aggregates in families by examining the rate of disorder in the relatives of affected individuals (probands) and comparing this with the rate of disorder in the general population or in a control group. Alternatively we can compare the frequency of disorder in the relatives of probands with the frequency among relatives of a control group of normal individuals or those with another disorder.

There are two types of family studies. The **family history** method is more economical in that the psychiatric history is taken from the proband. However, given that most individuals are unlikely to know as much about family members as about themselves, this method results in an underestimate of diagnoses in relatives. A more thorough but more time-consuming approach is the **family study** method where all available relatives are directly interviewed.

(b) Ascertainment

An important issue is how a family study sample is ascertained. Ideally, probands should be ascertained independently from each other. This is unlikely to pose a problem for rare disorders. However, for more common conditions where a series of cases is collected, for example, by consecutive referrals of the disorder to a particular hospital, it is possible that families included in a family study contain more than one proband. This is known as multiple incomplete ascertainment. Complete ascertainment, where all affected individuals in a given population are included, is rarely possible and in most instances probands are identified after some selection process (e.g. referrals to a particular hospital). Thus, factors influencing selection, such as comorbidity and help seeking may also influence observed patterns of familial aggregation.

(c) Age correction

For genetic studies, we are interested in the proportion of individuals who have ever had the disorder (lifetime prevalence) rather than the proportion who show the disorder at one point in time (point prevalence). However, a difficulty encountered when carrying out family studies is that the observed rates of disorder will also depend on the age of the individual, the risk period for the disorder, and whether or not the individual has lived through that risk period. Thus, some members may not yet have reached the age of risk for the disorder, some are currently unaffected but will become affected at some later point, and others may have died whilst still unaffected. The most appropriate method is to correct for age and express the rate of disorder in relatives as the **morbid risk (MR)** or lifetime expectancy.

There are many methods of age correction, of which the Slater-Stromgen adaption of Weinberg's shorter method is the most straightforward. The MR of the disorder can be estimated as the number of affecteds (A) divided by the *bezugsziffer* (BZ) where the BZ is calculated as:

$$\Sigma_{\mathrm{i}}[\mathrm{a1}]w_i + A$$

and where w_i is the weight given to the ith unaffected individual based on their current age. The most accurate approach is to use an empirical age of onset distribution from a large separate sample, for example a national registry of psychiatric disorders, to obtain the cumulative frequency of disorder over a range of age bands, from which weights can be derived.

Another approach is to carry out life table analysis. The distribution of survival times (or times to becoming ill) is divided into a number of intervals. For each of these one can calculate the number and proportion of subjects who entered the interval unaffected and the number and proportion of cases that became affected during that interval as well as the number of cases that were lost to follow-up (because they had died or had otherwise 'disappeared from view'). Based on these, the numbers and proportions 'failing' or becoming ill over a certain time interval (usually taken as the entire period of risk) can be calculated. A further alternative is to use a Kaplan Meier product limit estimator. This allows one to estimate the survival function directly from continuous survival or failure times instead of classifying observed survival times into a life table. Effectively this means creating a life table in which each time interval contains exactly one case. It therefore has an advantage over a life table method in that the results do not depend on grouping of the data.

Twin studies

Identical or monozygotic twins, by virtue of arising from the fertilization of one egg, share 100 per cent of their genes. Non-identical or dizygotic twins are from two fertilized eggs and like full biological siblings share on average 50 per cent of their genes. Thus, assuming that monozygotic twins and dizygotic twins share environment to the same extent, monozygotic twins would share greater similarity than dizygotic twins for a disorder that is genetically influenced. Twin studies are an important method for disentangling the effects of genes and shared environment and can be used to estimate the contribution of genetic influences, shared environmental factors and non-shared environmental factors to the total variation for a given trait or disorder.

For continuous traits, twin similarity is expressed as an intraclass correlation coefficient where:

$$r_{\mathrm{mz}} = h^2 + c^2$$

$$r_{\mathrm{dz}} = 0.5h^2 + c^2$$

Thus, from observed monozygotic and dizygotic correlations for a given trait we can calculate heritability from the above equations where $h^2 = 2(r_{\mathrm{mz}} - r_{\mathrm{dz}})$, $c^2 = 2r_{\mathrm{dz}} - r_{\mathrm{mz}}$, and e^2 is the remaining variance $= 1 - h^2 - c^2$ (see path analysis below).

For dichotomous characteristics (e.g. affected with a disorder and unaffected), twin similarity is expressed as concordance rates. A **pairwise concordance rate** is estimated as the number of twin pairs who both have the disorder divided by the total number of pairs. However, where there has been systematic ascertainment, for example a twin register, it is preferable to report a **probandwise concordance rate** which is calculated as the number of affected twins divided by the total number of cotwins.

(a) Ascertainment

One potential source of bias in twin studies stems from ascertainment procedures. For example, affected twins referred to a specific study or volunteer samples are likely to include more twin pairs who are monozygotic and who are concordant. Ascertainment of twin pairs through hospital registers overcomes this problem to some extent, but for some disorders may be biased by the process of referral. Population-based samples overcome these biases, although when examining disorders rather than traits extremely large sample sizes are required to obtain an adequate number of affected individuals.

(b) Zygosity

A further potential source of error is in the assignment of zygosity. Ideally zygosity should be determined by DNA typing. However, it may be more practical to use a twin similarity questionnaire which includes questions such as whether the twins share the same hair/eye colour, and whether they look alike as two peas in a pod. This method of assigning zygosity is simple and inexpensive with a reported accuracy of over 90 per cent.

(c) Equal environments assumption

It is sometimes argued that a major drawback to the twin study method is that monozygotic twins may experience a more similar environment and may be treated more similarly than dizygotic twins. However, where there is evidence that monozygotic twins share greater environmental similarity than dizygotic twins it is difficult to infer whether this contributes to their similarity for the disorder or whether this is the consequence of greater genetic similarity. There have been several approaches adopted to further explore this issue.

In some studies questionnaire measures of environmental sharing (e.g. being dressed alike as children, sharing friends) have been used. These suggest that environmental sharing is indeed greater for monozygotic twins than for dizygotic twins. However, it appears that for many traits and disorders such as cognitive ability, personality, depressive symptoms, and depressive disorder this degree of similarity for childhood environment does not account for monozygotic twin similarity for the trait. One way of disentangling cause and effect is to use direct observational studies. Although this method has not been much used, one study of young twins suggested that the greater similarity of parental responses to monozygotic twins compared to dizygotic twins appeared to be elicited by the twins themselves.

An alternative method of examining the effects of environmental sharing is to study twins who are mistaken about their zygosity. However, most studies which have used this method suggest that perceived zygosity is a less important influence on twin similarity than true zygosity.

Finally, the most powerful means of examining the effects of environmental sharing is to look at monozygotic twins who have been reared apart. However, such twin pairs are rare and have mostly been ascertained in a biased fashion. Nevertheless, studies of reared-apart twins have informed us that there is a substantial genetic contribution to cognition, personality, and psychosis.

(d) Comparability of twins

The final potential criticism of the twin method is whether twins can be regarded as representative of the general population given some important differences. Twin births are relatively common (1 in 80 births), although the number of dizygotic twins varies in different countries and is influenced by factors such as maternal age and multiparity, a family history of twins and increasingly, the use of fertility drugs. Twins are more likely to experience greater intrauterine and perinatal adversity and the experience of being brought up as a twin is unusual in itself. There is also some evidence that depression is more common in mothers of young twins than among mothers of singletons. However, these differences are only important if they result in different rates of disorder or symptoms in twins compared to singletons. So far there is little evidence to suggest that the rate of psychiatric disorder in twins is any higher than amongst singletons.

Adoption studies

Adoption studies provide another means of teasing apart the effects of genes and environment. The basic method of the adoption study lies in comparing the rates of disorder in biological relatives and adoptive relatives. There are three main types of adoption study.

1 **The adoptee study**: Here the rate of disorder in the adopted-away offspring of affected individuals is compared with the rate of disorder in control adoptees whose biological parents are unaffected.

2 **The adoptee's family study**: In this design, the rate of disorder in the biological relatives of affected adoptees is compared with that among the adopted relatives.

3 **The cross-fostering study**: This allows us to examine gene-environment interaction by comparing the rate of disorder in adoptees who have unaffected biological parents and affected adoptive parents with the rate of disorder in adoptees who have affected biological parents and unaffected adoptive parents.

Although adoption studies allow us to examine the effects of both genes and environment, there are several potential drawbacks to the method. First, adoption is in itself an unusual event and there is a tendency for higher rates of some psychiatric difficulties such as antisocial personality traits amongst adoptees. Second, adoptive placements are not random in that adoption agencies are likely to attempt to match adoptive and biological parents for physical, social, and other characteristics. Nevertheless, despite these difficulties, adoption evidence has given much support to the role of both genes and environment for traits and behaviours such as cognitive ability and criminality.

Methods of analysis

Although the statistical methods used in quantitative genetics may seem complex, the principles are straightforward. We will now consider the methods of analyses that are most commonly used for examining the contribution of genetic and environmental factors, to psychiatric disorders and traits.

Path analysis

Path analysis provides a simple diagrammatic method of estimating the contribution of genetic and environmental factors. The basic path diagram in Fig. 2.4.1.3 shows the sources of resemblance for phenotypes (P_1 and P_2) in a pair of siblings. Using the rules of path analysis, the correlation between the siblings (r_{sib}) is derived by multiplying the path coefficients for each connecting path and then summing these coefficients. Thus

$$r_{sib} = h \times r_g \times h + c \times c.$$

The genetic correlation r_g is 1 for monozygotic twins who share 100 per cent of their genes in common and is 0.5 for full siblings or dizygotic twins. Thus, using path analysis we obtain the equations described earlier where

$$r_{mz} = h^2 + c^2$$

$$r_{dz} = 1/2h^2 + c^2$$

Model fitting

Although we can simply estimate h^2, c^2, and e^2 from the equations above for more complex data, solving multiple linear equations becomes difficult. We may also wish to test alternative models, for example one where there is no genetic contribution or one where shared environmental influences are dropped. Model fitting allows us to first statistically test how well a given model explains the observed data and to then compare different models.

Computer packages such as Mx[(2)] are all based on the same principles. The raw data are read into the program and the researcher supplies the initial starting values for the unknown parameters (*h*, *c*, and *e* for a full genetic model). The program then iterates with different parameter estimates until values are found which give an optimum fit (usually this involves maximizing a likelihood function or minimizing a χ^2). The goodness of fit of the model is then assessed by examining the χ^2 goodness of fit where a smaller value indicates a better fit.

The fit of a reduced model (*R*) can then be compared against the full model (*F*) by subtracting the χ^2 values ($R - F$). Alternatively the fit of models can be compared by using the likelihood ratio test where twice the difference between the log likelihoods for each model (this approximates a χ^2 distribution) is calculated.

(a) Application of model fitting

So far we have considered the influence of genes and environment on variation in a single phenotype using a traditional twin design. This type of analysis is known as univariate genetic analysis. However the most interesting questions in psychiatry are best addressed by more testing more complex models (See Kendler and Prescott[(3)] for excellent examples). Designs that involve measuring the same phenotype over time and several phenotypes at the same time (e.g. depression and anxiety) have been used to investigate comorbidity, the aetiological contribution to developmental changes over time and diagnostic boundaries. Studies that have employed such methods have yielded interesting findings. For example, there is evidence that the same set of genes, but different non-shared environmental factors influence anxiety and depressive disorders (and symptoms). The contribution of genetic factors to depressive symptoms and IQ has been found to increase in adolescence compared to childhood. Family and twin studies of autism suggest that there is familial and genetic loading for a broader cognitive and social phenotype in relatives of those with narrowly defined autism.

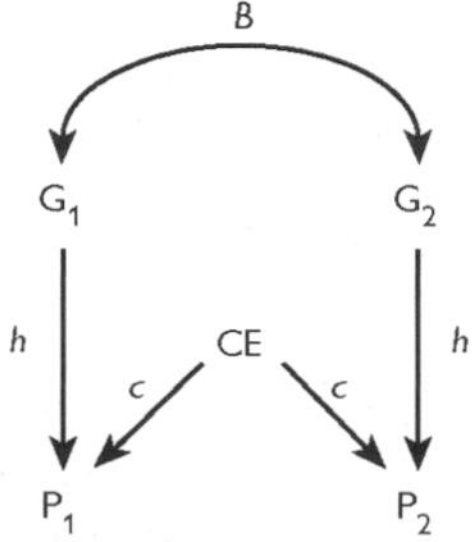

Fig. 2.4.1.3 A single path model of the sources of resemblance between twins or pairs of siblings. G_1 and G_2 are genotypes with correlation *B*, CE is common environment, P_1 and P_2 are phenotypes, and *h* and *c* are path coefficients.

There have also been imaginative extensions of the twin design that have allowed investigation of different questions. Each type of design has its own set of strengths and weaknesses. Thus having a variety of available methods is invaluable. Examples of different but related designs include studies of the children of twins,[(4)] studies combining twins, siblings, half siblings, step siblings, and families of twins.[(5)]

(b) Multiple regression analysis

Another commonly used method of analysing twin data is multiple regression analyses.[(6)] Here the score of the co-twin *C* is predicted by the score of the proband twin *P*, the coefficient of the relationship or zygosity *R* and an interaction term *PR*. The partial regression coefficients provide direct estimates of heritability and shared environment. The advantage of this method is that it can then also be used to test whether the magnitude of genetic contribution of extreme scores for a continuous trait differs from scores within the normal range. For example, such analyses suggest that the contribution of genetic factors to variation in very low IQ scores is low, unlike the contribution to IQ variation across the 'normal range'.

Twin and adoption study methods for investigating gene–environment interplay

Traditional twin study designs and analysis of MZ twin similarity and difference that include both measured aspects of the environment (e.g. reported life events) and phenotype (e.g. depression) can be used to test the extent to which the association of environmental factors with psychopathology is mediated by genetic and environmental pathways (gene–environment correlation). For example, one twin study showed environmentally mediated risk effects of childhood maltreatment on antisocial behaviour but different findings for corporal punishment where there were genetically mediated effects.[(7)] Twin studies have also been used to demonstrate the importance of G × E. Kendler and colleagues (1995)[(8)] showed that those at higher genetic risk of a major depressive disorder (inferred by lifetime ever diagnosis of major depression in MZ and DZ co-twins) were more sensitive to the depressogenic effects of adverse life events.

Adoption study designs provide a useful method for testing gene–environment interaction as post-natal environmental risk factors (apart from the very earliest) are experimentally separated from genetic risk. Such studies have shown evidence that the risk of antisocial behaviour is much higher in those who are not only at higher genetic risk (by virtue of having a parent with antisocial behaviour) but who are also exposed to adverse rearing environments in the adoptive home.

Gene mapping

A more direct approach to locating and identifying genes involved in psychiatric disorders is to attempt to map them. Gene mapping technology has advanced at an astonishing pace over the past 20 years. Early studies in psychiatric disorders such as schizophrenia[9] had to rely purely on 'classical' genetic markers such as HLA antigens blood groups and various protein polymorphisms. Capabilities in systematic gene mapping, which involves mounting a search throughout the whole genome (i.e. the 22 pairs of autosomes and the sex chromosomes), only became possible after the discovery of markers based on variation in DNA length. The first of these were the restriction fragment length polymorphisms and these have largely been supplanted by single nucleotide polymorphisms (SNPs). Informative combinations of markers are known as haplotypes. The Human Genome Project has led to a detailed map of common variation in the human genome. This public database of more than one million SNPs[10] provides information about the patterns of linkage disequilibrium between these markers that can guide selection of 'tagging SNPs' for gene mapping studies. Such marker maps allow the genes contributing to traits or diseases to be located. The methods for mapping are linkage and association. Gene mapping is discussed further in Section 2.4.2.

Gene regulation

The human genome is much more complex than previously thought.[11] Gene activity and expression (the process by which proteins are made) is regulated by inherited DNA and RNA, non-inherited mechanisms (epigenetics), endogenous biological factors such as hormones and environmental factors operating externally to the individual organism (e.g. toxins, psychosocial stress).

For example, non-coding sequences of DNA were previously thought to be 'junk DNA'. There is increasing evidence that this is not the case and that such regions may play an important role in regulating gene activity. Gene activity is also altered by environmental factors.[11] Animal studies have now shown that environmental factors can alter the genome through measurable biological mechanisms, that these changes can be passed onto the next generation and be subject to modification. For example, maternal care giving behaviour early in life, notably high levels of licking and grooming of rat pups, has an effect on brain glucocorticoid receptor expression and sensitivity to stress in the offspring.[12] This effect is observable even when non-genetically related pups are fostered to mothers who have low levels of licking. This 'programming effect' appears to be mediated by structural modifications of DNA. The molecular mechanisms explaining this 'epigenetic marking' are beginning to be identified and include DNA methylation and histone acetylation. These non-inherited effects persist over two generations and in animals appear to be possibly reversible.

Linkage

In linkage studies, rather than just studying the segregation of a disease in families, the co-segregation of the disease and a set of genetic markers is investigated. The aims are, first, to detect linkage, indicated by the disorder and the marker co-occurring more often than would be expected by chance (i.e. not showing Mendelian independent assortment) and, second, to estimate the distance between a linked marker and the gene conferring to susceptibility to the disorder.

It is possible to detect linkage only in families containing at least one parent who is a double heterozygote (i.e. heterozygous at both the marker and the disease loci). Technically such families are referred to as double back-cross or intercross/intercross matings but, for simplicity, we will just focus on the double back-cross type (Table 2.4.1.1). The table shows a double heterozygote parent where the alleles *A* and *B* are on one chromosome with *a* and *b* on the other. Consequently offspring of the types *aaBb* or *Aabb* result from recombination or crossing over between the homologous pair of chromosomes during meiosis. These types of offspring are called **recombinants**. Offspring of the same type as the parents (i.e. *AaBb aabb*) are non-recombinant. We can then simply define the recombination fraction, θ, as the number of recombinants divided by total number of offspring.

For two loci that are very widely separated on the same chromosome (and all pairs of loci carried on to two different chromosomes) independent assortment occurs and $\theta = 1/2$. When the two loci are close together dependent assortment may be observed indicated by a recombination fraction of less than a half. The size of the recombination fraction depends on the physical distance between the two loci and (within certain limits) is proportional to it, so that for loci that are very close together recombination rarely occurs and θ tends to zero. Genetic distances estimated by linkage studies are measured in centimorgans (cM) with 1 cM the equivalent of a recombination fraction of 0.01. For reasons that are not fully understood, recombination occurs more frequently in female than in male meioses. Hence, the size of the female human genome expressed in centimorgans is larger than the male genome. The sex-averaged size of the human genome is about 3700 cM. With reasonable sample sizes major gene effects can be confidently detected over distances of around 10 to 15 cM. Hence, a whole genome search can be carried out using 200 to 300 polymorphic markers, provided they are approximately evenly spaced. A **polymorphism** can be defined as a gene or sequence of DNA that occurs in two or more common forms. Classically, 'common' means an allele frequency of at least 1 per cent. SNP markers are common

Table 2.4.1.1 Double back-cross mating

		Parent 1	*x*	**Parent 2**
		AB/ab		ab/ab
Offspring	*AB/ab* Non-recombinant	*Ab/ab* Recombinant	*aB/ab* Recombinant	ab/ab Non-recombinant
No linkage	1/4	1/4	1/4	1/4
Linkage	$(1-\theta)/2$	$\theta/2$	$\theta/2$	$(1-\theta)/2$

and biallelic. Sometimes combinations of allelic variants across different markers (haplotypes) are analysed in gene mapping studies.

Linkage analysis

The standard method of carrying out linkage analysis in humans is the lod score approach devised by Morton.[9,13] Essentially, for a given set of data, lod scores are calculated over a range of values of θ between 0 and 0.5. Where the lod score reaches a maximum, provides the best (or maximum likelihood) estimate of θ. The lod score is so called because it is the common **l**og of the **od**ds that θ has a certain value θ'; rather than a value of 0.5, i.e.

$$\text{lod} = \log_{10}\frac{\text{probability }(\theta = \theta')}{\text{probability }(\theta = 0.5)}.$$

By convention, a lod of 3 or more is accepted indicating that linkage has been detected, while a lod of -2 or less indicates that linkage can be excluded at that particular value of θ. A lod of 3 corresponds to odds on linkage of 1000:1 and to a nominal P value of 0.0001. This therefore seems at first sight to be a very stringent criterion. However, linkage between two loci taken at random is inherently unlikely[13] and Morton's[9] original argument took into account the low prior probability of linkage to arrive at a criterion that gave a posterior probability, or reliability, of 95 per cent. More recently researchers have been concerned about the effects of carrying out many statistical tests in a genome-wide search for linkage and have sought to set an approp riate level of lod score to compensate for this. In fact, as it turns out, the original suggestion of a lod of about 3 is close to recent calculations of what lod is required to conclude in favour of genome-wide significance.[13]

As originally devised, the lod method deals purely with regular Mendelian traits. However, it can be readily adapted for detection of single genes that have incomplete penetrance by applying the general single major locus model discussed earlier. The main drawback is that the model (as specified by the penetrance values, and less critically the gene frequency) must be known accurately. Where the model is mis-specified there is a high risk that linkage will fail to be detected.

A further difficulty is that diseases may show locus heterogeneity, i.e. there may be two or more different (and unlinked) loci where mutations result in similar phenotypes. There are many instances of this among rare Mendelian diseases. A good example is Usher's syndrome causing deafness and retinitis pigmentosa, which can result from mutations in any one of six different genes. Subforms of common diseases can also show locus heterogeneity, the most relevant to psychiatry being early onset familial Alzheimer's disease where autosomal dominant forms can result from mutations in three different genes, called presenilin 1, presenilin 2, and amyloid precursor protein. Although methods exist for detecting linkage in the presence of heterogeneity these have not so far in practice been of great help in psychiatric or other common disorders. Rather, the most frequent general strategy has been to focus on multiplex families (i.e. those containing multiple members with the disorder under study) and to make the following simplifying assumptions.

1 There are major gene subforms of the disorder in at least some families.

2 Although the mode of transmission is unknown, a reasonable guess at the defining parameters can be made.

3 Although there may be locus heterogeneity in the disorder as a whole, within any given family there is likely to be homogeneity.

This has worked very well for several disorders, including, as we have just mentioned, Alzheimer's disease, but it initially produced a rather confusing set of results from studies of schizophrenia and bipolar disorder. The most likely cause of this is that assumption 1 is incorrect and that subforms of these conditions resulting from major genes are very rare or perhaps non-existent. Consequently most recent studies use other linkage methods that do not rely on any assumptions about the mode of transmission. These concentrate on affected siblings or other pairs of relatives both affected by the disorder.

Methods based on relative pairs

The underlying principle of the affected sib-pair approach is simple. For any given locus the probabilities that siblings share 0, 1, or 2 alleles that are identical by descent from their parents is respectively ¼, ½, ¼. On the other hand, if both members of a sib pair are affected by the same disease and we are studying a locus close to a gene that confers susceptibility to that disease, there will be increased allele sharing. This will occur irrespective of the mode of transmission of the susceptibility gene and hence simple non-parametric statistics can be used to test whether there is any perturbation of the expected identical-by-descent proportions. Affected sib-pair methods are therefore robust and are now generally considered to be the method of choice in detecting linkage in oligogenic or polygenic disorders. In order to be certain that a pair of siblings share alleles identical by descent, one needs to know their parents' genotypes. Otherwise it could be that a shared allele identical by state results from one of the pair having inherited it from the father and the other from the mother. However, an advantage of using highly polymorphic single sequence repeat polymorphisms is that it may not always be necessary to genotype parents, i.e. where the population is reasonably homogenous and where gene frequencies can be estimated, it is possible to compute the likelihood that a pair who share one or two alleles identical by state are truly identical by descent. This means that in return for a fairly modest reduction in power (because one is now dealing with a probability rather than a certainty of counting alleles that are identical by descent) there is a halving in the amount of genotyping that needs to be done.[20] In our own experience, the other advantage of being able to make do without parental genotypes is that they are often difficult to obtain in adult-onset disorders such as schizophrenia. Significant regions of genetic linkage for disorders, notably schizophrenia, bipolar disorder, and autism that have been shown across different studies or found in pooled analyses have now been identified. Another use of sib-pair methods is in studying continuous traits (e.g. height, weight, personality test scores) to attempt to detect the quantitative trait loci that contribute to their heritability.[14] One approach is to select probands who have extreme scores on some quantitative measure and investigate the extent to which marker allele sharing by siblings predicts the regression to the population mean of the siblings' scores.[14] This has been successfully used in mapping a quantitative trait locus contributing to reading ability in children. Unfortunately the drawback of such methods and of sib-pair linkage approaches generally is that they are only capable of detecting moderately large effects. This means that a quantitative trait locus contributing less than about

10 per cent of the variance, or a disease susceptibility locus conferring a relative risk of less than 2, will probably require very large samples running into several hundreds, perhaps thousands, of pairs. If we assume that most common diseases and complex behaviours involve the combined action of many genes of small effect, complementary strategies based on allelic association are required.

Association

In their classic form, allelic association studies are more straightforward to carry out than linkage studies. A sample of cases affected by a disorder (or subjects who have scores higher than a given threshold on a quantitative measure) is compared with controls who do not have the disorder (or subject whose scores are near average). The frequency of alleles at the marker locus is then compared in the two groups. The significance of the difference can then be compared in the usual way for contingency table analysis using a χ^2 test (or Fisher's exact test if expected frequencies are small). In addition to significance it is useful to have a measure of the strength of association. A variety of statistics can provide this but probably the most useful and intuitively appealing is the **relative risk**, i.e. the proportion of cases among those carrying the marker allele or risk factor, P_1, divided by the proportion of cases among those not carrying the factor, P_2. As we can calculate from Table 2.4.1.2, RR = $P_1/P_2 = (a/(a+b))/(c/(c+d))$. If the disorder is uncommon, i.e. a and c are small relative to b and d, RR can be approximated by another, easier-to-obtain statistic, the odds ratio, OR = $a \times d/(b \times c)$. If a positive marker disease association has been found the odds ratio will be significantly greater than 1.

Before the current era of molecular genetics many association studies of disease with classical markers were carried out most notably with blood groups and with the HLA system. One of the earliest well-replicated findings was an association between blood group O and duodenal ulcer. The odds ratio was less than 2 in most studies and Edwards(15) pointed out that the proportion of variance in liability to the disorder explained by the association was only about 1 per cent. Even though later disease association studies on HLA, with other diseases such as type I diabetes and various auto immune disorders were stronger, it has been pointed out that here too only a small proportion of variance is accounted for. Although this could in one respect be considered disappointing, it demonstrates that allelic association can detect small gene effects in polygenic or multifactorial traits and may therefore prove to be more useful than linkage.

How does allelic association arise and what does its detection tell us? There are three principal mechanisms of association. The first is linkage disequilibrium. Normally pairs of alleles at two different loci occur together no more often than would be expected by chance (i.e. they are in 'equilibrium'). In most cases this is the result of independent assortment. However, even if loci are linked they will usually approach equilibrium very rapidly with the proportion of associated alleles decreasing by $1 - \theta$ each generation. Only where the two loci are very close together does disequilibrium tend to persist. For example, where the distance is 1 cM corresponding to a recombination rate of one meiosis in 100, the time taken for an association to go half way to equilibrium is 69 generations. For a distance of 0.1 cM the time taken is 693 generations, or about 20 000 years. The second cause of association is when a polymorphism within a gene itself has a functional effect which results in susceptibility to a disease. The third, and in most cases least interesting, phenomenon is population stratification. This occurs where there has been recent admixture of populations or two or more ethnically distinct populations living side by side with little interbreeding. If the populations differ in terms of the frequency of alleles of the genetic markers and in the frequency of the disease being studied, marker disease associations can arise if there is not careful ethnic matching of patients and controls.

Table 2.4.1.2 Case-control allelic association

Marker	*N* affected	*N* unaffected
Present	*a*	*b*
Absent	*c*	*d*

Another way of overcoming stratification is not to study unrelated cases and controls but to study families and derive the controls 'internally'. The most familiar method in current use is the transmission disequilibrium test.(16) This requires affected individuals to have at least one parent who is heterozygous at the test locus. The affecteds can therefore each receive one of two alleles from such parents. A 2 × 2 contingency table can then be constructed on whether a particular allele is the transmitted or the non-transmitted allele. This is illustrated in Table 2.4.1.3 for a marker with two alleles, A_1 and A_2. The entries in each cell of the table, a, b, c, and d are counts of the number of parents transmitting or not transmitting each allele to their affected offspring. The significance of the transmission disequilibrium test is simply assessed by a McNemar χ^2 test.

Finally, it is becoming increasingly accepted to actually test for population stratification in the laboratory by examining whether random gene variants not thought to be involved in disease, differ in cases and controls. Assuming that stratification can be overcome there are broadly two ways to proceed with association studies. The first is candidate gene association studies and the second is whole genome association studies.

(a) Candidate gene association studies

Functional candidate gene studies concentrate on polymorphisms in or near genes that encode for proteins that are likely to be involved in the disorder. This has so far been the commonest type of association study in psychiatry as in most other common diseases, and there are some interesting early results relating to, for example, polymorphisms at the serotonin *5-HT$_{2a}$* receptor gene in schizophrenia(17) and the dopamine *D4* receptor gene in attention-deficit-hyperactivity disorder.(18) Positional candidate gene studies involve selecting genes that are in regions implicated by linkage.

Table 2.4.1.3 Transmission disequilibrium test: affected subjects with at least one parent heterozygous for allele A

	Non-transmitted	
Transmitted	A_1	A_2
A_1	*a*	*b*
A_2	*c*	*d*

X^2.1 df = $(b-c)^2/(b+c)$

This approach, fine mapping using association to narrow down a region discovered by linkage, has for example resulted in identification of a susceptibility locus, *KIAA0319*,[19] involved in reading disability. Another positional strategy involves obtaining clues about the potential position of a susceptibility gene from individual families who present with a disorder and have a specific region of a chromosome disrupted. For example, a study of Scottish families with translocations involving a region on chromosome 1 and schizophrenia and bipolar disorder led to identification of a susceptibility gene *DISC1* for schizophrenia.[20]

(b) Whole genome association (WGA) studies

The second approach, which has only recently become technically feasible, is to attempt a systematic search through the entire genome with the aim of detecting linkage disequilibrium or direct association. It follows from what we have discussed earlier that a genome-wide search for linkage disequilibrium or direct association has a particular attraction in the study of polygenic disorders in that it should be capable of detecting genes of small effect. Very high throughput genetic analysis involves hydridizing DNA into many thousands of oligonucleotides on microarrays and allows a very large number of biallelic single nucleotide polymorphisms (SNPs) to be tested very rapidly and at comparatively low cost. Cost can be reduced even further by performing the initial screening by DNA pooling. Such methods[21] combine samples from groups of patients and groups of controls processing them in batches. Positive findings can then be followed up by doing individual genotyping. Thus if pools consist of say 100 individuals, the initial cost of genotyping is reduced 100-fold. Against this, some information is lost by DNA pooling and accurate construction of pools is difficult and time consuming. The problem of multiple testing can be overcome either (as in the DNA pooling approach), by carrying out a two-stage analysis with fairly liberal test criteria in the first stage followed by stringent criteria in the second stage, or by simply setting a very stringent criterion at the beginning. It has been shown for example that, even with an alpha level set at 1×10^{-6}, detection of linkage disequilibrium with genes of small effect is feasible with realistic sample sizes.

As we write, WGA studies are being completed using commercially available microarrays containing 500 000 SNPs.[22] Such studies present formidable challenges including the need for very large samples of subjects to provide adequate power of detection and problems of multiple testing and handling of huge amounts of data. Nevertheless, WGA studies have already led to the identification of susceptibility genes for common non psychiatric disorders (e.g. macular degeneration and diabetes) and the initial results of several WGA studies of psychiatric disorders including schizophrenia, bipolar disorder, and ADHD will soon be available or have already been published.[23]

Molecular genetic studies investigating gene–environment interplay and intermediate phenotypes

Genetic variants do not necessarily confer risk for a psychiatric disorder unless in the presence of a specific environmental risk factor. Molecular genetic studies allow a direct test of whether the association of a specific gene variant with disorder is contingent upon exposure to a specific environmental factor. There are a number of important methodological issues that need to be considered when investigating G × E.[24] Most importantly, in testing for G × E, there is the problem of multiple testing given the potential for testing a large number of gene variants and environmental risk factors. Thus, there need to be good *a priori* hypotheses before selecting a specific gene variant and environmental measure. Despite these caveats, there is increasing evidence of the likely importance of G × E in psychiatry as a number of findings have now been replicated. The presence of G × E also provides one potential explanation (amongst others) for non-replication of genetic association findings across different studies.

To date the strongest evidence of G × E has been for a gene variant that affects MAOA enzymatic activity and which appears to increase the risk of antisocial behaviour only in the presence of childhood maltreatment.[25] There is also evidence to suggest that possession of a gene variant that affects function of the serotonin transporter (5HTT) increases the risk of depression in the presence of life events.[26,27] A potentially clinically important type of G × E research is pharmacogenetics. Here the aim is to identify genetic variants that influence clinical response and the risk of side-effects upon exposure to specific types of medication. The hope is that such approaches may lead to a more individually tailored approach to prescribing.

As gene variants associated with psychiatric disorder are identified, and variants that affect gene function recognized, there is an increasing need to identify the intermediate biological pathways and mechanisms. This has led to an increasing amount of research on potential intermediate phenotypes that may account for the link between risk factor and psychiatric outcome. Most interest to date has focused on measures of brain function and structure, assessed through imaging studies[28] as well as neurocognitive, biochemical, and physiological traits. For example, the functional variant in the 5HTT that is associated with depression in the presence of adverse life events appears to be associated with amygdala hyper-responsivity to stress. There is also some evidence that a functional COMT gene variant plays an important role in dopamine clearance in the prefrontal cortex and is associated with prefrontal cortical functioning, assessed through cognitive task performance and fMRI. It is hoped that this new era of imaging genetics together with other areas of neurobiological research will help elucidate the risk pathways that lead from genetic and environmental risk factors to psychiatric disorder.

Further information

Kendler, K.S. and Prescott, C.A. (2006). *Genes, environment and psychopathology: understanding the causes of psychiatric and substance use disorders*. Guilford Publications. New York.

Rutter, M. (2006). *Genes and behavior: nature-nurture interplay explained*. Blackwell, Oxford.

Institute of Medicine Board on Health Sciences Policy. (2006). *Genes, behaviour and the social environment: moving beyond the nature nurture debate*. The National Academies Press, Washington DC (http://www.nap.edu).

References

1. Rutter, M., Moffitt, T.E. and Caspi, A. (2006). Gene-environment interplay and psychopathology: multiple varieties but real effects. *Journal of Child Psychology and Psychiatry, and Allied Disciplines*, **47**(3–4), 226–61.

2. Neale, M.C. and Cardon, L R. (1991). *Methodology of genetic studies of twins and families*. Kluwer, Dordrecht, The Netherlands.
3. Kendler, K.S. and Prescott, C.A. (2006). *Genes, environment, and psychopathology: understanding the causes of psychiatric and substance use disorders*. Guilford Press, New York.
4. D'Onofrio, B.M., Turkheimer, E.N., Eaves, L.J., *et al.* (2003). The role of the children of twins design in elucidating causal relations between parent characteristics and child outcomes. *Journal of Child Psychology and Psychiatry, and Allied Disciplines*, **44**(8), 1130–44.
5. Plomin, R., DeFries, J.C., Craig, I.W., *et al.* (eds.) (2003). *Behavioral genetics in the postgenomic era*. APA Books, Washington, DC.
6. De Fries, J.C. and Fulker, D.W. (1988). Multiple regression analysis of twin data: etiology of deviant scores versus individual differences. *Acta Geneticae Medicae et Gemellolologiae*, **37**, 205–16.
7. Jaffee, S.R., Caspi, A., Moffitt, T.E., *et al.* (2004). The limits of child effects: evidence for genetically mediated child effects on corporal punishment but not on physical maltreatment. *Developmental Psychology*, **40**(6), 1047–58.
8. Kendler, K.S., Kessler, R.C., Walters, E.E., *et al.* (1995) Stressful life events, genetic liability, and onset of an episode of major depression in women. *American Journal of Psychiatry*, **152**(6), 833–42.
9. Morton, N.E. (1982). *Outline of genetic epidemiology*. Karger, Basel.
10. International HapMap Consortium. (2005). A haplotype map of the human genome. *Nature*, **437**(7063), 1299–320.
11. Rutter, M. (2006). *Genes and behaviour. Nature-nurture interplay explained*. Blackwell, Oxford.
12. Meaney, M.J. and Szyf, M. (2005). Maternal care as a model for experience-dependent chromatin plasticity? *Trends in Neurosciences*, **28**(9), 456–63.
13. Morton, N.E. (1955). Sequential tests for the detection of linkage. *American Journal of Human Genetics*, **7**, 277–318.
14. Fulker, D.W. and Cardon, L.R. (1994). A sib-pair approach to interval mapping of quantitative trait loci. *American Journal of Human Genetics*, **54**, 1092–103.
15. Edwards, T.H. (1965). The meaning of the associations between blood groups and disease. *Annals of Human Genetics*, **29**, 77–83.
16. Spielman, R.S., McGinnis, R.E., and Ewenst, W.J. (1993). Transmission test for linkage disequilibrium: the insulin gene region and insulin-dependent diabetes mellitus (IDDM). *American Journal of Human Genetics*, **52**, 506–16.
17. Owen, M.J., Craddock, N., and O'Donovan, M.C. (2005). Schizophrenia: genes at last? *Trends in Genetics*, **21**(9), 518–25.
18. Thapar, A., O'Donovan, M., and Owen, M.J. (2005). The genetics of attention deficit hyperactivity disorder. *Human Molecular Genetics*, **14**(Spec No. 2), R275–82.
19. Cope, N., Harold, D., Hill, G., *et al.* (2005). Strong evidence that KIAA0319 on chromosome 6p is a susceptibility gene for developmental dyslexia. *American Journal of Human Genetics*, **76**(4), 581–91.
20. Porteous, D.J., Thomson, P., Brandon, N.J., *et al.* (2006). The genetics and biology of DISC1—an emerging role in psychosis and cognition. *Biological Psychiatry*, **60**(2), 123–31.
21. Daniels, J.P., Holmans, P., Williams, N., *et al.* (1998). A simple method for analysing microsatellite allele image patterns generated from DNA pools and its application to allelic association studies. *American Journal of Human Genetics*, **62**, 1189–97.
22. Carlson, C.S., Eberle, M.A., Kruglyak, L., *et al.* (2004). Mapping complex disease loci in whole-genome association studies. *Nature*, **429**(6990), 446–52.
23. Wellcome Trust Case Control Consortium (2007). Genome-wide association study of 14, 000 cases of seven common diseases and 3,000 shared controls. *Nature*, **447**(7145), 661–78.
24. Moffitt, T.E., Caspi, A., Rutter, M. (2005). Strategy for investigating interactions between measured genes and measured environments. *Archives of General Psychiatry*, **62**(5), 473–81.
25. Kim-Cohen, J., Caspi, A., Taylor, A., *et al.* (2006). MAOA, maltreatment, and gene-environment interaction predicting children's mental health: new evidence and a meta-analysis. *Molecular Psychiatry*, **11**(10), 903–13.
26. Caspi, A., Sugden, K., Moffitt, *et al.* (2003). Influence of life stress on depression: moderation by a polymorphism in the 5-HTT gene. *Science*, **301**(5631), 386–9.
27. Kendler, K.S., Kuhn, J.W., Vittum, J., *et al.* (2005). The interaction of stressful life events and a serotonin transporter polymorphism in the prediction of episodes of major depression: a replication. *Archives of General Psychiatry*, **62**(5), 529–35.
28. Meyer-Lindenberg, A. and Weinberger, D.R. (2006). Intermediate phenotypes and genetic mechanisms of psychiatric disorders. *Nature Reviews. Neuroscience*, **7**(10), 818–27.

2.4.2 Molecular genetics

Jonathan Flint

Introduction

The transformation of the LOD score (an acronym for log of the odds ratio), from obscurity as a footnote in medical genetics, to celebrity as multiple choice test item in professional examinations in psychiatry, epitomizes the invasion of genetics, and particularly molecular genetics into psychiatric research. Moreover, like other celebrities caught up in fast moving fields, LOD scores are likely to return to their humble origins within a few years. As molecular genetic approaches to mental health move away from simply identifying genes and DNA sequence variants towards functional studies of increasing complexity, newcomers to the field have to master an expanding literature that covers diverse fields: from quantitative genetics to cell biology, from LOD scores to epigenetics. This chapter takes on the task of making the reader sufficiently familiar with the broad range of subjects now required to follow the progress of psychiatric genetics in the primary literature.

A number of achievements have to be highlighted. Foremost among these is the completion of the human genome project. Announced annually from 2001[1–3] and thereby begging the question as to what constitutes completion, the human genome project is now an essential biological resource. As expected, the ability to sequence whole genomes has transformed the way genetics is carried out, perhaps most egregiously with the rise of bioinformatics as a core discipline: discovery now takes place using the internet rather than the laboratory. Anyone with an interest in human biology should look at the frequently updated information at http://www.ensembl.org or http://genome.ucsc.edu.

Without the human genome two other critical developments would have been impossible: the ability to analyse the expression of every gene in the genome and the ability to analyse (theoretically at least) every sequence variant. Both developments also depend on miniaturization technologies that enable the manufacture and interrogation of initially thousands and then millions of segments of DNA. In addition, results from the International Haplotype Map (HapMap) project,[4] which catalogues common variation in the human genome have been crucial in making it possible to take apart the genetic basis of common, complex disorders such as depression, schizophrenia, and anxiety.

Few disciplines are more burdened with jargon than molecular genetics. This is partly due to the proliferation of molecular techniques, but it is also partly intrinsic to the subject; the only unifying principle is evolution, which often operates in a very ad hoc fashion. Biological solutions to the problems posed by selection result in the adaptation of existing structures to new uses, rather than to the invention of purpose-built systems. Consequently there are few general lessons to be learnt and the novice simply has to become adept at recognizing the acronyms and neologisms that decorate the literature. The material in this chapter aims to equip the reader with the necessary terminology. It begins with the structure and function of DNA, an essential starting place for a number of reasons.

Nucleic acid structure and function

The chemical constituents of genetic information are deoxyribonucleic acid (**DNA**) and ribonucleic acid (**RNA**). Both molecules consist of linear chains of nitrogenous bases bound to a sugar (ribose) and a phosphate backbone. Because of the way the sugars are joined together, one end of each nucleic acid strand will have a terminal sugar residue in which the carbon atom at position number 5 of the ribose molecule is not linked; the other end has a free carbon atom at position 3. These two ends are termed the 5′ (5 prime) and 3′ (3 prime) ends respectively.

It is usual to describe a DNA or RNA sequence by writing the order of bases in a single strand, in the 5′ to 3′ direction. DNA contains four nitrogenous bases: adenine (A), guanine (G), cytosine (C), and thymine (T). RNA differs in that it contains uracil instead of thymine.

Two structural differences between DNA and RNA are important for understanding nucleic acid function. First, DNA has a hydroxyl group on part of its sugar constituent whereas RNA has a hydrogen atom. The result is that, in most biological environments, RNA is much more unstable than DNA. Second, RNA normally exists as a single molecule, whereas DNA is a double helix in which two strands are held together by weak hydrogen bonds between opposed base pairs (**bp**), C joined to G and A to T. The sequence of one strand can therefore be inferred from the other. The two strands are said to be complementary to each other, and this property is exploited whenever DNA is copied (during meiosis, mitosis, or *in vitro* processes such as amplification of DNA using a polymerase chain reaction).

As befits an unstable molecule, RNA mediates the expression of genetic information; its production and degradation are tightly controlled. RNA is translated into a linear order of amino acids in proteins according to a three-letter code (e.g. GAA encodes the amino acid glutamine). DNA acts as a template for the production of RNA in a process termed as transcription. But DNA is more than a stable repository of encoded protein sequence information; it also contains information that controls the transcription of RNA.

Disorders of the template function of DNA are the molecular basis of inherited dispositions and illness, and are the subject matter of genetics. By contrast, gene expression (the transcription and translation of RNA) is not entirely genetically predetermined. It is highly regulated, but in response to changes in the cellular environment which in turn reflect changes in the state of the organism. Disorders of gene regulation are now emerging as important causes of disease.

Genome organization

DNA within cells is packaged into chromosomes in the cell nucleus, with a tiny amount (16 569 bases containing 37 genes) in the mitochondria. Since mitochondria in the fertilized egg are maternally derived, mitochondrial inheritance is through the female lineage. Although small, mitochondrial disorders contribute substantially to degenerative disorders including ageing. More important is nuclear DNA.

As of 2007, the size of the nuclear genome is 3 253 037 807 bp (3.3 gigabases) containing 21 662 known and 1064 novel genes (http://www.ensembl.org). Packing such a large molecule into a cell is done at a number of levels, with profound consequences for gene function. At the first level, 147 bp lengths of DNA are wrapped around octamers of proteins known as histones. These nucleosomes are the fundamental units of the state of packaged DNA known as chromatin.

Packaged DNA is itself organized into 22 autosomal chromosomes, one inherited from the mother and one from the father, and two sex chromosomes, X and Y. Each chromosome pair exchanges stretches of DNA during sexual division (meiosis) in a process called recombination (without which genetic mapping, the basic method of finding disease genes, would be impossible). Chromosomes have three functional elements: origins of replication, centromeres, and telomeres. Replication origins are required to initiate DNA replication and maintain chromosome copy number. Their molecular structure is unknown. Centromeres are responsible for the segregation of chromosomes during cell division. Their molecular nature is also not understood, but they are visible in light microscopy as a constriction where the duplicated chromosomes (called chromatids) are held together. Chromosomes are said to have two arms, separated by the centromere which, despite its name, is not always at the centre. Short arms are termed p (*petit*) and long arms q (*queue*). Telomeres are the ends of chromosomes and their molecular nature is well understood. They consist of long stretches of the sequence TTAGGG without which the chromosome is unstable, tending to break apart and fuse with itself or to other chromosomes.

No one has found any general principles that organize genetic material within chromosomes. Rather than being an efficiently organized plan of the organism consisting of precise drawings, the genome resembles a working copy written over countless rough drafts and discarded versions, among which there are literally thousands of jottings and scribbles, most irrelevant to the final structure. While there are examples of gene families clustered in the same chromosomal location (for instance genes involved in immune regulation are clustered on chromosome 6p), more commonly the position of genes on chromosomes does not reflect functional similarity. For example, genes expressed only in one tissue, or at one stage of development, are often immediately adjacent to widely expressed housekeeping genes.

Genes and the regulation of gene expression

DNA is transcribed into RNA, which in turn is translated into protein. Transcription involves the excision of large portions of transcribed RNA (by RNA splicing enzymes) and modifications to the ends of the RNA molecule (capping of one end and polyadenylation of the other). The final product, messenger RNA (**mRNA**), contains a central section, translated into protein, and flanking non-coding regions. The consequence of these manipulations is that DNA and mRNA are not coterminous; sections of DNA that encode mRNA (termed exons) are interrupted by often very large stretches of DNA that are not translated (termed introns) (Fig. 2.4.2.1).

Gene expression is controlled in a number of ways, predominantly at the level of transcription (but posttranscriptional processing and translational control are important for some genes). While knowledge in this area is still rudimentary, but advancing fast, it has already led to new insights in disease aetiology: understanding theories of the neurobiology of depression now requires familiarity with chromatin remodelling; epigenetic effects are often invoked in molecular biology of intellectual disability. Below I summarize information about the relevant molecular processes.

1. **Transcription factors:** transcription factors exercise control over gene expression. Transcription occurs when RNA polymerases manufacture RNA from the template DNA, a process that requires the help of transcription factors, proteins that recognize and bind to specific DNA sequences (note that transcription factors can also repress transcription). Although transcription factor-binding sites are found close to a gene, at a 5′ region known as the promoter (see Fig. 2.4.2.1), they may also be situated far away, sometimes within other genes. The characterization of these control elements remains a major challenge for genome research and is currently a focus of the ENCODE project, a continuation of the human genome project whose aim is the comprehensive identification of all the functional elements in our genome (http://genome.ucsc.edu/ENCODE/).

   Transcription factors typically control the expression of a number of genes, reflecting the presence of a hierarchical structure of coordinated gene expression. Consequently mutations in transcription factors have effects on different, seemingly unrelated phenotypes, a phenomenon called pleiotropy. The constellation of phenotypic abnormalities seen in intellectual disability syndromes can be explained in this way. For example mutations in the X-linked ATRX gene result in an anaemia (α-thalassaemia), a characteristic facial appearance, profound developmental delay, neonatal hypotonia, and genital abnormalities.[5] The gene contains sequence motifs indicating that it belongs to a group of proteins that bind to chromatin and is involved in chromatin remodelling, discussed below.[6]

2. **DNA methylation:** gene inactivation is associated with DNA methylation, predominantly the addition of methyl groups to cytosine bases. DNA methylation occurs almost always at CpG dinucleotides, and most CpGs in the genome are methylated.[7] DNA methylation represses gene expression in two ways: first, modification of cytosine inhibits the association of some DNA-binding factors with their DNA recognition sequences, and second proteins that recognize methyl-CpG can repress transcription from the methylated DNA. Methylation of DNA does not change the DNA sequence itself, as it is reversible, but the methylation status is maintained when cells divide. Consequently the change is referred to as epigenetic modification.

   DNA methylation is critical for imprinting, a form of gene regulation in which transcripts are expressed from only one of the two parental chromosomes. Although there are relatively few imprinted genes (about 60 are currently documented, although sequence features in the region of known imprinted promoters implicate 600) imprinting is an important phenomenon in neurobiology for three reasons[8]: (i) There is evidence from studies of embryos that maternally expressed genes enhance and paternally expressed genes reduce brain size, indicating that at least some imprinted genes are likely to be involved in neurodevelopment.[9] (ii) Disorders of imprinting are important in intellectual disability syndromes: Rett syndrome, Prader–Willi syndrome, Turner syndrome, and Angelman syndrome.[10] (iii) Imprinting is involved in X chromosome inactivation, the mechanism by which cells compensate for males having just one copy of the X chromosome while females have two.[11] The X chromosome contains a disproportionately high density of loci affecting cognition and since males always inherit their X chromosome from their mother, the presence of X-linked imprinted genes is believed to contribute to sexually dimorphic effects.

   The biology of imprinting is complex and not fully understood. In germ cells and in pre-implantation embryos, all methylation

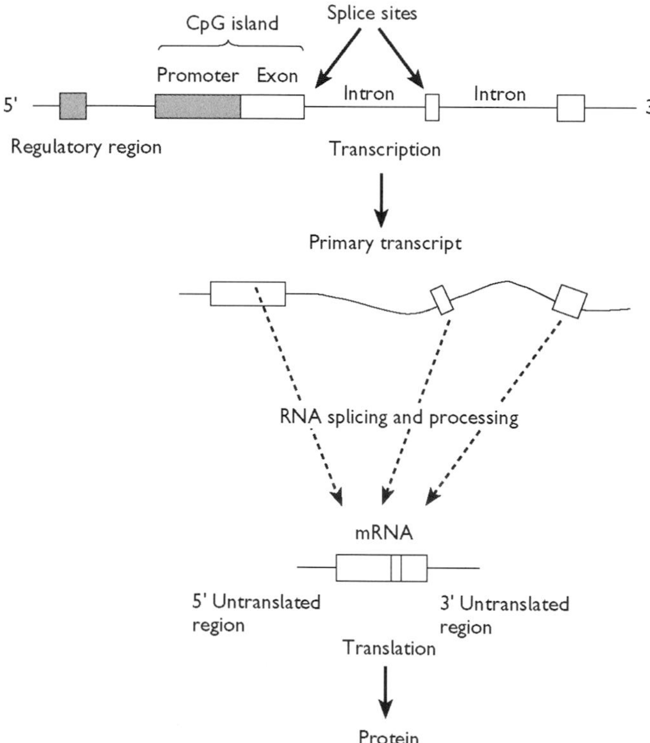

Fig. 2.4.2.1 At the top of the figure the organization of a gene in genomic DNA is shown. Unshaded boxes correspond to coding regions (exons) and the two shaded boxes correspond to control regions. The control region immediately 5′; of the first exon, where transcription is initiated, is known as the promoter and often has a characteristic sequence composition. In almost all ubiquitously expressed genes (and in many tissue-specific genes) it is unmethylated, GC rich, and has a relative excess of the dinucleotide CpG. The region, which typically contains the first exon as well as the promoter, is called a CpG island. The boundaries between exons and introns are called splice sites and are conserved; introns virtually always start with the sequence GT and end with the sequence AG. The entire genomic region is transcribed into a primary transcript (bold arrow) which is then processed to excise the introns. Many human genes undergo alternative splicing to yield a number of different mRNA products. Mature mRNA is then translated into a protein product.

patterns are removed, and then re-established.[12] About half of identified imprinted genes are clustered within imprinting centres (IC) which carry the allele-specific methylation marks established at this developmental stage. Most maternally silenced imprinted genes are repressed by promoter methylation. No protein-coding imprinted gene has been found that is repressed by paternal methylation derived from the sperm (presumably because of active demethylation of the paternal genome). Importantly, paternal repression is achieved, at least in some cases, by using a transcript on the opposite strand (an antisense transcript). Promoter methylation of the antisense transcript (usually resulting from oocyte-derived methylation) represses its transcription and thus activates the protein-coding gene epigenetically.

Some evidence, obtained by examining females with a single X chromosome (Turner syndrome females), indicates that imprinted genes on the sex chromosomes influence brain structure and function.[13] Since the single X chromosome is inherited from either the mother or father, it is possible to compare the effects attributable to a maternally or paternally imprinted chromosome. Maternally expressed X-linked genes have been reported to influence hippocampal development, while paternally expressed genes influence the normal development of the caudate nucleus and thalamus in females. Using Turner syndrome patients, Skuse and colleagues have suggested that a paternally expressed allele is associated with enhanced social–cognitive abilities.[14] A similar observation has been found in a mouse model of Turner syndrome, lending weight to the view that imprinted genes are involved in cognitive processes.[15]

3. **Chromatin remodelling:** the nucleosome forms a barrier to transcription, primarily because DNA has to be free of nucleosomes for it to be accessible to transcription factors and the large complex of proteins that constitutes RNA polymerase. To some extent the organizational information of where nucleosomes are positioned is embedded within DNA sequence, in a nucleosome code; but the nucleosome is not a static unit. It too has dynamic properties and exerts an effect on transcription. Furthermore, like methylation, the effects are heritable, providing a second form of epigenetic modification to DNA (X inactivation also involves this form of epigenetic modification).

   Histones (the proteins that constitute nucleosomes) are subject to a large number of modifications (acetylation, ubiquitination, methylation, ADP-ribosylation, and sumolation of lysine residues; and phosphorylation of serines and threonines) of which two, lysine acetylation and methylation, have been most heavily studied. Histone modifications can influence each other and may also interact with DNA methylation, in part through the activities of protein complexes that bind modified histones or methylated cytosines. These, and other proteins that remodel chromatin, control genes involved in the development and activity of the central nervous system.

   Chromatin remodelling has attracted attention as a possible mechanism for bringing about persistent change subsequent to an environmental stressor.[16] Two examples are relevant. Meaney and colleagues have reported that heritable differences in stress reactivity in rats depend on variation in parenting, not variation in DNA.[17] Adult offspring of mothers that show higher levels of licking, grooming, and arched-back nursing (high-LG-ABN) are less fearful and show more modest hypothalamic-pituitary axis responses to stress than offspring of 'low-LG-ABN' mothers.[18] How are these maternal effects, or other forms of environmental programming, sustained over the lifespan of the animal?

   Variations in maternal care were found to alter the methylation status of a promoter of the glucocorticoid receptor gene. Central infusion of a histone de-acetylase inhibitor enhanced histone acetylation of the glucocorticoid receptor promoter in the offspring of the low-LG-ABN mothers. Analysis of the promoter showed that CpG dinucleotides were hypomethylated. In consequence, the maternal effect on hippocampal glucocorticoid receptor expression and the hypothalamic-pituitary axis response to stress were both eliminated.[19] This finding suggests that there is a causal relation between epigenetic modifications, glucocorticoid receptor expression, and the maternal effect on stress responses.[20]

   Nestler's group invoked chromatin remodelling as an explanation for the long-lasting behavioural change induced by antidepressants.[21] Chronic defeat stress in rodents is reversed by chronic (but not acute) antidepressant treatment, a model for the action of antidepressant action in our own species. Chronic defeat stress and chronic antidepressant treatment are associated with reciprocal, long-lasting changes in expression levels of brain derived neurotrophic factor (BDNF). This is in turn associated with lasting changes in chromatin architecture at the corresponding BDNF gene promoter. Furthermore, down-regulation of a histone de-acetylase (Hdac5) by chronic antidepressant treatment was necessary for the therapeutic efficacy of the antidepressant.

4. **Small RNAs:** small RNAs include micro RNAs (miRNAs) and small interfering RNAs (siRNAs) directly or indirectly alter gene transcription.[22,23] siRNAs, derived from double-stranded RNAs (dsRNAs), control cleavage of other transcripts and can themselves direct the production of dsRNA by RNA-dependent RNA polymerase; they are also implicated in recruiting heterochromatic modification that leads to transcriptional silencing.

   The extent of siRNA involvement in eukaryotic gene regulation is still unclear. Micro RNAs specify posttranscriptional gene repression by base pairing to the messages of protein-coding genes. They represent nearly 1–5 per cent of all genes in higher eukaryotes and have been implicated in developmental timing and neuronal patterning. They are believed to facilitate the transition between developmental stages and therefore are likely to have an effect on the expression and evolution of most mammalian mRNAs.

   Only 3 per cent of the genome codes for protein.[24] However, that is not to say that the remaining 97 per cent is inactive; in fact the number of transcripts is at least 10 times as great as the number of genes.[25,26] What this means in terms of function is not clear, but along with the discovery of small RNAs it has forced a re-evaluation of what is meant by a gene. The idea that a gene is a section of DNA transcribed into RNA, which in turn encodes a protein, fails to capture the gamut of RNA species, some of known function (such miRNAs), some with only suspected function. The emerging complexity of gene function and the multiple species that need to be included in any definition of a gene has dramatically increased our understanding of molecular pathogenesis.

Genetics and genotyping

Chromosomes are not stable structures. They rearrange during meiosis, recombining material between the paternal and maternal chromosomes. The mechanisms of recombination are not relevant for understanding neurobiology, but without recombination we would not be able to track mutations. This section describes the basic methodologies currently used. To follow it, and the many reports in the literature, it is essential to be familiar with genetic terminology. A brief reminder is provided next.

A position on a chromosome is called a locus, a general term which can refer to a gene or a segment of DNA with no known function. DNA sequences that differ at the same locus are called allelic variants. Since we have two copies of each chromosome, by definition we have two alleles at each locus. If these alleles are identical the individual is said to be a homozygote; if they are different, the individual is a heterozygote. It follows that for a locus with two alleles (that is one which is di-allelic, as are the single nucleotide polymorphisms that form the basis of almost all genetic mapping experiments), then there are three possible genotypes. For example, if the alleles are either C or T, the possible genotypes are CC, CT, and TT, whose frequencies in a population, in the absence of migration, mutation, natural selection, and assortative mating, are a simple function of allele frequencies (this phenomenon is termed Hardy–Weinberg equilibrium).

The relationship between alleles at different loci is important for genetic mapping. Assume there are two loci on the same chromosome, separated by approximately 1 megabase (Mb). The loci are again di-allelic, the first with alleles C and T, the second with alleles A and G, so that there are nine possible two-locus genotypes: ATCC, TTCG, AAGG etc. Consequently, the chromosomes of an individual with the two-locus genotype ATCG could be any of the following four: A-C, A-G, T-C, or T-G. This combination of alleles along a chromosome is known as a haplotype. If recombination occurs between the two loci it will break-up the haplotype, so that the offspring of someone with the haplotype A-C on one chromosome and T-G on the other may inherit the novel haplotype A-G. The probability at which this occurs depends on the genetic distance between the two loci. For 1 Mb in the human genome this probability is approximately 1 per cent per meiosis, or 1 cM.

Molecular mapping depends on the availability of genetic markers across the genome. The genome is replete with DNA sequence polymorphisms whose only known use is to enable geneticists to map disease genes. On average, every 1000 bp will contain 1.4 bases that differ between two randomly chosen individuals, almost all of which have no phenotypic consequence. In addition, there are small runs of repeated sequence (most commonly CA) which differ in length between individuals. At least one of these short tandem repeats (**STR**s), or **microsatellites**, is found every 50 kilobases (**kb**) and they also have no known phenotypic consequences. There are other more complex sequence polymorphisms, but single nucleotide polymorphisms (**SNP**s) and microsatellites are the most useful for identifying disease genes.

Genotyping of genetic markers almost always starts by amplifying DNA using the polymerase chain reaction (PCR). PCR requires the following reagents: a DNA polymerase; a pair of oligonucleotides (also referred to as primers), which are synthetic single-stranded DNA, usually between 15 and 25 bases long, complementary to two sequences on opposite strands of the target DNA; the target DNA itself; all four nucleotides, usually present in excess; appropriate buffer and cofactors for the reaction. The reaction proceeds in a cycle of three steps: (1) the mixture is heated to over 90°C for 1 min to separate the complementary strands of target DNA, (2) the mixture is cooled, to about 50°C, so that the oligonucleotides anneal to their complementary sequence in the target DNA and allow the DNA polymerase to bind (oligonucleotides are required to prime the polymerase), and (3) the temperature is adjusted to allow the polymerase to function in the extension component of the reaction. Typically the polymerase is from a thermophilic bacterium with a permissive temperature of 72°C. Products from the first cycle serve as targets for a second round of amplification and so on, for up to about 40 cycles.

The method used to genotyping the PCR product depends on the nature of the sequence variant. Microsatellite genotyping involves discriminating the length of the PCR products, usually accomplished by separating the fragments by electrophoresis, in which an electrical current causes smaller fragments to migrate more quickly than larger fragments through a matrix. Typically a fluorescent label is incorporated into the amplified DNA allowing the PCR products to be detected by a laser, a method that allows automated analysis.

SNP genotypes can also be worked out from differences in molecular weight. For example, the nucleotide added to a primer complementary to sequence immediately preceding a SNP in the PCR fragment will depend on the genotype of the individual. The small difference between a primer with a C nucleotide added to its end (reflecting the presence of a G nucleotide in the PCR fragment) compared to the same primer with the addition of a T nucleotide, can be determined using a mass spectrometer. However, most high-throughput genotyping methodologies (required for whole genome association studies) exploit the specificity of DNA hybridization: while two complementary single strands of DNA stick (or hybridize) together (ATTGAC will anneal to TAACTG) a single base mismatch will prevent hybridization (ATTGAC will not anneal to ATAGAC). Consequently, a SNP can be detected by determining whether primers hybridize to the PCR fragment. By labelling the primers, for example, with a fluorescent dye, the hybridization can be visualized, and, using the same technology that builds computer semiconductors, millions of primers can be manufactured on a small piece of glass, allowing the simultaneous detection of millions of SNPs.

Genetic mapping: linkage and association

For genetic disorders that arise from a mutation in a single gene, behaving in a Mendelian fashion (dominant, recessive, or sex-linked inheritance), disease gene identification is conceptually straightforward. Marker alleles follow Mendelian laws of segregation so that it is possible to determine if a marker is co-segregating with a disease in a family and to test the result statistically using methods described in Chapter 2.4.1. The expected result is an estimate of the probability that an allele and a disease locus will recombine; the lower the probability, the closer together the two loci are on the chromosome. The statistical test gives the likelihood that the estimate of recombination distance between a marker and a mutation is correct. If the likelihood is acceptably high, then the next task is to reduce the genetic interval as much as possible and to identify a causative mutation. Access to the human genome makes it straightforward to identify all genes within a given interval (go to one of the two websites mentioned above) and the ease of DNA sequencing (many companies make this service available) makes it possible to screen candidates by a brute force approach: enough is known about sequence codes to recognize a mutation that will disrupt gene expression, and this can be experimentally verified by looking at the production and structure of mRNA.

A good example of the success of gene mapping in pedigrees is the identification of a mutation in the FOXP2 gene in a family that has a language disorder. The phenotype is complex, including both verbal and non-verbal cognitive impairments. However, the inheritance pattern is straightforward: it fits a model in which a single mutation in one copy of the gene is sufficient to cause disease. By using markers from across the genome, a region on chromosome 7 was identified that co-segregated with the defect and a mutation in a transcription factor, FOXP2, subsequently identified.[27,28]

Pedigree-based linkage works well when the disease follows Mendelian laws of segregation and has led to the identification of many genes involved in intellectual disability and dementia. However, pedigree-based methods for disorders where the genetics does not fit a simple Mendelian pattern have been much less successful. The methods (described in Chapter 2.4.1) typically ask whether affected siblings in a family (usually just a pair) share the same allele at a locus: the more often sharing is observed, the closer the markers locus is inferred to be to the disease gene. The relative failure of the affected sibling pair strategy is almost certainly because of the small contribution that each locus contributes to disease susceptibility.

Neil Risch and Kathleen Merikangas pointed out in 1996 that if the genetic effect size attributable to a single locus is small (that is to say it would increase the risk of developing the disease less than two-fold) then the number of families required using a pedigree method would be impractically large.[29] However, a direct test of association between genetic marker and disease gene had much greater power. Simply by genotyping a marker and determining whether the distribution of genotypes was significantly different between a set of unrelated cases and unrelated controls, small effects could be detected with relatively small sample sizes. The drawback was the need to test variants in every gene, possibly requiring researchers to genotype a million individual markers. Surprisingly, Risch and Merikangas showed that the objection to mounting such a study was not statistical, but technological.

Two advances made whole genome association studies feasible. First, as described above, technologies are available for genotyping on an appropriate scale. Second, an enormous catalogue of SNPs has been compiled. As of April 2007, 11 577 475 SNPs have been identified and mapped on the human genome. Fortunately, not all these variants need to be genotyped for mapping disease genes. It was found that many SNPs were highly correlated with each other, because recombination is less likely to disrupt haplotypes of closely linked markers than of more distantly spaced markers (a phenomenon termed linkage disequilibrium (LD)). Consequently, aetiological variants can be expected to be in LD with one or more SNPs. By genotyping a carefully selected set of markers (called 'tagged SNPs') most of the common variation in the genome can be assayed. However, for this strategy to be practical, a haplotype map of the genome was first required that catalogues the distribution of LD in different populations (since LD patterns are a product of population history, as well as of recombination distance). Genotyping on an immense scale in multiple populations was undertaken by the International Haplotype Map (HapMap) consortium,[4] and the results, regularly updated, are available on the internet (http://www.hapmap.org).

The molecular basis of psychiatric disorders: Mendelian disorders

There are a number of conditions in psychiatry that arise from mutations in single genes (Mendelian mutations). As a rule, such disorders are rare and, importantly, they account for very few, if any, instances of common disorders: depression has never been attributed to a Mendelian mutation (though some single mutations, such as Huntington disease, do include a mood disorder in their phenotype). Nevertheless, rare single gene mutations can provide important clues to the aetiology of more common conditions: for example, mutations in neuroligins, identified as a rare cause of autism, suggest that the pathophysiology lies in abnormalities of synaptic function.

In general, the molecular basis of Mendelian mutations in psychiatry is typical of other human genetic disorders in that they arise primarily from changes to one, or a few, nucleotides. These are described below under the heading point mutations. However, there are two exotica: triplet repeats and imprinting defects.

Point mutations

Changes in a single base pair (e.g. from C to T) of the coding sequence of the gene may alter the function of the protein (**mis-sense mutations**), result in premature termination of the protein product (**non-sense mutations**), or create or destroy a splice site. In addition, deletions (of a single base pair or many megabases of DNA) and insertions (again of any size) disrupt transcription and translation of a gene. Deletions or insertions that do not affect a multiple of three bases alter the way that the message is translated and are known as frame-shift mutations. While none of these mechanisms is special to psychiatric genetics, describing the mutational basis of a genetic disorder is an initial step in understanding how the disorder arises; what the DNA sequence change does to the protein gives a clue to the protein's function (if unknown) and to the pathogenesis of the condition. Analysis of mutants causing dementia, isolated by positional molecular cloning, are an example.

The presenilins are ubiquitously expressed transmembrane proteins in which mutations give rise to about 40 per cent of familial Alzheimer's disease.[30] More than 160 mutations in the presenilin genes have been identified. Almost all are mis-sense mutations. Why are there no frame-shift or non-sense mutants? Mis-sense mutants alter an amino acid in the protein and therefore can alter its function. One clue about the nature of the functional change comes from looking at where mutations occur within the protein, thereby discerning whether some parts of the molecule are more frequently involved than others. The distribution of mutations in the presenilins is indeed non-random; mutations occur at residues which are the same in both presenilin genes, lying on one side of the α helix in transmembrane domains, predominantly in exon 8. Thus the mutational spectrum highlights key residues for understanding the protein's functions.(31,32) The mutations in presenilin result in a gain of function: they alter the ratio of the two forms of amyloid that constitute neuritic plaques, one of the histological hallmarks of the Alzheimer's disease.(33,34)

Where a gene's function is known, the distribution of mutations may reveal the likely pathogenesis. For example, mutations in the tau gene cause frontotemporal dementia with Parkinsonism (Pick's disease).(35,36) The most common mutation occurs in the 5′ splice site of exon 10, resulting in overproduction and accumulation of one form of tau; mutations in other regions of the gene lead to accumulation of a different form of the protein. The position of the mutations in tau indicate that they cause disruption of tau microtubule binding, which may cause cell death by the degeneration of microtubules or through an increase in unbound tau.

Triplet repeats

One mutational mechanism is unusual and deserves special comment: expansion of trinucleotide repeats.(37) Its importance in psychiatry is that it occurs in at least 16 neurological disorders, some with behavioural phenotypes (such as Huntington disease). No one knows why trinucleotide repeat expansions tend to be found in disorders of the central nervous system. The mechanism was first discovered in 1991 as the cause of fragile X syndrome,(38,39) a common form of inherited X-linked intellectual disability.

The mechanism is important because it explains some otherwise unusual features of the phenotype. Table 2.4.2.1 lists the diseases associated with triplet repeats. At each locus there is a normal range of copy numbers above which the repeat array becomes unstable: the larger the number of copies, the more unstable the allele and in general the more severe the disease. Repeats increase and decrease in size both in somatic and germ line tissues, with two important consequences. First, it may not be possible to infer the severity of the condition from a blood test, since the repeat length in the brain may not be the same as in the lymphocytes (this is an example of somatic mosaicism). Second, as the repeat length increases in successive generations, the age of onset may decrease (this is called anticipation). For instance the age of onset of myotonic dystrophy ranges from birth to adulthood.

Genomic rearrangements and gene dosage effects

A number of disorders, primarily those associated with intellectual disability, have been found to be due to chromosomal rearrangements. Down syndrome (trisomy 21) is by far the most common, accounting for about a third of all cases with moderate to severe retardation.(40) Chromosomal rearrangements can be extremely complex, like the nomenclature used to describe them.

Abnormalities of the number of chromosomes result in aneuploidy. Deletion of part or an entire chromosome is termed a monosomy (or haploinsufficiency); an extra copy of either part of or an entire chromosome is called trisomy. A general term to describe either loss or excess of chromosomal material is aneusomy. Most chromosomal abnormalities involve small regions of aneusomy and consequently are known as segmental aneusomy syndromes or contiguous gene syndromes.(41)

Table 2.4.2.1 Triplet repeat diseases

Disease		Repeat unit	Gene	Normal repeat	Expanded repeat	Mechanism
Fragile X syndrome	FRAXA	(CGC)n	FMRP	6–60	>200	Loss of function
Fragile XE syndrome	FRAXE	(CCG)n	FMR2	4–39	200–900	Loss of function
Friedrich ataxia	FRDA	(GAA)n	Frataxin	6–32	>200	Loss of function
Myotonic dystrophy type 1	DM1	(CTG)n	DMPK	5–37	50–10 000	RNA-mediated
Myotonic dystrophy type 2	DM2	(CCTG)n	ZNF9	10–26	>75	RNA-mediated
Fragile X–associated tremor ataxia syndrome	FXTAS	(CGG)n	FMR1	6–60	60–200	RNA-mediated
Huntington disease	HD	(CAG)n	Huntingtin	6–34	36–121	Polyglutamine expansion
Spinocerebellar ataxia	SCA1	(CAG)n	Ataxin1	6–44b	39–82	Polyglutamine expansion
Spinocerebellar ataxia	SCA2	(CAG)n	Ataxin2	15–24	32–200	Polyglutamine expansion
Spinocerebellar ataxia	SCA3	(CAG)n	Ataxin3	13–36	61–84	Polyglutamine expansion
Spinocerebellar ataxia	SCA6	(CAG)n	CACNA1A	4–19	10–33	Polyglutamine expansion
Spinocerebellar ataxia	SCA7	(CAG)n	Ataxin7	4–35	37–306	Polyglutamine expansion
Spinocerebellar ataxia	SCA17	(CAG)n	TBP	25–42	47–63	Polyglutamine expansion
Spinobulbar muscular atrophy	SBMA	(CAG)n	Androgen receptor	9–36	38–62	Polyglutamine expansion
Dentatorubral-pallidoluysian atrophy	DRPLA	(CAG)n	Atrophin	7–34	49–88	Polyglutamine expansion
Spinocerebellar ataxia	SCA8	(CTG)n	SCA8	16–34	>74	Unknown
Spinocerebellar ataxia	SCA10	(ATTCT)n	10–20	500–4500		Unknown
Spinocerebellar ataxia	SCA12	(CAG)n	PPP2R2B	7–45	55–78	Unknown
Huntington disease-like 2	HDL2	(CTG)n	Junctophilin	7–28	66–78	Unknown

The distribution of rearrangements in the genome is not random, reflecting instead the involvement of higher-order architectural features.[42] Regions susceptible to rearrangement are frequently flanked by, or contain, region-specific repeat sequences, or low-copy repeats. In general, recurrent rearrangements, or those of common size and having clustered breakpoints, most frequently result from homologous recombination between repeats.[43]

Chromosomal rearrangements in psychiatric patients other than those with intellectual disabilities are rare, but their occurrence has led to some important discoveries. Deletions on the end of chromosome 22q cause a syndrome that includes a psychosis often indistinguishable from schizophrenia, thus prompting an intense investigation of this region of the genome.[44] Characterization of patients with translocations and psychosis also led to the identification of a gene called DISC1 (for **d**isrupted **in** **sc**hizophrenia)[45] and screening for chromosomal rearrangements in patients with Tourette's syndrome led to the identification of mutations in a Slit and Trk-like family member 1 (SLITRK1) gene.[46]

The phenotypes of chromosomal rearrangements are thought to arise because of the loss, in the case of monosomy, or addition, in the case of trisomy, of dosage-sensitive genes, of unrelated function, that happen to lie next to each other on the chromosome. However this is not always the case, as the examples of Prader–Willi syndrome and Angelman syndrome show.

Imprinting defects

A number of diseases can be attributed to a failure to establish, maintain, or recognize methylation. Rett syndrome is a progressive neurodevelopmental disorder that occurs almost exclusively in females, with an incidence of between 1/10 000 and 1/15 000 live births.[47] Most females with Rett syndrome are usually heterozygous for a *de novo* mutation in methyl-CpG-binding protein MeCP2, a protein that induces the recruitment of protein complexes involved in histone modifications and chromatin remodelling. Prader–Willi syndrome and Angelman syndrome are both caused by loss of function of imprinted genes on the proximal long arm of human chromosome 15.[48] Prader–Willi syndrome occurs if the paternal chromosome 15 is missing, Angelman syndrome if the maternal. In a few per cent of patients the disorder is due to aberrant imprinting and gene silencing.

Non-coding RNA

The discovery that small RNA molecules regulate gene expression has occurred too recently for us to know the importance of mutations in this system as a cause of disease. Examples are however beginning to be reported: a point mutation was shown to create a new promoter, driving a novel transcript that in turn silenced a neighbouring gene.[49] There is one example from neuropsychiatric genetics, in which mutations in the binding site for microRNA hsa-miR-189 have been identified as a cause of Tourette's syndrome.[46] These complex mechanisms are difficult to detect without a detailed understanding of gene regulation, which is likely to come in future years.

The molecular basis of psychiatric disorders: complex disorders

Genetic attempts to dissect common psychiatric conditions have been very slow to yield robust results. For every paper that reports a positive association between a genetic variant and schizophrenia, anxiety or alcohol abuse, another can be found that fails to replicate the finding.[50] There are at least three explanations for the difficulties in arriving at agreement. One is that scientific journals afford more importance to positive than negative results; for example, there have been more than 40 studies investigating the relationship between a variant of the dopamine D2 receptor and alcohol abuse. By plotting the effect size of each study against the year of publication, a clear and statistically significant negative correlation is found: studies with the largest effects are published first.[51] Publication bias almost certainly exists in other studies, but has rarely been systematically examined.

Second, a number of commentators have pointed out that the sparse success of genetic linkage and association studies in complex traits can be explained by the low power of individual studies.[52] Meta-analytic techniques that make it possible to combine data from many individual studies have revealed that the odds ratios attributable to individual susceptibility loci are commonly less than 1.3.[53] Analysis of obesity, Type 2 diabetes and breast cancer shows that it is possible to obtain association results that replicate, but that tens of thousands of subjects are required.[54,55] There is no reason to believe that psychiatric disorders will be any different in this respect; it is simply that no study has reported data from enough cases.

A third reason for the inconsistencies is that interaction between genes can obscure the signal attributable to the main effect of the locus.[56] Gene interaction, or epistasis, means that the phenotype depends on the allelic configuration of a number of loci. For example, if there are two alleles (i and j) at a susceptibility locus on chromosome 1 and two alleles at a susceptibility locus on chromosome 2 (l and m) then in an epistatic interaction disease will only manifest in those individuals with allele i on chromosome 1 and allele m on chromosome 2. Imagine a population in which allele i on chromosome 1 is common. Genetic association tests of the effect of allele m on chromosome 2 will detect an effect. But the same test, when carried out in a population where allele i is rare, will not detect an effect, even though allele m is present at equivalent frequencies in both populations.

Epistasis is suspected to be important, but there are currently no well-documented examples in psychiatric genetics. More attention, and more information, is available for a similar phenomenon called gene by environment interaction (GXE). Interaction between genes and environment is said to occur if disease manifests only when specific alleles are exposed to a given environment. For example, individuals with one allele (called *s* (for short)) at the promoter of the serotonin transporter may have an increased chance of developing depression, but only if they have been exposed to stressful life events.[57] Individuals with the *l* (for long) allele are protected against the effect of this environmental stressor and are less likely to become depressed. GXE hides genetic association in the same way as epistasis. In the presence of GXE, unless differences in the environmental stresses experienced by subjects are taken into consideration, contradictory results may be obtained from testing a genetic association between the serotonin transporter polymorphism and depression in different populations.

The advent of whole genome association studies applied to large case-control cohorts is beginning to unravel the molecular basis of common complex diseases. These studies are proving to be successful, in that they are identifying small numbers of loci that can be replicated in independent samples. However, since most studies find at best a handful of loci contributing to disease susceptibility, the results show that the bulk of the genetic predisposition to complex disease is almost certainly due to loci with much smaller effects than those found to date. There are also indications that many of the variants will be extremely rare, possibly even private to individual families.

One important indicator of the importance of rare variants is the poor coincidence between the location of whole genome association hits and those from linkage studies. It is important to bear in mind that linkage and association are detecting different signals: linkage will detect an effect when there are multiple different variants in the same gene (allelic heterogeneity). However, allelic heterogeneity dramatically reduces the power of genetic association, so that signals will be missed. Re-sequencing of genes has also led to a greater appreciation of the role of rare variants. Although individually rare, non-synonymous sequence variants in certain genes are cumulatively frequent and are known to influence quantitative traits, such as plasma lipoprotein levels[(58)]; it may prove to be true also for behavioural phenotypes.

Finding rare non-synonymous variants in genes should not obscure the importance of aetiological variants that lie outside genes. It had been thought that the spectrum of sequence variants in complex disease would be similar to mutations found from the analysis of Mendelian conditions: that is to say variants in the coding regions of genes, the splice sites, or the promoters. However, SNPs with robust, replicated results for association with complex disease are usually found nowhere near coding regions; they are located outside genes, in regions not known to have any function. Furthermore, when genes implicated by genetic association in psychiatric disease have been entirely sequenced, no obvious abnormalities are seen. This is true, for example, of the genes believed to be involved in schizophrenia (dysbindin and neuregulin).

Genome-scanning technologies have also uncovered an unexpectedly large amount of structural variation in the human genome, including deletions, duplications, and large-scale copy-number variants, as well as insertions, inversions, and translocations. A global survey of copy-number variants identified 1447 regions, covering 360 Mb (a remarkable 12 per cent of the genome), revealing a considerable contribution to overall genetic heterogeneity.[(59)] Critically, these variants were found in supposedly disease-free populations. It is possible that copy-number variants play an important part in the aetiology of common psychiatric disorders. For example, genome-scanning of autism has found copy-number variants in 10 per cent of cases of sporadic autism and in only 1 per cent of controls.[(60)]

Functional analysis

The armamentarium of molecular genetics tools wielded in the onslaught on the genetic basis of psychiatric disorders is impressive, expensive, and at the same time relatively uninformative about the neurobiology of the illnesses. As genes are identified an equally complex technology is being applied to working out what those genes do. The last section of this chapter provides a guide to the relevant molecular biology.

One of the most fruitful ways of investigating gene function is through genetic manipulation of animals, for example, by introducing a copy of the gene into a mouse or mutating the mouse version of the gene. Both approaches work because exogenous DNA can integrate into chromosomes. If the site of integration can be targeted, rather than being random, the exogenous DNA can be used to create mutations in specific genes.

Transgenic mice are made by injecting DNA (usually, but not necessarily, human) into fertilized mouse oocytes. Integration is a rare and random event and almost always involves multiple copies entering at a single site, making interpretation of some transgenic experiments difficult. More specific genetic manipulation is achieved by exploiting homologous recombination in embryonic stem (**ES**) cells. DNA containing a mutated copy of the gene of interest in tandem with a selectable marker (e.g. an antibiotic resistance gene) is introduced into ES cells. In a small number of cases the exogenous DNA recombines with, and consequently replaces, the cell's copy of the gene. ES cells are isolated from embryos and can be grown in flasks while retaining the potential to develop into any tissue. Once they have been genetically manipulated and re-injected back into a pregnant mouse, the resulting embryo is a mixture of mutant and normal cells. If some of the ES cells contribute to the germ line of the embryo, then its offspring will be heterozygote mutants, from which homozygotes can be bred.

One important reservation should be borne in mind when assessing studies that have used gene targeting: the genetic background of a mutant can have an effect on the mutant.[(61)] Most targeting experiments use the ES stem cells derived from substrain 129 mice, which are crossed with another inbred line. The choice of inbred line into which the mutation is bred can be critical because many inbred lines have specific behavioural phenotypes; for instance, the inbred strain DBA/2 shows poor hippocampal-dependent learning and C57BL/6 mice are poor avoidance learners.[(62)]

Improvements in knockout technology have had a major impact on neurobiology. Rather than simply knockout genes, homologous recombination can be used to change part of a gene, for example, by substituting one amino acid to another, a process referred to as a knock-in technology. The development of binary systems, where two engineered lines are crossed, has given experimenters remarkable control over gene expression: genes can now be turned on, or off, by feeding the animal a compound that penetrates to the cell nucleus, such as tetracycline.[(63)] The tetracycline transactivator (tTA) is used as a transcriptional switch to drive the expression of a gene of interest. The tTA system requires the use of two lines of transgenic mice. In one line the expression of the tTA protein is driven by a tissue or cell-type-specific promoter; in the second, a gene of interest is placed downstream of the tet operator (tetO) and a promoter. The tTA protein binds to the tetO sequence and induces transcription. However, when the tetracycline is present, it binds to tTA and prevents it from binding to tetO and this halts transcription.

Binary systems also make it possible to generate mutations that are restricted to specific cell or tissue-types. This is done by introducing sequences recognized by an enzyme, cre recombinase, on either side of the gene of interest. Cre is a site-specific DNA recombinase derived from a bacteriophage that recognizes 34 bp sequences termed loxP sites. Cre catalyses the deletion of DNA flanked by a pair of loxP sites (the DNA is said to be floxed). Again the experimental system requires two lines: in one the gene of interest is floxed; in the other, cre is driven by a tissue-specific promoter so that its expression is restricted to the cells of interest. Consequently, the gene is only deleted in that subset of cells.

Targeted homologous recombination, combined with conditional control, has proved so successful a method for investigating gene function, that three major mouse knockout programmes are underway worldwide, working together to mutate every gene in the mouse genome using this technology. I have chosen a few examples on the application of the technology to illustrate the remarkable power of the approach and reveal why it has generated such interest in the neuroscience research community.

One of the earliest was the genetic demonstration of the effect of a brain-subregion-restricted NMDA receptor knockout on spatial memory.[64] Following the discovery that high-frequency stimulation of the hippocampal input fibres can result in long-lasting enhancement of synaptic transmission, long-term potentiation (LTP) has been subject to extensive investigation. The induction of LTP is blocked by amino-phosphonovaleric acid (AP5), an antagonist of the NMDA subset of glutamate receptors. A voltage-dependent magnesium block and high calcium permeability mean that the receptor can be opened by glutamate only when the postsynaptic neurone is depolarized, thereby allowing the receptor to function as a detector and integrator of coincident activity at the synapse. Unsurprisingly, the demonstration that infusion of AP5 into the ventricles of rats impaired spatial learning generated intense interest in the potential role of the NMDAR as a crucial component of memory. Furthermore, since disorders of working memory have been documented in schizophrenia, NMDAR dysfunction has attracted the attention of psychosis researchers. The genes encoding the receptor were identified in the early 1990s. There are seven subunits (NR1, NR2A–D, and NR3A and B), of which the NR1 subunit is the only one that is indispensable for the formation of a functional receptor.

Functional investigation of the NR1 receptor using gene knockout technology proved to be impossible because NR1-knockout mice do not survive for more than a day after birth: the receptor has a crucial role in the midbrain for breathing. This is a general problem with constitutive knockout technology: lethality before, or just after birth is common. Tonegawa and colleagues used the conditional technology to get over this problem. They floxed the NR1 receptor and crossed the mouse to a line in which cre recombinase was under the control of a promoter of a gene expressed in the hippocampus.[65] Because the recombinase was predominantly active in the CA1 region of the hippocampus, the NR1 gene could be knocked out postnatally in CA1 pyramidal cells.

The mouse strain had apparently normal growth and was fertile, but was severely impaired in a test of spatial learning.[65] Furthermore, recording of neuronal activity indicated a loss of coherent spatial representation in the hippocampus.[66] The conditional knockout provided strong evidence that NMDAR activity and NMDAR-dependent synaptic plasticity in the hippocampus are crucial for spatial learning. The importance of CA1 NMDARs in the acquisition of hippocampus-dependent memory was subsequently extended to various non-spatial tasks, including recognition of novel objects, and fear conditioning.

Advances in genetic engineering have also been critical in shaping views of the neurobiology of anxiety and depression. There are a large number of publications reporting anxiety phenotypes associated with constitutive knockouts, implicating so many genes that as one reviewer points out 'the overall message one takes away from these studies is that normal anxiety requires normal neuronal functioning. Disrupt such functioning in any of a number of different ways and anxiety-like behaviour is likely to be disrupted—not a very specific or informative conclusion'.[67] Application of the more focused molecular technology has been more informative.

Benzodiazepines bind the α-subunit of the pentameric receptor, enhancing the efficacy of GABA in activating the receptor. By introducing a histidine to arginine mutation into the genes encoding each of the α1, α2, and α3 subunits and by testing mutants for behavioural abnormalities, it has been possible to determine that the α2 isoform is responsible for the anxiolytic effects, but not the sedative or amnesic, effects of benzodiazepines in mice.[68–70] These results have encouraged a search for isoform-specific medications, since a drug specific for the α2 subunit might reduce anxiety while having little or no sedative effects.

The importance of developmental, as well as tissue-specific effects, has also emerged from the use of conditional knockouts. While knockouts of the 5-HT1A serotonin receptor indicated the importance of this gene in anxiety, the mechanism by which it exerts an effect was not appreciated until Hen and colleagues developed a tissue-specific, inducible rescue of the 5-HT1A knockout.[71] A mutant line, in which the 5-HT1A promoter was replaced with a tTA responsive element, was crossed with a line in which the tTA protein was under the control of a promoter expressed in the hippocampus and cortex (the CaMKII promoter). The tTA protein induced expression of the 5-HT1A receptor in postsynaptic target tissues, but not in the serotonergic neurones of the dorsal raphe nucleus. Rescue of the knockout restored normal anxiety-like behaviour, demonstrating that the lack of postsynaptic receptors, rather than presynaptic, causes the anxiety phenotype. Furthermore, by giving tetracycline only during adulthood, so that the 5-HT1A receptor was expressed only during development, it was found that the mice behaved like wild type animals. By contrast, when 5-HT1A receptor expression was ablated during development, it was not possible to rescue the phenotype in the adult, demonstrating that stimulation of postsynaptic 5-HT1A receptors during a developmental critical period is required to establish normal patterns of anxiety-like behaviour that then persist into adulthood.

The creation of knockouts should not obscure an equally important application of molecular genetic methods in neuroscience: to augment existing functional tools or to create entirely novel ones. The developments can be categorized into visualization tools and, more recently, tools for intervention.

The ability to visualize proteins in cells has transformed cellular neurobiology. Visualization is made possible by attaching a fluorescent tag, usually green fluorescent protein or one of its congeners, to the DNA encoding the relevant protein. The genome projects have made available complete libraries of cloned DNA, so that it is possible to obtain cloned DNA of any gene. By using homologous recombination in bacteria, any gene can be tagged, and then inserted into the mouse genome, either by targeting or random transgenesis.[72,73] This genetic tagging has made it possible to track gene products spatially and temporally at the highest level of resolution (fluorescently tagged genes expressed in the mouse brain can be seen at http://www.gensat.org). One immediate application of this technology is the identification of sequences that confer tissue-specific gene expression, revealed by the expression of the fluorescent protein. Genes expressed in a specific brain region can then be replaced, rather than tagged, making it possible to target proteins to brain regions.[74] This is one of the key technical requirements for mounting an interventionist approach to neurobiology.

Interventionist tools are set to transform neurobiology from a discipline in which function is inferred by observing the connectivity of the nervous system, into one in which a function can be directly tested by activating its component parts. Sensor proteins, that detect changes in the physiological states of neurones through the emission of light, and actuator proteins that effect such changes in response to an exogenous signal, can be genetically engineered and inserted into organisms using genetic targeting technologies.(75,76) The ability to activate specific cell types through genetically encoded sensors responsive to light will undoubtedly facilitate the exploration of neuronal circuits. These techniques, though still in their infancy and currently most useful in invertebrate model organisms, are likely to have broad applications in neurobiology and will be a critical tool for understanding the function of genes involved in psychiatric disease.

Further information

Strachan, T. and Read, A. (2003). *Human molecular genetics* (3rd Revises edn). Garland Publishing Inc., US.

Alberts, B. (ed.) (2002). *Molecular biology of the cell* (4th Revises edn). Garland Publishing Inc., US.

http://www.genome.ucsc.edu/

http://www.ensembl.org/index.html

http://www.hapmap.org/

References

1. Lander, E.S., Linton, L.M., Birren, B., *et al.* (2001). Initial sequencing and analysis of the human genome. *Nature*, **409**, 860–921.
2. Venter, J.C., Adams, M.D., Myers, E.W., *et al.* (2001). The sequence of the human genome. *Science*, **291**, 1304–51.
3. International-Human-Genome-Sequencing-Consortium. (2004). Finishing the euchromatic sequence of the human genome. *Nature*, **431**, 931–45.
4. Altshuler, D., Brooks, L.D., Chakravarti, A., *et al.* (2005). A haplotype map of the human genome. *Nature*, **437**, 1299–320.
5. Gibbons, R.J., Picketts, D.J., Villard, L., *et al.* (1995). Mutations in a putative global transcriptional regulator cause X-linked intellectual disability with í-thalassemia (ATR-X Syndrome). *Cell*, **80**, 837–45.
6. Gibbons, R.J. and Higgs, D.R. (2000). Molecular-clinical spectrum of the ATR-X syndrome. *American Journal of Medical Genetics*, **97**, 204–12.
7. Klose, R.J. and Bird, A.P. (2006). Genomic DNA methylation: the mark and its mediators. *Trends in Biochemical Sciences*, **31**, 89–97.
8. Wood, A.J. and Oakey, R.J. (2006). Genomic imprinting in mammals: emerging themes and established theories. *PLoS Genetics*, **2**, e147.
9. Ferguson-Smith, A.C. and Surani, M.A. (2001). Imprinting and the epigenetic asymmetry between parental genomes. *Science*, **293**, 1086–9.
10. Raymond, F.L. and Tarpey, P. (2006). The genetics of intellectual disability. *Human Molecular Genetics*, **15** (Spec. no. 2), R110–16.
11. Reik, W. and Lewis, A. (2005). Co-evolution of X-chromosome inactivation and imprinting in mammals. *Nature Reviews. Genetics*, **6**, 403–10.
12. Reik, W., Dean, W., and Walter, J. (2001). Epigenetic reprogramming in mammalian development. *Science*, **293**, 1089–93.
13. Davies, W., Isles, A.R., Burgoyne, P.S., *et al.* (2006). X-linked imprinting: effects on brain and behaviour. *BioEssays*, **28**, 35–44.
14. Skuse, D.H., James, R.S., Bishop, D. V. *et al.* (1997). Evidence from Turner's syndrome of an imprinted X-linked locus affecting cognitive function. *Nature*, **387**, 705–8.
15. Davies, W., Isles, A., Smith, R., *et al.* (2005). Xlr3b is a new imprinted candidate for X-linked parent-of-origin effects on cognitive function in mice. *Nature Genetics*, **37**, 625–9.
16. Tsankova, N., Renthal, W., Kumar, A., *et al.* (2007). Epigenetic regulation in psychiatric disorders. *Nature Reviews. Neuroscience*, **8**, 355–67.
17. Francis, D., Diorio, J., Liu, D., *et al.* (1999). Nongenomic transmission across generations of maternal behavior and stress responses in the rat. *Science*, **286**, 1155–8.
18. Meaney, M.J. (2001). Maternal care, gene expression, and the transmission of individual differences in stress reactivity across generations. *Annual Review of Neuroscience*, **24**, 1161–92.
19. Weaver, I.C., Cervoni, N., Champagne, F.A., *et al.* (2004). Epigenetic programming by maternal behavior. *Nature Neuroscience*, **7**, 847–54.
20. Meaney, M.J. and Szyf, M. (2005). Maternal care as a model for experience-dependent chromatin plasticity? *Trends in Neurosciences*, **28**, 456–63.
21. Tsankova, N.M., Berton, O., Renthal, W., *et al.* (2006). Sustained hippocampal chromatin regulation in a mouse model of depression and antidepressant action. *Nature Neuroscience*, **9**, 519–25.
22. Zaratiegui, M., Irvine, D.V., and Martienssen, R.A. (2007). Noncoding RNAs and gene silencing. *Cell*, **128**, 763–76.
23. Nilsen, T.W. (2007). Mechanisms of microRNA-mediated gene regulation in animal cells. *Trends in Genetics*, **23**, 243–9.
24. Carninci, P., Kasukawa, T., Katayama, S., *et al.* (2005). The transcriptional landscape of the mammalian genome. *Science*, **309**, 1559–63.
25. Cheng, J., Kapranov, P., Drenkow, J., *et al.* (2005). Transcriptional maps of 10 human chromosomes at 5-nucleotide resolution. *Science*, **308**, 1149–54.
26. Cawley, S., Bekiranov, S., Ng, H.H., *et al.* (2004). Unbiased mapping of transcription factor binding sites along human chromosomes 21 and 22 points to widespread regulation of noncoding RNAs. *Cell*, **116**, 499–509.
27. Fisher, S.E., Vargha-Khadem, F., Watkins, K.E., *et al.* (1998). Localisation of a gene implicated in a severe speech and language disorder. *Nature Genetics*, **18**, 168–70.
28. Lai, C.S., Fisher, S.E., Hurst, J.A., *et al.* (2001). A forkhead-domain gene is mutated in a severe speech and language disorder. *Nature*, **413**, 519–23.
29. Risch, N. and Merikangas, K. (1996). The future of genetic studies of complex human diseases. *Science*, **273**, 1516–17.
30. Tandon, A. and Fraser, P. (2002). The presenilins. *Genome Biology*, **3**, 1–9.
31. Hardy, J. (1997). Amyloid, the presenilins and Alzhheimer's disease. *Trends in Neurosciences*, **20**, 154–9.
32. Hardy, J., Duf, K., Hardy, K.G., *et al.* (1998). Genetic dissection of Alzheimer's disease and related dementias: amyloid and its relationship to tau. *Nature Neuroscience*, **1**, 355–8.
33. Goedert, M. and Spillantini, M.G. (2006). A century of Alzheimer's disease. *Science*, **314**, 777–81.
34. Shen, J. and Kelleher, R.J. III. (2007). The presenilin hypothesis of Alzheimer's disease: evidence for a loss-of-function pathogenic mechanism. *Proceedings of the National Academy of Sciences of the United States of America*, **104**, 403–9.
35. Hutton, M., Lendon, C.L., Rizzu, P., *et al.* (1998). Association of missense and 5'-splice-site mutations in tau with the inherited dementia FTDP-17. *Nature*, **393**, 702–5.
36. Spillantini, M.G., Murrell, J.R., Goedert, M., *et al.* (1998). Mutation in the tau gene in familial multiple system tauopathy with presenile dementia. *Proceedings of the National Academy of Sciences of the United States of America*, **95**, 7737–41.
37. Orr, H.T. and Zoghbi, H.Y. (2007). Trinucleotide repeat disorders. *Annual Review Neuroscience*, **30**, 575–621.

38. Yu, S., Pritchard, M., Kremer, E., *et al.* (1991). Fragile X genotype characterized by an unstable region of DNA. *Science*, **252**, 1179–81.
39. Verkerk, A.J., Pieretti, M., Sutcliffe, J.S., *et al.* (1991). Identification of a gene (FMR-1) containing a CGG repeat coincident with a breakpoint cluster region exhibiting length variation in fragile X syndrome. *Cell*, **65**, 905–14.
40. Antonarakis, S.E. and Epstein, C.J (2006). The challenge of Down syndrome. *Trends in Molecular Medicine*, **12**, 473–9.
41. Budarf, M.L. and Emanuel, B.S. (1997). Progress in the autosomal segmental aneusomy syndromes (SASs): single or multi-locus disorders? *Human Molecular Genetics*, **6**, 1657–65.
42. Sharp, A.J., Cheng, Z., and Eichler, E.E. (2006). Structural variation of the human genome. *Annual Review of Genomics and Human Genetics*, **7**, 407–42.
43. Lee, J.A. and Lupski, J.R. (2006). Genomic rearrangements and gene copy-number alterations as a cause of nervous system disorders. *Neuron*, **52**, 103–21.
44. Karayiorgou, M. and Gogos, J.A. (2004). The molecular genetics of the 22q11-associated schizophrenia. *Brain Research. Molecular Brain Research*, **132**, 95–104.
45. Mackie, S., Millar, J.K., and Porteous, D.J. (2007). Role of DISC1 in neural development and schizophrenia. *Current Opinion in Neurobiology*, **17**, 95–102.
46. Abelson, J.F., Kwan, K.Y., O'Roak, B.J., *et al.* (2005). Sequence variants in SLITRK1 are associated with Tourette's syndrome. *Science*, **310**, 317–20.
47. Bienvenu, T. and Chelly, J. (2006). Molecular genetics of Rett syndrome: when DNA methylation goes unrecognized. *Nature Reviews. Genetics*, **7**, 415–26.
48. Horsthemke, B. and Buiting, K. (2006). Imprinting defects on human chromosome 15. *Cytogenetic and Genome Research*, **113**, 292–9.
49. De Gobbi, M., Viprakasit, V., Hughes, J.R., *et al.* (2006). A regulatory SNP causes a human genetic disease by creating a new transcriptional promoter. *Science*, **312**, 1215–17.
50. Ioannidis, J.P., Ntzani, E.E., Trikalinos, T.A., *et al.* (2001). Replication validity of genetic association studies. *Nature Genetics*, **29**, 306–9.
51. Munafo, M.R., Matheson, I.J., and Flint, J. (2007). Association of the DRD2 gene Taq1A polymorphism and alcoholism: a meta-analysis of case-control studies and evidence of publication bias. *Molecular Psychiatry*, **12**, 454–61.
52. Ioannidis, J.P., Trikalinos, T.A., and Khoury, M.J. (2006). Implications of small effect sizes of individual genetic variants on the design and interpretation of genetic association studies of complex diseases. *American Journal of Epidemiology*, **164**, 609–14.
53. Ioannidis, J.P., Trikalinos, T.A., Ntzani, E.E., *et al.* (2003). Genetic associations in large versus small studies: an empirical assessment. *Lancet*, **361**, 567–71.
54. Wellcome Trust Case Consortium (2007). Genome–wide association study of 14,000 cases of seven common disease and 3,000 shared controls. *Nature*, **447**, 661–78.
55. Cox, A., Dunning, A., Garcia-Closas, M., *et al.* (2007). A common coding variant in CASP8 is associated with breast cancer risk. *Nature Genetics*, **39**, 352–7.
56. Carlborg, O. and Haley, C.S. (2004). Epistasis: too often neglected in complex trait studies? *Nature Reviews. Genetics*, **5**, 618–25.
57. Caspi, A., Sugden, K., Moffitt, T.E., *et al.* (2003). Influence of life stress on depression: moderation by a polymorphism in the 5-HTT gene. *Science*, **301**, 386–9.
58. Cohen, J.C., Kiss, R.S., Pertsemlidis, A., *et al.* (2004). Multiple rare alleles contribute to low plasma levels of HDL cholesterol. *Science*, **305**, 869–72.
59. Redon, R., Ishikawa, S., Fitch, K.R., *et al.* (2006). Global variation in copy number in the human genome. *Nature*, **444**, 444–54.
60. Sebat, J., Lakshmi, B., Malhotra, D., *et al.* (2007). Strong association of *de novo* copy number mutations with autism. *Science*, **316**, 445–9.
61. Gerlai, R. (2000). Targeting genes and proteins in the analysis of learning and memory: caveats and future directions. *Reviews in the Neurosciences*, **11**, 15–26.
62. Crawley, J.N., Belknap, J.K., Collins, A., *et al.* (1997). Behavioral phenotypes of inbred mouse strains: implications and recommendations for molecular studies. *Psychopharmacology (Berl)*, **132**, 107–24.
63. Lewandoski, M. (2001). Conditional control of gene expression in the mouse. *Nature Reviews. Genetics*, **2**, 743–55.
64. Nakazawa, K., McHugh, T.J., Wilson, M.A., *et al.* (2004). NMDA receptors, place cells and hippocampal spatial memory. *Nature Reviews. Neuroscience*, **5**, 361–72.
65. Tsien, J.Z., Huerta, P.T., and Tonegawa, S. (1996). The essential role of hippocampal CA1 NMDA receptor-dependent synaptic plasticity in spatial memory. *Cell*, **87**, 1327–38.
66. McHugh, T.J., Blum, K.I., Tsien, J.Z., *et al.* (1996). Impaired hippocampal representation of space in CA1-specific NMDAR1 knockout mice. *Cell*, **87**, 1339–49.
67. Gordon, J.A. and Hen, R. (2004). Genetic approaches to the study of anxiety. *Annual Review of Neuroscience*, **27**, 193–222.
68. Low, K., Crestani, F., Keist, R., *et al.* (2000). Molecular and neuronal substrate for the selective attenuation of anxiety. *Science*, **290**, 131–4.
69. Rudolph, U., Crestani, F., Benke, D., *et al.* (1999). Benzodiazepine actions mediated by specific gamma-aminobutyric acid(A) receptor subtypes. *Nature*, **401**, 796–800.
70. McKernan, R.M., Rosahl, T.W., Reynolds, D.S., *et al.* (2000). Sedative but not anxiolytic properties of benzodiazepines are mediated by the GABA(A) receptor alpha1 subtype. *Nature Neuroscience*, **3**, 587–92.
71. Gross, C., Santarelli, L., Brunner, D., *et al.* (2000). Altered fear circuits in 5-HT(1A) receptor KO mice. *Biological Psychiatry*, **48**, 1157–63.
72. Copeland, N.G., Jenkins, N.A., and Court, D.L. (2001). Recombineering: a powerful new tool for mouse functional genomics. *Nature Reviews. Genetics*, **2**, 769–79.
73. Gong, S., Zheng, C., Doughty, M.L., *et al.* (2003). A gene expression atlas of the central nervous system based on bacterial artificial chromosomes. *Nature*, **425**, 917–25.
74. Hatten, M.E. and Heintz, N. (2005). Large-scale genomic approaches to brain development and circuitry. *Annual Review of Neuroscience*, **28**, 89–108.
75. Lima, S.Q. and Miesenbock, G. (2005). Remote control of behavior through genetically targeted photostimulation of neurons. *Cell*, **121**, 141–52.
76. Arenkiel, B.R., Peca, J., Davison, I.G., *et al.* (2007). *In vivo* light-induced activation of neural circuitry in transgenic mice expressing channelrhodopsin-2. *Neuron*, **54**, 205–18.

2.5

The contribution of psychological science

Contents

2.5.1 Developmental psychology through infancy, childhood, and adolescence
William Yule and Matt Woolgar

2.5.2 Psychology of attention
Elizabeth Coulthard and Masud Husain

2.5.3 Psychology and biology of memory
Andreas Meyer-Lindenberg and Terry E. Goldberg

2.5.4 The anatomy of human emotion
R. J. Dolan

2.5.5 Neuropsychological basis of neuropsychiatry
L. Clark, B. J. Sahakian, and T. W. Robbins

2.5.1 **Developmental psychology through infancy, childhood, and adolescence**

William Yule and Matt Woolgar

Introduction

The child is father to the man. This saying seems so obviously true that it may surprise some people that it needs to be analysed and certain assumptions inherent in it need to be challenged if psychiatric practice across the lifespan is to be properly informed by findings from developmental psychology. This chapter examines different conceptualizations of children and childhood through the ages and the ideas and theoretical models that have shaped popular, as well as professional, views on how children develop. It notes that there are no overarching theories of child development, but rather a pot-pourri of smaller models, most of which address disparate aspects of development.

Developmental psychology is not just about charting the norms of development, although knowledge of such is essential in all clinical practice. Rather, there are many issues that need to be critically examined in trying to understand how individuals develop. Taking a developmental perspective is about integrating this knowledge and understanding the patient's presenting problems within such a framework.

The significance that the clinician will place on a particular piece of behaviour will depend not only on the child's socio-cultural background, but also on the child's developmental age. Cox and Rutter[1] note four reasons for taking a developmental perspective:

1 Children behave differently at different ages. The clinician must be familiar with the range of behaviours and their age-appropriateness in separating the normal from the abnormal. For instance, simple consonant substitutions are widespread in the speech of pre-school children, but indicate some delay or deviation in the speech of teenagers.

2 Many aspects of behaviour can be viewed as progressing through a normal sequence. Admittedly, discrete stages are over-emphasized by stage theorists such as Freud, Piaget, and Bowlby, whereas the continuities in development are more emphasized by social-learning theorists such as Staats, Bijou, and Baer. Either way, an understanding of the normal sequences and ages permits a judgement as to whether the child has deviated in his or her development.

3 Different stages of development are associated with different stresses and different developmental tasks. Bladder and bowel training are normally achieved between the ages of 2 and 4 years. Major stresses on the child or the family at the time may interfere with the achievement of proper bladder and bowel control. Mood swings are very common in adolescence, making it difficult to diagnose the severity of depression at this stage.[2,3]

4 An understanding of the processes which underlie both normal and abnormal development will help in the understanding of how the problems have arisen.[4] Such an historical perspective can help explain to the parents why a particular problem developed, as well as give possible clues for future programmes for prevention. A major implication of this for clinical practice is that it is always necessary to obtain a good account of the child's developmental history.

5 A better understanding of the *processes* underlying a child's development will lead to far better interventions and prevention.

Once we have a better understanding of the *distal* and *proximal* causes of behaviour, better targeted interventions will follow.

Developmental theories and views

There is a bewildering set of mini-models and mini-theories of developmental processes, each trying to deal with changes in children's functioning either at different periods in their lives or in different psychological functions such as perception, language, and memory. By and large, the different theories seem to ignore each other's work—and many also seem keener on theories than on data that might test the theories.

For example, Piaget's theories predominantly address how children develop a cognitive understanding of their world. His was a biological view of development, and his cross-sectional methodology emphasized the separation between the stages he posited. Staats[(5)] argued that most of the phenomena described by Piaget and his followers could be interpreted within a social learning theory framework that instead emphasized the continuity of development across stages.

Kohlberg's theory of moral judgement is a stage theory that differs radically from Piaget's in that the different forms of reasoning said to typify different stages can coexist. However, the way in which children (or adults for that matter) judge an ethical dilemma does not necessarily determine how they behave. Most financiers would have little difficulty in providing sophisticated moral judgements on Kohlberg type tasks, but many financiers also present the unacceptable face of capitalism in their ruthless dealings. It is not the case that the older we are, the wiser we behave.

In Freud's theory of psychosexual development, children are seen as passively passing through stages, their development being impeded by obstacles or even regressing in the face of trauma. This view owes more to literature than to science, and the evidence on children's psychosexual development clearly shows that whatever Freud was unaware of during the latency period, children are certainly far from inactive.[(6)]

Apart from being stage theories, these three sets of influential theories really have very little in common. The psychological mechanisms determining growth of cognitive understanding bear little relationship to any that supposedly underlie socio-emotional behaviour. None of the theories take into account all of the work done in perceptual development, language development, development of memory, development of peer relationships, development during adolescence, and so on. They pay little attention to the work on individual differences in personality or temperament, or to biological development generally.

A totally biological, determinist view of development was anathema to the new theorists of behaviour modification and behaviour therapy in the 1960s. It was seen as too pessimistic, offering little hope of change. By ignoring the biological basis of behaviour and seeking explanations solely in the here-and-now (proximal) influences on behaviour, they undoubtedly broke through to a much more optimistic era of interventions.

Simultaneously, child developmentalists were recognizing the contributions the child brought to all aspects of development. The child has increasingly been seen as an active participant in development. The direction of influence was not all one way: the child helped shape the environment. Thus, parents react to individual differences in children. Different children call out different responses from their social environment. As parents have known all along, children do have different temperaments from birth, and these shape how they develop.[(7,8)]

The implications of this for child psychiatry are many. For example, it implies that clinicians must take into account a child's temperament when planning treatment.[(7,9)] Children who are extremely introvert react differently to praise and punishment than children who are extremely extrovert.[(9,10)] They also respond to different teaching styles in the classroom. Such differences need to be accommodated in setting up individualized treatment programmes.

With young infants, it can be very reassuring to a parent to be told that anyone would find their unpredictable child difficult to rear. It can boost parental self-confidence to be told (when true) that their parenting style is perfectly adequate for most children—just not effective with this particular one. This reassurance should greatly alter the way such a parent participates in parent training programmes that are increasingly part of primary and secondary level child mental health services.[(11)]

All this is not to say that stage theories carry no implications for child mental health services. Far from it. It is very helpful to remember that young children think and reason about their worlds differently from older children. This has to be borne in mind when interviewing children, when trying to elicit their own understanding of their problem, and, equally, when giving them instructions, feedback, or explanations. However, it must again be emphasized that the stages should only ever be regarded as rough guidelines. We know that there are such wide individual differences in the rate at which children develop that we should never make assumptions about the individual child knowing only his chronological age.

Let us take one example that increasingly confronts clinicians—the issue of helping children deal with bereavement. It is not until around the age of 10 or 11 that *most* children appreciate that death is both universal and irreversible.[(11–14)] This helps explain why some younger children show an almost casual, matter-of-fact interest in death of a loved one and are less upset by it than adults are.[(13)] But it would be wrong to assume that all younger children fail to have an adult appreciation of the significance of death, and indeed some children as young as 4 years old have been found to have a mature understanding. Knowledge of the broad outline of the development of the conceptualization of death helps clinicians formulate their questions, but the onus must always be on the clinician to check whether or not the individual child conforms to the average. The adult's task may not be finished when they have helped a young child to understand bereavement at the level the child can cope with. That same child will probably want to revisit the issue when she is older and can understand it in a more mature way.[(15)] What is true of bereavement also holds true for understanding any other major life event and its effects on the child.

Critical issues in development

When one takes a closer look at how children develop, one cannot help but be amazed at the complexities of the process. Children the world over start using words around their first birthday and within a couple of years more, they are talking in complex sentences using complicated ideas. The contrast between the language development of most children and the minority who suffer a severe mental handicap is devastating. Likewise, blind children start to smile at the same time as sighted children; deaf children start to use a similar range of phonemes; children in Japan, France, and Britain all start uttering the same range of sounds only to have them narrowed down to those they need in their native language—with the later consequence that they may not even be able to discriminate some of the unused sounds, let alone incorporate them when learning a foreign language. The broad developmental trajectory seems very similar across cultural groups, but particular children do not always follow the average in a smooth, predictable way.

Rutter and Rutter[16] draw attention to a number of issues that need to be considered when trying to understand developmental processes. Clinicians are understandably focused on trying to make sense of cases where something has gone wrong in development. Mostly in child psychiatry, abnormal behaviours of children are quantitatively different from normal rather than being qualitatively different. Disorders following brain damage or genetic/chromosomal abnormalities and many involving very severe degrees of mental handicap, including infantile autism, are increasingly recognized as being qualitatively different. Most of the other disorders seen in child and adolescent mental health services are probably best viewed as deviations lying at the extreme of a continuum. But why do some children break down under stress while others do not? Why are some more resilient than others? What factors protect children against environmental and social stressors? Is it really the case that severe depression in late adolescence is just the extreme end of a continuum ranging from happiness through sadness to suicidality? In order to tackle these issues, it is necessary to clarify some of the concepts of development.

1 One should not assume that the same mechanisms underlie both normal and abnormal development.

2 A biological perspective is necessary to understand human development fully. The brain is clearly the most important organ concerned—the genetic inheritance, insults during critical periods of brain growth, hormonal changes—all these have considerable influence on how children develop.

3 One has to expect both *continuities* and *discontinuities* in development. At times, continuities are intrinsic to the particular process as in language development; at other times, continuities—as in academic attainment—are in large part influenced by continuities imposed by the social environment. Parents concerned about education influence the choice of schools and provide support for learning.

4 The *timing* of an experience is as important as its nature. The brain is most vulnerable to insult when it is developing most rapidly, at and shortly after birth. Severe disruptions in caretaking have their greatest effects from around 9 months to 2 or 3 years. Before then, the infant does not show the same quality of selective attachments; after language is well established, the child can better hold the memory of a loved one, and that may act as a protection against the separation.

5 Children are *active* creatures. Not only do they call out responses from others, but as they develop cognitively and linguistically, they actively seek to make sense of their world. They appraise threat from others, even if they do not always get it right. When they are involved in a major catastrophe, their assumptive world[17] can be literally turned upside down and they take a long time to reconstruct the world as a safe place. The way the child interprets experience will come to determine in part how similar experiences are responded to in the future.

6 'Continuity may be heterotypic as well as homotypic'[16] (p. 8). The brilliant idea developed in the New York Longitudinal Study[18] of temperament was that rather than seeking evidence for predictability and continuity in particular infant behaviours across times when behaviour was developing rapidly, the investigators looked instead at how a variety of topographically different behaviours were expressed and found considerable continuities in such aspects as regularity of functions, strength of response, and predominant reaction to new stimuli. Thus, they adduced evidence of temperamental characteristics that were independent of the specific behaviours shown, and moreover, these temperamental characteristics proved to be predictive of later behaviour and adjustment.[16]

7 Both risk and protective factors, and the interactions between them, must be considered. Not all apparently adverse experiences are necessarily wholly bad for healthy development. In the same way that exposure to a virus or infection can boost resistance to infection, so exposure to mild stressors may boost resistance to other stressful experiences later. In part, this is the basis for stress inoculation therapy.[19] Some would argue that young children should have practice in separating from parents under enjoyable conditions so that in the event of a sudden, unexpected, or traumatic separation being necessary, the effects of experience will be mitigated.

8 As noted earlier, continuities may arise indirectly in that the way parents or society in general support attainment and in turn entry to the job market. The moderately high correlations between early attainment and later earning power are thereby in part determined and supported environmentally.

9 Similarly, the achievement of a particular behaviour may set in motion a chain of events. It is important to understand the processes underlying such a sequence. Too often studies are short-term and cross-sectional in nature and despite being aware of the pitfall of confusing correlation with causality, investigators remain prone to identifying a correlate as being a causal agent. For example, in the early days of studies of reading difficulties, it was noted that poor readers did badly on tests of visual perception. It was assumed that they therefore had a visual-perceptual deficit and generations of poor readers were subjected to hours of mindless tracing of lines and walking along benches. The end result was that they performed better on the particular visual-perceptual test but they were no better at reading! A different experimental design was needed to demonstrate causal relationships between psychological processes and poor reading,[20] and when that was understood, the way was open for better remedial work based on a proper understanding of causal mechanisms.

This can also be viewed as an error in confusing a risk *indicator* with a risk *process*. Forty years ago, studies of the dehumanizing effects of institutionalization on adults and children[21] found that poor living conditions and block treatment of residents were related to a greater risk of behavioural and emotional problems. In one set of studies, a good *indicator* of block treatment was whether patients had their own toothbrushes. Clearly, providing individual toothbrushes to all would not make much difference if all the other aspects of institutionalization remained in force. A fuller understanding of the *process* of institutionalization is needed in order to be able to develop more humane care that improves development.

These critical issues demonstrate just how complicated the relationship between nature, experience, and development can be. But human beings are indeed very complicated, thank goodness, and so a proper appreciation of all these factors is needed in order to be able to understand how a particular child reached a particular point in development; to be able to predict what the future may hold for a child and to be able to develop rational interventions that have a hope of making a real difference to children's lives.

Developmental psychopathology

Developmental psychopathology emerged in the 1980s to bridge the rift between academic and clinical child psychology.[22,23] 'The developmental psychopathologist is concerned with the time course of a given disorder, its varying manifestations with development, its precursors and sequelae, and its relation to non-disordered patterns of behaviour' (p. 18).[23] Developmental psychopathologists, like social learning theorists, look to normal development to illuminate pathological development. They are interested in continuities and changes in behaviour across time. This fits in well with the tradition of risk research[24] and attempts to answer questions not only about why some children are more vulnerable than others, but also about what protective factors operate to lessen the impact of stressors.

Sroufe and Rutter,[23] following Santostefano,[25] articulated several propositions that are broadly agreed across the many different theories alluded to above:

(a) Holism

'The meaning of behaviour can only be determined within the total psychological context' (p. 20).[23] Thus, behaviour such as crying can only be evaluated according to the age of the child and the circumstances in which it occurs. Crying on separation would be seen as usual for a 3-year-old, but unusual in a 15-year-old. One cannot simply judge the significance of a behaviour simply on the basis of its physical, stimulus properties, but one has to evaluate it within the broader social context.

(b) Directedness

Children are not passive reactors to the demands of the environment. Development consists of a reorganization of previous elements, skills, and behaviour, not just a linear addition of skills.

(c) Differentiation of modes and goals

Over time, children's reactions to their environment become both more flexible and increasingly complex in organization. Thus, one sign of pathology is for children to get stuck in a particular way of trying to solve a problem.

(d) Mobility of behavioural functions

Earlier behaviour becomes integrated into later patterns, and 'the individual does not operate only in terms of behaviours that define a single stage. Especially in periods of stress, early modes of functioning may become manifest' (p. 21).[23] In other words, under stress, those patterns of behaviour that have most recently become integrated into the child's repertoire are most susceptible of disruption. This is very different from the unsatisfactory concept of regression in which all skills achieved remain available in the child's repertoire; some earlier ones also manifest at times of stress.

(e) The problem of continuity and change

Above all, development is seen as lawful, even though we are still far from understanding the processes involved in these laws. Sroufe and Rutter[23] emphasize: 'the continuity lies not in isomorphic behaviours over time but in lawful relations to later behaviour, however complex the links' (p. 21). As noted, Thomas, Chess, and Birch[18] were among the first to demonstrate continuities in the *style* of behaviour (temperament) rather than continuities of behaviour *per se*.

It is now recognized that there are many complex ways in which child behaviour is related to later and even adult adjustment.[26] One of the most powerful predictors of later adult psychopathology is inadequate peer relations. The mechanism by which these work may be due to two interacting processes: (1) Poor peer relations are signs of failure to adapt during childhood, and that failure persists; (2) social support later acts as a buffer against adult stressors.[23]

Clearly, this view of development, with its implications for psychopathology, is far removed from the lessons learned from the Skinner box. Yet what has been learned from the paradigms of classical and operant conditioning must also be integrated into ways that child therapists assess children's problems if we are to provide better treatments. This holistic view manages to incorporate ideas on the biological basis for behaviour and the notion of the child as an active participant interacting with his or her effective social environment within a broad social learning framework.[27,28] Understanding how a problem has arisen may provide useful guidance on what aspects to focus on, but the treatment will still focus on the present. There will be implications for maintaining treatment gains and preventing future problems, as well as implications for preventing such problems arising in other children.

For clinicians more used to working with adult patients, it is worth pointing out that children differ in many ways from their grown up counterparts. This has implications for improving diagnostic classificatory systems in that both DSM and ICD are still too adult oriented and pay insufficient attention to developmental aspects of disorders.[29–31]

Garber[32] makes the point that children differ from adults in cognition, language, physiology, and emotions. Such maturational differences may impact children's abilities to experience or express certain affects, cognitions, or behaviours, and thus the manner in which symptoms are expressed may differ over the course of development (p. 32). Recent work on the effects of major disasters and acute stress on children's adjustment, it became evident that children as young as 8 years old showed most of the symptoms of post-traumatic stress disorder (**PTSD**)—with unpleasant thoughts, poor concentration, and sleep disorders predominating.[33,34] Parents and teachers were often unaware of the nature and extent of the children's subjective distress, and only sympathetic but direct questioning elicited the full spectrum of symptomatology.

The criteria for PTSD are less appropriate for children under 8 years of age. Pre-school children often react with more repetitive play and drawing than older ones. Even the youngest children will report very disturbing, intrusive thoughts about the disaster. Scheeringa *et al.*[35] suggest varying criteria for making the diagnosis of PTSD in young children. Leaving aside the logical problem of altering criteria but keeping the same name for the supposed underlying condition, this clearly is one aspect of the isomorphism mentioned earlier. It is also interesting to speculate whether the repetitive play seen in 6-year-olds is functionally equivalent to the intrusive thoughts seen in 10 year olds, and when the one changes into the other.

Garber also notes that some disorders, such as mental handicap and autism, first manifest in childhood and persist into adulthood. Others, such as encopresis and enuresis manifest in childhood, but rarely persist into adulthood unless part of a more global developmental delay. Some, such as anorexia and bulimia, are more typical of adolescence. Suicide, although rare before puberty, is rapidly becoming the major cause of death in adolescence, but peaks in old age. Major depression and schizophrenia are rare in childhood, although precursors are being more firmly established. While the wish to treat disorders in childhood so as to prevent them continuing to adulthood is laudable, treating them to improve adjustment during childhood is equally valid.

Linking developmental psychopathology to developing children

These exciting ideas need to be brought out of experimental settings and into clinics—the aim of developmental psychopathology theorists. In the second half of this chapter, some of the key aspects of child development relevant to clinical practice will be highlighted in this framework.

(a) Individual differences

Children differ in their personality, character, or temperament. European psychologists have always emphasized these individual differences and adduced evidence that many were based on biologically determined ways of responding to the world. While the three factor structure of personality developed by Eysenck evolved into the big five structure of today, an issue remained as to how one could demonstrate *continuity* in personality from a very early age. The same issue bedevilled studies seeking to establish continuity in differences in intellectual functioning—simply put, little babies show such a different repertoire of behaviour from mobile, talking pre-school children that it was impossible to test the same behaviours at different ages.

In part, the problem was solved in the New York Longitudinal Study[18] (see Box 2.5.1.1 One) by looking at differences in *style* of behaviour rather than differences in content or topography. By avoiding talking of biologically based personality, the findings reawakened interest in the genetics of individual differences.

In the original sample of 78 babies, the investigators were able to demonstrate considerable individual differences in temperament. There was good inter-rater reliability in making these judgements and direct observations agreed well with reports from parents. The temperamental characteristics were found to be stable over both the short (2 years) and medium term and even predicted reasonably well into late childhood.

Three broad types of temperament were characterized—children who were regular, predictable, and showed generally positive reactions—the easy babies; those who were almost the opposite—whom Chess called the mother killers and a sizeable minority who were slow to warm up to new situations but who adjusted eventually. The difficult children were over represented in those who developed behavioural problems in later childhood.

Box 2.5.1.1 Temperamental characteristics

The repertoire of infant behaviour is so different from that of the pre-school child that it proved very difficult to examine whether there were any continuities of behaviour across the ages. Thomas *et al.*[18] and their collaborators in the New York Longitudinal Study were among the earliest to show continuities across the age, but continuities in *style* of behaviour rather than *content*. Through a mixture of observation and exhaustive interviews with mothers, they originally developed nine different categories of behavioural style or *temperament*.

Mainly

1. Active	1. Passive
2. Regular: (e.g. in feeding and sleeping habits)	2. Irregular
3. Reacts intensely (strongly)	3. Reacts mildly
4. Shows approach behaviour to new people, places, toys, foods, etc.	4. Shows withdrawal behaviour
5. Adaptive—adapts fairly easily to change	5. Non-adaptive
6. Reacts easily to small changes	6. Reactions slow
7. Predominantly good moods—happy, contented disposition	7. Predominantly bad disposition—fretful, hard to please
8. Persistent in what she/he is doing as regards time, and in the face of difficulties	8. Non-persistent
9. Easily distracted from whatever she/he is doing	9. Not easily distracted

(b) Cognitive development

One of the major aspects of development that exercises parents and teachers alike is how best to improve the intellectual functioning of children, be that in language, reading, memory, or general intelligence. To what extent individual differences in these areas are predominantly related to heredity or to environment continues to be a popular, if sterile, source of argument. Clearly, the end result comes from an interaction between genetic predisposition and experience, but there remain issues of how best to manipulate the environment so as to help children gain their maximum potential. To that end, an understanding of modern behavioural genetics is essential. Here, some of the methodological issues in assessing babies' cognitive processes and findings in cognitive development, language, and memory are considered.

(c) Getting inside the baby's head

Until a baby starts to speak, it is difficult to know what they are thinking. Fond parents interpret wind-driven grimaces as smiling; every child is seen as recognizing people and being smart from a young age. But how can one tell what really goes on inside a baby's head?

Robert Fantz[36] studied infants' eye movements and used fixation time as a measure of preference for different stimuli. Film recordings were made of light reflected off the baby's eyes. In a study of 30 infants tested weekly from 1 to 15 weeks of age, it was shown that the infants spent longer looking at complex than simple patterns. This demonstration of a clear perceptual preference in the first few weeks after birth gave the lie to the view that all begins as a big, booming confusion. Infants as young as one week show clear preference for human faces over other shapes presented to them some 10 in. away.

Fantz took advantage of the technology of the day. Since then, others have utilized measures of changes in temperature, in galvanic skin response and in heartbeat to provide behavioural indices of preferences. In addition, investigators have used various indices from learning and conditioning paradigms.

Results from such studies highlight the extent to which infants enter the world ready for social interaction. Infants are highly dependent on their parents because of the cortical developments and increase in brain volume required to allow the special human cognitive characteristics to develop that take place *after* the baby has made its way down the birth canal. Infant's readiness to be part of a social interaction, imbued with intentionality, appears to serve a survival function.

The neonate has remarkable hard-wired skills that can be detected from within moments of birth, while the neonate is in a period of alert inactivity. However, there are limits to the extent of the early ability. Eyesight acuity is about 1/30th of adults at birth and develops over the next 4 years, although significant improvements arise by the second month. Despite problems with visual acuity and focusing, even neonates can track objects, albeit jerkily, and scan for simple, visual features, such as linearity, luminance, and symmetry when stimuli are within about 10 in. of their face.[37] These intrinsic visual abilities combine with preferences for certain spatial forms found in the human face, e.g. a preference for vertical over horizontal symmetry. Fagan[38] tested visual preference in 7-month-old babies and later measured their intelligence when they were 3 and 5 years old. The time spent looking at the novel stimulus when a baby correlated 0.42 with performance on the later Picture Vocabulary Test. Thus, it is getting easier to measure various indices of baby's reactions and some of these are found to be usefully predictive of later development and adjustment.

Hearing is pretty much complete by the 5th or 6th week of foetal life, with sophisticated auditory discrimination abilities along the dimensions of pitch, volume, tone, and duration. Hence neonates may come into the world already familiar with soap opera theme tunes, but so too are they familiar with their mother's voice and are able to orientate towards them from the start. Neonates have a preference for women's voices over men's and unlike the specificity shown towards the mother, appear to show little preference for their father's voice compared with other men.[39]

Bathed in amniotic fluid in the womb, it is unclear whether the foetus has strictly speaking *smelled* the mother before birth, although their olfactory system is well-developed *in utero*. Nonetheless, within hours of birth neonates demonstrate a preference for their mother's smell and, within days, can reliably orient their head towards breast pads worn by their mothers over those worn by other women.[40]

Meltzoff and colleagues have demonstrated that a neonate's social sensitivity is not just a passive turning to stimuli, they can also actively imitate them.[41] Indeed, within moments of birth, neonates are able to mirror adult's facial expressions such as tongue protrusions or mouth openings. Quite how this process operates at a cognitive level is unclear. One can speculate on its function as a way to provide a satisfying contingency for a parent that helps imbue the infant with a sense of communication, agency, and personhood. Overall, neonate's abilities to discriminate between stimuli and their hard-wired preferences for some constellations over others lead them to orient towards their caregivers, as the very beginnings of a selective attachment.

(d) Piaget and cognitive development

Piaget was a biologist who studied amoebas for his doctoral work. Biological models found useful for that purpose clearly influenced the way he regarded cognitive development. He held to a sort of moving homeostasis—children develop a model of the world. New information that challenges that model is gradually assimilated and eventually the model accommodates the new ways of thinking—a bit like an amoeba reaching out to a piece of food, surrounding it and assimilating it.

According to this theory, the child passes through three broad stages of thinking (see Box 2.5.1.2): A sensori-motor stage, a long stage where they think in terms of what he called concrete operations, and finally a stage where they can think logically.

Piaget's stage theory has been very influential and helpfully sparked off a great deal of research which has led to a much better understanding of how children develop cognitively. However, his original models were somewhat simplistic and to have seen only three major stages covering a period of such rapid development

Box 2.5.1.2 Piaget's stages of cognitive development

Birth to 18 months: sensori-motor stage

Cognition is based mainly on the child's actions and six sub-stages were described. A key concept at this stage is that of object permanence—the ability to understand that an object continues to exist even when it is out of sight. Infants of 12 months will continue to look for an object where an experimenter hides it, even when they watch the experimenter move it. It is as if the object belongs only in a particular place.

18 months to 12 years: concrete operations

This is the stage of concrete operations. At the early stage, language develops rapidly. Children begin to demonstrate symbolic play, showing that they have memories and internal representations. Many ingenious little experiments were developed to illustrate how children's thinking about their world develops. Various other conservation tasks—of length, mass, and number for instance—convince teachers that children think differently about the world than adults and this has had a major—if not always beneficial—effect on ways of teaching.

12 years and over: formal operations

From around puberty onwards, the child is able to formulate and test hypotheses about the world. The child realizes that mass and volume can be altered in many ways, but they remain essentially unchanged. Children can examine their own thought processes and can begin to reason more logically.

strikes one as inadequate. Moreover, for the clinician, the question one often wants to raise is how can one use this understanding to bolster the reasoning of a child who is developmentally delayed—what Piaget witheringly dismissed as the American question. Piaget tended to argue that children could not be hurried through the stages. However, critics soon argued that some of the regularities that were apparently replicated in his work owed more to the manner in which the tasks were presented to the child than to any necessary underlying cohesion in types of thinking.

A typical experiment is to give a child two pieces of clay that are identical. Then one is rolled out into a sausage and the child is asked if they remain the same. Alternatively, the child is shown two test tubes of differing diameters. The same amount of liquid is poured into each, but, of course, reaches different heights. Which test tube has more liquid? Not surprisingly, younger children make more errors than older ones and it has been shown that conservation of mass (seeing that the quantity of material remains the same in spite of changes in shape) is acquired around 7 to 8 years, while conservation of *weight* is not achieved until 9 or 10 years. It is not until 11 or 12 that the child typically thinks that each shape also occupies the same amount of space (i.e. achieves conservation of *volume*).

Bruner was one of the earliest to demonstrate that children's judgements could be radically manipulated by small changes in the ways the tasks were presented. For example, in the studies on conservation of volume, a screen was placed between the child and the test tubes so that only the tops showed but not the levels reached by the liquid. This simple change meant that many younger children now understood that by pouring liquid from one container to another—perhaps something done daily in the bath—nothing had changed. Some children as young as 4 years were able to perform the revised task, but once they had to make the judgement again without the screen, they reverted to the more primitive form of reasoning. In other words, young children are more at the mercy of their perceptual impressions, a finding that needs to be taken on board in many circumstances.

(e) Language development

Children communicate from the beginning. They signal their basic needs, often by crying. Parents soon learn to respond to the differing signals. Their own child's crying can be very aversive to most parents and so they quickly learn how to switch the noise off! Autistic and brain damaged children produce grossly abnormal cries, but often parents with little experience do not recognize the unusual nature of the cry. Whilst lower primates and other animals can communicate, none use language in the flexible way that human infants come to do. Language—both spoken and written—is truly the most human of attributes.

Sophisticated social interaction is a precursor to the development of language. Though the infant is hard-wired for social interaction, it is not clear that these behaviours are strictly communicative in the sense of being intentional acts. What appears to be an early communicative competence may be best understood in terms of a *social releaser* model, where caregivers' interactions are triggers that release hard-wired reflexes from the infant, little different from the familiar palmar grasp reflex of the first month that causes an infant to grip an adult's thumb, even in their sleep. In this formulation there is no sense of a two-way communicative interaction being shared between carer and infant.

From approximately 2 months of age, infants appear to be active participants in the interactions that caregivers and their babies regularly play. When carers adjust their speech to the infant's preferences for high-pitched, rhythmic, and repetitive speech, often referred to as *motherese* and hold their face about 12 in. away, within the infants optimal focal range, a dynamic dance of turn-taking between carer and infant can be observed. The infant's attention is held, shared smiling can occur, the pitch and tone of utterances becomes matched and the infant can be observed to make distinctive formations with their lips referred to as 'pre-speech'. Caregiver and infant certainly appear to be experiencing social reciprocity. Some clever experiments based on perturbing the reciprocal nature of the infant caregiver interaction have challenged the notion of a social releaser model and given support to the infant's sophisticated early developing sensitivity to social reciprocity.

The still face paradigm requires the infant's partner to disturb the relationship by substituting their dynamic interaction by holding a still, expressionless face.[42] Presented with this perturbation, infants will initially increase their gesturing, as if to draw the adult back in, but become increasingly distressed, crying, or grimacing as this unnatural state continues. Of course, this is a relatively gross perturbation and technological advances have allowed developmentalists to alter more subtle aspects of the real-time contingency between an infant and its mother using a video link. Murray and colleagues filmed mothers and infants interacting over a video link and then altered the contingency by replaying a segment of the mother's interaction to the infant.[43] Infants as young as 8 weeks were able to detect this perturbation, and initially showed reduced levels of engagement followed by distress and protest. The levels of engagement rose again when the link was switched back to a live interaction. The replay condition demonstrated that simply presenting caregiver behaviours that had been previously adequate to elicit sustained interaction were no longer appropriate when they were taken out of the context of the dynamic flow between infant and caregiver. Thus it was not simply the presentation of maternal signals that triggered the release of infant communicative behaviours, but like a dance or a conversation, it was the to and fro sequence of behaviours between infant and caregiver that set the context of the flow of behaviours.

Language has not been the subject of serious study until the past 50 years. Beginning with simple descriptive studies of the acquisition of words, the complexities of grammar and cross-cultural comparisons, studies of language development now encompass many other dimensions from neuropsychological, brain imaging, and genetics. What stands out is just how difficult it is to affect the onset of language by manipulating the environment. It takes extraordinarily environmental deprivation to interfere with language development and even then, when the environment is normalized, considerable catch up occurs.

The grunts and single syllables of the first couple of months soon give way to the production of the full range of phonemes and babbling between 2 and 4 months. States of feelings are communicated clearly by 3 to 7 months. From 6 months, the baby begins to imitate simple sounds and unreinforced phonemes disappear from the vocabulary. By 8 months, the baby begins to utter two syllable combinations such as ma-ma and da-da—amongst the easiest to produce physically and, perhaps not coincidentally, the most emotionally evocative words parents want to hear. At around 12 months, the first true word appears, usually as the infant takes his first

Box 2.5.1.3 Language development

Vocabulary grows astronomically from 1 to 3 years and beyond. Children's sentences get longer and more complex. A good working approximation is that the average length of sentences is in keeping with the number of years of age:

Average length of sentences—2–5 years							
Age in months	24	30	36	42	48	54	60
Average number of words per sentence	1.7	2.4	3.3	4.0	4.3	4.7	4.6

From Smith.(46)

step—girls reaching the milestone slightly ahead of boys. Vocabulary grows astronomically from one to three years and beyond. Children's sentences get longer and more complex. A good working approximation is that the average length of sentences is in keeping with the number of years of age.(46)

Studies in the 1960s and 1970s established that language development followed complicated underlying rules. The idea that children learned language by successive approximations to adult speech being differentially reinforced was quickly laid to rest. Such techniques have an important place in remedial intervention for children with deviant language development, but for ordinary children the sheer inevitability, speed, and beauty of acquisition is overwhelming. This led many to postulate that there is a genetically encoded Language Acquisition Device that guides communication, although not the particular form of language that a particular child will develop. That still depends on what language they are exposed to.

Early sentences are telegraphic with some words acting as pivots on which other words hang to form flexible sentences. Thus, the pivot, 'all-gone' can have 'sock', 'milk', or 'daddy' added to create a whole range of meaningful simple sentences. Children develop rules for expression. A common error is for them to extract a rule and then overgeneralize it to a situation that is an exception in their particular language. For example, the present tense is used before the past tense. Instead of saying 'I went' children often form past participles by adding -ed to a stem and come up with the often heard 'I goed'. This shows they are learning a rule, even though they make some mistakes on the way.

Different ways of describing and classifying language disorders have been proposed in the past few years.(44) Bishop's(45) twin study finds that when language disorder is defined as a discrepancy between non-verbal IQ and language score the heritability is far less than when language delay and disorder are considered without reference to IQ. This is important for clinicians in identifying children with such difficulties .

(f) Memory

One of the most intriguing observations in the current child development literature is the contrast between the ever increasing evidence of just how complicated children's cognitive development is and the phenomenon known as infantile amnesia. Basically, people have very few memories before the age of 3 years. Clearly from all that has been described earlier about the differential reactions of babies to specific stimuli, to their recognizing their mother's voice or holding out their arms to their father rather than to a stranger, children increasingly have some form of central representations that they can work on. Yet, these early memories are not accessible in later life. It is really not until language is well established that people have what is ordinarily termed memory for past events.

Clearly, infantile amnesia poses a major challenge to any theory of child development or personality that tries to link very early experiences with later adjustment. Yet, early experience does affect the way in which relationships are formed, so what are the mechanisms? As the different types of memory (See Box 2.5.1.4) are better understood, so better assessment of these functions is possible.

Some very recent work has looked at implicit and explicit memory as well as attentional processes in children with generalized anxiety disorder, PTSD and depression. Broadly speaking, the preliminary findings are in accord with the voluminous findings with adult patients, namely that depressed children tend to have biases in memory for sad things, while anxious children do not. In contrast, children with anxiety disorders (including PTSD) have biases in attention that make them attend more to threatening cues in their environment—or at least to threatening words projected on computer screens. Studies using these adult-generated paradigms but utilized within a developmental framework should greatly increase our understanding of why some children break down under stress and others do not. Biases in cognitive processing of

Box 2.5.1.4 Memory

Goswami(48) summarizes many ingenious experiments that establish the parameters of children's memory. While parents and teachers often talk about children having problems with memory and even short-term memory, developmental psychologists have worked on much more complex paradigms and identified a number of different memory systems:

Recognition memory is simply the ability to realize that a particular stimulus has been encountered before. Recognition is always easier than recall—as those learning a foreign language can testify. Once established in the first year of life, recognition memory does not change much.

Implicit memory is another term for memory without awareness. Although not able to put it into words, people can act differently to previously exposed stimuli than to novel ones. This seems to be fully developed by around 4 years of age.

Episodic memory involves awareness. It is this memory system that organizes memories into stories or scripts concerning similar activities. These scripts contain both temporal and causal information. The ability to learn sequences in a particular chain of events does develop with age. It is now that one realizes that there needs to be some mechanism to get rid of many of the memories for everyday activities, otherwise the whole memory will get clogged up with non-essential information. In other words, memory processes are seen as being very active with some memory traces remaining in (technically) short-term memory for only a few seconds unless operated upon and stored in long-term store.

Eye witness memory has taken on a special importance as children are expected to testify in court on things they have witnessed happening to themselves or to others. Children can recall things fairly accurately, as long as deliberate leading questions are not put to them.(49) Three-year olds are more suggestible than 5-year olds. Experienced adults—such as psychiatrists or judges—evaluate children's responses to questioning about a real event using the child's behaviour while giving their answer. Where children gave firm answers with lots of supporting details, they were judged to have clear and accurate memories. Where children were uncertain and hesitant, they were seen as fabrication whereas they were hesitating because the questioner was asking the wrong questions—ones that were in conflict with what had actually happened—they were the ones who were actually telling the truth. The younger, confident children were often telling the adult what they wanted to hear! A great deal more needs to be done in relation to helping children recall what has happened to them without using leading questions.

Working memory was seen by Baddeley and his co-workers as consisting of a central executive processing linked to two separate subsystems: a phonological loop and a visuospatial sketch pad. Information decays in the phonological loop in 1 or 2 s, unless it is actively rehearsed. It is thought that children predominantly use a visuospatial encoding until they switch to the phonological/verbal system around the age of 5 years. Deaf children continue to rely on the visual encoding for much longer.

emotional reactions are implicated and can now be studied more readily.(47)

Social and emotional development

Alongside cognitive development, children are developing both socially and emotionally. It has been recognized for years that children brought up in institutions, away from their natural parents, often develop serious and subtle problems in social interactions and emotional development.

Arising in part from his studies of infants in institutions and his collaborative studies of children's reactions to being in hospital, as well as his dissatisfaction with contemporary psychoanalytic theory, Bowlby turned to ethology for an understanding of early infant relationships. He came to view the intense relationship between the infant and the caretaker, usually but not always the biological mother, as serving a biological survival value and as having been produced by natural selection. Bowlby proposed an attachment system that served to keep the child safe during the extended dependency of human infancy, by ensuring proximity to specific and reliable caregivers.(50)

As memory develops in the first year of life, and as the infant becomes more able to express emotion and to move independently, so there is evidence for selective attachment. This is shown round about 6 to 8 months onwards by the upset at leaving the attachment figure, by seeking comfort when threatened and by a general wariness of strangers.

The idea that attachments were simply associative learning—the baby comes to love the person who feeds him—was quickly dismissed by the evidence from Harlow's studies of infant monkeys. They attached to the cuddly terry-towelling surrogate rather than the wire surrogate where they were fed. Rather, selective attachments in the human served to protect the infant during the prolonged period of helplessness. The function of attachment changes over the years, with children using an attachment figure as a secure base from which to explore. Thus, almost paradoxically, the well attached toddler may move away from the attachment figure more than the insecurely attached counterpart. Attachment is not the same as clinginess.

The attachment system is just one amongst several innate systems proposed to operate in infancy, and it is the interplay between competing behavioural systems that led to the gold standard measure of attachment in infancy. Mary Ainsworth's based her Strange Situation Procedure (**SSP**) around observations of infants in Uganda.(51) The SSP pits the attachment system against the fear and exploration systems, in a structured, unfamiliar situation comprised of increasing levels of stress (e.g. strange room, strange adult, and separation from the caretaker). Observations are focused primarily on proximity seeking and contact maintaining behaviours during reunions with the caregiver. This measure is made possible by the development of stranger fear and mobility around the age of 9 months, and loses its validity by about 18 months as the infant's cognitive development permits different responses to separation, e.g. symbolic representation and language. After this point attachment assessments become less about observed behaviours and more about language and play.(52,53)

The SSP originally suggested three types of infant classification, representing organized responses to the prevailing environment: Insecure Avoidant (A) infants whose behaviour implied an attempt to minimize the importance of the attachment relationship and whose impoverished play and exploration functioned as a distraction from their need of comfort from the caretaker; Secure (B) infants who sought sufficient comfort from the caretaker to be able to quickly return to play and exploration; Insecure-Ambivalent, or Insecure-Resistant (C) infants whose behaviour suggested a maximization of the attachment relationship and an ambivalent

Box 2.5.1.5 Attachment

Ainsworth developed the theory and a method for detecting individual differences in attachment. She introduced the strange situations test in which an infant is left in the care of a stranger for a few minutes. The observer then notes how the infant copes both with the separation and with the reunion. These observations led to a tripartite classification of attachments:

- **Secure attachment:** The infant tends to seek proximity and contact with the attachment figure, shows a preference for the mother over a stranger, and shows very little distress before and after separation.
- **Avoidant insecure:** The baby does not cling when held, avoids the mother (or caretaker) during the reunion, and does not differentiate greatly between the caretaker and a stranger.
- **Resistant insecurity:** The infant resists contact and interaction with the mother. There is great distress at reunion.
- **Disorganized or avoidant insecurity:** This category had to be introduced when it was found that infants of severely depressed and abusive mothers showed a mixed pattern of attachments. The child shows contradictory patterns and unusual patterns of negative emotions.

preoccupation with the caretaker, at the expense of returning to play and exploration. Mary Main's observations of children in high-risk environments, particularly those exposed to maltreatment or parental psychopathology, led to an additional coding category, independent of, but complementing the tripartite Ainsworth system. Main noted a high rate of bizarre infant behaviours in the SSP of some children, which seemed to denote a lack of a clear, organized adaptation to separation from the caregiver. There was also evidence of apprehension and fearful behaviour in the presence of the caregiver, these infants seemed disorganized/disoriented, and were categorized as an Insecure-Disorganized (D) attachment pattern.(54)

A second innovation that Bowlby's attachment theory brought to the study of child development was the notion that the experience of the caregiving environment becomes represented as a cognitive heuristic or *internal working model of attachment* (**IWM**). This model is a dynamic, lifelong *work-in-progress*, which evolves as environmental experience accumulates but which also guides the selection of current behaviour on the basis of past experiences. Thus the infant's model of attachment is shaped by the experience of their caregiving environment, but simultaneously influences interactions with the infant's environment by selecting the behaviours most likely to achieve the goals, of say, proximity, based on what was previously successful. The IWM reflects an adaptation to the current environment, but the flexibility to adapt to changes in the environment is weighted by the accumulation of previous experience. So the possibility of fundamental change in attachment style is always possible but more difficult the longer the old environment prevailed.

Bowlby proposed that as time goes on the IWM becomes less about selecting the appropriate behaviours to protect the dependent infant via maintaining proximity to a safe and reliable caretaker, but moves to a level of representation of the self in relation to others. There is evidence to support the idea that the quality of attachment in infancy has some degree of influence over a range of social and emotional outcomes in early childhood, with peers, teachers and even stretching into later adolescence and early adulthood with partners and, as parents, their own offspring.(55) There is good evidence of some degree of continuity across the lifespan, but as Bowlby's original thesis would predict, expectations of continuity should not be overstated, and the degree of continuity is particularly low in high-risk samples.(56)

By the age of 3 to 4 years, most children show good evidence of having multiple attachment figures. By this age, their memories are so much greater that they are less dependent on the physical presence of the attachment figure to provide security and comfort. Bowlby saw good attachments in infancy as laying the basis for future social and intimate relationships and there is currently an explosion of work re-examining psychiatric conditions from an attachment perspective. Thus, Bowlby saw the child as developing a cognitive model of his effective social world, in keeping with the views of other cognitive theorists such as George Kelly, Aaron Beck, and Ronnie Janoff-Bulmann.

(a) Attachment, psychopathology, and 'reactive attachment disorder'

There is sometimes confusion surrounding the ideas of the relationship between insecure attachment and psychopathology. An organized-insecure attachment is an appropriate response to a particular environment. At most an organized-insecure attachment might be a vulnerability factor for later problems, in the context of other risks, but by no means would it be a major risk factor for pathology in itself. In terms of outcomes such as behaviour problems, the greatest influences still appear to be social risk factors, although attachment may confer some small additional risk.(57) There is stronger evidence for insecure-disorganized attachments predicting psychopathology. Aggressive behaviour problems in preschool are associated with insecure-disorganized classifications in infancy.(58) One study has suggested some degree of homotypic continuity into late adolescence with elevated rates of dissociative phenomena echoing the bizarre stilling and freezing behaviours typical of a insecure disorganized classification in infancy.(59) Of course, disorganized classifications most often occur in high-risk environments, so it is not always obvious if consequent psychopathology is a result of the attachment classification or of the continuing impact of a high-risk environment. Clearer evidence for the enduring impact of disorganized attachment could be collected when the high-risk environment that has led to the disorganization is terminated.

A negative aspect of the focus on attachments has been the emergence of an ill defined disorder described as reactive attachment disorder which seems to be diagnosable by the presence of any or all of a long list of symptoms and signs that haunted previous generations under such labels as Minimal Brain Dysfunction and the like. This has been associated in some countries with the use of assaultative holding therapies intended to break the child's resistance to forming attachments. Clearly, more careful studies need to be undertaken to try to pinpoint the subtle social difficulties presented by children whose early lives have been disrupted in fostering and adoption, but care also needs to be taken to adduce evidence for appropriate interventions.

Having good, supportive social relationships has been shown to be a major protective factor in the aetiology and maintenance of many psychiatric disorders. The ability to make and maintain friends—initially of the same age and later of any age—is often related to the existence of disorders such as personality disorders, social anxiety disorders, depression, and even post-traumatic stress disorders. The emphasis on social skills training for socially inadequate persons points to the early basis for such deficits even though they may have their greatest impact in adulthood. Some children are less sensitive to social cues than others, and some children misinterpret the intentions of other people. Both lead to difficulties, albeit of different sorts.

Boys and girls tend to develop different types of social relationships. It may be inconveniently politically incorrect to note that children tend to prefer playing with others of the same gender when freed from adult influence. Boys tend to play in larger, looser groups in which issues of dominance and play fighting predominate; girls relate in smaller groups of more intense relationships, with best friends often changing.

Concluding comments

Taking a developmental perspective to mental health issues should apply across the lifespan. Psychiatrists working with adults need to understand where their clients are coming from and where they are going to. They need to understand the pleasures and pressures that children bring to their parents, and where appropriate they should be considering the impact of parental illness on the children. The institutionalized separation of child and adult psychiatry (in terms of service delivery) should not lead to a separation in ways of considering the developmental context of presenting problems.

This chapter has shown that there are many small, focused models of development that deal with discrete areas of development. Stage theories emphasize differences at different stages; social learning theories emphasize continuities on processes of development. As long as practitioners are aware that when they say a child is at a particular stage, this is but a rough guide to describing the child, which may be fine. It is when such models are taken literally, that oversimplification leads to poor practice. There is no one overarching theory of child development and while this may be inconvenient for examiners, it truly reflects the rich diversity of human development. By paying more attention to the interactions between biological, social, and psychological factors, a better understanding of healthy, normal development will emerge. Empirical studies will help identify risk and protective factors which in turn will lead to better mental health promotion and more effective interventions when mental disorders manifest.

Further information

Field, T. (2007). *The amazing infant*. Oxford, Blackwell.

Grossman, K.E., Waters, E., and Grossman, K. (2006). *Attachment from infancy to adulthood: the major longitudinal studies*. Guilford, New York.

http://www.apa.org/topics/topicchildren.html

http://www.devpsy.org/links/index.html

References

1. Cox, A. and Rutter, M. (1985). Diagnostic appraisal and interviewing. In *Child psychiatry: modern approaches* (2nd edn) (eds. M. Rutter and L. Hersov). Blackwell, Oxford.
2. Rutter, M., Graham, P., Chadwick, O., *et al.* (1975). Adolescent turmoil: fact or fiction? *Journal of Child Psychology and Psychiatry*, **17**, 35–56.
3. Harrington, R. (1993). *Depressive disorder in childhood and adolescence*. Wiley, Chichester.
4. Rutter, M. (1975). *Helping troubled children*. Penguin Books, Harmondsworth.
5. Staats, A.W. (1971). *Child learning, intelligence and personality: principles of a behavioral interaction approach*. Harper & Row, New York.
6. Rutter, M. (1980). Psychosexual development. In *Scientific foundations of developmental psychiatry* (ed. M. Rutter), pp. 322–39. Heinemann Medical, London.
7. Berger, M. (1985). Temperament and individual differences. In *Child psychiatry: modern approaches* (2nd edn) (eds. M. Rutter and L. Hersov). Blackwell, Oxford.
8. Kagan, J. (1997). Temperament. In *Handbook of child and adolescent psychiatry*, Vol. 1: *Infants and preschoolers* (ed. J.D. Noshpitz), pp. 268–75, Chapter 27. Wiley, New York.
9. Keogh, B.K. (1982). Children's temperament and teachers' decisions. In *Temperamental differences in infants and young children* (eds. R. Porter and G.M. Collins), pp. 269–78. Pitman, London.
10. Eysenck, H.J. and Eysenck, S.B.G. (1969). *Personality structures and measurement*. Routledge and Kegan Paul, London.
11. Scott, S. (2003). Integrating attachment theory with other approaches to developmental psychopathology. *Attachment and human development*, **5**, 307–12.
12. Childers, P. and Wimmer, M. (1971). The concept of death in early childhood. *Child Development*, **42**, 1299–301.
13. Koocher, G.P. (1974). Talking with children about death. *The American Journal of Orthopsychiatry*, **44**, 404–11.
14. Wolff, S. (1969). *Children under stress*. Allen Lane, Penguin Press, London.
15. Monroe, B. and Kraus, F. (eds.) (2005). *Brief interventions with bereaved children*. Oxford University Press, Oxford.
16. Rutter, M. and Rutter, M. (1993). *Developing minds: challenge and continuity across the life span*. Basic Books, New York.
17. Janoff-Bulman, R. (1985). The aftermath of victimization: rebuilding shattered assumptions. In *Trauma and its wake*, Vol. 1 (ed. C.R. Figley). Brunner/Mazel, New York.
18. Thomas, A., Chess, S., and Birch, H.G. (1968). *Temperament and behavior disorders in children*. University of London Press, London.
19. Meichenbaum, D. (1993). Stress inoculation training: a 20-year update. In *Principles and practice of stress management* (2nd edn) (eds. P.M. Lehrer and R.L. Woolfolk). Guilford, New York.
20. Bradley, L. and Bryant, P.E. (1983). Categorizing sounds and learning to read B a causal connection. *Nature*, **301**, 419–21.
21. King, R.D., Raynes, N.V., and Tizard, J. (1971). *Patterns of residential care: sociological studies in institutions for handicapped children*. Routledge & Kegan Paul, London.
22. Cicchetti, D. (1984). The emergence of developmental psychopathology. *Child Development*, **55**, 1–7.
23. Sroufe, L.A. and Rutter, M. (1984). The domain of developmental psychopathology. *Child Development*, **55**, 17–29.
24. Garmezy, N. (1974). Children at risk: the search for the antecedents of schizophrenia. I: conceptual models and research methods. *Schizophrenia Bulletin*, **8**, 14–90.
25. Santostefano, S. (1978). *A biodevelopmental approach to clinical child psychology*. John Wiley & Sons, New York.
26. Rutter, M. (1983). Continuities and discontinuities in socioemotional development: empirical and conceptual perspectives. In *Continuities and discontinuities in development* (eds. R. Harmon and R. Emde). Plenum Press, New York.
27. Bandura, A. (1973). *Aggression: a social learning analysis*. Prentice-Hall, London.
28. Yule, W. (1978). Behavioural treatment of conduct disorder. In *Child psychiatry: modern approaches* (eds. M. Rutter and L. Hersov). Blackwell, Oxford.
29. Cantwell, D.P. (1988). DSM-III Studies. In *Assessment and diagnosis in child psychopathology* (eds. M. Rutter, A.H. Tuma., and I.S. Lann), pp. 3–36. David Fulton Publishers, London.
30. Rutter, M. and Shaffer, D. (1980). A step forward or back in terms of the classification of child psychiatric disorders? *Journal of the American Academy of Child Psychiatry*, **19**, 371–94.
31. Yule, W. (1981). The epidemiology of child psychopathology. In *Advances in clinical child psychology*, Vol. 4 (eds. B.B. Lahey and A.E. Kazdin), pp. 1–51. Plenum, New York.
32. Garber, J. (1984). Classification of childhood psychopathology: a developmental perspective. *Child Development*, **55**, 30–48.
33. Yule, W. and Williams, R. (1990). Post traumatic stress reactions in children. *Journal of Traumatic Stress*, **3**, 279–95.
34. Yule, W., Perrin, S., and Smith, P. (1999). Post-traumatic stress disorders in children and adolescents. In *Post-traumatic stress disorders: concepts and therapy* (ed. W. Yule), pp. 25–50. Wiley, Chichester.
35. Scheeringa, M.S., Zeanah, C.H., Drell, M.J., *et al.* (1995). Two approaches to the diagnosis of Posttraumatic Stress Disorder in infancy and early childhood. *Journal of the American Academy of Child and Adolescent Psychiatry*, **34**, 191–200.
36. Fantz, R.L. (1961). *The origin of form perception*. Scientific American, Reprint 459.
37. Morton, J. and Johnson, M. (1991). CONSPEC and CONLERN: a two-process theory of infant face-recognition. *Psychological Review*, **98**, 164–81.

38. Fagan, J.F. (1984). The relationship of novelty preferences during infancy to later intelligence and later recognition memory. *Intelligence*, **8**, 339–46.
39. DeCasper, A.J. and Spence, M.J. (1986). Prenatal maternal speech influences newborns' perception of speech sounds. *Infant Behavior & Development*, **9**(2), 133–50.
40. Porter, R.H., Makin, J.W., Davis, L.B., *et al.* (1992). Breast-fed infants respond to olfactory cues from their own mother and unfamiliar lactating females. *Infant Behavior & Development*, **15**(1), 85–93.
41. Meltzoff, A. and Moore, M. (1989). Imitation in newborns: exploring the range of gestures imitated and the underlying mechanisms. *Developmental Psychology*, **25**, 954–62.
42. Tronick, E.Z., Als, H., Adamson, L., *et al.* (1978). The infants' response to entrapment between contradictory messages in face-to-face interactions. *Journal of the American Academy of Child Psychiatry*, **16**, 1–13.
43. Murray, L. and Trevarthen, C. (1986). The infant's role in mother-infant communications. *Journal of Child Language*, **13**(1), 15–29.
44. Yule, W. and Rutter, M. (eds.) (1987). *Language development and disorders*. MacKeith Press, London.
45. Bishop, D.V.M. (1998). In *Perspectives on the classification of specific developmental disorders* (eds. J. Rispens, T. van Yperen, and W. Yule). Kluwer Academic, Dordrecht, The Netherlands.
46. Smith, M.E. (1926). An investigation of the development of the sentence and extent of vocabulary in young children. *University of Iowa Studies in Child Welfare*, **3**(5).
47. Dalgleish, T., Taghavi, M.R., Neshat-Doost, H.T., *et al.* (2003). Patterns of processing bias for emotional information across clinical disorders: a comparison of attention, memory and prospective cognition in children and adolescents with depression, generalized anxiety and Posttraumatic Stress Disorder. *Journal of Clinical Child and Adolescent Psychology*, **32**(1), 10–21
48. Goswami, U. (1998). *Cognition in children*. Psychology Press, Hove.
49. Bruck, M., Ceci, S., and Hembrooke, H. (1998). Reliability and credibility of young children's reports. *American Psychologist*, **53**(2), 136–51.
50. Bretherton, I. (1992). The origins of attachment theory: John Bowlby and Mary Ainsworth. *Developmental Psychology*, **28**, 759–75.
51. Ainsworth, M.D.S., Blehar, M.C., Waters, E., *et al.* (1978). *Patterns of attachment: a psychological study of the strange situation*. Lawrence Erlbaum, Hillsdale NJ.
52. Main, M. and Cassidy, J. (1988). Categories of response to reunion with the parent at age 6: predictable from infant attachment classifications and stable over a 1-month period. *Developmental Psychology*, **24**, 415–26.
53. Green, J., Stanley, C., Smith, V., *et al.* (2000). A new method of evaluating attachment representations in the young school-age children: the Manchester Child Attachment Story Task (MCAST). *Attachment & Human Development*, **2**(1), 48–70.
54. Main, M. and Solomon, J. (1990). Procedures for identifying infants as disorgainzed/disoriented during the Ainsworth Strange Situation. In *Attachment in the preschool years: theory, research and intervention* (eds. M.T. Greenberg, D. Cicchetti, and E.M. Cummings), pp. 121–60. University of Chicago Press, Chicago.
55. Grossmann, Klaus E., Grossmann, Karin, Waters, and Everett. (2005). Attachment from infancy to adulthood: the major longitudinal studies. Guilford Press, New York, US.
56. Weinfield, N.S., Sroufe, L.A., and Egeland, B. (2000). Attachment from infancy to early adulthood in a high-risk sample: continuity, discontinuity, and their correlates. *Child Development*, **71**(3), 695–702.
57. Belsky, J. and Fearon, R.M.P. (2002). Infant-mother attachment security, contextual risk, and early development: a moderational analysis. *Development and Psychopathology*, **14**(2), 293–310.
58. Lyons Ruth, K., Easterbrooks, M.A., and Cibelli, C.D. (1997). Infant attachment strategies, infant mental lag, and maternal depressive symptoms: predictors of internalizing and externalizing problems at age 7. *Developmental Psychology*, **33**(4), 681–92.
59. Carlson, E.A. (1998). A prospective longitudinal study of attachment disorganization/disorientation. *Child Development*, **69**(4), 1107–28.

2.5.2 Psychology of attention

Elizabeth Coulthard and Masud Husain

Introduction

Attention is generally taken to be the process by which people are able to concentrate on certain information or processes, while ignoring other events. It appears to be a fundamental attribute of human brain processing, although difficult to pin down in terms of mechanism. Psychologists have attempted to fractionate attention in many different ways, using ingenious behavioural paradigms. In this section we, too, will consider different aspects of attention: selective, phasic and sustained, divided and executive control of attention. However, it would be fair to say that all these aspects of attention do not normally operate in isolation. Instead they interact, and deficiencies in one aspect of attention, for example, in a patient population, often to do not occur in isolation. Functional imaging and lesion studies of attention have proliferated in recent years, attempting to place a neurobiological framework to these varied processes. In general, these studies also tend to confirm the view that attention is likely an emergent property of widespread brain networks, with a special emphasis on frontal and parietal regions of the human brain (Fig. 2.5.2.1). In this discussion we illustrate several aspects of attention with examples particularly from literature on visual attention, which is the most widely studied area, but it should be appreciated that many of the concepts discussed here extend to other domains. In fact, there is a good deal of evidence to suggest that several aspects of attention operate at a supra- or cross-modal level allowing integration of information from different sources.

Recent studies suggest there are two fronto-parietal networks: (Fig. 2.5.2.1) a *dorsal* parieto-frontal network involving the superior parietal lobe (SPL) and dorsal frontal regions such as the frontal eye field (FEF); and a *ventral* network involving the inferior parietal lobe (IPL), temporoparietal junction (TPJ) and inferior frontal gyrus (IFG). In addition, dorsomedial frontal areas, including the anterior cingulate cortex (ACC) and pre-supplementary area (pre-SMA) may play a key role in flexible control of attention for strategic behaviour.

Selective attention

Selective attention refers to the processes involved in selecting relevant information and filtering out irrelevant items from the vast array of information we are exposed to. The brain has limited capacity: it simply cannot process everything it is exposed to. Nor would it be sensible for it do so because the majority of sensory input to which it is exposed is not behaviourally relevant. Therefore there is a need for mechanisms to select the

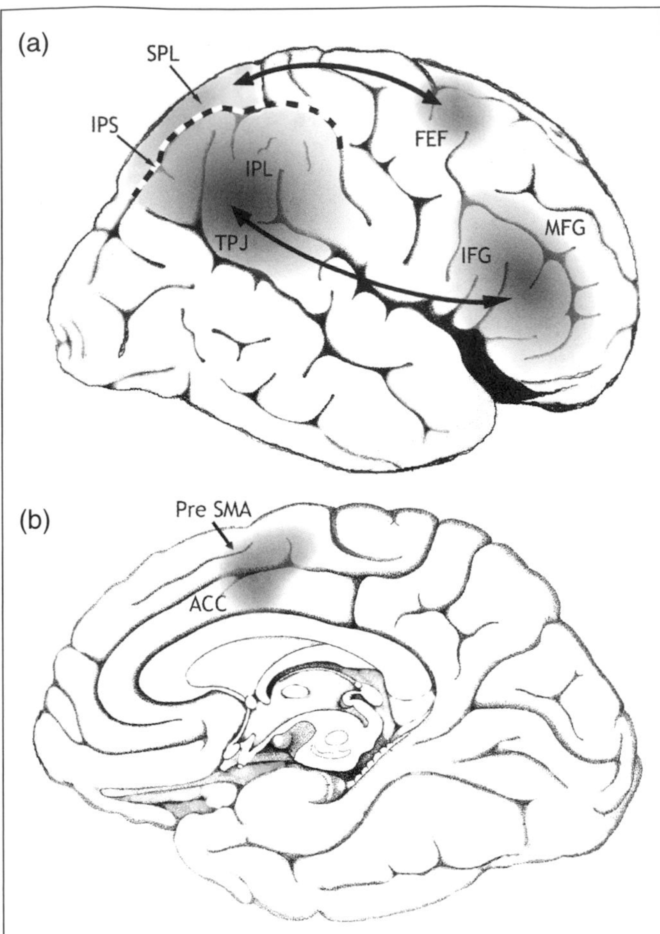

Fig. 2.5.2.1 Lateral (a) and medial (b) regions in the right hemisphere involved in attention. (IPS intraparietal sulcus; MFG, middle frontal gyrus.)

most behaviourally significant and important material, and dispose of trivial, unimportant information. Such selection may occur 'bottom-up', driven by competition between sensory inputs, or 'top-down',
guided by the goals that an individual might have at any moment in time.[1]

Thus if a ball is unexpectedly hurled towards an observer, his attention is likely to be captured—'bottom-up'—by the sensory input of a projectile moving at high velocity towards his head. In this case, selection has been driven by the most perceptually salient item in the external environment. 'Top-down' attention mechanisms, on the other hand, concern selection that is biased by internal goals. For example, consider the processes involved in looking for a friend in a busy, crowded train station. Here the selection process is driven by the features you are searching for: your friend's hair colour, facial features, height all play a role in guiding this search. Importantly, under these circumstances, even perceptually very salient items may be filtered out—or not attended—if they are irrelevant to the task.

But when does selection occur? Is it early or late in the processing of sensory information? This is an issue that dominated attention research for many years. Some investigators proposed that selection occurs early, directly after analysis of the physical characteristics or features of sensory stimuli, but before they are fully identified. According to this view, unattended information receives little or no further processing from this point on. By contrast, others argued that *all* stimuli are analysed up to the point that they are identified. Selection occurs only after this, late in the processing stream. So items that are eventually ignored or unattended, i.e. those that are not selected, actually receive considerable processing before they are discarded. Note that this late selection model allows for the possibility that items which are eventually ignored may nevertheless be processed to a deep level. Thus, even though they may not be attended to, they have the potential to influence our actions subliminally. Most researchers would now agree that there is good evidence for *both* early and late selection systems in the human brain. In fact, whether selection occurs early or late is likely to be influenced by the specific demands of the task.

Two highly influential experimental paradigms used to study selective attention in healthy humans and patients have both focused on *spatial* attention in the visual system. Posner first developed a spatial cueing task in which subjects view a display consisting of a central cross on which they are asked to maintain fixation throughout the trial. On either side of the cross, there are two square boxes. Participants are instructed to ignore a cue which consists of transient illumination of either the left or right box. At varying intervals after the cue, a target stimulus (an asterisk) appears in either left or right box and subjects are required to press a response button as quickly as possible. In 80 per cent of trials the cue is 'valid' in that it occurred at the location of the subsequent target. However, in the remaining 20 per cent of trials the cue is 'invalid', appearing in the box opposite that in which the target subsequently appeared. In healthy volunteers, reaction times to targets appearing where valid cues appear are significantly shorter than when invalid cues are presented.

This critical finding suggests that attention can be spatially localized like a beam or 'spotlight'. Moreover, attention can be captured by the abrupt onset of the cue so that visual processing is selectively oriented towards it, thereby improving responses if a target subsequently appears there. On invalid trials, Posner argued, attention would first have to disengage from the invalidly cued location and then shift to the correct location before engaging it. Note that such shifts occur covertly in the absence of overt eye movements; they represent shifts of visual processing from one location to another across a representation of space in the brain. Subsequent studies have shown that the orienting of attention to a spatial location not only appears to speed up detection of a visual stimulus, as measured by reaction times, but also can improve discrimination of items from non-targets. The neurophysiological mechanisms underlying such boosting of performance are currently the subject of intense scrutiny.[2]

The second experimental task that has proven to be extremely important in selective attention research is the visual search paradigm developed by Treisman. In this task, subjects have to find a target shape embedded among distractors. In simple so-called 'feature search', a target may be defined by a unique feature, e.g. a red circle among green circles is defined uniquely by its colour and therefore 'pops-out' among the distractors. Treisman has considered that such feature searches can occur *pre-attentively* in parallel across the visual scene, without the need for a spotlight of visual attention. She argued that attention needs to be deployed in more complex tasks where a target may share one or more features with distractors, e.g. finding a red circle among green circles and red squares. In this case, a single feature (colour or shape) is not sufficient to define the target. Instead, the visual system has to find the unique conjunction of red colour and circular shape, and the target does not pop-out to the observer. Such 'conjunction searches', Treisman argued, requires the spotlight of attention to shift serially from one location to the next, inspecting each item in turn. In her model, spatial attention acts to bind or glue together features occupying the same location in space, e.g. the colour, form, luminance, and other attributes that belong to an object at one location in space.

Both the Posner cueing task and Triesman's conjunction task have been used in neuroimaging studies of healthy volunteers and patients with focal lesions on the brain.(3) The results of such studies suggest that regions within the parietal and frontal cortex play a critical role in deploying spatial attention (Fig. 2.5.2.1). In general, dorsal regions of this parieto-frontal network have been implicated in the spatial shifts of processing attention that occupy such a key role in the models of selective attention developed by Posner and Treisman.

Phasic, sustained, and vigilant attention

Several groups have made a distinction between phasic alertness, sustained attention, and vigilance. In general, 'phasic alertness' is used to refer to improvements in performance that follow a warning signal, e.g. an auditory tone or visual cue. The tasks used in such studies are often very simple, comparing the time to respond to a particular stimulus when it is preceded, or not, by a warning tone. Over the course of a few hundred milliseconds after such a warning signal, performance can alter appreciably, with reaction times first declining in the interval from 100 to 500–1000 ms after the tone, and then increasing again thereafter. Thus, this attentional facilitation is limited to a very narrow window in time and refers to the ability of the brain to respond better when warned to expect an upcoming cue to act.

By contrast, 'vigilance' is the term used to refer to the ability to be in a state of readiness to detect small, infrequent changes in the environment which occur at random intervals over *prolonged* periods of time (often hours or tens of minutes). The early studies on vigilance were conducted to assess the ability of radar operators to detect infrequent signals on their screens in the Second World War. Over long 'vigils' the ability to detect rare changes falls—the so-called 'vigilance decrement'—and this may be modulated by the frequency of target and non-target (distractor) stimuli as well as the memory load imposed on observers.

'Sustained attention' is best considered to be at the other end of the continuum from vigilance. Here, too, observers may have to respond over a prolonged period, but the information flow is rapid, with a high frequency of events to monitor and respond to. An everyday, extreme example may be the interpreter who has to give a simultaneous translation of a press conference. In the laboratory, sustained attention may be studied using stimuli presented at a rapid rate, as in many continuous performance tests (CPTs). Such experiments reveal that even healthy subjects may show 'lapses of attention' under such circumstances, with errors of omission (failing to respond to a target stimulus) or errors of commission (responding to a non-target), or increase in mean response time. Another measure that has attracted interest, of late, particularly in patient populations, is the variability of reaction times in such tests.

Functional imaging and lesion studies of patients have emphasized the role of the right lateral frontal lobe in aspects of vigilance and sustained attention. However, it is clear that the inferior parietal lobe of the right hemisphere also has a critical role to play in these functions. The distinction between frontal and parietal contributions remains to be established but, unlike spatial attention studies, investigations of non-spatial vigilance and sustained attention suggest that *ventral*—and not dorsal—frontal and parietal regions of the right hemisphere have a special role in these processes (Fig. 2.5.2.1).(4)

Divided attention

Divided attention is the ability to concentrate on more than one activity at once. Although we often execute two tasks simultaneously ('dual task'), performance on one or both tasks may be impaired compared to doing either alone, e.g. when driving and having a phone conversation. Experimental findings that demonstrate such decrements in performance raise important questions regarding the mechanisms underlying attention. Many investigators have proposed that if a second task leads to deterioration in performance of the first, one may conclude that the two tasks depend on the same brain resources. Because such resources are limited, there will be a decrement in performance once resource limits are reached. Some authors have argued for a single, central resource while others have presented evidence for multiple resources, but the basic concept is the same across these accounts: tasks compete for finite brain resources and if they share those resources, performance suffers.

Other investigators have raised the possibility that it is not just 'resources' that we need to consider but also processing limitations. Two tasks might be difficult to perform simultaneously because they both use a single processing channel or because the tasks interfere with each other. Different paradigms have suggested 'bottlenecks'—mechanisms that are dedicated serially to only one task at a time or have limited resources to spread over two tasks. Such bottlenecks may exist at the level of attentional focus, storage in visual short-term memory (VSTM), and motor preparation.(5) Consider first the issue of processing bottlenecks.

The attentional blink paradigm is used to investigate temporal limitations of attentional processing. Subjects view a stream of individually presented letters and are required to report when they see either of the two target letters (say X and Y). People generally struggle to report a second target if it falls within 360 ms of the first, despite being able to report the second target when not attending to the first. Processing the first object before being free to process the next item appears to require up to 360 ms. Thus speed of attentional processing may act as a limiting factor in dual task processes. Functional imaging studies suggest, once again, that a fronto-parietal network is critical in this regard. Activity in fronto-parietal areas occurs only when the second stimulus is reported. In contrast, even when the second stimulus is undetected, there is still activity in the early visual areas. These findings point to a bottleneck in attentional processes which occurs after basic visual processing has begun, but before conscious perception, consistent with pre-attentive and attentive stages of visual processing as discussed in the section on selective attention above.

The amount of information we can encode at any one time is also limited. The capacity for holding objects in visual short-term memory (VSTM) is around four objects. Diversion of attention away from an object reduces the accuracy with which it can be encoded suggesting that attention is an important limiting factor in the number of items held in VSTM. Both electrophysiological and functional imaging experiments have suggested that the capacity for storage of objects in VSTM is related to posterior parietal and occipital cortex activity.

As well as these perceptual and memory limitations in capacity, there are limits at the motor selection stage of processing. The psychological refractory period (PRP) refers to the delay in the second response when a subject has to respond to two stimuli one after the other. The shorter the time difference between the two stimuli, the greater the delay in the second response. This bottleneck may be at the level of response selection rather than a pure perceptual or attentional slowing. However, although it is often the case that performing two simultaneous responses with a single effector (e.g. the hand) may be impossible, the PRP cannot simply be explained in terms of a motor selection bottleneck.

When subjects are asked to make two responses to the same attribute of an object (name the colour and press a button for the colour), they can select the appropriate responses at the same time. In addition the PRP is much longer when required to make an incongruent response (e.g. saying 'A' in response visual presentation of the number 1) than a congruent response (e.g. saying 'one' in response to visual presentation of number 1) to the second stimulus. Pashler has proposed that at any time we have a number of response selection rules, with each rule specifying condition-action linkages or associations, i.e. which condition is associated with which action. According to this view, the bottleneck is at the level of rule application, but each rule can specify multiple motor responses.

But how and where rules are selected and maintained? Many studies have suggested a critical role for frontal—so-called 'executive'—control systems when rules need to be applied, as we shall discuss in the next section. Performing two *well learned* or relatively *automatic* tasks together might not lead to performance impairment because these tasks do not require input from such 'executive' control systems to implement rules and select appropriate responses.

In summary, there are multiple possible levels at which processing capacity may be limited. Both the speed of attentional processing and the number of items that can be attended to at once and held in memory are limited. In addition, supervisory or executive control regions may regulate motor output perhaps by implementing goals or strategies. Whether these bottlenecks are due to one resource being serially applied to each stimulus or a limited capacity system shared simultaneously by two processes, but perhaps with a bias toward one, is currently unclear.

Executive control of attention

How are the subtypes of attention mentioned above organized so that they are activated at the appropriate time? Events in our environment reflexively engage attentional networks and this type of stimulus-driven or bottom-up activation may underlie some processes such as rapid shifts in spatial attention to highly salient events. However, everyday experience tells us that rather than always reacting to our surroundings, we are able to generate and implement plans to complete complex tasks and sometimes ignore highly salient events. This has led to the idea of a supervisory or executive attentional control system. Evidence for the presence of such a system comes from patients with brain damage, particularly those with frontal damage.

Patients with frontal lesions have difficulty maintaining attention on a task. They may be highly distractable, or find it difficult to divide attention between competing task demands in an optimal way. Some patients also encounter problems shifting from one task type or task rule to another, often demonstrating perseveration—

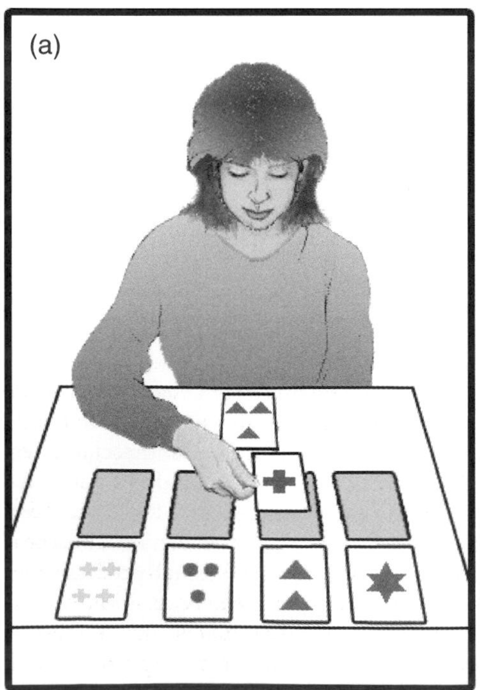

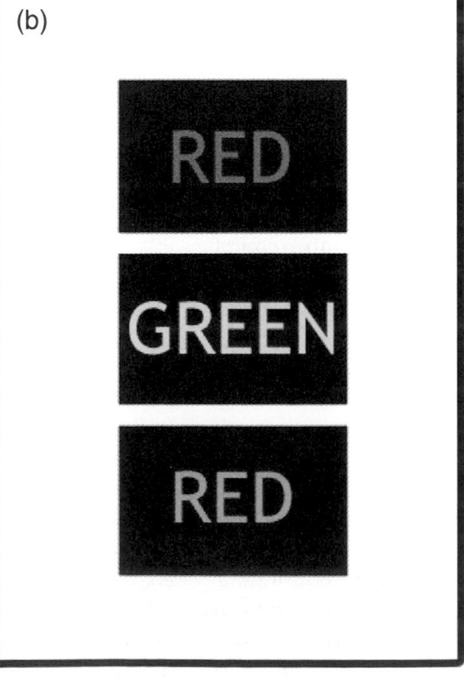

Fig. 2.5.2.2 In the Wisconsin card sorting test (a), the patient has to place a new card alongside one of the visible cards according to a rule to match colour, suit or number. The rule changes during the task and the learning occurs by trial and error. Patients with frontal lobe damage fail to update the new rule. The Stroop task (b) requires subjects to give the colour of the text. In the first box this is easy because the colour of the text and the meaning of the word are congruent (both red). The second and third boxes illustrate the incongruent condition. This is more difficult because the text colour is different from the meaning of the word. Normal individuals are slower to respond in the incongruent than congruent conditions.

applying the 'old' task rule inappropriately when they should be applying the 'new' one. For example, on tasks such as the Wisconsin card sorting task, where subjects establish the criteria for grouping playing cards into sets (according to either colour, or suit, or number) and then have to change to a new grouping rule, such individuals have great difficulty shifting to a new rule (Fig. 2.5.2.2a). Multiple components of executive control including flexible task-switching and response inhibition, as well as vigilance and error monitoring, are required to successfully sort the cards when the rule is switched.

Norman and Shallice developed a model of attention control called the supervisory attention system that conceptualized how this behaviour might be organized. They proposed that routine or well-learned behaviour occurs because perceptual information activates a set of schemas that then triggers appropriate motor output. However, these perceptual-motor associations would no longer be appropriate when the rule changed, for example when one had to sort according to suit rather than number in the Wisconsin card sorting task (Fig. 2.5.2.2a). Under these circumstances, they proposed that the supervisory attention network alters the bias of the schemas so that different motor outputs are triggered by perceptual events. Therefore, rather than processing simple stimulus-response associations such as always signalling the right foot to move from the brake to the accelerator when a green traffic light appears, brain regions within the supervisory network would respond to information at a more abstract level. When driving, for example, one might want to *inhibit* the prepotent response associated with the green traffic light (to press the accelerator) if confronted by a variety of visual inputs such as someone still crossing the road or a car stalled in front. *Response inhibition* in this and other contexts is thought to be one of many abstract functions undertaken by the supervisory control systems.

What are these abstract processes and which regions of the brain perform these supervisory operations? Both lesion studies and functional imaging work have contributed to understanding executive functions. Functional imaging studies provide information about areas activated in association with certain processes while lesion investigations show which regions are critical for normal behaviour. In paradigms such as the Stroop task, subjects are asked to report either the colour of print used to type a word or read the word which can be the same (congruent) or a different (incongruent) colour to the print (Fig. 2.5.2.2b). To avoid making errors in the incongruent condition one is required to focus attention on the target information and suppress the unwanted response. This is usually associated with a reaction time delay in the incongruent compared to the congruent condition. The delay is greater when subjects have to report the colour of the print and inhibit their reading of the word, presumably because word reading is a more hard-wired or automatic than colour naming. Functional imaging and lesion data from subjects performing the Stroop tasks show that medial and lateral frontal as well as parietal areas appear to form a network for executive control of attention.

There is recent evidence that each of these regions has a distinct role within the executive control network. Specifically, the left lateral frontal cortex is thought to maintain and flexibly update task rules, whereas, right lateral prefrontal cortex is critically involved in *inhibiting* the prepotent response associated with a stimulus. Dorsomedial frontal regions (Fig. 2.5.2.1b) reliably activate when executive control is required and are thought perhaps to play a key role in monitoring errors. In addition, part of this area—the anterior cingulate cortex—is considered by some investigators to be important for mediating the physiological autonomic response to demanding circumstances. More posterior regions including parietal cortex, may also contribute to attentional control but, to date, their role has been less well investigated. Research into how areas involved in executive control act and interact to modulate attention is a rapidly expanding area of cognitive neuroscience, likely to yield important insight into mechanisms behind flexible and efficient behaviour.

Acknowledgements

This work is funded by the Wellcome Trust.

Further information

Johnson, A. and Proctor, R.W. (2004). *Attention theory and practice.* Sage Press, California.

Styles, E.A. (2006). *The psychology of attention.* (2nd edn). Psychology Press, New York.

Ward, A. (2004). *Attention a neuropsychological approach.* Psychology Press, Hove.

References

1. Desimone, R. and Duncan, J. (1995). Neural mechanisms of selective visual attention. *Annual Review of Neuroscience*, **18**, 193–222.
2. Treue, S., (2001). Neural correlates of attention in primate visual cortex. *Trends in Neurosciences*, **24**(5), 295–300.
3. Corbetta, M. and Shulman, G.L. (2002). Control of goal-directed and stimulus-driven attention in the brain. *Nature Reviews Neuroscience*, **3**, 215–29.
4. Husain, M. and Nachev, P. (2007). Space and the parietal cortex. *Trends in Cognitive Sciences*, **11**, 30–36.
5. Marois, R. and Ivanoff, J. (2005) .Capacity limits of information processing in the brain. *Trends in Cognitive Sciences*, **9**, 296–305.

2.5.3 **Psychology and biology of memory**

Andreas Meyer-Lindenberg and Terry E. Goldberg

Memory in psychiatric practice

Memory is the ability to store, retain, and retrieve information. This cognitive function plays a key role in psychiatry. Dementia and the amnesic disorders have memory dysfunction as a defining feature. Intrusive and recurrent emotional memories are one of the most distressing symptoms in post-traumatic stress disorder. Although not as obvious, problems with memory are also commonly revealed on testing in schizophrenia. Remembered episodes are often a focus in psychotherapy, as is the acquisition of new habits and response patterns. An ability to understand and assess memory is therefore important for the practising psychiatrist. In this chapter, basic neurobiological and psychological information on memory will be reviewed. We have tried to cover a very broad field in a concise manner and give the interested reader a sense of the key memory systems and subsystems that are thought to be important for human information processing in health and in disease. We have emphasized the conceptual over the theoretical and key findings over the experimental details where possible. At times, we have not carefully separated the cognitive and neuroanatomical levels of analysis, both because they are sometimes almost inextricably bound and because it made our explanations clearer not to do so. Necessarily but not happily, we have omitted many important and active areas of investigation.

Forms of memory

One of the key discoveries of cognitive neuroscience is that 'memory' is not an unitary function, but consists of several forms that can be dissociated neurally and are differentially impacted by psychiatric disorders.[1] Several approaches can be taken to subdivide memory. One of the most straightforward is by the duration over which information is retained. In this way, ultrashort-term, short-term, and long-term memory can be distinguished. **Ultrashort-term**, also called **sensoric** or **echoic/iconic** memory, lasts from milliseconds to seconds and consists of a brief and modality-specific retention of sensory information. For example, most people are able to 'replay' the auditory trace of the last second or so of a conversation, or briefly maintain a scene visualized after they close their eyes. In contradistinction, **short-term memory** has been shown to be relevant to a large number of psychiatric disorders. In short-term memory, information is briefly (over a period from seconds to minutes) held in mind, often through a process of rehearsal. A typical example is remembering a phone number from reading it to dialing without writing it down. A key feature of short-term memory is capacity limitation: most people are able to retain about seven items in short-term memory.[2] A specific form of short-term memory that has received considerable interest is **working memory**: the ability to hold information in mind that is necessary for a task at hand, but not present in the environment. This faculty is often regarded as a 'mental workspace' that is critical for information manipulation and goal-directed adaptive behavior, and the association of working memory with specific brain systems and psychiatric disorders has been widely studied. Rehearsal is also one important mechanism by which material is being transferred into **long-term memory**, which refers to the ability to retain information for time periods lasting from minutes up to the life span of the individual. This form of memory, which is also of major clinical importance, is not clearly capacity limited and is thought to depend on more enduring changes in neuronal structure and connectivity, raising the question of where in the brain these enduring memory traces, or 'engrams', are stored, how they are encoded for storage and how they are retrieved from it.

A second important subdivision is whether the content of memory can be consciously and intentionally retrieved (this is called explicit or **declarative** memory) or not (nondeclarative or **implicit** memory) (**Fig. 2.5.3.1**). Declarative memory is further subdivided in memory of facts and memory of events. Memory of events, which often includes recollection of temporal, spatial and emotional circumstances, is called **episodic** memory. Questions such as 'What did you have for breakfast this morning?' or 'Where did you go to school?' access episodic memory. Several features of episodic memory bear mention for their clinical relevance. For example, people can often say that they have seen a specific item before or that it 'feels familiar' without being able to recall the specifics of where and when (the episodic context). As discussed below, some evidence suggests that familiarity and recall may be supported by different brain regions. Intense feelings of familiarity without recall are experienced as *déjà vu* in a psychiatric context. People can also be convinced to remember events that did not, in fact, happen. These so-called **false memories** are also encountered in psychiatry. There has been much work on paradigms that produce false memories in normal individuals that address how they develop and how and why they might be successfully rejected. In one canonical account of episodic memory, the medial temporal lobe system (MTL) stores or indexes contextual markers that serve to bind feature information of a memory into an episodic configuration.

In contradistinction to episodic memory, memory of facts is not connected to specific experience. It is called **semantic** memory, and recollection of facts or vocabulary are examples of information that has become independent of episodic memory. Over time such material is thought to be stored in neocortex and can be retrieved without engagement of medial temporal lobe structures (MTL). Various models of the distinctions between semantic and episodic memory have proposed that while learning in the episodic system is rapid and can be based on a single trial or exposure, storage of information in the semantic system occurs slowly over time and only after multiple exposures or activations [3]. Some accounts suggest that the MTL may also be involved in semantic memory, for example for separation or 'decompression' of stimuli previously learned as a unit.[4,5] We have chosen not to review semantic memory in further detail because of space limitations and its complex overlap with psycholinguistics.

Whereas the subdivision of declarative memory is comparatively simple, implicit memory encompasses quite a heterogeneous group of functions that are supported by different brain systems. Among them are **procedural memory**, which refer to the gradual acquisition of sensorimotor, perceptual or cognitive skills through repeated exposure, **priming** (the facilitation of a response to an item if it was previously encountered), **conditioning** as well as various phenomena wherein a previously acquired response is gradually reduced or lost, such as **extinction**. Since the distinction between declarative and implicit depends on whether or not a memory process supports conscious recollection, clinicians must be careful not to confuse this with the properties of a given neuropsychological test; for example, a test of sentence completion requires conscious

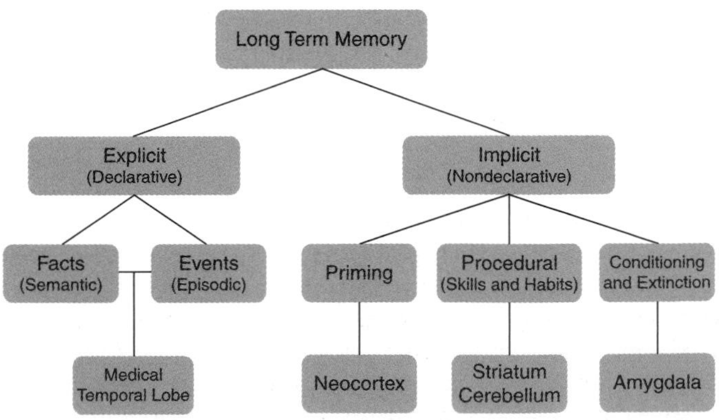

Fig. 2.5.3.1 Classification of memory and associated neural systems

production of words, but performance may strongly depend on implicit processes such as priming.

Although a taxonomy of memory systems is useful, many everyday tasks require functionality from several memory domains, and even relatively subtle changes in task demands may disrupt the balance among those cognitive systems. More refined analysis of learning tasks suggests that a variety of learning systems may mediate performance,[6] and that a given neural system participates in several forms of memory. For example, the hippocampal formation (HF), which is critical for episodic memory, is also thought to play a role in learning sequences so that indirect relations can be specified.[7] Thus, the HF becomes critical not during a>b, b>c, and c>d discriminations, but for the discrimination of the critical indirect b>d probe (e.g. if John is taller than Bill and Bill is taller than Mary and Mary is taller than Ellen, then Bill must be taller than Ellen).

Cellular and molecular mechanisms of memory

Memory is one of the most impressive examples of neural plasticity: the ability of the nervous system for enduring change triggered by external events. Arguably the best-studied cellular mechanisms underlying plasticity are long-term potentiation (LTP) and long-term plasticity (LTD), which mediate enduring changes on the level of the synapse.[8] Both have been best characterized in the hippocampus, one of the key structures for declarative memory.

By stimulating presynaptic fibres in the hippocampus (especially the CA1 section) with a brief pulse of high-frequency electric impulses, a long-lasting increase in responsiveness of the postsynaptic cells to low-frequency stimulation is reliably observed that can last for weeks (**Fig. 2.5.3.2**). This is called LTP. Initiation of this process depends on multiple second messenger mechanisms (**Fig. 2.5.3.2**). One of the best studied pathways starts with calcium influx into the presynapse through a glutamate receptor, NMDA, which activates further molecular cascades involving cAMP and protein kinases such as CamKII (other receptors, such as the glutamate receptors AMPA and mGluR, also play a role). LTP is then maintained by changes in gene transcription factors, such as CREB, and changed patterns of protein synthesis and phosphorylation, probably also dependent on protein kinase cascades. The time course of these processes can be used for a distinction between early phase LTP (the cellular signature of learning that occurs over seconds to minutes) and late phase LTP, which involves protein synthesis and occurs over minutes to hours and is thought to be critical for consolidation of new memoranda and would be linked to memory consolidation.[9,10]

LTD is a closely related process that is triggered when presynaptic stimulation is lower, causing less calcium influx (again through NMDA receptors) and preferential activation of calcineurin, a protein phosphatase. Together, LTP and LTD allow bidirectional enduring modulation of synaptic strength that could underlie formation and reversal of experience-dependent coupling in neural assemblies. Linking these synaptic changes to validated mechanisms underlying the complexities of human memory remains a challenge. However, the active field of neural network modeling has shown that, in principle, such changes in synaptic efficacy can produce efficient mechanisms to encode, store and retrieve information, a proposal first made by the neurophysiologist Donald Hebb.

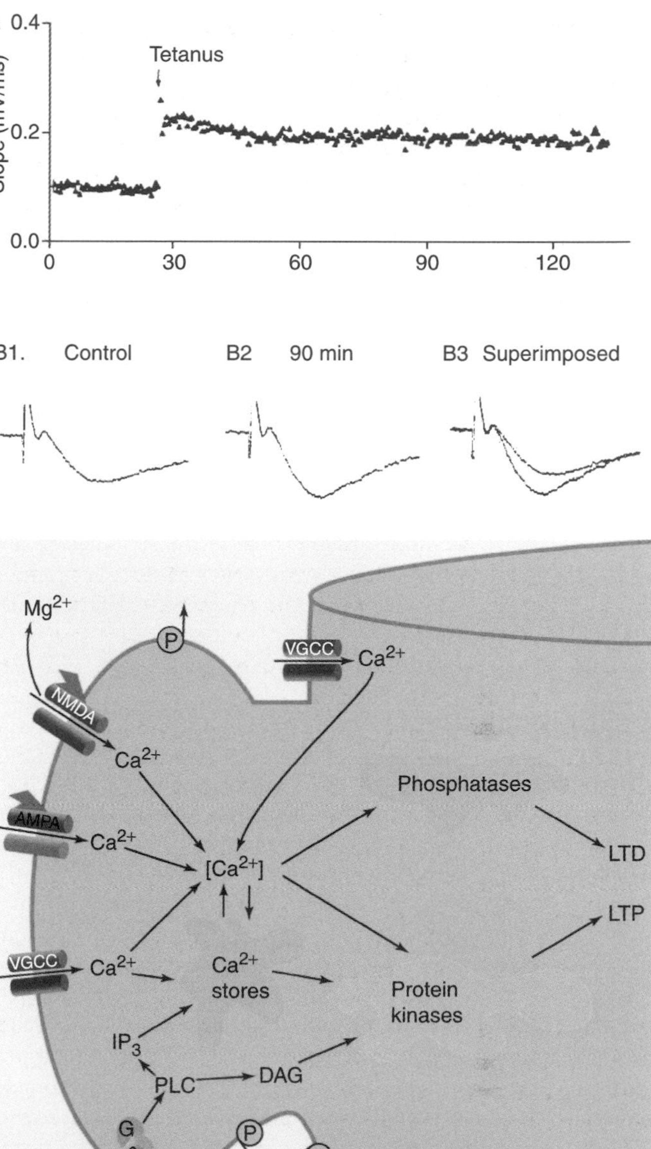

Fig. 2.5.3.2 Top: Long-term potentiation after a tetanic stimulation in the HF. Bottom: molecular mediators of long-term potentiation.

Declarative/episodic memory

(a) Neural systems

Current evidence indicates that the HF and linked regions of the medial temporal lobe (MTL), in interactions with parts of the prefrontal cortex, play a critical role in the encoding and retrieval of episodic memories, whereas engrams are stored in neocortex[11] (**Fig. 2.5.3.3**). Interactions of the HF with amygdala are important for emotional memories. The HF consists of the hippocampus proper, the entorhinal cortex, which provides the main port of entry for connections with the cortex, and the adjacent perirhinal and parahippocampal cortices, which interact with the entorhinal cortex and in turn receive projections from all other neocortical areas, with parietal, dorsal occipital and prefrontal regions primarily projecting to parahippocampal gyrus and temporal cortex to

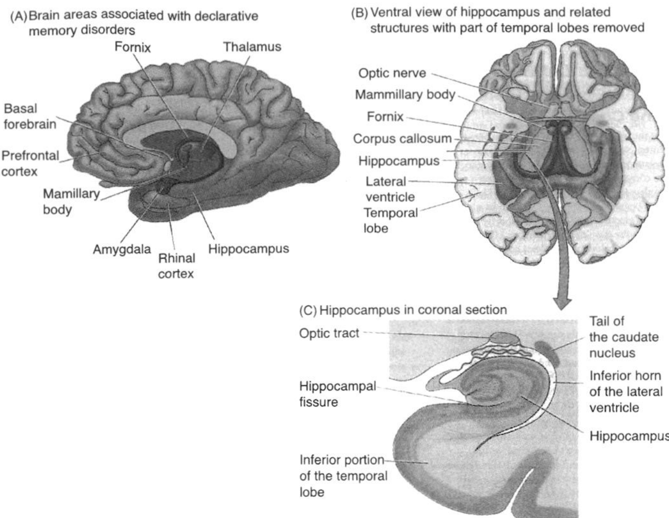

Fig. 2.5.3.3 (A) brain regions associated with dysfunction in episodic memory. (B) the hippocampal formation, view from below. (C) coronal section through the hippocampal formation.

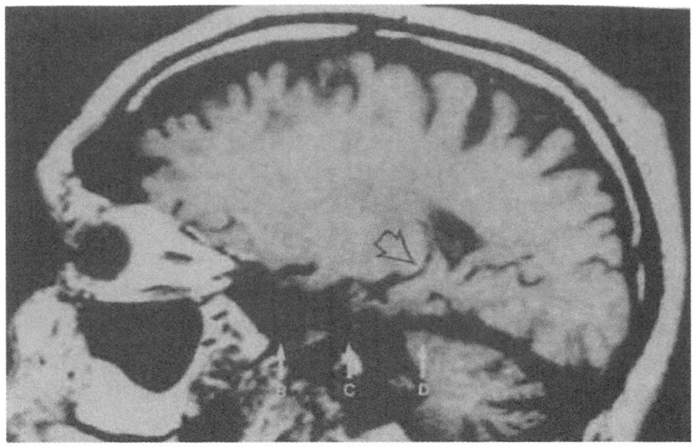

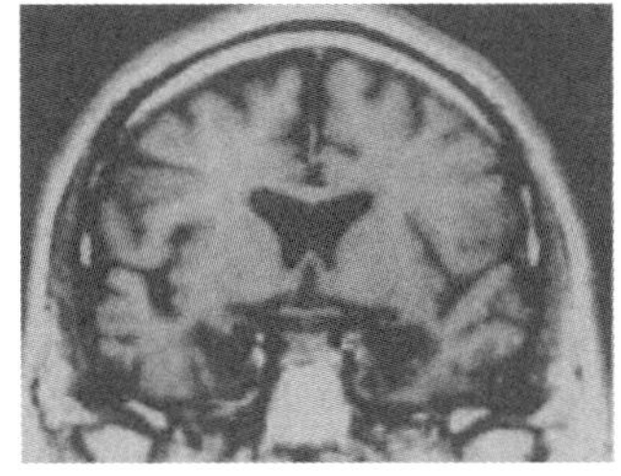

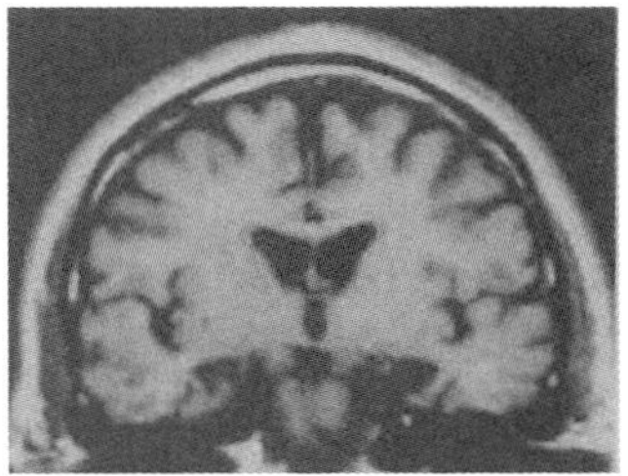

Fig. 2.5.3.4 Hippocampal damage in patient H.M., shown on a sagittal (top) and two coronal slices (below) of the patient's MRI.

perirhinal cortex. In this way, the HF is bidirectionally connected with the rest of the brain. Although pertinent observations were already made at the end of the 19th century by Bechterew, the importance of the hippocampal formation for episodic memory was dramatically shown in 1953 by the case of patient H.M., in whom the HF and amygdala were resected bilaterally as a treatment for drug-resistant epilepsy[(12)] (**Fig. 2.5.3.4**). This led to complete and enduring **anterograde** amnesia (inability to form new episodic memories). In addition, he has some degree of **retrograde** amnesia (i.e. an inability to retrieve episodic information stored before the operation), while his working and procedural memory, as well as priming, is unimpaired. A similar pattern of memory impairment is observed in Wernicke encephalopathy/Korsakov's syndrome or other neurological processes impacting on diencephalic structures, including the medial thalamus, mamillary body and the fornix, which project to the HF. This indicates that these structures may be viewed as a system that is critical for assigning a spatiotemporal (episodic) context. In rodents, a major role of the HF is indeed to function as a neural map of the environment;[(13)] it is controversial to what degree this applies to humans. Neuroimaging studies confirm that activation of the HF is observed during successful encoding and retrieval of episodic information.[(14)]

A neurocognitive model system for examining the computational role of MTL subsystems involved in episodic memory may help the reader gain a sense of the interplay among various subprocessing modules.[(15)] In this model, the MTL binds memories and their instance-specific context and then stores their code for later retrieval. The model described here is based on studies showing that the bulk of hippocampal (HC) cortical input is segregated over two pathways. One of these may convey spatial information; the other may convey information regarding items and objects. The two streams are interconnected at various levels within entorhinal cortex, which likely contributes to the integration of cortical inputs into a representation of their co-occurrence. The hippocampus proper may quickly associate a code to the conjunction of cortical inputs, such that similar entorhinal patterns come to be separated via their associated hippocampal patterns. These hippocampal patterns are thus not directly associated with individual features, but serve to separate the large number of overlapping entorhinal patterns, which is important to ensure that retrieval will be unambiguous. The representational overlap in entorhinal cortex, combined with the pattern separation system in the hippocampus proper, enormously increases the storage capacity of the memory store and allows accurate recall of episodic memories. In this model, retrieval in this memory system can be sampled using cues, consisting of *partial* input patterns; for instance, part of a context representation from a previously experienced episode. Initially, such a cue may activate only part of an associated entorhinal pattern, but if the set of activated entorhinal nodes sufficiently resembles a stored representation, their combined firing will tend to activate associated hippocampal nodes, through previously strengthened connections with these nodes. The hippocampal nodes, in turn, will recruit missing nodes of the entorhinal representation. This pattern completion process will reinstate the original pattern in the entorhinal layer, which, in turn, can reinstate associated information in the input layers, namely, item representations that have been experienced in that particular context (feature extraction). Thus, all features of an episode can be recalled, even when only part of the input layers is cued.

The model was shown to be sensitive to various types of simulated lesions including reductions of nodes ('neurones'), addition of noise to the system, and perhaps most relevant for the modeling of schizophrenia, marked reductions in connectivity between the various modules. At the network level, this reduced connectivity led to compromised cross-association of episodic features (i.e. item and context) and a superimposed, mild reduction of pattern separation in the system. The latter malfunction made some patterns irretrievable, affecting all memory tasks including recognition, albeit to a mild degree. The cross-association problem also attenuated 'searching' of the memory store, particularly with single-source cues. This preferentially affected tasks with a large retrieval demand, such as free recall. From an information processing standpoint, what appeared to be disproportionate failures in retrieval were due to compromised encoding.

Recent work has indicated that recollection is predominantely mediated by the hippocampus proper, whereas familiarity has been linked to perirhinal cortex.(16) While this distinction is supported by functional neuroimaging studies of healthy individuals (e.g. Eldridge *et al.*[17]), studies of patients with circumscribed lesions of the hippocampus have nevertheless found severe familiarity-based recognition memory impairments.(18) These results do not necessarily contradict a dual process distinction, but could rather suggest that MTL regions comprise an integrated network that supports both processes.

There has been much interest in the precise role of episodic memory systems in the formation of associations between items that are entering memory. Several new studies suggest that the hippocampus is engaged preferentially when inter-item associations are formed in memory. While there have been several compelling accounts that specific subsystems in the MTL complex play different roles in single item encoding and associative encoding, the distinction between the two may be relative, not absolute.(11,19)

Neuroimaging and lesion studies have suggested that interactions between the HF and the amygdala are relevant for emotional memories, especially if these have a fearful or aversive character.(20) Neuroimaging has also demonstrated that encoding and especially retrieval is associated with activation of the lateral prefrontal cortex, as well as with increased functional interactions of these regions with the HF that are supported by anatomical tracts such as the uncinate fascicle. In some studies, left prefrontal cortex is differentially more involved than right in encoding information into episodic memory, whereas right prefrontal cortex is differentially more involved than left in episodic memory retrieval.(21) Compared to encoding and retrieval, the evidence is much less clear with regard to the storage of the engrams themselves. Cases such as H.M. and the clinical picture of Korsakov's syndrome show that the HF and diencephalic structures cannot be the store, since most episodic and semantic memories laid down before the onset of illness are spared. Current evidence suggests that the neocortex is the ultimate store of memories and that engrams reside in regions that are also specialized in processing stimuli to which they pertain. For example, circumscribed cortical lesions can result in category-specific impairments in retrieving object information, the so-called anomias, which have been described for classes such as people, tools, or living things, and neuroimaging studies show that similar regions are differentially activated during naming of these object classes. In each case, engrams are assumed to be stored in a distributed pattern of synaptic connections over a large group of neurones. It is an open question how the interaction of the HF and cortex accomplishes the encoding, and retrieval of information from these neural assemblies (but see above for a model). On the molecular level, glutamatergic neurotransmission is crucial to support the LTP mechanisms that support the neural plasticity essential for memory formation. In addition, acetylcholine is a neurotransmitter associated with declarative memory function since it is known that muscarinic receptor blockade impairs episodic memory and degeneration of cholinergic neurones in the basal nucleus (of Meynert) is a prominent finding in Alzheimer's disease. It is likely that cholinergic mechanisms act on declarative memory by modulating glutamate-dependent LTP and LTD in MTL regions.

(b) Assessment and neuropsychology

Clinical assessment of memory systems is an important facet of neuropsychiatric and neuropsychologic test batteries. Assessments may vary widely in their depth and breadth and systematic approach. There are numerous tests of episodic memory that can be used for clinical purposes. Well known batteries include the Wechsler Memory Scale-III, which involves verbal memory for stories, verbal paired associates, and word lists, and visual memory for scenes, faces, and designs. Immediate and delayed recall of these tests is assessed. There are also many standardized verbal list learning tests that involve differing degrees of semantic relatedness among words (and perhaps requiring different degrees of strategic encoding) and minor differences in administration. These include the California Verbal Learning Test, the Hopkins Verbal Learning Test, and the Selective Reminding Test. These tests have alternate but equivalent forms that reduce practice effects when tests are administered repeatedly. A comprehensive evaluation of memory should include multiple trials of a word list to assess learning rate or slope; measures of immediate and delayed memory (e.g. recall after 30 minutes); a recognition test in which a subject must decide whether an item had been studied or not (was old or new in order to minimize effortful retrieval); and tests of visual memory and verbal memory that preferentially engage the right or left MTL systems, which are thought to be material specific, at least to some degree.

Cognitively, there are several distinctions or processes in episodic memory that bear special comment. Most are still being actively investigated. One of the earliest and best replicated findings in processing oriented theories of memory suggests that the level at which an item is encoded is an important predictor of later recall.(22) Thus, words that are encoded deeply (for example, after a semantic judgment about animacy) are remembered better than words encoded superficially (for example, after a judgment about whether the word contains a specific orthographic feature). The exact cognitive mechanism by which this occurs is unclear, but could involve the creation of more cue-item associations so that a wider variety of different searches might have yield.

Another important area involves the distinction between a sense of familiarity with an item at recall versus the recollection of an item, which implies knowledge about the spatiotemporal context in which the item was encoded. It is thought that memories may be retrieved through either of these two processes: recollection of a memory that involves adjunctive contextual information; or the feeling of knowing that an item, face, thing, etc. has been encountered before without memory of the surrounding context.(23,24)

Rate of forgetting reflects the degree to which memories that were once successfully retrieved can no longer be retrieved after a delay. For healthy individuals savings (the inverse of rate of forgetting) may be at 80–90 per cent for several hours or more after initial recall. Several amnesic conditions, as well as a form of frontal temporal dementia, have been associated with increased rates of forgetting. In Alzheimer's disease and Korsakov's syndrome, savings may be less than 50 per cent after delays of several minutes. Nevertheless, the situation is undoubtedly more complex psychometrically and cognitively than presented here.(25,26)

Implicit memory

(a) Neural systems

(i) Procedural memory

Clinical experience shows that the acquisition of new visuomotor skills is often unimpaired in patients with deep amnesia due to medial temporal lobe lesions. Conversely, skill learning, but not declarative memory, is often impaired in patients with degenerative or vascular lesions of the basal ganglia (for example in Huntington's) or cerebellum. Neuroimaging has confirmed the importance of basal ganglia and cerebellum for procedural memory[1] and has also demonstrated time-variant activation of primary and secondary motor cortex during skill learning. The basal ganglia receive excitatory glutamatergic projections from the cortex and thalamus, integrate them with monoaminergic inputs and sends them via the globus pallidus and substantia nigra pars reticulata to the thalamus, which projects back to prefrontal cortex.[27] These parallel processing loops are critical for the integration of sensorimotor, cognitive and emotional information.[27] It is usual to distinguish between a dorsal and a ventral subdivision of the striatum, and it is the dorsal striatum (caudate nucleus, putamen and globus pallidus) that is strongly interconnected with cortical areas relevant for motor planning and execution. The learning of repetitive sequence, as well as so-called 'open loop' tasks, in which visual feedback is delayed, especially depends on the integrity of the dorsal striatum and its interactions with cortex.[28] This extends to skills that are not motor, for example the prediction of probabilistic sequences or the planning of complex tasks. Conversely, the importance of the cerebellum lies with 'closed loop' tasks that require continuous visuomotor feedback, as well as fast error control. The cerebellum has also been proposed to play a role in creating new stimulus-response mappings.

(ii) Priming

Neuroimaging suggests that the neural substrate of priming lies in neocortex. Specifically, a reduction of activation to a primed stimulus is consistently found, either in modality-specific regions (such as visual areas for visual repetition priming) or in 'amodal' cortical areas such as lateral temporal cortex for semantic priming. It has been hypothesized that this reduced activation represents neural assemblies that are optimized, by 'pruning' of unnecessary connections, for easier activation, and that this may underlie the facilitated response to a primed stimulus.[29] Clinically, this leads to the prediction that priming should be altered in disorders that impair the integrity of the cortical regions involved, such as semantic priming in Alzheimer's disease.

(iii) Fear conditioning and extinction

Conditioned fear is of high relevance in psychiatry in disorders ranging from simple phobias and generalized anxiety disorder to major depression. In conditioning, a fear response to an unconditional stimulus (for example, an electric shock) is transferred to a conditional stimulus with which it is paired (CS, for example, a tone regularily preceding this shock). A large body of research has established a key role for the amygdala in this memory process.[30] Different subnuclei of this complicated structure are implicated in establishing and storing fear conditioning memory traces. An area of recent research interest concerns extinction, the process in which a conditioned fear response is gradually lost if the conditioned stimulus is repeatedly presented without adverse consequences. It is now clear that extinction is not a passive process, but depends on interactions between amygdala and the cingulate cortex.[31] This circuit has been implicated in depression and anxiety in humans, in which dysphoric mood and affect are abnormally maintained, i.e. not extinguished.[32]

(b) Assessment and neuropsychology

Despite at least 20 years of cognitive science research in implicit memory, procedural memory, or habit formation, there are no commercially available versions of these tests. In part, this may have to do with lack of psychometric evaluation of test-retest reliability, ceiling or floor effects, etc. or unclear relations to functional status or outcome. It might be possible to adapt some instrumentation used experimentally (e.g. rotor pursuit) if there are adequate local normative data for the test. There are several forms of implicit learning, all of which are thought to involve learning or memory without conscious awareness of recall. Various motor skills can be learned incrementally, such as rotor pursuit or mirror tracing. Others involve motor sequences. Probabilistic learning can occur when there is acquisition of information or representations that reflect underlying structural regularities in the input, i.e. when there are statistical regularities between stimuli and responses.[33] This can occur in tasks as seemingly disparate as the so-called weather prediction task (characterized by probabilistic relationships between specific stimulus configurations and a response, in this case 'sunshine' or 'rain') and artificial grammar. Critically, implicit learning can occur even when the episodic system of recollection is dysfunctional.

Other types of implicit memory may be item specific, including some types of priming. Priming is thought to be an instance of memory without awareness. Such priming can be reflected in improvements in accuracy or reaction time during testing. It can be demonstrated in a variety of tasks, some rather rarefied, like word stem completion, and some rather simple and robust, like so-called repetition priming. In the latter paradigm, an item is repeated and access to it (usually measured in reaction time) is speeded at the second presentation, while concomitantly, physiological measures, ranging from single cell activity to BOLD activation, demonstrate reductions in neocortical areas (e.g. for words, inferior prefrontal cortex). Some of these effects may be quite long, lived.

The degree to which episodic memory may also support some types of priming is sometimes unclear and may depend on the paradigm and experimental manipulations. Perhaps the best evidence that priming reflects a dissociable memory system comes from amnesic patients in whom there is little chance that the episodic system is supporting priming (e.g. studies of priming in the amnesic patient HM [34]). Additionally, an important and critical review[35] has proposed that some priming may not reflect changes in the abstract representation of an item, but rather response learning.

Finally, conditioning (especially classical or Pavlovian) has also been considered a type of implicit learning. The neurobiological literature on this phenomenon is quite extensive.[36] The phenomenon itself might be relevant for understanding a wide range of behaviors, including anxiety (as a result of fear conditioning) and preferences.

(c) Working memory

(i) Neural systems

A large body of work has established the importance of dorsolateral prefrontal cortex (DLPFC) for working memory. Both the simple maintenance of information over a delay and the manipulation of that information require DLPFC function. In the influential model of Baddeley, a 'central executive' component of working memory works together with modality-specific storage systems, the 'visuospatial scratchpad' for visual information and the 'phonological loop' for auditory information.[37] While the details of how this cognitive account reflects neural organization are being debated, it is clear from a multitude of studies that DLPFC activation is usually observed in conjunction with activity of posterior cortical areas that receive input from a variety of specialized sensory cortices.[38] Chief among those is the inferior parietal lobule, a brain region strongly and bidirectionally connected with DLPFC that is likely to be important for item storage during working memory. Within DLPFC proper, some models propose a regional differentiation based on the modality of information stored (with more dorsal activation associated with visual, ventral with semantic items), while others propose a specialization based on cognitive operations (manipulation of memory items being performed more dorsally than pure maintenance). Clinically, large lesions of DLPFC are invariably associated with working memory impairment, however, problems of similar magnitude are also observed in schizophrenia, where only subtle structural abnormalities are found in this (as in any other) brain region.[39] The association of working memory impairment with schizophrenia has driven an extensive programme of research aimed at understanding mechanisms underlying memory impairments in this disorder. One well-validated finding from this work is the importance of the neurotransmitter, dopamine, for DLPFC function, which has been found to exhibit an 'inverted u' shaped relationship with working-memory related activation of DLPFC neurones and dopaminergic, especially D1-receptor, stimulation.[40] It is believed that dopaminergic tone is essential for optimizing signal to noise ratio, or tuning, in DLPFC, an essential network property for working memory maintenance. This is further supported by a modulation of working memory by a functional variant in the COMT gene which alters the protein's thermolability and hence its ability to degrade dopamine in cortex, the impact of dextroamphetamine on N Back driven BOLD activation in fMRI, and the COMT inhibitor tolcapone's impact on N Back RT.[41–43]

Interactions between DLPFC and hippocampus may also be disturbed in schizophrenia and reflect an inability to disengage episodic memory processes during working memory.[44]

(ii) Assessment and neuropsychology

The classic test of simple working memory is digit span, which involves repetition of short sequences of digits. Span is assessed by increasing the length of the sequence that can be recalled. Nonverbal working memory often involves short sequences of locations (as in Visual Span in the WMS-R and the so-called Corsi blocks.) Tests thought to depend on simultaneous storage and manipulation of information are generally considered executive in nature. The Letter-Number Span is a good example of this class of tests. In it, the subject is asked to order a short random sequence of letters or numbers numerically and alphabetically. Interestingly, the test is highly correlated with a nonverbal, formally dissimilar, problem solving task, the Wisconsin Card Sort, providing evidence that both these tests engage executive processes. The Card Sort itself may be the best known executive test administered in clinical test batteries. It calls upon such executive abilities as abstraction, set shifting, and response to examiner feedback.

An exceptionally well validated computerized battery of 'frontal lobe tests' called the CANTAB is based on the comparative and pharmacologic challenge literature, as well as human lesion studies. All tests are nonverbal and may involve problem solving (as in Tower of London), various levels of set shifting (in the ID/ED task), and self-ordered pointing that demands that the subject remember his/her own actions.

A widely used test of cognitive control is the Stroop, for which there are several commercially available versions. In the critical interference condition, the subject must respond to words printed in incongruent colors (e.g. red) by naming the colour of the ink and simultaneously suppressing the prepotent response to read the word.

There are many experimental tests of working memory and executive that could in theory be adapted for clinical purposes provided these have adequate local normative data and adequate validity and psychometric characteristics. In general, many of the paradigms that have interested cognitive neuroscientists have not yet become part of routine clinical assessment.

The working memory (WM) system is thought to be a limited capacity system that holds information on line when the stimulus is no longer present (perhaps up to 40 seconds, as demonstrated in densely amnesic patients). The idea that WM is a capacity limited system comes from the work of G. Miller.[2] Several compelling accounts now suggest that it may under some circumstance be smaller than Miller's canonical '7±2.' For instance, in studies of visual stimuli, Luck *et al.*[45] have suggested that a visual store may hold only four items. Subsystems include a slave system for short term memory of phonological information. This system includes an articulatory rehearsal mechanism and a phonological store. A visual spatial scratchpad processes visual, non-linguistic information. An episodic memory buffer is thought to play a role in the interface between working and episodic memory. A central executive is involved in the allocation of cognitive resources during dual tasks and in the manipulation or transformation of information. The central executive may be involved in cognitive control, such that when there is response conflict (e.g. during response selection in the Stroop task or Eriksen flanker task) more resources can be made available for biasing decisions.[46] More specifically, in this account, cognitive conflict is detected (by the anterior cingulate) and signals are sent to executive areas (in DLPFC) that increase processing resources. The increase in resources is used to bias a response to one or another aspect of the stimulus' features. Importantly, various computational models of this process have shown that a homunculus (i.e. a director or decider) is not necessary for a correct response to be made. There is ongoing interest in how best to characterize operations in the WM system. One view that posits a single algorithm that maintains a stable representation over a delay (although subsystems may be dedicated to spatial, object or verbal information) can be used to characterize the basic function of this system. Goldman Rakic and colleagues provided much neurobiological evidence in favor of this argument. Another view holds that multiple computational algorithms perform a variety of tasks.[47,48] Such functions as attentional set shifting, planning, and monitoring of sequences of responses (self or externally generated) can be brought to bear on a task, depending on its demands and are separable from basic mnemonic maintenance functions.

Updating of information in WM (i.e. registering information and dumping information from a buffer) and suppression of interference may also engage the executive system and may be critical for refining goal-directed behavior.[49] In one version of a task that makes continual demands for updating and resistance to interference, a restricted set of numbers are displayed successively (and approximately every two seconds) and the subject views one while responding by pressing a button corresponding to a stimulus 'one back'. Thus, the subject must continuously update his/her working memory buffer in that a target-to-be must be shifted in status to a target prior to being 'dumped' from a computational buffer and interference from other similar stimuli must be suppressed. Recent data (see below) suggest that dopaminergic tone at the cortical level may be particularly important in this specific aspect of cognitive control.

Finally, there are several integrative accounts of goal directed behaviour that are dependent on various working and executive functions. In perhaps the best known of these, a 'script' that engages multiple short-term and long-term memories bridges the temporal gap for projects that may be quite long temporally.[50]

Future directions

As our understanding of neural systems involved in memory dysfunction in a variety of psychiatric disorders matures, it will be important to leverage that knowledge to identify new molecular treatment targets. One important recent development in this direction is the identification of genes impacting on memory function. Genetic variation in the neurotrophic factor BDNF, for example, has been shown to impact on hippocampal function and episodic memory,[51] as have several risk genes for schizophrenia.[52] COMT, a gene that impacts on cortical dopamine concentrations, affects working memory performance and prefrontal activation.[41,53] Risk genes for depression and anxiety may affect amygdala-cingulate and amygdala-hippocampal interactions that are important for fear extinction and emotional memory, respectively, providing neural mechanisms for gene by environment interactions mediating the effects of early adverse experience on risk for psychiatric disorders.[32,54] Translational strategies for drug development can arise from these findings. The COMT inhibitor tolcapone has been shown to improve working memory in normals.[43] Data suggesting an impact of stress hormones such as corticosteroids on hippocampal integrity in posttraumatic stress disorder suggest neuroprotective strategies to prevent development of disease before anticipated exposure, for example in battle. Finally, it has become clear that memory impairment is an important predictor for treatment response in psychiatry, schizophrenia being an important example, and neurorehabilitative programs to improve memory are being explored. The study of the neurobiology of memory is therefore a promising avenue towards improved and specific therapies in psychiatry.

Further information

Miyake, A. and Shah, P. (eds.) (1999) *Models of Working Memory: Mechanisms of Active Maintenance and Executive Control.* Cambridge University Press, New York.

Squire, L.R. and Schachter, D.L. (eds.) (2002), *Neuropsychology of Memory.* The Guildford Press, New York.

Hippocampus (the journal).

Wikipedia (wikipedia.org) entry 'memory'.

References

1. Gabrieli, J.D. (1998). Cognitive neuroscience of human memory. *Annual Review of Psychology*, **49**, 87–115.
2. Miller, G.A. (1956). The magical number seven plus or minus two: some limits on our capacity for processing information. *Psychological Review*, **63**(2), 81–97.
3. O'Reilly, R.C. and Norman, K.A. (2002). Hippocampal and neocortical contributions to memory: advances in the complementary learning systems framework. *Trends in cognitive sciences*, **6**(12), 505–10.
4. Gluck, M.A., Meeter, M. and Myers, C.E. (2003). Computational models of the hippocampal region: linking incremental learning and episodic memory. *Trends in cognitive sciences*, **7**(6), 269–76.
5. Moscovitch, M., *et al.* (2005). Functional neuroanatomy of remote episodic, semantic and spatial memory: a unifi ed account based on multiple trace theory. *Journal of Anatomy*, **207**(1), 35–66.
6. Ashby, F.G. and Maddox, W.T. (2005). Human category learning. *Annual Review of Psychology*, **56,** 149–78.
7. Eichenbaum, H. (2006). Remembering: functional organization of the declarative memory system. *Current Biology*, **16**(16): R643–5.
8. Miller, S. and Mayford, M. (1999). Cellular and molecular mechanisms of memory: the LTP connection. *Current Opinion in Genetics & Development*, **9**(3), 333–37.
9. Hawkins, R.D., Kandel, E.R. and Bailey, C.H. (2006). Molecular mechanisms of memory storage in Aplysia. *The Biological Bulletin*, **210**(3), 174–91.
10. Izquierdo, I., *et al.* (2006). Different molecular cascades in different sites of the brain control memory consolidation. *Trends in Neurosciences*, **29**(9), 496–505.
11. Squire, L.R., Stark, C.E. and Clark, R.E. (2004). The medial temporal lobe. *Annual Review of Neuroscience*, **27**, 279–306.
12. Scoville, W.B. and Milner, B. (1957). Loss of recent memory after bilateral hippocampal lesions. *Journal of Neurology, Neurosurgery, and Psychiatry*, **20**(1), 11–21.
13. O'Keefe, J. and Dostrovsky, J. (1971). The hippocampus as a spatial map. Preliminary evidence from unit activity in the freely-moving rat. *Brain Research*, **34**(1), 171–75.
14. Squire, L.R., *et al.* (1992). Activation of the hippocampus in normal humans: a functional anatomical study of memory. *Proceedings of the National Academy of Sciences of the United States of America*, **89**(5), 1837–41.
15. Talamini, L.M., *et al.* (2005). Reduced parahippocampal connectivity produces schizophrenia-like memory deficits in simulated neural circuits with reduced parahippocampal connectivity. *Archives of General Psychiatry*, **62**(5), 485–93.
16. Suzuki, W.A. and Eichenbaum, H. (2000). The neurophysiology of memory. *Annals of the New York Academy of Sciences*, **911**, 175–91.
17. Eldridge, L.L., *et al.* (2000). Remembering episodes: a selective role for the hippocampus during retrieval. *Nature Neuroscience*, **3**(11), 1149–52.
18. Wais, P.E., *et al.* (2006). The hippocampus supports both the recollection and the familiarity components of recognition memory. *Neuron*, **49**(3), 459–66.
19. Davachi, L. and Wagner, A.D. (2002). Hippocampal contributions to episodic encoding: insights from relational and item-based learning. *Journal of Neurophysiology*, **88**(2), 982–90.
20. Cahill, L., *et al.* (1996). Amygdala activity at encoding correlated with long-term, free recall of emotional information. *Proceedings of the National Academy of Sciences of the United States of America*, **93**(15), 8016–21.
21. Habib, R., Nyberg, L. and Tulving, E. (2003). Hemispheric asymmetries of memory: the HERA model revisited. *Trends in Cognitive Sciences*, **7**(6), 241–5.
22. Craik, F.I.M. and Tulving, E. (1975). Depth of processing and the retention of words in episodic memory. *Journal of Experimental Psychology: General*, **104**, 268–94.

23. Cipolotti, L. and Bird, C.M. (2006). Amnesia and the hippocampus. *Current Opinion in Neurology*, **19**(6), 593–98.
24. Yonelinas, A.P. (2001). Components of episodic memory: the contribution of recollection and familiarity. *Philosophical Transactions of the Royal Society of London. Series B, Biological sciences*, **356**(1413), 1363–74.
25. Greene, J.D., Baddeley, A.D. and Hodges, J.R. (1996). Analysis of the episodic memory deficit in early Alzheimer's disease: evidence from the doors and people test. *Neuropsychologia*, **34**(6), 537–51.
26. Murre, J.M., Graham, K.S. and Hodges, J.R. (2001). Semantic dementia: relevance to connectionist models of long-term memory. *Brain*, **124**(Pt 4), 647–75.
27. Alexander, G.E., DeLong, M.R. and Strick, P.L. (1986). Parallel organization of functionally segregated circuits linking basal ganglia and cortex. *Annual Review of Neuroscience*, **9**, 357–81.
28. Packard, M.G. and Knowlton, B.J. (2002). Learning and memory functions of the Basal Ganglia. *Annual Review of Neuroscience*, **25**, 563–93.
29. Wiggs, C.L. and Martin, A. (1998). Properties and mechanisms of perceptual priming. *Current Opinion in Neurobiology*, **8**(2), 227–33.
30. Phelps, E.A. and LeDoux, J.E. (2005). Contributions of the amygdala to emotion processing: from animal models to human behavior. *Neuron*, **48**(2), 175–87.
31. Quirk, G.J., *et al.* (2003). Stimulation of medial prefrontal cortex decreases the responsiveness of central amygdala output neurons. *The Journal of Neuroscience*, **23**(25), 8800–807.
32. Pezawas, L., *et al.* (2005). 5-HTTLPR polymorphism impacts human cingulateamygdala interactions: a genetic susceptibility mechanism for depression. *Nature Neuroscience*, **8**(6), 828–34.
33. Forkstam, C. and Petersson, K.M. (2005). Towards an explicit account of implicit learning. *Current Opinion in Neurology*, **18**(4), 435–41.
34. Corkin, S. (2002). What's new with the amnesic patient H.M.? *Nature Reviews. Neuroscience*, **3**(2), 153–60.
35. Schacter, D.L., Dobbins, I.G. and Schnyer, D.M. (2004). Specificity of priming: a cognitive neuroscience perspective. *Nature Reviews. Neuroscience*, **5**(11), 853–62.
36. Thompson, R.F. (1990). Neural mechanisms of classical conditioning in mammals. *Philosophical Transactions of the Royal Society of London. Series B, Biological sciences*, **329**(1253), 161–70.
37. Baddeley, A. (1992). Working memory. *Science*, **255**(5044), 556–9.
38. Smith, E.E. and Jonides, J. (1997). Working memory: a view from neuroimaging. *Cognitive Psychology*, **33**(1), 5–42.
39. Weinberger, D.R., *et al.* (1992). Evidence of dysfunction of a prefrontal-limbic network in schizophrenia: a magnetic resonance imaging and regional cerebral blood flow study of discordant monozygotic twins. *The American Journal of Psychiatry*, **149**(7), 890–97.
40. Williams, G.V. and Goldman-Rakic, P.S. (1995). Modulation of memory fields by dopamine D1 receptors in prefrontal cortex. *Nature*, **376**(6541), 572–75.
41. Goldberg, T.E., *et al.* (2003). Executive subprocesses in working memory: relationship to catechol-O-methyltransferase Val158Met genotype and schizophrenia. *Archives of General Psychiatry*, **60**(9), 889–96.
42. Mattay, V.S., *et al.* (2003). Catechol O-methyltransferase val158-met genotype and individual variation in the brain response to amphetamine. *Proceedings of the National Academy of Sciences of the United States of America*, **100**(10), 6186–91.
43. Apud, J.A., *et al.* (2007). Tolcapone improves cognition and cortical information processing in normal human subjects. *Neuropsychopharmacology*, **32**(5), 1011–20.
44. Meyer-Lindenberg, A.S., *et al.* (2005). Regionally specific disturbance of dorsolateral prefrontal-hippocampal functional connectivity in schizophrenia. *Archives of General Psychiatry*, **62**(4), 379–86.
45. Luck, S.J. and Vogel, E.K. (1997). The capacity of visual working memory for features and conjunctions. *Nature*, **390**(6657), 279–81.
46. Botvinick, M.M., Cohen, J.D. and Carter, C.S. (2004). Conflict monitoring and anterior cingulate cortex: an update. *Trends in Cognitive Sciences*, **8**(12), 539–46.
47. Petrides, M. (2005). Lateral prefrontal cortex: architectonic and functional organization. *Philosophical Transactions of the Royal Society of London. Series B, Biological sciences*, **360**(1456), 781–95.
48. Robbins, T.W. (1996). Dissociating executive functions of the prefrontal cortex. *Philosophical Transactions of the Royal Society of London. Series B, Biological sciences*, **351**(1346), 1463–70; discussion 1470–1.
49. Smith, E.E. and Jonides, J. (1999). Storage and executive processes in the frontal lobes. *Science*, **283**(5408), 1657–61.
50. Wood, J.N., *et al.* (2005). Neural correlates of script event knowledge: a neuropsychological study following prefrontal injury. *Cortex*, **41**(6), 796–804.
51. Egan, M.F., *et al.* (2003). The BDNF val66met polymorphism affects activitydependent secretion of BDNF and human memory and hippocampal function. *Cell*, **112**(2), 257–69.
52. Callicott, J.H., *et al.* (2005). Variation in DISC1 affects hippocampal structure and function and increases risk for schizophrenia. *Proceedings of the National Academy of Sciences of the United States of America*, **102**(24), 8627–32.
53. Egan, M.F., *et al.* (2001). Effect of COMT Val108/158 Met genotype on frontal lobe function and risk for schizophrenia. *Proceedings of the National Academy of Sciences of the United States of America*, **98**(12), 6917–22.
54. Meyer-Lindenberg, A., et al. (2006). From the Cover: Neural mechanisms of genetic risk for impulsivity and violence in humans. *Proceedings of the National Academy of Sciences of the United States of America*, **103**(16), 6269–74.

2.5.4 The anatomy of human emotion

R. J. Dolan

Introduction

Emotions, uniquely among mental states, are characterized by psychological and somatic referents. The former embody the subjectivity of all psychological states. The latter are evident in objectively measurable stereotyped behavioural patterns of facial expression, comportment, and states of autonomic arousal. These include unique patterns of response associated with discrete emotional states, as for example seen in the primary emotions of fear, anger, or disgust often thought of as emotion proper. Emotional states are also unique among psychological states in exerting global effects on virtually all aspects of cognition including attention, perception, and memory. Emotion also exerts biasing influences on high level cognition including the decision-making processes that guide extended behaviour. An informed neurobiological account of emotion needs to incorporate how these wide ranging effects are mediated.

Although much of what we can infer about emotional processing in the human brain is derived from clinic-pathological correlations, the advent of high resolution, non-invasive functional neuroimaging techniques such as functional magnetic resonance imaging (fMRI) and positron emission tomography (PET) has greatly expanded this knowledge base. This is particularly the case for emotion, as opposed to other areas of cognition, where normative studies have provided a much richer account of the underlying neurobiology than that available on the basis of observations from pathology as in classical neuropsychology.

Emotion has historically been considered to reflect the product of activity within the limbic system of the brain. The general utility of the concept of a limbic-based emotional system is limited by a lack of a consensus as to its precise anatomical extent and boundaries, coupled with knowledge that emotion-related brain activity is, to a considerable degree, configured by behavioural context. What this means is that brain regions engaged by, for example, an emotion of fear associated with seeing a snake can have both distinct and common features with an emotion of fear associated with a fearful recollection. Consequently, within this framework emotional states are not unique to any single brain region but are expressed in widespread patterns of brain activity, including activity within early sensory cortices, shaped by the emotion eliciting context. This perspective emphasizes a global propagation of emotional signals as opposed to a perspective of circumscribed limbic-mediated emotion-related activity.

The amygdala and emotion

The above considerations aside, the structure most closely affiliated with emotional processing is the amygdala. This structure is an anatomically and functionally heterogeneous, bilateral, collection of nuclei located in anterior medial temporal cortex. The importance of the amygdala in emotional control was first highlighted by reports that rhesus monkeys with bilateral temporal lobe ablations no longer show appropriate fear or anger responses.(1) The role of the amygdala in emotion has been subsequently extended by findings that humans with lesions to this structure have impaired emotional recognition, particularly for fear, and no longer acquire Pavlovian conditioned responses(2) (see below). Finally, functional neuroimaging findings show activation of amygdala in responses to face stimuli that depict a range of emotions, particularly fear but also other primary emotions.(3, 4)

The importance of the amygdala in emotion derives in part from its extensive anatomical connections with all sensory processing cortices, as well as hippocampus, basal ganglia, cingulate cortex and the homeostatic regulatory regions of hypothalamus and brain stem.(5) This widespread anatomical connectivity means that this structure can access information processing in multiple brain regions and, in turn, can exert diffuse modulatory influences, including influences on effector autonomic and motor output systems. In this way activation of the amygdala by a sensory based emotional stimulus influences widespread brain regions including those that mediate homeostatic regulatory responses as expressed in altered autonomic state, such as change in heart rate, blood pressure and respiration.

Learning predictive emotional responses

A central role for emotion is to index value, specifically whether present or future sensory events or states of the environment that are likely to be associated with reward or punishment. From this perspective, all emotions are to a greater or lesser degree valanced. For example, an emotion of joy signals a likelihood of reward while an emotion of fear signals a likelihood of punishment. The fact that signals that predict such emotional occurrences are to some degree arbitrary means that the brain must have some means of associating sensory cues with potential emotional outcomes, an ability that seems crucial for adaptive behaviour.

Associative learning provides a phylogenetically highly conserved means to predict future events of value, such as the likelihood of food or danger, on the basis of predictive sensory cues. The amygdala plays a crucial role in mediating this form of emotional learning as evidenced by deficits seen with animal lesion data and learning-related effects seen in human functional neuroimaging experiments.(6, 7) In its simplest form, Pavlovian conditioning is expressed when a previously neutral sensory stimulus (the conditioned stimulus, or CS+) acquires emotional predictive significance through pairing with a biologically salient reinforcer (the unconditioned stimulus, or UCS). With conditioning, the predictive stimulus (CS+) comes to elicit behaviour previously associated with the UCS, but in the absence of UCS presentation. There is a wealth of animal and human data which now shows that the amygdala has a key role in this form of associative learning, for both appetitive and aversive outcomes.

How the brain updates predictions of emotional outcomes

While contingencies acquired on the basis of associative learning provide a basis for generation of predictions of future event of value in response to sensory cues, this form of learning lacks flexibility in optimizing future behaviour. For example, the value of future states associated with predictive cues may change in the absence of subsequent pairing with these cues. Thus, a cue that is associated with a particular food that is valued when a person is hungry has diminished relevance when the person is sated with that same food. Consequently, it is important for optimal adaptive behaviour to be able to maintain an updated representation of the current value of such sensory-predictive cues that does not slavishly depend on new learning in relation to that cue.

Reinforcer devaluation is a standard experimental methodology for examining how value representations accessed by predictive cues are updated. As indicated, in the case of food, its value can be decreased through what is termed sensory-specific satiety. In this type of manipulation, the reward value of a food eaten to satiety is reduced (devalued) relative to foods that are not eaten to satiety. In humans, functional neuroimaging measured brain responses elicited by predictive stimuli (such as a CS+), that have been subject to devaluation, are associated with significant response decrements in the OFC paralleling the behavioural effects of satiation.(8) This response pattern within OFC indicates that this region is involved in representing reward value of predictive stimuli in a flexible manner, observations that also accord with extensive evidence from animal lesion data.(9, 10)

The observation that neural responses evoked by a food predictive conditioned stimulus (a CS+) in OFC are directly modulated by hunger states can inform an understanding of the behavioural impact of pathologies that impact on orbital-frontal cortex, especially the feeding abnormalities observed in both the Kluver-Bucy syndrome and fronto-temporal dementias. Patients with these conditions frequently show increased appetite, indiscriminate eating, food cramming, and change in food preference, hyperorality, and even attempts to eat non-food items. A dysfunctional network involving OFC and amygdala would mean that food cues, and other predictive cues, are unable to recruit motivationally appropriate representations of food-based reward value.

A computational account of emotional learning

Learning to predict reward or danger is a basic and highly conserved form of learning, as embodied in Pavlovian or associative learning. However, to be maximally adaptive, it is important that this form of learning is used not only to predict but also to shape optimal actions. The computational principles that underpin what is now referred to as value learning, involving prediction and optimization of action with respect to likely future outcomes, is more than an abstract issue and speaks to the critical issue of optimal control in decision-making.

One classical solution as to how associative learning is implemented is by means of a signal, referred to as a prediction error, which registers a difference between a predicted and actual outcome. This type of solution to predictive learning has been formalized within what is known as the Rescorla-Wagner learning rule. Temporal difference learning (TD) provides a more sophisticated computational extension of this learning rule that accounts in a precise manner for how an organism learns to make predictions, as well as select optimal actions, in response to states of the environment so as to maximize long-term reward or avoid long-term punishment.[(11)] As in the case of the Rescorla-Wagner model, when a positive (or negative outcome) is not predicted there is a large prediction error which reduces to zero when this same outcome is fully predicted. The function of the prediction error is to act as a teaching signal that can both update future predictions as well as shape optimal policies or action choices. In temporal difference learning (TD), credit is assigned by means of the difference between temporally successive predictions, rather than between a predictive stimulus and an outcome, such that learning occurs whenever there is a change in prediction over time.

The importance of the above theoretical considerations rests upon empirical observations that TD error-like responses have now been demonstrated in the response pattern of dopamine neurones recorded in monkeys during associative learning.[(12)] Consequently, in a classical conditioning context where a stimulus is followed by an unexpected reward it can be shown that dopamine neurones respond with a burst of action potentials after actual reward receipt. Over the course of learning, with repeated presentations of a predictive stimulus and reward, dopamine neurones no longer respond to receipt of the reward. In this latter case, the reward is accurately predicted because of the occurrence of the preceding predictive stimulus. What is now observed is a prediction error at the time of the earliest predictor of this reward, for example at time of presentation of a predictive CS stimulus. Prediction error type brain responses have also been shown to occur in the human striatum and orbital-prefrontal cortex during both Pavlovian and Instrumental learning in humans, as measured by fMRI.[(13,14)] Indeed, a crucial link between a dopamine prediction error signal, human striate activity and reward-related choice behaviour in humans has also been shown using fMRI techniques. In this latter case, a reward outcome prediction error signal was enhanced by boosting the impact of dopamine using L-dopa (a precursor of dopamine), while a dopaminergic blocker Haloperidol led to an attenuation of a prediction error signal. Crucially, the former manipulation was associated with enhanced reward learning while the latter was associated with impaired reward learning in a manner that indicates that a reward outcome prediction error is involved in shaping optimal behaviour.[(15)]

How emotion influences memory

The cognitive domain where the modulatory influences of emotion have been best characterized is with respect to episodic memory, the type of memory that underpins autobiographical experience. Emotion enhances episodic memory function as seen in an enhancement for material that encompasses personal autobiographical, picture, and word based-items, an effect best seen in free recall tasks.[(16)] The critical role played by the amygdala in this modulation is illustrated by functional neuroimaging experiments where amygdala activity during encoding predicts a benefit in later recall of emotional material relative to neutral material.[(17)] Thus, enhanced amygdala activity at encoding for both positive and negative stimuli is predictive of later episodic memory function, during free recall tasks.

During encoding of emotional items there are bi-directional interactions between amygdala and hippocampus, the latter structure being a region essential for episodic memory formation. The bi-directional interaction between amygdala and hippocampus is inferred from the fact that an enhanced amygdala response, measured using functional neuroimaging, to presentation of emotional items is dependent on influence from hippocampus. Conversely, an enhanced hippocampal response to emotional items is dependent on influences from the amygdala.[(18)] While these studies were carried out at encoding it is important to acknowledge a role for the amygdala during retrieval of emotional items and contexts.

How emotion influences perception

Emotion often signals an environmental event of value. From an evolutionary perspective, it is important that such occurrences are amenable to privileged perceptual processing. There appears to be two distinct mechanisms by which emotion can influence perception of such event. One of these is through emotion grabbing attention, leading to enhanced deployment of attention to an emotional eliciting stimulus. This would result in preferential detection of emotional events enabling appropriate adaptive responses to be enacted.

There is also evidence for a second means by which emotion can influence perception that appears to operate independent of attention. For example, in visual backward masking paradigms, a target presented for a brief instance can be rendered invisible if it is immediately followed by a second 'masking stimulus'. In situations where the hidden target stimulus is an emotional item, for example, a conditioned angry face or a spider, there is preserved processing. This is evident in differential skin conductance responses (SCRs) to fear-relevant compared to fear-irrelevant unseen targets.[(19)] Similar findings are reported using what is referred to as an attentional blink paradigm. The latter refers to a situation where detection of an initial target stimulus, in a stimulus stream, leads to impaired awareness, or inattentional blindness, for a successive second target. Critically, when this second target has emotional content there is an increased probability of its detection as opposed to the default attentional blindness.[(20)]

In terms of anatomical substrates of these modulatory effects, there is compelling evidence to implicate the amygdala. In functional neuroimaging experiments, using visual backward masking paradigms, an amygdala response discriminates between unseen emotional and unseen non-emotional target.[19] In other experiments that involve overt stimulus presentation, but where attention is systematically manipulated, such that emotional items are presented out of the window of attention, an amygdala response to emotional stimuli is independent of the concurrent attentional focus.[21] Likewise, in studies of patients with either blindsight (loss of primary visual cortex resulting in visual field blindness) or visual extinction (a situation following a lesion to the right inferior parietal cortex whereby subjects cannot consciously represent stimuli in the contra-lesional visual field) demonstrate an amygdala response to emotional stimuli presented out of awareness in the damaged hemifield.[22]

How pre-attentive processing of emotional events influence, and enhance, perception is an important mechanistic question. One possibility is that inputs from emotional processing regions, in particular the amygdala, modulate the very regions involved in object perceptual processing, specifically when this relates to an emotion eliciting object or event. Anatomically, the amygdala receives visual inputs from ventral visual pathways and sends feedback projections to all levels of this pathway. Neuroimaging data provide evidence for enhancement of the strength of connectivity between amygdala and extra-striate visual regions during processing of an emotional visual input. In patients with amygdala lesions, the enhancement of activity seen in early extra-striate visual areas during encoding of emotional items, for example faces, is no longer expressed. Crucially, neuropsychological data from patients with amygdala damage indicate that a perceptual enhancement seen in extra-striate visual cortex for emotional items is abolished following damage to this structure.[23] This type of evidence is consistent with a proposal that boosting of activity in early sensory cortices, when an emotional stimulus is encountered, reflects a direct modulatory influence from the amygdala.

The neurobiology of subjective feeling states

Human emotion research often conflates the neurobiological mechanisms that index the perception or occurrence of an emotional event (representational aspects of emotion) with their subjective experiential counterparts, usually referred to as feeling states. Feelings can be formally defined as mental representations of physiological changes that characterize, and are consequent upon, processing an emotion eliciting object event or image.[24] This definition assigns an important causal role in the genesis of subjective feeling states to afferent feedback to the brain from the body, both sensory and neurochemical. At a broader level, feeling states can be thought of as reflecting the operation of homeostatic mechanisms that underlie survival of the organism. In a recent theoretical model, based on neurological observations, prime emphasis is given to the cerebral representation of bodily states as providing the substrate for the conscious awareness of feeling states.[25]

A key neurobiological question is whether brain systems supporting emotional perception are distinct from those supporting feelings states. Candidate structures that mediate feeling states encompass those involved in bodily homeostasis and that process information regarding the bodies internal milieu including brain stem peri-acqueductal grey (PAG) and parabrachial nuclei, tegmentum, hypothalamus, insula, somatosensory and cingulate cortices. Functional neuroimaging provides strong evidence that feeling states are mediated by distinct neuronal systems to those that support emotional perception.[26] Thus, functional neuroimaging studies of volunteer subjects have shown that the central generation and re-representation of peripheral autonomic states involve structures such as anterior cingulate and insular cortex. For example, recall of subjective feeling states associated with past emotional experiences engages regions encompassing the upper brainstem nuclei, hypothalamus, somatosensory, insular and orbitofrontal cortices. In subjects with pure autonomic failure (PAF), where there is absence of visceral afferent and information regarding the peripheral body state due to selective acquired peripheral autonomic damage, there is attenuation of subjective emotional feelings as well as emotion evoked neuronal activity in regions implicated in mediating feeling states, such as anterior cingulate and insula cortex.[27]

Among the regions most strongly implicated in mediating subjective feeling states is the insula cortex, an extensive region of cortex enfolded from the cortical surface within temporal lobes. Direct evidence for its role in representing subjective feeling states comes from investigations that tap awareness of internal bodily states, such as that required in performing a heartbeat detection task.[28] In this task, subjects who have the ability to detect and accurately report their own heartbeat, which is seen as evidence of somatic awareness, show enhanced activity in the anterior insula cortex when performing such a task.[29]

The proposal that the insula cortex area mediates subjective feeling states is bolstered by evidence that empathetic awareness of the subjective feeling states of others, for example, that engendered when one observes another person receiving pain, is reflected in enhanced activity within anterior insula and cingulated cortex.[30] These same regions are also engaged when a subject is exposed to a pain eliciting stimulus suggesting the same neural matrix that represents subjective feeling states is engaged when representing the subjective feeling states of another person.

(a) Imaging emotional influences on decision-making

Emotion is frequently invoked as influencing decision-making, often detrimentally, a view that tends to pit a hot 'irrational' emotional decision system in opposition to a cold 'rational' cognitive decision-making system. This dichotomy almost certainly represents a simplification and there are compelling neurobiological reasons to suggest multiple decision-making systems in the human brain with emotion in many instances facilitating optimal decision-making.

Real-life decision-making often involves choices between actions which yield potential rewards or punishments, albeit with some element of uncertainty, for example, as manifest in varying probabilities and magnitudes of outcomes. Adaptive decisions that seek to optimize goal-oriented behaviour require an estimation of expected future reward that will follow from choosing a particular action. This behaviour can be described as utility maximization. As outlined previously, reward prediction based on expected reward value can be studied through classical conditioning, in which an arbitrary cue (or conditioned stimulus) takes on predictive value by association with subsequent delivery of an affectively significant or unconditioned stimulus (which can be a reward or punishment, or strictly speaking, an appetitive or aversive stimulus).

Neuroimaging studies implicate OFC alongside structures such as amygdala and ventral striatum in prediction for reward and punishment.[31] As described above, human neuroimaging studies of classical conditioning for reward have highlighted a prediction error signal in prominent target areas of dopamine neurones, including the striatum and OFC. The finding that a neural reward prediction error signal is expressed, present in OFC and striatum, and indeed throughout the reward network, is consistent with the idea that this signal provides a basis for flexible learning and updating of stimulus-reward associations.[33]

Accounts of human decision-making emphasize rationalistic perspectives which invoke analytic processes mediated by an executive prefrontal cortex. An emotional or value based contribution to high level decision-making is evident following ventromedial prefrontal cortex damage where, despite the absence of intellectual deficits, such patients often make real life decisions that are disadvantageous.[33] The types of deficits seen in these patients have been conceptualized as a myopia for the future, in which current needs (as opposed to an integration of current and future needs) dominate decision-making. Observations from patients with this type of lesion has led to the suggestion that this ventromedial OFC provides access to feeling states evoked by past decisions during contemplation of future decisions of a similar nature. Thus, evocation of past feeling states biases the decision-making process, towards or away from a particular behavioural option.[34] However, alternative frameworks that might explain behavioural deficits seen following damage to this region include an inability to represent the value of competing options for action or extreme discounting of future rewards (a myopia for the future), leading to an overvaluing of current as opposed to future rewards.

It is well recognized that normative human decision-making does not always accord with rationalistic perspectives of utility maximization. An influence of prior emotional experience on decision processes is captured by the consequences of an emotion such as regret. Regret is an emotion generated by counter-factual thinking involved in comparing an obtained and foregone outcome which indicates to the subject that the latter, if chosen, would have been more advantageous. In this sense, regret is also a prototypical example of a secondary or higher order emotion, meaning that it emerges out of cognitive or higher order processing as opposed to being stimulus elicited as in the case of fear or disgust (prototypical exemplars of primary emotions). It is known that subjects who experience regret as a consequence of a choice show a subsequent bias away from a rationalistic imperative that invokes a maximization of expected value when making similar choices, an effect that can be explained as regret minimization. This behavioural bias is associated with engagement of the amygdala and orbitofrontal cortices regions, that are also engaged by the actual experience of regret.[35] This pattern of brain response is consistent with theories that suggest evocation of past emotions in the context of decision-making, providing a biasing influence on rational decision processes.

An additional tenet of rational behaviour is the idea that human decisions should be consistent regardless of how choices are presented. One notable deviation from this axiom is described as a framing effect. In simple terms, the framing effect describes a bias in decision-making observed when choices are presented in terms of gain, leading to choices of a sure as opposed to a risky option, versus the same choices presented in a loss where subjects are biased to choose a risky option. Functional neuroimaging data show that a framing engendered bias in human decision-making, risk averseness in the gain and risk seeking in the loss frame, is associated with enhanced amygdala activity at the point of decision-making.[36] The suggestion here is that an emotional heuristic, mediated via key emotion processing brain regions, is invoked when humans make decisions under situations where information is incomplete or overly complex.

Conclusions

The neurobiology of human emotion has now undergone a radical revision with the development of sophisticated neuroimaging technologies. There is a clear evidence that it no longer makes sense to think of the brain in terms of simple dichotomies such as limbic and non-limbic. Emotion engages widespread regions of the brain with the precise regions being dynamically con ured as a function of behavioural context. Thus, patterns of brain activity evoked by the seeing a fear eliciting stimulus, such as a snake, are distinct from those evoked when seeing another person in pain. The former situations involve activation of the amygdala and through its modulatory effects it influences widespread interconnected regions, including early sensory cortices. The latter situation results in engagement of distinct structures such as the insula and cingulate cortex. Learning about likely emotional occurrences involves a distinct teaching signal, a prediction error, expressed in widespread brain regions including the striatum and OFC, the latter region mediating a flexible representation of the value of emotional occurrences including reward.

Further information

Glimcher, P. W. and Rustichini, A. (2004). Neuroeconomics: the consilience of brain and decision. *Science,* **306**, 447–52.

Dayan, P. and Balleine, B.W. (2002). Reward, motivation, and reinforcement learning. *Neuron,* **36**, 285–98.

Schultz, W. and Dickinson, A. (2000). Neuronal coding of prediction errors. *Annual Review Neuroscience,* **23**, 473–500.

References

1. Weiskrantz, L. (1956). Behavioural changes associated with ablation of the amygdaloid complex in monkeys. *Journal of Comparative Physiology and Psychology*, **49**, 381–391.
2. Bechara, A., Tranel, D., Damasio, H., *et al.* (1995). Double dissociation of conditioning and declarative knowledge relative to the amygdala and hippocampus in humans. *Science*, **269**, 1115–8.
3. Morris, J.S., Frith, C.D., Perrett, D.I., *et al.* (1996). A differential neural response in the human amygdala to fearful and happy facial expressions. *Nature*, **383**, 812–5.
4. Winston, J.S., O'Doherty, J., Dolan, R.J. (2003). Common and distinct neural responses during direct and incidental processing of multiple facial emotions. *Neuroimage*, **20,** 84–97.
5. Amaral, D.G., Price, J.L., Pitkanen, A. *et al.* (1992). Anatomical organization of the primate amygdaloid complex. In *The amygdala: neurobiological aspects of emotion, memory and mental dysfunction* (ed. J. Aggleton), New York, Wiley_Liss.
6. Buchel, C., Morris, J., Dolan, R.J., *et al.* (1998). Brain systems mediating aversive conditioning: an event-related fMRI study. *Neuron*, **20**, 947–57.
7. LaBar, K.S., LeDoux, J.E., Spencer, D.D., *et al.* (1995). Impaired fear conditioning following unilateral temporal lobectomy in humans. *J Neurosci*, **15**, 6846–55.

8. Gottfried, J.A. and Dolan, R.J. (2004). Human orbitofrontal cortex mediates extinction learning while accessing conditioned representations of value. *Nat Neurosci*, **7**, 1144–52.
9. Hatfield, T., Han, J.S., Conley, M., *et al.* (1996). Neurotoxic lesions of basolateral, but not central, amygdala interfere with Pavlovian second-order conditioning and reinforcer devaluation effects. *J Neurosci*, **16**, 5256–65.
10. Malkova, L., Gaffan, D. and Murray, E.A. (1997). Excitotoxic lesions of the amygdale fail to produce impairment in visual learning for auditory secondary reinforcement but interfere with reinforcer devaluation effects in rhesus monkeys. *J Neurosci*, **17**, 6011–20.
11. Sutton, R. and Barto, A. (1998). *Reinforcement Learning; An Introduction* (Adaptive Computation & Machine Learning). Cambridge, MA: MIT Press.
12. Schultz, W. (1997). Dopamine neurons and their role in reward mechanisms. *Curr Opin Neurobiol*, **7**, 191–7.
13. O'Doherty, J., Dayan, P., Schultz, J., *et al.* (2004). Dissociable roles of ventral and dorsal striatum in instrumental conditioning. *Science*, **304**, 452–4.
14. O'Doherty, J.P., Dayan, P., Friston, K., *et al.* (2003). Temporal difference models and reward-related learning in the human brain. *Neuron*, **38**, 329–37.
15. Pessiglione, M., Seymour, B., Flandin, G., *et al.* (2006). Dopaminedependent prediction errors underpin reward-seeking behaviour in humans. *Nature*, **442**, 1042–5.
16. Cahill, L., Prins, B., Weber, M., *et al.* (1994). Beta-adrenergic activation and memory for emotional events. *Nature*, **371**, 702–4.
17. Canli, T., Zhao, Z., Brewer, J., *et al.* (2000). Event-related activation in the human amygdala associates with later memory for individual emotional experience. *J Neurosci*, **20**, RC99.
18. Richardson, M.P., Strange, B.A. and Dolan, R.J. (2004). Encoding of emotional memories depends on amygdala and hippocampus and their interactions. *Nat Neurosci*, **7**, 278–85.
19. Morris, J.S., Ohman, A. and Dolan, R.J. (1998). Conscious and unconscious emotional learning in the human amygdala [see comments]. *Nature*, **393**, 467–70.
20. Anderson, A.K. and Phelps, E.A. (2001). Lesions of the human amygdala impair enhanced perception of emotionally salient events. *Nature*, **411**, 305–9.
21. Vuilleumier, P., Armony, J.L., Driver, J., *et al.* (2001). Effects of Attention and Emotion on Face Processing in the Human Brain. An Event-Related fMRI Study. *Neuron*, **30**, 829–41.
22. Vuilleumier, P., Armony, J.L., Clarke, K., *et al.* (2002). Neural response to emotional faces with and without awareness: event-related fMRI in a parietal patient with visual extinction and spatial neglect. *Neuropsychologia*, **40**, 2156–66.
23. Vuilleumier, P., Richardson, M.P., Armony, J.L., *et al.* (2004). Distant influences of amygdala lesion on visual cortical activation during emotional face processing. *Nat Neurosci*, **7**, 1271–8.
24. Damasio, A. (1999). *The Feeling of What Happens*. New York, Harcourt Brace.
25. Damasio, A.R. (1996). The somatic marker hypothesis and the possible functions of the prefrontal cortex. *Philos Trans R Soc Lond B Biol Sci*, **351**, 1413–20.
26. Critchley, H.D., Mathias, C.J. and Dolan, R.J. (2001). Neuroanatomical basis for fi rst- and second-order representations of bodily states. *Nat Neurosci*, **4**, 207–12.
27. Damasio, A.R., Grabowski, T.J., Bechara, A., *et al.* (2000). Subcortical and cortical brain activity during the feeling of self-generated emotions. *Nat Neurosci*, *3*, 1049–56.
28. Critchley, H.D., Mathias, C.J. and Dolan, R.J. (2002). Fear conditioning in humans: the infl uence of awareness and autonomic arousal on functional neuroanatomy. *Neuron*, **33**, 653–63.
29. Critchley, H.D., Wiens, S., Rotshtein, P., *et al.* (2004). Neural systems supporting interoceptive awareness. *Nat Neurosci*, **7**, 189–95.
30. Singer, T., Seymour, B., O'Doherty, J., *et al.* (2004). Empathy for pain involves the affective but not sensory components of pain. *Science*, **303**, 1157–62.
31. Knutson, B., Adams, C.M., Fong, G.W., *et al.* (2001). Anticipation of increasing monetary reward selectively recruits nucleus accumbens. *J Neurosci*, **21**, RC159.
32. Elliott, R., Dolan, R.J. and Frith, C.D. (2000). Dissociable functions in the medial and lateral orbitofrontal cortex: evidence from human neuroimaging studies. *Cereb Cortex*, **10**, 308–17.
33. Anderson, S.W., Bechara, A., Damasio, H., *et al.* (1999). Impairment of social and moral behaviour related to early damage in human prefrontal cortex. *Nat Neurosci*, **2**, 1032–7.
34. Bechara, A., Damasio, H., Tranel, D., *et al.* (1997). Deciding advantageously before knowing the advantageous strategy. *Science*, **275**, 1293–5.
35. Coricelli, G., Critchley, H.D., Joffily, M., *et al.* (2005). Regret and its Avoidance: A Neuroimaging Study of Choice Behaviour. *Nature Neuroscience*, **8**, 1255–1262.
36. De Martino, B., Kumaran, D., Seymour, B., *et al.* (2006). Frames, biases, and rational decision-making in the human brain. *Science*, **313**, 684–7.

2.5.5 Neuropsychological basis of neuropsychiatry

L. Clark, B. J. Sahakian, and T. W. Robbins

Introduction

Neuropsychology makes an essential contribution to neuropsychiatry. It seeks objectively to characterize mental competence in component cognitive functions such as perception, attention, spatial cognition, memory, learning, language, thinking, and 'executive' function. Executive function is often associated with the functions of the frontal lobes, although these are not at all synonymous; we will pay special attention to this domain below, as it may be crucial to the understanding of several neuropsychiatric disorders. Neuropsychology is often conveniently divided into clinical neuropsychology and cognitive neuropsychology. The former is primarily concerned with the methodology and psychometric theory that lies behind the selection, administration, and interpretation of standardized psychological tests aimed at assessing deviation from the norm and an individual patient's profile of strengths and weaknesses with a view to optimizing functional outcome and quality of life. Cognitive neuropsychology, by contrast is more concerned with the elucidation of cognitive processes through the study of patients, using both classical and newly devised tasks.[1] Neuropsychology also forms part of cognitive neuroscience, which has as its major goal the understanding of normal, as well as abnormal cognitive function, not only through the neuropsychological study of patients and healthy controls, but also using other techniques, including functional neuroimaging and the use of transcranial magnetic stimulation or psychopharmacology. In practical terms, a neuropsychological assessment is often made together with a psychiatric examination; in addition to contributing to diagnosis it also helps to define the functional status of the patient.

Functions of neuropsychological assessment

These are perhaps easiest to define when there has been an organic brain injury causing a lesion; for example, due to a stroke, removal of a tumour, or a closed or penetrating head injury. It is clearly vital to have an accurate evaluation of a patient's cognitive status so that his or her care can be optimized. This applies equally in neuropsychiatric disorders. In conditions like attention-deficit/hyperactivity disorder (ADHD) or prodromal Alzheimer's disease, the cognitive examination provides essential information for making a diagnosis. Whilst acquired brain damage can lead to neuropsychiatric symptoms (e.g. depression or apathy), it may also be associated with specific patterns of cognitive deficit. However, most neuropsychiatric disorders are not associated with clearly defined brain injuries, but are instead hypothesized to result from the cumulative effects of neurodegenerative disease, neurotransmitter malfunctions, developmental hypoplasias, diffuse white matter lesions, or brain volume gains and losses. This is an important point, as it may require more sensitive new methodologies to characterize deficits produced by regional *overactivity*, or deficits associated with changes in regional *connectivity*, as distinct from brain lesions per se. In these examples, neuropsychology offers the opportunity to examine underlying pathophysiological mechanisms, in combination with other methods such as structural and functional brain imaging and evoked brain potentials.

Cognitive deficits (e.g. of memory) can exist in parallel to, and independently of, psychiatric symptoms (e.g. of melancholia) but they may also be intrinsic to them. For example, part of the psychiatric description of anxiety may emphasize abnormal attentional biases paid to threatening stimuli, which can be objectively assessed using cognitive testing.[2] Furthermore, some psychological factors may influence performance across a number of distinct cognitive domains, producing a broad profile of impairments from a relatively specific form of deficit. For example, patients with depression may show a 'catastrophic response' to receiving error feedback during testing, such that they are then more likely to respond incorrectly on the subsequent trial.[3] This interaction of emotional and social factors with cognitive processes forms an especially important part of neuropsychology as applied to psychiatry. Neuropsychology also enables the impact of neuropsychiatric symptoms to be assessed on functional status—whether the patient will be able to function in everyday life, and return to paid employment, and how rehabilitation may be best achieved. It is becoming clear that the effective treatment of certain symptoms (e.g. psychotic symptoms) can sometimes unmask profound cognitive impairments that are actually the main barrier to rehabilitation, as has recently been shown in schizophrenia.[4,5] Taking into account the corollary finding that cognitive status may be the best predictor of functional outcome and return to paid employment, this has made cognitive disabilities a new target for pharmaceutical treatment. Of course, with schizophrenia again in mind, it is also necessary to ascertain that medication is not associated with significant cognitive toxicity, for example in terms of sedation, distractibility, or impaired judgement. Neuropsychology must play a major role in providing such evidence. Sometimes neuropsychology may substantially contribute to the diagnosis itself of a psychiatric state, for example in dissociative disorders and in the study of fatigue disorders and malingering.

Principles of neuropsychological testing

Neuropsychological scores on most tests are standardized with respect to overall age, IQ, and ideally gender. Parallel forms of tests exist in different languages although cultural and ethnic factors are still difficult to take account of adequately. Testing is generally done in a quiet room without distraction by an experienced clinical neuropsychologist. Most tests have generally been shown to give consistent results when given by different testers and on different occasions to the same patient, when using standardized instructions. These 'inter-tester' and 'test–retest' forms of reliability are often critical factors in situations where testing has to be repeated, for example, in drug trials, or epidemiological studies.[6] Good test–retest reliability (i.e. $r > 0.8$) can be hindered by practice effects that markedly change how subjects approach the tasks. Such factors typically affect measures of executive function, where the subject may evolve strategies for dealing with the task over repeated test sessions. The various cognitive domains are usually tested in one or two sessions that contain an assortment of tests drawn from the types described above to provide a cognitive profile of the patient. The duration of the test sessions should be carefully considered in view of the concentration span and distractibility, or apathy of many patients. Neuropsychological test batteries normally comprise a selection of paper and pencil tests which are being supplemented increasingly with computerized elements. Computerized tasks benefit from the ease and accuracy of recording and analysing complex data (e.g. reaction times), and of standardizing the presentation of the test materials and trial-by-trial feedback. The Cambridge Neuropsychological Test Automated Battery (CANTAB), for example, utilizes a touch sensitive screen that allows the subject to interact directly with the test materials and obviates the need for divided attention between a video monitor screen and keyboard or desktop. Other possible advantages of computerized testing include the removal of the 'confrontational' or 'interrogative' elements of conventional testing, which may be especially advantageous when testing, for example, schizophrenic patients. The construction of batteries may also be affected by other factors such as the need to translate findings, presumably through the use of non-verbal tests, across species, based on the extensive knowledge of underlying neurobiological mechanisms gained through studies of non-human primates. Alternatively, there is a trend to customize neuropsychological batteries so as to focus on typical deficits in a given disorder, as illustrated by the recent derivation of the MATRICS battery for cognitive deficits in schizophrenia.[7]

Domains and neuropsychological tests of cognitive function

Neuropsychological assessment is made generally with respect to the overall profile of cognitive performance. For example, it is difficult to interpret an apparent memory deficit if the subject has a profound impairment in perception or attention. An important index of overall performance is the intelligence quotient, or IQ. The structure of intelligence is still being debated; whether there is a distinction for example between Cattell's fluid and concrete intelligence, and the possible existence of a general factor, Spearman's *g* versus Thurstone's more specific components.[8] Regardless of these theoretical issues, it is still useful to classify an individual in terms of their overall intelligence with a mean scaled score of 100 and a standard deviation of 15. IQ is often measured using sub-tests from the Wechsler Adult Intelligence Scale (or the child equivalent, the WISC), which broadly subdivides into verbal and non-verbal ('performance') components. The individual sub-tests include such categories as vocabulary, information, comprehension, arithmetic, digit span, similarities, block design, picture arrangement, picture completion, object assembly, and digit symbol, which thus probe a range of abilities from general knowledge and basic language skills to memory span, working memory, visuo-spatial construction, and psychomotor speed. As the time taken to make all these assessments can be prohibitive, a 'prorated' score based on a smaller selection of the tests is often employed, justified by the relatively high inter-correlation of performance among the 12 sub-tests. Intelligence is also measured effectively by the Raven's Matrices, a set of visuo-spatial problems based on analogies.

Frequently, it is useful to be able to gauge the patient's premorbid intelligence level, before the onset of psychiatric symptoms. One way of estimating this is from years of education, as frequently employed in the United States. A second method depends on the National Adult Reading Test (NART), an instrument that depends on the subject's ability to pronounce infrequent words; this correlates with educational level, and its utility was realized when it became apparent that patients with Alzheimer's disease showed relative sparing of reading abilities, thus enabling their premorbid IQ to be captured by this test.[9] Alongside its US analogue, the Wechsler Test of Adult Reading (WTAR), the NART is now widely used to estimate premorbid intelligence in neuropsychiatric disorders including schizophrenia.

Superimposed on this general assessment of IQ is performance on tests of more specific abilities. The Wechsler Memory scale provides a method by which memory can be assessed in the context of overall intelligence. Some of its components, such as the Logical Memory test are still much used. However, with our burgeoning theoretical understanding of the components of cognition has come the introduction of ever more sophisticated instruments for measuring sub-components of cognitive performance. This brief chapter can but summarize some of the consequences of this, and encyclopaedic compilations of the various tests are now available, together with details of their mode of administration and interpretation.[10] However, the main domains of function that are generally evaluated are now outlined.

Over and above basic clinical sensory testing, measures of higher order perception in either the auditory or the visual modalities are available—for example, the Visual Object and Space Perception Battery.[11] Memory function is a controversial and complicated area of assessment. Most rapid batteries include tests of recognition memory, simply deciding whether or not a stimulus is familiar or not. Recent evidence, for example from the animal literature, suggests that such memory is relatively independent of hippocampal function, and depends instead on such regions as the perirhinal cortex.[12] Verbal recall, particularly a free recall, is considered to be a more demanding form of memory, thought to require the coordinated functioning of medial temporal lobe and frontal lobe structures. The frontal lobes are also implicated in retrieval of the temporal sequence or order of events, or the source of a particular memory in the past. Tulving's distinction between episodic and semantic memory is still influential.[13] Episodic memory generally refers to the subjective reminiscence of an event that has 'what, where, and when' qualities, almost invariably associated with a person's autobiographical memory. By contrast, semantic memory reflects memory for facts that may well have a different form of representation within the temporal lobe and is importantly influenced by verbal processes. In addition to these various modalities of memory material, are specific memory processes that have to be evaluated, such as encoding and retrieval. The latter is often assessed efficiently by the so-called verbal fluency tests, in which subjects have to retrieve words from a semantic category (e.g. animals) or beginning with a specific letter (e.g. F) in a set time period, usually of 60 s. Standardized tests of learning of verbal or non-verbal forms of material are provided by the California Verbal Learning Test (CVLT), the Rey Auditory Verbal Learning Test (RAVLT), and the CANTAB Paired Associate Learning (PAL) test. Emotional memory, which almost certainly implicates such structures as the amygdala, is another area of memory research that requires urgent development for application to psychiatry, for such conditions as Post-Traumatic Stress Disorder (PTSD). However, it is difficult to see how the current tests of traditional neuropsychology can be of much assistance here when the problem is to quantify the disruptive effect of a specific memory that has become over-salient rather than inaccessible.

Working memory is another important component of memory that refers to the coordination of various short-term memory stores to provide more permanent representations and aid in the solution of ongoing activities such as planning and discourse. Working memory comprises short-term visuo-spatial and verbal memory stores, with postulated rehearsal processes (e.g. the articulatory 'loop') and a 'central executive' system. Perhaps a simple way of understanding what working memory accomplishes is to contrast digit span in a forward and backward modes (e.g. repeat back the sequence '5 2 3 7 1' in either the same order, or in the reverse order). In the former case, it represents the buffer capacity of the verbal store, whereas in the latter case, the response sequence requires manipulation at output. Working memory reflects the active ('conscious') processing of memory traces whether at the encoding or retrieval stages and is clearly dependent on such factors as attention and arousal level.

Attention is a complex theoretical construct that has gained much in recent years from its analysis in terms of underlying neural systems.[14] Unfortunately, despite the interest in attention from experimental psychology, there are not many standardized tests of attention in general use. A common distinction is between the automatic forms of 'covert' attention mediated by posterior cortical structures and voluntary forms engaged by anterior cortical (cingulate and prefrontal cortices).[15] In practical terms, tests are usually provided of *sustained attention*, which might include detecting infrequent visual or auditory targets in 'continuous performance' tasks over a protracted period of several minutes. *Vigilance*, the capacity to detect rare targets over very long time periods, is rarely assessed, for obvious practical reasons. The capacity for *selective attention* is very important to assess in psychiatry because of the evident distractibility of patients with anxiety, psychosis, or attentional deficit/hyperactivity disorder. Selective attention can be assessed with a variety of tests including the Stroop task, the Eriksen Flanker paradigm, or the Posner covert spatial attentional task. In the Stroop test, for example, the subject is required to name the ink colour of congruent or incongruent colour words (e.g. the word GREEN prinked in red ink). Resolution of response conflict is a key feature of this test, which has been associated with anterior cortex function through extensive investigation with functional brain imaging.[16] The Stroop test has been much used in psychiatry, both in its standard form and in various adapted forms with disorder-relevant stimuli. In the Alcohol Stroop, for example, alcohol-related stimuli (e.g. BOTTLE in red ink) may also interfere with naming of the ink colour in patients with alcohol-dependency problems.

There is, in fact, considerable overlap between tests of working memory, attention, and what is termed executive function. The notion of a set of control functions that optimize performance is controversial but seemingly necessary in accounting for performance on complex tests involving planning and decision-making. Planning is generally measured by such tests as the 3-disc Tower of London task, which requires subjects to move discs in one array to match the goal arrangement of another. The test is especially useful in its form where the subjects are not allowed to move the discs but are required to visualize and plan the solution in their 'mind's eye'. Validation of this test as being sensitive to frontal lobe function has come from the study of patients with neurosurgical lesions of the frontal lobe and also functional brain imaging.[17] However, it should be realized that there is no such thing as a 'frontal lobe' test; this is evident for example from studies of patients with basal ganglia lesions and also from the demonstration of an extensive neural network that is activated during spatial planning performance. The Tower of London is a planning task where there is one goal only, whereas many real life situations that overwhelm psychiatric patients require the optimization of performance on several task simultaneously. This requires high level planning and scheduling of behaviour, as tapped by the 'Six Elements Test' in which six different tasks have to be completed.

A further cluster of executive tasks tap into higher-level emotional and affective processes, which appear to be associated with the inferior parts of the frontal lobes including the ventromedial prefrontal cortex. Famous neurological case studies like Phineas Gage and EVR displayed profound changes in personality, social behaviour, and judgement after lesions to this brain area. These processes are also often defective in psychiatric disorders such as bipolar disorder and schizophrenia, which resemble in some respects, the problems in everyday life encountered by patients with ventromedial prefrontal cortex lesions. The Iowa Gambling Task is a measure of emotional decision-making that was developed for the assessment of such patients. The Iowa task allows subjects to 'play' with four decks of cards which vary in their pay-offs, such that two risky decks are associated with attractive short-term gains but with heavy occasional penalties over time. Typically, patients with ventromedial frontal lesions persist in selecting from these 'dangerous' decks, despite accruing considerable debt, and comparable neuropsychological deficits have also been seen in neuropsychiatric conditions, particularly drug dependence.[18] These tasks also draw on concepts of inhibitory control over behaviour, as there is a requirement to suppress responses that have either become dominant through repeated practice, or that are superficially attractive by virtue of immediate reinforcement.

Specific applications of neuropsychological tests to psychiatric disorders

(a) Standardization of neuropsychological assessment in schizophrenia

Now that cognitive deficits have been realized to be a core problem in schizophrenia, there is increasing attention being focused on the nature of these cognitive deficits and how to remediate them, for example by novel pharmacological treatments. In order to facilitate this process, NIH funded researchers to perform a meta-analysis of the cognitive deficits in schizophrenia in order to determine a profile of deficits and to construct a battery that would be sensitive to those deficits and to possible remediation.[19] They provided a principal component analysis suggesting cognitive impairments to be present in seven major domains: attention and vigilance, visual long-term memory, verbal long-term memory, working memory, reasoning and problem solving, psychomotor speed, and social cognition.[7] In fact, there was not very much published evidence for prominent deficits in the latter, but the investigators felt that it was justified to include it on the basis of clinical judgement. This led secondarily to the construction of a test battery for those domains, with a major requirement being its test–retest reliability. This battery is being used now in clinical trials and so it is too early to assess its utility. As with many other initiatives to provide a standard battery, this carries with it both advantages and disadvantages. A consensus battery is clearly of enormous value and aids the collection of data across multiple sites. Hard decisions do have to be made about the trade-off of reliability with validity and sensitivity and committees have to make compromises because of the difficulties of addressing these sometimes intangible issues. For example, the Wisconsin Card Sort test is clearly sensitive to deficits in schizophrenia, but it does have relatively poor test–retest reliability because of its intrinsic changes of contingency and requirement for cognitive shifting, and so has been excluded. However, it is possible that performance on such a test would be sensitive to cognitive enhancing drugs. Similarly, all tests using verbal material are problematic because of the need to provide translated versions whose reliability and relationship to the existing test has to be reassessed to determine its validity. Once batteries such as MATRICS are adopted it is sometimes difficult for innovative methods based on other theoretical perspectives, such as contemporary cognitive neuroscience to be developed. However, the recognition of a domain of cognitive function, social cognition, for which there are relatively few standardized instruments available has been useful for motivating new research and test development in that area. The final crucial issue, which has a much more general applicability than the MATRICS battery, is the need to relate the profile of deficits obtained to sensitive and reliable measures of functional outcome.

(b) Early detection of Alzheimer's disease

Alzheimer's Disease (AD) is a chronic and severe form of dementia that is increasing in prevalence as improved health care extends life expectancy. AD patients typically present with deficits in episodic memory; that is, memory for specific events or experiences that can be defined in time and space. AD poses an important challenge to neuropsychologists, to facilitate the early detection of the illness, so that future generations of pharmacological interventions may be administered to patients at the earliest opportunity, so that the rapid decline may be slowed, or eventually, halted. Individuals in the prodrome of AD often report subjective memory problems but do not fulfil clinical criteria for AD, in that activities of daily living and non-memory cognitive faculties are intact. This condition is referred to as Mild Cognitive Impairment (MCI) or 'Questionable Dementia'. There is accumulating evidence that the Paired Associates Learning test in the CANTAB assessment may be sensitive to the early stages of AD. PAL is a non-verbal test of learning and memory that requires the subject to associate abstract visual patterns with a series of box locations on a computer screen. Successful performance relies on learning the conjunction of shape and location; the task cannot be solved by learning either shape or location alone. The task increases in difficulty from one to eight patterns, and the task is terminated if the subject fails repeatedly at a given stage.

PAL performance was previously shown to be defective in patients with mild Alzheimer's disease, and test scores could discriminate AD from other neuropsychiatric conditions with similar symptom presentation, including Fronto-Temporal Dementia and unipolar depression.[20] Recent studies of 'at risk' older adults with MCI or Questionable Dementia have reliably isolated a subgroup of cases who have an increased likelihood of converting to a full AD diagnosis by the time of a follow-up assessment. PAL performance in the baseline assessment could be used to accurately predict the conversion from Questionable Dementia to an AD diagnosis.[21] Through a combination of age, PAL score, and performance on the Graded Naming test, subjects with Questionable Dementia could be classified with 100 per cent accuracy into those who did or did not convert to probable AD at a 32-month follow-up.[22] These neuropsychological measures display both sensitivity, in reliably detecting the progression to AD in a subclinical sample, as well as specificity, in differentiating AD from depression. A strong programme of translational research with the PAL task suggests this utility may stem from the critical role of medial temporal lobe structures in visuo-spatial associative learning.

(c) Relating neuropsychiatric disorders to specific impairments in executive function: ADHD, OCD, and mania

Recent biological analyses of such disorders as bipolar illness, ADHD, and OCD have focused on the importance of providing objective measures of performance that relate strongly to the clinical symptoms themselves, but that also provide sensitive indices of the underlying pathophysiology. These markers are often referred to as endophenotypes, a term that draws a further link to the putative genetic susceptibility to these conditions. One example is the profound deficit in thinking and decision-making that is a characteristic symptom of mania—a recent study has been able to demonstrate deficits in decision-making in patients with mania in the context of a gambling task.[23] What was especially striking about that study was that one of the main measures of quality of decision-making correlated significantly with symptom ratings on the Young Mania scale.

ADHD is a spectrum disorder with several sub-types that are characterized by the prominence of different clusters of symptoms that may be related to different underlying psychological constructs, neural and neurochemical substrates, and genetic factors.[24] Prominent among these is the so-called hyperactive/impulsive sub-type, which then requires sensitive and reliable measures of behavioural inhibition. One commonly used test is the Go-No-Go type task. In perhaps its most sophisticated form, this task measures the capability to countermand a speeded response (the 'stop signal reaction time (SSRT) task). The speed of the SSRT has been related to the volume of damage in the right inferior frontal gyrus in patients with frontal damage.[25] The task is also robustly impaired in children and adults with ADHD, and this deficit can be remediated by psychostimulant treatment with drugs such as methylphenidate.[26]

OCD may also relate to pathology in executive functions. The compulsive component in particular may arise from the repeated selection of a response option long after that option has ceased to be beneficial or contextually appropriate. This symptom may be operationalized in a neuropsychological setting in two complementary ways. First, there may be a failure to suppress a previously reinforced response, comparable to the deficit reported above in ADHD. Second, there may be a failure to flexibly shift responding to the newly-relevant mode. These processes can be assessed with some further tasks that are frequently employed in the assessment of psychiatric patients. For example, the Wisconsin Card Sorting test requires subjects to learn a rule on the basis of trial-and-error feedback and then to shift that rule according to altered feedback. OCD patients, like neurosurgical patients with frontal lobe lesions, display perseveration where they continue to sort cards according to the previously reinforced rule. Performance on a similar set-shifting test has been shown to be impaired not only in patients with OCD, but also in their first-degree relatives, implying that this capacity for cognitive flexibility may provide a suitable endophenotype for this disorder. Structural and functional neuroimaging data support a neuropsychological account that implicates the orbitofrontal region and interconnected (ventral) striatal circuitry in the pathophysiology of this condition.[27]

Conclusion

Psychiatry is the science of psychopathology, and as such, the measurement of behaviour and cognition is central to its theory and methodology. Neuropsychology provides such measures, which can be used to augment the psychiatric interview and other clinical instruments, as well as to provide an interface with other important approaches including functional brain imaging (see Dolan, this volume), functional genomics, and clinical psychopharmacology. Clinical neuropsychology has developed via the need to assess brain-damaged patients, whereas in most neuropsychiatric disorders, such damage is much less well defined if it is present at all. Thus, whilst there is growing information about specific brain abnormalities in many forms of neuropsychiatric disorder, the lesion model is not necessarily the most appropriate. Moreover, some of the deficits in disorders such as depression and anxiety involve subtle interactions between specific emotional and attentional mechanisms with cognitive function. Therefore, the study of neuropsychiatric patients has also enriched our understanding of clinical neuropsychology. We predict that these aspects of the discipline will develop considerably in the next few years, particularly in combination with data from other domains such as functional brain imaging and pharmacogenetics. Indeed, the specification of specific neural systems implicated in core behavioural or cognitive processes may well aid the enterprise of psychiatric genetics by providing more precise definitions of phenotypes (or endophenotypes) than are currently feasible in nosology (e.g. as defined by the Diagnostic and Statistical Manual).

A further theme for the future that can readily be envisaged is the development of neuropsychological methods for children and adolescents that are more suitable in a psychiatric context. We can predict that there will be an increasing emphasis on 'lifespan' studies that potentially will enable the origins of many psychiatric disorders and prodromal states to be identified. Thus, it will be necessary to examine cognitive function, including under-researched areas such as 'social cognition', in longitudinal terms with tests that can be administered appropriately at different points in the lifespan. Allied to this will be pressure to make tests less 'laboratory-bound' and more predictive of everyday functioning at school or in the workplace. One technological advance that may facilitate all of these requirements would be through the use of 'virtual reality' software, and also the collection of norms on a massive scale by utilizing web-based data collection. It is to be hoped that psychiatry will encourage and embrace such developments, rather than rely on the traditional methods.

Further information

Baddeley, A.D. (2007). *Working memory, thought and action*. Oxford University Press, New York.

Gottesman, I.I. and Gould, T.D. (2003). The endophenotype concept in psychiatry: etymology and strategic intentions. *The American Journal of Psychiatry*, **160**, 636–45.

Lezak, M.D., Howieson, D.B., and Loring, D.W. (2004). *Neuropsychological assessment* (4th edn). Oxford University Press, New York.

Robbins, T.W. (2007). Shifting and stopping: fronto-striatal substrates, neurochemical modulation and clinical implications. *Philosophical Transactions of the Royal Society of London (Biological Sciences)*, **362**, 917–32.

Ron, M.A. and Robbins, T.W. (2004). *Disorders of brain and mind*, Vol. 2. Cambridge University Press, Cambridge.

References

1. Shallice, T. (1988). *From neuropsychology to mental structure*. Cambridge University Press, Cambridge.
2. Williams, J.M., Mathews, A., and MacLeod, C. (1996). The emotional stroop task and psychopathology. *Psychological Bulletin*, **120**, 3–24.
3. Elliott, R., Sahakian, B.J., Herrod, J.J., *et al.* (1997). Abnormal response to negative feedback in unipolar depression: evidence for a diagnosis specific impairment. *Journal of Neurology, Neurosurgery, and Psychiatry*, **63**, 74–82.
4. Green, M.F. (1996). What are the functional consequences of neurocognitive deficits in schizophrenia? *The American Journal of Psychiatry*, **153**, 321–30.
5. Turner, D.C. and Sahakian, B.J. (2006). Analysis of the cognitive enhancing effects of modafinil in schizophrenia. *Progress in Neurotherapeutics and Neuropsychopharmacology*, **1**, 133–47.
6. Ferris, S.H., Lucca, U., Mohs, R., *et al.* (1997). Objective psychometric tests in clinical trials of dementia drugs. Position paper from the international working group on harmonization of dementia drug guidelines. *Alzheimer's Disease and Associated Disorders*, **11**(Suppl. 3), 34–8.
7. Green, M.F., Nuechterlein, K.H., Gold, J.M., *et al.* (2004). Approaching a consensus cognitive battery for clinical trials in schizophrenia: the NIMH-MATRICS conference to select cognitive domains and test criteria. *Biological Psychiatry*, **56**, 301–7.
8. Mackintosh, N.J. (1998). *IQ and human intelligence*. Oxford University Press, New York.
9. Crawford, J.R., Parker, D.M., and Besson, J.A. (1988). Estimation of premorbid intelligence in organic conditions. *The British Journal of Psychiatry*, **153**, 178–81.
10. Spreen, O. and Strauss, E. (1991). *A compendium of neuropsychological tests*. Oxford University Press, New York.
11. Warrington, E.K. and James, M. (1991). *The visual object and space perception battery*. Harcourt Assessment, San Antonio, TX.
12. Murray, E.A., Bussey, T.J., and Saksida, L.M. (2007). Visual perception and memory: a new view of medial temporal lobe function in primates and rodents. *Annual Review of Neuroscience*, **30**, 99–122.
13. Tulving, E. (2002). Episodic memory: from mind to brain. *Annual Review of Psychology*, **53**, 1–25.
14. Desimone, R. and Duncan, J. (1995). Neural mechanisms of selective visual attention. *Annual Review of Neuroscience*, **18**, 193–222.
15. Posner, M.I. and Petersen, S.E. (1990). The attention system of the human brain. *Annual Review of Neuroscience*, **13**, 25–42.
16. Bush, G., Luu, P., and Posner, M.I. (2000). Cognitive and emotional influences in anterior cingulate cortex. *Trends in Cognitive Sciences*, **4**, 215–22.
17. Robbins, T.W. (1998). Dissociating executive functions of the prefrontal cortex. In *The prefrontal cortex: executive and cognitive functions* (eds. A.C. Roberts, T.W. Robbins, and L. Weiskrantz). Oxford University Press, Oxford.
18. Bechara, A. and Damasio, H. (2002). Decision-making and addiction. I. Impaired activation of somatic states in substance dependent individuals when pondering decisions with negative future consequences. *Neuropsychologia*, **40**, 1675–89.
19. Kern, R.S., Green, M.F., Nuechterlein, K.H., *et al.* (2004). NIMH-MATRICS survey on assessment of neurocognition in schizophrenia. *Schizophrenia Research*, **72**, 11–19.
20. Swainson, R., Hodges, J.R., Galton, C.J., *et al.* (2001). Early detection and differential diagnosis of Alzheimer's disease and depression with neuropsychological tasks. *Dementia and Geriatric Cognitive Disorders*, **12**, 265–80.
21. Blackwell, A.D., Sahakian, B.J., Vesey, R., *et al.* (2004). Detecting dementia: novel neuropsychological markers of preclinical Alzheimer's disease. *Dementia and Geriatric Cognitive Disorders*, **17**, 42–8.
22. De Jager, C., Blackwell, A.D., Budge, M.M., *et al.* (2005). Predicting cognitive decline in healthy older adults. *The American Journal of Geriatric Psychiatry*, **13**, 735–40.
23. Murphy, F.C., Rubinsztein, J.S., Michael, A., *et al.* (2001). Decision-making cognition in mania and depression. *Psychological Medicine*, **31**, 679–93.
24. Castellanos, F.X. and Tannock, R. (2002). Neuroscience of attention-deficit/hyperactivity disorder: the search for endophenotypes. *Nature Reviews Neuroscience*, **3**, 617–28.
25. Aron, A.R., Fletcher, P.C., Bullmore, E.T., *et al.* (2003). Stop-signal inhibition disrupted by damage to right inferior frontal gyrus in humans. *Nature Neuroscience*, **6**, 115–16.
26. Lijffijt, M., Kenemans, J.L., Verbaten, M.N., *et al.* (2005). A meta-analytic review of stopping performance in attention-deficit/hyperactivity disorder: deficient inhibitory motor control? *Journal of Abnormal Psychology*, **114**, 216–22.
27. Chamberlain, S.R., Blackwell, A.D., Fineberg, N.A., *et al.* (2005). The neuropsychology of obsessive compulsive disorder: the importance of failures in cognitive and behavioural inhibition as candidate endophenotypic markers. *Neuroscience and Biobehavioral Reviews*, **29**, 399–419.

2.6

The contribution of social sciences

Contents

2.6.1 Medical sociology and issues of aetiology
George W. Brown

2.6.2 Social and cultural anthropology: salience for psychiatry
Arthur Kleinman

2.6.1 Medical sociology and issues of aetiology

George W. Brown

Introduction

David Mechanic, in his pioneering textbook, *Medical Sociology*,[1] views human activity within an adaptive framework—as a struggle of human beings to control their environment and life situation. While this view informs the research to be outlined, there are a number of ways it differs in emphasis from much medical sociology. First, by its concern with particular disorders defined in medical terms. Second, by its use of the investigator rather than respondent to characterize phenomena—to decide, for example, whether an incident should be classified as a life event. Third, by the importance placed on context. In order, for example, for an investigator to make a judgement about the likely meaning of an event such as a loss of a job it is essential to know whether it cast the person in a bad light; its impact on the person's family; her chance of getting another job, and so on. It is such circumstances surrounding an event that usually give it meaning via the emotion they create. Finally, by recognizing that where appropriate such emotion should be taken into account: 'A world experienced without any affect would be a pallid, meaningless world, and it is what gives us feedback about what is what is good or bad about our lives'.[2]

Context and measurement

Concern with context in the social sciences was central to the problem of meaning discussed widely in Germany in the late nineteenth century; and the ideas were introduced into sociology by Max Weber[3] and into psychiatry by Karl Jaspers,[4] although no one showed how to apply the methods systematically to concrete examples.[5] Jaspers, in his *Allegemeine Psychopathologie*, emphasized the way in which *Verstehen*, or understanding, on the part of an investigator 'depends primarily on the tangible facts' (i.e. verbal contents, cultural factors, people's acts, ways of life, and expressive gestures) in terms of which the connection is understood, and which provides the objective data.[4] While this view influenced the approach to meaning in what follows, there is a critical difference. No attempt has been made to make a judgement about the presence of a causal link between a set of circumstances and a psychiatric episode. The investigator has to judge only the likely meaning of a set of circumstances in the light of 'tangible facts' about a person's past and present. Any link with disorder is explored using established scientific procedures.

As noted by Jaspers, it is possible to take note of cultural factors; for example, when rating the likely implications of a birth, as part of research among women in a black township in Zimbabwe, investigators took into account the cultural importance on a wife producing a male child for her husband and his family.[6]

A second, more limited, use of context deals with the actual observation of emotion. For example, the Camberwell Family Interview, by taking account of vocal (in contrast to verbal) aspects of speech, for example, establishes how far a parent's talk about a child conveys 'criticism' rather than 'dissatisfaction'.[7] The approach can be extended to deal with core sociological concepts such as role commitment. For example, mothers in North London have been shown to differ substantially in commitment to roles such as 'mother' or 'wife' judged by how enthusiastically associated activities are discussed.[8] The relevant context is limited to the interview itself and what this conveys about a person's emotional style. In everyday life we automatically make allowances for the fact, for example, that some people show warmth in a more open way and, by taking this into account, makes it is possible for different expressive styles to be treated as equivalent.

Some methodological considerations

These developments have enabled 'soft' variables to be quantified. It has also been possible to make a reasonably persuasive case that significant bias has not followed the use of the investigator as the measuring instrument. For example, Creed[9] in a study of appendectomy found a relationship between severely threatening events rated contextually and the onset of non-inflamed but not inflamed conditions. This result was persuasive for two reasons. First, on the basis of a detailed description of the event and surrounding circumstances a consensus rating team reached agreement about the likely degree of threat, blind to what the person conveyed she felt and to whether she was a patient. Second, Creed, who provided the team with this edited account, was blind to clinical details. (He consulted medical records after the ratings had been made.) Such flexibility is difficult, if not impossible, with a questionnaire-based instrument which hands over the task of measurement to the respondent.

There are now a number of investigator-based instruments developed to deal with psychiatric issues covering areas ranging from 'expressed emotion' (e.g. critical comments, warmth, etc.), attitudes to self (e.g. self-esteem), plans and concerns (e.g. commitment to various roles), behavioural systems (e.g. styles of attachment), experience of adversity in childhood (e.g. sexual and physical abuse), and characteristics of non-family groups (e.g. restrictiveness of a psychiatric ward regimen). Around each a fair amount of replicable and theoretically relevant findings have emerged. Particularly important was the development in the 1960s of the clinically informed interview-based Present State Examination (**PSE**) by Wing *et al.*[10] later amended to deal with a 12-month period,[11] and psychosocial measures such as that of 'expressed emotion'[12] and the Life Events and Difficulties Schedule.[13] Part of the strength of the resulting research has been due to the levels of inter-rater reliability achieved and the ability of the approach to deal with time order. It is often overlooked that even with longitudinal designs it can be important to be able to establish what has happened between interviews.

Life events and building aetiological models

The characteristic features of the aetiological studies that have emerged can be illustrated by those dealing with life events. The significance of findings concerning depression is enhanced by the fact that most studies have produced broadly consistent findings about the role of events.[14–16] Indeed, for some years the challenge has been not so much to establish the presence of an effect, but to learn more about the nature of the events involved and to integrate findings into a more comprehensive aetiological model.[17]

The role of life events in the aetiology of depression

(a) Measurement and meanings

The original version of the Life Events and Difficulties Schedule was developed to study schizophrenic episodes[18] and there has since been a good deal of research dealing with psychotic patients.[19] An early achievement in the study of depression was to make clear that the amount of change in activity as such appears to be irrelevant and that the impact of events results from their meaning.[13] It has also been clear that attention needs to be given to ongoing difficulties that can either be brought about by an event (e.g. the death of husband leading to financial problems) or lead to an event (e.g. a marital difficulty eventually ending in a separation).

In dealing with meaning, two perspectives have proved productive. The first is summed up by the statement that we cannot fully know the meaning of an event until we relate it in some manner to our concerns. One way of conceiving of these is in terms of the impact of a particular event on plans and purposes that stem from role activity caught up in the crisis: how, for example, being turned down for rehousing by a local authority thwarts a woman's wish to move from an overcrowded and damp flat to give her children 'a better start in life'.

A second perspective concerning meaning assumes the likely presence of evolutionary-based response patterns that help to guide us in terms of what to want or to avoid, and that such systems are sensitive to a particular range of stimuli. The attachment system and fear responses are obvious examples.[20, 21] Of course, such responses will be influenced by individual differences of various kinds and by cultural display rules concerning emotions, but there is good reason to believe that such systems are often involved in the development of psychiatric disorders. For example, the central importance in a number of cultures of 'critical comments' of a close relative rather than 'dissatisfaction' in a schizophrenic relapse probably reflects an evolutionary-based sensitivity to emotionally toned criticism interacting with some constitutional predisposition to the disorder.[22]

The Life Events and Difficulties Schedule deals with both kinds of meaning. Blind consensus ratings usually based on four-point scales, made by several members of a team are employed to rule out reporting artifacts using 'edited' accounts supplied by the person who carried out the interview as discussed earlier in relation to the study of appendectomy. General as well as specific kinds of threat are rated in this way. They are contextual in the sense of taking into account a person's likely concerns of relevance for the event insofar as these can be assessed from a person's current circumstances and biography. In making such ratings no account is taken of reported feelings or whether a disorder followed the event. It deals not only with possible bias on the part of raters, but also with the problem that the cognitive processes involved in the appraisal of an event are not necessarily ones a person is willing or able to report.[23] General guidelines for rating severity of threat are given in an extensive manual containing thousands of examples listed in terms of a number of event categories (such as 'demotion at work' and 'unplanned pregnancy'). A similar procedure is followed for ongoing difficulties.

Some findings concerning depression

The first use of the Life Events and Difficulties Schedule to study depressive conditions took place in the early 1970s and involved a patient series seen at the Maudsley Hospital together with a sample of women from the local Camberwell population. A threshold of 'caseness' reflected what an outpatient psychiatrist would accept as a 'case'.[13] This enquiry, and a number made later, have established that the majority of episodes of clinical relevance are preceded by a severely threatening event.[14–16] These at a minimum had to be judged to continue to convey threat for at least a further 10 to 14 days. Nothing emerged to suggest that events with only short-term threat play a role.

Table 2.6.1.1 gives a typical result from a prospective enquiry of 400 women living in Islington in North London with at least one child at home. The table shows that 29 of the 32 onsets in the first

Table 2.6.1.1 Onset of depression within 6 months of a severe event or a severe difficulty among 303 women in Islington

	Percentage onset
Severe event	22 (29/130)
Severe difficulty and no severe event	5 (1/20)
Neither	1 (2/153)
Total	11 (32/303)

follow-up year were preceded by at least one severe event in the prior 6 months with most occurring within a matter of weeks.(8,23) For example, a woman experiencing a second miscarriage after persistent attempts to have her first child would probably have the event rated severe, but a first miscarriage shortly after marriage would most likely be rated upsetting but not severely so.

This finding emerged despite the use of contextual ratings that, as made clear, are based on a limited amount of information and deliberately designed to be approximate and probabilistic. It was also possible to obtain more direct evidence about the relevance of plans and purposes by a measure of emotional commitment to various roles made at the time of the first interview based on how they were talked about. Where a severe event (e.g. a child's delinquency) in the follow-up year 'matched' an area of high emotional commitment (e.g. to motherhood), risk of an onset was considerably increased when compared with a non-matching severe event.(8)

The contextual approach has also been used to take account of more specific aspects of meaning. Severe events preceding an onset of depression generally involve loss, if this is defined broadly not only in terms of loss of a person but loss of a role or a cherished idea—the latter about oneself or someone close.(24) (In contrast, events preceding the onset of anxiety tend to involve 'danger'—the threat of future loss.(25)) However, although loss is typically present it may not be the factor of central aetiological importance. Table 2.6.1.2 illustrates this by the development of a more comprehensive rating scheme—again carried out by the investigator. Four overall types of meaning are considered, covering in all nine categories. The ratings are hierarchical. Where more than one rating is possible the highest on the scale is taken. The first three categories concern possible types of **humiliation**, i.e. the likelihood of the event provoking a sense of being put down or a marked devaluation of self. The first category, for example, covers separating from a partner or a lover where they either took the initiative or the respondent was 'forced' to leave or break off a relationship because of violence or the discovery of infidelity.

Table 2.6.1.2 Onset by type of severe event over 2-year period in the Islington community series

Hierarchical event classification	No. of onsets	Percentage onset rate
(a) All 'humiliation' events	31/102	30
Humiliation: separation	12/34	35
Humiliation: other's delinquency	7/36	19
Humiliation: put down	12/32	38
(b) All 'trapped' alone events (i.e. not (a))	10/29	34
(c) All 'loss' alone events (i.e. not (a) or (b))	14/157	9
Death	7/24	29
Separation: subject initiated	2/18	11
Other key loss	4/58	7
Lesser loss	1/57	2
(d) All 'danger' alone events (i.e. not (a), (b), or (c))	3/89	3
All severe events	58/377	15

Events associated with **entrapment**, the second main type, had to have failed to meet criteria for one of the three humiliation categories. Such events emphasized the fact of being imprisoned in a punishing situation that had gone on for some time. The third type deals with four kinds of **loss** (in the absence of humiliation or entrapment) with the final type, **danger**, involving threat of a future loss.(24)

The table shows whether a particular severe event (or sequence of closely related events) was followed by an onset of depression, taking the event (or sequence) nearest to the onset when there was more than one event within 6 months of onset. Using a 2-year period for the Islington women, it shows that there were large differences in risk by event type. If events involving humiliation are combined with those of entrapment, risk was increased threefold.(24) The relatively low risk of depression associated with loss alone, except following a severe event involving a death, suggests that while the majority of events involve loss, something more than this is usually involved and that the experience of humiliation or entrapment associated with the loss is often critical.

Diagnostic issues

So far I have discussed only studies dealing with depressive onsets in the general population, almost entirely of a 'neurotic' kind. In the Camberwell enquiry of psychiatric patients, while events were rather less frequent before 'melancholic' than before 'neurotic' depression, there was considerable overlap between the two types. This lack of a clear link between the presence of a provoking life event and type of diagnosis had been reported earlier(26) and also in several subsequent studies.(27,28)

A recent study of North London psychiatric depressive patients has thrown possible light on this somewhat unexpected picture. When episode number was taken into account, those patients with both a melancholic/psychotic diagnosis and a prior episode of depression had a much smaller chance of experiencing a severe event before onset.(29) A patient series from Pittsburgh produced consistent findings.(30) These results, if confirmed, may also help to explain inconsistencies in published results since the proportion with a melancholic/psychotic picture and a prior episode is bound to vary by type of treatment centre. It is also of note that this same London study concluded that, despite detailed questioning, as many as one-tenth of *patients* with a 'neurotic' depressive disorder gave no hint of being provoked by social adversity of any kind.(24)

It is of interest that the smaller number with provoking events as episode number rises has also been found to relate to the course of bipolar conditions where there is some evidence for a sensitization or kindling mechanism.(31) Important research continues to emerge about psychosocial risk factors and bipolar conditions(32) and other psychiatric conditions.(33) However, for this brief review I will continue to focus on common depressive disorders.

Course and remission

Life-event research has also thrown some light on the processes involved in remission from depression. Evidence has begun to emerge that these often involve the reverse of the process leading to onset. A 'positive' event or the reduction in the level of a severe difficulty (with or without an event) is commonly found to have been present in the 20-week period before any remission (or marked improvement). However, it is of interest that although the events involved were rated contextually as likely to have given renewed hope about the future, one-third were at the same time judged as severely threatening.(34)

In the Islington general population series somewhat over half of the remissions of episodes that had lasted 20 weeks or more were preceded by such an event. There was no such link with episodes lasting less than this. In the patient series the result was much the same, although the chances of a positive event or difficulty reduction for those on antidepressant medication was somewhat less.(35)

A different approach to the issue of outcome concerns determinants of the length of a particular episode. Here the presence of severe interpersonal difficulty at the point of onset (but no other difficulty) was an important predictor of whether a depressive episode would go on to last for at least 1 year, and this held for a general population and patient series.(36, 37) Ongoing difficulties therefore need to be taken into account in terms both remission and in terms of whether an episode takes a chronic course.

Psychosocial vulnerability

The part played by severe events in depression has proved to be a particularly effective platform for exploring psychosocial vulnerability. The importance of this question was, in fact, illustrated in Table 2.6.1.1 where, despite the fact that the majority of onsets were preceded by a severe event, only one-fifth of those who experienced a severe event developed depression. While, as already discussed, taking account of event type increases this to one-third, it is still necessary to ask why only a minority go on to develop clinically relevant depression following a severe event.

In the Islington series, two background factors present at the time of the first interview proved highly predictive of onset: a negative environmental factor (negative interaction with others in the home and in addition, for single mothers, lack of a close confidant seen fairly often) and a negative psychological factor (negative evaluation of self). (The presence of chronic anxiety or subclinical depressive symptoms has often been included in the latter index, but findings are broadly similar with only negative evaluation of self.)

Their predictive power can be judged by the fact that, while only 23 per cent of the women without depression at the time of first contact had both, three-quarters of onsets in the 12-month follow-up occurred among these women.(38) The result has recently been confirmed in a second prospective enquiry.(39)

In terms of an overall aetiological model, the predictive power of the two indices appears to be largely a result of relating to a greater chance of a severe event occurring and to a lack of effective emotional support from a close confidant once the event has occurred.(40–43) Consideration of social support, of course, links the research, with social science concepts such as 'social integration', 'social bond', and 'social alienation'.(5) The topic is too complex to pursue in any detail in the present brief review. Research has so far underlined the need to recognize that support at one point in time does not necessarily predict what will occur in a subsequent crisis and, indeed, that a significant aspect of a number of severe events is the fact they involve the withdrawal of social support that up to that point had largely been taken for granted.(43, 44) There is also some indication that the ability of a woman to make supportive ties that can be used in a future crisis, and also to use them in such circumstances, is adversely influenced by the early experience of childhood abuse and neglect.(45, 46)

Figure 2.6.1.1, dealing with the Islington series, sums up research on the issue of vulnerability. It takes into account both event type and vulnerability and it shows that a severe event, however threatening, was not enough to provoke depression without the presence of at least one of the two vulnerability risk factors. Subsequent research has confirmed this general picture.

Gender differences

Most research on depression using the Life Events and Difficulties Schedule has dealt with women, although in the original Camberwell enquiry a small series of men gave similar results, as did a subsequent population enquiry.(24) However, recent research has gone further to suggest that the well recognized greater risk of a depressive onset among women may relate to their greater sensitivity to severe events involving their role as mothers. In a study of couples experiencing a severe event in common, women were twice as likely to develop a depressive episode following events involving procreation, children, and housing; for other events, risk was much the same.(47) While this study requires replication, it does support the increasingly held opinion that the large gender difference in the experience of 'neurotic' depression is likely to have an essentially psychosocial explanation.(48)

A lifespan perspective

So far only current environmental circumstances have been taken into account. The Camberwell research also identified loss of a mother before the age of 11 as a risk factor.(43) While there has been a good deal of controversy about this finding,(49, 50) two further population studies produced equally clear evidence with the added suggestion that such a loss between 11 and 17 may also increase

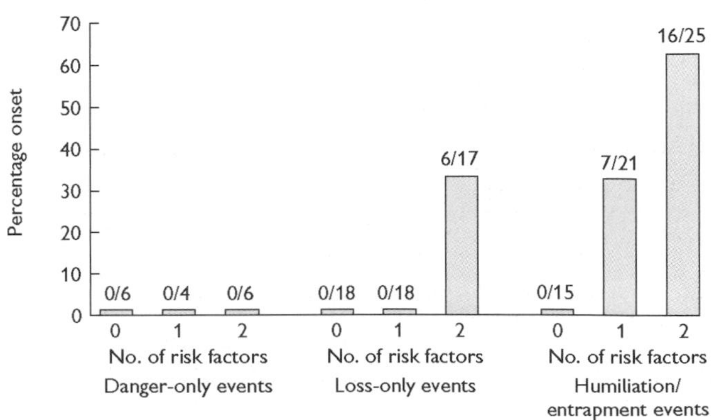

Fig. 2.6.1.1 Onset rate among 130 Islington women with a severe event by type of event and number of background risk factors.

risk.(51,52) The mode of the impact of such an early loss of mother for women is undoubtedly complex, but several studies have now established the critical importance of untoward experiences during childhood *after* the loss and have downplayed the role of loss as such.(51) More important than the loss of the mother itself was the quality of replacement parental care (in terms of an index of parental indifference or lax control). Risk of adult depression was doubled for those positive on the index.In order to understand its link with later adult depression it has been necessary to trace the history of a woman from the loss itself to such depression in a way that makes it possible to gain some sense of a life trajectory. Certain early experiences are particularly associated with the chance of experiencing the kind of adult factors already discussed.(53)

A factor playing a critical mediating role was the experience of a premarital pregnancy, and, like the care index itself, this was found to be associated with the subsequent experience of severe events. What seemed to be crucial about these premarital pregnancies was that they often trapped women in relationships which they might well not otherwise have chosen and which became a source of ongoing problems—such as severe housing and financial difficulties consequent upon a couple starting a family too young to have built up adequate savings, or marital difficulties with undependable partners. These women also emerged as less upwardly mobile, in terms of social class, than their peers without such pregnancies. In interpreting this complex of experiences, a conveyor belt of adversities was outlined, on which some women often appeared to move inexorably from one crisis to another, starting with lack of care in childhood and passing via premarital pregnancy to current working-class status, lack of social support and high rates of severe events.(53)

Although it was often hard to see from the women's accounts of their lives how they could have left this conveyor belt once their childhood had located them on it, a more personal element is likely to have played a role in many instances. Here the work of Quinton and Rutter(54–57) has been particularly significant in developing a lifespan perspective in this regard, and over this issue the results of the two research programmes have largely complemented each other.

The kind of early adverse experience just outlined was subsequently incorporated into a broader index of childhood adversity that included severe physical abuse within the family and also severe sexual abuse in any setting.(58) This index not only relates to a doubling of the risk of a depressive onset in adult life, but also to a number of other adverse outcomes, for example to the quadrupling of risk of an episode taking a chronic course(59) and also to the risk of a depressive condition comorbid with anxiety disorder defined by DSM-IIIR criteria (excluding simple phobias and mild agoraphobia).(60) It can be added that the retrospectives measures of early maltreatment used in these enquiries appear to be sufficiently free of bias to enable the findings to be taken seriously.(61, 62)

A population perspective

It is useful also to consider 'neurotic' conditions that form the bulk of depressive disorders, even in patient series, in terms of a population perspective. Figure 2.6.1.2 summarizes the findings of six population studies of women aged between 18 and 65 carried out in a comparable manner, using the same semi-structured interview-based measures as in the Islington survey, including the Present State Examination. The bottom half of Fig. 2.6.1.2 shows the rate of depressive 'caseness' in a 12-month period. Between the two extreme populations there is a 10-fold difference—3 per cent in a rural Basque-speaking population in Spain(63) and 30 per cent in a black urban population in Zimbabwe.(6, 64) In addition these rates are fairly closely paralleled by differences in the experience of severe events particularly likely to provoke depression (see top half of Fig. 2.6.1.2).

One of the implications of these results becomes clear in the context of a behavioural genetic perspective. A key point about the concept of heritability is that it is specific to a particular population and based on consideration of individual discrepancies from a population mean. While there may well be a genetic contribution in each of the six populations, this would reflect individual variability in risk within each population. Even if large, the genetic contribution would only be likely to be of relevance for explaining the substantial population differences in rates of depression if there were large population differences in the frequency of relevant genes. On present evidence the most plausible interpretation of such differences is that they are the result of psychosocial factors.(65)

There is, however, no inherent conflict between the two perspectives—they refer to different ways of looking at the 'variance' of a condition.(66) The general point is that the study of individual variability within particular populations cannot rule out the possibility that the mean level of disorder is largely under environmental control; that it can be increased or decreased markedly by external changes quite uninfluenced by the genetic make-up of a population.

A population perspective is also concerned with variability in rates of disorder within populations in terms of social categories such as socio-economic status. Thus, the survey in Camberwell in South London in the early 1970s found that, while the rate of severe events was related to social class position, this explained comparatively little of the large class difference in prevalence of depression; of greater importance were background vulnerability factors such as an unsupportive marriage.(13) However, the picture has recently become more complex with the finding that severe events involving

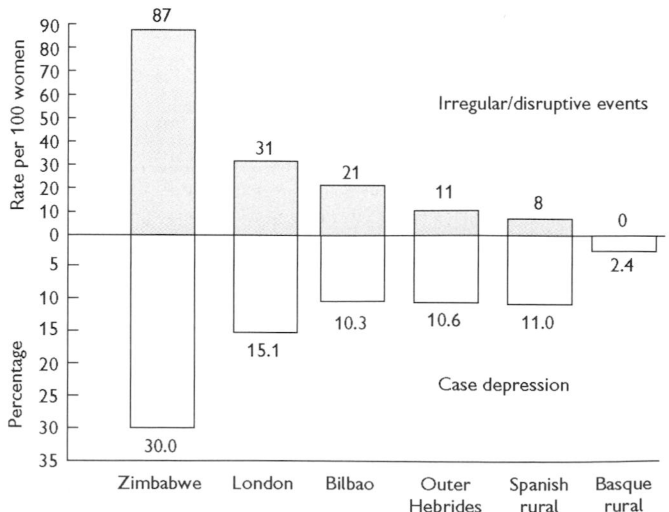

Fig. 2.6.1.2 Yearly rate of irregular or disruptive severe events per 100 women in six populations and prevalence of caseness of depression in year.

humiliation and entrapment are not only especially depressogenic but particularly common in high-risk populations (such as Harare) and within populations in high-risk subgroups (such as working-class women in London). In Islington such events were common among single mothers, a social category that has expanded dramatically in most western populations in recent years and among whom there is a high risk of depression.(67)

Final comments

There are two ways of looking at the findings that have been reviewed. First, that the study of life events has been an effective way of opening up wider issues concerning psychosocial factors and the aetiology of depression. This has been possible because, given the presence of a substantial causal link, a platform is provided for the study of a whole range of other experiences. As research has progressed it has pushed back in time to consider the aetiological role of early experiences of neglect and abuse which can have event-like characteristics. In more general terms the study of events has led to consideration of issues of vulnerability and protection, event production, chronicity, and course of particular episodes, and also issues not covered in this account such as coping and social support. It can be added that the work has also led to a good deal of research on other psychiatric conditions that have not been reviewed.(9,18,68,69)

The second contribution of the findings reviewed involves the stimulation of cross-disciplinary research concerning the depression—event link itself. This is a complex issue because life events correlate with factors ranging from genetic/personality(70) to macrolevel/societal.(65) The growing literature on the role of the serotonin transporter gene in depression is of particular interest as evidence has emerged for an important interplay with life events. A recent study has documented an interaction of the *s* allele variant of 5-HTTLPR polymorphism and life events with young adults. It also reported that childhood maltreatment predicted depression only among those with the *s* allele.(71) A somewhat similar finding with adult twins concerning life events has also been reported.(72) It is intriguing that there is a possibility of an important developmental contribution: that the critical gene-environmental interplay occurs early in life perhaps involving experiences such as parental maltreatment.(73) However, other studies have had more mixed findings with some showing no evidence of an interactive effect.(74,75) It is clearly too soon to review findings with any confidence—for example, some of the mix findings may well relate to the general failure to utilize the kind of detailed investigator-based measure of life events reviewed earlier and a failure to restrict consideration to events occurring not long before onset. In most studies the environmental measures fall a good way short of current best practice, although optimizing such assessments is essential for the detection of gene x environment interaction.(76,77) Nonetheless the research is an exciting development and it seems possible that well-established findings will emerge. But here my earlier comments about the likely critical importance of psychosocial factors in explaining differences in *rates* of disorder across populations should be kept in mind, although here there is some evidence that the genotype for 5-HTTLPR polymorphism may differ across populations.(78) It will also be important to take into account diagnostic issues. For example, it would be interesting to explore the fact, mentioned earlier, that it has been possible to isolate a small group of 'endogenous' neurotic depressive episodes.(24) Also it should be borne in mind that while this short review has largely restricted itself to work on depression, the life-event approach has been successfully employed with a number of other psychiatric and physical conditions and the possibility for collaborative research may well be much wider. For example, the *s* variant of 5-HTTLPR polymorphism also appears to be relevant for other psychiatric conditions.(74) There are other relevant biological considerations. The findings concerning life events involving humiliation and entrapment may need to be viewed from an evolutionary perspective, that is, that in some way a response pattern closely linked to issues surrounding defeat and exclusion, which has developed in group-living animals, may have functioned to promote survival.(78,79) It is possible that clinically relevant depressive conditions are often a complication of essentially non-pathological submission and appeasement responses to defeat in group-living mammals. Therefore, the high rates of clinically relevant depression that appear to be possible in some populations may well be a result of the more highly developed cognitive developments of *Homo sapiens* together with the event-creating potential of many societies experiencing periods of marked social change due to factors such as war, industrialization, technological development, urbanization, changing sexual mores.(80)

Further information

Brown, G.W. and Harris, T.O. (1989). *Life events and illness*. Guilford Press, New York.

Goldberg, D. and Goodyer, I. (2005). *The origins and course of common mental disorders*. Routledge, London and New York.

Monroe, S.M. and Hadjiyannakis, K. (2002). The social environment and depression: focusing on severe events. In *Handbook on depression* (eds. I.H. Gotlib and C.L. Hammen), pp. 314–40. Guilford Press, New York.

References

1. Mechanic, D. (1978). *Medical sociology* (2nd edn). Free Press, New York.
2. Tomkins, S.S. (1979). Script theory: differential magnification of affects. In *Nebraska symposium on motivations*, Vol. 26 (eds. H.E. Howe and R.A. Dienstbier), pp. 201–36. University of Nebraska Press, Lincoln, NE.
3. Weber, M. (1964). *The theory of social and economic organisation* (ed. and trans. T. Parsons). Collier-Macmillan, London.
4. Jaspers, K. (1962). *General psychopathology* (trans. J. Hoenig and M.W. Hamilton). Manchester University Press, Manchester.
5. Scheff, T.J. (1990). *Microsociology: discourse, emotion and social structure*. University of Chicago, Chicago.
6. Broadhead, J.C. and Abas, M.A. (1998). Life events, difficulties and depression among women in an urban setting in Zimbabwe. *Psychological Medicine*, **28**, 29–38.
7. Brown, G.W. (1985). The discovery of 'Expressed Emotion': induction or deduction? In *Expressed emotion in families: its significance for mental illness* (eds. J. Leff and C. Vaughn), pp. 7–27. Guilford Press, New York.
8. Brown, G.W., Bifulco, A., and Harris, T.O. (1987). Life events, vulnerability and onset of depression: some refinements. *The British Journal of Psychiatry*, **150**, 30–42.
9. Creed, F. (1981). Life events and appendectomy. *Lancet*, **i**, 1381–5.
10. Wing, J.K., Cooper, J.E., and Sartorious, N. (1974). *The measurement and classification of psychiatric symptoms: an instruction for the Present State Examination and CATEGO Programme*. Cambridge University Press, Cambridge.

11. Finlay-Jones, R., Brown, G.W., Duncan-Jones, P., *et al.* (1980). Depression and anxiety in the community. *Psychological Medicine*, **10**, 445–54.
12. Brown, G.W., Birley, J.L.T., and Wing, J.K. (1972). The influence of family life on the course of schizophrenia. *Journal of Health and Social Behavior*, **9**, 203–14.
13. Brown, G.W. and Harris, T.O. (1978). *Social origins of depression: a study of psychiatric disorder in women.* Tavistock Publications, London.
14. Jenaway, A. and Paykel, E.S. (1997). Life events and depression. In *Depression: neurobiological psycho-pathological and therapeutic advances* (eds. A. Honig and H.M. van Praag), pp. 279–96. Wiley, Chichester.
15. Bebbington, P., Hurry, J., Tennant, C., *et al.* (1981). Epidemiology of mental disorders in Camberwell. *Psychological Medicine*, **11**, 561–79.
16. Surtees, P.G., Miller, P.M., Ingham, J.G., *et al.* (1986). Life events and the onset of affective disorders: a longitudinal general population study. *Journal of Affective Disorders*, **10**, 37–50.
17. Bebbington, P., Wilkins, S., Sham, P.I., *et al.* (1996). Life events before psychotic episodes: do clinical and social variables affect the relationship? *Social Psychiatry and Psychiatric Epidemiology*, **31**, 122–8.
18. Brown, G.W. and Birley, J.L.T. (1968). Crises and life changes and the onset of schizophrenia. *Journal of Health and Social Behaviour*, **9**, 203–14.
19. Ventura, J., Nuechterlein, K.H., Subotnik, K.L., *et al.* (2000). Life events can trigger depressive exacerbations in early course of schizophrenis. *Journal of Abnormal Psychology*, **109**, 139–44.
20. Gilbert, P. (1989). *Human nature and suffering*. Erlbaum, Hove.
21. Ohman, A. (1986). Face the beast and fear the face: animal social fears as prototypes for evolutionary analysis of emotion. *Psychophysiology*, **23**, 123–45.
22. Martins, C.M, de Lemos, A.I., and Bebbington, P.E. (1992). A Portuguese/Brazilian study of expressed emotion. *Social Psychiatry and Psychiatric Epidemiology*, **27**, 22–7.
23. Brown, G.W. (1989). Depression. In *Life events and illness* (eds. G.W. Brown and T.O. Harris), pp. 49–94. Guilford Press, New York.
24. Brown, G.W., Harris, T.O., and Hepworth, C. (1995). Loss, humiliation and entrapment among women developing depression. A patient and non-patient comparison. *Psychological Medicine*, **25**, 7–21.
25. Finlay-Jones, R. and Brown, G.W. (1981). Types of stressful life event and the onset of anxiety and depressive disorders. *Psychological Medicine*, **11**, 803–15.
26. Paykel, E.S., Prusoff, B.A., and Klerman, G.L. (1971). The endogenous-neurotic continuum in depression, rater independence and factor distributions. *Journal of Psychiatric Research*, **8**, 73–90.
27. Katschnig, H., Pakesch, G., and Egger-Zeidner, E. (1986). Life stress and depressive subtypes: a review of present diagnostic criteria and recent research results. In *Life events and psychiatric disorders: controversial issues* (ed. H. Katschnig), pp. 201–45. Cambridge University Press, Cambridge.
28. Bebbington, P. and McGuffin, P. (1989). Interactive models of depression. In *Depression, an integrative approach* (eds. E. Paykel and K. Herbst), pp. 65–80. Heinemann Medical Books, London.
29. Brown, G.W., Harris, T.O., and Hepworth, C. (1994). Life events and endogenous depression: a puzzle re-examined. *Archives of General Psychiatry*, **51**, 525–34.
30. Frank, E., Anderson, B., Reynolds, C.F., *et al.* (1994). Life events and research diagnostic criteria endogenous subtype. *Archives of General Psychiatry*, **51**, 519–24.
31. Post, R.M., Rubinow, D.R., and Ballenger, J.C. (1986). Conditioning and sensitisation in the longitudinal course of affective illness. *The British Journal of Psychiatry*, **149**, 191–201.
32. Kim, E.Y., Miklowitz, D.J., Biuckians, A., *et al.* (2007). Life stress and the course of early-onset bipolar disorder. *Journal of Affective Disorder*, **99**, 37–44.
33. Hatcher, S. and House, A. (2003). Life events, difficulties and dilemmas in the onset of chronic fatigue syndrome: a case-control study. *Psychological Medicine*, **33**, 1185–92.
34. Brown, G.W., Lemyre, L., and Bifulco, A. (1992). Social factors and recovery from anxiety and depressive disorders: a test of the specificity hypothesis. *The British Journal of Psychiatry*, **161**, 44–54.
35. Brown, G.W. (1993). Life events and affective disorder: replications and limitations. *Psychosomatic Medicine*, **55**, 248–59.
36. Brown, G.W. and Moran, P. (1994). Clinical and psychosocial origins of chronic depressive episodes. I. A community survey. *The British Journal of Psychiatry*, **165**, 447–56.
37. Brown, G.W., Harris, T.O., Hepworth, C., *et al.* (1994). Clinical and psychosocial origins of chronic depressive episodes. II. A patient enquiry. *The British Journal of Psychiatry*, **165**, 457–65.
38. Brown, G.W., Bifulco, A., and Andrews, B. (1990). Self-esteem and depression. 3. Aetiological issues. *Social Psychiatry and Psychiatric Epidemiology*, **25**, 235–43.
39. Bifulco, A., Brown, G.W., Moran, P., *et al.* (1998). Predicting depression in women. The role of past and present vulnerability. *Psychological Medicine*, **28**, 39–50.
40. Harris, T.O. (1992). Some reflections of the process of social support: and nature of unsupportive behaviors. In *The meaning and measurement of social support* (eds. H.O.F. Veiel and U. Baumann), pp. 171–89. Hemisphere, Washington, DC.
41. Edwards, A.C., Nazroo, J., and Brown, G.W. (1998). Gender difference in marital support following a shared life event. *Social Science & Medicine*, **46**, 1077–85.
42. Veiel, H.O.F. and Baumann, U. (eds.) (1992). *The meaning and measurement of social support*. Hemisphere, Washington, DC.
43. Brown, G.W., Andrews, B., Harris, T.O., *et al.* (1986). Social support, self-esteem and depression. *Psychological Medicine*, **16**, 813–31.
44. Andrews, B. and Brown, G.W. (1998). Marital violence in the community. A biographical approach. *The British Journal of Psychiatry*, **153**, 305–12.
45. Harris, T.O., Brown, G.W., and Bifulco, A. (1986). Loss of parent in childhood and adult psychiatric disorder. The role of lack of adequate parental care. *Psychological Medicine*, **16**, 641–59.
46. Harris, T.O., Brown, G.W., and Bifulco, A. (1990). Loss of parent in childhood and adult psychiatric disorder: a tentative overall model. *Development and Psychopathology*, **2**, 311–28.
47. Nazroo, J.Y., Edwards, A.C., and Brown, G.W. (1997). Gender differences in the onset of depression: a study of couples. *Psychological Medicine*, **27**, 9–19.
48. Bebbington, P. (1996). The origins of sex differences in depressive disorder: bridging the gap. *International Review of Psychiatry*, **8**, 295–332.
49. Tennant, C., Bebbington, P., and Hurry, J. (1980). Parental death in childhood and risk of adult depressive disorders; a review. *Psychological Medicine*, **10**, 289–99.
50. Harris, T.O. and Brown, G.W. (1985). Interpreting data from aetiological studies: pitfalls and ambiguities. *The British Journal of Psychiatry*, **147**, 5–15.
51. Harris, T.O., Brown, G.W., and Bifulco, A. (1987). Loss of parent in childhood and adult psychiatric disorder: the role of social class position and premarital pregnancy. *Psychological Medicine*, **17**, 163–83.
52. Bifulco, A., Brown, G.W., and Harris, T.O. (1987). Childhood loss of parent, lack of adequate parental care and adult depression: a replication. *Journal of Affective Disorders*, **12**, 115–28.
53. Harris, T.O. (1988). Psycho-social vulnerability to depression: the biographical perspective of the Bedford college studies. In *Handbook of social psychiatry* (eds. A.S. Henderson and G.D. Burrows), pp. 55–71. Elsevier, Amsterdam.

54. Quinton, D. and Rutter, M. (1984). Parents with children in care. 1. Current circumstances and parenting skills. *Journal of Child Psychology and Psychiatry*, **25**, 211–29.
55. Quinton, D. and Rutter, M. (1984). Parents with children in care. 2. Intergenerational continuities. *Journal of Child Psychology and Psychiatry*, **25**, 231–50.
56. Pawlby, S.J., Mills, A., and Quinton, D. (1997). Vulnerable adolescent girls: opposite-sex relationships. *Journal of Child Psychology*, **38**, 909–20.
57. Quinton, D., Pickle, A., Maughan, B., *et al.* (1993). Partners, peers and pathways: assertive pairing and continuities in conduct disorder. *Development and Psychopathology*, **5**, 763–83.
58. Bifulco, A., Brown, G.W., and Harris, T.O. (1994). Childhood Experience of Care and Abuse (CECA): a retrospective interview measure. *Child Psychology and Psychiatry*, **35**, 1419–35.
59. Brown, G.W., Craig, T.K.J., Harris, T.O., *et al.* (2007). Development of a retrospective interview measure of parental maltreatment using the Childhood Experience of Care and Abuse (CECA) instrument—a life-course study of adult chronic depression—1. *Journal of Affective Disorders*, **103**, 205–15.
60. Brown, G.W. and Harris, T.O. (1993). Aetiology of anxiety and depressive disorders in an inner-city population. 1. Early adversity. *Psychological Medicine*, **23**, 143–54.
61. Brown, G.W. (2006). Childhood maltreatment and adult psychopathology: some measurement options. In *Relational processes and DSM-V: Neuroscience, Assessment, Prevention and Intervention* (eds. S.R.H Beach, M. Wamboldt, N. Kaslow, *et al.*), pp. 107–22. American Psychiatric Association, Washington, DC.
62. Brown, G.W., Craig, T.K.J., Harris, T.O., *et al.* (2007). Validity of retrospective measures of early maltreatment and depressive episodes using CECA (Childhood Experience of Care and Abuse)—a life-course study of adult chronic depression—2. *Journal of Affective Disorders*, **103**, 217–24.
63. Gaminde, I., Uria, M., Padro, D., *et al.* (1993). Depression in three populations in the Basque country—a comparison with Britain. *Social Psychiatry and Psychiatric Epidemiology*, **28**, 243–51.
64. Abas, M.A. and Broadhead, J.C. (1997). Depression and anxiety among women in an urban setting in Zimbabwe. *Psychological Medicine*, **27**, 59–71.
65. Brown, G.W. (1998). Genetic and population perspectives in life events and depression. *Social Psychiatry and Psychiatric Epidemiology*, **33**, 363–72.
66. Weizmann, F. (1971). Correlational statistics and the nature-nurture problem. *Science*, **171**, 589.
67. Brown, W. and Moran, P. (1997). Single mothers, poverty and depression. *Psychological Medicine*, **27**, 21–33.
68. Craig, T.K.J., Drake, H., Mills, K., *et al.* (1994). The South London somatisation study. II. Influence of stressful life events, and secondary gain. *The British Journal of Psychiatry*, **165**, 248–58.
69. Harris, T.O. (1989). Disorders of menstruation. *Life events and illness* (eds. G.W. Brown and T.O. Harris), pp. 261–94. Guilford Press, New York.
70. Owens, M.J. and McGuffin, P. (1997). Genetics and psychiatry. *The British Journal of Psychiatry*, **171**, 201–2.
71. Caspi, A., Sugden, K., Moffitt, T.E., *et al.* (2003). Influence of life stress on depression: moderation by a polymorphism in the 5-HTT gene. *Science*, **301**, 386–9.
72. Kendler, K.S., Kuhn, J.W., Vittum, J., *et al.* (2005). The interaction of stressful life events and a serotonin transporter polymorphism in the prediction of episodes of major depression: a replication. *Archives of General Psychiatry*, **62**, 529–35.
73. Sibille, E. and Lewis, D.A. (2006). SERT-ainly involved in depression, but when. *The American Journal of Psychiatry*, **163**, 8–11.
74. O'Hara, R., Schroder, C.M., Mahadevan, R., *et al.* (2007). Serotonin transporter polymorphism, memory and hippocampal volume in the elderly: association and interaction with cortisol. *Molecular Psychiatry*, **12**, 544–55.
75. Surtees, P.G., Wainwright, N.W.J., Willis-Owen, S.A.G., *et al.* (2006). Social adversity, the serotonin transporter (5-HTTLPR) polymorphism and major depressive disorder. *Biological Psychiatry*, **59**, 224–9.
76. Kaufman, J. (2007). Failure to replicate gene-environment interactions in psychopathology: a reply. *Biological Psychiatry*, **62**, 545.
77. Nestler, E.J., Alreja, M., and Aghajanian, G.K. (1999). Molecular control of locus coeruleus neurotransmission. *Biological Psychiatry*, **46**, 1131–9.
78. Williams, R.B., Marchuk, D.A., Gadde, K.M., *et al.* (2003). Sertonin-related gene polymorphisms and central nervous system serotonin function. *Neuropsychopharmacology*, **28**, 533–41.
79. Gilbert, P. (2006). Evolution and depression: issues and implications. *Psychological Medicine*, **36**, 287–97.
80. Brown, G.W. (2002). Social roles, context and evolution in the origins of depression. *Journal of Health and Social Behavior*, **43**, 255–76.

2.6.2 Social and cultural anthropology: salience for psychiatry

Arthur Kleinman

Social and cultural anthropology

One of the social sciences (together with history, economics, political science, sociology, and social psychology), social and cultural anthropology is principally concerned with the study of society, in almost all of its aspects. Together with linguistics, archaeology, and biological anthropology, social and cultural anthropology formed the classic (and now considered overly ambitious) four-field base of anthropology, the science of man. Yet still, in many universities, anthropology departments bridge the traditional divisions of the humanities, social sciences, and natural sciences. From the outset, anthropologists defined their subject in holistic terms meant to contextualize women and men in a nested hierarchy of influential environments that ran from the human body to the social body, and that assumed that these levels were related to each other, so that individual and collective processes (biological, psychological, social relational, and cultural) intersected in some way. Social and cultural anthropology, in particular, took as its subject matter studies of communities, ranging from small-scale preliterate groups to neighbourhoods or institutions in megacities. Comparison of different societies, or different structures and processes in those societies, is still seen as a defining approach, as is the analysis of cultural symbol systems (from languages to aesthetics), history of kinship, and other systems of social relationship, as well as research on large-scale social changes such as our era's globalization, ethnonationalism, and resurgence of religious fundamentalism.

Anthropology's chief research methodology is ethnography, the close study of a local world—a village, an urban neighbourhood, an institution, a network. Ethnography privileges local language, conceptual categories, values, and practices. Its procedure is to begin with local definitions and perceptions of reality (sometimes called 'emics', from phonemics), and only when these experience—near patterns are understood in a particular context of everyday life (with the larger political, economic, and cultural forces that influence it) are comparisons made with other local worlds in the framework of experience-distant scientific definitions of reality (referred to as 'etics', from phonetics). Knowledge is generated by participant observation, informal interviews, and the use of more formal procedures from structured interviews to questionnaires. Cross-cultural comparison is another core mode of knowledge production. Both ethnography and cross-cultural comparisons draw on empirical data to engage larger questions in social theory, which itself is constantly being reorganized in this dialectical engagement.

In this century, social and cultural anthropology's division of labour has spun off at least two subfields that are of particular relevance for psychiatry: psychological anthropology and medical anthropology.

Psychological anthropology

This subfield grew out of the culture and personality school (ca. 1930–1950), when psychoanalysts and anthropologists sought to collaborate to understand how mental processes differed or were similar across greatly different societies. Margaret Mead, Ruth Benedict, and Irving Hallowell are those anthropologists most often associated with this school. Although, most anthropologists became critical of the basis of the field in psychoanalysis and a correlation of individuals with entire cultures, a small group of social and cultural anthropologists continue, none the less, to pursue this direction, and over time they have developed broader ties with psychology, as can be readily seen by their leading research interests in cognition, lifecycle development, and ethnopsychological categories. Anthropologists working in this tradition have studied self-concepts and self-images, emotion terms, interpersonal processes and their relation to personhood, as well as experiences of childhood, child rearing, adolescence, midlife, and ageing. Psychological anthropology has been influential in recent years in psychology, where a sister subdiscipline called cultural psychology has started up in close connection to it.

Medical anthropology

Physicians were among the founders of anthropology, and some, like the British polymath W.H.R. Rivers, combined medicine and anthropology. Another source of medical anthropology was social medicine and public health; indeed the great German pathologist and social medicine advocate, Rudolph Virchow, was one of the first to use the term 'medical anthropology'. Thus, medical anthropology's early roots were applied. After the Second World War, the field took off as anthropologists developed an interest in the theoretical and empirical aspects of non-Western medical traditions, religious healing and its relation to medicine, and increasingly in experiences of suffering. In more recent years, medical anthropologists, of whom there are several thousand worldwide, have developed special interests in infectious diseases (especially diarrhoeal disease, malaria, tuberculosis, and AIDS), female reproductive lifecycle problems, the health problems of children and the aged, substance abuse, cancer, diabetes, disabilities, medical ethics, and the economic and social transformation of health care. One of the earliest and abiding interests has been in psychiatric diagnosis, disorders, and treatments. This subfield of social and cultural anthropology has many ongoing relationships to cultural psychiatry (see Chapter 2.6.1) and has been active in recent years in the effort to introduce mental health concerns into international health (see Chapter 1.3.2 and 7.3). Indeed, the cultural sections of the DSM-IV were contributed by a taskforce that included both medical anthropologists and cultural psychiatrists, in equal numbers.

Major contributions of anthropology to psychiatry

Cultural critique of biomedicine

One of the crucial contributions of anthropology is theoretical, namely a critique of the theoretical biases inherent in psychiatric science and clinical practice. This may seem self-evident because unlike any other branch of medicine, there is no blood test, biopsy, or radiograph to diagnose psychiatric disorder (leaving aside Alzheimer's disease, which is after all a neurological disorder). That means that psychiatric diagnosis is based on the establishment of symptom and syndromal criteria, which are based in turn in language, lay categories, and everyday social experience. Cultural bias can enter this process in several ways. Anthropologists have shown that this can happen when diagnostic criteria that have been developed in one society are applied to another where they lack validity. This is called a 'category fallacy', a term introduced by Kleinman.(1) Classic examples include trance and possession states in many non-Western societies, which are frequently normative and normal experiences. Failure to recognize this phenomenon, and therefore the diagnosis of persons in religious trance as psychotic, creates a category fallacy in the application of the diagnostic criteria of psychosis to normal people. The cultural critique has been applied to personality disorders as well, because this category of disorder models self-processes on a Euro-American, middle-class, and usually male behavioural type and lifestyle. Anthropologists argue for a much more flexible and interactive understanding of subjectivity that changes in basic ways in response to different social circumstances.

In the 1990s, cultural critique has been important in highlighting the influence of institutional racism in psychiatric diagnosis, referral, and treatment. Leading examples are the overdiagnosis of African-Americans and African-Caribbean Britons with schizophrenia, the tendency to perceive them as more dangerous and less amenable to psychotherapy, and differences in the way their discharge and aftercare are organized. Anthropologists have examined how racism is unwittingly built into psychiatric categories and infiltrates the model cases used to illustrate diagnostic criteria, and also the way that psychiatrists are trained to replicate such patterns in the practice of triage.

Cultural critique, informed by the cross-cultural and international data, is the basis for anthropologists' doubts about the validity of many of the psychiatric conditions detailed in DSM-IV and ICD-10. The ethnographic database strongly suggests that, apart from brain tumours and infections, Alzheimer's disease, metabolic encephalopathy, substance abuse, and other well-documented brain-based disorders such as certain sleep disorders, only six psychiatric syndromes of adults can be found cross-culturally; i.e. only these have stability as syndromes outside the cultural mainstream of Euro-American societies. The conditions are schizophrenia, brief reactive psychoses, major depression, bipolar disease, a range of anxiety disorders from panic states through phobias to obsessive–compulsive disorder, and trauma, whether understood as PTSD or in other categories. Most of the other hundreds of conditions described in DSM-IV, for example, are culture bound to Euro-America.

Related to these contributions of cultural critique, anthropologists have also contributed to the development of culturally informed diagnostic criteria, questionnaires, structured interviews, and guidelines for working with translators. Globalizing and indigenizing psychiatric approaches is an even more general emphasis in anthropology. Anthropology contains numerous concepts and methods that might be tried out, but relatively few have been experimented with or adopted. Besides those described below, several examples of the concepts, methods, and findings from anthropology that await trial in psychiatry are listed in Table 2.6.2.1.

Local moral worlds: interpersonal basis of illness experience

Ethnographies—hundreds of them, including many on psychiatric topics—demonstrate, with great consistency, that most people and most patients are not isolated individuals but rather live their lives as active members of local worlds. By local worlds, ethnographers mean villages, neighbourhoods, networks, and families, as well as particular social institutions, including hospitals and outpatient systems. These local worlds are differentiated by class, ethnicity, gender, age cohort, political faction, religious ties, and still other social differences. In any given local world crucial things are at stake that orient the attention and actions of participants. What is at stake may be shared (status, resources, survival, transcendence), but it also can be as distinctive as the different meanings of ultimacy that make religions distinguishable from each other.

Illness experience and experiences of treatment are as much caught up these stakes as experiences of normality. Thus, for anthropology how a person's illness is encountered, coped with, understood, and lived is crucial for understanding the illness and the treatment. Therefore, anthropologists write about the social course of illness: meaning that local worlds shape the course of illness so thoroughly that the same disease process (diabetes, AIDS, depression, schizophrenia) can take different trajectories. When sick people go for treatment, who they first seek out, whether they comply with the therapeutic regime, how they assess their experience of treatment—all are in one way or another influenced by what is most at stake for communities, families, networks, and individuals. The anthropological contribution here is to highlight the processes through which individuals relate to collectives. Thus, Estroff[2] shows that collective and individual definitions of identity affect how schizophrenic patients live their schizophrenia as an illness identity, which in turn affects their careers as patients and their experiences in other domains (family, workplace, etc.).

Table 2.6.2.1 Anthropological concepts, methods, and findings that await trial in psychiatry

Ethnography
Ethnography as a research strategy in clinical and epidemiological research. For example, as a means of studying the clustering of psychiatric conditions with social problems. Ethnography also has uses in evaluation research, in generating categories and questions in epidemiological studies, and in sociosomatic research. It is also a means of training researchers.
Ethnographic database
Ethnographic database as a routine source of knowledge about communities (foreign and domestic) for clinicians, mental health planners, and researchers.
Cross-cultural comparisons
Cross-cultural comparisons as a routine form of knowledge production. For example, cross-cultural comparisons of psychotherapy might help (a) to clarify what is common among religious, moral, and medical healing, (b) to determine how culture influences psychotherapeutic practice, and (c) to develop psychotherapeutic techniques for use with patients and families from different minority, ethnic, and international populations.
Social theory
Systematic reading of social theory as a source of hypotheses for research in social psychiatry and as a means of preparing clinicians to practise community psychiatry. Concepts such as social and symbolic capital, globalization, marginalization. ethnic identity, and institutional racism, among many others, can be used to frame psychiatric research and clinical intervention.

Practical clinical relevance

Immigration processes have so altered national demographic patterns that most nation states today have plural populations representing distinctive ethnic backgrounds. In 1900, the population of the United States, for example, included only 13 per cent categorized as ethnic minority members. By 1990 that figure was greater than 25 per cent. The percentage is projected to be one-third in 2010, and by mid-century to reach an astonishing 50 per cent. In California, the largest American state, non-Hispanic white Americans are already in a minority.

Ethnic background has been shown empirically to influence epidemiological rates of disease, patterns of access to health care, help-seeking, and patient–doctor interactions, often with negative outcomes such as delayed treatment, misdiagnosis, non-compliance, and treatment failure. Taking ethnicity into account in the provision of services means a variety of things, such as making translators available, putting up signs in several languages, holding clinics at times when working-class patients can attend, and paying attention to differences in cultural meanings and practices. The now popular idea of providing culturally informed and sensitive care is premised on anthropological concepts and methods. Several of these have been elaborated in the literature.

1. The distinctions between illness and disease: for medical anthropologists illness is the patient's experience of symptoms in the context of family, work, and community; disease is the practitioner's model of the pathological process. Help-seeking is usually orientated around the illness experience with respect to what is most at stake for the patient and significant others. Care can founder when the patient's primary concerns with the illness experience conflicts with or is entirely different from the physician's focus on disease. Thus, many patients with chronic pain experience interrogation of the disease process by the sceptical physician as delegitimizing their illness experience. This leads to high rates of dissatisfaction with care among this group of patients. When patients and families are from ethnic minority backgrounds, differences in cultural meanings and practices intensify conflicts between patient and physician models.

2 Medical anthropology sponsors a method to reduce this explanatory gap and thereby to improve clinical relationships. Called the explanatory models' methodology, it involves three steps.[3]

(a) Elicitation of patient and family explanatory models of the illness experience and treatment, which can be accomplished by asking the following questions:

- What do you call your problem?
- What do you think caused it?
- Why did it start when it did?
- What course will it take from here on?
- How does it work in your body?
- What do you most fear about the illness?
- What kind of treatment do you desire for this illness?
- What do you most fear about the treatment?

(b) Presentation of the clinician's explanatory model of the disease process.

(c) Negotiation of a mutually acceptable understanding of the clinical problem across patient, family, and physician models.

Closely related to this technique is the development of a mini-ethnography. This is a brief description, based on interviewing the key parties about the impact of family and work context on the illness experience and vice versa. The mini-ethnography and the explanatory models' elicitation generally give rise to patient stories of the illness experience. The influence of cultural categories, values and practices on the illness and treatment can be assessed from this standpoint.[4]

Revised cultural formulation

Appendix I to DSM-IV contains an outline of how psychiatric cases can be culturally formulated. This has recently been updated[6] and includes:

- the ethnic identity of the individual
- what is at stake as patients and their loved ones face an episode of illness
- the illness narrative
- psychosocial stresses and social supports
- cultural elements of the relationship between the individual and the clinician
- an examination of the efficacy of a cultural competency approach in the particular case

This is a feasible approach to routine patient care with members of ethnic minorities and recent immigrants and refugees that has a high likelihood of making that care culturally informed and culturally sensitive. Key to it, as it is to anthropology's core methodology, ethnography, is the display of genuine respect for patients, families, and their meanings and practices. That respect for the person and his or her illness experience is the indispensable condition of anthropologically informed care. It includes, as its first step, the ethical act of acknowledging the suffering of the other in his or her own terms as the basis for diagnosis and treatment. In this sense, it reverses the cultural preoccupation of the biomedical practitioner with the disease process, and establishes the interpersonal relationship as the grounds of knowledge as well as caregiving.

Conclusions

Anthropology's chief contribution to psychiatry is to emphasize the importance of the social world in diagnosis, prognosis, and treatment, and to provide concepts and methods that psychiatrists can apply (the appropriate cross-disciplinary translation first being made, however). But that is not the only contribution that anthropology offers. Ethnographers are aware that knowledge is positioned, facts and values are inseparable, and experience is simply too complex and robust to be easily boxed into tight analytical categories. Hence a sense of the fallibility of understanding, the limitation of practice, and irony and paradox in human conditions is the consequence of ethnography as a method of knowledge production.

Anthropology also complements the idea of psychosomatic relationships with evidence and theorizing about sociosomatic relationships. Here moral processes—namely what is at stake in local worlds—are shown to be closely linked with emotional processes, which are frequently about experiences of loss, fear, vexation, and betrayal of what is collectively and individually at stake in interpersonal relationships. Change in the former can change the latter, and this can at times work in reverse as well. Examples include the way symptoms intensify or even arise in response to fear and vexation concerning threats perceived as serious dangers to what is most at stake.

The relationship of poverty to morbidity and mortality is a different example of sociosomatic processes. Poverty correlates with increased morbidity and mortality. Psychiatrists have often had trouble getting the point that public health and infectious disease experts have long understood. But it is not just diarrhoeal disease, tuberculosis, AIDS, heart disease, and cancer that demonstrate this powerful social epidemiological correlation—so do psychiatric conditions. Depression, substance abuse, violence, and their traumatic consequences not only occur at higher rates in the poorest local worlds, but also cluster together (much as do infectious diseases), and those vicious clusters define a local place, usually a disintegrating inner-city community. Hence the findings of the National Co-Morbidity Study in the United States of America that most psychiatric conditions occur as comorbidity is a step toward this ethnographic knowledge—that in the most vulnerable, dangerous, and broken local worlds, psychiatric diseases are not encountered as separate problems but as part of these sociosomatic clusters.

Finally, anthropology is also salient for policy and programme development in psychiatry. Against an overly narrow neurobiological framing of psychiatric conditions as brain disorders, anthropology in psychiatry draws on cross-national, cross-ethnic, and disintegrating community data to emphasize the relationship of increasing rates of mental health problems, especially among underserved, impoverished populations worldwide, and increasing problems in the organization and delivery of mental health services to fundamental transformations in political economy, institutions, and culture that are remaking our epoch. In so doing, anthropology projects a vision of psychiatry as a discipline central to social welfare and health policy. It argues as well against the profession's ethnocentrism and for the field as a larger component of international health. Anthropology (together with economics, sociology, and political science) also provides the tools for psychiatry to develop policies and programmes that address the close ties between social conditions and mental health conditions, and social policies and mental health policies.[5] In this sense, anthropology urges psychiatry in a global direction, one in which psychiatric knowledge and practice, once altered to fit in more culturally salient ways in local worlds around the globe, have a more important place at the policy table.[6,7]

Further information

Jenkins, J. and Barrett, R. (eds.) (2004). *Schizophrenia, culture, and subjectivity: the edge of experience.* Cambridge University Press, Cambridge.

Kleinman, A. and Good, B. (eds.) (1985). *Culture and depression.* University of California Press, Berkeley, CA.

Kleinman, A. (ed.) (2006). *What really matters: living a moral life amidst uncertainty and danger.* Oxford Press, Oxford.

Luhrmann, T. (2000). *Of two minds: the growing disorder in American psychiatry.* Knopf, New York.

References

1. Kleinman, A. (1977). Depression, somatization and the new cross-cultural psychiatry. *Social Science and Medicine*, **11**, 3–10.
2. Estroff, S.E. (1993). Disability and schizophrenia. In *Knowledge, power and practice: the anthropology of medicine and everyday life* (eds. S. Lindenbaum and M. Lock), pp. 247–86. University of California Press, Berkeley, CA.
3. Kleinman, A. (1988). *The illness narratives.* Basic Books, New York.
4. Kleinman, A. (1988). *Rethinking psychiatry: from cultural category to personal experience.* Free Press, New York.
5. Lee, S. and Kleinman, A. (1997). Mental illness and social change in China. *Harvard Review of Psychiatry*, **5**, 43–5.
6. Kleinman, A. and Benson, P. (2006). Anthropology in the clinic: The problem of cultural competency and how to fix it. *PLoS Medicine*, **3**, e294. www.plosmedicine.org.
7. Desjarlais, R., Eisenberg, L., Good, B., *et al.* (ed.) (1995). *World mental health: problems and priorities in low-income countries.* Oxford University Press, New York.

2.7

The contribution of epidemiology to psychiatric aetiology

Scott Henderson

Introduction

Epidemiology deals with the overall patterns of disease. On one hand, people are unique with their own genetic endowment and life experiences. This idiographic paradigm is balanced by the nomothetic in which recurrent and predictable patterns are sought in the whole of humankind. It is the business of psychiatric epidemiology to determine the distribution of mental disorders in populations, the factors determining that distribution, and measures that may help in their prevention.

From their undergraduate years onward, clinicians see patients who have a disorder and who at the same time give a history of certain experiences from birth to their present. It may be tempting for both patient and doctor to accept that the patient's recent experiences have some role in the onset of symptoms. But if the principles of epidemiology are brought into play, some questions need to be asked first. Being unwell may itself bias the recall of recent or distant experiences. What proportion of the general population have had the same experiences but not developed the disorder? What proportions have the same disorder but have not had these experiences? What proportions have the same disorder but have not reached health services? A simple two-by-two table is the simplest way to think this through (Table 2.7.1).

The columns are made up of persons in a population who have or do not have a particular disorder. The rows are the numbers who have or have not had a certain exposure. That exposure is being considered as a putative risk factor. It may be biological or psychosocial and may have taken place at any time from conception to the present.

Table 2.7.1 Cases and exposure: a two-by-two table

		Case	
		Yes	**No**
Exposed	Yes	*a*	*b*
	No	*c*	*d*

Letters refer to numbers of persons.

To establish a causal link between some factor and a disorder is a demanding but most engaging exercise. It is well worth reading the classic expositions by Hill[1] and Susser[2] on how a cause can reasonably be inferred from the data.

The uses of epidemiology

In his celebrated monograph bearing this title, Morris[3] described seven uses of epidemiology. It continues to give us a framework for assessing the state of psychiatric epidemiology in relation to the biological and psychosocial conditions of the contemporary world. Morris's list can be reinterpreted for our use as follows.

Completing the clinical picture

This means knowing about all the ways in which a disorder may present and what its usual course is. But it also means relating subclinical cases to fully developed ones. An excellent example here would be the anxiety, depressive, or somatization states seen in general practice or field surveys compared to the more severe syndromes specified in the international criteria and encountered by psychiatrists.

Community diagnosis

Here one obtains estimates of morbidity as it occurs at the general population level, not just in persons who have reached primary care or mental health services. Only by having such estimates of prevalence or incidence for whole populations can the size of the nation's disease burden be determined. This is because community-based measures of morbidity include not only persons with treated conditions but also those who are symptomatic yet have not reached services.

Secular changes in incidence

This refers to the rise and fall of diseases in populations. For example, there is some evidence that schizophrenia has been dropping in incidence and becoming more benign in its clinical course; and it is likely that in many Western countries, depressive disorder has become more frequent in persons born since the Second World

War.[4] The suicide rate of young persons has indisputably increased in many industrialized countries. It is likely that eating disorders have increased in frequency and it is certain that the use of illegal drugs and AIDS are new arrivals and will be a continuing burden.

The search for causes

Here, epidemiology is looking for aetiological clues. It is the substance of this chapter.

Applying population data to individual risk

In this, the focus moves from the population back to the individual. For example, if the annual incidence rate for schizophrenia is known in a population and if this information is age-specific, it is possible to estimate the probability that a person in a given age group will develop the disorder within the next year. This is the base rate, before one starts to consider risk factors such as family history. Next, by aggregating data on the course of schizophrenia, it is possible to estimate the chances of recovery for persons who are currently having their first episode. The common principle is that data based on large numbers of persons are used to make probability estimates for individuals.

Delineation of syndromes

This is done by examining the distribution of clinical phenomena as they occur in the population. It fits well with recent experience of repetitive strain injury, chronic fatigue syndrome, and post-traumatic stress disorder or its congeners.

Health services research

This begins with a determination of needs and of resources, then an analysis of services currently in action, and ends with attempts to evaluate them, including the costs. Research activity in this area has expanded greatly in recent years, driven by the forces of economic rationalism.

Prevention

To Morris's seven uses of epidemiology should be added prevention, which Gruenberg[5] said was its 'ultimate service'. All other uses are subsidiary to this. Examples are the current activity in the prevention of suicide in young persons and of alcohol or drug abuse. In these, the traditional medical approach of targeting high-risk groups should be contrasted with the epidemiological and population-based approach described by Rose.[6] One under-recognized fact is that knowledge about factors that determine the duration of a disorder can lead to prevention. This is because prevalence is the incidence rate times the duration. So shortening the duration will lower the prevalence. For example, if people with depressive disorder were treated earlier in primary care, the prevalence should fall. The prevention of a mental disorder is greatly helped by knowledge about aetiology, but it is not essential. For example, Snow did not know about the cholera vibrio when he had the water supply changed. Prevention is discussed further by Bertolotte in Chapter 7.4, prevention in child psychiatry by Lenroot in Chapter 9.1.4, and in intellectual disability by Kaski in Chapter 10.3.

Research on aetiology: three levels

Epidemiological methods can be applied at any of the three levels: to disorders as these present in hospitals and specialist health services, in primary care, or in the general population. These are represented diagrammatically in Fig. 2.7.1 as a three-dimensional cone, derived from the seminal volume on pathways to care by Goldberg and Huxley.[7] The base of the cone consists of those in the general population who have clinically significant psychological symptoms (Stage 1). When these symptoms become unmanageable to self or to others, people seek help from their doctor or other health practitioners (Stage 2). But only some of them are recognized by the professional to have significant mental health problems (Stage 3). A small proportion may be referred to mental health services (Stage 4), of whom an even smaller fraction are admitted to inpatient care (Stage 5). Note that most teaching and the diagnostic criteria in international use are largely based on their authors' experience in Stages 4 and 5, where patients are more severely ill!

There are two very different ways to express morbidity. The most common, and easiest to obtain, is prevalence, either at the time of assessment (point prevalence), 1-month, 1-year, or lifetime prevalence. The other is incidence, the number of new or fresh onset cases in a given period. For aetiological research, incident cases are emphatically preferable.

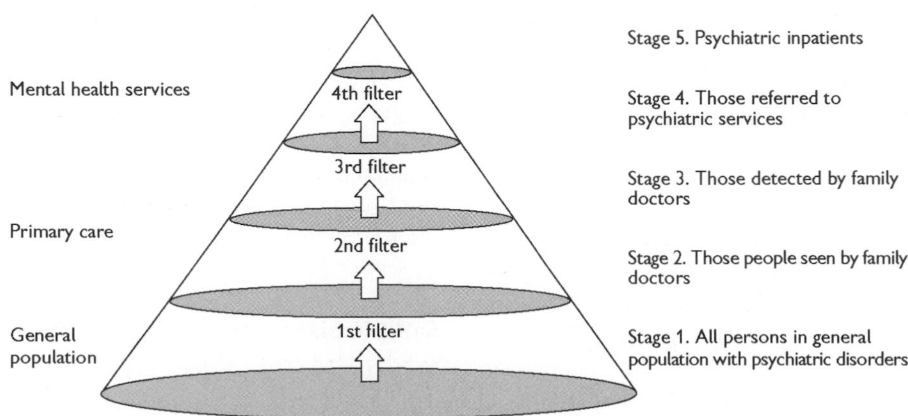

Fig. 2.7.1 Pathways to care. (Reproduced from D.P. Goldberg and P. Huxley, *Mental illness in the community,* Copyright © 1980, The Tavistock Institute.)

Three main designs

At any of these levels, research directed at aetiology uses one of three designs: cross-sectional, prospective longitudinal, or case-control. A cross-sectional study is often an excellent start, because it provides a picture of how much morbidity is present at one point in time and the variables most closely associated with this. But because it is only a 'snapshot', the cross-sectional study can rarely allow much to be said about causes. For example, in a community sample of several thousand adults, the data will show that persons with symptoms of anxiety or depression will tend to report having had more adversities. But it would be unwise to conclude that adversity contributes to the onset of symptoms. First, persons with anxiety or depression may be more inclined to report that they have had many troubles. This may be through selective recall of unpleasant events, because it is known that depressed people are more likely to remember bad times than good times.(8) Another mechanism is effort after meaning, whereby people try to account for feeling psychologically unwell. Next, symptomatic persons may be more likely to have unpleasant things happen to them as a consequence of their mental state. Lastly, persons with anxiety or depression may have certain personality traits or lifestyles that make them more likely to have troubled lives and also be vulnerable to common mental disorders.

Such problems in methodology can be resolved to some extent by using a *prospective longitudinal design* or cohort study. In this, a population sample is assessed at the start when most persons are psychologically well. In one type of cohort study, the sample may deliberately include a group who have had a particular exposure, such as a head injury or disaster, and an equivalent number who have not. At the start, data are obtained on personality, lifestyle, past health, and family history. The cohort is then re-examined at least once after an appropriate interval. Some will have developed symptoms. The research question is whether the putative risk factors that were assessed at the start were more frequently present in those who later developed symptoms. A design of this type yields considerably more information about the causal processes likely to be at work, either those leading to mental disorders or protecting against them. It also overcomes the problem of a putative risk factor really being a consequence rather than an antecedent of a disorder. But it is obviously very demanding in resources—human, administrative, and financial. It also takes a long time. For these reasons, epidemiologists often use the *case-control* method as a more practicable alternative.

Case-control designs have been underused in psychiatric research, but they can be a powerful strategy for identifying risk factors for a specified disorder.(9,10) The essence of the case-control design lies in obtaining data to complete the cells in Table 2.7.1. The aim is to find a sample of all persons in a population who have reached case level for a particular disorder and an equivalent number of persons who are similar in age, gender, and other variables, but who do not have the disorder, at least not yet. The cases should ideally be 'incident' or recent in onset. If instead, the study has to have recourse to all the cases of the disorder known to the service, that is, the prevalent cases, some will be long-standing and some more recent. This could lead to misleading results because a putative risk factor may show up as 'positive' not because it is a cause or true risk factor, but because it is associated with chronicity through prolonging the duration of the disorder. This problem can be avoided only by recruiting recent-onset or incident cases for case-control studies. The cases and controls are then asked about the various possible exposures. If the cases are unable to give information because they are cognitively impaired (as in dementia), at least one informant has to be found for each case, usually a partner or close family member.

In Table 2.7.1, the important question is whether there are more persons in cell a than would occur by chance. We do not know the incidence of the disorder in all persons in the population who were exposed to each risk factor, nor do we know the number not exposed. Likewise, we do not know how many people in the population have recently developed the disorder. As a consequence, we cannot compare the incidence in those exposed and not exposed for the whole population. All we have are the data from the cases examined, who are necessarily only a fraction of all incident cases in the population; and data from a fraction of all healthy persons. But we can proceed as follows. First, the relative risk is calculated from Table 2.7.1. The relative risk is $a/(a + b)$ divided by $c/(c + d)$

i.e. $\dfrac{a/(a+b)}{c/(c+d)}$

By simple algebra, this becomes

$$\frac{a(c+d)}{c(a+b)}$$

Then something very helpful can be done. Where a disorder is fairly uncommon in the general population, a will be very small compared with b, and c will be small compared with d. If we assume a negligible contribution by a in the term $a + b$, and by c in the term $c + d$, the relative risk will be nearly equal to

$$\frac{ad}{bc}$$

This is the odds ratio, which is an expression of the strength of a risk factor.

Whom to study: principles of sampling

The essential principle is that everyone in the true denominator (usually the total population within a defined geographical or administrative area) *must have an equal probability* of being included in the numerator. If this is not achieved, there is a likelihood of bias whereby the achieved sample may be systematically different in ways that could be important in the analysis. For example, the sample of cases should not differ from all the incident cases in that population in attributes such as level of education, age, or likelihood of having been exposed to a candidate exposure or risk factor. So in a study of the association between, say, sexual abuse in childhood and depressive disorder in adult life, the cases of depression should ideally be representative of all those with depressive disorder in that community and not just those reaching a particular service. See also Chapter 2.2 by Dunn.

Sample bias

In field surveys, it has long been accepted that not everyone who is in the 'target sample' will agree to be interviewed or will be available at the time the interviewer calls. It is common to find that only 70 to 90 per cent are actually assessed. Furthermore, those who refuse or are repeatedly not available are known to be more likely to have the mental disorder under investigation. For this reason, the prevalence that is found will often be an underestimate. A putative risk factor may itself increase the chances of a person's not being in a sample in the first place, of dropping out, or of dying during the study. Statistical methods are available for estimating how much error may have occurred due to refusals and how to correct for this in the conclusions drawn.

The other occasion when non-response is a problem is in longitudinal studies, where a sample is followed over several years. If a disorder with an increased mortality is the topic, such as dementia or schizophrenia, it is recognized that some cases will be lost at follow-up. This means that those who are successfully re-examined are a survival élite and are different in important ways from the original cohort. These distortions could lead to mistaken conclusions if the losses are not allowed for. Various techniques have been developed to handle these difficulties, including Bayesian methods which adjust final estimates on the basis of prior knowledge.[(11)]

Specifying the disorders

Diagnostic categories

The epidemiology of mental disorders could have made no real progress without methods for specifying the disorders to be investigated, then measuring these. Only in this way can research data be comparable between research teams, within and between countries. Having consistency in diagnosis has been made much easier through the development of the diagnostic criteria now in wide international use. The two systems are the International Classification of Diseases (10th Revision) (**ICD-10**) with its *Classification of Mental and Behavioural Disorders*; and the *Diagnostic and Statistical Manual*, fourth edition (**DSM-IV**) of the American Psychiatric Association. These classifications are described further in Chapter 1.9. Both are under revision.

Continuous measures of morbidity

Reliable and valid case ascertainment might be assumed to be the *sine qua non* for any progress in the epidemiology of mental disorders. But to use the traditional expression 'case ascertainment' nicely illustrates the very problem that has to be re-thought, because it implies a categorical structure in the morbidity that we wish to study. In a population, there are traditionally cases and non-cases. But this is not really how morbidity shows itself. As expressed by Pickering,[(12)] 'Medicine in its present state can count up to two, but not beyond'. He was referring to hypertension, but others have argued that mental disorders also have dimensional properties.[(6)] The frequency distribution of their component symptoms such as anxiety, depression, or cognitive impairment is usually a reversed J-shape, with most people having none or only a few symptoms and progressively fewer persons having higher counts. A committee of clinicians in Geneva or Washington, whose experience is largely derived from teaching hospitals, has decided by consensus where the cut-point should be placed for persons to be 'cases'. While this is entirely appropriate for some purposes, it may not always be a true representation of the underlying pathology. In statistical terms, it loses information.

It is not disputed that mental disorders exist in categorical states and that these have some utilitarian value: a depressive episode, Alzheimer's disease, anorexia nervosa, or alcohol dependency are clinically realistic entities. What is proposed here is that, in epidemiological studies at the general population level, hypotheses about the aetiology require large numbers of respondents, solely because the base rates for such conditions are not large. But it is possible to identify persons with *some* symptoms of depression, of cognitive impairment, of abnormal eating, or of alcohol misuse. The score on a scale of these symptoms can become the dependent variable in an analysis of candidate risk factors. So it is usually more powerful statistically to look for associations between a putative risk factor and morbidity expressed as a continuous variable, rather than as a dichotomy of cases and non-cases.

When a continuous measure of common psychological symptoms such as the General Health Questionnaire (**GHQ**)[(13)] (*vide infra*) is applied to a population, a unimodal distribution curve is found, with no break between so-called cases and normals. Rose[(6)] argued that there are three important consequences from this approach to studying morbidity. First, a characteristic of the community as a whole emerges. This is the mean and standard deviation of its GHQ scores. Second, this collective characteristic may show significant differences between men and women, geographical regions, social strata, and income groups. These differences are based on shifts of the entire distribution. The third consequence is that differences between these groups in the prevalence of probable cases (those with a score above a threshold) are related to different average scores in these groups. As Rose[(6)] concisely put it, 'The visible part of the iceberg (prevalence) is a function of its total mass (the population average)'.

He suggested that '*Psychiatrists, unlike sociologists, seem generally unaware of the existence and importance of mental health attributes of whole populations, their concern being only with sick individuals*' (emphasis added). It is an appealing notion that populations, while they are made up of individuals, take on properties of their own, much as molecules acquire attributes not found in their constituent atoms. The concept of populations having different frequency distributions of dimensional morbidity, not just different prevalence rates for clinical cases, carries with it the implication that some factors are shifting the overall distribution in some populations but not in others. An example is the societal forces that Durkheim[(14)] proposed were related to national suicide rates.

Disablement

There is yet a further advantage in considering morbidity as a continuum in a population. Morbidity refers to symptoms, syndromes, or disorders. But there is a universe of discourse closely linked to this, namely disablement. This is the collective noun now used to refer to the impairment, disability, and social role handicap in daily life that disorders bring with them. The main categories of mental disorder, especially the psychoses, affective disorders, and dementias, are almost always associated with substantial disablement. But subclinical levels of mental disorders also carry with them a certain amount of disablement. From the point of view of a whole population, the cumulative amount of disablement from subclinical or milder conditions is considerable because such conditions have a high point prevalence. Therefore, from a public health perspective, the significance of milder mental disorders is not trivial.

Measurement of disablement

The most comprehensive measure is the Disability Assessment Schedule (DAS)[15] that assesses an individual's functioning in daily life. Its short form is suitable for survey use. Self-completion instruments are the Brief Disability Questionnaire (BDQ)[16] and the SF-36[17] or its briefer version, the SF-12.

The measurement of psychiatric symptoms

Instruments for epidemiological research fall into two types: self-completed questionnaires and standardized interviews.

Questionnaires

The more simple type is a symptom scale which can be completed by respondents themselves or administered by an interviewer. The best-known instrument is the GHQ. The briefest version, the GHQ-12, is a highly efficient screening tool. A score of 2 or more indicates that the person is likely to have one of what Goldberg and Huxley[18] have usefully termed common mental disorders. Another screening instrument is the Hopkins Symptom Checklist.[19] For depressive states specifically, examples are the Center for Epidemiologic Studies Depression Scale (**CES-D**)[20] and the Beck Depression Inventory.[21]

The Alcohol Use Disorders Identification Test (**AUDIT**) was developed by the WHO for population screening. This 10-item test has been shown to have satisfactory psychometric and predictive properties. The total score is 40 and a score of 8 or more (7 for women) is recommended for identifying persons likely to have adverse consequences of drinking.[22]

For cognitive impairment, the Mini-Mental State Examination (**MMSE**)[23] gives a score for a person's current cognitive function, or by applying a cut-point to that score, it can be used to identify persons who are likely to have a dementia. Like any other cognitive test, it cannot itself make a diagnosis of dementia. It detects cognitive impairment, not cognitive decline, which requires a history. The MMSE is known to be sensitive to education, in that persons with limited intelligence or education may have low scores without their having had any cognitive decline.

All these instruments can be used in two ways: by applying a cut-point to identify persons who are likely to be clinically significant cases; or by using the score as a continuous variable. When a questionnaire or self-rated instrument is used in research, the investigators have to be confident about its psychometric properties. In addition to validity and reliability, there are two others: its sensitivity and specificity. These refer to its performance when compared with a criterion or 'gold standard', such as a comprehensive psychiatric examination or a consensus diagnosis amongst experts. In Table 2.7.2, a sample of persons has been examined with both the screening instrument and a full examination. We consider the number of persons who are 'cases' according to both assessments (a), according to one but not the other (b or c), and according to neither (d).

Sensitivity is the proportion who screen positive and who are indeed cases by the criterion; that is: $a/(a + c)$, while specificity is the number who screen negative and who are indeed not cases: $d/(b + d)$.

The sensitivity and specificity of a test are expressed as a percentage and vary according to where the cut-point is placed on the scores.

Table 2.7.2 Screening a population sample

		Criterion (cases by full psychiatric assessment)		
		Yes	**No**	
Cases by screening test	Yes	a	b	$a+b$
	No	c	d	$c+d$
		$a+c$	$b+d$	

Letters refer to numbers of persons.

As sensitivity increases, specificity tends to decrease, so that an appropriate balance between the two has to be determined. For some purposes, such as in screening for depression, it is more important to identify as many as possible of the true cases, but it does not matter if there are quite a few false-positives because these can be corrected by a more extensive second-stage examination. Under these conditions, one would want a highly sensitive screening test that placed most of the true cases in cell a and few in c. It matters rather less if quite a few of the true non-cases are incorrectly placed in b. See also Chapter 2.2 by Dunn.

Standardized psychiatric interviews

Even the best-designed questionnaires with the best psychometric properties cannot be a substitute for a psychiatric interview. Only it can obtain the information that leads to a diagnosis, reached according to the international criteria. What is termed information variance is reduced by having interviewers ask about symptoms in the same way. Next is the reduction of criterion variance, where the symptoms or signs elicited are, like building bricks, assembled in exactly the same way, both within and across studies. This is achieved by applying to the data an algorithm that is a precise expression of the diagnostic criteria in ICD or DSM. The algorithm can be computerized so that the responses to each item in the interview are assembled automatically and invariably.

There are two types of standardized psychiatric examination. The Schedule for Clinical Assessment in Neuropsychiatry (**SCAN**) is a clinician's instrument, requiring familiarity with the phenomenology of mental disorders. It assumes that interviewers are comfortable in examining persons with a mental disorder. The second type, exemplified by the Composite International Diagnostic Interview (**CIDI**) is fully scripted and has been automated for interviewing on laptop computers so that it can be administered by laypersons after only a few days' training. A very large body of survey data has now been collected using it. These instruments are fully described by Cooper and Oates in Chapter 1.8.1.

Validity issues

The quality of information these instruments obtain is clearly of central importance. We know that they do not obtain the same information as each other, nor do they identify the same persons as cases of a particular diagnostic category in the same sample. Their validity and the practical significance is therefore important for administrators using the data obtained in large surveys to guide planning. But it is also a matter of interest for aetiological research.

Typical prevalence estimates

The above instruments have been used in a large number of surveys of the prevalence of the main mental disorders in the general population. Examples are shown in Table 2.7.3. The rates vary markedly, but little is known about why this is so. The differences may be due to differences in methods of case ascertainment; or they may indicate actual variation between countries. What is important is that they all *attempt* to estimate the prevalence in the community of syndromes familiar to psychiatrists working in clinics and hospitals. Prevalence estimates provide evidence for the public health significance of mental illnesses and their associated disablement. Their administrative impact has been considerable. So far, however, they have brought little to advance knowledge about aetiology.

(a) Possible causes of mental disorders: the domains

Having specified the psychiatric disorder to be studied and having developed methods to measure it, the next task is to identify whatever factors might contribute to its onset or to its course. These lie in the traditional three domains: the biological, social, and psychological. But in epidemiology, any variable is rarely specific to one domain. Some biological, some social, and some psychological factors are often conflated. For example, gender expresses biological differences but also different social experiences in the past, different social contexts in the present, and different psychological or intrapersonal differences in personality traits and behaviour. Likewise, age groups can reflect social role, educational opportunities in the past, marital status, financial concerns, and physical health. It is therefore important not to be misled into thinking that a variable is tapping only what one is primarily interested in. Confounding is ever present.

(b) Sociodemographic variables

The level of psychiatric morbidity in a population may differ significantly between age groups, gender, marital status, ethnic

Table 2.7.3 Some 12-month prevalence rates per 100 of population, all by DSM-IV criteria

	Any disorder* (%)	Anxiety disorder	Mood disorder	Alcohol or substance use disorder
Australia	20.3	5.6	6.6	7.9
Canada	10.9	5.2	5.8	–
China (Beijing)	9.1	3.2	2.5	2.6
Colombia	17.8	10.0	6.8	2.8
European countries (six)	9.6	6.4	4.2	1.0 (alcohol only)
Iran†	17.1	8.4	4.3	nil
Lebanon	16.9	11.2	6.6	1.3
New Zealand	20.7	14.8	8.0	3.5
Nigeria	4.7	3.3	0.8	0.8
Ukraine	20.5	7.1	9.1	6.4
USA	26.4	18.2	9.6	3.8

*Includes disorders other than those listed.
†Only lifetime estimates were published.

background, and socio-economic or educational level. Depressive disorders are consistently more prevalent in women[24] and dementia has a higher prevalence, not only with increasing age, but also in those with lower education.[25] Furthermore, there may be important interaction effects between variables in their relation to morbidity. For example, the average age of onset in schizophrenia is different in men and in women. This has proved to be a clue to causal processes.

(c) The social environment

This can be considered in two parts: first is the individual's immediate social environment—what the sociologist Cooley[26] called the primary group—consisting of those around a person with whom there is both interaction and commitment. There is then the wider community with its standard of living, lifestyle, and cultural values. Plausibly, both may have some influence on the incidence of mental disorders and on their course. The hypothesis that social support protects against depression and other common mental disorders has proved hard to investigate.[27, 28] This is because social support is probably influenced by some intrapersonal factors rather than being a product solely of the individual's environment. Here is a good example of confounding: a major variable concerning the social environment of individuals turns out to be determined not solely by environmental factors, but partly by their own personality attributes. The evidence suggests that social support, stripped of these confounding factors, is not a powerful factor in aetiology.[29] A separate issue is whether social support influences the outcome of psychiatric disorders once these have developed.

Societal (macrosocial) variables have long been suspected of playing an important role in aetiology. It was such a hypothesis that was investigated in the celebrated Stirling County Study in Canada by Dorothea and Alexander Leighton *et al.*[30] with their concept of sociocultural disintegration. The current increase in depression and suicide in the young is popularly attributed to such macrosocial variables. On the other hand, work opportunities, diet and use of drugs and alcohol have also changed appreciably over the last 50 years. There is no certain explanation so far.

Experiential variables

'Experiential' is a useful term to refer inclusively to all that individuals have been exposed to, from conception to death. In epidemiological research, it includes intrauterine exposures—such as maternal influenza or malnutrition—and perinatal events. In infancy and childhood, social and interpersonal experiences have been the main focus of research. Maternal deprivation was intensively studied in both clinical and community samples for two decades. The expectation from Bowlby's attachment theory was that loss or separation from the mother would be pathogenic for depression and possibly personality disorders.[31] This hypothesis has proved very hard to test because of confounding by other factors. Rutter[32] concluded that '... the residual effects of early experiences on adult behaviour tend to be quite slight because of both the maturational changes that take place during middle and later childhood and also the effects of beneficial and adverse experiences during all the years after infancy ... '

Migration and schizophrenia

Migration is an excellent example of how epidemiological data lead to aetiological clues, straddling both the biological and social. People who have moved from one country to another have offered opportunities for aetiological research on schizophrenia for a long time, starting with the celebrated study in 1932 by Ödegaard. He found that Norwegian migrants to Minnesota had more mental disorders than those at home. Since then, migration has become increasingly common and some striking findings have been made. An integrative review[33] has found a relative risk of 2.7 for first-generation migrants and 4.5 for the second-generation. While a family history is the largest risk factor for schizophrenia, migration is the next compared with most others. It is not due to an artefact in diagnosis. The effect is unlikely to be due to any single factor. Both biological and social factors are probably implicated. In the latter, perception of social inequality is thought to be a plausible mechanism.

Parental style

Promising findings have been obtained on the association between parenting style and depressive disorders in adulthood. Parker[34] developed the Parental Bonding Instrument (**PBI**) to measure two fundamental dimensions of the manner in which parents behave towards their children: care and affection as one dimension and protectiveness as the other. The PBI is too lengthy for epidemiological research on community samples where the interview is often already extensive. Parker and his colleagues have subsequently developed a briefer instrument, the Measure of Parenting Style (**MOPS**), which includes the experience of physical and sexual abuse.[35] MOPS is likely to prove useful in case-control and prospective studies of psychiatric disorders for systematically obtaining information on exposures of theoretical relevance.

(a) Childhood abuse

It seems intuitively likely that children who have been physically or sexually abused have an increased risk of having anxiety, depression, or other psychiatric disorders in adulthood. The findings from epidemiological studies on unreferred samples (people in the community) point to the many other adverse experiences that accompany childhood sexual abuse, including physical violence, unstable and untrustworthy relationships with parents, and emotional deprivation. This topic is further considered in Chapter 9.3.3.

(b) Recent exposure to adversity

Adverse experiences have been very extensively studied for their contribution to the onset and course of psychiatric disorders. In epidemiological research, much attention has been accorded to issues that arise in the measurement of adversity. Some of these issues are equally relevant in clinical practice. They include the following:

- The duration of the stressor: acute or long-standing.
- Its magnitude and how to determine this independently of the person's reaction to it.
- The independence of the event from the individual: some events are entirely independent while others may have come about because of the individual's own behaviour or psychiatric state.
- The personal context of the experience may augment or reduce its psychological impact.
- Confounding by personality traits that may be independently associated with psychiatric morbidity.
- The additive effect of multiple events, some of which may be causally linked in a chain.
- The quality of the event itself: a loss or a threat.
- Effort after meaning, whereby patients and doctors may attribute symptoms to a particular experience as a way to explain the onset of illness.

These issues are fully discussed in Chapter 2.6.1.

Personality variables

Although personality traits may contribute to how vulnerable individuals are to adverse experiences, it has not often been possible to measure personality traits in general populations, then follow the sample prospectively to demonstrate if the incidence of specific disorders is indeed higher in some types. Many measures of personality are too lengthy to be used in surveys. One exception is the Eysenck Personality Questionnaire (**EPQ-R**) in which the trait of neuroticism has been found to confer increased risk of anxiety, depression or later schizophrenia.[36] The assessment of personality is considered in Chapter 1.8.2.

Molecular genetics and epidemiology

In the next few years, it can be expected that some personality traits will be found to occur more often in people with particular alleles in genes related to brain function. Amongst these, a preferred group of candidates are genes with known polymorphisms that alter the function of neurotransmitter systems, either by affecting the metabolism of a transmitter or some aspect of its function such as transport, receptor binding, or signal transduction. The attraction for psychiatric epidemiology is twofold: the promise of introducing to population studies a biological variable of fundamental significance; and the possibility of looking for interaction between biologically based vulnerability and life experiences. The finding by Caspi *et al.*[37] sparked great interest by reporting an association between a 5-HTT polymorphism and depression, but only on persons who had been exposed to recent adversity. The finding has not been consistently replicated. Furthermore, the relevant polymorphisms may be rather more complicated than at first assumed. What is significant is that it is now feasible to study genotype and environment at the population level.

How epidemiologists think

We can now look back on the strategies used to find causes of mental disorders and how epidemiologists go about the task. To find aetiological clues, they look firstly for associations, some of which may later be shown to have a causal influence. This is often best done by working not with individual patients, nor even with a series of patients in one clinic. Instead it is better to have data that represent *all* cases of a disorder in a defined population. The way in which a candidate risk factor comes to be proposed is itself very interesting. There are three:

Table 2.7.4 The search for causes: a matrix for epidemiological studies

		Child psychiatric disorders	Anxiety disorders	Affective disorders	Schizophrenia	Dementias	Personality disorders	Eating disorders	Alcohol and substance abuse	Suicide	Parasuicide	Intellectual disability	Psychological well being
Sociodemographic factors	Gender												
	Age												
	Marital status												
	Social class												
	Education												
	Employment status												
	Urban/rural												
	World region												
Experiential factors	Season of birth												
	Parental age												
	Childhood separation												
	Parental style												
	Cultural or subcultural beliefs and attitudes												
	Adverse experiences												
	Extreme experiences												
	Bereavement												
	Expressed emotion (for relapse)												
	Social support												
	Secular changes in society												
	Other macrosocial factors (economic depression, war, social cohesion)												
	Migration												
	Climate and daylight												
	Noise												
	Environmental toxins												
	Diet												
	Alcohol and drugs												
	Medication												
	Infections												
	Physical illness												
	Interaction of two or more factors												
	Comorbidity												
	Genetics: major genes quantitative trait loci												

No attempt has been made to be exhaustive in either the classes of morbidity or the putative causal factors.

1 **The inspired hypothesis**. A sharp-eyed clinician develops the idea that some factor—in any of the three domains—is present more often than by chance in a certain disorder; and that factor may contribute to the onset of the disorder. This is exactly what happened to the ophthalmologist Sir Norman Gregg in Sydney when he noticed that many disabled children had mothers who had contracted rubella during the pregnancy. The association was later confirmed and shown to be causal. So here a hypothesis arising in the course of clinical work was taken out of the clinic and tested by epidemiological methods, then the knowledge applied in prevention.

2 **A coarse observation**. A second pathway to a hypothesis starts with a coarse observation of a link between a disorder and, say, some demographic variable. Here are two examples. In the aetiology of schizophrenia, a slight excess in winter birthdates was noticed in persons who later developed schizophrenia. Work on the 1946 birth cohort in Britain showed that persons who later developed schizophrenia had been recorded as children to have had more speech and educational problems, more social anxiety, and a preference for solitary play. Both observations point to a neurodevelopmental hypothesis for schizophrenia.

3 **The enquiry is theory driven**. A good example is what came from attachment theory. In epidemiological research on Alzheimer's disease, it was theory that led to a search for putative risk factors such as a family history of Down syndrome, aluminium in drinking water, maternal age at the patient's birth, and a history of previous head injury. It was also theory that led Jenkinson *et al.* to find an inverse association between Alzheimer's disease and rheumatoid arthritis. This subsequently led to studies of people who had been treated with long-term anti-inflammatory drugs.

4 **The search for causes: a matrix for epidemiological studies**. All these three approaches can be brought together, and then used as the building material to construct a matrix. This can then drive a systematic search. In Table 2.7.4, the main categories of mental disorders are listed across the top to form the columns, while the rows are made up of those variables that may contribute to the onset or course of morbidity. The matrix proves to be a tidy way of organizing what information is already available; but it also acts heuristically by proposing associations that call for investigation but might not otherwise have been considered. The variables can be placed in categories: sociodemographic, experiential, intrapersonal (psychological), and biological. The alert observer will notice that interactions between two or more variables should be considered, because these can be of the greatest importance.

Conclusion

The epidemiology of psychiatric disorders has shown the extent to which these are present in all human populations. It has also provided a large body of knowledge about aetiology. Now that biological including genetic information can be added to data on environmental exposures, opportunities for further advancement carry much promise.

Further information

Burger, H. and Neeleman, J. (2007). A glossary on psychiatric epidemiology. *Journal of Epidemiology Comm Health*, **61**, 185–9.

Hybels, C.F. and Blazer, D.G. (2003). Epidemiology of late-life mental disorders. *Clinics in Geriatric Medicine*, **19**, 663–96.

Henderson, A.S. (1988). *An introduction to social psychiatry*. Oxford University Press, Oxford.

References

1. Hill, A.B. (1965). The environment and disease: association or causation? *Proceedings of the Royal Society for Medicine*, **58**, 295–300.
2. Susser, M. (1973). *Causal thinking in the health sciences*. Oxford University Press, New York.
3. Morris, J.N. (1964). *Uses of epidemiology*. Williams and Wilkins, Baltimore, MD.
4. Klerman, G.L. (1988). The current age of youthful melancholia: evidence for increase in depression among adolescents and young adults. *British Journal of Psychiatry*, **152**, 4–14.
5. Gruenberg, E.M. (1966). Epidemiology of mental illness. *International Journal of Psychiatry*, **2**, 78–134.
6. Rose, G. (1993). Mental disorder and the strategies of prevention. *Psychological Medicine*, **23**, 553–5.
7. Goldberg, D.P. and Huxley, P. (1980). *Mental illness in the community: the pathway to psychiatric care*. Tavistock Publications, London.
8. Neugebauer, R. and Ng, S. (1990). Differential recall as a source of bias in epidemiologic research. *Journal of Clinical Epidemiology*, **43**, 1337–41.
9. Schlesselman, J.L. (1982). *Case-control studies: design, conduct, analysis*. Oxford University Press, New York.
10. Anthony, J.C. (1988). The epidemiologic case-control strategy, with applications in psychiatric research. In *Handbook of social psychiatry* (eds. A.S. Henderson and G.D. Burrows), pp. 157–71. Elsevier, Amsterdam.
11. Best, N.G., Spiegelhalter, D.J., Thomas, A., *et al.* (1996). Bayesian analysis of realistically complex models. *Journal of the Royal Statistical Society*, **159**, 323–42.
12. Pickering, G.W. (1968). *High blood pressure*. Churchill Livingstone, London.
13. Goldberg, D.P. and Williams, P. (1988). *A user's guide to the GHQ*. NFER/Nelson, London.
14. Durkheim, E. (1897). *Le Suicide: Etude de Sociologie*. Felix Alcan, Paris.
15. World Health Organization. (1988). *Psychiatric disability assessment schedule* (*WHO/DAS*). World Health Organization, Geneva.
16. Von Korff, M., Üstün, T.B., Ormel, J., *et al.* (1996). Self-report disability in an international primary care study of psychological illness. *Journal of Clinical Epidemiology*, **49**, 297–303.
17. Brazier, J.E., Harper, R., Jones, N.M.B., *et al.* (1992). Validating the SF-36 health survey questionnaire, new outcome measure for primary care. *British Medical Journal*, **305**, 160–4.
18. Goldberg, D. and Huxley, P. (1992). *Common mental disorders*. Tavistock Publications/Routledge, London.
19. Derogatis, L.R., Lipman, R.S., Rickels, K., *et al.* (1974). The Hopkins Symptom Checklist (HSCL): a self-report symptom inventory. *Behavioral Science*, **19**, 1–15.
20. Radloff, L.S. (1977). The CES-D scale: a self-report depression scale for research in the general population. *Applied Psychological Measurement*, **1**, 385–401.
21. Beck, A.T. (1967). *Depression: clinical, experimental and theoretical aspects*. Harper and Row, New York.
22. Conigrave, K.M., Hall, W.D., and Saunders, J.B. (1995). The AUDIT questionnaire: choosing a cut-off score. *Addiction*, **90**, 1349–56.
23. Folstein, M.F., Folstein, S.E., and McHugh, P.R. (1975). 'Mini-Mental State': a practical method for grading the cognitive state of patients for the clinician. *Journal of Psychiatric Research*, **12**, 189–98.
24. Bebbington, P. (1998). Sex and depression. *Psychological Medicine*, **28**, 1–8.

25. White, L., Katzman, R., Losonczy, K., *et al.* (1994). Association of education with incidence of cognitive impairment in three established populations for epidemiologic studies of the elderly. *Journal of Clinical Epidemiology*, **47**, 363–74.
26. Cooley, C.H. (1909). *Social organization: a study of the larger mind.* Scribner, New York.
27. Henderson, S., Byrne, D.G., and Duncan-Jones, P. (1981). *Neurosis and the social environment.* Academic Press, Sydney.
28. Henderson, A.S. and Brown, G.W. (1988). Social support: the hypothesis and the evidence. In *Handbook of social psychiatry* (eds. A.S. Henderson and G.D. Burrows), pp. 73–85. Elsevier, Amsterdam.
29. Henderson, A.S. (1998). Social support: its present significance for psychiatric epidemiology. In *Adversity, stress and psychopathology* (ed. B.P. Dohrenwend), pp. 390–7. Oxford University Press, New York.
30. Leighton, D.C., Harding, J.S., Macklin, D.B., *et al.* (1963). *The character of danger.* Basic Books, New York.
31. Bowlby, J. (1977). The making and breaking of affectional bonds. I. Aetiology and psychopathology in the light of attachment theory. *British Journal of Psychiatry*, **130**, 201–10.
32. Rutter, M. (1981). *Maternal deprivation reassessed*, p. 197. Penguin, Harmondsworth.
33. Cantor-Graae, E. and Selten, J.P. (2005). Schizophrenia and migration: a meta-analysis and review. *The American Journal of Psychiatry*, **162**, 12–24.
34. Parker, G. (1992). Early environment. In *Handbook of affective disorders* (2nd edn) (ed. E.S. Paykel), pp. 171–83. Guilford Press, New York.
35. Parker, G., Roussos, J., Hadzi-Pavlovic, *et al.* (1997). The development of a refined measure of dysfunctional parenting and assessment of its relevance in patients with affective disorders. *Psychological Medicine*, **27**, 1193–203.
36. Fergusson, D.M., Horwood, L.J., and Lawton, J.M. (1989). The relationships between neuroticism and depressive symptoms. *Social Psychiatry and Psychiatric Epidemiology*, **24**, 275–81.
37. Caspi, A., Sugden, K., Moffitt, T.E., *et al.* (2003). Influence of life stress on depression: moderation by a polymorphism in the 5-HTT gene. *Science*, **301**(5631), 386–9.

SECTION 3

Psychodynamic Contributions to Psychiatry

3.1 **Psychoanalysis: Freud's theories and their contemporary development** *293*
Otto F. Kernberg

3.2 **Object relations, attachment theory, self-psychology, and interpersonal psychoanalysis** *306*
Jeremy Holmes

3.3 **Current psychodynamic approaches to psychiatry** *313*
Glen O. Gabbard

3.1

Psychoanalysis: Freud's theories and their contemporary development

Otto F. Kernberg

Psychoanalysis is:

1 A personality theory, and, more generally, a theory of psychological functioning that focuses particularly on unconscious mental processes;

2 A method for the investigation of psychological functions based on the exploration of free associations within a special therapeutic setting;

3 A method for treatment of a broad spectrum of psychopathological conditions, including the symptomatic neuroses (anxiety states, characterological depression, obsessive–compulsive disorder, conversion hysteria, and dissociative hysterical pathology), sexual inhibitions and perversions ('paraphilias'), and the personality disorders.

Psychoanalysis has also been applied, mostly in modified versions, i.e. in psychoanalytic psychotherapies, to the treatment of severe personality disorders, psychosomatic conditions, and certain psychotic conditions, particularly a subgroup of patients with chronic schizophrenic illness.

All three aspects of psychoanalysis were originally developed by Freud(1–3) whose theories of the dynamic unconscious, personality development, personality structure, psychopathology, methodology of psychoanalytic investigation, and method of treatment still largely influence the field, both in the sense that many of his central ideas continue as the basis of contemporary psychoanalytic thinking, and in that corresponding divergencies, controversies, and radical innovations still can be better understood in the light of the overall frame of his contributions. Freud's concepts of dream analysis, mechanisms of defence, and transference have become central aspects of many contemporary psychotherapeutic procedures.

Freud's ideas about personality development and psychopathology, the method of psychoanalytic investigation, and the analytic approach to treatment gradually changed in the course of his dramatically creative lifespan. Moreover, the theory of the structure of the mind that he assumed must underlie the events that he observed clinically changed in major respects, so that an overall summary of his views can hardly be undertaken without tracing the history of his thinking. The present overview will lead up to summaries of his final conclusions as to the structure of the mind and how this is reflected in personality development and psychopathology. Psychoanalysis will then be described as a method of treatment, as seen from the point of view of resolution of conflict between impulse and defence, and from that of object-relations theory. We shall explore significant changes that have occurred in all these domains, and conclude with an overview of contemporary psychoanalysis, with particular emphasis upon the presently converging tendencies of contemporary psychoanalytic approaches, and new developments that remain controversial.

Freud's theory of the mental apparatus: motivation, structure, and functioning

Unconscious mental processes: the topographic theory; defence mechanisms

Freud's starting point(4) was his study of hysterical patients and the discovery that, when he found a way to help these patients piece together a coherent account of the antecedents of their conversion symptoms, dissociative phenomena, and pathological affective dispositions, all these psychopathological phenomena could be traced to traumatic experiences in their past that had become unconscious. That is, these traumatic experiences continued to influence the patients' functioning despite an active defensive mechanism of 'repression' that excluded them from the patient's conscious awareness. In the course of a few years, Freud abandoned his early efforts to recover repressed material by means of hypnosis, and replaced hypnosis with the technique of 'free association', an essential aspect of psychoanalytic technique until the present time. Freud instructed his patients to eliminate as much as possible all 'prepared agendas', and to try to express whatever came to mind, while attempting to exert as little censorship over this material as they could. He provided them with a non-judgemental and stable setting in which to carry out their task, inviting them to recline on a couch while he sat behind it. The sessions lasted for an hour and were conducted five to six times a week. There has been little change in the essentials of this format, except that sessions have been shortened to 45 to 50 min and are carried out three to five times a week. The method of free association led to the gradual recovery of repressed memories of traumatic events. Originally, Freud thought that the recovery of such events into consciousness would permit their abreaction and elaboration, and thus resolve the patients' symptoms.

Practicing this method led Freud to several lines of discovery. To begin, he conceptualized unconscious mechanisms of defence that opposed the recovery of memories by free association. He described these mechanisms, namely, repression, negation, isolation, projection, introjection, transformation into the opposite, rationalization, intellectualization, and most important, reaction formation. The last of these involves overt chronic patterns of thought and behaviour that serve to disguise and disavow opposite tendencies linked to unconscious traumatic events and the intrapsychic conflicts derived from them. The discovery of reaction formations led Freud to the psychoanalytic study of character pathology and normal character formation, and still constitutes an important aspect of the contemporary psychoanalytic understanding and treatment of personality disorders (for practical purposes, character pathology and personality disorders are synonymous concepts).

A related line of development in Freud's theories was the discovery of the differential characteristics of conscious and unconscious thinking. Freud differentiated conscious thinking, the 'secondary process', invested by 'attention cathexis' and dominated by sensory perception and ordinary logic in relating to the psychosocial environment, from the 'primary process' of the 'dynamic unconscious'. That part of the unconscious mind he referred to as 'dynamic' exerted constant pressure or influence on conscious processes, against the active barrier constituted by the various defensive operations, particularly repression. The dynamic unconscious, Freud proposed, presented a general mobility of affective investments, and was ruled by the 'pleasure principle' in contrast to the 'reality principle' of consciousness. The 'primary process' thinking of the dynamic unconscious was characterized by the absence of the principle of contradiction and of ordinary logical thinking, the absence of negation and of the ordinary sense of time and space, the treatment of a part as if it were equivalent to the whole, and a general tendency towards condensation of thoughts and the displacement of affective investments from one to another mental content.

Finally, Freud proposed a 'preconscious', an intermediate zone between the dynamic unconscious and consciousness. It represented the storehouse for retrievable memories and knowledge and for affective investments in general, and it was the seat of daydreaming, in which the reality principle of consciousness was loosened, and derivatives of the dynamic unconscious might emerge. Free association, in fact, primarily tapped the preconscious as well as the layer of unconscious defensive operations opposing the emergence of material from the dynamic unconscious.

This model of the mind as a 'place' with unconscious, preconscious, and conscious 'regions' constituted Freud's[1] 'topographic theory'. He eventually replaced it with the 'structural theory' namely, the concept of three interacting psychic structures, the ego, the superego, and the id.[5] This tripartite structural theory is still the model of the mind that dominates psychoanalytic thinking. A major determinant of the shift from the topographic to the structural model was Freud's recognition that the 'regions' of conscious, preconscious, and unconscious were fluid, and that the defence mechanisms directed against the emergence in consciousness of the dynamic unconscious were themselves unconscious. Another consideration was Freud's[6] discovery of a specialized unconscious system of infantile morality, the superego. What follows is a summary of the characteristics and contents of these structures, an analysis that will lead us directly into contemporary psychoanalytic formulations.

The structural theory, the dual-drive theory, and the Oedipus complex

The id: infantile sexuality and the Oedipus complex

The id is the mental structure that contains the mental representatives of the 'drives', that is, the ultimate intrapsychic motivations that Freud[7] described in his final, 'dual-drive theory' of libido and aggression, or metaphorically, the sexual or life drive and the destruction or death drive to be examined below. Behind this categorical formulation lies a complex set of discoveries regarding the patients' unconscious experiences that Freud came across in the course of the application of the psychoanalytic method to the treatment of neurotic and characterological symptoms. In exploring unconscious mental processes, what at first appeared to be specific traumatic life experiences turned out to reflect surprisingly consistent, repetitive intrapsychic experiences of a sexual and aggressive nature.

Freud[4] was particularly impressed by the regularity with which his patients reported the emergence of childhood memories reflecting seductive and traumatic sexual experiences on one hand, and intense sexual desires and related guilt feelings, on the other. He discovered a continuity between the earliest wishes for dependency and being taken care of (the psychology, as he saw it, of the baby at the mother's breast) during what he described as the 'oral phase' of development; the pleasure in exercising control and struggles around autonomy in the subsequent 'anal phase' of development (the psychology of toilet training); and, particularly, the sexual desire towards the parent of the opposite gender and the ambivalent rivalry for that parent's exclusive love with the parent of the same gender. He described this latter state as characteristic of the 'infantile genital stage' (from the third or fourth to the sixth year of life) and called its characteristic constellation of wishes and conflicts the positive Oedipus complex. He differentiated it from the negative Oedipus complex, i.e. the love for the parent of the same gender, and the corresponding ambivalent rivalry with the parent of the other gender. Freud proposed that Oedipal wishes came to dominate the infantile hierarchy of oral and anal wishes, becoming the fundamental unconscious realm of desire.

Powerful fears motivated the repression of awareness of infantile desire: the fear of loss of the object, and later of the loss of the object's love was the basic fear of the oral phase, directed against libidinal wishes to possess the breast; the fear of destructive control and annihilation of the self or the object was the dominant fear of the anal phase directed against libidinal wishes of anal expulsion and retentiveness, and the fear of castration, 'castration anxiety', the dominant fear of the Oedipal phase of development, directed against libidinal desire of the Oedipal object. Unconscious guilt was a dominant later fear, originating in the superego and generally directed against drive gratification (see under superego). Unconscious guilt over sexual impulses unconsciously equated with Oedipal desires constitute a major source of many types of pathology, such as sexual inhibition and related character pathology.

Prototypical intrapsychic infantile experiences linked to the Oedipus complex were fantasies and perceptions around the sexual intimacy of the parents (the 'primal scene'), and unconscious fantasies derived from experiences with primary caregivers ('primal seduction'). In all these phases of infantile development of drive motivated wishes and fears, powerful aggressive strivings accompanied the libidinal ones, such as cannibalistic impulses during the oral phase of physical dependency on the breast and psychological dependency on mother, sadistic fantasies linked to the anal phase, and parricidal wishes and phantasies in the Oedipal stage of development.

Freud described the oral phase as essentially coinciding with the infantile stage of breast feeding, the anal phase as coinciding with struggles around sphincter control, and the Oedipal stage as developing gradually during the second and through the fourth years, and culminating in the fourth and the fifth years of life. This latter phase would then be followed by more general repressive processes under the dominance of the installation of the superego, leading to a 'latency phase' roughly corresponding to the school years, and finally, to a transitory reactivation of all unconscious childhood conflicts under the dominance of Oedipal issues during puberty and early adolescence.

The id: drives

The drives represent for human behaviour what the instincts constitute for the animal kingdom, i.e. the ultimate biological motivational system. The drives are constant, highly individualized, developmentally shaped motivational systems. Under the dominance of the drives and guided by the primary process, the id exerts an ongoing pressure towards gratification, operating in accordance with the pleasure principle. Freud initially equated the drives with primitive affects. After discarding various other models of unconscious motivation, he ended up with the dual-drive theory of libido and aggression.

He described the libido or the sexual drive as having an 'origin' in the erotogenic nature of the leading oral, anal, and genital bodily zones; an 'impulse' expressing the quantitative intensity of the drive by the intensity of the corresponding affects; an 'aim' reflected in the particular act of concrete gratification of the drive; and an 'object' consisting of displacements from the dominant parental objects of desire.

The introduction of the idea of an aggressive or 'death' drive, arrived at later in Freud's[7, 8] writing, stemmed from his observations of the profound self-destructive urges particularly manifest in the psychopathology of major depression and suicide, and of the 'repetition compulsion' of impulse-driven behaviour that frequently seemed to run counter to the pleasure principle that supposedly governed unconscious drives. He never spelled out the details of the aggressive drive as to its origins. This issue was taken up later by Klein,[9] Fairbairn,[10] Winnicott,[11] Jacobson,[12] and Mahler and her colleagues.[13] Freud described drives as intermediate between the body and the mind; the only thing we knew about them, Freud suggested,[14] were 'representations and affects'.

The structure and functions of the ego

While the id is the seat of the unconscious drives, and functions according to the 'primary process' of the dynamic unconscious, the ego, Freud[5] proposed, is the seat of consciousness as well as of unconscious defence mechanisms that, in the psychoanalytic treatment, appear as 'resistances' to free association. The ego functions according to the logical and reality-based principles of 'secondary process', negotiating the relations between internal and external reality. Guided by the reality principle, it exerts control over perception and motility; it draws on preconscious material, controls 'attention cathexes' and permits motor delay as well as selection of imagery and perception. The ego is also the seat of basic affects, particularly anxiety as an alarm signal against the danger of emergence of unconscious, repressed impulses. This alarm signal may turn into a disorganized state of panic when the ego is flooded with external perceptions that activate unconscious desire and conflicts, or with overwhelming, traumatic experiences in reality that resonate with such repressed unconscious conflicts, and overwhelm the particularly sensitized ego in the process. The fact that the ego was seen by Freud as the seat of affects, and that affects had previously been described by him as discharge phenomena reflecting drives (together with their mental representations) tended to dissociate affects from drives in psychoanalytic theory, in contrast to their originally being equated in Freud's early formulations. As we shall see, this issue, the centrality of affects in psychic reality and interactions, has gradually re-emerged as a major aspect of contemporary psychoanalytic thinking.

Freud originally equated the 'I', i.e. the categorical self of the philosophers, with consciousness; later, once he established the theory of the ego as an organization of both conscious and unconscious functions, he at times treated the ego as if it were the subjective self, and at other times, as an impersonal organization of functions. Out of this ambiguity evolved the contemporary concept of the self within modern ego psychology as well as in British and American object relations and cultural psychoanalytic contributions.[15] An alternative theory of the self was proposed by Kohut[16] the originator of the self-psychology approach within contemporary psychoanalysis.

Nowadays, an integrated concept of the self as the seat of subjectivity is considered an essential structure of the ego, and the concept of 'ego identity' refers to the integration of the concept of the self: because of developmental processes in early infancy and childhood better understood today, an integrated self-concept usually goes hand-in-hand with the capacity for an integrated concept of significant others. An unconscious tendency towards primitive dissociation or 'splitting' of the self-concept and of the concepts of significant objects runs counter to such integration: we shall return to this process later. Already Freud,[17] in one of his last contributions, described a process of splitting in the ego as a way of dealing with intolerable intrapsychic conflict, thus opening up the road for considering splitting processes of the ego as an alternative, pathological defence against intolerable intrapsychic conflict (alternative, that is, to the repression of that conflict and to drawing important related ego functions into repression as well).

Character, from a psychoanalytic perspective, may be defined as constituting the behavioural aspects of ego identity (the self-concept) and the internal relations with significant others (the internalized world of 'object relations'). The sense of personal identity and of an internal world of object relations, in turn, reflect the subjective side of character. It was particularly the ego psychological approach—one of the dominant contemporary psychoanalytic schools—that developed the analysis of defensive operations of the ego, and of pathological character formation as a stable defensive organization that needed to be explored and resolved in the psychoanalytic treatment. In the process, ego psychology contributed importantly to the psychoanalytic treatment of personality disorders.

Personality disorders reflect typical constellations of pathological character traits derived from abnormal developmental processes under the influence of unconscious intrapsychic conflicts. The description of 'reaction formation' as one of the defences of the ego led Freud to the description of the 'oral', 'anal', and 'genital' characters, particularly to the description of the obsessive–compulsive personality as a typical manifestation of reaction formations against anal drive derivatives. This was followed by the description by Abraham[18] of the hysterical personality as a consequence of multiple reaction formations against the female castration complex. Over the years, psychoanalytic explorations led to the description of a broad spectrum of pathological character constellations, which today are a part of the spectrum of personality disorders.

Perhaps the most important psychoanalytic contribution to character pathology and the personality disorders is the clinical description of the narcissistic personality disorder. While Freud provided the basic elements that led to its eventual description, psychoanalytic understanding and treatment, it was not he who crystallized the concepts of normal and pathological narcissism. Freud[19] conceptualized narcissism as the libidinal investment of the ego or self, in contrast to the libidinal investment of significant others ('objects'). In proposing the possibility of a withdrawal of libidinal investment from others with an excessive investment in the self as the basic feature of narcissistic pathology, he pointed to a broad spectrum of psychopathology, and thus first stimulated the contribution of Abraham,[20] and later those of Klein,[21] Rosenfeld,[22] Grunberger,[23] Kohut,[16] Jacobson,[12] and Kernberg.[24] Thus, crystallized the description of the narcissistic personality as a disorder derived from a pathological integration of a grandiose self as a defence against unbearable aggressive conflicts, particularly around primitive envy.

The superego in normality and pathology

In his analysis of unconscious intrapsychic conflicts between drive and defence, Freud regularly encountered unconscious feelings of guilt in his patients, reflecting an extremely strict, unconscious infantile morality, which he called the superego. This unconscious morality could lead to severe self-blame and self-attacks, and particularly, to abnormal depressive reactions, which he came to regard as expressing the superego's attacks on the ego. It was particularly in studying normal and pathological mourning, where Freud[6] arrived at the idea of excessive mourning and depression as reflecting the unconscious internalization of the representation of an ambivalently loved and hated lost object. In unconsciously identifying the self with that object introjected into the ego, the individual now attacked his or her own self in replacement of the previous unconscious hatred of the object; and the internalization of aspects of that object into the superego reinforced the strictness of the individual's pre-existing unconscious infantile morality.

Freud traced the origins of the superego to the overcoming of the Oedipus complex via unconscious identification with the parent of the same gender: in internalizing the Oedipal parent's prohibition against the rivalry with him or her and the unconscious death wishes regularly connected with such a rivalry, and against the incestuous desire for the parent of the other gender, this internalization crystallized an unconscious infantile morality. The superego, thus based upon prohibitions against incest and parricide, and a demand for submission to, and identification with the Oedipal rival, became the guarantor of the capacity for identification with moral and ethical values in general. In simple terms, the little boy renounces mother out of fear and love of father, takes father's fantasized prohibition against the little boy's sexuality into the superego as a fundamental prohibition, and establishes an identification with his father in the consolidation of his character structure. The little boy thus enacts the unconscious fantasy that, in identifying with father, he will gradually grow into his role, and satisfy his sexual desire in the distant future, by choosing another woman who, unconsciously and symbolically, will represent mother. The superego thus introduces a new time perspective into the functioning of the psychic apparatus.

Freud also described the internalization of the idealized representations of both parents into the superego in the form of the 'ego ideal'. He suggested that the earliest sources of self-esteem, derived from mother's love, gradually fixated by the baby's and small child's internalizations of the representations of the loving mother into the ego ideal, led to the parental demands becoming internalized as well. In other words, normally self-esteem is maintained both by living up to the expectations of the internalized idealized parental objects, and by submitting to their internalized prohibitions. This consideration of self-esteem regulation leads to the clinical concept of narcissism as normal or pathological self-esteem regulation, in contrast to the theoretical concept of narcissism as the libidinal investment of the self.

The superego, in summary, is a mental structure constituted by the internalized demands and prohibitions from the parental objects of childhood, the 'heir to the Oedipal complex'. This unconscious structure is of fundamental importance in determining unconscious 'fixations' to infantile prohibitions against drive derivatives and the corresponding unconscious motivation for the activation of a broad spectrum of ego defences against them, thus preventing the ego from responsibility-examining and reintegrating unresolved pathogenic conflicts from early childhood. In health, this internal sense of unconscious morality is the underpinning of moral and ethical systems. Excessive superego severity, usually derived from excessive parental strictness, determines excessive repressive mechanisms and ego inhibitions, irrational moralistic behaviour, or pathological activation of depression and loss of self-esteem.

Having thus summarized the basic psychoanalytic theory of motivation (drives), of development (the stages of development from the early oral phase to the dominance of the Oedipal complex), of structure (the tripartite model), and their implications for psychopathology, I shall now describe more specifically the contemporary psychoanalytic theory of psychopathology and of psychoanalytic treatment.

Psychoanalytic treatment

The psychoanalytic theory of psychopathology

The psychoanalytic theory of psychopathology proposes that the clinical manifestations of the symptomatic neuroses, character pathology, perversions, sexual inhibitions, and selected types of psychosomatic and psychotic illness reflect unconscious intrapsychic conflicts between drive derivatives following the pleasure principle, defensive operations reflecting the reality principle, and the unconscious motivations of the superego. Unconscious conflicts between impulse and defence are expressed in the form of structured conflicts between the agencies of the tripartite structure: there are ego defences against impulses of the id; the superego motivates inhibitions and restrictions in the ego; at times the repetitive, dissociated expression of id impulses ('repetition compulsion') constitutes an effective id defence against superego pressures. The resolution of unconscious conflicts implies the analysis of all these intersystemic conflicts.

All these conflicts are expressed clinically by three types of phenomena:

1 inhibitions of normal ego functions regarding sexuality, intimacy, social relations, work, and affect activation;

2 compromise formations between repressed impulses and the defences directed against them;

3 dissociative expression of impulse and defence.

The last category implies a dominance of the splitting mechanisms referred to before; these have acquired central importance in the understanding of severe character pathology as reflected in contemporary psychoanalytic thinking.

The structural formulation of the psychoanalytic method

Psychoanalytic treatment consists, in essence, in facilitating the reactivation of the pathogenic unconscious conflicts in the treatment situation by means of a systematic analysis of the defensive operations directed against them. This leads to the gradual emergence of repressed impulses, with the possibility of elaborating them in relation to the analyst, and their eventual adaptive integration into the adult ego. Freud[(25)] had described the concept of 'sublimation' as an adaptive transformation of unconscious drives: drive derivatives, converted into a consciously tolerable form, are permitted gratification in a symbolic way while their origin remains unconscious. The result of this process is an adaptive, non-defensive compromise formation between impulse and defence. In analysis, the gradual integration into the patient's conscious ego of unconscious wishes and desires from the past and the understanding of the phantasized threats and dangers connected with them, facilitates their gradual elaboration and sublimatory expression in the consulting room and in everyday life as well.

The object-relations theory formulation of psychoanalytic treatment

In the light of contemporary object-relations theory, the formulation based upon the structural theory (resolution of unconscious conflicts between impulse and defence) has changed, in the sense that all unconscious conflicts are considered to be imbedded in unconscious internalized object relations. Such internalized object relations determine both the nature of the defensive operations and of the impulses against which they are directed. These internalized object relations constitute, at the same time, the 'building blocks' of the tripartite structure of id, ego, and superego. Object-relations theory proposes that the gradual analysis of intersystemic conflicts between impulse and defence (structured into conflicts between ego, superego, and id) decomposes the tripartite structure into the constituent conflicting internalized object relations. These object relations are reactivated in the treatment situation in the form of an unconscious relation between self and significant others replicated in the relation between patient and analyst, i.e. the 'transference'.

The transference is the unconscious repetition in the 'here and now' of unconscious, conflicting pathogenic relationships from the past. The transference reflects the reactivation of the past conflict not in the form of a memory, but in the form of a repetition. This repetition provides essential information about the past, but constitutes, at the same time, a defence in the sense that the patient repeats instead of remembering. Therefore, transference has important informative features that need to be facilitated in their development, and defensive features that need to be therapeutically resolved once their nature has been clarified. Transference analysis is the fundamental ingredient of the psychoanalytic treatment.

The psychoanalytic treatment process

The psychoanalytic treatment consists of the creation of an atmosphere of safety in which a patient is willing to try to express whatever comes to mind. In 45 to 50 min sessions, three to five times per week, the patient usually reclines on a couch while the analyst, generally sitting behind the patient, helps the patient become aware of his or her defensive operations ('resistances') by means of interpretations. The systematic interpretation of resistances gradually permits an ever-growing freedom of free association, and helps the patient to become aware of his or her unconscious desires and fears, phantasies and terrors, traumatic situations, and unresolved mourning. Defensive operations are usually classified as ego defences (in the form of the mechanisms listed earlier), superego defences in the form of excessive guilt feelings activated during the treatment, id resistances in the form of repetition compulsion, the development of secondary gain from symptoms as a powerful resistance, and, last and most importantly, the transference as the dominant resistance and source of information.

Gill,[(26)] in a classical definition that is still relevant today, proposed the definition of psychoanalysis as a treatment that facilitates the development of a 'regressive transference neurosis' and its resolution by means of interpretation alone, carried out by the analyst from a position of technical neutrality. Let us define these concepts.

'Regression' refers to the patient's return to earlier experiences (temporal regression), and modes of functioning (structural and formal regression) under the effect of the analysis of resistances, and is an expression of the reactivation of his unconscious conflicts from the past in the transference. In essence, the patient activates or enacts earlier object relations in the transference. Certain past stages of development where particular traumatic experiences occurred act as gathering points ('fixations') that foster regression towards them. The concept of a regressive transference neurosis refers to the gradual gathering into the relationship with the analyst of the patient's most important past pathogenic experiences and unconscious conflicts. The concept of a regressive transference neurosis has been largely abandoned in practice because, particularly in patients with severe character pathology, transference regression occurs so early and consistently that the gradual development of a regressive transference neurosis is no longer a useful concept.

Gill's proposal that the resolution of the transference be achieved 'by interpretation alone', refers to 'interpretation' as a set of the psychoanalyst's interventions that starts with 'clarification' of the patient's subjective experiences communicated by means of free association, expands with the tactful 'confrontation' of aspects of the patient's patterns of behaviour that are expressed in a dissociated or split-off manner from his subjective awareness, and thus complements the total expression of his intrapsychic life in the treatment situation, and finally evolves into 'interpretation per se'. Interpretation per se implies the formulation of hypotheses regarding the unconscious meanings in the 'here and now' of the patient's material, and the relation of these unconscious meanings with the 'there and then' of the patient's unconscious, past pathogenic experiences. The analysis of the transference is 'systematic', in the sense that all emerging transference dispositions are interpreted, ideally, in the natural sequence of their emergence in the analytic situation. Gill's phrase, 'by interpretation alone', implies that the psychoanalyst abstains from measures other than helping the patient to fully understand the unconscious conflicts activated in the here and now. Thus, providing guidance about life decisions, or attempting to modify the patient's behaviour or state by means of praise, prohibition, or reward is not part of the psychoanalytic method of treatment.

The concept of 'technical neutrality' refers to the analyst's impartiality regarding both impulse and defence, with a concerned objectivity that provides a helpful collaboration with the patient's efforts to come to grips with his intrapsychic conflicts.

This definition of the nature of psychoanalytic treatment needs to be complemented with the contemporary concepts of 'transference', 'countertransference', 'acting out', and 'working through'.

An object-relations theory model of the transference and countertransference

Modern object-relations theory, further explored below, and presented in more detail in terms of particular schools in Chapter 3.2, proposes that, in the case of any particular conflict around sexual or aggressive impulses, the conflict is imbedded in an internalized object relation, i.e. in a repressed or dissociated representation of the self ('self-representation') linked with a particular representation of another who is a significant object of desire or hatred ('object representation'). Such units of self-representation, object representation, and the dominant sexual, dependent or aggressive affect linking them are the basic 'dyadic units', whose consolidation will give rise to the tripartite structure. Internalized dyadic relations dominated by sexual and aggressive impulses will constitute the id; internalized dyadic relations of an idealized or prohibitive nature the superego, and those related to developing psychosocial functioning and the preconscious and conscious experience, together with their unconscious, defensive organization against unconscious impulses, the ego. These internalized object relations are activated in the **transference** with an alternating role distribution, i.e. the patient enacts a self-representation while projecting the corresponding object representation onto the analyst at times, while at other times projecting his self-representation onto the analyst and identifying with the corresponding object representation. The impulse or drive derivative is reflected by a dominant, usually primitive affect disposition linking a particular dyadic object relation; the associated defensive operation is also represented unconsciously by a corresponding dyadic relation between a self-representation and an object representation under the dominance of a certain affect state.

For example, a conflict between unconscious aggression and unconscious guilt feelings, respectively located in id and superego, is clinically represented by manifestations of a guilt-provoking object representation relating to a guilty self (the superego defence), and an enraged self-representation attempting to attack a threatening or frustrating object representation (the id impulse). The development of the transference, therefore, consists of a sequence of activation of such impulsively determined and defensively determined internalized object relations and their systematic clarification, confrontation, and interpretation by the analyst.

The concept of **countertransference**, originally coined by Freud as the unresolved, reactivated transference dispositions of the analyst is currently defined as the total affective disposition of the analyst in response to the patient and his or her transference, shifting from moment to moment, and providing important data of information to the analyst. The countertransference, thus defined, may be partially derived from unresolved problems of the analyst, but stems as well from the impact of the dominant transference reactions of the patient, from reality aspects of the patient's life, and sometimes from aspects of the analyst's life situation that are emotionally activated in the context of the transference developments. In general, the stronger the transference regression, the more the transference determines the countertransference; thus the countertransference becomes an important diagnostic tool. The countertransference includes both the analyst's empathic identification with a patient's central subjective experience ('concordant identification') and the analyst's identification with the reciprocal object or self-representation ('complementary identification') unconsciously activated in the patient as part of a certain dyadic unit, and projected onto the analyst.[27] In other words, the analyst's countertransference implies an identification with what the patient cannot tolerate in him- or herself, and must dissociate, project, or repress.

At this point, it is important to refer to certain primitive defensive operations that were described by Klein[9] and her school in the context of the analysis of severe character pathology. Primitive defensive operations are characteristic of patients with severe personality disorders, and emerge in other cases during periods of regression. They include splitting, projective identification, denial, omnipotence, omnipotent control, primitive idealization, and devaluation (contempt). All these primitive defences centre around splitting, i.e. an active dissociation of contradictory ego (or self) experiences as a defence against unconscious intrapsychic conflict. They represent a regression to the phase of development (the first 2 to 3 years of life) before repression and its related mechanisms mentioned are established.

Primitive defensive operations present important behavioural components that tend to induce behaviours or emotional reactions in the analyst, which, if the analyst manages to 'contain' them, permit him to diagnose in himself projected aspects of the patient's experience. Particularly 'projective identification' is a process in which:

1 the patient unconsciously projects an intolerable aspect of self-experience onto (or 'into') the analyst;

2 the analyst unconsciously enacts the corresponding experience ('complementary identification');

3 the patient tries to control the analyst, who now is under the effect of this projected behaviour;

4 the patient meanwhile maintains empathy with what is projected.

This scenario is in contrast to the more mature mechanism of 'projection', secondary to repression, where there is no longer any conscious emotional contact with what is projected. Such complementary identification in the countertransference permits the analyst to identify him- or herself through his own experience with the aspects of the patient's experience communicated by means of projective identification. This information complements what the analyst has discovered about the patient by means of clarification and confrontation, and permits the analyst to integrate all this information in the form of a 'selected fact' that constitutes the object of interpretation. Interpretation is thus a complex technique that is very much concerned with the systematic analysis of both transference and countertransference.

Contemporary trends of the psychoanalytic method

Contemporary psychoanalytic technique can be seen as having evolved from a 'one person psychology' into a 'two person psychology' and then into a 'three person psychology'. The concept of 'one person psychology' refers to Freud's original analysis of the patient's unconscious intrapsychic conflicts by analysing the intrapsychic defensive operations that oppose free association. The 'two person psychology' refers to the central focus on the analysis of transference and countertransference. In the views of the contemporary intersubjective, interpersonal, and self-psychology psychoanalytic schools, the relationship between transference and countertransference is mutual, in the sense that the transference is at least in part a reaction to reality aspects of the analyst, who therefore must be acutely mindful of his contribution to the activation of the transference. The so-called 'constructivist' position regarding transference analysis assumes that it is impossible for the analyst to achieve a totally objective position outside the transference/countertransference bind.

In contrast, the contemporary 'objectivist' position, represented by the 'three person psychology' approaches of the Kleinian school, the French psychoanalytic mainstream, and significant segments of contemporary ego psychology proposes that the analyst has to divide him- or herself between one part influenced by transference and countertransference developments, and another part that, by means of self-reflection, maintains him- or herself outside this process, as an 'excluded third party', who, symbolically, provides an early triangulation to the dyadic regression that dominates transference developments. This triangulation in the treatment situation becomes particularly important in the treatment of severe personality disorders.

The 'enactment' of pathogenic past internalized object relations in the form of both transference and countertransference developments needs to be differentiated from **acting out**, the replacement of self-awareness by often dramatic, and at times, violent action. It is characteristic of patients with severe character pathology, and may occur in both patient and analyst under the influence of regression. Acting out may occur both during and outside the sessions. While it reflects an intense defensive operation and resistance, it also offers the opportunity for a very fundamental exploration of a primitive conflict, if dealt with by consistent interpretations in as much depth as possible. Acting out may also be considered an extreme, behavioural manifestation of 'enactment' as the usual experience of transference/countertransference manifestations.

The **repetition compulsion** as a resistance of the id is most probably a form of acting out as a defence against emotional containment of an extremely painful or traumatic set of experiences. **Working through** refers to the repeated elaboration of an unconscious conflict in the psychoanalytic situation. It is a major task for the analyst, who has to be alert to the subtle variation in meanings and implications of what on the surface may appear to be an endless repetition of the same conflict in the transference. The patient elaboration of the conflict that presents itself with these repetitive characteristics also implies the function of 'holding' originally described by Winnicott.[(11)] It consists of the analyst's capacity to withstand the onslaught of primitive transferences without retaliation, abandonment of the patient, or a self-devaluing giving up, and the maintenance of a working relationship (or 'therapeutic alliance') that addresses itself consistently to the healthy part of the patient, even when the latter is under the control of his most conflicting behaviours. Bion's concept[(28)] of 'containing' is complementary to 'holding', in the sense that holding deals mostly with the affective disposition of the analyst, and containing with his cognitive capacity to maintain a concerned objectivity and focus on the 'selected fact', permitting the integration in the analyst's mind what the patient can only express in violently dispersed or split-off behaviour patterns.

Dream analysis developed in the context of the method of free association, and constituted, in Freud's[(29)] view, a 'royal road to the unconscious'. Freud's discovery of primary process thinking derived from his method of dream analysis. By now, psychoanalytic thinking has evolved into the view that there are many 'royal roads' to the unconscious. The analysis of character defences, for example, or of particular transference complications, may be equally important avenues of entry into the patient's unconscious mind.

The technique of dream analysis consists, in essence, in asking the patient to free associate to elements of the 'manifest content' of the dream, in order to arrive at its 'latent' content, the unconscious wish defended against and distorted by the unconscious defensive mechanisms that constitute the 'dream work', and have transformed the latent content into the manifest dream. The latent content is revealed with the help of the simultaneous analysis of the way in which the dream is being communicated to the analyst, the 'day residuals' that may have triggered the dream, the unconscious conflicts revealed in it, and the dominant transference dispositions in the context of which the dream evolved. Dreams also provide some residual, universal symbolic meanings that may facilitate the total understanding of the latent content.

The **analysis of character** may be the single most important element of the psychoanalytic method in bringing about fundamental characterological change. Character analysis is facilitated by the patient's use of reaction formations, i.e. his defensively motivated character traits, as transference resistances. Thus, the activation of defensive behaviours in the transference, reflecting the patient's characterological patterns in all interpersonal interactions, facilitates both the analysis of the underlying unconscious conflicts, and in the process, the resolution of pathological character patterns. The result is an increase in the patient's autonomy, flexibility, and capacity for adaptation. Character analysis was originally developed by Reich[(30)] within an ego-psychology perspective, but has re-emerged in the work of Rosenfeld[(31)] and Steiner[(32)] in the analysis of 'pathological organizations' in the transference, within the Kleinian school. Gray[(33)] and Busch[(34)] within an ego-psychological perspective, have enriched further the technique of character analysis by means of detailed exploration of particular characterological defences in the transference.

Character analysis, although not always referred to under this specific heading, constitutes a major focus of contemporary psychoanalytic treatment. In essence, its technique addresses repetitive, ego syntonic behaviour patterns in the transference, raising the patient's curiosity about their function in the relationship with the analyst, and inviting the patient to associate about this behaviour. Gradually, their exploration makes character resistances ego dystonic, and facilitates the discovery of the underlying internalized object relations condensed in these pathological character traits, both in their defensive and impulsive meanings. The question, to what extent such rigid behaviours should be analysed first, in order to free the patient's capacity for analytic work, or to what extent they should be left for later, until more fluid conflicts have been resolved, has been settled in favour of the general psychoanalytic technical principle of focusing interpretations upon what is affectively dominant in each hour.[35] Affective dominance refers once more to the 'selected fact',[36] to be interpreted. All interpretations are usually carried out from surface to depth, which in practice means first analysing the object relation activated by the need for defence before analysing the corresponding object relation activated by impulse.

The overall objective of psychoanalytic treatment is not only the resolution of symptoms and pathological behaviour patterns or characteristics, but fundamental, structural change, that is the expansion and enrichment of ego functions as the consequence of resolution of unconscious conflict and the integration of previously repressed and dynamically active id and superego pressures into ego potentialities. Such change is reflected in the increasing capacity for both adaptation to and autonomy from psychosocial demands and expectations, and an increased capacity for gratifying and successful functioning in love and work.

Derived modalities of treatment

One of the most important contributions of psychoanalytic theory and technique to the contemporary treatment of a broad spectrum of patients with severe psychopathology who, for various reasons, cannot benefit from psychoanalytic treatment proper, is the development of psychoanalytic psychotherapy, also called expressive or exploratory psychotherapy, and of supportive psychotherapy (SP) based on psychoanalytic principles. These treatments are explored below.

Psychoanalytic psychotherapy

Psychoanalytic psychotherapy may be characterized by the same basic techniques as psychoanalysis, but with quantitative modifications that, in combination, result in a qualitative shift in the nature of the treatment. Any given session of psychoanalytic psychotherapy may be indistinguishable from a psychoanalytic session, but over time, the differences emerge quite clearly. Psychoanalytic psychotherapy utilizes interpretation, but with patients with severe psychopathology, a good deal of time must be devoted to clarification and confrontation before interpretation can be effective; and interpretations of unconscious meanings in the 'here and now' occupy the foreground until late in the treatment, when genetic interpretations in the 'there and then' become useful.[15, 37]

In the treatment of patients with severe character pathology, transference analysis is the essential focus of psychoanalytic psychotherapy from the very beginning; it must be modified, however, by active interpretive connection of transference analysis with exploration in depth of the patient's daily life situation, an approach made necessary by the predominance of primitive defence operations in these patients. Splitting operations in particular tend to dissociate the therapeutic situation from the patient's external life, and may lead to severe, dissociated acting out either in the sessions or outside the sessions. Therefore, interpretive linkage between the patient's external reality and transference developments in the hours becomes central.

In order to enable the therapist to analyse transference developments in sufficient depth, psychoanalytic psychotherapy requires a minimum frequency of two sessions per week. It is usually carried out in 'face-to-face' sessions.

Technical neutrality is an essential feature of analysis in general, but in the treatment of patients with severe character pathology, the need to set limits may necessitate abandoning neutrality again and again, in order to control life- or treatment-threatening acting out. The self-perpetuating nature of acting out in these cases may prove impossible to resolve interpretively without such structuring or setting limits. Whenever the analyst has to abandon technical neutrality to protect the patient or the treatment, it is essential to explore the episode immediately. The transference implications of the therapist's structuring behaviour must be laid out, followed by the analysis of the transference implications of the patient's behaviour that necessitated the imposition of limits or the initiation of a new structure in the treatment; this in turn is followed by the gradual resolution of the structure or limit setting by interpretive means, thus restoring technical neutrality. In short, technical neutrality in psychoanalytic psychotherapy is an ideal working state that is again and again preventively abandoned and interpretively reinstated.[15, 37, 38]

Supportive psychotherapy

Supportive psychotherapy based on psychoanalytic theory may also be defined in terms of the three major techniques of interpretation, transference analysis, and technical neutrality. Supportive psychotherapy utilizes the preliminary steps of interpretive technique, i.e. clarification and confrontation, but rarely uses interpretation per se. It seeks to strengthen the ego by bolstering adaptive compromises between impulse and defence through the provision of cognitive support in the form of information, persuasion and advice, and emotional support via suggestion, reassurance, encouragement, and praise. Supportive psychotherapy may call upon direct environmental intervention by the therapist, relatives, or other mental health personnel engaged in auxiliary therapeutic functions.[39]

While the transference is seldom interpreted in supportive psychotherapy, it is not ignored either. Careful attention to transference developments helps the therapist to analyse any maladaptive transference developments, to call the patient's attention to the reproduction with the therapist of pathological interactions the patient generally engages in with significant others, and to encourage the patient to reduce such pathological behaviours. Pointing out the distorted, unproductive, destructive, or confusing nature of the patient's behaviour is accompanied by clarifying the patient's conscious reasons for his behaviour, followed by the transfer or 'export' of the knowledge thus achieved to the patient's relationships outside the treatment. In short, supportive psychotherapy includes the clarification, reduction, and 'export' of the transference, thus contributing to the re-educative functions of supportive psychotherapy together with the direct cognitive and affective support of adaptive combinations of impulse and defence, and direct supportive environmental interventions.

Technical neutrality is systematically abandoned in supportive psychotherapy, the therapist taking a stance alternatively on the side of the ego, superego, id, or external reality, according to which agency represents, at a certain point, the more adaptive potential for the patient. The main dangers, of course, in supportive psychotherapy are, on the one hand, infantilizing the patient by an excessively supportive stance, and, on the other, countertransference acting out as a consequence of the abandonment of the position of technical neutrality. The therapist carrying out supportive psychotherapy, therefore, needs a heightened awareness of the risk of these complications. Like psychoanalytic psychotherapy, supportive psychotherapy is carried out in 'face-to-face' sessions. It has the advantage of considerable flexibility regarding its frequency, from several sessions per week, to one session a week, or one or two sessions per month, according to the urgency of the patient's present difficulties, the long-range objectives of the treatment, and the patient's ability to tolerate and use the relationship with the therapist.

Indications and contraindications for psychoanalysis and derived psychotherapies

The **indications** for these three modalities of treatment remain controversial: with the recognition of the limitations of psychoanalysis in many cases with severe, chronic, life-threatening self-destructive behaviour, such as chronic suicidal behaviour, severe eating disorders, dependence upon drugs or alcohol, and severely antisocial behaviour, psychoanalytic psychotherapy has proven to be a highly effective treatment for many but by no means all patients with these conditions. The differential diagnosis of a spectrum of severity of antisocial behaviour and those cases of severe self-destructive and antisocial behaviour who are amenable to treatment with psychoanalytic psychotherapy has been one of the important side-products of the psychoanalytic exploration of these cases.[37]

Supportive psychotherapy, originally conceived of as the treatment of choice for patients with severe personality disorders, now may be considered the alternative treatment for those patients with severe personality disorders who are unable to participate in psychoanalytic psychotherapy. The Menninger Foundation Psychotherapy Research Project showed that patients with the least severe psychopathological disturbances tend to respond very positively to all three modalities derived from psychoanalytic theory, although best to standard psychoanalysis.[40]

Standard psychoanalysis is the treatment of choice for patients with neurotic personality organization, that is with good identity integration and a repertoire of defences centring on repression along with sufficient severity of illness to warrant such a major therapeutic intervention. Psychoanalysis has also expanded its scope to some of the severe personality disorders, particularly a broad spectrum of patients with narcissistic personality disorders, patient with mixed hysterical-histrionic features, and selected cases of patients with severe paranoid, schizoid, and sado-masochistic features.

We are still lacking systematic studies of the relationship between particular types of psychopathology and outcome with the various psychotherapeutic treatments derived from psychoanalytic theory. As a tentative generalization it may be stated that there is a definite relationship between outcome and the severity of illness in any diagnostic category. The least severe cases will respond favourably to either brief psychoanalytic psychotherapy, supportive psychotherapy, or psychoanalysis. Psychoanalysis represents the opportunity for most improvement if the severity of the case warrants psychoanalytic treatment. For cases of neurotic personality organization of moderate severity, psychoanalysis is the treatment of choice; definitely less can be expected in these cases from psychoanalytic psychotherapy. For the most severely ill patients (those with severe identity diffusion, predominance of primitive defences centring on splitting, and general 'ego weakness') psychoanalytic psychotherapy is the treatment of choice, with supportive psychotherapy a second choice if psychoanalytic psychotherapy is contraindicated. A few such cases may be able to participate in psychoanalysis and benefit from it.

In all cases, individualized **contraindications** for the respective treatment are important: in the case of psychoanalysis, individual contraindications depend on the questions of ego strength, motivation, introspection or insight, secondary gain of illness, intelligence, and age. In the case of psychoanalytic psychotherapy, secondary gain, the impossibility of control of life- or treatment-threatening acting out, limited intelligence, significant antisocial features, and a desperate life situation may constitute individual contraindications, particularly when they occur in combination. When psychoanalytic psychotherapy is contraindicated for such reasons, supportive psychotherapy becomes the treatment of choice. Participation in supportive psychotherapy requires a sufficient capacity for commitment to an ongoing treatment arrangement, and the absence of severe antisocial features as minimal individual requirements. This is not meant to be a complete list, but an illustration of the kind of criteria that become dominant in the individual decisions regarding the selection of the treatment and its contraindications.

Psychoanalytic object-relations theories: overview and critique

Given the centrality of object-relations theory in practically all contemporary psychoanalytic formulations and treatment approaches, the following summary is included. It should help the reader to further clarify the references made earlier to this theory.

Psychoanalytic object-relations theories may be defined as those that place the internalization, structuralization, and reactivation in the transference and countertransference of the earliest dyadic object relations at the centre of their clinical formulations, and of their thinking about motivation, pathogenesis, development, and psychic structure. Internalization of object relations refers to the concept that, in all interactions of the infant and child with the significant parental figures, what the infant internalizes is not merely an image or representation of the other ('the object' of fear, hatred, or desire), but the relationship between the self and the other, in the form of a self-image or self-representation linked to an object image or object representation by the affect that dominates their interaction. This internal structure replicates in the intrapsychic world both real and phantasied relationships with significant others.

Several major issues separate different object-relations theories, the most important of which is the extent to which the theory is perceived as harmonious with or in opposition to Freud's traditional drive theory: i.e. whether object relations are seen as replacing drives as the motivational system for human behaviour. From this perspective, Klein,[9,21] Mahler *et al.*,[13] and Jacobson[12] occupy one pole.

They combine Freud's dual-drive theory with an object-relations theory. For Fairbairn,[10] and Sullivan,[41] on the other hand, object relations themselves replace Freud's drives as the major motivational system. Here, the establishment of gratifying object relations in itself constitutes the major motivational system. Contemporary interpersonal psychoanalysis as represented by Greenberg and Mitchell,[42] based upon an integration of principally Fairbairnian and Sullivanian concepts, asserts the essential incompatibility between drive- and object relations-based models of psychic motivational systems. Winnicott,[11] Loewald,[43] Sandler,[44] and Sandler and Sandler,[45] (each for different reasons) maintain an intermediate posture; they perceive the affective frame of the infant–mother relationship as a crucial determinant in shaping the development of drives. While adhering to Freud's dual-drive theory, Kernberg[15] considers drives supraordinate motivational systems, while affects are their constituent components.

A related controversy has to do with the origin and role of aggression as motivator of behaviour. Those theoreticians who reject the idea of inborn drives,[41] or equate libido with the search for object relations,[10] conceptualize aggression as secondary to the frustration of libidinal needs, particularly traumatic experiences in the early mother–infant dyad. Theoreticians who adhere to Freud's dual-drive theory, in contrast, believe aggression is inborn and plays an important part in shaping early interactions: this group includes Klein in particular, and to some extent Winnicott, and ego-psychology object-relations theoreticians such as Kernberg.[37] Finally, contrast may be made between object-relations theories and French approaches, both Lacanian and (non-Lacanian) mainstream psychoanalysis. The French psychoanalytic mainstream,[46, 47] has maintained close links with traditional psychoanalysis, including the British object-relations theories. Insofar as Lacan[48] conceptualizes the unconscious as a natural language and focuses on the cognitive aspects of unconscious development, he underemphasizes affect—a dominant element of object-relations theories. At the same time, however, in postulating a very early Oedipal structuralization of all infant–mother interactions, Lacan emphasizes archaic Oedipal developments, which implicitly links his formulations with those of Kleinian object-relations theory in general. French mainstream analysis also focuses on archaic aspects of Oedipal developments, but places a traditional emphasis on Freud's dual-drive theory and on the affective nature of the early ego-id. As neither French mainstream nor Lacanian psychoanalysis spells out specific structural consequences of dyadic internalized object relations, however, neither would fit the definition that frames the field of object-relations theory as proposed in this chapter.

All object-relations theories focus heavily on the enactment of internalized object relations in the transference, and on the analysis of countertransference in the development of interpretive strategies. They are particularly concerned with severe psychopathologies, including those psychotic patients who are approachable with psychoanalytic techniques, borderline conditions, severe narcissistic character pathology, and the perversions ('paraphilias'). Object-relations theories explore primitive defensive operations and object relations both in cases of severe psychopathology and at points of severe regression with all patients, regarding such exploration as essential in facilitating transference analysis and conflict resolution.

The contemporary re-evaluation of Freud's dual-drive theory that has occurred mostly in France is relevant to the relationship between object-relations theory and drive theory. Perhaps particularly the work of Laplanche[49] and Green[46] has emphasized the central importance of unconscious destructive and self-destructive drive manifestations in the form of attacks on object relations, and the central role of unconscious erotization in the mother–infant relationship in libidinal development, all of which tends to link drive theory and object-relations theory in intimate ways.

Another important development within psychoanalytic theory has been the growing emphasis on affects as primary motivators, and the centrality of the communicative functions of affects in early development, particularly the infant–mother relationship.[50] This emphasis has linked affect theory and object-relations theory quite closely, despite the persistent controversy between those who see affect, particularly peak affect states, as essential representatives of the drives,[50] and those who stress the psychophysiological nature of the affective response, and attempt to replace drive theory with an affect theory.[51]

The basic (self-representation–object representation) units of internalized object relations include the representative affects, or else, the constituent affective components of the drives. One might say that the affect of sexual excitement is the central affect of libido, in the same way as the affect of primitive hatred constitutes the central affect of the aggressive or death drive. The id is conceptualized in this object-relations theory model as the sum total of repressed, desired, and feared primitive object relations. The gradual integration of successive layers of persecutory and idealized, prohibitive and demanding, internalized object relations become part of the primitive superego, while internalized object relations activated in the service of defence consolidate as part of an integrated self-structure surrounded by integrated representations of significant others. In short, the id or dynamic unconscious, the superego, and the ego are constituted by different constellations of internalized object relations, so that the development of the drives and the development of the psychic apparatus—the tripartite structure—occur hand in hand.

Perhaps the most important practical implication of object-relations theory is the conception of identification as a series of internalization processes of dyadic units of self-representation and object representation linked by a dominant affect state, ranging from earliest introjections to identifications per se, to the development of complex identity formation. Each step includes the internalizing of both self and object representations and their affective interactions under the conditions that prevail at different developmental levels.

In the transference of healthier patients, with a well-consolidated ego identity, the diverse self-representations are relatively stable in their coherent mutual linkage. This fosters the relatively consistent projection onto the analyst of the object representation aspect of the enacted object relationship. In contrast, patients with severe identity diffusion lack such linkage of self-representations into an integrated self. They tend to alternate rapidly between projection of self and object representations in the transference, so that the analytic situation seems chaotic. Systematic interpretation of how the same internalized object relation is enacted again and again with rapid role reversals between patient and analyst makes it possible to clarify the nature of the unconscious object relation, and the double splitting of self-representation from object representation and idealized from persecutory object relations. This process of interpretation promotes integration of the split representations, which characterize severe psychopathology and account for the marked instability of the emotions, behaviour, and interpersonal relationships of these patients.

Kernberg[37] proposes that affects are the primary motivational system and that, internalized or fixated as the very frame of internalized 'good' and 'bad' object relations, affects are gradually integrated into libidinal and aggressive drives to form hierarchically supraordinate motivational systems. In other words, primitive affects are the 'building blocks' of the drives. He sees unconscious intrapsychic conflicts as always between the following:

1 certain units of self and object representations under the impact of a particular drive derivative (clinically, a certain affect disposition reflecting the drive derivative side of the conflict);

2 contradictory or opposing units of self and object representations and their respective affect dispositions reflecting the defensive structure.

Unconscious intrapsychic conflicts are never simply between impulse and defence; rather, both impulse and defence find expression, respectively, through certain internalized object relations.

In patients with borderline personality organization and severe conflicts around early aggression, splitting mechanisms stabilize such dynamic structures within an ego-id matrix and permit the contradictory aspects of these conflicts to remain at least partially conscious, in the form of primitive, mutually split-off, idealized, and persecutory transferences. In contrast, patients with neurotic personality organization present impulse–defence configurations that contain specific unconscious wishes of an integrated though infantile self, reflecting sexual and aggressive drive derivatives embedded in unconscious phantasies relating to the Oedipal objects. Repressed unconscious wishes, however, always come in the form of corresponding units composed of self-representation and object representation and affect linking them.

Patients with neurotic personality organization present well-integrated superego, ego, and id structures; within the psychoanalytic situation, the analysis of resistances brings about the activation, in the transference, first of relatively global characteristics of these structures, and later, the internalized object relations of which they are composed. Oedipal conflicts dominate the dynamic unconscious of these patients. The analysis of drive derivatives occurs in the context of the analysis of the relation of the patient's infantile self to significant parental objects as projected onto the analyst.

Patients with severe personality disorders or borderline personality organization, in contrast, show a predominance of psychic representations of pre-Oedipal conflicts, with pre-Oedipal aggression, in particular, condensed with representations of the Oedipal phase. Conflicts are not predominantly repressed and therefore unconsciously dynamic: rather, they are avoided by being represented in mutually dissociated ego states reflecting the defence of primitive dissociation or splitting. The activation of primitive object relations that predate the consolidation of ego, superego, and id is manifest in the transference as apparently chaotic affect states, which have to be analysed in sequential steps as follows:

1 the clarification of a dominant primitive object relation in the transference, with its corresponding self and object representation, and the dominant affect linking them;

2 the analysis of the alternative projection of self and object representation onto the therapist, while the patient identifies with a reciprocal self or object representation of this object relationship, leading to the patient's gradual capacity to become aware of his identification with an object in that relationship;

3 the interpretive integration of mutually split-off, idealized and persecutory 'part object' relations with the characteristics mentioned.

This analysis may gradually bring about a transformation of mutually split, ('part object') relations into 'total object' relations, or of primitive transferences (largely reflecting Mahler's stages of development that predate object constancy) into the advanced transferences of the Oedipal phase. In other words, a gradual integration of self-representations into an integrated self-concept, and a parallel integration of significant object representations into integrated concepts of significant others develop first in the transference, and later generalize in the patient's relations with significant others. The analyst's exploration of his or her countertransference, including concordant and complementary identifications in the countertransference,[27] facilitates transference analysis; and the analysis of primitive defensive operations, particularly splitting and projective identification in the transference, also contributes to strengthening the patient's ego.

Treatment results: research on outcome

The psychoanalytic profession has been slow in developing systematic research on treatment process and results, let alone controlled randomized comparison of treatment methods evaluating efficacy and efficiency. The reasons are multiple: the complexity of the psychoanalytic treatment, and the changes in its technique; the long duration of treatment, making systematic research, and controlled comparison with other treatment methods difficult; the private nature of psychoanalytic exploration in the context of patients' regression, and the related concerns over disturbing the therapeutic relationship by recording or direct observation. In addition, the general methodology of psychotherapy research evolved to a degree of sophistication applicable to the evaluation of psychoanalytic treatment only in recent decades. With all these reservations, significant progress has been made, and outcome studies are beginning to be available.

The Menninger Psychotherapy Research Project, a naturalistic study comparing psychoanalysis, psychoanalytic psychotherapy, and SP, showed psychoanalysis to be the most effective of these approaches with patients presenting relatively good ego strength, while patients with severe ego weakness—what nowadays would be described as presenting severe personality disorders or borderline personality organization—improved most with psychoanalytic psychotherapy.[39] This research also showed how important supportive elements were throughout all modalities of treatment.[52] A comprehensive review of outcome studies on psychoanalytic psychotherapy and psychoanalysis by Bachrach *et al.*[53] concluded that the improvement rates are in the 60 to 90 per cent, but it also pointed to limitations and problems in the methodology utilized.

Recently, studies regarding the treatment process and outcome of psychoanalysis and psychoanalytic psychotherapy have become more precise in defining the specific treatment variables of psychotherapeutic and psychoanalytic treatments, and several systematic studies on psychoanalytic psychotherapies and psychoanalysis are in progress.[54] A recent study by the Stockholm Outcome of Psychoanalysis and Psychotherapy Project has found, on the basis of a relatively large patient population, that psychoanalytic treatment, in comparison with psychoanalytic psychotherapy, obtained a significantly higher degree long-range symptomatic improvement.[55] The extent to which the psychotherapist had years of experience linked with appropriate, long-term supervisory experiences, i.e. an 'experiential learning cluster', was related to treatment outcome, in the sense that those therapists with long experiences in doing teaching or supervision of psychotherapy had a significantly better outcome than therapists who only had been in supervision or personal therapy for long periods. It also appeared that the maintenance of a rigid 'psychoanalytic' attitude as part of a psychoanalytic psychotherapy was not as effective as a more flexible shift in techniques in psychotherapy, but not in analysis proper.[56] A manualized psychoanalytic psychotherapy for a specific patient population, namely, the psychotherapy research project of the Cornell Personality Disorders Institute's manualized treatment for borderline patients has provided evidence for the efficacy of the treatment with severely ill patients. This treatment, called Transference Focused Psychotherapy (TFP) was found to be more effective than treatments as usual (TAU) for borderline patients,[38] and, compared to dialectic behaviour therapy (DBT), and supportive psychotherapy (SP) in a randomized controlled study, proved as effective as DBT and SP in improving depression, anxiety, global functioning, and social adjustment at the end of 1 year of treatment. It also was more effective in reducing aggression than DBT and SP, and the only one to improve reflective function (RF), an index of mentalization, that is the patient's capacity for self-reflection and appropriate assessment of others in depth.[57,58] (Bateman and Fonagy[59,60] have found that mentalization-based therapy (MBT), another form of psychoanalytic psychotherapy was more effective than treatment as usual (TAU) in the treatment of borderline patients in a day hospital setting. Further developments of MBT research will be referred to in Sections 3, 5, and 6.

In summary, process research has predated outcome research on psychoanalysis and derived psychotherapies; major efforts at outcome research are being made, and should contribute to clarify the effects, not only of psychoanalysis proper, but also of the derived psychotherapeutic approaches now being carried out in clinical practice.

Further information

Cooper, A.M. (ed.) (2006). *Contemporary psychoanalysis in America: leading analysts present their work.* American Psychiatric Publishing, Washington, DC.

Kernberg, O.F. (2004). *Contemporary controversies in psychoanalytic theory, techniques, and their applications.* Yale University Press, New Haven.

Laplanche, J. and Pontalis, J.-B. (2006). *The language of psychoanalysis.* Karnac Books, London.

Skelton, R.M. (ed.) (2006). *The Edinburgh international encyclopedia of psychoanalysis.* Edinburgh University Press, Edinburgh.

References

1. Freud, S. (1963). *Introductory lectures on psycho-analysis. Standard edition*, Vol. 16, pp. 243–463. Hogarth Press, London.
2. Freud, S. (1964). *An outline of psycho-analysis. Standard edition*, Vol. 23, pp. 141–207. Hogarth Press, London.
3. Breuer, J. and Freud, S. (1955). *Studies on hysteria. Standard edition*, Vol. 2, pp. 3–311. Hogarth Press, London.
4. Freud, S. (1953). *Three essays on the theory of sexuality. Standard edition*, Vol. 7, pp. 125–245. Hogarth Press, London.
5. Freud, S. (1961). *The ego and the id. Standard edition*, Vol. 19, pp. 3–66. Hogarth Press, London.
6. Freud, S. (1957). *Mourning and melancholia. Standard edition*, Vol. 14, pp. 237–58. Hogarth Press, London.
7. Freud, S. (1955). *Beyond the pleasure principle. Standard edition.* Hogarth Press, London.
8. Freud, S. (1961). *Civilization and its discontents. Standard edition*, Vol. 21, pp. 57–145. Hogarth Press, London.
9. Klein, M. (1952). Notes on some schizoid mechanisms. In *Developments in psycho-analysis* (ed. J. Riviere), pp. 292–320. Hogarth Press, London.
10. Fairbairn, W.R.D. (1954). *An object-relations theory of the personality.* Basic Books, New York.
11. Winnicot, D. (1965). *The maturational processes and the facilitating environment.* International Universities Press, New York.
12. Jacobson, E. (1964). *The self and the object world.* International Universities Press, New York.
13. Mahler, M., Pine, F., and Bergman, A. (1975). *The psychological birth of the human infant.* Basic Books, New York.
14. Freud, S. (1957). *Instincts and their vicissitudes. Standard edition*, Vol. 14, pp. 109–40. Hogarth Press, London.
15. Kernberg, O. (1984). *Severe personality disorders. Psychotherapeutic strategies.* Yale University Press, New Haven.
16. Kohut, H. (1971). *The analysis of the self.* International Universities Press, New York.
17. Freud, S. (1964). *Splitting of the ego in the process of defense. Standard edition*, Vol. 23, pp. 273–4. Hogarth Press, London.
18. Abraham, K. (1920). Manifestations of the female castration complex. In *Selected papers on psycho-analysis*, pp. 338–69. Brunner/Mazel, New York.
19. Freud, S. (1957). *On narcissism. Standard edition*, Vol. 14, pp. 69–102. Hogarth Press, London.
20. Abraham, K. (1979). A particular form of neurotic resistance against the psychoanalytic method. In *Selected papers on psycho-analysis.* (1919), pp. 303–11. Brunner/Mazel, New York.
21. Klein, M. (1957). *Envy and gratitude.* Basic Books, New York.
22. Rosenfeld, H. (1964). On the psychopathology of narcissism: a clinical approach. *International Journal of Psycho-Analysis*, **45**, 332–7.
23. Grunberger, B. (1979). *Narcissism: psychoanalytic essays.* International Universities Press, New York.
24. Kernberg, O.F. (1975). *Borderline conditions and pathological narcissism.* Jason Aronson, Inc., New York.
25. Freud, S. (1953). *Fragment of an analysis of a case of hysteria. Standard edition*, Vol. 7, pp. 3–122. Hogarth Press, London.
26. Gill, M. (1954). Psychoanalysis and exploratory psychotherapy. *Journal of American Psychoanalytic Association*, **2**, 771–97.
27. Racker, H. (1957). The meaning and uses of countertransference. *Psychoanalytic Quarterly*, **26**, 303–57.
28. Bion, W.R. (1967). *Second thoughts. Selected papers on psychoanalysis.* Basic Books, New York.
29. Freud, S. (1953). *The interpretation of dreams. Standard edition*, Vol. 4, pp. 1–338; Vol. 5, pp. 339–625. Hogarth Press, London.
30. Reich, W. (1972). *Character analysis.* Farrar, Straus, & Giroux, New York.
31. Rosenfeld, H. (1987). *Impasse and interpretation.* Tavistock, New York.
32. Steiner, J. (1993). *Psychic retreats*, Routledge, London.
33. Gray, P. (1994). *The ego and analysis of defense.* Aronson, Northvale, NJ.
34. Busch, F. (1995). *The ego at the center of clinical technique.* Jason Aronson, Northvale, NJ.
35. Fenichel, O. (1941). *Problems of psychoanalytic technique.* Psychoanalytic Quarterly, Inc., Albany.
36. Bion, W.R. (1967). *Second thoughts. Selected papers on psychoanalysis.* Basic Books, New York.
37. Kernberg, O.F. (1992). *Aggression in personality disorders and perversion.* Yale University Press, New Haven.
38. Clarkin, J.F., Foelsch, P.A., Levy, K.N., *et al.* (2001). The development of a psychodynamic treatment for patients with borderline personality

disorder: a preliminary study of behavioral change. *Journal of Personality Disorders*, **15**, 487–95.

39. Rockland, L.H. (1989). *Supportive therapy: a psychodynamic approach*. Basic Books, New York.
40. Kernberg, O.F., Burnstein, E., Coyne, L., *et al.* (1972). Psychotherapy and psychoanalysis: final report of the menninger foundation's psychotherapy research project. *Bulletin Menninger Clinic*, **36**, 1–275.
41. Sullivan, H. (1953). *The interpersonal theory of Psychiatry*. Norton, New York.
42. Greenberg, J.R. and Mitchell, S.A. (1983). *Object relations in psychoanalytic theory*. Harvard University Press, Cambridge, MA.
43. Loewald, H.W. (1960). On the therapeutic action of psycho-analysis. *International Journal of Psycho-Analysis*, **41**, 16–33.
44. Sandler, J. (1987). *From safety to superego: selected papers of Joseph Sandler*. Guilford Press, New York.
45. Sandler, J. and Sandler, A.M. (1998). *Internal objects revisited*. Karnac Books, London.
46. Green, A. (1993). *Le Travail du Négatif*. Paris: Les Editions de Minuit.
47. Laplanche, J. (1992). *Seduction, translation, drives*. Psychoanalytic Forum. Institute of Contemporary Arts, London.
48. Lacan, J. (1966). *Ecrits*. Editions du Seuil, Paris.
49. Laplanche, J. (1987). *Nouveaux fondements pour la psychanalyse*. Presses Universitaires de France.
50. Krause, R. (1998). *Allgemeine Psychoanalytische Krankheitslehre*, Vols 1 and 2. Kohlhammer, Stuttgart.
51. Mitchell, S. (1988). *Relational concepts in psychoanalysis*. Harvard University Press, Cambridge, MA.
52. Wallerstein, R. (1986). *Forty-two lives in treatment: A study of psycho-analysis and psychotherapy*. Guilford Press, New York.
53. Bachrach, H.M., Weber, J.J., and Murray, S. (1985). Factors associated with the outcome of psychoanalysis. Report of the Columbia Psychoanalytic Research Center (IV). *International Review of Psychoanalysis*, **12**, 379–89.
54. Fonagy, P., Kächele, H., Krause, R., *et al.* (eds.) (1998). *An open door review of outcome studies in psychoanalysis*. International Psychoanalytic Association, London.
55. Sandell, R., Blomberg, J., and Lazar, A. (1997). When reality doesn't fit the blueprint: doing research on psychoanalysis and long-term psychotherapy in a public health service program. *Psychotherapy Research*, **7**, 333–44.
56. Sandell, R., Schubert, J., Blomberg, J., *et al.* (1997). The influence of therapist factors on outcomes of psychotherapy and psychoanalysis in the Stockholm Outcome of Psychotherapy and Psychoanalysis Project (STOPP). Paper presented at the Annual Meeting of the Society for Psychotherapy Research, Geilo, Norway.
57. Clarkin, J. F., Levy, K.N., and Schiavi, J.M. (2005). Transferenced focused psychotherapy: development of a psychodynamic treatment for severe personality disorders. *Clinical Neuroscience Research*, **4**, 379–86.
58. Clarkin, J.F., Yeomans, F., and Kernberg, O.F. (2006). *Psychotherapy for borderline personality: focusing on object relations*. American Psychiatric Publishing, Washington, DC.
59. Bateman, A. and Fonagy, P. (2004a). *Psychotherapy for borderline personality disorder: Mentalization-based treatment*. Oxford University Press, New York.
60. Bateman, A. and Fonagy, P. (2004b). Mentalization-based treatment of BPD. *Journal of Personality Disorders*, **18**, 36–51.

3.2

Object relations, attachment theory, self-psychology, and interpersonal psychoanalysis

Jeremy Holmes

Despite many splits and schisms, dating back to Adler and Jung's early break with Freud, there has been an enduring attempt within psychoanalysis to hold to a central psychodynamic vision and to find common ground between differing theoretical and clinical approaches. The aim of this chapter is to describe the work of some of the major figures who have extended and developed Freud's ideas, pointing to areas of both conflict and convergence, and, wherever possible, to relate their concepts to the everyday practice of psychiatry.

From drive theory to object relations

Psychoanalysis started its life as a 'drive theory' or 'dual instinct' theory—the idea that mental life and its pathologies could be understood in terms of the interplay between the erotic and death drives, and the ways in which these were repressed, or expressed either covertly via 'conversion', or directly. As Freud's thought evolved, so new paradigms began to emerge. Drive theory had little to say about relationships: other people appear merely as satisfiers or thwarters of an individual's instinctual needs. Freud began to ask how children, and later adults, reconciled their own wishes and desires—their drives or instincts—with those of their care-givers and peers. Struggling with this problem, while remaining within the confines of drive theory, he now differentiated between self-love, or narcissism, and other, or 'anaclitic', love, directed outwards. In this model, the individual gradually emerges from egg-like self-absorption and healthy narcissism into the world of relationships.

A further push towards a more relational theory came from Abraham, later to become Melanie Klein's analyst, who noticed the parallels between the phenomena of grief and depression. The intense psychic pain and disruption associated with a loss suggested a much more intimate connection between relationships and the architecture of the psyche than drive theory would allow. 'The unconscious' is not so much a repository of drives and desires, but an inner world populated by significant others or 'objects'. The self is forged out of these 'objects' with whom the individual has or has had important relationships: 'the shadow of the object falls on the ego'.[1] A further theoretical move arose from considering the origins of conscience and ideals. It is a matter of observation that much of development depends on processes of imitation and identification. The developing child internalizes, or 'introjects', his or her parent's values and standards. How, and where in the psyche, does this process take place? In Freud's 'tripartite model', the 'superego', alongside the ego (i.e. executive and experienced self) and the id (the locus of desire and dreaming), is the focus for these internalized parental values and aspirations. The inner world now contained not just 'objects', but value-based relations between them: prohibitions, encouragements, injunctions, and gratifications. Much of post-Freudian theory consists of attempts to develop and elaborate these ideas.

Object relations 1: Klein, Fairbairn, and their successors

This was the state of theoretical play in psychoanalysis when **Melanie Klein** first burst on to the scene in the late 1920s. Like Freud, her work can be divided into a number of phases.[2,3]

Psychoanalysis is concerned with early mental life, which it sees as the basis for much adult psychopathology. But how do we gain access to the thought processes of small children, whose verbal and introspective capacities are limited or non-existent? Klein's great technical innovation was the introduction of play therapy. She provided her little patients with play materials—paper and pencils, a doll house with figures, a sandpit, and farmyard animals—and observed the pictures and games which the children set-up, making her interpretations around them. She used the methods of dream interpretation to formulate her ideas. What she observed in play—movement of figures in and out; bringing things together, often violently; separation and disruption—she took to represent the workings of the child's mind. Still deeply influenced by drive theory, and by Freud's insistence on the pre-eminence of sexuality and castration anxiety, she found sexual and aggressive meanings in all that was presented to her. Every vertical line or orifice-shaped circle drawn had a sexual significance; every conjoining or emitted sound stood for parental intercourse, by which the child was both fascinated and frightened. Exploration and the drive to know were seen as an expression of the desire to possess the mother's body, and inhibitions of learning as manifestations of castration anxiety.

Here Klein began to depart from Freud. For him the Oedipus complex arose around the age of three, when the child begins to observe his or her parents' relationship and to feel such emotions as passionate love, envy, fear, and jealous vengefulness. Klein, by contrast, saw Oedipal phenomena as arising much earlier in development. For example, the infant may experience weaning as a punishment or symbolic castration, and believe that his mother's breast in his mouth has been displaced by the paternal penis in her vagina. Two other aspects of Kleinian thought emerge from this. First, in Klein's schema the infant has an instinctual knowledge of the body and its relationships. There appears to be a reservoir of unconscious phantasy, which she saw as the mental accompaniment of bodily function: phantasies about the breast, the mouth, the penis, the vagina, and their relationships that could not have arisen from direct observation, and therefore must be present from within, as correlates of the child's bodily sensations, which Klein saw as dominating the early years of life. Unconscious phantasies are akin to Jungian archetypes or perhaps the 'language acquisition devise' postulated by linguists: preformed mental constructs unconsciously shaping experience and patterns of relationship.

Second, and closely related to unconscious phantasy, is the idea of internal objects—initially body parts, and later 'whole objects' that are salient to emotional life—the mother and her breast, the father and his penis, bellies and their contents such as unborn babies, faeces, and sphincters. These objects are endowed with motivational properties reflecting the infant's emotional life, which Klein saw as dominated by persecutory fears. The 'death instinct' ensures that the child reacts to frustration with overwhelming feelings of hatred and destructiveness. These feelings are then projected outwards on to the objects in the child's emotional environment, which are in turn reintrojected to populate the inner world. To preserve good feelings from these terrifying bad objects, the child also projects goodness outwards. Thus a radical split arises between good and bad experiences, which are attributed to good and bad objects: 'in the very earliest stage every unpleasant stimulus is related to the 'bad', denying, persecuting breasts, every 'good' experience to the 'good' gratifying breasts'.[(2)]

Klein depicts early emotional life as dominated by the infant's fears of annihilation from without, and the use of the mechanisms of splitting and projection to reduce these fears. She postulated the onset of a new type of anxiety towards the end of the first year of life. Here the infant is beginning to bring the image of the 'good' and the 'bad' breast together, and to realize that they are one and the same. With weaning, the child experiences his first major loss. Now 'depressive' anxiety comes into the picture. The child believes that he is responsible for the loss, and that he has destroyed the good object with his aggression and sadism. He begins to feel guilt and remorse, and wants to repair the damage he believes he has inflicted on his objects. His attempts at creation, the gifts he offers, and the charm with which he approaches his caregivers are all motivated by this sense of depressive despair and the wish to make reparation.

Klein thus described a developmental sequence: inherent aggression, annihilation anxiety, projection and splitting of the object into good and bad, loss, bringing together the split objects, depressive despair, concern for the object, and finally reparation. For her this was a description of normal development, and she saw pathological states as resulting from developmental arrest along this line. The fulcrum of this sequence is the movement from what, drawing on Fairbairn's term (see below) Klein now called the **'paranoid–schizoid' position** (**PSP**) to the **'depressive' position** (**DP**), a movement from splitting, blaming, and avoidance, to integration, responsibility, and concern for the object (see Hobson *et al.*[(4)] for objective evidence of the validity of the PSP–DP distinction). Klein saw the struggle between PSP and DP as a lifelong process, an equilibrium driven one way or the other depending on life experience and constitutional endowment.

Klein was generally rather unconcerned about the impact of external reality on psychological development (a point which, as we shall see, stimulated Bowlby's divergence from her ideas). To the extent that she did consider the real as opposed to the phantasized role of the parents, it was as benign figures whose job it is to mitigate the strength of the infant's need to hate, project, and split. An important late theoretical contribution, however, concerned the role of envy in psychic life. One of the strengths of a psychoanalytical approach to psychotherapy is that it takes seriously the phenomenon of resistance, and the fact that psychic growth is usually hard-won, often with much backsliding and self-defeatingness. With her emphasis on the dark side of human nature, Klein realized that the infant may feel persecuted not just by frustration and separation, but also by the very capacity of the caregiver to satisfy his needs. The breast upon which the baby depends for satisfaction and pleasure can also be a source of envy and hatred in its plenitude and ability to create dependency. This **envy** then becomes a basis for destructiveness within psychotherapy, and more generally: an explanation, perhaps, for the graffiti which inevitably appear on beautiful buildings, or, at times, the fact that patients attack and seem to want to destroy the very help that is offered to them.

Another key Kleinian concept is that of **projective identification** (**PI**), a difficult and perhaps misnamed concept, coined almost casually by Klein in an attempt to describe how parts of the ego may be split-off and projected not just *on to* objects in the environment as visualized in Freud's notion of projection, but *into* them. As originally conceived by Klein PI referred to the solipsistic world of the infant described above, in which unbearable feelings of rage and hatred are split-off, projected into the breast, which is then perceived by the child as 'having' properties that in fact originated in the self. Projective identification here is a form of misperception or delusional perception, which can be used both to explain the fact that normal adults' experience of the world is inevitably coloured by their emotional state (the gloomy or rose-tinted spectacles with which we view the world), and to account for delusional ideas in psychosis, such as paranoid feelings of persecution which, it is hypothesized, originate in the subject's own aggressive phantasies but are attributed, via projective identification, to persecutors.

Projective identification differs from simple projection in that the objects of PI are induced or controlled by the projection in such a way that they then *enact* the phantasy, which has been transferred into them. Paranoid people have the capacity to make those around them behave in suspicious or hostile ways, and thus projective identification can be thought of as a form of communication in which the recipient of the projection is induced to think or feel in ways that properly 'belong' to the projector. Post-Kleinian authors, notably Bion,[(5)] Heimann,[(6)] and Ogden,[(7)] have extended the concept of projective identification, with an emphasis on this communicative aspect, in that PI requires a recipient as well as a projector.

Bion, an analysand of Klein, realized that projective identification also underlies normal empathy and fellow feeling. PI is 'primitive' in the sense that preverbal children rely on it almost exclusively to communicate their feelings, but this denotes immaturity rather than pathology. Bion went on to develop his **container-contained** theory of early emotional communication. Here the mother, or 'breast', acts, via PI, as a recipient or container for the infant's unmanageable feelings of fear, hatred, annihilation, etc. These feelings are contained or held by the mother, and 'detoxified' before they are 'returned' to the infant through her understanding and empathic handling. She knows intuitively—through projective identification—when her child cries whether it is hungry or cold, or bored or wet, etc., and responds appropriately. In this way the infant begins to build-up a sense of himself through the **reflective awareness** of the mother. Disruptions of this process, for example through maternal depression or the violent use by the parent of the infant as a container (**role reversal**) as occurs in child abuse, may sow the seeds of disorders of identity found in borderline personality disorder in later life.

PI is important in the contemporary understanding of **countertransference**. Paula Heimann pointed out that the therapist's reactions to the patient, while no doubt coloured to some extent by her own conflicts (Freud's classical conceptualization of countertransference), also represent feelings induced by contact with the patient, that is to say they are a manifestation of projective identification. By attending to these thoughts and feelings the therapist gains clues about the patient's state of mind, which can then be put into words as interpretations. Here the therapist's mind is the container for the patient's split-off feelings. Sometimes this container-contained relationship fails, and the therapist is induced to enact some aspect of the patient's inner world, for instance by forgetting an appointment with a patient who has felt neglected and overlooked as a child, or by expressing anger or boredom in his tone of voice, being himself moved by feelings which properly belong to the patient.

The firm boundaries of psychotherapy are, in part, designed to minimize these occurrences (although they are unavoidable, and often, if reflected on, can be put to good use in the form of deepened understanding), but in the much more uncontained setting of general psychiatric wards or community mental health centres such enactments are widespread. A common example would be the polarization which disturbed people with borderline personality disorder can induce in their carers, some seeing the patient as manipulative and demanding, others feeling intense sympathy, and the wish to repair past hurts on the patient's behalf. Each perspective represents a split-off aspect of the patient's inner world that has been picked up via PI by different staff members. This is an essentially interactive process, since, no doubt, what determines which aspect depends on the carers' own developmental history and defensive strategies.

Working in the relative isolation of Scotland, and coming to essentially similar conclusions to Klein about the importance of splitting, W.R.D. Fairbairn[(8)] further developed this interpersonal perspective. For him drives were 'a signpost to the object', the glue that held human beings together. Sex is what gets us close to those who matter, rather than vice versa, as originally conceived by Freud. Like Bion later, Fairbairn also placed great emphasis on the role of the mother and of environmental failure as a source of psychopathology. Frustration plays a central part in his schema. With a perfectly responsive mother, the child has no need to think or develop an inner world. When separation and frustration come into play, the child then builds up an image of the object, which is split into three parts: the **ideal object** (one that would never cause frustration), the **libidinal object** (one that could satisfy the child's drive-related needs), and the **anti-libidinal object** (the one that frustrates). This in turn sets up a split of the self into three corresponding parts—ideal self, libidinal self, and anti-libidinal self. The Fairbairnian model provides clarity in understanding some typical phenomena found in severe personality disturbance: the swing between idealization and denigration of therapists and partners (who become the anti-libidinal withholding object at that point), the self-destructiveness of the anti-libidinal self, or 'internal saboteur', and the split-off search for pure libidinal satisfaction unrelated to persons represented by substance abuse and promiscuity.

Fairbairn's notion of schizoid withdrawal was conceptualized as a typical interpersonal strategy in the face of frustration. John Steiner[(9)] has developed a similar idea in his notion of the psychic retreat, an inner place to which individuals with borderline personality may repair in the face of environmental trauma, and which may make them relatively inaccessible in therapy. Another important neo-Kleinian development has been Ronald Britton's[(10)] attempt to link the Oedipus complex with the tolerance of separateness and loss implicit in the depressive position. Britton sees the ability, at times, to let go of the mother as the Oedipal stage is successfully negotiated—in which the child comes to see that his mother and father are sexually involved with one another and he is necessarily excluded—as an important developmental step towards the establishment of an inner world and the ability to see things from varying perspectives. This can be linked with Bion's idea of creative thought in which ideas are brought together to create 'conceptions', in contrast to the destructiveness of schizoid thinking in which, as a way of reducing anxiety, the links between things and ideas are attacked, and the world emptied of meaning. The restoration of meaning is a central task of psychotherapy. The dialectic of close involvement and repeated separation inherent in the therapeutic relationship fosters this capacity, enabling disturbed patients first to **find their experience mirrored** by the responsive therapist, then gradually to **tolerate loss and envy**, and so to gain the capacity to think and to feel more autonomously.

Object relations 2: Balint and Winnicott

The 'Object relations' school of psychoanalysis is a broad church. Klein's view of the mind and of psychopathology was essentially a **conflictual** model: difficulty arises out of the inherent conflict in an immature mind between love and hate, and attempts to avoid the inevitability of loss. For her, such conflict was characteristic of normal development, and pathology merely an exaggeration of normal conflict in which the environment has failed to mitigate its potentially destructive effects. By contrast, the non-Kleinian members of the 'object relations' school tend to espouse some variety of a **deficit** model, in which normal and abnormal development are more sharply differentiated, and the basis for psychopathology is a failure of the environment to provide the conditions needed for healthy psychic growth.

Michael Balint[(11)] is perhaps best known for his work in raising psychological awareness among general practitioners through the use of 'Balint groups', but he was also a significant figure in psychoanalysis, introducing a number of key terms and concepts. In contrast to Klein, who saw the newborn infant as wracked with fear and conflict, Balint proposed a state of **primary love** characterizing the early mother–infant relationship—which he described as a 'harmonious interpenetrative mix-up'. Where, however, parenting was inadequate, due to neglect, overintrusiveness, aggression, or abuse he claimed that the child would be permanently scarred at the level of the '**basic fault**'. His model of therapy implied a **remedial**, rather than purely **interpretative** approach, with the therapist's role including both quiet acceptance, and on occasion therapeutic 'acting in': Balint would sometimes gently hold the patient's hand, and, famously, once encouraged a patient who stated that she had never had the courage to do a somersault to try one out in the consulting room then and there (behaviour therapy meets psychoanalysis!).

Donald Winnicott,[12] visualized an intermediate zone in the early years of life that was neither the realm of pure phantasy (as described by Klein), nor that of reality (to which adaptation by the ego was required, as described by Freud), although it partakes of both. In this intermediate, or **transitional** zone the infant learns, with the help of the mother, to play (another key Winnicottian theme). Here phantasies can become reality, at least for the duration of the interactive play. In this transitional space Winnicott saw the origins of creativity and culture generally, and of a nascent sense of self. He suggested that the mother's face is a kind of mirror in which the child sees his own feelings reflected, and through this recognition begins to gain a sense of who he is. This process is disrupted if the mother is depressed or abusive, and here perhaps are the germs of borderline personality disorder, characterized by a deficient sense of self, and feelings of inner emptiness and sterility. Winnicott saw 'learning to play' as a key task in therapy in helping patients to regain their sense of self.

A related phenomenon is that of the **transitional object**—the special handkerchiefs, teddy bears, and precious playthings that toddlers often need for comfort and to help them sleep. Winnicott saw these as buffers against loss, objects that are invested with the properties of the primary object (the mother and her breast) but remain under the control of the child. They are 'transitional' in the sense that they lie between the ideal object of phantasy and the real, but potentially unreliable, objects of external reality.

The subtlety of Winnicott's thought is exemplified by his notion of the **good-enough mother**. Unlike some psychoanalytical writers he did not attribute all the evils of mankind to parental failure. Winnicott realized that a 'perfect' mother, intrusively aware of her infant's needs could inhibit rather than foster the development of a sense of oneself as a separate and autonomous being. Mothers (and presumably fathers) should be 'good enough', not perfect, not least because through healthy protest about parental failure the child learns his own strength and finds limits, which reassure him that his parents can withstand his aggression and still love him.

Winnicott realized that developmental deficit does not always take the form of neglect or overt violence. He noticed the ways in which parents, driven by their own unconscious needs, may subtly impose their will on a compliant child, thereby inhibiting the growth of a robust and distinct sense of self. The **false-self-real-self** distinction tries to capture the ways in which children, and later personality disordered adults, may present an acceptable face to the world that is radically at variance with inner feelings of terror, emptiness, or rage. In his seminal, but today largely forgotten, classic *The Divided Self*, R.D. Laing[13] took Winnicott's false-self-real-self distinction as a central theme in his psychodynamic account of schizophrenia, seeing delusions as representing a way of holding together, albeit 'falsely', a disintegrating 'real' self and its inner world.

John Bowlby and attachment theory

Winnicott's contemporary John Bowlby[14] life's work was an attempt to bring logical and scientific rigour to psychoanalytical thought. Attachment theory, an empirically validated version of object relations theory, starts from Freud's[15] revised theory of anxiety, in which, rather than viewing it as the result of incomplete repression of incestual wishes, **anxiety is conceptualized in interpersonal terms as a response to the threat of the loss of a loved one**. Based on his observations of delinquent youths, many of whom had suffered the loss of a parent during early childhood, and the depressive reactions of small children to separation from their parents on entering hospital, Bowlby saw that protection from danger was a key component of the parent–child relationship, and that there were built-in psychological mechanisms to ensure the maintenance of attachment bonds.

Attachment theory[16] postulates that, when faced with threat, illness, or exhaustion, children will seek proximity to their caregivers, or '**secure base**'. A protective response from the caregiver assuages the child's attachment needs, who can then return to play or exploratory behaviour, secure in the knowledge that help will once more be at hand if needed. This provides the conditions for **secure attachment**, and the child builds up an **internal working model** (Bowlby's preferred term for the inner world) of a secure robust self and responsive others.

Secure attachment arises out of **responsive and sensitive parenting** and is contrasted with **insecure attachment**, which Bowlby saw as a factor predisposing to adult neurosis. Bowlby's collaborator, Mary Ainsworth, and her students, have researched different patterns of insecure attachment and the conditions under which they arise.[17] They delineate three main types of insecure attachment: **insecure-avoidant, insecure-ambivalent, and insecure-disorganized**. The avoidant child has experienced brusque or aggressive parenting, and tends to avoid close contact with people, hovering near caregivers rather than openly expressing need when faced with threat. The ambivalent child clings to his inconsistent parents, and finds exploratory play difficult, even when the danger has past. Disorganized children behave in bizarre ways when threatened, and tend to have parents who are either emotionally intrusive or absent, often in the context of a parental history of abuse in their childhood. Disorganization is thought to be a severe form of insecure attachment and a possible precursor of severe personality disorder and dissociative phenomena in adolescence and early adulthood.

Mary Main[18] has developed a psychodynamic interview schedule, the Adult Attachment Interview (**AAI**), which is rated for the interviewee's narrative style, and, in long-term follow-up studies of children whose attachment patterns have been classified in infancy, yields significant links with these earlier patterns of attachment. As with response to threat in childhood, adults' ways of talking about themselves and their lives vary enormously. Some, in the **secure-autonomous** style, talk freely about themselves and their past pain in a coherent and apposite way. The **insecure-dismissive** style minimizes problems and is characterized by unelaborated speech lacking in metaphor or vividness. The **insecure-preoccupied** style is rambling and emotionally laden, while an **insecure-unresolved** pattern has evident breaks in continuity and logical flow. These insecure speech patterns are, it is suggested, manifestations of the underlying psychobiological relational dispositions, which the various theories of object relations attempt to capture. The way we speak about ourselves reveals the state of our inner world. Peter Fonagy[19] has suggested that the capacity to represent experience, which he calls **reflexive function**, (a contemporary version of the classical psychoanalytic notion of 'insight'), is a buffer against psychiatric disturbance. Once pain is represented in the mind the sufferer can distance himself from it, and consider alternative ways of responding. Enhancement of reflexive function is a generic psychotherapeutic strategy and applies as much to cognitive therapy (becoming aware of negative cognitions and automatic thoughts) as psychodynamic therapies.

Bowlby objected to what he saw as the hijacking of the term 'biological' by organic psychiatry, since he believed the attachment relationship and its vicissitudes, adaptively shaped by evolutionary pressures, was no less 'biological' than the neurochemistry which presumably mediates it. For him human psychology was fundamentally relational. He saw attachment needs as existing throughout the life cycle, and put separation and loss as central to his view of the origins of psychiatric disturbance. In the attachment model, separation from a caregiver is a threat: we are biologically programmed to respond with shock, denial, anger, and searching behaviours when separated from a loved person or object. Loss is an irrevocable separation, and the early phases of the bereavement response are all vain attempts to restore the status quo. Despair and depression come with the recognition that separation is final, and, beyond that, reorganization of internal working models, the recognition that although the loved one is lost in reality, good memories live on in the inner world.

The attachment perspective has implications for the day-to-day practice of psychiatry. One function of the psychiatric facilities and of mental health workers is to provide the patient with a 'secure base', which in itself goes some way to reducing anxiety. Appropriate dependency is integral to the supportive psychotherapeutic relationship, which is such a key part of the psychotherapeutic dimension of psychiatry. Short-term, unresponsive, or rejecting relationships with psychiatrists and other mental health workers reinforce insecure attachment and may lead patients to redouble their efforts to cling on to the psychiatric institution—an all too familiar vicious circle.

The ego and its defences: Anna Freud, Hartmann, and Lacan

The role of the ego and of defence mechanisms was a particular concern of Anna Freud,[20] who represented a parallel tendency to the object relations school. She elaborated a taxonomy of defences used by the ego to maintain its integrity in the face of both internal threat from the id, and the demands and impingements of external reality. Valliant[21] groups Anna Freud's defences into those that are **immature** (like projective identification and splitting), **neurotic defences** (which include intellectualization, reaction formation, and identification with the aggressor), and **mature** ones (such as humour and sublimation).

Reaction formation describes the ways in which the ego counteracts unconscious desires or impulses that threaten its equilibrium by consciously held views directly contrary to these: the militant pacifist who is out of touch with any feelings of aggression for example. **Identification with the aggressor** is frequently invoked in discussions of the psychological effects of childhood abuse. One way of dealing with the horror of abuse is to 'dis-identify' with oneself (a form of dissociation), and to put oneself in the place of the person who is attacking, thereby reducing feelings of pain and helplessness. This idea helps to explain how those who have been abused in childhood may become abusers themselves in adult life. A frequent experience in working with severely disturbed patients, many of whom are abuse survivors, is that health care workers may themselves feel attacked or symbolically 'abused' by these patients—seeing how the patient may have unconsciously identified with their aggressor can help carers to a greater understanding of their patients' problems and to respond less defensively to these attacks.

Valliant has found that men who use more mature defence mechanisms are less vulnerable to physical and psychological illness, and an important aim of psychotherapy would be to help the patient move from the use of more- to less-primitive defence mechanisms. Defences are therefore legitimately seen as adaptive, and, from a developmental perspective, the earlier the presumed psychic trauma, the more likely are primitive defence mechanisms to be employed.

David Malan's[22] **triangular model** of anxiety, defence, and 'hidden impulse' is another variety of ego psychology, which has found favour in psychiatric circles. It provides a clear formula for thinking about neurotic difficulties: for example people suffering from agoraphobia commonly defend against anxiety by avoidance and dependency; underlying this there may be hidden feelings of dissatisfaction and aggression, immediately towards a spouse, and in the past towards a controlling but unaffectionate mother. For Malan, the task of therapy is to allow the ego to tolerate and express the hidden feelings; note that cognitive therapy (q.v.) similarly helps the patient to become aware of and then counteract the automatic thoughts (equivalent to hidden feelings) that undermine the ego's attempts to achieve conflict-free functioning.

The self, meaning, and interpersonal psychoanalysis: Sullivan, Horney, and Kohut

Freud's models of the mind were essentially intrapsychic, and couched in quasi-scientific language. Object relations retained this perspective but introduced a relational dimension never fully developed by Freud. **Interpersonal psychoanalysis** in the United States was even more radically interpersonal than object relations. Harry Stack Sullivan[23] was a free thinker who emphasized this existential aspect of psychotherapy, while remaining within the psychoanalytical tradition. He worked particularly with people suffering from schizophrenia. Sullivan believed in close involvement with his psychotic patients. His mission was always to find meaning in their experience, rather than dismiss it as an unintelligible manifestation of organic illness. He was a major influence on a generation of psychoanalytically informed psychiatrists including Harold **Searles**, Freida **Fromm-Reichman**, and Karen Horney.[24]

The latter, like Sullivan, was critical of the patriarchal bias of psychoanalysis. For her, castration complex and penis envy were social rather than biological phenomena, manifestations of social relations that subjugated women, and from which, by appropriate action, including psychotherapy, they could be liberated. Horney's contemporary, Eric **Fromm**, brought a Marxist influence into psychoanalysis, emphasizing the part played by capitalist production methods in contributing to isolation and anomie of modern men and women and their psychological troubles.

Although conventional psychoanalytical treatment for schizophrenia is now largely discredited, there is increasing interest in the role of psychosocial interventions in psychosis. Here the Sullivanian principles of respect for the patient's experience and its meaning, the need for a long-term supportive psychotherapeutic relationship, attention to the social precipitants of psychosis, and a focus on the ways in which the therapist may, through countertransference, foster recovery or reinforce pathology, are all highly relevant to contemporary psychiatry.

Heinz Kohut(25) was concerned not so much with schizophrenia, but with that intermediate world between neurosis and psychosis which psychoanalysts call 'borderline' pathology, and which has entered the DSM as Borderline Personality Disorder. Like Sullivan, Kohut puts **self-esteem and its disorders** at the centre of his psychology, seeing the origins of self-esteem in the empathic responsiveness of caregivers in the early years of life. For him there is a core of **healthy narcissism**, which is based on the grandiosity and omnipotence of the young child ('his majesty the baby', as Freud put it), which is both accepted and fostered by effective parenting. Parents at this stage are '**self-objects**', a concept akin to Winnicott's transitional objects, who partake both of the self and of the responsive environment, and which the infant believes, in his state of healthy delusion, to be there exclusively for his benefit.

Like Winnicott, Kohut emphasizes 'mirroring' as a key interpersonal theme. For Winnicott parental mirroring helps the child to own his emotions and begin to know who he is. Kohut, by contrast, takes up the narcissistic aspect of the mirror: the child sees his reflected glory in the eyes of his admiring parents, and this contributes towards his own positive self-regard. As development proceeds there is a process of 'optimal disillusionment', similar to the resolution of the Oedipus complex, in which the child gradually learns that his objects have a life of their own. By this time, however, his sense of a valued and effective self will be sufficiently developed, and residual narcissism will serve the useful functions of ambition, aspiration to success and admiration, a sense of duty and concern for others, and the capacity to invest in ones offspring.

Where the environment is unempathic, mirroring is deficient, fragile grandiosity squashed, or disillusionment traumatic, the stage is set for borderline pathology, in which self-absorption, and the use of others as self-objects, appropriate to the infantile years, persists into adult life. Self-injurious behaviour such as drug abuse, eating disorders, and deliberate self-harm are 'breakdown products' of a disintegrated self, trying to use the environment as a self-object that will provide momentary and illusory satisfaction and self-affirmation.

A therapeutic implication of Kohut's approach is that the therapist is more supportive than in classical analysis, tolerant of the patient's grandiose designs, especially in the early stages of treatment. This contrasts with the approach of Otto Kernberg(26) who synthesizes classical and Kleinian concepts, and advocates rigorous interpretation, especially of destructive and self-defeating behaviour in borderline patients. Kohut's and Kernberg's theories reflect the typical polarization that such patients evoke in clinical settings, perhaps mirroring an inner world rigidly split into good and bad objects. Effective treatment requires a synthesis: empathy and tolerance is needed to form a working alliance, but firm limit-setting and confrontation of destructiveness is also essential. Another interpersonal synthesis is to be found in the work of Stephen Mitchell(27) whose approach reminds the therapist of the reciprocity of the therapeutic relationship in what Robert Lang calls the 'bipersonal field': patient and therapist form a system of mutual influence, the job of the therapist being both to participate in this, and at the same time to be sufficiently detached to be able to reflect upon it.

The shift in interpersonal psychoanalysis away from the analyst as an objective and privileged observer to a co-participant has given rise to a contemporary interest in narrative or hermeneutic explanations in psychotherapy,(28) in contrast to the scientific psychology, which Freud originally hoped to establish. These authors argue the case for psychoanalysis as a hermeneutic discipline whose aim is to explore meaning rather than objective truth. If Freud is one of the intellectual founding fathers of modernism, their approach is 'postmodern' in the sense that it stresses the relativism of values and meanings, and the importance of power in determining one's view of the world. Here is a link—albeit so far rather distant—with the emerging 'user' movement in psychiatry, and the importance of giving as much weight to the client's voice as to that of the professional. Psychological truths are inherently contextual, and without awareness of the social context they can be obfuscatory.

Conclusions

Many new perspectives have emerged in the century since psychoanalysis was conceived. Emphasis has shifted from the intrapsychic to the interpersonal. Kleinian psychoanalysis offers a unique vision of the ways in which interpersonal reality is inescapably coloured by the emotional state of the participants. Attachment theory provides an account of human psychological development that both takes account of meaning and is empirically based. Psychoanalysis is emerging from its isolation and bridges have begun to be built with cognitive science: the inner world of phantasy is not unlike the world of schemata and assumptions that are the focus of cognitive therapy. There are, through modern neuroimaging techniques links to be forged with neurobiology: the impact of effective therapeutic interventions on brain architecture can now be visualized. Progress will depend on further theoretical syntheses and technological advances, while holding firm to the humanistic emphasis on personal meaning and inner experience that is the fundamental contribution of psychoanalysis to contemporary psychiatry.

Further information

Bateman, A. and Holmes, J. (1995). *Introduction to psychoanalysis: contemporary theory and practice*. Routledge, London.

Cassidy, J. and Shaver, P. (eds.) (2007). *Handbook of attachment* (2nd edn). Guilford, New York.

Fonagy, P. and Target, M. (2002). *Psychoanalytic theories. Perspectives from developmental psychopathology*. Whurr, London.

Gabbard, G., Beck, J., and Holmes, J. (2005). *Oxford textbook of psychotherapy*. Oxford University Press, Oxford.

Mayes, L., Fonagy, P., and Target, M. (eds.) (2007). *Developmental science and psychoanalysis*. Karnac, London.

References

1. Freud, S. (1917). Mourning and melancholia. In *Standard edition of the complete psychological works of Sigmund Freud*, Vol. 14 (ed. J. Strachey), pp. 239–58. Hogarth Press, London, 1957.
2. Klein, M. (1986). *The selected Melanie Klein* (ed. J. Mitchell). Penguin, Harmondsworth.
3. Spillius, E. (1988). *Melanie Klein today*. Routledge, London.
4. Hobson, R.P., Patrick, M., and Valentine, J. (1998). Objectivity in psychoanalytic judgements. *The British Journal of Psychiatry*, **173**, 172–7.
5. Bion, W. (1988). Attacks on linking. In *Melanie Klein today* (ed. E. Spillius), pp. 178–86. Routledge, London.
6. Heimann, P. (1950). On countertransference. *International Journal of Psychoanalysis*, **31**, 81–4.
7. Ogden, T. (1979). On projective identification. *International Journal of Psychoanalysis*, **60**, 357–73.
8. Fairbairn, W.R. (1952). *Psychoanalytic studies of the personality*. Routledge, London.
9. Steiner, J. (1993). *Psychic retreats*. Routledge, London.
10. Britton, R., Feldman, M., and O'Shaughnessy, E. (1989). The Oedipus complex todsay. Karnac Press, London.
11. Balint, M. (1968). *The basic fault*. Tavistock Press, London.
12. Winnicott, D. (1971). *Playing and reality*. Penguin, Harmondsworth.
13. Laing, R. (1961). *The divided self*. Penguin, Harmondsworth.
14. Bowlby, J. (1988). *A secure base: clinical applications of attachment theory*. Routledge, London.
15. Freud, S. (1926). Inhibitions, symptoms, and anxiety. In *Standard edition of the complete psychological works of Sigmund Freud*, Vol. 20 (ed. J. Strachey). Hogarth Press, London.
16. Cassidy, J. and Shaver, P. (eds.) (2007). *Handbook of attachment* (2nd edn). Guilford, New York.
17. Holmes, J. (2001). The search for the secure base: attachment theory and psychotherapy. Routledge, London.
18. Main, M. (1995). In *Attachment theory: social, development and clinical perspective* (eds. S. Goldbery, R. Muir and J. Kerr), pp. 407–74. Analytic Press. New York.
19. Fonagy, P. (1995). In Attachment theory: social, development and clinical perspective (eds S. Goldbery, R. Muir and J. Kerr), pp. 233–78. Analytic Press. New York.
20. Freud, A. (1936). *The ego and the mechanisms of defense*. Hogarth Press, London.
21. Valliant, G. (1992). *Ego mechanisms of defense: a guide for clinicians and researchers*. American Psychiatric Press, Washington, DC.
22. Malan, D. and Coughlin Della Selva, P. (2006). *Lives transformed*. Karnac, London.
23. Sullivan, H.S. (1962). *Schizophrenia as a human process*. Norton, New York.
24. Horney, K. (1939). *New ways in psychoanalysis*. Norton, New York.
25. Kohut, H. (1977). *The restoration of the self*. International Universities Press, New York.
26. Kernberg, O. (1996). A psychoanalytic theory of personality disorders. In *Major theories of personality disorder* (eds. J. Clarkin and M. Lenzenweger), pp. 116–137. Guilford Press, New York.
27. Mitchell, S. (1988). *Relational concepts in psychoanalysis: an integration*. Harvard Universities Press, Cambridge, MA.
28. Roberts, G. and Holmes, J. (eds.) (1998). *Healing stories: narrative in psychiatry and psychotherapy*. Oxford University Press, Oxford.

3.3

Current psychodynamic approaches to psychiatry

Glen O. Gabbard

Psychodynamic psychiatry is broadly defined today. In fact, the term psychodynamic is now used almost synonymously with psychoanalytical. Freud originally used the term psychodynamic to emphasize the conflict between opposing intrapsychic forces: a wish was opposed by a defence, and different intrapsychic agencies, such as ego, id, and superego, were in conflict with one another. Indeed, for much of the twentieth century psychoanalytical theory was dominated by the drive-defence model, often referred to as ego psychology.

In the last decades of the twentieth century, however, psychoanalytical theory expanded beyond the notion of conflict among intrapsychic agencies. Internal object relations became paramount in models deriving from these sources. In addition, a deficit model of symptomatology arose from the work of the British object-relation theorists, such as Balint and Winnicott. In the United States, Kohut's self-psychology also developed a model based on developmental deficits. In other words, disturbed patients who came to treatment were seen as suffering from absent or weakened psychic structures based on developmental failures by parents or caretakers in the early childhood environment. (See Chapter 3.1 for an account of the development and modern practice of psychoanalysis.)

The typical psychodynamic psychiatrist then uses multiple models to assist in the understanding of a particular patient. Developments in neuroscience must also be taken into account. Moreover, the diagnostic and treatment approach to an individual patient is psychodynamically informed even when a decision has been made to forego psychodynamic psychotherapy. Psychodynamic thinking provides a conceptual framework within which all treatments are prescribed, including pharmacotherapy, psychotherapy, inpatient or partial hospital treatment, and group or family modalities. Psychodynamic psychiatry is not synonymous with psychodynamic psychotherapy.

A comprehensive definition of current psychodynamic psychiatry is the following:[1]

Psychodynamic psychiatry is an approach to diagnosis and treatment characterized by a way of thinking about both patient and clinician that includes unconscious conflict, deficits, and distortions of intrapsychic structures, and internal object relations, and that integrates these element with contemporary findings from the neurosciences.

Basic principles

A set of time-honoured basic principles, all derived from psychoanalytical technique and theory, define the overall approach of the dynamic psychiatrists (Table 3.3.1).

The unconscious

A fundamental premise of psychodynamic psychiatry is that mental activity going on outside our awareness can be profoundly influential. Freud saw signs of the unconscious in two major types of clinical evidence: parapraxes and dreams. Parapraxes, commonly referred to as slips of the tongue or 'Freudian slips', involve substituting one word for another. For example, a patient who intends to say 'Protestant', may unwittingly say 'prostitute'. Parapraxes may also involve actions, such as forgetting, or executing one action when intending to do another.

Freud regarded dreams as the 'Royal Road' to the understanding of the unconscious. Another primary way that the unconscious manifests itself in the clinical setting is the patient's behaviour toward the clinician. Certain characteristic patterns of relatedness to others set in childhood become internalized and are manifested automatically and unconsciously as part of the patient's character. Hence certain patients may consistently act deferentially toward the clinician, while others will behave in a highly rebellious way. This type of procedural memory is closely linked to Squire's[2] notion of implicit memory, which occurs outside the realm of verbal narrative memory.

While declarative or autobiographical memory involves remembered events and narratives of one's life, procedural memory

Table 3.3.1 Basic principles of psychodynamic psychiatry

The unconscious
Psychic determinism
Developmental orientation
Emphasis on the uniqueness of the individual rather than how the individual is like others
Transference
Countertransference
Resistance

stores the 'how' of executing sequences of actions, such as motor skills. Once guitar-playing or bicycle-riding has been mastered, no conscious recall is necessary when one sits down with a guitar or jumps on a bicycle. The schema referred to as unconscious internal object relations are to some extent procedural memories repeated again and again in a variety of interpersonal situations. They are non-conscious, but not dynamically unconscious, in the sense of being defensively banished from conscious awareness.

The notion that much of mental life is unconscious is one that is often challenged by psychoanalytical critics, but it is also one that is extensively validated by literature from experimental psychology.[3] Repression of memory has even been demonstrated in fMRI research.[4] The active effort to 'forget' unwanted past experiences involves a novel form of reciprocal interaction between the prefrontal cortex and the hippocampus. When subjects control unwanted memories, there is increased dorsolateral prefrontal activation associated with reduced hippocampal activation. The magnitude of forgetting is predicted by prefrontal, cortical, and right hippocampal activations.

Psychic determinism

The notion of psychic determinism is intimately linked with the construct of the unconscious. Freud felt that behaviour and mental life were related to multiple and complex causation.[5] The term overdetermination implies that a variety of intrapsychic and unconscious factors come together to produce specific symptoms or behaviours. The notion of multiple causation implies that there can be alternate sets of sufficient conditions, some involving primarily unconscious conflicting forces, others stemming from biological and environmental influences that ultimately produce similar symptoms or behaviours.

Developmental orientation

Regardless of which psychoanalytical theory seems to fit best with a particular patient, the dynamic psychiatrist always thinks in terms of developmental models. Patterns of relatedness established in childhood are repeated in adult relationships. Modern dynamic psychiatrists avoid the early psychoanalytical reductionism that attempted to link an adult psychopathological syndrome to a specific developmental arrest or fixation in childhood. Today, full account is taken of genetic contributions to personality and to psychiatric disorders. Environmental influences and genetic factors interact with one another reciprocally to shape the human being in health and illness. Still, the wisdom of the psychodynamic approach is that within each of us is a child yearning to complete some unfinished business from earlier in life.

Emphasis on the uniqueness of the individual

In much of descriptive psychiatry the major focus is on taxonomy—specifically: How do groups of patients fit together under one classification? In psychodynamic psychiatry, by contrast, there is great interest in how a particular patient is unique—in other words, different from others. The subjective experience of the individual has been forged through an idiosyncratic narrative that is different from all other life stories and involves a specific interaction between genetic predisposition, intrapsychic factors, and environmental influence.

Transference

Intrinsic to the developmental model of mental organization is that adults are constantly repeating childhood patterns in the present. Transference is the best-known example of this phenomenon. The patient unconsciously experiences the doctor as a significant figure from the past and reacts to the doctor based on a set of unconscious attributions based on those past experiences. Transference has undergone considerable revision in more recent writings, so that today much more emphasis is placed on the clinician's contributions to the patient's transference. In other words, if a clinician is silent and remote, the patient may experience that clinician as disengaged and cold. While an internal template of past experiences with authority figures may correlate with that perception, we would also recognize that the clinician's real behaviour contributes to that precise transference paradigm. In that regard, a more contemporary view of transference would be that every treatment relationship is a mixture of new features based on real characteristics of the clinician and old experiences from the patient's past. Psychodynamic clinicians also recognize a bidimensional quality to transference: while one dimension involves repetition of the past, another dimension is seeking an experience with a new object to facilitate further emotional growth.

Countertransference

Central to the psychodynamic viewpoint is that the clinician and the patient bring their own separate subjectivities to an encounter, and mutually influence one another. Countertransference, in this respect, is the counterpart of transference. In other words, as Freud originally used the term, it referred to the analyst's attribution of certain qualities to the patient based on the analyst's past experiences with similar figures. This perspective, often referred to as the narrow view of countertransference, regarded the phenomenon as an obstacle to be removed because it interfered with the analyst's objectivity.

Subsequent contributors to the literature on countertransference[6, 7] noted that countertransference with severely disturbed patients often involves an objective component. The patient behaves in such a provocative manner that virtually anyone would respond with a certain set of emotional reactions to that patient. This way of looking at countertransference is often regarded as the broad or totalistic view. Inherent in this perspective is that the clinician's reaction has much less to do with his or her own individual past than with the specific characteristics of the patient and that patient's capacity to induce strong reactions in others.

As the definition has continued to evolve, countertransference is now generally regarded as involving both the narrow and the broad characteristics. In other words, most theoretical perspectives view countertransference as entailing a jointly created reaction in the clinician that stems, in part, from contributions of the clinician's past and, in part, from feelings induced by the patient's behaviour.[8] In some cases the emphasis may be more on the contributions of the clinician than the patient, while in other cases the reverse may be true. This model also regards countertransference as something of a unique construction that varies depending on the two subjectivities involved (see Box 3.3.1). In this contemporary perspective, countertransference is both a source of valuable information about the patient's internal world and something of an interference with the treatment.

Box 3.3.1 Changing views of countertransference

Narrow The original Freudian view connoting the analyst's transference to the patient: an obstacle to be removed through careful analysis of the clinician.
Broad or totalistic All the feelings experienced towards the patient, some of which are induced by the patient's behaviour.
Joint creation The contemporary perspective that emphasizes mutual contributions from the patient's behaviour toward the clinician and the clinician's past experiences with similar figures. This perspective emphasizes countertransference as a source of valuable information in addition to being an interference.

Resistance

In 1912 Freud[9] wrote, 'The resistance accompanies the treatment step by step. Every single association, every act of the person under treatment must reckon with the resistance and represents a compromise between the forces that are striving towards recovery and the opposing ones'. The patient's resistance defends the patient's illness from the clinician's attempt to treat it and change it. Resistance may be conscious, preconscious, or unconscious. It may take many forms, including not taking medication as prescribed, forgetting appointments with the psychiatrist, changing the subject in the middle of an appointment to something trivial, and discounting every insight the psychiatrist offers. The patient's characteristic defence mechanisms are often transformed into resistances in the treatment situation. The dynamic psychiatrist knows that all progress will be accompanied by some degree of resistance, and the exploration of resistance is a major part of therapeutic work. Resistance is intimately related to transference because the patient often rebels against the doctor resulting from unconscious transference configurations that lead the patient to oppose the doctor's help.

The mind–brain interface

The psychodynamic psychiatrist eschews reductionism. Recognizing that mental life and psychiatric symptoms are both overdetermined and multiply caused, psychodynamic clinicians are always interested in the interface between the biological and the psychosocial. Psychodynamic psychiatry is not antibiological. The psychodynamic psychiatrist is the integrator par excellence. Avoiding Cartesian dualism, the mind is seen as the expression of the activity of the brain.[10] Subjective experience affects the brain just as mental phenomena arise from the brain. Every treatment intervention is seen as being biopsychosocial in nature. Medications have psychological effects. Psychotherapeutic interpretations affect the brain. Moreover, psychodynamic psychotherapy and medications may work synergistically to provide better outcomes for patients. For example, a patient with a bipolar disorder who is denying that he has an illness and refusing to take lithium may ultimately have better compliance with the medication if the clinician explores the meaning of his denial and his reluctance to consider himself as someone requiring treatment.

The comprehensive mind–brain strategy of the contemporary psychodynamic psychiatrist fits well with our growing knowledge of the interaction between genes and the environment. In an inspired series of experiments with the marine snail *Aplysia*, Kandel[11,12] has demonstrated that synaptic connections are strengthened and permanently altered through regulation of gene expression connected with learning from the environment. In *Aplysia* the number of synapses actually double or triple as a result of learning. Kandel has suggested that psychotherapy might make similar neuroanatomical changes in the synapses. He argues that just as representations of self and others are malleable, the brain itself is a dynamic and plastic structure. He postulates that psychotherapy is a form of learning that produces alteration of gene expression and thereby alters the strength of synaptic connections. While the template function or the sequence of the gene is not affected by environmental experience, the transcriptional function of the gene (namely the ability of a given gene to direct the manufacture of specific proteins) is highly regulated and responsive to environmental factors.

Antisocial personality disorder may be a model disorder with which to examine the interaction of genes and environment. In a perspective study based in Dunedin,[13] a birth cohort of 1037 children was followed prospectively. By the age of 26, 96 per cent of the sample was contacted and evaluated. Between the ages of 3 and 11 years, 8 per cent experienced 'severe' maltreatment, 28 per cent experienced 'probable' maltreatment, and 64 per cent experienced no maltreatment. The investigators determined that a functional polymorphism in the gene responsible for the neurotransmitter metabolizing enzyme monoamine oxidase-A (MAO-A) was found to moderate the effect of maltreatment. Males with low MAO-A activity genotype who were maltreated in childhood had elevated antisocial scores. Males with high MAO-A activity did not have elevated antisocial scores, even when they had experienced childhood maltreatment. Of males with both low MAO-A activity genotype and severe maltreatment, 85 per cent developed antisocial behaviour.[13]

The research summarized here points to the dynamic interplay between genetic expression and the environment. Gene expression cannot be considered static. It is a dynamic phenomenon that interacts with and reacts to environmental experiences. Heritable characteristics of children actually shape their relationships with their parents and siblings.[14] In turn, the response of family members to the child affect the genetic expression. Hence genetic influences on some types of psychopathology may be dependent on the mediation of social processes. A child's genetic endowment will influence the way parents relate to a child, and the way the parents treat the child will then influence that child's developing brain. Biological and psychosocial processes are constantly intertwined, and neither is prior.

In many major psychiatric disorders, such as depression, genetic factors appear to influence whether a stressor produces an episode of illness.[15] From a psychodynamic perspective, the meaning of stressors must also be incorporated. Some stressors that may seem mild to one individual are overwhelming to another because of their idiosyncratic conscious or unconscious meaning. In addition, the presence of biologically generated symptoms in no way diminishes the importance of meaning. Pre-existing psychodynamic conflicts may attach themselves to biologically driven symptoms, and the symptoms then function as a vehicle for the expression of the conflicts.[16] Auditory hallucinations are generated by alterations in neurotransmitters in persons with schizophrenia, but the content of the hallucination often has specific meanings based on the patient's psychodynamic conflicts. Hence a patient who is being told that he is a failure and should kill himself by a hallucinated voice may be tormented by a sense that his life is shattered by his illness and that he no longer has any purpose in living.

Development of personality

Another key component of the psychodynamic approach is that the clinician treats the person and not just the illness. In practice, that perspective means taking the personality into account in every case. The interface of the biological and the psychosocial is particularly apparent in the area of personality. The psychobiological model of personality developed by Cloninger *et al.*[17] recognizes an equal contribution of biological and environmental factors (see Table 3.3.2). The four dimensions of temperament are roughly 50 to 60 per cent heritable independently of one another. They all manifest themselves early in life, and they involve preconceptual biases, habit formation, and perceptual memory. They include the following:

1 novelty-seeking: characterized by active avoidance of frustration, quick loss of temper, impulsive decision-making, frequent exploratory activity in response to novelty, and extravagance in the approach to cues and rewards

2 harm-avoidance: which involves pessimistic worry about the future, passive avoidant behaviour such as fear of uncertainty, shyness regarding strangers, and rapid fatiguability

3 reward-dependence: characterized by sentimentality, social attachment, and dependence on the approval of others

4 persistence: which refers to the capacity to persevere despite fatigue and frustration

Certain of these temperament dimensions appear to correlate with specific types of personality disorders. The cluster A personalities in DSM-IV, for example, are strongly associated with low reward-dependence. Cluster B personality disorders have been shown to be high in novelty-seeking, while cluster C personality disorder patients tend to rate high in harm-avoidance.

The other component of personality in this model is character. While temperament is genetically based, character is shaped by environmental experiences, such as family relationships, peer relationships, trauma, and neglect. These dimensions appear to make up about 50 per cent of personality. There have been three dimensions of character identified that appear to mature in adulthood. These dimensions influence social and personal effectiveness by insight-learning about self-concepts. The three character dimensions are self-directedness, cooperativeness, and self-transcendence.

Table 3.3.2 Development of personality

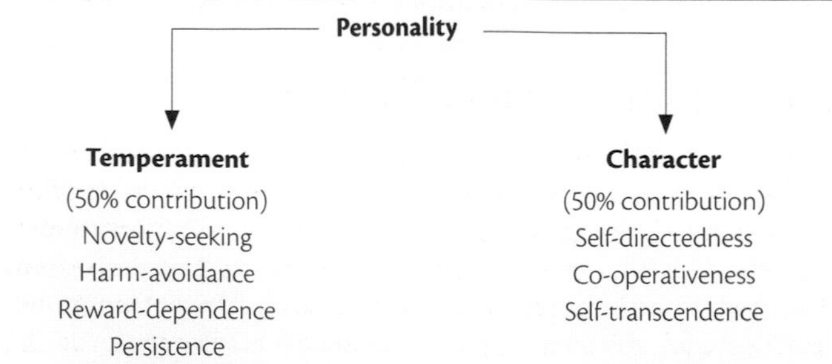

Reproduced from Cloniger, C.R., Svarik, D.M. and Pryzbeck, T.R. (1993). A Psychobiological model of temperament and character. *Archives of General Psychiatry*, **50**, 975–90. Copyright 2003, The American Medical Association.

Low self-directedness and low cooperativeness are associated with all categories of personality disorder in the DSM-IV system.[17] Self-transcendence, on the other hand, does not differentiate patients with personality disorders from those without personality disorders.

Self-directedness and cooperativeness reflect two fundamental tasks in personality development as defined by Blatt *et al.*[18]: the achievement of a stable, differential, realistic, and positive identity, and the establishment of enduring, mutually gratifying relationships with others. These two dimensions evolve in a dialectical and synergistic relationship to one another throughout the life cycle. Patients with character pathology tend to divide into two groups: introjective types, who are primarily focused on self-definition; and anaclitic types, who are more concerned about relatedness.

The character dimensions readily lend themselves to typical psychodynamic constructs. The self-directedness dimension is closely linked to what are often called ego functions or self-structures. The dimension of cooperativeness is a direct measure of a person's characteristic pattern of internal object relations as they are externalized in relationships with others. In one's assessment of a patient's personality, the transference–countertransference dimensions of the clinical interaction provide a privileged glimpse of the typical patterns of relatedness that cause difficulties in the patient's outside relationships.[19] The patient is involved in an ongoing attempt to actualize certain patterns of relatedness that reflect various wishes in the patient's unconscious. Through the patient's behaviour, he or she subtly tries to impose on the clinician a certain way of responding and experiencing.[20]

An individual internalizes a self-representation in interaction with an object representation connected by an affect through a series of repetitive interactions in childhood. This pattern ultimately leads to an internalized set of self- and object representations in interaction with one another. The adult individual repeats these patterns again and again as an effort to fulfill an unconscious wish. Even abusive or painful relationships involving a 'bad' or tormenting object may be wished for because of the safety and affirmation such relationships provide. In other words, a child who has been abused has internalized a highly conflictual abusive relationship as a predictable and familiar pattern. Having an abusive object may be preferable to having no object at all or being abandoned. Many patients with histories of an abusive childhood become convinced that the only way to remain connected to a significant person is to maintain an abuser–victim relationship.

The repetitive interactions seen in patients with personality disorder may reflect actual relationships with real objects in the past, but they may also involve wished-for relationships, such as those often seen in patients with childhood trauma who seek a rescuer. Clinicians who are influenced by the patient's interpersonal pressure to respond in a particular way may unconsciously accept the role in which they have been cast. When this phenomenon occurs, it is often referred to as projective identification.[8] In other words, the patient may 'nudge' the therapist into assuming the role of an abuser in response to the patient's 'victim' role, and the therapist may feel countertransference hate or anger and begin to make sarcastic or demeaning comments to the patient.

In addition to this pattern of object relations, the other major component of character, from a psychodynamic perspective, is the particular constellation of defence mechanisms that characterizes the individual patient.[21] While defences were traditionally regarded as intrapsychic mechanisms designed to prevent awareness of unconscious aggressive or sexual wishes, the current understanding of defence mechanisms has been expanded far beyond Freud's dual-drive theory. We now understand that defences also preserve a sense of self-esteem in the face of narcissistic vulnerability, assure safety when one feels dangerously threatened by abandonment, and serve to insulate one from external dangers through, for example, denial or minimization.

Different personality types or disorders use characteristic sets of defence mechanisms. For example, the paranoid personality may typically use projection as a way of disavowing unacknowledged feelings and attributing them to others. Patients with obsessive–compulsive personality disorder may use defensive operations such as isolation of affect, intellectualization, and reaction formation to control affective states that are highly threatening. In the relationship with the clinician, as noted previously, these defences will manifest themselves as resistances. Hence, if a patient with an obsessive–compulsive personality disorder uses intellectualization as a defence against painful affects, when the patient comes to treatment, intellectualization will be used as a resistance to avoid getting at feelings in psychotherapy.

Dynamic pharmacotherapy

The commonly used psychodynamic constructs, such as therapeutic alliance, transference, countertransference, and resistance apply to all modalities of psychiatric treatment, even though their usage is generally associated with psychodynamic psychotherapy. In a study of the relationship between the therapeutic alliance and the outcome of 250 depressed outpatients in the National Institute of Mental Health Treatment of Depression Study,[22] the therapeutic alliance was found to be of extraordinary importance. The patients had been randomly assigned to one of four conditions: brief interpersonal therapy, brief cognitive behavioural therapy, imipramine plus clinical management, or placebo plus clinical management. The researchers found that the therapeutic alliance was just as important for drug therapy as for psychotherapy. In all four treatment cells, the therapeutic alliance counted for more of the variance of treatment outcome than the treatment method itself. This was the first empirical study to show the importance of the therapeutic alliance in psychotherapy, pharmacotherapy, and placebo outcome.

Non-compliance is one of the most challenging problems facing psychiatric practitioners. Many factors go into compliance. Although many patients blame side effects, they often unconsciously undermine the treatment plan. The patient may have a negative transference to the prescribing clinician related to attitudes toward parents and other authority figures that lead the patient to rebel and defy the doctor's orders. Some clinicians may have countertransference reactions to specific patients that lead them to prescribe in a highly authoritarian manner or a tentative and ambivalent manner, giving unconscious messages to the patient that reflect the doctor's attitude about the medication. Patients who feel the doctor is bullying them to take the medication may not comply. Similarly, patients who sense their doctor is ambivalent about the value of the medication may also choose not to fill the prescription. Unconscious resistance is frequently a major factor in non-compliance. Medications may have idiosyncratic meanings to patients based on unconscious identifications with family members who have taken the same medication, views of psychiatric illness as moral weakness, or fears about the effects of the medication. Sometimes a pill or capsule may serve as a transitional object that substitutes for the person of the prescriber when the physician is unavailable. The colour or shape of a tablet may take on special significance for some patients, making them reluctant to change dosage or switch to another medication.

Multiple-treater settings

In inpatient units and partial hospital settings, psychodynamic concepts are of considerable value in understanding the patient's psychopathology as it unfolds in a group setting. Patients re-create their internal object relations in the inpatient or partial hospital milieu.[23] The conflicts that occur in their family context will re-emerge in their relationships with hospital staff members. Through projective identification the patient subtly pressures various staff members to play the roles that are in keeping with the patient's internal world. Hence a patient who has been physically and/or sexually abused by a parent will behave in such a way toward a certain nurse, for example, that the nurse begins to feel abusive toward the patient. The same patient may treat another nurse as an idealized rescuer figure, eliciting loving and protective feelings from that nurse. This form of splitting[23] may create extraordinary conflicts between staff members over the best treatment approach to the patient. Therefore failure to attend to the transference–countertransference dimensions of the milieu treatment may lead to a total disruption of the staff members' capacity to be effective with certain patients.

Moreover, individual patients often act out covert staff conflicts. Psychodynamically informed hospital treatment may help to identify these conflicts and allow staff to process them in such a way that the patients no longer need to enact them. When covert conflicts between staff members become overt and open to discussion, the patient's disruptive behaviour often settles down.[23] This observation reflects how the dynamics of the patient group and staff group often parallel each other. The psychodynamic clinician also understands that individuals behave differently in groups than they do alone or in a one-to-one context. Powerful group forces, such as scapegoating, can be recognized and processed so they do not become destructive to treatment. Similarly, the patient's recurrent problems in groups can be diagnosed, in part, by a careful study of the transference and countertransference responses.

Two-person context of treatment

One of the major shifts in psychodynamic thinking in recent years has been a greater acknowledgement of the influence of the clinician's perspective on the observations about the patient. Postmodern contributions from intersubjectivity and social constructivism have challenged the view that the clinician assesses the patient from a detached and objective frame of reference. Fundamental to this perspective is that clinicians can never transcend their irreducible subjectivity.[24] The psychiatrist in this context can never fully know how his or her subjectivity is influencing the diagnostic assessment or the treatment process. Countertransference is viewed as both unconscious and continuous, so that a therapist cannot possibly be capable of keeping up with every emotional reaction of the patient.[25]

This two-person model of the treatment situation has contributed to the demise of the classical psychoanalytical view of the therapist or analyst as a blank screen or a dispassionate observer. The influence of the clinician's biases and unconscious feelings toward the patient may have far-reaching implications for a variety of situations in psychiatry. Frustration about a patient's non-responsiveness to treatment, for example, can lead a clinician to recommend electroconvulsive therapy as a reaction to despair, rather than as a result of systematic decision trees or algorithms about refractory depression. Even in the case of physician-assisted suicide, countertransference may play a major, though hidden, role.[26] Within this context the patient's wish to die may stem from a self-concept as worthless and a burden to others that is, in part, a reflection of what the physician brings to the encounter. Similarly, the doctor's death-anxiety might underlie an omnipotent need to triumph over death through the prescription of physician-assisted suicide that strives to preserve an illusion of control and mastery. In the worst scenario, a clinician's intense countertransference hate toward a patient may lead to a wish to kill that is transposed into a recommendation for physician-assisted suicide.

Psychodynamic psychotherapy for specific disorders

A psychodynamic approach is relevant to the treatment of the vast majority of psychiatric disorders encountered in clinical practice. Depending on the nature of the illness, the setting in which the illness is treated, and the psychological mindedness of the patient, psychodynamic strategies may be the major emphasis in the treatment plan or a relatively minor contribution. Psychodynamic psychotherapy per se is generally divided into short-term psychodynamic psychotherapy (STPP) and long-term psychodynamic psychotherapy (LTPP). The former is generally regarded as involving fewer than 24 sessions or 6 months' duration, while the latter is viewed as a therapy lasting more than 6 months.[27] Psychodynamic psychotherapy, whether long-term or short-term, is often defined as 'a therapy that involves careful attention to the therapist–patient interaction, with thoughtfully timed interpretation of transference and resistance embedded in the sophisticated appreciation of the therapist's contribution to the two-person field'.[28] This form of psychotherapy is also conceptualized as operating on an expressive-supportive continuum. The highly expressive forms of psychodynamic psychotherapy offer more interpretation of unconscious conflict, while the forms that are more supportive focus on bolstering adaptive defences and building self-esteem. The continuum of interventions from the most expressive to the most supportive (see Table 3.3.3) guide the psychotherapist in how to intervene with any given patient.

Short-term psychodynamic psychotherapy

A recent meta-analysis of STPP[29] found that this modality made significant changes in general psychiatric symptoms, target problem, and social functioning. The treatment also yielded significant and large pre-treatment—post-treatment effect sizes. The effect sizes were stable and tended to increase at follow-up. No significant differences were found between STPP and other forms of psychotherapy. Evidence from randomized controlled trials supports the use of STPP for major depressive disorder, panic disorder, social phobia, and post-traumatic stress disorder. In addition, the treatment has also been efficacious in somatoform disorders, bulimia nervosa, and substance-related disorders in association with drug counseling.

Long-term psychodynamic psychotherapy

Research on LTPP has been more limited than for STPP because the gold standard of the randomized controlled trial is more difficult to implement when studying LTPP. One must find a suitable control group where an alternative extended treatment or a placebo condition can be implemented. The most rigorous controlled condition is an alternative extended treatment, although some investigations have used treatment as usual as well.[30] The dropout rate can also be problematic in long-term studies. In addition, intervening life events, Axis I conditions, and medication shifts can influence outcome. Nevertheless, despite the obstacles to designing and implementing rigorous research on LTPP, there are a number of studies that have appeared in recent years that suggest that LTPP is an efficacious treatment.

Two randomized controlled trials have shown LTPP to be efficacious with Cluster C personality disorders. Included in this group are avoidant, dependent, and obsessive–compulsive personality disorders. One study compared 40 sessions of psychodynamic therapy to control patients on a waiting list and found substantially better outcomes than those who received the dynamic therapy.[31] In a more rigorously designed study,[32] 40 sessions of dynamic psychotherapy were compared to 40 sessions of cognitive behaviour therapy. While both treatments were effective, the dynamic therapy resulted in continued improvement after termination of treatment, suggesting that patients internalized the therapeutic dialogue and used it to deal with problems as they arose.

Borderline personality disorder has also been subjected to rigorous trials of long-term psychodynamic psychotherapy. In one head-to-head comparison between a form of LTPP known as transference-focused psychotherapy (TFP), dialectical behaviour therapy (DBT), and supportive psychotherapy (SPT),[33,34] all three modalities

Table 3.3.3 An expressive–supportive continuum of interventions

Expressive	Interpretation	Observation	Confrontation	Clarification	Encouragement to Elaborate	Empathic Validation	Advice and Praise	Supportive

(Data modified from Gabbard, G.O. (2004), *Long-term psychodynamic psychotherapy: a basic text*, American Psychiatric Publishing, Arlington, VA.)

showed general improvement. However, TFP showed improvements that were not demonstrated by either SPT or DBT. Participants in the study who received TFP were more likely to move from an insecure attachment classification to a secure one, show greater changes in mentalizing capacity, and have more extensive symptomatic improvement than the other two groups. Only TFP made significant changes in impulsivity, irritability, verbal assault, and direct assault. Suicidality was reduced to an equal extent by TFP and DBT.

A psychoanalytically oriented partial hospitalization treatment for patients with borderline personality disorder was compared to a treatment-as-usual approach.[35,36] In the treatment group, the major difference was the provision of individual and group psychotherapy compared to the control condition. The treatment lasted a maximum of 18 months, and was significantly superior to standard psychiatric care, both at the end of therapy and at the 18-month follow-up.

A randomized controlled trial for children with learning disabilities[37] compared intensive psychodynamic therapy (four times a week) to once-a-week sessions. This trial on featured treatments had lasted longer than 1 year. In the follow-up assessment, children who had sessions four times a week showed much greater improvement.

Future directions

The psychodynamic model continues to enrich the patient's understanding and the psychiatrist's practice. The time-honoured principles elaborated here serve as windows into the murky recesses of the unconscious and illuminate human motivation. They also provide the clinician with a 'second sight' that helps make sense out of bewildering and complex clinical situations.

The evidence regarding the impact of psychotherapy on the brain opens up new lines of investigation to enhance our understanding of psychopathology and treatment. These include the following:

1 the mechanisms of action of psychotherapy

2 the interrelationships between the mechanisms of action of psychotherapy and medication

3 a clearer understanding of pathogenesis itself and the malleability of some components of the pathogenetic mechanisms of major psychiatric disorder

Research is sorely needed on psychodynamic treatments because there is only a modest empirical base for psychodynamic therapy. Many more studies are needed, especially those with a randomized controlled design targeted at specific disorders. Studies investigating extended dynamic therapy of a year or more are needed to demonstrate which patients benefit from the additional investment of time and money. In the current climate of cost containment, practitioners of psychodynamic therapy must take cost-effectiveness into account.

The optimal treatment for many psychiatric patients involves a combination of medication and psychotherapy, but research support for this view is also rather modest. Controlled studies of combined treatment versus single modalities are needed for personality disorders and anxiety disorders. In addition, the role of psychodynamic thinking in compliance problems needs rigorous investigation.

In the meantime, the psychodynamic model continues to focus on the uniqueness of the individual patient. Psychodynamic psychiatry, above all, is interested in the person with illness rather than the illness alone.

Further information

Gabbard, G.O. (2004). *Long-term psychodynamic psychotherapy: a basic text.* American Psychiatric Publishing, Arlington, VA.

Gabbard, G.O. (2005). *Psychodynamic psychiatry in clinical practice* (4th edn). American Psychiatric Publishing, Arlington, VA.

Leichsenring, F., Rabung, S., and Liebing, E. (2004). The efficacy of short-term psychodynamic therapy in specific psychiatric disorders: a meta-analysis. *Archives of General Psychiatry*, **61**, 1208–16.

References

1. Gabbard, G.O. (2005). *Psychodynamic psychiatry in clinical practice* (4th edn). American Psychiatric Publishing, Arlington, VA.
2. Squire, L.R. (1987). *Memory and brain.* Oxford University Press, New York.
3. Westen, D. (1999). The scientific status of unconscious processes: is Freud really dead? *Journal of the American Psychoanalytic Association*, **47**, 1061–106.
4. Anderson, M.C., Ochsner, K.N., Kuhl, B., *et al.* (2004). Neural systems underlying the suppression of unwanted memories. *Science*, **303**, 232–5.
5. Sherwood, M. (1969). *The logic of explanation in psychoanalysis.* Academic Press, New York.
6. Winnicott, D.W. (1949). Hate in the countertransference. *International Journal of Psycho-analysis*, **30**, 69–74.
7. Kernberg, O.F. (1965). Notes on countertransference. *Journal of the American Psychoanalytic Association*, **13**, 38–56.
8. Gabbard, G.O. (1995). Countertransference: the emerging common ground. *International Journal of Psycho-analysis*, **76**, 475–85.
9. Freud, S. (1912). The dynamics of transference. In *The standard edition of the complete works of Sigmund Freud*, Vol. 12 (ed. J. Strachey), pp. 97–108. Hogarth Press, London, 1958.
10. Andreasen, N.C. (1997). Linking mind and brain in the study of mental illness: a project for a scientific psychopathology. *Science*, **275**, 1587–93.
11. Kandel, E.R. (1983). From metapsychology to molecular biology: explorations into the nature of anxiety. *The American Journal of Psychiatry*, **140**, 1277–93.
12. Kandel, E.R. (1998). A new intellectual framework for psychiatry. *The American Journal of Psychiatry*, **155**, 457–69.
13. Caspi, A., McClay, J., Moffitt, T.E., *et al.* (2002). Role of genotype in the cycle of violence in maltreated children. *Science*, **297**, 851–4.
14. Reiss, D., Plomin, R., and Hetherington, E.M. (1991). Genetics and psychiatry: an unheralded window on the environment. *The American Journal of Psychiatry*, **148**, 283–91.
15. Kendler, K.S., Kessler, R.C., Walters, E.E., *et al.* (1995). Stressful life events, genetic liability, and onset of an episode of major depression in women. *The American Journal of Psychiatry*, **152**, 833–42.
16. Gabbard, G.O. (1992). Psychodynamic psychiatry in the decade of the brain. *The American Journal of Psychiatry*, **149**, 991–8.
17. Cloninger, C.R., Svrakic, D.M., and Pryzbeck, T.R. (1993). A psychobiological model of temperament and character. *Archives of General Psychiatry*, **50**, 975–90.
18. Blatt, S.J., Ford, R.Q., Berman, W.H. Jr., *et al.* (1994). *Therapeutic change: an object relations perspective.* Plenum Press, New York.
19. Gabbard, G.O. (1997). Finding the 'person' in personality disorders. *The American Journal of Psychiatry*, **154**, 891–3.
20. Sandler, J. (1981). Character traits and object relationships. *The Psychoanalytic Quarterly*, **50**, 694–708.
21. Gabbard, G.O. (1999). Psychoanalysis and psychoanalytic therapy. In *The DSM-IV personality disorders* (ed. W.J. Livesley). Guilford Press, New York.

22. Krupnick, J.L., Sotsky, S.M., Simmens, S., *et al.* (1996). The role of the therapeutic alliance in psychotherapy and pharmacotherapy outcome: findings in the National Institute of Mental Health treatment of depression collaborative research program. *Journal of Consulting and Clinical Psychology*, **64**, 532–9.
23. Gabbard, G.O. (1989). Splitting in hospital treatment. *The American Journal of Psychiatry*, **146**, 444–51.
24. Renik, O. (1993). Analytic interaction: conceptualizing technique in light of the analyst's irreducible subjectivity. *The Psychoanalytic Quarterly*, **62**, 553–71.
25. Hoffman, I.Z. (1998). *Ritual and spontaneity in the psychoanalytic process: the dialectical constructivist view*. Analytic Press, Hillsdale, NJ.
26. Varghese, F.T. and Kelly, B. (1999). Countertransference and assisted suicide. In *Review of psychiatry*, Vol. 18 (eds. J. Oldham and M. Riba), *Countertransference in psychiatric treatment* (ed. G. Gabbard), pp. 85–118. American Psychiatric Press, Washington, DC.
27. Gabbard, G.O. (2004). *Long-term psychodynamic psychotherapy: a basic text*. American Psychiatric Publishing, Arlington, VA.
28. ibid., p. 2.
29. Leichsenring, F., Rabung, S., and Liebing, E. (2004). The efficacy of short-term psychodynamic therapy in specific psychiatric disorders: a meta-analysis. *Archives of General Psychiatry*, **61**, 1208–16.
30. Gabbard, G.O., Gunderson, J.G., and Fonagy, P. (2002). The place of psychoanalytic treatments within psychiatry. *Archives of General Psychiatry*, **59**, 505–10.
31. Winston, A., Laikin, M., Pollack, J., *et al.* (1994). Short-term psychotherapy of personality disorders. *The American Journal of Psychiatry*, **151**, 190–4.
32. Svartberg, M., Stiles, T.C., and Seltzer, M.H. (2004). Effectiveness of short-term dynamic psychotherapy and cognitive therapy for cluster C personality disorders: a randomized controlled trial. *The American Journal of Psychiatry*, **161**, 810–17.
33. Clarkin, J.F., Levy, K.N., Lenzenweger, M.F., *et al.* (2007). Evaluating three treatments for borderline personality disorder: a multiwave study. *The American Journal of Psychiatry*, **164**, 922–28.
34. Levy, K.N., Meehan, K.B., Clarkin, J.F., *et al.* (2006). Change in attachment patterns and reflective function in a randomized control trial of transference-focused psychotherapy for borderline personality disorder. *Journal of Consulting and Clinical Psychology*, **74**, 1027–74.
35. Bateman, A. and Fonagy, P. (1999). The effectiveness of partial hospitalization in the treatment of borderline personality disorder: a randomized control trial. *The American Journal of Psychiatry*, **156**, 1563–9.
36. Bateman, A. and Fonagy, P. (2001). Treatment of borderline personality disorder with psychoanalytically oriented partial hospitalization: an 18-month follow-up. *The American Journal of Psychiatry*, **158**, 36–42.
37. Heinicke, C.M. and Ramsey-Klee, D.M. (1986). Outcome of child psychotherapy as a function of frequency of sessions. *Journal of the American Academy of Child Psychiatry*, **25**, 247–53.

SECTION 4

Clinical Syndromes of Adult Psychiatry

4.1 Delirium, dementia, amnesia, and other cognitive disorders 325

4.1.1 Delirium *325*
David Meagher and Paula Trzepacz

4.1.2 Dementia: Alzheimer's disease *333*
Simon Lovestone

4.1.3 Frontotemporal dementias *344*
Lars Gustafson and Arne Brun

4.1.4 Prion disease *351*
John Collinge

4.1.5 Dementia with Lewy bodies *361*
I. G. McKeith

4.1.6 Dementia in Parkinson's disease *368*
R. H. S. Mindham and T. A. Hughes

4.1.7 Dementia due to Huntington's disease *371*
Susan Folstein and Russell L. Margolis

4.1.8 Vascular dementia *375*
Timo Erkinjuntti

4.1.9 Dementia due to HIV disease *384*
Mario Maj

4.1.10 The neuropsychiatry of head injury *387*
Simon Fleminger

4.1.11 Alcohol-related dementia (alcohol-induced dementia; alcohol-related brain damage) *399*
Jane Marshall

4.1.12 Amnesic syndromes *403*
Michael D. Kopelman

4.1.13 The management of dementia *411*
John-Paul Taylor and Simon Fleminger

4.1.14 Remediation of memory disorders *419*
Jonathan J. Evans

4.2 Substance use disorders *426*

4.2.1 Pharmacological and psychological aspects of drugs abuse *426*
David J. Nutt and Fergus D. Law

4.2.2 Alcohol use disorders *432*

4.2.2.1 Aetiology of alcohol problems *432*
Juan C. Negrete and Kathryn J. Gill

4.2.2.2 Alcohol dependence and alcohol problems *437*
Jane Marshall

4.2.2.3 Alcohol and psychiatric and physical disorders *442*
Karl F. Mann and Falk Kiefer

4.2.2.4 Treatment of alcohol dependence *447*
Jonathan Chick

4.2.2.5 Services for alcohol use disorders *459*
D. Colin Drummond

4.2.2.6 Prevention of alcohol-related problems *467*
Robin Room

4.2.3 Other substance use disorders *472*

4.2.3.1 Opioids: heroin, methadone, and buprenorphine *473*
Soraya Mayet, Adam R. Winstock, and John Strang

4.2.3.2 Disorders relating to the use of amphetamine and cocaine *482*
Nicholas Seivewright and Robert Fung

4.2.3.3 Disorders relating to use of PCP and hallucinogens *486*
Henry David Abraham

4.2.3.4 Misuse of benzodiazepines *490*
Sarah Welch and Michael Farrell

4.2.3.5 Disorders relating to the use of ecstasy and other 'party drugs' *494*
Adam R. Winstock and Fabrizio Schifano

4.2.3.6 Disorders relating to the use of volatile substances *502*
Richard Ives

4.2.3.7 The mental health effects of cannabis use *507*
Wayne Hall

4.2.3.8 Nicotine dependence and treatment *510*
Mª Inés López-Ibor

4.2.4 Assessing need and organizing services for drug misuse problems *515*
John Marsden, Colin Bradbury, and John Strang

4.3 Schizophrenia and acute transient psychotic disorders *521*

4.3.1 Schizophrenia: a conceptual history *521*
Nancy C. Andreasen

4.3.2 Descriptive clinical features of schizophrenia *526*
Peter F. Liddle

4.3.3 The clinical neuropsychology of schizophrenia *531*
Philip D. Harvey and Christopher R. Bowie

4.3.4 Diagnosis, classification, and differential diagnosis of schizophrenia *534*
Anthony S. David

4.3.5 Epidemiology of schizophrenia *540*
Assen Jablensky

4.3.6 Aetiology *553*

4.3.6.1 Genetic and environmental risk factors for schizophrenia *553*
R. M. Murray and D. J. Castle

4.3.6.2 The neurobiology of schizophrenia *561*
Paul J. Harrison

4.3.7 Course and outcome of schizophrenia and their prediction *568*
Assen Jablensky

4.3.8 Treatment and management of schizophrenia *578*
D. G. Cunningham Owens and E. C. Johnstone

4.3.9 Schizoaffective and schizotypal disorders *595*
Ming T. Tsuang, William S. Stone, and Stephen V. Faraone

4.3.10 Acute and transient psychotic disorders *602*
J. Garrabé and F.-R. Cousin

4.4 Persistent delusional symptoms and disorders *609*
Alistair Munro

4.5 Mood disorders *629*

4.5.1 Introduction to mood disorders *629*
John R. Geddes

4.5.2 Clinical features of mood disorders and mania *632*
Per Bech

4.5.3 Diagnosis, classification, and differential diagnosis of the mood disorders *637*
Gordon Parker

4.5.4 Epidemiology of mood disorders *645*
Peter R. Joyce

4.5.5 Genetic aetiology of mood disorders *650*
Pierre Oswald, Daniel Souery, and Julien Mendlewicz

4.5.6 Neurobiological aetiology of mood disorders *658*
Guy Goodwin

4.5.7 Course and prognosis of mood disorders *665*
Jules Angst

4.5.8 Treatment of mood disorders *669*
E. S. Paykel and J. Scott

4.5.9 Dysthymia, cyclothymia, and hyperthymia *680*
Hagop S. Akiskal

4.6 Stress-related and adjustment disorders *693*

4.6.1 Acute stress reactions *693*
Anke Ehlers, Allison G. Harvey, and Richard A. Bryant

4.6.2 Post-traumatic stress disorder *700*
Anke Ehlers

4.6.3 Recovered memories and false memories *713*
Chris R. Brewin

4.6.4 Adjustment disorders *716*
James J. Strain, Kimberly Klipstein, and Jeffrey Newcorm

4.6.5 Bereavement *724*
Beverley Raphael, Sally Wooding, and Julie Dunsmore

4.7 Anxiety disorders *729*

4.7.1 Generalized anxiety disorders *729*
Stella Bitran, David H. Barlow, and David A. Spiegel

4.7.2 Social anxiety disorder and specific phobias *739*
Michelle A. Blackmore, Brigette A. Erwin, Richard G. Heimberg, Leanne Magee, and David M. Fresco

4.7.3 Panic disorder and agoraphobia *750*
James C. Ballenger

4.8 Obsessive–compulsive disorder *765*
Joseph Zohar, Leah Fostick, and Elizabeth Juven-Wetzler

4.9 Depersonalization disorder *774*
Nick Medford, Mauricio Sierra, and Anthony S. David

4.10 Disorders of eating *777*

4.10.1 Anorexia nervosa *777*
Gerald Russell

4.10.2 Bulimia nervosa *800*
Christopher G. Fairburn, Zafra Cooper, and Rebecca Murphy

4.11 Sexuality, gender identity, and their disorders *812*

4.11.1 Normal sexual function *812*
Roy J. Levin

4.11.2 **The sexual dysfunctions** *821*
Cynthia A. Graham and John Bancroft

4.11.3 **The paraphilias** *832*
J. Paul Fedoroff

4.11.4 **Gender identity disorder in adults** *842*
Richard Green

4.12 Personality disorders *847*

4.12.1 **Personality disorders: an introductory perspective** *847*
Juan J. López-Ibor Jr.

4.12.2 **Diagnosis and classification of personality disorders** *855*
James Reich and Giovanni de Girolamo

4.12.3 **Specific types of personality disorder** *861*
José Luis Carrasco and Dusica Lecic-Tosevski

4.12.4 **Epidemiology of personality disorders** *881*
Francesca Guzzetta and Giovanni de Girolamo

4.12.5 **Neuropsychological templates for abnormal personalities: from genes to biodevelopmental pathways** *886*
Adolf Tobeña

4.12.6 **Psychotherapy for personality disorder** *892*
Anthony W. Bateman and Peter Fonagy

4.12.7 **Management of personality disorder** *901*
Giles Newton-Howes and Kate Davidson

4.13 Habit and impulse control disorders *911*

4.13.1 **Impulse control disorders** *911*
Susan L. McElroy and Paul E. Keck Jr.

4.13.2 **Special psychiatric problems relating to gambling** *919*
Emanuel Moran

4.14 Sleep–wake disorders *924*

4.14.1 **Basic aspects of sleep–wake disorders** *924*
Gregory Stores

4.14.2 **Insomnias** *933*
Colin A. Espie and Delwyn J. Bartlett

4.14.3 **Excessive sleepiness** *938*
Michel Billiard

4.14.4 **Parasomnias** *943*
Carlos H. Schenck and Mark W. Mahowald

4.15 Suicide *951*

4.15.1 **Epidemiology and causes of suicide** *951*
Jouko K. Lonnqvist

4.15.2 **Deliberate self-harm: epidemiology and risk factors** *957*
Ella Arensman and Ad J. F. M. Kerkhof

4.15.3 **Biological aspects of suicidal behaviour** *963*
J. John Mann and Dianne Currier

4.15.4 **Treatment of suicide attempters and prevention of suicide and attempted suicide** *969*
Keith Hawton and Tatiana Taylor

4.16 Culture-related specific psychiatric syndromes *979*
Wen-Shing Tseng

4.1

Delirium, dementia, amnesia, and other cognitive disorders

Contents

4.1.1 Delirium
David Meagher and Paula Trzepacz

4.1.2 Dementia: Alzheimer's disease
Simon Lovestone

4.1.3 Frontotemporal dementias
Lars Gustafson and Arne Brun

4.1.4 Prion disease
John Collinge

4.1.5 Dementia with Lewy bodies
I. G. McKeith

4.1.6 Dementia in Parkinson's disease
R. H. S. Mindham and T. A. Hughes

4.1.7 Dementia due to Huntington's disease
Susan Folstein and Russell L. Margolis

4.1.8 Vascular dementia
Timo Erkinjuntti

4.1.9 Dementia due to HIV disease
Mario Maj

4.1.10 The neuropsychiatry of head injury
Simon Fleminger

4.1.11 Alcohol-related dementia (alcohol-induced dementia; alcohol-related brain damage)
Jane Marshall

4.1.12 Amnesic syndromes
Michael D. Kopelman

4.1.13 The management of dementia
John-Paul Taylor and Simon Fleminger

4.1.14 Remediation of memory disorders
Jonathan J. Evans

4.1.1 Delirium

David Meagher and Paula Trzepacz

Introduction

Delirium is an acute or subacute, usually reversible syndrome of impaired higher cortical functions hallmarked by generalized cognitive disturbance and caused by one or more aetiologies. It is most common in medical-surgical patients, especially in intensive care units, and those in hospice and nursing homes. The term 'delirium' derives from the Latin '*lira*' meaning literally to wander from the furrow. Prior to DSM-III (1980) such disturbances were described by a plethora of labels (acute organic brain syndrome, acute confusional state, brain failure, toxic encephalopathy, intensive care psychosis), before Lipowski advocated for the umbrella term delirium to subsume these multiple synonyms. This engendered a more scientific research effort and consistent approach to detection and management. Though delirium has been recognized for at least two millenia, it is only now beginning to receive the attention that it warrants, with increasing appreciation of the considerable impact upon outcomes and independent need for treatment as a brain disorder beyond only treating its underlying aetiological precipitants.

Inattention is the cardinal disturbance, including distractibility, reduced vigilance or concentration, and impaired environmental awareness. This contrasts with dementia, another disorder of generalized cognitive deficits, where memory deficits are cardinal. While full-blown episodes are easier to diagnose, its prodrome, subclinical presentation, and potential persistence present unresolved dilemmas regarding diagnostic boundaries of delirium. Further, comorbidity with dementia presents challenges for detection and attribution of progressive impairments in the elderly. Though delirium occurs at any age, there is a dearth of research in younger age groups such that it is unclear whether research findings from geriatric studies can be generalized to other age groups (e.g. regarding risk factors and outcomes). Studies that clarify common features such as phenomenology, neural circuitry or electrophysiology are thus critical.

Clinical features

Delirium is a complex neuropsychiatric syndrome with a broad range of cognitive and neurobehavioural symptoms which is why it can be misattributed to other psychiatric disorders by nonspecialists. Symptoms involve cognition, thought, language, sleep-wake cycle, perception, affect, and motor behaviour. The constellation of symptoms—along with the cardinal symptom of inattention and acute onset and fluctuating temporal course—are characteristic of delirium and when comorbid with dementia, delirium dominates the clinical presentation.[1] Phenomenology studies (mostly cross-sectional) suggest that 'core' symptoms occur with greater frequency while other less consistent 'associated' symptoms may reflect the biochemical influence of particular aetiologies or genetic, neuronal or physiological vulnerabilities (see Table 4.1.1.1). Accumulating evidence indicates three core domains of delirium phenomenology: 'Cognition' comprising of inattention and other cognitive deficits; 'Higher Level Thinking Processes' including impaired executive function, semantic expression, and comprehension; and 'Circadian Rhythm' including fragmented sleep-wake cycle.[2] The underlying neural support for these domains is consistent with neuroanatomical findings in lesion and functional neuroimaging studies that implicate certain brain regions and neural circuitry.

Table 4.1.1.1 Symptoms of delirium

Symptoms of delirium
Diffuse cognitive deficits
Attention
Orientation (time, place, person)
Memory (short- and long-term; verbal and visual)
Visuoconstructional ability
Executive functions
Temporal course
Acute/abrupt onset
Fluctuating severity of symptoms over 24-hr period
Usually reversible
Subclinical syndrome may precede and/or follow the episode
Psychosis
Perceptual disturbances (especially visual), including illusions, hallucinations, metamorphosias
Delusions (usually paranoid and poorly formed)
Thought disorder (tangentiality, circumstantiality, loose associations)
Sleep-wake disturbance
Fragmented throughout 24-hr period
Reversal of normal cycle
Sleeplessness
Psychomotor behavior
Hyperactive
Hypoactive
Mixed
Language impairment
Word-finding difficulty/dysnomia/paraphasia
Dysgraphia
Altered semantic content
Severe forms can mimic expressive or receptive aphasia
Altered or labile affect
Any mood can occur, usually incongruent to context
Anger or increased irritability common
Hypoactive delirium often mislabeled as depression
Lability (rapid shifts) common
Unrelated to mood preceding delirium

(Reproduced from Trzepacz, P.T., Meagher, D.J. *Delirium, Chapter 11 in American Psychiatric Publishing Textbook of Neuropsychiatry*, (5th edn) eds. S. Yudofsky and R. Hales, copyright 2007, American Psychiatric Publishing, Inc., Washington DC.)

Delirium occurs as a stage of consciousness in the continuum between normal awakeness/alertness and stupor or coma. During the 20th century, delirium was described as a 'clouding of consciousness' but this rather nebulous concept has been replaced by a better understanding of the components of phenomenology that culminate in severely impaired higher order brain functions. Specifically, a disproportionate disturbance of attentional processes, including environmental awareness difficulties, along with impaired higher level thinking reflected in irrelevant, unfocused or illogical thought processes and impaired abstraction and comprehension (i.e. executive cognition and semantic language function) typifies the delirious state. Sleep-wake cycle fragmentation belies a circadian disturbance that may contribute to the abnormal level of consciousness and alterations in motor behaviour, where hypoactivity contributes to difficulties in differential diagnosis of delirium from stupor. Delirium is distinguished from stuporose states by the presence of arousability. The majority of intensive care unit patients emerging from comatose states experience a period of diagnosable delirium.[3]

Inattention is the cardinal and required symptom to diagnose delirium and is noticeable on interview by distractibility, spatial inattention, and inability to sustain attention. More formal testing can be assessed using months of the year backwards or digit span. The Cognitive Test for Delirium (CTD)[4] allows for separate visual digit span and vigilance testing. Memory impairment—of both short and long term—can be affected by inattention but appears to be independently impaired. Visuospatial impairment can be assessed by observing patient behaviour in their immediate environment e.g. losing their way or getting lost. Constructional ability can be tested formally by copying figures; clock face drawing assesses not only proportions and details but also involves prefrontal executive functions for placing the minute hand correctly. Delirious patients have executive dysfunction affecting abstraction, initiation/perseveration, switching mental sets, working memory, temporal sequencing and organization, insight and judgment. Poor performance on the Trailmaking Part B test distinguishes delirious from nondelirious patients and requires not only spatial attention and concentration but also switching mental sets. Though none of these cognitive deficits is specific to delirium, the array and pattern is highly suggestive.

Thought process abnormalities in delirium range from circumstantiality and tangentiality to frank loose associations in more severe cases. Naming impairment is common though more severe cases can mimic fluent dysphasia with semantic deficits being characteristic such that communication is wrought with deficits of meaningfulness. Interestingly, the dysphasia can be mistaken for Wernicke's aphasia and possible stroke but is reversible when the delirium clears. Careful assessment can usually distinguish between semantic deficits (language impairment) and loose associations (thought process disorder) except with word salad.

Disruption of sleep-wake cycle is essentially ubiquitous in delirium except in the briefest episodes (e.g. concussion) and often predates the appearance of a full-blown episode. Minor disturbances with insomnia or excessive daytime somnolence may be hard to distinguish from other medically ill patients without delirium, but more substantial alterations involve sleep fragmentation or even complete sleep-wake cycle reversal that reflect disturbed circadian rhythm regulation. The relationship of circadian disturbances to the characteristic fluctuating severity of delirium symptoms over a 24 hr period or to motor disturbance is unknown.

Motor activity alterations are very common in delirium. They have been used to define clinical subtypes (hypoactive, hyperactive, mixed) though studies are inconsistent as to the prevalence of these subtypes and often include nonmotor symptoms in descriptions. Cognitive impairments and EEG slowing are comparable in hyperactive and hypoactive patients though other symptoms may vary. Psychotic symptoms occur in both although the prevailing stereotype suggests that they only occur in hyperactive cases. Hypoactive cases are prone to non detection or misdiagnosis as depression. A range of studies suggest that motor subtypes differ regarding underlying pathophysiology, treatment needs, and prognosis for function and mortality though inconsistent subtype definitions and delayed/poorer detection of hypoactives impacts interpretation of these findings.

Psychotic symptoms occur in up to 50 per cent of patients with delirium. Thought content abnormalities include suspiciousness, overvalued ideation and frank delusions. Delusions are typically poorly-formed and less stereotyped than in schizophrenia or Alzheimer's disease. They usually relate to persecutory themes of impending danger or threat in the immediate environment (e.g. being poisoned by nurses), and less commonly to grandiose themes. Misperceptions include depersonalization, delusional misidentifications, illusions and hallucinations. Hallucinations and illusions are primarily visual though they can be tactile and auditory whereas auditory modalities tend to dominate in psychosis in mood and primary psychotic disorders. Formications suggest dopamine or anticholinergic toxicity.

Delirium may be abrupt as with concussion, drug intoxication or stroke, or can be preceded by a prodromal period characterized by anxiety, sleep disturbance, cognitive impairments and increased levels of perceived distress. Symptom profile appears similar across age groups[5] but delirium is understudied in pediatric patients. The propensity for particular aetiologies to shape clinical presentation is also understudied. Unfortunately, delirium tremens (with florid psychosis and agitation) is the dominant clinical stereotype even though many cases present with relative hypoactivity especially in the elderly, those with concomitant dementia, or where delirium is related to metabolic causes or organ failure. This misleading stereotype is one of the reasons for the poor recognition of delirium where typically 50 per cent of cases are missed in routine clinical practice.

Diagnosis and differential diagnosis

ICD-10 and DSM-IV share key features used to diagnose delirium (i.e. acute onset, fluctuating course, inattention, and disorganized thinking) although the ICD-10 description gives better account of the breadth of symptoms that can occur (e.g. disturbances of sleep and motor activity). DSM IV is more inclusive and preferred in research studies, though may be less rigorous than ICD-10 when used by less skilled clinicians. DSM-IV classifies cases according to presumed aetiological cause, though a single aetiology occurs in less than half of cases and no aetiology is identified in around 10 per cent. Delirium is also subclassified according to its relationship to dementia.

Delirium is poorly detected in clinical practice by nonpsychiatrists with more than 50 per cent of cases missed, misdiagnosed, or diagnosed late. This is due to multiple factors: the complex and fluctuating nature of delirium symptoms, inadequate education and interview skills of nonpsychiatrists, underappreciation of the prognostic significance of delirium, and inadequate routine cognitive screening in real world practice. Delirium can be the first indicator of serious physical morbidity (e.g. stroke) and represents a medical emergency. It is not surprising therefore that nondetection is associated with poorer outcomes that include elevated mortality.[6] Poor outcomes in hypoactive patients may be in part due to nondetection.

The course of delirium is highly variable reflecting the heterogeneity of aetiology and patient populations in which delirium occurs, with recent studies emphasizing that it is frequently not the benign and transient condition that was previously thought. While in many cases, delirium is brief (hours to days), represents a transitional state from unconsciousness or is a benign reaction to treatment exposures, in other cases it can be more prolonged (e.g. after traumatic brain injury) or associated with serious complications and persistent cognitive difficulties where differentiation from dementia becomes difficult. Rudberg *et al.*[7] studied elderly medical-surgical inpatients with delirium and found that episode duration was 24 hrs or less in over two-thirds of patients. Conversely, Sylvestre *et al.*[8] studied elderly medical admissions over two-month follow-up and identified five separate patterns of recovery, with fast improvement in only 11 per cent of patients. Greater clarity regarding the factors that shape these varying courses is needed.

Delirium diagnosis is complicated by *comorbidity* where over 50 per cent of cases are superimposed on dementia or other preexisting cognitive impairments. Distinguishing delirium from the neuropsychiatric symptoms of dementia can be challenging but acute onset, fluctuating course, temporal relationship to an identifiable physical precipitant, prominent inattention and altered level of consciousness usually allow differentiation. Third party informants and previous medical charts can be crucial in clarifying the trajectory of cognitive impairment. Studies comparing symptoms of delirium and dementia indicate that where they coexist, delirium symptoms dominate the clinical picture. Given the poor prognostic implications of delirium, a management hierarchy applies with delirium taking diagnostic precedence over other neuropsychiatric disorders so that any acute alteration in mental state is presumed to be delirium until otherwise established.

Some symptoms of delirium also *overlap with primary psychiatric disorders*. Major depressive disorder can be misdiagnosed in hypoactive presentations or when affective lability includes tearfulness and sad mood. Agitated depression or severe mania ('Bell's mania') can mimic hyperactive delirium but the affective lability and incongruent moods of delirium contrast with more sustained alterations in mood and effect in major mood disorders. The character of psychotic symptoms in delirium differs from primary psychotic illness (see above). Acute schizophrenic psychosis involves disorganized thoughts with delusions and hallucinations but inattention is less prominent. Acute schizophrenia can include marked cognitive impairment with perplexity that can mask or be mistaken for comorbid delirium and in such cases the EEG can be helpful. Table 4.1.1.2 describes key clinical features for differentiating delirium from other neuropsychiatric conditions.

Table 4.1.1.2 Differential diagnosis of delirium vs other common neuropsychiatric conditions

	Delirium	Dementia	Depression	Schizophrenia
Onset	Acute	Insidious[a]	Variable	Variable
Course	Fluctuating	Often progressive	Diurnal variation	Variable
Reversibility	Frequently[b]	Not usually	Usually but can be recurrent	Chronic relapsing and remitting course typical
Level of consciousness	Impaired	Unimpaired until late stages	Generally unimpaired	Unimpaired (perplexity in acute stage)
Attention/memory	Inattention is primary with poor memory	Poor memory without marked inattention except in end-stage illness	Mild attention problems, inconsistent pattern – depressive pseudodementia, memory intact with formal testing	Poor attention, inconsistent pattern, memory intact
Affect	Lability	No clear pattern	Flattening	Incongruity
Hallucinations	Usually visual; can be auditory, tactile, gustatory, olfactory	Can be visual or auditory	Usually auditory	Usually auditory
Delusions	Fleeting, fragmented, and usually persecutory often relate to immediate environment or impending danger	Paranoid, often fixed, relate to misconceptions	Complex and mood congruent e.g. themes of guilt or nihilism	Frequent, complex, systematized, and often paranoid

[a]Except for large strokes that can be abrupt and Lewy Body Dementia which can be subacute.

[b]Can be chronic (paraneoplastic syndrome, central nervous system adverse events of medications, severe brain damage).

Nondetection of delirium is particularly common in older patients with comorbid dementia, multiple medical problems and hypoactive motor presentations. Chronic subsyndromal delirium in the elderly is commonly related to low grade infections or medication adverse effects, where adjusting medications can significantly improve cognition. Monitoring for any acute deterioration from baseline function coupled with regular formal assessment with simple cognitive tests such as the digit span, months of year backwards, serial sevens or clock drawing enables delirium detection. Unfortunately, over-reliance on orientation as a measure of cognition precludes more accurate detection. The emphasis on orientation, inconsistent administration, and ceiling effects limit the usefulness of the (MMSE) in measuring delirium. The Cognitive Test for Delirium was designed specifically for delirium and emphasizes attention, semantic comprehension, and nonverbal, right hemisphere cognitive functions. It is particularly useful in critically medically ill persons.

The *Confusion Assessment Method* (CAM)[(9)] is a screening tool to assess the presence or absence of four items from DSM-III-R delirium criteria to make a provisional diagnosis of delirium. It is especially suited to epidemiological studies and screening in high risk populations where neuropsychiatric differential diagnosis or broad phenomenological measurements are not needed. Its accuracy is enhanced if ratings are anchored by formal testing as in the CAM-ICU[(10)] but is substantially reduced when used by nurses because they frequently miss inattention when it is present.

Psychiatrists and delirium specialists use *more detailed instruments* for more specific and sensitive detection of a broader range of symptoms. The Delirium Rating Scale-Revised-98 (DRS-R98)[(11)] and the Memorial Delirium Rating Scale (MDAS)[(12)] are the most widely used rating scales, and include measures of a wide breadth of symptoms. The MDAS is a severity scale used in conjunction with a DSM or ICD diagnosis whereas the DRS-R98 is both a diagnostic and severity instrument where each item rating is anchored by phenomenological descriptions.

In clinically challenging situations, an *EEG* can be used to help differentiate delirium from other neuropsychiatric disorders where generalized slowing of the dominant posterior rhythm is characteristic. Additionally, clues for specific disorders like complex partial status epilepticus can be identified.

Epidemiology and outcomes

Epidemiological studies have focused on elderly hospitalized populations with far less research in younger age groups or the general population. Delirium occurs in all age groups but those at age extremes, with pre-existing cognitive impairment, cancer, and the critically ill have especially high rates. It is estimated that around 10 per cent to–15 per cent of general hospital patients have delirium upon admission with a further 10–40 per cent developing delirium during hospitalization. Overall frequency is estimated at 11 per cent to–42 per cent[(13)] with the clinical rule of thumb that one in five general hospital inpatients experience delirium at some time during hospitalization. Delirium incidence is expected to increase as demographics of the general population shift toward older ages and with higher prevalence of dementia and cerebrovascular and cardiovascular disorders, although improved medical care for elderly persons may offset this pattern. Presence of APOE-4 alleles may confer increased risk for poorer recovery from delirium, reflecting vascular and neurodegenerative influences.

Delirium episodes are associated with elevated morbidity, longer hospital stays, greater costs of care, and higher frequency of complications.[(14)] Moreover, in the elderly, reduced post hospital independence and elevated one year mortality rates occur. Although the latter is partly due to the effects of age, frailty, comorbid dementia, severity of medical comorbidities, and medication exposure, some epidemiological studies identify delirium as an independent predictor of poorer outcomes in the elderly. However, most studies have not adequately accounted for premorbid vulnerability and cognition, burden of medical problems, and pharmacological effects such that delirium may simply be a marker of underlying pathology causing poor outcomes. Delirium incidence or severity in the elderly can be improved by earlier specialist intervention including the judicious use of haloperidol and more comprehensive delirium care, though the magnitude of this effect remains unclear.

Many report a new diagnosis of *dementia after an episode of delirium.* Some evidence suggests that persistent cognitive impairment can occur after delirium even in those thought to be premorbidly cognitively intact[15,16], while others find that baseline status or medical burden predicts outcome and follow-up reveals progression of an incipient dementing process. Contributors to post delirium cognitive decline include baseline CNS vascular or neurodegenerative pathology, physical problems that also caused the delirium, toxic effects of or inability to comply and benefit from treatments, unresolved delirium, an accelerating effect of delirium on cognitive decline, or possibly a direct neurotoxic effect of the delirious state itself. However, it is still unclear whether delirium plays a causal role or is simply a marker of medical morbidity and preexisting baseline vulnerabilities both of which are associated with delirium. Pharmacological effects (beneficial or adverse effects) are unaccounted for in most studies. The possibility that delirium itself is neurotoxic remains unproven, though could theoretically involve the effects of neurochemical abnormalities associated with delirium (e.g. dysfunctional cellular metabolism or glutamatergic surges). Studies in younger age groups are needed to disentangle confounds from aging.

Elevated mortality rates (ranging from 4 per cent to–65 per cent) during the index admission may reflect a variety of factors including the impact of underlying physical causes of delirium, the consequences of reduced ability to cooperate with medical care, the complications that occur due to the delirium symptoms (e.g. pressure sores, infections, falls). Critical review of methodology suggests that delirium mostly carries an associated increased mortality risk during the year following an episode. Mortality risk is related to agedness, severity of underlying physical illness, presence of dementia, timing of diagnosis, motor presentation and delirium symptom severity. Mortality is elevated even when the confounding effects of age, medical morbidity, and medication exposure are accounted for.[17,18] Mortality is also elevated in hospitalized patients with up to four selected delirium symptoms ('subsyndromal') but without meeting syndromal criteria,[19] highlighting the need for careful assessment and monitoring of patients at risk.

Table 4.1.1.3 Factors associated with an increased risk for delirium

1. Patient vulnerabilities
Age extremes
Pre-existing cognitive impairment e.g. dementia
CNS disorder
Genetic factors e.g. APOE genotype
Visual deficit
Hearing deficits
Poor nutritional status
Previous episode of delirium
2. Environmental
Social isolation
Sensory extremes
Immobility
Novel environment
Stress
Use of restraints
ICU stay
3. Medical
Severe medical illness
Burns
HIV / AIDS
Organ insufficiency
Infection (e.g. UTI)
Hypoxemia
Fracture
Hypothermia / fever
Metabolic disturbances
Dehydration
Elevated BUN
Low serum albumin
Nicotine withdrawal
Increased blood-brain barrier permeability
Uncontrolled pain
4. Procedure-related
Peri-operative
Type of surgery (e.g. hip)
Emergency procedure
Duration of operation
Urinary Catheterization
Artificial respiration
5. Drug-related
Polypharmacy
Drug / alcohol dependence
Psychoactive drug use
Specific agents (e.g. anticholinergics / opiates/ benzodiazepines)

Risk factors

Delirium is a multifactorial condition. A typical episode reflects the cumulative effects of predisposing risk factors, individual patient vulnerabilities (including genetic), and precipitating aetiological insults. A wide range of patient, illness, and treatment variables increase the likelihood of developing delirium but preexisting cognitive impairment, any CNS disorder, age extremes, low serum albumin, and exposure to particular medications are particularly robust predictors of delirium across populations. Geriatric and paediatric medically ill patients may share risk factors such as more vulnerable cholinergic neurotransmission—related to aging effects and developmental immaturity, respectively. Some risk factors are also considered aetiologies (e.g. UTI, anticholinergic medications). Table 4.1.1.3 lists a variety of reported risk factors across a number of reports.

The interaction between predisposition (baseline vulnerability) and precipitating insults account for delirium incidence. Inouye and Charpentier[20] developed a model of four common predisposing and five precipitating factors that predicted a 17-fold variation in delirium risk in elderly medical patients, which has been replicated in post-operative elderly patients.[21] To date most genetic studies have focussed on genotyes related to increased risk of alcohol withdrawal delirium, though APOE-4 allele genotype has been linked to longer duration of delirium in ICU patients.[22]

Aetiology

Single-aetiology delirium is the exception with typically 3–4 significant causative factors relevant during any single episode which interact and overlap sequentially to produce or sustain delirium symptoms. It is crucial that potential aetiologies are constantly reevaluated throughout a delirium episode and even after a single cause is identified, efforts to unearth other factors should continue. Categories of delirium aetiologies include drug intoxication, drug withdrawal, metabolic/endocrine, traumatic brain injury, seizures, intracranial infection, systemic infection, intracranial neoplasm, extracranial neoplasm, cerebrovascular disorder, organ insufficiency, other CNS disorder, and other systemic factors (heat stroke, radiation, hypothermia, etc). Table 4.1.1.4 lists clinical investigations recommended in routine evaluation of delirium and additional tests indicated in particular cases.

Among the most common causes are infections and those related to illicit and prescribed drugs and alcohol, either in toxicity or withdrawal. Additionally, when serum albumin levels are low, more unbound drug is available to cause adverse events. Increased blood-brain barrier permeability (e.g. uremia, sepsis) can allow passage of drugs that ordinarily do not cross into the brain and delirium can result.

Neuropathogenesis

Delirium reflects a generalized disturbance of brain function as evidenced by the broad range of neuropsychiatric symptoms, diffuse slowing on EEG, and widespread alterations in cerebral blood flow.[23] Despite the range of underlying aetiologies, delirium presents with a relatively consistent clinical profile and is thus considered a unitary syndrome reflecting a final common neural pathway for multiple diverse causes and pathophysiologies.[24,25] When studying delirium pathophysiology, it is important to distinguish between physiological mechanisms of aetiologies and neural pathology in the CNS that leads to characteristic delirium symptoms. Figure 4.1.1.1 offers examples of areas to distinguish.

Many functions are typically not disturbed in delirium (e.g. primary motor or sensory functions) and certain neuropsychological functions are disproportionately impaired (e.g. attention) suggesting that particular neurobiological underpinnings are relevant to delirium neuropathogenesis. Neuroimaging and neuropsychological studies suggest involvement of prefrontal cortex, thalamus, nondominant posterior parietal and fusiform cortices, and subcortical regions, especially right-sided pathways.[24] Additionally, anterior and posterior portions of cingulate cortex may be involved in Cognition and Higher Level Thinking domains, while subcortical regions including thalamus, hypothalamus, basal forebrain and brainstem may be involved in the Circadian Rhythm domain. Other features may be related indirectly to the underlying brain disturbances that cause domain abnormalities.

Evidence from preclinical studies, causation (e.g. exposure to anticholinergic and dopaminergic deliriogenic agents), direct studies of pathophysiology, and treatment with dopamine blockers point to a relative cholinergic deficit and dopaminergic excess as the principal neurochemical disturbances underpinning delirium although other neurochemical systems (e.g. serotonergic, glutamateric, GABAergic, noradrenergic) are clearly implicated in delirium due to particular aetiologies, perhaps through their interactions with dopaminergic and cholinergic systems. Synaptic, axonal and glial abnormalities are implicated.

Altered oxidative metabolism, stress axis activation, and neuroinflammatory mechanisms may acutely impact neurotransmission. Further, neurostructural derangements previously thought to occur in chronic neurodegenerative disorders can occur acutely and transiently, and may underlie delirium. These include traumatic hyperphosphorylation during anaesthesia or traumatic elevations of Abeta inducing synaptic morphological and functional alterations.

Table 4.1.1.4 Clinical investigations recommended for delirium

1. Mandatory (recommended for all patients)
Full blood count and differential
Urea and electrolytes to include Mg, Ca, Po4
Renal function
Liver function tests to include serum albumin
Urinalysis
Random blood glucose
Electrocardiogram
Chest X-Ray
2. As indicated (according to particular clinical circumstances—list not exhaustive)
Drug screen (therapeutic and illicit)
Blood alcohol concentration
Blood cultures
Cardiac enzymes
Arterial blood gases
Serum Folate / B12
Thyroid function tests
Erythrocyte sedimentation rate
Cerebrospinal fluid examination
Syphilis serology
CT brain
MRI brain
Electroencephalography (with nasopharyngeal leads)
Polysomnography
Prothrombin time
Urinary porphyrins
Screen for heavy metals and insecticides

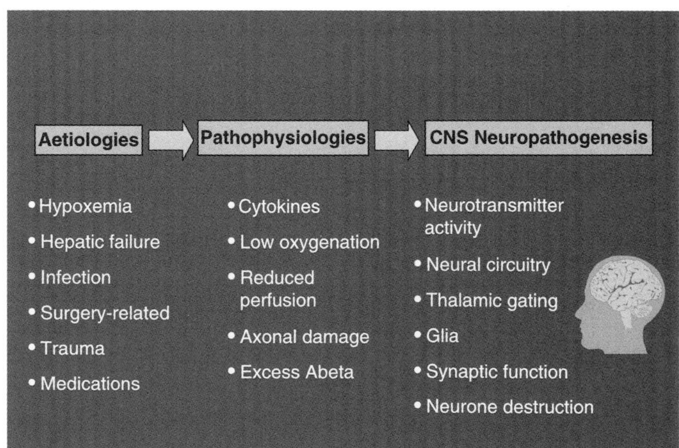

Fig. 4.1.1.1. Examples of different aetiologies for delirium and a variety of pathophysiological mechanisms that can then alter brain function. The neuropathogenesis of delirium involves dysfunction of brain regions and circuitry which may ultimately result in characteristic symptoms of delirium despite a wide variety of aetiologies and pathophysiological insults to the brain.

The broad disturbance of CNS function that occurs in delirium inevitably involves alterations to many cortical and subcortical regions and their neural circuitry, via both direct and indirect (diaschesis) effects.

Management

Delirium is a medical urgency, yet the value of timely intervention in limiting the many deleterious effects of a delirium episode is underappreciated. Optimal management requires the collaborative efforts of primary treating physicians and nursing staff with delirium specialists. Both the underlying causes and the brain disorder need simultaneous assessment and treatment. Careful attention to reorientation strategies (e.g. clearly visible clock/calendar), safety in immediate surroundings and optimal level of environmental stimulation (e.g. natural levels of diurnal lighting) are fundamental to the management of delirium across treatment settings and populations.[26] Relatives / loved ones can report changes in behaviour and mental state ('not themselves') and provide collateral information about baseline cognitive and independent functioning and risk factor exposure.

Delirium prevention using multicomponent interventions to address modifiable risk factors can reduce the frequency and severity of delirium in elderly medical and post-operative populations.[27,28] Common elements include elimination of unnecessary medications, careful attention to hydration and nutritional status, pain relief, correction of sensory deficits, sleep enhancement, early mobilization, and cognitive stimulation. Careful attention to reorientation strategies (e.g. clearly visible clock/calendar), safety in immediate surroiundings and optimal level of environmental stimulation (e.g. natural levels of diurnal lighting) are key elements of delirium care.[26]

Recent studies of pharmacological prophylaxis of delirium in high-risk populations have been encouraging. Controlled studies using haloperidol,[29] olanzapine,[30] donepezil[31] and rivastigmine[32] report significant reductions in delirium incidence, severity and/or duration.

(a) Pharmacological management

Pharmacological management of delirium addresses the brain dysfunction itself while the underlying medical problems are being separately considered. This is akin to acute heart failure where treatment of cardiac function is concurrent with management of the aetiologies for the organ failure. Pharmacological management of delirium is based on empirical knowledge drawn from case reports, open label prospective studies and a small number of randomized trials some of which are comparator studies. Adequately powered double blind randomized placebo-controlled efficacy trials are needed because there is currently no medication with an indication for delirium treatment by any regulatory authority. The inherent fluctuating nature, varying duration, spontaneous recovery rate, and impact of medical treatments upon underlying causes render placebo-controlled studies especially important in evaluating therapeutic interventions. Nevertheless, there are over 20 well-conducted prospective studies of antipsychotic agents used in acute treatment of delirium where more than two-thirds of treated delirious patients experience clinical improvement, typically within a week.[33] A randomized controlled trial of haloperidol vs olanzapine vs non-drug treatment in elderly patients indicated similar response rates in those receiving haloperidol (87.5 per cent) and Olanzapine (82 per cent), which was significantly greater than those in the non-drug treatment group (31 per cent).[34] Treatment response includes improved cognitive and noncognitive symptoms of delirium and does not appear to be closely linked to antipsychotic effect or sedative action. Younger patients with hyperactive presentations and patients without comorbid dementia respond more robustly to antipsychotics, but hypoactive patients also improve and deserve treatment given that delirium comprises many serious symptoms besides challenging motor behaviour.[35,36]

Most pharmacological strategies are based upon the prevailing notion of a relative dopaminergic excess and cholinergic deficiency as the principal neurochemical aberrations underlying delirium, and agents with either procholinergic or antidopaminergic effects are favoured. *Haloperidol* remains the standard agent used to treat delirium and is available in oral, intramuscular, and intravenous preparations. However, intravenous haloperidol does not have any indicated use by a regulatory agency and carries a high risk for QTc prolongation and torsades de pointes tachyarrhythymia that can lead to sudden death. Suggested haloperidol doses are 1–2 mg every four hours as needed but with lower doses (e.g. 0.25–0.5 mg every four hours) in the elderly, very frail, or populations with neuroleptic sensitivity—APA guidelines, 1999.[37] Uncontrolled agitated delirium can be life threatening especially in critically ill intensive care unit patients where substantially higher doses have been reported without major adverse effects. Careful monitoring of ECG (telemetry with intravenous haloperidol), and maintaining normal serum potassium, calcium, and magnesium levels are recommended.

Accumulating evidence supports the use of *atypical antipsychotic agents* in delirium (risperidone, olanzapine, quetiapine, aripirazole, ziprasidone, amisulpiride). Comparison studies suggest similar response rates to haloperidol for both risperidone and olanzapine but with reduced extrapyramidal side effects. In highly agitated patients where sedation is desirable, more sedative agents or combination with lorazepam may be considered. Given the importance of sleep-wake cycle disturbances in delirium, dose scheduling should encourage recovery of normal sleeping patterns.

Benzodiazepines can act as either an alleviating or as a risk factor for delirium depending on the circumstances of exposure. Benzodiazepines can be associated with worsening of mental state[38] and increase delirium risk in ICU[39] and cancer patients.[40] Moreover, therapeutic effects vary from anxiolytic to sedative to hypnotic with ascending doses. Conversely, benzodiazepines are first line treatment for delirium related to sedative and alcohol-withdrawal or seizures. Benzodiazepines can allow for lower neuroleptic doses where intolerance is a problem or where extra sedation is desired. Lorazepam is preferred due to its short acting nature and relatively predictable bioavailability when given intramuscularly. Lower doses are required in the elderly and those with respiratory or hepatic compromise or receiving drugs that undergo extensive hepatic oxidative metabolism. Unwanted effects of benzodiazepines can be rapidly reversed with flumazenil.

The use of *procholinergic agents* such as intravenous physostigmine has long been advocated for delirium due to toxicity with anticholinergic drugs, but routine delirium use is limited by gastrointestinal side effects, cardiac arrythmia and seizures. To date there has been limited study of newer procholinergics in part because their long half-lives preclude reaching steady state for use in acute conditions, in contrast to parenteral physostigmine's fast onset of action.

Anecdotal evidence also exists for the use of mianserin, trazadone, melatonin, psychostimulants, and even ECT in the treatment of delirium but these strategies are not well-studied or applied in routine clinical practice.

(b) Risks, benefits, and dosing

Adequate drug treatment of delirium is limited by concerns over potential toxic effects in highly morbid, frail elderly whose delirium may actually herald bad outcome from medical illness. In assessing the risk-benefit ratio of medication use one must consider the risk of nontreatment of delirium given its grave consequences. Dosing needs to take into account structural degenerative changes, reduced neurochemical flexibility, less robust counter-regulatory homeostatic mechanisms, reduced renal and hepatic function, lower water to fat ratio with reduced muscle mass, and reduced plasma esterase activity. In hypoactive or mechanically ventilated patients careful dose titration can be assisted by regular monitoring of sedation. With sedation, a beneficial effect of catching up from sleep deprivation also needs to be considered. Adverse events such as Parkinsonism or akathisia can be misattributed to agitation of delirium, though are uncommon in treatment studies perhaps reflecting a protective effect of the hypocholinergic state that frequently underpins delirium. The potential for cardiac arrythmias can be reduced with ECG monitoring in high dose or intravenous haloperidol use or where patients have a cardiac history or baseline ECG shows QTc interval >450 mSec.

(c) Patients with concomitant dementia

Both pharmacological[(35)] and non-pharmacological strategies[(28)] appear less effective in patients with concomitant dementia perhaps reflecting the inherently poor outcome of elderly demented populations with high physical comorbidity. There are concerns regarding the small but increased risk of cerebrovascular events in demented patients chronically receiving neuroleptics, but the relative risks of short-term use in delirium must be proportionalized against potential benefits. Lower doses should be used with careful monitoring for adverse effects and more prolonged use should not occur in the absence of clear benefits.

(d) Management after recovery

Depending on the degree of memory imprinting during an episode, patients experience significant emotional distress after recovery[(41)] and many continue to have distressing recollections of delirium six months later, especially where the episode has involved psychotic symptoms. For families, disturbing recollections of final contacts with loved ones can be enduringly distressing and associated with complicated bereavement reactions. Some patients minimize their experiences fearing that they represent emerging senility or loss of competence. Explicit recognition allows clarification of the causes of delirium and reduction of future risk factors.

Conclusion

Delirium is a complex neuropsychiatric syndrome that occurs commonly across all age groups and healthcare settings. Significant adverse outcomes of delirium are increasingly recognized and can be reduced by a more consistent approach to detection that emphasizes disturbances of attention. Optimal management requires the collaborative efforts of carers and healthcare staff and judicious use of pharmacological and nonpharmacological strategies that concurrently manage underlying physical causes and the delirium itself. Greater clarity is needed regarding the prognostic relationship to dementia, phenomenology of prodromal, subsyndromal and syndromal delirium, and how risk factors, vulnerabilities, and treatment may vary across populations and treatment settings.

Further information

The *European Delirium Association* advocates for better research and aims to foster research activity across all disciplines. Annual meeting details, educational materials and a discussion forum are available at www.europeandeliriumassociation.com

A US-based delirium organization aims to foster delirium care and research in critically ill patients and includes various teaching resources including protocols for assessment and treatment at www.icudelirium.org

The American Psychiatric Association website includes detailed delirium treatment guidelines, a quick reference guide as well as a patient and family guide (see www.psych.org/psych_pract/treatg/quick_ref_guide/DeliriumQRG_4-15-05.pdf)

References

1. Trzepacz, P.T., Mulsant, B.H., Dew, M.A., *et al.* (1998). Is delirium different when it occurs in dementia? A study using the Delirium Rating Scale. *J Neuropsychiatry Clin Neurosci*, **10**, 199–204.
2. Meagher, D.J., Moran, M., Raju, B., *et al.* (2007): Phenomenology of 100 consecutive adult cases of delirium. *British Journal of Psychiatry*, **190**, 135–41.
3. McNicoll, L., Pisani, M.A., Zhang, Y. *et al.* (2003). Delirium in the intensive care unit: occurrence and clinical course in older patients. *J Am Geriatr Soc*, **51**, 591–98.
4. Hart, R.P., Levenson. J.L., Sessler, C.N., *et al.* (1996). Validation of a cognitive test for delirium in medical ICU patients. *Psychosomatics*, **37**, 533–46.
5. Turkel, S.B., Trzepacz, P.T., Tavare, C.J. (2006). Comparison of delirium in adults and children. *Psychosomatics*, **47**, 320–24
6. Kakuma, R., du Fort, G.G., Arsenault, L., *et al.* (2003). Delirium in older emergency department patients discharged home: effect on survival. *J Am Geriatr Soc*, **51**, 443–50.
7. Rudberg, M.A., Pompei, P., Foreman, M.D., *et al.* (1887). The natural history of delirium in older hospitalized patients: a syndrome of heterogeneity. *Age Ageing*, **26**, 169–74.
8. Sylvestre, M.P., McCusker, J., Cole, M., *et al.* (2006). Classification of patterns of delirium severity scores over time in an elderly population. *Int Psychogeriatr*, **18**, 667–80.
9. Inouye, S.K., van Dyke, C.H., Alessi, C.A., *et al.* (1990). Clarifying confusion: the Confusion Assessment Method. *Ann Intern Med*, **113**, 941–48.
10. Ely EW, Gordan S, Francis J, *et al.* (2001). Evaluation of delirium in critically ill patients: validation of the Confusion Assessment Method for the intensive care unit (CAM-ICU). *Crit Care Med*, **29**, 1370–79.
11. Trzepacz, P.T., Mittal, D., Torres, R., *et al.* (2001). Validation of the Delirium Rating Scale–Revised-98: comparison to the Delirium Rating Scale and Cognitive Test for Delirium. *J Neuropsychiatry Clin Neurosci*, **13**, 229–42.
12. Breitbart, W., Rosenfeld, B., Roth, A., *et al.* (1997).The Memorial Delirium Assessment Scale. *J Pain Symptom Manage*, **13**, 128–37.
13. Siddiqi, N., House, A.O., Holmes, J.D., *et al.* (2006). Occurrence and outcome of delirium in medical in-patients: a systematic literature review. *Age Ageing*, **35**, 350–64.

14. Fick, D.M., Kolanowski, A.M., Waller, J.L., *et al.* (2005). Delirium superimposed on dementia in a community-dwelling managed care population: a three-year retrospective study of occurrence, costs and utilization. *J Gerontol Med Sci*, **60A**, 748–53.
15. Gruber-Baldini, A.L., Zimmerman, S., Morrison, R.S., *et al.* (2003). Cognitive impairment in hip fracture patients: timing of detection and longitudinal follow-up. *J Am Geriatr Soc*, **51**, 1227–36.
16. Lundstrom, M., Edlund, A., Bucht, G., *et al.* (2003). Dementia after delirium in patients with femoral neck fractures. *J Am Geriatr Soc*, **51**, 1002–6.
17. Ely, E.W., Shintani, A., Truman, B., *et al.* (2004). Delirium as a predictor of mortality in mechanically ventilated patients in the intensive care unit. *JAMA*, **291**, 1753–62.
18. Pitkälä, K.H., Laurila, J.V., Strandberg, T.E., *et al.* (2005). Prognostic signifi cance of delirium in frail older people. *Dement Geriatr Cogn Disord*, **19**, 158–63.
19. Cole, M., McCusker, J., Dendukuri, N., *et al.* (2003). The prognostic signifi cance of subsyndromal delirium in elderly medical inpatients. *J Am Geriatr Soc*, **51**, 754–60.
20. Inouye, S.K. and Charpentier, P.A., *et al.* (1996): Precipitating factors for delirium in hospitalized elderly patients: predictive model and interrelationships with baseline vulnerability. *JAMA*, **275**, 852–57.
21. Kalisvaart, K.J., Vreeswijk, de Jonghe, J., *et al.* (2005b) Risk factors and prediction of post-operative delirium in elderly hip surgery patients. Implementation and validation of the Inouye risk factor model. *Int Psychogeriatrics*, **17** (S2), 261.
22. Ely, E.W., Girard, T.D., Shintani, A.K., *et al.* (2007). Apolipoprotein E4 polymorphism as a genetic predisposition to delirium in critically ill patients. *Crit Care Med*, **35**, 112–7.
23. Yokota, H., Ogawa, S., Kurokawa, A., *et al.* (2003). Regional cerebral blood fl ow in delirious patients. *Psychiatry Clin Neurosci*, **57**, 337–9.
24. Trzepacz, P.T. (1994). Neuropathogenesis of delirium: a need to focus our research. *Psychosomatics*, **35**, 374–91.
25. Trzepacz, P.T., Meagher, D.J. (2007). Delirium. In *American Psychiatric Publishing Textbook of Neuropsychiatry* (5th edn). (eds S. Yudofsky and R. Hales). American Psychiatric Publishing, Inc, Washington, DC.
26. Meagher, D. (2001). Delirium: optimising management. *British Medical Journal*, **7279**, 144–9.
27. Inouye, S.K., Bogardus, S.T., Charpentier, P.A., *et al.* (1999). A multicomponent intervention to prevent delirium in hospitalized older patients. *N Engl J Med*, **340**, 669–76.
28. Marcantonio, E.R., Flacker, J.M., Wright, R.J., *et al.* (2001). Reducing delirium after hip fracture: a randomized trial. *J Am Geriatr Soc*, **49**, 516–22.
29. Kalisvaart, K.J., de Jonghe, J.F.M., Bogaards, M.J., *et al.* (2005). Haloperidol prophylaxis for elderly hip surgery patients at risk for delirium: a randomized, placebo-controlled study. *J Am Geriatr Soc*, **53**, 1658–66.
30. Larsen, K., Kelly, S., Stern, T., *et al.* (2007). A double-blind, randomized, placebocontrolled study of perioperative administration of olanzapine to prevent postoperative delirium in joint replacement patients. Academy of Psychosomatic medicine 54th Annual meeting proceedings.
31. Sampson, E.L., Raven, P.R., Ndhlovu, P.N., *et al.* (2006). A randomized, double-blind, placebo-controlled trial of donepezil hydrochloride (Aricept) for reducing the incidence of postoperative delirium after elective total hip replacement. *Int J Geriatr Psychiatry*, **22**, 343–9.
32. Moretti, R., Torre, P., Antonello, R.M., *et al.* (2004). Cholinesterase inhibition as a possible therapy for delirium in vascular dementia: a controlled, open 24-month study of 246 patients. *Am J Alzheimers Dis Other Demen*, **19**, 333–9.
33. Meagher, D. and Leonard, M. (2008). The active management of delirium: improving detection and treatment. *Advances in Psychiatric Treatment*, **14**, 292–301.
34. Hua, H., Wei, D., Hui, Y., *et al.* (2006). Olanzapine and haloperidol for senile delirium: a randomised controlled observation. *Chinese Journal of Clinical rehabilitation*, **10**, 188–90.
35. Breitbart, W., Tremblay, A., Gibson, C., *et al* (2002). An open trial of olanzapine for the treatment of delirium in hospitalized cancer patients. *Psychosomatics*, **43**, 175–82.
36. Platt, M.M., Breitbart, W., Smith, M., *et al.* (1994). Efficacy of neuroleptics for hypoactive delirium. *J Neuropsychiatry Clin Neurosci*, **6**, 66–67.
37. American Psychiatric Association (1999). Practice guidelines for the treatment of patients with delirium. *Am J Psychiatry*, **156**(suppl), 1–20.
38. Breitbart, W., Marotta, R., Platt. M.M., *et al.* (1996). A double-blind trial of haloperidol, chlorpromazine, and lorazepam in the treatment of delirium in hospitalized AIDS patients. *Am J Psychiatry*, **153**, 231–37.
39. Pandharipande, P., Shintani, A., Peterson, J., *et al* (2006). Lorazepam is an independent risk factor for transitioning to delirium in intensive care unit patients. *Anesthesiology*, **104**, 21–6.
40. Gaudreau, J.D., Gagnon, P., Harel, F., *et al.* (2005). Psychoactive medications and risk of delirium in hospitalized cancer patients. *J Clin Oncol*, **23**, 6712–8.
41. Breitbart, W., Gibson, C. and Tremblay, A., *et al.* (2002b). The delirium experience: delirium recall and delirium-related distress in hospitalized patients with cancer, their spouses/caregivers, and their nurses. *Psychosomatics*, **43**, 183–94.

4.1.2 **Dementia: Alzheimer's disease**

Simon Lovestone

Introduction

Alzheimer's disease (**AD**) and other dementias incur huge costs to society, to the families of those affected, and to the individuals themselves. Costs to society include both direct costs to health and social services and indirect economic costs in terms of lost productivity, as carers are taken out of the workplace, and the economic costs to those families caring for or funding the care of their relative. Increasingly, as treatments become available, these costs are targets for change and are part of the cost–benefit analysis of new compounds, especially the largest single direct cost, that of the provision of nursing and other forms of continuing care. Apart from the financial cost to families there is the emotional impact resulting in distress and psychiatric morbidity.

As the population ages, these costs pose substantial social and economic problems. Although lifespan itself has remained static, the numbers of elderly in both developed and developing societies is increasing rapidly. In the developed world the sharpest projected growth is in the very elderly cohort—precisely the one that is at most risk of AD. Within the developing world, the total number of elderly people is projected to rise substantially, reflecting to a large part better child health and nutrition. For countries in South America and Asia, with large and growing populations, the costs involved in caring for people with dementia in the future will become an increasing burden on health and social services budgets. In the absence of such services families will inevitably shoulder the main part of providing care, although the very process of development is associated with increasing urbanization and, to some degree, a diminution of the security provided by extended family structures.

From discovery towards understanding

In the early part of the twentieth century, Alois Alzheimer described his eponymous disorder in a middle-aged woman who suffered not only cognitive deterioration and functional decline but psychotic experiences, including delusions and auditory hallucinations. Neuropathology included gross atrophy and plaques and tangles on microscopy. Although all the important features of AD were described at this stage, two important developments came much later. First, in the 1960s with the studies of Roth and colleagues in Newcastle[1] and others elsewhere, it was appreciated that much dementia in the elderly has an identical neuropathological appearance to that of AD in younger people. The other development was the rediscovery that AD has a rich phenomenology. The non-cognitive symptomatology of AD is integral to the clinical manifestation of this disease, and is a major cause of carer burden and medical intervention. This second phase of research—the recognition that both the neuropathology and clinical phenomenology described by Alzheimer occur in what had previously been though of as senile dementia or, worse, just ageing, was accompanied by a growing understanding of the neurotransmitter deficits in AD. The cholinergic hypothesis provided the first glimpse of possible interventions, and remains the most important finding from this period of AD investigations. The third phase of AD research encompasses the use of molecular approaches to understanding pathogenesis. The techniques of molecular biology have been applied to understanding the formation of plaques and tangles, to a growing understanding of the genetic aetiology of much of AD, and, through the use of transgenic approaches, to developing animal and cellular models of pathogenesis.

Just as research can broadly be seen to have three phases—discovery, neuropathology, and molecular aspects—so too does the clinical response to AD. For many years cognitive impairment in the elderly was perceived as senility. As a process thought to be an inevitable consequence of ageing it was difficulty to establish medical-care models. Hence the needs of the elderly with AD were not seen as requiring specialist intervention, carers needs were not realized, and public appreciation of the impact of dementia on the elderly themselves or on the family was negligible. The change in perception of AD from 'just ageing' to a disease was accompanied, and to some degree led, by the development of 'old-age psychiatry' as a specialism on the one hand and by the rapid growth of the AD societies on the other. During this second phase of AD treatment, the goals have been to ensure that the care needs of patients are met, that families' concerns are addressed, and that behavioural disturbance is minimized. The third phase of AD treatment began with the arrival of specifically designed interventions. Compounds have been introduced that were designed to ameliorate some of the deficits incurred by the disease process, and other approaches are being developed to treat those disease processes themselves.

Clinical features

Cognitive impairment

Dementia is acquired cognitive decline in multiple areas resulting in functional impairment; AD is one cause of dementia and the core clinical symptom of AD is cognitive loss. However, as noted above, AD is clinically heterogeneous and includes diverse non-cognitive symptoms. Cognitive decline is manifested as **a**mnesia, **a**phasia, **a**gnosia, and **a**praxia (the 4As).

(a) Amnesia

Memory loss in AD is early and inevitable. Characteristically, recent memories are lost before remote memories. However, there is considerable individual variation, with some patients able to recall specific and detailed events of childhood and others apparently having few distant memories accessible. With disease progression, even remote and emotionally charged memories are lost. The discrepancy between recent and remote memory loss suggests that the primary problem is of acquisition or retrieval of memory rather than a destruction of memory, and this is confirmed in early AD,[2] although as the disease progresses it is likely that all memory processes are impaired. Retrieval of remote memory is assumed to be preserved for longer because of rehearsal over life.

(b) Aphasia

Language problems are found in many patients at presentation, although the language deficits in AD are not as severe as those of the fronto-temporal degenerations[3] and may only be apparent on detailed examination. Word-finding difficulties (nominal dysphasia) are the earliest phenomena observed and are accompanied by circumlocutions and other responses, for example repetitions and alternative wordings. As the disorder progresses, syntax is affected and speech becomes increasingly paraphasic. Although harder to assess, receptive aphasia, or comprehension of speech, is almost certainly affected. In the final stages of the disorder, speech is grossly deteriorated with decreased fluency, preservation, echolalia, and abnormal non-speech utterances.

(c) Agnosia

Patients with AD may have difficulty in recognizing as well as naming objects. This can have implications for care needs and safety if the unrecognized objects are important for daily functioning. One particular agnosia encountered in AD is the loss of recognition of one's own face (autoprosopagnosia). This distressing symptom is the underlying cause of perhaps the only clinical sign in AD—the mirror sign. Patients exhibiting this will interpret the face in the mirror as some other individual and respond by talking to it or by apparent fearfulness. Autoprosopagnosia can present as an apparent hallucinatory experience, until it is realized that the 'hallucination' is fixed in both content and space, occurring only when self-reflection can be seen.

(d) Apraxia

Difficulties with complex tasks that are not due to motor impairment become apparent in the moderate stages of AD. Typically, difficulties with dressing or tasks in the kitchen are noticed first, but these are inevitably preceded by loss of ability for more difficult tasks. Strategies to avoid such tasks are often acquired as the disease progresses, and it is only when these fail that the dyspraxia becomes apparent.

Other cognitive impairment

There appear to be no cognitive functions that are truly preserved in AD. Visuospatial difficulties commonly occur in the middle stages of the disorder and may result in topographical disorientation, wandering, and becoming lost. Difficulties with calculation, attention, and cognitive planning all occur.

Functional impairment

Although the cognitive decline in AD is the core symptom, it is the functional deterioration that has the most impact on the person themselves and it is the functional loss that necessitates most of the care needs of patients with AD, including nursing-home residency.(4) Increasingly, abilities to function in ordinary life (activities of daily living (**ADLs**)) are lost, starting with the most subtle and easily avoided and progressing to the most basic and essential. In general, functional abilities decline alongside cognitive abilities. However, the precise correlation between these functions is not perfect, suggesting that factors other than disease severity account for part of the variance between patients.(5) Functional abilities are related to gender; for example, cooking abilities are rehearsed more frequently in women, and home-improvement skills in men. However, the overall pattern shows some similarities between groups of patients with similar disease severity. This is exploited in the Functional Assessment Staging (**FAST**) Scale;(6) in the original form, this is a seven-point scale of functional impairment, with stage 1 as no impairment and stage 7 as severe AD. A sequential decline is mapped by descriptions of the abilities that are lost: stage 2, difficulties with language and finding objects; stage 4, difficulties with finances; stage 6, incontinence and inability to dress or wash oneself.

ADLs are divided into those that relate to self-care and those that concern instrumental activities. Instrumental ADLs, those related to the use of objects or the outside world, are lost first and can be subtle.(7) A change in the ability to use the telephone properly or to handle finances accurately may not be apparent. Self-care ADLs include dressing and personal hygiene and are also lost gradually; for example, untidiness in clothing progresses to difficulties in dressing. Personal hygiene becomes poor as dentures are not cleaned and baths taken less often, before finally assistance is required with all self-care tasks.

Neuropsychiatric symptoms

(a) Mood

The relationship between AD and depression is complex. Depression is a risk factor for AD, depression can be confused with dementia (pseudodementia), depression occurs as part of dementia, and cognitive impairments are found in depression. Depression occurring as a symptom of dementia will be considered here. Assessing the mood of a person with dementia is difficult for obvious reasons. However, psychomotor retardation, apathy, crying, poor appetite, disturbed sleep, and expressions of unhappiness all occur frequently. The rates of depression found in cohorts of patients with AD vary widely, reflecting changes in prevalence at different levels of severity and difficulties in the classification of symptoms suggestive of depression in those with cognitive loss. A major depressive episode is found in approximately 10 per cent of patients, minor depressive episode in 25 per cent, some features of depression in 50 per cent, and an assessment of depression by a carer in up to 85 per cent.(8–12) It is commonly believed that depression is more common in the early than in the later stages of AD, although this may reflect the difficulties of assessing depression in the more severely affected and least communicative patients. Indeed, severely affected patients in nursing homes may be particularly prone to depression.(13) Elation, disinhibition, and hypomania all occur in AD but are relatively infrequent, elevated mood being found in only 3.5 per cent of patients by Burns *et al.*(10)

The underlying cause of mood change in AD is not known. However, loss of serotonergic and noradrenergic markers accompanies cholinergic loss; some studies have found a greater loss of these markers at post-mortem in AD patients with depression than in non-depressed patients.(14–16)

(b) Psychosis

Psychotic symptoms occur in many patients, although, as with depression, there is an inherent difficulty in determining the presence of delusions or hallucinatory experiences in the moderately to severely demented. In community-based surveys, between 20 and 70 per cent are reported to suffer from some form of psychotic symptom with delusions being more common than hallucinations.(11,17,18) Delusions are frequently paranoid and the most common delusion is one of theft. In the context of the confusion and amnesia of dementia, it is easy to appreciate how the experience of mislaying an object becomes translated into conviction of a theft. Other patients become convinced that someone, often a family member, is trying to harm them.

Hallucinations are only somewhat less frequent than delusions—the median of one series of studies being 28 per cent.(19) Visual hallucinations are reported more commonly than auditory ones, and other modalities are rare. Most studies of the non-cognitive symptomatology of AD precede the wide recognition and accepted criteria of dementia with Lewy bodies, one of the cardinal symptoms of which is visual hallucinations. It is probable that a large number of those AD patients experiencing visual hallucinations reported in the studies would now be classified as having dementia with Lewy bodies.

Phenomena falling short of delusions or hallucinations, such as persecutory ideas or intrusive illusionary experiences, are common in AD as are misidentification syndromes. Capgras' syndrome may occur, but frequently the symptom is less fully evolved with the patient mistaking one person for another. Failure to recognize one's own face may be due to visuospatial difficulties or to a true misidentification syndrome—distinguishing between the two is difficult.

Various factors have been associated with psychosis in AD, but few have been substantiated in multiple studies. Burns *et al.*(20) found that more men than women suffered delusions of theft, although others find that psychosis occurs more often or earlier in women. An association with polymorphic variation in serotonin receptors has been reported.(21–23) The relationship between psychosis and dementia severity is not as clear cut as that between functional ability and dementia severity. Psychosis can occur at any stage of the disease process, although most studies find the maximal rate of psychosis in those with at least moderate dementia.

Although the biological basis of psychosis within AD is not fully understood,(14) it is clear that psychosis symptoms impact upon carers causing increased distress,(24,25) and that underlying psychosis accounts for much of the behavioural disturbance and aggression encountered in AD.(26)

(c) Personality

Changes in personality are an almost inevitable concomitant of AD. Indeed, it is difficult to envisage how profound cognitive impairment resulting in the loss of recognition of loved ones, and an understanding of and ability to react with the outside world, could not result in a change in personality. Family members have described the loss of personality as a 'living bereavement'—the body remains, but the person once known has gone. Personality change is most frequently one of loss of awareness and normal responsiveness to the environment. Individuals may become more anxious or fearful, there is a flattening of affect, and a withdrawal from challenging situations. Catastrophic reactions are short-lived emotional reactions that occur when the patient is confronted, and cannot avoid, such a challenging situation. Less commonly, personality changes may be of disinhibition with inappropriate sexual behaviours or inappropriate affect. Aggressiveness is, as noted above, often accompanied by psychosis, but it may be part of a more general personality change.

(d) Other behavioural manifestations

Behavioural complications in AD have become a target of therapy. However, the term encompasses a wide range of behaviours, some of which include neuropsychiatric syndromes, some caused by neuropsychiatric syndromes, and some of which have little apparent relationship to mood or to thought content. Behavioural complication is itself a largely subjective term that relies to a great extent on informer evaluation: but behaviour may be a complication in one context, although not in another.

Behaviours exhibited in AD include wandering, changes in eating habit, altered sleep or circadian rhythms, and incontinence. These behaviours are closely linked to disease severity and occur to some extent in the majority of patients with AD. Wandering may be a manifestation of topographical confusion, a need for the toilet, or it may reflect hunger, boredom, or anxiety. Sleep is frequently disturbed, with many patients exhibiting altered sleep–wake cycles and others experiencing increased confusion towards evening ('sundowning'). A central defect in the regulation of circadian rhythms underlying these phenomena is postulated.(27) Excessive or inappropriate vocalizations (grunting and screaming) occur in the late stages.

Classification

Alzheimer's disease is classified, as with all other disorders, by DSM-IV and by ICD-10. In addition, it also has a specialized classification system resulting from the National Institute of Neurological and Communicative Disorders and Stroke–AD and Related Disorders Association (**NINCDS–ADRDA**).(28) This clinical diagnostic system is internationally accepted and widely observed. There are also classification systems for neuropathological diagnosis, most notably the Consortium to Establish a Registry for AD (**CERAD**) criteria.(29)

DSM-IV stipulates that a dementia syndrome is characterized by deterioration in multiple cognitive deficits, including amnesia, resulting in functional impairment. A gradual onset and decline in the absence of other conditions sufficient to cause dementia indicates AD. ICD-10 shares with DSM-IV the definition of a dementia syndrome and notes that an insidious onset and slow decline in the absence of other disorders sufficient to cause dementia indicates AD. The NINCDS–ADRDA criteria defines possible, probable, and definite categories; the latter being restricted to neuropathological confirmation of a clinical diagnosis.(28) It is important to note that both clinical and neuropathological data are required—no single neuropathological lesion is pathognomonic of AD, and it is still uncertain how often or to what extent the neuropathological lesions of AD also occur in normal ageing.(30) Probable AD, according to NINCDS–ADRDA, requires a dementia with progressive decline in memory and other cognitive areas, cognitive impairment established by formal testing, no disturbance of consciousness, and absence of other disorders sufficient to cause dementia. Supporting features include decline in function, change in behaviour, positive family history, and decline in specific cognitive areas including aphasia, apraxia, and agnosia. Non-specific change on electroencephalography (**EEG**) and progressive changes on CT are supporting, but not necessary, features. Possible AD should be diagnosed if there are variations in the clinical presentation, another disorder sufficient to cause a dementia (even if it is not thought to do so in this case), or a restricted cognitive decline.

A number of studies have attempted to determine the accuracy of diagnostic criteria against post-mortem diagnosis. One of the difficulties in these studies is that because AD is the most common dementia (by some way), such studies are very likely to find a high-positive predicative value. Kukull *et al.*(31) found the specificity of DSM-III to be higher than NINCDS–ADRDA (0.8 versus 0.65), but NINCDS–ADRDA had a higher sensitivity (0.92 versus 0.76), Mok *et al.* find broadly similar findings for both primary care physicians and for neurologists;(32) some others find an even lower specificity.(33)

Diagnosis

Alzheimer's disease is the most common of the dementias, occurring in some 60 to 70 per cent of cases. However, this oft-stated figure must be treated with some caution for two reasons. First, cases that come to post-mortem represent a biased sample and in the community a large proportion (up to a third) of non-demented individuals have pathological signs of AD such as neuritic plaques.(30) Second, even at post-mortem the distinction between different dementias is not clear cut—many AD brains show the presence of Lewy bodies and others have considerable evidence of vascular damage. The proportion of mixed pathologies is actually rather high, between 15 and 30 per cent of all dementias. Thirdly, even the gold-standard of neuropathological diagnosis is not infallible. Neuropathologists show a very high degree of inter-rater agreement on the diagnosis of probable AD and Dementia with Lewy Bodies (DLB) but a rather lower rate of agreement when there is vascular damage, when the diagnosis is of fronto-temporal dementia (FTD) and on the more equivocal cases of AD.(34)

History

Making a clinical diagnosis of AD is a positive process and not one of exclusion. The most valuable diagnostic assessment is a careful informant history, paying attention to the pattern and timing of onset and progression. In the research context, a family history interview conducted by telephone provides a degree of accuracy compatible with a full clinical assessment.(35) Detailed semi-structured family informant diagnostic schedules are available, such as Cambridge Mental Disorders of the Elderly Examination (CAMDEX).(36) A history should be taken for the presence of risk factors for AD (e.g. a positive family history) and vascular and other risk factors (e.g. hypertension and head injury). Taking a family history for late-onset disorders such as AD requires special attention. Because of attrition due to other illness, many elderly people have had too few relatives reach the age of onset of dementia to make a pedigree analysis informative. The ages at death of all relatives should be established, together with cause of death and the presence or absence of dementia or memory problems in late life. The term 'sporadic' dementia should be avoided, and is misleading when applied to an individual with a dementia where one parent died young and where no sibling reached the age of 65 to 70 years. The history should also screen for the presence of other illnesses sufficient to cause a dementia and for systemic health in general. The presence of any significant physical illness, from chronic pain to delirium, may significantly alter cognitive abilities in the elderly, and especially so in those with AD.

A careful history should also establish the presence of any behavioural disturbance that has occurred. The relationship of aggression, wandering, agitation, or other behaviours to care tasks and other recent changes in the provision of the care package should be established. As the mainstay of the management of behavioural disturbance in all dementias is behavioural, establishing the antecedents to behaviour is an absolute prerequisite to effective management.

Examination

In addition to an examination of the mental state to establish the presence of disorders of mood and thought content, the examination will establish the specific pattern of cognitive impairment and the degree of impairment. Screening tests used to establish the presence of cognitive impairments include the Mini Mental State Examination;(37) this is a 30-point scale routinely used in all clinical trials of drugs for the treatment of AD, which is also a useful proxy measure for severity. It should be accompanied by other cognitive testing, including supplementary examination for aphasia and apraxias. Other cognitive and physical examinations will be necessary where the differential diagnosis is between a lobar dementia (e.g. FTD) or a subcortical dementia (e.g. that accompanying Huntington's disease).

In addition to the cognitive examination, a physical examination should be conducted in all patients with AD, although this might not be most effectively and conveniently performed at the initial assessment. Physical illness, including chronic pain, infection, cardiac insufficiency, or anaemia are all common in the elderly and can both complicate the diagnosis of AD and increase confusion in those known to have AD.

Assessment of function

Clinical assessment of function can be performed by informant history and by direct observation. Key to an assessment of function is a careful informant history seeking to establish where there has been a functional decline and remembering that instrumental ADLs are lost before basic activities. Instrumental ADLs are highly individual and require careful interviewing to assess—one patient may have a modest decline in their ability to use information technology whilst another may have trouble using all the appropriate settings on the central heating. The occupational therapist fulfils an invaluable role in establishing the detailed functional ability of those with AD, in addition to implementing changes in the home designed to maximize function. The FAST Scale(6) is based on the premise that the pattern of decline in function is relatively uniform in AD, and hence establishes a staging of severity on function rather than cognition. As in most instances functional severity is of more relevance for the provision of services, there is much to recommend such an approach. Scales used in research that can also be usefully employed in the clinic include the Bristol ADL Scale(38) and the Disability Assessment for Dementia.(39)

Global assessment

Driven largely by the United States Food and Drugs Administration, global assessment has become part of the assessment of all patients with AD in clinical trials and is finding its way into clinical practice. The underlying premise is that an assessment by a clinician, often supplemented by an informant history, provides information on severity that neither a cognitive assessment nor a functional assessment alone can provide. Two scales, the Clinicians Interview of Change,(40) and the Clinical Dementia Rating,(41) have become widely used in this context.

Investigations

At the initial assessment, patients with dementia should be investigated for other disorders that could complicate, exacerbate, or be confused with AD. A dementia screen might include routine biochemistry, thyroid function tests, vitamin B_{12} and folate estimations, and a full blood count; many would also include syphilis serology, although the frequency of abnormal findings is low. Neuroimaging is recommended in all cases by expert guidelines,(42) and serves two purposes—to exclude reversible causes of dementia and to contribute towards a definitive diagnosis. Thus using structural imaging with CT or, increasingly, with magnetic resonance imaging (MRI), the hippocampal atrophy of AD, the frontal predominant atrophy of FTD and the lesions of vascular dementia can be identified, adding to the specificity of diagnosis. In practice, neuroimaging is often omitted particularly when patients present with a typical history of a slowly progressive dementia of many years standing. Functional scanning (single-photon emission CT (SPECT) in particular) can be useful where regional dementias are suspected, and MRI should be the imaging modality of first choice where vascular dementia is a possibility. An EEG is nearly always non-specifically abnormal even in the early stages of AD, in contrast with fronto-temporal degenerations where an EEG remains unaffected at a broadly equivalent severity. This can help to distinguish the conditions, particularly where there is neuroimaging evidence of regional insufficiency.

Aetiology and molecular neurobiology

Alzheimer's disease is the most common dementia, affecting more than 20 per cent of the population over the age of 85 years. Epidemiological evidence has suggested risk factors and putative protective factors, but the greatest advances in understanding its pathogenesis have come from the combination of molecular and epidemiological approaches.

Neuropathology

At post-mortem, the brain in AD is lighter than aged-unaffected controls with more prominent sulci and a larger ventricular volume. Microscopic examination reveals the most prominent lesions described by Alzheimer—the extracellular plaque and intracellular neurofibrillary tangle. No consensus has developed regarding which of these lesions is responsible for the cognitive impairment of AD. Plaques, or more precisely amyloid load, might correlate with the degree of cognitive impairment,[43] although a significant amyloid deposition is also found in normal, unimpaired, aged individuals.[30] However, there is a high degree of correlation between dementia severity and neurofibrillary tangle formation,[44] although it is possible that some of the features of AD are more stable than others; for example, extracellular neurofibrillary tangles persist after the neurone has died, whereas extracellular Lewy bodies are not found.

The plaque consists of an amyloid core surrounded by dystrophic neurites, which are themselves filled with highly phosphorylated tau protein. Studies of Down syndrome brains have suggested a temporal course to plaque formation. First, peptides derived from the amyloid precursor protein (**APP**) are deposited in a diffuse plaque.[45] Over time this becomes organized as the amyloid peptides become fibrillar and form the amyloid deposit, neuritic change then occurs, and the plaque becomes fully mature.

Neurofibrillary tangles are composed of paired helical filaments, structures which are also found in the dystrophic neurites around mature plaques, and together with straight filaments, in neuropil threads. These filaments are themselves composed of the microtubule-associated protein, tau, which is present in a stably and highly phosphorylated state.[46,47] Tau is a neuronal-specific protein, found predominantly in the axon that functions to stabilize microtubules, a property that is regulated by phosphorylation. Phosphorylated tau is less effective in promoting tubulin polymerization into microtubules; normal adult brain a proportion of tau is highly phosphorylated, but this proportion is considerably greater in AD. Tau deposits are a feature of other disorders, such as progressive supranuclear palsy and some fronto-temporal degenerations[48] and together these tau-related disorders have been grouped together as the 'tauopathies'. Mutations have been found in fronto-temporal degenerations with parkinsonism (FTDP-17), and in other tauopathies thereby emphasizing the importance of this molecule to neurodegeneration.[49]

Braak and Braak[50] studied large numbers of brains from individuals who died at various ages and at different stages of dementia severity, which has resulted in the wide acceptance of the neuropathological staging of AD. The very earliest stages, before the clinical manifestation of dementia, are characterized by the appearance of highly phosphorylated tau in the hippocampus. In later stages, neurofibrillary tangles appear in the same brain regions and then become more widely distributed.

(a) The cholinergic hypothesis

The pathological changes in AD are localized both structurally and functionally. Plaques and tangles first occur in the hippocampus before spreading to involve other regions. Some areas of the brain are relatively preserved—the occipital lobe is affected relatively late and the cerebellum appears to be spared from neuritic change (neurofibrillary tangles and the fully matured plaques, although diffuse amyloid deposits do occur). Functional localization was demonstrated by evidence of the relatively greater and earlier loss of cholinergic neurotransmission. At post-mortem there is evidence of significantly greater neuronal loss in the cholinergic nucleus basalis of Meynert and loss of cholinergic markers.[51] These observations led to the cholinergic hypothesis, which stated that the cognitive impairment of AD was due to a disorder predominantly affecting cholinergic neurones. It was this hypothesis that led to the development of pharmacological strategies to rectify cholinergic loss and the introduction of the first compounds specifically designed for and efficacious in AD. However, the cholinergic hypothesis was something of a simplification as other neurotransmitter systems (e.g. serotonergic and noradrenergic) are also affected in AD.

(b) The amyloid cascade hypothesis

In 1984, the protein deposited in blood vessels (congophilic angiopathy) in AD was shown to be a 4-kDa peptide known as β-amyloid. This peptide, which is identical to the amyloid in plaques, is derived from a larger peptide, APP, the gene for which is coded on chromosome 21. Subsequently, mutations in the *APP* gene were found in a family with autosomal dominant early onset AD. These two discoveries—the identification of β-amyloid and the discovery of mutations in the parent *APP* gene—led the way to the amyloid cascade hypothesis, which has remained the dominant molecular model of the disorder (reviewed in Refs[52–54]). Many subsequent molecular observations have been consistent with this model, which posits the formation of β-amyloid as the initiating, or at least early event, leading to all the other changes observed including tau aggregation and phosphorylation, neuronal loss, cholinergic deficits, and clinical symptoms. Perhaps the most convincing evidence that there is such a unidirectional cascade comes from the observation that mutations in the *APP* gene give rise to plaque formation and also to neurofibrillary tangle pathology, whereas mutations in the tau gene give rise to tangle formation but not to plaque formation in the tauopathies.

Much subsequent research has concentrated upon understanding the metabolism of APP and the formation of β-amyloid peptide. APP is a ubiquitous single-pass cell-membrane protein expressed in many cell lines with a high degree of evolutionary conservation. At least three putative secretases cleave APP[55] and the metabolic products can be detected in individuals unaffected by AD; the processing is not pathological in AD, but the balance between different metabolic routes may be shifted in the disease state. α-Secretase cleaves APP at the outer cell-membrane surface at a site within the β;-amyloid moiety itself. Clearly, α-secretase cannot therefore yield intact β-amyloid, and this metabolic route, resulting in a secreted product, APPs, and other fragments, is termed non-amyloidogenic. On the other hand, amyloidogenic metabolism is the result of β-secretase (also known as Beta Amyloid Cleaving Enzyme or BACE) cleaving APP beyond the amino terminus of β-amyloid and of γ-secretase cleaving the resulting peptides at the carboxy terminus in the cell. The β-amyloid products vary in length, with predominant species having a length of 40 or 42 amino acids. The longer peptides are somewhat more prone to forming aggregates *in vitro* and it is probable that a relative increase in the longer peptides is critical in pathogenesis, and that mutations in the *APP* gene increase these longer amyloid peptides. Transgenic mice overexpressing the mutated *APP* gene also produce more β-amyloid peptide and have amyloid deposits in brain.[56] Interestingly, these animals do not develop other aspects of AD pathology, in particular they lack tangle formation. The nature of the toxicity of β-amyloid peptide is not fully understood but increasingly it appears that it is small aggregates (oligomers) that damage neurones rather than the longer fibrils that form the core of the plaque.[57]

(c) The presenilin genes

Mutations in *presenilin-1 (PS-1)* and *presenilin-2 (PS-2)*, two very similar genes on chromosome 14 and chromosome 1 respectively, also cause early onset autosomal dominant AD. The proteins encoded by these genes are part of the γ-secretase complex that metabolizes APP to β-amyloid. In fact these unique proteins turn out to have very many substrates and function in relation to many of these to release an intracellular component of a membrane bound protein that then translocates to the nucleus and triggers gene transcription events.[58] This is certainly the case for APP and also for Notch protein, which is also implicated in some other neurodegenerative conditions, for example. Mutations in the presenilin genes result in an increase in the production of β-amyloid probably through interfering with the normal γ-secretase complex.

Tangle formation and tau phosphorylation

Tangles are composed of paired helical filaments, themselves composed of aggregated and highly phosphorylated tau.[59–62] There are other post-translational modifications in tau, including truncation, and it is not fully determined which of these are primary events. However, in post-mortem studies, neuropathological evidence does suggest that highly phosphorylated tau accumulates in the brain before the formation of tangles, and before the clinical manifestation of AD suggesting that it is a early change in the pathological process.[63]

Protein phosphorylation is a product of kinase and phosphatase activity. It is likely that many such enzymes may participate in the regulation of tau phosphorylation in the brain, but two have been shown to be predominant. In cells, and *in vitro*, glycogen synthase kinase-3 and cyclin-dependent kinase 5 (CDK5) seem to be the predominant tau-kinases and protein phosphatase 2A is probably the predominant tau phosphatase.[64,65]

Molecular genetics

Mutations in three genes have been found to cause early onset familial AD, which is inherited in an autosomal dominant fashion.[66,67] Mutations in the *APP* gene (on chromosome 21) are the least common, only affecting perhaps 20 families worldwide. Mutations in *PS-1* (on chromosome 14) are somewhat more frequent, although are still a rare cause of AD. Mutations in *PS-2* (on chromosome 1) appear to be largely restricted to an ethnic German people residing in the United States, suggesting an individual founder effect. Individuals with Down's syndrome are at extremely high risk of AD, with neuropathological evidence being present in virtually all individuals living to middle age, probably because of trisomy APP (on chromosome 21). Mutations in other genes gives rise to disorders showing similarities to AD and much has been learnt from these findings about the overlap between neurodegenerative disorders. These genes include *tau* and *progranulin*, mutations in which give rise to FTD and related disorders.

The genetic component of late-onset AD has been demonstrated by epidemiological studies, showing that a family history of dementia is the largest single risk factor for AD.[68] However many, perhaps most, patients with AD do not have a positive family history, thus giving rise to the idea of 'sporadic' AD with a separate aetiology to 'familial' AD. For late-onset AD this concept is outmoded and redundant. Many patients with AD do not have a family history because of attrition of family members due to death by other causes. For the cohort currently suffering from AD their parents were born in the latter part of the nineteenth century or early years of the twentieth, lived through two major world wars, and reached adulthood before the discovery of antibiotics. It is not surprising that few patients with late-onset AD have two parents and more than one sibling living to the age of onset of AD, and if one parent died young and there are no elderly siblings then the family history is non-informative. Risk figures for relatives of probands with late-onset AD have been calculated and can be useful in counselling families.[69]

One gene has been unequivocally associated with late-onset AD, although even this gene accounts for only something like 50 per cent of the genetic variance.[70] The *apolipoprotein E* gene (*APOE*, gene; apoE, protein) on chromosome 19 has three common alleles, coding for three protein isoforms that differ by the substitution of an amino acid at just two positions. Of the three alleles ε3 is the most frequent and ε2 the least; following linkage to chromosome 18 it was demonstrated that the ε4 allele confers risk, whilst the ε2 may be protective.[71,72]

The mechanism of action of the *APOE* gene in increasing the risk of AD is not known. As *APOE* variation is a major genetic influence on serum cholesterol (people with the *APOE* ε4/* genotype have higher serum cholesterol levels), it is possible that an altered lipid metabolism—either peripherally or locally—might affect the pathogenesis of AD.[73,74] Alternative theories arise from *in vitro* studies, which show a differential binding of APOE protein isoforms both to amyloid protein and to tau protein.

Other genes have been associated with AD, but none have been replicated in as many studies as *APOE*. It is likely that a combination of linkage and association studies using large populations will identify the other genes that influence AD, either alone or in interactions with other genes or the environment.

Treatment

For many conditions the goals of treatment or intervention are self-evident—cure, prevention of relapse, and resolution of symptoms. For AD, however, the goals of treatment can be less obvious and differ between patients and for individual patients over time. Ultimately, the quality of life of the patient should be improved, but assessing quality of life is difficult in those with dementia, and given the early loss of insight who is to judge such issues?[75] Quality of life may appear poor—patients may have diminished emotional repertoires, few pleasurable activities, and considerable handicap—but they may share none of the negative cognitions experienced by others with a similarly questionable quality of life induced by different illnesses. Other patients may appear content or happy, despite the loss of the autonomy and self-awareness normally considered an essential component of a good quality life. The needs of the patient can be difficult to ascertain.[76] Equally, the treatment unit in AD includes carers, and there are times when the patient's quality of life is in conflict with the quality of life for other members of the family.[77] Resolving such conflicts of interest and other moral and ethical issues is part of the treatment process in AD. With the arrival of specific treatments for AD and the prospect of disease-modifying therapies, an even harder question arises regarding prolonging life for those with dementia: if quality of life appears poor to observers, is it right to prolong the process, can quality of life in those with dementia truly be assessed, or should carers and families be allowed to assess for themselves the benefits and costs of treatment?

There is no single model of management of patients with AD. In many countries management is the role of the gerontologist or neurologist. In others, as in the United Kingdom, the old-age psychiatry team provides the core specialist services. Many, perhaps even the majority, of those with AD are managed within primary care with the support of social services. Referral from primary care to specialist services will be according to local agreements, but most would concur that behavioural disturbance or the use of specific drugs to treat AD warrant referral to secondary care. Interventions for AD, whether provided in primary or secondary care, can be thought of as directed towards the patient, the patient's family, and the patient's environment. Guidelines on the identification and management of patients with dementia have been produced and may be a constructive approach to ensuring best clinical practice.[78]

Managing the patient

Management of the patient with dementia is discussed in greater detail in Chapter 4.1.13. Management starts with the assessment and diagnosis, and perhaps the difficult dilemma is how much of the diagnosis and prognosis to discuss with the patient.[79–81] Most practitioners do not discuss the diagnosis with the patient themselves, although practice is changing and especially in the early stages a frank consultation can be beneficial.

A large part of managing the patient is directed towards managing mood and behavioural disturbance. Accurate assessment of the disturbance is critical, and includes determining the antecedents and responses to the behaviour as well as a full description of the behaviour and any associated abnormalities in the mental state. Treatments of behavioural disturbance in AD are most often behavioural and sometimes restricted to giving information to carers. Evidence overwhelmingly suggests that anti-psychotic medication is relatively ineffective and has frequent adverse effects in dementia.[82,83] They should be a treatment of last resort, if at all.

Specific treatments for AD have been developed, concentrating in clinical trials on ameliorating the core symptom of cognitive impairment. The first to be licensed were the cholinesterase inhibitors followed by memantine. Drug treatments for AD are described in Chapter 6.2.7.

Managing the family

Although patients may not appreciate or be able to follow a detailed discussion of the diagnosis and prognosis, their relatives, spouses, and other carers will. This is an important part of the treatment process; as the carer provides the main interventions for much of the period of the disease process, care should be taken to ensure that appropriate and sufficiently complete information is given.

Caring for a patient with AD can be difficult and stressful and some carers suffer accordingly and need, and may benefit from support.[84] The characteristics of both carers and patients influence the impact that this 'burden' of caring has on the carers themselves. Men in general, and husbands in particular, seem to be less vulnerable to the adverse effects of caring, possibly because of the response seen in many male carers of rapidly and effectively recruiting outside help.[85] Women may be socialized into accepting more caring roles themselves and therefore seek less help. Non-white carers appear to suffer from less adverse consequences of caring, perhaps because of cultural differences in the perception of family bonds.[86] Patient characteristics that increase the burden of caring include behavioural disturbances,[25] depression, and unawareness of cognitive impairment but not the cognitive impairment itself. Although the core outcome variable in clinical trials of AD drugs is the severity of cognitive impairment, it is not the variable that induces most stress in relatives nor is it the variable that predicts entry to residential care. Other variables are almost certainly protective, and caring for a loved one with dementia is not a universally negative experience. Much caring is done willingly, effectively, with love, and without complaint.

Carer support groups offer much to a person with a relative afflicted by AD. Through support groups, and especially through the national AD societies and the umbrella group—AD International—carers can obtain up-to-date and useful information regarding all aspects of AD. A support group can help individuals practically and emotionally through difficult times. Many carers talk of the support group as a lifeline, although little empirical evidence exists as to the impact on carer well being.

One particular intervention for the family is that of genetic counselling. Many relatives are worried about inheriting AD. This concern might arise from two sources—the frequent discussion of genes 'for' AD in the media and the observation of familial occurrence of AD in many individual families. For families with clinically apparent familial AD, advice, information, and where appropriate, genetic testing can be arranged through a genetics centre. Where predictive testing is contemplated for genes causing autosomal dominant, early onset AD this will adhere to guidelines established for Huntington's disease. Genetic testing in late-onset AD is not recommended at the present time but is the subject of an ongoing research programme.[87]

Managing the environment

The mainstay of interventions for AD are provided by social services. The goal of the provision of social care in people with AD is to provide an environment that is comfortable, stimulating, and, above all, safe. For most patients, and for all patients in the early stages, this means care at home, perhaps with the support of home-meal delivery and home-helps to provide shopping and cleaning assistance. Further home care may become necessary as the patient requires assistance with basic self-care tasks such as washing and dressing. The carer may require a sitting service, either for periods during the day to allow them time to themselves or in the evening to allow them to attend a carers group or for socializing. Safety issues are especially important for those with dementia living alone. There are inherent risks to the patient themselves if they wander out of the home and risks to others if the gas can be left on or fires started.

Day care is appropriate for many patients, ideally in a specialist unit. In a generic facility for elderly people those with early dementia can receive little input and those with moderate or advanced dementia can necessitate too much input from the day-centre staff. A good dementia specialist day-care facility will provide the staffing ratio appropriate to patients with a range of 70s, in addition to providing a varied programme of group and recreational facilities to maintain interest and stimulation. Day centres, where patients are arrayed around the edge of the room with a television as a focal point, are, or should be, consigned to history. Day care provides essential respite to many carers, and longer periods of occasional or regular respite can prolong the period a patient can remain in their own home.

The multidisciplinary team consisting of care workers, social services, community psychiatric nurse occupational therapist, and psychologist can maintain patients at home more effectively and for longer periods than can clinicians alone. However, long-term care becomes a necessity for many patients at some point. The costs of providing nursing-home care are huge and far outweigh the costs of providing relatively intensive community care or relatively costly drugs. If treatments were shown to reduce the total length of stay in nursing homes then this would affect the cost–benefit ratio of these compounds considerably.

Translational research in AD

The rapid and comprehensive advances in understanding the molecular basis of AD has led to the promise of advances in health care—translational or bench to bedside research. Most importantly are potential disease modifying therapies. These are distinguished from symptomatic therapies in that they are designed to halt or slow down the disease process itself. Designing trials to assess efficacy of a potential treatment that might only slow down deterioration, and differentiating symptomatic effects from disease-modifying effects is not easy.(88) Two broad approaches are suggested—either a comparison of slopes of decline in which case a disease-modifying therapy would result in divergent slopes whereas a symptomatic therapy would result in parallel slopes, or strategies such as delayed start where in the case of a disease-modifying therapy the treatment arm of the delayed group never do quite as well as the early start group.(89)

Many approaches to disease modification are being pursued including therapeutics designed to alter APP processing—BACE inhibitors and γ-secretase inhibitors for example—or therapeutics designed to prevent β-amyloid from aggregating or for increasing the clearance of β-amyloid.(90) Many such compounds are in early stages of development and some were in phase III trials in 2007. Other potential therapies attempt to reduce tau phosphorylation or aggregation and yet other approaches are predicated on epidemiological findings such as the observation that non-steroidal anti-inflammatory drugs reduce risk of AD or that diabetes increases risk. Primary preventative therapies are probably even further away than disease-modification therapies but modifying cardiovascular risk or other approaches have been suggested. Secondary prevention, possibly in those with memory impairments not amounting to dementia (minimal cognitive impairment), is a more realistic prospect rendering the determination of the very earliest signs of disease or evidence of a prodromal state a high priority.

A second significant translational target in AD research close to clinical utility is that of biomarkers.(91,92) A marker is sought that might help in diagnosis, prediction or disease monitoring. For diagnosis a biomarker is sought that would make early or differential diagnosis more accurate, for prediction a biomarker that would help in predicting which elderly people were more likely to suffer from dementia or, more likely, which of those with mild cognitive impairment are more likely to convert to dementia. A marker of disease progression is sought that could supplement clinical assessments of deterioration. Of the many approaches to biomarkers, biochemical assays of tau and β-amyloid in CSF(91,93) and serial quantitative MRI(94) are the most promising although markers in plasma appear promising.(95,96)

Conclusions

For the foreseeable future, AD will remain a disorder afflicting a large proportion of the world's elderly. The impact on developing countries especially will be considerable. Care for these patients will continue to be provided from many sources, with specialist services being necessary to compliment primary and generic services, particularly for those patients exhibiting the complex psychiatric phenomenology described by Alzheimer and for those patients where specific drugs are indicated. As the molecular pathogenesis of AD is increasingly understood it is to be hoped that this is translated into treatments ever more effective in modifying or preventing the disease process itself.

Further information

http://www.alzforum.org/
http://www.alzheimers.org.uk/
http://alzheimers-research.org
http://www.alz.org/

References

1. Tomlinson, B.E., Blessed, G., and Roth, M. (1970). Observation on the brains of demented old people. *Journal of the Neurological Sciences*, **11**, 205–42.
2. Petersen, R.C., Smith, G.E., Ivnik, R.J., *et al.* (1988). Memory function in very early Alzheimer's disease. *Neurology*, **44**(5), 867–72.
3. Neary, D., Snowden, J.S., Northen, B., *et al.* (1988). Dementia of frontal lobe type. *Journal of Neurology, Neurosurgery, and Psychiatry*, **51**, 353–61.
4. Riter, R.N. and Fries, B.E. (1992). Predictors of the placement of cognitively impaired residents on special care units. *The Gerontologist*, **32**, 184–90.
5. Reed, B.R., Jagust, W.J., and Seab, J.P. (1989). Mental status as a predictor of daily function in progressive dementia. *The Gerontologist*, **29**, 804–7.
6. Reisberg, B. (1988). Functional assessment staging (FAST). *Psychopharmacology Bulletin*, **24**, 653–9.
7. Green, C.R., Mohs, R.C., Schmeidler, J., *et al.* (1993). Functional decline in Alzheimer's disease: a longitudinal study. *Journal of the American Geriatrics Society*, **41**, 654–61.
8. Levy, M.L., Cummings, J.L., Fairbanks, L.A., *et al.* (1996). Longitudinal assessment of symptoms of depression, agitation, and psychosis in 181 patients with Alzheimer's disease. *The American Journal of Psychiatry*, **153**(11), 1438–43.
9. Rovner, B.W., Broadhead, J., Spencer, M., *et al.* (1989). Depression and Alzheimer's disease. *The American Journal of Psychiatry*, **146**, 350–3.
10. Burns, A., Jacoby, R., and Levy, R. (1990). Psychiatric phenomena in Alzheimer's disease. III: disorders of mood. *The British Journal of Psychiatry*, **157**, 81–6, 92.
11. Tractenberg, R.E., Weiner, M.F., Patterson, M.B., *et al.* (2003). Comorbidity of psychopathological domains in community-dwelling persons with Alzheimer's disease. *Journal of Geriatric Psychiatry and Neurology*, **16**(2), 94–9.
12. Weiner, M.F., Doody, R.S., Sairam, R., *et al.* (2002). Prevalence and incidence of major depressive disorder in Alzheimer's disease: findings from two databases. *Dementia Geriatric and Cognitive Disorders*, **13**(1), 8–12.
13. Payne, J.L., Sheppard, J.M., Steinberg, M., *et al.* (2002). Incidence, prevalence, and outcomes of depression in residents of a long-term care facility with dementia. *International Journal of Geriatric Psychiatry*, **17**(3), 247–53.

14. Meeks, T.W., Ropacki, S.A., and Jeste, D.V. (2006). The neurobiology of neuropsychiatric syndromes in dementia. *Current Opinion in Psychiatry*, **19**(6), 581–6.
15. Zubenko, G.S., Moossy, J., and Kopp, U. (1990). Neurochemical correlates of major depression in primary dementia. *Archives of Neurology*, **47**, 209–14.
16. Forstl, H., Burns, A., Levy, R., *et al.* (1992). Neuropathological correlates of behavioural disturbance in confirmed Alzheimer's disease. *The British Journal of Psychiatry*, in press.
17. Holtzer, R., Tang, M.X., Devanand, D.P., *et al.* (2003). Psychopathological features in Alzheimer's disease: course and relationship with cognitive status. *Journal of the American Geriatrics Society*, **51**(7), 953–60.
18. Steinberg, M., Sheppard, J.M., Tschanz, J.T., *et al.* (2003). The incidence of mental and behavioral disturbances in dementia: the cache county study. *Journal of Neuropsychiatry and Clinical Neurosciences*, **15**(3), 340–5.
19. Wragg, R.E. and Jeste, D.V. (1989). Overview of depression and psychosis in Alzheimer's disease. *The American Journal of Psychiatry*, **146**, 577–87.
20. Burns, A., Jacoby, R., and Levy, R. (1990). Psychiatric phenomena in Alzheimer's disease. I: disorders of thought content. *The British Journal of Psychiatry*, **157**, 72–6, 92.
21. Assal, F., Alarcon, M., Solomon, E.C., *et al.* (2004). Association of the serotonin transporter and receptor gene polymorphisms in neuropsychiatric symptoms in Alzheimer disease. *Archives of Neurology*, **61**(8), 1249–53.
22. Nacmias, B., Tedde, A., Forleo, P., *et al.* (2001). Association between 5-HT(2A) receptor polymorphism and psychotic symptoms in Alzheimer's disease. *Biological Psychiatry*, **50**(6), 472–5.
23. Holmes, C., Arranz, M.J., Powell, J.F., *et al.* (1998). 5-HT_{2A} and 5-HT_{2C} receptor polymorphisms and psychopathology in late onset Alzheimer's disease. *Human Molecular Genetics*, **7**, 1507–9.
24. Coen, R.F., Swanwick, G.R., O'Boyle, C.A., *et al.* (1997). Behaviour disturbance and other predictors of carer burden in Alzheimer's disease. *International Journal of Geriatric Psychiatry*, **12**, 331–6.
25. Donaldson, C., Tarrier, N., and Burns, A. (1998). Determinants of carer stress in Alzheimer's disease. *International Journal of Geriatric Psychiatry*, **13**, 248–56.
26. Gormley, N., Rizwan, M.R., and Lovestone, S. (1998). Clinical predictors of aggressive behaviour in Alzheimer's disease. *International Journal of Geriatric Psychiatry*, **13**, 109–15.
27. Volicer, L., Harper, D.G., Manning, B.C., *et al.* (2001). Sundowning and circadian rhythms in Alzheimer's disease. *The American Journal of Psychiatry*, **158**(5), 704–11.
28. McKhann, G., Drachman, D., Folstein, M., *et al.* (1984). Clinical diagnosis of Alzheimer's disease: report of the NINCDS–ADRDA Work Group under the auspices of Department of Health and Human Services Task Force on Alzheimer's Disease. *Neurology*, **34**, 939–44.
29. Gearing, M., Mirra, S.S., Hedreen, J.C., *et al.* (1995). The Consortium to Establish a Registry for Alzheimer's Disease (CERAD). Part X. Neuropathology confirmation of the clinical diagnosis of Alzheimer's disease. *Neurology*, **45**, 461–6.
30. MRC CFAS. (2001). Pathological correlates of late-onset dementia in a multicentre, community-based population in England and Wales. Neuropathology Group of the Medical Research Council Cognitive Function and Ageing Study (MRC CFAS). *Lancet*, **357**(9251), 169–75.
31. Kukull, W.A., Larson, E.B., Reifler, B.V., *et al.* (1990). The validity of 3 clinical diagnostic criteria for Alzheimer's disease. *Neurology*, **40**, 1364–9.
32. Mok, W., Chow, T.W., Zheng, L., *et al.* (2004). Clinicopathological concordance of dementia diagnoses by community versus tertiary care clinicians. *American Journal of Alzheimer's Disease and Other Dementias*, **19**(3), 161–5.
33. Nagy, Z., Esiri, M.M., Hindley, N.J., *et al.* (1998). Accuracy of clinical operational diagnostic criteria for Alzheimer's disease in relation to different pathological diagnostic protocols. *Dementia and Geriatric Cognitive Disorders*, **9**(4), 219–26.
34. Halliday, G., Ng, T., Rodriguez, M., *et al.* (2002). Consensus neuropathological diagnosis of common dementia syndromes: testing and standardising the use of multiple diagnostic criteria. *Acta Neuropathologica*, **104**(1), 72–8.
35. Devi, G., Marder, K., Schofield, P.W., *et al.* (1998). Validity of family history for the diagnosis of dementia among siblings of patients with late-onset Alzheimer's disease. *Genetic Epidemiology*, **15**, 215–23.
36. Roth, M., Tym, E., Mountjoy, C.Q., *et al.* (1986). CAMDEX. A standardised instrument for the diagnosis of mental disorder in the elderly with special reference to the early detection of dementia. *The British Journal of Psychiatry*, **149**, 698–709.
37. Folstein, M.F., Folstein, S.E., and McHugh, P.R. (1975). Mini-mental state: a practical method of grading the cognitive state of patients for the clinician. *Journal of Psychiatric Research*, **12**, 189–98.
38. Bucks, R.S., Ashworth, D.L., Wilcock, G.K., *et al.* (1996). Assessment of activities of daily living in dementia: development of the Bristol Activities of Daily Living Scale. *Age Ageing*, **25**(2), 113–20.
39. Gelinas, I., Gauthier, L., McIntyre, M., *et al.* (1999). Development of a functional measure for persons with Alzheimer's disease: the disability assessment for dementia. *The American Journal of Occupational Therapy*, **53**(5), 471–81.
40. Knopman, D.S., Knapp, M.J., Gracon, S.I, *et al.* (1994). The Clinician Interview-Based Impression (CIBI): a clinician's global change rating scale in Alzheimer's disease. *Neurology*, **44**, 2315–21.
41. Hughes, C.P., Berg, L., Danziger, W.L., *et al.* (1982). A new clinical scale for the staging of dementia. *The British Journal of Psychiatry*, **140**, 566–72.
42. Waldemar, G., Dubois, B., Emre, M., *et al.* (2007). Recommendations for the diagnosis and management of Alzheimer's disease and other disorders associated with dementia: EFNS guideline. *European Journal of Neurology*, **14**(1), e1–26.
43. Cummings, B.J. and Cotman, C.W. (1995). Image analysis of β-amyloid load in Alzheimer's disease and relation to dementia severity. *Lancet*, **346**, 1524–8.
44. Nagy, Z., Esiri, M.M., Jobst, K.A., *et al.* (1995). Relative roles of plaques and tangles in the dementia of Alzheimer's disease: correlations using three sets of neuropathological criteria. *Dementia*, **6**, 21–31.
45. Mann, D.M., Brown, A., Prinja, D., *et al.* (1989). An analysis of the morphology of senile plaques in Down's syndrome patients of different ages using immunocytochemical and lectin histochemical techniques. *Neuropathology and Applied Neurobiology*, **15**, 317–29.
46. Lovestone, S. and Reynolds, C.H. (1997). The phosphorylation of tau: a critical stage in neurodevelopmental and neurodegenerative processes. *Neuroscience*, **78**(2), 309–24.
47. Avila, J. (2006). Tau phosphorylation and aggregation in Alzheimer's disease pathology. *FEBS Letters*. **580**(12), 2922–7.
48. Buee, L. and Delacourte, A. (1999). Comparative biochemistry of tau in progressive supranuclear palsy, corticobasal degeneration, FTDP-17 and Pick's disease. *Brain Pathology*, **9**(4), 681–93.
49. Heutink, P. (2000). Untangling tau-related dementia. *Human Molecular Genetics*, **9**(6), 979–86.
50. Braak, H. and Braak, E. (1991). Neuropathological staging of Alzheimer-related changes. *Acta Neuropathologica*, **82**, 239–59.
51. Francis, P.T., Palmer, A.M., Snape, M., *et al.* (1999). The cholinergic hypothesis of Alzheimer's disease: a review of progress. *Journal of Neurology, Neurosurgery, and Psychiatry*, **66**, 137–47.
52. Hardy, J. (2006). Alzheimer's disease: the amyloid cascade hypothesis: an update and reappraisal. *Journal of Alzheimer's Disease*, **9**(Suppl. 3), 151–3.
53. Hardy, J. and Selkoe, D.J. (2002). The amyloid hypothesis of Alzheimer's disease: progress and problems on the road to therapeutics. *Science*, **297**(5580), 353–6.

54. Selkoe, D.J. (2000). Toward a comprehensive theory for Alzheimer's disease. Hypothesis: Alzheimer's disease is caused by the cerebral accumulation and cytotoxicity of amyloid beta-protein. *Annals of the New York Academy of Sciences*, **924**, 17–25.
55. Esler, W.P. and Wolfe, M.S. (2001). A portrait of Alzheimer secretases—new features and familiar faces. *Science*, **293**(5534), 1449–54.
56. Emilien, G., Maloteaux, J.M., Beyreuther, K., *et al.* (2000). Alzheimer disease: mouse models pave the way for therapeutic opportunities. *Archives of Neurology*, **57**(2), 176–81.
57. Walsh, D.M. and Selkoe, D.J. (2007). A beta Oligomers—a decade of discovery. *Journal of Neurochemistry*, **101**(5), 1172–84.
58. Parks A.L. and Curtis, D. (2007). Presenilin diversifies its portfolio. *Trends in Genetics*, **23**(3), 140–50.
59. Lace, G.L., Wharton, S.B., and Ince, P.G. (2007). A brief history of tau: the evolving view of the microtubule-associated protein tau in neurodegenerative diseases. *Clinical Neuropathology*, **26**(2), 43–58.
60. Mi, K. and Johnson, G.V. (2006). The role of tau phosphorylation in the pathogenesis of Alzheimer's disease. *Current Alzheimer Research*, **3**(5), 449–63.
61 Binder, L.I., Guillozet-Bongaarts, A.L., Garcia-Sierra, F., *et al.* (2005). Tau, tangles, and Alzheimer's disease. *Biochimica et Biophysica Acta*, **1739**(2–3), 216–23.
62. Iqbal, K., Alonso, A.C., Chen, S., *et al.* (2005). Tau pathology in Alzheimer disease and other tauopathies. *Biochimica et Biophysica Acta*, **1739**(2–3), 198–10.
63. Braak, E., Braak, H., and Mandelkow, E.-M. (1994). A sequence of cytoskeleton changes related to the formation of neurofibrillary tangles and neuropil threads. *Acta Neuropathologica*, **87**, 554–67.
64. Jope, R.S. and Johnson, G.V. (2004). The glamour and gloom of glycogen synthase kinase-3. *Trends in Biochemical Sciences*, **29**(2), 95–102.
65. Trojanowski, J.Q. and Lee, V.M. (1995). Phosphorylation of paired helical filament tau in Alzheimer's disease neurofibrillary lesions, focusing on phosphatases. *The FASEB Journal*, **9**(15), 1570–6.
66. Blacker, D. and Lovestone, S. (2006). Genetics and dementia nosology. *Journal of Geriatric Psychiatry and Neurology*, **19**(3), 186–91.
67. Bertram, L. and Tanzi, R.E. (2004). The current status of Alzheimer's disease genetics: what do we tell the patients? *Pharmacological Research*, **50**(4), 385–96.
68. van Duijn, C.M., Clayton, D.G., Chandra, V., *et al.* (1994). Interaction between genetic and environmental risk factors for Alzheimer's disease: a reanalysis of case-control studies. *Genetic Epidemiology*, **11**, 539–51.
69. Cupples, L.A., Farrer, L.A., Sadovnick, A.D., *et al.* (2004). Estimating risk curves for first-degree relatives of patients with Alzheimer's disease: the REVEAL study. *Genetics in Medicine*, **6**(4), 192–6.
70. Owen, M., Liddell, M., and McGuffin, P. (1994). Alzheimer's disease. *British Medical Journal*, **308**, 672–3.
71. Raber, J., Huang, Y., and Ashford, J.W. (2004). ApoE genotype accounts for the vast majority of AD risk and AD pathology. *Neurobiology of Aging*, **25**(5), 641–50.
72. Cedazo-Minguez, A. and Cowburn, R.F. (2001). Apolipoprotein E: a major piece in the Alzheimer's disease puzzle. *Journal of Cellular and Molecular Medicine*, **5**(3), 254–66.
73. Hatters, D.M., Peters-Libeu, C.A., and Weisgraber, K.H. (2006). Apolipoprotein E structure: insights into function. *Trends in Biochemical Sciences*, **31**(8), 445–54.
74. Martins, I.J., Hone, E., Foster, J.K., *et al.* (2006). Apolipoprotein E, cholesterol metabolism, diabetes, and the convergence of risk factors for Alzheimer's disease and cardiovascular disease. *Molecular Psychiatry*, **11**(8), 721–36.
75. Ettema, T.P., Droes, R.M., de, L.J., *et al.* (2005). The concept of quality of life in dementia in the different stages of the disease. *International Psychogeriatrics*, **17**(3), 353–70.
76. van der Roest, H.G., Meiland, F.J., Maroccini, R., *et al.* (2007). Subjective needs of people with dementia: a review of the literature. *International Psychogeriatrics*, **19**(3), 559–92.
77. Glozman, J.M. (2004). Quality of life of caregivers. *Neuropsychology Review*, **14**(4), 183–96.
78. Waldemar, G., Dubois, B., Emre, M., *et al.* (2000). Diagnosis and management of Alzheimer's disease and other disorders associated with dementia. The role of neurologists in Europe. European Federation of Neurological Societies. *European Journal Neurology*, **7**(2), 133–44.
79. Derksen, E., Vernooij-Dassen, M., Gillissen, F., *et al.* (2006). Impact of diagnostic disclosure in dementia on patients and carers: qualitative case series analysis. *Aging & Mental Health*, **10**(5), 525–31.
80. Elson, P. (2006). Do older adults presenting with memory complaints wish to be told if later diagnosed with Alzheimer's disease? *International Journal of Geriatric Psychiatry*, **21**(5), 419–25.
81. Lin, K.N., Liao, Y.C., Wang, P.N., *et al.* (2005). Family members favor disclosing the diagnosis of Alzheimer's disease. *International Psychogeriatrics*, **17**(4), 679–88.
82. Schneider, L.S., Tariot, P.N., Dagerman, KS., *et al.* (2006). Effectiveness of atypical antipsychotic drugs in patients with Alzheimer's disease. *The New England Journal of Medicine*, **355**(15), 1525–38.
83. Schneider, L.S., Dagerman, K.S., and Insel, P. (2005). Risk of death with atypical antipsychotic drug treatment for dementia: meta-analysis of randomized placebo-controlled trials. *The Journal of American Medical Association*, **294**(15), 1934–43.
84. Thompson, C.A., Spilsbury, K., Hall, J., *et al.* (2007). Systematic review of information and support interventions for caregivers of people with dementia. *BMC Geriatrics*, **7**, 18.
85. Bedard, M., Molloy, D.W., Pedlar, *et al.* (1997). Associations between dysfunctional behaviors, gender, and burden in spousal caregivers of cognitively impaired older adults. *International Psychogeriatrics*, **9**, 277–90.
86. Connell, C.M. and Gibson, G.D. (1997). Racial, ethnic, and cultural differences in dementia caregiving: review and analysis. *The Gerontologist*, **37**, 355–64.
87. Roberts, J.S., Barber, M., Brown, T.M., *et al.* (2004). Who seeks genetic susceptibility testing for Alzheimer's disease? Findings from a multisite, randomized clinical trial. *Genetics in Medicine*, **6**(4), 197–203.
88. Vellas, B., Andrieu, S., Sampaio, C., *et al.* (2007). Disease-modifying trials in Alzheimer's disease: a European task force consensus. *Lancet Neurology*, **6**(1), 56–62.
89. Leber, P. (1996). Observations and suggestions on antidementia drug development. *Alzheimer Disease and Associated Disorders*, **10**(Suppl. 1), 31–35.
90. Pangalos, M.N., Jacobsen, S.J., and Reinhart, P.H. (2005). Disease modifying strategies for the treatment of Alzheimer's disease targeted at modulating levels of the beta-amyloid peptide. *Biochemical Society Transactions*, **33**(Pt 4), 553–8.
91. Sunderland, T., Hampel, H., Takeda, M., *et al.* (2006). Biomarkers in the diagnosis of Alzheimer's disease, are we ready? *Journal of Geriatric Psychiatry and Neurology*, **19**(3), 172–9.
92. Lovestone, S. (2006). Biomarkers in Alzheimer's disease. *The Journal of Nutrition Health & Aging*, **10**(2), 118–22.
93. Wiltfang, J., Lewczuk, P., Riederer, P., *et al.* (2005). Consensus paper of the WFSBP task force on biological markers of dementia: the role of CSF and blood analysis in the early and differential diagnosis of dementia. *The World Journal of Biological Psychiatry*, **6**(2), 69–84.
94. Fox, N.C., Black, R.S., Gilman, S., *et al.* (2005). Effects of Abeta immunization (AN1792) on MRI measures of cerebral volume in Alzheimer disease. *Neurology*, **64**(9), 1563–72.
95. van, O.M., Hofman, A., Soares, H.D., *et al.* (2006). Plasma Abeta(1-40) and Abeta(1-42) and the risk of dementia: a prospective case-cohort study. *Lancet Neurology*, **5**(8), 655–60.
96. Hye, A., Lynham, S., Thambisetty, M., *et al.* (2006). Proteome-based plasma biomarkers for Alzheimer's disease. *Brain*, **129**(Pt 11), 3042–50.

4.1.3 Frontotemporal dementias

Lars Gustafson and Arne Brun

Introduction

Nosological classification of organic dementia is based on current knowledge and theories of aetiology, including genetics, clinical picture, the pathological substrate, and the predominant location of brain damage. This chapter is concerned with dementia syndromes caused by a degenerative disease primarily affecting the frontal and temporal lobes, named frontal-lobe dementia[1] or frontotemporal dementia (**FTD**).[2] The terminology should be viewed from a historical perspective. The relationship between localized cortical atrophy in dementia and symptoms of aphasia was first reported by Pick in 1892.[3] The pathological account of this lobar degeneration by Alzheimer in 1911 described 'ballooned' neurones (Pick cells) and argentophilic globes (Pick bodies),[4] and the clinicopathological entity was named **Pick's disease**.

In the 1980s, attention was drawn to a larger group of frontal-lobe dementias associated with frontotemporal cortical degeneration.[5–7] The Lund–Manchester consensus of 1994 delineated the prototypical clinical syndrome of FTD with three neuropathological constituents, frontal lobe degeneration of non-Alzheimer type (**FLD**),[5] (alternatively designated '**dementia lacking distinctive histology**'),[8] Pick's disease, and motor neurone disease (**MND**) with dementia (**FTD-MND**).[2] The 1998 consensus on clinical diagnostic criteria for frontotemporal lobar degeneration (**FTLD**)[9] encompassed two additional dementia syndromes; progressive non-fluent aphasia (**PA**),[10,11] and **semantic dementia**.[12] Corticobasal degeneration (**CBD**) and progressive supranuclear palsy (**PSP**) have also been associated with FTLD.[13] A changing clinical classification is shown in Fig. 4.1.3.1. The addition of important genetic and histochemical characteristics has further added to the complex classification of FTD and FTLD with a risk of developing numerous and partly competing definitions. FTLD may be further subclassified into forms positive or negative for tau and ubiquitin. The ubiquitinated form will be referred to as **FTD-U**, which is synonymous to **FLTD-U**.[14]

Neuropathology

On a neuropathological basis about two-thirds of the FTLD cases are of the type with ubiquitinated inclusions (FTD-U) or of FTD type without such inclusions (FLD), both lacking tau pathology.[14,15] In an attempt to classify FTD forms from a structural point of view, FLD might be appointed as a basic form, showing type and distribution of main pathological changes common to the majority of FTLD forms. To this set of alterations are added further features proceeding in the description of frontotemporal degenerative disorders (Table 4.1.3.1).

In FLD, the cortex is the site of a *simple* degenerative process resulting in a cortical atrophy which is frontotemporal with or without asymmetries, moderate or even at times mild. It involves cortical layers 1–3, showing neuronal loss, gliosis, and microvacuolation, seen also in the striatum in a small proportion of cases as well as a mild-to-moderate degeneration of the substantia nigra.[5] DLDH has essentially the same pathology as FLD.[8]

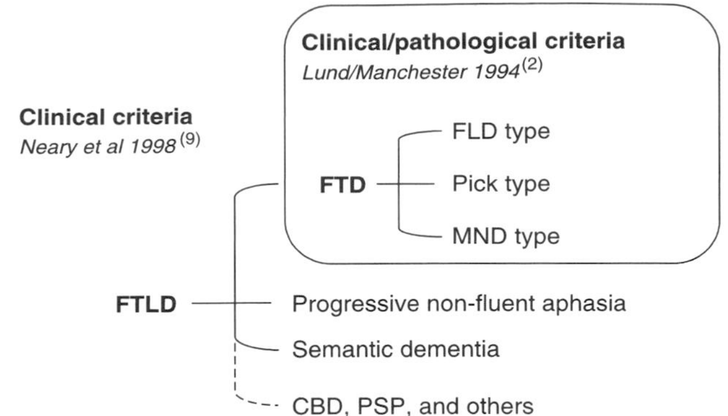

Fig. 4.1.3.1 Clinical classification of frontotemporal dementias.

In FTD-U the ubiquitin-positive inclusions and dystrophic neurites supplement the picture of FLD, as also described in FTD, linked to chromosome 3.[16] The inclusions contain a ubiquitinated protein, also identified in some other varieties of FTD such as FTD-MND.[17] Here there is also a degeneration of motor neurones and paths. The language variants of FTLD show a mainly temporal degeneration in semantic dementia and an asymmetric frontotemporal degeneration with left-sided predominance in PA.

With a mainly frontal or frontotemporal including anterior cingulate gyrus involvement FTD differs markedly from Alzheimer's disease (AD) with its posterior temporal parietal, posterior cingulate, and severe hippocampal involvement and also with Lewy bodies, amyloid, and plaque pathology not seen in FTD. So far mentioned FTD forms belong in the same histopathological group of non-tauopathies and further share a frequent and individually varyingly severe white-matter sclerosis, which is often predominantly frontal and may be primary or secondary.[18] It is also seen in the tauopathy group and in forms of vascular dementia.

The remaining, less common forms comprise the FTD-tau group. In Pick's disease the degenerative process is more intense and partly involves all cortical layers, creating a severe circumscribed or lobar frontotemporal atrophy referred to as 'knife blade atrophy'. Microscopically there are tau-positive neuronal inclusions and sometimes glial tangles and often ballooned nerve cells. The FTD with Parkinsonism (FTDP-17) group with a number of familial disorders shares basic pathological features with the FLD but is

Table 4.1.3.1 Organic dementia with frontotemporal lobar degeneration (FTLD)

Frontal lobe degeneration of non-Alzheimer type (FLD) (Dementia lacking distinctive histology) without ubiquitinated inclusions
FTD with ubiquitin-positive inclusions (FTD-U)
Familial FTD with chromosome 3 mutation (FTD-3)
FTD with motor neurone disease (FTD-MND)
Progressive non-fluent aphasia (PA)
Semantic dementia
Pick's disease
FTD with Parkinsonism (FTDP-17)
Corticobasal degeneration (CBD)
Progressive supranuclear palsy (PSP)

regularly more severe in the basal ganglia and substantia nigra.[19] Glial cells and neurones contain various types of tau-positive inclusions. CBD is structurally and clinically heterogeneous, resulting in overlap with other diseases, especially PSP.[20] These two may represent varieties of the same pathological process, less obviously belonging in the FTD group even if a similar laminar frontal cortical degeneration and related symptoms are part of the presentation. In CBD ballooned neurones, tau-positive inclusions in neuronal and glial cells, white-matter rarefaction and nigral degeneration may be found. For PSP different forms and patterns are noted but it basically affects more widely the striatum, basal ganglia, and hypothalamus. It also involves the brain stem including the substantia nigra as well as the cerebellum, again with silver- or tau-positive inclusions and tangles in neurones and glial cells.[21]

Epidemiology

Most demographic data concern the grouping of FTD, not separating FLD and Pick's disease. Pick's disease is rare, estimated at 24–60/100 000 in Minnesota and 30–60 in Switzerland.[22] The calculated prevalence of FTD in the Netherlands is 10.7 per million between 50 and 60 years of age and 28 between 60 and 70 years.[23] The prevalence of FTD in the province Zuid-Holland in the Netherlands was 3.6/100 000 at age 50–59, 9.4 at age 60–69 years, and 3.8 at age 70–79 years.[24] Pasquier *et al.*[25] diagnosed FTD in 4.8 per cent of all types of dementia. The marked geographic variation of the prevalence might be due to genetic and environmental factors, but also influenced by differences in the diagnostic process and the age group studied. In a clinical study of a total catchments area of 20 million people in Germany the relative proportion of FTLD was 1.9 per cent.[26] The prevalence of dementia in motor neurone disease has been estimated to 2–6 per cent.[27] The proportion of FTD in relation to all types of dementia in different clinicopathological studies varies between 5 and 18.9 per cent.[7, 8, 28–30]

Clinical features

The first clinical manifestations of FTD usually appear in the presenium, in some cases as early as 35 and seldom after 70 years of age. The mean age at onset in post-mortem verified FLD cases is 56 ± 7.6 years with a mean duration of 8 ± 3.4 years (range 3–17 years).[31] The mean age of onset in Pick's disease is similar, 62 years, with a range of 40–80 years and a mean survival of 9.8 years with a range of 4.8–21.2 years.[22] The large variations of the duration of FLD and Pick's disease are similar to that of early-onset AD. The clinical onset of MND dementia is usually in the sixth decade and the mean duration is about 30 months. Age at onset is similar in familial and sporadic cases of FTD and sometimes past 80 years.[32] The Lund–Manchester consensus on clinical criteria for FTD is summarized in Table 4.1.3.2.

Disordered behaviour

The early stage of FLD and Pick's disease is characterized by changes of personality and behaviour, affective symptoms, and a progressive reduction of expressive speech. The clinical onset is insidious with slow progression without ictal events. The changes of personality and behaviour are rather non-specific and easily misinterpreted as a non-organic mental disease such as mood disorder, stress reaction, schizophrenia, or other psychotic reaction. Loss of insight concerning the mental changes is an early and alarming manifestation of the disease. FTD patients may, however, consult a doctor referring to symptoms such as anxiety, tiredness, and strange somatic complaints combined with bizarre hypochondriacal ideas.

Table 4.1.3.2 The Lund–Manchester consensus (1994) on clinical criteria for frontotemporal dementia (slightly modified)[2]

Core diagnostic features
Behavioural disorder
Insidious onset and slow progression
Early loss of insight into changes of own mental state
Early loss of personal and social awareness
Early signs of disinhibition and lack of judgement
Mental rigidity and inflexibility
Stereotyped, repetitive, and imitating behaviour
Hyperorality, oral/dietary changes
Utilization behaviour
Distractibility, impulsivity, and impersistence
Affective symptoms
Depression, anxiety, excessive sentimentality
Hypochondriasis, bizarre somatic complaints
Emotional bluntness, apathy, and lack of empathy
Amimia
Speech disorder
Progressive reduction of speech output
Stereotypy of speech, perseveration
Echolalia
Late mutism
Spatial orientation, receptive speech, and praxis preserved
Physical signs
Early primitive reflexes
Early incontinence
Late akinesia, rigidity, and tremor
Low and labile blood pressure
Investigations
Normal EEG despite clinically evident dementia
Brain imaging (structural and/or functional): predominant frontal and/or anterior temporal abnormality
Neuropsychology: profound failure on 'frontal-lobe' tests in the absence of severe amnesia, or perceptual spatial disorder
Supportive diagnostic features
Onset before 65
Positive family history of similar disorder in a first-degree relative
Bulbar palsy, muscular weakness and wasting, fasciculations (motor neurone disease)

(Reproduced from A. Brun, E. Englund, L. Gustafson, *et al.* Consensus statement—clinical and neuropathological criteria for frontotemporal dementia, *Journal of Neurology, Neurosurgery, and Psychiatry*, **57**, 416–18, copyright 1994, BMJ Publishing Group Ltd.)

The early loss of personal and social awareness is seen as neglect of personal hygiene and grooming, and tactlessness and antisocial behaviour.[6,9] The impaired control of behaviour is seen as increased sentimentality, inadequate smiling, inappropriate joking, irritability, and acts of aggressiveness, leading to conflicts at home and work. Craving for affection and sexual contact may be easily provoked, but usually expressions of sexual disinhibition are possible to divert. Impulse buying, shoplifting, indecency, and other disinhibited behaviour may, however, lead to rejection by the family and society. Such unpredictable and pseudopsychopathic behaviour imposes severe strain on the patient's family, leading in some cases to economic problems, divorce, and even suicide in the family.[33] Complications of this type are uncommon in families with an AD patient. FTD patients tend to become inattentive and careless and a danger to traffic. Changes in drinking behaviour are sometimes reported. The patient starts to drink more frequently and in larger quantities than before. The changes of behaviour, which may lead to misdiagnosis of alcohol-induced dementia, can often be controlled by a firm attitude from relatives.

Affective symptoms

The FTD patient becomes emotionally shallow and blunt, showing less concern about family and friends. The patient is described as egocentric, rigid, and lacking empathy. The early emotional changes may be difficult to differentiate from non-organic personality disorders and affective disorder. Mood changes towards euphoria, especially when associated with press of speech and overactivity, may at first be mistaken for a hypomanic or manic state. Slowly developing apathy, in combination with sparse mimical movements and verbal aspontaneity, may be misdiagnosed as depression. During the depressive reactions, which are mostly of short duration, the patient may become dysphoric, and dwell on suicidal thoughts. FTD patients are often diagnosed as depressed and treated with antidepressant medication during the early stage of the disease.[32]

Early symptoms of dementia must be judged against information about the patient's premorbid personality, education, and social background. The vast majority of cases show normal premorbid personality although a few have previously manifested anxiety and restlessness. The emotional features in FTD do not seem primarily related to premorbid personality traits but rather to the distribution of brain pathology as shown at autopsy and brain imaging.[34]

Other symptoms

A striking feature of FTD is the **stereotyped and perseverative behaviour** seen as wandering, clapping, humming, dancing, and hoarding of objects, as well as complex rituals involving washing and dressing. Such behaviour sometimes reaches psychotic intensity. Imitative behaviour is frequent in FTD and occurs more often than in AD.

Hallucinations and delusions are reported in about 20 per cent of FTD and early-onset AD cases. The psychotic symptoms in FTD are often bizarre and the combination with emotional changes and stereotypy of speech and behaviour gives the impression of functional psychosis with schizophrenia as an early tentative diagnosis.[6–8] The psychotic symptoms in early-onset AD seem more strongly related to the cognitive failure with memory failure, impaired recognition, and disorientation, and the degeneration of the temporoparietal association cortex.[6]

The **human counterpart of the Klüver–Bucy syndrome** has been reported in FLD and in Pick's disease. The hyperorality and changes of oral/dietary behaviour are seen as overeating, food fads, excessive smoking, and alcohol consumption. Utilization behaviour, defined as an irresistible impulse to explore and use objects in the visual environmental, shows important similarity to the hypermetamorphosis and distractibility of the Klüver–Bucy syndrome.[35] The Klüver–Bucy syndrome in AD is usually less complete than in FTD with less hypersexuality and utilization behaviour, supporting the suggestion that frontal as well as temporal limbic involvement is needed to produce the syndrome in humans.[6]

Dissolution of language

A core feature of FTLD is progressive impairment of speech and language. In FTD, this has been described as *dissolution du langage* or *Sprachverödung*.[6] Speech becomes aspontaneous with word-finding difficulties and frequent use of stereotyped comments and set phrases. During the early stage there may also be increased pressure of speech. The language dysfunction in FTD is dominated by dynamic expressive failure, which is in agreement with damage in the frontal cortex especially premotor areas. Echolalia is observed in about 50 per cent of FTD and Pick cases.[31] Finally the patients become mute which in combination with the amimia makes communication extremely difficult. The ability to understand information and instructions usually remains until comparatively late in the course of FTD, as does the ability to write. The handwriting may, however, change in magnitude, spelling, and speed of writing. These disturbances are unlike the temporoparietal type of dysgraphia and global dysphasia observed in AD. The symptom constellation of palilalia (stereotypy of speech), echolalia, mutism, and amimia (PEMA syndrome of Guiraud) is typical of FTD and seldom found in AD.

There are important similarities between the speech disorder of early FTD and the clinical spectrum of PA,[10] characterized by effortful speech production in the context of preserved word comprehension and relative preservation of memory and practical abilities. Dementia often develops later in the course, and the underlying degenerative process may be similar to that of FLD, with a predominant and early involvement of the speech-dominant hemisphere. Semantic dementia, the fluent language variant of FTLD is characterized by progressive loss of word retrieval and understanding, and recognition of sensory stimuli.[36] The pathological substrate is bilateral, often asymmetric temporal lobe degeneration.

Physical signs

Few pathological somatic findings including neurological symptom are reported early in FTD. However, primitive reflexes may appear early, while akinesia, rigidity, and tremor may emerge later in the course. Increased muscular tension is, however, significantly more common in AD.[6] The spectrum of FTLD also includes the syndrome of the disinhibition–dementia–parkinsonism–amyotrophy complex linked to chromosome 17 also named FTD-17.[37]

Generalized epileptic seizures may appear in FTD although less prevalent than in AD, and myoclonic twitchings and logoclonia which are prevalent in early-onset Alzheimer's cases are rare in FTD. Urinary incontinence, which is reported early in about 50 per cent of FTD cases, is a comparatively late feature in uncomplicated early-onset AD.

FTD patients in general have low and labile blood pressure with a high prevalence (50 per cent) of orthostatic blood pressure drops and syncopal attacks. These symptoms are, however, also reported in early-onset AD (40 per cent) and late in the course of vascular dementia (50 per cent). The relationship between blood pressure changes and brain damage especially the white-matter changes in FTD is still unclear.[18]

Dementia in motor neurone disease

The clinical picture of the dementia in motor neurone disease is similar to that in FLD with early changes of personality and behaviour, emotional changes such as euphoria and apathy, and signs of disinhibition and hyperorality.[38] Speech becomes stereotyped and perseverative, later developing into mutism. Receptive speech function, orientation, and practicable abilities remain relatively untouched by the degenerative process. The mental changes may appear early and even precede development of typical neurological features.

Investigations

EEG

The EEG may be normal or only slightly pathological in FTD at a stage when dementia is strongly suspected or clinically evident, but it is usually pathological late in the course. This has been shown in FLD, Pick's disease, and FTD-MND.[39] By contrast, EEG is almost always pathological in AD even at an early stage. Quantitative EEG mapping and repeated recordings may strongly improve the differential diagnosis between FTD and AD.[32]

Brain imaging and other investigations

Structural and functional brain imaging has strongly improved the diagnosis and differential diagnosis of FTD, AD, and other dementias. Cortical atrophy with more or less frontal focal accentuation, sometimes asymmetrical, is shown with CT and magnetic resonance imaging (**MRI**).[8,40] MRI may show significantly more prevalent and severe frontal periventricular white-matter lesions in FTD patients than in matched normal controls. The anterior–posterior gradient of the atrophic changes may, however, contribute to the differentiation from AD.[18,40] The differential diagnosis from vascular dementia with frontal subcortical lesions, but lacking large cortical infarctions, may be difficult.

Functional brain imaging measuring regional cerebral blood flow (rCBF) and metabolism with SPECT, PET, and other techniques show frontal and frontotemporal flow pathology in FTD with better preserved perfusion in posterior areas.[41,42] PET studies have indicated the ventromedial frontal cortex as the earliest site of imaging pathology.[43] These changes may at an early stage be mild and asymmetric in accordance with the clinical picture.

Recently several biomarkers in the cerebrospinal fluid (CSF) have been developed for differential diagnosis of dementia. Riemenschneider *et al.*[44] reported significantly higher CSF tau concentrations in FTD compared to healthy controls, but significantly lower than in AD, while CSF Abeta42 levels were significantly lower in FTD than in controls, but significantly higher than in AD. Early diagnosis of FTD might in the future be based on a combination of profile and levels of CSF biomarkers such as tau, β-amyloid, and neurofilaments.[45] Interestingly tau levels are dependent on lobar localization but independent of the degree of cerebral atrophy.[44,46]

Assessment of cognitive impairment

The cognitive changes, which appear early in FTD, may be difficult to evaluate due to the patient's emotional and behavioural changes. Distractibility and slightly reduced recent memory are common findings and remote memory is also impaired although to a lesser extent than in AD. The patients show significant impairment on 'frontal-lobe' tests such as the Wisconsin card sorting test, word fluency test, and the Stroop and trail-making tests. The early test profile is characterized by slow verbal production and relatively intact visuospatial ability, reasoning, and memory, while intellectual and motor speed are reduced.[10,47] Early AD usually shows a relatively preserved verbal ability and simultaneous impairment of reasoning ability, verbal and spatial memory dysfunction, dysphasia, and dyspraxia.[10,48,49] Difficulties in understanding instructions are found early only in a minority of FTD cases. Misspelling and dyscalculia are sometimes reported early in FTD.

Discrimination between FTD and AD can be based on a short test-battery (verbal ability, visuospatial ability, and verbal memory), when used in the context of a neuropsychological evaluation of qualitative as well as quantitative aspects of test performance.[47,49,50] Using a screening instrument based on frontal release signs, awareness of social/ethical dilemma in a short story, and the number of preservation errors, FTD was classified correctly in 83 per cent, validated against clinical diagnosis.[51] The Mini-Mental State Examination does not reflect the FTD patient's true competence because of influence of motivational and behavioural factors.[52]

Differential diagnosis

Differential diagnosis between FTD and AD and other dementias is often possible based on a careful clinical history and examination, supported by diagnostic tests and brain imaging. Detailed neuropathology remains a gold standard for definite diagnosis of FTD and other disorders presenting with FTD-like clinic (Table 4.1.3.3).

The clinical differences between FTD and AD are often obvious at an early stage. The initial stages of FTD are dominated by emotional and personality changes, and progressive reduction of speech. Consequently severe dyspraxia, memory failure, and spatial disorientation develop comparatively late with the relative sparing of the temporoparietal occipital cortical areas. In contrast, early-onset AD is characterized by memory failure, dyspraxia, dysgnosia, and impaired sense of locality, whereas habitual personality traits, social competence, and insight are better preserved in agreement with the consistent pattern of cortical involvement.[6] A minority of AD cases, about 5 per cent, show a marked frontal-lobe involvement at an early stage and consequently also present a frontal-lobe clinical pattern in addition to the temporoparietal symptoms.

The Lund–Manchester consensus[2] is recommended as a guideline for clinical recognition and differential diagnosis of FTD.[53–55]

Table 4.1.3.3 Clinical diagnostic alternatives to FTD

Alzheimer's disease (AD) with frontal emphasis
Vascular dementia with frontal emphasis
Selective white-matter infarction
Binswanger's disease
Multiinfarct dementia with frontal emphasis
Strategic infarct dementia (striatal, thalamic)
Huntington's disease
Creutzfeldt–Jacob disease
General paresis

The NINCDS–ADRDA criteria for AD were originally formulated with the aim to differentiate between AD and vascular dementia. Varma *et al.*[56] found a high sensitivity for probable AD, but also a low specificity since 77 per cent of pathologically confirmed FTD cases fulfilled the NINCDS–ADRDA criteria for AD.

Vascular dementia with frontal emphasis may be caused by selective incomplete white-matter infarction, Binswanger's disease, and frontal and strategic thalamic infarctions. The frontal-lobe dysfunction caused by vascular lesions may closely mimic the course of FTD, when developing gradually without dramatic onset or fluctuations.

The clinical distinction between FTD and Huntington's disease may be difficult when personality changes and psychotic features dominate, and when neurological characteristics are less obvious or appear late in the course. Brain imaging showing striatal involvement and genetic analysis may contribute to the diagnosis.

PSP and the rare progressive subcortical gliosis may also show a frontal-lobe clinical and imaging pathology. CBD may also present with a dementia of frontal-lobe type in addition to the typical asymmetric akinetic-rigid dystonic syndrome.[20] These three diseases have grown increasingly important because of studies suggesting a linkage to chromosome 17.[19]

Dementia of the frontal and frontal subcortical type is also found in Creutzfeldt–Jakob disease, in the AIDS dementia complex, and in general paresis.

Classification dilemma

Classification of frontotemporal dementias must be viewed in a historical perspective. The various clinicopathological entities have been identified by presence of certain and absence of other clinical and pathological features. The current classification and terminology of FTD illustrates, however, the difficulties of most one-dimensional diagnostic systems. A classification on pure clinical grounds is unsatisfactory since symptoms depend more on the starting point in the brain or topography than type of changes, and also on the progression pattern of the disease among brain areas, factors which may vary between cases with structurally identical disorders. A diagnostic classification should be clinically useful and valid, flexible and open to new ideas. There is a need for combination of classifications such as one based on phenomenological syndrome kept apart from, and combined with, aetiological including genotypical classification. Hopefully new generations of classifications and new diagnostic techniques and treatment strategies will further increase the awareness of FTD in clinical practice and research.

DSM-IV[1] and ICD-10[57] do not introduce the concepts of frontal-lobe dementia or FTD. DSM-IV presents Pick's disease as 'One of the pathologically distinct aetiologies among the heterogeneous group of dementing processes that are associated with frontotemporal brain atrophy'. ICD-10 describes 'dementia in Pick's disease' as an early-onset non-Alzheimer degenerative brain disease.

Aetiology and pathogenesis

The FTD is a heterogeneous disease group, but with important clinical features and probably also aetiological factors in common. The clinical and pathological similarities between familial and sporadic cases are, however, striking. About 40–50 per cent of patients with FLD have a history of similar disorder in a first-degree relative.[23,31] A family history study on 478 first-degree relatives of 74 index patients suffering from FTD reported a 10-fold increase in the incidence of FTD compared with the incidence of FTD in a population study.[58] A Swedish pedigree with FTD in 10 out of 21 family members in three generations has been described.[59]

Several genetic loci for FTD have been identified at human chromosomes 3, 9, and 17 in familial forms of the disease. One FTDP-17 locus has been mapped to a region of chromosome 17 where the tau gene is located. So far 35 different mutations in around 100 families have been identified.[36] However, tau mutations seem to be a rare cause of FTD. Dementia of frontal-lobe type has also been linked to chromosome 3p11–12 in a Danish family.[16] Conflicting results exist concerning the relation of FTD-MND to a locus on chromosome 9[60] and to chromosome 19 and the ApoE-allele pattern.[61] There is no solid proof of an autosomal-dominant inheritance in the majority of studies with Pick disease.

Several research groups have recently found mutations in the progranulin (PGRN) gene close to the tau gene to result in a loss of function of the growth or maintenance factor PGRN. This leads to a shortage of PRGN and degenerative dementia of the FTD type, including autosomal-dominant FTLD-U linked to chromosome 17 as well as further tau-positive and tau-negative forms.[17,62] Further research has shown that this mechanism may operate also in other neurodegenerative brain disorders including CBD and MND. MND is often linked to FTD-U by a common ubiquitinated protein[17] and by a frequent concurrence. This protein TDP-43 forms inclusions in a wide variety of functional brain areas in close correspondence to the symptomatology in the FTD spectrum, the clinical expression of which depends on the individual anatomical starting point and spread of the degeneration. The identification of mutations in PGRN explains why multiple families linked to chromosome 17 lack tau mutations.[62]

The pattern of degeneration in FTD may be related to a selective vulnerability of different brain regions to factors such as oxidative stress, environmental toxins, neurotransmitter dysfunction, and certain mutations. A retrospective study of risk for sporadic FTD reported a significantly higher prevalence of head trauma and thyroid disease.[63] A prion aetiology has been excluded in FLD and also in FTDP-17.

Neurochemical post-mortem studies of FTD have indicated abnormalities in serotonin metabolism but no alterations in cholinergic markers have been found.[64,65]

Treatment and care

Early diagnosis is a prerequisite for adequate treatment and care of the patient and support for the family and other carers involved. It is essential to explain the nature of the patients' changed behaviour and current problems. It is important not to forget the children who may still be at school age. It is especially in the social interaction that the earliest signs of the brain disease emerge.[33] Alternative optimal placements must be arranged when the patient can no longer be taken care of at home because of disturbing symptoms and lack of insight. Temporary and prolonged hospital admissions may be needed to make it possible for the family to cope with the situation. Being a spouse is both physically and emotionally exhausting, causing ill health and socio-economic problems for the family. FTD patients are often restless and stereotyped with a strong need for physical activity such as walking long distances, which, as well as the comparatively preserved memory, spatial and practical abilities should be channeled in a meaningful way rather than restricted. A well-structured programme for daily activities considering the patients premorbid personality and interests, 'routinizing therapy'[(66)] may be rewarding and minimize the need for pharmacological treatment. Prevailing psychotic features and unpredictable aggressive behaviour should be managed by a special psychiatric or psychogeriatric services[(33)] also responsible for support to the spouse and family members who often suffer from social isolation and loneliness.

There is presently no specific pharmacological treatment for the underlying degenerative disease in FTD but symptomatic treatment with serotonin-boosting antidepressants may be effective in treating some behavioural disturbances.[(67)] There are no reports that acetylcholinesterase inhibitors improve cognition or behaviour in FTD, and clinical experience is that the FTD patient may be extremely sensitive to psychotropic medication with disturbing side effects and paradoxical reactions. Various ways to improve progranulin levels may offer future pharmacological treatment for the FTD disorders.

Further information

Neary, D., Snowden, J., and Mann, D. (2005). Frontotemporal dementia. *Lancet Neurology*, **4**, 771–80 [review].

Alzheimer Research Forum: http://www.alzforum.org/

Referencest

1. American Psychiatric Association. (1994). *Diagnostic and statistical manual of mental disorders* (4th edn). American Psychiatric Association, Washington, DC.
2. Brun, A., Englund, E., Gustafson, L., *et al.* (1994). Consensus statement–clinical and neuropathological criteria for frontotemporal dementia. *Journal of Neurology, Neurosurgery, and Psychiatry*, **57**, 416–18.
3. Pick, A. (1892). Über die Beziehungen der senilen Hirnatrophie zur Aphasie. *Prager Medizinische Wochenschrift*, **17**, 165–7.
4. Alzheimer, A. (1911). Über eigenartige Krankheitsfälle des späteren Alters. *Zeitschrift für die Gesamte Neurologie und Psychiatrie*, **4**, 356–85.
5. Brun, A. (1987). Frontal lobe degeneration of non-Alzheimer type. I. Neuropathology. *Archives of Gerontology and Geriatrics*, **6**, 193–207.
6. Gustafson, L. (1987). Frontal lobe degeneration of non-Alzheimer type. II. Clinical picture and differential diagnosis. *Archives of Gerontology and Geriatrics*, **6**, 209–23.
7. Neary, D., Snowden, J.S., Northern, B., *et al.* (1988). Dementia of frontal lobe type. *Journal of Neurology, Neurosurgery, and Psychiatry*, **51**, 353–61.
8. Knopman, D.S., Mastri, A.R., Frey, *et al.* (1990). Dementia lacking distinctive histologic features. A common non-Alzheimer degenerative dementia. *Neurology*, **40**, 251–6.
9. Neary, D., Snowden, J.S., Gustafson, L., *et al.* (1998). Frontotemporal lobar degeneration. A consensus on clinical diagnostic criteria. *Neurology*, **51**, 1546–54.
10. Snowden, J.S., Neary, D., and Mann, D.M.A. (1996). *Frontotemporal lobar degeneration: frontotemporal dementia, progressive aphasia, semantic dementia.* Churchill Livingstone, London.
11. Mesulam, M.M. (1982). Slowly progressive aphasia without generalised dementia. *Annals of Neurology*, **11**, 592–8.
12. Hodges, J.R., Patterson, K., Oxbury, S., *et al.* (1992). Semantic dementia. Progressive fluent aphasia with temporal lobe atrophy. *Brain*, **115**, 1783–806.
13. Kertesz, A., McMonagle, P., Blair M., *et al.* (2005). The evaluation and pathology of frontotemporal dementia. *Brain*, **128**, 1996–2005.
14. Shi, J., Shaw, C.L., Du Pleiss, D., *et al.* (2005). Histopathological changes underlying frontotemporal lobar degeneration with clinicopathological correlation. *Acta Neuropathologica*, **110**, 501–12.
15. Josephs, K.A., Holton J.L., Rossor, M.N., *et al.* (2004). Frontotemporal lobar degeneration and ubiquitin immunohistochemistry. *Neuropathology and Applied Neurobiology*, **30**, 369–73.
16. Brown, J., Asworth, A., Gydesen, S., *et al.* (1995). Familial non-specific dementia maps to chromosome 3. *Human Molecular Genetics*, **4**, 1625–8.
17. Neumann, M., Sampathu, D.M., Kwong L.K., *et al.* (2006). Ubiquitinated TDP-43 in frontotemporal lobar degeneration and amyotrophic lateral sclerosis. *Science*, **314**, 130–3.
18. Larsson, E.M., Passant, U., Sundgren, P.C., *et al.* (2000). Magnetic resonance imaging and histopathology in dementia, clinically of frontotemporal type. *Dementia and Geriatric Cognitive Disorders*, **11**, 123–34.
19. Hutton, M., Lendon, C.L., Rizzu, P., *et al.* (1998). Association of missense and 5;-splice-site mutation in tau with the inherited dementia FTDP-17. *Nature*, **393**, 702–5.
20. Boeve, B.F., Lang, A.E., and Litvan, I. (2003). Corticobasal degeneration and its relationship to progressive supranuclear palsy and frontotemporal dementia. *Annals of Neurology*, **54**, S15–19.
21. Cairns, N.J., Lee, V.M., and Trojanowski, J.Q. (2007). Genetics and neuropathology of frontotemporal dementia. In *The human frontal lobes. Function and disorders* (eds. B. Miller and J.L. Cummings), pp. 382–407. The Guilford Press, NY, London.
22. Markesbery, W.R. (1998). Pick's disease. In *Neuropathology of dementing disorders* (ed. W.R. Markesbery), pp. 142–57. Arnold, London.
23. Stevens, M., Van Duijn, C.M., Kamphorts, W., *et al.* (1998). Familial aggregation in fronto-temporal dementia, *Neurology*, **50**, 1541–5.
24. Rosso, S.M., Donker Kaat, L., Baks T., *et al.* (2003). Frontotemporal dementia in the Netherlands: patient characteristics and prevalence estimates from a population-based study. *Brain*, **126**, 2016–22.
25. Pasquier, F., Lebert, F., and Amouyel, P. (1995). In *Les démences frontotemporales, épidémiologie* (eds. F. Pasquier and F. Lebert), pp. 23–9. Masson, Paris.
26. Ibach, B., Koch, H., Koller, M., *et al.* (2003). Hospital admission circumstances and prevalence of frontotemporal lobar degeneration: a multicenter psychiatric state hospital study in Germany. *Dementia and Geriatric Cognitive Disorders*, **16**, 253–64.
27. Lopez, O.L., Becker, J.T., and De Kosky, S.T. (1994). Dementia accompanying motor neuron disease. *Dementia*, **5**, 42–7.
28. Barker, W.W., Luis, C.A., Kashuba, A., *et al.* (2002). Relative frequencies of Alzheimer's disease, Lewy body, vascular and frontotemporal dementia, and hippocampal sclerosis in the state of Florida Bank. *Alzheimer Disease and Associated Disorders*, **16**, 203–12.
29. Giannakopoulos, P., Hof, P.R., and Bouras, C. (1995). Dementia lacking distinctive histopathology: clinicopathological evaluation of 32 cases. *Acta Neuropathologica*, **89**, 346–55.

30. Kertesz, A., McMonagle, P., Blair, M., *et al.* (2005). The evaluation and pathology of frontotemporal dementia. *Brain*, **128**, 1996–2005.
31. Gustafson, L. (1993). Clinical picture of frontal lobe degeneration of non-Alzheimer type. *Dementia*, **4**, 143–8.
32. Passant, U., Rosén, I., Gustafson, L., *et al.* (2005a). The heterogeneity of frontotemporal dementia with regard to initial symptoms, qEEG and neuropathology. *International Journal of Geriatric Psychiatry*, **20**, 983–8.
33. Passant, U., Elfgren, C., Englund, E., *et al.* (2005b). Psychiatric symptoms and their psychosocial consequences in frontotemporal dementia. *Alzheimer Disease and Associated Disorders*, **19**, S15–18.
34. Lebert, F., Pasquier, F., and Petit, H. (1995). Personality traits and frontal lobe dementia. *International Journal of Geriatric Psychiatry*, **10**, 1046–9.
35. Cummings, J.L. and Duchen, L.W. (1981). Klüver–Bucy syndrome in Pick's disease: clinical and pathological correlations. *Neurology*, **31**, 1415–22.
36. Neary, D., Snowden, J., and Mann, D. (2005). Frontotemporal dementia. *Lancet Neurology*, **4**, 771–80.
37. Lynch, T., Sano, M., Marder, K.S., *et al.* (1994). Clinical characteristics of a family with chromosome 17-linked disinhibition–dementia–parkinsonism–amyotrophy complex. *Neurology*, **44**, 1878–84.
38. Neary, D., Snowden, J.S., and Mann, D.M.A. (1990). Frontal lobe dementia and motor neuron disease. *Journal of Neurology, Neurosurgery, and Psychiatry*, **53**, 23–32.
39. Rosén, I., Gustafson, L., and Risberg, J. (1993). Multichannel EEG frequency analysis and somatosensory-evoked potentials in patients with different types of organic dementia. *Dementia*, **4**, 43–9.
40. Förstl, H., Besthorn, C., Hentschel, F., *et al.* (1996). Frontal lobe degeneration and Alzheimer's disease: a controlled study on clinical findings, volumetric brain changes and quantitative electroencephalography data. *Dementia*, **7**, 27–34.
41. Risberg, J., Passant, U., Warkentin, S., *et al.* (1993). Regional cerebral blood flow in frontal lobe dementia of non-Alzheimer type. *Dementia*, **4**, 186–7.
42. Foster, N.L. (2003). Validating FDG-PET as a biomarker frontotemporal dementia. *Experimental Neurology*, **184**, S2–8.
43. Salmon, E., Garaux, G., Delbeuck, X., *et al.* (2003). Predominant ventromedial frontopolar metabolic impairment in frontotemporal dementia. *Neuroimage*, **20**, 435–40.
44. Riemenschneider, M., Wagenpfeil, S., Diehl, J., *et al.* (2002). Tau and Abeta42 protein of patients with frontotemporal degeneration. *Neurology*, **11**, 1622–8.
45. Engelborghs, S., Maertens, K., Vloeberghs, E., *et al.* (2006). Neuropsychological and behavioural correlates of CSF biomarkers in dementia. *Neurochemistry International*, **48**, 286–95.
46. Pijnenburg, Y.A.L., Schoonenboom, S.N.M., Barkhof, F., *et al.* (2006). CSF biomarkers in frontotemporal lobar degeneration: relations with clinical characteristics, apolipoprotein E genotype, and neuroimaging. *Journal of Neurology, Neurosurgery, and Psychiatry*, **77**, 246–8.
47. Johanson, A. and Hagberg, B. (1989). Psychometric characteristics in patients with frontal lobe degeneration of non-Alzheimer type. *Archives of Gerontology and Geriatrics*, **8**, 29–137.
48. Frisoni, G.B., Pizzolato, G., Geroldi, C., *et al.* (1995). Dementia of the frontal type: neuropsychological and (99Tc)-HMPAO SPET features. *Journal of Geriatric Psychiatry and Neurology*, **8**, 42–8.
49. Elfgren, C., Brun, A., Gustafson, L., *et al.* (1994). Neuropsychological tests as discriminators between dementia of Alzheimer type and frontotemporal dementia. *International Journal of Geriatric Psychiatry*, **9**, 635–42.
50. Thompson, J.C., Stopford, C.L., Snowden, J.S., *et al.* (2005). Qualitative neuropsychological performance characteristics in frontotemporal dementia and Alzheimer's disease. *Journal of Neurology, Neurosurgery, and Psychiatry*, **76**, 920–7.
51. Gregory, C.A., Orrell, M., Sahakian, B., *et al.* (1997). Can frontotemporal dementia and Alzheimer's disease be differentiated using a brief battery of tests? *International Journal of Geriatric Psychiatry*, **12**, 375–83.
52. Pasquier, F. (1996). Neuropsychological features and cognitive assessment in frontotemporal dementia. In *Frontotemporal dementia* (eds. D. Pasquier, F. Lebert, and P. Scheltens), pp. 46–69. ICG, the Netherlands.
53. Miller, B.L., Ikone, C., Ponton, M., *et al.* (1997). A study of the Lund–Manchester research criteria for frontotemporal dementia: clinical and single-photon emission CT correlations. *Neurology*, **48**, 937–42.
54. Bathgate, D., Snowden, J.S., Varma, A., *et al.* (2001). Behaviour in frontotemporal dementia, Alzheimer's disease and vascular dementia. *Acta Neurologica Scandinavica*, **103**, 367–78.
55. Ikeda, M., Brown, J., Holland, A.J., *et al.* (2002). Changes in appetite, food preference, and eating habits in frontotemporal dementia and Alzheimer's disease. *Journal of Neurology, Neurosurgery, and Psychiatry*, **73**, 371–6.
56. Varma, A.R., Snowden, J.S., Lloyd, J.J., *et al.* (1999). Evaluation of the NINCDS-ADRDA criteria in the differentiation of Alzheimer's disease and frontotemporal dementia. *Journal of Neurology, Neurosurgery and Psychiatry*, **66**, 184–8.
57. World Health Organization. (1992). *The ICD-10 classification of mental and behavioural disorders. Clinical descriptions and diagnostic guidelines.* World Health Organization, Geneva.
58. Gräsbeck, A., Horstmann, V., Nilsson, K., *et al.* (2005). Dementia in first-degree relatives of patients with frontotemporal dementia. *Dementia and Geriatric Cognitive Disorders*, **19**, 145–53.
59. Passant, U., Gustafson, L., and Brun, A. (1993). Spectrum of frontal lobe dementia in a Swedish Family. *Dementia*, **4**, 160–2.
60. Vance, C., Al-Chalabi, A., Ruddy, D., *et al.* (2006). Familial amyotrophic lateral sclerosis with frontotemporal dementia is linked to a locus on chromosome 9p13.2-21.3. *Brain*, **129**, 868–76.
61. Pickering-Brown, S.M., Siddons, M., Mann, D.M.A., *et al.* (1995). Apolipoprotein E allelic frequencies in patients with lobar atrophy. *Neuroscience Letters*, **188**, 205–7.
62. Baker, M., Mackenzie, I.R., Pickering-Brown, S.M., *et al.* (2006). Mutations in progranulin cause tau-negative frontotemporal dementia linked to chromosome 17. *Nature*, **442**, 916–9.
63. Rosso, S.M., Landweer, E.J., Houterman, M., *et al.* (2003). Medical and environmental risk factors for sporadic frontotemporal dementia: a retrospective case-control study. *Journal of Neurology, Neurosurgery, and Psychiatry*, **74**, 1574–6.
64. Francis, P.T., Holmes, C., Webster, M.-T., *et al.* (1993). Preliminary neurochemical findings in non-Alzheimer dementia due to lobar atrophy. *Dementia*, **4**, 172–7.
65. Huey, E.D., Putnam, K., and Grafman, J. (2006). A systematic review of neurotransmitter deficits and treatments in frontotemporal dementia. *Neurology*, **66**, 17–22.
66. Tanabe, H., Ikeda, M., and Komori, K. (1999). Behavioral symptomatology and care of patients with frontotemporal lobe degeneration—based on the aspects of the phylogenetic and ontogenetic processes. *Dementia and Geriatric Cognitive Disorders*, **10**, S50–4.
67. Lebert, F., Stekke, W., Hasenbroekx, C., *et al.* (2004). Frontotemporal dementia: a randomised, controlled trial with trazodone. *Dementia and Geriatric Cognitive Disorders*, **17**, 355–9.

4.1.4 Prion disease

John Collinge

Introduction

The human prion diseases, also known as the subacute spongiform encephalopathies, have been traditionally classified into Creutzfeldt–Jakob disease (**CJD**), Gerstmann–Sträussler syndrome (**GSS**) (also known as Gerstmann–Sträussler–Scheinker disease), and **kuru**. Although rare, affecting about 1–2 per million worldwide per annum, remarkable attention has been recently focused on these diseases. This is because of the unique biology of the transmissible agent or prion, and also because bovine spongiform encephalopathy (**BSE**), an epidemic bovine prion disease, appears to have transmitted to humans as variant CJD (**vCJD**), opening the possibility of a significant threat to public health through dietary exposure to infected tissues.

The transmissibility of the human diseases was demonstrated with the transmission, by intracerebral inoculation with brain homogenates into chimpanzees, of first kuru and then CJD in 1966 and 1968, respectively.[1,2] Transmission of GSS followed in 1981. The prototypic prion disease is **scrapie**, a naturally occurring disease of sheep and goats, which has been recognized in Europe for over 200 years and which is present in the sheep flocks of many countries. Scrapie was demonstrated to be transmissible by inoculation in 1936[3] and the recognition that kuru, and then CJD, resembled scrapie in its histopathological appearances led to the suggestion that these diseases may also be transmissible.[4] Kuru reached epidemic proportions amongst the Fore linguistic group in the Eastern Highlands of Papua New Guinea and was transmitted by ritual cannibalism. Since the cessation of cannibalism in the 1950s the disease has declined but a few cases still occur as a result of the long incubation periods in this condition, which may exceed 50 years.[5] The term Creutzfeldt–Jakob disease was introduced by Spielmeyer in 1922 bringing together the case reports published by Creutzfeldt and Jakob. Several of these cases would not meet modern diagnostic criteria for CJD and indeed it was not until the demonstration of transmissibility allowed diagnostic criteria to be reassessed and refined that a clear diagnostic entity developed. All these diseases share common histopathological features; the classical triad of spongiform vacuolation (affecting any part of the cerebral grey matter), astrocytic proliferation, and neuronal loss, may be accompanied by the deposition of amyloid plaques.

Aetiology

Prion diseases of both humans and animals are associated with the accumulation in the brain of an abnormal, partially protease-resistant, isoform of a host-encoded glycoprotein known as prion protein (PrP). The disease-related isoform, PrP^{Sc}, is derived from its normal cellular precursor, PrP^{C}, by a post-translational process that involves a conformational change. PrP^{C} is rich in α-helical structure while PrP^{Sc} appears to be predominantly composed of β-sheet structure. According to the 'protein-only' hypothesis,[6] an abnormal PrP isoform[7] is the principal, and possibly the sole, constituent of the transmissible agent or prion. PrP^{Sc} is hypothesized to act as a conformational template, promoting the conversion of PrP^{C} to further PrP^{Sc}. PrP^{C} appears to be poised between two radically different folding states, and α- and β-forms of PrP can be inter-converted in suitable conditions.[8] Soluble β-PrP aggregates in physiological salt concentrations to form fibrils with morphological and biochemical characteristics closely similar to PrP^{Sc}. A molecular mechanism for prion propagation can now be proposed.[8] Prion replication, with recruitment of PrP^{C} into the aggregated PrP^{Sc} isoform, may be initiated by a pathogenic mutation (resulting in a PrP^{C} predisposed to form β-PrP) in inherited prion diseases, by exposure to a 'seed' of PrP^{Sc} in acquired cases, or as a result of the spontaneous conversion of PrP^{C} to β-PrP (and subsequent formation of aggregated material) as a rare stochastic event in sporadic prion disease.

The human PrP gene (*PRNP*) is a single copy gene located on the short arm of chromosome 20 and was an obvious candidate for genetic linkage studies in the familial forms of CJD and GSS, which both showed an autosomal dominant pattern of disease segregation. A turning point in understanding the human prion diseases was the identification of mutations in the prion protein *gene* in familial CJD and GSS in 1989. The first mutation to be identified in *PRNP* was in a family with CJD and constituted a 144 bp insertion into the coding sequence.[9] A second mutation was reported in two families with GSS and genetic linkage was confirmed between this missense variant at codon 102 and GSS, confirming that GSS was an autosomal dominant Mendelian disorder.[10] Uniquely, these diseases are therefore both inherited and transmissible. Current evidence suggests that around 15 per cent of prion diseases are inherited and over 30 coding mutations in *PRNP* are now recognized.

With the exception of the rare iatrogenic CJD cases mentioned above, most prion disease occurs as sporadic CJD. While, by definition, there will not be a family history in sporadic cases, mutations are seen in occasional apparently sporadic cases, as with a late-onset disease the family history may not be apparent or non-paternity may occur. However, in the majority of sporadic CJD cases there is neither a coding mutation nor a history of iatrogenic exposure. Human prion diseases can therefore be subdivided into inherited, sporadic, and acquired forms. However, a common PrP polymorphism at residue 129, where either methionine or valine can be encoded, is a key determinant of genetic susceptibility to acquired and sporadic prion diseases, the large majority of which occur in homozygous individuals.[11,12] This protective effect of *PRNP* codon 129 heterozygosity is also seen in some of the inherited prion diseases.

The aetiology of sporadic CJD remains unclear. It has been speculated that these cases might arise from somatic mutation of *PRNP* or spontaneous conversion of PrP^{C} to PrP^{Sc} as a rare stochastic event. The alternative hypothesis, in which such cases arise as a result of exposure to an environmental source of either human or animal prions, is not supported by epidemiological evidence.[13]

A major problem for the 'protein-only' hypothesis of prion propagation has been how to explain the existence of multiple isolates or strains of prions, with distinct biological properties. Understanding how a protein-only infectious agent could encode such phenotypic information has been of considerable biological interest. However, it is now clear that prion strains can be distinguished by differences in the biochemical properties of PrP^{Sc}. Prion strain diversity appears to be encoded by differences in PrP conformation and pattern of glycosylation.[14] A molecular strain typing approach based on these characteristics has allowed the identification of four main types amongst CJD cases, sporadic and iatrogenic CJD being of PrP^{Sc} types 1–3, while all vCJD cases are associated with a distinctive type 4 PrP^{Sc} type.[14,15] A similar PrP^{Sc} type to that seen in vCJD is seen in BSE and BSE when transmitted to several other species. Such molecular strain typing strongly supported the hypothesis that vCJD was human BSE. This conclusion was strengthened by subsequent transmission studies of vCJD into both transgenic and conventional mice which argued that cattle BSE and vCJD were caused by the same strain.[16,17] Such studies are allowing a molecular classification of human prion diseases. Two such classifications are in use: no internationally agreed classification has yet emerged and it is likely that additional PrP^{Sc} types or strains will be identified.[15,18] Molecular classification may well open new avenues of epidemiological investigation and offer insights into causes of 'sporadic' CJD. The ability of a protein to encode a disease phenotype has important implications in biology, as it represents a non-Mendelian form of transmission. It would be surprising if this mechanism had not been used more widely during evolution such that prion biology may prove to be of far wider relevance.

Transmission of prion diseases between different mammalian species is limited by a so-called 'species barrier'. Early studies of the molecular basis of the species barrier argued that it principally resided in differences in PrP primary structure between the species from which the inoculum was derived and the inoculated host. Transgenic mice expressing hamster PrP were, unlike wild-type mice, highly susceptible to infection with hamster prions.[19] That most sporadic and acquired CJD occurred in individuals homozygous at *PRNP* polymorphic codon 129 supported the view that prion propagation proceeded most efficiently when the interacting PrP^{Sc} and PrP^{C} were of identical primary structure.[12] However, it has been long recognized that prion strain type affects ease of transmission to another species. Interestingly, with BSE prions the strain component to the barrier seems to predominate, with BSE not only transmitting efficiently to a range of species, but maintaining its transmission characteristics even when passaged through an intermediate species with a distinct PrP gene.[20] The term 'species-strain barrier' or simply 'transmission barrier' may be preferable.[21] Both PrP amino acid sequence and strain type affect the 3D structure of glycosylated PrP which will presumably, in turn, affect the efficiency of the protein–protein interactions thought to determine prion propagation.

Mammalian PrP genes are highly conserved. Presumably only a restricted number of different PrP^{Sc} conformations (that are highly stable and can therefore be serially propagated) will be permissible thermodynamically and will constitute the range of prion strains seen in mammals. While a significant number of different such PrP^{Sc} conformations may be possible amongst the range of mammalian PrPs, only a subset of these would be allowable for a given single mammalian PrP. Substantial overlap between the favoured conformations for PrP^{Sc} derived from species A and species B might therefore result in relatively easy transmission of prion diseases between these two species, while two species with no preferred PrP^{Sc} conformations in common would have a large barrier to transmission (and indeed transmission would necessitate a change of strain type). According to such a *conformational selection model*[21] of a prion transmission barrier, BSE may represent a thermodynamically highly favoured PrP^{Sc} conformation that is permissive for PrP expressed in a wide range of different species, accounting for the remarkable promiscuity of this strain in mammals. Contribution of other components to the species barrier are possible and may involve interacting co-factors which mediate the efficiency of prion propagation, although no such factors have yet been identified.

Additional data has further challenged our understanding of transmission barriers.[22] The assessment of species barriers has relied on the development of a clinical disease in inoculated animals. However, it is now clear that *subclinical prion infections* are sometimes established on prion inoculation of a second species.[23] Such animals harbour high levels of prion infectivity but do not develop clinical disease during a normal lifespan. The existence of such subclinical carrier states of prion infection has important potential animal and public health implications and argues against direct neurotoxicity of prions.

The transmission barrier between cattle BSE and humans cannot be directly measured but can be modelled in transgenic mice expressing human PrP^{C}, which produce human PrP^{Sc} when challenged with human prions. Long-term transmission studies have been carried out using such 'humanized' mice to both to characterize the distinct prion strains causing human disease and to model human susceptibility to infection with BSE and other prions.[24] While these transgenic mouse models have been able to faithfully propagate human prion strains[14,16,25] and recapitulate the characteristic neuropathology of vCJD,[26] there are important caveats in extrapolating from such animal models to human susceptibility. However, these studies have found a much higher infection rate in transgenic mice expressing human PrP M129 than mice expressing human PrP V129 when challenged with either BSE or vCJD prions, and demonstrated that BSE prion infection can produce disease phenotypes resembling sporadic CJD infection of these mice and also novel prion strain phenotypes. Most recently, these studies have argued that the vCJD phenotype may only be expressed in the presence of the M form of human PrP.[27] While this would imply that only those humans expressing human PrP M129 may develop the vCJD phenotype, this does not mean that VV individuals are completely resistant to BSE prion infection—but rather that if infected they would show a different phenotype.[27] Modelling of susceptibility of the MV genotype suggests that several different phenotypes, all distinct from vCJD, may be possible when infected with BSE or vCJD prions.[28]

Clinical features and diagnosis

The human prion diseases can be divided aetiologically into inherited, sporadic, and acquired forms with CJD, GSS, and kuru now seen as clinicopathological syndromes within a wider spectrum of disease. Kindreds with inherited prion disease have been described with phenotypes of classical CJD, GSS, and also with other neurodegenerative syndromes including fatal familial insomnia. Some kindreds show remarkable phenotypic variability which can encompass both CJD- and GSS-like cases as well as other cases which do not conform to either CJD or GSS phenotypes and which indeed readily mimic, and are frequently misdiagnosed as, many other neurodegenerative conditions. Inherited prion diseases are a frequent cause of pre-senile dementia and a family history is not always apparent: *PRNP* should be analysed in all suspected cases of CJD, and considered in all early-onset dementia and ataxias. Cases diagnosed by *PRNP* analysis have been reported which are not only clinically atypical but which lack the classical histological features entirely. Significant clinical overlap exists with familial Alzheimer's disease, Pick's disease, frontal lobe degeneration of non-Alzheimer type, and amyotrophic lateral sclerosis with dementia. Although classical GSS is described below it now seems more sensible to designate the familial illnesses as inherited prion diseases and then to subclassify these according to mutation. Acquired prion diseases include iatrogenic CJD, kuru, and now vCJD. Sporadic prion diseases at present consist of CJD and atypical variants of CJD. Cases lacking the characteristic histological features of CJD have been transmitted. As there are at present no equivalent aetiological diagnostic markers for sporadic prion diseases to those for the inherited diseases, it cannot yet be excluded that more diverse phenotypic variants of sporadic prion disease exist. The key clinical features and investigations for the diagnosis of prion disease are given in the Table 4.1.4.1.

Table 4.1.4.1 Diagnosis of prion disease

Sporadic (classical) CJD

- Rapidly progressive* dementia with two or more of myoclonus, cortical blindness, pyramidal signs, cerebellar signs, extrapyramidal signs, akinetic mutism
- Most cases age 45–75
- Serial EEG shows pseudoperiodic complexes in most cases
- CSF 14-3-3 protein usually positive
- CT normal or atrophy, MRI may show high signal in the striatum and/or cerebral cortex in FLAIR or diffusion-weighted images
- *PRNP* analysis: no pathogenic mutations, most are 129 MM (VV and MV may be longer duration, clinically atypical and EEG less often positive)
- Brain biopsy in highly selected cases (to exclude treatable alternative diagnoses): PrP immunocytochemistry or Western blot for PrP^{Sc} types 1–3

Iatrogenic CJD

- Progressive cerebellar syndrome and behavioural disturbance or classical CJD-like syndrome with history of iatrogenic exposure to human prions (pituitary-derived hormones, tissue grafting, or neurosurgery)
- May be young
- EEG, CSF, and MRI generally less helpful than in sporadic cases
- *PRNP* analysis: no pathogenic mutations, most are 129 homozygotes
- Brain biopsy in highly selected cases (to exclude treatable alternative diagnoses): PrP immunocytochemistry or Western blot for PrP^{Sc} types 1–3

Variant CJD

- Early features: depression, anxiety, social withdrawal, peripheral sensory symptoms
- Cerebellar ataxia, chorea, or athetosis often precedes dementia, advanced disease as sporadic CJD
- Most in young adults; however, age at onset 12–74 years seen
- EEG non-specific slow waves, CSF 14-3-3 may be elevated or normal
- MRI: pulvinar sign usually present (particularly using FLAIR sequence) but may be late feature
- *PRNP* analysis: no mutations, all 129 MM to date
- Tonsil biopsy: characteristic PrP immunostaining and PrP^{Sc} on Western blot (type 4t)

Iatrogenic vCJD

- Has occurred in recipients of blood transfusion from a donor who subsequently developed clinical vCJD
- Known recipients of implicated blood or blood products in the UK have been notified of their risk status
- Clinical features and investigations as for primary vCJD

Inherited prion disease

- Varied clinical syndromes between and within kindreds: should consider in all pre-senile dementias and ataxias irrespective of family history
- *PRNP* analysis: diagnostic, codon 129 genotype may predict age at onset in pre-symptomatic testing

*Clinical duration typically 6 months or less but high variability: type 1 PrP^{Sc} associated with short duration (~8 weeks); ~10% have duration >2 years.

Sporadic prion disease

CJD

The core clinical syndrome of classic CJD is of a rapidly progressive multifocal dementia usually with myoclonus. The onset is usually in the 45–75-year age group with peak onset between 60 and 65 years. The clinical progression is typically over weeks progressing to akinetic mutism and death often in 2–3 months. Around 70 per cent of cases die in under 6 months. Prodromal features, present in around a third of cases, include fatigue, insomnia, depression, weight loss, headaches, general malaise, and ill-defined pain sensations. In addition to mental deterioration and myoclonus, frequent additional neurological features include extrapyramidal signs, cerebellar ataxia, pyramidal signs, and cortical blindness. About 10 per cent of cases present initially with cerebellar ataxia.

Routine haematological and biochemical investigations are normal although occasional cases have been noted to have raised serum transaminases or alkaline phosphatase. There are no immunological markers and acute phase proteins are not elevated. Examination of the cerebrospinal fluid is normal 14-3-3 protein is usually elevated in CJD and is a useful adjunct to diagnosis in the appropriate clinical context.[29] It is also positive in recent cerebral infarction or haemorrhage and in viral encephalitis, although these conditions do not usually present diagnostic confusion with CJD. It may also be elevated in rapidly progressive Alzheimer's disease, which may be difficult to clinically distinguish from CJD. Neuronal specific enolase (NSE) and S-100b may be also elevated although also are not specific for CJD and represent markers of neuronal injury[30,31] Neuroimaging with CT or MRI is crucial to exclude other causes of subacute neurological illness but MRI has become increasingly useful in diagnosis of sporadic CJD, showing high signal in the striatum and/or cerebral cortex in FLAIR or diffusion-weighted images.[32] Cerebral and cerebellar atrophy may be present in longer duration cases. The electroencephalogram (EEG) may show characteristic pseudoperiodic sharp wave activity, which is very helpful in diagnosis but present only in around 70 per cent of cases. To some extent demonstration of a typical EEG is dependent on the number of EEGs performed and serial EEG is indicated to try and demonstrate this appearance.

Prospective epidemiological studies have demonstrated that cases with a progressive dementia, and two or more of the following: myoclonus; cortical blindness; pyramidal, cerebellar, or extrapyramidal signs; or akinetic mutism in the setting of a typical EEG nearly always turn out to be confirmed as histologically definite CJD if neuropathological examination is performed.

Neuropathological confirmation of CJD is by demonstration of spongiform change, neuronal loss, and astrocytosis. PrP amyloid plaques are usually not present in CJD although PrP immunohistochemistry, using appropriate pre-treatments, will nearly always be positive. Protease resistant PrP, seen in all the currently recognized prion diseases, can be demonstrated by immunoblotting of brain homogenates. *PRNP* analysis is important to exclude pathogenic mutations. Genetic susceptibility to CJD has been demonstrated in that most cases of classical CJD are homozygous with respect to the common 129 polymorphism of PrP (see aetiology).

Atypical forms of CJD

Atypical forms of CJD are well recognized. Around 10 per cent of cases of CJD have a much more prolonged clinical course with a disease duration of over 2 years. These cases may represent the occasional occurrence of CJD in individuals heterozygous for PrP polymorphisms. Around 10 per cent of CJD cases present with cerebellar ataxia rather than cognitive impairment, so-called ataxic CJD. Heidenhain's variant of CJD refers to cases in which cortical blindness predominates with severe involvement of the occipital lobes. The panencephalopathic type of CJD refers to cases with extensive degeneration of the cerebral white matter in addition to spongiform vacuolation of the grey matter and has been predominately reported from Japan.

Amyotrophic variants of CJD have been described with prominent early muscle wasting. However, most cases of dementia with amyotrophy are not experimentally transmissible and their relationship with CJD is unclear. Most cases are probably variants of motor neurone disease with associated dementia. Amyotrophic features in CJD are usually seen in late disease when other features are well established.

Acquired prion diseases

While human prion diseases can be transmitted to experimental animals by inoculation, they are not contagious in humans. Documented case to case spread has only occurred during ritual cannibalistic practices (kuru) or following accidental inoculation with prions during medical or surgical procedures (iatrogenic CJD).

Kuru

Kuru reached epidemic proportions amongst a defined population living in the Eastern Highlands of Papua New Guinea.[(33)] The earliest cases are thought to date back to the early part of the century. Kuru affected the people of the Fore linguistic group and their neighbours with whom they intermarried. Kuru predominantly affected women and children (of both sexes), with only 2 per cent of cases in adult males and was the commonest cause of death amongst women in affected villages. It was the practice in these communities to engage in consumption of dead relatives as a mark of respect and mourning. Women and children predominantly ate the brain and internal organs, which is thought to explain the differential age and sex incidence. Preparation of the cadaver for consumption was performed by the women and children such that other routes of exposure may also have been relevant. It is thought that the epidemic related to a single sporadic CJD case occurring in the region some decades earlier. Epidemiological studies provided no evidence for vertical transmission, since most of the children born after 1956 (when cannibalism had effectively ceased) and all of those born after 1959 of mothers affected with or incubating kuru were unaffected. From the age of the youngest affected patient, the shortest incubation period is estimated as 4.5 years, although may have been shorter, since time of infection was usually unknown. The disease has gradually declined in incidence although a small number of cases have been documented in recent years with incubation periods which may exceed 50 years.[(5)]

Kuru affects both sexes and onset of disease has ranged from age 5 to over 60. The mean clinical duration of illness is 12 months with a range of 3 months to 3 years; the course tends to be shorter in children. The central clinical feature is progressive cerebellar ataxia. In sharp contrast to CJD, dementia is usually absent, even in the latter stages, although in the terminal stages many patients have their faculties obtunded. The occasional case in which gross dementia occurs is in marked contrast to the clinical norm. Detailed clinical descriptions have been given by a number of observers and the disease does not appear to have changed in features at different stages of the epidemic. A prodrome and three clinical stages are recognized:

(a) Prodromal stage

Kuru typically begins with prodromal symptoms consisting of headache, aching of limbs, and joint pains, which can last for several months.

(b) Ambulatory stage

Kuru was frequently self-diagnosed by patients at the earliest onset of unsteadiness in standing or walking, or of dysarthria or diplopia. At this stage there may be no objective signs of disease. Gait ataxia however worsens and patients develop a broad-based gait, truncal instability, and titubation. A coarse postural tremor is usually present and accentuated by movement; patients characteristically hold their hands together in the midline to suppress this. Standing with feet together reveals clawing of toes to maintain posture. This marked clawing response is regarded as pathognomonic of kuru. Patients often become withdrawn at this stage and occasionally develop a severe reactive depression. Prodromal symptoms tend to disappear. Astasia and gait ataxia worsen and the patient requires a stick for walking. Intention tremor, dysmetria, hypotonia, and dysdiadochokinesis develop. Although eye movements are ataxic and jerky, nystagmus is rarely seen. Strabismus, usually convergent, may occur particularly in children. This strabismus does not appear to be concomitant or paralytic and may fluctuate in both extent and type sometimes disappearing later in the clinical course. Photophobia is common and there may be an abnormal cold sensitivity with shivering and piloerection even in a warm environment. Tendon reflexes are reduced or normal and plantar responses are flexor. Dysarthria usually occurs. As ataxia progresses the patient passes from the first (ambulatory) stage to the second (sedentary) stage. The mean clinical duration of the first stage is around 8 months and correlates closely with total duration.

(c) Sedentary stage

At this stage patients are able to sit unsupported but cannot walk. Attempted walking with support leads to a high steppage, wide-based gait with reeling instability, and flinging arm movements in an attempt to maintain posture. Hyperreflexia is seen although plantar responses usually remain flexor with intact abdominal reflexes. Clonus is characteristically short-lived. Athetoid and choreiform movements and Parkinsonian tremors may occur. There is no paralysis, although muscle power is reduced. Obesity is common at this stage but may be present in early disease associated with bulimia. Characteristically, there is emotional lability and bizarre uncontrollable laughter, which has led to the disease being referred to as 'laughing death'. There is no sensory impairment. In sharp contrast to CJD, myoclonic jerking is rarely seen. EEG is usually normal or may show non-specific changes. This stage lasts around 2–3 months. When truncal ataxia reaches the point where the patient is unable to sit unsupported, the third or tertiary stage is reached.

(d) Tertiary stage

Hypotonia and hyporeflexia develop and the terminal state is marked by flaccid muscle weakness. Plantar responses remain flexor and abdominal reflexes intact. Progressive dysphagia occurs and patients become incontinent of urine and faeces. Inanition and emaciation develop. Transient conjugate eye signs and dementia may occur. Primitive reflexes develop in occasional cases. Brainstem involvement and both bulbar and pseudobulbar signs occur. Respiratory failure and bronchopneumonia eventually lead to death. The tertiary stage lasts 1–2 months.

Iatrogenic CJD

Iatrogenic transmission of CJD has occurred by accidental inoculation with human prions as a result of medical procedures. Such iatrogenic routes include the use of inadequately sterilized neurosurgical instruments, dura mater and corneal grafting, and use of human cadaveric pituitary-derived growth hormone or gonadotrophin. It is of considerable interest that cases arising from intracerebral or optic inoculation manifest clinically as classical CJD, with a rapidly progressive dementia, while those resulting from peripheral inoculation, most notably following pituitary-derived growth hormone exposure, typically present with a progressive cerebellar syndrome, and are in that respect somewhat reminiscent of kuru. Unsurprisingly the incubation period in intracerebral cases is short (19–46 months for dura mater grafts) as compared to peripheral cases (typically 15 years or more). There is evidence for genetic susceptibility to iatrogenic CJD with an excess of codon 129 homozygotes[(11)] (see aetiology).

Epidemiological studies have not shown increased risks of particular occupations that may be exposed to human or animal prions, although individual CJD cases in two histopathology technicians, a neuropathologist, and a neurosurgeon have been documented. While there have been concerns that CJD may be transmissible by blood transfusion, extensive epidemiological analysis in the UK has found that the frequency of blood transfusion and donation was no different in over 200 cases of CJD and a matched control population.[(34)] Recipients of blood transfusions who developed CJD had clinical presentations similar to those of sporadic CJD patients and not to the more kuru-like iatrogenic cases arising from peripheral exposure to human prions. Furthermore, experimental transmission studies have shown only weak evidence for infectivity in blood, even when inoculated via the most efficient (intracerebral) route. Iatrogenic (secondary) vCJD related to blood transfusion has however been recognized (see below).

Variant CJD

In late 1995, two cases of sporadic CJD were reported in the UK in teenagers.[(35)] Only four cases of sporadic CJD had previously been recorded in teenagers, and none of these cases occurred in the UK. In addition, both cases were unusual in having kuru-type plaques, a finding seen in only around 5 per cent of CJD cases. Soon afterwards a third very young sporadic CJD case occurred. These cases caused considerable concern and the possibility was raised that they might suggest a link with BSE. By March 1996, further extremely young onset cases were apparent and review of the histology of these cases showed a remarkably consistent and unique pattern. These cases were named 'new variant' CJD although it was clear that they were also rather atypical in their clinical presentation; in fact most cases did not meet the accepted clinical diagnostic criteria for probable CJD. Extensive studies of archival cases of CJD or other prion diseases failed to show this picture and it seemed that it did represent the arrival of a new form of prion disease in the UK. The statistical probability of such cases occurring by chance was vanishingly small and ascertainment bias seemed most unlikely as an explanation. It was clear that a new risk factor for CJD had emerged and appeared to be specific to the UK. The UK Government advisory committee on spongiform encephalopathy (SEAC) concluded that, while there was no direct evidence for a link with BSE, exposure to specified bovine offal (SBO) prior to the ban on its inclusion in human foodstuffs in 1989, was the most likely explanation. A case of vCJD was soon after reported in France. Direct experimental evidence that vCJD is caused by BSE was provided by molecular analysis of human prion strains and transmission studies in transgenic and wild-type mice (see aetiology). While it is now clear that vCJD is caused by infection with BSE prions, it is unclear why this particular age group should be affected and why none of these cases had a pattern of unusual occupational or dietary exposure to BSE. However, very little is known of which foodstuffs contained high-titre bovine offal. It is possible that certain foods containing particularly high titres were eaten predominately by younger people. An alternative is that young people are more susceptible to BSE following dietary exposure or that they have shorter incubation periods. A possible age-related co-factor could be coexistent infection involving lymphoid tissue, for example tonsillar infection. It is important to appreciate that BSE contaminated feed was fed to sheep, pigs, and poultry and that although there is no evidence of natural transmission to these species, it would be prudent to remain open minded about other dietary exposure to novel animal prions.

vCJD has an insidious clinical onset and its early features are highly non-specific. The clinical presentation is often with behavioural and psychiatric disturbances and in some cases with sensory disturbance. Initial referral has frequently been to a psychiatrist and the most prominent feature is depression but anxiety, social withdrawal, and behavioural change is frequent. Suicidal ideation is infrequent and response to antidepressants poor. Delusions, which are complex and unsustained, are common. Other features include emotional lability, aggression, insomnia, and auditory and visual hallucinations. A prominent early feature in some is dysaesthesiae or pain in the limbs or face or pain, which is persistent rather than intermittent and unrelated to anxiety levels. A minority of cases have been noted to have forgetfulness or mild gait ataxia from an early stage but in most cases overt neurological features are not apparent until some months into the clinical course. In most patients a progressive cerebellar syndrome develops with gait and limb ataxia. Overt dementia then occurs with inevitable progression to akinetic mutism. Myoclonus is seen in most patients, and chorea is often present which may be severe in some patients. Cortical blindness develops in a minority of patients in the late stages of disease. Upgaze paresis, an uncommon feature of classical CJD, has been noted in some patients. The age at onset in the initial 14 cases reported ranged from 16 to 48 years (mean 29 years) and the clinical course was unusually prolonged (9–35 months, median 14 months). The age range of cases has since broadened, with ages at onset ranging from 12 to 74 years, although the mean remains around 28 years. The EEG is abnormal, most frequently showing generalized slow wave activity, but without the pseudoperiodic pattern seen in most sporadic CJD cases. Neuroimaging by CT is either normal or shows only mild atrophy. The most useful non-invasive investigation in advanced cases is MR neuroimaging, particularly the FLAIR sequence.[36] Early case reports noted bilateral increased signal in the posterior thalamus (pulvinar) on T2-weighted images.[37] A retrospective review of 36 histologically confirmed cases of vCJD suggested that the 'pulvinar sign' occurred frequently in advanced cases of vCJD[38] with a sensitivity and specificity of up to 86 and 96 per cent, respectively. However, this sign appears a late feature of the disease process. Histologically confirmed cases of vCJD with minimal or absent pulvinar changes at a mean 10.5 months during an illness of mean 15 months duration were identified in this series. Figures of 81 per cent sensitivity and 94 per cent specificity have also been reported in a series including 27 cases of vCJD diagnosed by tonsil biopsy.[39] As these studies suggest, the pulvinar sign is not specific for vCJD. These MRI appearances are described in sporadic CJD and paraneoplastic limbic encephalitis, both of which are important considerations in the differential diagnosis of patients with suspected vCJD. Pulvinar signal change on MRI is also reported in a number of rare conditions, which might otherwise be distinguished from vCJD on clinical grounds such as benign intracranial hypertension, status epilepticus associated with cat scratch disease, Alpers' disease, and post-infectious encephalitis. The absence of pulvinar sign does not exclude a diagnosis of vCJD.

Tonsillar biopsy remains the most sensitive and specific diagnostic procedure for vCJD.[39–43] Tonsillar PrP^{Sc} is uniformly present in clinically affected cases of vCJD but not in other forms of human prion disease, including iatrogenic CJD associated with use of human cadaveric-derived pituitary hormones, arguing that this distinctive pathogenesis relates to effect of prion strain rather than to a peripheral route of infection.[41–43] As infection of lymphoreticular tissues is thought to precede neuroinvasion, and indeed has been detected in archived surgical samples removed prior to development of vCJD,[44,45] it is likely to allow firm diagnosis at the early clinical stage or indeed pre-clinically.[46] The PrP^{Sc} type detected on Western blot in vCJD tonsil has a characteristic pattern designated type 4t. A positive tonsil biopsy obviates the need for brain biopsy, which may otherwise be considered in such a clinical context to exclude alternative, potentially treatable diagnoses. CSF 14-3-3 protein may be elevated or normal. *PRNP* analysis is essential to rule out pathogenic mutations, as the inherited prion diseases present in younger patients and may clinically mimic vCJD. It is particularly important to exclude mutations prior to tonsil biopsy. Remarkably, to date all clinical cases of vCJD have been of the *PRNP* codon 129 MM genotype (see aetiology).

The neuropathological appearances of vCJD are striking and relatively consistent, generally allowing differentiation from other forms of prion disease. While there is widespread spongiform change, gliosis and neuronal loss, most severe in the basal ganglia and thalamus, the most remarkable feature is abundant PrP amyloid plaques in cerebral and cerebellar cortex. These consist of kuru-like, 'florid' (surrounded by spongiform vacuoles) and multicentric plaque types. The 'florid' plaques, seen previously only in scrapie, are a consistent feature. There is also abundant pericellular PrP deposition in the cerebral and cerebellar cortex. A further unusual feature is extensive PrP deposition in the molecular layer of the cerebellum. Western blot analysis (molecular strain typing, see aetiology) of brain tissue demonstrates PrP^{Sc} type 4, which is pathognomonic of vCJD.

Some of the features of vCJD are reminiscent of kuru, in which behavioural changes and progressive ataxia predominate. In addition, peripheral sensory disturbances are well recognized in the kuru prodrome. Kuru plaques are seen in around 70 per cent of cases and are especially abundant in younger kuru cases. The observation that iatrogenic prion disease related to peripheral exposure to human prions has a more kuru-like than CJD-like clinical picture may well be relevant and would be consistent with a peripheral prion exposure.

The relatively stereotyped clinical presentation and neuropathology of vCJD contrasts sharply with sporadic CJD. This may be because vCJD is caused by a single prion strain and may also suggest that a relatively homogeneous genetically susceptible subgroup of the population with short incubation periods to BSE has been selected to date.

Secondary (iatrogenic) vCJD

The prominent lymphoreticular involvement raised early concerns that vCJD may be transmissible by blood transfusion. Indeed the tissue distribution is similar to that of ovine scrapie where prionaemia has been demonstrated experimentally. In 2004, two transfusion-associated cases of vCJD prion infection were reported amongst a small cohort of patients identified as having received blood from a donor who subsequently developed vCJD. One patient had a typical clinical course of vCJD although the diagnosis was not made until autopsy, and had the *PRNP* codon 129 MM genotype. The second, who died of an unrelated condition, was found to have prion infection at autopsy. This patient had the *PRNP* codon 129 MV genotype which is associated with relative resistance to prion disease. Subsequently two further patients have been diagnosed with vCJD during life from this group of 23 known surviving recipients of implicated blood. That 4/23 patients have been infected, three dying of vCJD, in each case following transfusion with a single unit of implicated red cells, suggests the risk to recipients of blood from a silently infected donor is very substantial. The incubation period in the clinical cases was 6–7 years. Since 2003, all known recipients of implicated blood have been notified of their status. Over 6000 individuals in the UK have been exposed to blood products prepared from large donor pools containing blood from a donor who went on to develop vCJD. None of these individuals, predominantly haemophiliacs, have yet developed vCJD.

Inherited prion diseases

Gerstmann–Sträussler–Scheinker disease

The first case was described by Gerstmann in 1928 and was followed by a more detailed report on seven other affected members of the same family in 1936. The classical presentation of GSS is with a chronic cerebellar ataxia accompanied by pyramidal features, with dementia occurring later in a much more prolonged clinical course than that seen in CJD. The mean duration is around 5 years, with onset usually in either the third or fourth decades. Histologically, the hallmark is the presence of multicentric amyloid plaques. Spongiform change, neuronal loss, astrocytosis, and white matter loss are also usually present. Numerous GSS kindreds from several countries (including the original Austrian family described by Gerstmann, Sträussler, and Scheinker in 1936) have now been demonstrated to have mutations in the PrP gene. GSS is an autosomal dominant disorder which can now be classified within the spectrum of inherited prion disease.

Inherited prion diseases

The identification of one of the pathogenic PrP gene mutations in a case with neurodegenerative disease allows not only molecular diagnosis of an inherited prion disease but also its subclassification according to mutation (see Fig. 4.1.4.1). Over 30 pathogenic mutations are reported in the human PrP gene and consist of two groups: (1) point mutations within the coding sequence resulting in amino acid substitutions in PrP or production of a stop codon resulting in expression of a truncated PrP; (2) insertions encoding additional integral copies of an octapeptide repeat present in a tandem array of five copies in the normal protein (octapeptide repeat insertion [OPRI]). A suggested notation for these diseases is 'Inherited prion disease (PrP mutation)', for instance: Inherited prion disease (PrP 6 OPRI) or Inherited prion disease (PrP P102L). Brief details of the more commonly seen types are given below, for a more comprehensive review see Ref.[47] *PRNP* analysis should be considered in all early-onset dementing or ataxic disorders and is available from the UK National Prion Clinic (see websites).

(a) PrP P102L

This mutation was first reported in 1989 in a UK and US family and has now been demonstrated in many other kindreds worldwide. Progressive ataxia is the dominant clinical feature, with dementia and pyramidal features. However, marked variability both at the clinical and neuropathological level is apparent in some families. A family with marked amyotrophic features has also been reported and cases with severe dementia in the absence of prominent ataxia are also recognized.

(b) PrP A117V

This mutation has been described in families from France, United States, and UK. The clinical features are pre-senile dementia associated with pyramidal signs, parkinsonism, pseudobulbar features, and cerebellar signs. Parkinsonian features may predominate in the early stages and mimic Parkinson's disease.

(c) PrP D178N

This mutation was originally described in two Finnish families with a CJD-like phenotype and has since been demonstrated in families in Hungary, the Netherlands, Canada, Finland, France, and the UK. This mutation was also reported in two unrelated families with fatal familial insomnia (FFI).[48] The first case described had a rapidly progressive disease characterized clinically by untreatable insomnia, dysautonomia and motor signs, and neuropathologically by selective atrophy of the anterior-ventral and medio-dorsal thalamic nuclei. Proteinase K treatment of extracted PrP^{Sc} from FFI cases has shown a different sized PrP band on Western blots than PrP^{Sc} from CJD cases suggesting that FFI may be caused by a distinct prion strain type. Goldfarb *et al.*[49] reported that in all the codon 178 families they studied with a CJD-like disease the codon 178 mutation was encoded on a valine 129 allele while all FFI kindreds encode the same codon 178 mutation on a methionine 129 allele. They suggested that the genotype at codon 129 determines phenotype. Insomnia is not uncommon in CJD patients and FFI and CJD may represent extremes of a spectrum of related disease phenotypes. An inherited case with the E200K

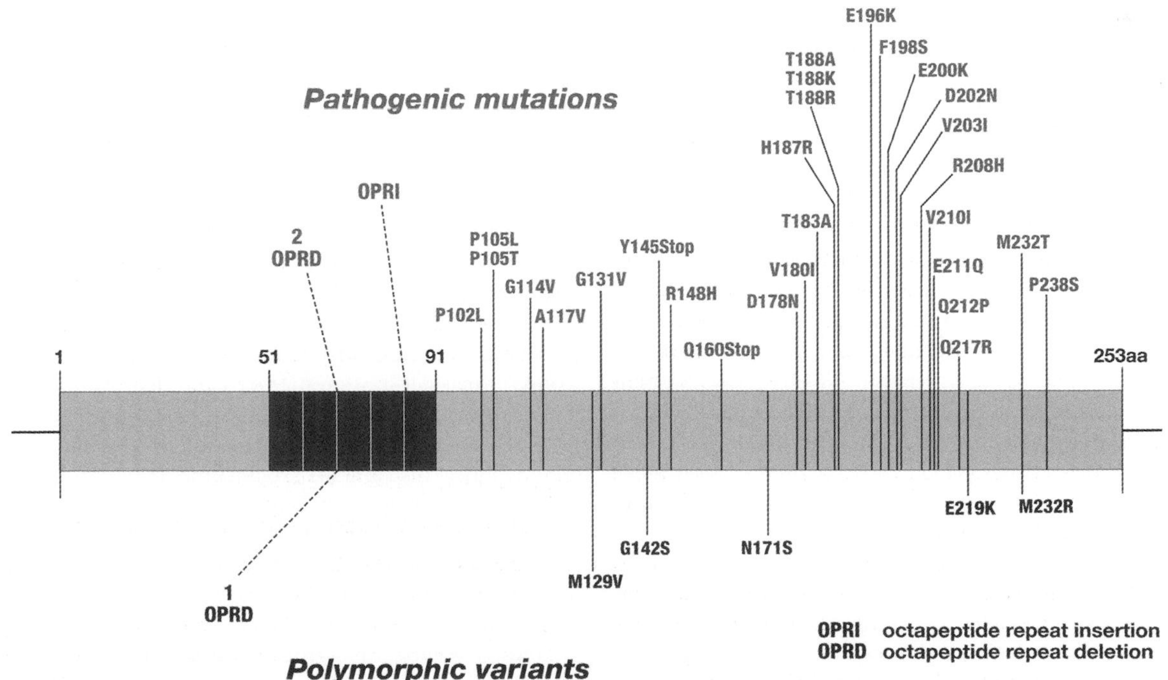

Fig. 4.1.4.1 Pathogenic mutations (above) and polymorphic variants of the human prion protein gene.

mutation, which is normally associated with a CJD-like phenotype, has been reported with an FFI phenotype. An Australian family has also been reported with the FFI genotype but in which affected family members have a range of phenotypes encompassing typical CJD, FFI, and an autosomal dominant cerebellar ataxia-like illness.

(d) PrP E200K

This mutation was first described in families with CJD. Affected individuals develop a rapidly progressive dementia with myoclonus and pyramidal, cerebellar or extrapyramidal signs, and a duration of illness usually less than 12 months. In marked contrast to other variants of inherited prion disease, the EEG usually shows the characteristic pseudoperiodic sharp wave activity seen in sporadic CJD. Interestingly, this mutation accounts for the three reported ethnogeographic clusters of CJD where the local incidence of CJD is around 100-fold higher than elsewhere (amongst Libyan Jews and in regions of Slovakia and Chile).[50,51] Now that cases can be diagnosed by PrP gene analysis, atypical forms of this condition are being detected with phenotypes other than that of classical CJD. Of interest also are reports that peripheral neuropathy can occur in this disease. Elderly unaffected carriers of the mutation have been reported. Patients with this condition have now been reported in several other countries outside the well-recognized clusters, including the UK. At least one of the UK cases does not appear to related to the ethnogeographic clusters mentioned above suggesting a separate UK focus for this type of inherited prion disease.

(e) PrP 6 OPRI

This was the first PrP mutation to be reported and was found in a small UK family with familial CJD[9] now known to form part of a the largest known kindred with an inherited prion disease caused by an OPRI mutation. The diagnosis in the family had been based on an individual who died in the 1940s with a rapidly progressive illness characteristic of CJD. The reported duration of illness was 6 months. Pathologically there was gross status spongiosis and astrocytosis affecting the entire cerebral cortex, and this case is used to illustrate classic CJD histology in Greenfield's *Neuropathology*. However, other family members had a much longer duration GSS-like illness. Histological features were also extremely variable. This observation led to screening of various case of neurodegenerative disease and to the identification of a case classified on clinical grounds as familial Alzheimer's disease.[52] More extensive screening work identified further families with the same mutation which were then demonstrated by genealogical studies to form part of an extremely large kindred.[53–55] Clinical information has been collected on over 80 affected individuals over seven generations. Affected individuals develop in the third to fourth decade onset of a progressive dementia associated with a varying combination of cerebellar ataxia and dysarthria, pyramidal signs, myoclonus and occasionally extrapyramidal signs, chorea and seizures. The dementia is often preceded by depression and aggressive behaviour. A number of cases have a long-standing personality disorder, characterized by aggression, irritability, antisocial and criminal activity, and hypersexuality, which may be present from early childhood, long before overt neurodegenerative disease develops. The histological features vary from those of classical spongiform encephalopathy (with or without PrP amyloid plaques) to cases lacking any specific features of these conditions.[56] Age at onset in this condition can be predicted according to genotype at polymorphic codon 129. Since this pathogenic insertional mutation occurs on a methionine 129 PrP allele, there are two possible codon 129 genotypes for affected individuals, methionine 129 homozygotes or methionine 129/valine 129 heterozygotes. Heterozygotes have an age at onset which is about a decade later than homozygotes.[53]

Pre-symptomatic and antenatal testing

Direct gene testing allows unequivocal diagnosis in patients with inherited forms of the disease and pre-symptomatic testing of unaffected but at-risk family members, as well as antenatal testing.[57] Because of the effect of *PRNP* codon 129 genotype on the age of onset of disease associated with some mutations it is possible to determine within a family whether a carrier of a mutation will have an early or late onset of disease. Most of the mutations appear to be fully penetrant, however experience with some is extremely limited. In some families, for example with E200K or D178N (fatal familial insomnia), there are examples of elderly unaffected gene carriers who appear to have escaped the disease. Genetic counselling is essential prior to pre-symptomatic testing and follows a protocol similar to that established for Huntington's disease. A positive PrP gene analysis has important consequences for other family members, and it is preferable to have discussed these issues with others in the immediate family before testing. Following the identification of a mutation the wider family should be referred for genetic counselling. It is vital to counsel both those testing positive for mutations and those untested but at-risk that they should not be blood or organ donors and should inform surgeons, including dentists, of their risk status prior to significant procedures as precautions may be necessary to minimize risk of iatrogenic transmission.

Prevention

While prion diseases can be transmitted to experimental animals by inoculation, it is important to appreciate that they are not contagious in humans. Documented case-to-case spread has only occurred by cannibalism (kuru) or following accidental inoculation with prions. Such iatrogenic routes include the use of inadequately sterilized intracerebral electrodes, dura mater, and corneal grafting, and from the use of human cadaveric pituitary-derived growth hormone or gonadotrophin. As discussed above, there is now evidence that vCJD prion infection is transmissible by blood transfusion. UK policy for some time has been to leucodeplete all whole blood and to source plasma for plasma products from outside the UK. A further possible route of transmission of vCJD is via contaminated surgical and medical instruments. Prions resist conventional sterilization methods and neurosurgical instruments are known to be able to act as a vector for prion transmission: several cases of iatrogenic transmission of sporadic CJD prions via neurosurgical instruments are documented.[58,59] Recent evidence suggests that classical CJD may also be transmitted by other surgical procedures.[60] The wider tissue distribution of prions in vCJD[42] together with the potential that significant numbers in the population may be silently infected has considerably increased these concerns.

Certain occupational groups are at risk of exposure to human prions, for instance neurosurgeons and other operating theatre staff, pathologists and morticians, histology technicians, as well as an increasing number of laboratory workers. Because of the prolonged incubation periods to prions following administration to sites other than the central nervous system (CNS), which is associated with clinically silent prion replication in the lymphoreticular tissue, treatments inhibiting prion replication in lymphoid organs may represent a viable strategy for rational secondary prophylaxis after accidental exposure. A preliminary suggested regimen is a short course of immunosuppression with oral corticosteroids in individuals with significant accidental exposure to human prions.(61)

Prognosis and treatment

All recognized prion diseases are invariably fatal following a progressive course.

The duration of illness in sporadic patients is very short with a mean duration of 3–4 months. However, in some of the inherited cases the duration can be 20 years or more. However, there have been significant recent advances in understanding prion propagation and neurotoxicity and clear proof of principle studies of several therapeutic or secondary prophylactic approaches in animal models suggesting effective therapeutics for human disease is realistic.(62)

A variety of drugs have been tried in individual or small numbers of patients over many years. There is no clear evidence of efficacy of any agent, and controlled clinical trials are needed. Such trials are highly challenging. Prion diseases are rare, often rapidly progressive and always fatal which may make randomization to placebo unacceptable. Patterns of disease overall extremely variable with clinical durations varying from weeks to more than 2 years in sporadic CJD, and more than 20 years in some inherited prion diseases. As 'first generation' treatments proposed for prion disease are likely, at best, to have only a modest effect on disease progression, even using survival duration as an outcome measure requires study of large numbers to reliably assess efficacy. There is a lack of systematic natural history studies of disease progression and an absence of biological markers of disease activity. In the United Kingdom, at the request of the Government's Chief Medical Officer, a clinical trial protocol (http://www.controlled-trials.com/ISRCTN06722585/prion1) and infrastructure has been developed to rigorously assess the drug quinacrine(63) and to provide a framework for assessment of novel therapeutics as these become available: the MRC PRION-1 trial. Importantly under these circumstances, a formal consultation with patient's representatives was organized to refine the protocol so that it would be acceptable to the majority of potential participants http://www.mrc.ac.uk/prn/pdf-cjd_workshop.pdf). Pentosan polyphosphate is another candidate anti-prion drug and has shown some efficacy in animal models. Unlike quinacrine, it does not enter the CNS readily and has been administered by intraventricular infusion in several patients. Major toxicity has been reported by this route in animal studies and such treatment was not supported by the UK's Committee of Safety on Medicines or CJD Therapy Advisory Group. A report summarizing clinical experience to date with this treatment has been produced (http://www.mrc.ac.uk/Utilities/Documentrecord/index.htm?d=MRC003453).

While the precise molecular events in prion propagation are not clear, it is clear that PrP^C is the essential substrate. Interference with PrP^C expression in adult brain is without serious effect and blocks onset of neurological disease in animal models.(61) It should be possible to identify small molecules, which penetrate the CNS to bind to PrP^C and to prevent its recruitment into prions, or to use one of a number of emerging technologies to reduce PrP^C expression in brain. If such methods are able to reduce prion propagation rates to below those of natural clearance mechanisms it ought to be possible to cure prion infection. New methods for early diagnosis—and their timely use—will be crucial, as such methods will not reverse neuronal cell loss which is appreciable or severe by the time clinical diagnosis is typically reached. Proof of principle studies in animal models suggest that humanized anti-PrP monoclonal antibodies could be used for passive immunization in the early pathogenesis to block neuroinvasion. This treatment could be considered for known iatrogenically infected individuals.(64)

Further information

UK National Prion Clinic, National Hospital for Neurology and Neurosurgery, London, http://www.nationalprionclinic.org

Medical Research Council Prion Unit, Institute of Neurology, London, http://www.prion.ucl.ac.uk/

UK CJD Surveillance Unit, Western General Hospital, Edinburgh, http://www.cjd.ed.ac.uk/

UK Department of Health, http://www.dh.gov.uk/PolicyAndGuidance/HealthAndSocialCareTopics/CJD/fs/en

CJD Support Network, http://www.cjdsupport.net/

References

1. Gajdusek, D.C., Gibbs, C.J. Jr, and Alpers, M.P. (1966). Experimental transmission of a kuru-likc syndrome to chimpanzees. *Nature*, **209**, 794–6.
2. Gibbs, C.J. Jr, Gajdusek, D.C., Asher, D.M., *et al.* (1968). Creutzfeldt-Jakob disease (spongiform encephalopathy): transmission to the chimpanzee. *Science*, **161**, 388–9.
3. Cuillé, J. and Chelle, P.L. (1936). La maladie dite tremblante du mouton est-elle inocuable? *C R Acad Sci*, **203**, 1552–4.
4. Hadlow, W.J. (1959). Scrapie and kuru. *Lancet*, **2**, 289–90.
5. Collinge, J., Whitfield, J., McKintosh, E., *et al.* (2006). Kuru in the 21st century—an acquired human prion disease with very long incubation periods. *Lancet*, **367**, 2068–74.
6. Griffith, J.S. (1967). Self replication and scrapie. *Nature*, **215**, 1043–4.
7. Prusiner, S.B. (1982). Novel proteinaceous infectious particles cause scrapie. *Science*, **216**, 136–44.
8. Jackson, G.S., Hosszu, L.L.P., Power, A., *et al.* (1999). Reversible conversion of monomeric human prion protein between native and fibrilogenic conformations. *Science*, **283**, 1935–7.
9. Owen, F., Poulter, M., Lofthouse, R., *et al.* (1989). Insertion in prion protein gene in familial Creutzfeldt-Jakob disease. *Lancet*, **1**, 51–2.
10. Hsiao, K., Baker, H.F., Crow, T.J., *et al.* (1989). Linkage of a prion protein missense variant to Gerstmann–Straussler syndrome. *Nature*, **338**, 342–5.
11. Collinge, J., Palmer, M.S., and Dryden, A.J. (1991). Genetic predisposition to iatrogenic Creutzfeldt-Jakob disease. *Lancet*, **337**, 1441–2.
12. Palmer, M.S., Dryden, A.J., Hughes, J.T., *et al.* (1991). Homozygous prion protein genotype predisposes to sporadic Creutzfeldt-Jakob disease. *Nature*, **352**, 340–2.
13. Brown, P., Cathala, F., Raubertas, R.F., *et al.* (1987). The epidemiology of Creutzfeldt-Jakob disease: conclusion of a 15-year investigation in France and review of the world literature. *Neurology*, **37**, 895–904.
14. Collinge, J., Sidle, K.C.L., Meads, J., *et al.* (1996). Molecular analysis of prion strain variation and the aetiology of 'new variant' CJD. *Nature*, **383**, 685–90.

15. Hill, A.F., Joiner, S., Wadsworth, J.D., *et al.* (2003). Molecular classification of sporadic Creutzfeldt-Jakob disease. *Brain*, **126**(Pt 6), 1333–46.
16. Hill, A.F., Desbruslais, M., Joiner, S., *et al.* (1997). The same prion strain causes vCJD and BSE. *Nature*, **389**, 448–50.
17. Bruce, M.E., Will, R.G., Ironside, J.W., *et al.* (1997). Transmissions to mice indicate that 'new variant' CJD is caused by the BSE agent. *Nature*, **389**, 498–501.
18. Parchi, P., Giese, A., Capellari, S., *et al.* (1999). Classification of sporadic Creutzfeldt-Jakob disease based on molecular and phenotypic analysis of 300 subjects. *Annals of Neurology*, **46**, 224–33.
19. Prusiner, S.B., Scott, M., Foster, D., *et al.* (1990). Transgenetic studies implicate interactions between homologous PrP isoforms in scrapie prion replication. *Cell*, **63**, 673–86.
20. Bruce, M., Chree, A., McConnell, I., *et al.* (1994). Transmission of bovine spongiform encephalopathy and scrapie to mice: strain variation and the species barrier. *Philosophical Transactions of the Royal Society of London. Series B, Biological Sciences*, **343**, 405–11.
21. Collinge, J. (1999). Variant Creutzfeldt-Jakob disease. *Lancet*, **354**, 317–23.
22. Hill, A.F., Joiner, S., Linehan, J., *et al.* (2000). Species barrier independent prion replication in apparently resistant species. *Proceedings of the National Academy of Sciences of the United States of America*, **97**, 10248–53.
23. Hill, A.F. and Collinge, J. (2003). Subclinical prion infection. *Trends in Microbiology*, **11**, 578–84.
24. Collinge, J. (2001). Prion diseases of humans and animals: their causes and molecular basis. *Annual Review of Neuroscience*, **24**, 519–50.
25. Collinge, J., Palmer, M.S., Sidle, K.C.L., *et al.* (1995). Unaltered susceptibility to BSE in transgenic mice expressing human prion protein. *Nature*, **378**, 779–83.
26. Asante, E.A., Linehan, J.M., Desbruslais, M., *et al.* (2002). BSE prions propagate as either variant CJD-like or sporadic CJD-like prion strains in transgenic mice expressing human prion protein. *The EMBO Journal*, **21**, 6358–66.
27. Wadsworth, J.D., Asante, E.A., Desbruslais, M., *et al.* (2004). Human prion protein with valine 129 prevents expression of variant CJD phenotype. *Science*, **306**, 1793–6.
28. Asante, E.A., Linehan, J.M., Gowland, I., *et al.* (2006). Dissociation of pathological and molecular phenotype of variant Creutzfeldt-Jakob disease in transgenic human prion protein 129 heterozygous mice. *Proceedings of the National Academy of Sciences of the United States of America*, **103**, 10759–64.
29. Collinge, J. (1996). New diagnostic tests for prion diseases. *The New England Journal of Medicine*, **335**, 963–5.
30. Otto, M., Stein, H., Szudra, A., *et al.* (1997). S-100 protein concentration in the cerebrospinal fluid of patients with Creutzfeldt-Jakob disease. *Journal of Neurology*, **244**, 566–70.
31. Zerr, I., Bodemer, M., Räcker, S., *et al.* (1995). Cerebrospinal fluid concentration of neuron-specific enolase in diagnosis of Creutzfeldt-Jakob disease. *Lancet*, **345**, 1609–10.
32. Macfarlane, R.G., Wroe, S.J., Collinge, J., *et al.* (2006). A review of the neuroimaging findings in human prion disease. *Journal of Neurology, Neurosurgery, and Psychiatry*.
33. Alpers, M.P. (1987). Epidemiology and clinical aspects of kuru. In *Prions: novel infectious pathogens causing scrapie and Creutzfeldt-Jakob disease* (eds. S.B. Prusiner and M.P. McKinley), pp. 451–65. Academic Press, San Diego.
34. Esmonde, T.F., Will, R.G., Slattery, J.M., *et al.* (1993). Creutzfeldt-Jakob disease and blood transfusion. *Lancet*, **341**, 205–7.
35. Britton, T.C., Al-Sarraj, S., Shaw, C., *et al.* (1995). Sporadic Creutzfeldt-Jakob disease in a 16-year-old in the UK. *Lancet*, **346**, 1155.
36. Collie, D.A., Summers, D.M., Sellar, R.J., *et al.* (2003). Diagnosing variant Creutzfeldt-Jakob disease with the pulvinar sign: MR imaging findings in 86 neuropathologically confirmed cases. *AJNR. American Journal of Neuroradiology*, **24**, 1560–9.
37. Chazot, G., Broussolle, E., Lapras, C.I., *et al.* (1996). New variant of Creutzfeldt-Jakob disease in a 26-year-old French man. *Lancet*, **347**, 1181.
38. Zeidler, M., Sellar, R.J., Collie, D.A., *et al.* (2000). The pulvinar sign on magnetic resonance imaging in variant Creutzfeldt-Jakob disease. *Lancet*, **355**, 1412–8.
39. Siddique, D., Kennedy, A., Thomas, D., *et al.* (2005). Tonsil biopsy in the investigation of suspected variant Creutzfeldt-Jakob disease—a cohort study of 50 pts. *Journal of the Neurological Sciences*, **238**(Suppl. 1), S1–570.
40. Hill, A.F., Zeidler, M., Ironside, J., *et al.* (1997). Diagnosis of new variant Creutzfeldt-Jakob disease by tonsil biopsy. *Lancet*, **349**, 99–100.
41. Hill, A.F., Butterworth, R.J., Joiner, S., *et al.* (1999). Investigation of variant Creutzfeldt-Jakob disease and other human prion diseases with tonsil biopsy samples. *Lancet*, **353**, 183–9.
42. Wadsworth, J.D.F., Joiner, S., Hill, A.F., *et al.* (2001). Tissue distribution of protease resistant prion protein in variant CJD using a highly sensitive immuno-blotting assay. *Lancet*, **358**, 171–80.
43. Hilton, D.A., Sutak, J., Smith, M.E., *et al.* (2004). Specificity of lymphoreticular accumulation of prion protein for variant Creutzfeldt-Jakob disease. *Journal of Clinical Pathology*, **57**, 300–2.
44. Hilton, D.A., Fathers, E., Edwards, P., *et al.* (1998). Prion immunoreactivity in appendix before clinical onset of variant Creutzfeldt-Jakob disease. *Lancet*, **352**, 703–4.
45. Hilton, D.A., Ghani, A.C., Conyers, L., *et al.* (2004). Prevalence of lymphoreticular prion protein accumulation in UK tissue samples. *The Journal of Pathology*, **203**, 733–9.
46. Collinge, J. (2005). Molecular neurology of prion disease. *Journal of Neurology, Neurosurgery, and Psychiatry*, **76**, 906–19.
47. Collinge, J. (2005). Creutzfeldt-Jakob disease and other prion diseases. In *Dementia* (ed. J.T. O'Brien), pp. 763–76.
48. Medori, R., Montagna, P., Tritschler, H.J., *et al.* (1992). Fatal familial insomnia: a second kindred with mutation of prion protein gene at codon 178. *Neurology*, **42**, 669–70.
49. Goldfarb, L.G., Petersen, R.B., Tabaton, M., *et al.* (1992). Fatal familial insomnia and familial Creutzfeldt-Jakob disease: disease phenotype determined by a DNA polymorphism. *Science*, **258**, 806–8.
50. Goldfarb, L.G., Korczyn, A.D., Brown, P., *et al.* (1990). Mutation in codon 200 of scrapie amyloid precursor gene linked to Creutzfeldt-Jakob disease in Sephardic Jews of Libyan and non-Libyan origin. *Lancet*, **336**, 637–8.
51. Brown, P., Galvez, S., Goldfarb, L.G., *et al.* (1992). Familial Creutzfeldt-Jakob disease in Chile is associated with the codon 200 mutation of the PRNP amyloid precursor gene on chromosome 20. *Journal of Neurological Sciences*, **112**, 65–7.
52. Collinge, J., Harding, A.E., Owen, F., *et al.* (1989). Diagnosis of Gerstmann-Straussler syndrome in familial dementia with prion protein gene analysis. *Lancet*, **2**, 15–17.
53. Poulter, M., Baker, H.F., Frith, C.D., *et al.* (1992). Inherited prion disease with 144 base pair gene insertion. I. Genealogical and molecular studies. *Brain*, **115**, 675–85.
54. Mead, S., Poulter, M., Beck, J., *et al.* (2006). Inherited prion disease with six octapeptide repeat insertional mutation—molecular analysis of phenotypic heterogeneity. *Brain*, **129**(Pt 9), 2297–317.
55. Collinge, J., Brown, J., Hardy, J., *et al.* (1992). Inherited prion disease with 144 base pair gene insertion. II. Clinical and pathological features. *Brain*, **115**, 687–710.
56. Collinge, J., Owen, F., Poulter, M., *et al.* (1990). Prion dementia without characteristic pathology. *Lancet*, **336**, 7–9.
57. Collinge, J., Poulter, M., Davis, M.B., *et al.* (1991). Presymptomatic detection or exclusion of prion protein gene defects in families with inherited prion diseases. *American Journal of Human Genetics*, **49**, 1351–4.

58. Bernoulli, C., Siegfried, J., Baumgartner, G., *et al.* (1977). Danger of accidental person-to-person transmission of Creutzfeldt-Jakob disease by surgery [letter]. *Lancet*, **1**, 478–9.
59. Blattler, T. (2002). Implications of prion diseases for neurosurgery. *Neurosurgical Review*, **25**, 195–203.
60. Collins, S., Law, M.G., Fletcher, A., *et al.* (1999). Surgical treatment and risk of sporadic Creutzfeldt-Jakob disease: a case-control study. *Lancet*, **353**, 693–7.
61. Aguzzi, A., and Collinge, J. (1997). Post-exposure prophylaxis after accidental prion inoculation. *Lancet*, **350**, 1519–20.
62. Mallucci, G. and Collinge, J. (2005). Rational targeting for prion therapeutics. *Nature Reviews. Neuroscience*, **6**, 23–34.
63. Korth, C., May, B.C., Cohen, F.E., *et al.* (2001). Acridine and phenothiazine derivatives as pharmacotherapeutics for prion disease. *Proceedings of the National Academy of Sciences of the United States of America*, **98**, 9836–41.
64. Wroe, S., Pal, S., Siddique, D., *et al.* (2006). Clinical presentation and pre-mortem diagnosis of variant Creutzfeldt-Jakob disease associated with blood transfusion: a case report. *Lancet*, **368**, 2061–7.

4.1.5 Dementia with Lewy bodies

I. G. McKeith

Introduction

Lewy bodies are spherical neuronal inclusions, first described by the German neuropathologist Friederich Lewy while working in Alzheimer's laboratory in Munich in 1912. In 1961, Okazaki published case reports about two elderly men who presented with dementia and died shortly after with severe extrapyramidal rigidity. Autopsy showed Lewy bodies in their cerebral cortex.[1] Over the next 20 years, 34 similar cases were reported, all by Japanese workers. Lewy body disease was thus considered to be a rare cause of dementia, until a series of studies in Europe and North America, in the late 1980s, identified Lewy bodies in the brains of between 15 and 20 per cent of elderly demented cases reaching autopsy.[2,3] Dementia with Lewy bodies (DLB) is unlikely to be a newly occurring disorder, since re-examination of autopsy material collected from elderly demented patients in Newcastle during the 1960s, reveals cortical Lewy bodies in 17 per cent of cases. The recent recognition of DLB as the second most common form of degenerative dementia in old age is largely due to the widespread use of improved neuropathological techniques, initially antiubiquitin immunocytochemistry, and more recently specific staining for alpha-synuclein which is a core constituent of Lewy bodies and related lesions.

The spectrum of Lewy body disease

The presence of Lewy bodies probably indicates neuronal dysfunction which is usually indicative of neurological disease. The clinical presentation varies according to the site of Lewy body formation and associated neuronal loss. Three main clinicopathological syndromes have been described.

- Parkinson's disease, an extrapyramidal movement disorder—associated with degeneration of subcortical neurones, particularly in substantia nigra.
- Dementia with Lewy bodies, a dementing disorder with prominent neuropsychiatric features—associated with degeneration of cortical neurones, particularly in frontal, anterior cingulate, insular, and temporal regions.
- Autonomic failure with syncope and orthostatic hypotension—associated with degeneration of sympathetic neurones in spinal cord.

In clinical practice, elderly patients often have heterogenous combinations of parkinsonism, dementia, and autonomic failure, reflecting pathological involvement at multiple locations.

Clinical features

Dementia is usually, but not always, the presenting feature of DLB. A minority of patients present with parkinsonism alone, some with psychiatric disorder in the absence of dementia, and others with orthostatic hypotension, falls, or transient disturbances of consciousness. Episodes of confusion, progressive cognitive decline, and dementia follow in due course. Fluctuation in cognitive performance and functional abilities, which is based in variations in attention and level of consciousness, is the most characteristic feature of DLB and the one which causes greatest diagnostic difficulties. It is usually evident on a day-to-day basis, and often apparent within much shorter periods. The marked amplitude between best and worst performance distinguishes it from the minor day-to-day variations that commonly occur in dementia of any aetiology. Transient disturbances of consciousness, in which patients are found mute and unresponsive for periods of several minutes, may represent the extreme of fluctuation in attention and arousal and are often mistaken for transient ischaemic attacks despite a lack of focal neurological signs. Repeated visual hallucinations are present in about two-thirds of patients. They take the form of vivid, colourful, and sometimes fragmented figures of people and animals, which are usually described in great detail. Emotional responses vary from intense fear to indifference or even amusement. Although patients may respond to their hallucinations, for example, trying to feed an imaginary dog, they later often have good insight into their unreality. Others develop elaborate systematized delusions, usually persecutory or of a phantom boarder. Auditory hallucinations are much less frequent, and only a minority of patients have olfactory or tactile experiences. Depressive symptoms are common and about 40 per cent of patients will have a major depressive episode, similar to the rate in Parkinson's disease and significantly greater than in Alzheimer's disease (AD). The frequency and severity of spontaneous motor features of parkinsonism varies from one clinical setting to another due to referral biases. Postural instability and gait difficulty are the most common manifestations, tremor dominant symptoms occurring in only 20 per cent or less.[4] Less than half of DLB cases have parkinsonism at presentation and a quarter continue to have no evidence at any point in their illness. Clinicians must therefore be prepared to make the diagnosis of DLB in the absence of extrapyramidal motor features. If they do not, their case detection rates will be unacceptably low. Severe neuroleptic sensitivity reactions can precipitate irreversible parkinsonism, further impair consciousness level, and induce autonomic disturbances reminiscent of neuroleptic malignant syndrome. They occur in 40 to 50 per cent of neuroleptic-treated DLB cases and are associated with a two- to threefold increased mortality.[5] Acute D_2 receptor blockade is thought to mediate these effects; and, despite initial reports, atypical antipsychotics seem to be as likely to cause neuroleptic sensitivity reactions as older drugs.[6] Sleep disorders have more recently been recognized as common in DLB with daytime somnolence and rapid eye movement sleep behaviour disorder as prodromal features.[7] Recurrent falls and syncope occur in up to a third of DLB cases, reflecting autonomic nervous system involvement which may also be evident as early urinary incontinence, constipation, and sexual dysfunction.

Pathological classification

Lewy bodies are composed of intermediate neurofilament proteins, which are abnormally truncated and phosphorylated. Their presence indicates that a neurone is attempting to eliminate damaged proteins from its cytoplasm, a process which is usually followed by cell death. Ubiquitin, α-synuclein, α- and β-crystalin, and associated enzymes are the main chemical constituents. Subcortical Lewy bodies have a dense hyaline core surrounded by a halo of radiating filaments, and are easily seen with conventional histopathological techniques. Cortical Lewy bodies are more easily visualized using antiubiquitin staining but this lacks specificity and immunohistochemical staining for alpha-synuclein, is now the most sensitive and specific method currently available for detecting Lewy bodies and Lewy-related pathology. Current thinking is that Lewy bodies form within neurones as a cytoprotective response in an attempt to sequester toxic alpha-synuclein oligomers. Widely distributed aggregates of alpha-synuclein (Lewy neurites) probably represent an earlier stage in the neurodegenerative process than Lewy body formation itself. Lewy neurites are seen in the substantia nigra, hippocampal region CA2/3, dorsal vagal nucleus, basal nucleus of Meynert, and transentorhinal cortex. Ubiquitin immunocytochemistry and α-synuclein-specific monoclonal antibody stains are beginning to reveal the extensive nature of these neuritic changes, which are probably more relevant for symptom formation than the relatively sparsely distributed Lewy bodies. The presence of Lewy neurites in presynaptic terminals is thought to have a particularly severe impact on synaptic function.[8]

Recommendations have been made[9] about which brain regions to examine for the presence of Lewy bodies and Lewy neurites and a simple semi-quantitative scoring system devised. These scores are added to generate three pathological categories:

1 Brainstem-predominant DLB: predilection sites are substantia nigra, locus coeruleus, and dorsal nucleus of vagus.

2 Limbic (or transitional) DLB: predilection sites are anterior cingulate and transtentorhinal cortex.

3 Neocortical DLB: predilection sites are frontal, temporal, and parietal cortex.

Of DLB cases presenting via psychiatric clinics, 69 per cent have extensive neocortical Lewy body pathology,[10] but this is not essential for the development of dementia or other psychiatric symptoms, both of which may occur in the presence of disease limited to limbic structures (24 per cent of cases) or the brainstem (7 per cent).

Interpretation of the significance of coexistent Alzheimer-type pathology is a major issue in the pathological assessment of DLB cases. High senile plaque counts are found in 80 to 90 per cent of DLB cases, diffuse and neuritic β-amyloid plaques occurring in similar proportions as in pure AD. Significant tau pathology is absent, however, in 80 to 90 per cent whether measured biochemically or by counting neocortical neurofibrillary tangles. Most DLB cases are therefore classified as 'the Lewy body variant of AD'[2] if AD is defined by increased plaque density. Conversely, if AD is defined by frequent neocortical neurofibrillary tangles, equivalent to Braak stages 5 and 6, then 85 to 90 per cent of DLB cases will not fulfil such criteria.[11] (The pathological classification of AD is also discussed in Chapter 4.1.2.) The most recent revision of pathological diagnostic criteria for DLB suggests that both Lewy and Alzheimer pathologies should be fully reported. A probability matrix (see Table 4.1.5.1) is then used to predict the likelihood of the patient having presented with a DLB clinical syndrome, this being directly related to the severity of Lewy-related pathology, and inversely related to the severity of concurrent AD-type pathology.[9] Minor vascular pathology is additionally present in 30 per cent of DLB cases[10] and this is also likely to impact upon the clinical manifestations.

Table 4.1.5.1 Pathological criteria for DLB taking into account the relative contributions of Lewy body and Alzheimer type pathology as predictors of a probable DLB clinical presentation–high, intermediate, or low probability.

		Alzheimer type pathology		
		NIA–Reagan Low (Braak stage 0-II)	**NIA–Reagan Intermediate (Braak stage III-IV)**	**NIA–Reagan High (Braak stage V-VI)**
Lewy Body type pathology	**Brainstem-predominant**	Low	Low	Low
	Limbic (transitional)	High	Intermediate	Low
	Diffuse neocortical	High	High	Intermediate

The relationship between DLB and Parkinson's disease dementia

There has been extended debate about the classification of patients who present with motor symptoms of Parkinson's disease and later develop the typical features of DLB, sometimes after many years of severe motor disability. This is a common outcome reported in up to 78 per cent of PD patients followed over an 8-year period. No major differences between DLB and Parkinson's disease dementia have been found in any variable examined including cognitive profile, neuropsychiatric features, sleep disorders, autonomic dysfunction, type and severity of parkinsonism, neuroleptic sensitivity, and responsiveness to cholinesterase inhibitors. It has been suggested that DLB should be diagnosed when dementia occurs before or concurrently with parkinsonism and Parkinson's disease dementia should be used to describe dementia that occurs in the context of well-established Parkinson's disease.[9,12] This distinction between DLB and Parkinson's disease dementia has two distinct clinical phenotypes, based solely on the temporal sequence of appearance of symptoms that has been criticized by those who regard the different clinical presentations as simply representing different points on a common spectrum of LB disease, itself underpinned by abnormalities in alpha-synuclein metabolism.

The neurobiological basis of dementia in Parkinson's disease is discussed in detail in Chapter 4.1.6.

Clinical diagnosis of DLB

Patients with DLB may present to psychiatric services (cognitive impairment, psychosis, or behavioural disturbance), internal medicine (acute confusional states or syncope), or neurology (movement disorder or disturbed consciousness). The details of clinical assessment and differential diagnoses will, to a large extent, be shaped by these symptom and specialty biases. In all cases, a detailed history from the patient and reliable informants should document the time of onset of relevant key symptoms, the nature of their progression, and their effects on social, occupational, and personal function.

The recent consensus criteria for the clinical diagnosis of DLB are shown in Table 4.1.5.2. Particular emphasis needs to be given to recognizing the characteristic dementia syndrome. Attentional deficits and prominent frontosubcortical and visuo-perceptual dysfunction are the main features—symptoms of persistent or prominent memory impairment are not always present early in the course of illness, although they are likely to develop in most patients with disease progression. Patients with DLB perform better than Alzheimer's disease on tests of verbal recall, but relatively worse on tests of copying and drawing. With the progression of dementia, the selective pattern of cognitive deficits may be lost, making differential diagnosis based on clinical examination difficult during the later stages.

It is the evaluation of fluctuation which causes greatest difficulty in clinical practice.[13] Questions such as, 'are there episodes when his/her thinking seems quite clear and then becomes muddled?' were previously suggested as useful probes, but two recent studies found 75 per cent of both AD and DLB carers to respond positively.[14,15] More detailed questioning and qualitative analysis of carers' replies is therefore needed. The Clinician Assessment of Fluctuation Scale[16] requires an experienced clinician to judge the severity and frequency of 'fluctuating confusion' or 'impaired consciousness' over the previous month. The semi-structured One Day Fluctuation Assessment Scale[16] can be administered by less experienced raters and generates a cut-off score to distinguish DLB from AD or VaD. The Mayo Fluctuations Composite Scale[15] requires three or more 'yes' responses from caregivers to structured questions about the presence of daytime drowsiness and lethargy, daytime sleep >2 h, staring into space for long periods or episodes of disorganized speech, as suggestive of DLB rather than AD. Recording variations in attentional performance using a computer-based test system offers an independent method of measuring fluctuation, which is also sensitive to drug treatment effects.[17] The assessment of extrapyramidal motor features may be complicated by the presence of cognitive impairment. A simple, five-item subscale of the Unified PD Rating Scale[18] contains only those items that can reliably be assessed in DLB independent of severity of dementia (tremor at rest, action tremor, body bradykinesia, facial expression, rigidity). Standardized methods of assessing visual hallucinations and other visual pathologies in DLB are under development.[19]

(a) Consensus criteria for DLB

Probable DLB can be diagnosed (Table 4.1.5.2) if any two of the three core features (fluctuation, visual hallucinations, spontaneous

Table 4.1.5.2 Consensus criteria for the clinical diagnosis of probable and possible dementia with Lewy bodies (DLB) (Reproduced from McKeith I., Dickson, D., Emre, M., *et al.* Dementia with Lewy bodies, 3rd report of the dementia consortium, *Neurology*, **65**, 1863–72, copyright 2005, AAN Enterprises, Inc.)

1	**Central feature** (*essential for a diagnosis of possible or probable DLB*) Dementia defined as progressive cognitive decline of sufficient magnitude to interfere with normal social or occupational function. Prominent or persistent memory impairment may not necessarily occur in the early stages but is usually evident with progression. Deficits on tests of attention, executive function and visuo-spatial ability may be especially prominent.
2	**Core features** (*two core features are sufficient for a diagnosis of probable DLB, one for possible DLB*) Fluctuating cognition with pronounced variations in attention and alertness Recurrent visual hallucinations that are typically well formed and detailed Spontaneous features of parkinsonism
3	**Suggestive features** (*if one or more of these is present in the presence of one or more core features, a diagnosis of probable DLB can be made. In the absence of any core features, one or more suggestive features is sufficient for possible DLB. Probable DLB should not be diagnosed on the basis of suggestive features alone*) REM sleep behaviour disorder Severe neuroleptic sensitivity Low dopamine transporter uptake in basal ganglia demonstrated by SPECT or PET imaging
4	**Supportive features** (*commonly present but not proven to have diagnostic specificity*) Repeated falls and syncope Transient, unexplained loss of consciousness Severe autonomic dysfunction e.g. orthostatic hypotension, urinary incontinence Hallucinations in other modalities Systematized delusions Depression Relative preservation of medial temporal lobe structures on CT/MRI scan Generalised low uptake on SPECT/PET perfusion scan with reduced occipital activity Abnormal (low uptake) MIBG myocardial scintigraphy Prominent slow wave activity on EEG with temporal lobe transient sharp waves
5	**A diagnosis of DLB is less likely** In the presence of cerebrovascular disease evident as focal neurological signs or on brain imaging In the presence of any other physical illness or brain disorder sufficient to account in part or in total for the clinical picture If parkinsonism only appears for the first time at a stage of severe dementia
6	**Temporal sequence of symptoms** DLB should be diagnosed when dementia occurs before or concurrently with parkinsonism (if it is present). The term Parkinson's disease dementia (PDD) should be used to describe dementia that occurs in the context of well-established Parkinson's disease. In a practice setting the term that is most appropriate to the clinical situation should be used and generic terms such as LB disease are often helpful. In research studies in which distinction needs to be made between DLB and PDD, the existing one-year rule between the onset of dementia and parkinsonism DLB continues to be recommended. Adoption of other time periods will simply confound data pooling or comparison between studies. In other research settings that may include clinico-pathologic studies and clinical trials, both clinical phenotypes may be considered collectively under categories such as LB disease or alpha-synucleinopathy.

motor features of parkinsonism) are present. Probable DLB can also be diagnosed if one core feature is accompanied by one or more suggestive features (REM sleep behaviour disorder, severe neuroleptic sensitivity, low dopamine transporter uptake in basal ganglia demonstrated by SPECT or PET imaging). Possible DLB can be diagnosed if there is one core feature alone or one or more suggestive features in the absence of any core features. Suggestive features are not in the light of current knowledge considered sufficient, even in combination, to warrant a diagnosis of probable DLB in the absence of any core feature.

Differential diagnosis

There are four main categories of disorder that should be considered in the differential diagnosis of DLB (Table 4.1.5.3).

(a) Other causes of dementia

Of autopsy-confirmed DLB cases, 65 per cent meet the NINCDS-ADRDA clinical criteria for probable or possible AD,[20] and this is the most frequent clinical misdiagnosis of DLB patients presenting with a primary dementia syndrome. This suggests DLB should routinely be excluded when making the diagnosis of AD. Up to one-third of DLB cases are additionally misclassified as vascular dementia by virtue of items such as the fluctuating nature and course of illness. Pyramidal and focal neurological signs are, however, usually absent. The development of myoclonus in patients with a rapidly progressive form of DLB may lead the clinician to suspect Creutzfeldt–Jakob disease.

(b) Other causes of delirium

In patients with intermittent delirium, appropriate examination and laboratory tests should be performed during the acute phase to maximize the chances of detecting infective, metabolic, inflammatory, or other aetiological factors. Pharmacological causes are particularly common in elderly patients. Although the presence of any of these features makes a diagnosis of DLB less likely, comorbidity is not unusual in elderly patients and the diagnosis should not be excluded simply on this basis.

Table 4.1.5.3 Conditions to be considered in the differential diagnosis of dementia with Lewy bodies

Other causes of dementia
Alzheimer's disease
Vascular dementia
Creutzfeldt–Jakob disease
Other causes of delirium
Infective/pharmacological/metabolic/inflammatory
Other neurological syndromes
Parkinson's disease
Progressive supranuclear palsy (Steele–Richardson–Olszewski syndrome)
Multisystem atrophy
Corticobasal degeneration
Rapid eye movement sleep behaviour disorder (RBD)
Recurrent syncope/unexplained falls
Transient disturbances of consciousness
Comlex partial seizures
Late-onset psychiatric disorders
Delusional disorder (late paraphrenia/late-onset schizophrenia)
Depressive psychosis

(c) Other neurological syndromes

In patients with a prior diagnosis of Parkinson's disease, the onset of visual hallucinations and fluctuating cognitive impairment may be attributed to side-effects of antiparkinsonian medications, and this must be tested by dose reduction or withdrawal. Other atypical parkinsonian syndromes associated with poor levodopa response, cognitive impairment, and postural instability include progressive supranuclear palsy and multi-system atrophy. Syncopal episodes in DLB are often incorrectly attributed to transient ischaemic attacks, despite an absence of focal neurological signs. Recurrent disturbances in consciousness accompanied by complex visual hallucinations may suggest complex partial seizures (temporal lobe epilepsy), and vivid dreaming with violent movements during sleep may meet criteria for REM sleep behaviour disorder. Both these conditions have been reported as uncommon presenting symptoms of autopsy-confirmed DLB.[21,22]

(d) Late-onset functional psychiatric disorder

DLB should be considered if a patient spontaneously develops parkinsonian features or cognitive decline (or shows excessive sensitivity to neuroleptic medication) in the course of late-onset delusional disorder, depressive psychosis, or mania.[21]

Laboratory investigations including neuroimaging

Systemic and pharmacological causes of delirium need to be excluded. The standard EEG may show early slowing, epoch by epoch fluctuation, and transient temporal slow wave activity.[23] There are as yet no clinically applicable genotypic or CSF markers to support a DLB diagnosis.[24] There are, however, sufficient studies to conclude that neuroimaging investigations may be helpful in supporting the clinical diagnosis. Changes associated with DLB include preservation of hippocampal and medial temporal lobe volume on MRI[25,26] and occipital hypo-perfusion on SPECT.[27] Other features such as generalized atrophy, white matter changes,[28] and rates of progression of whole brain atrophy[29] appear to be unhelpful in differential diagnosis. Dopamine transporter loss in the caudate and putamen, a marker of nigro-striatal degeneration can be detected by pre-synaptic dopaminergic SPECT. Preliminary studies suggesting high specificity and sensitivity for predicting clinical[30] and pathological diagnoses of DLB have been confirmed in a large multi-centre trial which found 78 per cent sensitivity and 90 per cent specificity for identifying probable DLB versus non-DLB dementia.[31] Diagnostic sensitivity based upon the presence of the three core clinical features alone has been estimated at below 50 per cent and specificity at >90 per cent which suggests that dopaminergic imaging is most useful when significant clinical diagnostic uncertainty exists.

Epidemiology

In population-based clinical studies, prevalences of around 0.7 per cent for DLB in the 65+ age group have been reported suggesting that it could account for up to 10 per cent of all dementia cases, a figure consistent with DLB rates of 10–15 per cent from hospital-based autopsy series. A recent community study of 85+ year olds found 5.0 per cent to meet consensus criteria for DLB (3.3 per cent probable, 1.7 per cent possible) representing 22 per cent of all demented cases,[32] similar to other clinical estimates and consistent with estimates of Lewy body prevalence in a dementia case register followed to autopsy.[33] One population-based, autopsy study found Lewy bodies to be evenly distributed between the demented and the non-demented, and this may be interpreted as evidence of a substantial pool of pre-clinical cases.[34] Classical epidemiological studies to determine age and sex variation and potential risk factors for DLB have not yet been reported.

Genetics

It is clear from several case studies that familial cases of DLB occur[35,36] and that Lewy bodies are commonly seen in familial cases of Alzheimer's disease.[37] There are recent reports that triplication of the alpha-synuclein gene (SNCA) can cause DLB, Parkinson's disease, and Parkinson's disease dementia whereas gene duplication is associated only with motor Parkinson's disease suggesting a gene dose effect.[38] However, SCNA multiplication is not found in most Lewy body disease patients.

Course and prognosis

Rate of cognitive decline in DLB is generally reported as similar to Alzheimer's disease[39] and survival from onset to death is reduced with self-reports of depression and the presence of extrapyramidal signs as important adverse predictors.[40] The end stage is typically one of profound dementia and parkinsonism. Even in the early stages, personal and social function and performance in daily living skills may be markedly impaired by a combination of cognitive, psychiatric, and neurological disability to a degree significantly greater than in patients with Alzheimer's disease and comparable mental test scores.[41] Psychotic symptoms, particularly visual hallucinations, tend to be very persistent throughout the whole course of illness. There have been three overlapping stages of the illness described.[21]

The first stage is often recognized only in retrospect, and may extend back 1 to 3 years' prepresentation with occasional minor episodes of forgetfulness, sometimes described as lapses of concentration or 'switching off'. A brief period of delirium is sometimes noted for the first time, often associated with genuine physical illness and/or surgical procedures. Disturbed sleep, nightmares, and daytime drowsiness often persist after recovery.

Progression to the second stage frequently prompts psychiatric or medical referral. A more sustained cognitive impairment is established, albeit with marked fluctuations in severity. Recurrent confusional episodes are accompanied by vivid hallucinatory experiences, visual misidentification syndromes, and topographical disorientation. Extensive medical screening is usually negative. Attentional deficits are apparent as apathy, and daytime somnolence and sleep behaviour disorder[17] may be severe. Gait disorder and bradykinesia are often overlooked, particularly in elderly subjects. Frequent falls occur due to either postural instability or syncope.

The third and final stage often begins with a sudden increase in behavioural disturbance, leading to requests for sedation or hospital admission by perplexed and exhausted carers. The natural course from this point is variable and obscured by the high incidence of adverse reactions to neuroleptic medication. For patients not receiving, or not tolerating, neuroleptics a progressive decline into severe dementia with dysphasia and dyspraxia occurs over months or years, with death usually due to cardiac or pulmonary disease. During this terminal phase patients show continuing behavioural disturbance including vocal and motor responses to hallucinatory phenomena. Lucid intervals with some retention of recent memory function and insight may still be apparent. Neurological disability is often profound, with fixed flexion deformities of the neck and trunk and severe gait impairment. Parkinsonian signs and paraplegia in flexion may also occur in advanced AD and other dementias. Parkinsonism occurring for the first time late in the course of a dementia is therefore consistent with a diagnosis of DLB, but not specific for it.

Advice about management

Patient management in DLB is complex and includes: early detection, investigation, diagnosis, and treatment of cognitive impairment; assessment and management of neuropsychiatric and behavioural symptoms; treatment of the movement disorder and monitoring and management of autonomic dysfunction, and sleep disorders. The evidence base for making recommendations about the management of DLB is limited and what follows is based upon consensus opinion of clinicians experienced in treating DLB.[9] The most important practice point in the management of a patient with DLB is caution in (or preferably avoidance of) the use of neuroleptic medications, which are the mainstay of antipsychotic treatment in other patient groups. Severe neuroleptic sensitivity reactions[5,6] can precipitate irreversible parkinsonism, further impair consciousness level, and induce autonomic disturbances reminiscent of neuroleptic malignant syndrome. They occur in 40 to 50 per cent of neuroleptic-treated DLB cases and are associated with a two- to threefold increased mortality. Acute D_2 receptor blockade is thought to mediate these effects; and despite initial reports, atypical antipsychotics seem to be as likely to cause neuroleptic sensitivity reactions as older drugs. A scheme for the management of the neuropsychiatric symptoms of DLB is suggested in Fig. 4.1.5.1.

Until safe and effective medications become available, there is no doubt that the mainstay of clinical management is to educate patients and carers about the nature of their symptoms and to suggest coping strategies. The clinician must ascertain which symptoms are most troublesome for the sufferer and explain the risks and benefits associated with changes in medication. In these circumstances where the clinician is walking a therapeutic tightrope between parkinsonism and psychosis, the best outcome is invariably a compromise between a relatively mobile but psychotic patient and a non-psychotic but immobile individual. The patient and his carers may only be able to decide which is the lesser of these evils after experiencing both states.

Non-pharmacological interventions

Non-pharmacological interventions have the potential to ameliorate many of the symptoms and functional impairments associated with DLB, but none have yet been systematically evaluated. Cognitive dysfunction and associated symptoms such as VH can for example, be exacerbated by low levels of arousal and attention and strategies to increase these by social interaction and environmental novelty may reduce their presence and impact.

Pharmacological treatments

Pharmacological treatment strategies are based upon our knowledge of the neurochemical deficits underlying specific symptoms in DLB. The most clearly established is a correlation between

Explain hallucinations, delusions, and other neuropsychiatric symptoms of DLB to patient and carer as an intrinsic part of the disorder.
EDUCATION ↓

Establish the nature and extent of cognitive impairment, neuropsychiatric features, sleep disorder, autonomic dysfunction and motor parkinsonism by interview with patient and carer.
Determine the extent to which of these impairs quality of life and requires active treatment.
Record pretreatment scores for each using appropriate rating scales.
BASELINE ASSESSMENT ↓

Gradually reduce, and if possible stop, antiparkinsonian medications in the following order:
- anticholinergics
- L-deprenyl
- amantadine
- direct dopamine agonists
- COMT inhibitors
- levodopa

Gradually reduce, and if possible stop other anticholinergics, sedatives and drugs which may exacerbate confusional symptoms.
REDUCE ANTI-PARKINSONIAN MEDICATIONS ↓

After each drug change, repeat measures in all relevant symptom domains to monitor for beneficial or adverse responses.
MONITOR RESPONSE ↓

If psychotic symptoms persist despite the reduction or withdrawal of unwanted medications a cholinesterase inhibitor should be gradually introduced in standard dose. Improvements are generally seen within the first few weeks and rapid relapse may occur if the drug is stopped abruptly.
CHOLINESTERASE INHIBITOR TRIAL ↓

If psychotic symptoms still persist a cautious trial of an antipsychotic may be justified as long as the patient and carer understand the potential risks of severe adverse side-effects. Since most neuroleptic sensitivity reactions occur during the first 2 weeks of treatment, it may be wise to admit patients into hospital during initiation of neuroleptic therapy. Since side-effects are dose related, treatment should start with the lowest possible dose and slow titration. Approximately 50% of patients are expected to tolerate medication.
NEUROLEPTIC TRIAL—VERY LOW DOSE AND SLOW TITRATION ↓

Neuroleptics should be discontinued if parkinsonism appears for the first time in a DLB patient, and the dose substantially reduced or stopped in patients whose pre-existing parkinsonism worsens. Severe neuroleptic sensitivity reactions should be treated as a medical emergency similar to neuroleptic malignant syndrome.
STOP IF NEUROLEPTIC SENSITIVITY IS SUSPECTED ↓

Other psychotropic medications may offer short-term benefits. Clonazepam can help nocturnal hallucinations and behavioural disturbance. SSRIs and SRNIs may improve mood disorders.
CONSIDER ALTERNATIVE MEDICATIONS

Fig. 4.1.5.1 Management of the neuropsychiatric symptoms of DLB.

substantia nigra neurone loss and severity of parkinsonism. Levodopa responsiveness is less predictable in DLB than in Parkinson's disease. Activity of the cholinergic enzyme choline acetyltransferase is lower in DLB than AD, particularly in temporal and parietal cortex.(42) Clouding of consciousness, confusion, and visual hallucinations are recognized effects of anticholinergic drug toxicity, and the summative effects of subcortical and cortical cholinergic dysfunction probably play a major role in the spontaneous generation of similar fluctuating symptoms in DLB. Reductions in choline acetyltransferase activity are correlated with the severity of cognitive impairment, and hallucinations may be related to hypocholinergic and (relatively) hypermonoaminergic neocortical neurotransmitter function.

Levodopa can be used for the motor disorder of both DLB and PDD.(43,44) Medication should generally be introduced at low doses and increased slowly to the minimum required to minimize disability without exacerbating psychiatric symptoms. Anticholinergics should be avoided. Visual hallucinations are the most commonly experienced psychiatric symptom and are often accompanied by delusions, anxiety and behavioural disturbance. When pharmacological intervention is required the options include cholinesterase inhibitors or atypical antipsychotic medications. Open label studies have demonstrated the effectiveness of all three generally available cholinesterase inhibitors in DLB but placebo controlled trial data is only available to date for rivastigmine.(45) The reported reduction in symptom frequency and intensity of VH appears to be mediated at least in part by improved attentional function and the presence of VH is associated with greater cognitive improvement. Cholinesterase inhibitors also improve cognitive impairment with an effect size that is generally larger than seen with the same drugs when used in AD.(46) There is a risk of symptom of rebound on sudden withdrawal,(47) limited data on long term effects,(48) and none about possible disease modifying effects.

Side effects of cholinesterase inhibitors in DLB include hypersalivation, lacrimation, and urinary frequency, in addition to the usual gastro-intestinal symptoms and a dose dependent exacerbation of extrapyramidal motor features may occur in a minority.(49) There is no evidence that any one cholinesterase inhibitor is better than others.(50) If they are ineffective or if more acute symptom control of behaviour is required, it may be difficult to avoid a cautious trial of an atypical antipsychotic. The clinician should warn both the carer and patient of the possibility of a severe sensitivity reaction.[5] Second generation atypicals with potentially more favourable pharmacological properties, such as quetiapine, clozapine, and aripiprazole may have theoretical advantages over traditional agents in LB disease but controlled clinical trial data is lacking and clinicians should remain vigilant to the possibility of adverse side effects.

Depression is common in DLB and there have been no systematic studies of its management. At the present time SSRI and SNRIs are probably preferred pharmacological treatment. Tricylic antidepressants and those with anticholinergic properties should generally be avoided. Apathy is also common and may improve with cholinesterase inhibition. Sleep disorders are frequently seen in LB disease and may be an early feature. Rapid eye movement sleep behaviour disorder can be treated with clonazepam 0.25 mg at bedtime, melatonin 3 mg at bedtime, or quetiapine 12.5 mg at bedtime and titrated slowly monitoring for both efficacy and side effects.[7]

Further information

http://www.lewybodydementia.org/—US-based carer organization

http://lewybody.org/—UK-based carer organization

http://www.nlm.nih.gov/medlineplus/lewybodydisease.html—MEDLINE PLUS information site

John O'Brien, Ian McKeith, David Ames, Edmond Chiu. (eds.) (2006). *Dementia with Lewy bodies and Parkinson's disease dementia*. Taylor and Francis, London—the first multidisciplinary textbook covering DLB and related disorders.

References

1. Okazaki, H., Lipkin, L.E., and Aronson, S.M. (1961). Diffuse intracytoplasmic ganglionic inclusions (Lewy type) associated with progressive dementia and quadriparesis in flexion. *Journal of Neuropathology and Experimental Neurology*, **20**, 237–44.
2. Hansen, L., Salmon, D., Galasko, D., *et al.* (1990). The Lewy body variant of Alzheimer's disease: a clinical and pathologic entity. *Neurology*, **40**, 1–8.
3. Perry, R.H., Irving, D., Blessed, G., *et al.* (1990). Senile dementia of Lewy body type. A clinically and neuropathologically distinct form of Lewy body dementia in the elderly. *Journal of the Neurological Sciences*, **95**, 119–39.
4. Burn, D.J., Rowan, E.N., Minett, T., *et al.* (2003). Extrapyramidal features in Parkinson's disease with and without dementia and dementia with Lewy bodies: a cross-sectional comparative study. *Movement Disorders*, **18**, 884–9.
5. McKeith, I., Fairbairn, A., Perry, R., *et al.* (1992). Neuroleptic sensitivity in patients with senile dementia of Lewy body type. *British Medical Journal*, **305**, 673–8.
6. Aarsland, D., Ballard, C., Larsen, J.P., *et al.* (2005). Marked neuroleptic sensitivity in dementia with Lewy bodies and Parkinson's disease. *The Journal of Clinical Psychiatry*, **66**(5), 633–7.
7. Boeve, B.F., Silber, M.H., and Ferman, T.J. (2004). REM sleep behavior disorder in Parkinson's disease and dementia with Lewy bodies. *Journal of Geriatric Psychiatry and Neurology*, **17**, 146–57.
8. Kramer, M.L. and Schulz-Schaeffer, W.J. (2007). Presynaptic alpha-synuclein aggregates, not Lewy bodies, cause neurodegeneration in dementia with Lewy bodies. *The Journal of Neuroscience*, **27**, 1405–10.
9. McKeith, I., Dickson, D., Emre, M., *et al.* (2005). Dementia with Lewy bodies: diagnosis and management: third report of the DLB consortium. *Neurology*, **65**, 1863–72.
10. McKeith, I.G., Ballard, C.G., Perry, R.H., *et al.* (2000). Prospective validation of consensus criteria for the diagnosis of dementia with Lewy bodies. *Neurology*, **54**, 1050–8.
11. Lippa, C.F. and McKeith, I. (2003). Dementia with Lewy bodies improving diagnostic criteria. *Neurology*, **60**, 1571–2.
12. Lippa, C., Duda, J.E., Grossman, M., *et al.* (2007). DLB and PDD boundary issues: diagnosis, treatment, molecular pathology, and biomarkers. *Neurology*, **68**, 812–19.
13. Cummings, J.L. (2004). Fluctuations in cognitive function in dementia with Lewy bodies. *Lancet Neurology*, **3**, 266.
14. Bradshaw, J., Saling, M., Hopwood, M., *et al.* (2004). Fluctuating cognition in dementia with Lewy bodies and Alzheimer's disease is qualitatively distinct. *Journal of Neurology, Neurosurgery, and Psychiatry*, **75**, 382–7.
15. Ferman, T.J., Smith, G.E., Boeve, B.F., *et al.* (2004). DLB fluctuations: specific features that reliably differentiate from AD and normal aging. *Neurology*, **62**, 181–7.
16. Walker, M.P., Ayre, G.A., Cummings, J.L., *et al.* (2000). The clinician assessment of fluctuation and the one day fluctuation assessment scale. Two methods to assess fluctuating confusion in dementia. *The British Journal of Psychiatry*, **177**, 252–6.
17. Walker, M.P., Ayre, G.A., Cummings, J.L., *et al.* (2000). Quantifying fluctuation in dementia with Lewy bodies, Alzheimer's disease and vascular dementia. *Neurology*, **54**, 1616–24.
18. Ballard, C., McKeith, I., Burn, D., *et al.* (1997). The UPDRS scale as a means of identifying extrapyramidal signs in patients suffering from dementia with Lewy bodies. *Acta Neurologica Scandinavica*, **96**, 366–71.
19. Mosimann, U.P., Rowan, E.N., Partington, C.E., *et al.* (2006). Characteristics of visual hallucinations in Parkinson disease dementia and dementia with Lewy bodies. *The American Journal of Geriatric Psychiatry*, **14**, 153–60.
20. McKeith, I.G., Fairbairn, A.F., Perry, R.H., *et al.* (1994). The clinical diagnosis and misdiagnosis of senile dementia of Lewy body type (SDLT). *The British Journal of Psychiatry*, **165**, 324–32.
21. McKeith, I.G., Perry, R.H., Fairbairn, A.F., *et al.* (1992). Operational criteria for senile dementia of Lewy body type (SDLT). *Psychological Medicine*, **22**, 911–22.
22. Boeve, B., Silber, M., Ferman, T., *et al.* (2001). Association of REM sleep behavior disorder and neurodegenerative disease may reflect an underlying synucleinopathy. *Movement Disorders*, **16**, 622–30.
23. Briel, R.C.G., McKeith, I.G., Barker, W.A., *et al.* (1999). EEG findings in dementia with Lewy bodies and Alzheimer's disease. *Journal of Neurology, Neurosurgery, and Psychiatry*, **66**, 401–3.
24. McKeith, I., Mintzer, J., Aarsland, D., *et al.* (2004). Dementia with Lewy bodies. *Lancet Neurology*, **3**, 19–28.
25. Barber, R., Ballard, C., McKeith, I.G., *et al.* (2000). MRI volumetric study of dementia with Lewy bodies. A comparison with AD and vascular dementia. *Neurology*, **54**, 1304–9.
26. Barber, R., Gholkar, A., Scheltens, P., *et al.* (1999). Medial temporal lobe atrophy on MRI in dementia with Lewy bodies. *Neurology*, **52**, 1153–8.
27. Lobotesis, K., Fenwick, J.D., Phipps, A., *et al.* (2001). Occipital hypoperfusion on SPECT in dementia with Lewy bodies but not AD. *Neurology*, **56**, 643–9.
28. Barber, R., Gholkar, A., Scheltens, P., *et al.* (2000). MRI volumetric correlates of white matter lesions in dementia with Lewy bodies and Alzheimer's disease. *International Journal of Geriatric Psychiatry*, **15**, 911–16.
29. O'Brien, J.T., Paling, S., Barber, R., *et al.* (2001). Progressive brain atrophy on serial MRI in dementia with Lewy bodies, AD, and vascular dementia. *Neurology*, **56**, 1386–8.
30. O'Brien, J.T., Colloby, S., Fenwick, J., *et al.* (2004). Dopamine transporter loss visualized with FP-CIT SPECT in the differential diagnosis of dementia with Lewy bodies. *Archives of Neurology*, **61**, 919–25.

31. McKeith, I., O'Brien, J., Walker, Z., *et al.* (2007). Sensitivity and specificity of dopamine transporter imaging with (123)I-FP-CIT SPECT in dementia with Lewy bodies: a phase III, multicentre study. *Lancet Neurology*, **6**, 305–13.
32. Rahkonen, T., Eloniemi-Sulkava, U., Rissanen, S., *et al.* (2003). Dementia with Lewy bodies according to the consensus criteria in a general population aged 75 years or older. *Journal of Neurology, Neurosurgery, and Psychiatry*, **74**, 720–4.
33. Holmes, C., Cairns, N., Lantos, P., *et al.* (1999). Validity of current clinical criteria for Alzheimer's disease, vascular dementia and dementia with Lewy bodies. *The British Journal of Psychiatry*, **175**, 45–50.
34. The Neuropathology Group MRC CFAS. (2001). Pathological correlates of late-onset dementia in a multicentre, community-based population in England and Wales. *Lancet*, **357**, 169–75.
35. Tsuang, D.W., DiGiacomo, L., and Bird, T.D. (2004). Familial occurrence of dementia with Lewy bodies. *The American Journal of Geriatric Psychiatry*, **12**, 179–88.
36. Gwinn-Hardy, K. and Singleton, A.A. (2002). Familial Lewy body diseases. *Journal of Geriatric Psychiatry and Neurology*, **15**, 217–23.
37. Trembath, Y., Rosenberg, C., Ervin, J.F., *et al.* (2003). Lewy body pathology is a frequent co-pathology in familial Alzheimer's disease. *Acta Neuropathologica*, **105**, 484–8.
38. Singleton, A. and Gwinn-Hardy, K. (2004). Parkinson's disease and dementia with Lewy bodies: a difference in dose? *Lancet*, **364**, 1105–7.
39. Ballard, C., O'Brien, J., Morris, C.M., *et al.* (2001). The progression of cognitive impairment in dementia with Lewy bodies, vascular dementia and Alzheimer's disease. *International Journal of Geriatric Psychiatry*, **16**, 499–503.
40. Williams, M.M., Xiong, C.J., Morris, J.C., *et al.* (2006). Survival and mortality differences between dementia with Lewy bodies vs Alzheimer disease. *Neurology*, **67**, 1935–41.
41. McKeith, I.G., Rowan, E., Askew, K., *et al.* (2006). More severe functional impairment in dementia with Lewy bodies than Alzheimer disease is related to extrapyramidal motor dysfunction. *The American Journal of Geriatric Psychiatry*, **14**, 582–8.
42. Perry, E.K., Haroutunian, V., Davis, K.L., *et al.* (1994). Neocortical cholinergic activities differentiate Lewy body dementia from classical Alzheimer's disease. *Neuroreport*, **5**, 747–9.
43. Molloy, S., McKeith, I.G., O'Brien, J.T., *et al.* (2005). The role of levodopa in the management of dementia with Lewy bodies. *Journal of Neurology, Neurosurgery, and Psychiatry*, **76**, 1200–3.
44. Bonelli, S.B., Ransmayr, G., Steffelbauer, M., *et al.* (2004). L-dopa responsiveness in dementia with Lewy bodies, Parkinson disease with and without dementia. *Neurology*, **63**, 376–8.
45. McKeith, I., Del-Ser, T., Spano, P.F., *et al.* (2000). Efficacy of rivastigmine in dementia with Lewy bodies: a randomised, double-blind, placebo-controlled international study. *Lancet*, **356**, 2031–6.
46. Samuel, W., Caligiuri, M., Galasko, D., *et al.* (2000). Better cognitive and psychopathologic response to donepezil in patients prospectively diagnosed as dementia with Lewy bodies: a preliminary study. *International Journal of Geriatric Psychiatry*, **15**, 794–802.
47. Minett, T.S.C., Thomas, A., Wilkinson, L.M., *et al.* (2003). What happens when donepezil is suddenly withdrawn? An open label trial in dementia with Lewy bodies and Parkinson's disease with dementia. *International Journal of Geriatric Psychiatry*, **18**, 988–93.
48. Grace, J., Daniel, S., Stevens, T., *et al.* (2001). Long-term use of rivastigmine in patients with dementia with Lewy bodies: an open-label trial. *International Psychogeriatrics*, **13**, 199–205.
49. Thomas, A.J., Burn, D.J., Rowan, E.N., *et al.* (2005). A comparison of the efficacy of donepezil in Parkinson's disease with dementia and dementia with Lewy bodies. *International Journal of Geriatric Psychiatry*, **20**, 938–44.
50. Bhasin, M., Rowan, E., Edwards, K., *et al.* (2007). Cholinesterase inhibitors in dementia with Lewy bodies-a comparative analysis. *International Journal of Geriatric Psychiatry*, **22**, 890–5.

4.1.6 Dementia in Parkinson's disease

R. H. S. Mindham and T. A. Hughes

Introduction

Parkinson's disease has been regarded as a neurological condition mainly affecting motor function and arising from specific lesions in the brain stem. The recognition of dementia in Parkinson's disease is of importance in management but the possibility that motor and cognitive functions may be located in the same region of the brain is of theoretical importance.

The nature of dementia in Parkinson's disease

There have been numerous reports of the impairment of specific cognitive functions in patients with Parkinson's disease. Mortimer and colleagues reported cognitive impairment in 93 per cent of a substantial group of patients with Parkinson's disease.[1] Their data showed neither a clear distinction between impaired groups nor the presence of subtypes of Parkinson's disease in which cognitive impairment is a more frequent occurrence. They proposed that cognitive impairment in Parkinson's disease lay on a continuum of severity, rather than as a feature of particular subgroups. The impairments identified included deficits in memory, language, visuospatial functioning, abstract reasoning, slowness in intellectual tasks, and difficulty in shifting from task to task. These deficits are widespread among patients with Parkinson's disease and can occur at an early stage of the disorder.

A proportion of patients with Parkinson's disease show impairment of a range of cognitive functions akin to the global impairment seen in Alzheimer's disease.[2] However, the pattern of impairment is frequently less severe than in Alzheimer's disease where the pathological changes in the brain are known to be widespread. Cognitive impairment in a range of disorders of movement where the main neuropathological changes reside in the subcortical region of the brain led to the concept of 'subcortical dementia', a form of intellectual impairment of lesser degree than in Alzheimer's disease, but affecting several cognitive functions. Albert described a syndrome of which the main features were: emotional or personality changes, impaired memory, defective ability to manipulate acquired knowledge, and a striking slowness in the rate of information processing.[3]

Many issues arose as to the nature of 'subcortical dementia'. Was it a clinical or a pathological concept? Was the difference between this and other forms of dementia simply one of degree? Did the pathological changes occur in the subcortical region of the brain alone? Was the syndrome of cognitive impairment distinctly different from other dementias or did the presence of motor features of the disorder simply give the intellectual impairment a distinct character? Was subcortical dementia a stable condition or a transitional state leading eventually to global dementia? Opinion has ranged from full acceptance of the concept to scepticism.[4,5]

McHugh[6] suggested that the subcortical region subserves functions not only in motor control and cognitive function but also in the control and display of mood. He suggested that these form a 'subcortical triad' of symptoms most convincingly seen in Huntington's disease. A notable difference between this concept and that of subcortical dementia was that the pathological disturbance of mood is only intermittently present, whereas the motor and cognitive changes are persistent.

Cummings[7] suggested that cognitive impairment in Parkinson's disease takes three forms: one which is relatively mild and meets the criteria for subcortical dementia, a more severe form showing wider impairment of cognitive function but neuropathologically distinct from Alzheimer disease and a severe form which shows neuropathological changes in both the subcortical region of the brain, and in the cortex, the latter of Alzheimer type. This proposal provides a basis for viewing cognitive changes in Parkinson's disease, albeit provisional.

Many reports have suggested that global dementia occurs in Parkinson's disease. Whether such a severe change in cognitive function can be regarded as an intrinsic feature of this disease, whether it implies an extension of a neuropathological process more widely in the brain, or whether it suggests a different neuropathology from the outset is, as yet, uncertain. More recently the debate has shifted to whether dementia in Parkinson's disease, dementia with Lewy bodies and Alzheimer's disease should be viewed as a spectrum, or as separate conditions with varying degrees of clinical and pathological overlap.

The methodology of studies of dementia in Parkinson's disease

Research to establish the status of dementia in Parkinson's disease has confronted a range of methodological issues.[8] A major problem is in the diagnosis of Parkinson's disease itself. The original description of paralysis agitans by Parkinson was the identification of a syndrome rather than of a disease. The part played by such agents as heavy metals, infections, and vascular disease was subsequently recognized. In spite of the use of standardized methods, a substantial proportion of patients diagnosed as suffering from Parkinson's disease in life do not show the expected findings in the brain post-mortem. In a follow-up study, 80 per cent of cases were shown to have neuropathological changes of Parkinson's disease after death but over 20 per cent were diagnosed as having suffered from progressive supranuclear palsy, multiple system atrophy, or Alzheimer's disease.[9] Furthermore, some dementing illnesses may show disorder of movement as a clinical feature.

Studies of dementia in Parkinson's disease

Cases of dementia in Parkinson's disease have been reported for over a hundred years. The frequency of dementia reported in cross-sectional or prevalence studies ranges from 0 to over 80 per cent. A recent review found a prevalence of between 28 and 44 per cent in community studies but in older samples of subjects the prevalence was much higher.[10]

Follow-up studies have great advantages in studying the frequency of dementia in Parkinson's disease as they allow the diagnosis of Parkinson's disease to be checked, repeated assessment reduces errors in the recognition of dementia, the pattern of evolution of dementia may be followed, the underestimation of dementia by selective loss through death is avoided, and they reveal the incidence rather than the prevalence of the condition. The choice of methods of diagnosis and assessment that will remain appropriate throughout the period of the follow-up remains a problem.

A prospective, controlled study in the United Kingdom reported an incidence of dementia of 19 per cent after 4.5 years observation. A later report on the same cohort of subjects showed an incidence of dementia of 38 per cent after 10 years of observation. The control group showed cases of cognitive impairment but none amounting to dementia.[11,12] A community based, prospective, controlled study, in Norway, showed the risk of dementia was 5.9 times greater than in the control group.[13] A prospective, controlled study in the United States showed that dementia was 3.7 times greater in the Parkinson's disease group with severely affected, elderly patients especially at risk (Table 4.1.6.1).[14,15]

Prediction of dementia in Parkinson's disease

Those most likely to develop dementia are: older people, patients with Parkinson's disease of longer duration, subjects who have a greater severity of motor symptoms and signs of Parkinson's disease, and those who show greater physical disability.[11–15] Some studies have shown that male sex or late onset are associated with dementia. The apparent association between Parkinson's disease treated with levodopa and dementia is probably due to improved survival.

Neuropathology

The basic lesions are the degeneration of the pigmented neurones in the pars compacta of the substantia nigra in the brain stem; the presence of **Lewy bodies** which are intracytoplasmic neuronal inclusions composed of abnormally phosphorylated neural filament proteins aggregated with ubiquitin and alpha-synuclein; gliosis; and the formation of **Lewy neurites** which are degenerating neurites containing ubiquitin and alpha-synuclein. Alpha-synuclein may play an important role in the pathological process leading to the formation of Lewy bodies, but conclusive proof is lacking. Clinical Parkinson's disease is not apparent until about 80 per cent of the nigro-striatal dopaminergic neurones have died. Lewy bodies had come to be regarded as pathognomonic of Parkinson's disease, but are now known to be present in other diseases. An agreed though arbitrary difference between dementia in Parkinson's disease and dementia with Lewy bodies is that in the latter, parkinsonian symptoms must not precede the occurrence of dementia by more than 12 months.

The degenerative changes in the substantia nigra are known to be closely linked with decreased dopaminergic neurotransmission in the brain, and this deficiency leads to the main motor features of the disease, although other neurotransmitters are also deficient. Some of these deficiencies, which have been associated with cognitive impairment in other disorders, include a deficiency in acetylcholinesterase in the cortex, a deficiency of noradrenaline in the cortex, and a deficiency of serotonin in both striatum and cortex. The concentrations of a range of neuropeptides may also be altered.

The neuropathology of cases of Parkinson's disease showing dementia is inconsistent; some show neuropathological changes

Table 4.1.6.1 Some prospective studies of dementia in Parkinson's disease, using control subjects and employing standardized methods of diagnosis and assessment

Study	PD subjects (N)	Control subjects (N)	Length of follow-up (years)	Diagnostic criteria for dementia	% of PD demented	Number demented per 1000 person years	Dementia in PD v controls: relative risk (95% CI), †odds ratio, ‡hazard ratio
1. Biggins *et al.* 1992 (UK)	87	50	4.5	DSM-III-R	19	47.6	–
2. Hughes *et al.* 2000 (UK)	83	50	10	DSM-III-R	38	42.6	–
3. Aarsland *et al.* 2001 (Norway)	171	3062	4.2	DSM-III-R	33	95.3	†5.9 (3.9–9.1)
4. Levy *et al.* 2002 (USA)	180	180	3.6	DSM-III-R	28.9	79.9	‡3.7 (2.1–6.3)
5. Aarsland *et al.* 2003 (Norway)	224	3295	8	DSM-III-R	78.2	–	2.8
6. Hobson & Meara 2004 (UK)	86	102	4	DSM-IV	35.3	107.1	5.1 (2.1–12.5)
7. de Lau *et al.* 2005 (Holland)	139	6512	9	DSM-III-R	15.1	–	‡2.8 (1.8–4.4)

Notes on studies:

1. Prevalent cases of dementia at entry to study excluded from analysis; PD & controls assessed concurrently; DSM-III-R criteria assessed blind; PD sample drawn from neurological clinics.
2. Same PD cohort and controls, same method of assessment as study 1.
3. Community sample in Norway; controls from community sample in Demark assessed by different instruments and at different intervals. Prevalent cases of dementia excluded from entry to study. DSM-III-R criteria (dementia diagnosis) not assessed blind.
4. Community sample. Prevalent cases of dementia at entry to study excluded from analysis. Concurrent examination of PD and control groups using same instruments; DSM-III-R criteria not assessed blind.
5. Same PD cohort and controls, similar method of assessment, same method of diagnosis of dementia as study3. % PD demented includes 26% cases prevalent at entry to study. Relative risk is for dementia in PD subjects at 4 years versus control subjects at 5 years.
6. Prevalent cases of dementia excluded from entry to study. Elderly sample. DSM-IV criteria not assessed blind.
7. Community sample. Prevalent cases of dementia at entry to study excluded from analysis. DSM-III-R criteria not assessed blind.

extending beyond the subcortical region, whereas in others neuropathological changes are restricted to the subcortical region. Some studies have shown a correlation between the extent of Lewy body pathology and the severity of dementia, but others have not. Lewy bodies may be found in individuals without cognitive impairment and dementia may develop with only minimal cortical Lewy bodies.[16] In some patients with dementia the neuropathological diagnosis is of Alzheimer's disease or of other recognized degenerative conditions of the brain.

Just as there are difficulties in isolating Parkinson's disease from other conditions, there are problems in understanding the interrelationships of dementing disorders. Several distinct neurodegenerative diseases share some aetiological factors, which may represent an interaction between environmental factors and the ageing process but with differing end results arising from factors specific to the process.[17–19] Problems in the diagnosis of Parkinson's disease, the shrinking category of idiopathic Parkinson's disease, and the difficulties occasionally encountered in explaining the development of dementia in the disease, suggests that the interrelationship between causative agents, the clinical features of disorders of movement, the occurrence of cognitive impairment, and the neuropathology of this group of disorders requires substantial further work before it is understood.

The influence of dementia on mortality

Dementia is associated with increased mortality. In Parkinson's disease increased mortality is associated with age, late age of onset of the disease, cognitive impairment, dementia, and, in some studies, male sex. Many of the studies that have been carried out have been methodologically faulty, making comparisons between studies and the identification of the effect of particular factors, including dementia, problematic. One study showed a hazard ratio for Parkinson's disease compared with controls of 1.64, in general, and of 1.94 for to Parkinson's disease with dementia.[20] In another study of mortality almost 50 per cent of those who died were demented compared with a quarter of those who survived.[21]

Clinical aspects of Parkinson's disease with dementia

The most important step in the recognition of dementia in Parkinson's disease is to suspect its presence. The typical blank facial expression seen in Parkinson's disease may obscure a decline in intellectual activity, slowness in movement may conceal intellectual slowness, and sadness may suggest that morbid depression of mood is the reason for a reduction in liveliness. The clinical picture can usually be clarified by careful examination of the mental state. Standardized psychological tests may be useful in some cases.

The clinical importance of dementia in Parkinson's disease is that there is a marked increase in disability, with problems arising in areas of functioning not previously affected by motor impairment alone. Dementia may be accompanied by an increased liability to confusional episodes from the toxic effects of drugs and other causes.[22]

Management of dementia is similar to that for patients suffering from other dementing disorders (Chapter 4.1.3). Controlled trials suggest rivastigmine and donepezil have a moderate effect on cognitive function, but tolerability can be a problem, with worsening of parkinsonism and gastrointestinal upsets.[23] Rivastigmine is started at 1.5 mg twice daily, and increased by 3 mg per day at intervals of 4 weeks upto a maximum of 12 mg daily. Donepezil should be started at 5 mg in the evenings, increasing to 10 mg after 6 weeks, if tolerated.

Further information

http://www.mrw.interscience.wiley.com/cochrane/clsysrev/articles/CD004747/frame.html

References

1. Pirozzolo, F.J., Hansch, E.C., Mortimer, J.A., *et al.* (1982). Dementia in Parkinson's disease: a neuropsychological analysis. *Brain and Cognition*, **1**, 71–83.
2. Pollack, M. and Hornabrook, R.W. (1966). The prevalence, natural history and dementia of Parkinson's disease. *Brain*, **89**, 429–48.
3. Albert, M.L., Feldman, R.G., and Willis, A.L. (1974). The 'subcortical dementia' of progressive supranuclear palsy. *Journal of Neurology, Neurosurgery, and Psychiatry*, **37**, 121–30.
4. Mayeux, R., Stern, Y., Rosen, J., *et al.* (1983). Is 'subcortical dementia' a recognisable clinical entity? *Annals of Neurology*, **14**, 278–83.
5. Brown, R.G. and Marsden, C.D. (1988). Subcortical dementia: the neuropsychological evidence. *Neuroscience*, **25**, 363–87.
6. McHugh, P.R. (1990). The basal ganglia: the region, the integration of its systems and implications for psychiatry and neurology. In *Function and dysfunction in the basal ganglia* (ed. A.J. Franks, J.W. Ironside, R.H.S. Mindham, R.J. Smith, E.J.S. Spokes, and W. Winlow), pp. 259–69. Manchester University Press, Manchester.
7. Cummings, J.L. (1988). The dementias of Parkinson's disease: prevalence, characteristics, neurobiology, and comparison with dementia of the Alzheimer type. *European Neurology*, **28**(Suppl 1), 15–23.
8. Mindham, R.H.S. (1999). The place of dementia in Parkinson's disease: a methodologic saga. In *Advances in neurology*, Vol. 80 (ed. G.M. Stern), pp. 403–8. Lippincott, Williams & Wilkins, Philadelphia.
9. Hughes, A.J., Daniel, S.E., Kilford, L., *et al.* (1992). Accuracy of clinical diagnosis of idiopathic Parkinson's disease: a clinico–pathlolgical study of 100 cases. *Journal of Neurology, Neurosurgery, and Psychiatry*, **55**, 181–4.
10. Emre, M. (2003). Dementia associated with Parkinson's disease. *Lancet Neurology*, **2**, 229–37.
11. Biggins, C.A., Boyd, J.L., Harrop, F.M., *et al.* (1992). A controlled longitudinal study of dementia in Parkinson's disease. *Journal of Neurology, Neurosurgery, and Psychiatry*, **55**, 566–71.
12. Hughes, T.A., Ross, H.F., Musa, S., *et al.* (2000). A 10-year study of the incidence of and factors predicting dementia in Parkinson's disease. *Neurology*, **54**, 1596–602.
13. Aarsland,D., Andersen, K., Larsen, J.P., *et al.* (2001). Risk of dementia in Parkinson's disease: a community based, prospective study. *Neurology*, **56**, 730–6.
14. Levy, G., Schupf, N., Tang, M.X., *et al.* (2002). Combined effect of age and severity on the risk of dementia in Parkinson's disease. *Annals of Neurology*, **51**, 722–9.
15. Hobson, P. and Meara, J. (2004). Risk and incidence of dementia in a cohort of older subjects with Parkinson's disease in the United Kingdom. *Movement Disorders*, **19**, 1043–9.
16. Braak, H., Rüb, U., Jansen Steur, E.N.H., *et al.* (2005). Cognitive status correlates with neuropathologic stage in Parkinson's disease. *Neurology*, **64**, 1404–10.
17. Appel, S.H. (1981). A unifying hypothesis for the cause of amyotrophic lateral sclerosis, parkinsonism and Alzheimer's disease. *Annals of Neurology*, **10**, 499–505.
18. Calne, D.B., McGeer, E., Eisen, E., *et al.* (1986). Alzheimer's disease, Parkinson's disease and motor neurone disease: abiotrophic interactions between aging and environment. *Lancet*, **328**, 1067–70.
19. Ben-Shlomo, Y., Whitehead, A.S., and Smith, G.D. (1996). Parkinson's, Alzheimer's, and motor neurone disease. Clinical and pathological overlap may suggest common genetic and environmental factors. *Lancet*, **312**, 728.
20. Hughes, T.A., Ross, H.F., Mindham, R.H.S., *et al.* (2004). Mortality in Parkinson's disease and its association with dementia and depression. *Acta Neurologica Scandinavica*, **110**, 118–23.
21. de Lau, L.M.L., Schipper, C.M.A., Hofman, A., *et al.* (2005). Prognosis of Parkinson's disease. Risk of dementia and mortality: the Rotterdam study. *Archives of Neurology*, **62**, 1265–9.
22. Aarsland, D., Brønnick, K., Ehrt, U., *et al.* (2007). Neuropsychiatric symptoms in patients with Parkinson's disease and dementia: frequency, profile and associated care-giver stress. *Journal of Neurology, Neurosurgery, and Psychiatry*, **78**, 36–42.
23. Maidment, I.D., Fox, C., and Boustani, M. (2005). A review of studies describing the use of acetylcholinesterase inhibitors in Parkinson's disease dementia. *Acta Psychiatrica Scandinavica*, **111**, 403–9.

4.1.7 Dementia due to Huntington's disease

Susan Folstein and Russell L. Margolis

Introduction

Huntington's disease (HD) was first described in 1872 by an American physician living on Long Island, New York. His father and grandfather practised medicine in the same community, so he had access to case notes from several generations of families who lived there. This long period of record keeping allowed him to document a hereditary form of chorea, similar to 'common (Sydenham's) chorea', but progressing over many years to death. Its sufferers had a tendency to insanity and suicide. Huntington's brief essay, which also included a clear description of autosomal dominant inheritance, remains one of the classical descriptions of a medical disorder.[1]

Clinical features and course of illness

Huntington's disease is an inherited neuropsychiatric disorder mainly affecting the striatum and its direct connections. It is characterized by a triad of clinical features that are common to diseases of this region: a non-aphasic *dementia*, *depression* and other disorders of mood, and a variety of *dyskinesias*, most typically chorea.[2,3] Chorea, from the Greek word for 'dance', describes involuntary non-stereotyped jerky movements. The illness, insidious in onset, may begin with all or any one of these three features. Patients who present initially to psychiatrists usually have dementia, loss of temper, or depression, often with suicidal thoughts or attempts. Symptoms may appear at any time from early childhood to old age, most frequently between 35 and 45 years of age. Once the illness begins, sufferers gradually deteriorate over many years in their cognitive and motor functioning and end in a persistent vegetative state with almost complete loss of voluntary motor function. Death occurs after about 16 years and is usually caused by inanition or aspiration pneumonia. Some patients die earlier from suicide or subdural haematoma caused by a fall. Patients with early onset progress more rapidly than those whose symptoms begin later in life.

Pathology and genetics

The earliest visible neuropathology is in the striosomes of the caudate/putamen,[4] followed by a dorsal-to-ventral progressive loss of almost all striatal output neurones. The deep layers of multiple cortical regions are also prominently affected, and there can also be milder neuronal loss in some brainstem nuclei. Protein aggregates, most easily detectable in neuronal nuclei, are prominent. Neuroimaging studies have shown that neuropathological changes typically begin before the onset of clinically detectable disease. In particular, the extent of striatal loss in presymptomatic individuals, as measured by MRI, correlates with the predicted time until disease onset.[5] Cortical thinning[6] and white matter loss and disorganization[7,8] have also been detected in presymptomatic gene carriers. Subtle changes that may be related to abnormal brain development have also been reported.

The disorder, with a point prevalence of about 6/100 000,[9] is caused by the expansion of an unstable triplet repeat sequence (CAG) in the first exon of a gene near the telomere of chromosome 4p.[10] It is transmitted as an autosomal dominant trait; if one parent is affected, each offspring (regardless of sex) has an independent 50 per cent chance of inheriting the abnormal gene. Normal repeat lengths range from about 7 to 28 triplets. Individuals with 29–35 triplets will not develop HD but may pass an expanded allele to an offspring, while individuals with 40 or more triplets will develop HD. Repeat lengths of 36–39 triplets may or may not cause disease. The rate of mutation from a normal-length allele to an expanded one is low, so that most patients have an affected parent. Family history, however, can be obscured by multiple factors, including misdiagnosis of the parent, death of the parent before disease onset, adoption, and incorrect paternity. The repeat length does not remain stable at meiosis. In HD, the number of CAG triplets is more likely to increase when the gene is transmitted by fathers. As the number of repeats increases, the age at onset is earlier. Thus, paternal transmission is often associated with 'anticipation', earlier onset in the subsequent generation; most individuals with childhood onset have affected fathers.[11]

The pathogenesis of HD is not well understood but appears to be multifaceted. The gene, *huntingtin*, with the expanded repeat is expressed as a protein, huntingtin. The CAG repeat expansion is translated as an expanded polyglutamine tract, which appears to have neurotoxic properties. The region of the huntingtin protein with the polyglutamine tract may be cleaved from the rest of the protein and adopt an abnormal configuration. This in turn is thought to lead to disruption of cellular functions, including transcriptional machinery, protein degradation processes, and cellular transport. It is also possible that the expansion mutation results in a partial loss of the normal functions of huntingtin, one of which is the stimulation of the neurotrophic factor BDNF; decreased BDNF may contribute to neurotoxicity.[12]

Diagnosis

The most difficult aspect of diagnosis is to think of HD in the differential. Diagnosis remains dependent on a thorough psychiatric history, including a detailed family history and history of changes in social adjustment, mental state examination, including a cognitive examination, and neurological examination. The features vary, depending on how long the patient has been ill.[13] Once the disease is suspected, genetic testing, available through many commercial laboratories, provides the definitive diagnosis.

Diagnosis of patients with early symptoms

Patients with HD who initially consult psychiatrists present with a variety of psychiatric syndromes, including depression, bipolar disorder, obsessive–compulsive disorder, schizophrenia, or excessive anxiety. Irritability is common with any of these or may appear outside the context of another syndrome. These psychiatric syndromes are clinically indistinguishable from idiopathic disorders and may be the only manifestation of HD for several years. It is during this prodromal phase that patients often commit suicide; this may occur even if the patient is unaware of his risk for HD.[14] Presenting symptoms and problems with functioning at work or at home must often be elicited from an informant; the patient may minimize them, be embarrassed, or even unaware of them. These include declines in work speed or accuracy, which may have resulted in demotion or warnings from superiors; a tendency to become irritated or physically aggressive in response to annoying stimuli that would not have elicited such a response in the past; and a decreased interest in activities. Most of these symptoms and behaviours are common in psychiatric disorders, but the cognitive inefficiency and irritability may seem to be out of proportion, relative to the patient's other symptoms. On cognitive examination, the patient may have difficulty recalling dates of important life events and more difficulty than expected with 'serial sevens'. Usually, the cognitive changes are easier to notice after the psychiatric disorder is treated, which can usually be accomplished using standard medications. However, unlike idiopathic disorders, cognitive inefficiency and difficulties at work, apathy (if present), and sometimes irritability remain even after the patient's mood, energy, and sleep patterns have improved. When this happens in the course of treatment of depression, a dementia work-up should be considered and the family history further scrutinized through hospital records and other family informants.

On neurological examination, motor restlessness is usually present but is easily misinterpreted as a manifestation of anxiety. Motor signs may be subtle: slightly slow saccadic eye movements,[15] writhing movements of the protruded tongue or of the fingertips when the arms are held at 90°, or mild disdiadochokinesis.

Diagnosis can be further complicated by the apparent lack of a family history of HD. The family may not have been informed about the affected parent's diagnosis, or may know only that a parent died in a psychiatric institution or committed suicide. In other cases the paternity is uncertain. If the family history is actually negative (this is quite uncommon) or unobtainable (often the case for adopted individuals who frequently present in childhood), the diagnosis may be confirmed by testing for the HD gene expansion.

(a) Diagnosis in childhood and adolescence

When HD starts in childhood or early adolescence,[16] motor signs include parkinsonian-like motor slowness of voluntary movement, with lead pipe or cogwheel rigidity and very slow saccades. Occasional children have a coarse tremor; later myoclonus is seen. Cognitively, the rate of learning in school slows, handwriting deteriorates, and interest in school and social activities declines.[17] Of the patients who present with a schizophrenic syndrome, most are adolescents. Psychosis and loss of cognitive capacity may be the only clinical features for several years before motor impairment begins. Children with HD often have seizures, which are usually grand mal. Sometimes myoclonus is mistaken for seizures.

(b) The importance of early diagnosis

Even though it can be difficult, it is important to make the diagnosis of HD as early as possible, particularly in employed persons. Poor function at work (or in schoolwork or household duties) occurs early, and patients can lose their jobs, often on suspicion of drug or alcohol abuse. This is usually avoided if the diagnosis is made known to the family and employer, allowing modification of the work environment or retirement on the basis of disability. Prompt diagnosis does not mean that the patient needs to be informed of the diagnosis at that same time. Some patients are too depressed to do this safely; others indicate that they do not wish to be told. Treatment can usually proceed despite the patient's reluctance to label the disorder.

Diagnosis of patients with well-established signs and symptoms

After a few years of illness, diagnosis is easier. The signs and symptoms will have worsened, and usually the motor disorder is obvious. A typical patient who has been ill for about 5 to 7 years is unable to work or manage finances, but lives at home and is able to manage personal needs. Some patients remain active and energetic, continuing to participate as fully in life as their cognitive and motor disabilities allow; others are apathetic most of the time, but irritable when disturbed; still others have severe depression with delusions, obsessions, or compulsions, and most are anxious and easily upset by changes of routine. An uncommon, but very troublesome, feature of HD is sexual abnormality. While most patients become impotent or uninterested in sex, a few are hypersexual and may develop paraphilias.[18] It is important to inquire about these specifically because neither the patient nor spouse will likely mention it.

Cognitively, patients complain of forgetfulness and becoming easily distracted. Thinking is slow; patients have difficulty following a conversation and cannot complete a multistaged task. On cognitive examination, Mini Mental State Examination scores[19] may still be above the 23 cut-off score, but serial sevens will be very poor, and one or two items will be missed on recalling words after a distraction. On neuropsychological testing, IQ will be lower than expected for education, and there will be difficulty learning word lists and performing tests that require changing sets.

Most patients will have obvious involuntary choreic movements, as well as difficulty with control of voluntary motor movements, as seen by clumsiness, slowness, dysarthria, and an unsteady gait. The involuntary movements will wax and wane with the level of arousal; it can be worsened by performing serial 7 s or by fine motor tasks. Speech will have an irregular staccato, often laboured, quality. Saccadic eye movements will be slow or irregular, and the patient will be obviously clumsy on diadochokinesis and finger-thumb tapping, although finger-to-nose testing is normal. Gait will be wide based and irregular, with difficulty with tandem walking. Reflexes are usually brisk, and a history of falls can be elicited.

Diagnosis of patients with advanced disease

After 10 years of illness, dementia is more severe, with poor performance on all aspects of the cognitive examination except naming. Speech is dysfluent with long lapses between the examiner's question and the patient's reply, rather like Brocca's aphasia. Some patients will be almost unable to speak, although language comprehension is relatively preserved. Patients (if they are cooperative) can carry out simple commands and will recognize relatives and nursing staff. Patients may be irritable, particularly when their verbal requests cannot be understood or when routines are altered. Psychiatric syndromes are more difficult to discern, but most can be diagnosed by observing behaviour such as hoarding, sleeplessness, or diurnal variation in mood. Physical disabilities are much worse. Patients often need to be fed, toileted, and helped with most daily needs. They have difficulty walking and may fall, causing further disability through broken limbs or subdural haematomas. Chorea often stabilizes or subsides,[13] but the ability to carry out voluntary movements becomes seriously handicapping. If they survive long enough, patients become unable to initiate speech, swallow with great difficulty, are unable to walk, and have such severely rigid muscle tone that they may be nearly unable to move their bodies. Clonus and positive Babinski signs are present. Patients in this sort of 'persistent vegetative state'[20] are difficult to distinguish from individuals with other advanced movement disorders or dementias; as in early disease, diagnosis will depend on eliciting a family history or genetic testing.

Differential diagnosis

The differential diagnosis of HD is extensive,[3] but only a few of the disorders for which it can be mistaken are common.[2] These include other dementias, other movement disorders, and other psychiatric disorders. The most frequent subcortical dementia is **Parkinson's disease**, which has a similar motor slowness, but a pill-rolling tremor and festinating gait are rare in HD. The dementia associated with **late-life depression** can look very similar to HD, including motor slowness. **Alzheimer's disease** is easily distinguished by the lack of motor signs during the first several years of illness and more prominent difficulty with memory and language, as opposed to attention and calculation. Perhaps most difficult to distinguish clinically are the **frontotemporal dementias**, which present with prominent behavioural disturbances and a positive family history. The clinical presentation may be insufficient to distinguish these various dementias in patients with advanced disease, since they all progress to a persistent vegetative state. The family history and the duration of illness (which is longer for HD than for Alzheimer's disease or frontotemporal dementia) can be helpful.

Several other diseases classified as **movement disorders** include all the features of the subcortical triad. They often have an autosomal dominant inheritance pattern and expansion of unstable trimeric repeat sequences. These include Fahr's syndrome (calcification of the striatum), some forms of spinocerebellar degeneration, chorea acanthocytosis, Huntington's disease-like 2 (HDL2), and dentatorubropallidolusian atrophy (DRPLA). The latter three disorders, while much rarer than HD, can look so similar that they can only be distinguished by genetic testing and by a blood smear for acanthocytes. The most common movement disorder that resembles HD is **tardive dyskinesia**. Patients with HD occasionally have several years of hallucinations and delusions before the movement disorder begins. If they have been treated with neuroleptics, the subsequent onset of involuntary movements can be mistaken for tardive dyskinesia. On the other hand, the choreoathetotic involuntary movements of severe tardive dyskinesia may involve the trunk and extremities as well as the face and can be mistaken for HD. Usually, it is possible to distinguish the patients with tardive dyskinesia by their normal saccadic eye movements, normal tandem gait, and fluid and fluent speech.[21] However, genetic testing may be necessary in some cases. Wilson's disease also presents with the subcortical triad and should be considered when neither of the parent is affected. It is recessively inherited, so that the only affected relatives are siblings. Very late-onset HD may be diagnosed as 'senile chorea' because the family history appears to be negative. Family members will also present symptoms only late in life and may have died before their manifestation.

The differential diagnosis of nearly all **psychiatric disorders** includes HD, as described above.

Treatment and management

Currently, no treatment influences the course of illness of HD, but based on research on likely genetic mechanisms, clinical trials of agents protective against oxidants, excitotoxicity, and metabolic stress are underway. No agent yet tested has had a dramatic benefit. The development of biochemical assays and cell and animal models that mimic various aspects of HD can be used to screen for effective therapies.

It is possible to alleviate some of the symptoms of HD. Small doses of neuroleptics can be helpful in decreasing involuntary movements in the first stages of the illness, as can tetrabenazine and occasionally benzodiazepines. Doses of more than 5 mg. of haloperidol do not further decrease chorea and may worsen cognition and cause motor stiffness and slowing.[22] Persons with the advanced form of the disease are often unresponsive to neuroleptics. Treatment of psychiatric manifestations significantly improves quality of life for the patients and their families. Clinical experience suggests that depression, anxiety, and obsessive–compulsive disorder associated with HD usually respond to the pharmacological treatments used for the similar idiopathic disorders. SSRIs can be particularly helpful. Because some patients seem unaware of their depressed mood (just as they can be unaware of their involuntary movements) an informant is often needed to elicit the symptoms. It is also important to distinguish depression (from which the patient is miserable and sleepless) and apathy, which does not cause distress. Occasionally, mood and anxiety disorders are chronic and unresponsive to treatment. Severe, unresponsive depression can be treated successfully with electroconvulsive therapy.[23] Bipolar disorder in patients with HD does not usually respond to lithium, but may improve with carbamazepine or valproic acid. Valproic acid, serotonin specific reuptake inhibitors, and low dose antipsychotic agents may also be helpful in the treatment of irritability. Lithium is difficult to administer because patients require high fluid intake and easily become lithium toxic if fluid intake is insufficient. In one case report, high doses of sertraline were effective for intractable aggression.[24] Schizophrenic symptoms can be difficult to treat. Sometimes a combination of an antipsychotic, including clozaril, with an antidepressant will prove helpful. Muscle rigidity and consequent contractions occur in late HD, causing pain and difficulty in positioning the patient to avoid pressure sores. Amantadine (which also has a positive effect on mood) can somewhat decrease the rigidity; chairs and beds must be padded and tailored to each patient's specific needs.

Family and environment

As with most dementias, psychopathology influences, and is influenced by, the patient's environment. Patients do best in a calm, highly predictable environment where cognitive expectations are not too complicated. When the environment is too taxing, patients become irritable, especially towards their family. HD seriously damages family relationships, which in turn affects the patient. The well spouse becomes responsible for supporting the family, caring for children and the patient, and making family and financial decisions. Spouses' lives are further complicated by patients' unwillingness to relinquish financial and family decision-making; patients usually make poor decisions that damage family relationships and finances. Some patients neglect their children or treat them badly. If the other parent cannot prevent this, it is wisest to remove the patient from the home. There is no research on the treatment of sexual aggression, which occasionally occurs in males, but the author has successfully treated a few males with depot progesterone. Supportive psychotherapy for the patient should focus on minimizing demoralization at lost abilities. Spouses can be helped to reorganize family life in ways that maximize the predictability of the patient's environment, diplomatically decrease patients' domestic responsibilities. It is crucial that the spouse has time away from the patient.

Helping persons at risk for HD

People at risk for HD vary in their abilities to deal with the burden of uncertainty, depending on their personal attributes and their experience with the illness in a relative. A few consult physicians for reassurance, but most avoid doctors unless they become ill, and even then many resist medical attention, claiming against all evidence that they are perfectly well. Currently, a minority of asymptomatic persons at risk for HD decide to have genetic testing, but these individuals, skewed towards those whose anxiety is lessened by planning for the future, have usually handled the test results well, regardless of its outcome.[25] When clinical trials are launched for individuals with the HD mutation who are without detectable symptoms, the incentive for presymptomatic testing will likely increase, with a concomitant change in the nature of individuals seeking testing. Foetal and pre-implantation genetic testing are now available in some centers, each with its own set of potentially complicated ethical and practical issues to be sorted out prior to testing.

Presymptomatic genetic testing of any sort should always be preceded by genetic counselling, provided either by a genetic counselor or by a clinician familiar with HD genetics and the potential practical and psychological consequences of both positive and negative test results. Counselling should include a discussion of the motivations for seeking testing, which may include decisions about childbearing, education, employment, finances, participation in clinical trials, or the potential at-risk status of offspring. Many individuals who come for testing have not seriously considered the possibility that they will test positive for the mutation, so that role playing about various outcome scenarios is important. Occasionally, persons request testing who have learned only recently that they are at risk for HD. Others apply who are depressed or under unusual stress for other reasons. Such persons should be encouraged to delay testing until their situation becomes more settled. Finally, some people who request testing already have symptoms of HD, yet do not wish to have a diagnosis. Considerable care is required to decide how best to support such individuals, and family members or close friends of the person should be consulted.[26]

Further information

Wells, R. and Ashizawa, T. (2006). *Genetic Instabilities and Neurologic Diseases* (2nd edn). Academic Press, San Diego.

Bates, G. Harper, P. and Jones, L. (2002). *Huntington's disease* (3rd edn). Oxford University Press, Oxford.

Walker, F.O. (2007). Huntington's disease. *Lancet*, **369**, 218–28.

References

1. Huntington, G. (1872). On chorea. Reprinted in *Advances in Neurology*, **1**, 33–5 (1973).
2. Folstein, S. (1989). *Huntington's disease. A disorder of families*. Johns Hopkins University Press, Baltimore, MD.
3. Harper, P. (ed.) (1991). *Huntington's disease*, Vol. 22. W.B. Saunders, London.
4. Hedreen, J.C. and Folstein, S.E. (1995). Early loss of neostriatal striosome neurons in Huntington's disease. *Journal of Neuropathology and Experimental Neurology*, **54**, 105–20.
5. Aylward, E.H, Codori, A.M., Rosenblatt, A., *et al.* (2000). Rate of caudate atrophy in presymptomatic and symptomatic stages of Huntington's disease. *Movement Disorders*, **15**, 552–60.
6. Rosas, H.D., Hevelone, N.D., Zaleta, A.K., *et al.* (2005). Regional cortical thinning in preclinical Huntington disease and its relationship to cognition. *Neurology*, **65**, 745–7.
7. Paulsen, J.S., Magnotta, V.A., Mikos, A.E., *et al.* (2006). Brain structure in preclinical Huntington's disease. *Biological Psychiatry*, **59**, 57–63.
8. Reading, S.A., Yassa, M.A., Bakker, A., *et al.* (2005). Regional white matter change in presymptomatic Huntington's disease: a diffusion tensor imaging study. *Psychiatry Research*, **140**, 55–62.
9. Folstein, S.E, Chase, G.A., Wahl, W.E., *et al.* (1987). Huntington disease in Maryland: clinical aspects of racial variation. *American Journal of Human Genetics*, **41**, 168–79.
10. Huntington's Disease Collaborative Research Group. (1993). A novel gene containing a trinucleotide repeat that is expanded and unstable on Huntington's disease chromosomes. *Cell*, **72**, 971–83.
11. Ranen, N.G., Stine, O.C., Abbott, M.H., *et al.* (1995). Anticipation and instability of (CAG)*n* repeats in IT-15 in parent–offspring pairs with Huntington's disease. *American Journal of Human Genetics*, **57**, 593–602.
12. Ross, C.A., Russell, L.M., Becher, M.W., *et al.* (1998). Pathogenesis of neurodegenerative diseases associated with expanded glutamine repeats: new answers, new questions. *Progress in Brain Research*, **117**, 398–419.
13. Folstein, S.E., Leigh, R., Parhad, I.M., *et al.* (1986). The diagnosis of Huntington's disease. *Neurology*, **36**, 1279–83.
14. Folstein, S.E., Abbott, M.H., Franz, M.L., *et al.* (1983). The association of affective disorder with Huntington's disease in a case series and in families. *Psychological Medicine*, **13**, 537–42.
15. Lasker, A.D. and Zee, D.S. (1994). Ocular motor abnormalities in Huntington's disease. *Vision Research*, **34**, 3639–45.
16. Kosky, R. (1981). Children and Huntington's disease: some clinical observations of children at risk. *The Medical Journal of Australia*, **1**, 405–7.
17. Nance, M. (1997). Genetic testing of children at risk for Huntington's disease. *Neurology*, **49**, 1048–53.
18. Federoff, J.O., Peyser, C.E., Franz, M.L., *et al.* (1994). Sexual disorders in Huntington's disease. *The Journal of Neuropsychiatry and Clinical Neuroscience*, **6**, 147–53.
19. Folstein, M.F., Folstein, S.E., and McHugh, P.R. (1975). 'Mini-Mental State': a practical method for grading the cognitive state of patients for the clinician. *Journal of Psychiatric Research*, **2**, 189–98.
20. Walshe, T.M. and Leonard, C. (1985). Persistent vegetative state: extension of the syndrome to include chronic disorders. *Archives of Neurology*, **42**, 1045–7.
21. David, A.S., Jeste, D.V., Folstein, M.F., *et al.* (1987). Voluntary movement dysfunction in Huntington's disease and tardive dyskinesia. *Acta Neurologica Scandinavia*, **75**, 130–9.
22. Barr, A.N., Fischer, J.H., Koller, W.C., *et al.* (1988). Serum haloperidol concentration and choreiform movements in Huntington's disease. *Neurology*, **38**, 84–8.
23. Ranen, N.G., Peyser, C.E., and Folstein, S.E. (1994). ECT as a treatment for depression in Huntington's disease. *Journal of Neuropsychiatry and Clinical Neurosciences*, **6**, 154–9.
24. Ranen, N.G., Lipsey, J.R., Treisman, G., *et al.* (1996). Sertraline in the treatment of severe aggressiveness in Huntington's disease. *The Journal of Neuropsychiatry and Clinical Neuroscience*, **8**, 338–40.
25. Almqvist, E.W., Brinkman, R.R., Wiggins, S., *et al.* (2003). Psychological consequences and predictors of adverse events in the first 5 years after predictive testing for Huntington's disease. *Clinical Genetics*, **64**, 300–309.
26. Scourfield, J., Soldan, J., Gray, J., *et al.* (1997). Huntington's disease: psychiatric practice in molecular genetic prediction and diagnosis. *The British Journal of Psychiatry*, **170**, 146–9.

4.1.8 Vascular dementia

Timo Erkinjuntti

Introduction

Vascular dementia is the second most frequent cause of dementia.[1,2] Because vascular causes of cognitive impairment are common, may be preventable, and the patients could benefit from therapy, early detection, and accurate diagnosis of vascular dementia is desirable.[3]

Vascular dementia is not only multi-infarct dementia, but is related to other vascular mechanisms and pathological changes in the brain, and has other causes and clinical manifestations. Vascular dementia is not a disease, but a syndrome. The origin of this syndrome reflects complex interactions between vascular aetiologies (cerebrovascular disorders and vascular risk factors), changes in the brain (infarcts, white-matter lesions, atrophy), host factors (age, education), and cognition.[4–8]

Conceptual issues related to of vascular dementia include the definition of the cognitive syndrome (type, extent, and combination of impairments in different cognitive domains), and the vascular causes (vascular aetiologies and changes in the brain). Variations in these definitions has led to different estimates of point prevalence, to different groups of patients, and to reports of different types and distribution of brain lesions.[9–11] The cognitive syndrome of vascular dementia is characterized by predominate executive dysfunction rather than deficits in memory and language function.[12] Although the course of cognitive decline may be stepwise, it is often slowly progressive, and may include periods of stability or even some improvement.

The relationship between vascular lesions in the brain and cognitive impairment is important, but which type, extent, side, site, and tempo of vascular lesions in the brain relates to different types of vascular dementia is not established in detail.[4–6,13]

Current criteria for vascular dementia are based on the concept of cerebral infarcts. For example the widely used NINDS-AIREN criteria include dementia, cerebrovascular disease, and a relationship between these two disorders. The main tools for the diagnosis include detailed history, neurological examination, mental state examination, relevant laboratory examinations, and preferably magnetic resonance imaging of the brain.

Vascular dementia research, until recently overshadowed by that into Alzheimer's disease, is now developing rapidly. There is great promise for intervention. Developments in classification, diagnosis, and treatment are likely.

Aetiology and pathophysiology

Aetiology

The main causes of vascular dementia are cerebrovascular disorders and their risk factors. The prevalent cerebrovascular disorders include large artery disease (artery-to-artery embolism, occlusion of an extra- or intracranial artery), cardiac embolic events, small-vessel disease (lacunar infarcts, ischaemic white-matter lesions) and haemodynamic mechanisms.[13–15] Less frequent causes include specific arteriopathies including cerebral autosomal dominant arteriopathy with subcortical infarcts and leucoencephalopathy (CADACIL) and cerebral amyloid angiopathy (CAA), haemorrhage (intracranial haemorrhage, subarachnoidal haemorrhage), haematological factors, venous disease, and hereditary disorders. There may be as yet undiscovered causes.

In most patients diagnosed with vascular dementia, several aetiological factors are involved. However, the roles these factors play have not been identified in detail, and it is not certain which of these mechanisms distinguish vascular dementia from cerebrovascular disease without dementia.[4,5,7,16,17]

Risk factors for vascular dementia can be divided into vascular factors (e.g. arterial hypertension, atrial fibrillation, myocardial infarction, coronary heart disease, diabetes, generalized atherosclerosis, lipid abnormalities, smoking), demographic factors (e.g. age, education), genetic factors (e.g. family history, individual genetic features), and stroke-related factors (e.g. type of cerebrovascular disease, site and size of stroke).[18,19] Hypoxic ischaemic events (cardiac arrhythmias, congestive heart failure, myocardial infarction, seizures, pneumonia) may be an important risk factor for incident dementia in patients with stroke.[20]

Changes in the brain

Vascular dementia is related to both ischaemic and non-ischaemic changes in the brain.[4,5,13,14] The ischaemic lesions include arterial territorial infarct, distal field (watershed) infarct, lacunar infarct, ischaemic white-matter lesions, and incomplete ischaemic injury. Incomplete ischaemic injury incorporates laminar necrosis, focal gliosis, granular atrophy, and incomplete white-matter infarction.[21,22] In addition, both focal (around the ischaemic lesion) and remote (disconnection, diaschisis) functional ischaemic changes relate to vascular dementia, and the volume of functionally inactive tissue exceeds that of focal ischaemic lesions in vascular dementia.[23] Limitation in current clinical methods have hampered the detection of both incomplete ischaemic injury and functional ischaemic changes related to vascular dementia. Atrophy is the non-ischaemic factor related to vascular dementia. However, there are no methods to distinguish between ischaemic and degenerative causes of atrophy clinically.

Brain imaging findings

Work on the relationship between brain lesions and cognition in vascular dementia has used varying definitions and measures of cognitive impairment, varying techniques to reveal brain changes, and varying criteria for the selection of patients.[17]

CT and magnetic resonance imaging (**MRI**) studies on vascular dementia have shown that bilateral ischaemic lesions are important.[4,5,7,17] Some studies emphasize deep infarcts in the frontal and limbic areas, while others report cortical lesions especially in the temporal and parietal areas. There is disagreement about the number and volume of the infarcts, as well as the extent and location of atrophy. Diffuse and extensive white-matter lesions have been suggested as an important factor leading to functional disconnection of cortical brain areas. Some general conclusions on brain lesions in vascular dementia may be drawn.

1 There is no single pathological feature, but a combination of infarcts, ischaemic white-matter lesions of varying size and type, and atrophy of varying degree and site.

2 Infarcts associated with vascular dementia tend to be bilateral, multiple (more than two), and located in the dominant hemisphere and in the limbic structures (frontolimbic or prefrontal–subcortical and medial–limbic or medial–hippocampal circuits).

3 White-matter lesions on CT or magnetic resonance imaging (MRI) associated with vascular dementia are extensive, extending in periventricular white matter, and confluent to extending in the deep white matter.

4 It is doubtful whether a single small lesion on imaging can be accepted as evidence for vascular dementia.

5 Absence of cerebrovascular lesions on CT or MRI is contrary to a diagnosis of vascular dementia.

Pathophysiology

The extent to which pathological changes in the brain cause, compound, or only coexist with the vascular dementia syndrome is still uncertain. The vascular changes in the brain can be the main cause of cognitive impairment (as assumed in vascular dementia[24,25]), they can contribute to the clinical picture of other dementia syndromes including Alzheimer's disease (AD),[7,26] or they may be coincidental. The occurrence of infarcts may cause an earlier presentation of clinical symptoms in a brain in which there is existing and progressive Alzheimer's disease pathology.[26]

It is not certain which are the critical changes in the brain leading to the clinical picture of vascular dementia. The syndrome has been related to the volume of brain infarcts (with a critical threshold), the number of infarcts, the site of infarcts (bilateral, in strategic cortical or subcortical, or affecting white matter), to other ischaemic factors (incomplete ischaemic injury, delayed neuronal death, functional changes), to the atrophic changes (origin, location, extent), and finally to the additive effects of other pathologies

(Alzheimer's disease, Lewy body dementia, frontal lobe dementias). But it is uncertain which type, extent, side, site, and tempo of vascular lesions in the brain, and which combination with other pathologies, relate to vascular dementia.(4–6,13)

Classification and clinical criteria

Classification

Vascular dementia has been divided into subtypes on the basis of clinical, radiological, and neuropathological features. It is uncertain whether these subtypes are distinct disorders, with separate pathological and clinical features, and responses to therapy.(27) If homogenous subtypes could be identified the comparability of research studies would be greater and multicentre studies easier.(28)

The subtypes of vascular dementia included in most classifications include multi-infarct dementia (cortical lesions), small-vessel dementia or subcortical ischaemic vascular disease and dementia (SIVD) (subcortical deep lesions), and strategic infarct dementia.(12,14,27,29–33) Many include also hypoperfusion dementia.(12,14,30,34) Further suggested subtypes include haemorrhagic dementia, hereditary vascular dementia, and combined or mixed dementia (Alzheimer's disease with cerebrovascular disease).

DSM-IV(35) does not specify subtypes. ICD-10(36) includes six subtypes (acute onset, multi-infarct, subcortical, mixed cortical and subcortical, other, and unspecified). The NINDS-AIREN criteria(30) include, without detailed description, cortical vascular dementia, subcortical vascular dementia, Binswanger's disease, and thalamic dementia. In addition separate research criteria for subcortical vascular dementia, the SIVD, have been proposed.(37)

Main subtypes

Multi-infarct dementia or cortical vascular dementia, and small-vessel dementia or subcortical vascular dementia are the two common subtypes, although their frequencies vary in different series.(12,14,31)

Cortical vascular dementia relates to large-vessel disease, cardiac embolic events, and hypoperfusion. Infarcts are predominantly in the cortical and corticosubcortical arterial territories, and their distal fields (watershed). Typical clinical features are lateralized sensorimotor changes and the abrupt onset of cognitive impairment and aphasia.(31) A combination of different cortical neuropsychological syndromes has been suggested to occur in cortical vascular dementia.(38)

Subcortical vascular dementia, small-vessel dementia, the SIVD(33,37) incorporates the entities 'lacunar state' and 'Binswanger's disease'. It relates to small-vessel disease and hypoperfusion, with predominately lacunar infarcts, focal and diffuse ischaemic white-matter lesions, and incomplete ischaemic injury.(31,33,37–39) Clinically, small-vessel dementia is characterized by pure motor hemiparesis, bulbar signs, dysarthria, depression, and emotional lability, and especially deficits in executive functioning.(38–41)

Clinical criteria

Since the 1970s several clinical criteria for vascular dementia have been published.(11,42,43) The most widely used include those in DSM-IV,(35) ICD-10,(36) and NINDS-AIREN.(30)

The two cardinal elements of any clinical criteria for vascular dementia are the definition of the cognitive syndrome(44) and the definition of the cause.(11,43,45) All clinical criteria are consensus criteria, derived neither from prospective community-based studies on vascular factors affecting the cognition, nor on detailed natural histories.(28,30,42,43,46) All these criteria are based on the concept of ischaemic infarcts. They are designed to have high specificity, but have been poorly validated.(42,46) An important consequence of the different definitions of the dementia syndrome,(9,44) and the vascular cause,(10,11) is that the different diagnostic criteria identify different populations.

The DSM-IV definition of vascular dementia (Table 4.1.8.1) requires focal neurological signs and symptoms or laboratory evidence of focal neurological damage clinically judged to be related to the disturbance.(35) The course is specified by sudden cognitive and functional losses. The DSM-IV criteria do not detail brain imaging requirements. The DSM-IV definition of vascular dementia is reasonably broad and lacks detailed clinical and radiological guidelines.

The ICD-10 criteria(36) (Table 4.1.8.2) require unequal distribution of cognitive deficits, focal signs as evidence of focal brain damage, and significant cerebrovascular disease judged to be aetiologically related to the dementia. The criteria do not detail brain imaging requirements. The ICD-10 criteria specify six subtypes of vascular dementia (Table 4.1.8.3). The ICD-10 criteria for vascular dementia have been shown to be highly selective and only some of those fulfilling the general criteria for ICD-10 vascular dementia

Table 4.1.8.1 The DSM-IV definition of vascular dementia

Focal neurological signs and symptoms (e.g. exaggeration of deep tendon reflexes, extensor plantar response, pseudobulbar palsy, gait abnormalities, weakness of an extremity, etc.) or Laboratory evidence of focal neurological damage (e.g. multiple infarctions involving cortex and underlying white matter)
The cognitive deficits cause significant impairment in social or occupational functioning and represent a significant decline from a previously higher level of functioning
The focal neurological signs, symptoms, and laboratory evidence are judged to be aetiologically related to the disturbance
The deficits do not occur exclusively during the course of delirium
Course characterized by sustained periods of clinical stability punctuated by sudden significant cognitive and functional losses

Table 4.1.8.2 The ICD-10 criteria for vascular dementia

Unequal distribution of deficits in higher cognitive functions with some affected and others relatively spared. Thus, memory may be quite markedly affected while thinking, reasoning, and information processing may show only mild decline
There is evidence for focal brain damage, manifest as at least one of the following: unilateral spastic weakness of the limbs, unilaterally increased tendon reflexes, an extensor plantar response, pseudobulbar palsy
There is evidence from the history, examination, or test of significant cerebrovascular disease, which may reasonably be judged to be aetiologically related to the dementia (history of stroke, evidence of cerebral infarction)

Table 4.1.8.3 Characteristics of the vascular dementia subtypes in ICD-10

Subtype	Characteristics
Acute onset (F01.0)	The dementia develops rapidly (i.e. usually within 1 month but within no longer than 3 months) after a succession of strokes, or (rarely) after a single large infarction
Multi-infarct (F01.1)	The onset of the dementia is more gradual (i.e. within 3-6 months) following a number of minor ischaemic episodes. Comments: it is presumed that there is an accumulation of infarcts in the cerebral parenchyma. Between the ischaemic episodes there may be periods of actual clinical improvement
Subcortical (F01.2)	A history of hypertension, and evidence from clinical examination and special investigations of vascular disease located in the deep white matter of the cerebral hemispheres, with preservation of the cerebral cortex.
Mixed cortical and subcortical (F01.3)	Mixed cortical and subcortical components of vascular dementia may be suspected from the clinical features, the results of investigation, or both
Other (F01.8) **Unspecified (F01.9)**	In the ICD-10 criteria no specific diagnostic guidelines are given for these two vascular dementia sybtypes

can be classified into one of the subtypes.(11,45) The shortcoming of these criteria include lack of detailed guidelines (e.g. of unequal cognitive deficits and changes on neuroimaging), lack of aetiological criteria, and heterogeneity.(11,45)

The NINDS-AIREN research criteria for vascular dementia(30) include a dementia syndrome, cerebrovascular disease, and a relationship between these (Table 4.1.8.4). Cerebrovascular disease is defined by the presence of focal neurological lesions and brain imaging evidence of ischaemic changes in the brain. A relationship between dementia and cerebrovascular disorder is inferred from the onset of dementia within 3 months following a recognized stroke, or on abrupt deterioration in cognitive functions, or fluctuating stepwise progression of cognitive deficits. The criteria include a list of features consistent with the diagnosis, as well as a list of features that make the diagnosis uncertain or unlikely. Also, different levels of certainty of the clinical diagnosis (probable, possible, definite) are included. The NINDS-AIREN criteria recognize heterogeneity(47) of the syndrome and variability of the clinical course in vascular dementia, and highlight detection of ischaemic lesions and a relationship between lesion and cognition, as well as stroke and dementia onset.

The NINDS-AIREN criteria are currently most widely used in clinical drug trials on vascular dementia. In a neuropathological series, sensitivity of the NINDS-AIREN criteria was 58 per cent and specificity 80 per cent.(48) The criteria successfully excluded Alzheimer's disease in 91 per cent of cases, and the proportion of combined cases misclassified as probable vascular dementia was 29 per cent.(48) The inter-rater reliability of the NINDS-AIREN criteria is moderate to substantial ($\kappa = 0.46$–0.72).(49)

These three sets of criteria for vascular dementia are not interchangeable; they identify different numbers and clusters of patients. The DSM-IV criteria are less restrictive than the ICD-10 and NINDS-AIREN criteria.(11,50)

Table 4.1.8.4 The NINDS-AIREN criteria for probable vascular dementia

(I) The criteria for the clinical diagnosis of PROBABLE vascular dementia include *all* of the following

1 *Dementia*
2 *Cerebrovascular disease*, defined by the presence of focal signs on neurological examination, such as hemiparesis, lower facial weakness, Babinski sign, sensory deficit, hemianopia, dysarthria, etc. consistent with stroke (with or without history of stroke), and evidence of relevant CVD by brain imaging (CT or MRI) including multiple large-vessel strokes or a single strategically placed infarct (angular gyrus, thalamus, basal forebrain, PCA or ACA territories), as well as multiple basal ganglia and white-matter lacunes or extensive periventricular white-matter lesions, or combinations thereof
3 *A relationship between the above two disorders*, manifested or inferred *by* the presence of one or more of the following
   (a) Onset of dementia within 3 months following a recognized stroke
   (b) Abrupt deterioration in cognitive functions, or fluctuating stepwise progression of cognitive deficits

(II) Clinical features consistent with the diagnosis of PROBABLE vascular dementia include the following
   (a) Early presence of a gait disturbance (small-step gait or *marche a petits-pas*, apraxic–ataxic or parkinsonian gait)
   (b) History of unsteadiness and frequent unprovoked falls
   (c) Early urinary frequency, urgency, and other urinary symptoms not explained by urological disease
   (d) Personality and mood changes, abulia, depression, emotional incontinence, other subcortical deficits including psychomotor retardation and abnormal executive function

(III) Features that make the diagnosis of vascular dementia uncertain or unlikely include the following
   (a) Early onset of memory deficit and progressive worsening of memory and other cognitive functions such as language (transcortical sensory aphasia), motor skills (apraxia), and perception (agnosia), in the absence of corresponding focal lesions on brain imaging
   (b) Absence of focal neurological signs, other than cognitive disturbance
   (c) Absence of cerebrovascular lesions on brain CT or MRI

CVD, cerebrovascular disease; PCA, posterior cerebral artery; ACA, anterior cerebral artery.

Vascular cognitive impairment

Vascular cognitive impairment (VCI) is currently considered the most recent modification of the terminology to reflect the all-encompassing effects of vascular disease or lesions on cognition and incorporates the complex interactions between vascular aetiologies, risk factors, and cellular changes within the brain and cognition.(51,52)

VCI refers to all aetiologies of CVD including vascular risks which can result in brain damage leading to cognitive impairment. The impairment encompasses all levels of cognitive decline, from the earliest deficits to a severe and broad dementia-like cognitive syndrome.(51,53) VCI cases that do not meet the criteria for dementia can also be labelled as VCI with no dementia, vascular CIND.(54)

VCI may include cases with cognitive impairment related to hypertension, diabetes, or atherosclerosis, transient ischaemic attacks, multiple corticosubcortical infarcts, silent infarct, strategic infarcts, small-vessel disease with white-matter lesions an lacunae, as well as AS pathology with coexisting CVD.[55] The concept and definitions of VCI and vascular CIND are still evolving, but it seems clear that the diagnosis should not be confined to a single aetiology comparable to the traditional 'pure AD' concept.[51,52]

Clinical features

Cognitive syndrome

The cognitive syndrome of vascular dementia is characterized by memory deficit, dysexecutive syndrome, slowed information processing, and mood and personality changes. These features are found especially among patients with subcortical lesions. Patients with cortical lesions often have additional cortical neuropsychological syndromes.[38]

The memory deficit in vascular dementia is often less severe than in Alzheimer's disease. It is characterized by impaired recall, relatively intact recognition, and more benefit from cues.[56] The dysexecutive syndrome in vascular dementia includes impairment in goal formulation, initiation, planning, organizing, sequencing, executing, set-sifting and set-maintenance, as well as in abstracting.[12,38,56] The dysexecutive syndrome in vascular dementia relates to lesions affecting the prefrontal subcortical circuit including prefrontal cortex, caudate, pallidum, thalamus, and the thalamocortical circuit (capsular genu, anterior capsule, anterior centrum semiovale, and anterior corona radiata).[57] Typically, personality and insight are relatively preserved in mild and moderate cases of vascular dementia.

Features that make the diagnosis of vascular dementia disease uncertain or unlikely include early and progressive worsening of episodic memory, and other cognitive cortical deficits in the absence of corresponding focal lesions on brain imaging.[30]

Neurological findings

Frequent neurological findings indicating focal brain lesion early in the course of vascular dementia include mild motor or sensory deficits, decreased co-ordination, brisk tendon reflexes, Babinski's sign, visual field loss, bulbar signs including dysarthria and dysphagia, extrapyramidal signs (mainly rigidity and akinesia), disordered gait (hemiplegic, apraxic–ataxic, or small-stepped), unsteadiness, unprovoked falls, and urinary frequency and urgency.[30,31,39–41] Features that make the diagnosis of vascular dementia uncertain or unlikely include absence of focal neurological signs, other than cognitive disturbance.[30]

In cortical vascular dementia, typical clinical features are lateralized sensorimotor changes and abrupt onset of cognitive impairment and aphasia, and in subcortical vascular dementia disease pure motor hemiparesis, bulbar signs, dysarthria, disordered gait and unsteadiness.[31]

Behavioural and psychological symptoms of dementia

Depression, anxiety, emotional lability and incontinence, and other psychiatric symptoms are frequent in vascular dementia. Depression, abulia, emotional incontinence, and psychomotor retardation are especially frequent in subcortical vascular dementia disease.[12,38]

(a) Ischaemic scores

Cardinal features of vascular dementia disease are incorporated in the Hachinski Ischaemia Score[58] (Table 4.1.8.5). In a neuropathological series, stepwise deterioration (odds ratio, 6.0), fluctuating course (odds ratio, 7.6), history of hypertension (odds ratio, 4.3), history of stroke (odds ratio, 4.3), and focal neurological symptoms (odds ratio, 4.4) differentiated patients with definite vascular dementia from those with definite Alzheimer's disease.[59] Nocturnal confusion and depression did not discriminate. However, the ischaemia score was unable to differentiate the Alzheimer's disease patients with cerebrovascular disease from those with vascular dementia.

Table 4.1.8.5 Hachinski ischaemia score

Item	Score value
Abrupt onset	2
Stepwise deterioration	1
Fluctuating course	2
Nocturnal confusion	1
Relative preservation of personality	1
Depression	1
Somatic complaints	1
Emotional incontinence	1
History of hypertension	1
History of strokes	2
Evidence of associated atherosclerosis	1
Focal neurological symptoms	2
Focal neurological signs	2

Course and prognosis

Traditionally, vascular dementia has been characterized by a relative abrupt onset (days to weeks), a stepwise deterioration (some recovery after worsening), and fluctuating course (e.g. differences between days) of cognitive functions. These features are seen in patients with repeated lesions affecting cortical and corticosubcortical brain structures, i.e. large-vessel multi-infarct vascular dementia, and with watershed infarcts related to haemodynamic problems. However, in patients with small-vessel dementia, i.e. subcortical vascular dementia, the onset is more insidious and course more slowly progressive.[28,30,39,60]

The mean duration of vascular dementia is around 5 years.[2] In most studies survival is less than for the general population or those with Alzheimer's disease.[61,62] Surprisingly little is known about the rate and pattern of cognitive decline, either overall or among different subgroups of vascular dementia.[63] This underlines the lack of studies detailing the natural history of vascular dementia.

Diagnosis and differential diagnosis

The clinical evaluation of patients with memory impairment has two stages, the symptomatic diagnosis, i.e. evaluation of the type and extent of cognitive impairment, and the aetiological diagnosis, i.e. evaluation of vascular cause(s) and related factors. The symptomatic categories other than dementia include the more mild cognitive stages, i.e. VCI or vascular CIND, delirium, circumscribed neuropsychological syndromes (e.g. aphasia) and functional psychiatric disorders (e.g. depression).[46] Stages of aetiological diagnosis include diagnosis of the specific causes, especially the potentially treatable conditions, evaluation of secondary factors able to affect the cognitive functioning, and more detailed differentiation between specific causes, especially that between vascular dementia disease and Alzheimer's disease.

Clinical evaluation

The cornerstone in the evaluation of a patient with suspected vascular dementia is detailed clinical and neurological history and examination, including interview of a close informant. Assessment of social functions, activities of daily living, as well as psychiatric and behavioural symptoms, is part of the basic evaluation. These patients are challenging and enough time should be allocated time for the consultation, often 40 to 60 min.

Mental status examination

Bedside mental status examination includes the Mini-Mental State Examination.[64] However, this has limitations as it emphasizes language, does not include timed elements and the recognition portion of the memory tests, is insensitive to mild deficits, and is influenced by education and age. Other proposed screening instruments for vascular dementia include a 10-word memory test with delayed recall, cube drawing test for copy, verbal fluency test (number of animals named in 1 min), Luria's alternating hand sequence, or finger rings and letter cancellation test (neglect).[30] Other test include the Clox and Exit designed to screen the dysexecutive features.[65]

Frequently a more detailed neuropsychological test is needed. It should cover the main cognitive domains including memory functions (working memory, episodic memory, semantic memory), abstract thinking, judgement, aphasia, apraxia, agnosia, orientation, attention, executive functions, and speed of information processing.[44,66]

Brain imaging

Brain imaging should be performed at least once during the initial diagnostic workout. MRI is preferred because it has high sensitivity and the ability to demonstrate medial temporal lobe and basal forebrain areas. Depending on the criteria of vascular dementia used, focal brain infarcts have been revealed in 70 to 100 per cent, and more extensive white-matter lesions in 70 to 100 per cent of cases.[13,25,30,67,68]

Single-photon emission CT and positron-emission tomography may reveal patchy reduction of regional blood flow and metabolism, as well as decreased white-matter flow and metabolism.[69]

Other investigations

Chest X-ray, electrocardiography, and screening laboratory tests are part of the basic evaluation.[15,70,71] In selected cases extended laboratory investigations, analysis of the cerebrospinal fluid, and EEG are performed, as well as examinations of the extra- and intracranial arteries and detailed cardiological investigations.[15,70,71]

In vascular dementia EEG is more often normal than in Alzheimer's disease, and if abnormal more frequently suggests a focal abnormality. Abnormalities increase with more severe intellectual decline both in vascular dementia disease and Alzheimer's disease.[60]

At present there is no specific laboratory test for vascular dementia. Tests may reveal risk factors and concomitant disorders such as hyperlipidaemia, diabetes, and cardiac abnormality.[60] Apolipoprotein E_4 is a established risk factor for Alzheimer's disease, but its relationship to vascular dementia has not been consistent.[72] Determination of apolipoprotein E status is currently not part of clinical evaluation in vascular dementia.

Differential diagnosis of vascular dementia disease

(a) Alzheimer's disease

Typical Alzheimer's disease is characterized by insidious onset and slowly progressive intellectual deterioration, absence of symptoms and signs indicating focal brain damage, and absence of any other specific disease affecting the brain.[73] Alzheimer's disease has typical clinical stages ranging from early changes to profound dementia.[74,75]

When patients with vascular dementia have a clinical history, neurological examination, and brain imaging findings compatible with ischaemic changes of the brain, the differentiation from Alzheimer's disease can be made clinically.[25]

Diagnostic problems arise when Alzheimer's disease is combined with cerebrovascular disease. Difficult clinical problems include stroke unmasking Alzheimer's disease in patients with post-stroke dementia, insidious onset, and/or slow progressive course in vascular dementia patients, and cases where it is difficult to assess the role of white-matter lesions or of infarcts found on neuroimaging. A solution to recognize patients with Alzheimer's disease and cerebrovascular disease would be to discover reliable biological markers for clinical AD. Other potential markers include early prominent episodic memory impairment, early and significant medial temporal lobe atrophy on magnetic resonance imaging, bilateral parietal hypoperfusion on single-photon emission computed tomography and low concentrations of cerebrospinal fluid amyloid peptides with high tau protein concentrations. The distinction would be also less difficult if there were more detailed knowledge of the sites, type, and extent of ischaemic brain changes critical for vascular dementia, and the extent and type of medial temporal lobe atrophy critical for Alzheimer's disease.

Other important conditions to be differentiated from vascular dementia include normal pressure hydrocephalus,[76] frontal lobe tumours and other intracranial masses,[15] Lewy body disease,[77] frontotemporal degenerations,[78] Parkinson's disease and dementia,[79] progressive supranuclear palsy,[80] and multisystem atrophy.[81]

Epidemiology

Vascular dementia is the second most common cause of dementia accounting for 10 to 50 per cent of cases, depending on the geographic location, patient population, and clinical methods used.[1,2] The prevalence of vascular dementia is from 1.2 to 4.2 per cent of persons aged 65 years and older, and the incidence is 6 to 12 cases per 1000 persons aged over 70 years per year.[2] The prevalence and the incidence of vascular dementia disease increases with increasing age, and men seem to have a higher prevalence of vascular dementia than women. Epidemiology of vascular dementia has been affected by variations in the definition of the disorder, the clinical criteria used, and the clinical methods applied.[18,82,83]

The frequency of vascular dementia disease has been higher than previously reported in recent series comprising older subjects.[10] Stroke and cerebrovascular disorders relate also to a high risk of cognitive impairment and dementia.[24,84] Finally, vascular factors such as stroke and white-matter lesions have a clinical effect on Alzheimer's disease.[26] Thus, vascular factors may even be the leading cause of cognitive impairment worldwide especially when cognitive impairment as opposed to dementia is considered.[51,85]

Treatment

The objectives of targeted treatment of vascular dementia include symptomatic improvement of core symptoms (e.g. cognitive, behavioural), slowing progression of the disorder, and treatment of secondary factors affecting cognition (e.g. depression, anxiety, agitation).

A number of drugs have been studied in the symptomatic treatment of vascular dementia including cerebro- and vasoactive drugs, nootropics, and some calcium antagonists, but largely these studies have shown negative results.[86] Studies on symptomatic improvement in vascular dementia have mostly had small numbers, short treatment periods, variations in diagnostic criteria and tools, mixed populations, and have had variation in clinical endpoints applied.

First nimodipine,[87] memantine,[88] and propentofylline[89] raised expectations for a symptomatic treatment of vascular dementia. However, all the studies failed to fulfil the current requirement by the regulators for and treatment indication in vascular dementia.[90,91]

More recently cholinesterase inhibitors (donepezil, galantamine, rivastigmine) have been tested in large randomized controlled trials in patients with probable vascular dementia. All showed significant cognitive improvement compared to placebo, but failed to show significantly better global outcome with the Alzheimer-type measures. Accordingly, none of the acetylcholinesterase inhibitors have received marketing authorization for the treatment of vascular dementia.[91] Patients with Alzheimer's disease with coexisting cerebrovascular disease show good benefit from galantamine.[92]

Possibilities for prevention

For primary prevention the target is the brain at risk of cerebrovascular disease and cognitive impairment. The methods relate to the treatment of putative risk factors of vascular dementia, and the promotion of potential protective factors. Risk factors include those related to cerebrovascular disorders and stroke, to vascular dementia, to post-stroke dementia, to white-matter lesions, and to cognitive impairment or dementia, and also those related to Alzheimer's disease.[8] The vascular risk factors include arterial hypertension, atrial fibrillation, myocardial infarction, coronary heart disease, diabetes, generalized atherosclerosis, lipid abnormalities, and smoking. The demographic factors include age and education. One putative protective factor is oestrogen.[93]

Knowledge of effects of primary prevention on these risk factors in populations free of cognitive impairment is still scant.[8,94] In a European study, treatment of mild systolic hypertension decreased the incidence of dementia.[95] Positive effects in primary prevention of stroke support the idea that action on vascular risk factors could reduce the numbers of patients with vascular dementia.

For secondary prevention the target is the brain already affected by cerebrovascular disease and at risk of vascular dementia. Actions include diagnosis and treatment of acute stroke in order to limit the extent of ischaemic brain changes, prevention of recurrence of stroke, and treatment of risk factors. Treatment is guided by the aetiology of cerebrovascular disorder such as large artery disease (e.g. aspirin, dipyridamole, carotid endarterectomy), cardiac embolic events (e.g. anticoagulation, aspirin), small-vessel disease (e.g. antiplatelet therapy), and haemodynamic mechanisms (e.g. control of hypotension and cardiac arrhythmias).[15,29,46] A recent large study showed some benefit from perindopril and indapamide in the prevention of post-stroke dementia.[96] Hypoxic ischaemic events (cardiac arrhythmias, congestive heart failure, myocardial infarction, seizures, pneumonia) are an important risk factor for incident dementia in patients with stroke and should be taken into account in the secondary prevention of vascular dementia.[20]

Detailed knowledge of the effects of secondary prevention of vascular dementia is lacking. In a small series of patients with established vascular dementia, control of high arterial blood pressure,[97] cessation of smoking,[97] and use of aspirin[98] improved or stabilized cognition. It has been suggested that lowering of plasma viscosity could also have an effect in vascular dementia.[99] The absence of progressive cognitive decline in patients receiving placebo in treatment trials of vascular dementia may also reflect an effect of intensified risk factor control.[89]

Further information

Erkinjuntti, T., and Gauthier, S. (eds). (2002). *Vascular cognitive impairment*. Martin Duniz Publishers, London, England.

Vascular burden of the brain. *International Psychogeriatrics* (Suppl 1) 2003.

Bowler, J. and Hachinski, V. (eds.) (2003). *Vascular cognitive impairment preventable dementia*. pp. 176–92, Oxford University Press, Oxford, UK.

Mohr, J.P., Choi, D.W., Grotta, J.C., *et al.* (2004). *Stroke: Pathophysiology, Diagnosis, and Management*, (4th edn), Philadelphia, Elsevier.

Burns, A., O'Brien, J. and Ames, D. (2005). *Dementia* (3rd edn). Edward Arnold (Publishers), London, UK.

Growdon, J.H. and Rossor, M.N. (eds.) (2007). *Blue books of practical neurology, The Dementias 2*. Butterworth Heineman Elsevier, Philadephia, PA.

Ritchie, C.W., Ames, D., Masters, C.L., *et al.* (2007). *Therapeutic strategies dementia*. Clinical Publishing, Atlas Medical Publishing Ltd, Oxford, UK.

References

1. Rocca, W.A., Hofman, A., Brayne, C., *et al.* (1991). The prevalence of vascular dementia in Europe: facts and fragments from 1980–1990 studies. EURODEM-prevalence research group. *Annals of Neurology*, **30**, 817–24.
2. Hebert, R. and Brayne, C. (1995). Epidemiology of vascular dementia. *Neuroepidemiology*, **14**, 240–57.
3. Bowler, J.V. and Hachinski, V. (1995). Vascular cognitive impairment: a new approach to vascular dementia. *Baillières Clinical Neurology*, **4**, 357–76.
4. Tatemichi, T.K. (1990). How acute brain failure becomes chronic. A view of the mechanisms and syndromes of dementia related to stroke. *Neurology*, **40**, 1652–9.
5. Chui, H.C. (1989). Dementia: a review emphasizing clinicopathologic correlation and brain–behavior relationships. *Archives of Neurology*, **46**, 806–14.

6. Desmond, D.W. (1996). Vascular dementia: a construct in evolution. *Cerebrovascular and Brain Metabolism Reviews*, **8**, 296–325.
7. Pasquier, F. and Leys, D. (1997). Why are stroke patients prone to develop dementia? *Journal of Neurology*, **244**, 135–42.
8. Skoog, I. (1998). Status of risk factors for vascular dementia. *Neuroepidemiology*, **17**, 2–9.
9. Pohjasvaara, T., Erkinjuntti, T., Vataja, R., *et al.* (1997). Dementia three months after stroke. Baseline frequency and effect of different definitions of dementia in the Helsinki Stroke Aging Memory Study (SAM) cohort. *Stroke*, **28**, 785–92.
10. Skoog, I., Nilsson, L., Palmertz, B., *et al.* (1993). A population-based study of dementia in 85-year-olds. *New England Journal of Medicine*, **328**, 153–8.
11. Wetterling, T., Kanitz, R.D., and Borgis, K.J. (1996). Comparison of different diagnostic criteria for vascular dementia (ADDTC, DSM-IV, ICD-10, NINDS-AIREN). *Stroke*, **27**, 30–6.
12. Cummings, J.L. (1994). Vascular subcortical dementias: clinical aspects. *Dementia*, **5**, 177–80.
13. Erkinjuntti, T. (1996). Clinicopathological study of vascular dementia. In *Vascular dementia. Current concepts* (eds I. Prohovnik, J. Wade, S. Knezevic, T.K. Tatemichi, and T. Erkinjuntii), pp. 73–112. Wiley, Chichester.
14. Brun, A. (1994). Pathology and pathophysiology of cerebrovascular dementia: pure subgroups of obstructive and hypoperfusive etiology. *Dementia*, **5**, 145–7.
15. Amar, K. and Wilcock, G. (1996). Vascular dementia. *British Medical Journal*, **312**, 227–31.
16. Pantoni, L. and Garcia, J.H. (1995). The significance of cerebral white matter abnormalities 100 years after Binswanger's report. A review. *Stroke*, **26**, 1293–301.
17. Erkinjuntti, T. and Hachinski, V.C. (1993). Rethinking vascular dementia. *Cerebrovascular Disease*, **3**, 3–23.
18. Skoog, I. (1994). Risk factors for vascular dementia: a review. *Dementia*, **5**, 137–44.
19. Gorelick, P.B. (1997). Status of risk factors for dementia associated with stroke. *Stroke*, **28**, 459–63.
20. Moroney, J.T., Bagiella, E., Desmond, D.W., *et al.* (1996). Risk factors for incident dementia after stroke. Role of hypoxic and ischemic disorders. *Stroke*, **27**, 1283–9.
21. Pantoni, L. and Garcia, J.H. (1997). Pathogenesis of leukoaraiosis: a review. *Stroke*, **28**, 652–9.
22. Englund, E., Brun, A., and Alling, C. (1988). White matter changes in dementia of Alzheimer's type. Biochemical and neuropathological correlates. *Brain*, **111**, 1425–39.
23. Mielke, R., Herholz, K., Grond, M., *et al.* (1992). Severity of vascular dementia is related to volume of metabolically impaired tissue. *Archives of Neurology*, **49**, 909–13.
24. Tatemichi, T.K., Paik, M., Bagiella, E., *et al.* (1994). Risk of dementia after stroke in a hospitalized cohort: results of a longitudinal study. *Neurology*, **44**, 1885–91.
25. Erkinjuntti, T., Haltia, M., Palo, J., *et al.* (1988). Accuracy of the clinical diagnosis of vascular dementia: a prospective clinical and post-mortem neuropathological study. *Journal of Neurology, Neurosurgery, and Psychiatry*, **51**, 1037–44.
26. Snowdon, D.A., Greiner, L.H., Mortimer, J.A., *et al.* (1997). Brain infarction and the clinical expression of Alzheimer disease. The Nun Study. *Journal of the American Medical Association*, **277**, 813–17.
27. Wallin, A. and Blennow, K. (1994). The clinical diagnosis of vascular dementia. *Dementia*, **5**, 181–4.
28. Chui, H.C., Victoroff, J.I., Margolin, D., *et al.* (1992). Criteria for the diagnosis of ischemic vascular dementia proposed by the State of California Alzheimer's disease diagnostic and treatment centers. *Neurology*, **42**, 473–80.
29. Konno, S., Meyer, J.S., Terayama, Y., *et al.* (1997). Classification, diagnosis and treatment of vascular dementia. *Drugs & Aging*, **11**, 361–73.
30. Roman, G.C., Tatemichi, T.K., Erkinjuntti, T., *et al.* (1993). Vascular dementia: diagnostic criteria for research studies. Report of the NINDS-AIREN International Work Group. *Neurology*, **43**, 250–60.
31. Erkinjuntti, T. (1987). Types of multi-infarct dementia. *Acta Neurologica Scandinavica*, **75**, 391–9.
32. Loeb, C. and Meyer, J.S. (1996). Vascular dementia: still a debatable entity? *Journal of the Neurological Sciences*, **143**, 31–40.
33. Roman, G.C., Erkinjuntti, T., Wallin, A., *et al.*(2002). Subcorticalischaemic vascular dementia. *Lancet Neurology*, **1**, 426–36.
34. Sulkava, R. and Erkinjuntti, T. (1987). Vascular dementia due to cardiac arrhythmias and systemic hypotension. *Acta Neurologica Scandinavica*, **76**, 123–8.
35. American Psychiatric Association. (1994). *Diagnostic and statistical manual of mental disorders* (4th edn). American Psychiatric Association, Washington, DC.
36. World Health Organization. (1993). *ICD-10 classification of mental and behavioural disorders: diagnostic criteria for research*. World Health Organization, Geneva.
37. Erkinjuntti, T., Inzitari, D., Pantoni, L., *et al.* (2000). Research criteria for subcortical vascular dementia in clinical trials. *Journal of Neural Transam*, **59**, 23–30.
38. Mahler, M.E. and Cummings, J.L. (1991). The behavioural neurology of multi-infarct dementia. *Alzheimer's Disease and Associated Disorders*, **5**, 122–30.
39. Roman, G.C. (1987). Senile dementia of the Binswanger type. A vascular form of dementia in the elderly. *Journal of the American Medical Association*, **258**, 1782–8.
40. Babikian, V. and Ropper, A.H. (1987). Binswanger's disease: a review. *Stroke*, **18**, 2–12.
41. Ishii, N., Nishihara, Y., and Imamura, T. (1986). Why do frontal lobe symptoms predominate in vascular dementia with lacunes? *Neurology*, **36**, 340–5.
42. Rockwood, K., Parhad, I., Hachinski, V., *et al.* (1994). Diagnosis of vascular dementia: consortium of Canadian centres for clinical cognitive research consensus statement. *Canadian Journal of Neurological Sciences*, **21**, 358–64.
43. Erkinjuntti, T. (1994). Clinical criteria for vascular dementia: the NINDS-AIREN criteria. *Dementia*, **5**, 189–92.
44. Erkinjuntti, T., Ostbye, T., Steenhuis, R., *et al.* (1997). The effect of different diagnostic criteria on the prevalence of dementia. *New England Journal of Medicine*, **337**, 1667–74.
45. Wetterling, T., Kanitz, R.D., and Borgis, K.J. (1994). The ICD-10 criteria for vascular dementia. *Dementia*, **5**, 185–8.
46. Erkinjuntti, T. (1997). Vascular dementia: challenge of clinical diagnosis. *International Psychogeriatrics*, **9**(Suppl. 1), 51–8.
47. Erkinjuntti, T. (1994). Clinical criteria for vascular dementia: the NINDS-AIREN criteria. *Dementia*, **5**, 189–92.
48. Gold, G., Giannakopoulos, P., Montes-Paixao, J.C., *et al.* (1997). Sensitivity and specificity of newly proposed clinical criteria for possible vascular dementia. *Neurology*, **49**, 690–4.
49. Lopez, O.L., Larumbe, M.R., Becker, J.T., *et al.* (1994). Reliability of NINDS-AIREN clinical criteria for the diagnosis of vascular dementia. *Neurology*, **44**, 1240–5.
50. Verhey, F.R., Lodder, J., Rozendaal, N., *et al.* (1996). Comparison of seven sets of criteria used for the diagnosis of vascular dementia. *Neuroepidemiology*, **15**, 166–72.
51. O'Brien, J.T. (2003). Vascular cognitive impairment. *Lancet Neurology*, **2**, 89–98.
52. Roman, G.C., Sachdev, P., Royall, D.R., *et al.* (2004). Vascular cognitive disorder: a new diagnostic category updating vascular cognitive impairment and vascular dementia. *Journal of Neurol Sc*, **226**, 81–7.
53. Bowler, J.V., Steenhuis, R., and Hachinski, V. (1999). Conceptual background of vascular cognitive impairment. *Alzheimer Disease and Associated Disorders*, **13**, S30–7.

54. Rockwood, K., Wenzel, C., Hachinski, V., *et al.* (2000). Prevalence and outcomes of vascular cognitive impairment. *Neurology*, **54**, 447–51.
55. Kalaria, R.N., Kenny, R.A., Ballard, C.G., *et al.* (2004). Towards defining the neuropathological substrates of vascular dementia. *Journal of Neurol Sci*; **226**, 75–80.
56. Desmond, D.W., Erkinjuntti, T., Sano, M., *et al.* (1999). *The cognitive syndrome of vascular dementia: implications for clinical trials. Alzh Dis Assoc Disord*, **13** (Suppl 3), S21-S9. (Review).
57. Cummings, J.L. (1993). Fronto-subcortical circuits and human behavior. *Archives of Neurology*, **50**, 873–80.
58. Hachinski, V.C., Iliff, L.D., Zilhka, E., *et al.* (1975). Cerebral blood flow in dementia. *Archives of Neurology*, **32**, 632–7.
59. Moroney, J.T., Bagiella, E., Desmond, D.W., *et al.* (1997). Meta-analysis of the Hachinski ischemic score in pathologically verified dementias. *Neurology*, **49**, 1096–105.
60. Erkinjuntti, T. (1987). Differential diagnosis between Alzheimer's disease and vascular dementia: evaluation of common clinical methods. *Acta Neurologica Scandinavica*, **76**, 433–42.
61. Mölsä, P.K., Marttila, R.J., and Rinne, U.K. (1995). Long-term survival and predictors of mortality in Alzheimer's disease and multi-infarct dementia. *Acta Neurologica Scandinavica*, **91**, 159–64.
62. Skoog, I., Nilsson, L., Palmertz, B., *et al.* (1993). A population-based study on dementia in 85-year-olds. *New England Journal of Medicine*, **328**, 153–8.
63. Chui, H.C., and Gonthier, R. (1999). Natural history of vascular dementia. *Alzheimer Dis Assoc Disord*, **13** (Suppl 23), S124–S30.
64. Folstein, M.F., Folstein, S.E., and McHugh, P.R. (1975). 'Mini-Mental State': a practical method for grading the cognitive state of patients for the clinician. *Journal of Psychiatric Research*, **12**, 189–98.
65. Royall, D. and Roman, G. (1999). Executive control function: a rational basis for the diagnosis of vascular dementia. *Alzheimer Disease and Associated Disorders*, **13**(Suppl. 3), 69–80.
66. Pohjasvaara, T., Erkinjuntti, T., Ylikoski, R., *et al.* (1998). Clinical determinants of poststroke dementia. *Stroke*, **29**, 75–81.
67. Erkinjuntti, T., Ketonen, L., Sulkava, R., *et al.* (1987). Do white matter changes on MRI and CT differentiate vascular dementia from Alzheimer's disease? *Journal of Neurology, Neurosurgery, and Psychiatry*, **50**, 37–42.
68. Erkinjuntti, T., Ketonen, L., Sulkava, R., *et al.* (1987). CT in the differential diagnosis between Alzheimer's disease and vascular dementia. *Acta Neurologica Scandinavica*, **75**, 262–70.
69. Launes, J., Sulkava, R., Erkinjuntti, T., *et al.* (1991). 99mTC-HM-PAO SPECT in suspected dementia. *Nuclear Medicine Communications*, **12**, 757–65.
70. Orrell, R.W. and Wade, J.P.H. (1996). Clinical diagnosis: how good is it and how should it be done? In *Vascular dementia. Current concepts* (eds I. Prohovnik, J. Wade, S. Knezevic, T.K. Tatemichi, and T. Erkinjuntii), pp. 143–63. Wiley, Chichester.
71. Erkinjuntti, T. and Sulkava, R. (1991). Diagnosis of multi-infarct dementia. *Alzheimer Disease and Associated Disorders*, **5**, 112–21.
72. Slooter, A.J., Tang, M.X., van Duijn, C.M., *et al.* (1997). Apolipoprotein E epsilon4 and the risk of dementia with stroke. A population-based investigation. *Journal of the American Medical Association*, **277**, 818–21.
73. McKhann, G., Drachman, D., Folstein, M., *et al.* (1984). Clinical diagnosis of Alzheimer's disease: report of the NINCDS-ADRDA work group under the auspices of Department of Health and Human Services Task Force on Alzheimer's disease. *Neurology*, **34**, 939–44.
74. Petersen, R.C. (1995). Normal aging, mild cognitive impairment, and early Alzheimer's disease. *Neurologist*, **1**, 326–44.
75. Braak, H. and Braak, E. (1991). Neuropathological staging of Alzheimer-related changes. *Acta Neuropathologica*, **82**, 239–59.
76. Roman, G.C. (1991). White matter lesions and normal-pressure hydrocephalus: Binswanger disease or Hakim syndrome? *American Journal of Neuroradiology*, **12**, 40–1.
77. McKeith, I.G., Galasko, D., Kosaka, K., *et al.* (1996). Consensus guidelines for the clinical and pathologic diagnosis of dementia with Lewy bodies (DLB): report of the consortium on DLB international workshop. *Neurology*, **47**, 1113–24.
78. Anonymous (1994). Clinical and neuropathological criteria for frontotemporal dementia. The Lund and Manchester groups. *Journal of Neurology, Neurosurgery, and Psychiatry*, **57**, 416–18.
79. Marder, K., Tang, M.X., Cote, L., *et al.* (1995). The frequency and associated risk factors for dementia in patients with Parkinson's disease. *Archives of Neurology*, **52**, 695–701.
80. Erkinjunti, T., Roman, G.C., Gauthier, S., *et al.* (2004). Emerging therapies for vascular dementia and vascular cognitive impairment. *Stroke*, **35**, 1010–17.
81. Wenning, G.K., Be-Sholomon, Y., Magalhaes, M., *et al.* (1995). Clinicopathological study of 35 cases of multiple system atrophy. *Journal of Neurology, Neurosurgery, and Psychiatry*, **58**, 160–6.
82. Jorm, A.F., Korten, A.E., and Henderson, A.S. (1987). The prevalence of dementia: a quantitative integration of the literature. *Acta Psychiatrica Scandinavica*, **76**, 465–79.
83. Rocca, W.A., Hofman, A., Brayne, C., *et al.* (1991). The prevalence of vascular dementia in Europe: facts and fragments from 1980–1990 studies. *Annals of Neurology*, **30**, 817–24.
84. Tatemichi, T.K., Desmond, D.W., Mayeux, R., *et al.* (1992). Dementia after stroke: baseline frequency, risks, and clinical features in a hospitalized cohort. *Neurology*, **42**, 1185–93.
85. Hachinski, V. (1992). Preventable senility: a call for action against the vascular dementias. *Journal of the American Geriatrics Society*, **340**, 645–8.
86. Knezevic, S., Labs, K.H., Kittner, B., *et al.* (1996). The treatment of vascular dementia: problems and prospects. In *Vascular dementia. Current concepts* (eds I. Prohovnik, J. Wade, S. Knezevic, T.K. Tatemichi, and T. Erkinjuntii), pp. 301–12. Wiley, Chichester.
87. Pantoni, L., Carosi, M., Amigoni, S., *et al.* (1996). A preliminary open trial with nimodipine in patients with cognitive impairment and leukoaraiosis. *Clinical Neuropharmacology*, **19**, 497–506.
88. Görtelmeyer, R. and Erbler, H. (1992). Memantine in treatment of mild to moderate dementia syndrome. *Drug Research*, **42**, 904–12.
89. Rother, M., Erkinjuntti, T., Roessner, M., *et al.* (1998). Propentofylline in the treatment of Alzheimer's disease and vascular dementia. *Dementia*, **9**(Suppl. 1), 36–43.
90. Erkinjuntti, T. (1999). Cerebrovascular dementia: a guide to diagnosis and treatment. *CNS Drugs*, **12**, 35–48.
91. Erkinjunti, T., *et al.* (2004). Emerging therapies for vascular dementia and vascular cognitive impairment. *Stroke*, **35**, 1010–17.
92. Erkinjuntti, T., *et al.* (2002). Efficacy of galantamine in probable vascular dementia and Alzheimer's disease combined with cerebrovascular disease: a randomised trial. *Lancet*, **359**, 1283–90.
93. Mortel, K.F. and Meyer, J.S. (1995). Lack of postmenopausal estrogen replacement therapy and the risk of dementia. *Journal of Neuropsychiatry and Clinical Neurosciences*, **7**, 334–7.
94. Skoog, I. (1997). The relationship between blood pressure and dementia: a review. *Biomedicine and Pharmacotherapy*, **51**, 367–75.
95. Forette, F., Seux, M.L., Staessen, J.A., *et al.* (1998). Prevention of dementia in randomised double-blind placebo-controlled Systolic Hypertension in Europe (Syst-Eur) trial. *Journal of the American Geriatrics Society*, **352**, 1347–51.
96. Tzourio, C., *et al.* (2003). Effects of blood pressure lowering with perindopril and indapamide therapy on dementia and cognitive decline in patients with cerebrovascular disease. *Archives of Internal Medicine*, **163**, 1069–75.

97. Meyer, J.S., Judd, B.W., Tawaklna, T., *et al.* (1986). Improved cognition after control of risk factors for multi-infarct dementia. *Journal of the American Medical Association*, **256**, 2203–9.
98. Meyer, J.S., Rogers, R.L., McClintic, K., *et al.* (1989). Randomized clinical trial of daily aspirin therapy in multi-infarct dementia. A pilot study. *Journal of the American Geriatrics Society*, **37**, 549–55.
99. Lechner, H. (1998). Status of treatment of vascular dementia. *Neuroepidemiology*, **17**, 10–13.

4.1.9 Dementia due to HIV disease

Mario Maj

Introduction

The first description of a syndrome consisting of cognitive, motor, and behavioural disturbances in patients with AIDS was published in 1986.[1] The syndrome was named 'AIDS dementia complex'. In 1990, the World Health Organization (WHO) introduced the term 'HIV-associated dementia',[2] pointing out that subclinical or mild cognitive and/or motor dysfunctions without impairment of performance in daily living activities cannot be subsumed under the term 'dementia'. The expression 'mild cognitive/motor disorder' was proposed for those conditions. The same distinction was made in 1991 by the American Academy of Neurology,[3] which identified an 'HIV-associated dementia complex' and an 'HIV-associated minor cognitive/motor disorder'. The present chapter focuses on the dementia syndrome associated with HIV infection.

Clinical features

The onset of HIV-associated dementia is usually insidious. Early cognitive symptoms include forgetfulness, loss of concentration, mental slowing, and reduced performance on sequential mental activities of some complexity (the subject misses appointments, or needs lists to recall ordinary duties; loses track of conversations or his or her own train of thought; needs additional time and effort to organize thoughts and to complete daily tasks). Early behavioural symptoms include apathy, reduced spontaneity and emotional responsivity, and social withdrawal (the subject becomes indifferent to his or her personal and professional responsibilities; his or her work production decreases, as well as the frequency of social interactions; the subject complains of early fatiguability, malaise, and loss of sexual drive). Depression, irritability or emotional lability, agitation, and psychotic symptoms may also occur. Early motor symptoms include loss of balance and coordination, clumsiness, and leg weakness; the subject is less precise in normal hand activities, such as writing and eating, drops things more often than usual, trips and falls more frequently, and perceives the need to exercise more care in walking.[1,4]

Routine mental status tests, in this early stage, may be normal or show only slowing in verbal or motor responses and/or difficulty in recalling a series of objects after 5 min or more. Neurological examination may show tremor (best seen when the patient sustains a posture, such as holding the arms and fingers outstretched), hyperreflexia (particularly of the lower extremities), ataxia (usually seen only on rapid turns or tandem gait), slowing of rapid alternating movements (of the fingers, wrists, or feet), frontal release signs (snout reflex, palmar grasp), dysarthria. Tests of ocular motility may show interruption of smooth pursuits, and slowing or inaccuracy of saccades.

In the late stages of the disease, there is usually a global deterioration of cognitive functions and a severe psychomotor retardation. Speech is slow and monotonous, with word-finding difficulties and possible progression to mutism. Patients become unable to walk, due to paraparesis, and usually lie in bed indifferent to their illness and their surroundings. Bladder and bowel incontinence are common. Myoclonus and seizures may occur. Pedal paraesthesias and hypersensitivity may appear, due to concurrent sensory neuropathy. The level of consciousness is usually preserved, except for occasional hypersomnolence.

Classification

The WHO criteria for HIV-associated dementia[2] are as follows:

1 The research criteria for dementia of the ICD-10 are met, with some modifications:
   (a) decline in memory may not be severe enough to impair activities of daily living;
   (b) decline in motor function may be present, and is verified by clinical examination and, when possible, formal neuropsychological testing;
   (c) the minimum requested duration of symptoms is 1 month;
   (d) aphasia, agnosia, and apraxia are unusual.
2 Laboratory evidence for systemic HIV infection is present.
3 No evidence of another aetiology from history, physical examination, or laboratory tests should be present (specifically, cerebrospinal fluid analysis and either computed tomography (CT) or magnetic resonance imaging (MRI) should be done to exclude active central nervous system opportunistic processes).

The American Academy of Neurology criteria[3] require the following:

1 Laboratory evidence for systemic HIV infection.
2 Acquired abnormality in at least two of the following cognitive abilities (present for at least 1 month): attention/concentration, speed of processing of information, abstraction/reasoning, visuospatial skills, memory/learning, and speech/language.
3 At least one of the following:
   (a) acquired abnormality in motor function or performance;
   (b) decline in motivation or emotional control or change in social behaviour.
4 Absence of clouding of consciousness during a period long enough to establish the presence of 2.
5 Absence of evidence of another aetiology.

Both the WHO and the American Academy of Neurology criteria distinguish three levels of severity of the dementia syndrome (mild, moderate, and severe), on the basis of the degree of the impairment in activities of daily living.

Diagnosis and differential diagnosis

Neuropsychological tests

Neuropsychological examination supports the clinical diagnosis of HIV-associated dementia, by providing evidence of cognitive and motor dysfunction. Moreover, it may be useful in the differential diagnosis with a depressive syndrome.

The most prominent impairment is observed on tests of fine motor control (finger tapping, grooved pegboard), rapid sequential problem solving (trail-making A and B, digit symbol), visuospatial problem solving (block design), spontaneity (verbal fluency), and visual memory (visual reproduction). In contrast, naming and vocabulary skills are largely preserved even in the most advanced cases.

The signs that should alert to the possible presence of a depressive 'pseudodementia' are as follows:[5]

1 the intratest variability of performance (i.e. missing easy items and then correctly answering more difficult questions);

2 mood-congruent complaints, which are at odds with objective performance (i.e. the subject complains of having difficulties with a test, whereas his or her performance is near perfect);

3 responses of 'I don't know' or giving up, which are followed by the correct answer, when the subject is further urged to respond.

It should be considered, however, that dementia and depression may coexist in HIV-seropositive subjects.

Brain imaging

Brain imaging provides additional support to the diagnosis of HIV-associated dementia, especially by excluding central nervous system opportunistic processes, in particular cerebral toxoplasmosis and primary central nervous system lymphoma.

The predominant finding in HIV-associated dementia is cerebral atrophy: both CT and MRI demonstrate widened cortical sulci and, less commonly, enlarged ventricles. Furthermore, MRI frequently shows high-intensity signal abnormalities on the T_2-weighted image (diffuse widespread involvement, patchy localized involvement, focal distinct areas of involvement, or punctuate white-matter hyperdensities). These lesions are without mass effect and are most commonly located in the periventricular white matter and the centrum semiovale (less frequently, in the basal ganglia or in the thalamus).

As to differential diagnosis, both CT and MRI are able to demonstrate the multiple bilateral ring-enhancing lesions that are characteristic of cerebral toxoplasmosis, and the contrast-enhancing mass lesions of primary central nervous system lymphoma.

Cerebrospinal fluid analysis

Cerebrospinal fluid analysis can support the clinical diagnosis of HIV-associated dementia, especially by excluding several central nervous system opportunistic infections, in particular cryptococcal meningitis.

The most frequent cerebrospinal fluid findings in HIV-associated dementia are the increase of total proteins and of the IgG fraction and index. A mononuclear pleocytosis may occur. The presence of the HIV core antigen p24 can be detected, although this finding is possible also in neurologically normal subjects. HIV RNA can be demonstrated in the cerebrospinal fluid by using the polymerase chain reaction. Increased cerebrospinal fluid levels of neopterin, β_2-microglobulin, and quinolinic acid (non-specific markers of immune activation), soluble Fas and Fas ligand (associated with apoptosis), as well as several cytokines (interleukin 1β, interleukin 6, tumour necrosis factor-α), have been reported, but may be detected also during central nervous system opportunistic infections.

As to differential diagnosis, Indian ink staining, cryptococcal antigen titres, and fungal culture can be decisive for the identification of cryptococcal meningitis. Other central nervous system opportunistic infections that can be identified by cerebrospinal fluid analysis include central nervous system tuberculosis, cytomegalovirus encephalitis, and neurosyphilis.

Epidemiology

There has been a decrease in the incidence of HIV-associated dementia after the introduction of highly active antiretroviral therapy (HAART): while between 1990 and 1992 the mean incidence was 21.1 cases per 1000 person-years, between 1996 and 1998 it decreased to 10.5 cases per 1000 person-years.[6] However, the incidence seems to have increased again in 2003.[7] A post-mortem neuropathologic study reported that, while severe HIV encephalopathy was not detected anymore in the HAART era, the prevalence of mild and moderate encephalopathy increased, probably reflecting the longer survival time after initial HIV infection.[8]

Pathogenesis

HIV crosses the blood-brain barrier by a Trojan-horse-type mechanism, using the macrophages it infects.[9] Once in the brain, it infects glial cells. Infected and activated macrophages and microglia release neurotoxins which lead to neuronal damage and apoptosis.[10] It is possible that direct effects of viral proteins on neurones also contribute to neurodegeneration. Post-mortem studies have revealed the presence of HIV in frontal lobes, subcortical white matter and the basal ganglia.[11]

Course and prognosis

In the pre-HAART era, HIV-associated dementia often progressed rapidly to severe deterioration and death, especially in patients with advanced systemic disease. Today, many patients present an attenuated form which is slowly progressive or static. The mean survival, which was 5 months in 1993–1995, increased to 38.5 months in 1996–2000.[12] Prominent psychomotor slowing, a history of intravenous drug use and low CD4 T-lymphocyte count seem to predict a more rapid progression.[13]

Available treatments

Antiretrovirals are not always successful in crossing the blood-brain barrier, but, as mentioned above, have been able to reduce the incidence and modify the course of HIV-associated dementia. There is evidence that they can improve specific aspects of cognitive functioning, such as psychomotor speed performance, in people with HIV-associated dementia.[14] The optimal HAART regimen for the treatment of HIV-associated dementia has not been established.

Neuroprotective drugs whose beneficial effect on cognitive performance in patients with HIV infection has been preliminarily documented include the monoamine oxidase inhibitor deprenyl (a putative antioxidant and antiapoptotic agent) and peptide T (which blocks the HIV gp120 envelope protein). Other investigational drugs include memantine and nitroglycerin (which are *N*-methyl-D-aspartate receptor antagonists), nimodipine (a calcium-channel blocker), pentoxifylline (an inhibitor of the production and activity of tumour necrosis factor-α), and lexipafant (an antagonist of platelet-activating factor).

The psychostimulant methylphenidate has been found to be useful in treating apathy and cognitive slowing in patients with HIV-associated dementia, with relatively mild side effects. Only anecdotal evidence is available concerning the usefulness of cholinesterase inhibitors such as donepezil.

Patients with AIDS, when treated with typical antipsychotic drugs for the presence of psychotic symptoms or behavioural dyscontrol, are particularly prone to develop extrapyramidal side effects and neuroleptic malignant syndrome. According to preliminary research evidence, some atypical antipsychotics are well tolerated even by patients who had to stop standard neuroleptics due to extrapyramidal side effects.

AIDS patients with depressed mood have been found to respond to tricyclic antidepressants and selective serotonin reuptake inhibitors (SSRIs) as well as HIV-seronegative subjects. There is a preliminary evidence that SSRIs (or at least some of them) are better tolerated than tricyclic antidepressants, except in patients with diarrhoea.

Management

Patients with HIV-associated dementia often have additional disease processes which may aggravate the cognitive impairment, including secondary infections and metabolic disturbances. These conditions should be adequately diagnosed and managed.

An appropriate HAART regimen should be implemented and constantly monitored (taking into account that cognitive dysfunction may have a negative impact on adherence to treatment). If psychotic symptoms, behavioural dyscontrol, or mood disturbances are present, the same strategies which are used for other people with these problems should be implemented, taking into account that HIV-infected patients have an increased sensitivity to the side effects of antipsychotics and antidepressants, and that adverse interactions may occur between psychotropic drugs and antiretrovirals (for instance, the administration of St. John's Wort induces the metabolism of the protease inhibitor indinavir, thus decreasing its serum concentration to levels which may cause treatment failure).[15] Methylphenidate (5–20 mg/day) may be used to reduce apathy and psychomotor slowing.

Psychosocial interventions in HIV-associated dementia should include maintenance of a structured daily schedule, titration of external stimuli, restriction to familiar environments, frequent orienting interactions with significant others, and monitoring of personal and financial affairs. Psychoeducational intervention with families and significant others is also essential.

The care of patients with HIV-associated dementia will make increasing demands on health services, as well as on volunteer and community support systems. It is uncertain, at present, whether such care is best provided in specialized units (e.g. inpatient AIDS units), or within general psychiatric or medical services. Special management problems may arise when the behavioural disturbance (e.g. poor impulse control, sexual acting-out behaviour) is such as to constitute a risk for other patients or staff members. Placement of patients in the terminal stage of the disease may also represent a problem: the lack of appropriate options in the community may obstruct their timely and humane discharge from the hospital.

Further information

Dougherty, R.H., Skolasky, R.L., and McArthur, J.C. (2002). Progression of HIV-associated dementia treated with HAART. *The AIDS Reader*, **12**, 69–74.

Kaul, M. and Lipton, S.A. (2006). Mechanisms of neuronal injury and death in HIV-1 associated dementia. *Current HIV Research*, **4**, 307–18.

Maj, M., Starace, F., and Sartorius, N. (1993). *Mental disorders in HIV-1 infection and AIDS*. Hogrefe and Huber, Bern.

References

1. Navia, B.A., Jordan, B.D., and Price, R.W. (1986). The AIDS dementia complex: I. clinical picture. *Annals of Neurology*, **19**, 517–24.
2. World Health Organization. (1990). Report of the Second Consultation on the Neuropsychiatric Aspects of HIV-1 Infection, Geneva, 11–13 January 1990. World Health Organization, Geneva.
3. American Academy of Neurology AIDS Task Force. (1991). Nomenclature and research case definitions for the neurological manifestations of human immunodeficiency virus type-1 infection. *Neurology*, **41**, 778–85.
4. Maj, M. (1990). Organic mental disorders in HIV-1 infection. *AIDS*, **4**, 831–40.
5. Van Gorp, W.G., Satz, P., Hinkin, C., *et al.* (1989). The neuropsychological aspects of HIV-1 spectrum disease. *Psychiatric Medicine*, **7**, 59–78.
6. Sacktor, N., Lyles, R.H., Skolasky, R., *et al.* (2001). HIV-associated neurologic disease incidence changes: multicenter AIDS cohort study, 1990–1998. *Neurology*, **56**, 257–60.
7. McArthur, J.C. (2004). HIV dementia: an evolving disease. *Journal of Neuroimmunology*, **157**, 3–10.
8. Neuenburg, J.K., Brodt, H.R., Herndier, B.G., *et al.* (2002). HIV-related neuropathology, 1985 to 1999: rising prevalence of HIV encephalopathy in the era of highly active antiretroviral therapy. *Journal of Acquired Immune Deficiency Syndromes*, **31**, 171–7.
9. Lawrence, D.M. and Major, E.O. (2002). HIV-1 and the brain: connections between HIV-1-associated dementia, neuropathology and neuroimmunology. *Microbes and Infection*, **4**, 301–8.
10. Nath, A. (2002). Human immunodeficiency virus (HIV) proteins in neuropathogenesis of HIV dementia. *Journal of Infectious Diseases*, **186**(Suppl. 2), S193–8.
11. Kaul, M., Garden, G.A., and Lipton, S.A. (2001). Pathways to neuronal injury and apoptosis in HIV-associated dementia. *Nature*, **410**, 988–94.
12. Dore, G.J., McDonald, A., Li, Y., *et al.* (2003). Marked improvement in survival following AIDS dementia complex in the era of highly active antiretroviral therapy. *AIDS*, **17**, 1539–45.
13. Bouwman, F.H., Skolasky, R., Hes, D., *et al.* (1998). Variable progression of HIV-associated dementia. *Neurology*, **50**, 1814–20.
14. Sacktor, N.C., Lyles, R.H., Skolasky, R., *et al.* (1999). Combination antiretroviral therapy improves psychomotor speed performance in HIV-seropositive homosexual men. *Neurology*, **52**, 1640–6.
15. Piscitelli, S.C., Burstein, A.H., Chaitt, D., *et al.* (2000). Indinavir concentrations and St. John's Wort. *Lancet*, **355**, 547–8.

4.1.10 The neuropsychiatry of head injury

Simon Fleminger

Head injury 'imparts at a blow both physical and psychological trauma',[1] and the consequences are often devastating and enduring.[2] Not infrequently head injury leads to a psychiatric consultation, which will need to take into account the interplay between the brain and its injuries as well as the psychodynamic processes that follow from the injury.

In the immediate aftermath of the head injury, the management rests with the acute surgical and medical team.[3] The psychiatrist is usually not involved at this stage. Nevertheless, to understand the later neuropsychiatric effects of head injury it is first necessary to know what happens to the brain when it is injured.

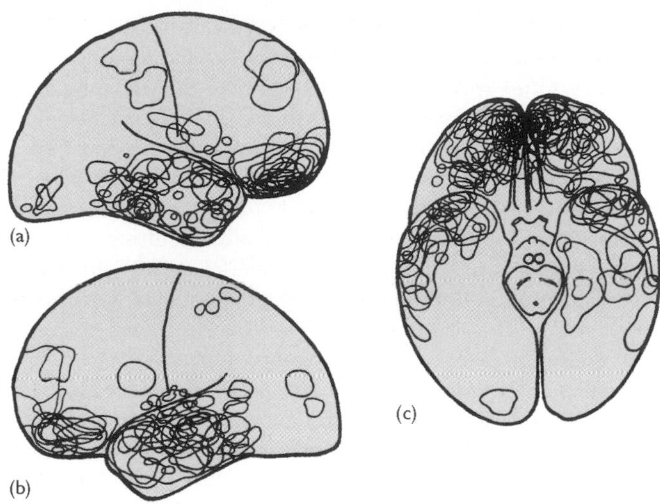

Fig. 4.1.10.1 A composite of the contusions found in 50 cases of people dying from head injury. (Reproduced with permission from Courville, C.B. (1937). *Pathology of the central nervous system*, Part IV. Pacific Press, Mountain View, CA)

Neuropathology

Open head injuries

In open head injuries there is penetration of the skull often with considerable destruction of brain tissue local to the trauma, but relatively less at a distance—particularly for lower velocity injuries such as stabbing. Open head injuries may therefore be associated with little, if any, loss of consciousness, which is generally a marker of diffuse brain injury.

Closed head injuries

(a) Contusions

In closed head injuries acceleration/deceleration forces and shearing forces damage the brain. The soft brain moves within its hard bony box and is damaged. Contusion of the brain occurs, ranging from slight localized small vessel bleeding into surrounding tissue to almost complete local destruction of the brain.

The medial orbital frontal cortex and the tips and undersurface of the temporal lobes are particularly vulnerable to contusions (Fig. 4.1.10.1). The brain becomes traumatized on adjacent bone of the floor of the skull. Contrecoup localization of contusions is sometimes evident.

(b) Intracerebral haemorrhage

Localized haemorrhage into the brain occurs at the site of a contusion. Scattered intracerebral haemorrhages found at the interface between grey and white matter are thought to be associated with diffuse axonal injury (see below). A large isolated haematoma suggests that a blood vessel has ruptured.

In very severe injury haemorrhages are also found round the aqueduct in the brainstem, perhaps caused by distortion of the brainstem as a result of cerebral herniation into the posterior fossa due to raised intracranial pressure. They are associated with prolonged coma or death.

(c) Extradural and subdural haemorrhage

Haemorrhage into the extradural or subdural space will act as a space-occupying lesion and contribute to raised intracranial pressure. The extradural haemorrhage, being under high pressure, can rapidly cause coma and death. The patient may 'talk and die', regaining consciousness after the head injury, only to lapse a few hours later into severe coma. Without acute neurosurgical intervention to drain the blood these patients will die.

Subdural haematomas tend to run a subacute course and as such are of more interest to the psychiatrist. They may present with a failure to improve, or fluctuating drowsiness, weeks or months after the head injury. They may regress spontaneously or may require surgical drainage, but they do have a propensity to recur.

(d) Diffuse axonal injury

Diffuse axonal injury occurs in the white matter tracts of the cerebral hemispheres, including the corpus callosum, and the brainstem, particularly the cerebellar peduncles. Axons break up over the course of the first 24 to 48 h following brain trauma with the formation of 'retraction balls'-globular structures at the end of transected axons.[4]

(e) Oedema and ischaemia

Oedema of damaged brain occurs over the first few hours following brain injury. The resulting raised intracranial pressure compromises the cerebral circulation and results in ischaemia, which may further contribute to brain injury. Cerebral oedema tends to resolve over the course of a few days or weeks.

(f) Neuronal death

Two fairly distinct processes result in neuronal death from traumatic brain injury.[4] Necrotic cell death occurs when there is massive cell disruption either from the direct effects of the trauma on the cell membrane or from anoxia. It is a relatively passive process though may involve toxic effects of high levels of intracellular calcium, excitatory transmitters, and free radicals. On the other hand apoptotic cell death, 'cell suicide', is a more active process triggered by various routes including ligand binding to cell death receptors. These activate, for example, endonucleases which attack cellular DNA. Markers of apoptotic cell death are elevated in the days and weeks after injury.

(g) Late effects

Ventriculomegaly may develop over the weeks and months following injury. Often it is the result of atrophy of the white matter of the cerebral hemispheres, usually attributed to diffuse axonal injury, and is associated with atrophy of the corpus callosum. More localized atrophy is observed when contusions resolve to leave a loss of brain tissue.

Of greater importance is hydrocephalus resulting from the residual effects of subarachnoid blood interfering with the normal cerebrospinal fluid flow and preventing it from escaping into the venous system. This may require insertion of a ventriculo-peritoneal shunt to prevent deterioration in cognitive function.

Fractures to the floor of the skull, particularly if they are associated with cerebrospinal fluid leaks, may allow infection into the subarachnoid space, causing meningitis sometimes years after injury. Cerebral abscesses may take months before they become clinically evident.

Box 4.1.10.1 Clinical indicators of head injury severity

- The duration of retrograde amnesia—the period leading up to the injury for which memories have been lost. Tends to shrink as the patient recovers.
- The depth of unconsciousness as assessed by the worst score on the Glasgow Coma Scale—a score of 3 indicates absent responses with severe coma, 15 is normal consciousness.
- The duration of coma—this may be difficult to ascertain because of routine sedation and ventilation following severe head injuries.
- Neurological evidence of cerebral injury—abnormality on neuroimaging or EEG.
- The duration of post-traumatic amnesia—interval between injury and the return of normal day-to-day memories.

Loss of consciousness following head injury

The mechanism of loss of consciousness after mild blows to the head is poorly understood. Based on animal work some researchers suggest it is produced by activation of cholinergic nuclei in the pons.(5)

Loss of consciousness lasting for more than a few minutes is likely to damage either cortical areas necessary for consciousness or the subcortical arousal systems. Raised intracranial pressure, partly as a result of compromising cerebral circulation, causes coma. Large or multiple haematomas are likely to be associated with a period of coma, particularly if they are associated with cerebral oedema.

Some patients, however, show prolonged coma with little to be found on brain scan apart from some evidence of generalized cerebral oedema. In these patients, diffuse axonal injury may be the cause of their coma, possibly by damaging the white matter tracts that carry arousal signals from the brainstem to the cortex.

Remember that the head injury may have been caused by an accident triggered by a loss of consciousness, for example, due to hypoglycaemia, alcohol intoxication, or an epileptic fit. Systemic effects (e.g. hypoxaemia or fat emboli) may exacerbate unconsciousness due to head trauma, as may drug intoxication.

Head injury severity

It is surprisingly difficult to predict the degree of brain injury from the size of the blow to the head. Some patients after a severe blow to the head sustain little injury to the brain. Others will suffer severe brain injury associated with prolonged unconsciousness, merely as a result of hitting their head on the ground by falling over from the standing position. Perhaps in the very occasional case significant brain injury occurs when there is no, or only momentary, loss of consciousness (see post-concussion syndrome below). The presence of a skull fracture says little about the severity of the brain injury incurred.

There are several clinical indicators of head injury severity (Box 4.1.10.1). Of these the duration of retrograde amnesia is probably the least valuable: it correlates very poorly with head injury severity.

The duration of post-traumatic amnesia is probably the best marker of outcome,(6) and is particularly useful because it can be assessed retrospectively. Most patients with a post-traumatic amnesia of less than 1 week will be left with little if any disability, while a duration of more than 1 month indicates that there is likely to be enduring and significant disability.

Predictors of a worse outcome after head injury are a previous head injury, older age, *APOE e4* positive status, and alcohol dependence.

There is no universally accepted classification of head injury severity. However, the most widely used grading system is based on the lowest rating of the Glasgow Coma Scale (**GCS**)(7) following injury.

- Mild: GCS score 13 to 15. Likely to be associated with a loss of consciousness of less than 30 min and a post-traumatic amnesia of less than 24 h. There must be clinical evidence of concussion.
- Moderate: GCS score 9 to 12. Likely to be associated with a loss of consciousness of more than a few minutes but less than 6 h and a post-traumatic amnesia of more than 1 day but less than 2 weeks.
- Severe: GCS score 3 to 8. Likely to be associated with a loss of consciousness of more than 6 h or a post-traumatic amnesia of more than 2 weeks.

Epidemiology

On average 200–300/100 000 population attend hospital with a head injury every year.(8) About one-sixth of those attending hospital will be admitted. This reflects the fact that about 80 per cent of head injuries are mild, 10 per cent moderate, and 10 per cent severe.

At greatest risk are 15- to 25-year-olds. The sex ratio is about two to three males to one female. Risk factors include alcohol misuse as well as lower socio-economic class. Road traffic accidents are the largest single cause of head injury in most civilian cohorts, followed by assaults and falls. A significant proportion will sustain their head injury as a result of deliberate self-harm.

The prevalence rate for those experiencing considerable disability as a result of head injury is in the order of 100 per 100 000.

Investigations

Neuroimaging

In the emergency room or on the trauma unit CT brain scanning is generally the preferred investigation, with its faster acquisition time and good visualization of subdural and extradural haematomas.

For later neuropsychiatric assessment magnetic resonance imaging (MRI) is preferred.[9] Cerebral contusions are often found near the bone–brain interface (see above) where the image quality of CT is reduced because of imaging artefacts from the adjacent bone. MRI has no such limitation and generally has better sensitivity and anatomical definition. MRI is able to detect, on T_2-weighted images, changes in signal associated with a diffuse axonal injury when the white matter would have appeared normal on CT brain imaging. Gradient echo MRI sequences should be performed to detect haemosiderin deposits from old small traumatic haemorrhages.

Despite its greater sensitivity a normal MRI does not rule out significant brain injury. On the other hand, particularly in the elderly, MRI may detect abnormalities unrelated to the head injury. It may not be possible to perform an MRI scan if there is magnetic material present in the body (e.g. a pacemaker).

The MRI scan can be normal and yet functional imaging of cerebral metabolism using single-photon emission computed tomography or positron-emission tomography will detect abnormalities. In general, changes on functional imaging correlate better with neuropsychological test performance than do lesions found on structural imaging.[10] However, abnormalities on functional imaging are not necessarily due to brain injury. Hypometabolism may be seen in mental illness without brain injury, for example in depression. Marked hypometabolism on positron-emission tomography imaging has been observed in a man with cognitive impairment occurring immediately after a psychological trauma.[11] He had sustained no head injury.

Electroencephalography

Electroencephalography (EEG) may be useful in the investigation of a deteriorating conscious level or unexpectedly prolonged unconsciousness, and in the investigation of unusual behavioural disturbances that may be attributable to epilepsy. However, EEG is not a good predictor of post-traumatic epilepsy and is generally not useful as a guide to prognosis.

Neuropsychological assessment

A neuropsychological assessment is an invaluable accompaniment to the psychiatric history and examination, and good liaison with the neuropsychologist is essential. Areas of impaired performance can be documented and quantified. This is often useful as a baseline for future assessments and to guide rehabilitation.

The National Adult Reading Test, for people whose first language is English, gives a good estimate of pre-injury IQ.[12] This can then be compared with the present performance on cognitive testing, to estimate the impairment produced by the head injury.

Subtle neuropsychological impairments, which are often not obvious clinically, suggest that the patient may have more problems when they return to work than would otherwise have been expected. On the other hand, if there is clinical evidence of underperformance, and yet standard neuropsychological test results are normal, then it is particularly important that executive function is tested.[13]

Function and health

Psychological symptoms far outstrip neurophysical symptoms (e.g. hemiparesis or dysarthria) as determinants of chronic disability and suffering, both of the patient and their carer, following brain injury.

The ideas encapsulated in the International Classification of Functioning, Disability and Health (ICF) (http://www3.who.int/icf/icftemplate.cfm) are important for understanding recovery from brain injury. ICF is so named because it wishes to emphasize health and functioning by moving away from a dichotomous distinction between those who are healthy and those who are disabled. ICF is a development of the earlier classification ICIDH based on:

- Impairments—abnormalities of structure, or physiological or psychological function.
- Disability—concerned with performance of activities.
- Handicap—reflects limitations fulfilling the person's normal social role and participation in society. It is very responsive to external, e.g. environmental and societal, factors.

In ICF an individual's position on the spectrum between health and disability is considered according to (i) functioning and disability and (ii) contextual factors. ICF details the environmental impacts on functioning, e.g. the consequences of living in an area prone to flooding in somebody who is wheelchair dependent. What a person can do in a standard environment (their capacity) is distinguished from what they actually do in their usual environment (their performance).

Recovery and long-term outcome from head injury

Most recovery takes place in the first year. As a general rule, the milder the head injury the sooner the patient achieves the asymptote of their recovery curve. After a mild head injury most patients will have fully recovered within 6 months. After very severe injury significant further improvements in impairment may be seen after the first year post-injury. Neuropsychological impairments tend to continue improving after neurophysical impairments are static. Nevertheless most of the recovery of cognitive function occurs within the first year.[14] Psychiatric symptoms, with their multifactorial aetiology, generally show no simple pattern of recovery.

Improvement in functioning and participation may continue long after the recovery of the underlying impairment has stopped. These further improvements often reflect improved coping strategies and environmental measures to facilitate independence. This will be the focus of the community rehabilitation team as they attempt to help minimize handicap, for example by improving access to local shops. Memory aids may enable the person to return to work. Continuing improvements in participation in social life and work can take place 5 to 10 years after head injury.[15]

But sometimes early gains are made, for example as a result of being in a return-to-work rehabilitation programme, which are subsequently lost over the longer term. In one study,[16] 25 per cent had deteriorated at 5 years follow-up, with a similar proportion improving compared with how they were at 6 months. Those who deteriorated were more depressed and anxious, had lower self-esteem and had more problems with alcohol than those who improved.

In the longer term, decades after injury, it has been suggested that the reduced reserve of the injured brain makes it particularly vulnerable to the effects of ageing. Some studies have found an accelerated cognitive decline compared with age matched controls, for example in head-injured soldiers 25 years later.[17] Head injury may be a risk factor for the development of Alzheimer's disease, particularly in men.[18] However the evidence, both for an accelerated cognitive decline and for an increased risk of Alzheimer's disease, is inconsistent.

Aetiology of psychological sequelae

To understand the mental symptoms that follow head injury it is necessary to know about the person who has been injured, what brain injuries they sustained, and the consequences. However, the interaction between these is complex and poorly understood.

Pre-traumatic factors

People who take risks or get into fights are more likely to sustain a head injury; therefore these personality traits, present before injury, are over-represented in head-injury survivors. Young men are at high risk, as are those who have already had a head injury or have cognitive dysfunction.[19]

The poor social adjustment of many patients before the head injury partly explains why so many run into behavioural problems afterwards. But premorbid characteristics do not strongly predict who will develop emotional and behavioural problems. Nevertheless, traumatic brain injury probably has the potential to turn pre-injury personality traits into post-injury personality disorders.

The trauma

The extent of brain injury probably explains less than 10 per cent of the variance in the amount of psychiatric morbidity that follows brain injury.[20] In general, early psychiatric symptoms, within weeks and months of the injury, correlate better with the extent and location of brain injury than do late psychiatric symptoms. Left hemisphere damage seems to be associated with greater psychiatric morbidity. Specific relationships between the location of brain injury and the psychiatric symptoms are discussed below.

But the head injury is also a psychological trauma. Amnesia for the event, as a result of the head injury, protects against post-traumatic stress disorder. However, it is a mistake to believe that amnesia for the event prevents a psychological stress reaction to the event itself.

- The meaning of the event may be distressing to the patient.[21] In the case of assaults, the head injury may signal the potential for further assaults. An accident may have been life-threatening and a shocking reminder to the patient that they are mortal. They may feel aggrieved by an employer's negligent action that caused the accident.
- The patient may be amnesic for the event, lacking explicit memories of what happened, but retain implicit memory of what happened. The consequences of these implicit memories may be akin to that observed in one of Claperède's amnesic patients.[22] The doctor shook the patient's hand, pricking it while doing so with a concealed drawing pin. The next day the patient could not remember having met the doctor, but flinched from shaking his hand when it was offered.
- They may have islets of intact memories that may be extremely frightening.[23]

Post-traumatic factors

Post-traumatic factors deserve special attention because they are most likely to be amenable to intervention. The psychiatrist needs to consider the patient's reaction to any disability, as well as the consequences of the disability on the role of the patient in the family and society. There may be reinforcing cycles of maladaptive behaviour, and compensation claims may complicate the picture.

Cognitive impairment

Cognitive impairment correlates with measures of head injury severity better than any of the other mental sequelae. For example, there is a strong correlation between the duration of post-traumatic amnesia and the severity of cognitive impairment.

Attention and concentration

Non-specific cognitive impairments include slowness and reduced concentration. The severely injured patient is likely to be stimulus bound, i.e. responding to each and every stimulus they are exposed to in a rather concrete way. At the same time they may show perseveration, with previous responses inappropriately interfering with the answers to subsequent questions, or when the topic of a conversation has been changed.

Dysexecutive syndrome

More specific impairments, generally referred to as the dysexecutive syndrome, result from a disturbance of the executive system responsible for organizing, planning, scheduling, prioritizing, and monitoring cognitive activities.[24] In some patients with isolated medial orbito-frontal lesions or dorso-lateral prefrontal lesions, the dysexecutive syndrome may stand alone. Disturbance of the executive system also results in difficulties in attending to two things at once, and distractibility.

Patients with the dysexecutive syndrome may be much more impaired in everyday life than is predicted by their performance on standard neuropsychological tests. They can manage with the clear instructions of the well-structured and constrained test situation. But in the real world these are absent; priorities have to be set, a strategy planned, decisions taken, and the unexpected dealt with, all without guidance. In the real world, impairment of the executive system may be catastrophic. Tests of the dysexecutive syndrome have been developed in order to be better predictors of these real-life problems. [13]

Memory impairment

Memory impairment is perhaps the most common cognitive impairment that follows head injury, and can be very disabling.[25] People will have problems remembering where they put things, what to do next, how to get home from the shops, or what they did yesterday. Anterograde amnesia refers to these enduring problems laying down new memories, and must be distinguished from retrograde and post-traumatic amnesia (see Box 4.1.10.1).

No consistent pattern of brain injury is associated with anterograde amnesia and it seems likely that it is the combined damage to several areas which causes the amnesia. Frontal injury may be particularly implicated perhaps by interfering with the executive processes required for normal memory, for example in memory retrieval. As with most amnesic states the amnesia following brain injury is for explicit memories, namely those which are consciously remembered. Implicit memory, for example remembering and learning a motor skill, is relatively well preserved.

Anterograde amnesia is often characterized by distortions and inaccurate recall with poor monitoring and insight. Confabulations are often seen.

Communication

Dysphasia is quite common after head injury, and may be rather different from that seen after stroke. The more diffuse and widespread injury of traumatic brain injury results in additional cognitive impairments which colour the picture. Monitoring of language errors is often particularly poor and the patient may demonstrate a jargon aphasia such that they are apparently unaware that their speech is completely incomprehensible. Dysphasia often continues to improve even many years post-injury.[26]

Dysprosody, in which the normal rhythms and intonations of speech are lost, is also seen, more so after right hemisphere damage. This interferes with social communication because the voice sounds flat and fails to convey emotion. Social communication is disrupted for other reasons, for example the patient fails in the turn-taking necessary for normal conversation. Word-finding difficulties are common.

Visuospatial impairments

Visuospatial impairments may contribute to spatial disorientation. Visual agnosia is easy to miss in someone with quite widespread cognitive impairments. Hemi-neglect can be troublesome.

Personality change

Personality change after head injury results in more suffering than any other single sequel.[27,28] In general, personality change goes hand in hand with cognitive impairment. However, a severe personality change is occasionally found in somebody with almost no impairment of cognitive function. Normal test scores for memory and intellect do not rule out brain injury as a cause of personality change after head injury.

Aetiology

It is not easy to predict who will develop a change in personality after head injury. Sometimes a personality trait present before the injury becomes much more troublesome, but often there is no obvious predisposition. The site of the brain injury may play a role.[29] Lesions of the medial and lateral surfaces of the frontal lobe can produce impairments of drive. Whereas orbito-frontal lesions, on the undersurface of the frontal lobe, may cause a more troublesome personality change with impairments in social behaviour.

Post-traumatic factors also need to be considered. Some patients seem to learn maladaptive patterns of behaviour; for example the response of the carers may unwittingly reinforce unwanted behaviours. Chronic mental illness, aggravated by chronic psychosocial stressors, may be manifest as personality change. Dependence on drugs, particularly alcohol, frequently confounds the picture.

Characteristics of the personality change

Changes in personality[27] include apathy and impairment of motivation and ambition. Patients are often described as childish; this covers a range of traits including impulsivity, poor tolerance of frustration, being demanding and self-centred, and generally lacking the ability to take on the adult role in terms of independent decision-making. Patients may be fatuous and facetious. Antisocial behaviours (see below) and disinhibition are severe handicaps that make integration back into the community difficult. Sexual disinhibition of any type is particularly worrisome. A spectrum of severity is seen, ranging from being inappropriately flirtatious through to indiscriminate sexual assaults. Head injury is probably a risk factor for borderline personality disorder.[30]

In acquired antisocial personality disorder the person is often self-centred and relatively oblivious to the needs of others. They are likely to be tactless and, on occasion, offensively rude. Irritability and aggression and impulsive behaviour are seen. They may show a lack of remorse for violent behaviour. These personality traits often are accompanied by the dysexecutive syndrome. Thus not only does the person show disturbed social decision-making, resulting in antisocial behaviours, but also disruption of the planning and organizational skills needed for cognitive tasks. For example, helpful and supportive friends may be alienated in favour of disreputable acquaintances, at the same time as money is impulsively spent and lost, on risky projects without any attempt to weigh up the options.

Effects on family and carers

Families find personality change particularly difficult to cope with.[31] Children may be ignored and the partner's needs, particularly emotional needs, forgotten. The healthy balance of the relationship with the partner may be destroyed, with the head-injured person now unable to take an effective part in the household. The partner becomes a carer and the change in roles may have a serious impact on the sexual relationship. Divorce not infrequently follows. However, parents may find the childish personality of the brain-injured person easier to cope with; they revert to taking on the parental role.

Personality change may deteriorate. Supportive social networks are lost and social isolation and financial problems may contribute to depression or alcohol abuse, which then cause a deterioration in the behavioural problems associated with the personality change. Follow-up studies lend some support to this argument. Some behavioural problems are found to have deteriorated at 5 years after head injury,[32] and family burden increases over this period.

Early mental symptoms following brain injury

On recovery of consciousness many patients after a severe head injury go through a period of delirium with clouding of consciousness. The clouding of consciousness may resolve, leaving a confusional state in clear consciousness with disorientation and thought disorder consisting of muddled thinking, rambling talk, and perseverations. This state is often dominated by misperceptions and misrecollections as the patient flits from one false observation to another.[33] Fear is common.

Distortions of memory

Confabulations, brief-lived false memories, emerge at about this time. Confabulations occur particularly in association with memory disturbance associated with frontal injury. The patient almost invariably shows poor insight into their memory problems, and is likely to be disorientated.

Occasionally after a severe head injury there are islets of memory in the dense amnesic period immediately around the time of the injury. These may be recollections of something that was consciously experienced at the time. On the other hand, the memories may have been fabricated from information subsequently given to the patient about what happened, or the memories may have no basis in reality and be properly described as a delusional memory.

Alterations of mood and perception

In the early recovery period oneroid states may be seen. The patient may be perplexed. He or she may feel that the trauma never occurred and that the whole event, including being in hospital, is a fabrication. Derealization/depersonalization may be associated with prominent anxiety, with the patient constantly asking for reassurance. Agitation occurs in about 10 per cent of patients with severe brain injury.[34]

Hallucinations, particularly visual, are occasionally observed, whereas illusions of familiarity are quite common after brain injury. The patient may have a sense of *déja vu*, or that he or she has met clinical staff or patients before. Distortions of the sense of familiarity seem to be implicated in many of the delusions observed early after brain injury.

Apathetic states

In many patients the recovery period lacks the positive features described above and is dominated by an apathetic withdrawn state.

Psychosis after brain injury

Early psychotic symptoms

The vast majority of the delusions and hallucinations occurring during the recovery period will themselves remit spontaneously and not relapse. However, it has been shown that, in some patients who have recovered from these early delusions, amylobarbitone can produce a return of symptoms.[35] This suggests that generalized disturbance of brain function plays an important part in the development of early delusions.

(a) Delusional misidentification

Delusional misidentifications of place, persons, objects, and events may be observed early in the course of recovery. Of these the one that is most pathognomonic of brain injury, and which is also associated with other causes of organic mental disorder, is reduplicative paramnesia. The term reduplicative paramnesia covers a range of phenomena which involve duplication of events or places. Pick,[36] who introduced the term, used it to describe a patient who believed she had visited a duplicate hospital.

Delusional disorientation for place may involve the belief that the current location is a duplicate of the true location or in some way displaced, for example that the hospital is in a different country. The patient may have two incompatible attitudes to orientation; this is sometimes referred to as a double orientation. For example, a patient who lives in Edinburgh acknowledges that he is in a hospital in London, but says that his home is just a few yards down the road. A common delusional disorientation is the patient's belief that they are still at work, despite the fact that they remain in hospital recovering from their injuries. Such patients lack insight into their injuries and report, for example, that they have been sent to complete some work assignment and that staff on the ward are colleagues from work.

Whereas isolated delusional misidentifications of place are rare in the absence of manifest organic brain disease, most cases of delusional misidentification of person (e.g. Capgras syndrome) are to be found in schizophrenia. Delusional misidentifications of person may also be observed following brain injury, often alongside a reduplicative paramnesia (see also Chapter 4.4).

Delusional misidentification syndromes can best be understood as the result of an interaction between organic brain disease and psychological disorder.[37] Lesions of the right hemisphere, often in combination with frontal injury or more diffuse evidence of brain disease, are particularly associated with delusional misidentification.

Late psychosis

(a) Schizophrenia-like psychosis

A psychotic illness may develop long after the acute confusional state has resolved. The patient may develop a typical schizophrenia indistinguishable from idiopathic schizophrenia. Would he or she have developed schizophrenia regardless of having had a head injury?

Davison and Bagley, almost 40 years ago,[38] estimated that patients after a head injury had a two- to three-fold increased risk of developing a schizophrenia-like psychosis compared with the general population. But there were large variations in the different studies they examined, and most were cohorts of war veterans who will have suffered open head injuries.

Any apparent association between head injury and schizophrenia might be explained by the fact that the period from late teens to early 20s is both the period of greatest risk of head injuries and the time when schizophrenia tends to start. In addition people at risk of schizophrenia may also be at increased risk of suffering a head injury ('reverse causality'[39]). Two large studies from Denmark[40] and Sweden,[41] based on linkage of nation wide hospital case registers, have shown that there appears to be no elevated risk of being admitted to hospital with a diagnosis of schizophrenia in those who have previously suffered a head injury. However, the second study did suggest that other non-affective psychoses, not diagnosed as schizophrenia, might be more common after a head injury. This fits with clinical experience; the patients whose psychosis seems most convincingly related to their head injury are those with more severe injuries. They would be diagnosed as suffering an organic psychosis, not schizophrenia.

(b) Paranoid psychosis

Paranoid psychoses may emerge after brain injury. Not infrequently this occurs relatively early and in a patient with severe cognitive impairment and personality change. Memory impairment will facilitate the development of persecutory ideas; for example, the patient believes that belongings have been stolen. Persecutory ideas or delusions of reference are a fairly common cause of aggression and may be hidden by communication difficulties.

Mood disorders, including anxiety disorders

Depression

The study of depression after head injury raises two fundamental questions about the nosological status of depression.[42] First, with a severe disability should the belief that life is not worth living be regarded as a symptom of depression or a 'rational' reaction to an intolerable predicament? Second, what is one to make of symptoms of apathy or anhedonia when the brain pathways involved in generating spontaneous behaviour or the experience of pleasure have been damaged? Most of the biological symptoms of depression can be produced by brain injury.

The diagnosis of depression therefore relies heavily on identifying a depressive mood. Symptoms like self-deprecation or guilt are also particularly helpful in diagnosis. Estimates of the prevalence of depression after head injury vary, partly because of the lack of uniformity in defining depression. Perhaps 25 per cent of patients meet DSM-IIIR criteria for major depression 1 month after injury.[43] A similar rate of depression at 1 year is described in several studies, though perhaps the more conservative figure of 14 per cent[44] is more realistic. Over the first year many who are initially depressed recover, to be replaced by those previously not depressed who become depressed.

Aetiological factors include a personal history of depression, which is twice as common in those who become depressed, and lack of social support. Depression after head injury interferes with rehabilitation, and is associated with aggression. It may exacerbate cognitive impairment and in some cases produce a pseudodementia.

Emotional lability may occur, particularly after severe head injury, and is frequently associated with the presence of depression.

Mania

Manic illness after head injury is much less common than depression. It needs to be distinguished from the neurobehavioural symptoms of, for example, disinhibition and fatuous behaviour that may follow frontal injury. Mania is particularly associated with aggressive and assaultative behaviour following brain injury.

Anxiety disorder

Symptoms of anxiety are common after head injury,[45] particularly in those who have suffered mild injury. Generalized anxiety disorder occurs in perhaps 10–15 per cent of cases.[46]

Early symptoms may be observed in relation to derealization/depersonalization symptoms, or perplexity. Early on, the amnesic period surrounding the injury may cause great distress. In the catastrophic reaction, which is observed in patients with moderate to severe cognitive impairment, sudden distress occurs when they fail to perform a task, or because of their inability to communicate.

Anxiety symptoms, particularly in those with a mild head injury, may develop over the weeks and months following a head injury. It is then more likely to be associated with depression, post-concussion syndrome, and with post-traumatic stress disorder. Phobic avoidance is seen, for example when there is travel anxiety following a road traffic accident. Apprehension is a common complaint, perhaps reflecting problems caused by cognitive impairments, and the person may be indecisive. Therefore anxiety symptoms may emerge on return to work. Anxiety symptoms will be inflated in the presence of financial or family stress.

Obsessive–compulsive disorder is recognized sequelae of head injury. This may partly reflect the inflexibility and rigidity of the brain-injured person, or a response to doubt resulting from memory disorder.

Suicide

The risk of suicide is increased following head injury occurring in about 1 per cent of cases over the first 15 years or so after injury.[47] This represents about a three-fold increase in suicide rate compared with the age matched population rates. There is no evidence of a specific at risk period. At least some of the increased risk is probably because those at increased risk of head injury also have a greater risk of suicide. Rates of attempted suicide are increased after head injury.

Agitation and aggression

The psychiatrist is more likely to be asked to advise about the management of agitation and aggression following head injury than any other mental symptom.

Agitation in the early recovery period after severe brain injury will generally spontaneously improve over the course of days or weeks.[34] Early agitation may be followed by more intractable aggressive behaviour.[48] A major predictor of aggression is antisocial behaviour before the head injury.

If the aggressive behaviour emerges early, namely during the confusional state or shortly after it resolves, then this suggest that the aetiology is largely organic. A pattern of aggression that is highly stereotyped, or erupts over seconds with no or trivial triggers, or is bizarre, and is against a background of calm behaviour, suggests the possibility of epilepsy.

Other causes need to be considered. It is important to rule out any medical or surgical complications of the head injury, for example a subdural haematoma. Likewise pain and sources of infection, for example a UTI. The patient's worries and fears need to be explored, and phobic anxiety disorder considered. Drugs may make agitation worse and paradoxical effects of sedative medication occur if the medication increases confusion or disinhibition, or results in akathisia. The patient may be in a withdrawal state having stopped a drug they were taking regularly before the head injury. Drug and alcohol dependence may be especially problematic. Symptoms of mental illness may not be immediately obvious because of communication difficulties. It is therefore necessary to search for evidence of persecutory delusions, mania, depression, and anxiety. Any mental illness should be treated before considering medication specifically to treat agitation (see below).

Alcohol and head injury

Alcohol dependence complicates the management of the head-injured person several-fold. The person may have suffered several previous head injuries, as well as the effects of alcoholic brain damage before the head injury. A blow to the head may result in much greater brain injury for reasons that are poorly understood.[49] Poor physical health is likely to prejudice immediate management after the head injury. Subdural haematomas may be problematic.

Alcohol craving may interfere with medical care and rehabilitation.[50] Social networks are often poor, thus complicating discharge from hospital.

Very occasionally a head injury seems to cure the alcohol dependence. Unfortunately alcohol dependence often gets worse, perhaps because the head injury has weakened impulse control. Indeed some patients develop alcohol dependence when they find that alcohol relieves their anxiety symptoms.

Post-concussion syndrome

The post-concussion syndrome is poorly defined.[51] The term is perhaps most usefully reserved to describe a constellation of symptoms that may result in surprisingly severe disability after mild head injury. These symptoms may be observed after moderate and severe head injuries, in which case they are likely to be in the company of other symptoms more readily understood as resulting from brain injury. There is no consistent relationship between the prevalence of post-concussion symptoms and injury severity.

Phenomenology

Early symptoms tend to have a more neurological flavour and include headache, dizziness, and for example diplopia. Mild head injury fairly consistently results, in the immediate aftermath, in impairment of speed of information processing and concentration. Fatigue is also evident from early on, along with symptoms of noise sensitivity. Anxiety, depression, and irritability are common and may appear after a latent period. The symptoms of post-concussion syndrome overlap with those of post-traumatic stress disorder, and chronic fatigue. Other symptoms occasionally reported include tinnitus, unsteadiness, and muscle pain.

In general after a mild to moderate injury symptoms will have recovered by 2 to 6 months. But a few patients, sometimes after a latent period, develop persistent symptoms that last for years. Psychological factors are likely to be important in such patients, particularly if their injury is mild.

Aetiology

(a) Brain injury

Several observations support the contribution of brain injury, even in those with mild injury. Microscopic lesions in the brain have been described at post-mortem, following mild head injury.[52] Imaging, particularly functional imaging with single-photon emission CT or positron-emission tomography, may show abnormalities. Early after mild head injury there is evidence of cerebral dysfunction. One month after a mild head injury patients undertaking a working memory task showed more widespread activation of cerebral cortex compared to controls, even though their actual performance on the task was normal.[53]

(b) Psychological factors

Psychosocial factors have also been found to play a part in post-concussion syndrome, more so in those with symptoms lasting longer than 1 year. If the accident occurs at work, particularly if the person blames their employer, symptoms are more likely. A meta-analysis of the effects of compensation on symptoms, any symptom, after head injury concluded that, on average, being involved in compensation claims increases symptoms by about 25 per cent.[54] This effect was larger in those with milder injuries.

(c) Model of interaction

Lishman has proposed a model in which early disturbance of brain function after mild head injury results in the early symptoms of post-concussion syndrome.[1] In most patients these gradually resolve and a good recovery is made. However, the post-concussion syndrome may develop if psychological effects interfere with the normal process of recovery. Anxiety is thought to play a large part in impeding recovery; the patient worries about the symptoms and focuses on them. These may be aggravated if the patient is vulnerable to somatization, or there are compensation issues at stake. The symptoms may cause secondary disability provoking yet more anxiety, which will be made worse if there are additional psychosocial stressors. The role of psychological factors is greatest in those with very mild head injuries and very chronic symptoms.

Post-traumatic epilepsy

Early fits, within the first week, are relatively benign, sensitive to prophylactic anti-convulsants, and are only weak predictors of later epilepsy.

Only about 5 per cent of closed head injuries go on to develop late seizures, compared with 30 per cent after an open head injury. The majority of these late seizures start in the few years following injury. By the time 5 to 10 years have elapsed without seizures any subsequent seizure development may be unrelated to the head injury.[55]

The likelihood of developing seizures in patients with a closed head injury is increased by the presence of a depressed skull fracture, intracranial haematoma, and early seizure, as well as by the severity of the injury. Mild head injuries result in only a small increased risk of epilepsy above population norms. The EEG is generally not a good predictor of post-traumatic epilepsy.

Post-traumatic epilepsy increases psychiatric morbidity, particularly mood disorders, and may increase the risk of late dementia.

Prophylactic anti-convulsants have no effect on reducing the incidence of late post-traumatic epilepsy.[56] Carbamazepine, rather than phenytoin, is the drug of choice if an anti-convulsant is needed because it has less effect on cognition.[57] Half of all patients with post-traumatic epilepsy from open head injuries are found to be in remission by 5 to 10 years.

Head injury in children

Children, compared with adults, are more likely to suffer cerebral oedema and early post-traumatic epilepsy. They tend to develop a relatively stereotyped pattern of changes in personality with emotional lability, overactivity, reduced attention span, and irritability with outbursts of temper and rage. Apart from personality changes the commonest psychiatric disorders that follow childhood head injuries are attention-deficit hyperactivity disorder, and obsessive–compulsive disorder.[58] Children who develop attention-deficit hyperactivity disorder after head injury tend to demonstrate less hyperactivity than is seen in the idiopathic form.

It is sometimes said that the greater potential for plasticity which may be present in the younger person's brain, results in a better outcome compared to adults. There is some evidence for this for mild and moderate head injuries. However, children with severe head injuries are likely to be left with persistent cognitive deficits and behavioural problems. Very young children with severe head injury suffer a double hazard[59] with both loss of acquired skills and interference with further development. This is often complicated by the fact that many of these children will have demonstrated pre-injury behavioural problems. The quality of parenting has a powerful effect on outcome; those with poor parenting are much more likely to develop behavioural problems.[60]

Boxing

In the past, when the average number of career bouts was about 300, 10 to 20 per cent of professional boxers went on to develop a chronic traumatic encephalopathy,[61] the punch-drunk syndrome. However now, with an average boxing career of 13 bouts, cases are much less frequently seen.[62]

Patients with chronic traumatic encephalopathy suffer damage to the extrapyramidal system as well as cerebellar and pyramidal pathways. They are slow and ataxic. Cognitive impairment, in particular memory impairment, is a frequent accompaniment and about 50 per cent have dementia. Upper brainstem lesions may explain the neurological symptoms, while cerebral atrophy, white matter changes, and damage to diencephalic structures may account for cognitive changes. Perforation of the septum pellucidum, which separates the two lateral ventricles, is a characteristic finding. *APOE e4* status increases vulnerability to the punch-drunk syndrome,[63] and this is consistent with the finding that amyloid is often present.

Professional footballers may show evidence of subtle impairments of thinking. This raises the possibility that repeated blows to the head from heading the ball may be sufficient to cause slight brain injury; but a more likely explanation for any injury is head-to-head contact.[64]

Management of early neurobehavioural problems

Interventions aimed at reducing the risk of enduring post-concussional symptoms after milder injuries, using brief educational, and supportive therapy in the early days post-injury, have been shown to be effective.[65]

But there is little evidence to guide the management of behavioural problems and mental symptoms arising in the days and weeks following a more severe brain injury. Such symptoms should be regarded as a flag to indicate the need to check on the progress of recovery. The history needs to be reviewed, paying attention to the period leading up to injury. The patient will need to be examined physically including a thorough neurological examination and checking for fever. It is essential to document the conscious level and orientation. Routine blood tests should be performed, and blood gases and a chest radiograph considered. Medication needs to be scrutinized. A neurological or neurosurgical opinion may be needed with a view to considering neuroimaging or an EEG. A lumbar puncture, for example looking for meningitis, should probably not be done without specialist advice.

Causes of deterioration after head injury are listed in Box 4.1.10.2. Once these have been excluded then the principle of care should be to allow recovery to take place in a safe environment, paying attention to the general principles of the care of the delirious or demented patient as indicated. Explanation to the patient and his or her family as to what is happening, is required.

Box 4.1.10.2 Causes of late deterioration in cognitive function after brain injury

Specific

- Subdural haematoma
- Hydrocephalus
- Epilepsy, particularly complex partial status
- Late intracranial infection, including cerebral abscess

Non-specific

- Systemic illness, including fat emboli and pain
- Drug intoxication
- Severe mental illness, in particular depression
- The patient 'gives up' as he or she gains insight
- Independent dementing process

Management of late mental sequelae

The reader is referred to Chapter 4.1.14 for many of the management principles relevant to patients with severe cognitive impairment after a head injury.

Psychological interventions

(a) Evidence of effectiveness

A small RCT has shown that cognitive behavioural treatment may be useful in those with persistent post-concussion syndrome.[66] Inpatient cognitive rehabilitation is probably needed only in those with more severe injuries.[46] Community therapy can improve handicap.[67] The evidence that behavioural strategies can improve behavioural problems, particularly aggression, in those with brain injury rests very largely on single case studies[68] or case series showing marked improvement in patients with very long-standing symptoms.[69]

(b) Principles of management

The first step, after medical issues have been excluded (Box 4.1.10.2), is to ensure that the patient has received adequate rehabilitation. In those with severe cognitive impairment once the patient is medically stable appropriate inpatient rehabilitation, perhaps on a locked unit, will probably be required. Problems arise if patients have to be sedated to ensure their safety, and the safety of other patients, while they remain inappropriately in an acute hospital bed. Timely access to rehabilitation is likely to reduce the risk of mental sequelae. Not infrequently psychological problems arise if any part of this process has not gone smoothly, or is perceived to have failed. Education, and access to information, is an important part of the care plan. Good advice on strategies for return to work can be invaluable, and some will require formal vocational rehabilitation. A social worker should be asked to undertake a community care assessment, which may identify the need for respite care or modifications to the home.

The management of any mental sequelae rests on a good understanding of the severity of the brain injury in order to estimate the likely contribution of brain damage to the mental sequelae.

A neuropsychological assessment, to determine injury severity and the pattern of impairments, may be needed. The severity of brain injury will suggest whether a particular symptom is mainly due to brain injury or to psychological processes. The degree of cognitive impairment may indicate whether or not the patient is capable of benefiting from certain psychological therapies. Those with less severe impairments should be offered CBT as appropriate, for example to treat travel anxiety or depression. In addition, the individual and their family should have access to support and guidance as they try to adjust to the changes forced on them by the head injury. Sometimes carers or family will need advice on how to manage challenging behaviours, particularly if their responses seem to be reinforcing the behaviour.

Pharmacological management

By and large patients should be given psychotropics only if absolutely necessary,[70] attending to the principles described in Box 4.1.10.3 and avoiding multiple drugs given concurrently. There is an emerging literature on drugs which may enhance cognition.[71]

(a) Agitation and aggression

Evidence—There are no good trials of medication for agitation and aggression after brain injury.[72] Only β-blockers have been exposed to randomized controlled trials. These studies showed a slight effect in favour of medication. But despite this β-blockers are rarely used in the management of agitation and aggression. In the RCTs very large doses of β-blockers were used that will almost inevitably cause worrying side effects in most patients.

Management—Because of the lack of controlled trials, prescribing for agitation and aggression after brain injury is very much trial and error, requiring good monitoring and documentation of the behaviour. If there is no evidence of benefit then the drug should be withdrawn and another drug tried. Be wary of responding to every episode of aggression by increasing the dose or adding a new drug.

For many psychiatrists, based on little more than anecdotal evidence, valproate, or carbamazepine are the drugs of first choice for aggression after brain injury. They have the advantage of anticonvulsant as well as mood-stabilizing effects. Perhaps a third of patients will respond.

Antipsychotics should be used if delusions or persecutory ideas of reference or fear are also present. But akathisia may perpetuate agitated behaviour which would otherwise have resolved spontaneously. Atypical antipsychotics, having less risk of motor side effects, are to be recommended.

Antidepressants may be helpful particularly if symptoms of anxiety or depression are present. Selective serotonin-reuptake inhibitors should be given in preference to tricyclics. Trazodone given at night may be useful if there is sleep disturbance.

Benzodiazepines should be considered for agitation and aggression during the early recovery from severe head injury. But be wary of increasing the confusion, and paradoxical violence due to disinhibition. Because of the potential for addiction, benzodiazepines should not be given to a patient with a chronic aggressive disorder.

Box 4.1.10.3 Prescribing psychotropics in brain injury

No knee jerk reaction—if possible wait to see if the problem goes away spontaneously
Small doses—start low, go slow
Only continue treatment if good evidence of effect
Drug profile—choose drugs with less potential for:

- Lowering seizure threshold—avoid clozapine
- Anticholinergic activity—to minimize potential for increasing confusion
- Extrapyramidal side-effects—especially akathisia, parkinsonism, and neuroleptic malignant syndrome
- Enzyme induction or other pharmacodynamic interaction with other drugs

Regular medication with long-acting anxiolytics, compared with short-acting drugs as required, is less likely to produce:

- Withdrawal syndrome
- Development of addiction
- Reinforcement of unwanted behaviour but may produce raised blood concentrations

(b) Mood disorders and psychosis

Evidence—Good studies evaluating the efficacy of medication for depression or psychosis after head injury are lacking.[71]

Management—Depression after a head injury is probably more difficult to treat than in those without brain injury.[73] However, some studies in head-injured depressed patients have found good response rates. The selection of an antidepressant is no different from that used to treat depression in the absence of brain injury, provided that the principles given in Box 4.1.10.3 are taken into account.

Confabulations and delusions early after brain injury should be allowed to resolve spontaneously where possible. For established psychotic symptoms atypical antipsychotics are probably to be recommended.

(c) Apathy

Bromocriptine and methylphenidate may be useful for treating apathetic states but controlled trials are lacking. Methylphenidate, with its risk of addiction and troublesome side effects, should only be prescribed if bromocriptine has not been successful, and under consultant supervision.

(d) Drugs which enhance memory and concentration

Evidence—Preliminary evidence supports the use of methylphenidate for deficits in attention and speed of information processing,[74] donepezil for attention and memory problems[75] and bromocriptine for executive problems.[76]

Management—There is now a case for considering medication to enhance cognitive function after brain injury. Drugs are available that may result in small improvements in attention, memory, and executive function. However in almost every case the evidence relies heavily on a single fairly small randomized controlled trial. Longer-term adverse consequences are uncertain. These drugs should only be considered:

- for patients with definite moderate to severe brain injury to account for their cognitive complaints,

- after discussion with the patient and their family about the uncertainties of treatment,
- if there is good reason to believe that a small increase in cognitive function can result in significant improvement in handicap,
- with close monitoring of response and side effects.

Insight, capacity, and detention in hospital

Insight and capacity to consent to treatment should be assessed in all patients. Lack of awareness of deficits is a common problem for the head-injured person[77] and affects compliance with, and capacity to consent to treatment. The Mental Capacity Act, 2005 (http://www.opsi.gov.uk/acts/acts2005/20050009.htm or http://www.dca.gov.uk/menincap/legis.htm) governs decision-making on behalf of adults in England and Wales who lack capacity to consent to treatment and manage their affairs. In these patients if there is no family or friend to act on their behalf, an independent advocate may be needed. The clinical team will need to ensure that all reasonable measures have been taken to enable the patient to take part in any decision-making. Any decision to act in the patient's 'best interests' should take into account what is known about their previous views and opinions. Very occasionally advance decisions may be in place which dictate how the patient wishes to be treated.

The psychiatrist may be called when the patient demands to leave hospital against medical advice. Only the very exceptional patient who is demanding to leave hospital following a head injury, and who as a result would be putting his or her health severely at risk, will be found to be competent. If they are not, it may be necessary to consider detention under the Mental Health Act, 1983 (England and Wales) or equivalent.

Patients will also need to be assessed to see if they are capable of managing their finances and affairs. If they are not, appropriate legal arrangements should be made; in the United Kingdom a receiver may need to be appointed to protect their interests. The prospect of compensation should be considered and, if appropriate, they should be enabled to pursue a personal injury claim.

Further information

http://www.ninds.nih.gov/disorders/tbi/tbi.htm National Institute of Neurological Disorders and Stroke—Traumatic brain injury information page.

http://www.dh.gov.uk/en/Healthcare/NationalServiceFrameworks/Long-termNeurologicalConditionsNSF/index.htm The National Service Framework on Long term (neurological) conditions. This provides guidance for health and social services on therapy and support for people with long term neurological conditions. The guidance is very relevant to patients with traumatic brain injury.

Silver, J.M., McAllister, T.W., and Yudofsky, S.C. (2005). *Textbook of traumatic brain injury.* American Psychiatric Publishing Inc., Washington, DC. A large multi-author textbook on all aspects of traumatic brain injury.

Damasio, A.R. (1994). *Descartes' error: emotion, reason and the human brain.* Grosset/Putnam, New York.

Lishman, W.A. (1998). *Organic psychiatry: the psychological consequences of cerebral disorder* (3rd edn). Blackwell Science, Oxford.

References

1. Lishman, W.A. (1988). Physiogenesis and psychogenesis in the 'post-concussional syndrome'. *The British Journal of Psychiatry*, **153**, 460–9.
2. Kapur, N. (1997). *Injured brains of medical minds: views from within.* Oxford University Press, Oxford.
3. National Collaborating Centre for Acute Care. (2003). *Head injury: triage, assessment, investigation and early management of head injury in infants, children and adults.* Guideline commissioned by the National Institute for Clinical Excellence. http://www.nice.org.uk/guidance/CG4
4. Povlishock, J.T. and Katz, D.I. (2005). Update of neuropathology and neurological recovery after traumatic brain injury. *The Journal of Head Trauma Rehabilitation*, **20**, 76–94.
5. Hayes, R.L., Lyeth, B.G., and Jenkins, L.W. (1989). Neurochemical mechanisms of mild and moderate head injury; implications for treatment. In *Mild head injury* (eds. H. S. Levin, H. M. Eisenberg, and A. L. Benton), pp. 54–79. Oxford University Press, Oxford.
6. Bishara, S., Partridge, F., Godfrey, H., *et al.* (1992). Post-traumatic amnesia and Glasgow Coma Scale related to outcome in survivors in a consecutive series of patients with severe closed head injury. *Brain Injury*, **6**, 373–80.
7. Teasdale, G. and Jennett, B. (1974). Assessment of coma and impaired consciousness. A practical scale. *Lancet*, **2**, 81–4.
8. Kraus, J.F. and Chu, L.D. (2005). Epidemiology. In *Textbook of traumatic brain injury* (eds. J.M. Silver, T.W. McAllister, and S.C. Yudofsky), pp. 3–26. American Psychiatric Publishing, Washington, DC.
9. Parizel, P.M., Van Goethem, J.W., Ozsarlak, O., *et al.* (2005). New developments in the neuroradiological diagnosis of craniocerebral trauma. *European Radiology*, **15**, 569–81.
10. Goldenberg, G., Oder, W., Spatt, J., *et al.* (1992). Cerebral correlates of disturbed executive function and memory in survivors of severe closed head injury: a SPECT study. *Journal of Neurology, Neurosurgery, and Psychiatry*, **55**, 362–8.
11. Markowitsch, H.J., Kessler, J., Van Der Van, C., *et al.* (1998). Psychic trauma causing grossly reduced brain metabolism and cognitive deterioration. *Neuropsychologia*, **36**, 77–82.
12. Nelson, H.E. and Willison, J.R. (1991). *National adult reading test* (2nd edn). NFER–Nelson, Windsor.
13. Wilson, B.A., Alderman, N., Burgess, P.W., *et al.* (1996). *Behavioural assessment of the dysexecutive syndrome.* Thames Valley Test Co., Bury St Edmunds, Suffolk.
14. Ruff, R.M., Young, D., Gautille, T., *et al.* (1991). Verbal learning deficits following severe head injury: heterogeneity in recovery over 1 year. *Journal of Neurosurgery*, **75**, S50–8.
15. Wilson, B. (1992). Recovery and compensation strategies in head injured memory impaired people several years after insult. *Journal of Neurology, Neurosurgery, and Psychiatry*, **55**, 177–80.
16. Whitnall, L., McMillan, T.M., Murray, G.D., *et al.* (2006). Disability in young people and adults after head injury: 5–7 year follow up of a prospective cohort study. *Journal of Neurology, Neurosurgery, and Psychiatry*, **77**, 640–5.
17. Corkin, S., Rosen, J., Sullivan, E.V., *et al.* (1989). Penetrating head injury in young adulthood exacerbates cognitive decline in later years. *Journal of Neuroscience*, **9**, 3876–83.
18. Fleminger, S., Oliver, D.L., Lovestone, S., *et al.* (2003). Head injury as a risk factor for Alzheimer's disease: the evidence 10 years on; a partial replication. *Journal of Neurology, Neurosurgery, and Psychiatry*, **74**, 857–62.
19. Teasdale, T.W. and Engberg, A. (1997). Duration of cognitive dysfunction after concussion, and cognitive dysfunction as a risk factor: a population study of young men. *British Medical Journal*, **315**, 569–72.
20. Lishman, W.A. (1968). Brain damage in relation to psychiatric disability after head injury. *The British Journal of Psychiatry*, **114**, 373–410.
21. Pilowsky, I. (1985). Cryptotrauma and 'accident neurosis'. *The British Journal of Psychiatry*, **147**, 310–11.

22. Claparède, E. (1911). Récognition et moiïté. *Archives of Psychology (Genève)*, **11**, 79–90.
23. Whitty, C.W.M. and Zangwill, O.L. (1966). Traumatic amnesia. In *Amnesia* (eds. C.W.M. Whitty and O.L. Zangwill), pp. 92–108. Butterworths, London.
24. Shallice, T. and Burgess, P.W. (1991). Deficits in strategy application following frontal lobe damage in man. *Brain*, **114**, 727–41.
25. Brooks, D.N. (1975). Long and short term memory in head injured patients. *Cortex*, **11**, 329–40.
26. Thomsen, I.V. (1984). Late outcome of very severe blunt head trauma: a 10–15 year second follow-up. *Journal of Neurology, Neurosurgery, and Psychiatry*, **47**, 260–8.
27. Lezak, M.D. (1978). Living with the characterologically altered brain injured patient. *The Journal of Clinical Psychiatry*, **39**, 592–8.
28. Parker, R.S. (1996). The spectrum of emotional distress and personality changes after minor head injury incurred in a motor vehicle accident. *Brain Injury*, **10**, 287–302.
29. Blumer, D. and Benson, D.F. (1978). Personality changes with frontal and temporal lobe lesions. In *Psychiatric aspects of neurologic disease* (eds. D.F. Benson and D. Blumer), pp. 151–70. Grune and Stratton, New York.
30. Hibbard, M.R., Bogdany, J., Uysal, S., *et al.* (2000). Axis II psychopathology in individuals with traumatic brain injury. *Brain Injury*, **14**, 45–61.
31. Thomsen, I.V. (1974). The patient with severe head injury and his family: a follow-up study of 50 patients. *Scandinavian Journal of Rehabilitation Medicine*, **6**, 180–3.
32. Olver, J.H., Ponsford, J.L., and Curran, C.A. (1996). Outcome following traumatic brain injury: a comparison between 2 and 5 years after injury. *Brain Injury*, **10**, 841–8.
33. Symonds, C.P. (1937). Mental disorder following head injury. *Proceedings of the Royal Society of Medicine*, **30**, 1081–94.
34. Brooke, M.M., Questad, K.A., Patterson, D.R., *et al.* (1992). Agitation and restlessness after closed head injury: a prospective study of 100 consecutive admissions. *Archives of Physical Medicine & Rehabilitation*, **73**, 320–3.
35. Weinstein, E.A. and Kahn, R.L. (1951). Patterns of disorientation in organic brain disease. *Journal of Neuropathology and Clinical Neurology*, **1**, 214.
36. Pick, A. (1903). Clinical studies. III: on reduplicative paramnesia. *Brain*, **26**, 260–7.
37. Fleminger, S. and Burns, A. (1993). The delusional misidentification syndromes in patients with and without evidence of organic cerebral disorder: a structured review of case reports. *Biological Psychiatry*, **33**, 22–32.
38. Davison, K. and Bagley, C.R. (1969). Schizophrenia-like psychoses associated with organic disorders of the central nervous system: a review of the literature. In *Current problems in neuropsychiatry: schizophrenia, epilepsy, the temporal lobe* (ed. R.N. Herrington), *The British Journal of Psychiatry*, Special Publication No. 4, pp. 113–84. Headley Brothers, Ashford.
39. David, A.S. and Prince, M. (2005). Psychosis following head injury: a critical review. *Journal of Neurology, Neurosurgery, and Psychiatry*, **76**(Suppl. 1), i53–60.
40. Nielsen, A.S., Mortensen, P.B., O'Callaghan, E., *et al.* (2002). Is head injury a risk factor for schizophrenia? *Schizophrenia Research*, **55**, 93–8.
41. Harrison, G., Whitley, E., Rasmussen, F., *et al.* (2006). Risk of schizophrenia and other non-affective psychosis among individuals exposed to head injury: case control study. *Schizophrenia Research*, **88**, 119–26.
42. Fleminger, S., Oliver, D.L., Williams, W.H., *et al.* (2003). The neuropsychiatry of depression after brain injury. *Neuropsychological Rehabilitation*, **13**, 65–87.
43. Jorge, R.E., Robinson, R.G., Arndt, S.V., *et al.* (1993). Depression following traumatic brain injury: a 1 year longitudinal study. *Journal of Affective Disorder*, **27**, 233–43.
44. Deb, S., Lyons, I., Koutzoukis, C., *et al.* (1999). Rate of psychiatric illness 1 year after traumatic brain injury. *The American Journal of Psychiatry*, **156**, 374–8.
45. Warden, D.L. and Labbate, L.A. (2005). Posttraumatic stress disorder and other anxiety disorders. In *Textbook of traumatic brain injury* (eds. J.M. Silver, T.W. McAllister, and S.C. Yudofsky), pp. 231–44. American Psychiatric Publishing, Washington, DC.
46. Salazar, A.M., Warden, D.L., Schwab, K., *et al.* (2000). Cognitive rehabilitation for traumatic brain injury: a randomized trial. Defense and Veterans Head Injury Program (DVHIP) study group. *The Journal of the American Medical Association*, **283**, 3075–81.
47. Teasdale, T.W. and Engberg, A.W. (2001). Suicide after traumatic brain injury: a population study. *Journal of Neurology, Neurosurgery, and Psychiatry*, **71**, 436–40.
48. Mysiw, W.J. and Sandel, M.E. (1997). The agitated brain injured patient. Part 2: Pathophysiology and treatment. *Archives of Physical Medicine and Rehabilitation*, **78**, 213–20.
49. Rönty, H., Ahonen, A., Tolonen, U., *et al.* (1993). Cerebral trauma and alcohol abuse. *European Journal of Clinical Investigation*, **23**, 182–7.
50. Sparadeo, F.R. and Gill, D. (1989). Effects of prior alcohol use on head injury recovery. *The Journal of Head Trauma Rehabilitation*, **4**, 75–82.
51. Ryan, L.M. and Warden, D.L. (2003). Post concussion syndrome. *International Review of Psychiatry*, **15**, 310–6.
52. Povlishock, J.T. and Coburn, T.H. (1989). Morphological change associated with mild head injury. In *Mild head injury* (eds. H.S. Levin, H.M. Eisenberg, and A.L. Benton), pp. 37–53. Oxford University Press, New York.
53. McAllister, T.W., Saykin, A.J., Flashman, L.A., *et al.* (1999). Brain activation during working memory 1 month after mild traumatic brain injury: a functional MRI study. *Neurology*, **53**, 1300–8.
54. Binder, L.M. and Rohling, M.L. (1996). Money matters: a meta-analytic review of the effects of financial incentives on recovery after closed-head injury. *The American Journal of Psychiatry*, **153**, 7–10.
55. Annegers, J.F., Grabow, J.D., Groover, R.V., *et al.* (1980). Seizures after head trauma: a population study. *Neurology*, **30**, 683–9.
56. Schierhout, G. and Roberts, I. (1998). Prophylactic antiepileptic agents after head injury: a systematic review. *Journal of Neurology, Neurosurgery, and Psychiatry*, **64**, 108–12.
57. Wroblewski, B.A., Glenn, M.B., Whyte, J., *et al.* (1989). Carbamazepine replacement of phenytoin, phenobarbital and primidone in a rehabilitation setting: effects on seizure control. *Brain Injury*, **3**, 149–56.
58. Max, J.E. (2005). Children and adolescents. In *Textbook of traumatic brain injury* (eds. J.M. Silver, T.W. McAllister, and S.C. Yudofsky), pp. 477–94. American Psychiatric Publishing, Washington, DC.
59. Anderson, V., Catroppa, C., Morse, S., *et al.* (2005). Functional plasticity or vulnerability after early brain injury? *Pediatrics*, **116**, 1374–82.
60. Max, J.E., Robin, D.A., Lindgren, S.D., *et al.* (1997). Traumatic brain injury in children and adolescents: psychiatric disorders at two years. *Journal of the American Academy of Child and Adolescent Psychiatry*, **36**, 1278–85.
61. Roberts, A.H. (1969). *Brain damage in boxers*. Pitman, London.
62. Clausen, H., McCrory, P., and Anderson, V. (2005). The risk of chronic traumatic brain injury in professional boxing: change in exposure variables over the past century. *British Journal of Sports Medicine*, **39**, 661–4.
63. Jordan, B.D., Relkin, N.R., Ravdin, L.D., *et al.* (1997). Apolipoprotein E e4 associated with chronic traumatic brain injury boxing. *The Journal of the American Medical Association*, **278**, 136–40.
64. McCrory, P.R. (2003). Brain injury and heading in soccer. *British Medical Journal*, **327**, 351–2.
65. Wade, D.T., King, N.S., Wenden, F.J., *et al.* (1998). Routine follow up after head injury: a second randomised controlled trial. *Journal of Neurology Neurosurgery, and Psychiatry*, **65**, 177–83.

66. Tiersky, L.A., Anselmi, V., Johnston, M.V., *et al.* (2005). A trial of neuropsychologic rehabilitation in mild-spectrum traumatic brain injury. *Archives of Physical Medicine and Rehabilitation*, **86**, 1565–74.
67. Powell, J., Heslin, J., and Greenwood, R. (2002). Community based rehabilitation after severe traumatic brain injury: a randomised controlled trial. *Journal of Neurology, Neurosurgery, and Psychiatry*, **72**, 193–202.
68. Alderman, N., Davies, J.A., Jones, C., *et al.* (1999). Reduction of severe aggressive behaviour in acquired brain injury: case studies illustrating clinical use of the OAS-MNR in the management of challenging behaviours. *Brain Injury*, **13**, 669–704.
69. Eames, P. and Wood, R. (1985). Rehabilitation after severe brain injury: a follow-up study of a behaviour modification approach. *Journal of Neurology, Neurosurgery, and Psychiatry*, **48**, 613–9.
70. Goldstein, L.B. (1995). Prescribing of potentially harmful drugs to patients admitted to hospital after head injury. *Journal of Neurology, Neurosurgery, and Psychiatry*, **58**, 753–5.
71. Neurobehavioral Guidelines Working Group. Warden, D.L., Gordon, B., McAllister, T.W., *et al.* (2006). Guidelines for the pharmacologic treatment of neurobehavioral sequelae of traumatic brain injury. *Journal of Neurotrauma*, **23**, 1468–501.
72. Fleminger, S., Greenwood, R.J., and Oliver, D.L. (2006). Pharmacological management for agitation and aggression in people with acquired brain injury. *Cochrane Database of Systematic Reviews*, **4**, CD003.
73. Dinan, T.G. and Mobayed, M. (1992). Treatment resistance of depression after head injury: a preliminary study of amitriptyline response. *Acta Psychiatrica Scandinavica*, **85**, 292–4.
74. Whyte, J., Hart, T., Vaccaro, M., *et al.* (2004). Effects of methylphenidate on attention deficits after traumatic brain injury: a multidimensional, randomized, controlled trial. *American Journal of Physical Medicine & Rehabilitation*, **83**, 401–20.
75. Zhang, L., Plotkin, R.C., Wang, G., *et al.* (2004). Cholinergic augmentation with donepezil enhances recovery in short-term memory and sustained attention after traumatic brain injury. *Archives of Physical Medicine and Rehabilitation*, **85**, 1050–5.
76. McDowell, S., Whyte, J., and D'Esposito, M. (1998). Differential effect of a dopaminergic agonist on prefrontal function in traumatic brain injury patients. *Brain*, **121**, 1155–64.
77. Prigatano, G.P. and Schacter, D.L. (1991). *Awareness of deficit after brain injury: clinical and theoretical issues*. Oxford University Press, New York.

4.1.11 **Alcohol-related dementia (alcohol-induced dementia; alcohol-related brain damage)**

Jane Marshall

Introduction

Long-term heavy alcohol consumption causes significant brain abnormalities and impairs cognitive functioning. A number of terms have been used to describe these effects, including: 'alcohol-related dementia', 'alcohol-induced dementia', and 'alcoholic dementia'.(1) The more pragmatic umbrella term 'alcohol-related brain damage' (ARBD) is also used. The literature is beset with limitations, in particular the lack of a diagnostic gold standard, and the difficulty in making a clinical diagnosis. Many individuals labelled as having an alcohol-related dementia are, in fact, suffering from the Wernicke–Korsakoff syndrome (WKS).(2) (This is a specific neuropathological disease caused by thiamine deficiency, which can occur secondary to alcohol misuse. It is considered in Chapter 4.1.12.) When considering the topic of 'alcohol-related dementia' it is probably sensible to take a broad clinically-based diagnostic view that includes both WKS and other cases of 'dementia' that appear to be alcohol-related.(3)

Diagnostic criteria

Diagnostic criteria for 'substance-induced persisting dementia' are included in DSM-IV(4) (Table 4.1.11.1), which also states that there must be evidence from the history, physical examination, or laboratory findings that the deficits are aetiologically related to the persisting effects of substance use (in this case alcohol). No specific inclusion criteria are offered to distinguish alcohol-related dementia from other dementias. In ICD-10,(5) the Korsakoff syndrome is listed separately under the amnesic syndrome heading (F10.6) whereas alcohol-induced 'dementia' and 'other persisting cognitive impairment' are included under the 'residual and late-onset psychotic disorder' category (F10.73 and F10.74 respectively), where diagnostic guidelines can be found.

Diagnostic criteria for establishing a diagnosis of 'alcohol-related dementia' have been proposed, conceiving it as a spectrum of alcohol-related intellectual and neurological syndromes, ranging from moderate deficits to the more severe Wernicke–Korsakoff syndrome.(3) 'Alcohol-related dementia' is thus defined as a syndrome that results from several aetiological mechanisms including the direct neurotoxic effects of alcohol, metabolic dysfunction during intoxication and withdrawal, trauma, vascular injury and thiamine or other nutritional deficiencies.

Table 4.1.11.1 DSM-IV diagnostic criteria for substance-induced persisting dementia

A. The development of multiple cognitive deficits manifested by both (1) memory impairment (impaired ability to learn new information or to recall previously learned information) (2) one (or more) of the following cognitive disturbances: (a) aphasia (language disturbance) (b) apraxia (impaired ability to carry out motor activities despite intact motor function) (c) agnosia (failure to recognize or identify objects despite intact motor sensory function) (d) disturbance in executive functioning (i.e. planning, organization, sequencing, abstracting)
B. The cognitive deficits in criteria A1 and A2 each cause significant impairment in social or occupational functioning and represent a significant decline from a previous level of functioning.
C. The deficits do not occur exclusively during the course of a delirium and persist beyond the usual duration of substance intoxication or withdrawal
D. There is evidence from the history, physical examination, or laboratory findings that the deficits are aetiologically related to the persisting effects of substance use (e.g. a drug of abuse, a medication)

Prevalence

Adequate epidemiological studies to determine the size of the problem have not been carried out. It has been estimated that 'alcohol-related dementia' accounts for 10 per cent of the dementia population.[1] Indeed alcohol misuse may contribute to as many as 21–24 per cent of all cases of cognitive impairment in mid-adulthood.[6] The prevalence is likely to be higher in areas of socio-economic deprivation, with most cases presenting between the ages of 50 and 60 years.[7] Early onset has been associated with poorer prognosis and potential for recovery. Recent evidence suggests that the prevalence of the Wernicke–Korsakoff syndrome, caused by thiamine deficiency, may be increasing.[8,9] Early identification and intervention can help to maximize optimum recovery.

Causal mechanisms

There is no single cause of 'alcohol-related dementia'. Individual susceptibility may be influenced by age; age of onset of drinking and the drinking history; gender; genetic background; family history of alcohol dependence; nutrition; alcohol exposure before birth; and general health status.[10] Causal mechanisms include: the neurotoxic effect of alcohol and its metabolite acetaldehyde; repeated episodes of intoxication and withdrawal; dietary neglect and vitamin deficiencies; repeated episodes of head trauma; cerebrovascular events; and liver damage. In particular, thiamine depletion, and metabolic factors, such as hypoxia, electrolyte imbalance, and hypoglycaemia, all of which result from acute or chronic intoxication and withdrawal, are important and interrelated. It is difficult to determine the relative contributions of these mechanisms. A number of theories have been advanced by Lishman and others to explain the mechanisms by which chronic alcohol use might lead to dementia.[1,6]

- The brain might be vulnerable to both thiamine depletion and alcohol neurotoxicity, the former affecting the basal brain regions and the latter both the basal brain and the frontal cortex.[1] Individual genetic vulnerability is likely to have a role in influencing these processes.
- Wernicke–Korsakoff pathological processes in the basal brain have the potential to damage nearby cholinergic fibres projecting to the cerebral cortex: the so-called cholinergic hypothesis.[1,6]
- Alcohol-induced brain pathology couples with other processes including 'ageing, trauma, vascular changes, and hepatic dysfunction' leading to cognitive decline: the coupling hypothesis.[1,6]
- Ethanol stimulates pituitary corticotrophin leading to elevated corticosteroid levels and possible injury to the hippocampus.
- Recurrent alcohol withdrawal has been hypothesized to have a kindling effect.[11] During alcohol withdrawal there is increased *N*-methyl-d-aspartate (NMDA) function which is postulated to lead to increased neuronal excitability and to glutamate-induced neurotoxicity.[12] The way in which alcohol interferes with glutamatergic neurotransmission, especially through the NMDA receptor, is probably central to an understanding of its long-term effects on the brain.
- Alcohol might lead to an accelerated ageing process.

Areas of the brain affected

There is evidence that the frontal lobes and sub-cortical areas such as the limbic system, the thalamus and the basal forebrain are particularly vulnerable to alcohol-related damage. The cerebellum is also vulnerable. Alcohol-related brain changes in the frontal lobes become more prominent with age.[13] Emotional processing is affected by long-standing heavy alcohol use and dependence, and probably reflects abnormalities in the limbic system and the frontal lobes.[14] This is manifested as difficulty with interpreting non-verbal emotional cues and recognizing facial expressions of emotion.

Alcohol-related brain damage has been studied using a variety of methods, ranging from the neuropathology of the post-mortem alcoholic brain to neuro-imaging techniques focusing on structural, functional and biochemical changes. There is also a considerable neuropsychological literature.

Neuropathology

Early neuropathological studies of the alcoholic brain described fairly uniform cerebral atrophy, mainly over the dorso-lateral frontal regions, widened sulci, a narrowed cortical ribbon, and enlargement particularly of the anterior horns of the lateral ventricles.[1]

The reduction in cerebral volume seen in the alcoholic brain is due mainly to the loss of white matter in the cerebral hemispheres.[15] The reduced white matter is not related to changes in hydration or changes in the chemical structure of the myelin. Selective neuronal loss in the superior frontal cortex was reported in one study[15] but not confirmed in another.[16] However, there is evidence that individual neurones are shrunken in regions where neuronal numbers are normal, such as the superior frontal, cingulate, and motor cortices.[15,16]

Animal research suggests that alcohol has a direct neurotoxic effect on the brain. Chronic ingestion of ethanol by well-nourished rats has been shown to be toxic to cholinergic projection neurones[17] and to reduce the complexity of dendritic arborization in hippocampal pyramidal neurones.[18] In the former study, transplantation of cholinergic neurones into the hippocampus and neocortex corrected the cholinergic deficits and memory abnormalities. In the latter, abstinence led to an increase in dendritic arborization.

Structural neuroimaging

Neuroimaging studies (CT and magnetic resonance imaging (MRI)) have compared recently detoxified alcoholics without obvious cognitive impairment with age-matched controls. CT studies confirmed diffuse atrophy of brain tissue, with the frontal lobes showing most extensive shrinkage.[19] Follow-up studies showed that abstinence was associated with reversibility of brain shrinkage,[19] particularly in younger individuals and in women.[20]

Structural MRI studies have reported reduced volume of both grey and white matter in the cerebral cortex, especially the frontal lobes, which are used for reasoning, judgement, and problem solving,[13] particularly in older age groups. Changes have also been shown in other structures involved in memory, such as the hippocampus (in adolescents and adults), mammillary bodies, thalamus and cerebellar cortex.[21–24] Other abnormalities include thinning of the corpus callosum and reduced volume in the pons.[25] Reduced white-matter volume is also seen in the temporal lobes (in alcohol dependent subjects with seizures) and in the cerebellar vermis where the loss is associated with deficits in postural stability.[26] More recent MRI studies have not supported the idea of increased vulnerability among women. [27] Abstinence is associated with recovery of tissue volume.

Functional neuroimaging

Functional neuroimaging studies have reported hypometabolism in the frontal and parietal cortices of chronic alcoholics without major neurological impairment, when compared with normal controls.[28–31] These abnormalities improve following abstinence,[31,32] mainly during the 16 to 30 days after the last use of alcohol. Metabolic recovery is most marked in the frontal area.[31]

Proton magnetic resonance spectroscopy can be combined with MRI, allowing ***in vivo*** insight into brain metabolism.[33–35] The metabolic changes observed in the few magnetic resonance spectroscopy studies that have been carried out suggest neuronal loss and compensatory gliosis.

Neuropsychology

Many individuals with a history of chronic excessive alcohol consumption show evidence of moderate impairment in short- and long-term memory, learning, visuoperceptual abstraction, visuospatial organization, the maintenance of cognitive set, and impulse control.[36] This tendency for alcoholics to show proportionally greater visuospatial than language-related impairments suggests that alcohol might have a selective effect on the right hemisphere: the so-called 'right hemisphere hypothesis'.[37] However, right hemisphere functions also decline with ageing and the current view is that the functional lateralities of 'alcoholics' and ageing individuals are similar to normal controls.[37]

Neuropsychological performance improves with abstinence. However, impairments can be detected in apparently healthy, abstinent alcohol dependent individuals[38] and are still detectable even after 5 years of abstinence.[39] Performance on neuropsychological tests has generally been poorly correlated with structural imaging changes,[19,40] particularly with changes in grey-matter volume. However, one MRI study reported significant correlations between cortical (sulcal) and subcortical (ventricular) fluid volumes and some cognitive measures.[22] Another study, using a combination of structural (CT or MRI) and functional imaging (positron emission tomography) together with neuropsychological tests in older alcohol-dependent patients who were abstinent, found a significant correlation between degree of atrophy/metabolic functioning in the cingulate gyrus, and performance on the Wisconsin Card Sort Test.[41]

Neuropsychological test scores do not predict outcome in alcohol-dependent patients.[42, 43]

Management

Difficulties in establishing a diagnosis of alcohol-related dementia/brain damage mean that it remains an 'invisible disability'[7], usually goes unrecognized, and is often masked by other problems such as continuing alcohol consumption and withdrawal, physical ill-health, depression and associated traumatic brain damage.

All dementia work-ups should include a history of past and present alcohol use, confirmed with a collateral history.[6] Appropriate treatment of alcohol withdrawal syndromes, assessment and re-assessment should be carried out over a two-year period. Ongoing assessment and care planning are important as these patients have the capacity to improve with abstinence. The possibility of Wernicke–Korsakoff pathology in cognitively impaired patients with an alcohol use disorder should prompt swift and appropriate treatment with parenteral thiamine.[44] Oral B vitamins should be continued long-term.

The mainstay of long-term treatment in alcohol-related dementia is abstinence. This can be facilitated by a supportive non-drinking social network, and cognitive behavioural methods to teach recognition of factors that predispose to relapse and alternative coping strategies.[6] Families and care-givers facilitate success and must be actively educated and supported. A rehabilitation approach to activities of daily living and occupation is also a key factor.

Patients with alcohol-related dementia are younger and more physically active than the usual dementia population. They do not fit neatly into any category of care and are at risk of falling 'through the net'. Services lack the capacity to manage this population so they are passed between services and find it difficult to access specialist assessment or care.

Conclusions

Alcohol-related dementia should be recognized as a preventable condition. However, identification is hampered by a lack of clarity in terminology, and a lack of standardized and specialized screening instruments and assessment procedures.[45] These individuals make repeated use of Accident and Emergency Departments, general medical, and long stay wards. Early identification would reduce their need for these services. Abstinence is the key to recovery. Treatment services should be integrated and flexible.

Further information

Baddeley, A.D., Kopelman, M/D., Wilson, B.A. (2003). *The Handbook of Memory Disorders*, (2nd edn.) Chichester: John Wiley and Sons Ltd.

Edwards, G., Marshall, E.J., Cook, C.C.H. (2003). *The Treatment of Drinking Problems: a Guide for the Helping Professions*, (4th edn.) Cambridge: Cambridge University Press

Lishman, W.A. (1998). *Organic Psychiatry. The Psychological Consequences of Cerebral Disorder*, (3rd edn). Oxford: Blackwell Science.

The National Institute of Alcohol Abuse and Alcoholism website has a portal which supports researchers and practitioners searching for information relating to alcohol research. It has a number of links to other databases: http://etoh.niaaa.nih.gov/

References

1. Lishman, W.A. (1990). Alcohol and the brain. *British Journal of Psychiatry*, **156**, 635–44.
2. Victor, M. (1993) Persistent altered mentation due to ethanol. *Neurologic Clinics*, **11**, 639–61.
3. Oslin, D., Atkinson, R.M, Smith, D.M., *et al* (1998). Alcohol related dementia: proposed clinical criteria. *International Journal of Geriatric Psychiatry*, **13**, 203–12.
4. American Psychiatric Association (1994). *Diagnostic and statistical manual of mental disorders* (4th edn). American Psychiatric Association, Washington, DC.

5. World Health Organization (1992). *International statistical classification of diseases and related health problems, 10th revision*. WHO, Geneva.
6. Smith, D. and Atkinson, R. (1995). Alcohol and dementia. *International Journal of Addictions,* **30**, 1843–69.
7. MacRae, S. and Cox, S. (2003). *Meeting the needs of people with alcohol-related brain damage: a literature review on the existing and recommended service provision and models of care*. University of Stirling, Scotland.
8. Smith, I. and Flanigan, C. (2000). Korsakoff's psychosis in Scotland. Evidence for increased prevalence and regional variation. *Alcohol and Alcoholism,* **35**, Suppl 1, 8–10.
9. Ramayya, A. and Jauher, P. 1997). Increasing incidence of Korsakoff's Psychosis in the east end of Glasgow. *Alcohol and Alcoholism*, **32**, 281–85.
10. Oscar-Berman M., Marinkovic, K. (2003) Alcoholism and the brain: an overview. *Alcohol Research and Health,* **27**, 125–33.
11. Ballenger, J.C. and Post, R.M. (1978). Kindling as a model for alcohol withdrawal syndromes. *British Journal of Psychiatry*, **33**, 1–14.
12. Tsai, G., Gastfriend, D.R., and Coyle, J.T. (1995). The glutamatergic basis of human alcoholism. *American Journal of Psychiatry*, **152**, 332–40.
13. Pfefferbaum, A., Sullivan, E.V., Mathalon, D.H., *et al.* (1997). Frontal lobe volume loss observed with magnetic resonance imaging in older chronic alcoholics. *Alcoholism: Clinical and Experimental Research*, **21**, 521–9.
14. Kornreich, C., Philippot, P., Foisy, M.L. (2002) Impaired emotional facial expression recognition is associated with interpersonal problems in alcoholism. *Alcohol and Alcoholism,* **37**, 394–400.
15. Kril, J.J. and Harper, C.G. (1989). Neuronal counts from four cortical regions in alcoholic brains. *Acta Neuropathologica*, **79**, 200–4.
16. Jensen, G.B. and Pakkenburg, B. (1993). Do alcoholics drink their neurones away? *Lancet*, **342**, 1201–4.
17. Arendt, T.A., Allen, Y., Sinden, J., *et al.* (1988). Cholinergic–rich brain transplants reverse alcohol–induced memory deficits. *Nature*, **332**, 448–50.
18. McMullan, P.A., Saint–Cyr, J.A., and Carlen, P.L. (1984). Morphological alterations in rat CA1 hippocampal pyramidal cell dendrites resulting from chronic ethanol consumption and withdrawal. *Journal of Comparative Neurology*, **225**, 111–18.
19. Ron, M.A. (1983). *The alcoholic brain: CT scan and psychological findings*. Psychological Medicine Monograph 3. Cambridge University Press.
20. Carlen, P.L. and Wilkinson, D.A. (1987). Reversibility of alcohol–related brain damage: clinical and experimental observations. *Acta Medica Scandinavica*, **222** (Suppl 717), 19–26.
21. Sullivan, E.V., Marsh, L., Mathalon, D.H., *et al* (1995). Anterior hippocampal volume deficits in nonamnesic, ageing chronic alcoholics. *Alcoholism: Clinical and Experimental Research*, **19**, 110–22.
22. Davila, M.D., Shear, P.K., Lane, B., *et al.* (1994). Mammillary body and cerebellar shrinkage in chronic alcoholics: an MRI and neuropsychological study. *Neuropsychology*, **8**, 433–44.
23. Shear, P.K., Sullivan, E.V., Lane, B.J., *et al.* (1996). Mammillary body and cerebellar shrinkage in chronic alcoholics with and without amnesia. *Journal of the International Neuropsychological Society*, **2**, 34–5.
24. De Bellis, M.D., Clark, D. B., Beers, S.R. *et al.* (2000). Hippocampal volume in adolescent-onset alcohol use disorders. *American Journal of Psychiatry,* **157**, 737–44.
25. Pfefferbaum, A., Lim, K.O., Desmond, J.E., *et al.* (1996). Thinning of the corpus callosum in older alcoholic men: a magnetic resonance imaging study. *Alcoholism: Clinical and Experimental Research*, **20**, 752–7.
26. Rosenbloom, M., Sullivan, E.V., Pfefferbaum A. (2003). Using magnetic resonance and diffusion tensor imaging to assess brain damage in alcoholics. *Alcohol Research and Health,* **27**, 146–52.
27. Pfefferbaum, A., Rosenbloom, M.J., Deshmukh, A., *et al.* (2002). Sex differences in the effects of alcohol on brain structure. *American Journal of Psychiatry,* **158**, 188–97.
28. Sachs, H., Russell, J.A.G., Christman, D.R., and Cook, B. (1987). Alteration of regional cerebral glucose metabolic rate in non–Korsakoff chronic alcoholism. *Archives of Neurology*, **44**, 1242–51.
29. Volkow, N.D., Hitzemann, R., Wang, G.–J., *et al.* (1992). Decreased brain metabolism in neurologically intact healthy alcoholics. *American Journal of Psychiatry*, **149**, 1016–22.
30. Volkow, N.D., Wang, G.–J., Hitzemann, R., *et al.* (1994). Recovery of brain glucose metabolism in detoxified alcoholics. *Americal Journal of Psychiatry*, **151**, 178–83.
31. Nicolas, J.M., Catafau, A.M., Estruch, R., *et al.* (1993). Regional cerebral blood flow—SPECT in chronic alcoholism: relation to neuropsychological testing. *Journal of Nuclear Medicine*, **34**, 1452–9.
32. Fein, G., Meyerhoff, D.J., Di Sclafani, V., *et al.* (1994). 1H magnetic resonance spectroscopic imaging separates neuronal from glial changes in alcohol–related brain atrophy. In *Alcohol and glial cells*, pp. 227–41. Research Monograph 27. National Institutes of Health, Bethesda, MD.
33. Martin, P.R., Gibbs, S.J., Nimmerrichter, A.A., *et al.* (1995). Brain proton magnetic resonance spectroscopy studies in recently abstinent alcoholics. *Alcoholism: Clinical and Experimental Research*, **4**, 1078–82.
34. Seitz, D., Widmann, U., Seeger, U., *et al.* (1999). Localised proton magnetic resonance spectroscopy of the cerebellum in detoxifying alcoholics. *Alcoholism: Clinical and Experimental Research*, **23**, 158–63.
35. Bloomer, C.W., Langleben, D.D., Meyerhoff, D.J. (2004) Magnetic resonance detects brainstem changes in chronic, active heavy drinkers. *Psychiatry Research,* **30**, 209-18.
36. Oscar–Berman, M. (2000). Neuropsychological vulnerabilities in chronic alcoholism. In: Noronha, A., Eckardt, M.J., and Warren, K., eds. *Review of NIAAA's Neuroscience and Behavioural Research Portfolio*. National Institute on Alcohol Abuse and Alcoholism (NIAAA) Research Monograph No 34. Bethesda, MD: NIAAA, pp. 437–71.
37. Ellis, R.J. and Oscar-Berman, M. (1989). Alcoholism aging, and functional cerebral asymmetries. *Psychological Bulletin*, **106**, 128–47.
38. Davies, S.J.C., Pandit, S.A., Feeney, B., *et al.* (2005). Is there impairment in clinically 'healthy' abstinent alcohol dependence? *Alcohol and Dependence,* **40**, 498–503.
39. Brandt, J., Butters, N., Ryan, C., *et al.* (1983). Cognitive loss and recovery in long term alcohol abusers. *Archives of General Psychiatry*, **40**, 435–42.
40. Carlen, P.L., Wilkinson, D.A., and Wortzman, G., *et al.* (1981). Cerebral atrophy and functional deficits in alcoholics without clinically apparent liver disease. *Neurology*, **31**, 377–85.
41. Adams, K.M., Gilman, S., Koeppe, R.A., *et al.* (1993). Neuropsychological deficits are correlated with frontal hypometabolism in positron emission tomography studies of older alcoholic patients. *Alcoholism: Clinical and Expeimental Research,* **17,** 205–10.
42. Alterman, A.I., Kushner, H., and Holahan, J.M. (1990). Cognitive functioning and treatment outcome in alcoholics. *Journal of Nervous and Mental Disorders*, **178**, 494–9.
43. Leenane, K.J. (1988). Patients with alcohol–related brain damage: therapy and outcome. *Australian Drug and Alcohol Review*, **7**, 89–92.
44. Thomson A. D. and Marshall, E.J (2006) The treatment of patients at risk of developing Wernicke's Encephalopathy in the community. *Alcohol and Alcoholism*, **41**, 159–67.
45. Smith I., Hillman A (1999). Management of the alcoholic Korsakoff syndrome. *Advances in Psychiatric Treatment,* **5**, 271–75.

4.1.12 Amnesic syndromes

Michael D. Kopelman

Introduction

Amnesic disorders can be broadly classified across two orthogonal dimensions. Along the first dimension, there can be transient or discrete episodes of amnesia as opposed to persistent memory impairment. On the second dimension, memory loss can result from either neurological damage or psychological causation, although admixtures of these factors are, of course, very common. The notion of confabulation has traditionally been associated with amnesic syndromes, particularly the Korsakoff syndrome, although it may have a separate basis, and false memories are now known to arise in a number of different situations. With the advent of drugs purporting to influence memory, there is increasing interest in the psychopharmacology of memory disorders. This chapter will consider findings from investigations of patients with memory disorders and a few selected psychopharmacological studies of relevance. It will not review the extensive literature on functional imaging in normal subjects.

Transient amnesias

Transient global amnesia

Transient global amnesia (TGA) most commonly occurs in the middle-aged or elderly, more frequently in men, and it results in a period of amnesia lasting several hours. It is characterized by repetitive questioning, and there may be some confusion, but patients do not report any loss of personal identity (they know who they are). It is sometimes preceded by headache or nausea, a stressful life event, a medical procedure, or vigorous exercise. Hodges and Ward[1] found that the mean duration of amnesia was 4 h and the maximum was 12 h. In 25 per cent of their sample, there was a past history of migraine, which was considered to have a possible aetiological role. In a further 7 per cent of the sample, the patients subsequently developed unequivocal features of epilepsy (there had been no focal signs or features of epilepsy during the original attack) and the memory loss was therefore attributed, in retrospect, to previously undiagnosed epilepsy. There was no association with either a past history of vascular disease, clinical signs suggestive of vascular pathology, or known risk factors for vascular disease. In particular, there was no association with transient ischaemic attacks. In 60 to 70 per cent of the sample, the underlying aetiology was unclear.

More recently, Quinette *et al.*[2] reviewed the findings in 1353 patients reported in the clinical literature since 1956 and their own data from 142 patients, seen between 1994 and 2004. In general, the findings were consistent across the two sources. There was no sex bias, and the vast majority of attacks occurred between the ages of 50 and 80 (mean = 60.3 ± 9.6). Most patients had a single attack, but the annual rate of recurrence ranged from 2.9 per cent to 26.3 per cent (6.3 per cent in their own study). In the literature, the duration of attacks ranged from 15 min to 24 h and, in their own investigation, the range was 30 min to 16 h (mean = 5.6 h). These authors investigated putative predisposing and precipitating factors in great detail, concluding that TGA may encompass at least three different groups of patients: (i) younger patients with a history of migraine, in whom spreading neurochemical depression may be implicated, (ii) women who have experienced acute emotional or physical stress, and often have a history of anxiety or depression, and (iii) men who, following physical exertion, develop venous congestion in the context of insufficient jugular vein valves and a precipitating Valsalva manoeuvre.

In instances of TGA where neuropsychological tests have been administered to patients during the acute episode of memory loss,[1,3] the patients show a profound anterograde amnesia, as expected, on tests of both verbal and non-verbal memory. However, performance on tests of retrograde memory is variable. Follow-up studies show either complete or almost complete recovery of memories, several weeks to months after the acute attack. In general, retrograde amnesia recovers before anterograde amnesia; the degree of shrinkage of retrograde amnesia is heterogeneous; and anterograde memory (new learning) recovers gradually.

The general consensus is that the amnesic disorder results from transient dysfunction in limbic-hippocampal circuits, crucial to memory formation. Medial temporal abnormalities have been reported bilaterally in terms of single-photon emission CT (SPECT) measures of perfusion, positron emission tomography (PET) measures of metabolism, diffusion weighted imaging (DWI), and small hippocampal cavities on T2 reversed magnetic resonance imaging (MRI) images.[4,5] In addition, venous duplex sonography has shown jugular vein valve insufficiency in a proportion of cases.[5]

Transient epileptic amnesia

This term was coined by Kapur,[6] and it refers to the minority of patients with transient global amnesia in whom epilepsy appears to be the underlying cause of the syndrome.[1] Where epilepsy has not previously been diagnosed, the main predictive factors for an epileptic aetiology are brief episodes of memory loss (an hour or less) with multiple attacks.[1] It is important to note that standard electroencephalography (EEG) and CT findings are often normal. However, an epileptic basis to the disorder may be revealed on sleep EEG recordings.[1,7]

Patients with transient epileptic amnesia may show residual deficits in between their attacks, associated with their underlying neuropathology. Kopelman *et al.*[7] found a moderate degree of residual anterograde memory impairment in their patient, related to subsequent (unpublished) findings of small foci of MRI signal alteration and PET hypometabolism bilaterally in the medial temporal lobes. Several authors have reported patients who describe 'gaps' in past personal memories, and Manes *et al.*[8] have reported disproportionate inter-ictal retrograde amnesia. The latter group also reported abnormal long-term forgetting of verbal material, but whether these gaps in memory result from faulty encoding (because of subclinical ictal activity), impaired consolidation (giving rise to accelerated forgetting), or deficits in retrieval remains controversial.

Epilepsy may, of course, give rise to automatisms or post-ictal confusional states. Where there is an automatism in such circumstances, there is always bilateral involvement of the limbic structures involved in memory formation, including the hippocampal and parahippocampal structures bilaterally as well as the mesial diencephalon. Consequently, amnesia for the period of automatic behaviour is always present and is usually complete.

Head injury

In head injury, it is important to distinguish between a brief period of retrograde amnesia, which may last only a few seconds or minutes but can be weeks or months, a longer period of post-traumatic amnesia, and islands of preserved memory within the amnesic gap.[9] Occasionally post-traumatic amnesia may exist without any retrograde amnesia, although this is more common in cases of penetrating lesions. Sometimes there is a particularly vivid memory for images or sounds occurring immediately before the injury, on regaining consciousness, or during a lucid interval between the injury and the onset of post-traumatic amnesia. These vivid memories may become the intrusive flashbacks of a post-traumatic stress disorder (PTSD) syndrome.

Post-traumatic amnesia (PTA) is generally assumed to reflect the degree of underlying diffuse brain pathology, in particular rotational forces giving rise to axonal tearing and generalized cognitive impairment. The length of PTA is predictive of eventual cognitive outcome, psychiatric outcome, and social outcome.[10] However, the duration of PTA is often not well documented in medical records, and these relationships are often weaker than is generally assumed. In addition, contusion to the frontal and anterior temporal lobes is a common consequence of head injury. The clinical features and underlying pathophysiology of head injury have recently been well described elsewhere.[11]

Post-traumatic amnesia needs to be distinguished from the persisting anterograde memory impairment, which may be detected on clinical assessment or cognitive testing long after the period of PTA has ended. Moreover, forgetfulness is a common complaint within the context of a post-traumatic syndrome, which may include anxiety, irritability, poor concentration, and various somatic complaints. Commonly, these complaints persist long after the settlement of any compensation issues.[11]

Alcoholic blackouts

Alcoholic blackouts are discrete episodes of memory loss for significant events, which should not be confused with withdrawal seizures or other ictal phenomena. Alcoholic blackouts are associated with severe intoxication, usually in the context of a history of prolonged alcohol abuse. Goodwin *et al.*[12] described two types of blackout—the *fragmentary* and the *en bloc*. However, alcohol-induced state-dependent experiences can be viewed as related phenomena, and it has been suggested that the three represent gradations of alcohol-induced memory impairment. In state-dependent effects, subjects when sober cannot remember events or facts from an episode of intoxication, which they recall easily when they again become intoxicated. In fragmentary blackouts, the subjects are aware of their memory loss on being told later of an event; there are islands of preserved memory; and the amnesia tends to recover partially through time by shrinkage of the amnesic gap. In *en bloc* blackouts there is an abrupt beginning and end to the period of memory loss, and the lost memories are very seldom recovered. Blackouts may be more common in binge drinkers, because they are related to a high blood alcohol level. Hypoglycaemia may also be a contributory factor, and blackouts are more common where there is a history of previous head injuries.

After electroconvulsive therapy

This is an iatrogenic form of transient amnesia. Benzodiazepines and anticholinergic agents can also give rise to transient memory loss in more moderate form.[13]

Subjects tested within a few hours of electroconvulsive therapy (ECT) show a retrograde impairment for information from the preceding 1 to 3 years, a pronounced anterograde memory impairment on both recall and recognition memory tasks, and an accelerated rate of forgetting.[14] When retested approximately 6 to 9 months after completion of a course of ECT, memory generally returns to normal on objective tests. However, complaints of memory impairment can persist, and they may be evident three or more years after a course of ECT has been completed.[15] It seems that patients with persistent complaints of memory loss tend to be those who have recovered least well from their depression,[14,15] although their complaints tend to focus upon the period for which there was an initial retrograde and anterograde amnesia. A recent American study suggested that sine wave stimulation induces cognitive slowing in terms of reaction time, and that multiple bilateral ECT administrations can produce impairments in autobiographical memory retrieval 6 months following treatment.[16]

Verbal memory appears to be particularly sensitive to disruption. Unilateral electroconvulsive therapy to the non-dominant hemisphere produces considerably less memory impairment than bilateral ECT, although it is important to identify the non-dominant hemisphere by a valid procedure. Attempts to minimize memory disruption by either making changes in premedication or the concomitant administration of other substances—such as glycopyrrolate, physostigmine, thyroxine, dexamethasone, or acetylcholine—have produced limited or no benefit.

Post-traumatic stress disorder

This clinically important syndrome is described in Chapter 4.6.2. Post-traumatic stress disorder (PTSD) is characterized by vivid, intrusive thoughts and memories ('flashbacks'), avoidance and anxiety phenomena, and hyper-arousal and hyper-vigilance symptoms. However, there may be instances of brief memory loss, distortions, or even frank confabulations. For example, a victim of the *Herald of Free Enterprise* disaster at Zeebruge described trying to rescue a close friend still on board the ship, when other witnesses reported that the close friend had, in fact, not been seen by the victim from the moment the ship turned over. Cases of PTSD may, of course, be confounded by other factors, such as head injury. Nevertheless, it is of interest that PTSD symptoms can occur even when a subject is completely amnesic for an episode.[17] PTSD victims can show deficits in anterograde memory on formal tasks many years after the original trauma, and there is also evidence that they may show loss of hippocampal volume on magnetic resonance imaging (MRI) brain scan, which has been attributed by some to a surge in glucocorticoid secretion. Brewin[18] has recently reviewed four controversies in autobiographical memory for trauma. He found that qualitative and quantitative differences do exist between trauma and non-trauma memories in PTSD victims, and that memories for trauma can be either better or worse than non-trauma memories. In other words, some incidents may be recalled particularly vividly, and others may be forgotten.

Psychogenic fugue

A fugue state is a syndrome consisting of a sudden loss of all autobiographical memories and knowledge of personal identity, usually associated with a period of wandering, for which there is a subsequent amnesic gap on recovery. Characteristically, fugue states last a few hours or days, up to about 3 weeks. There are also descriptions in the literature of persisting autobiographical memory loss, in which personal identity has been 're-learned', and these are better known as 'psychogenic focal retrograde amnesia'.[19] However, whenever such complaints persist, the suspicion of simulation must arise. Fugue states differ from transient global amnesia or transient epileptic amnesia in that the subject does not know who he or she is, and repetitive questioning is not a characteristic feature in fugues.

As discussed elsewhere,[20] fugue states are always preceded by a severe precipitating stress. Second, depressed mood is also an extremely common antecedent for a psychogenic fugue state, and may be associated with manifest suicidal ideas just before or following recovery from the fugue. Third, various authors have noted that there is often a past history of a previous transient neurological amnesia, such as epilepsy or head injury. In brief, it appears that patients who have experienced a previous transient organic amnesia, and who become depressed and/or suicidal, are particularly likely to go into a fugue in the face of a severe, precipitating stress. That stress may consist of marital or emotional discord, bereavement, financial problems, a criminal charge, or stress during wartime. Fugues have been described as a 'flight from suicide'. Recent neuro-imaging investigations have examined people purportedly in a fugue state with very inconsistent results, probably because the delay until imaging, the imaging techniques employed, and the clinical situations themselves have varied considerably across studies.

Amnesia for offences

This is a phenomenon commonly brought to the attention of psychiatrists, particularly forensic psychiatrists, although the empirical literature on this disorder is scanty. Amnesia is claimed by 25 to 45 per cent of offenders in cases of homicide, approximately 8 per cent of perpetrators of other violent crimes, and a small percentage of non-violent offenders.[21] It is necessary to exclude underlying neurological or endocrine factors such as an epileptic automatism, post-ictal confusional state, head injury, sleepwalking, or hypoglycaemia. Underlying medical disorder can be grounds for a so-called 'insane' automatism in English law (if the result of an internal brain disease) or a 'sane' automatism (if the consequence of an external agent), but otherwise amnesia per se does not constitute grounds for alleviation of responsibility for an offence.

Amnesia for an offence is most commonly associated with the following:

1 States of either extreme emotional arousal or peri-traumatic dissociation, in which the offence is unpremeditated, and the victim usually a lover, wife, or family member. This is most commonly seen in homicide cases ('crimes of passion').

2 Alcohol intoxication (sometimes in association with other substances), usually involving very high peak levels ('alcoholic blackout'), and often a long history of alcohol abuse. The victim is not necessarily related to the offender, and the offence may vary from criminal damage, through assault, to homicide.

3 Florid psychotic states or depressed mood. Occasionally offenders describe a delusional account of what has happened, quite at odds with what was seen by other observers, and sometimes resulting in confessions to crimes that the person could not actually have committed (a paramnesia or delusional memory). In many other cases, depressed mood is associated with amnesia for an offence, just as it is a common associate of psychogenic fugue.

Pyszora *et al.*[22] examined the psychiatric reports of all offenders given a life sentence in England and Wales in 1994, 29 per cent of whom claimed amnesia. Detailed, follow-up reports at 3 years were also examined, and these suggested that approximately one-third of those who had claimed amnesia at trial reported complete recovery, one-third showed partial recovery, and one-third reported no change in their amnesias. Only about 2 per cent were thought to have been malingering.

Persistent memory disorder

The amnesic syndrome can be defined as follows:

> An abnormal mental state in which memory and learning are affected out of all proportion to other cognitive functions in an otherwise alert and responsive patient.[23]

The Korsakoff syndrome can be defined in the same way but with the addition of the following phrase:

> . . . resulting from nutritional depletion, notably thiamine deficiency.

In fact, Victor *et al.*[23] used the first description as a definition of the Korsakoff syndrome, but it is important to distinguish between amnesic syndromes in general (for which the Victor *et al.* definition suffices) and the particular clinical condition described by Korsakoff,[24] whose cases can all be viewed (with hindsight) as having suffered nutritional depletion, whether of alcoholic or non-alcoholic causation. Various disorders can give rise to an amnesic syndrome.

The Korsakoff syndrome

As mentioned, this is the result of nutritional depletion, namely a thiamine deficiency. Korsakoff[24] described this condition as resulting from alcohol abuse or from a number of other causes, but by far the most common nowadays is alcohol abuse.

(a) Clinical

There are frequent misunderstandings about the nature of this disorder. 'Short-term memory', in the sense that psychologists employ it, is intact but learning over more prolonged periods is severely impaired, and there is usually a retrograde memory loss which characteristically extends back many years or decades.[20] Korsakoff himself noted that his patients 'reason about everything perfectly well, draw correct deductions from given premises, make witty remarks, play chess or a game of cards, in a word comport themselves as mentally sound persons'.[24] However, he also noted repetitive questioning, the extensive nature of the retrograde memory loss, and a particular problem in remembering the temporal sequence of events, associated with severe disorientation in time. As will be discussed below, he gave examples of confabulation reflecting the problem with the temporal sequence memory, such that real memories were jumbled up and retrieved inappropriately, out of temporal context.

Many cases of the Korsakoff syndrome are diagnosed following an acute Wernicke encephalopathy, involving confusion, ataxia, nystagmus, and opthalmoplegia. Usually, not all these features are present, and the opthalmoplegia in particular responds rapidly to treatment with high-dose vitamins. These features are often associated with a peripheral neuropathy. However, the disorder can also have an insidious onset, and such cases are more likely to come to the attention of psychiatrists; in these cases, there may be either no known history of or only a transient history of Wernicke features. There are also reports that the characteristic Wernicke–Korsakoff neuropathology is found much more commonly at autopsy in alcoholics than the diagnosis is made in life, implying that many cases are being missed.

Victor *et al.*(23) reported that 25 per cent of patients with the Korsakoff syndrome 'recover', 50 per cent show improvement through time, and 25 per cent remain unchanged. Whilst it is unlikely that any established patient shows complete recovery, the present author's experience is that substantial improvement does occur over a matter of years if the patient remains abstinent. It is probably correct to say that 75 per cent of these patients show a variable degree of improvement, whilst 25 per cent show no change.(20)

(b) Pathology

The characteristic neuropathology in what is often known as the Wernicke–Korsakoff syndrome consists of neuronal loss, microhaemorrhages, and gliosis in the paraventricular and periaqueductal grey matter.(23) However, there has been a debate as to which particular lesions are critical for the manifestation of chronic memory disorder. Victor *et al.*(23) pointed out that all 24 of their cases in whom the medial dorsal nucleus of the thalamus was affected had a clinical history of persistent memory impairment (Korsakoff syndrome), whereas five cases in whom this nucleus was unaffected had a history of Wernicke features without any recorded clinical history of subsequent memory disorder. By contrast, the mammillary bodies were implicated in all the Wernicke cases, whether or not there was subsequent memory impairment. However, Mair *et al.*(25) provided a careful pathological and neuropsychological description of two patients with the Korsakoff syndrome, whose autopsies showed lesions in the mammillary bodies, the midline, and anterior portion of the thalamus, but not in the medial dorsal nuclei. Mayes *et al.*(26) obtained very similar findings in two further patients with the Korsakoff syndrome, who had also been very carefully described both neuropsychologically and at autopsy. Harding *et al.*(27) reported that pathology in the anterior principal thalamic nuclei was the critical difference between eight patients who suffered a persistent Korsakoff syndrome, and five others who experienced only a transient Wernicke episode. Taken together, these findings suggest that the mammillary bodies, the mammillothalamic tract, and the anterior thalamus may be more important to memory dysfunction than the medial dorsal nucleus of the thalamus.

There is also evidence of general cortical atrophy particularly involving the frontal lobes in patients with the Korsakoff syndrome, and this is associated with neuropsychological evidence of 'frontal' or 'executive' test dysfunction in these patients.(20)

There have been a number of neuro-imaging studies of the Korsakoff syndrome. CT scan studies indicated a general degree of cortical atrophy, particularly involving the frontal lobes.(28) MRI studies have indicated more specific atrophy in diencephalic structures.(29) PET investigations show variable findings, but hypometabolism has been reported in thalamic, orbito-medial frontal, and retrosplenial regions.(30)

Herpes encephalitis

This can give rise to a particularly severe form of amnesic syndrome.(31) Many cases are said to be primary infections, although others may involve a reactivation of the virus. Characteristically, there is a fairly abrupt onset of acute fever, headache, and nausea. There may be behavioural changes. Seizures can occur. The fully developed clinical picture with neck rigidity, vomiting, and motor and sensory deficits seldom occurs during the first week. Moreover, some cases commence more insidiously with behavioural change or psychiatric phenomena, the confusion and neurological features becoming evident only later. Diagnosis is by the PCR test or a raised titre of antibodies to the virus in the cerebrospinal fluid. A presumptive diagnosis is sometimes made on the basis of the clinical picture as well as severe signal alteration, haemorrhaging, and atrophy in the temporal lobes on MRI brain imaging.

Neuropathological and neuro-imaging studies usually show extensive bilateral temporal lobe damage,(29,32) although occasionally the changes are surprisingly unilateral. There may be frontal changes, often in the orbito-frontal regions, and there may be focal changes elsewhere as well as a variable degree of general cortical atrophy. The medial temporal lobe structures are usually particularly severely affected, including the hippocampi, amygdalae, entorhinal, and perirhinal cortices, and other parahippocampal structures. Encephalitis, like head injury, can also implicate basal forebrain structures which give cholinergic outputs to the hippocampi; this may further exacerbate the damage.

The chronic memory disorder in herpes encephalitis is often very severe,(31) but it shows many resemblances to that seen in the Korsakoff syndrome, consistent with the fact that there are many neural connections between the thalami, mammillary bodies, and the hippocampi. Patients with herpes appear to have better 'insight' into the nature of their disorder, and a 'flatter' temporal gradient to their retrograde memory loss (i.e. less sparing of early memories), and they may have a particularly severe deficit in spatial memory when the right hippocampus is involved.(20) However, the similarities in the episodic memory disorder tend to outweigh the differences.

On the other hand, a more extensive involvement of semantic memory is characteristic in herpes encephalitis, and this results from the widespread involvement of the lateral, inferior, and posterior regions of the temporal lobes. Semantic memory refers to a knowledge of facts, concepts, and language (see Chapter 2.5.3). Left temporal lobe pathology in herpes encephalitis commonly gives rise to an impairment in naming, reading (a so-called 'surface dyslexia'), and other aspects of lexico-semantic memory. Right temporal lobe damage may lead to a particularly severe impairment in face recognition memory or knowledge of people.

Severe hypoxia

Severe hypoxia can give rise to an amnesic syndrome following carbon monoxide poisoning, cardiac and respiratory arrests, or suicide attempts by hanging or poisoning with the exhaust gases from a car. Drug overdoses may precipitate prolonged unconsciousness and cerebral hypoxia, and this quite commonly occurs in heroin abusers. Zola–Morgan *et al.*(33) described a patient with repeated episodes of hypoxia and/or cardiovascular problems who developed a moderately severe anterograde amnesia. At autopsy 6 years later, this patient was shown to have a severe loss of pyramidal cells in the CA1 region of the hippocampi bilaterally, with the rest of the brain appearing relatively normal. Hippocampal atrophy on MRI has found in hypoxic, amnesic patients,(29) and also thalamic hypometabolism on FDG–PET scanning.[34] In brief, the memory disorder is likely to result from a combination of hippocampal and thalamic changes, related to the many common neural pathways between these two structures. However, Caine and Watson[35] in an important review reported that less than 20 per cent of hypoxic patients described in the literature show either a specific amnesic syndrome (in the absence of other cognitive deficits) or damage solely confined to the hippocampi.

Vascular disorders

Two types of specific vascular lesions can particularly affect memory, as opposed to general cognitive functioning, namely thalamic infarction and subarachnoid haemorrhage. However, memory disorder may be the first manifestation of the vascular form of 'mild cognitive impairment'.

In an elegant CT scan study, von Cramon *et al.*[36] showed that damage to the anterior thalamus was critical in producing an amnesic syndrome. When the pathology was confined to the more posterior regions of the thalamus, memory function was relatively unaffected. The anterior region of the thalamus is variably supplied by the polar or paramedian arteries in different individuals, both of which are, ultimately, branches of the posterior cerebral artery that also supplies the posterior region of the hippocampi. When there is a relatively pure lesion of the anterior thalamus, anterograde amnesia without an extensive retrograde memory loss commonly results. However, cases in whom there is also retrograde memory loss, or even a generalized dementia, have been described following thalamic infarction, and this presumably relates to the extent to which thalamic projections are also implicated in the infarction.

Subarachnoid haemorrhage following rupture of a berry aneurysm can result in memory impairment, whether the anterior cerebral or posterior cerebral circulation from the Circle of Willis is involved. Most commonly described in the neuropsychological literature have been ruptured aneurysms from the anterior communicating arteries, because these affect ventro-medial frontal structures and the basal forebrain. Gade[37] has argued that it is whether or not the septal nuclei of the basal forebrain are implicated in the ischaemia which determines whether a persistent amnesic syndrome occurs in such patients. Others have attributed the florid confabulation, which these patients often exhibit, to concomitant orbito-frontal damage.[38]

Head injury

As discussed above, severe head injury can produce a persistent amnesia which may or may not be associated with generalized cognitive impairment. There may be direct trauma to the frontal and anterior temporal lobes, resulting in contusion and haemorrhaging, contrecoup damage, intracranial haemorrhage, and axonal tearing and gliosis following acceleration-deceleration or rotational forces. Memory function is commonly the last cognitive function to improve following an acute trauma, and patients can show the characteristic features of an amnesic syndrome. The phenomenon of 'isolated retrograde amnesia' has been described: in such cases, it seems likely that a mild head injury has precipitated a more purely psychiatric phenomenon. Traumatic head injury is considered in more detail in Chapter 4.1.10 and by Fleminger.[11]

Other causes of an amnesic syndrome

Deep midline cerebral tumours can give rise to an amnesic syndrome, and this may be exacerbated by surgical or irradiation treatment for pituitary tumours. Other infections, such as tuberculous meningitis or HIV, may, on occasion, give rise to an amnesic syndrome. Mild cognitive impairment and the very early stages of Alzheimer dementia may manifest themselves as a focal amnesic syndrome. Surgical treatment to the temporal lobes for epilepsy can result in profound amnesia, if there is bilateral involvement. There is increasing evidence that focal lesions in the frontal lobes can also produce severe memory impairment on aspects of anterograde and retrograde memory.[20] This can occur even in the absence of basal forebrain involvement, but it probably results from particular aspects of memory being implicated, including planning and organization, source and context monitoring, and particular aspects of retrieval processes.[39]

Neuropsychological aspects

The terms 'short-term' and 'long-term' memory should be abolished from psychiatric discourse, as they cause confusion across disciplines. It is more useful to consider current or recent memory versus remote (or autobiographical) memory. In addition, 'prospective memory' refers to remembering to do something.

Concepts of memory are considered in Chapter 2.5.3. As described in that chapter, a distinction is generally drawn between so-called 'working memory', which holds information for brief periods (a matter of several seconds) and allocates resources, and secondary memory, which holds different types of information on a permanent or semi-permanent basis. Secondary memory, in turn, can be subdivided into an episodic (or 'explicit') component, semantic memory, and implicit memory. Episodic memory refers to incidents or events from a person's past, such that he/she can 'travel back mentally in time'; this is characteristically severely affected in the amnesic syndrome. As mentioned previously, semantic memory refers to knowledge of facts, concepts, and language. The learning of new semantic memories is variably affected in the amnesic syndrome, although there is now some evidence that new facts can be learned even in the presence of severe, bilateral medial temporal lobe damage. Other aspects of semantic memory, including naming, reading, and comprehension, are affected in disorders where there is concomitant widespread temporal lobe pathology, such as herpes encephalitis, Alzheimer dementia, or semantic dementia (a form of frontotemporal dementia). Implicit memory refers to procedural or perceptuomotor skills, and to the facilitation of responses in the absence of explicit memory, known as 'priming'. Both these aspects are characteristically spared in the amnesic syndrome,[40] although the precise extent of sparing does depend on particular features in the experimental design.[41]

Over the years, there has been extensive debate concerning whether the primary deficit in the amnesic syndrome lies in the initial encoding of information, or some kind of physiological 'consolidation' into secondary memory, or accelerated forgetting of that information, or in retrieval processes.[20] There is still very little agreement about this debate, but, if anything, the consensus is that retrieval problems are secondary to initial acquisition and consolidation impairments, at least in anterograde amnesia. Retrieval deficits may be more important where there is an extensive retrograde memory loss,[20] which might account for why there is generally a poor correlation between scores on anterograde memory measures and retrograde memory measures.

Much recent research has focused on the specific function of the hippocampi, and how there their role is distinct from other structures within the medial temporal lobes, more lateral temporal lobe regions, and the frontal lobes. Suggestions include a particular contribution to the binding of complex associations, relational memory, the binding of the distributed features of an episode into a coherent trace, novel or incremental learning, and a contribution to retrieval processes.[20,42] Aggleton and Brown[43] have suggested that the hippocampi are critical to the recall of contextual richness and detail, involved in 'remembering' or 'recollection', whereas the perirhinal cortex is particularly implicated in the familiarity judgements essential in recognition memory. The frontal lobes are generally thought to contribute to planning and organization in memory, aspects of context and source memory, awareness of memory performance (metamemory), prospective memory, and to particular aspects of retrieval processes.[20,39]

There are also many controversies concerning the nature of the extensive retrograde memory loss found in many of the above disorders. Modern neuropsychological studies have confirmed that this retrograde memory loss can extend back many years or decades, but that it often shows a 'temporal gradient' with relative sparing of early memories. The gradient is characteristically steeper in the amnesic syndrome than in dementing disorders such as Alzheimer dementia or Huntington's disease. Differing patterns of retrograde memory loss can occur; left temporal lobe damage seems to affect memory for facts and for the more linguistic components of remote memory, whereas right temporal lobe damage may affect memory for the incidents in a person's life.[20] One theory of retrograde amnesia and of the temporal gradient is that, as memories become 'consolidated' through time, they become independent of the medial temporal lobes and are relatively protected against brain injury to these structures. A second theory is that, through time, episodic memories adopt a less vivid, more 'semantic' form, and this protects earlier memories from the effects of brain injury. A third theory suggests that the hippocampi are always involved in the retrieval and reactivation of memories, and that every time a memory is retrieved, a new trace is laid down, resulting in 'multiple traces' protecting against the effects of brain injury.[44] These three theories make differing predictions and, at present, the underlying basis of retrograde amnesia remains hugely controversial.

Confabulation disorders

Confabulation can be subdivided into 'spontaneous' confabulation, in which there is a persistent, unprovoked outpouring of erroneous memories, and 'momentary' or 'provoked' confabulation, in which fleeting intrusion errors or distortions are seen in response to a challenge to memory, such as a memory test.[20,45]

Confabulation is widely believed to be particularly associated with the Korsakoff syndrome, but this is incorrect. Spontaneous confabulation arises in confusional states and in frontal lobe disease.[45] The link with frontal lobe pathology, particularly in the ventro-medial region, has been established in many investigations.[20,38] Spontaneous confabulation is often seen in the confusional state of a Wernicke encephalopathy, but it is rare in the more chronic phases of the Korsakoff syndrome. On the other hand, fleeting intrusion errors or distortions ('momentary confabulation') do occur in the chronic phase of a Korsakoff syndrome, when memory is challenged. However, such intrusion errors are also seen in healthy subjects when memory is 'weak' for any reason, such as a prolonged delay until recall.[45] They are also seen in Alzheimer dementia and other clinical amnesic syndromes, and they are certainly not specific to the Korsakoff syndrome.

There has been considerable interest of late in the nature of spontaneous confabulations. Confabulation can extend across episodic, personal semantic, and more general semantic memories.[46] A theory put forward by Korsakoff himself, as well as other authorities,[24] emphasizes problems in the temporal ordering of memories. In a particularly elegant study, Schnider *et al.*[47] found that a group of 'spontaneous confabulators' could be differentiated from other amnesic patients and controls on the basis of their errors on a temporal context memory task, but not on other memory or executive tests. More recently Schnider[48] has interpreted these findings in terms of a failure in 'reality monitoring'. Somewhat similarly, Johnson *et al.*[49] has argued that confabulation may reflect an interaction between a vivid imagination, an inability to retrieve autobiographical memories systematically, and source or context monitoring deficits. By contrast, Gilboa *et al.*[38] found that a failure to make fine-grained distinctions within memory could account for Schnider's observations. They argued that a failure in strategic retrieval and post-retrieval monitoring, related to ventromedial and orbito-frontal pathology, is critical for spontaneous confabulation to arise. Somewhat similar hypotheses have been put forward by Burgess and Shallice[50] It has also been argued that the content of confabulations may be heavily influenced by motivational factors.[51]

The notion of 'confabulation' or 'false memory' has now been extended to a variety of other disorders, including delusional memory, confabulation in schizophrenia, false confessions, apparently false memories for child sexual abuse, pseudologia fantastica, and dissociative identity disorder. Whilst each of these can potentially be accounted for in terms of a general model of memory and executive function, provided that the social context and some notion of 'self' is incorporated, there are likely to be differing mechanisms which give rise to these different types of false memory.[20]

Neurochemistry and neuropharmacology of memory disorders

The Korsakoff syndrome is relatively unusual among memory disorders in that there is a distinct neurochemical pathology with important implications for treatment. Since animal studies in the 1930s and 1940s, and the important observations of De Wardener and Lennox[52] and others in malnourished prisoners of war, it has been known that **thiamine depletion** is the mechanism which gives rise to the acute Wernicke episode, followed by a Korsakoff memory impairment. However, the genetic factor that predisposes a minority of heavy drinkers to develop this syndrome before they develop hepatic or gastrointestinal complications of alcohol abuse remains unclear. Transketolase is the enzyme which requires thiamine pyrophosphate (TPP) as a cofactor. Thiamine depletion affects six neurotransmitter systems (including acetylcholine, glutamate, aspartate, and GABA), either by reduction of TPP-dependant enzyme activity or by direct structural damage. Direct genomic PCR sequences of a high-affinity thiamine transporter gene

(SLC19A2) have identified three genetic variants in the Wernicke–Korsakoff syndrome.[53] Whatever the underlying genetic mechanism, treatment as soon as possible with high doses of parenterally administered multivitamins is essential in patients with the Wernicke–Korsakoff syndrome. The Wernicke features respond well to high-doses of vitamins, and such treatment can prevent the occurrence of a severe, chronic Korsakoff state.[20,23] The small risk of anaphylaxis is completely outweighed by the high risk of severe brain damage and the appreciable risk of litigation if such treatment is not administered.

There has been an extensive literature on the effects of **cholinergic antagonists** (such as scopolamine) upon memory. Kopelman and Corn[54] found a pattern of impairment in anterograde memory that closely resembled that seen in the amnesic syndrome. It has been argued that cholinergic blockade produces an effect upon the 'central executive' component of working memory, but Rusted[55] has concluded that this is not sufficient to account for the drug effect upon memory processes. Although some have argued that the predominant effect of scopolamine is on attention, it has been found that covarying for the sedation or psychomotor effects of the drug did not eliminate the strong drug effects on episodic memory tests.[13,54] The anticholinesterases, donepezil, rivastigmine, and galantamine are now widely used in the management of Alzheimer dementia.

Despite their very different pharmacological actions, the effects of the **benzodiazepines** upon memory and attention are remarkably similar to those of scopolamine. When recall or recognition is tested after a delay, benzodiazepines produce a marked anterograde impairment in explicit or episodic memory, similar to scopolamine.[13] As with scopolamine, however, once learning has been accomplished, the rate of forgetting is normal, and benzodiazepines do not produce any retrograde deficits.[13] Procedural learning tasks after both benzodiazepine and scopolamine administration show similar effects, with learning curves on the active drug generally paralleling those for placebo.[13,54] Benzodiazepine effects can be attenuated by coadministration of the benzodiazepine antagonist, flumazenil.

The effects of **catecholamines** upon memory have been studied for many years, but the general consensus is that they act upon 'tonic attentional processes' rather than directly upon the storage or retrieval of memories. In an elegant study, Cahill *et al.*[56] examined the effects of the β-adrenergic receptor antagonist propranolol on memory for an emotionally arousing story, compared with a carefully matched neutral story. As expected, subjects given a placebo recalled more of the emotional than the neutral story, when tested 1 week later. Subjects given propranolol recalled the neutral story as well as the placebo subjects, but were impaired on the emotional story, whereas stimulation of noradrenaline (with yohimbine) produced some enhancement of the emotional elements, and benzodiazepines impaired memory equally for both the neutral and emotional elements of the story.[13]

Some years ago, there was interest in the **serotonergic system** and alcohol-induced memory impairment. Early reports suggested that zimelidine, a serotonin reuptake inhibitor, reversed the memory impairment in healthy volunteers after the administration of ethanol. Later, it was claimed that fluvoxamine improved memory performance in five patients with the Korsakoff syndrome, and that the improvements correlated significantly with reductions in a cerebrospinal fluid breakdown product. The samples were small, and the benefits were minor. Nevertheless, 3,4-methylenedioxymethamphetamine (ecstasy) has been reported to produce memory impairments either by direct or indirect effects.[57] Some of the apparent cognitive effects of serotonergic agents may be the by-product of their effects on mood.[13]

Of forensic psychiatric importance are agents which produce transient but profound amnesia, and may be implicated in offences such as 'date rape'. These include flunitrazepam (Rohypnol) and gammahydroxybutyrate (GHB), and this topic has recently been reviewed by Curran.[58]

Conclusions

Systematic clinical descriptions of amnesic disorders and their underlying pathology have become more detailed and rigorous over the years. In particular, recent advances in neuro-imaging (structural, metabolic, and activation) have provided the opportunity to relate particular cognitive abnormalities to specific changes in brain function. The use of pharmacological agents, in parallel with such imaging techniques, may promote the development of pharmacological agents more potent than the meagre array that we have at present for the treatment of severe memory disorder.

Further information

Baddeley, A.D., Kopelman, M.D., and Wilson, B.A. (eds.) (2002). *The handbook of memory disorders* (2nd edn). John Wiley & Sons Ltd, Chichester.

Kopelman, M.D. (2002). Disorders of memory. *Brain*, **125**, 2152–90.

Squire, L.R. and Schacter, D.L. (eds.) (2002). *Neuropsychology of memory* (3rd edn). The Guilford Press, New York.

References

1. Hodges, J.R. and Ward, C.D. (1989). Observations during transient global amnesia: a behavioural and neuropsychological study of five cases. *Brain*, **112**, 595–620.
2. Quinette, P., Guillery-Girard, B., Dayan, V., *et al.* (2006). What does transient global amnesia really mean? Review of the literature and thorough study of 142 cases. *Brain*, **129**, 1640–58.
3. Kritchevsky, M., Squire, L.R., and Zouzounis, J.A. (1988). Transient global amnesia: characterization of anterograde and retrograde amnesia. *Neurology*, **38**, 213–9.
4. Nakada, T., Kwee, I.L., Fujii, Y., *et al.* (2005). High-field, T2 reversed MRI of the hippocampus in transient global amnesia. *Neurology*, **64**, 1170–4.
5. Sander, K. and Sander, D. (2005). New insights into transient global amnesia: recent imaging and clinical findings. *Lancet Neurology*, **4**, 437–44.
6. Kapur, N. (1993). Transient epileptic amnesia—a clinical update and a reformulation. *Journal of Neurology, Neurosurgery, and Psychiatry*, **56**, 1184–90.
7. Kopelman, M.D., Panayiotopoulos, C.P., and Lewis, P. (1994). Transient epileptic amnesia differentiated from psychogenic 'fugue': neuropsychological, EEG and PET findings. *Journal of Neurology, Neurosurgery, and Psychiatry*, **57**, 1002–4.
8. Manes, F., Graham, K.S., Zeman, A., *et al.* (2005). Autobiographical amnesia and accelerated forgetting in transient epileptic amnesia. *Journal of Neurology, Neurosurgery, and Psychiatry*, **76**, 1387–91.
9. Russell, W.R. and Nathan, P.W. (1946). Traumatic amnesia. *Brain*, **69**, 280–300.

10. Brooks, N. (1984). Cognitive deficits after head injury. In *Closed head injury: psychological, social and family consequences* (ed. N. Brooks), pp. 44–73. Oxford University Press, Oxford.
11. Fleminger, S. (in press). Head injury. In *Lishman's organic psychiatry* (4th edn) (eds. A. David, S. Fleminger, M.D. Kopelman, S. Lovestone, and J. Mellers). Blackwell, Oxford,.
12. Goodwin, D.W., Crane, J.B., and Guze, S.E. (1969). Phenomenological aspects of the alcoholic 'blackout'. *The British Journal of Psychiatry*, **115**, 1033–8.
13. Curran, H.V. and Weingartner, H. (2002). Psychopharmacology of human memory. In *The handbook of memory disorders* (2nd edn) (eds. A.D. Baddeley, M.D. Kopelman, and B.A. Wilson), pp. 123–41. John Wiley & Sons Ltd., Chichester.
14. Frith, C.D., Stevens, M., Johnstone, E.C., *et al.* (1983). Effects of ECT and depression on various aspects of memory. *The British Journal of Psychiatry*, **142**, 610–7.
15. Squire, L.R. and Slater, P.C. (1983). ECT and complaints of memory dysfunction: a prospective three-year follow–up study. *The British Journal of Psychiatry*, **142**, 1–8.
16. Sackeim, H.A., Prudic, J., Fuller, R., *et al.* (2007). The cognitive effects of electroconvulsive therapy in community settings. *Neuropharmacology*, **32**, 244–54.
17. Harvey, A.G., Brewin, C.R., Jones, C., *et al.* (2003). Coexistence of posttraumatic stress disorder and traumatic brain injury: towards a resolution of the paradox. *Journal of the International Neuropsychological Society*, **9**, 663–76.
18. Brewin, C.R. (2007). Autobiographical memory for trauma: update on four controversies. *Memory*, **15**, 227–48.
19. Kopelman, M.D. (2000). Focal retrograde amnesia and the attribution of causality: an exceptionally critical review. *Cognitive Neuropsychology*, **17**, 585–621.
20. Kopelman, M.D. (2002). Disorders of memory. *Brain*, **125**, 2152–90.
21. Taylor, P.J. and Kopelman, M.D. (1984). Amnesia for criminal offences. *Psychological Medicine*, **14**, 581–8.
22. Pyszora, N.M., Barker, A.F., and Kopelman, M.D. (2003). Amnesia for criminal offences: a study of life sentence prisoners. *Journal of Forensic Psychiatry and Psychology*, **14**, 475–90.
23. Victor, M., Adams, R.D., and Collins, G.H. (1971). *The Wernicke–Korsakoff syndrome*. F.A. Davis, Philadelphia, PA.
24. Korsakoff, S.S. (1889). Psychic disorder in conjunction with peripheral neuritis. Translated and republished by M. Victor and P.I. Yakovlev (1955). *Neurology*, **5**, 394–406.
25. Mair, W.G.P., Warrington, E.K., and Weiskrantz, L. (1979). Memory disorder in Korsakoff's psychosis; a neuropathological and neuropsychological investigation of two cases. *Brain*, **102**, 749–83.
26. Mayes, A.R., Meudell, P.R., Mann, D., *et al.* (1988). Location of lesions in Korsakoff's syndrome: neuropsychological and neuropathological data on two patients. *Cortex*, **24**, 367–88.
27. Harding, A., Halliday, G., Caine, D., *et al.* (2000). Degeneration of anterior thalamic nuclei differentiates alcoholics with amnesia. *Brain*, **123**, 141–54.
28. Jacobson, R.R. and Lishman, W.A. (1990). Cortical and diencephalic lesions in Korsakoff's syndrome: a clinical and CT scan study. *Psychological Medicine*, **20**, 63–75.
29. Colchester, A., Kingsley, D., Lasserson, D., *et al.* (2001). Structural MRI volumetric analysis in patients with organic amnesia, 1: methods and findings, comparative findings across diagnostic groups. *Journal of Neurology, Neurosurgery, and Psychiatry*, **71**, 13–22.
30. Reed, L.J., Lasserson, D., Marsden, P., *et al.* (2003). ^{18}FDG–PET findings in the Wernicke–Korsakoff syndrome. *Cortex*, **39**, 1027–45.
31. Hokkanen, L. and Launes, J. (2007). Neuropsychological sequelae of acute-onset sporadic viral encephalitis. *Neuropsychological Rehabilitation*. **17**, 429–49.
32. Reed, L.J., Lasserson, D., Marsden, P., *et al.* (2005). Correlations of regional cerebral metabolism with memory performance and executive function in patients with herpes encephalitis or frontal lobe lesions. *Neuropsychology*, **19**, 555–65.
33. Zola–Morgan, S., Squire, L.R., and Amaral, D.G. (1986). Human amnesia and the medial temporal region: enduring memory impairment following a bilateral lesion limited to field CA1 of the hippocampus. *The Journal of Neuroscience*, **6**, 2950–67.
34. Reed, L.J., Lasserson, D., Marsden, P., *et al.* (1999). FDG-PET analysis and findings in amnesia resulting from hypoxia. *Memory*, **7**, 599–612.
35. Caine, D. and Watson, J.D. (2000). Neuropsychological and neuropathological sequelae of cerebral anoxia: a critical review. *Journal of International Neuropsychological Society*, **6**, 86–99.
36. von Cramon, D.Y., Hebel, N., and Schuri, U. (1985). A contribution to the anatomical basis of thalamic amnesia. *Brain*, **108**, 997–1008.
37. Gade, A. (1982). Amnesia after operations on aneurysms of the anterior communicating artery. *Surgical Neurology*, **18**, 46–9.
38. Gilboa, A., Alain, C., Stuss, D.T., *et al.* (2006). Mechanisms of spontaneous confabulations: a strategic retrieval account. *Brain*, **129**, 1399–1414.
39. Baldo, J.V. and Shimamura, A.P. (2002). Frontal lobes and memory. In *The handbook of memory disorders* (2nd edn) (eds. A.D. Baddeley, M.D. Kopelman, and B.A. Wilson), pp. 363–79. John Wiley & Sons Ltd., Chichester.
40. Schacter, D.L. (1987). Implicit memory: history and current status. *Journal of Experimental Psychology. Learning, Memory and Cognition*, **13**, 501–18.
41. Ostergaard, A.L. (1994). Dissociations between word priming effects in normal subjects and patients with memory disorders: multiple memory systems or retrieval? *Quarterly Journal of Experimental Psychology. A, Human Experimental Psychology*, **47**, 331–64.
42. Cohen, N.J., Poldrack, R.A., and Eichenbaum, H. (1998). Memory for items and memory for relations in the procedural/declarative memory framework. *Memory*, **6**, 6689–99.
43. Aggleton, J. P. and Brown, M.W. (1999). Episodic memory, amnesia and the hippocampal-anterior thalamic axis. *The Behavioural and Brain Sciences*, **22**, 425–44.
44. Moscovitch, M., Nadel, L., Winocur, G., *et al.* (2006). The cognitive neuroscience of remote episodic, semantic and spatial memory. *Current Opinion in Neurobiology*, **16**, 179–90
45. Kopelman, M.D. (1987). Two types of confabulation. *Journal of Neurology, Neurosurgery, and Psychiatry*, **50**, 1482–7.
46. Kopelman, M.D., Ng, N., and Van den Brouke, O. (1997). Confabulation extending across episodic memory, personal and general semantic memory. *Cognitive Neuropsychology*, **14**, 683–712.
47. Schnider, A., von Däniken, C., and Gutbrod, K. (1996). The mechanisms of spontaneous and provoked confabulations. *Brain*, **119**, 1365–1375.
48. Schnider, A. (2003). Spontaneous confabulation and the adaptation of thought to ongoing reality. *Nature Reviews. Neuroscience*, **4**, 662–71.
49. Johnson, M.K., O'Connor, M., and Cantor, J. (1997). Confabulation, memory deficits, and frontal dysfunction. *Brain and Cognition*, **34**, 189–206.
50. Burgess, P.W. and Shallice, T. (1996). Confabulation and the control of recollection. *Memory*, **4**, 359–411.
51. Fotopoulou, A., Solms, M., and Turnbull, O. (2004). Wishful reality distortions in confabulations: a case study. *Neuropsychologia*, **42**, 727–44.
52. De Wardener, H.E. and Lennox, B. (1947). Cerebral beriberi (Wernicke's encephalopathy): review of 52 cases in Singapore prisoner-of-war hospital. *Lancet*, **1**, 11–7.
53. Guerrini, I., Thomson, A.D., Cook, C., *et al.* (2005). Direct genomic PCR sequencing of the high affinity thiamine transporter (SLC19A2) gene identifies three genetic variants in Wernicke–Korsakoff syndrome (WKS). *American Journal of Medical Genetics*, **137B**, 17–19.

54. Kopelman, M.D. and Corn, T.H. (1988). Cholinergic 'blockade' as a model for cholinergic depletion: a comparison of the memory deficits with those of Alzheimer-type dementia and the alcoholic Korsakoff syndrome. *Brain*, **111**, 1079–110.
55. Rusted, J. (1994). Cholinergic blockade and human information processing: are we asking the right questions? *Journal of Psychopharmacology*, **8**, 54–9.
56. Cahill, L., Prins, B., Weber, M., *et al.* (1994). Beta-adrenergic activation and memory for emotional events. *Nature*, **3H**, 702–4.
57. Kopelman, M.D., Reed, L.J., Marsden, P., *et al.* (2001). Amnesic syndrome and severe ataxia following the recreational use of MDMA ('ecstasy') and other substances, *Neurocase*, **7**, 423–32.
58. Curran, H.V. (2006). Effects of drugs on witness memory. In *Witness testimony—psychological, investigative and evidential perspectives* (eds. A. Heaton-Armstrong, E. Shepherd, G. Gudjonsson, and D. Wolchover), pp 77–87. Oxford University Press, New York.

4.1.13 The management of dementia

John-Paul Taylor and Simon Fleminger

Introduction

The term dementia is used in two different ways. First there are the **dementias**. These are **diseases** that cause progressive and diffuse cerebral damage, of which Alzheimer's disease is the most common. Second, dementia can be used to refer to a **clinical syndrome**. Thus dementia is 'an acquired global impairment of intellect, memory, and personality, but without impairment of consciousness'.(1) For clinicians this is the preferred usage, and the one adopted in this chapter. It demands that the cause of the dementia is explored, and makes no comment on the likely prognosis.

This chapter will focus on the management of dementia regardless of the cause; however given the burden of dementia in older age, the discussion will be invariably, but not exclusively, slanted towards the management of dementia in this age group. Aspects of management specific to individual diseases which produce dementia will be avoided. In addition, a discourse on the management of cognitive and memory problems is excluded as these are described elsewhere (see Chapters 2.5.4 and 6.2.7). Patients who suffer the dementia before 18 years of age will, by and large, not be included; their needs are often best met by services provided for people with intellectual disability.

The newly diagnosed patient with dementia

Given that it is now possible to diagnose dementia early in the course of the disease it is important to consider when and how to disclose the diagnosis. This is often seen by clinicians as a difficult task and one to be avoided until the diagnosis is absolutely certain. Stigma is associated with the diagnosis of dementia; it is perceived as a chronic debilitating illness, with a progressive deterioration in mental faculties that ultimately leads to a loss of self-identity and an unpleasant death. The clinician may believe there is not much to offer until later in disease, and so there is not much point in disclosing the diagnosis at an early stage. Furthermore, they may find it difficult to break 'bad news', particularly when an individual with dementia may not understand or retain information.

Nevertheless, leaving these discussions until the diagnosis is certain may be too late; the patient's ability to take part in decisions about their future treatment, and their family's future, may by then be jeopardized by cognitive decline. Only early in the course of the illness will they be able to make a power of attorney, settle their will, and discuss with their doctors how they wish to be treated once the disease is well advanced.

The way in which the diagnosis is given will affect how patients and their families cope and deal with the diagnosis in long-term. Although there are no specific strategies for disclosure of a dementia diagnosis, techniques developed for breaking bad news in disclosure of cancer diagnosis are probably applicable; for example, the excellent protocol devised by Baile *et al.*(2)

Formal psychotherapy and counselling may help patients and their families come to terms with the diagnosis.(3) Clear simple pamphlets or information sheets should be available so that patients and their families can assimilate the diagnosis and its consequences outside of the interview. Referrals can also be made to dementia support groups and local dementia societies; these can provide psychoeducation, befriending services, and networking groups for patients and their families.

After initial meeting and disclosure, it is important that a follow-up meeting is arranged; this will allow patients and families to take on board the diagnosis and formulate any questions they might have. Detailed management strategies are probably best discussed during follow-up appointments, as patients and their families might be overwhelmed at the initial appointment.

Genetic counselling and testing for dementia

Many patients and their families are concerned about the heritability of the condition and will ask if any genetic tests can be performed. But such a request needs to be considered carefully.

In only about 5–10 per cent of cases is the dementia directly due to a high penetrance genetic mutation (for example, early-onset Alzheimer's, frontotemporal dementia, and dementia associated with Huntington's disease). Low penetrance gene variants, such as the apolipoprotein E (APOE) genotype, while modulating, for example, the risk of development of Alzheimer's dementia, do not adequately predict disease development. Consensus groups have therefore advised against using APOE predictive testing.(4–6)

There are also significant social ramifications of genetic testing for the relatives of patients with dementia; positive tests could have serious implications for employment, family planning, and insurance. Therefore access to appropriate pre-test counselling is important.

Box 4.1.13.1 shows a current modus operandi, based on United Kingdom guidelines produced by the National Institute of Clinical Excellence in dealing with this difficult subject.(4) However, the clinician is advised to keep abreast of current best practice given the likely rapid advances in this area.

The younger patient with dementia

The incidence of dementia under the age of 65 is rare. However dementia in younger people has significant additional consequences. Often the younger person with dementia has dependents and considerable financial commitments. Spouses may have to give up

Box 4.1.13.1 Guidelines for genetic testing for dementia

- People likely to have a genetic cause for their dementia (for example, familial autosomal dominant Alzheimer's disease or frontotemporal dementia, cerebral autosomal dominant arteriopathy with subcortical infarcts and leukoencephalopathy [CADASIL], or Huntington's disease) and their unaffected relatives should be offered referral for genetic counselling and testing.
- All patients referred for testing should have appropriate counselling in helping deal with psychological and social consequences.
- If a specific genetic cause for dementia is not suspected, as is the case in late-onset dementia, genotyping should not be undertaken for clinical purposes.

work to care for their partners and there are very high rates of caregiver burn-out.

Specialist service provision for the younger patient with dementia is often lacking. These patients have different life expectations than their elderly counterparts. Many will be physically fit and often do not fit easily into the service models provided for their elderly counterparts. Specialist multidisciplinary teams allied to traditional dementia services have been advocated[4] although actual implementation is still required.

Driving

Decisions about whether or not a person with dementia should be allowed to drive are often difficult. The patient's right to autonomy needs to be balanced against their social and legal responsibilities. The clinician has a duty to consider the safety of other people on the road, as well as the patient themselves. But there is no clear consensus on the best way of making the decision, although a number of regulatory authorities have issued guidance. As a rule of thumb, patients with moderate or severe dementia should not be driving; patients with mild dementia need a careful assessment.

Advice: Begin with a history from family and relatives; this may need to be done while the patient is not present. Have there been any accidents or near accidents? Do they feel the patient is unsafe and shouldn't be driving? A cognitive assessment (especially of executive and visuospatial function, and psychomotor speed) and physical examination of the patient is of some value although not definitive. The gold standard is a driving assessment on the road; a driving simulator test is an alternative.

Often, as in the United Kingdom, patients are legally obliged to inform their driving licensing authority about their diagnosis. The clinician should advise the patient and their relative of this, and document the discussion. Difficulties arise when a patient who is not fit to drive fails to inform the authority and continues to drive. A written warning to stop driving is often sufficient, particularly if the patient and their relatives are reminded that their car insurance policy is no longer valid. In some cases where the patient presents a real risk the clinician may need to break confidentiality and inform the authorities.

If the patient is deemed fit to continue driving, then they should be advised about risk reduction, for example keep to well-known routes and avoid busy roads, driving in bad weather conditions, or at night. They should be regularly reassessed with regard to their fitness to drive. Often this has to happen in any case because they will only be issued a short-term license (e.g. 1 year).

Behavioural and neuropsychiatric symptoms in dementia

Background

Behavioural and Psychological Symptoms in Dementia (BPSDs) have been defined by the International Psychogeriatric Association (1996) as 'signs and symptoms of disturbed perception, thought content, mood, or behaviour that frequently occur in patients with dementia'.[7]

Identification, assessment, and management of BPSDs are central to good dementia care. These heterogeneous symptoms are highly prevalent in dementia; one study[8] found that 61 per cent of 329 patients with dementia exhibited BPSDs, with the most common symptoms being apathy (27 per cent), depression (24 per cent), and agitation/aggression (24 per cent). The presence of BPSDs is cited by carers and relatives as being the most significant determinant in generating carer stress,[9] carer burden,[10] and increasing the likelihood of subsequent institutionalization.[11]

There appears to be only a weak correlation between the level of cognitive impairment and the occurrence and severity of BPSDs. Stronger associations have been noted between the presence of BPSDs and the degree of impairment in activities of daily living.[12]

A complex interplay of factors can give rise to these symptoms and include intrinsic host attributes and extrinsic environmental influences (Fig. 4.1.13.1). Therefore the same symptom in different individuals may be due to different causes. For example, aggression may be the response to a delusion in one individual, and the reaction to a change in caregiver in another. Often several different problem behaviours are seen in the same patient, such as wandering and sleep disturbance. There may be causal links between different BPSDs, for example the presence of distressing auditory hallucinations and persecutory delusions is strongly associated with consequent aggression.[13] Particular constellations of BPSDs are often associated with specific dementia syndromes (Table 4.1.13.1). BPSDs will change over time; for example aggression and psychosis tend to occur in the early to middle stages of Alzheimer's dementia whereas incontinence is invariably a feature of late disease.

Of all the symptoms that patients with dementia suffer, it is the problems caused by BPSDs that are most likely to trigger a pharmacological intervention or institutionalization. But whether or not a BPSD is reported as being a problem depends heavily on the informant and the situation. For example, night-time wandering may be tolerated by the spouse with the patient in their own home, but not by nursing staff in an acute medical ward.

Assessment

Assessment of a BPSD begins with a carefully taken informant history to assess the nature, history, and severity of the BPSD, and to garner the background medical, psychiatric, and social history. For example, there may be a history of phobic disorder, which is now manifest as agitation, or a lifelong tendency to aggression. Alcohol or other drug abuse must be addressed. The effect of recently prescribed, and recently stopped, medications needs to be

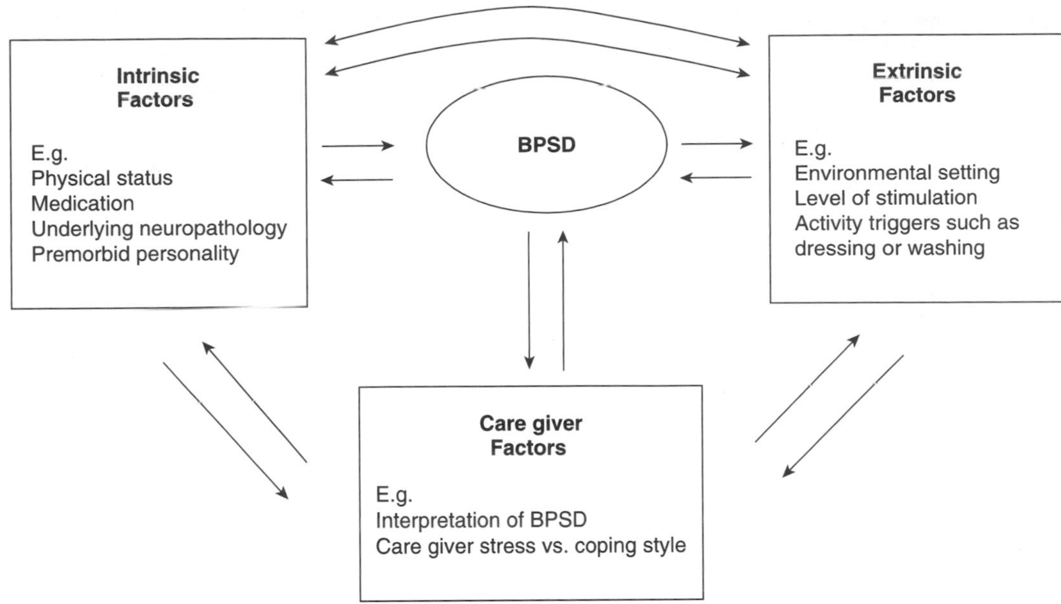

Fig. 4.1.13.1 Interaction between intrinsic host factors, extrinsic factors, and caregiver factors in the aetiology of BPSDs.

considered. The impact of the BPSD on the patient and the carer should be determined. Consider environmental influences; ask when the BPSD first occurred and whether it now occurs at any specific time, and whether it is related to any prior activity or antecedents. This will aid in formulation of specific behavioural management strategies (see below).

The mental state examination will look for evidence of anxiety, depression, or psychosis and persecutory delusions, and ascertain the patient's insight and understanding of their behavioural/neuropsychiatric symptoms. With specific problem behaviours direct observation of the behaviour can be very useful. A thorough physical examination will be needed to exclude physical illnesses; if suspected then appropriate medical investigations should be considered such as a midstream urine sample or chest X-ray. In agitated behaviours, sources of pain and fear should be considered, as well as the possibility of sleep loss or constipation, cold, or hunger. The presence of any sensory deprivation (e.g. hearing loss) should be looked for. Conversely the patient may be over-stimulated, as commonly occurs on general medical or surgical wards because of the noise and hustle and bustle.

Table 4.1.13.1 Common BPSDs in major dementia syndromes

Dementia	Common BPSDs
Alzheimer's dementia	Agitation, apathy, depression, anxiety, delusions
Vascular dementia	Depression, apathy
Dementia with Lewy bodies	Visual hallucinations, delusions, depression
Frontotemporal dementia	Disinhibition, repetitive behaviours, altered eating patterns, apathy

Assessment scales

A range of objective instruments for the measurement of BPSDs now exist.(14) Some measure multiple domains, for example the Behavioural Pathology in Alzheimer's Disease rating scale.(15) Other instruments are specific for one symptom, such as the Cohen–Mansfield Agitation Inventory(16) or Cornell scale for depression in dementia.(17) There are several caveats to the use of such scales, including the large intra-individual variations in scale scores which reflects the dynamic nature of BPSDs and variable reporting patterns of different observers. Some scales take a long time to complete or require training to administer. Nevertheless in clinical practice, the judicious use of such scales can allow for more reliable assessment of the response to a specific behavioural or pharmacological intervention.

Management of agitation and challenging behaviour

Agitation includes behaviour that is aggressive or abusive and occurs at an inappropriate frequency or is socially inappropriate.(18) Challenging behaviour has been used as a 'catch all' for a number of different behaviours including aggression, combativeness and disruptive vocalizations and may or may not be associated with agitation.

(a) Behavioural interventions

Evidence: Research into the effectiveness of behavioural techniques for agitation and challenging behaviour is based largely on studies using A–B–A–B or single-case design, and case series. Recent systematic reviews suggest that individually tailored behavioural interventions are effective.(19–22)

Advice: An intervention programme would start with a situational, or ABC, analysis:

- Antecedents—what was happening before the behaviour started?
- Behaviour—a clear description of the behaviour.

- Consequences—what happened as a result of the behaviour, particularly looking for possible reinforcers of the behaviour?

The frequency and severity of the behaviour then need to be charted as a baseline before introducing the specific intervention. Many programmes rely on the differential reinforcement of other behaviour (**DRO**); this involves positive reinforcement of other, appropriate behaviours, with the hope that these will then replace the challenging behaviour. A useful technique to be used alongside DRO is 'time out on the spot' (**TOOTS**), in which the unwanted behaviour is met with immediate withdrawal of social contact; appropriate behaviours receive warm social contact.

Unfortunately the limiting factor in use of behavioural interventions in dementia is the lack of trained individuals; often behavioural programmes can only be implemented in specialist units. In addition, the whole nursing/multidisciplinary team must be aware of the principles of reinforcement and extinction of behaviour, because behavioural programmes are unlikely to be effective unless consistently applied across the team. Evidence for the effectiveness of educating carers/family members in behaviour management techniques is currently inconclusive.[22] An alternative view which is gaining prominence is that while some challenging behaviours may not be amenable to interventions, it is possible to change the caregiver perception of the problem; this can lead to a reduction in caregiver distress and often by improving an aberrant interaction between caregiver and patient, there is a reduction in the challenging behaviour itself.

(b) Psychosocial and environmental interventions

Evidence: Despite numerous studies there is still a paucity of high quality evidence for the effectiveness of psychosocial and environmental interventions.[19,20,22] Some interventions have shown some promise helping ameliorate aggressive or disruptive behaviours in dementia. A non-exhaustive selection of the major psychosocial interventions that have been used is shown in Table 4.1.13.2.

Advice: The interventions should be tailored to the individual person taking account of their level of function and response to the approach. Psychosocial interventions are best applied when there is no clear cause for the disruptive behaviour; they should be only considered when a thorough assessment of the behaviour has be carried out to exclude treatable causes, for example, pain or psychosis. Even though certain psychosocial approaches may only have modest efficacy in decreasing disruptive behaviour, they may still be useful care adjuncts in improving general patient well-being.

(c) Antipsychotics

Evidence: Short-term treatment with atypical antipsychotics is of benefit in treating aggression, agitation, and psychosis, although the effect size is modest.[4,23,24] With regard to typical antipsychotics, meta-analyses have suggested that haloperidol might improve symptoms of aggression.[25,26] There is no evidence for benefit of longer term treatment (i.e. greater than 3 months).

Adverse effects of antipsychotics may be troublesome, particularly in the elderly; indeed outcomes from the Clinical Antipsychotic Trials of Intervention Effectiveness for Alzheimer's disease suggested that the adverse effects of atypical antipsychotics offset treatment

Table 4.1.13.2 Psychosocial interventions in dementia

Intervention	Description	Evidence for effectiveness
Psychoeducation to staff	Educating staff about dementia, neuropsychiatric symptoms, and reduced use of restraint	Possibly effective—might have sustained benefits
Reminiscence therapy	Uses materials related to patient and their era for example, old photographs and news articles, to stimulate memories and allow sharing of experiences	Possibly effective
Cognitive stimulation	Similar to reality orientation therapy, based on information processing rather than orientation knowledge	Possibly effective—might have sustained benefits
Music therapy	Can consistent of playing music as part of activity sessions or at specific times of the day. Music often of patient's era	Possibly effective—but no evidence of prolonged benefit
Snoezelen/multi-sensory therapy	Combined relaxation and use of sensory stimuli e.g. sounds, lights, touch	Possibly effective—but benefit wears off quickly. Also time/staff intensive
Aromatherapy	Mostly using lemon balm oil and lavender oil either inhaled or applied by massage	Possibly effective for agitation and restlessness
Bright light therapy	Sustained exposure to high levels of light (up to 10 000 lux)	Possibly effective (may be more benefit in sleep disturbance than behavioral disturbance). Time/staff intensive
Pet therapy	Contact with animals	Inconclusive
Exercise	Walking or light exercise sessions	Inconclusive
Simulated presence	Audiotape recorded by caregiver/family member played to patient where positive autobiographical memories are reiterated	Not effective
Reality orientation	Regular provision of orientating information e.g. time, date, etc.	Not effective
Validation therapy	Rogerian-based therapy; allowing resolution of unfinished conflicts, the acceptance of the reality and the expression of feelings	Not effective

advantages in patients with Alzheimer's disease.[24] Antipsychotic use is also an independent risk factor for falls in people with dementia.[27] Confusion may deteriorate, particularly with drugs with anticholinergic effects, and sedation may be problematic. In addition, the risk of emergent extra-pyramidal symptoms appears to be significantly increased with the use of haloperidol and risperidone;[28] these side-effects manifest even at low doses (for example, 1–2 mg of risperidone). Neuroleptic sensitivity is particularly evident in dementia with Lewy bodies; severe neuroleptic reactions can occur in up to 50 per cent of these patients.[29]

There is some evidence for an increased mortality risk for olanzapine and risperidone. There may be an increased risk of cerebrovascular adverse events in people with dementia taking these medications.[30] It is unclear whether this is drug specific or a class effect. Meta-analyses have indicated that there is a 1.5- to 1.7-fold increase in mortality risk for people with Alzheimer's disease treated with atypical neuroleptics. In 2005, the FDA asked the manufacturers of olanzapine, risperidone, aripiprazole, quetiapine, clozapine, and ziprasidone to include warning labels indicating increased risk of death on their products.[31] In the United Kingdom, the Committee for the Safety of Medicines (2004) advised that risperidone and olanzapine should not be used for the treatment of behavioural symptoms of dementia.[30] More recently, Wang *et al.* (2005), reported increased mortality rates in patients over the age of 65 treated with typical neuroleptics compared with atypicals; the risk was greatest shortly after initiation of the treatment and when higher doses were used.[32] Neuroleptic use has also been suggested to hasten cognitive decline although a more recent study refutes this.[33]

Advice: A high level of caution needs to applied to the use of antipsychotics in dementia. A careful weighing of benefits versus the risks is required. General principles for the use of antipsychotics (and other psychotropics) in dementia are similar to psychotropic prescribing for people with head injury (Box 4.1.10.3 in Chapter 4.1.10). Additionally, in dementia:

- Use drugs only if psychosocial or behavioural strategies have failed, and only if absolutely necessary.
- Review prescriptions regularly looking for side-effects. Patients with dementia often have physical co-morbidities and as a consequence take multiple medications; do not allow cocktails to build up.
- Do not prescribe for prolonged periods. Regularly reassess the need for the drug; can alternative interventions be applied now the situation is containable?
- For mild to moderate behavioural disturbances, consider the use of cholinesterase inhibitors or memantine (see below).

(d) Benzodiazepines

Benzodiazepines can be effective in agitation, particularly if it is associated with anxiety, sleep disturbance, or restlessness. However side effects are frequently associated with benzodiazepine use in people with dementia including sedation, worsening of cognitive function, paradoxical increased agitation, and increased risk of falls. The use of benzodiazepines should therefore be judicious and on a needs only basis. Short-acting benzodiazepines, for example oxazepam or lorazepam, are recommended by some, particularly in the elderly, because they are less likely to result in steadily accumulating blood levels.

(e) Mood stabilizers

There is limited evidence that carbamazepine may be beneficial in the treatment of agitation, although there are concerns about its safety in elderly patients given its propensity to induce haematological abnormalities.[23] High dose valproate does appear to reduce agitation, but, again, there is a significant risk of serious side effects.[34]

(f) Cholinesterase inhibitors and memantine

Evidence: In addition to providing benefits for cognition in dementia (see Chapter 6.2.7), cholinesterase inhibitors may help reduce BPSDs in people with dementia (see Ballard and Howard, 2006, for discussion).[28] However in most studies behaviour improvements have been secondary outcomes and a recent multi-centre 12-week trial of donepezil in patients with Alzheimer's disease found that donepezil was no more effective than placebo in treating agitation.[35] One group who do appear to gain clear benefit from cholinesterase inhibitor use is people with Lewy body dementia. Rivastigmine at a dose of up to 12 mg/day for 20 weeks appeared to significantly reduce psychotic symptoms in this group.[36] There is conflicting evidence for the use of memantine for the treatment of behavioural symptoms.

Advice: In terms of prescribing, it is probably worth considering the use of cholinesterase inhibitors and memantine in BPSDs, given their low propensity for serious adverse side effects.

(g) Other agents

Trazodone, a sedative medication, in preliminary findings appeared to be helpful in the treatment of behavioural disturbances. However more recent randomized control trials (RCTs) have refuted the benefits of this medication in dementia.[28]

Citalopram, aside from its antidepressant properties may have some beneficial effects on irritability and restlessness.[37] Propranolol has been considered; however, most trials for its effectiveness are from old, open label trials. If used, blood pressure and the ECG need to be closely monitored.

(h) Wandering

Many people with dementia will wander, and others will abscond or demand to leave. A risk assessment may be needed to determine their safety outside, for example assessing road safety and their ability to find their way back home.

Evidence: The use of two-dimensional grid patterns by the door of the ward, environmental sign-posting, or concealing the exit by use of a mirror may possibly reduce inappropriate exiting behaviour; however the evidence for these strategies is relatively weak.[22] There is probably better evidence for behavioural interventions (see above).[21]

Advice: Number entry locks which the patient with dementia cannot use can be helpful although it may frustrate the patient. The use of identification bracelets or tagging systems which sound an alarm if the patient leaves the unit is controversial and the subject of ethical debate. An inpatient or residential unit will need both an 'absent without leave' policy, which will include the protocol for informing family and police, and a locked door policy which must take into account what happens if there is a fire. Detention under a mental health or mental capacity act may need to be considered.

Mood disturbance

(a) Depression and apathy

Depression in people with dementia is quite common. Therefore it is important to consider depression as a cause for almost any change in function or behaviour, and to look for risk factors for depression, for example a recent bereavement, in the history. A screening test to detect depression may be appropriate (see above). Apathy, another common symptom in dementia, may be both a symptom of depression and a consequence of organic brain disease affecting those brain systems involved in motivation.

If the patient is depressed then review the general medical state, including any drugs that may produce depression. Make sure that all general psychosocial issues have been addressed, for example appropriate support services, leisure activities, and housing. Specific psychological therapy, for instance cognitive therapy, for depression in people with dementia is generally unavailable. However there is some limited evidence that a cognitive behavioural approach may help in treating depressive symptoms in people with dementia and be of benefit to carers.(38)

(i) *Evidence for pharmacological treatment*

There is some suggestion that antidepressant treatment of depression in patients with dementia is effective, although the evidence is limited.(39) The treatment of apathy in the absence of depression is less clear. The is some evidence that cholinesterase inhibitors improve apathy(40) and case series suggest that bromocriptine and methylphenidate are effective, though clinical experience indicates that the effects may be short-lived.

(ii) *Advice on pharmacological treatment*

The choice of which antidepressant drug to use will depend heavily on their side-effect profile. Newer antidepressants such as the serotonin reuptake inhibitors, having less anticholinergic activity and less cardiotoxicity, are generally preferred. Some method to evaluate the effectiveness of the treatment needs to be in place, preferably before treatment is started to get a baseline measure. For example, a measure of activities of daily living may be the target outcome to see whether it improves with antidepressant treatment.

Mania

Mania is rare in dementia, though there is possibly a specific association with Huntington's chorea. There is no evidence to suggest that mania treatment in a person with dementia be any different from normal protocols.

Psychotic symptoms

The phenomenology of psychotic symptoms influences treatment choice. For example, the occurrence of auditory hallucinations with secondary persecutory delusions may be more responsive to antipsychotic therapy whereas delusions of theft, founded on memory impairment, may respond better to psychosocial interventions such as strategies to help the person keep tags on where they put things.

Evidence: There are few hard data on which to base decisions about pharmacological treatment for relieving psychotic symptoms in dementia although there is reasonable evidence that cholinesterase inhibitors are successful in treating visual hallucinations in dementia with Lewy bodies.(36)

Advice: The choice of which antipsychotic to use is likely to be determined by its profile of side-effects. The same cautions and advice given for antipsychotic use in agitation in dementia (above) need to be applied for their use in treating psychotic symptoms.

Disorders of sexual behaviour

(a) Impotence or reduced libido

Reduced sexual activity and interest is the most common disorder of sexual behaviour associated with dementia, though it is the least likely to come to the attention of the clinician. It probably plays a part in the high rates of divorce seen, for example, in young couples after one partner has sustained a brain injury. Psychological effects, in particular the change in the patient's role in the partnership as a result of dementia, as well as the physiological effects of brain dysfunction on erectile function, contribute to impotence and reduced libido.

The first and most important step is to recognize the problem and talk about it. The couple may wish to be referred to a sexual disorders clinic. If reduced libido is part of a more generalized apathy or depression then it may respond when these features are appropriately treated (see above). Erectile dysfunction may respond to oral phosphodiesterase inhibitors such sildenafil.

(b) Sexual disinhibition and overactivity

Any display of sexual disinhibition, although uncommon in dementia, is likely to become a major management issue and needs a thorough behaviour assessment. Occasionally it may be part of a Klüver–Bucy-like syndrome with hyperorality and excessive eating.

Sexual disinhibition may respond to behavioural/psychosocial strategies. It may, for example, be necessary to ensure that only men nurse the patient if all the sexual disinhibition is directed towards female staff. A full behavioural programme to try to extinguish the behaviour may be effective, but if the behaviour involves touching and groping then it is essential to discuss and monitor the programme with those involved in the hands-on care of the patient. Staff often find such behaviour particularly upsetting.

Antipsychotics may reduce sexually disinhibited behaviour. The antiandrogens, cyproterone acetate, and medroxyprogesterone (Depo-Provera), may need to be tried if all else fails.

Sleep disturbance

Patients with dementia often have a disturbed sleep pattern and this is most troublesome when the sleep–wake cycle is inverted, with the patient asleep during the day but awake at night.

(a) Assessment

It is worth considering restless legs or rapid eye movement (REM-sleep) behaviour disorder as a cause of sleep disturbance. REM-sleep behaviour disorder, often a feature of dementia with Lewy bodies can be successfully treated with low dose clonazepam. Does the patient have to get up at night to empty his or her bladder because of prostatism or bladder dysfunction? Are there other medical reasons why the patient may be waking at night, for example because of pain from a duodenal ulcer? Sleep apnoea, more common in the elderly, produces sleep disturbance and is a contra-indication for benzodiazepines and other drugs that may suppress respiration. Is the sleep disturbance due to depression? Has there been any recent change to the sleeping arrangements? If so any sleep disturbance may be self-limiting.

(b) Management

Hypnotics are likely to have deleterious effects on cognition and functional abilities, and increase the risk of falls; these drugs should only be considered after techniques to improve sleep hygiene have been tried.

If sleep hygiene techniques fail, there is little definitive evidence to guide the clinician as to which hypnotic to select in patients with dementia. Benzodiazepines should, if possible, not be given indefinitely; particular caution is needed if the patient already shows disinhibition. Trazodone has been tried, particularly if there is co-morbid depression, although the evidence for its efficacy is questionable (see above). It has been suggested that bright light therapy (Table 4.1.13.2) can resynchronize aberrant circadian rhythms, but there is no definite evidence that it is effective.

Incontinence

Dementia in the elderly roughly doubles the risk of urinary incontinence. To minimize incontinence, toilets should be easily identifiable and readily accessible. Clothing may need attention to ensure that it is easy to remove. For urinary incontinence reversible causes, such as urinary tract infection, constipation, and medication (such as diuretics or drugs with anticholinergic side-effects causing urinary retention and overflow) should be excluded.

A diary recording frequency of voiding on the toilet and frequency of incontinence should be kept to see if toileting times can be adjusted to minimize incontinence. Prompted voiding (asking the person hourly if they want to go to the toilet and giving praise for successful toileting) is effective for some individuals. A behavioural programme may be needed for the patient who urinates or defecates in inappropriate places.

If incontinence persists get the advice of a continence advisor before considering drug treatment.

Risk management in dementia

Risk assessment is an important part of the management of patients with dementia and Table 4.1.13.3 suggests various areas of risk that need to be considered. A good history from carers and others involved in the patient's care is essential for a full risk assessment, which is rarely complete without an assessment by an occupational therapist.

It is important to use the outcome of risk assessment to facilitate independence. This is done by introducing appropriate strategies to minimize risk. In addition, a risk–benefit analysis may demonstrate that it is appropriate to run a risk of some adverse event happening if there are clear benefits of doing so. For example, a patient may be at risk of wandering and getting lost from his or her home; however, if the strategy to prevent this involves moving the patient to new accommodation away from family and familiar surroundings, then this may itself be regarded as a sufficiently adverse event to make transfer inappropriate. But before implementing such a strategy discuss it with other clinicians involved in the case, and with the carers, family and, if possible, the patient. Document the outcome of these discussions as well as the rationale for the management plan.

Table 4.1.13.3 Risk assessment in dementia

Consider the following areas:	
Anti-social and other behaviour	
◆ *Violence/aggression*	—towards others —towards self
◆ *Sexual disinhibition/assault*	
◆ *Other antisocial behaviours*	—which may provoke assaults e.g. argumentative, spitting, etc.
◆ *Wandering/agitation*	
Safety associated with impaired memory and cognition and poor judgement	
◆ *Home safety*	—leaving kettles, fires, etc., on. —leaving doors/windows, etc. open —cigarettes
◆ *Out and about*	—getting lost —road safety —pedestrian —driving
◆ *Financial*	—not able to handle money, loses money —inapproriately spends money, poor judgement
◆ *Work*	—fails to monitor and check for errors —unsafe with dangerous machinery
◆ *Supervising others*	—especially children (and consider aggression/sexual behaviour)
Vulnerability to	
◆ *Abuse by others*	—physical, sexual, emotional, and financial
◆ *Self neglect*	—including not eating, squalor
Physical health	
◆ *Falls*	
◆ *Managing their illness*	—e.g. diabetes, diet —taking their medication—note risk of abruptly stopping anticonvulsants, or steroids —drug dependence
◆ *Epilepsy*	

Caregivers

The impact and burden of dementia on family and caregivers is profound. In addition to the burden of caring, caregivers may experience adverse financial consequences, loss of independence, and social isolation. As a result, caregivers often exhibit high levels of psychological and physical morbidity.

The role of caregivers needs be acknowledged in maintaining individuals with dementia in the community. Significant caregiver burden and stress drastically increases the likelihood of care home admission. Therefore support of the caregiver is intrinsic to good dementia care.

Evidence: There have been a large number of studies examining the effectiveness of interventions to support the caregiver. Even though these various studies rarely used the same outcome measures a recent meta-analysis was able to show that caregiver interventions can be beneficial in reducing caregiver psychological morbidity and, importantly, might also delay nursing home admission.[41] Intensive interventions that focus on psychoeducation, stress management, and include the person with dementia, seem particularly effective.

Advice: Support for the family and carers should consist of several components.[4] Start with education about the cause of the dementia, the possible prognosis, and the symptoms—both current and those that may develop. Family and friends need to understand that cognitive and behavioural symptoms arise from damage to the brain and are part of the illness. Caregivers need advice on the principles of care and skills training, for example ensuring that communication is simple and direct, avoiding changes to routine, not arguing with the patient, but on the other hand not endorsing false beliefs. They will need guidance on when and how to call on professional advice. Caregivers may also need help in obtaining social services input, additional care at home (including cleaning, nursing, and meals-on-wheels), as well as legal and financial advice. Voluntary organizations such as Alzheimer's Society UK (http://www.alzheimers.org.uk) and local self-help groups are often excellent sources of information and support for caregivers.

The burden of caring for someone with a dementia may result in depression and other signs of stress. The carer should have the opportunity of talking about any problems they have, if necessary getting their own psychiatric care.

Caregivers who are under stress are probably more likely to abuse, either physically or emotionally, the person with dementia. Try to ensure that any physical and emotional abuse of the demented person is picked up early. It helps if everybody involved in the person's care knows how to report any concerns they may have about what is happening.

Management of end-stage dementia

Previously, little attention was given to the end stages of the neurodegenerative dementias; most patients would die in hospital or long-term care facilities. However palliative care strategies are increasingly being used in dementia care. These emphasize physical, psychological, social, and spiritual aspects of care, with non-curative interventions aimed at maximizing quality of life. An important principle of treatment in palliative care is proportionality; any treatment should only be implemented if the balance of clinical benefit outweighs the burden such a treatment imposes.

For patients with dementia good palliative care includes management of BPSDs. In addition there are a number of end of life issues relevant to dementia:

Swallowing difficulties and aspiration pneumonia: These are common in end-stage dementia. Ethical consensus has indicated that the use of nasogastric and percutaneous endoscopic gastrostomy (PEG) tubes is seldom warranted in end-stage dementia although there may be individual cases in which the use of feeding tubes is not futile.[42] The use of antibiotics is more controversial. Certainly in other branches of palliative care there is evidence that even in the terminal stages of illness, antibiotics can relieve the distress caused by infected bronchial secretions.

Pain: Patients with dementia are often unable to communicate their distress. Be alert to the possibilities of pain; indeed always consider if a behavioural symptom is manifestation of pain. The management of pain in dementia is similar to pain management in other conditions. The aetiology of the pain should direct the choice of treatment. Adequate doses of analgesics to achieve good pain relief should be prescribed.

Further information

National Institute of Clinical Excellence. (2006). Dementia: supporting people with dementia and their carers in health and social care. National Clinical Practice Guideline Number 42. London. Available online: http://guidance.nice.org.uk/cg42.

Burns, A.B., O'Brien, J.T., and Ames, D. (2005). *Dementia* (3rd edn). Hodder Arnold, London.

Lovestone, S. and Gauthier, S. (2001). *Management of dementia* (1st edn). Martin Dunitz, London.

References

1. Lishman, W.A. (1998). *Organic psychiatry: the psychological consequences of cerebral disorder* (3rd edn). Blackwell Science, Oxford.
2. Baile, W.F., Buckman, R., Lenzi, R., *et al.* (2000). SPIKES-a six-step protocol for delivering bad news: application to the patient with cancer. *The Oncologist*, **5**, 302–11.
3. Cheston, R., Jones, K., and Gilliard, J. (2003). Group psychotherapy and people with dementia. *Aging & Mental Health*, **7**, 452–61.
4. National Institute of Clinical Excellence. (2006). Dementia: supporting people with dementia and their carers in health and social care. National Clinical Practice Guideline Number 42. London.
5. Brodaty, H., Conneally, M., Gauthier, S., *et al.* (1995). Consensus statement on predictive testing for Alzheimer disease. *Alzheimer Disease and Associated Disorders*, **9**, 182–7.
6. Post, S.G., Whitehouse, P.J., Binstock, R.H., *et al.* (1997). The clinical introduction of genetic testing for Alzheimer disease. An ethical perspective. *Journal of the American Medical Association*, **277**, 832–6.
7. Finkel, S.I., Costa, E., Silva, J., *et al.* (1996). Behavioral and psychological signs and symptoms of dementia: a consensus statement on current knowledge and implications for research and treatment. *International Psychogeriatrics*, **8** (**Suppl. 3**), 497–500.
8. Lyketsos, C.G., Steinberg, M., Tschanz, J.T., *et al.* (2000). Mental and behavioral disturbances in dementia: findings from the cache county study on memory in aging. *The American Journal of Psychiatry*, **157**, 708–14.
9. Victoroff, J., Mack, W.J., and Nielson, K.A. (1998). Psychiatric complications of dementia: impact on caregivers. *Dementia and Geriatric Cognitive Disorders*, **9**, 50–5.
10. Robert, F. Coen. (1997). Behaviour disturbance and other predictors of care burden in Alzheimer's disease. *International Journal of Geriatric Psychiatry*, **12**, 331–6.
11. Cohen, C.A., Gold, D.P., Shulman, K.I., *et al.* (1993). Factors determining the decision to institutionalize dementing individuals: a prospective study. *The Gerontologist*, **33**, 714–20.
12. Tekin, S., Fairbanks, L.A., O'Connor, S., *et al.* (2001). Activities of daily living in Alzheimer's disease: neuropsychiatric, cognitive, and medical illness influences. *The American Journal of Geriatric Psychiatry*, **9**, 81–6.
13. Aarsland, D., Cummings, J.L., Yenner, G., *et al.* (1996). Relationship of aggressive behavior to other neuropsychiatric symptoms in patients with Alzheimer's disease. *The American Journal of Psychiatry*, **153**, 243–7.
14. Burns, A., Lawlor, B., and Craig, S. (2003). *Assessment scales in old age psychiatry* (2nd edn). Martin Dunitz Ltd., London.
15. Reisberg, B., Borenstein, J., Salob, S.P., *et al.* (1987). Behavioral symptoms in Alzheimer's disease: phenomenology and treatment. *Journal of Clinical Psychiatry*, **48** (Suppl.), 9–15.

16. Cohen-Mansfield, J., Billig. (1986). Agitated behaviours in the elderly. A conceptual review. *Journal of the American Geriatric Society*, **34**, 711–21.
17. Alexopoulos, G.S., Abrams, R.C., Young, R.C., *et al.* (1988). Cornell scale for depression in dementia. *Biological Psychiatry*, **23**, 271–84.
18. Cohen-Mansfield, J., Werner, P., Watson, V., *et al.* (1995). Agitation among elderly persons at adult day-care centers: the experiences of relatives and staff members. *International Psychogeriatrics*, **7**, 447–58.
19. Ayalon, L., Gum, A.M., Feliciano, L., *et al.* (2006). Effectiveness of nonpharmacological interventions for the management of neuropsychiatric symptoms in patients with dementia: a systematic review. *Archives of Internal Medicine*, **166**, 2182–8.
20. Doody, R.S., Stevens, J.C., Beck, C., *et al.* (2001). Practice parameter: management of dementia (an evidence-based review). Report of the Quality Standards Subcommittee of the American Academy of Neurology. *Neurology*, **56**, 1154–66.
21. Spira, A.P. and Edelstein, B.A. (2006). Behavioral interventions for agitation in older adults with dementia: an evaluative review. *International Psychogeriatrics*, **18**, 195–225.
22. Livingston, G., Johnston, K., Katona, C., *et al.* (2005). Systematic review of psychological approaches to the management of neuropsychiatric symptoms of dementia. *The American Journal of Psychiatry*, **162**, 1996–2021.
23. Sink, K.M., Holden, K.F., and Yaffe, K. (2005). Pharmacological treatment of neuropsychiatric symptoms of dementia: d review of the evidence. *Journal of the American Medical Association*, **293**, 596–608.
24. Schneider, L.S., Tariot, P.N., Dagerman, K.S., *et al.* (2006). Effectiveness of atypical antipsychotic drugs in patients with Alzheimer's disease. *The New England Journal of Medicine*, **355**, 1525–38.
25. Lanctot, K.L., Best, T.S., Mittmann, N., *et al.* (1998). Efficacy and safety of neuroleptics in behavioral disorders associated with dementia. *Journal of Clinical Psychiatry*, **59**, 550–61.
26. Schneider, L.S., Pollock, V.E., and Lyness, S.A. (1990). A metaanalysis of controlled trials of neuroleptic treatment in dementia. *Journal of the American Geriatric Society*, **38**, 553–63.
27. Kallin, K., Gustafson, Y., Sandman, P.O., *et al.* (2004). Drugs and falls in older people in geriatric care settings. *Aging Clinical and Experimental Research*, **16**, 270–6.
28. Ballard, C. and Howard, R. (2006). Neuroleptic drugs in dementia: benefits and harm. *Nature Reviews. Neuroscience*, **7**, 492–500.
29. McKeith, I., Fairbairn, A., Perry, R., *et al.* (1992). Neuroleptic sensitivity in patients with senile dementia of Lewy body type. *British Medical Journal*, **305**, 673–8.
30. Committee of the Safety of Medicines. (2004). Atypical antipsychotic drugs and stroke. [online] accessed: 13/03/07, http://www.mhra.gov.uk.
31. United States Food and Drug Agency: Center for Drug Evaluation and Research. (2005). Deaths with antipsychotics in elderly patients with behavioral disturbances. [online] accessed: 13/03/07, http://www.fda.gov/cder/drug/advisory/antipsychotics.html.
32. Wang, P.S., Schneeweiss, S., Avorn, J., *et al.* (2005). Risk of death in elderly users of conventional vs. atypical antipsychotic medications. *The New England Journal of Medicine*, **353**, 2335–41.
33. Livingston, G., Walker, A.E., Katona, C.L.E., *et al.* (2007). Antipsychotics and cognitive decline in Alzheimer's disease: the LASER-Alzheimer's disease longitudinal study. *Journal of Neurology Neurosurgery, and Psychiatry*, **78**, 25–9.
34. Lonergan, E.T., Cameron, M., and Luxenberg, J. (2004). Valproic acid for agitation in dementia. *Cochrane Database Systematic Reviews*, (2), CD003945.
35. Howard, R.J., Juszczak, E., Ballard, C.G., *et al.* (2007). Donepezil for the treatment of agitation in Alzheimer's disease. *New England Journal of Medicine*, **357**, 1382–92.
36. McKeith, I., Del Ser, T., Spano, P., *et al.* (2000). Efficacy of rivastigmine in dementia with Lewy bodies: a randomised, double-blind, placebo-controlled international study. *Lancet*, **356**, 2031–6.
37. Nyth, A.L. and Gottfries, C.G. (1990). The clinical efficacy of citalopram in treatment of emotional disturbances in dementia disorders. A Nordic multicentre study. *The British Journal of Psychiatry*, **157**, 894–901.
38. Teri, L., Logsdon, R.G., Uomoto, J., *et al.* (1997). Behavioral treatment of depression in dementia patients: a controlled clinical trial. *Journal of Gerontology: Psychological Sciences and Social Sciences*, **52**, P159–66.
39. Bains, J., Birks, J.S., and Dening, T.R. (2002). The efficacy of antidepressants in the treatment of depression in dementia. *Cochrane Database Systematic Reviews*, (4), CD003944.
40. Cummings, J.L. (2003). Use of cholinesterase inhibitors in clinical practice: evidence-based recommendations. *The American Journal of Geriatric Psychiatry*, **11**,131–145.
41. Brodaty, H., Green, A., and Koschera, A. (2003). Meta-analysis of psychosocial interventions for caregivers of people with dementia. *Journal of the American Geriatrics Society*, **51**, 657–64.
42. Gillick, M.R. (2000). Rethinking the role of tube feeding in patients with advanced dementia. *The New England Journal of Medicine*, **342**, 206–10.

4.1.14 **Remediation of memory disorders**

Jonathan J. Evans

Introduction

Memory problems are a feature of the majority of psychiatric and neurological conditions. Any condition that affects the physical or functional integrity of the brain is likely to have an impact on some aspect of a person's ability to remember, as successful remembering involves many different interacting cognitive systems (see Chapter 2.5.3 on the neuropsychology of memory and Chapter 4.1.12 on the amnesic syndromes). Furthermore, mood disorders such as anxiety or depression, which impair concentration, also reduce the efficiency of memory.

Remembering difficulties disrupt the ability to participate effectively in activities of daily living, as well as social, leisure, and vocational activities. For some, memory problems will be mild and cause only minor inconvenience in everyday life. Others, such as those with the amnesic syndrome that accompanies dysfunction in limbic system structures, may be severely disabled by their memory impairment. People forget to do things (e.g. take medication, turn-off the cooker, pay bills, attend appointments, pass on messages), forget what they have been told, forget people's names, forget where they left things (e.g. keys, the car in the car park), find it difficult to remember routes or learn new procedures, have difficulty recollecting personal experiences, and so on. Such problems lead to frustration, lowered self-confidence, and dependence on others. As such they represent an important therapeutic target.

Assessment of the nature of the memory disorder and the functional consequences for the individual should precede remediation intervention planning. As far as remediation of memory is concerned, although the future in terms of biological treatments is promising,[1] for the present time pharmacological options remain limited (see Chapter 6.2.7). The most effective treatments are cognitive rehabilitation techniques. These include use of memory aids, which function as cognitive prostheses, and methods of learning that promote more effective acquisition of knowledge or skills.

Planning memory remediation—assessment

The World Health Organization International Classification of Functioning, Disability and Health[2] provides a helpful framework for the assessment and remediation of cognitive deficits including memory impairment.[3] ICF, which complements the diagnostic approach of ICD, emphasizes that health (or illness) and functioning can be considered at the level of body structure (pathology), body function (impairment), activities, and participation. Application of this framework in relation to assessment of memory is illustrated in Box 4.1.14.1.

An assessment of memory should therefore address both the impairment *and* the functional consequences for the individual patient. This is important because treatment interventions will differ depending on the form and severity of the memory impairment and the nature of the everyday problems. Such an assessment will of course typically be just one part of a broader assessment of cognition—memory impairment is the focus here, but the same principles apply to all other cognitive impairments.

Box 4.1.14.1 The WHO ICF model and its relationship to assessment of memory

ICF classification	Example in relation to assessment of memory	Approaches to assessment/ investigation
Body structure (*Pathology*)	Loss of cholinergic neurones in basal forebrain region affecting functioning of medial temporal lobe limbic system (Alzheimer's disease)	Physical investigations (e.g. routine medical and brain imaging investigations)
Body function (*Impairment*)	Episodic memory deficit	Standardized neuropsychological assessment tools (e.g. Wechsler Memory Scales III; Rivermead Behavioural Memory Test)
Activities (*Disability*)	Failure to remember to do important tasks, failure to remember events that have happened, or things previously told	Clinical interview with patient and significant other, questionnaires, and observation
Participation (*Handicap*)	Inability to work; increased dependence on others; inability to participate in leisure activities	Clinical interview; quality of life measures

Assessment of memory impairment

Memory impairment is assessed through the use of standardized neuropsychological assessment tools (see Chapter 1.8.3).

Assessment of functional consequences of memory impairment

Activity limitations arising from memory disorders can be assessed through clinical interview with the patient and proxy, but it can also be helpful to use a standardized questionnaire to aid information gathering. Several questionnaires exist for this purpose. The Prospective and Retrospective Memory Questionnaire[4] is one example of a useful, brief questionnaire with self-rating and proxy-rating forms that address both prospective remembering (e.g. Do you fail to do something you were supposed to do a few minutes later even though it's there in front of you, like take a pill or turn off the kettle?) and retrospective remembering (e.g. Do you fail to recall things that have happened to you in the last few days?). This questionnaire also has normative data for self-rating and proxy-ratings.[5,6]

Awareness of the functional consequences of memory impairment may be limited on the part of the patient and the carer (see section on assessment of awareness below). It is possible that functional consequences will also be minimized (again by patient and under some circumstances the carer). In some cases there may be significant impairment of memory and associated limitations of activity, but a spouse/family may take on most or all of the remembering responsibility and hence the significant disability on the part of the patient may not represent a problem for patient or spouse/family. In this circumstance it is important to investigate whether there is adequate awareness of rehabilitation options.

Assessment of use of memory aids and strategies

Pre-morbid and current use of memory aids and strategies should also be discussed as part of the clinical interview. Given that the most effective approaches to memory rehabilitation are those that enable people with memory dysfunction to compensate for their impairment, it is important to understand what past experience of use of memory aids the patient has, and which aids/strategies are used currently. Some people will have made extensive use of memory aids and strategies throughout their life, and continue to do so in response to onset of memory problems. Others may have used aids and strategies in the past, but then do not use them despite the onset of memory problems. Others have little previous experience. Some examples of aids and strategies to investigate, drawn from a survey of use of memory aids by people with memory impairment,[7] are shown in Box 4.1.14.2.

Assessment of awareness of memory deficits

Awareness of impairment should also be examined as this will impact on the approach to remediation that will follow. To what extent is the patient aware of his or her memory (and any other cognitive) problems? Insight and awareness is a complex issue. Clare[8] presents a biopsychosocial model of the construction of awareness in Alzheimer's disease, though the principles of the

Box 4.1.14.2 Assessment of pre-morbid and current use of memory aids and strategies

Use of memory aids and strategies is a central component of memory rehabilitation. Investigation of prior experience, and current use, of aids and strategies is an important part of the assessment process. Below are examples of aids and strategies that are most commonly used by people with memory impairment.[3] This list is not exhaustive and it is important to ask whether any other aids/strategies are used.

- Wall calendar/chart/memo board
- Notebook
- Lists (e.g. things to do/shopping)
- Checklists (e.g. instructions for how to operate washing machine)
- Appointment diary/personal organizer (e.g. Filofax)
- Asking others to remind you to do something or of things that have happened
- Mental retracing (e.g. of steps when lost an object)
- Placing objects in unusual places (e.g. by door if need to take it when leaving or as reminder to do something)
- Leaving notes in special places
- Dosett box or other pill reminder
- Repetitive practice (learning something new by frequent repetition)
- Making associations
- Watch with date/alarm
- Having a daily routine
- Journal (a daily diary record of personal experiences)
- Daily timetable
- Alarm clock/timer
- Mobile phone (e.g. with alarm reminder/GPS navigation function)
- Electronic organizer (Personal Digital Assistant—PDA)
- NeuroPage (paging-based reminding system)

model apply to most neurological and indeed many psychiatric conditions. Another simple model, but one that is useful in clinical practice, is the hierarchical model of Crosson and colleagues[9] which suggests that awareness may be *intellectual*, *emergent*, or *anticipatory*. Intellectual awareness refers to knowing that you have an impairment, but not necessarily recognizing the occurrence of problems as they occur. Emergent awareness refers to 'online' awareness of problems as they occur, whilst anticipatory awareness refers to using knowledge of deficits to anticipate problems and taking steps to prevent problems occurring. This tripartite model of awareness can be helpful in formulating a patient's level of awareness of memory problems. The extent to which the patient's reporting of problems is discrepant from their relative's account (in interview or on questionnaires), or from what might be expected on the basis of standardized test results will give some indication of level of awareness. In addition it is useful to establish the extent to which the patient is aware of the type of memory problems that arise and the extent to which s/he makes attempt to compensate for the problems. Bear in mind that severe memory impairment may itself impact on awareness—patients may have difficulty remembering that, or what, they forget.

Planning memory remediation—treatment approaches

Memory remediation interventions must take account of several factors, including the form and severity of memory impairment, the presence/absence of additional cognitive impairment, and awareness of the deficit. With regard to form of impairment, the major distinction that is drawn is between primary/working memory and secondary/-term memory.

Remediation of primary/working memory

Primary/working memory refers to the process of briefly holding verbal or visuospatial information in mind, and in the case of working memory, manipulating information in the mental workspace. Primary/working memory processes are reflected in tasks such as digit span, with backward digit span seen as taxing working memory. Working memory is considered to be crucial for effective mental control and executive functions such as problem solving. There is some evidence, primarily from studies of patients with a diagnosis of schizophrenia that cognitive training (involving extensive practice on tasks, sometimes computerized, which make demands on working memory) improves working memory performance over and above control conditions.[10,11] Intervention for working memory problems as part of a more comprehensive cognitive remediation programme should therefore be given serious consideration, at least for patients with schizophrenia.[12] Perhaps ironically, given the acknowledgement that cognitive rehabilitation for schizophrenia has its roots in neurorehabilitation for traumatic brain injury,[10] there is a much more limited evidence base relating to the effectiveness of this type of intervention with other neurological conditions.[13]

Remediation of secondary/long-term memory problems

Secondary or long-term memory refers to the process of encoding, storage, and retrieval of memories after a delay, where 'delay' means anything from a few minutes to a lifetime. Secondary memory is what is used to recall episodes, to acquire knowledge and to remember to do things. It is secondary memory that is impaired in amnesia. Box 4.1.14.3 provides a decision tree that reflects some of the processes involved in identifying memory remediation interventions.

(a) Are there contributory factors?

As part of the assessment and formulation of memory disorders and their functional consequences, one must consider whether a range of other factors are contributing to the functional disability. If so, then one should include intervention for these factors in the treatment plan. This includes treatment of mood disorders, sleep disorders, management of fatigue and pain, or adjustment of medication where possible. In some patients, memory problems will be secondary to

Box 4.1.14.3 Guidelines for genetic testing for dementia

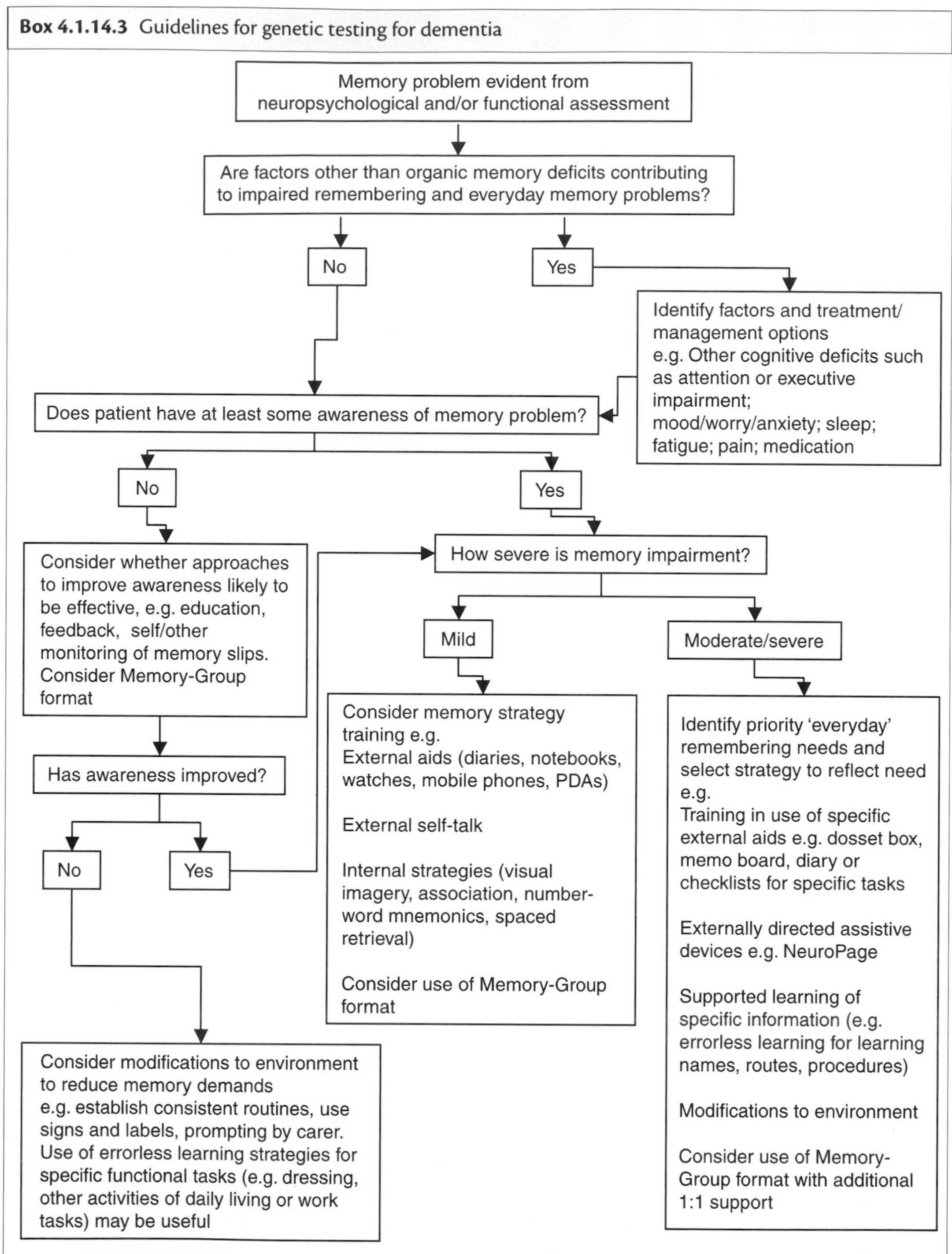

impaired attention and concentration and if this is the case, then interventions to address these problems should be considered.

(b) Is the person aware of the problem?

The question of the patient's awareness of memory problems should be addressed. If there is no awareness then it is important to consider means of improving awareness before pressing on with specific remediation strategies. Improving awareness is sometimes straightforward and a question of providing basic information and feedback, but often it is more complex. Use of education and self/other monitoring of memory slips in conjunction with feedback can help. This must be done sensitively as minimizing of problems may be a psychological coping mechanism and insensitive confrontation may be threatening. Working with patients in a group format can contribute to improving awareness—patients can be supported to provide feedback to each other. Patients may feel more able to acknowledge problems if others are also doing this in the group context.[14] *If awareness cannot be improved* (which may be the case if memory problems are occurring in the context of more global and severe cognitive impairment) then the strategy of modifying the environment to reduce memory demands on the patient must be considered. Environmental modifications include the use of prominent signs/labelling (e.g. of toilets, cupboards, draws, rooms) to support orientation in the physical environment. Establishing very fixed daily routines can also help develop behavioural habits. It may be the case that the patient requires prompting from carers. If this is the case then the minimal level of prompting required should be established and regularly monitored, and if possible prompting can be gradually reduced as behavioural sequences are learned.

(c) Strategies for mild problems

If the patient demonstrates at least some awareness of memory problems then the severity of the memory problem should be considered. Systematic reviews of cognitive rehabilitation[15,16] have recommended that different approaches are required for different levels of severity of memory disorder. There is no evidence that 'drill and repetitive practice' without additional strategy training is effective in improving memory.[17,18] However, in the context of mild memory impairment then memory strategy training is recommended.[15] Memory strategy training can be carried out on a 1:1 basis or in a group. The aim is to provide information and training in the use of a range of memory strategies which the patient learns to apply independently in specific situations in their own life, via homework tasks, over the course of the training programme. The patient is provided with a range of strategy options that s/he can select according to personal needs. This includes training in the use of external memory aids, such as many of those listed in Box 4.1.14.2. Internal memory strategies are also trained. These include strategies to aid deeper encoding of information. It is a well-established principle that deeper (more meaningful, personally relevant, emotionally salient), multi-modal (i.e. visual and verbal) processing of information results in more effective learning and recollection of that information.[19] For those with severe amnesia whether or not the information is processed deeply will make little difference, but for those with more mild impairment, strategies to enhance processing are more relevant. Strategies include visual imagery, categorization, association with established knowledge, motor movement (e.g. rehearsing in mind an action that has to be carried out at some later time) and spaced retrieval/expanding rehearsal (gradually increasing the time between successive trials of testing recollection of material to be learned). Craik and colleagues[20] and Evans[1] discuss internal strategies further.

(d) Strategies for more severe problems

For those with more severe memory impairment general strategy training is unlikely to be effective as the demands of learning a range of strategies and applying them when required are too great.[18] The approach recommended in this context is to try to map specific everyday remembering priorities to specific strategies. In other words, rather than providing a tool box of strategies and relying on the patient independently selecting the right tools for the right task when needed, the clinician establishes with the patient and carer what is essential to be learned/remembered and then considers how can this be achieved. For some this will be just one task for which one remembering strategy will be established. For others a more complex 'memory system' can be constructed to allow several remembering tasks to be achieved. Some of the commonly used external aids (memory notebooks, diaries, memo boards) will be used. For people with more severe impairment, formal training in learning how to use these aids consistently is required. A number of studies have shown that comprehensive training approaches can lead to effective use of memory journals, even in people with severe amnesia.[21–23] Kime[24] provides instruction on devising needs-led practical approaches to compensating for memory deficits.

(e) Electronic memory aids

These aids offer the major advantage of having the facility to prompt an action using alarms and so are particularly valuable in relation to prospective memory (remembering to do things). They also provide a means of combining a number of different memory aid functions (e.g. alarmed reminders, schedule, contact information, to-do list) into one portable tool. The most extensively evaluated electronic reminding system is NeuroPage.[25] Reminder messages are sent to standard alpha-numeric pagers worn by people with memory and/or planning problems, according to a pre-arranged schedule. This system has now been evaluated in randomized clinical trials and single case studies and shown to be very effective.[25,26] In recent years there has been a massive worldwide increase in use of mobile phones such that the vast majority of people acquiring cognitive impairment now will have had exposure to this technology before the onset of their memory deficit. This opens up the possibility of much greater use of portable reminding technology delivered via mobile phones, including the use of SMS text messaging.[27,28]

(f) Errorless learning

Another approach to remediation can be applied when there is a need to learn specific information or a procedure. Errorless learning is based on the principle that for those with severe memory impairment, learning will be most effective if errors can be avoided during the learning process. This is because memory-impaired patients may be more likely to repeat errors (as a result of intact *implicit* memory processes), but are unable to recollect that a response was an error. Thus errors become reinforced. Errorless learning techniques have been used for many years to teach new skills to people with learning disabilities and more recently this technique has been used with people with acquired neurological impairment and with schizophrenia. Baddeley and Wilson[29] published the first study demonstrating that people with amnesia learn better when prevented from making mistakes during the learning process. This finding has been replicated with people with a diagnosis of schizophrenia.[30] These were theoretical studies of word list learning. However, several single case and group studies have shown the benefit of errorless learning methods in teaching more practical, everyday information including learning names of people important in a person's life,[31] work tasks.[32] Kessels and de Haan's[33] meta-analysis concluded that errorless learning was more effective than standard, 'trial and error' conditions.

Many of the treatment interventions described here are relatively labour-intensive requiring a significant amount of clinician/therapist time for them to be successfully implemented. Occupational Therapists and Clinical Psychologists specializing in neuropsychology have relevant training in the assessment and treatment of memory disorders and hence memory remediation should be considered within the interdisciplinary context.

Summary and conclusions

Memory disorders are frequently encountered in clinical practice and cause significant disability. Memory should therefore be carefully assessed as part of routine clinical assessment. Restoration of normal functioning is not typically possible and remediation is therefore usually concerned with compensating for impaired memory. A range of treatment approaches is available, and the treatment of choice will depend on the form and severity of memory disorder and the functional problems faced by the patient.

Further information

Clare, L. and Wilson, B.A. (1997) *Coping with memory problems: a practical guide for people with memory impairments, their relatives, friends and carers.* Harcourt, London.

Evans, J.J. (2004). Disorders of memory. In *Clinical neuropsychology: a practical guide to assessment and management* (eds. L.H. Goldstein and J. McNeil), pp. 143–63. John Wiley & Sons, Chichester.

Kapur, N., Glisky, E., and Wilson, B.A. (2004). External memory aids and computers in memory rehabilitation. In *The essential handbook of memory disorders for clinicians* (eds. A.D. Baddeley, M. Kopelman, and B.A. Wilson). John Wiley & Sons, Chichester.

Information on managing memory impairment is also available in booklets from Headway, the brain injuries association (www.headway.org.uk/).

References

1. Evans, J.J. (2006). Memory dysfunction. In *Textbook of neural repair and rehabilitation* (eds. M.E. Selzer, M.D. Clarke, L.G. Cohen, P.W. Duncan, and F.H. Gage), pp. 461–74. Cambridge University Press, Cambridge.
2. World Health Organization. (2001). International classification of functioning, disability and health (ICF). WHO, Geneva.
3. Wade, D. (2003). Applying the WHO ICF framework to the rehabilitation of patients with cognitive deficits. In *The effectiveness of rehabilitation for cognitive deficits* (eds. P. Halligan and D. Wade). Oxford University Press, Oxford.
4. Smith, G., Della Sala, S., Logie, R.H., *et al.* (2000). Prospective and retrospective memory in normal ageing and dementia: a questionnaire study. *Memory*, **8**, 311–21.
5. Crawford, J.R., Smith, G., Maylor, E.A., *et al.* (2003). The Prospective and Retrospective Memory Questionnaire (PRMQ): normative data and latent structure in a large non-clinical sample. *Memory*, **11**, 261–75.
6. Crawford, J.R., Henry, J.D., Ward, A.L., *et al.* (2006). The Prospective and Retrospective Memory Questionnaire (PRMQ): latent structure, normative data and discrepancy analyses for proxy-ratings. *The British Journal of Clinical Psychology*, **45**, 83–104.
7. Evans, J.J., Needham, P., Wilson, B.A., *et al.* (2003). Which memory impaired people make good use of memory aids? Results of a survey of people with acquired brain injury. *Journal of the International Neuropsychological Society*, **9**, 925–35.
8. Clare, L. (2004). The construction of awareness in early stage Alzheimer's disease: a review of concepts and models. *The British Journal of Clinical Psychology*, **43**, 155–75.
9. Crosson, B., Barco, P.P., Velozo, C.A., *et al.* (1989). Awareness and compensation in post-acute head injury rehabilitation. *The Journal of Head Trauma Rehabilitation*, **4**, 46–54.
10. Twamley, E.W., Jeste, D.V., *et al.* (2003). A review of cognitive training in schizophrenia. *Schizophrenia Bulletin*, **29**, 359–82.
11. Kurtz, M.M., Seltzer, J.C., Shagan, D.S., *et al.* (2007). Computer-assisted cognitive remediation in schizophrenia: what is the active ingredient? *Schizophrenia Research*, **89**, 251–60.
12. Wykes, T. and Reeder, C. (2005). *Cognitive remediation therapy for schizophrenia.* Routledge, London.
13. Cicerone, K., Levin, H., Malec, J., *et al.* (2006). Cognitive rehabilitation interventions for executive function: moving from bench to bedside in patients with traumatic brain injury. *Journal of Cognitive Neuroscience*, **18**, 1212–22.
14. Evans, J.J. and Wilson, B.A. (1992). A memory group for individuals with brain injury. *Clinical Rehabilitation*, **6**, 75–81.
15. Cicerone, K.D., Dahlberg, C., Malec, J., *et al.* (2005). Evidence-based cognitive rehabilitation: updated review of the literature from 1998 through 2002. *Archives of Physical Medicine and Rehabilitation*, **86**, 1681–92.
16. Cappa, S., Benke, T., Clark, S., *et al.* (2005). EFNS guidelines on cognitive rehabilitation: report of an EFNS task force. *European Journal of Neurology*, **12**, 665–80.
17. Cicerone, K.D., Dahlberg, C., Kalmar, K., *et al.* (2000). Evidence-based cognitive rehabilitation: recommendations for clinical practice. *Archives of Physical Medicine and Rehabilitation*, **81**, 1596–615.
18. Clare, L., Woods, R.T., Moniz Cook, E.D., *et al.* (2003). Cognitive rehabilitation and cognitive training for early stage Alzheimer's disease and vascular dementia (Cochrane Review). In *The cochrane library*, (4). John Wiley & Sons, Chichester, UK.
19. Craik, F.I.M. and Lockhart, R.S. (1972). Levels of processing: a framework for memory research. *Journal of Verbal Learning and Verbal Behavior*, **11**, 671–84.
20. Craik, F.I.M., Winocur, G., Palmer, H., *et al.* (2007). Cognitive rehabilitation in the elderly: effects on memory. *Journal of the International Neuropsychological Society*, **13**, 132–42.
21. Sohlberg, M.M. and Mateer, K. (1989). *Introduction to cognitive rehabilitation: theory and practice.* The Guilford Press, New York.
22. Donaghy, S. and Williams, W. (1998). A new protocol for training severely impaired patients in the usage of memory journals. *Brain Injury*, **12**, 1061–77.
23. Kime, S.K., Lamb, D.G., and Wilson, B.A. (1996). Use of a comprehensive programme of external cueing to enhance procedural memory in a patient with dense amnesia. *Brain Injury*, **10**, 17–25.
24. Kime, S.K. (2006). *Compensating for memory deficits using a systematic approach.* AOTA Press, Bethesda MD. (www.aota.org)
25. Wilson, B.A., Emslie, H., Quirk, K., *et al.* (2001). Reducing everyday memory and planning problems by means of a paging system: a randomised control crossover study. *Journal of Neurology, Neurosurgery, and Psychiatry*, **70**, 477–82.
26. Evans, J.J., Emslie, H., and Wilson, B.A. (1998). External cueing systems in the rehabilitation of executive impairments of action. *Journal of the International Neuropsychological Society*, **4**, 399–408.
27. Pijnenborg, G.H.M., Withaar, F.K., Evans, J.J., *et al.* (2007). SMS text messages as a prosthetic aid in the cognitive rehabilitation of schizophrenia. *Rehabilitation Psychology*, **52**(2), 236–40.
28. Fish, J., Evans, J.J., Nimmo, M., *et al.* (2007). Rehabilitation of executive dysfunction following brain injury: Content-free cueing improves everyday prospective memory performance. *Neuropsychologia*, **45**, 1318–30.

29. Baddeley, A.D. and Wilson, B.A. (1994). When implicit learning fails: amnesia and the problem of error elimination. *Neuropsychologia*, **32**, 53–68.
30. Pope, J.W. and Kern, R.S. (2006). An 'errorful' learning deficit in schizophrenia? *Journal of Clinical and Experimental Neuropsychology*, **28**, 101–10.
31. Clare, L., Wilson, B.A., Breen, K., *et al.* (1999). Errorless learning of face-name associations in early Alzheimer's disease. *Neurocase*, **5**, 37–46.
32. Kern, R.S., Green, M.F., Mintz, J., *et al.* (2003). Does 'errorless learning' compensate for neurocognitive impairments in the work rehabilitation of persons with schizophrenia? *Psychological Medicine*, **33**, 433–42.
33. Kessels, R.P.C. and DeHaan, E.H.F. (2003). Implicit learning in memory rehabilitation: a meta analysis on errorless learning and vanishing cues methods. *Journal of Clinical and Experimental Neuropsychology*, **25**, 805–14.

4.2

Substance use disorders

Contents

4.2.1 Pharmacological and psychological aspects of drugs abuse
David J. Nutt and Fergus D. Law

4.2.2 Alcohol use disorders

4.2.2.1 Aetiology of alcohol problems
Juan C. Negrete and Kathryn J. Gill

4.2.2.2 Alcohol dependence and alcohol problems
Jane Marshall

4.2.2.3 Alcohol and psychiatric and physical disorders
Karl F. Mann and Falk Kiefer

4.2.2.4 Treatment of alcohol dependence
Jonathan Chick

4.2.2.5 Services for alcohol use disorders
D. Colin Drummond

4.2.2.6 Prevention of alcohol-related problems
Robin Room

4.2.3 Other substance use disorders

4.2.3.1 Opioids: heroin, methadone, and buprenorphine
Soraya Mayet, Adam R. Winstock, and John Strang

4.2.3.2 Disorders relating to the use of amphetamine and cocaine
Nicholas Seivewright and Robert Fung

4.2.3.3 Disorders relating to use of PCP and hallucinogens
Henry David Abraham

4.2.3.4 Misuse of benzodiazepines
Sarah Welch and Michael Farrell

4.2.3.5 Disorders relating to the use of ecstasy and other 'party drugs'
Adam R. Winstock and Fabrizio Schifano

4.2.3.6 Disorders relating to the use of volatile substances
Richard Ives

4.2.3.7 The mental health effects of cannabis use
Wayne Hall

4.2.3.8 Nicotine dependence and treatment
Mª Inés López-Ibor

4.2.4 Assessing need and organizing services for drug misuse problems
John Marsden, Colin Bradbury, and John Strang

4.2.1 Pharmacological and psychological aspects of drugs abuse

David J. Nutt and Fergus D. Law

Drug abuse, misuse, and addiction are major issues in society because of their enormous personal, social, and economic costs and their important psychiatric components.[1] Many drug treatment programmes are run by psychiatrists, and the evidence strongly supports the notion that a significant proportion of severe drug abusers are psychiatrically ill. Moreover, drug misuse appears to be becoming more frequent in patients with other psychiatric disorders, where it can lead to problems in treatment and poorer outcomes. It is therefore essential for all psychiatrists and related health professionals to have a good understanding of the basis of drug misuse.

Why do people take drugs?

A very common misconception is that drug misuse is simply a **search for fun**. In fact, people take drugs for many reasons other than to get the buzz or high. Indeed, studies have shown that straightforward pleasure seeking is the primary reason for initiation of drug use in fewer than 20 per cent of individuals. Whilst the high or buzz is the most obvious pleasurable effect, many people also describe using drugs to feel comfortably numb, pleasantly drowsy, or full of energy and confidence. Many others will be chasing the high or buzz that they first experienced, always seeking the intensity of their first experience. Still others will be self-medicating for anxiety, anger, pain, boredom, lack of motivation, lack of self-confidence, and many other aversive states including drug withdrawal.

The main reason to try to ascertain the reasons for drug use is that in many cases identification of the cause can lead to effective interventions. For example, many **alcoholics** will point to **anxiety** as their reason for drinking;[2] indeed, social anxiety is one of the most common causes of alcoholism in young men.[3] If this can be treated (e.g. by selective serotonin reuptake inhibitors) then they are frequently able to become abstinent or even drink normally. **Social anxiety** and **attention-deficit disorder** are common reasons for the use of stimulants. **Depression**, is particularly likely to lead to excess alcohol intake, and a vicious cycle can develop because both alcohol and its withdrawal are depressogenic. Alcohol is also one of the most serious risk factors for suicide. There is increasing use of **stimulants** and **cannabis** by **schizophrenic** patients. In part this reflects the behaviour of their peer group but in part is because they can offset some of the more negative aspects of the illness and medication side effects. As both these types of drugs can worsen psychotic illness, dealing with drug misuse in this group is a priority.

Other factors affecting drug use may be less amenable to psychiatric intervention, such as **pressure from peers** or others. For instance, female opiate addicts often have a male partner who also uses drugs or even deals drugs. Should she stop use, relapse is almost certain to occur if she continues to live with this partner. Another reason for drug use is to reduce **pain** or **boredom**, the latter being a common reason given by disadvantaged youth in areas of high unemployment and poor environmental quality such as inner cities or out-of-town housing estates. Other reasons for drug use, especially with the psychedelics, include the **search for meaning** or for **mystical experiences**. Whilst not directly relevant to psychiatry, this use can precipitate psychotic episodes in susceptible individuals and may trigger schizophrenia.

Finally, it is important to remember that the reasons for use of a specific drug are not static. An opiate addict may use the same dose of **heroin** to get going in the morning, to 'top off' a pleasant experience later in the day, to deal with angry feelings when they occur, and to promote sleep at night. Similarly during a **drug-using career** different motivations may become dominant. This has been well characterized in opiate users where for many the initial use was for pleasure or escape. Over months, as physical dependence becomes increasingly apparent, use becomes driven by the need to avoid withdrawal and to feel normal at almost any cost.

Drug use and misuse

It is possible to view the issue of drug abuse from different perspectives, which range from the molecular and genetic through the pharmacological to the psychological and social. Each view has its merits and is important, but there is little doubt that an integrated view is necessary, because for most drugs and for most societies no one perspective can explain all the known features of drug abuse. However, for the purpose of this chapter we have concentrated on the psychological and pharmacological.[1,4–6]

Problem use, addiction, dependence, and craving

These are some of the most commonly used terms regarding drug misuse but at the same time they are also the most problematic. The use of drugs in any circumstance, therapeutic, or otherwise, can be associated with problems, although the nature and scale of this varies (see Table 4.2.1.1). The terms problem use and misuse usually refer to use of drugs (prescription or otherwise) for pleasure but with disregard for the personal or social dangers. For example, alcohol misuse can lead to irresponsible behaviour whilst intoxicated and, if prolonged, to liver, gastric, and nervous system damage without the individual necessarily being addicted or dependent.

Table 4.2.1.1 Potential problems with drug use

Type of drug use and associated issues	Examples/effects
Therapeutic use	
Adverse effects	Sedation, poor driving
Drug interactions	Increased drug levels
Withdrawal	Convulsions, delirium tremens
Drug use with pain	Difficulty reducing opiate dose
Misuse/problem use	
Illegality	Criminal records; social stigmatization
Intoxication	Physical/social damage
Excessive regular use	Physical/social damage
Injecting drug use	Infections, thromboses, Hepatitis C
Dependence	
Tolerance	Dose escalation
Withdrawal	Physical dependence
Urge to use/cannot abstain	Psychological dependence
Craving/drug seeking	Drug dominates life
Drug becomes dominant life goal	Personal/social decline
Reinstatement on relapse	Cycles of dependency

Addiction is a term that had become so misused in general parlance and had acquired such a pejorative edge, that in the past two decades attempts have been made to remove it from the psychiatric lexicon. Unfortunately, the replacement terminology of **dependence**, or the dependence syndrome, has been similarly devalued by popular usage. In fact there exists a spectrum of dependence ranging from physiological supplementation (as with insulin in diabetes mellitus) through to life-altering dependence on illicit drugs such as heroin (see Table 4.2.1.1). Addiction is still a useful construct if it is reserved for the collection of phenomena that occur at the extreme end of the dependence spectrum, and includes the concept of social and personal decline associated with drug use, as well as **craving, tolerance**, and **withdrawal** symptoms (cf. DSM-IV and ICD-10).

Another area of some confusion is the distinction between **physical and psychological dependence**. When originally conceived, this distinction was helpful in that it emphasized that drug dependence was more than just physical adaptation to drugs as manifest by withdrawal symptoms, and that psychological processes, especially drug liking, were also important. However, drugs without obvious physical withdrawal syndromes (e.g. stimulants) also result in measurable physiological withdrawal changes in sleep and activity as well as measurable psychological changes such as those in mood. In addition, new neuroimaging techniques such as **PET, SPECT,** and **functional MRI** are beginning to reveal the brain circuits underlying the pleasurable effects of drugs, and this has resulted in a blurring of the distinction between physical and psychological processes. For example, the plate shows a PET scan of heroin addicts in which the brain regions showing increased blood flow activated by craving for heroin are illuminated using the radiotracer oxygen-15 (Plate 4.2.1.1). Similar studies have revealed the brain regions involved in the pleasurable effects of opiates and stimulants.[7] Thus there is a clear convergence in terms of mechanisms, but in terms of treatment regimens the distinction between physical and psychological remains.

Craving is also a term that is widely used yet ill-defined. Craving is a desire, which most commonly is taken to mean a strong and sometimes irresistible desire to use a drug. The emotional valence of craving is not necessarily pleasurable. Craving can reliably be elicited in situations of negative valence. It is commonly found in withdrawal, when it can lead to relapse. Craving can also be present as an urge or desire to use a drug although the sufferer may be actively denying or resisting its presence. The complex interplay of physical and psychological processes is well exemplified by the physical responses that craving can produce. For example when opiate-dependent subjects are shown drug-related paraphernalia they may experience emotions that range from pleasurable anticipation to early withdrawal (shaking, tearing of the eyes, pupil dilatation, etc.). Each one of these experiences can lead to a desire to use the drug, that is craving.

Studies in both animals and humans have demonstrated that **conditioning** occurs to both the positive and negative aspects of craving.[8] **Tolerance** is to a large extent a conditioned response, particularly related to the environmental context in which a drug has been taken.[9] Thus an environmental context which is drug familiar results in physiological changes in the brain in preparation for the drug effect, and thus less actual drug effect occurs (i.e. tolerance). However, in a novel context, such preparatory changes do not occur so that a standard drug dose will result in a larger drug effect and a potentially fatal outcome. Thus the lethality of a drug is largely dependent on the environment in which it is taken.

Attempts have been made to dissect out the subcomponents of craving using questionnaires. The best known of these are the set designed by Tiffany *et al.*[10] who independently rate the five main subcomponents of craving—urges and desires to use, intention and planning to use, anticipation of positive outcome, anticipation of relief from withdrawal or negative outcome, and loss of control over use. Ongoing neuroimaging studies are beginning to support this multiprocess view of craving by revealing activation or inhibition of different brain regions to be correlated with individual symptom clusters.

There is also increasing evidence that the particular **cognitions** of patients may be important for treatment, especially during withdrawal. Just as panic disorder patients have catastrophic cognitions, addicted patients may have a high fear of craving and other withdrawal symptoms in association with related catastrophic cognitions. This detoxification fear has been measured in opiate addicts, and shown to predict outcome.[11] Withdrawal expectations also play a significant role,[12] and a 15 to 30 min explanation of what the opiate detoxification involves may reduce the measured withdrawal distress by over one-third. Indeed, such is the strength of psychological factors in addiction treatment, there is little doubt that drug treatments should always be combined with the appropriate psychological interventions.

Psychological processes and treatment implications

One of the most influential models in addiction treatment is known as the **stages of change model.**[13] The stage of change that a person can be identified as being at determines the therapeutic approach and type of treatment offered. Thus at the precontemplation stage where there is no recognition of a need for treatment, there is no point in offering intensive treatment interventions. Similarly, at the contemplation stage when treatment is being considered, the appropriate intervention is to help the person clarify their views and build their motivation to change rather than offering active treatment. Indeed, it is only in the decision and action stages that treatment should be actively offered and facilitated.

The brief counselling technique of **motivational interviewing**[14–16] has been proved to improve outcome effectively, and ties in well with the stages of change model. In the early stages the therapy is focused on encouraging the patient to reduce or resolve their ambivalence, which acts as their psychological barrier to treatment. The patient in this client-centred but focused therapy is facilitated to discover the solutions to their own problems themselves. This approach of accepting the client's current level of thinking (rather than offering ready-made solutions, or confronting them, or trying to argue them into the solution) has been shown to be surprisingly effective in the clinical trials.[16] The effectiveness of this technique has resulted in a new understanding of motivation, which is seen as a dynamic state rather than as a fixed state, and one which can be influenced by the therapeutic stance.

Other cognitive therapies also make significant contributions to treatment. **Relapse prevention** involves the teaching of cognitive and behavioural strategies for dealing with high-risk situations and mental states.[17,18] **Other cognitive behavioural therapies**, including extinction of conditioning, contingency management, community reinforcement techniques,[19] and indeed Beck's cognitive therapy,[20] have been effectively applied to substance misuse. The very large Project MATCH (matching alcoholism treatments to client heterogeneity) study of alcohol treatments compared three types of treatment and found that motivational enhancement, 12-step facilitation, and cognitive behavioural therapy were equally effective overall, although each therapy excelled in certain subgroups.[21,22] Based on these results it seems likely that specific therapies targeted at specific issues of importance in patients with addiction are roughly equally effective overall, but that we do not yet know enough to confidently match specific patient subtypes to specific therapies.

A number of **other therapies** have also been shown to be effective, particularly in the alcohol field, including self-control training, self-help groups, marital and family therapy, coping and social skills training, anxiety and stress management, aversion therapies, and brief intervention strategies.[23,24] The Cochrane reviews found that there was insufficient evidence to prove the effectiveness of psychosocial interventions used alone, but that there was added benefit from combining such interventions with pharmacological treatments in both maintenance and detoxification.[4–6]

Personality variables and the genetics of addiction

The role of personality in addiction is a major issue, with some believing in an 'addictive personality' and others suggesting different personality types might predispose to different aspects or forms of drug misuse.(1) In this highly controversial field a few facts are generally agreed. Predisposition to experiment with both licit and illicit drugs is more likely in those with sensation-seeking or impulsive behaviour traits, and in extroverts rather than introverts. However, once drug dependence is established, those with obsessional, dependent, or anxious characteristics find it hardest to stop.(1)

The genetics of drug abuse are beginning to be unravelled and already these studies have thrown up some important insights in relation to personality. The best studied dependence is that on alcohol, where the Scandinavian adoption studies have found the risk of alcoholism in male children of male alcoholics is the same regardless of whether the child is reared with the alcoholic father or by a non-drinking adoptive family. Building on these data, Cloninger(25) has identified two main forms of alcoholism. Type I is the late-onset form that has low inheritance and is associated with anxiety and stress which drinking is used to relieve, often in binges. In contrast, Type II alcoholism starts at a younger age with a heavy regular intake and is associated with antisocial personality traits and criminality. This form is male limited, is associated with impulsivity, and may be related to underfunctioning of brain 5-hydroxytryptamine systems, as genetic polymorphisms of 5-hydroxytryptamine receptors and enzymes have been found in these subjects.(26)

How abused substances affect the brain

The brain works by transmitting information between neurones using the primary neurotransmitters. The **primary neurotransmitters** are glutamate, which is stimulatory (i.e. it turns neurones on), and the closely related amino acid γ-aminobutyric acid (GABA), which is inhibitory (i.e. it turns neurones off). The appropriate balance between these neurotransmitters leads to the brain processes underlying action, sensation, learning, and memory. **Secondary transmitters** are the monoamines and peptides such as dopamine, 5-hydroxytryptamine, noradrenaline (norepinephrine), acetylcholine, and endogenous opiates. These add the tone, valence, and emotion to the primary processes, and some such as noradrenaline are important in memory formation. All 'drugs' (probably even solvents through indirect effects) act by interfering with these neurotransmitters in ways summarized in Table 4.2.1.2. However, it is important to realize that the brain has its own **endogenous 'addictive' neurotransmitters**. The best known are the endogenous opioid peptides such as the endorphins and enkephalins, but there are also endogenous cannabinoids (anandamide) and probably others. It is not yet known whether these endogenous substances are mediators of addiction to cannabis or other drugs, although this would certainly seem possible.(27–29)

What is certain is that some of the most addictive agents (especially the full agonist opiates such as heroin/morphine) act on the endogenous **opioid neurotransmitter pathway**, but with a much greater effect than the natural transmitter. The profound ability of opiates such as heroin to produce addiction is because these drugs highjack the natural transmitter system leaving normal levels of stimulation seeming tame by comparison. Treatment with partial agonist opiates such as **buprenorphine** offer a compromise in that they are less addicting than heroin yet restore some of the

Table 4.2.1.2 Drugs and transmitters

Drug class	Endogenous transmitter	Treatment implications
Mimic natural transmitters		
Opiates (alcohol)	Endorphins/enkephalins	Antagonists (naltrexone) Partial agonists (buprenorphine)
Cannabis	Anandamide/others	Antagonists
Alcohol	GABA	GABA modulator (? acamprosate)
Benzodiazepines/barbiturates	GABA	Partial benzodiazepine agonists Antagonists (flumazenil)
Nicotine	Acetylcholine	Antagonists (mecamylamine) Partial agonist (varenicline)
Release transmitters		
Cocaine (buproprion)	DA	Other uptake site blockers
Amphetamines	DA	D2-receptor antagonists/partial agonists As cocaine
Nicotine	DA	As cocaine
Ecstasy	5-HT/DA	5-HT uptake blockers/antagonists
Alcohol, solvents?	NA/DA	NA/DA uptake blockers
Block transmitters		
Alcohol	Glutamate	Glutamate modulators (acamprosate)
Barbiturates	Glutamate	Glutamate modulators
LSD/other psychedelics	5-HT	Antagonists

DA, dopamine; GABA, γ-aminobutyric acid; 5-HT, 5-hydroxytryptamine; NA, noradrenaline.

brain's deficiency of opiate tone. They also have the advantage of being much safer than full agonists in overdose and rarely cause death from respiratory depression.[30] Other drugs, in particular alcohol, seem to act in part by indirectly stimulating the endogenous opioid system, which is why opioid antagonists such as naltrexone can be useful treatments.[31]

Other drugs act on the natural stimulant transmitter **dopamine**. Dopamine deficiency (for instance in Parkinson's disease) has long been known to limit motor behaviour. Stimulant drugs increase energy and stamina by increasing the synaptic levels of dopamine, either by increasing the release or by blocking its reuptake in the basal ganglia. Many drugs of addiction can also increase dopamine availability in other brain regions, the two most important being the nucleus accumbens and the prefrontal cortex.[32] A huge body of evidence points to the nucleus accumbens as being a critical gateway in drug misuse. Most abused substances (with possible exceptions of opiates and benzodiazepines) act to increase dopamine release in this region. How they do this varies—cocaine and nicotine act at the level of the dopamine terminals, whilst cannabis and alcohol activates the cell bodies in the brain stem. The net effect is to increase dopamine transmission out of the nucleus accumbens into the basal ganglia and thalamus, frontal cortex, amygdala, and hypothalamus.[1]

This circuit is the one that was shown by Olds in the 1950s to sustain electrical self-stimulation in rats and is the brain's own **reward circuit**. It is normally activated by positive reinforcers, such as food, water, and sex that are critical to survival. Because drugs of abuse produce greater effects than the natural reinforcers, the resultant effect is that the brain directs its normal drives away from the natural reinforcers and towards the more pleasurable drugs. In severe addiction, which frequently occurs with the most powerful reinforcers (such as heroin and cocaine), all natural drives may be subsumed to an overwhelming search for and use of the drug. Thus addicts may give up sex, grooming, hygiene, relationships, work, hardly eat or drink, and ignore health problems.

The routes and risks of addiction

In addition to its impact on the social aspects of life, drug misuse can lead to significant medical problems. The dangers of drug abuse relate to two main factors; the route of use of the drug and the effects the drug has outside of the reinforcement circuit of the brain.

For most drugs of abuse the faster the drugs reach their target site in the brain the better they are liked and the more psychologically reinforcing they are. Indeed, the 'pharmaceutical' history of most abused drugs illustrates the progressive refinement of their preparation, in order to accelerate their rate of entry into the brain. A good example is **cocaine**. The Andean Indians originally experienced its effects from chewing coca leaves, which released low levels of cocaine slowly. An increase in vigour and a resistance to fatigue is produced, but little pleasure. Over the centuries cocaine has become more refined, first to paste and then to cocaine hydrochloride powder (snow) which when taken nasally produces high levels in the brain within 5 to 10 min and a clear 'high'. Further refinement to the free base produces a more lipophilic form (crack) that can be smoked, resulting in entry into the brain in seconds. Intravenous drug use also serves the same purpose of getting the drug to the active site very fast.

A similar process of pharmaceutical refinement to accelerate brain entry has taken place with the **opiates**. Smoking opium is a method of delivering morphine and related substances reasonably quickly but in low amounts. Refining opium into its active constituents (e.g. morphine) means that higher doses are more easily ingested. However, morphine crosses the blood–brain barrier relatively slowly and has therefore been largely supplanted by opiates such as heroin that cross more rapidly. Heroin is a diacetylated synthetic derivative of morphine that is more lipophilic, meaning that it is able to enter the brain more rapidly and give a better rush. Interestingly, the active form of heroin is morphine; heroin has to be deacetylated before it can act, which proves that pharmacokinetic differences are the critical variable with opiate preference. Similarly, codeine is also inactive until metabolized to morphine, but because this happens very slowly codeine has less abuse potential than morphine.

The **benzodiazepines** were abused relatively rarely until the advent of gel-filled capsules of temazepam. These provided experienced intravenous opiate users with a convenient source of a concentrated drug, which they began to experiment with in the late 1980s. In an attempt to stop this, the drug was reformulated in wax, which led to users heating up the caplets until they melted and then injecting the hot solution into their veins (hot lining). Unfortunately at body temperature the wax solidified, blocking the veins and arteries into which it was administered, leading to severe ischaemia that often lead to gangrene and the loss of the limb. Since there are no therapeutic advantages of temazepam over other benzodiazepines that are much less abusable, this drug has recently been put under a higher degree of regulatory control in the United Kingdom in order to deter its prescription and misuse.

As well as affecting the relative reinforcing actions of abused drugs, **the rate of brain entry** also contributes to risk. A very rapid drug entry makes dose adjustments difficult or impossible and so predisposes to overdose. This is most obvious for intravenous use of opiates where respiratory depression is the main cause of death, but is less common with smoked opiates as intake can more easily be titrated to the desired effect.

The **route of use** also affects risk, most notably with the risk of infection from intravenous use, especially when needles are not cleaned or are shared. The majority of current intravenous users are Hepatitis C positive and we can therefore expect cirrhosis to become a major cause of their death in the next decade or so. This also raises ethical and economic issues; interferon treatment significantly reduces the progression of the disease but is costly and its routine use in addicts would be massively expensive and likely to cause public disquiet. The other main infections are hepatitis B and AIDS. The frightening rise of AIDS in drug abusers, where it occurred faster than in any other group, was the main impetus to the harm-reduction approach becoming the treatment style of the 1990s. Needle-exchange programmes and increased methadone availability were both proven to reduce the spread of AIDS and have become the cornerstone of treatment in many countries.

Relative risks of abused drugs

This is a critical issue in relation to directing legal as well as medical inputs into drug abuse. There are four main factors, which have to be taken into account in determining relative risk:[33]

- risk due to the route of use
- risk of the drug itself

- extent to which the drug controls behaviour (addictiveness)
- ease of stopping

The risks due to the route have been covered above. The risks of the drugs themselves are determined by standard tests and clinical experience and can be encapsulated in concepts such as the **therapeutic index**. This is the ratio of toxic dose to therapeutic (or usual) dose. The ratio is very low for heroin and similar opiates, for cocaine especially crack, and for intravenous temazepam and oral ecstasy. It is quite high for psychedelics, cannabis, benzodiazepines, and orally used stimulants such as amphetamines. Another important consideration is the **health complications** of long-term use, which by and large reflects the therapeutic index. An exception to this is the opiates, which, provided sterile administration is used, are thought to have little detrimental effect, even when used chronically and intravenously. Chronic cocaine can lead to cardiac damage, and heavy cannabis smoking causes precancerous change in the same way as tobacco smoking, as well as causing greater levels of chronic bronchitis.

The degree of **control over behaviour** that the drug elicits is a major factor in drug dependence, and is the closest concept to addictiveness. Although the route of administration is another critical variable, we can make some reasonable generalizations. Strong opiates and cocaine are the most addictive, being overall as addictive as nicotine. The benzodiazepines, ecstasy, and psychedelics are the least addictive, and are significantly less addictive than alcohol.

There are three main factors contributing to drugs gaining control over behaviour, all of which affect the ease with which a drug may be stopped. The first is the pleasure a drug produces—the positive drive for use (pleasure giving and seeking). The others both involve the pain of abstinence—withdrawal in both physical and psychological terms—which leads to drug use to relieve it (discomfort escape). The pattern of drug use during an addiction career generally begins with the quest for pleasure and progressively evolves into the escape from withdrawal pain as neuroadaptive processes develop. In this context it may be thought that withdrawal discomfort is best limited to symptoms with a clear physical symptomatology, that is the autonomic symptoms indicative of physical dependence. But in terms of addictiveness, psychological withdrawal may in fact be more important than physical withdrawal. This is illustrated by the finding that those dependent on opiates for medical reasons, although physically dependent, experience little craving and risk of relapse once detoxified, provided the reason for being on the opiate resolves. The ease of stopping the drug thus depends on both the physical and psychological withdrawal symptoms, as well as the ability of the drug to provide positive reinforcement.

It is possible to provide rough guides for these three processes for each drug, so that the overall addictiveness potential can be gauged (Table 4.2.1.3). For completeness, the main licit drugs are also shown as well as another highly motivated behaviour which can produce a state of addiction/dependence, that is gambling.

Table 4.2.1.3 Addictiveness of various agents and activities

	Pleasure giving	Physical withdrawal problems	Psychological withdrawal problems
Opiates	+++	+++	+++
Amphetamines	++	+	+
Crack/cocaine	+++	++	+++
Cannabinoids	+	+	+
Barbiturates	++	+++	++
Benzodiazepines	+	++	++
Ecstasy	++	+	0
Psychedelics	++	+	0
Cigarettes	+++	+	+++
Alcohol	++	+++	++
Caffeine	+	+	+
Gambling	++	0	++

0 none; + slight; ++ moderate; +++ strong.

Further information

Nutt, D.J., Robbins, T.W., Stimson, G.V., *et al.* (2006). *Drugs and the future: brain science, addiction and society*. Elsevier, Burlington, MA.

NIDA (National Institute on Drug Abuse) www.nida.nih.gov

SAMHSA (Substance Abuse and Mental Health Services Administration) www.samhsa.gov

References

1. Nutt, D.J., Robbins, T.W., Stimson, G.V., *et al.* (2006). *Drugs and the future: brain science, addiction and society*. Elsevier, Burlington, MA.
2. George, D.T., Nutt, D.J., Dwyer, B.A., *et al.* (1990). Alcoholism and panic disorder: is the comorbidity more than coincidence? *Acta Psychiatrica Scandinavica*, **81**, 97–107.
3. Marshall, J.R. (1994). The diagnosis and treatment of social phobia and alcohol abuse. *Bulletin of the Menninger Clinic*, **58**, 58–66.
4. Amato, L., Minozzi, S., Davoli, M., *et al.* (2004). Psychosocial and pharmacological treatments versus pharmacological treatments for opioid detoxification. *Cochrane Database of Systematic Reviews*, (4), CD005031.
5. Amato, L., Minozzi, S., Davoli, M., *et al.* (2004). Psychosocial combined with agonist maintenance treatments versus agonist maintenance treatments alone for treatment of opioid dependence. *Cochrane Database of Systematic Reviews*, (4), CD004147.
6. Mayet, S., Farrell, M., Ferri, M., *et al.* (2004). Psychosocial treatment for opiate abuse and dependence. *Cochrane Database of Systematic Reviews*, (4), CD004330.
7. Schlaepfer, T.E., Strain, E.C., Greenberg, B.D., *et al.* (1998). Site of opioid action in the human brain: mu and kappa agonists' subjective and cerebral blood flow effects. *The American Journal of Psychiatry*, **155**, 470–3.
8. O'Brien, C.P., Testa, T., O'Brien, T.J., *et al.* (1997). Conditioned narcotic withdrawal in humans. *Science*, **195**, 1000–2.
9. Siegel, S., Hinson, R.E., Krank, M.D., *et al.* (1982). Heroin overdose death: contribution of drug–associated environmental cues. *Science*, **216**, 436–7.
10. Tiffany, S.T., Singleton, E., Haertzen, C.A., *et al.* (1993). The development of a cocaine craving questionnaire. *Drug and Alcohol Dependence*, **34**, 19–28 (erratium at 2004, **16**, 326).
11. Schumacher, J.E., Milby, J.B., Fishman, B.E., *et al.* (1992). Relation of detoxification fear to methadone maintenance outcome: 5-year follow-up. *Psychology of Addictive Behaviors*, **6**, 41–6.

12. Phillips, G.T., Gossop, M., and Bradley, B. (1986). The influence of psychological factors on the opiate withdrawal syndrome. *The British Journal of Psychiatry*, **149**, 235–8.
13. Prochaska, J.O. and DiClemente, C. (1983). Stages and processes of self-change of smoking: towards a more integrative model of change. *Journal of Consulting and Clinical Psychology*, **51**, 390–5.
14. Rollnick, S. and Miller, W.R. (1995). What is motivational interviewing? *Behavioral and Cognitive Psychotherapy*, **23**, 325–34.
15. Miller, W.R. and Rollnick, S. (2002). *Motivational interviewing: preparing people for change* (2nd edn). Guilford Press, New York.
16. Noonan, W.C. and Moyers, T.B.(1997). Motivational interviewing. *Journal of Substance Misuse*, **2**, 8–16.
17. Marlatt, G.A. and Gordon, J.R. (eds.) (1985). *Relapse prevention: maintenance strategies in the treatment of addictive behaviors*. Guilford Press, New York.
18. Wanigaratne, S., Wallace, W., Pullin, J., *et al.* (eds.) (1990). *Relapse prevention for addictive behaviours: a manual for therapists*. Blackwell, London.
19. Stitzer, M.L. and Higgins, S.T. (1995). Behavioral treatment of drug and alcohol abuse. In *Psychopharmacology: the fourth generation of progress* (eds., F.E. Bloom and D.J. Kupfer), pp. 1807–19. Raven Press, New York.
20. Beck, A.T., Wright, F.D., Newman, C.F., *et al.* (eds.) (1993). *Cognitive therapy of substance abuse*. Guilford Press, New York.
21. Project MATCH Research Group. (1997). Matching alcoholism treatments to client heterogeneity: project MATCH posttreatment drinking outcomes. *Journal of Studies on Alcohol*, **58**, 7–29.
22. Project MATCH Research Group. (1997). Project MATCH secondary *a priori* hypotheses. *Addiction*, **92**, 1671–98.
23. Miller, W.R., Brown, J.M., Simpson, T.L., *et al.* (1995). What works? A methodological analysis of the alcohol treatment outcome literature. In *Handbook of alcoholism treatment approaches: effective alternatives* (2nd edn) (eds. R.K. Hester and W.R. Miller), pp. 12–44. Allyn and Bacon, Boston, MA.
24. Edwards, E. and Dare, C. (eds.) (1996). *Psychotherapy, psychological treatments and the addictions*. Cambridge University Press, Cambridge.
25. Cloninger, C.R. (1987). Neurogenetic adaptive mechanisms in alcoholism. *Science*, **236**, 410–16.
26. Nielsen, D.A., Goldman, D., Virkkunen, M., *et al.* (1994). Suicidality and 5–hydroxyindoleacetic acid concentration associated with a tryptophan hydroxylase polymorphism. *Archives of General Psychiatry*, **51**, 34–8.
27. Nutt, D.J. (1997). Neuropharmacological basis for tolerance and dependence. In *Drug addiction and its treatment: nexus of neuroscience and behavior* (eds. B.A. Johnson and J.D. Roache), pp. 171–86. Raven Press, New York.
28. Nutt, D.J. (1999). Alcohol and the brain: pharmacological insights for psychiatrists. *The British Journal of Psychiatry*, **174**, 114–19.
29. Lingford-Hughes, A. and Nutt, D. (2003). Neurobiology of addiction and implications for treatment. *The British Journal of Psychiatry*, **182**, 97–100.
30. Law, F., Daglish, M.R.C., Myles, J.S., *et al.* (2004). The clinical use of buprenorphine in opiate addiction: evidence and practice. *Acta Neuropsychiatrica*, **16**, 246–74. (Erratum (2004), **16**, 326.)
31. Volpicelli, J.R., Alterman, A.I., Hayashida, M., *et al.* (1993). Naltrexone in the treatment of alcohol dependence. *Archives of General Psychiatry*, **49**, 876–80.
32. Di Chiara, G. (1995). The role of dopamine in drug abuse viewed from the perspective of its role in motivation. *Drug and Alcohol Dependence*, **38**, 95–137.
33. Nutt, D.J., King, L.A., Saulsbury, W., *et al.* (2007). Developing a rational scale for assessing the risks of drugs of potential misuse. *Lancet*, **369**, 1047–53.

4.2.2 Alcohol use disorders

Contents

4.2.2.1 Aetiology of alcohol problems
Juan C. Negrete and Kathryn J. Gill

4.2.2.2 Alcohol dependence and alcohol problems
Jane Marshall

4.2.2.3 Alcohol and psychiatric and physical disorders
Karl F. Mann and Falk Kiefer

4.2.2.4 Treatment of alcohol dependence
Jonathan Chick

4.2.2.5 Services for alcohol use disorders
D. Colin Drummond

4.2.2.6 Prevention of alcohol-related problems
Robin Room

4.2.2.1 Aetiology of alcohol problems

Juan C. Negrete and Kathryn J. Gill

Introduction

Approximately 8 out of every 10 persons living in Europe and the Americas would report consuming alcoholic beverages in their lifetime,[1] and the norm is for drinking to start in adolescence: in 2003 the average age of first drink in the United States was 14 years old.[2] Also in the year 2003, 79.3 per cent of persons aged 15 years or more in Canada reported to be current users of alcohol, and 22.6 per cent admitted to having exceeded the country's safe drinking guidelines (i.e. no more than 14 units/week for males and 12 units/week for females). The same survey elicited a rate of 'hazardous drinkers' of 13.6 per cent, defined as all respondents who scored 8+ on the AUDIT screening questionnaire.[3]

Epidemiological data in the United States indicates that roughly one in seven persons who start drinking will develop an alcohol dependence disorder in the course of their lives.[4] The figure is higher among men when compared to women. Of course it is also higher if other clinical forms of alcohol misuse (i.e. alcohol abuse/harmful drinking) are included in the rates in addition to dependence.

A moderate level of alcohol use appears to be relatively harmless; and there exist public health guidelines on 'safe' drinking practices. The recommendations vary considerably from country to country, but they all assume a greater vulnerability to alcohol effects in the female gender. In the United Kingdom, for instance, hazardous drinking is thought to start at 21 units/week for men and 16 units/week for women;[5] and in the United States the equivalent guidelines are 14 and 7 drinks per week.[6] It is among alcohol users who exceed such guidelines that the prevalence of dependence is the highest; up to 40 per cent of the more frequent violators.[7]

The expression 'alcohol problems' encompasses a wide range of untoward occurrences, from maladaptive, impaired, or harmful behaviour, to health complications and the condition of alcohol dependence. Alcohol problems are not incurred just by chronic excessive drinkers, but also by persons who drink heavily on isolated occasions (e.g. accidents, violence, poisoning, etc.). Given their high frequency and social costs, these consequences of acute inebriation represent the most significant public health burden of drinking.[8] This section focuses rather on the causes of problems of a clinical nature, the ones presented by individuals who engage in patterns of repeated excessive drinking, i.e. 'alcohol dependence' and 'alcohol abuse' (DSM-IV nomenclature) or 'harmful drinking' (ICD-10 nomenclature).

The causality of alcohol misuse

Alcoholism is a bio-psychosocial phenomenon par excellence; it results from the contribution of multiple individual and environmental risk factors. The complex dynamics influencing its development have been well acknowledged in the literature. Theories have taken many disparate facts into consideration, from the effects of alcohol policy to the influence of familial and sociocultural environments across cultures and over time. Some ethnic groups, for instance, have traditionally had low rates of alcoholism (Asians, Jews, and some North American Aboriginals) and the prevalence is generally higher in males across both age cohorts and ethnicities. Another layer of complexity lies in the fact that alcoholism is a clinically heterogeneous disorder with variable age of onset, drinking patterns, severity, and comorbidity with other mental disorders. In general, alcoholics have one or more clinical diagnoses in addition to alcohol dependence, including drug abuse, antisocial personality disorder, anxiety, and depression. The course of the disorder is variable with high rates of remission and relapse; its manifestation changing in pattern and severity in response to life events (stressors) and other aspects of the environment. A summary of the etiological factors that have been shown to influence the development of alcoholism is shown in Box 4.2.2.1.1.

Box 4.2.2.1.1 A bio-psychosocial model of the aetiology of alcoholism

The comunity/sociocultural environment

- policies affecting availability and price (temperance, prohibition, taxation)
- cultural patterns of consumption, social acceptability of drinking/drunkenness
- availability of other reinforcers (sources of pleasure/recreation)
- employment and/or educational opportunities (anomie/marginalization)
- peer influences/role models (affiliation with deviant subculture)

The family environment

- marital breakdown (lower socio-economic status, poor parental monitoring)
- family attitudes (availability of drugs/alcohol, modelling of siblings/parents)
- intrauterine exposure to alcohol/drugs (potential effects of alcohol, nicotine and other drugs on behaviour and cognition)
- familial substance abuse (poverty, violence, and increased rates of early life trauma including neglect and physical/sexual abuse)

Individual/host factors

- heritable genetic factors (genetic loading for alcohol/drug dependence, depression, anxiety disorders in first-degree relatives)
- differences in response to alcohol (low sensitivity in terms of physiological responses and subjective effects)
- metabolic differences (thiamine deficiency, alcohol metabolizing enzymes)
- high risk taking behaviours (male sex)
- childhood psychopathology (conduct disorder, untreated ADHD)
- psychiatric disorders (bipolar, depression, anxiety, schizophrenia)

Sociocultural factors

Macrocultural influences such as values, beliefs, and mores; social role functions; local economy; customs and dietary habits; rapid social change; and cultural stress do shape and dictate the way alcohol is used in human societies. But even within a single society, there is variance in the alcohol problems profile of different subgroups. For instance, drinking, heavy drinking, alcohol use disorders, and treatment for alcoholism are more frequently recorded in men than women,[1] the risk of hospital admission for alcoholic psychosis, acute intoxication, and liver cirrhosis is elevated in unskilled and blue-collar workers when compared with higher occupational categories; alcoholics are over-represented in occupations with flexible work schedules, in those less supervised, and in the ones which facilitate access to alcohol,[9,10] and although there are a larger proportion of regular alcohol users among the older, the wealthier, and the better educated, frequency of heavy drinking (i.e. episodes of intoxication, 5+ drinks at a time) is inversely correlated with age, income, and level of education.[3]

Cultural beliefs about drinking and related social norms largely determine the manner in which alcohol is used. Disorderly conduct and drunken violence are more likely to occur in societies which, while allowing drinking, do view alcohol as an evil substance. Similar consequences can be expected if drunkenness is culturally considered as a 'time out', when socially unacceptable behaviours are tolerated or excused.[11] In fact, the social condoning of drunkenness is considered as an epidemiological risk factor. The availability of alcohol and the social promotion of frequent or heavy drinking are examples of social risk. But environmental facilitation *per se* does not explain the genesis of an alcohol dependence disorder in specific individuals. This disorder is best understood as the result of social prompting and individual vulnerabilities.

Psychological factors

Alcoholics do not present a homogeneous premorbid personality profile. However, some distinctive trait clusters have been identified which seem to characterize different types of alcoholics.[12] One such group (type 1) tend to score low in novelty seeking and high in harm avoidance and reward dependence. Another group (type 2) is formed by the natural thrill seekers, who appear to ignore harmful consequences and punitive responses. This latter cluster, which prevails mostly in males with early-onset alcoholism, is also typical of antisocial personalities. Of all personality features, conduct disorder and antisocial behaviour are the strongest predictors of alcohol misuse.[13]

(a) Psychodynamic processes

Early psychodynamic writings portrayed alcoholism and other addictions as regressive behaviours caused by unconscious conflicts over libidinal pleasures, homosexuality, and aggression. More recent formulations emphasize ego and self-developmental problems, and consider psychoactive substance abuse as a response to psychological suffering; an attempt at re-establishing homeostasis. This is known as the *self-medication hypothesis* of addictions,[14] according to which, persons with self-regulatory deficiencies in the areas of self-care, self-esteem, self-object relations, and affect tolerance, would drink to palliate their distress.

(b) Learning

Alcohol abuse as seen by some as a behavioural pattern which has been learned through mechanisms of classical (i.e. Pavlovian) and operant conditioning. According to this interpretation, the perpetuation of heavy drinking results from its association with conditioned stimuli (cues), and from the action of positive (pleasant effects) or negative (stress reduction) behavioural reinforcement. Additional components of this equation are the so-called alcohol 'expectancies'. Alcohol abusers tend to overemphasize the pleasant aspects of drinking and to ignore the negative ones; the learning theory of alcoholism assumes that such a cognitive set is also acquired through social exposure. The Social Learning Theory posits that the positive expectancy of relaxation following a drink can facilitate more frequent alcohol use and thus contribute to the development of dependence.[15]

(c) Psychiatric comorbidity

Community and clinical epidemiology findings point to the presence of other psychiatric disorders as one of the most significant psychological risk factors in alcoholism.[16] The co-occurrence is sometimes sequential, with the psychiatric disorder preceding alcoholism; in which case a causal role in the development of heavy/frequent drinking is attributed to the former. While this is often observed in cases of conduct disorder, social phobia, attention deficit-hyperactivity (untreated) and depression, there are other psychiatric disturbances such as panic disorder, generalized anxiety and dysthymia that often become clinically significant only after the person has been abusing alcohol for sometime. These *alcohol-induced* mood and anxiety disorders represent a sizeable proportion of the comorbidity rates.[17] Whether or not it is 'primary', psychological stress is a widely recognized factor in alcoholism treatment failure and relapse.

Yet the comorbidity of some psychiatric disorders (e.g. bipolar disorder, schizophrenia) and alcoholism appears to develop in no predictable sequence, so that if not random, their co-occurrence could be assumed to result from common genetic influences (see below) and pathophysiological mechanisms. One such interpretation is the 'reward deficiency syndrome' hypothesis; it purports that both psychiatric disturbances (e.g. negative symptoms of schizophrenia) and the tendency to abuse addictive substances arise from a basic dysfunction of the dopamine mesocorticolimbic reward system.[18] The 'primary addiction' theory is another such explanation for comorbidity; it contends that a single neurobiological deficiency—primary abnormalities in the hippocampus and the frontal cortex—facilitate the development of schizophrenic symptoms and the person's toxicophilia in a parallel manner.[19]

Genetic factors in the development of alcoholism

In recent decades the biological perspective on the aetiology of alcoholism has gained considerable ground. Findings from family, twin and adoption studies demonstrate that there is significantly higher risk for alcoholism among individuals with an alcoholic biological parent or first-degree relative.[20–23] Meta-analysis has been used to jointly analyze data from twin and adoption studies grouped by country of origin (Scandinavian versus United States of America). Based on all available data, genetic factors accounted for between 40 and 60 per cent of the variance in alcoholism risk, with the effects of environment (shared and non-shared) estimated between 15 and 33 per cent. In a methodologically rigorous study, Prescott and Kendler[24] examined the concordance for alcoholism among a population-based sample from the Virginia Twin Registry. Monozygotic (MZ, $n = 861$) and dizygotic (DZ, $n = 653$) male twins were diagnosed using structured interviews and DSM criteria. Concordance rates for alcohol dependence were significantly higher for MZ (48 per cent) compared to DZ (32 per cent) twins, and analyses indicated that 48–58 per cent of the variation in alcoholism liability could be attributed to additive genetic factors.

Alcoholic males with family history of alcoholism (FHP) have been reported to have greater severity of alcoholic symptoms and poorer outcomes than alcoholics that are family history negative (FHN). Box 4.2.2.1.2 describes some characteristics of familial alcoholism. Onset of drinking prior to age 15 is associated higher rates of alcoholism,[25] ADHD, conduct and anxiety disorders, as well as a host of other negative events including unintentional injuries, physical fights, nicotine/drug dependence, and poor school performance. Children of alcoholics are significantly more likely to be exposed to high-risk environments that include poor prenatal care (alcohol/nicotine exposure, nutritional deficiencies), as well as homes in which there is more poverty and violence. Overall, it

Box 4.2.2.1.2 Characteristics of familial alcoholism

Family history positive (FHP) alcoholism is associated with:

- Earlier onset (<15 at age first drink is associated with increased rates of alcoholism, nicotine dependence, drug use, and conduct disorder. Early age of alcohol use is familial, heritable and may be related to transmission of disinhibitory psychopathology in males)
- Behavioural disturbances during childhood (conduct disorder, emotional lability, aggressivity, low attention span, low soothability)
- More severe alcohol dependence (higher levels of physical dependence, negative consequences)
- Lower educational and occupational achievement
- Deficits in executive cognitive functioning (poor problem solving, abstraction, and perceptual-motor skills)

appears likely that there are common genetic and environmental influences on a host of externalizing disorders—as well as gene–environment interactions.

Linkage studies to identify the genes underlying the heritability of alcoholism

A number of large-scale international linkage studies are currently underway that are aimed at mapping genes for alcoholism including the Irish Affected Sib Pair Study,[26] and the Collaborative Study on the Genetics of Alcoholism (COGA).[27] COGA is a multi-center program designed to detect and map susceptibility genes for alcoholism that is currently underway in the United States. Using a family-based linkage strategy, the study is examining a number of quantitative intermediary phenotypes (endophenotypes) including P300 evoked potentials, alcohol sensitivity, and personality traits (harm avoidance, novelty seeking, and reward dependence) in relation to both alcohol consumption, and alcohol dependence. In addition, the study is examining the association between polymorphisms in specific candidate genes such as alcohol dehydrogenase (ADH), monoamine oxidase (MAO_B), and the serotonin transporter and alcohol-related phenotypes. In early work, COGA-reported associations between alcoholism and regions on chromosomes 4 and 15 that encode genes for the inhibitory neurotransmitter, gamma-aminobutyric acid ($GABA_A$). Most recently, linkage and association genome scans for a broader 'addiction' vulnerability phenotype provided strong evidence for linkage to chromosome 4. Further assessment of single nucleotide polymorphism (SNP) genotypes within the chromosome 4 region provided strongest support for the involvement of the $GABA_A$ receptor α2 subunit (GABRA2 gene).[28] $GABA_A$ has been implicated in mediating some of the psychopharmacological effects of alcohol,[29] and the genetic studies provide convergent evidence suggesting that the predisposition to alcoholism may be inherited as a general state of CNS disinhibition/hyperexcitability that results from an altered responsiveness to GABA. However, this remains to be confirmed by additional genetic and experimental studies.

Other candidate genes and processes

It has been shown that genetic factors may influence a number of important processes such as initial sensitivity to the effects of alcohol, as well as the development of tolerance, sensitization, and physical dependence (including withdrawal complications such as seizures and delirium tremens). Several lines of research have suggested that sensitivity to alcohol may influence the propensity to abuse. Sensitivity refers to drug effects such as intoxication, physiological reactivity, and activation (tendency towards stimulation versus depression following ingestion). For example, Schuckit[30,31] found that individuals with low sensitivity to alcohol as measured by lower psychomotor responses and less subjective intoxication following alcohol dosing were *more* likely to be alcohol dependent at follow-up 10 years later.

Peripheral and central levels of alcohol metabolizing enzymes may be important modulators of the psychopharmacological response to alcohol. Ethyl alcohol (ethanol) is converted to acetaldehyde via the actions of alcohol dehydrogenase (ADH). There is evidence for linkage of gene(s) located on chromosome 4 (as discussed above) and two ADH genes closely linked on chromosome 4 (ADH1B and ADH1C) that encode for isozymes that differ in their kinetic properties. The allele ADH1B*2 (found largely in individuals of East Asian and Jewish descent) encodes a more active isozyme that has been associated with protection from alcohol dependence. Most recently Edenberg *et al.*[32] genotyped 110 SNPs across seven ADH genes in a COGA sample. There was strong evidence that variations in ADH4 were associated with alcoholism, and among African-Americans there was evidence that the ADH1B*3 allele was protective. Acetaldehyde produced by ethanol oxidation is rapidly metabolized by the enzyme aldehyde dehydrogenase (ALDH). A single base pair substitution in mitochondrial ALDH, termed the 'oriental' mutation (ALDH2*2 allele), is present in a large percentage of the Asian population. This mutation renders the enzyme inactive and produces a flushing response (warm-flushed face, tachycardia, nausea) following ingestion of small quantities of alcohol due to the buildup of acetaldehyde, particularly among ALDH2*2 homozygotes. Due to the aversive nature of the flushing response, the ALDH2*2 mutation is a significant protective factor against alcoholism.

Box 4.2.2.1.3 Potential candidate genes and markers for alcoholism

- Brain waves (P300 event-related brain potential)
- Brain enzymes (e.g. monoamine oxidase, adenylate cyclase)
- Alcohol and aldehyde metabolizing enzymes (ADH, catalase, ALDH, cytochrome P450IIE1)
- Opioids (e.g. kappa OPRK1receptor and prodynorphin ligand)
- Serotonin (e.g. polymorphisms of the 5-HT transporter and receptors (e.g. 5-HT1B, 5-HT2A, 5-HT2C), tryptophan hydroxylase TPH (218AC))
- Dopamine (polymorphisms of D_2, D_3, D_4 receptors and the dopamine transporter (DAT))
- GABA (polymorphisms in receptor subunits, variants in glutamate decarboxylase-2 (*GAD2*))

Note that this list is not exhaustive. For a more complete review consult references 32–5.

In addition to the examination of metabolic factors that may account for some of the genetic variance in the development of alcohol dependence, there is an intense search for other neurogenetic factors related to the effects of alcohol in the brain. As shown in Box 4.2.2.1.3, a large number of candidate markers and putative genetic loci that have been investigated to date. For example, abstinent alcoholics and approximately 35 per cent of sons of alcoholics have been shown to have lower amplitude of a P300 event-related brain potential. Analyses of COGA data indicate that P300 amplitude reduction (P3-AR) is heritable, but more recent analyses have demonstrated that the P3-AR is associated with risk for substance dependence generally (e.g. frequent use of cannabis).[33]

The analysis of various neurotransmitters (including synthesis, release, receptor density, second messengers, polymorphisms) in relation to alcoholism and other alcohol-related endophenotypes is a well-developed area of research. The high degree of comorbidity between alcoholism and other mental disorders suggests that there may be common neurobiological pathways, including those that modulate reward, compulsive behaviour, anxiety, depression, and stress responses.[34] In this context, dysregulation of the serotonin (5HT) system has been implicated in the aetiology of a number of psychiatric disorders (depression, OCD, eating disorders) and alcoholism. In particular, polymorphisms in the promoter region of the 5HT transporter (5HTTLPR) producing the short ('S' allele) or long ('L' allele) variants differentially modulate transcriptional activity of the promoter, yielding differences in 5HT uptake activity in human platelets and brain. Most recently analyses conducted in the COGA sample have failed to find an association between the 5HTTLPR polymorphism and alcohol dependence. In a family-based association analyses (n = 1913 Caucasians) there was evidence for association of the S allele with depression, but not with alcohol dependence.[27]

Numerous studies have examined the association between alcohol dependence and the A1 allele of the dopamine D2 receptor (DRD2), however results have been debated for more than a decade. In general, the A1 allele is not consistently associated with alcoholism, and it does not consistently co-segregate in families with alcoholism. The effect size of this allele is likely to be very small. The human genes for the dopamine D3 and D4 receptors are polymorphic and studies are currently underway examining the potential relationship between various alleles of these receptors and substance dependence.

As noted above, synaptic actions of GABA have been implicated in the psychopharmacological effects of alcohol. Associations between variants in glutamate decarboxylase-2 (*GAD2*), a gene encoding for a major enzyme in the synthesis of GABA have been reported. In particular a functional promoter *GAD2* -243 A > G variant may influence risk for alcohol dependence in populations exhibiting severe alcoholism.[35]

In summary, plausible candidate genes for alcoholism include loci associated with alcohol and aldehyde metabolism, as well as variants within the GABA, opiate, and serotonin systems. The strongest candidate to date is for the involvement of the $GABA_A$ receptor $\alpha 2$ subunit (GABRA2 gene) on chromosome 4. Notably, associations between various loci and alcoholism reported in the literature have not been consistently replicated. Discrepancies in the literature have beesn attributed to variations in sampling (ethnicity, diagnostic criteria, severity of alcoholism, sample sizes), as well as to the clinical and genetic heterogeneity of alcoholism. Thus in this context, it is important to note that possible mechanisms for indirect transmission of an alcoholism phenotype include personality traits, and comorbid psychopathology including anxiety, depression, and conduct disorder.

Further information

Sartor, C.E., Lynskey, M.T., Heath, A.C., *et al.* (2006). The role of childhood risk factors in initiation of alcohol use and progression to alcohol dependence. *Addiction*, **102**, 216–25.

References

1. Edwards, G., Anderson, P., Babor, T.F., *et al.* (1994). *Alcohol policy and the public good.* Oxford University Press, Oxford, UK.
2. Newes-Adeyi, G., Chen, C.M., Williams, G.D., *et al.* (2003). *Trends in underage drinking in the United States, 1991–2003. Surveillance Report No. 74.* National Institute on Alcohol Abuse and Alcoholism, Bethesda, MD.
3. Health Canada and the Canadian Executive Council on Addictions. (2004). *Canadian addiction survey.* Canadian Centre on Substance Abuse, Ottawa.
4. Anthony, J.C., Chen, C.Y., and Storr, C.L. (2005). Drug dependence epidemiology. *Clinical Neuroscience Research*, **5**, 55–68.
5. Royal College of General Practitioners. (1986). *Alcohol-a balanced view.* Royal College of General Practitioners, London.
6. National Institute on Alcohol Abuse and Alcoholism. (2004). *Helping patients with alcohol problems: a health practitioner's guide.* NIAAA, Bethesda, MD.
7. Dawson, D.A., Grant, B.F., and Li, T.K. (2005). Quantifying the risks associated with exceeding recommended drinking limits. *Alcoholism: Clinical and Experimental Research*, **29**, 902–8.
8. Rhem, J., Baliunas, D., Brochu, S., *et al.* (2006). *The costs of substance abuse in Canada 2002.* Canadian Centre on Substance Abuse, Ottawa.
9. Hemmingsson, T., Lundberg, I., Romelsjo, A., *et al.* (1997). Alcoholism in social classes and occupations in Sweden. *International Journal of Epidemiology*, **26**, 584–91.
10. Mandell, W., Eaton, W.W., Anthony, J.C., *et al.* (1992). Alcoholism and occupations: a review of 104 occupations. *Alcohol: Clinical and Experimental Research*, **16**, 734–46.
11. Heath, D.B. (1993). Recent developments in alcoholism: anthropology. *Recent Developments in Alcoholism*, **11**, 29–43.
12. Cloninger, C.R. (1987). Neurogenetic adaptive mechanisms in alcoholism. *Science*, **236**, 410–16.
13. Driessen, M., Veltrup, C., Wetterling, T., *et al.* (1998). Axis I and Axis II comorbidity in alcohol dependence and the two types of alcoholism. *Alcoholism: Clinical and Experimental Research*, **22**, 77–86.
14. Khantzian, E.J. (1985). The self-medication hypothesis of addictive disorders. *The American Journal of Psychiatry*, **142**, 1259–64.
15. Rotgers, F., Keller, D.S., and Morgenstern, J. (eds.) (1996). *Treating substance abuse: theory and technique.* Guilford Press, New York.
16. Kessler, R.C., McConagle, K.A., Zhao, S., *et al.* (1994). Lifetime and 12 month prevalence of DSM-III-R psychiatric disorders in the United States. *Archives of General Psychiatry*, **51**, 8–19.
17. Schuckit, M.A. (2006). Comorbidity between substance use disorders and psychiatric conditions. *Addiction*, **101**(Suppl. 1), 76–88.
18. Bowirrat, A. and Oscar-Berman, M. (2005). Relationship between dopaminergic neurotransmission, alcoholism and reward deficiency syndrome. *American Journal of Medical Genetics B Neuropsychiatric Genetics*, **132**, 29–37.
19. Chambers, R.A., Krystal, J.H., and Self, D.W. (2001). A neurobiological basis for substance abuse comorbidity in schizophrenia. *Biological Psychiatry*, **50**, 71–83.
20. Cotton, N.S. (1979). The familial incidence of alcoholism: a review. *Journal of Studies on Alcoholism*, **40**, 89–116.
21. Cloninger, C.R., Bohman, M., and Sigvardsson, S. (1981). Inheritance of alcohol abuse: cross-fostering analysis of adopted men. *Archives General Psychiatry*, **38**, 861–8.
22. Van den Bree, M.B.M., Johnson, E.O., Neale, M.C., *et al.* (1998). Genetic and environmental influences on drug use and abuse/dependence in male and female twins. *Drug and Alcohol Dependence*, **52**, 231–41.
23. Edenberg, H.J. and Foroud, T. (2006). The genetics of alcoholism: identifying specific genes through family studies. *Addiction Biology*, **11**, 386–96.
24. Prescott, C.A. and Kendler, K.S. (1999). Genetic and environmental contributions to alcohol abuse and dependence in a population-based sample of male twins. *The American Journal of Psychiatry*, **156**, 34–40.
25. Grant, B.F. and Dawson, D. (1997). Age at onset of alcohol use and its association with DSM-IV alcohol abuse and dependence: results from the national longitudinal alcohol epidemiologic survey. *Journal of Substance Abuse*, **9**, 103–10.

26. Kendler, K.S., Kuo, P.H., Todd Webb, B., *et al.* (2006). A joint genomewide linkage analysis of symptoms of alcohol dependence and conduct disorder. *Alcoholism: Clinical and Experimental Research*, **30**, 1972–7.
27. Dick, D.M., Plunkett, J., Hamlin, D., *et al.* (2007). Association analyses of the serotonin transporter gene with lifetime depression and alcohol dependence in the Collaborative Study on the Genetics of Alcoholism (COGA) sample. *Psychiatric Genetics*, **17**, 35–8.
28. Johnson, C., Drgon, T., Liu, Q.R., *et al.* (2006). Pooled association genome scanning for alcohol dependence using 104,268 SNPs: validation and use to identify alcoholism vulnerability loci in unrelated individuals from the collaborative study on the genetics of alcoholism. *American Journal of Medical Genetics: Part B Neuropsychiatric Genetics*, **141**, 844–53.
29. Krystal, J.H., Staley, J., Mason, G., *et al.* (2006). γ-Aminobutyric acid type A receptors and alcoholism. *Archives General Psychiatry*, **63**, 957–68.
30. Schuckit, M.A. and Smith, T.L. (1997). Assessing the risk for alcoholism among sons of alcoholics. *Journal of Studies on Alcohol*, **58**, 141–5.
31. Schuckit, M.A. (1994). Low level of response to alcohol as a predictor of future alcoholism. *The American Journal of Psychiatry*, **151**, 184–9.
32. Edenberg, H.J., Xuei, X., Chen, H.J., *et al.* (2006). Association of alcohol dehydrogenase genes with alcohol dependence: a comprehensive analysis. *Human Molecular Genetics*, **15**, 1539–49.
33. Yoon, H.H., Iacono, W.G., Malone, S.M., *et al.* (2006). Using the brain P300 response to identify novel phenotypes reflecting genetic vulnerability for adolescent substance misuse. *Addictive Behaviors*, **31**, 1067–87.
34. Lesch, K.P. (2005). Alcohol dependence and gene x environment interaction in emotion regulation: is serotonin the link? *European Journal of Pharmacology*, **526**, 113–24.
35. Lappalainen, J., Krupitsky, E., Kranzler, H.R., *et al.* (2006). Mutation screen of the *GAD2* gene and association study of alcoholism in three populations. *American Journal of Medical Genetics: Part B Neuropsychiatric Genetics*, **144**, 183–92.

4.2.2.2 Alcohol dependence and alcohol problems

Jane Marshall

Introduction

The problem of excessive alcohol consumption is a major cause of public health concern in most countries of the world today. Heavy consumption, which involves far more than 'dependence', can cause untold misery to the individual, who is usually affected by other physical, psychological, and social disabilities as well.

As early as 1950, the World Health Organization (WHO) viewed the lack of a commonly accepted terminology as a serious obstacle to international action in the alcohol field.[1]

Definitions of 'alcoholism' have been proposed by a range of professional and other bodies, from biomedical scientists, medical doctors and psychiatrists, psychologists, sociologists, patients in treatment, to the general public.[2] Terms such as 'alcoholism', 'addiction', and 'chemical dependence', have passed into everyday speech, becoming 'popularly enriched' and 'technically impoverished'.[2] These terms mean different things to different people and often have pejorative connotations. The lack of a precise definition of 'drinking problems' has hampered interdisciplinary communication.

In this section, the evolution of the term 'alcohol dependence' will be traced and put into context as but one aspect of a wider spectrum of alcohol-related problems. The concept of the alcohol dependence syndrome (ADS)[3] will be introduced and its influence on the 10th revision of the *International Classification of Diseases* (ICD-10)[4] and the fourth edition of the *Diagnostic and Statistical Manual of Diseases* (DSM-IV) will be reviewed.[5] The terms 'harmful use' (ICD-10) and 'alcohol abuse' (DSM-IV) will also be discussed. Finally 'alcohol-related problems' will be considered.

The development of classification systems for alcohol use disorders

From the time of its inception in 1948, WHO played a major role in formulating public health definitions of 'alcoholism', 'addiction', and 'dependence' through a series of expert committees. Early definitions stressed the sociological rather than the physical aspects of dependence, and thus had limited utility for biological research and psychiatric classification.

'Alcoholism' was classified under 'Other non-psychotic mental disorders' in ICD-8.[6] This definition of 'alcoholism' was generic, and included the subcategories of episodic excessive drinking, habitual excessive drinking, and alcohol addiction. Alcohol addiction was defined as:[6]

> a state of physical and emotional dependence on regular or periodic, heavy, and uncontrolled alcohol consumption, during which the person experiences a compulsion to drink. On cessation of alcohol intake there are withdrawal symptoms, which may be severe.

In ICD-9 the term 'alcoholism' was dropped in favour of the 'alcohol dependence syndrome'.[7] It was, however, still classified under the category 'Other non-psychotic mental disorders'.

At the same time as WHO was formulating public health definitions of 'alcoholism', 'addiction', and 'dependence', a trend towards formal diagnostic criteria was emerging in the United States. This was driven by practical considerations such as the need for better communication between clinicians, researchers, and the general public. Other influential factors included the growing need to categorize persons in an objective fashion for legal, medical, or psychiatric reasons, to collect and communicate accurate public health information, and to standardize practice nationally and internationally. The first two editions of the *Diagnostic and Statistical Manual (DSM-I and DSM-II)*, published in 1952 and 1968 respectively, classified 'alcoholism' as a category of personality disorder. In DSM-III,[8] it was included under a new and separate category of 'Substance use disorders'. The terms 'alcoholism' and 'addiction' were dropped and the terms 'dependence' and 'alcohol abuse' were used instead. Dependence was distinguished from abuse by the presence of tolerance or withdrawal symptoms.

By the mid-1980s, DSM-III and ICD-9 were undergoing reviews for the purposes of revision. The diagnostic criteria for dependence were broadened in DSM-IIIR[9] to incorporate the elements of the alcohol dependence syndrome as hypothesized by Edwards and Gross.[3] The essential feature of the DSM-IIIR dependence category was defined in the text as a 'cluster of cognitive, behavioural, and physiological symptoms, indicating that the person has impaired control over drinking and continues to drink despite adverse consequences'.

The alcohol dependence syndrome

Clinical description

In 1976, Edwards and Gross proposed the existence of alcohol dependence within a syndrome model.(3) Their description was based on the clinical observation that certain heavy drinkers manifested an interrelated clustering of signs and symptoms. They hypothesized that dependence was not an all-or-nothing phenomenon but existed in degrees of severity. The elements of the syndrome, as originally formulated, are summarized in Table 4.2.2.2.1. Not all the elements need always be present, nor always present with the same intensity. Edwards and Gross(3) also acknowledged the fact that not everyone who drinks too much is necessarily dependent on alcohol. They hypothesized that alcohol dependence should be conceptually distinguished from alcohol-related problems.

By drawing a clear distinction between the alcohol dependence syndrome and alcohol-related problems, Edwards and Gross introduced the concept of a bi-axial model. This was described further in the report of a WHO scientific group published in 1977.(10) Alcohol-related problems are defined as comprising those physical, psychological, and social problems that are a consequence of excessive drinking and dependence. Consumption may be viewed on a third axis.

The alcohol dependence syndrome was proposed in the first instance as an empirical formulation that would require research to confirm its assumptions. Unlike previous models of 'alcoholism' that had observational elements but no theoretical input, the alcohol dependence syndrome was influenced by psychological theory and proposed as a synthesis of both general learning theory and specific conditioning models of dependence.(11,12)

Establishment of the validity of the alcohol dependence syndrome

A considerable amount of scientific research evaluating the ADS has been carried out over the past 30 years, much of it supporting its validity.(13) Studies have focused on the degree to which the elements of the syndrome co-occur.(14,15) Other areas of research have included construct validity,(16) concurrent validity,(15,17,18) and predictive validity.(19,20) Field trials conducted as background to the preparation of ICD-10, DSM-IIIR, and DSM-IV, have all contributed to the body of research evidence.(5, 21–25) Difficulties have been encountered in operationalizing elements such as narrowing of repertoire, subjective change, and reinstatement.(25)

These studies have shown a remarkable similarity in terms of the coherence and dimensionality of the syndrome, and are particularly impressive because of the diversity of methods and populations used.(11)

Table 4.2.2.2.1 Key elements of the alcohol dependence syndrome

Narrowing of repertoire
Salience of drinking
Increased tolerance to alcohol
Withdrawal symptoms
Relief or avoidance of withdrawal symptoms by further drinking
Subjective awareness of compulsion to drink
Reinstatement after abstinence

Reproduced from G. Edwards and M. M. Gross (1976). Alcohol dependence: provisional description of a clinical syndrome. *British Medical Journal* **1**, 1058–61, copyright 1976, BMJ Publishing Group Ltd.

Individual elements of the alcohol dependence syndrome

(a) Narrowing of the drinking repertoire

Most drinkers vary their alcohol consumption from day to day and week to week. The pattern of their drinking is influenced by a range of internal cues and external circumstances. Heavy drinkers may initially widen their drinking repertoire. As dependence advances, so a diminished variability in drinking behaviour emerges. The dependent person begins to drink in the same manner every day. The daily pattern established ensures that a relatively high blood-alcohol level is maintained and that symptoms of alcohol withdrawal are avoided. As drinking becomes stereotyped with advanced dependence, dependent drinkers are able to describe their drinking day in minute detail.

(b) Salience of drinking-seeking behaviour

With advancing dependence, individuals give priority to maintaining their alcohol intake. Alcohol consumption is maintained despite painful direct consequences such as physical illness, rejection by family, and lack of money. They will 'beg, borrow, or steal' to obtain money for alcohol.(3)

(c) Increased tolerance to alcohol

Regular drinkers become tolerant to the central nervous system effects of alcohol and can sustain blood alcohol levels that would incapacitate the non-tolerant drinker. In short, they can 'drink others under the table'. Tolerance may decrease in the later stages of dependence, with individuals becoming intoxicated on much less alcohol than would previously have affected them. Cross-tolerance extends to other drugs, notably barbiturates and benzodiazepines.

(d) Withdrawal symptoms

The term 'alcohol withdrawal' describes a broad range of symptoms and signs, from the relatively trivial to the life-threatening. At first the symptoms are intermittent and mild, but as the degree of dependence increases, so do the frequency and intensity of withdrawal symptoms. Symptoms vary from person to person and do not require abstinence to appear; they can occur when blood-alcohol concentrations are falling. When the picture is fully developed, the dependent drinker typically has severe multiple symptoms every morning on waking; these symptoms may wake him in the middle of the night. Those who are severely dependent usually experience mild withdrawal symptoms during the day whenever their alcohol levels fall.

Withdrawal symptoms cannot occur without a high degree of central nervous system tolerance, but tolerance can occur without clinically manifest withdrawal symptoms.(3)

The spectrum of symptoms is wide, but the four key symptoms are tremor, nausea, sweating, and mood disturbance. A range of other symptoms can also occur, including sensitivity to sound (hyperacusis), ringing in the ears (tinnitus), itching, muscle cramps, sleep disturbance, perceptual distortion, hallucinations, generalized (grand mal) seizures, and delirium tremens.

The four key symptoms will be described in further detail.

(i) Tremor

The first experience of alcohol withdrawal tremor may be recalled vividly: 'One afternoon I went to cut the grass at a friend's house. She gave me a cup of tea and my hands kept shaking. I kept rattling the cup on the saucer and couldn't put the cup to my mouth. I had to put them down and pretend that I had finished.' Men often find it difficult to shave first thing in the morning and merely getting the first drink of the day to the mouth may be an ordeal in itself.

(ii) Nausea

Dependent drinkers commonly say that their bodies want to vomit first thing in the morning, but that they have nothing to bring up. This may be described as 'dry retching' or 'the dry heaves'. Typically they find it difficult to eat breakfast and to brush their teeth. The first drink of the day is often vomited back.

(iii) Sweating

Dependent drinkers commonly describe waking up in the early morning (3 a.m. or 4 a.m.) to find the bed sheets 'drenched'. In the earlier stages of dependence they may report feeling clammy.

(iv) Mood disturbance

This is an important feature of the withdrawal syndrome. Mildly dependent individuals may feel 'a bit edgy'. Severely dependent individuals may present with clinically significant symptoms of anxiety and depression.

(e) Relief or avoidance of withdrawal symptoms by further drinking

In the early stages of dependence, individuals may find that they need a lunchtime drink to alleviate discomfort. As dependence progresses there emerges the need for an early morning drink to relieve the symptoms of alcohol withdrawal coming on after a night's abstinence. Later, individuals may wake in the middle of the night for a drink, and alcohol is often kept by the bed. If they have to go for 3 or 4 hr without a drink during the day, they value the next drink for its relief effect.

Clues to the degree of dependence can be obtained by taking a detailed history of the first drink of the day. The person drinking from a bottle kept by the side of the bed before they get up is more dependent than the person who has breakfast and reads the paper first. The woman who pours whisky into her first cup of tea is more dependent than the librarian who slips out to the lavatory at midday to drink from a quarter bottle of vodka hidden in her handbag.

(f) Subjective awareness of compulsion to drink

This describes an altered subjective experience of an inability to limit drinking to an acceptable level. Although the familiar term 'loss of control' has been used to denote this element, it is more likely that control has been 'impaired' rather than lost.

Another complex experience is that of 'craving', the subjective experience of which is greatly influenced by environment. Individuals can experience craving of very different intensities on different occasions. Cues for craving include the experience of intoxication, the withdrawal syndrome, mood (anger, depression, elation), or situational cues (being in a pub or (bar), passing an off-licence (liquor store).

Here the key experience may best be described as a compulsion to drink. The desire for a further drink is seen as irrational, and is resisted, but despite this a further drink is taken.

(g) Reinstatement after abstinence

Alcohol dependent individuals who begin to drink again after a period of abstinence invariably relapse back into the previous stage of the dependence syndrome. This process occurs over a variable time course, with moderately dependent individuals perhaps taking weeks or months and severely dependent individuals taking a couple of days.

Influence of the alcohol dependence syndrome on ICD-10 and DSM-IV

Both DSM-IV and ICD-10 diagnostic approaches have drawn on the original concept of the alcohol dependence syndrome.[26,27] Although they have undoubtedly contributed to the standardization of psychiatric practice nationally and internationally, they picture dependence as an all-or-nothing phenomenon rather than as a dimensional state.[28]

ICD-10[4]

ICD-10 includes six items under dependence, most of which are similar to DSM-IV. For a diagnosis of dependence, three or more items should have occurred in the past year. The 'strong desire or sense of compulsion to take the substance' is viewed as a central descriptive characteristic of dependence in ICD-10. This compulsive-use indicator is not included in the DSM-IV concept of dependence (Table 4.2.2.2.2).

DSM-IV[5]

In view of the major changes in criteria that had occurred between 1980 and 1987, the DSM-IV Substance Use Disorders Work Group was reluctant to make any additional major changes to DSM-IIIR. The repetitive nature of the problem was highlighted in that three or more of the items should have occurred during the same 12-month period and the associated difficulties must have led to clinically significant impairment or distress. DSM-IV also uniquely allows for the subtyping of dependence with and without physiological dependence (Table 4.2.2.2.2).

Alcohol abuse and harmful use

Alcohol abuse

DSM-III; DSM-IIIR; DSM-IV

The term 'alcohol abuse' appeared infrequently in the American literature before 1970, when the United States National Institute on Alcohol Abuse and Alcoholism was formed. It was adopted as a formal diagnostic category by DSM-III,[8] which defined abuse as a behavioural concept: 'A pattern of pathological use for at least a month that causes impairment in social or occupational functioning'. Although enshrined in DSM-IIIR and DSM-IV, the term 'abuse' has been variously regarded as 'unscientific and pejorative'[29] and 'oppobrious' and 'vindictive'.[30]

The DSM-IV Substance Use Disorders Workgroup carried out extensive analysis in an effort to define abuse more precisely. Accordingly, in DSM-IV, four separate items, not included in dependence, are listed for the diagnosis of abuse, focusing on social, physical, legal, and interpersonal problems associated with alcohol use. These problems must have occurred repeatedly over a 12-month period, and caused 'clinically significant impairment or distress' (Table 4.2.2.2.3). In practice, the DSM-IV alcohol abuse definition includes a mixture of dependence and harm criteria which could be scaled along a single continuum of severity of alcohol dependence.

Table 4.2.2.2.2 Comparison of ICD-10 and DSM-IV criteria for substance dependence

ICD-10	DSM-IV
A diagnosis of dependence should usually be made only if three or more of the following have been experienced or exhibited at some time during the previous year:	A maladaptive pattern of substance use, leading to clinically significant impairment or distress, as manifested by three (or more) of the following at any time in the same 12-month period
Evidence of tolerance such that increased doses of the psychoactive substance are required in order to achieve effects originally produced by lower doses	Tolerance as defined by either of the following: ◆ need for markedly increased amounts of the substance to achieve intoxication or desired effect ◆ markedly diminished effect with continued use of the same amount of substance
A physiological withdrawal state when substance use has ceased or been reduced, as evidenced by: ◆ the characteristic withdrawal syndrome for the substance or ◆ use of the same (or a closely related) substance with the intention of relieving or avoiding withdrawal symptoms	Withdrawal as manifested by either of the following: ◆ the characteristic withdrawal syndrome for the substance ◆ the same (or closely related) substance is taken to relieve or avoid withdrawal symptoms
A strong desire or sense of compulsion to take the substance	No equivalent criterion
No equivalent criterion	There is a persistent desire or unsuccessful efforts to cut down or control substance use
Difficulties in controlling substance-taking behaviour in terms of its onset, termination, or levels of use	The substance is often taken in larger amounts or over a longer period than was intended
Progressive neglect of alternative pleasures or interests because of psychoactive substance use	Important social, occupation or recreational activities are given up or reduced because of substance use
Increased amount of time necessary to obtain or take the substance or recover from its effects	A great deal of time is spent in activities necessary to obtain the substance, use the substance, or recover from its effects
Persisting with substance use despite clear evidence of overtly harmful consequences. Efforts should be made to determine that the user was actually, or could be expected to be, aware of the nature and extent of the harm	The substance use is continued despite knowledge of having a persistent or recurrent physical and psychological problem likely to have been caused or exacerbated by the substance.
	Specify if: *With Physiological Dependence:* evidence of tolerance or withdrawal (either item is present) *Without Physiological Dependence:* no evidence of tolerance or withdrawal

Reproduced from ICD-10 and DSM-IV.[4, 5]

Table 4.2.2.2.3 Comparison of criteria for abuse or harmful use of substances

ICD-10 criteria for harmful use
A pattern of psychoactive substance use that is causing damage to health, either physical or mental. The diagnosis requires that actual damage should have been caused to the mental or physical health of the user. Socially negative consequences, or the disapproval of others are not in themselves evidence of harmful use. Harmful use should not be diagnosed if dependence syndrome, a psychotic disorder or another specific form of alcohol-related disorder is present.
DSM-IV criteria for substance abuse
A. A maladaptive pattern of substance use leading to clinically significant impairment or distress by one (or more) of the following occurring within a 12-month period: ◆ Recurrent substance use resulting in a failure to fulfill major role obligations at work, school or home ◆ Recurrent substance use in situations in which it is physically hazardous ◆ Recurrent substance-related legal problems ◆ Continued substance use despite having persistent or recurrent social or interpersonal problems caused or exacerbated by the effects of the substance B. The symptoms have never met criteria for substance dependence

Reproduced from ICD-10 and DSM-IV.[4, 5]

Harmful use

(a) ICD-10

The ICD-10 criteria for harmful use of alcohol differ significantly from the DSM-IV abuse classification. An ICD-10 diagnosis of harmful drinking requires a pattern of drinking that has caused actual physical or psychological harm to the user. This definition excludes social harms such as marital problems and does not overlap with the DSM-IV definition of alcohol abuse.

The future

Revision of the DSM and ICD classification systems must address the fact that the current systems do not address the continuum of severity of alcohol use disorders (AUDs). Research is needed to explore the relationship between AUDs and the quantity, frequency, and pattern of drinking.[31] Further refinements of the alcohol dependence diagnosis should focus on the essential or core features of the disorder.

Alcohol-related problems

Not everyone experiencing an alcohol problem or alcohol-related disability will be suffering from alcohol dependence. Both dependent and non-dependent drinkers, particularly binge drinkers, are at risk of problems related to heavy alcohol consumption. Indeed, epidemiological evidence supports the view that most alcohol-related harm in the general population occurs in heavy non-dependent drinkers.

Alcohol-related problems are extremely diverse. They have been defined as 'those problems that may arise in individuals around their use of beverage alcohol, and that may require an appropriate treatment response for their optimum management'.[32] The phrases 'alcohol problems' or 'alcohol-related problem' contain an assumption of causality.[33] This issue is a complex one, involving individual differences and the social context of drinking as well as the pattern, duration, and intensity of alcohol use.

Alcohol-related problems can be related to the acute or chronic consumption of alcohol. A fractured ankle sustained by falling over while acutely intoxicated is an example of the former category. Cirrhosis of the liver is an example of a chronic problem. An individual who drinks in binges will experience different problems compared with someone who drinks the same amount of alcohol spread out over a week or a month or a year. The way in which a person behaves while intoxicated is another important factor determining the nature of alcohol-related problems. The social consequences of drinking such as job loss, imprisonment, marital and family break-up, and drunk-driving have profound effects on the well being of the drinker, their family, and society.[33]

Types of alcohol-related problems

Although somewhat artificial, it is helpful to classify alcohol-related problems in individuals into physical, psychological, and social categories. There is often considerable overlap between these three areas. The more severe the dependence, the greater the likelihood of problems of all three kinds.[18]

Alcohol-related physical and psychological problems are discussed in the next section. Some of the social problems can be included here, for example the acute adverse consequences of drinking such as trauma resulting from road traffic accidents, injuries from fights, and death from overdose.[33]

The social problems that can result from drinking are legion. Alcohol is involved in all types of accidents and contributes to traffic deaths, home, and leisure injuries.[33] It is associated with domestic violence, child abuse, crime, homicide, and suicide and is also related to poor work performance, dismissal, unemployment, debt and housing problems, and crimes of violence.

There is a continuity between moderate and excessive drinking and between harmless drinking and drinking that results in harm or in problems. Such problem-clustering may reflect alcohol dependence, certainly amongst a proportion of these drinkers. Given this heterogeneity, no one form of treatment is likely to be effective for all individuals with alcohol problems.[32] A range of treatments is required and it should be possible for non-specialists to offer brief interventions (see Chapter 4.2.2.4).

The study of alcohol-related problems remains underdeveloped, compared with the study of alcohol dependence.[34] There may be several reasons for this, not least the difficulties inherent in measuring alcohol-related problems. Another important issue, central to these difficulties, is the extent to which alcohol is causally related to the problem.

Several questionnaires, measuring a variety of alcohol-related problems, have been developed. The Alcohol Problems Questionnaire (APQ)[34] is a standardized inventory, which includes 46 items covering eight problem domains: physical, psychological, friends, finances, police, marital, children, and work. All questions apply to the 6-month period prior to the completion of the questionnaire. The shorter or core version includes the first five domains (23 items). This questionnaire can make a useful contribution to the overall assessment, and is of potential value in outcome research.

Conclusions

An understanding of the concepts of alcohol dependence and alcohol-related problems is central to the therapeutic process with individual patients.

The development of diagnostic criteria has helped to standardize practice nationally and internationally, and aided interdisciplinary communication. The diagnostic criteria for dependence are imperfect because they view the syndrome as an all-or-nothing phenomenon rather than as a dimensional state. The concepts of abuse and harmful use need further refinement. The totality of alcohol problems is a vast area with major implications for the general population, not just dependent drinkers.

Further information

Reports and reviews

Raistrick D., Heather N., Godfrey, C (2006). *Review of the effectiveness of treatment for drinking problems*. London: National Treatment Agency for Substance Misuse. This review is eminently readable summary of the published international research literature on alcohol interventions and treatment. Chapter 2 describes the categories of alcohol misuse, and sets them in the context of treatment and interventions to reduce alcohol-related harm.

Room, R., Babor, T., Rehm, J. (2005). Alcohol and public health. *Lancet*, **365**, 510-530

Compilation of articles

Saunders, J. B.and Schuckit, M. A. (2006). Diagnostic issues in substance use disorders: refining the research agenda. *Addiction* (Suppl 1), **101**, 1–173. A series of 18 articles commissioned by the Substance Use Disorders Workgroup to inform the research agenda for the development of the Vth edition of the Diagnostic and Statistical Manual of Mental Disorders (DSM-V).

Marshall E. J, Farrell, M. Chapter editors. Addiction Psychiatry. *Psychiatry*, **5**, 421–63. Straightforward account of the classification and epidemiology of substance use disorders.

Book

Edwards, G. (2006). *Alcohol: the ambiguous molecule*. Harmondsworth, Penguin.

References

1. World Health Organization (1951). *WHO technical report series*, No 42. WHO, Geneva.
2. Babor, T.F. (1990). Social, scientific and medical issues in the definition of alcohol and drug dependence. In *The nature of drug dependence* (ed. G. Edwards and M. Lader), pp. 19–36. Oxford Medical Publications, Oxford.
3. Edwards, G. and Gross, M.M. (1976). Alcohol dependence: provisional description of a clinical syndrome. *British Medical Journal*, **1**, 1058–61.
4. World Health Organization (1992). *International statistical classification of diseases and related health problems, 10th revision*. WHO, Geneva.

5. American Psychiatric Association (1994). *Diagnostic and statistical classification of diseases and related health problems* (4th edn). American Psychiatric Association, Washington, DC.
6. World Health Organization (1974). *Glossary of mental disorders and guide to their classification: for use in conjunction with the International Classification of Diseases* (8th revision). WHO, Geneva.
7. World Health Organization (1978). *Mental disorders: glossary and guide to their classification in accordance with the Ninth Revision of the International Classification of Diseases*. WHO, Geneva.
8. American Psychiatric Association (1980). *Diagnostic and statistical manual of mental disorders* (3rd edn). American Psychiatric Association, Washington, DC.
9. American Psychiatric Association (1987). *Diagnostic and statistical manual of mental disorders* (3rd edn, revised). American Psychiatric Association, Washington, DC.
10. Edwards, G., Gross, M.M., Keller, M., Moser, J., and Room, R. (1977). *Alcohol–related disabilities*. WHO Offset Publication No. 32. WHO, Geneva.
11. Edwards, G. (1986). The alcohol dependence syndrome: a concept as stimulus to enquiry. *British Journal of Addiction*, **81**, 171–83.
12. Babor, T.F., Cooney, N.L., and Lauerman, R.J. (1987). The dependence syndrome concept as a psychological theory of relapse behaviour: an empirical evaluation of alcoholic and opiate addicts. *British Journal of Addiction*, **82**, 393–405.
13. Li, T.K., Hewitt, B.G., Grant, B.F (2007). The alcohol dependence syndrome, 30 years later: a commentary. *Addiction*, **102**, 1522–30.
14. Chick, J. (1980). Alcohol dependence: methodological issues in its measurement, reliability of the criteria. *British Journal of Addiction*, **75**, 175–86.
15. Stockwell, T., Murphy, D., and Hodgson, R. (1983). The severity of alcohol dependence questionnaire: its use, reliability and validity. *British Journal of Addiction*, **78**, 145–55.
16. Feingold, A. and Rounsaville, B. (1995). Construct validity of the dependence syndrome as measured by DSM–IV for different psycho–active substances. *Addiction*, **90**, 1661–9.
17. Kivlahan, D., Sher, K.J., and Donovan, D.M. (1989) The Alcohol Dependence Scale: a validation study among inpatient alcoholics. *Journal of Studies on Alcohol*, **50**, 170–5.
18. Caetano, R. (1993). The association between severity of DSM–III–R alcohol dependence and medical and social consequences. *Addiction*, **88**, 631–42.
19. Hodgson, R., Rankin, H.J., and Stockwell, T. (1979). Alcohol dependence and the priming effect. *Behaviour Research and Therapy*, **17**, 379–87.
20. Rankin, H., Stockwell, T., and Hodgson, R. (1982). Cues for drinking and degrees of alcohol dependence. *British Journal of Addiction*, **77**, 287–96.
21. Grant, B.F., Harfold, T.C., Chou, P., *et al.* (1992). DSM–III–R and the proposed DSM–IV alcohol use disorders. United States 1988. A methodological comparison. *Alcoholism, Clinical and Experimental Research*, **16**, 215–21.
22. Cottler, L.B. (1993). Comparing DSM–III–R and ICD–10 substance use disorders. *Addiction*, **88**, 689–96.
23. Rapaport, M.H., Tipp, J.E., and Schuckit, M.A. (1993). A comparison of ICD–10 and DSM–III–R criteria for substance abuse and dependence. *American Journal of Drug and Alcohol Abuse*, **19**, 143–51.
24. Rounsaville, B.J., Bryant, K., Babor, T., *et al.* (1993). Cross system agreement for substance use disorders: DSM–III–R, DSM–IV and ICD–10. *Addiction*, **88**, 337–48.
25. Cottler, L.B., Phelps, D.L., and Compton, W.M. (1995) Narrowing of the drinking repertoire criterion: should it have been dropped from ICD–10? *Journal of Studies on Alcohol*, **56**, 173–6.
26. Saunders, J.B. (2006). Substance dependence and non-dependence in the Diagnostic and Statistical Manual of Mental Disorders (DSM) and the International Classification of Diseases (ICD): can an identical conceptualization be achieved? *Addiction*,**101**, 48–58.
27. Grant, B. (1996). DSM–IV, DSM–III–R, ICD–10 alcohol and drug abuse/harmful use and dependence, United States, 1992: a nosological comparison. *Alcoholism, Clinical and Experimental Research*, **8**, 1481–8.
28. Edwards, G., Marshall, E.J., and Cook, C.C.H. (2003). *The treatment of drinking problems* (4th edn). Cambridge University Press.
29. Edwards, G., Arif, A., and Hodgson, R. (1981). Nomenclature and classification of drug– and alcohol–related problems: a WHO memorandum. *Bulletin of the World Health Organization*, **50**, 225–42.
30. Keller, M. (1982). On defining alcoholism: with comment on some other relevant words. In *Alcohol, science and society revisited* (ed. E.L. Gomberg, H.R. White, and J.A. Carpenter), pp. 119–33. University of Michigan Press, Ann Arbor, MI.
31. Hasin, D.S., Liu, X., Alderson, D., *et al.* (2006) DSM-IV alcohol dependence: a categorical or dimensional phenotype? *Psychological Medicine*, **36**, 1695–1705.
32. Institute of Medicine (1990). *Broadening the base of treatment for alcohol problems: report of a study by a Committee of the Institute of Medicine, Division of Mental Health and Behavioural Medicine*. National Academy Press, Washington, DC.
33. Babor, T.F., Caetano, R., Casswell, S., *et al.* ((2003). *Alcohol: No ordinary commodity. Research and Public Policy*. Oxford University Press.
34. Drummond, D.C. (1990). The relationship between alcohol dependence and alcohol–related problems in a clinical population. *British Journal of Addiction*, **85**, 357–66.

4.2.2.3 **Alcohol and psychiatric and physical disorders**

Karl F. Mann and Falk Kiefer

Intoxication

Clinical symptoms of alcohol intoxication are associated with both, blood alcohol concentration (**BAC**), and the individual's level of tolerance. Whereas in healthy persons without alcohol tolerance mild intoxication (BAC ≤ 100 mg per cent), medium intoxication (BAC 100–200 mg per cent), and severe intoxication (BAC >200 mg per cent) differ clinically, this schema does not work in patients suffering from alcoholism. In these people, different levels of tolerance can lead to completely different clinical pictures despite their having similar blood alcohol concentrations. Thus, psychopathology is more important than blood alcohol concentrations for estimating the severity of an acute intoxication state. With increasing BAC we observe elated mood, disinhibition, impaired judgement, belligerence, impaired social and occupational functioning, mood lability, cognitive impairment, reduced attention span, slurred speech, incoordination, unsteady gait, nystagmus, and stupor or coma.

The term 'pathological intoxication' can still be found in the older literature (reviewed by Lishman[1]). It was described as an outburst of aggression and uncontrollable rage, which might have led to serious destructions. As a rule, this behaviour, which was not typical for the individual, ended in terminal sleep and subsequent amnesia. However, since there is not enough empirical evidence for the existence of this syndrome, it was no longer considered in DSM-IV.[2]

Alcohol-induced amnesias ('blackouts')

This term refers to a transient state of amnesia after drinking excess. Usually patients' behaviour is no different from their behaviour during other periods of intoxication without blackouts. Nevertheless, the memory gap usually lasts for hours, but may be as long as a day or more. In extreme cases, patients find themselves in strange places with no recollection of how they got there.

Withdrawal

Withdrawal without complications

When alcohol is used regularly and withdrawn rapidly, a characteristic withdrawal syndrome can develop. It includes autonomic hyperactivity like hand tremor, insomnia, sweating, tachycardia, hypertension, and anxiety. The symptoms generally occur between 6 and 12 h after the last alcohol consumption. Depending on their severity they may last for up to 4 or 5 days. The neurobiological basis for withdrawal is a gradual upregulation of *N*-methyl-D-aspartate receptors under the influence of chronic alcohol use. As soon as the alcohol, which acts as a central nervous system depressant, is withdrawn, an overwhelming excitatory action in the brain mediated by the glutamatergic system is observed.

Withdrawal with perceptual disturbances

The individual usually experiences more discomfort and anxiety if transient visual, tactile, or auditory hallucinations or illusions are present. In this state, reality testing is still intact: the person still knows that the hallucinations are induced by the substance. If this is no longer true, a substance-induced psychotic disorder or a delirium tremens is likely.

Withdrawal with grand mal seizures (alcoholic convulsions, 'rum fits')

In about 30 per cent of the cases the typical grand mal seizures are followed by a delirium tremens. The electroencephalograph picture is only abnormal at the time of the fits, hence, alcohol convulsions differ pathophysiologically from latent epilepsy.

Alcohol-induced psychosis (delirium tremens)

In delirium tremens the symptoms of alcohol withdrawal described earlier are accompanied by a reduced level of consciousness, disorientation in time and place, impairment of recent memory, insomnia, and perceptual disturbances. The latter include misinterpretation of sensory stimuli and hallucinations; most are visual, but auditory and haptic hallucinations also occur. The hallucinations may be Lilliputian or of normal size, and may be of complex, frightening, and extremely realistic scenes. The patient is restless and fearful, and may become severely agitated. There is marked tremor, and ataxia when standing. Some patients experience vestibular disturbance. Autonomic disturbance includes sweating, tachycardia, raised blood pressure, and dilated pupils. There may be a mild pyrexia. Patients are usually dehydrated, often with abnormal electrolytes, leucocytosis, and impaired liver function. As in other forms of delirium, symptoms are worse at night.

Delirium tremens is the most severe of the states following withdrawal of alcohol, with a reported mortality of up to 5 per cent. In its fully developed form it is uncommon; the more frequent states are acute tremulousness, transient hallucinations with tremor, and uncomplicated fits. Delirium tremens usually begins after 3 to 4 days of abstinence from alcohol, although occasionally it starts while drinking continues. In the latter cases it is assumed that alcohol levels have fallen below a critical level. It is not known by what mechanism alcohol withdrawal leads to the clinical syndrome. Delirium tremens often appears to start suddenly, although close enquiry may reveal a prodromal stage of restlessness, anxiety, and insomnia. It usually lasts for 2 to 3 days, often ending with deep and prolonged sleep from which thepatient wakes symptom free and with little memory of the period of delirium. Rarely, the patient is left with an amnesic syndrome, perhaps the consequence of previous undetected Wernicke's encephalopathy.

Treatment is by sedation, usually with a benzodiazepine, together with fluid replacement under close observation. The possibility of accompanying head injury or infection should be investigated. Sedation should be adequate to prevent withdrawal seizures, with frequent monitoring of the response. High-potency vitamins are usually given to prevent Wernicke's encephalopathy. An anticonvulsant is given when there have been withdrawal seizures in the past. Cardiovascular collapse and hyperthermia occur occasionally and require urgent medical treatment.

Hallucinosis

Alcoholic hallucinosis is a rare condition in which auditory hallucinations are present in clear consciousness and without autonomic overactivity, usually in a person who has been drinking excessively for many years. The hallucinations often begin as simple noises, but are gradually replaced by voices, which may threaten, abuse, or reproach the person. Usually the voices speak to the person, but sometimes they discuss him or her in the third person. The voices may be occasional or relentlessly persistent. They may command the patient, who may respond with unrestrained or suicidal behaviour. Delusions are secondary interpretations of the hallucinations. Autochthonous hallucinations suggest schizophrenia, as do thought disorder or incongruity of affect. The patient is usually distressed, anxious, and restless.

In both ICD-10 and DSM-IV, the disorder is classified as a substance-induced psychotic disorder and not, as has been suggested in the past, a form of schizophrenia (released by heavy drinking). The differential diagnosis includes transient auditory hallucinations occurring during withdrawal from a period of heavy drinking, and delirium tremens in which auditory hallucinations may accompany the more prominent visual ones. In both conditions the auditory hallucinations are transient and disorganized, and in the latter consciousness is impaired. In contrast, the auditory hallucinations of an alcoholic hallucinosis are persistent and organized, and occur in clear consciousness. Other differential diagnoses are depressive disorder with psychotic symptoms and schizophrenia, both of which can be accompanied by heavy drinking.

The hallucinations usually respond rapidly to antipsychotic medication. The prognosis is good; usually the condition improves within days or a couple of weeks provided that the person remains abstinent. Symptoms that last for 6 months generally continue for years.(3)

Psychiatric disorders

Alcohol-dependent patients often present with symptoms of anxiety or depression. These states are generally referred to as comorbid disorders or dual diagnosis. Alcoholism can be a consequence of anxiety and mood disorders ('secondary alcoholism'). It can develop independently after anxiety and depression, or it can precede anxiety and depressive symptoms ('primary'). As the former are discussed elsewhere in this textbook, here we concentrate on the latter.

Alcohol-induced mood disorders

Alcohol is a central nervous system depressant. Taken regularly in high doses it may provoke feelings of sadness. Episodes of withdrawal or relative withdrawal can lead to excitability and nervousness, including anxiety. The more a person drinks, the more likely it is that these symptoms will occur. Finally in the stage of alcohol dependence, up to 80 per cent of people report depressive symptoms at some time in their life. About one-third of male patients and up to 50 per cent of female patients have experienced longer periods of severe depression.[4] These high prevalence rates are noteworthy, since more than 20 per cent of alcoholics have attempted suicide once or more and about 15 per cent die in their attempt. Besides depressive features, alcohol-induced mood disorders may also comprise manic symptoms or mixed features. However, the diagnosis should only be used when the symptoms cause clinically significant impairment or distress in social, occupational, or other areas of functioning.

Concerning treatment, it is interesting to note that despite the vast majority of patients who present with depressive symptoms at the beginning of treatment for alcoholism, only very few need specific antidepressant medication or specific psychotherapy. In most other cases depressive symptoms disappear within weeks of controlled abstinence.[5]

Alcohol-induced anxiety disorders

This diagnosis should only be used when anxiety symptoms are thought to be related to the direct physiological effects of alcohol. The symptomatology may involve anxiety, panic attacks, and phobias. Both alcohol-induced anxiety disorders and mood disorders can develop during intoxication, withdrawal, or up to 4 weeks after cessation of alcohol consumption. During intoxication or withdrawal, the diagnosis should only be given when the symptomatology clearly exceeds what would be expected from anxiety or depressive symptoms during a regular intoxication or withdrawal episode.

Anxiety disorders are among the most common groups of psychiatric disorders in the general population, with prevalence rates of up to 25 per cent.[6] In clinical studies between 20 and 70 per cent of patients with alcoholism also suffer from anxiety disorders.[7] On the other hand, between 20 and 45 per cent of patients with anxiety disorders also have histories of alcoholism.[8] However, it has been argued that the comorbidity figures are overestimated, because in some of the studies the focus was on drinking patterns rather than on alcohol dependence or they describe anxiety symptoms rather than disorders according to diagnostic criteria.[9] Family studies analysing the comorbidity of alcoholism and anxiety disorders might be a means of clarifying this controversy. For instance, in the Yale study the presence of anxiety disorders in the probands slightly increased the risk for alcohol dependence in their relatives, whereas alcohol dependence in the proband did not increase their relative's risk for anxiety disorders.[10] Similarly, Maier *et al.*[11] demonstrated an increased risk of alcoholism in probands with panic disorders, but not the reverse. Kendler *et al.*[12] in a study of female twins, found evidence that common genetic factors may underlie both alcoholism and panic disorder.

Effects on the brain

Cerebral cortex

Chronic alcohol consumption leads to structural and functional changes in the brain. Alcoholic dementia is dealt with in Chapter 4.1.11. Most of the tissue loss from the cerebral hemispheres in alcoholics is accounted for by a reduction in the volume of the cerebral white matter, additionally there is a slight reduction in the volume of the cerebral cortex. This has been demonstrated both pathologically[13] and using magnetic resonance imaging with quantitative morphometry.[14]

Harper *et al.*[15] documented neuronal loss in alcoholics. There was a 22 per cent reduction in the number of neurones in the superior frontal cortex (Brodmann's area 8), while surviving neurones showed shrinkage in the superior frontal, motor, and frontal cingulate cortices.[16] This finding of cortical damage in alcoholics is consistent with neuroradiological studies.[14]

Ferrer *et al.*[17] examined the dendritic tree of cortical neurones in alcoholic subjects using Golgi-apparatus impregnation techniques. They described a significant reduction in the basal dendritic tree of layer III pyramidal neurones in both the superior frontal and motor cortices. These studies suggest that, even though there is no significant reduction in the numbers of cortical neurones in the motor cortex, there are cellular structural abnormalities that could have important functional implications.

Wernicke's encephalopathy

The best-known features of heavy alcohol consumption in adults are Wernicke's encephalopathy and Korsakoff's syndrome. Wernicke's encephalopathy is directly caused by thiamine deficiency, which results from a combination of inadequate dietary intake, reduced gastrointestinal absorption, decreased hepatic storage, and impaired utilization. Only a subset of thiamine-deficient alcoholics develop Wernicke's encephalopathy, perhaps because they have inherited or acquired abnormalities of the thiamine-dependent enzyme transketolase, which reduces its affinity for thiamine. Wernicke's encephalopathy is characterized by degenerative changes, including gliosis and small haemorrhages in structures surrounding the third ventricle and aqueduct: namely, the mammillary bodies, hypothalamus, mediodorsal thalamic nucleus, colliculi, and midbrain tegmentum. Clinical features associated with the Wernicke–Korsakoff syndrome include memory deficits, ocular signs, ataxia, and global confusional states. Most can be related to damaged functional systems in the hypothalamus, midbrain, and cerebellum. In a large Scandinavian neuropathological study, 12.5 per cent of all alcoholics exhibited signs of Wernicke's encephalopathy.[18]

Korsakoff's syndrome

About 80 per cent of alcoholic patients recovering from Wernicke's encephalopathy develop Korsakoff's amnesic syndrome. It is characterized by marked deficits in anterograde and retrograde memory, apathy, an intact sensorium, and relative preservation of other intellectual abilities. Korsakoff's amnesic syndrome may also appear without an antecedent episode of Wernicke's encephalopathy. Acute lesions may be superimposed on chronic lesions, suggesting that subclinical episodes of Wernicke's encephalopathy may culminate in Korsakoff's amnesic syndrome. The memory disorder correlates best with the presence of histopathological lesions in the dorsomedial thalamus. (Amnesic syndrome is considered further in Chapter 4.1.12.)

Cerebellar degeneration

Many alcoholic patients develop a chronic cerebellar syndrome related to the degeneration of Purkinje cells in the cerebellar cortex. Quantitative studies revealed a significant loss of cerebellar Purkinje cells (by 10–35 per cent) and shrinkage of the cerebellar vermal, molecular, and granular cell layers.[19] Evidence for a direct toxic effect caused by ethanol is provided by animal models.[20] In neuroimaging studies, however, cerebellar ataxia in alcoholics does not correlate with the daily, annual, or lifetime consumption of ethanol. As in Wernicke's encephalopathy, thiamine deficiency due to poor nutrition has also been implicated. Cerebellar atrophy has been reported to occur in about 40 per cent of chronic alcoholics.[19] In a clinical study of alcoholic inpatients, 49 per cent had at least discrete clinical signs of cerebellar atrophy.[21]

The diagnosis of alcoholic cerebellar ataxia is based on the clinical history and neurological examination. The ataxia affects the gait most severely. Limb ataxia and dysarthria occur more often than in Wernicke's encephalopathy, whereas nystagmus is rare. Computed tomography or magnetic resonance imaging scans may show cerebellar cortical atrophy, but a considerable number of alcoholic patients with this finding are not ataxic on examination. Whether these represent subclinical cases in which symptoms will develop subsequently is unclear. It is interesting to note that impaired cerebellar function improves significantly when abstinence is maintained.[22]

Hepatocerebral degeneration

Hepatic encephalopathy develops in many alcoholics with liver disease, and is characterized by altered sensorium, frontal release signs, 'metabolic' flapping tremor, hyperreflexia, extensor plantar responses, and occasional seizures. Whereas some patients progress from stupor to coma and then death, others recover and suffer recurrent episodes. The brains of patients with hepatic encephalopathy show enlargement and proliferation of protoplasmic astrocytes in the basal ganglia, thalamus, red nucleus, pons, and cerebellum, in the absence of neuronal loss or other glial changes.[23]

Patients who do not recover fully after an episode of hepatic encephalopathy go on to develop a progressive syndrome of tremor, choreoathetosis, dysarthria, gait ataxia, and dementia. Hepatocerebral degeneration may progress in a stepwise fashion, with incomplete recovery after each episode of hepatic encephalopathy, or slowly and inexorably, without a discrete episode of encephalopathy.

Rare disorders

The **Marchiafava–Bignami syndrome** is a disorder of demyelination or necrosis of the corpus callosum and adjacent subcortical white matter. The course may be acute, subacute, or chronic, and is marked by dementia, spasticity, dysarthria, and an inability to walk. Patients may lapse into coma and die, survive for many years in a demential condition, or occasionally recover.

Central pontine myelinolysis is a disorder of the cerebral white matter that usually affects alcoholics, but it also occurs in non-alcoholics with liver disease including Wilson's disease, malnutrition, anorexia, burns, cancer, Addison's disease, and severe electrolyte disorders such as thiazide-induced hyponatraemia; however, the majority of cases occur in alcoholics, suggesting that alcoholism may contribute to the genesis of central pontine myelinolysis in, as yet, undefined ways.[23] Myelinolytic lesions can be reduced experimentally by rapid correction of chronic hyponatraemia. Symptoms include loss of pain sensation in the limbs, bulbar palsy, quadriplegia, disordered eye movements, vomiting, confusion, and coma.

Reversibility of brain damage

Alcohol-related neuroanatomical brain changes have been shown to be partially reversible. These findings created an ongoing debate on possible mechanisms and clinical correlates.[22]

Foetal alcohol syndrome

The first description of the foetal alcohol syndrome was given by French scientists in 1968.[24] As a research paradigm, it has a major impact on our understanding of alcohol's effects on the brain. Clinically the syndrome is characterized by: growth retardation involving height, weight, and head circumference; deficient intellectual and social performance and muscular coordination; minor structural anomalies of the face, together with more variable involvement of the limbs and the heart.

The basis of this pathology is a cascade of effects exerted by alcohol on the developing cell. Under normal conditions growth factors enhance the growth of cells and their differentiation, but alcohol can diminish these effects.[25] A second way of damaging the developing nerve cell is through the production of free radicals that allow calcium to accumulate in the cells.[26] The induction of a free-radical formation is induced by alcohol. The result of both pathogenic processes is a decrease in the overall size of the brain and a diminution in the thickness of the outer layers of the cortex, due to decreases in the total numbers of cells. Impaired nerve cell migration might also play a role in the development of the foetal alcohol syndrome.[27]

The effects of alcohol on the developing brain are clinically measured by assessing the head circumference, with a clear dose-dependent effect.

The foetal alcohol syndrome is considered further in Chapter 9.2.7.

Effects on the body

Malnutrition and vitamin deficiency

Malnutrition can be a consequence of deficient food intake. More important in alcoholics seem to be maldigestion and malabsorbtion ('secondary malnutrition'). Apart from the direct toxic effect of alcohol on most body tissues, malnutrition is an important contributor to organ damage in alcoholics.[28] Vitamin metabolism may be profoundly affected by chronic alcohol consumption. As a consequence, many alcoholics have deficiencies in vitamins B1 (thiamine), A, D, B6, and E, and folate. This can lead to a variety of physical consequences, including damage to different organs.

Peripheral neuropathy

Besides its effect on the central nervous system, alcohol also damages motor, sensory, and autonomic nerves that control muscles and internal organs. Symptoms are weakness, numbness, pain, and a prickly feeling or burning of the skin, especially the feet. Usually on neurological examination, the tendon reflexes are diminished or have completely disappeared and skin sensibility is reduced, especially in the feet and in the lower limbs. When patients abstain from alcohol, the progression of the symptoms can be stopped and even partial recovery is possible.

Muscle

Alcohol is toxic to skeletal muscles in a dose-dependent way. Alcoholics often suffer from malnutrition, which adds to the chronic changes in muscles. Chronic myopathy can be found in 40 to 60 per cent of alcohol-dependent patients.(29) Pathophysiological mechanisms of muscle damage include alterations in membrane fluidity, ion channels, and pumps, as well as protein synthesis and hormonal dysfunction. Patients complain of pain and weakness. Swelling of the muscle can be easily detected. In chronic states, muscle atrophy is evident. There is no acute treatment for alcoholic myopathy other than abstinence, when acute myopathy can rapidly disappear; chronic myopathy usually only improves, leaving persistent weaknesses.

Liver

The effects of ethanol on the liver are among the first and best-known symptoms of alcoholism. The first manifestation of alcoholic liver diseases is the fatty liver. It is followed by early fibrosis, which can be associated with alcoholic hepatitis. If the process continues, irreversible damage leading to severe fibrosis and to cirrhosis is observed.(30) These effects occur through heavy alcohol consumption even in the absence of dietary deficiencies.

Mortality from liver cirrhosis has long been an important correlate of the per capita consumption in a given population. Liver damage is also important because it produces an increase in liver enzymes such as aspartate transaminase, alanine transaminase, and γ-glutamyl transferase, which again are of great practical value as diagnostic markers of severe alcohol consumption. Alcohol accounts for more than 80 per cent of all cirrhosis deaths, a consequence that seems to be even more pronounced in women.(31)

Pancreas

About 5 per cent of alcoholics develop chronic pancreatitis. Ethanol seems to damage the pancreas slowly. In general, it takes between 10 and 15 years of heavy drinking before pancreatitis becomes clinically apparent. In the presomatic phase certain changes such as fibrosis, calcium deposits, and especially loss of functioning in enzyme- and hormone-producing cells can be demonstrated. The acute symptoms are abdominal pain and vomiting. Chronic complications include weight loss, steatorrhoea, and diabetes mellitus.(32)

Skin

Originally it was believed that skin alterations in alcoholics are due to alcoholic liver disease. However, more recent research has revealed that the skin may be affected much earlier by alcohol misuse.(33) Whereas the palmar erythema and spider naevi are well-known consequences of alcoholic liver disease, which also serve as diagnostic markers for alcoholism, psoriasis and facial erythema have less often been linked with high alcohol consumption. Alcohol clearly has to be on the list of agents known to exacerbate psoriasis. One possible mechanism of the action of alcohol on the skin could be a defect in the immune system.

Heart

Cardiac myopathy is one of the oldest known physical consequences of high alcohol consumption. Similar to ethanol's effects on skeletal muscles, the cells of the heart muscle are damaged by ethanol's influence on ion channels and pumps etc. Atrophy leads to a dilatation of the heart as a whole.

Recently, the effect of alcohol on coronary heart disease has been widely discussed. Indeed, it seems that there is a beneficial effect of moderate alcohol consumption. Although the reasons are currently under discussion, recent data suggest, that the combination of several actions including changes in lipid metabolism, antioxidant effects, changes in haemostasis and platelet aggregation, arterial vasodilatation mediated by NO release and the expression of cardioprotective proteins contribute to these 'French Paradox'.(34) It seems that an alcohol-induced increase in high-density lipoproteins and a decrease in low density lipoproteins may play a role in this process—an alteration in platelet aggregation could be one possible mechanism of action. Besides cardiomyopathy, cardiac arrhythmias are prominent consequences of alcohol consumption. Close to one-third of all cardiomyopathies can be attributed to alcohol consumption.

Hypertension

A dose-response relationship between drinking and diastolic and systolic blood pressure has been shown consistently.(31) In alcohol consuming population, the amount of alcohol consumption is significantly associated with hypertension and cardiovascular as well as all cause mortality. It is not clear, however, whether this relationship can only be seen above a threshold level of consumption.

Cancer

There is very clear evidence that alcohol increases the risk of cancer at the upper bronchodigestive tract. This includes cancer of the mouth, pharynx, larynx, and oesophagus. Additionally, alcohol consumption correlates with primary liver cancer. A possible link between alcohol and breast cancer is still a matter of debate: the association is not strong and not necessarily causative, at least for moderate consumption.(35) The same seems to be true for the correlation between beer drinking and cancer of the rectum.

Further information

Schuckit, M.A. (2006). *Drug and alcohol abuse: a clinical guide to diagnosis and treatment*. Springer, Berlin.

Erickson, C. (2007). *The science of addiction. From neurobiology to treatment*. W.W. Norton & Company, New York.

Icon Health Publications. (2004). *Alcohol addiction—a medical dictionary, bibliography, and annotated research guide to internet references*. Icon Group International, San Diego.

Spanagel, R. and Mann, K. (2005). *Drugs for relapse prevention of alcoholism*. Birkhäuser Verlag, Berlin.

References

1. Lishman, W.A. (1990). *Organic psychiatry. The psychological consequences of cerebral disorder* (2nd edn). Blackwell Science, Oxford.
2. American Psychiatric Association. (1994). *Diagnostic and statistical manual of mental disorders* (4th edn). American Psychiatric Association, Washington, DC.
3. Glass, I.B. (1989). Alcohol hallucinosis: a psychiatric enigma-2. Follow-up studies. *British Journal of Addiction*, **84**, 151–64.
4. Brown, S.A. and Schuckit, M.A. (1988). Changes in depression among abstinent alcoholics. *Journal of Studies on Alcohol*, **49**, 412–17.
5. Stetter, F., Rein, W., and Mann, K. (1991). How depressive are male alcoholic inpatients? Psychometric results from the Tübinger Alkoholismusprojekt. *European Psychiatry*, **6**, 243–9.
6. Kessler, R.C., McGonagle, K.A., Zhao, S., *et al.* (1994). Lifetime and 12-month prevalence of DSM-III-R psychiatric disorders in the United States: results from the National Comorbidity Survey. *Archives of General Psychiatry*, **51**, 8–19.
7. Merikangas, K.R. and Angst, J. (1995). Comorbidity and social phobia: evidence from clinical, epidemiologic, and genetic studies. *European Archives of Psychiatry and Clinical Neuroscience*, **244**, 297–303.
8. Kushner, M.G., Sher, K.J., and Beitman, B.D. (1990). The relation between alcohol problems and the anxiety disorders. *American Journal of Psychiatry*, **147**, 685–95.
9. Schuckit, M.A. and Hesselbrock, V. (1994). Alcohol dependence and anxiety disorders: what is the relationship? *American Journal of Psychiatry*, **151**, 1723–34.
10. Merikangas, K.R., Stevens, D., Fenton, B., *et al.* (1996). Comorbidity and co-transmission of anxiety disorders and alcoholism: results of the Yale Family Study. In *Proceedings of the American Psychiatric Association*, May 1996. American Psychiatric Association, Washington, DC.
11. Maier, W., Minges, J., and Lichtermann, D. (1993). Alcoholism and panic disorder: co-occurrence and co-transmission in families. *European Archives of Psychiatry and Clinical Neuroscience*, **243**, 205–11.
12. Kendler, K.S., Walters, E.E., Neale, M.C., *et al.* (1995). The structure of genetic and environmental risk factors for six major psychiatric disorders in women: phobia, generalized anxiety disorder, panic disorder, bulimia, major depression, and alcoholism. *Archives of General Psychiatry*, **52**, 374–83.
13. de la Monte, S.M. (1988). Disproportionate atrophy of cerebral white matter in chronic alcoholics. *Archives of Neurology*, **45**, 990–2.
14. Harper, C. (2007). The neurotoxicity of alcohol. *Human & Experimental Toxicology*, **26**, 251–7.
15. Harper, C., Kril, J., and Daly, J. (1987). Are we drinking our neurons away? *British Medical Journal*, **294**, 534–6.
16. Harper, C.G. and Kril, J.J. (1989). Patterns of neuronal loss in the cerebral cortex in chronic alcoholic patients. *Journal of Neurology Sciences*, **92**, 81–9.
17. Ferrer, I., Fabregues, I., Rairiz, J., *et al.* (1986). Decreased numbers of dendritic spines on cortical pyramidal neurons in human chronic alcoholism. *Neuroscience Letters*, **69**, 115–19.
18. Torvik, A., Lindbö, C.F., and Rodge, S. (1982). Brain lesions in alcoholics. *Journal of Neurological Sciences*, **56**, 233–48.
19. Torvik, A. and Torp, S. (1986). The prevalence of alcoholic cerebellar atrophy. A morphometric and histological study of an autopsy material. *Journal of Neurological Sciences*, **75**, 43–51.
20. Riley, J.N. and Walker, D.W. (1978). Morphological alterations in hippocampus after long term alcohol consumption in mice. *Science*, **201**, 646–8.
21. Mann, K. (1992). *Alkohol und Gehirn—über strukturelle und funktionelle veränderungen nach erfolgreicher therapie*. Springer, Berlin.
22. Mann, K., Mundle, G., Strayle, M., *et al.* (1995). Neuroimaging in alcoholism: CT and MRI results and clinical correlates. *Journal of Neural Transmission (General Section)*, **99**, 145–55.
23. Charness, M. (1993). Brain lesions in alcoholics. *Alcoholism, Clinical and Experimental Research*, **17**, 2–11.
24. Lemoine, P., Harousseau, H., Borteyru, J.-P., *et al.* (1968). Les enfants de parents alcooliques: anomalies observées à propos dc 127 cas. *Ouest Médical*, **25**, 477–82.
25. Dow, K.E. and Riopelle, R.J. (1985). Ethanol neurotoxicity: effects on neurite formation and neurotrophic factor production *in vitro*. *Science*, **228**, 591–3.
26. Manning, M.A. and Eugene Hoyme, H. (2007). Fetal alcohol spectrum disorders: a practical clinical approach to diagnosis. *Neuroscience and Biobehavioral Reviews*, **31**, 230–8.
27. Kumada, T., Jiang, Y., Cameron, D.B., *et al.* (2007). How does alcohol impair neuronal migration? *Journal of Neuroscience Research*, **85**, 465–70.
28. Estruch, R. (1996). Alcohol and nutrition. In *Alcohol misuse: a European perspective* (ed. T.J. Peters), pp. 41–61. Harwood Academic, London.
29. Urbano-Márquez, A. and Fernández-Solà, J. (1996). Musculo-skeletal problems in alcohol abuse. In *Alcohol misuse: a European perspective* (ed. T.J. Peters), pp. 123–44. Harwood Academic, London.
30. Lieber, C.S. (1998). Hepatic and other medical disorders of alcoholism: from pathogenesis to treatment. *Journal of Studies on Alcohol*, **59**, 9–25.
31. Huntgeburth, M., Ten Freyhaus, H., and Rosenkrank, S. (2005). Alcohol consumption and hypertension. *Current Hypertension Reports*, **7**, 180–5.
32. Niebergall-Roth, E., Harder, H., and Singer, M.V. (1998). A review: acute and chronic effects of ethanol and alcoholic beverages on the pancreatic exocrine secretion *in vivo* and *in vitro*. *Alcoholism, Clinical and Experimental Research*, **22**, 1570–83.
33. Higgins, E.M. (1996). Alcohol misuse and the skin. In *Alcohol misuse. A European perspective* (ed. T.J. Peters), pp. 77–87. Harwood Academic, London.
34. Providencia, R. (2006). Cardiovascular protection from alcoholic drinks: scientific basis of the French Paradox. *Revista Portuguesa de Cardiologia*, **25**, 1043–58.
35. Poschl, G. and Seitz, H.K. (2004). Alcohol and cancer. *Alcohol & Alcoholism*, **39**, 155–65.

4.2.2.4 Treatment of alcohol dependence

Jonathan Chick

A chronic relapsing disorder

Some people repeatedly put themselves or others at risk by drinking. One view is that such people could drink sensibly if they were more considerate and used more will power. Another increasingly accepted view is that many such individuals are in a state, existing in degrees of severity, in which the freedom to decide whether to change their drinking, and to adhere to that decision, is reduced compared with other drinkers. This state partly depends on perceived pay-offs for changing, and on acquired dispositions, which are less accessible to conscious control. Such persons become aware of a wish, or urge, to drink, which overcomes rational thought. They may then make up an explanation, for example, 'No wonder I feel like a drink, I've had a hard day'.

Such individuals benefit from help to unlearn those patterns, and to learn different approaches to problems. Discussion, care, and encouragement from others can bolster their will to do so. Assistance to set-up controls within or from outside themselves may help. Some people can do this without external help, and others with the help of Alcoholics Anonymous (**AA**) alone.[1]

This approach argues that dependence on alcohol should be managed like other relapsing disorders, such as diabetes and asthma,[2] by using long-term monitoring coupled with intermittent or continuous treatment.

Starting treatment

The initial interview

Assessment is the first step of intervention; clumsy interviewing alienates an ambivalent patient. The key to success is accepting that the patient is probably in two minds about the interview and about changing his or her drinking habits. Avoid confrontation. The drinking has probably already shown its resistance to deterrence by fear or pain. Gently nudge the matrix of conflicting motivations in the direction of action.

Patients may or may not have been referred for help with alcohol problems. Even if they have, the interview should begin with enquiry into the patient's current concerns. Reflective listening[3] helps the patient to clarify these concerns, conveys empathy, and avoids premature closure. A spirit of collaborative enquiry helps patients to reach their own conclusions about the role of alcohol in their troubles. This will be more convincing than a recitation of medical advice. People are more likely to believe what they hear themselves say than what others tell them. The interview is less likely to slip into confrontation if the doctor conveys recognition that, for the patient, drinking alcohol has been pleasurable. Therefore the assessment should not proceed in a series of closed questions, such as: 'Do you drink more than you intend to?' 'Does alcohol make you depressed?' Instead, ask open-ended questions: 'Tell me about your pattern of drinking. What are the good aspects . . . and what are the disadvantages?' 'How does alcohol fit in with these periods of hopelessness you describe?' The patient may want it understood that at times alcohol has dulled pain. Only then will there be a concession that the cumulative effect has been to worsen mood.

A comment such as 'I'm just a heavy social drinker, not an alcoholic' is not a gauntlet to be seized—an argument about definitions will distract from the work of clarifying and planning how to deal with the current problems. Instead, a response such as 'I gather you don't like labels' may reveal pertinent fears and prejudices (e.g. that alcoholics are failures, who get locked up in hospital).

Denial permits dismissal of unpleasant or unwanted facts and feelings. It hurts to admit that you have lost your family's respect, or that you will have to give up alcohol, which you enjoy. Alcohol problems still carry disgrace. In Islamic cultures, where alcohol is forbidden, denial from shame may be deepened by fear of punishment from the authorities.

Explain symptoms

Help the patient to understand withdrawal symptoms and how they can abort attempts to reduce consumption. Patients frequently attribute withdrawal symptoms to other causes; for example, waking at 4 a.m. with sweats and anxiety may be attributed to worry, and trembling hands in the morning to stress.

Informant

If the partner, a close friend, or a relative is present from the start, the salient points usually emerge more rapidly. However, the patient should also be seen alone because matters to do with the police, an employer, the bank, or a lover may still be unknown to the partner. Relatives should hear the exchange between doctor and patient, otherwise the version they hear later from the patient may be diluted: 'The doctor says I'm not an alcoholic'. This can leave relatives even angrier than before, convinced that no one understands their distress and that the drinker has once again deceived the doctor.

Assessments

The use of a breathalyser or saliva test to measure blood alcohol concentration puts alcohol consumption firmly into the objective arena. Use the test before the individual starts to detail recent drinking, there is nothing to be gained from showing that the patient sometimes minimizes the drinking.

Physical signs may be helpful. Heavy drinking may cause excessive capillarization in the conjunctivae or in the skin of the nose and cheeks. The liver may be enlarged. Look for tremor in the outstretched tongue, which is less commonly concealed (or exaggerated) than tremor in the fingers. Tachycardia is another useful sign of withdrawal. In a hyperaroused fearful patient, who has already been without a drink for 24 h, a pulse of over 110 beats/min may presage delirium tremens.

Clinicians vary in how structured an assessment they prefer, but at some point in the first one or two interviews the following should be noted: drinking patterns, history of withdrawal symptoms, previous attempts to stop drinking, use of drugs (prescribed and not prescribed), physical complications including head injuries, police, or Court involvement (past and current), dwelling arrangements, problems at home, trouble at work (specifying whether the employer has commented on drinking alcohol and/or started disciplinary action), psychiatric illness, family history, previous treatments, and experience of AA.

Medical assistance for withdrawal

Medical assistance to reduce the short-term discomfort of withdrawal can be the beginning of restructuring of thoughts and lifestyle towards long-term abstinence.

If dependence is severe, especially in an unplanned situation where a very heavy drinker is suddenly deprived of alcohol because of an accident, illness, or police arrest, care must be taken to prevent the life-threatening complications of convulsions or delirium. Anticipation is the key.

When dependence is less marked, withdrawal symptoms are mild and the person can stop drinking by gradual reduction, encouraged by the physician or a friend.

When the patient's aim is 'controlled drinking'(see below), this may also entail an initial stage of withdrawal, as the final goal is more likely to be achieved after abstinence for 2 or 3 months.

The setting

Controlled studies have shown that outpatient withdrawal is safe and effective for mild and moderately dependent alcoholics.[4,5] Advice for patients withdrawing at home is given in Box 4.2.2.4.1. Hayashida *et al.*[4] randomly allocated 164 mild to moderately affected patients to either inpatient or outpatient detoxification. Completion was successful in 95 per cent of the former and 72 per cent of the latter; inpatient care cost eight times more than outpatient care.

Box 4.2.2.4.1 Advice to patient on withdrawing from alcohol at home

If you have been chemically dependent on alcohol, stopping drinking causes you to become tense, edgy, perhaps shaky or sweaty, and unable to sleep. There can be vomiting or diarrhoea. This 'rebound' of the nervous system can be severe. Medication controls the symptoms while the body adjusts to being without alcohol. This usually takes 3 to 7 days from the time of your last alcoholic drink. If you did not take medication, the symptoms would be worst in the first 48 h, and then gradually disappear. This is why the dose starts high and then reduces.

You have agreed not to drink alcohol. You may become thirsty. Drink fruit juices and water but do not overdo it. You do not have to 'flush' alcohol out of the body. More than 3l of fluid could be too much. Do not drink more than three cups of coffee or five cups of tea. These contain caffeine, which disturbs sleep and causes nervousness.

Aim to avoid stress. The important task is not to give in to the urge to take alcohol. Help yourself relax by going for a walk, listening to music, or taking a bath.

Sleep. You may find that even people with capsules, or as they are reduced, your sleep is disturbed. You need not worry about this lack of sleep as it does not seriously harm you, but starting to drink again does. Your sleep pattern will return to normal in a month or so. It is better not to take sleeping pills so that your natural sleep rhythm returns. Try going to bed later. Take a bedtime snack or milky drink. The capsules may make you drowsy so you must not drive or operate machinery. If you become drowsy, miss out a dose.

Meals. Even when you are not hungry, try to eat something. Your appetite will return.

Admission to a hospital is indicated when the home social milieu is inimical to abstinence, or when there is a history of withdrawal convulsions or delirium; it is urgent when there are any signs of Wernicke's encephalopathy.

Medication

A benzodiazepine[6] is prescribed for two reasons: first, to reduce the risk of severe withdrawal symptoms with delirium or convulsions (indicated if recent consumption has been more than 15 units/day for more than 10 days); second, to assist the individual whose wish to abstain or reduce drinking is overcome by longing for alcohol (craving), shaking, anxiety, insomnia, or nausea and vomiting.

A typical outpatient regimen would be chlordiazepoxide 20 to 30 mg four times daily, reducing to zero over 5 days, with the larger doses given at night (Table 4.2.2.4.1). Medication is issued on the understanding that the patient does not also take alcohol. If there is any doubt that this instruction will be followed, medication is issued daily and a check made (ideally by breath or saliva tests) that drinking has not been resumed. Chlordiazepoxide is preferred to diazepam for outpatient use because it has a lower street value and is therefore less likely to be sold on. When managing severe withdrawal symptoms with marked agitation and tremor, or incipient delirium, diazepam (starting at 10 mg four times daily) is preferred

Table 4.2.2.4.1 Example of a fixed-dose regime for outpatient alcohol withdrawal using capsules of chlordiazepoxide 10 mg

	First thing	12 noon	6 p.m.	Bedtime
Day 1		3	3	3
Day 2	2	2	2	3
Day 3	2	1	1	2
Day 4	1	1		2
Day 5		1		1

because it has a more rapid action and can be given parenterally. A benzodiazepine with one metabolite only and a shorter half-life (e.g. oxazepam, lorazepam) is preferred if liver function is significantly impaired (i.e. there is jaundice, ascites, oedema, low serum albumin, or raised serum bilirubin).

For inpatients, a benzodiazepine such as diazepam 10 mg may be given every hour until symptoms are controlled (symptom-triggered dosing). This procedure leads to lower total prescription of benzodiazepine, less oversedation, and quicker discharge from hospital.[7]

If the patient is vomiting, give metoclopropamide 10 mg intramuscularly 30 min before the first benzodiazepine tablet and/or perhaps choose a benzodiazepine that can be administered parenterally; lorazepam 1 mg is absorbed adequately from the intramuscular site, or diazepam 10 mg can be given intravenously (or rectally).

Treating convulsions

With the aim of preventing further convulsions, the patient who has just had a fit or is in a fit is given 10 mg diazepam. Consider giving 15 to 20 mg in a patient who has been taking benzodiazepines regularly prior to this event, or is much above average weight. It is illogical to commence an anticonvulsant, which may take 2 to 3 days to reach a therapeutic serum level. Rather, increase the dose of the benzodiazepines. A convulsion may presage delirium.

Preventing convulsions

Deaths have occurred in hospital, prison, and police cells from repeated alcohol withdrawal fits. When withdrawal is planned in patients with a history of fits of any cause the risk can be reduced by commencing phenytoin (300 mg daily) 4 days before the cessation of drinking. In an acute situation, larger than normal doses of long-acting benzodiazepines are given in the first 36 h without waiting until the blood alcohol level has fallen to zero. The benzodiazepine should be started as soon as the blood alcohol level can be presumed to be falling, even though the patient still smells of alcohol or has a positive breath test, provided that he or she is sober enough to understand and cooperate with the procedure.

Treating delirium tremens

Increasing the dose of the benzodiazepine may be sufficient to control the agitation. If not, the slight epileptogenic effect of antipsychotic drugs should not deter their use, especially if delusions and hallucinations have developed, provided that anticonvulsant protection by a benzodiazepine is in place. Parenteral haloperidol plus parenteral lorazepam is usually effective. When a patient's behaviour is uncontrolled or dangerous, transfer to a secure unit may be needed. Authoritative calm nursing reduces the risk of aggression. Hospitals should have an emergency team of sufficient personnel to manage disturbed patients.

Preventing delirium tremens

If confusion and hallucinations develop, this usually occurs 48 to 72 h after the last drink. Sufficient benzodiazepine, given early in the withdrawal, reduces the risk, as does sensitive nursing in a quiet evenly-lit environment. Explaining symptoms and orientating the patient reduces anxiety, paranoia, and confusion.

Vitamin therapy

It is reasonable to prescribe thiamine 50 mg orally three times a day for 2 to 3 weeks, as thiamine stores may be depleted because of poor diet and alcohol-impaired gut absorption. Wernicke–Korsakoff syndrome is life-threatening and steps must be taken to avoid it developing.[8] The malnourished patient, or the patient who shows any sign of Wernicke's encephalopathy (confusion, ataxia, ophthalmoplegia, nystagmus—do not wait for the 'triad' of symptoms), must be given immediate parenteral B vitamins. Anaphylactic shock was a very rare complication of some older preparations. It is less likely with intramuscular than intravenous injection; infusion saline drip, when practicable, is probably preferable to slow bolus injection.

Interventions to reduce relapse

The evidence

With appropriate help, withdrawing from alcohol is not the dependent drinker's main difficulty. The main difficulty is avoiding relapse into further problematic drinking or dependence.

Before the era of randomized controlled trials, psychiatrists typically would explore with patients possible personality or psychological causes of their excessive drinking—trying to find out 'why?'. However, evidence that this reduced relapse was lacking. Indeed, it may have sometimes had an adverse effect by reinforcing the drinkers' perception of having a need to drink and by creating transference problems which might later trigger drinking.[9] Non-directive counselling may also sometimes have had negative effects, acting as a confessional, with a sense of absolution allowing further drinking.

In recent years, several systematic reviews and meta-analyses have been conducted of treatments to prevent relapse in alcohol dependence. Drawing on data from high quality trials a consensus has emerged.[10–12] Effective treatment are social skills training based on behavioural cognitive therapy principles,[13] motivational enhancement[14] albeit tested sometimes in less severe groups of patients, the community reinforcement approach,[15] behaviour contracting, and behavioural marital therapy[16] and the pharmacotherapies described below.

Abstinence or 'controlled drinking'?

Harmful or hazardous use of alcohol without severe dependence can sometimes revert to risk-free drinking. Patients with social supports (family and job) and without impulsive personalities and many social problems are most likely to succeed. For others, including most of those dependent on alcohol, the goal of abstinence is better.[29] Among patients attending specialized clinics,

Table 4.2.2.4.2 FRAMES: ingredients of a brief intervention

Feedback about personal risk or impairment
Responsibility: emphasis on personal responsibility for change
Advice to cut down or, if indicated because of severe dependence or harm, to abstain
Menu of alternative options for changing drinking pattern
Empathic interviewing
Self-efficacy: an interviewing style which enhances this

Reproduced with permission from T.H. Bein, *et al.* (1993), Motivational interviewing with alcoholic outpatients, *Behavioural and Cognitive Psychotherapy*, **21**, 347–56, copyright 1993, with permission from Cambridge University Press.

the proportion who can sustain problem-free drinking for at least 1 year is small—5 per cent is a typical finding.[17–19] A randomized trial comparing the goals of controlled drinking and abstinence did not favour controlled drinking.[20] However, for patients without established dependence, reduction programmes (whether or not towards abstinence) using FRAMES (Table 4.2.2.4.2) proved to be more effective than no intervention.[21–23] Interventions in primary care are discussed in Chapter 4.2.2.5.

If controlled drinking is the agreed goal, the patient and physician collaborate to monitor the amount and pattern of the drinking as follows:

1 Limit number of days of drinking and number of drinks on any occasion.

2 Slow the rate of drinking, and/or reduce alcoholic strength of drinks.

3 Develop assertiveness skills for refusing drinks.

4 Design reward system when goals are achieved.

5 Develop awareness of triggers to overdrinking.

6 Practise other ways of coping with triggers.

7 Record pattern and amount of drinking, for example in a diary.

8 Physician and patient monitor γ-glutamyl transferase blood test results.

Maintaining motivation and compliance

Enhancing motivation has a place not only at onset, but throughout the clinical contact. Treatment aimed only at enhancing motivation was for most outcome measures equal to cognitive behavioural therapy, and intensive intervention aimed at linking patients with AA.[24] Randomized controlled studies have shown the advantage of motivational interviewing over traditional supportive therapy.[10–12,25] The style of the opening interview using motivational interviewing techniques has already been discussed. The patient is encouraged not to forget the harm that drinking caused and the benefits of abstinence, but the losses and problems of being sober are not denied. Strategies for maintaining abstinence emerge from collaborative dialogue, and are owned by patients rather than offered as advice from the clinician. If medication is part of the treatment plan, unwanted effects are actively enquired into, and are recognized and not dismissed, and remedies are sought. Any discrepancies that patients reveal between their present view of themselves and how they would like to be, or between what patients say they believe and how they actually behave, are used as a fulcrum for shifting attitudes and testing alternative strategies. These techniques were elaborated by Miller and Rollnick[3] and enshrined as motivational enhancement therapy[26] by Project MATCH (see below).

Helping motivation: the social matrix

It is said that the only successful way to change your drinking is 'to do it for yourself'. Nevertheless, many of those dependent on alcohol start on the road to recovery because of pressure from outside. For example, if the person finds himself in Court, or has lost his driving licence, authorities may seek evidence that the offender has taken steps to alter harmful drinking patterns. Perhaps the partner is now being firmer, even demand a separation or divorce; or the employer has given a warning.

Friends, partners, colleagues at work, and even employers sometimes adopt an approach that they believe to be motivating but which has the opposite effect and enables the drinker to continue drinking. For example, they may cover-up, gloss over, make excuses, or even blame themselves for what is going wrong. This cushions drinkers from experiencing the harmful consequences of their drinking or allows them to believe that alcohol is not the chief problem, despite evidence that alcohol is in fact the critical common factor in their downward spiral.

A physician can help the parties improve communication so that important messages are not lost. If the message from the employer or partner, or even the children, is clear and positive, it can have a powerful motivating effect: 'We value our relationship with you. But the way you are drinking is harming that relationship and we will not tolerate it'.

Some physicians are overcautious about confidentiality in this situation. If a doctor is asked by a partner or an employer to comment on the patient's condition, he or she may or may not have permission, or feel it appropriate, to do so. But doctors can usefully help partners or employers clarify for themselves what they want, and then encourage a clear and firm, but positive message.

Sometimes doctors unwittingly collude in a cover-up. The smokescreen that can be set-up by a drinker who is severely dependent and ambivalent about change can be hard to penetrate: 'It's depression, doctor'; 'It's stress at work'; 'If only my wife was more understanding/my sleep was not so disturbed/I didn't get these memory blanks which I think are some kind of stroke'. The doctor may need to wait for that medical moment, perhaps a crisis, to help such an individual. Or, if the doctor has patience, the drip, drip of non-judgemental evidence, and perhaps some social pressure, may bring about the necessary change in the patient's understanding and thus the perceived motivational pay-offs. Understanding may lead to action. However, as Fig. 4.2.2.4.1 shows, that action may not be sustained and the process of helping understanding may need to be repeated many times.[27]

There are few randomized controlled studies allocating patients to different intensities of external motivation. However, alcoholics coerced into treatment have medium-term outcomes similar to those who attend voluntarily.[28]

Coping skills therapies

When incentives are powerful, many newly abstinent patients are able to abstain for short periods. Others lack the skills to cope with the triggers to drinking even when their motivation to abstain has been strong. Cognitive behavioural therapies seem to improve the

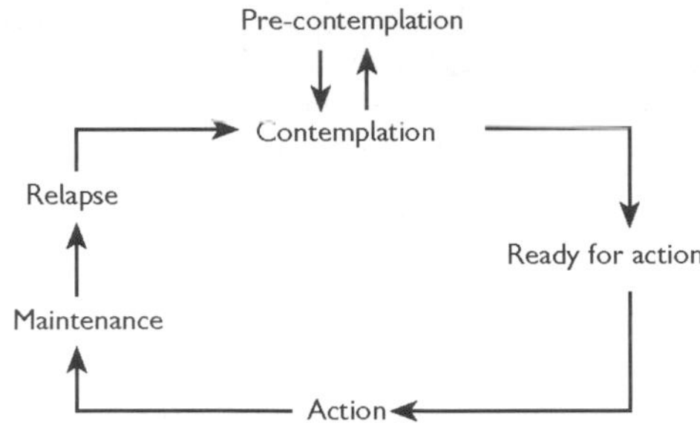

Fig. 4.2.2.4.1 Wheel of change. (Reproduced from J. Prochaska and C. DiClementi. Stages of change in the modification of problem behaviours. In *Progress in behavior modification*, Vol. 28 (eds. M. Hersen, R. Eisler, and P. Miller), pp. 183–218, copyright 1984, Sage Publishing, Sycamore, IL.

coping skills of these patients. If the triggers are in social situations, assertiveness, or conversation skills training can help. If the trigger is related to relationship of work problems, checking beliefs and attitudes, and reframing stressors may reduce the urge to use alcohol as a sedative.[13] Some patients are helped by learning to handle frustration and criticism without harbouring anger and resentments. Treatment can be in groups, where the opportunity to discuss these topics with others who have similar problems is appreciated. Groups also enable learning through role playing and by modelling on others. 'Relapse prevention therapy' as originally formulated has not stood up to meta-analytic critique.[11]

Cue exposure

The smell or sight of alcoholic drinks can be a powerful stimulus to drinking. Initial studies[30] found that 'deconditioning' by exposing inpatients to the sight and smell of their preferred drinks in a laboratory setting, without drinking, was associated in the coming 6 months with a longer period without a relapse. However, this is not a standalone treatment. Patients should not court danger by going into pubs and bars—these are places where people go to drink alcohol.

Couples should decide together whether or not to have alcohol in the house, but patients should not be encouraged to 'test themselves'.

Alcoholics Anonymous

There are many ingredients in the healing process of AA. Newcomers are helped to identify with others as members tell their stories. They see that it is possible to be frank about past errors and the hurt caused to others through the drinking. Telling their own story helps the members not to forget the harm that accrued from drinking. This reduces complacency, which is one of the most common precursors of relapse.

Alcoholism is viewed by AA as a physical, psychological, and spiritual illness, which can be arrested (by avoiding another drink) but cannot be cured. The meetings offer a new social network. Emotional openness is encouraged. Members learn to express warmth, and to accept that they and others have failings. The AA advice on coping with emotions and relationship difficulties has much in common with cognitive behavioural therapy and relapse prevention therapy. The method has some attractively simple concepts ('Just don't pick up that first drink'; 'HALT'—being alert to four of the most common triggers to relapse, i.e. hunger, anger,

Box 4.2.2.4.2 The 12 steps of Alcoholics Anonymous

Step 1 We admitted we were powerless over alcohol-that our lives had become unmanageable.
Step 2 Came to believe that a power greater than ourselves could restore us to sanity.
Step 3 Made a decision to turn our will and our lives over to the care of God *as we understood him.*
Step 4 Made a searching and fearless moral inventory of ourselves.
Step 5 Admitted to God, to ourselves, and to another human being the exact nature of our wrongs.
Step 6 Were entirely ready to have God remove all these defects of character.
Step 7 Humbly asked him to remove our shortcomings.
Step 8 Made a list of all persons we had harmed, and became willing to make amends to them all.
Step 9 Made direct amends to such people wherever possible, except when to do so would injure them or others.
Step 10 Continued to take personal inventory and when we were wrong promptly to admit it.
Step 11 Sought through prayer and meditation to improve our conscious contact with God *as we understood him*, praying only for knowledge of his will for us and the power to carry that out.
Step 12 Having had a spiritual awakening as a result of these steps, we tried to carry this message to practice these principles in our affairs.

loneliness, tiredness). There is a deeper aspect, which is to replace preoccupation with self by handing over to the group process, or to a 'Higher Power'.

Accepting that you are 'powerless' to control your drinking is the 'first step' in AA. This entails ceasing the struggle and letting the 'Higher Power' take over. Members vary in their interpretation of the 'Higher Power', and avowed atheists should not be deterred from sampling AA. Residential, outpatient, and day programmes, which teach the AA approach are sometimes called 12-step programmes (Box 4.2.2.4.2). One of their strengths is linking patients to the AA network. In Project MATCH,[24]

A psychiatrist can introduce patients to AA through a contact member who will tell the patient how AA works, will not ask personal details, and will extend an invitation to a meeting. Doctors are welcome to attend 'open' AA meetings to see how it works. A contact number is given in local telephone directories. AA does not work for everyone, but since it is difficult to predict who will be helped, it is good practice to offer contact to all patients with impaired control of their drinking.

A warning, often based on personal experience, may be given at AA meetings about transferring dependence from alcohol to other drugs. This usually refers to use of barbiturates or benzodiazepines, or to the danger of relying on a medication instead of adjusting one's way of living. The use of prescribed medication is not formally disapproved of by AA.

Evidence of efficacy

Naturalistic non-randomized studies have shown that treatment programmes using the AA approach are associated with outcomes in drinking and overall functioning similar to those of programmes using the cognitive behavioural approach. Patients in 12-step programmes improve on self-efficacy and coping skills scores much as patients treated by cognitive behavioural therapy.[31] Following the steps of AA is associated with improving drinking and psychosocial outcomes.[32]

Only two randomized controlled studies of 12-step programmes have been conducted. One compared inpatient treatment (with fewer hours of psychotherapy than many such programmes) with a 12-step inpatient programme (with slightly more hours of therapy). There was a non-significant trend towards a greater total abstinence programme and less relapse in the 12-step programme.[33] In Project MATCH, patients were randomly allocated to cognitive behavioural therapy, motivational enhancement therapy, or '12-step facilitation', which instructed patients in the tenets of AA, and assisted and encouraged them to attend AA meetings. The three treatments resulted in similar outcomes after 1 and 3 years. However, for those who had been relatively free of psychiatric problems at entry to the study, 12-step facilitation was associated with slightly better outcomes after 1 year. After 3 years the 12-step facilitation led to better outcome for patients who, at entry to the study, had family, social, or work environments bringing them into frequent contact with drinking.[34]

Help for the family

The family of someone with a drinking problem may suffer for years without recognition and can benefit from advice and understanding. They are a vital monitor of the patient's progress. Good family cohesion and low expressed emotion predict better outcome, even after controlling for the predictors of demographic variables and severity of alcohol dependence.

Life in the family becomes increasingly restricted. Finances dwindle. The children fear that the parent may be drunk, and so stop inviting friends to visit. They dread that arguments between mother and father will become violent. The drinker's behaviour becomes slovenly. He or she may wet the bed. Despite these hurts, the drinker may still make the family believe that they are the reason he or she drinks.

The invitation to a family member or partner to attend with the patient may be rejected if the drinker is the messenger, and the message is distorted to: 'The doctor says you're part of the problem'. A direct letter or telephone call from the clinician requesting 'your views on how I can assist' reduces the partner's fear of being burdened with extra guilt or responsibility.

The clinician can help reduce family behaviours, such as hostility or cover-up, that are damaging to the family and counterproductive for the drinker's recovery. Communication between the drinker and the spouse or children has often broken down. In many countries family groups, such as Al-Anon, provide help to families.

Behavioural marital therapy

When the patient is in a relationship, its quality can be motivating or demotivating. Reciprocal contracts are aimed at making the relationship more rewarding for each partner. Although abstinence is a prerequisite, specific agreements should not be contingent on the drinking[35]; otherwise, a relapse means that the partner ceases to work on the relationship. Another prerequisite might be that physical violence is excluded. Contracting could start thus: 'Although you are responsible for not drinking, is there anything that your partner could do more of, or less of, that would help you stick to the plan?' Check that the requests are reasonable and available before the partner is asked to agree. The partner makes reciprocal requests and negotiation follows. Even requests for small changes can start the process.

The partners should give clear messages, owning their statements: 'This is what I would like', 'It makes me feel good if you . . .'. They will need to be reminded to state the positives and to practise being good listeners, giving non-verbal signals that they are listening, and not butting in with unsolicited good advice.

Violence in the partnership may require specific attention. If the drinker is intoxicated, the partner is advised to back off and avoid argument. Sometimes each partner is asked to sign an agreement that neither will threaten nor hit the other. If they do, time-out in another room is agreed in advance to permit slow-breathing to aid calming down, or one of them will leave the house and go to a designated place for 36 to 72 h.

When the partner 'brings up the past', this can be a major irritant to the drinker. But this can be reframed as the partner 'helping the couple not repeat their past': the partner who feels heard and understood is more ready to look at changes that he or she might also make.

Efficacy

Behavioural marital therapy produces better outcomes of drinking and marital relations than individual counselling or similar control conditions. The superior effects last for 24 months after treatment. Outcome at 1 year is better if sessions of behavioural marital therapy continue after the end of treatment to reinforce what has been learnt and rehearse relapse prevention plans.[36]

Deterrent medication

Disulfiram

If taken in a sufficient dose for at least the preceding 3 to 4 days, disulfiram causes an unpleasant reaction to develop 15 to 20 min after alcohol enters the body. The reaction is due to accumulation of acetaldehyde, an intermediate metabolite of ethanol. The reaction includes flushing, headache, pounding in the chest or head, tightness in breathing, nausea, and sometimes vomiting. Hypotension can occur and is potentially dangerous. (In some countries, calcium carbimide, which has the same action is also available.) The disulfiram–ethanol reaction varies in intensity. It is recognized practice to increase the dose of disulfiram up to 400 mg daily if the patient has tested the alcohol reaction and it has not been severe enough to act as a deterrent.

Disulfiram is an aid, not a cure. The individual can become used to life without alcohol. This allows time for confidence to recover—in the family, at work, or in the social services if there have been concerns about the safety of children. Patients may object that it is weakness to take a deterrent, and they prefer to show that they can use will power. Explain to the patient that will power is not always there when most needed. With disulfiram a decision to drink or not still has to be made, but only once a day.

Unwanted effects which occur even when no alcohol is taken include drowsiness, bad breath, and headache. These make the drug unacceptable to some patients. Concerns that disulfiram can harm the liver are based on a few case reports (the risk is about 1 in 25 000 patient-years). It appears to be a hypersensitivity reaction, and if it is to occur it is likely to be in the first month. Overall, disulfiram is associated with improved liver function tests compared with control groups, presumably owing to reduction of drinking.[37] Peripheral neuropathy (almost always reversible) has been reported following several months at doses of over 250 mg: the risk maybe greater when the patient takes other drugs such as antidepressants which are metabolized in the liver. There are a few reports of psychosis induced by disulfiram, and psychotic illness has been a formal contraindication in the licensing in some countries. The risk is so low and the need to help schizophrenic patients with alcohol problems is sometimes so great that in other countries this contraindication has been changed to a 'caution'. There are many documented cases where improvement has occurred in psychotic patients while taking disulfiram, and in a dose of up to 250 mg daily there are no problems from unwanted actions or interactions with medication for the psychiatric illness.[38]

(a) Efficacy

Disulfiram will only aid recovery if it is taken regularly in a sufficient dose to deter. Earlier studies without attempts to increase adherence to the medication did not show efficacy unlike studies in which enhanced compliance was enhanced by arranging supervision. In some of these studies there was a degree of coercion; for example, if the patient ceased taking the disulfiram the partner might withdraw from some agreed item, or disciplinary action at work might be reinstated.

The disulfiram effect depends on the patient knowing that they have ingested the disulfiram, and so only single blind studies are appropriate to test its efficacy. Single blind studies over 1 year have shown, in patients with a family member to supervise the medication, that disulfiram is associated with less relapse than acamprosate[39] and naltrexone.[40]

(b) Suggested mode of use

Before prescribing, a physical examination and baseline liver function tests are performed. The patient is encouraged to ask the partner, a nurse, or welfare officer at work or at the health centre, or a pharmacist to see that the disulfiram is taken. This can be daily, or three times a week, provided that the total weekly dose is sufficient, i.e. at least 7 × 200 mg. Some specialist clinics have follow-up clinics thrice weekly to supervise disulfiram. A programme commencing for the first months with frequent clinic attendance, and thereafter encouragement to continue using disulfiram, reported abstinence rates of over 50 per cent in patients followed for up to 7 years.[41] The product is available in a dispersible form to be taken in water so that it can be seen to be swallowed.

There should be medical follow-up, but there is no consensus as to whether monitoring of liver function tests should be carried out beyond the first month. However, monthly follow-up is appropriate to check for signs of drinking and of any unwanted effects.

It is common to prescribe disulfiram for 6 months, but many patients ask to continue for longer and there may be slips when disulfiram is withdrawn, even after long periods of abstinence. Some patients keep a supply to use when they feel an increased risk of drinking, for example on a business trip or at a social event.

Specific neurotransmitter antagonists

(a) Acamprosate (calcium acetyl homotaurinate)

Acamprosate enhances γ-aminobutyric acid (**GABA**) transmission and antagonizes glutamate transmission, probably by antagonizing *N*-methyl-D-aspartate receptors (see Chapter 6.2.8). It reduces drinking in alcohol-dependent animals, and reduces the reinstatement of drinking behaviour in animals re-exposed to alcohol after a period of abstinence. Animals do not seek out acamprosate as they do addictive substances, and it does not have mood-altering or drug-abuse potential in humans.(42) It has no deterrent or disulfiram-like effect.

Acamprosate is excreted unchanged in the kidney. It has few unwanted effects; diarrhoea, and abdominal discomfort are the only ones reported in more than 10 per cent of patients (up to 20 per cent) and these are mild and transient. It does not exacerbate psychomotor impairment caused by alcohol. There are no known drug interactions. Systematic follow-up after the end of acamprosate treatment shows no sudden relapse and no discontinuation symptoms in patients who have received the medication for up to 1 year.

(i) Efficacy

Acamprosate has a dose-related effect of improving abstinence rates in recently detoxified patients. There are no studies comparing the advantages of differing lengths of treatment. Meta-analysis of published studies finds that acamprosate is associated with improvement in abstinence rate compared to placebo with an odds ratio of 1:88 and greater cumulative days of abstinence.(43)

Acamprosate has only been tested in patients who intend to abstain from alcohol. It has not been tested formally in patients aiming for controlled drinking. However, in literature, patients who resume drinking, consume less alcohol in subsequent days(44) if they had been allocated to acamprosate than to placebo.

(ii) Suggested mode of use

Acamprosate is indicated for patients who have withdrawal symptoms and relief drinking typical of severe alcohol dependence and requiring medical assistance to withdraw. It is started 2 to 7 days after the last drink (steady state pharmacokinetics are reached after 5 days). Patients who relapse while on acamprosate are advised to continue taking the medication and exert effort to limit the lapse. However, acamprosate is not normally continued in patients who relapse more than once despite regularly taking the drug. Those who appear to be benefiting from it should continue the drug for at least 6 months, and up to 1 year if there has been a history of repeated relapsing while in treatment.

Several studies have shown that acamprosate reduces self-reported craving for alcohol. Some newly abstinent patients experience strong craving, but others experience very little and there is no evidence that this should be a criteria for deciding to whom this medication should be offered.

Acamprosate may sometimes help prolong abstinence among patients who choose to take disulfiram.(45)

(b) Opiate antagonists

Endorphins are released in one of ethanol's many acute actions on the limbic system. It has been suggested that this effect contributes to loss of control.(46) Naltrexone (and nalmefene) antagonize the neurotransmitter action of endogenous endorphins. Naltrexone has been shown to reduce ethanol-seeking in alcohol-dependent animals. It does not exacerbate the psychomotor impairment caused by alcohol.

Some patients who drink alcohol while taking naltrexone report that they feel less of the ethanol 'high'. This could lead to less impulse to carry on drinking.(47,48) However, some studies have reported an increase in total abstinence as well as a reduction of drinking overall.(48,49) It is possible that the reduced craving for alcohol and the reduced likelihood of picking up the first drink occur because the strength of the previous triggers—emotional, cognitive, or environmental—is attenuated.

Nausea following the first few doses is the commonest unwanted effect, occurring in about 10 per cent of patients. Concerns in the 1970s that naltrexone might cause dysphoria seemed to be supported by statements from heroin addicts given naltrexone to help them abstain from opiates. However, laboratory studies and randomized controlled trials in subjects who have not been opiate dependent have not found evidence of dysphoria or loss of feelings of pleasure.(50)

(i) Efficacy

Short-term administration of naltrexone reduced the rate of relapse to heavy drinking (odds ratio 0:62 in the meta-analysis of Bouza *et al.*(43) but although individual studies have reported an advantage in rates of total abstinence, this is not upheld in meta-analysis.(43)

Even though the dose is once daily, adherence has been low in some studies, and a beneficial effect only demonstrable in compliant patients.(51) Developed partly to improve compliance, a long-acting injection given monthly has become available and found to be acceptable to patients. It was more effective in reducing relapse to heavy drinking than a monthly injection of the vehicle without active naltrexone.(49)

When supervised oral naltrexone was compared to supervised disulfiram it was found to be less effective in preventing relapse to heavy drinking.(40) However, when oral naltrexone has been compared to acamprosate it was more effective.(52–54)

(ii) Suggested mode of use

Opiate antagonists have a particular role in reducing relapse to heavy drinking in patients who will not or cannot attain abstinence. As well as prescribed as a daily dose, their targeted used has also been supported in patients trying to limit the amount consumed per session, when the patient takes a dose only on days when at risk of drinking or planning to drink.(55,56) Several studies have found that patient with a positive family history of alcohol dependence are more likely to benefit from an opiate antagonist than those without.

Interactions. Opiate antagonists such as naltrexone will precipitate an immediate opiate withdrawal syndrome if given to patients who are actively dependent on opiates, and will prevent pain relief of opiate analgesics.

Helping women with alcohol problems

It has been said that when a woman has an alcohol problem, there is a man in her life with a similar problem—usually her partner or her father. When the partner also drinks heavily, he should be invited to some joint therapy meetings. Some partners have adopted a controlling role, especially if the spouse has been unreliable in managing the children or the money, or has driven while intoxicated. The patient may allow her resentment at this to fuel her drinking, and it may need months to help her to see how this has come about.

Low self-esteem is very common in such women, even in those who were confident before the drinking became problematic. The partner, while remaining firm about the unacceptability of her drinking, may need help to be more caring and positive, to show interest in what concerns her, and to show appreciation.

When helping women with alcohol dependence to abstain some of the following may be relevant:

- Help her to stop feeling taken for granted, and to know that she has a right to set limits on what others expect of her.
- Although guilt may be proportional to what she has put her family through by her drinking, it may not help. It may prevent her from asking for the conditions at home or work that would make it easier for her to stop drinking.
- Help her let go of resentments.
- Help her find ways of recharging her batteries by, for example, taking up new interests or exercise.
- Talk with the partner, both alone and with her present. He may want to know that she acknowledges the strain on him. While still accepting complete responsibility for her drinking, she can let him know what he can do to help her.
- Self-help literature is available in many languages to help women improve self-confidence and self-assertion.(57)

Treatment of coexisting disorders

Affective disorder

Depression is common in patients who are dependent on alcohol. The drinking may have alienated friends, family, or employer, with resulting feelings of hopelessness, guilt, and lack of direction. Alcohol can reduce appetite, energy, and sexual drive. The drinker wakes in the small hours of the night feeling anxious owing to the rebound wakefulness of alcohol withdrawal. Those signs and symptoms suggesting depressive illness commonly clear with abstinence and help in tackling or tolerating personal problems and improving relationships.

Sometimes (more often in women than in men) a depressive episode precedes the alcohol dependence, the patient begins to use alcohol as self-medication. Sometimes depressive symptoms continue despite abstinence. In these cases, antidepressants should be offered in the usual way.(58,59) Relapsing alcoholism, secondary to depressive illness, is an indication for long-term antidepressants. Lithium is not a treatment for alcohol dependence itself, but is effective if alcohol dependence is secondary to manic–depressive disorder.

General practitioners and general psychiatrists often prescribe antidepressants to patients with alcohol dependence who are still drinking, because the patient has complained of low mood, insomnia, or anxiety. There is no evidence that this will improve the drinking problem, and the period of alcohol withdrawal under benzodiazepine cover can be an occasion to withdraw the antidepressant. Most depressive symptoms experienced while alcohol-dependent patients are drinking are alleviated with abstinence. Early-onset alcohol dependence, marked by novelty seeking and impulsivity, can be exacerbated by SSRIs.(60,61)

Anxiety and panic disorder

Some patients have had panic attacks for years before discovering that alcohol can end or prevent them. Others have a first panic attack during alcohol withdrawal, but the attacks continue independently even during sustained abstinence. In this case, cognitive behavioural therapy and/or medication are indicated. Anxiety symptoms, which persist are predictive of relapse in the coming year.(62) However, the majority of anxiety symptoms reported by alcohol-dependent patients resolve with abstinence(63,64) and the weight of evidence is that adding specific psychological therapy aimed at the anxiety symptoms does not improve the drinking or the anxiety outcomes beyond that achieved by the treatment for the alcohol dependence.(65,66) In Project MATCH, male patients with social phobia allocated to 12-step facilitation (i.e. encouragement to attend AA) improved their drinking as much or even slightly more than those patients allocated to cognitive behaviour therapy (CBT) who would have received specific treatment for their phobia, though an advantage to CBT showed in female socially phobic patients.(67)

One explanation for these findings could be that attending to the anxiety might, for some patients, distract attention from the drinking, or could even seem to 'justify' their continuing to drink. It is also the case that some phobic patients report that attending AA helped them to overcome their social phobia.

Three studies suggest that the serotonin agonist buspirone can help reduce both drinking and anxiety.(68) Tricyclic antidepressants and selective serotonin-reuptake inhibitors (**SSRIs**) are prescribed to patients whose anxiety disorder persists despite abstinence. Some patients with long histories of alcohol dependence and severe panic disorder fail to respond to these medications or to CBT. For these patients the risk of complications from a prescription for a long-acting benzodiazepine such as chlordiazepoxide may be less than the harm that might accrue if bouts of excessive drinking persisted. If prescribed (and to do so is controversial), the benzodiazepine should be dispensed in limited amounts. The prescription should be conditional on abstinence from alcohol, perhaps aided by disulfiram, if necessary. 'As-required' use (e.g. for travelling on public transport) helps to limit the development of tolerance, even though in theory it may perpetuate phobic beliefs. This method probably commits the patient to long-term use and an enduring risk of escalation.

Treating alcohol-dependent patients with antipsychotic medication when there is no psychotic illness may increase their drinking and should be avoided.(69,70)

Residential and inpatient treatment

It is debatable whether a period of inpatient treatment can improve the eventual outcome. Some studies have compared outcomes after patients have been randomly allocated to either inpatient or outpatient treatment. Usually no difference has been found. However, the interpretation of these results and their extrapolation to clinical reality has been debated. Finney *et al.*(71) concluded that the studies often lacked statistical power. Furthermore, the more seriously affected patients had sometimes been excluded before randomization.(72,73) While evidence that it is inpatient treatment rather than intensity of treatment which improves outcome is lacking,(74,75) admission to hospital can provide valuable respite for the drinker and the family when life is severely disorganized because drinking is out of control. Perhaps such respite need not be offered in a relatively expensive medical environment. However, if the patient has become suicidal as difficulties increase or has developed serious medical complications, then hospital admission may be indicated, ideally to specialized facilities. Longer stays in hospital are not supported by research. For example, Trent[76] found no evidence of worse outcome when the United States Navy reduced the length of its inpatient alcoholism treatment programme from 6 to 4 weeks. The role of inpatient treatment is considered further in Chapter 4.2.2.5.

Matching patients to treatments

It is recognized that people with alcohol dependence present a range of problems, come from various backgrounds, and have different personality characteristics. Some have no accompanying emotional disturbance; others have a psychiatric disorder. The poor outcomes of treatment for alcohol dependence have been attributed to their use with unsuitable patient, and better matching of patients to treatments has been sought. A North American study of 1726 outpatients (Project MATCH) set out to test hypotheses about matching treatments to patients. Three treatments were studied, each established in previous randomized controlled trials as more effective than 'supportive therapy': motivational enhancement therapy, cognitive behavioural therapy, and instruction in the AA approach with encouragement to take part in AA meetings ('12-step facilitation').

Few matching effects reached statistical significance. In patients recruited from outpatient clinics, those who scored high on anger at initial assessment averaged 85 per cent of abstinent days if they had been allocated to motivational enhancement therapy compared with 75 per cent if they had been allocated to 12-step facilitation or cognitive behavioural therapy.[77] In the first year of follow-up, patients with initially less severe psychiatric symptoms had more abstinent days after the 12-step facilitation than after cognitive behavioural therapy. Patients with critically high psychiatric severity did no better with cognitive behavioural therapy.[77]

Another marker of who benefits most from AA emerged in the 3-year Project MATCH data. Patients who came from a social milieu where they mixed a lot with other drinkers owing to family, neighbourhood, or work influences did better if they had received 12-step facilitation than with either cognitive behavioural therapy or motivational enhancement therapy.[34]

There are several reasons for the absence of evidence of other powerful predictors of treatment outcome in the Project MATCH data. Perhaps the key behaviour—not taking the first drink—can be arrived at in different ways.

Some clinical situations

Morbid jealousy

This is discussed in Chapter 4.4.

The homeless alcohol-dependent person

It is difficult to conduct randomized controlled studies with adequate follow-up to test the efficacy of interventions to reduce drinking and improve social conditions for the homeless, and few answers have been found. A brief hospital admission to 'dry out' and assessment for transfer to residential care may result in transient improvement in physical health and is more humane than prison. However, supporting evidence is lacking. The structured intensive outpatient intervention, 'community reinforcement approach', has been shown in a North American study to reduce drinking (corroborated by improvement in serum γ-glutamyl transferase) and increase the number of clients at work and in satisfactory housing.[78] The community reinforcement approach combined an offer of free housing, a place at a 'job club' to assist with finding employment, training in problem-solving skills, communication, goal-setting, refusal of drinks, and independent living. Patients had access to an alcohol-free social club. The housing offer was contingent on sobriety and some evidence of saving money. Continuation in the housing was contingent on sobriety checked by breathalyser. Disulfiram had been shown to improve the effects of the community reinforcement approach.[15,79]

Young people

There is a dearth of evaluation of programmes to help young people with alcohol problems. AA groups may have teenage members. When education or employment is in jeopardy, young people may accept disulfiram, supervised perhaps by the family. However, without the support of a non-drinking peer group (which they would have in AA), most young people will try again and again to resume 'social drinking'. Job or marriage commitments sometimes alter the pay-off matrix sufficiently for recovery to be sustained. Otherwise, it may not be until age 30 that the young person is sufficiently convinced that he or she cannot control drinking and takes serious steps to seek help.

Employment referrals

It is common for individuals to seek help when their drinking has put their job in jeopardy. Having a job helps recovery, and for the person to lose employment while paying only lip-service to treatment is common and disheartening for all. The psychiatrist should find out whether disciplinary procedures are in motion or threatened. It can be helpful if the psychiatrist and the patient are told this directly by the employer. If the consultation is part of an undertaking under a company 'alcohol and drugs policy', the patient may have given permission for the psychiatrist to answer the employer's request to know whether he or she is attending and following advice.

Patients who are on the point of dismissal may offer to take disulfiram supervised in the company's occupational health or welfare department. This can bring about recovery and employment for as long as the threat of dismissal remains, and sometimes afterwards.[80]

The liver transplant candidate

Some transplant centres require a demonstration of months of abstinence, to show commitment, before offering transplant to a patient with alcoholic liver disorder. Other centres have no such restrictions. From 6 to 80 per cent of transplant recipients, varying between centres, have recommenced drinking and exceeded safe limits by the end of the first year. Their eventual outcome in terms of quality of life and psychiatric health is no worse than for other transplant patients, and there is no evidence to support demanding lengthy preoperative abstinence. However, patients who relapse to problematic drinking are more likely to have had a history of definite alcohol dependence, and/or depressive illness.[81,82]

Physicians as patients

Alcohol dependence is commoner among doctors than among most other occupational groups, other than those groups who are employed in the alcohol beverage manufacturing or retailing. Doctors' outcome, once in treatment, tends to be good if they can return to their practice. This is probably partly due to the requirement by the licensing body that 'impaired physicians' accept monitoring by an independent specialist to corroborate that they are following advice and continuing to progress.[83,84]

Doctors' reluctance to accept help for their illnesses, and their tendency to treat themselves, is well known and true for substance misuse. Initial denial often means that problems escalate until there are disciplinary or Court proceedings and attempts to treat their own alcohol dependence may result in dependence on other substances. In some instances, where there is any risk to safety of the doctor's patients, the professional licensing body should be informed if not already involved.

The alcoholic doctor should be treated in the same way as a lay person. The partner should be invited to the interview. Ideally, information should be obtained from the employer or from a colleague about the nature of any problems at work or any disciplinary action, actual or threatened.

In some countries there are support groups for recovering doctors and dentists who meet together and are ready to offer advice and encouragement to individuals and their families.

Follow-up

Systematic follow-up has been shown to improve outcomes.[17,85] Early detection of relapse is important, and is aided by regular contact with the family or the workplace, a breathalyser test at interview, and tests for blood markers of drinking (γ-glutamyl transferase or carbohydrate-deficient transferrin).[86] Objective markers are required when a patient requests a report for a Court, the driving licence authority, or an employer.

Some guiding principles

Research into alcoholism spanning 50 years has shown that the attitudes of the agency and the therapist influence patients' outcome, as they may do for many illnesses. The therapeutic alliance is a strong predictor of outcome in the treatment of alcohol dependence.[87] However, agencies must also be prepared to set limits on drunken behaviour at the clinic and telephone calls when intoxicated. And for patients who repeatedly relapse, resumption of treatment should sometimes be made conditional on complying with a new treatment plan, such as supervision of medication.[88]

Showing respect, enhancing dignity, conveying accurate empathy, adopting objective and not moral criteria, involving the family, and reducing hurdles to seeking help have been shown to improve compliance, and often outcome, for alcohol dependence.

Further information

http://www.niaaa.nih.gov/Publications/AlcoholResearch/

References

1. Vaillant, G. (1997). *The natural history of alcoholism revisited*. Harvard University Press, Boston, MA.
2. O'Brien, C.P. and McLellan, A.T. (1996). Myths about the treatment of addiction. *Lancet*, **347**, 237–40.
3. Miller, W.R. and Rollnick, N. (2002). *Motivational interviewing* (2nd edn). Guilford Press, New York.
4. Hayashida, M., Alterman, A.I., McLellan, T., *et al.* (1989). Comparative effectiveness and costs of inpatient and outpatient detoxification with mild-moderate alcohol withdrawal syndrome. *The New England Journal of Medicine*, **320**, 358–65.
5. Bennie, C. (1998). A comparison of home detoxification and minimal intervention strategies for problem drinkers. *Alcohol and Alcoholism*, **33**, 157–63.
6. Mayo-Smith, M.F., for the American Society for Addiction Medicine Working Group. (1997). Pharmacological management of alcohol withdrawal: a meta-analysis and evidence-based practice guideline. *The Journal of the American Medical Association*, **278**, 144–61.
7. Foy, A., March, S., and Drinkwater, V. (1988). Use of an objective clinical scale in the assessment and management of alcohol withdrawal in a large general hospital. *Alcoholism, Clinical and Experimental Research*, **12**, 360–4.
8. Thomson, A.D. and Marshall, J. (2006). The treatment of patients at risk of developing Wernicke's encephalopathy in the community. *Alcohol and Alcoholism*, **41**, 159–67.
9. Vaillant, G.E. (1991). An alternative to psychotherapy. In *The international handbook of addiction behaviour* (ed. I.B. Glass), pp. 236–9. Routledge, London.
10. Raistrick, D., Heather, N., and Godfrey, C. (2006). *Review of the effectiveness of treatment for alcohol problems (full report for the (English)) NHS: National Treatment Agency for Substance Misuse*, http://www.nta.nhs.uk/publications/documents/nta_review_of_the_effectiveness_of_treatment_for_alcohol_problems_fullreport
11. Slattery, J., Chick, J., Craig, J., *et al.* (2003). *Prevention of relapse in alcohol dependence*, www.docs.scottishmedicines.org/docs/pdf/Alcohol%20Report.pdf
12. Berglund, M., Thelander, S., Salaspuro, M., *et al.* (2003). Treatment of alcohol abuse: an evidence-based review. *Alcoholism, Clinical and Experimental Research*, **27**, 1645–56.
13. Monti, P.M., Kadden, R.M., Rohsenow, D.J., *et al.* (2002). *Treating alcohol dependence: a coping skills training guide* (2nd edn). Guilford Press, New York.
14. Miller, W.R., Benfield, R.G., and Tonnegan, J.S. (1993). Enhancing motivation for change in problem drinkers: a comparative outcome study of three controlled drinking therapies. *Journal of Consulting and Clinical Psychology*, **61**, 455–61.
15. Azrin, N.H. (1976). Improvements in the community reinforcement approach to alcoholism. *Behavioural Research and Therapy*,**14**, 339–48.
16. O'Farrell, T.J., Choquette, K.A., and Cutter, H.S.G. (1998). Couples relapse prevention sessions after behavioural marital therapy for male alcoholics: outcomes during the three years after starting treatment. *Journal of Studies on Alcohol*, **59**, 357–70.
17. Chick, J., Connaughton, J., Ritson, B., *et al.* (1988). Advice versus extended treatment for alcoholism: a controlled study. *British Journal of Addiction*, **83**, 159–70.
18. Helzer, J.E., Robins, L.N., Taylor, J.R., *et al.* (1985). The extent of long-term moderate drinking among alcoholics discharged from medical and psychiatric treatment facilities. *The New England Journal of Medicine*, **312**, 1678–82.
19. Vaillant, G.E. (1996). A long-term follow-up of male alcohol abuse. *Archives of General Psychiatry*, **53**, 243–9.
20. Rychtarik, R.G., Foy, D.W., Scott, T., *et al.* (1987). Five year follow-up of broad spectrum behavioral treatment for alcoholism: effects of training controlled drinking skills. *Journal of Consulting and Clinical Psychology*, **55**, 106–8.
21. Sanchez-Craig, M., Leigh, G., Spivak, K., *et al.* (1989). Superior outcome of females over males after brief intervention for the reduction of heavy drinking. *British Journal of Addiction*, **84**, 395–404.

22. WHO Brief Intervention Group. (1996). A cross-national trial of brief intervention with heavy drinkers. *American Journal of Public Health*, **86**, 948–55.
23. Bien, T.H., Miller, W.R., and Tonigan, J.S. (1993). Brief interventions for alcohol problems: a review. *Addiction*, **88**, 315–36.
24. Project MATCH Research Group. (1997). Matching alcoholism treatments to client heterogeneity: project MATCH posttreatment drinking outcomes. *Journal of Studies on Alcohol*, **58**, 7–29.
25. Bien, T.H., Miller, W.R., and Boroughs, J.M. (1993). Motivational interviewing with alcoholic out-patients. *Behavioural and Cognitive Psychotherapy*, **21**, 347–56.
26. Miller, W.R., Zweben, A., DiClementi, C.C., *et al.* (1992). *Motivational enhancement therapy manual: a clinical research guide for therapists treating individuals with alcohol abuse and dependence*. NIAAA Project MATCH Monograph Series, Vol. 2. DHHS Publication No. (ADM) 92-1894. US Government Printing Office, Washington, DC.
27. Prochaska, J. and Di Clemente, C. (1992). Stages of change in the modification of problem behaviors. In *Progress in behavior modification*, Vol. 28 (eds. M. Hersen, R. Eisler, and P. Miller), pp. 183–218. Sycamore Publishing, Sycamore, IL.
28. Chick, J. (1998). Treatment of alcoholic violent offenders—ethics and efficacy. *Alcohol and Alcoholism*, **33**, 20–5.
29. Hall, S.M., Havassy, B.E., and Wasserman, D.A. (1990). Commitment to abstinence and acute stress in relapse to alcohol, opiates and nicotine. *Journal of Consulting and Clinical Psychology*, **58**, 175–81.
30. Drummond, C. and Glautier, S. (1994). A controlled trial of cue exposure treatment in alcohol dependence. *Journal of Consulting and Clinical Psychology*, **62**, 809–17.
31. Oiumette, P.C., Finney, J.W., and Moos, R.H. (1997). Twelve-step and cognitive–behavioural treatment for substance abuse: a comparison of treatment effectiveness. *Journal of Consulting and Clinical Psychology*, **65**, 230–40.
32. Suire, J.G. and Bothwell, R.K. (2006). The psychosocial benefits of alcoholics anonymous. *American Journal of Addiction*, **15**, 252–5.
33. Keso, L. and Salaspuro, M. (1990). In-patient treatment of employed alcoholics: a randomised clinical trial of Hazelden-type and traditional treatment. *Alcoholism, Clinical and Experimental Research*, **14**, 584–9.
34. Longabaugh, R., Wirtz, P.W., Zweben, A., *et al.* (1998). Network support for drinking: alcoholics anonymous and long-term matching effects. *Addiction*, **93**, 1313–34.
35. O'Farrell, T.J. (1995). Marital and family therapy. In *Handbook of alcoholism treatment approaches* (eds. R.K. Hester and W.R. Miller), pp. 195–220. Allyn and Bacon, Boston, MA.
36. O'Farrell, T.J., Choquette, K.A., and Cutter, H.S.G. (1998). Couples relapse prevention sessions after behavioural marital therapy for male alcoholics: outcomes during the three years after starting treatment. *Journal of Studies on Alcohol*, **59**, 357–70.
37. Chick, J. (1998). Safety aspects of disulfiram in the treatment of alcohol dependence. *Drug Safety*, **20**, 427–35.
38. Larson, E.W., Olincy, A., Rummans, T.A., *et al.* (1992). Disulfiram treatment of patients with both alcohol dependence and other psychiatric disorders: a review. *Alcoholism, Clinical and Experimental Research*, **16**, 125–30.
39. De Sousa, A. and De Sousa, A. (2005). An open randomized study comparing disulfiram and acamprosate in the treatment of alcohol dependence. *Alcohol and Alcoholism*, **40**, 545–8.
40. De Sousa, A. and De Sousa, A. (2004). A one-year pragmatic trial of naltrexone versus disulfiram in the treatment of alcohol dependence. *Alcohol and Alcoholism*, **39**, 528–31.
41. Krampe, H., Stawicki, S., Wagner, T.Y., *et al.* (2006). Follow-up of 180 alcoholic patients for up to 7 years after outpatient treatment: impact of alcohol deterrents on outcome. *Alcoholism, Clinical and Experimental Research*, **30**, 86–95.
42. Littleton, J. (1995). Acamprosate in alcohol dependence: how does it work? *Addiction*, **90**, 1179–88.
43. Bouza, C., Magro, A., Munoz, A., *et al.* (2004). Efficacy and safety of naltrexone and acamprosate in the treatment of alcohol dependence: a systematic review. *Addiction*, **99**, 811–28.
44. Chick, J., Lehert, P., and Landron, F. (2003). Does acamprosate improve reduction of drinking as well as aiding abstinence? *Journal of Psychopharmacology*, **17**, 387–92.
45. Besson, J., Aeby, F., Kasas, A., *et al.* (1998). Combined efficacy of acamprosate and disulfiram in the treatment of alcoholism: a controlled study. *Alcoholism, Clinical and Experimental Research*, **22**, 573–9.
46. Gianoulakis, C., Krishnan, B., and Thavundayil, J. (1996). Enhanced sensitivity of pituitary β-endorphin to ethanol in subjects at high risk of alcoholism. *Archives of General Psychiatry*, **53**, 250–7.
47. Volpicelli, J.R., Alterman, A.I., Hayashida, M., *et al.* (1992). Naltrexone in the treatment of alcohol dependence. *Archives of General Psychiatry*, **49**, 876–80.
48. O'Malley, S., Jaffe, A.J., Chang, G., *et al.* (1992). Naltrexone and coping skills therapy for alcohol dependence. *Archives of General Psychiatry*, **49**, 881–7.
49. Garbutt, J.C., Kranzler, H.R., O'Malley, S.S., *et al.* (2005). Efficacy and tolerability of long-acting injectable naltrexone for alcohol dependence: a randomized controlled trial. *The Journal of the American Medical Association*, **293**, 1617–25. [Erratum in *JAMA* 2005;293:1978; *JAMA* 2005;293:2864.]
50. Doty, P. and de Wit, H. (1995). Effects of naltrexone pretreatment on the subjective and performance effects of ethanol in social drinkers. *Behavioural Pharmacology*, **6**, 386–94.
51. Baros, A.M., Latham, P.K., Moak, D.H., *et al.* (2007). What role does measuring medication compliance play in evaluating the efficacy of naltrexone? *Alcoholism, Clinical and Experimental Research*, **31**, 596–603.
52. Anton, R.F., O'Malley, S.S., Ciraulo, D.A., *et al.* (2006). Combined pharmacotherapies and behavioral interventions for alcohol dependence: the COMBINE Study: a randomized controlled trial. *The Journal of the American Medical Association*, **295**, 2003–17.
53. Morley, K.C., Teesson, M., Reid, S.C., *et al.* (2006). Naltrexone versus acamprosate in the treatment of alcohol dependence: a multi-centre, randomized, double-blind, placebo-controlled trial. *Addiction*, **101**, 1451–62.
54. Kiefer, F., Jahn, H., Tarnaske, T., *et al.* (2003). Comparing and combining naltrexone and acamprosate in relapse prevention of alcoholism. *Archives of General Psychiatry*, **60**, 92–99.
55. Heinala, P., Alho, H., Kiianmaa, K., *et al.* (2001). Targeted use of naltrexone without prior detoxification in the treatment of alcohol dependence: a factorial double-blind, placebo-controlled trial. *Journal of Clinical Psychopharmacology*, **21**, 287–92.
56. Karhuvaara, S., Simojoki, K., Virta, A., *et al.* (2007). Targeted nalmefene with simple medical management in the treatment of heavy drinkers: a randomized double-blind placebo-controlled multicenter study. *Alcoholism, Clinical and Experimental Research*, **31**, 1179–87.
57. Jeffers, S. (1987). *Feel the fear and do it anyway*. Century Hutchinson, London.
58. McGrath, P.J., Nunes, E.V., Stewart, J.W., *et al.* (1996). Imipramine treatment of alcoholics with primary depression: a placebo controlled clinical trial. *Archives of General Psychiatry*, **53**, 232–40.
59. Cornelius, J.R., Salloun, I.M., Ehler, J.G., *et al.* (1997). Fluoxetine reduced depressive symptoms and alcohol consumption in patients with comorbid major depression and alcohol dependence. *Archives of General Psychiatry*, **54**, 700–5.
60. Kranzler, H.R., Burleson, J.A., Brown, J., *et al.* (1996). Fluoxetine treatment seems to reduce the beneficial effects of cognitive-behavioral therapy in type B alcoholics. *Alcoholism, Clinical and Experimental Research*, **20**, 1534–41.

61. Chick, J., Aschauer, H., and Hornik, K. (2004). Efficacy of fluvoxamine in preventing relapse in alcohol dependence: a one-year, double blind, placebo-controlled multicentre study with analysis by typology. *Drug and Alcohol Dependence*, **74**, 61–70.
62. Willinger, U., Lenzinger, E., Hornik, K., *et al.* (2002). Anxiety as a predictor of relapse in detoxified alcohol-dependent patients. *Alcohol and Alcoholism*, **37**, 609–12.
63. Driessen, M., Meier, S., Hill, A., *et al.* (2001). The course of anxiety, depression and drinking behaviours after completed detoxification in alcoholics with and without comorbid anxiety and depressive. *Alcohol and Alcoholism*, **36**, 249–55.
64. Allan, C.A., Smith, I., and Mellin, M. (2002). Changes in psychological symptoms during ambulant detoxification. *Alcohol and Alcoholism*, **37**, 241–4.
65. Bowen, R.C., D'Arcy, C., Keegan, D., *et al.* (2000). A controlled trial of cognitive behavioral treatment of panic in alcoholic inpatients with comorbid panic disorder. *Addictive Behaviors*, **25**, 593–7.
66. Randall, C.L., Thomas, S., and Thevos, A.K. (2001). Concurrent alcoholism and social anxiety disorder: a first step toward developing effective treatments. *Alcoholism, Clinical and Experimental Research*, **25**, 210–20.
67. Thevos, A.K., Roberts, J.S., Thomas, S.E., *et al.* (2000). Cognitive behavioral therapy delays relapse in female socially phobic alcoholics. *Addictive Behaviors*, **25**, 333–45.
68. Kranzler, H.R., Burleson, J.A., Boca, F.K., *et al.* (1994). Buspirone treatment of anxious alcoholics. *Archives of General Psychiatry*, **51**, 720–31.
69. Guardia, J., Segura, L., Gonzalvo, B., *et al.* (2004). A double-blind, placebo-controlled study of olanzapine in the treatment of alcohol-dependence disorder. *Alcoholism, Clinical and Experimental Research*, **28**, 736–45.
70. Wiesbeck, G.A., Weijers, H.-G., Lesch, O.M., *et al.* (2001). Flupenthixol decanoate and relapse prevention in alcoholics: results from a placebo-controlled study. *Alcohol and Alcoholism*, **36**, 329–34.
71. Finney, J., Hahn, A.C., and Moos, R.H. (1996). The effectiveness of inpatient and outpatient treatment for alcohol abuse: the need to focus on mediators and moderators of setting effect. *Addiction*, **91**, 1773–96.
72. Schuckit, M. (1998). Penny-wise, ton-foolish? The recent movement to abolish inpatient alcohol and drug treatment. *Journal of Studies on Alcohol*, **59**, 5–6.
73. Mattick, R.P. and Jarvis, T. (1994). Inpatient setting and long duration for the treatment of alcohol dependence? Outpatient care is as good. *Drug and Alcohol Review*, **13**, 127–35.
74. Annis, H.M. (1996). Inpatient versus outpatient setting effects in alcoholism treatment: revisiting the evidence. *Addiction*, **91**, 1804–7.
75. Rychtarik, R.G., Connors, G.J., Whitney, R.B., *et al.* (2000). Treatment settings for persons with alcoholism: evidence for matching clients to inpatient versus outpatient care. *Journal of Consulting and Clinical Psychology*, **68**, 277–89.
76. Trent, L.K. (1998). Evaluation of a four—versus six-week length of stay in the Navy's alcohol treatment program. *Journal of Studies on Alcohol*, **59**, 270–9.
77. Project MATCH Research Group. (1997). Project MATCH secondary a priori hypotheses. *Addiction*, **92**, 1671–98.
78. Smith, J.E., Meyers, R.I., and Delaney, H.D. (1998). The community reinforcement approach with homeless alcohol-dependent individuals. *Journal of Consulting and Clinical Psychology*, **66**, 541–8.
79. Azrin, N.H., Sisson, R.W., Meyers, R., *et al.* (1982). Alcoholism treatment by disulfiram and community reinforcement therapy. *Journal of Behavior Therapy and Experimental Psychiatry*, **13**, 105–12.
80. Robichaud, C., Strickland, D., Bigelow, G., *et al.* (1979). Disulfiram maintenance employee alcoholism treatment: a three phase treatment. *Behaviour Research and Therapy*, **17**, 618–21.
81. Kelly, M., Chick, J., Gribble, R., *et al.* (2006). Predictors of relapse to harmful alcohol consumption after orthotopic liver transplantation. *Alcohol and Alcoholism*, **41**, 278–83.
82. McCallum, S. and Masterton, G. (2006). Liver transplantation for alcoholic liver disease: a systematic review of psychosocial selection criteria. *Alcohol and Alcoholism*, **41**, 358–63.
83. Shore, J.H. (1987). The Oregon experience with impaired physicians: an eight year follow-up. *The Journal of the American Medical Association*, **257**, 2931–4.
84. Fowlie, D.G. (1999). The misuse of alcohol and other drugs by doctors: a UK report and one region's response. *Alcohol and Alcoholism*, **34**, 666–71.
85. Ahles, T.A., Schlundt, D.G., Prue, D.M., *et al.* (1983). Impact of aftercare arrangements on the maintenance of treatment success in abusive drinkers. *Addictive Behaviours*, **8**, 53–8.
86. Reynauld, M., Hourcade, F., Planche, F., *et al.* (1998). Usefulness of carbohydrate–deficient transferrin in alcoholic patients with normal gamma-glutamyl transferase. *Alcoholism, Clinical and Experimental Research*, **22**, 615–18.
87. Connors, G.J., Carroll, K.M., DiClemente, C.C., *et al.* (1997). The therapeutic alliance and its relationship to alcoholism treatment participation and outcome. *Journal of Consulting and Clinical Psychology*, **65**, 588–98.
88. Sereny, G., Sharma, V., Holt, S., *et al.* (1986). Mandatory supervised antabuse therapy in an out-patient alcoholism program: a pilot study. *Alcoholism, Clinical and Experimental Research*, **10**, 290–2.

4.2.2.5 **Services for alcohol use disorders**

D. Colin Drummond

A spectrum of disorders needing a range of services

The provision of services for alcohol use disorders has been driven by the prevailing view of their nature and prevalence. Following the Second World War, the disease concept of alcoholism gained increasing support in both the United States (US) and the United Kingdom (UK).[1] According to this concept, alcoholism is an all-or-nothing phenomenon affecting a relatively small subgroup of the population, and requires intensive specialist treatment. In the UK this led to the development of specialist alcohol treatment centres with an emphasis on intensive inpatient treatment involving group therapy, often with close affiliation to the Alcoholics Anonymous (**AA**) fellowship. Such programmes tended to be targeted at relatively socially stable men, and catering for the more severely alcohol dependent.[2]

In the 1970s and 1980s came a recognition that there existed a much wider range of alcohol-related problems in the population than would meet the narrow criteria of alcoholism or alcohol dependence, but which might nevertheless benefit from intervention. Research began to show that alcohol problems existed on a continuum of severity and thus might not necessarily require intensive specialist treatment with a lifelong goal of complete abstinence from alcohol. Screening and brief intervention with presymptomatic heavy drinkers in the primary care or general hospital medical ward setting could be effective in reducing excessive alcohol consumption and alcohol-related harm.[3,4] This led to the proposal that greater benefit could be accrued from less intensive approaches aimed at the large number of hazardous drinkers, than more intensive and expensive interventions catering for the minority of very heavy drinkers: the 'preventive paradox'.[5]

In a ground-breaking report, the US Institute of Medicine advocated 'broadening the base of treatment for alcohol problems'.[6] Recognizing the potential for increased prevention and treatment activity in health care personnel without specialist addiction training (e.g. general practitioners, physicians, social workers), and the limitations of expanding specialist treatment given the high prevalence of alcohol misuse, the report emphasized the need for an expanded range of locations and methods of intervention, across the spectrum of alcohol use disorders (see Fig. 4.2.2.5.1). Importantly however, the report also recognized that alcohol use disorders are heterogeneous, and different types of disorders are likely to require different types or intensities of treatment, that is, the need to match treatments to the nature of the presenting problem.

Since this report there has been some progress made towards increasing the range and accessibility of treatment. However, in some cases this has been disappointing. This chapter describes the range and organization of treatment approaches and explores the barriers to implementation of a comprehensive system of care for alcohol use disorders. The evidence suggests that we have a long way to go to deliver an optimal level of access to alcohol treatment for those in need. The evidence on the cost-effectiveness of alcohol treatment is discussed, and consideration is given to the needs of special groups in the population who may find access to treatment more difficult. The main conclusion is that on the basis of the existing research evidence there remain considerable opportunities to expand and improve treatment services for alcohol use disorders. This will require further training and dissemination initiatives and the political will and funding to achieve this throughout the health system.

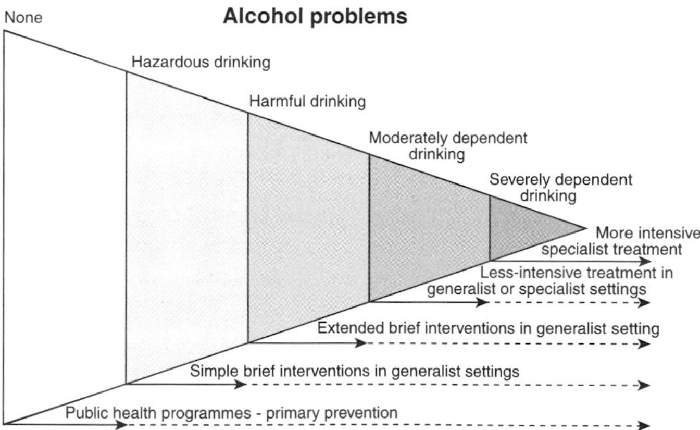

Fig. 4.2.2.5.1 A spectrum of responses to alcohol problems. (Reprinted from D. Raistrick, N. Heather, and C. Godfrey, (2006), *Review of the effectiveness of treatment for alcohol problems*, National Treatment Agency for Substance Misuse, London © 2001–2008 National Treatment Agency.) The triangle represents the general population, with the spectrum of alcohol problems experienced by the population shown along the upper side of the figure. Responses to these problems are shown along the lower side. The dotted lines suggest that primary prevention, simple brief intervention, extended brief intervention and less-intensive treatment may have effects beyond their main target area. Although the figure is not drawn to scale, the prevalence in the population of each of the categories of alcohol problem is approximated by the area of the triangle occupied; most people have no alcohol problems, a very large number show risky consumption but no current problems, many have risky consumption and less serious alcohol problems, some have moderate dependence and problems and a few have severe dependence or complicated alcohol problems.

Location and intensity of treatment

Brief interventions

There has been considerable research interest in the potential of brief interventions in primary care, and to a lesser extent in the general hospital.[7] There are several potential advantages in conducting treatment interventions in primary care. Patients with alcohol use disorders consult their general practitioner more frequently than other patients. Excessive drinkers identified by screening in primary care are largely at an earlier stage in their drinking career and are potentially more likely to benefit from brief early intervention than more severely dependent drinkers presenting to specialist treatment services. Further, primary care is often seen as less stigmatizing than a specialist clinic. Brief interventions typically involve opportunistic screening using tools such as the AUDIT questionnaire[8] or other shorter variants,[9] followed by 5–30 min. of brief intervention conducted by a practitioner who does not have training in specialist alcohol treatment.

Several studies have demonstrated the effectiveness of screening and brief intervention in hazardous drinkers in primary care. In a large randomized controlled trial, Wallace *et al.*[4] found that brief intervention was more effective than a control treatment in reducing alcohol consumption and γ-glutamyl transferase at 1-year follow-up. Similar findings were obtained in a large World Health Organization multicentre trial.[10]

Fewer screening and brief intervention studies have been conducted in the general hospital setting. A recent meta-analysis of this literature showed no difference between intervention and control in this setting.[11] However, some recent studies have shown benefits of screening and brief intervention in accident and emergency departments. One UK study showed reduced alcohol consumption and fewer reattendances in A&E attenders identified by screening and referred to an alcohol health worker.[12] Another UK study in young men with alcohol-related facial injuries found that brief intervention significantly reduced alcohol consumption and alcohol-related problems.[13]

Meta-analyses of brief interventions have mostly found advantages of brief intervention over control treatments with effect sizes of 10–20 per cent on reduced alcohol consumption at 1 year.[14–16] Some earlier reviews concluded that brief interventions are at least as effective as more intensive specialist treatments. However, the populations studied in brief intervention trials are heterogeneous.[17] Most trials have been conducted with opportunistic screening in non-treatment seeking populations in primary care. A smaller number have compared brief interventions to more intensive treatments in specialist alcohol treatment settings. A recent review found that brief interventions are effective only in less severe alcohol disorders in the context of opportunistic screening.[15]

There are barriers to implementation of brief intervention in non-specialist settings, which may limit its effectiveness. In a UK national survey,[18,19] it was found that general practitioners and primary care practice nurses were reluctant to engage in screening and brief interventions because of a perceived lack of training and support to carry-out this work. Effective implementation of large-scale screening and brief intervention programmes will require attention to the training and support needs of non-specialist personnel. Further, screening programmes will identify more severely alcohol dependent drinkers who may not respond to brief interventions alone. Thus, effective working arrangements between generalists and specialists are needed. Drummond[20] has also questioned the generalizability of brief intervention research findings in the typical clinical setting, given the large number of exclusions in research studies and a lack of pragmatic trials.

Specialist treatment in inpatient settings

The main treatment response to alcohol use disorders continues to be delivered by specialists, although this is mostly delivered in the community rather than in inpatient settings. There has been extensive research on the location and intensity of specialist treatment. An early influential study was that of Edwards *et al.*[21] in which 100 alcohol-dependent men referred to the Maudsley Hospital in London were randomized to receive either intensive specialist treatment, including specialist inpatient care, or a single session of counselling. At 1-year follow-up there was no difference in outcome between the two treatments. It was concluded that the reliance on intensive treatments up to that time was called into question by the findings. This controversial study gave rise to considerable debate and several studies have subsequently investigated the same issues. Another British study attempted to replicate the Edwards study and found only modest differences between advice only and extended treatment in a randomized controlled trial at 2 years' follow-up.[22] There were, however, no differences between treatments in abstinence rates or alcohol consumption level during follow-up. However, a later follow-up of the Edwards cohort found that more severely dependent drinkers benefited more from intensive treatment.[23]

In a larger study in the US, employees who were identified as drinking excessively were randomized to one of the three options: compulsory inpatient treatment, compulsory AA attendance, or a choice of these two options.[24] At 2-year follow-up there were no differences between the groups in terms of work-related outcome measures. However, drinking-related measures the inpatient group had the best, and the AA group the poorest outcome, with the choice group having an intermediate outcome. The compulsory AA group was more likely than the others to require subsequent inpatient treatment. However, the length of inpatient treatment does not appear to influence outcome significantly.[25,26]

Studies comparing inpatient versus outpatient alcohol detoxification have generally found the two approaches to be equally effective. For example, Hayashida *et al.*[27] randomized male military veterans to inpatient and outpatient detoxification. At 6 months' follow-up no differences in outcome were found between the two groups. Indeed, outpatient detoxification is generally regarded as the treatment of choice for the majority of patients. It should be noted, however, that studies comparing inpatient and outpatient treatment (including detoxification) have tended to exclude patients with particularly poor prognosis (e.g. poor social circumstances, severe psychiatric or physical comorbidity, those at risk of harm to themselves or others). Hence, the clinician needs to interpret the research evidence with caution in applying it to patients in the typical clinical setting. However, it is probably safe to assume that in less complicated alcohol dependence there is no evidence of an advantage of inpatient over outpatient treatment.

A recent randomized trial by Rychartic *et al.*[28] assigned alcohol dependent patients to inpatient, intensive outpatient, or standard outpatient treatment. Following treatment inpatients had reduced jail and subsequent inpatient episodes, and those with greater alcohol dependence or impaired cognitive function had better outcomes with inpatient treatment.

Overall, the majority of studies that have compared intensive specialist treatment with less intensive treatment have not supported the use of more intensive approaches. However, most of these studies excluded patients with more complex needs. Few studies have examined the interaction between treatment setting and problem severity. The emerging evidence now is that alcohol dependent patients with more complex needs (more severe alcohol dependence, psychiatric comorbidity, cognitive impairment, poor social circumstances, or support) are more likely to benefit from inpatient treatment.[9]

Community-based specialist treatments

The growth of studies questioning the value of specialist inpatient treatment and a move towards cost containment in health care have led to a shift in resources to treating alcohol use disorders in community settings. In the US for example 87 per cent of specialist alcohol treatment is delivered on an outpatient basis.[29] A similar survey in England found that 69 per cent of specialist alcohol treatment agencies were community based.[30]

Apart from the potential advantage of lower cost, community-based treatment provides the least social disruption for the individual and offers the opportunity to mobilize existing community resources to support sustained recovery. In the UK, the past 30 years have seen the widespread development of the community alcohol team (CAT) model of treatment following the original Maudsley Alcohol Pilot Project.[31] The main principle of the CAT model is that the specialist multi-disciplinary team (typically consisting of specialist medical, nursing, social work, and psychology staff) work to train and support generic teams, mainly in primary care, to manage alcohol use disorders more effectively. In practice, CATs have tended to find difficulty in avoiding becoming involved in a more traditional specialist role, often providing direct care for alcohol use disorders in the face of reluctance on the part of primary care personnel to take on this work.[32]

There has been remarkably little research conducted to evaluate the CAT model. One study randomly allocated 40 problem drinkers referred to the specialist alcohol treatment clinic at the Maudsley Hospital to receive either routine specialist treatment or 'shared care'.[33] Following specialist assessment, the shared care group was returned to the care of their general practitioner, who was then supported by the specialist CAT. Shared care within this model included advice and training for the general practitioner, a shared treatment plan, regular phone contact between specialist and general practitioner, and the offer of further specialist care should the patient remain unchanged or deteriorate. At 6 months' follow-up the specialist and shared care groups both showed significant improvements, but there was no difference in outcome between the two groups.

Another study in Scotland evaluated the efficacy of a home detoxification service compared with minimal intervention in a randomized controlled trial in 95 patients referred by their general practitioner.[34] At 6 months' follow-up the home detoxification group remained abstinent twice as long after treatment than the minimal intervention group.

The 'community reinforcement approach' has been demonstrated to have benefits in the treatment of alcohol dependence in the US.[35] This approach aims to provide reinforcers for abstinence from alcohol including positive family support, help in finding employment, membership of an alcohol-free social club, and alcohol counselling. The specialist treatment input aims to ensure that these supports are put in place. There is some evidence from small-scale controlled trials[35,36] that this approach is effective in reducing alcohol consumption and improving social adjustment compared to standard treatment, but it has not so far been fully evaluated, and has never been tested in the UK.

Another variant on the CAT approach has been the evaluation of community psychiatric nurse (CPN) aftercare following specialist inpatient treatment.[37] One study in the UK evaluated the effectiveness of regular CPN follow-up consisting of weekly 1 to 2 h visits to the patient's home for a period of 6 weeks post-discharge from inpatient care, followed by less frequent visits up to 1 year. The home-based sessions involved advice, support, counselling, partner involvement, and encouragement to attend AA. This was compared to routine 6-weekly hospital appointments. The study, which involved a non-randomized design, found significant improvements in abstinence and engagement in support in the CPN approach compared to the routine aftercare group.

There is growing interest in the potential application of Assertive Community Treatment (ACT) approaches for alcohol dependence, particularly for patients with more severe, complex and chronic problems who are difficult to engage in standard treatment approaches. This borrows from the experience of ACT in severe mental illness[38] and acknowledges that for some patients, alcohol dependence is a chronic disorder that in these cases may be more suited to a 'disease management' model of care, commonplace in treatment of many physical illnesses such as diabetes or hypertension. Assertive approaches appear promising in alcohol dependence,[39] but a definitive trial of ACT is needed.

In summary, the CAT model of alcohol service delivery has been widely implemented in the UK in advance of clear evidence of its effectiveness. Evidence is emerging showing at least the equivalence, and in some cases, the superiority, of outcome from community-based services compared with more traditional inpatient treatment approaches. However, the CAT approach is implemented in a range of ways in the UK, and encompasses many different models and specific interventions. More research is needed to evaluate the cost-effectiveness of community alcohol team approaches and to identify the specific elements and methods that contribute to treatment effectiveness.

Matching and stepped care

The Institute of Medicine report emphasized the need to match the level of intervention to the severity and nature of the presenting problems.[6] There is some empirical evidence of matching effects in relation to both inpatient and outpatient treatment.[40] Up until recently, however, matching effects have generally been explored in *post hoc* analyses in studies that lacked sufficient statistical power. The Project MATCH study in the US aimed to assess a wide range of matching hypotheses in a prospective design, but found no strong matching effects[42] (see Chapter 4.2.2.4). However, it should be noted that most controlled trials, including MATCH, excluded the more complex patients, including those with limited social support and those with severe psychiatric comorbidity. This tends to work against finding matching effects as the study sample lacked clinical heterogeneity.[43] Further, many of the patient and treatment programme characteristics likely to mediate treatment matching and treatment effectiveness, remain largely unresearched. The matching results of a similar trial in the UK are awaited.[43]

Stepped care is an alternative method of matching treatments to patient needs that has become accepted in the fields of smoking intervention and general medicine. Until now it has received relatively scant attention in the alcohol field. In essence, stepped care involves initially providing relatively low-intensity treatments, and only offering more intensive treatments to those who fail to respond.[44] This provides a potentially resource-efficient means of delivering treatment, and provides clinicians with clinical algorithms. A recent trial of alcohol screening in primary care compared stepped care intervention with minimal 5 min of advice delivered by a practice nurse.[45] In the stepped care group received an initial 40 min session of Behaviour Change Counselling delivered by a trained practice nurse who then followed up the patients (Step 1). Those who did not respond to Step 1 were referred to four sessions of Motivational Enhancement Therapy delivered by trained alcohol counsellors (Step 2). Finally those not responding to Step 2 were referred to more intensive treatment delivered by a CAT (Step 3). The study found no significant difference in alcohol consumption at 6 months, which may in part be due to a small sample size. However, the stepped care intervention was more cost-effective than minimal intervention, mainly through reduced health care and criminal justice costs.

Overall, few community-based studies have found significant treatment matching effects. But this may be in part due to exclusion of the most severe cases. Some studies have found advantages of inpatient compared with community treatment for patients with more severe and complex needs as described above. A more promising approach is stepped care, which is effectively pragmatic matching: that is patients not responding to less intensive treatments receive more intensive treatments. This now forms an important principle of the national framework for alcohol services in England.[46]

Cost-effectiveness of alcohol treatment

With a trend towards containment of health care costs in industrialized societies, there has been an increase in the application of health economic research in the alcohol treatment field. It has been estimated that the annual cost to society of alcohol misuse is in the region of US$184 billion in the US[47] and £20 billion in the UK.[48] In comparison, the direct treatment costs of alcohol use disorders by specialist treatment agencies amounted to approximately US$7.5 billion in the US and about £217 million in the UK.[47,30] Thus there is a need to demonstrate the cost-effectiveness of treatments for alcohol use disorders.

Until recently, research on cost-effectiveness has been largely speculative and not based on direct estimates of cost benefits. In a landmark study, Holder *et al.*[49] provided a 'first approximation' of the cost-effectiveness of treatment. In their analysis they used a combination of findings of efficacy from clinical trials, typical costs of different treatments, and recommendations from experts and treatment providers about appropriate treatment approaches. While noting the lack of studies directly assessing the cost-effectiveness of treatments, they concluded the cost of care was inversely correlated with evidence of effectiveness. They also noted that those treatments with the highest cost and lowest evidence of effectiveness were amongst the most prevalent in the North American treatment system. While this review has been criticized on methodological grounds, it has stimulated an important debate and has contributed to an increasing number of clinical trials including a health economic component in outcome evaluation.

Cost-effectiveness analysis, which takes a societal perspective rather than a narrow intervention cost perspective, provides a better measure of the overall impact of an intervention. These wider costs include patient out-of-pocket costs, lost productivity, unplanned health care utilization (e.g. admissions with alcohol-related physical and mental illnesses, primary care utilization), criminal justice costs, accidents, premature deaths, social work involvement, childcare costs, and costs associated with illnesses in relatives and carers.(50)

Also important in cost-effectiveness analysis is the estimation of improvements in quality of life following an intervention. This is beginning to be studied in the alcohol treatment field. Quality of life can be measured in a variety of ways (e.g. Euroqol, Short Form 36). In a randomized controlled trial an estimate of the difference in Quality Adjusted Life Years (QALYs) can be compared between treatment and control groups. The National Institute of Clinical Excellence (NICE) in the UK determines which treatments should be funded by the National Health Service (NHS) based on the available evidence. NICE regards a net cost per QALY, taking into account the costs of treatment and the savings to society, of £20 000 or less to be the maximum cost acceptable to implement the treatment in the NHS. Alcohol misusers typically have a much lower quality of life than non-alcohol misusers. One study compared quality of life in alcohol dependent drinkers before treatment with controls. Mean quality of life measured by the Euroqol (EQ5D) was 0.57 in the alcohol dependent group compared to age matched controls: 0.9 (1.0 being the best possible quality of life and 0 being death).(43) However, a recent review found that while treatment significantly reduces alcohol consumption and societal costs, it has a limited impact on quality of life.(9)

A recent review of cost-effectiveness examined the available literature on alcohol interventions.(9) In terms of intensive specialist alcohol treatment it was estimated that providing evidence-based alcohol interventions would result in a saving of £5 for the public sector for every £1 spent. However, it was noted that several studies showed an initial increase in costs in people newly entering alcohol treatment. This is likely to be because people not in treatment and in an active drinking phase find it harder to access services, and specialist alcohol services assist patients to address outstanding health and social care needs. Cost savings as a result of treatment therefore need to be examined over the longer term (>1 year). Comparing individual specialist interventions including pharmacotherapies and psychosocial interventions one review found the net health cost per death averted ranged from −£3073 to £2076 for most of the interventions that also provided significant clinical improvements.(51)

There is now good evidence that brief intervention in hazardous/harmful drinkers is highly cost-effective. Fleming *et al.*(52) found that, as well as reducing excessive drinking, there was a reduced length of hospitalization during the 12-month follow-up period. In addition, while brief intervention cost more than minimal intervention, this cost was more than offset by reductions in subsequent health care, criminal justice, and road traffic accident costs (US$56 000 savings per US$10 000 intervention costs). An analysis of several brief intervention studies found the cost per life year gained was approximately £2000, well within the NICE definition.(53)

There is considerable scope for further development of health economic research in the alcohol field. This will prove important in providing health care commissioners with appropriate information to make rational decisions in the provision of cost-effective evidence-based services for alcohol use disorders. (For a further account of cost-effectiveness analysis, see Chapter 7.7.)

The availability of alcohol services

The availability of alcohol services is likely to affect the overall impact of treatment at a whole population level. There is some evidence that the availability of alcohol treatment services is related to the prevalence of alcohol use disorders at a population level. Mann *et al.*(54) found that increased treatment services in Ontario, Canada, were associated with decreased hospital discharges for liver cirrhosis. A similar study in North Carolina examining the 20-year period between 1968 and 1987 found an association between increased alcohol treatment admissions and decreased cirrhosis mortality. Further, Mann *et al.*(55) found a relationship between AA membership and alcohol-related problems including cirrhosis mortality rates in the US, Canada, and other countries. They estimated that a 1 per cent increase in AA membership was associated with a 0.06 per cent decrease in cirrhosis mortality. These studies of course demonstrate associations rather than causal links between treatment availability and prevalence, but do provide support to the hypothesis that access to treatment could have an impact at a population level.

The National Drug and Alcohol Treatment Utilization Survey (**NDATUS**), which is a national census of public and private treatment programmes in the US, provides a unique data set to study treatment availability. It has been conducted intermittently since 1979 and provides a method to study trends over time. An analysis by the Institute of Medicine found large regional variations in the availability of treatment places.(6) There was no association found between treatment place availability and prevalence of alcohol misuse across states in the US. This points to the importance of 'needs assessment' in the rational allocation of public resources to fund treatment services. This involves a variety of data sources as indicators of alcohol use disorder prevalence in a particular locality, including general population surveys, mortality statistics (e.g. deaths from alcoholic liver disease), crime statistics (e.g. public drunkenness and driving whilst intoxicated arrests), and alcohol-related hospital admissions. Such indicators provide measures of relative 'need' in different localities, gaps between need and access to treatment, and can be used to direct resource allocation.

Examining data from NDATUS surveys between 1982 and 1993, Weisner *et al.*(56) found an increase in activity over this period of 147 per cent. In the US the impact of managed care organizations, which aim to limit access to treatment on the basis of individual need and cost, has yet to be fully established in relation to overall access to alcohol services. Such measures are likely to reduce the availability of inpatient services and to reduce the rate of readmission for those with chronic alcohol problems.

A recent national needs assessment in England examined *inter alia* the regional variation in the prevalence of alcohol use disorders and access to specialist alcohol treatment services.[30] The prevalence of alcohol dependence in adults was 3.6 per cent overall (men: 6 per cent; women: 2 per cent), varying from 1.6 per cent to 5.2 per cent across regions. The overall level of access to treatment also varied across regions. In England overall, 1 in 18 people with alcohol dependence gained access to treatment per annum (the Prevalence–Service Utilization Ratio). But this varied from 1 in 12, to 1 in 108 between the best and worst served regions. A ratio of 1 in 10 is regarded as a 'low' level of access and 1 in 5 a 'high' level in North America.[57] Factors associated with better access included a greater number of treatment agencies, greater overall spending on treatment, and shorter waiting times.

Special groups

Specialist alcohol treatment services typically attract younger, male, single patients of lower socio-economic and educational background, with more severe alcohol dependence. Relative to the prevalence of alcohol use disorders in the general population, women, older people, and people from ethnic minorities are typically under-represented, as are the homeless. Further, there are limited specialist alcohol services for young people. This is of particular concern as the prevalence of alcohol use disorders is increasing in young people in the UK.

Women

Thom and Green have identified three main factors that may account for the under-representation of women in alcohol treatment.[58] Women tend to perceive their problems differently from men, less often identifying themselves as 'alcoholic'. This may in part be related to negative public stereotypes of female drinking and negative attitudes towards female problem drinkers amongst professionals. Women have also been found to perceive the 'costs' of entering treatment differently from men. This is particularly in relation to the perceived social stigma as well as other costs, both financial, in relationships, and in terms of losing their children into the care system. Finally, women often find the services offered to be less appropriate in meeting their needs than do men. Often specialist alcohol services do not offer childcare or 'women-only' facilities. However, an increasing number of women are seeking help for alcohol use disorders, both in the US and the UK on the basis of general population surveys and surveys of treatment populations. In England we found that women with alcohol dependence were 1.6 times more likely to access treatment than men.[30] This suggests that some of the barriers to access identified by Thom and Green have been overcome. Nevertheless, more still needs to be done to provide alcohol treatment services that are sensitive to women's needs. Further, there is a need to develop services catering for pregnant women.[59]

Ethnic minority groups

The evidence concerning help-seeking in ethnic minority groups is complex (see Chapter 7.3). Harrison *et al.*[60] have provided a review of the evidence. In the US, Hispanics tend to be under-represented and African–Americans are over-represented in alcohol treatment compared with the general population prevalence. However, interpretation of the evidence is complicated by the fact that household surveys tend to under-represent socially disadvantaged individuals from ethnic minorities. Marmot *et al.*[61] found that cirrhosis mortality rates were elevated compared to the national average for men from the Asian subcontinent and from Ireland, but lower than average for African–Caribbean men. In women, cirrhosis mortality was lower than average in Asian and African–Caribbean women but higher in Irish women. However, there were few cirrhosis deaths in total in ethnic minorities, which may lead to large errors in extrapolation to the whole population alcohol misuse estimates. In terms of alcohol treatment populations, studies have tended to find higher rates of admission (per 100 000 population) in Indian-, Scottish- and Irish-born people than in those born in the Caribbean or Pakistan. Differences in culturally related health beliefs and help-seeking, as well as service factors such as the availability of interpreters or treatment personnel from appropriate ethnic minority groups, may account for some of these differences. There remain few specific services for people from ethnic minorities, although some examples of good practice exist in the UK.[60]

The homeless

There is a high prevalence of alcohol use disorders (as well as mental and physical health and social problems) amongst the homeless population, a group that is not typically well catered for by mainstream alcohol services (see Chapter 7.10.2). The prevalence of alcohol problems in the homeless has been found to be as high as 38 per cent in the UK[62] and between 2 and 86 per cent in the US; typically the prevalence is between 20 and 45 per cent in North American studies.[59] This has contributed to the development of specific alcohol services for the homeless and street drinkers, notably 'wet' hostels. In the 'wet' hostel, residents are able to continue drinking but are cared for in an environment that is designed to minimize the harm associated with heavy drinking and to tackle issues associated with homelessness.[59,62] Such facilities tend to be restricted to large urban centres and have restricted places compared to the number of street drinkers. Similarly, outreach services and 'crisis centres' have been developed to attract alcohol-misusing homeless people into treatment facilities.[63] Often those entering 'wet' hostels can subsequently be persuaded to undergo alcohol detoxification and progress to 'dry' (or alcohol-free) supported accommodation.

Young people

The prevalence of alcohol use disorders is increasing in young people, particularly young women in the UK.[48] The young are over-represented in alcohol-related road traffic accidents, and alcohol is a leading cause of accidental death in this group. Alcohol misuse is also associated with unprotected sexual activity. Nevertheless, there are few specialist alcohol services for young people. Most initiatives have been directed at prevention and health promotion in this group, but the evidence to support these is lacking. This has led to the proposal that individually targeted interventions, for example by the primary health care team or in accident and emergency departments, are more likely to be effective.[64]

Relatives and carers

Relatives and carers of people with alcohol use disorders often experience significant social and psychological problems related to the drinking of a 'significant other'. Alcohol use disorders are associated with a high level of domestic violence and child neglect and abuse. Many specialist treatment programmes provide help and support to relatives and carers, and Al-Anon (for adult carers and relatives) and Alateen (for the young), which are affiliates of AA, provide a widely available source of mutual aid for these groups.

Services for individuals with comorbidity

There is an increasing recognition of the problems associated with alcohol and other drug misuse and mental illness (see Chapter 4.2.2.3). Often alcohol misuse is complicated by multiple substance misuse. For example, in the Epidemiologic Catchment Area Study half of all patients with schizophrenia also had a substance use disorder,[65] and a recent British survey of psychiatric inpatients found that half had an alcohol use disorder.[66] However, there is currently no consensus on the most appropriate treatment services for patients with comorbidity.[67] Alcohol and substance misuse can be particularly problematic in the context of mental illness, and is associated with higher rates of violence and poor treatment outcome. Such patients are often poorly engaged with, and disruptive in mental health services, and typically have difficulty in engaging in alcohol or drug services. Assertive community outreach and integrated service models, covering both mental illness and substance misuse, have been advocated, but more research is needed to evaluate the cost-effectiveness of these approaches.

Conclusions

The alcohol treatment field has seen considerable change over the past 30 years. Some of this has been evidence based, and some has been largely politically driven, particularly in the pursuit of containing health care costs. On the positive side, a shift in policy from a limited number of treatment services catering only for the small minority of severely dependent drinkers, to more community orientated services with a greater emphasis on early identification and intervention, is to be broadly welcomed. However, in some places a move towards services catering for early stage 'at-risk' drinkers has been at the expense of losing services for those with more severe alcohol problems.[40] While the evidence in favour of matching treatments to individual needs is still at a relatively early stage of development, and clear evidence of matching effects is not yet available, clinical practice needs to be guided by pragmatic principles by which more intensive treatments are provided to more complex patients, and/or in a stepped care paradigm. It must be concluded that, despite a large research effort in evaluating intensive versus less intensive alcohol interventions, there is still a long way to go in developing pragmatic clinical trials that evaluate effectiveness and cost-effectiveness of treatment in a way that can best advise practitioners in the typical treatment setting.

On the positive side, research has begun to address fundamental health economic issues that are highly relevant to the rational funding of treatment services. Important in this is the development of health economic analysis in randomized controlled trials. The assessment of the impact of treatment availability on the prevalence of alcohol-related harm also represents a significant advance.

Health services research that does not influence clinical practice fails in its fundamental aim. For example, while there is a now considerable evidence base in support of brief intervention in the primary care setting, there is a resistance within primary care to adopt such approaches, often despite exhortations from governments and professional bodies. Part of the problem may lie in the disparity between the priorities of public health, which is directed towards population level benefits of an intervention, and the priorities of the individual practitioner, whose first duty is to the patient in his or her care.[17] If the individual practitioner remains unconvinced about the value of a particular intervention for the patient, such public health policies are likely to fail even if they are supported by research evidence.

Similarly, as Holder *et al.*[49] have pointed out, often treatment programmes continue to provide alcohol services that are not supported by research evidence. On occasions, but not exclusively, this criticism is levelled at private for-profit agencies, with the implication that their motivation is financial rather than being principally for the benefit of their patients. In many cases, however, the evidence base is lacking because the fundamental research has not yet been conducted. Or, as in the case of self-help organizations such as AA, the methodology necessary adequately to evaluate an intervention would be extremely complex, or perhaps impossible, to conduct to the standard typically expected in evidence-based medicine (i.e. a randomized controlled trial).

Nevertheless, treatment research cannot occur in a vacuum. Research needs to take account of the funding environment in which treatment takes place. Further, treatment research needs to provide answers to the key issues facing commissioners of health care. With the gradual improvement in the quality of treatment research over the past three decades[68] and the development of more advanced health economic methods to evaluate treatment, the treatment research community is in a much better position than ever before to provide evidence to guide the rational development of treatment services for alcohol use disorders.

While many differences between health care systems exist in different countries, the evidence points to the need for a wide spectrum of services to cater for different needs. The development of low-threshold community-based services should not occur at the expense of more specialized services for more severe alcohol use disorders. Similarly, a treatment system that provides only specialist services for the minority of severe cases misses a significant public health opportunity to reduce the prevalence of alcohol use disorders through early, brief interventions.

Further information

Edwards, G., Marshall, J., and Cook, C.C.H. (1997). *The treatment of drinking problems: a guide for the helping professions* (3rd edn). Cambridge University Press, Cambridge.

Institute of Medicine. (1990). *Broadening the base of treatment for alcohol problems.* National Academy Press, Washington, DC.

Raistrick, D., Heather, N., and Godfrey, C. (2006). *Review of the effectiveness of treatment for alcohol problems.* National Treatment Agency for Substance Misuse, London.

National Treatment Agency for Substance Misuse. (2006). *Models of care for alcohol misusers.* National Treatment Agency for Substance Misuse, London.

References

1. Jellinek, E.M. (1960). *The disease concept of alcoholism*. Hillhouse, New Haven, CT.
2. Edwards, G., Marshall, J., and Cook, C.C.H. (1997). *The treatment of drinking problems: a guide for the helping professions* (3rd edn). Cambridge University Press, Cambridge.
3. Chick, J., Lloyd, G., and Crombie, E. (1985). Counselling problem drinkers in medical wards: a controlled study. *British Medical Journal*, **290**, 965–7.
4. Wallace, P., Cutler, S., and Haines, A. (1988). Randomised controlled trial of general practitioner intervention in patients with excessive alcohol consumption. *British Medical Journal*, **297**, 663–8.
5. Kreitman, N. (1986). Alcohol consumption and the preventive paradox. *British Journal of Addiction*, **81**, 353–63.
6. Institute of Medicine. (1990). *Broadening the base of treatment for alcohol problems*. National Academy Press, Washington, DC.
7. Heather, N. (1998). Brief opportunities for change in medical settings. In *Treating addictive behaviors* (2nd edn) (eds. W.R. Miller and N. Heather), pp. 133–47. Plenum, New York.
8. Saunders, J.B., Aasland, O.G., Babor, T.F., *et al.* (1993). Development of the Alcohol Use Disorders Identification Test (AUDIT): WHO collaborative project on early detection of persons with harmful alcohol consumption—II. *Addiction*, **88**, 791–804.
9. Raistrick, D., Heather, N., and Godfrey, C. (2006). *Review of the effectiveness of treatment for alcohol problems*. National Treatment Agency for Substance Misuse, London.
10. Babor, T.F. and Grant, B. (eds.) (1992). *Programme on substance abuse: project on identification and management of alcohol related problems. Report on phase II: a randomised clinical trial of brief intervention in primary health care*. World Health Organization, Geneva.
11. Emmen, M.J., Schippers, G.M., Bleijenberg, G., *et al.* (2004). Effectiveness of opportunistic brief interventions for problem drinking in a general hospital setting: systemative review. *British Medical Journal*, **328**, 318–22.
12. Crawford, M.J., Patton, R., Touquet, R., *et al.* (2004). Screening and referral for brief intervention of alcohol misusing patients in an emergency department: a pragmatic randomized controlled trial. *Lancet*, **364**, 1334–9.
13. Smith, A.J., Hodgson, R.J., Bridgeman, K., *et al.* (2003). A randomized controlled trial of a brief intervention after alcohol-related facial injury. *Addiction*, **98**, 3–52.
14. Effective Health Care Team. (1993). *Brief interventions and alcohol use. Effective Health Care Bulletin 7*. Department of Health, London.
15. Moyer, A., Finney, J., Swearigan, C., *et al.* (2002). Brief interventions for alcohol problems: a meta-analytic review of controlled investigations in treatment seeking and non-treatment seeking populations. *Addiction*, **97**, 279–92.
16. Kaner, E.F.S., Beyer, F., Dickinson, H.O., *et al.* (2007). Effectiveness of brief alcohol interventions in primary care populations. *Cochrane Database of Systematic Reviews*, (2).
17. Heather, N. (1995). Interpreting the evidence on brief interventions for excessive drinkers: the need for caution. *Alcohol and Alcoholism*, **30**, 287–96.
18. Deehan, A., Templeton, L., Taylor, C., *et al.* (1998). Low detection rates, negative attitudes and the failure to meet 'Health of the Nation' targets: findings from a national survey of GPs in England and Wales. *Drug and Alcohol Review*, **17**, 249–58.
19. Deehan, A., Templeton, L., Taylor, C., *et al.* (1998). How do general practitioners manage alcohol misusing patients? Results from a national survey of GPs in England and Wales. *Drug and Alcohol Review*, **17**, 259–66.
20. Drummond, D.C. (1997). Alcohol interventions: do the best things come in small packages? *Addiction*, **92**, 375–9.
21. Edwards, G., Orford, J., Egert, S., *et al.* (1977). Alcoholism: a controlled trial of 'treatment' and 'advice'. *Journal of Studies on Alcohol*, **38**, 1004–31.
22. Chick, J., Ritson, B., Connaughton, J., *et al.* (1988). Advice versus extended treatment for alcoholism: a controlled study. *British Journal of Addiction*, **83**, 159–70.
23. Orford, J., Oppenheimer, E., and Edwards, G. (1976). Abstinence or control: the outcome for excessive drinkers two years after consultation. *Behaviour Research and Therapy*, **14**, 409–18.
24. Walsh, D.C., Hingson, R.W., Merrigan, D.M., *et al.* (1991). A randomised trial of treatment options for alcohol–abusing workers. *The New England Journal of Medicine*, **325**, 775–82.
25. Trent, L.K. (1998). Evaluation of a four–versus six–week length of stay in the navy's alcohol treatment program. *Journal of Studies on Alcohol*, **59**, 270–9.
26. Long, C.G., Williams, M., and Hollin, C.R. (1998). Treating alcohol problems: a study of programme effectiveness according to length and delivery of treatment. *Addiction*, **93**, 561–71.
27. Hayashida, M., Alterman, A.I., McLellan, A.T., *et al.* (1989). Comparative effectiveness and costs of inpatient and outpatient detoxification of patients with mild–to–moderate alcohol withdrawal syndrome. *The New England Journal of Medicine*, **320**, 358–65.
28. Rychartic, R., Connors, G., Whitney, R., *et al.* (2000). Treatment settings for persons with alcoholism: evidence for matching clients to inpatient versus outpatient care. *Journal of Consulting and Clinical Psychology*, **68**, 277–89.
29. Fuller, R.K. and Hiller-Sturmhofel, S. (1999). Alcoholism treatment in the US. *Alcohol Research and Health*, **23**, 69–77.
30. Drummond, C., Oyefeso, N., Phillips, T., *et al.* (2005). *Alcohol needs assessment research project: the 2004 national alcohol needs assessment for England*. Department of Health, London.
31. Shaw, S.J., Cartwright, A.K.J., Spratley, T.A., *et al.* (1978). *Responding to drinking problems*. Croom Helm, London.
32. Clement, S. and Stockwell, T. (eds.) (1987). *Helping the problem drinker: new initiatives in community care*. Croom Helm, London.
33. Drummond, D.C., Thom, B., Brown, C., *et al.* (1990). Specialist versus general practitioner treatment of problem drinkers. *Lancet*, **336**, 915–18.
34. Bennie, C. (1998). A comparison of home detoxification and minimal intervention strategies for problem drinkers. *Alcohol and Alcoholism*, **33**, 157–63.
35. Hunt, G.N. and Azrin, N.H. (1973). A community reinforcement approach to alcoholism. *Behaviour Research and Therapy*, **11**, 91–104.
36. Azrin, N.H., Sisson, R.W., Meyers, R., *et al.* (1982). Alcoholism treatment by disulfiram and community reinforcement therapy. *Journal of Behavior Therapy and Experimental Psychiatry*, **13**, 105–12.
37. Patterson, D.G., MacPherson, J., and Brady, N.M. (1997). Community psychiatric nurse aftercare for alcoholics: a five–year follow–up. *Addiction*, **92**, 459–68.
38. Marshall, M. and Lockwood, A. (1998). Assertive community treatment for people with severe mental disorders. *Cochrane Database of Systematic Reviews*, (2).
39. Hesse, M., Broekaert, E., Fridell, M., *et al.* (2006). Case management for substance use disorders. *Cochrane Database of Systematic Reviews*, (4).
40. Mattson, M.E., Allen, J.P., Longabaugh, R., *et al.* (1994). A chronological review of empirical studies matching alcoholic clients to treatment. *Journal of Studies on Alcohol*, **12**, 16–29.
41. Project MATCH Research Group. (1997). Matching alcoholism treatments to client heterogeneity: project MATCH post-treatment drinking outcomes. *Journal of Studies on Alcohol*, **58**, 7–29.
42. Drummond, D.C. (1999). Treatment research in the wake of Project MATCH. *Addiction*, **94**, 39–42.
43. UKATT Research Team. (2005). Effectiveness of treatment for alcohol problems: findings of the randomized UK Alcohol Treatment Trial (UKATT). *British Medical Journal*, **311**, 541–4.
44. Breslin, F.C., Sobell, M.B., Sobell, L.C., *et al.* (1997). Toward a stepped care approach to treating problem drinkers: the predictive utility of within treatment variables and therapist prognostic ratings. *Addiction*, **92**, 1479–89.

45. Drummond, D.C., James, D., Coulton, S., *et al.* (2003). *The effectiveness and cost effectiveness of screening and stepped care intervention for alcohol use disorders in the primary care setting.* Final Report to the Wales Office for Research and Development. St George's Hospital Medical School, London.
46. National Treatment Agency for Substance Misuse. (2006). *Models of care for alcohol misusers.* National Treatment Agency for Substance Misuse, London.
47. Harwood, H. (2000). *Updating estimates of the economic costs of alcohol abuse in the United States: estimates, update methods, and data.* National Institute of Alcohol Abuse and Alcoholism, Rockville, MD.
48. Prime Minister's Strategy Unit. (2004). *Alcohol harm reduction strategy for England.* Cabinet Office, London.
49. Holder, H.D., Longabaugh, R., Miller, W.R., *et al.* (1991). The cost effectiveness of treatment for alcohol problems: a first approximation. *Journal of Studies on Alcohol*, **52**, 517–40.
50. Drummond, M.F., O'Brien, B., Stoddard, G.L., *et al.* (1997). *Methods for the economic evaluation of health care programmes.* Oxford University Press, Oxford.
51. Slattery, J., Chick, J., Cochrane, M., *et al.* (2003). *Prevention of relapse in alcohol dependence.* Health technology assessment report 3. Health Technology Board for Scotland, Glasgow.
52. Fleming, M.F., Marlon, M.P., French, M.T., *et al.* (2000). Benefit cost analysis of brief physician advice with problem drinkers in primary care settings. *Medical Care*, **31**, 7–18.
53. Ludbrook, A., Godfrey, C., Wyness, L., *et al.* (2002). *Effective and cost effective measures to reduce alcohol misuse in Scotland.* Scottish Executive Health Department, Ediburgh.
54. Mann, R.E., Smart, R., Anglin, L., *et al.* (1988). Are decreases in liver cirrhosis rates a result of increased treatment for alcoholism? *British Journal of Addiction*, **83**, 683–8.
55. Mann, R.E., Smart, R., Anglin, L., *et al.* (1991). Reductions in cirrhosis deaths in the United States: associations with per capita consumption and AA membership. *Journal of Studies on Alcohol*, **52**, 361–5.
56. Weisner, C., Greenfield, T., and Room, R. (1995). Trends in the treatment of alcohol problems in the US general population, 1979 through 1990. *American Journal of Public Health*, **85**, 55–60.
57. Rush, B. (1990). A systems approach to estimating the required capacity of alcohol treatment services. *British Journal of Addiction*, **85**, 49–59.
58. Thom, B. and Green, A. (1996). Services for women with alcohol problems: the way forward. In *Alcohol problems in the community* (ed. L. Harrison), pp. 200–22. Routledge, London.
59. Institute of Medicine. (1988). *Homelessness, health, and human needs.* National Academy Press, Washington, DC.
60. Harrison, L., Harrison, M., and Adebowale, V. (1997). Drinking problems among black communities. In *Alcohol problems in the community* (ed. L. Harrison), pp. 223–40. Routledge, London.
61. Marmot, M., Adelstein, A., and Bulusu, L. (1984). *Immigrant mortality in England and Wales, 1970–78.* HMSO, London.
62. Harrison, L. and Luck, H. (1997). Drinking and homelessness. In *Alcohol problems in the community* (ed. L. Harrison), pp. 53–75. Routledge, London.
63. Freimanis, L. (1993). Alcohol and single homelessness: an outreach approach. In *Homelessness, health care and welfare provision* (eds. K. Fisher and J. Collins), pp. 44–51. Routledge, London.
64. May, C. (1993). Young heavy drinkers: is there a problem, is there a solution? *Health and Social Care*, **1**, 203–10.
65. Reiger, D.A., Farmer, M.E., Rae, D.S., *et al.* (1990). Co-morbidity of mental disorder with alcohol and other drug abuse: results from an Epidemiological Catchment Area (ECA) study. *The Journal of the American Medical Association*, **264**, 2511–18.
66. Barnaby, B., Drummond, D.C., McCloud, A., *et al.* (2003). Substance misuse in psychiatric inpatients: comparison of a screening questionnaire survey with case notes. *British Medical Journal*, **327**, 783–4.
67. Weaver, T., Renton, A., Stimson, G., *et al.* (1999). Severe mental illness and substance misuse. *British Medical Journal*, **318**, 137–8.
68. Moncrieff, J. and Drummond, D.C. (1998). The quality of alcohol treatment research: an examination of influential controlled trials and development of a quality rating system. *Addiction*, **93**, 811–23.

4.2.2.6 **Prevention of alcohol-related problems**

Robin Room

Alcohol consumption is widely distributed in the population in most parts of the world, with abstainers in a minority among adults in most developing societies but in a majority in many less developed societies.[1,2] Those qualifying to be diagnosed with an alcohol use disorder are usually a relatively small minority of drinkers.

On the other hand, alcohol is causally implicated in a wide variety of health and social problems. The WHO *Global Burden of Disease* (*GBD*) study for 2000 estimated that alcohol accounted globally for 4 per cent of the total health-related loss of disability-adjusted life years (DALYs), for 6.8 per cent in developed societies like those in Western Europe and North America, and for 12.1 per cent in Eastern Europe and Central Asia.[3] In terms of where this burden appears in the health system, while psychiatric conditions (including dependence) and chronic physical disease are both important, casualties often play a predominant role. The *GBD* 2000 study calculated that injuries accounted for 40 per cent of the DALYs lost worldwide due to alcohol.[3]

The public health importance of acute effects of a particular episode of intoxication underlies what is often described as the 'prevention paradox'. In many societies, a fairly substantial proportion of the population (particularly of males) gets intoxicated at least occasionally, and by that fact is at risk of experiencing and causing social and health harm from drinking.[4] Preventing alcohol problems thus requires looking beyond the considerably smaller segment of the population diagnosable with an alcohol use disorder, or the even smaller segment receiving treatment for such a disorder.

A complication in preventing alcohol problems is that there is also evidence of a health benefit from drinking in terms of reduced cardiovascular disease. This benefit is, however, important mainly for men over 45 and women past menopause, and can be attained with a pattern of very light regular drinking, as little as a drink every second day.[5] There is thus little potential conflict between taking alcohol as a preventive heart medication and any prevention policy short of total prohibition.

Simplifying somewhat, there are seven main strategies to minimize alcohol problems. One strategy is to educate or persuade people not to use or about ways to use so as to limit harm. A second strategy, a kind of negative persuasion, is to deter drinking-related behaviour with the threat of penalties. A third strategy, operating in the positive direction, is to provide alternatives to drinking or to drink-connected activities. A fourth strategy is in one way or another to insulate the use from harm. A fifth strategy is to regulate availability of the drug or the conditions of its use. Prohibition of supply may be regarded as a special case of such regulation. A sixth strategy is to work with social or religious movements oriented to reducing alcohol problems. And a seventh strategy is to treat or otherwise help people who are in trouble with their drinking. We will consider in turn these strategies and the evidence on their effectiveness in reducing rates of alcohol problems in the population.

Education and persuasion

In principle, education can be offered to any segment of the population in a variety of venues, but it is usually education of youth in schools, which first comes to mind in the prevention of alcohol problems. Community-based prevention programmes, which may be also directed at adults, often also include an educational component.

Education offers new information or ways of thinking about information, and leaves it to the listener to draw conclusions concerning beliefs and behaviour. However, most alcohol education programmes go beyond this. A commonplace of the North American evaluative literature on alcohol education is that 'knowledge-only' approaches do not result in changes in behaviour.(6) School-based alcohol education has thus usually had a persuasional element, aiming to influence students in a particular direction.

Persuasion is directly concerned with changing beliefs or behaviours, and may or may not also offer information. Mass-media campaigns aimed at persuasion have been a very common component of prevention programmes for alcohol-related problems, but persuasion can be pursued also through other media and modalities.

In most societies, public health-oriented persuasion about alcohol must compete with a variety of other persuasional messages, including those intended to sell alcoholic beverages. The evidence that alcohol advertising influences teenagers and young adults towards increased drinking and problematic drinking is becoming stronger.(7,8) Even where alcohol advertising is not allowed on the mass media, these messages are conveyed to consumers and potential consumers in a variety of other ways.

Evidence on effectiveness

The literature on effectiveness of educational approaches is dominated by studies from the United States on school-based education. This means that the alcohol education has usually been in the context of drug and tobacco education, and that the emphasis has been on abstention,(9) or at least on delaying the start of drinking, in cultural circumstances where the median age of actually starting drinking is about 13, while the minimum legal drinking age is 21. In general, despite the best efforts of a generation of researchers, this literature has had difficulty showing substantial and lasting effects.(10) There is a good argument from general principles for alcohol education in the context of consumer and health education, but there is little evidence from the formal evaluation literature at this point of its effectiveness beyond the short term.

Persuasional media campaigns have also been a favourite modality in many places in recent decades for the prevention of alcohol problems. In general, evaluations of such campaigns have been able to demonstrate impacts on knowledge and awareness about substance use problems, but little effect on drinking behaviour. As with school education approaches, there are hints in the literature that success may come more from influencing the community environment around the drinker—in terms of attitudes of significant others, or popular support for alcohol policy measures—than from directly persuading the drinker him/herself. Thus, media messages can be effective as agenda-setting mechanisms in the community, increasing or sustaining public support for other preventive strategies.(11)

Deterrence

In its broadest sense, deterrence means simply the threat of negative sanctions or incentives for behaviour—a form of negative persuasion. Criminal laws deter in two ways: by general deterrence, which is the effect of the law in preventing a prohibited behaviour in the population as a whole, and specific deterrence, which is the effect of the law in discouraging those who have been caught from doing it again.(12) A law tends to have a greater preventive effect and to be cheaper to administer to the extent it has a strong general deterrence effect.

Prohibitions on driving after drinking more than a specified amount are now in effect in most nations.(13) In many societies, there have also been laws against public drunkenness (being in a public place while intoxicated), and against obnoxious behaviour while intoxicated. Other common prohibitions are concerned with producing or selling alcoholic beverages outside state-regulated channels, and with aspects of drinking under a specified minimum age.

Evidence on effectiveness

Drinking-driving legislation, such as 'per se' laws outlawing driving while at or above a defined blood-alcohol level, has been shown to be effective in changing behaviour and reducing rates of alcohol-related problems (Babor *et al.*,[14] pp. 157–72). The effect is through both general and specific deterrence. The quickness and certainty of punishment, as well as its severity, are important in the deterrent value (too much severity tends to undercut its quickness and certainty). Drinking driving is an ideal area for applying general deterrence, since the gains from breaking the law are limited, and automobile drivers typically have something to lose by being caught.

Many English-speaking and Scandinavian countries have had a tradition of criminalizing drinking in public places or public drunkenness as such, but the trend has been to decriminalize public drunkenness. Though there are few specific studies, criminalizing public drunkenness is not very effective in changing behaviour, particularly of those who have little to lose (Parliament of Victoria, Drugs and Crime Prevention Committee,[15] pp. 309–20).

Providing and encouraging alternative activities

Another strategy, in principle involving positive incentives, is to provide and seek to encourage activities, which are an alternative to drinking or to activities closely associated with drinking. This includes such initiatives as making soft drinks available as an alternative to alcoholic beverages, providing locations for sociability as an alternative to taverns, and providing and encouraging recreational activities as an alternative to leisure activities involving drinking. Job creation and skill development programmes are other examples.

Evidence on effectiveness

'Boredom' and 'because there's nothing else to do' are certainly among the reasons that are given for drinking by some drinkers. And there are often good reasons of general social policy for providing and encouraging alternative activities. But it has been noted that the problem with alternatives to drinking is that drinking combines so well with so many of them. Soft drinks are indeed an alternative for quenching thirst, but they may also serve as a mixer in an alcoholic drink. Involvement in sports may go along with drinking as well as replace it. The few evaluation studies of providing alternative activities, again from a restricted range of societies, have generally not shown lasting effects on drinking behaviour,[(16,17)] though they undoubtedly often serve a general social purpose in broadening opportunities for the disadvantaged.[(18)]

Insulating use from harm

A major social strategy for reducing alcohol-related problems in many societies has been measures to separate the drinking, and particularly heavy drinking, from potential harm. This separation can be physical (in terms of distance or walls), it can be temporal, or it can be cultural (e.g. defining the drinking occasion as 'time-out' from normal responsibilities). These 'harm reduction' strategies, as they are called in the context of illicit drugs, are often built into cultural arrangements around drinking, but can also be the object of purposive programmes and policies (Moore and Gerstein,[19] pp. 100–11).

A variety of modifications of the driving environment affect casualties associated with drinking and driving, along with other casualties. These include mandatory use of seat belts, airbags, and improvements in the safety of road vehicles and roads. Many other practical measures tending to separate intoxication episodes from casualties and other adverse consequences have been put into practice, though usually without formal evaluation.

The main focus for self-conscious strategies of alcohol harm reduction in recent years has been on modifying the drinking environment, particularly in public drinking places, primarily by modifying the behaviour of alcohol servers through server training and enforcement of bans on serving those under age or already intoxicated (Babor *et al.*,[14] pp. 141–47).

Evidence on effectiveness

Drinking-driving countermeasures are a prime example of an approach in terms of insulating drinking behaviour from harm, since they seek to reduce alcohol-related traffic casualties without necessarily stopping or reducing alcohol use. There is substantial evidence of the success of a range of such countermeasures (Babor *et al.*,[14] pp. 159–68). Environmental measures which reduce road casualties in general—e.g. requiring wearing of seat belts in cars, providing sidewalks separated from the road—may prevent casualties associated with intoxication at least as much as other casualties. While there is also evidence for the effectiveness of some other harm reduction approaches, there are also many examples of well-meaning efforts which proved ineffective (Room *et al.*,[2] pp. 186–92).

Regulating the availability and conditions of use

In terms of the substantial harms to health and public order they can cause, alcoholic beverages are not ordinary commodities. Governments have thus often actively intervened in the markets for such beverages, far beyond usual levels of state intervention in markets for commodities.

Total prohibition can be viewed as an extreme form of regulation of the market. In this circumstance, where no one is licensed to sell alcohol, the state has no formal control over the conditions of the sales, which nevertheless occur, and there are no legal sales interests, controlled through licensing, to cooperate with the state in the market's regulation.

With a general prohibition, typically the consumption of alcohol does fall in the population, and there are declines also in the rates of the direct consequences of drinking such as cirrhosis or alcohol-related mental disorders.[(19,20)] But prohibition also brings with it characteristic negative consequences, including the emergence and growth of an illicit market, and the crime associated with this. Partly for this reason, prohibition is not now a live option in any developed society, although it is in some other societies.

The features of alcohol control regimes, regulating the legal market in alcohol, vary greatly. Special taxes on alcohol are very common, imposed often as much for revenue as for public health considerations. Many societies have minimum age limits forbidding sales to underage customers, and regulating forbidding sales to the already intoxicated. Often the regulations include limiting the number of sales outlets, restricting hours and days of sale, and limiting sales to special stores or drinking places. Rationing of alcohol purchases—limiting the amount individuals can buy in a given time-period—has also been used as a means of regulating availability. Regulations restricting or forbidding advertising of alcoholic beverages attempt to limit or channel efforts by private interests to increase demand for particular alcoholic beverage products. Such regulations potentially complement education and persuasion efforts. State monopolization of sales of some or all alcoholic beverages at the retail and/or wholesale level has also been commonly been used as a mechanism to minimize alcohol-related harm.[(21)]

The effectiveness of specific types of regulation of availability

The last 25 years have seen the development of a burgeoning literature on the effects of alcohol control measures. Specific types of regulation of the alcohol market, and the evidence on their effectiveness, are discussed below.

(a) Minimum age limits

A minimum age limit is a partial prohibition, applied to one segment of the population. There is a strong evaluation literature showing the effectiveness of establishing and enforcing minimum age limits in reducing alcohol-related problems (Babor *et al.*,[14] pp. 127–28). However, this literature has been primarily North America based, focuses mostly on youthful driving casualties, and mostly evaluates reduction from and increases to age 21 as the limit, a higher minimum age limit than in most societies. The applicability of the literature's findings in other societies and where youth cultures are less automobile-focused has been little tested.

(b) Taxes and other price increases

Generally, consumers show some response to the price of alcoholic beverages, as of all other commodities. If the price goes up, the drinker will drink less; data from developed societies suggests this is at least as true of the heavy drinker as of the occasional drinker (Babor *et al.*,[14] pp. 110–11). Studies have found that alcohol tax increases reduce the rates of traffic casualties, of cirrhosis mortality, and of incidents of violence.[22,23]

(c) Limiting sales outlets, and hours and conditions of sale

There is a substantial literature showing that levels and patterns of alcohol consumption, and rates of alcohol-related casualties and other problems, are influenced by such sales restrictions, which typically make the purchase of alcoholic beverages slightly inconvenient, or influence the setting of and after drinking (Babor *et al.*,[14] pp. 125–42). Enforcing rules influencing 'house policies' in drinking places on not serving intoxicated customers, etc., has also been shown to have some effect (Babor *et al.*,[14] pp. 142–45).

(d) Monopolizing production or sale

Studies of the effects of privatizing retail alcohol monopolies have often shown some increase in levels of alcohol consumption and problems, in part because the number of outlets and hours of sale typically increase with privatization.[24] From a public health perspective, it is the retail level which is important, while monopolization of the production or wholesale level may facilitate revenue collection and effective control of the market.

(e) Rationing sales

Rationing the amount of alcohol sold to an individual potentially directly impacts on heavy drinkers, and has been shown to reduce levels both of intoxication-related problems such as violence, and of drinking-history-related problems such as cirrhosis mortality.[25,26] But while a form of rationing—the medical prescription system—is well accepted in most societies for psychoactive medications, it has proved politically unacceptable nowadays for alcoholic beverages in developed societies.

(f) Advertising and promotion restrictions

Many societies have regulations on advertising and other promotion of sales of alcoholic beverages.[13] As noted, the evidence on the effects of advertising and promotion on overall demand has become stronger in the recent literature.[27] However, studies of the effects of advertising and promotion restrictions on alcohol consumption have so far found at best weak effects, at least in the short term (Babor *et al.*,[14] pp. 180–83).

Social and religious movements and community action

Substantial reductions in alcohol-related problems have often been the result of spontaneous social and religious movements, which put a major emphasis on quitting intoxication or drinking. In recent decades, there have also been efforts to form partnerships between state organizations and nongovernmental groups to work on alcohol problems, often at the level of the local community. There has been an active tradition of community action projects on alcohol problems, often using a range of prevention strategies.[28–31] School-based prevention efforts have also moved increasingly to try to involve the community, in line with general perceptions that such multifaceted strategies will be more effective.[32]

While some of the biggest historical reductions in alcohol problems rates have resulted from spontaneous and autonomous social or religious movements, support or collaboration from a government can easily be perceived as official cooptation or manipulation.[33] Thus there is considerable question about the extent to which such movements can or should become an instrument of government prevention policies.

Evidence on effectiveness

In the short term, movements of religious or cultural revival can be highly effective in reducing levels of drinking and of alcohol-related problems. Alcohol consumption in the United States fell by about one-half in the first flush of temperance enthusiasm in 1830–1845 (Moore and Gerstein,[19] p. 35). Rates of serious crime are reported to have fallen for a while to a fraction of their previous level in Ireland in the wake of Father Mathew's temperance crusade.[34] The enthusiasm which sustains such movements tends to decay over time, though they often leave behind new customs and institutions with much longer duration. For instance, though the days when the historic temperance movement in English-speaking societies was strong are long gone, the movement had the long-lasting effect of largely removing drinking from the workplace in these societies.

There are some good examples of well-evaluated community action projects with demonstrated effectiveness.[30,31] However, the strategies used in such projects should be guided by evidence on effectiveness; good intentions and effort in themselves offer no guarantee of effectiveness.

Treatment and other help

Providing effective treatment or other help for drinkers who find they cannot control their drinking can be regarded as an obligation of a just and humane society. The help can take several forms: a specific treatment system for alcohol problems, professional help in general health or welfare systems, or non-professional assistance in mutual-help movements. To the extent such help is effective, and it is also potentially a means of reducing rates of alcohol-related problems.

Treatments for alcohol problems need not be complex or expensive. The evaluation literature suggests that brief outpatient interventions aimed at changing cognitions and behaviour around drinking are as effective in most circumstances as longer and more intensive treatment.[35,36] Positive results from such interventions in a primary health care settings were shown in a WHO study including a number of countries.[37]

Evidence on effectiveness

In terms of the effects of treatment on those who come for it, there is good evidence of effectiveness of treatment for alcohol problem. Typically, the improvement rate from a single episode of treatment is about 20 per cent higher than the no-treatment condition. Further treatment episodes are often needed. Brief treatment interventions or mutual-help approaches usually result in net savings in social and health costs associated with the heavy drinker (at least where health care is not self-paid), as well as improving the quality of life.[38,39] However, evaluations of brief interventions by medical general practitioners have not always found effects.[40] Getting general practitioners to use the methods on a sustained basis has not proved easy,[41] and their patients are often unreceptive[42] or recalcitrant.[43] It remains to be seen whether and in what sociocultural circumstances making brief interventions for problematic drinking a routine part of general medical practice is a feasible and effective strategy.

The effectiveness of providing treatment as a strategy for reducing rates of alcohol problems in a society is more equivocal. In a North American context, it has been argued that the steep increase in alcohol problems treatment provision and mutual-help group membership in recent decades has contributed to reducing alcohol problems rates.[44] But the strength of the evidence for this contention is disputed.[45,46] A treatment system for alcohol problems is an important part of an integrated national alcohol policy, but as an instrument of prevention—of reducing societal rates of alcohol problems—it is probably not cost-effective.

Building an integrated societal alcohol policy

Often the different strategies for preventing alcohol problems appear to be synergistic in their effects.[47] Controls of availability, for instance, are more likely to be adopted, continued, and respected when the public has been successfully persuaded of their effects and effectiveness. But strategies can also work at cross-purposes: a prohibition policy, for instance, makes it difficult to pursue measures which insulate drinking from harm.

In a society where alcohol is a regular item of consumption, in view of the resulting rates of alcohol-related social and health problems, there is a strong justification for adopting a comprehensive policy concerning alcohol, taking into account production, marketing and consumption, and the prevention and treatment of alcohol-related problems. But while the adoption of overall alcohol strategies or policies has become common,[48] governments often tend to shy away from the most effective strategies.

In terms of strategies we have reviewed for managing and reducing the rates of alcohol problems in the society, there is clear evidence for effectiveness and cost-effectiveness of measures regulating the availability and conditions of use, and some such evidence for some measures which insulate use from harm. With respect to some aspects of alcohol problems, notably drinking-driving, deterrence measures also fall in the same category. The literature has begun to move beyond the question of effectiveness of these measures, and to consider questions of the relative cost-effectiveness of different measures in different societies.[49]

Despite their perennial popularity, evidence of the effectiveness of education/persuasion and treatment strategies in reducing societal rates of problems is limited at best. Education and treatment are good things for a society and a government to be doing about alcohol problems, but they do not constitute in themselves a public health policy on alcohol. These strategies will be nevertheless be pursued in most societies, and they can best pursued with attention to using cost-effective methods, and to integrating targets and messages with other aspects of alcohol policy.

Physicians and other health workers observe the adverse effects of alcohol in their daily practice, and are well-positioned to argue for public health approaches to reducing the burden of alcohol problems. Reports by colleges of psychiatrists and other physicians have played an important role in such countries as Britain[50] and Sweden[51] in putting a public health response to alcohol problems on the societal agenda.

Further information

References 2, 13, and 14 are useful also as sources of more general information.

Chikritzhs, T., Gray, D., Lyons, Z., *et al.* (2007). *Restrictions on the sale and supply of alcohol: evidence and outcomes. National Drug Research Institute, Curtin University of Technology, Perth,* http://www.ndri.curtin.edu.au/pdfs/publications/R207.pdf

WHO Expert Committee on Problems Related to Alcohol Consumption. (2007). *Second report.* WHO Technical Report Series, No. 944, http://www.who.int/substance_abuse/activities/expert_comm_alcohol_2nd_report.pdf

References

1. Rehm, J., Room, R., Monteiro, M., *et al.* (2004). Alcohol use. In *Comparative quantification of health risks. Global and regional burden of disease attributable to selected major risk factors,* Vol. 1 (eds. M. Ezzati, A.D. Lopez, A. Rodgers, and C.J.L. Murray), pp. 959–1108. World Health Organization, Geneva.
2. Room, R., Jernigan, D., Carlini-Marlatt, B., *et al.* (2002). *Alcohol and developing societies: A public health approach.* World Health Organization, Finnish Foundation for Alcohol Studies & Geneva, Helsinki.
3. Room, R., Babor, T., and Rehm, J. (2005). Alcohol and public health: a review. *Lancet,* **365**, 519–30.
4. Stockwell, T., Hawks, D., Lang, E., *et al.* (1996). Unravelling the preventive paradox. *Drug and Alcohol Review,* **15**, 7–16.
5. Bondy, S., Rehm, J., Ashley, M.J., *et al.* (1999). Low-risk drinking guidelines: the scientific evidence. *Canadian Journal of Public Health,* **90**, 272–6.
6. Botvin, G.J. (1995). Principles of prevention. In *Handbook on drug abuse prevention: a comprehensive strategy to prevent the abuse of alcohol and other drugs* (eds. R.H. Coombs and D. Ziedonis), pp. 19–44. Allyn and Bacon, Boston.
7. Ellickson, P.L., Collins, R.L., Hambarsoomians, K., *et al.* (2005). Does alcohol advertising promote adolescent drinking? Results from a longitudinal assessment. *Addiction,* **100**, 235–46.
8. Wyllie, A., Zhang, J.F., and Casswell, S. (1998). Positive responses to televised beer advertisements associated with drinking and problems reported by 18- to 29-year-olds. *Addiction,* **93**, 749–60.
9. Beck, J. (1998). 100 years of "just say no" versus "just say know". *Evaluation Review,* **22**, 15–45.
10. Foxcroft, D.R., Ireland, D., Lister-Sharp, D.J., *et al.* (2003). Longer-term primary prevention for alcohol misuse in young people: a systematic review. *Addiction,* **98**, 397–411.
11. Casswell, S., Gilmore, L., Maguire, V., *et al.* (1989). Changes in public support for alcohol policies following a community-based campaign. *British Journal of Addiction,* **84**, 515–22.
12. Ross, H.L. (1982). Deterring the drinking driver: legal policy and social control. Lexington Books, Lexington, MA.
13. WHO. (2004). *Global status report: alcohol policy.* World Health Organization, Geneva. http://www.who.int/substance_abuse/publications/en/Alcohol%20Policy%20Report.pdf
14. Babor, T., Caetano, R., Casswell, S., *et al.* (2003). *Alcohol: no ordinary commodity—research and public: policy.* Oxford University Press, Oxford.
15. Parliament of Victoria, Drugs and Crime Prevention Committee. (2006). *Report on inquiry into strategies to reduce harmful alcohol consumption.* Government Printer, Melbourne, http://www.parliament.vic.gov.au/dcpc/

16. Moskowitz, J.M., Mailvin, J., Schaeffer, G.A., *et al.* (1983). Evaluation of a junior high school primary prevention program, *Addictive Behaviors*, **8**, 393–401.
17. Norman, E., Turner, S., Zunz, S.J., *et al.* (1997). Prevention programs reviewed: what works? In *Drug-free youth: a compendium for prevention specialists* (ed. E. Norman), pp. 22–45. Garland Publishing, New York.
18. Carmona, M. and Stewart, K. (1996). *Review of alternative activities and alternatives programs in youth-oriented prevention*, CSAP Technical Report 13. Center for Substance Abuse Prevention, Rockville, MD.
19. Moore, M.H. and Gerstein, D.R. (eds.) (1981). *Alcohol and public policy: beyond the shadow of prohibition*. National Academy Press, Washington, DC.
20. Teasley, D.L. (1992). Drug legalization and the 'lessons' of prohibition. *Contemporary Drug Problems*, **19**, 27–52.
21. Room, R. (1993). The evolution of alcohol monopolies and their relevance for public health. *Contemporary Drug Problems*, **20**, 169–87.
22. Cook, P. (1981). Effect of liquor taxes on drinking, cirrhosis, and auto accidents. In *Alcohol and public policy: beyond the shadow of prohibition* (eds. M.H. Moore and D.R. Gerstein), pp. 255–85. National Academy Press, Washington, D.C.
23. Cook, P.J. and Moore, M.H. (1993). Violence reduction through restrictions on alcohol availability. *Alcohol Health and Research World*, **17**, 151–6.
24. Her, M., Giesbrecht, N., Room, R., *et al.* (1999). Privatizing alcohol sales and alcohol consumption: evidence and implications. *Addiction*, **94**, 1125–39.
25. Schechter, E.J. (1986). Alcohol rationing and control systems in Greenland. *Contemporary Drug Problems*, **13**, 587–620.
26. Norström, T. (1987). Abolition of the Swedish alcohol rationing system: effects on consumption distribution and cirrhosis mortality. *British Journal of Addiction*, **82**, 633–41.
27. Hastings, G., Anderson, S., Cooke, E., *et al.* (2005). Alcohol marketing and young people's drinking: a review of the research. *Journal of Public Health Policy*, **26**, 296–311.
28. Giesbrecht, N., Conley, P., Denniston, R., *et al.* (eds.) (1990). *Research, action and the community: experiences in the prevention of alcohol and other drug problems*. DHHS Publication No. (ADM) 89-1651, Office of Substance Abuse Prevention, Rockville, MD.
29. Greenfield, T. and Zimmerman, R. (eds.) (1993). *Experiences with community action projects: new research in the prevention of alcohol and other drug problems*. DHHS Publication No. (ADM) 93-1976, Center for Substance Abuse Prevention, Rockville, MD.
30. Holmila, M. (ed.) (1997). *Community prevention of alcohol problems*. Macmillan, Basingstoke, UK.
31. Holder, H.D. (1998). *Alcohol and the community: a systems approach to prevention*. Cambridge University Press, Cambridge, UK.
32. WHO Expert Committee on Problems Related to Alcohol Consumption. (2007). *Second report*. Technical Report Series, No. 944, WHO, Geneva.
33. Room, R. (1997). Voluntary organizations and the state in the prevention of alcohol problems. *Drugs & Society*, **11**, 11–23.
34. Room, R. (1983). Alcohol and crime: behavioral aspects. In *Encyclopedia of crime and justice*, Vol. 1 (ed. S. Kadish), pp. 35–44. Free Press, New York.
35. Finney, J.W. and Monahan, S.C. (1998). Cost-effectiveness of treatment for alcoholism: a second approximation. *Journal of Studies on Alcohol*, **57**, 229–43.
36. Long, C.G., Williams, M., and Hollin, C.R. (1998). Treating alcohol problems: a study of program effectiveness and cost effectiveness according to length and delivery of treatment. *Addiction*, **93**, 561–71.
37. Babor, T.F. and Grant, M. (1994). Randomized clinical trial of brief interventions in primary health care: summary of a WHO project (with commentaries and a response). *Addiction*, **89**, 657–78.
38. Holder, H.D., Lennox, R.D.L., and Blose, J.O. (1992). Economic benefits of alcoholism treatment: a summary of twenty years of research. *Journal of Employee Assistance Research*, **1**, 63–82.
39. Holder, H.D. and Cunningham, D.W. (1992). Alcoholism treatment for employees and family members: its effect on health care costs. *Alcohol Health and Research World*, **16**, 149–53.
40. Richmond, R., Heather, N., Wodak, A., *et al.* (1995). Controlled evaluation of a general practice-based brief intervention for excessive drinking. *Addiction*, **90**, 119–32.
41. Roche, A.M. and Freeman, T. (2004). Brief interventions: good in theory but weak in practice? *Drug and Alcohol Review*, **23**, 11–18.
42. Conigliaro, J., McNeil, M., Kraemer, K., *et al.* (1997). Are patients diagnosed with alcohol abuse in primary care ready to change their behavior? *Journal of General Internal Medicine*, **12**(Suppl. 1), 113.
43. Edwards, A.G.K. and Rollnick, S. (1997). Outcome studies of brief alcohol intervention in general practice: the problem of lost subjects. *Addiction*, **92**, 1699–704.
44. Smart, R.G. and Mann, R.E. (1990). Are increased levels of treatment and alcoholics anonymous large enough to create the recent reduction in liver cirrhosis? *British Journal of Addiction*, **85**, 1385–7.
45. Holder, H. (1997). Can individually directed interventions reduce population-level alcohol-involved problems? *Addiction*, **92**, 5–7.
46. Smart, R.G. and Mann, R.E. (1997). Interventions into alcohol problems: what works? *Addiction*, **92**, 9–13.
47. DeJong, W. and Hingson, R. (1998). Strategies to reduce driving under the influence of alcohol. *Annual Review of Public Health*, **19**, 359–78.
48. Crombie, I.K., Irvine, L., Elliott, L., *et al.* (2007). How do public health policies tackle alcohol-related harm? A review of 12 developed countries. *Alcohol and Alcoholism*, **42**, 492–9.
49. Chisholm, D., Rehm, J., van Ommeren, M., *et al.* (2004). Reducing the global burden of hazardous alcohol use: a comparative cost-effectiveness analysis. *Journal of Studies on Alcohol*, **65**, 782–93.
50. Baggott, R. (1990). *Alcohol, politics and social policy*. Avebury, Aldershot, UK.
51. Sutton, C. (1998). *Swedish alcohol discourse: constructions of a social problem*. Uppsala University Library, Studia Sociologica Upsaliensia 45, Uppsala.

4.2.3 Other substance use disorders

Contents

4.2.3.1 Opioids: heroin, methadone, and buprenorphine
Soraya Mayet, Adam R. Winstock, and John Strang

4.2.3.2 Disorders relating to the use of amphetamine and cocaine
Nicholas Seivewright and Robert Fung

4.2.3.3 Disorders relating to use of PCP and hallucinogens
Henry David Abraham

4.2.3.4 Misuse of benzodiazepines
Sarah Welch and Michael Farrell

4.2.3.5 Disorders relating to the use of ecstasy and other 'party drugs'
Adam R. Winstock and Fabrizio Schifano

4.2.3.6 Disorders relating to the use of volatile substances
Richard Ives
4.2.3.7 The mental health effects of cannabis use
Wayne Hall
4.2.3.8 Nicotine dependence and treatment
Mª Inés López-Ibor

4.2.3.1 Opioids: heroin, methadone, and buprenorphine

Soraya Mayet, Adam R. Winstock, and John Strang

Opium is derived from the seed of the opium poppy (Papaver somniferum) and has been used for thousands of years for its analgesic and euphoriant effects.

What are opioids?

Opioids are drugs which mimic endogenous opioid peptides (e.g. endorphins and enkephalins) and activate opioid receptors. Opioids include both naturally occurring opiates extracted from opium (morphine and codeine) and synthetic opioids (heroin and methadone). Heroin is the most common opioid to be misused partly because of its distinctive euphoriant effects.

Neurobiology of opioids

Opioid receptors are widely distributed throughout the central nervous system. Activation of opioid receptors inhibits activity of the dorsal horn. The three most important opioid receptors are μ-receptor, δ-receptor, and κ-receptor. The μ-receptor is concentrated in brain areas and is mostly involved in nocioception (pain sensation). μ-receptor and δ-receptor activation cause hyperpolarization of neurones by activating K+ channels involving G-proteins. Exogenous opioids such as heroin and methadone act at all opioid receptors but particularly at μ-receptors. Opioid receptor antagonists such as naloxone reverse the effects of opioid agonists.[(1)]

The precise mechanisms of tolerance and dependence to opioids are not clear. Short term use of opioids causing intoxication may not lead to neuroadaption of opioid receptors. However, continued use of opioids may lead to opioid receptor desensitization and dependency. Acutely, opioids lead to the inhibition of adenylate cyclase with reduced conversion of ATP to cAMP, resulting in reduced firing at noradrenergic neurones located on the locus coeruleus. Chronic opioid administration leads to compensatory upregulation of cAMP, returning levels towards baseline. On cessation of opioid use (or following opioid receptor antagonism), withdrawal ensues, characterized by a massive surge in unopposed noradrenergic activity (termed the 'noradrenergic storm') from the locus coeruleus. This noradrenergic hyperactivity is thought to underlie many symptoms of opioid withdrawal, and explains some of the efficacy of the presynaptic α2 agonists in the treatment of the symptoms of acute opioid withdrawal. Opioid receptors can readapt back to normal in the absence of opioids.[(2)]

Both glutamate and γ-aminobutyric acid (GABA) are also likely to be involved. Positive reinforcement is thought to be mediated via the dopaminergic mesolimbic system. In the ventral tegmental area, GABA inhibits dopaminergic neurones, which in turn are inhibited via μ-opioid receptor activation. Consequently, opioid use leads to increased dopaminergic activity which is thought to mediate the drive to use and its positive reinforcement.

Route of administration

Heroin may be administered by a number of routes including injecting (intravenous, intramuscular and subcutaneous 'skin popping'), snorting and 'chasing the dragon' (inhaling after heating on tin foil).[(3)] These different routes of administration have profound effects on bioavailability, speed of onset, severity of dependence and physical complications. Different types of heroin may be preferentially used by different routes of administration.[(4)] Brown heroin is poorly water soluble with a high oil content which 'runs' well on a heated foil making it better for 'chasing'. In contrast, white heroin tends to be more water soluble and better suited for intravenous use, although it may still be snorted or smoked after preparation.

Whilst smoking heroin ('chasing the dragon') is probably the most commonly used route of self-administration, it is not as effective or efficient as injecting. Consequently, as heroin users develop tolerance, many subsequently change to the intravenous route. Injecting heroin use is also associated with a greater risk of fatal overdose and hence reducing the transition from smoking to injecting may be associated with reduced harms. Although injecting in the upper limbs is the most common site for administration, as venous access becomes compromised increasingly risky sites such as the groin or neck my be used. However, non-injecting routes of administration are not without risks and may still result in dependence and similar treatment outcomes.

Opioid metabolism

The oral bioavailability of heroin (Diacetylmorphine) itself is poor due to complete first pass metabolism, which is the reason it is often administered by alternative routes. Following administration, heroin is rapidly metabolized to 6-monoacetylmorphine (6-MAM), which is the only metabolite that specifically indicates that heroin has been used. 6-MAM is metabolized to morphine, which is catalyzed in the liver. Morphine (either as a metabolite of heroin or given as a drug) is mostly metabolized by UDP-glucuronosyltransferase (UGT) to the inactive metabolite morphine-3-glucuronide (M3G) and in lesser amounts to the active morphine-6-glucuronide (M6G). Morphine is also ***N***-demethylated to normorphine by hepatic CYP3A4 and CYP2C8 enzymes (Fig. 4.2.3.1.1). Heroin and its metabolites can be monitored in the blood, hair, saliva and urine. 6-MAM is detectable up to 12 h post administration, whilst morphine can be detected in the urine for several days after use.[(5)] Methadone is primarily metabolized in the liver by CYP3A4 to the inactive metabolite 2-ethylidine-1,5-dimethyl-3,3-diphenylpyrrolidine (EDDP), then to 2-ethyl-5-methyl-3,3-diphenylpyraline (EMDP). Buprenorphine is metabolized to norbuprenorphine and to conjugated buprenorphine and norbuprenorphine. Codeine (3-methylmorphine) is synthesized from morphine and metabolized to codeine-6-glucuronide. Additionally codeine is

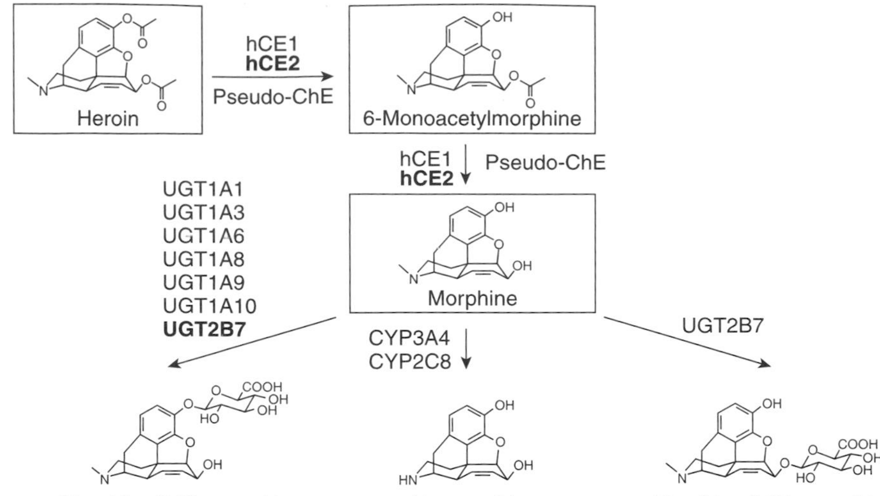

Fig. 4.2.3.1.1 Major metabolic pathways of heroin and morphine in humans.[6] Reproduced from Maurer, H.H., Sauer, C., Theobald, D.S. (2006). Toxicokinetics of drugs of abuse: current knowledge of the isoenzymes involved in the human metabolism of tetrahydrocannabinol, cocaine, heroin, morphine, and codeine. The Drug Monit. 2006 June; **28**(3), 447–53, copyright 2006, Lippincott Williams & Wilkins

metabolized to morphine by CYP2D6. Therefore a morphine positive result is possible after consuming codeine only.[5] Dihydrocodeine is metabolized to nordihydrocodeine and dihydromorphine and cannot normally be metabolized to codeine or morphine.

Epidemiology

The illicit nature of opioid use means that it is often difficult to estimate the exact prevalence. The European Monitoring Centre for Drugs and Drug Addiction reports that heroin use in the general population is less than one per cent.[6] Gender differences in opioid use have been reported with women accounting for approximately one third of all opioid users. Non-dependent recreational heroin use has been reported, but is rare. Dependence will often develop gradually over the first few years, most commonly in the late teens and early twenties. Treatment can alter the course of opioid dependence, by prolonging periods of abstinence and improving outcomes (see later sections). The risk of death from heroin dependence is approximately 12 times that of the general population, with most deaths occurring in males (> 80 per cent). Opioid use has a major effect on crime and it has been estimated that half of all crime is drug related, with estimated costs within the UK criminal justice system at £1 billion per annum in 1996.

The effects of opioids

The effects of opioids are outlined in Table 4.2.3.2.1. The effects vary depending on dose and route.

Opioid dependence and withdrawal

Opioid dependence may be classified according to the ICD-10 criteria (see appendix). Continued use of heroin (or other opioids) tends to lead to physiological dependence with the development of tolerance and withdrawal symptoms on discontinuing heroin. Tolerance occurs when the same dose gives a reduced effect or conversely, an increased opioid dose is required to have the same effect. Once physiological dependence is established, abrupt cessation or a marked reduction in dose will result in a withdrawal syndrome. During this time there is an 'undoing' of the neuroadaptation which had occurred during the development of tolerance. Withdrawal leads to 'gooseflesh' (piloerection) of the skin (which is the reason behind the term 'cold turkey'). Insomnia (with increase in Rapid Eye Movement sleep) and craving for the drug may persist for weeks. Most withdrawal symptoms appear within 4–12 h and peak at 48–72 h lasting 7–10 days. Longer acting opioids such as methadone may result in a more prolonged withdrawal. Opioid withdrawal is not usually considered to be life threatening.

Complications from opioid use

Complications may be biological, psychological, or social (Table 4.2.3.1.2).

Biological complications

Opioid overdose is the most common cause of death among opioid users, while blood-borne virus infection and other injecting related complications also contribute to increased morbidity and premature deaths.

(a) Opioid overdose

Opioid overdose occurs when the opioid dose exceeds the individual's tolerance to the respiratory depressant effect of the drug.

Table 4.2.3.1.1 Effects of opioids

Mood change (euphoria)
Analgesia
Drowsiness/Sleep
Respiratory depression
Cough reflex depression
Sensitization of the labyrinth with nausea and vomiting
Decreased sympathetic outflow (bradycardia and hypotension)
Lowering of the body temperature
Pupillary constriction
Constipation

Table 4.2.3.1.2 Complications of opioid use

Biological	Psychological	Social
Infections	Psychiatric complications	Criminal behavior
- hepatitis and HIV	- depression	- fund dependence
- bacterial endocarditis	- suicide	Loss of housing
- septicaemia		Unemployment
- abscesses		Loss of family
- cellulitis		- family breakdown
Cardiorespiratory		
- pulmonary emboli		
- aspiration		
- cardiac arrthymias		
- respiratory depression		
- overdose death		

It is more common when other Central Nervous System depressants are concurrently consumed. Respiratory depression is caused by the opioid action on the brain stem nuclei and death can follow within minutes of injecting excessive amounts. Risk factors for opioid overdose are injecting use, return to opioid use following recent abstinence (such as following detoxification and release from prison), during the early stages of dependence and starting opioid substitution treatment.(7) In addition, variability in opioid purity, increased central depressant effects following polysubstance use and high levels of psychiatric co-morbidity may increase the vulnerability for accidental or intentional overdose. Opioid overdose can be rapidly reversed if naloxone (opioid antagonist) is administered to the person who has overdosed. The management of an opioid overdose is described later in the chapter.

(b) Blood borne virus transmission

The risk of viral transmission is high among injecting drug users, and routine testing with counseling should be available to those at risk. Transmission of blood borne viruses is primarily related to sharing injecting equipment and involvement in the sex industry. Needle sharing appears to occur less frequently than sharing of spoons and filters, but any shared equipment may pose the risk of viral transmission. The prison population is particularly at risk, as injecting is more common likely to involve sharing injecting equipment.

Opioid substitution treatment is one of the most effective interventions for reducing the extent of injecting, thereby also reducing both the spread of and morbidity from blood borne viruses. Stabilization on methadone/buprenoprehine with abstinence from injecting, needle and other injecting equipment sharing, and unprotected sex should be encouraged among all dependent heroin users. Blood borne virus testing and referral to specialists for treatment is important. In addition, close liaison with medical and psychiatric services is important for improving outcomes and compliance with treatment.

(i) Human immunodeficiency virus (HIV)

Rates of HIV seropositivity amongst current injecting drug users in England and Wales although low, have recently increased, with an incidence of 1.5 per cent reported in 2004 (the highest since 1992), with higher rates reported in London.(8) The relatively low levels of HIV within the UK and elsewhere in Europe is believed to be due to the widespread availability of 'needle-exchange' services and provision of services focused towards 'harm minimization'.(9)

(ii) Hepatitis B & C

Screening of drug users in treatment has revealed prevalence rates of 20 per cent for Hepatitis B and more than 50 per cent for Hepatitis C. Intravenous drug users are likely to have higher rates estimated at 30 to 50 per cent (Hepatitis B) and up to 90 per cent (Hepatitis C).(10) Prognosis is worsened by high levels of alcohol consumption and therefore liaison with hepatitis/gastroenterology services is important. Screening for Hepatitis B and C and targeted vaccination for Hepatitis B, in addition to education and harm-reduction provision, should be provided.

Psychological complications

Numerous large epidemiological studies have identified that co-morbid psychiatric illness is common among those with opioid dependence, with prevalence rates of about 50 per cent.(11) Concurrent use of benzodiazepines, alcohol, and especially stimulant drugs increases psychiatric morbidity in addition to female gender, poor physical function, and difficulties in personal relationships.(12) Many of those with opioid dependence will have had childhood behavioural problems such as conduct disorder which may be a marker for subsequent drug use.(13) The rate of suicide among heroin users is estimated at 14 times that of age matched peers with reports of 3–35 per cent of deaths related to suicide. Risk factors include a history of depression, poly substance use in addition to generic risk factors.(14)

At entry into treatment, it may be difficult to make an accurate determination of an opioid user's psychiatric diagnosis and generally assessment should be repeated once stability on a substitution medication or detoxification has been achieved. Waiting to review a patient's mental health once they are out of crisis can prevent early misdiagnosis since much of psychiatric distress dissipates rapidly on cessation of illicit use and stabilization. In one follow up study of opioid users entering treatment, baseline levels of depression fell from 25 per cent at baseline to 11 per cent at 12 month follow up, with the observed decline being strongly related to treatment exposure.(15) Follow-up and provision of treatment for co-morbid disorders are thus essential. Enhancing compliance with prescribed medications through supervised dispensing or engagement of carers is useful. Treatment can be effective in reducing psychiatric distress observed on entry to treatment in this group. However, in a significant proportion, even on cessation of use or abstinence, major psychiatric illnesses can persist. If left untreated, co-morbid conditions can lead to a poorer prognosis particularly in respect to relapse and suicide.

Social complications

The ramifications of heroin dependence upon individual functioning and that individual's ability to relate and function within their family and community are immense. Although high rates of socioeconomic disadvantage often precede entry into heroin use, it is the other associated problems of relatively poorer premorbid functional and educational attainment that frequently compound later efforts at rehabilitation. High rates of criminal activity, homelessness, and unemployment are associated with opioid addiction, although treatment can improve socio-economic status.

Treatment of opioid dependence

Opioid maintenance treatment

Opioid maintenance treatment generally involves substituting heroin for an oral long-acting opioid, thereby reducing the plasma level variability and stopping injecting drug use. Oral methadone and buprenorphine have been licensed in several countries for use in the treatment of opioid dependence and both are approved in the UK.[16] The decision regarding whether methadone or buprenorphine is used should be based on individual factors estimating the risks and benefits and following discussion with the patient. If both drugs are equally suitable, cost-effectiveness examination by the National Institute of Clinical Excellence (NICE) concludes that methadone should be prescribed as the first choice.[16]

(a) Methadone maintenance treatment

Methadone is a synthetic orally active full opioid agonist with a half-life of 24–36 h, making it suitable for daily administration. This is an effective treatment for heroin dependence and has significantly better outcomes than non pharmacological substitution for retaining patients in treatment, decreasing heroin use, reducing crimes, reducing overdose deaths, reduced injecting and sharing of injecting equipment and consequent reduced risk behaviours leading to transmission of HIV.[17] Higher doses of methadone (60 to 120 mg/day) have been shown to be more effective than lower dosages[18] and doses greater than 80 mg daily are believed to provide a reasonable level of opioid receptor blockade such that euphoria from illicit opioids is diminished.

Methadone steady state plasma levels take approximately 4 to 5 days and so there is potential for methadone accumulation (and overdose) when initiating treatment. Deaths have been recorded during the induction phase onto methadone especially when the recipient is not as tolerant as believed or is using other opioids or substances.[19] Therefore, confirmation of the patient's dependent status is paramount as described in the chapter and it is safer to start treatment at low doses (not more than 30 mg daily). Treatment should be initiated under supervision with oral methadone liquid where consumption can be easily monitored. Doses should generally be increased slowly, and titrated against withdrawal symptoms. As methadone can accumulate, there should be increased observation over the first few weeks of treatment. Doses can then gradually be increased to within therapeutic levels (60–120 mg daily). Prescribing should follow the guidelines outlined later in the chapter.

(b) Buprenorphine maintenance treatment

Buprenorphine (Subutex) is a synthetic partial opioid agonist which is given as a sublingual tablet and has a high affinity at μ-opioid receptors. It is an effective treatment for use in maintenance treatment for heroin addiction, but is not more effective than methadone at adequate dosages.[20]

Buprenorphine undergoes extensive first metabolism. Therefore, it is administered as sublingual tablets (2 mg and 8 mg) with bioavailability of between 30–40 per cent. Optimizing sublingual absorption while minimizing diversion is a practical challenge that supervised dispensing points still need to address. Taking 5–7 minutes to dissolve, buprenorphine reaches a plateau on most physiological subjective effect at a daily dose of 4–16 mg. At higher doses, the duration of action increases, permitting less than daily dosing in about one-third of patients. Because of its high affinity for the opioid receptor, buprenorphine will precipitate withdrawal if administered to someone with an opioid agonist on board (typically within 8 h of heroin use or 24–36 h of methadone use). Therefore, patients are advised to wait until they are in mild withdrawal before commencing treatment. Finally, it is thought to be safer in overdose (with a 'ceiling' in the respiratory depression, unlike with full opioid agonists) and so induction can be quite rapid aiming for doses of between 8–16 mg by day 3.

It is an effective analgesic but may be less suitable than methadone for those with chronic pain. Although safer in overdose than methadone, fatal overdose can occur especially when taken in combination with other substances. As with methadone dose, reduction in someone stable on maintenance should be done gradually (typically 2 mg ever 2 weeks) and only supported when there is evidence of continued abstinence from illicit opioid use. Continued dose reduction in the face of return to illicit use is likely to further destabilize the patient. In some countries (e.g. many European countries since 2007), another preparation has become available (Suboxone), in which buprenorphine has been combined with naloxone in a ratio of 4:1 to reduce the desirability of injecting diverted medication. When taken as directed (sublingual), the bioavailability of naloxone is very poor, whereas when injected by a dependent opiate user, a severe withdrawal reaction may be precipitated.

(c) Other opioid maintenance treatments

Injectable methadone and injectable heroin are rarely prescribed in the United Kingdom and at present there is insufficient evidence to guide this use.[21] However, it may be considered in some patients as a 'second-line' treatment option for whom an adequate trial (e.g. at least 6 months) of optimized methadone maintenance treatment (e.g. doses > 80 mg daily, regular supervised dosing, regular appointments and appropriate management of medical or psychiatric co-morbidity) is ineffective in controlling illicit injecting heroin use. This should only be initiated by a specialist. Both long-acting morphine and dihyrocodeine have been compared to methadone in two randomized controlled trials which have revealed broadly equivalent outcomes between the groups.[23,23]

Opioid detoxification

Detoxification may be based on suppression of the 'nor-adrenergic storm' that accompanies opioid withdrawal, by prescribing either α2-receptor agonists or a gradual reduction of an opioid agonist. When a patient is stable and motivated, a gradual reduction in the dose of opioid maintenance dose can be an effective means for attaining abstinence. However, it must be noted that detoxification is generally associated with poor long term rates of abstinence and retention in treatment.

(a) Buprenorphine detoxification

Buprenorphine has been found to be more effective than clonidine (below) for the management of opioid withdrawal. In addition, there is no significant difference between buprenorphine and methadone in terms of completion of treatment, but withdrawal symptoms may resolve more quickly with buprenorphine.[24] This can be undertaken as an inpatient or outpatient. Buprenorphine should only be taken after cessation of heroin use as it can precipitate withdrawal. Withdrawal may be achieved by the burpenorphine dose being stabilized according to withdrawal over a 24–48 h period, after which a gradual dose reduction should occur over 5–21 days in the inpatient or outpatient setting.

(b) Methadone detoxification

Methadone detoxification can be used for pharmacologically assisted opioid detoxifications. A review revealed that withdrawal programs vary widely with regard to duration, design and treatment objectives. This review confirmed that slow tapering with temporary substitution of methadone accompanied by medical supervision and ancillary medications can reduce withdrawal severity. Nevertheless, the majority of patients relapsed to heroin use.(25)

(c) α2-Agonist assisted detoxification

α2-agonists, such as lofexidine and clonidine, reduce pre-synaptic nor adrenaline release alleviating many withdrawal symptoms associated with opioid withdrawal. The dose is titrated against the symptoms and signs of withdrawal whilst also avoiding hypotensive episodes. Detoxification can occur in both outpatient and inpatient settings. Lofexidine that has a lower incidence of hypotension than clonidine is the preferred non-opioid method of assisting opioid withdrawal. A review has concluded that there is no significant difference in efficacy for treatment regimes based on clonidine and lofexidine, compared to reducing doses of methadone over a period of around 10 days, for the management of opioid withdrawal.(26)

(d) Naltrexone assisted detoxification

Some research has been published suggesting that withdrawal may also be completed more quickly by additionally administering the long-acting opioid antagonist naltrexone. However, further research is still needed to confirm effectiveness and safety of this treatment.

Naltrexone for relapse prevention

Oral naltrexone has recently been recommended in the UK for the management of opioid dependence. Naltrexone is relevant for highly motivated patients who have completed an opioid detoxification. This may be combined with arrangements for supervision and should be given as part of a programme of supportive care. Regular reviews of effectiveness of naltrexone should be undertaken by the clinician and discontinuation of treatment should be considered if there is evidence of continued opiate misuse.(27)

Psychosocial interventions for opioid dependence

There are numerous psychosocial approaches that are currently used in the management of substance misuse. Treatment based on a holistic approach encompassing biological, psychological and social aspects of care is likely to improve outcomes. Psychosocial treatments such as relapse prevention, motivational interviewing and contingency management are often used in the addiction setting. Cognitive behaviour therapy and other types of psychotherapy are also used particularly for those with a specific psychiatric disorder such as depression and can be referenced elsewhere in the book.

Relapse Prevention looks at identification of triggers for craving (e.g. people, places, or moods) and uses learning techniques (distraction, relaxation) to handle high-risk situations.(28) Motivational interviewing techniques can help patients move along a 'cycle of change' from pre-contemplation (no interest in changing behaviour) to contemplator, to determination and action without confrontation.(29) This is based on five key principles (Table 4.2.3.1.3) which are often used in both addiction and eating disorders, but may also be used in any aspect of the doctor-patient relationship where the patient is ambivalent about change.(30) Although used rarely in the UK, Contingency Management (CM) has a stronger evidence base. This behavioural treatment uses rewards or other reinforcers to promote abstinence or other selected goals. Narcotics Anonymous is based on the 12-step program (the philosophy behind Alcoholics Anonymous) where the individual accepts they have a drug problem and uses 12 steps (Table 4.2.3.1.4) within the group setting, to attain abstinence.(31)

Table 4.2.3.1.3 Principles of motivational interviewing(30)

- express empathy
- help the client to see discrepancies in their behaviours
- avoid argument
- roll with resistance
- support the patient's sense of self-efficacy.

Reproduced from Miller, W. and Rollnick, S. Motivational Interviewing, copyright 1991, Guildford Press NY.

Psychosocial interventions alone have not been shown to be more effective than no treatment.(32) However psychosocial interventions combined with pharmacological interventions have been shown to lead to better outcomes.(33)

Educating the drug user about safe practices (including safer injecting, not sharing equipment) and harm-reduction techniques is important, as is appropriate liaison with other agencies such as social services or voluntary sector supports. Therapeutic communities, residential rehabilitation and 'concept houses' based on a religious or abstinent theme offer longer-term care.

Management of opioid dependence

The treatment plan should be made jointly between the clinician and patient. The actual management plan depends on whether the person has opioid dependence, the amount of opioids used, and the outcome of the mutually agreed treatment objectives and

Table 4.2.3.1.4 12 Steps of Narcotics Anonymous(31)

1. We admitted that we were powerless over our addiction, that our lives had become unmanageable.
2. We came to believe that a Power greater than ourselves could restore us to sanity.
3. We made a decision to turn our will and our lives over to the care of God as we understood Him.
4. We made a searching and fearless moral inventory of ourselves.
5. We admitted to God, to ourselves, and to another human being the exact nature of our wrongs.
6. We were entirely ready to have God remove all these defects of character.
7. We humbly asked Him to remove our shortcomings.
8. We made a list of all persons we had harmed, and became willing to make amends to them all.
9. We made direct amends to such people wherever possible, except when to do so would injure them or others.
10. We continued to take personal inventory and when we were wrong promptly admitted it.
11. We sought through prayer and meditation to improve our conscious contact with God as we understood Him, praying only for knowledge of His will for us and the power to carry that out.
12. Having had a spiritual awakening as a result of these steps, we tried to carry this message to addicts, and to practice these principles in all our affairs.

treatment plan. Opioid dependence management is sometimes based on 'abstinence', where the person refrains from taking drugs, but also needs to be based on the principles of harm reduction. Harm reduction aims to reduce harms from opioid use often in terms of reducing deaths, spread of blood-borne viruses or improving psychosocial outcomes. This may optimally be achieved through cessation of injecting illicit opioid use by stabilizing the person on an opioid replacement.

Assessment of opioid use and dependence

A comprehensive assessment of opioid use patterns and associated risks forms the basis of any treatment plan. A suggested plan of enquiry that allows both accurate diagnosis and risk assessment is outlined below.

(a) Clinical assessment

1 **Current consumption:** How much heroin (or other opioid) is consumed on a typical day, in terms of either weight or money spent, and for how long has consumption been at this level? Are opioids taken daily? What happens when no opioids are taken? The route of use (smoking, intravenous injection), number of administrations per day, and the minimum amount of opioid required each day to avoid withdrawal symptoms should also be assessed. Enquiry should be made to determine if more than one type of opioid is being used (e.g. prescribed medication or street methadone). All other substances being used should be identified (e.g. cocaine, benzodiazepines and alcohol) and their patterns of use.

2 **Typical day:** A systematic enquiry of the person's typical day and the use of opioids and other substances is particularly important for assessing evidence of withdrawal. This can also be useful for identifying risk activities that the user engages in to support their ongoing use, including criminal activity, high risk sex, or injecting practices.

3 **Drug use history:** A careful enquiry needs to be made to determine the temporal relationship between the onset of drug use and any psychological behaviors. The age of first use and the psychosocial precipitants of use should be established, as should the development of tolerance and craving through increased frequency of use, escalating dose, and where relevant, the onset of injecting.

4 **Biopsychosocial complications:** This should assess episodes of overdose (intentional or accidental), viral screening status and injecting behaviour including use of needle exchanges, sharing equipment and use of high-risk injection sites such as the groin and neck. Effects on family relationships, employment and criminal activity, and co-morbid psychiatric conditions related to opioid use should be assessed.

5 **Past treatments and abstinent periods:** Have they ever been in contact with treatment services, maintained on substitute medication or undertaken a detoxification? What was their longest period of abstinence? What has helped in the past? When and why did relapses occur? What are high-risk situations and other triggers for use?

6 **Motivation for change:** Why seek treatment now? What support is needed? Thinking of **L**ivelihood (financial), **L**ife (physical health), **L**ove life, **L**egal problems and **L**osing it (loss of control) can be helpful as these are often precipitants for seeking treatment and can be used to encourage behavioural change.

(b) Confirmation of dependence

Although a diagnosis of opioid dependence can be made by taking a full history; dependence and tolerance to opioids should be corroborated before commencing substitute treatment. Confirmation of dependence and tolerance prior to commencing treatment is important since the greatest risk associated with prescribing methadone is the possibility of overdose following consumption of methadone by a non-tolerant individual. Corroborative information may come from urine drug screens and other health care practitioners such as the GP or criminal justice worker. Physical examination is essential and may reveal stigmata of injecting drug use such as evidence of recent intravenous injection sites or the more long-term 'track marks' (linear scarring along veins from repeated intravenous use) on the drug user's limbs. All patients should be asked where they usually inject and recent injection sites should be examined. In those with poor upper limb veins, with evidence suggestive of ongoing illicit use, it may be appropriate to examine groin or neck sites.

Urines tests are supportive of use but not confirmatory of dependence. Sequential urine testing over a few days may allow the confirmation of regular opioid (although not necessarily heroin) consumption. Measurement of withdrawal by using withdrawal scales (Table 4.2.3.1.5) in addition to examining for presence of tachycardia and hypertension, following a period of abstinence, is helpful in confirming withdrawal. The Objective Opiate Withdrawal Scale (Table 4.2.3.1.5) is useful when assessing whether a person is in withdrawal before commencing opioid substitution treatment and useful after commencing treatment to aid assessing whether the opioid substitute dose is adequate. Partial or full reversal of withdrawal following a measured dose of opioids administered on site will provide some information of the patient's level of tolerance.

Table 4.2.3.1.5 Objective opiate withdrawal scale[27]

This is to be completed by clinician. A score should be given for each observation within a 5 minute observation period.

Observations	Scoring
1. Yawning	0 = no yawns 1 = ≥ 1 yawns
2. Rhinorrhoea	0 = <3 sniffs 1 = ≥3 sniffs
3. Piloerection (observe arm) 'gooseflesh'	0 = absent 1 = present
4. Perspiration	0 = absent 1 = present
5. Lacrimation	0 = absent 1 = present
6. Tremor	0 = absent 1 = present
7. Mydriasis	0 = absent 1 = ≥ 3mm
8. Hot and cold flushes	0 = absent 1 = shivering / huddling for warmth
9. Restlessness	0 = absent 1 = frequent shifts of position
10. Vomiting	0 = absent 1 = present
11. Muscle twitches	0 = absent 1 = present
12. Abdominal cramps	0 = absent 1 = Holding stomach
13. Anxiety	0 = absent 1 = mild – severe
TOTAL SCORE	

National Institute for Health and Clinical Excellence (NICE) (2005) TA115 Drug misuse–naltrexone. London: NICE. Available from www.nice.org.uk/ TA115 Reproduced with permission.

Investigations for patients with opioid dependence

Heroin dependence is associated with high rates of physical and psychiatric morbidity. Since access to primary health care may be difficult, basic physical health checks should be a fundamental part of all drug treatment. The core assessment should include history, physical examination, routine blood tests, blood borne virus screening and vaccination where appropriate, and assessment of nutritional status, mental and dental health. Referral to appropriate specialist services should be facilitated through coordinated care planning which should form the cornerstone of structured drug treatment delivery.

Management options for opioid dependence

Following a careful and thorough assessment which allows confirmation of dependence as outlined above, there are several treatment options. In the short term, opioid substitution treatments with methadone or buprenorphine may be offered. Opioid substitution treatment should be monitored closely, especially during the initial phase of treatment. Initiation of opioid substitution treatment usually takes place in the community setting, but may occur in an inpatient setting if there is a complicated history involving medical or psychiatric morbidity. Opioid maintenance treatment is continued in the community setting and can be continued as maintenance for the long term, with some patients continuing treatment for over 50 years. Treatment for opioid dependence is likely to be improved when framed within a comprehensive treatment package including psychosocial and pharmacological interventions.[32] Relapse prevention and motivational interviewing can be carried out during regular appointments with health professionals. Community substance misuse teams often use keyworking as a model of care for opioid dependent patients. This is where one healthcare professional looks after the patients care and provides the main source of contact, often following up referrals and ensuring medical and psychosocial needs are met. Opioid maintenance treatment within the community substance team may continue in the long term or be a prelude to starting abstinence based treatments, with the aim of stopping all illicit heroin use.

Abstinence can be achieved by pharmacologically assisted withdrawal from the opioid via a detoxification with either lofexidine or an opioid substitute such as methadone or buprenorphine (as above). This usually takes 10–21 days but may be longer if withdrawal from a longer acting opioid is required. Opioid detoxification may take place in the inpatient or community setting, depending on the level of medical and psychiatric morbidity. Following opioid detoxification patients may benefit from treatment within a therapeutic community or residential rehabilitation centre where life skills for dealing with a world without opioids may be developed. For patients who do not enter rehabilitation centres, regular sessions with keyworkers using relapse prevention and motivational interviewing may also be beneficial. Highly motivated patients may also benefit from naltrexone to prevent relapse (described above).

Prescribing opioids for opioid dependence

In the United Kingdom, all doctors may prescribe methadone or buprenorphine for the treatment of dependence, although prescribing should generally be initiated by a specialist or special interest general practitioner. Prescriptions for opioid dependence should ideally be dispensed daily with supervised doses, particularly for the first three months of treatment. After about three months, if a patient is stable (based on psychosocial outcomes and illicit substance use) the number of dispensings per week and level of supervision may be reduced, although this may be varied when there are extenuating circumstances. UK guidelines advocate that no more than a week's medication is dispensed at a time.

Liaison between the pharmacist, the general practitioner and the specialist is important to prevent double scripting, reduce diversion and improve safety. Clinicians in all specialties should be aware of the potential for all opioid-containing analgesics to be diverted for abuse or develop into iatrogenic dependence. Repeat prescriptions of such analgesics should be carefully reviewed. Prescriptions for controlled drugs can only be for 28 days in total and the total prescribed amount must be written in words and figures. It is recommended that the prescription should state the name of the pharmacy where the prescription is to be dispensed, how often the prescription should be dispensed and whether the dose should be consumed under supervision. Installment prescriptions for daily dispensing are available in the UK for burpenorphine and methadone. Only doctors in possession of a Home Office license are able to prescribe heroin for the treatment of opioid dependence.[34]

Opioid overdose management

Opioid overdose management training is particularly important as early recognition (Table 4.2.3.1.6) of an opioid overdose and prompt action (Table 4.2.3.1.7) can save lives. The antidote to heroin is naloxone and this should be given if an opioid overdose is suspected. Although intravenous naloxone is quicker acting, venous access may be difficult and therefore, intramuscular injection may be preferable and also results in a more gradual reversal of the overdose which may be less likely to provoke aggression. Hospital monitoring should always be recommended, since the plasma half-life of naloxone is shorter (<1 h) than the physiological effects of heroin (4–6 h) and methadone (24–36 h). In addition many overdoses are a result of concomitant substance use—the effects of which will not be reversed by naloxone alone. Opioid overdoses involving buprenorphine (partial agonist) will not be readily be reversed by naloxone; however buprenorphine is believed to have much less respiratory depressant effects.

The supply of 'take home' emergency naloxone may help reduce opioid related overdose deaths. It has, therefore, been advocated that providing take-home naloxone in combination with opioid overdose management training to opioid using patients and their families may help reduce deaths.[35]

Table 4.2.3.1.6 Recognition of an opioid overdose

Recognition
Respiratory Arrest with a pulse
Pinpoint pupils (unreactive to light)
Snoring giving way to shallow respiration
Respiratory Depression (<8 breaths per min)
Bradycardia and hypotension
Varying degrees of unconsiousness

Table 4.2.3.1.7 Management of an opioid overdose

Check area safe, then try to rouse overdose victim
If unrousable - Call for help/ambulance
Check airway and breathing a. If not breathing, give 2 rescue breaths b. If breathing — place in recovery position
Administer 0.4 mg Naloxone Intramuscularly — Increase dose until adequate reversal achieved
Consider use of high flow oxygen
Patient to have medical monitoring after naloxone, as opioid overdose may re-emerge. Patients may need additional doses of naloxone

Table 4.2.3.1.8 Aims of managing the pregnant drug user

- Engage and maintain contact with the patient and partner.
- Aim to reduce risk-taking behaviours (sharing needles, prostitution).
- Stabilize on oral methadone maintenance treatment (or extremely slow detoxification, if required).
- Ensure that other drug and alcohol use are assessed routinely.
- Provide health and psychosocial care including blood borne virus screening.
- Close liaison with multi-agency teams including possible social work assessment.
- Social stability and provisions for motherhood.

Special groups

Young people

Young people with opioid problems often have other emotional and/or behavioural problems, and frequently fall between the adult and child psychiatric services as well as addiction services, compounding the difficulties in providing effective services to this group. Increasingly dedicated services have recently been developed and these integrated services focus as much on the family and re-integration with education as they do on substance use issues. Approaches effective for the adult population may be less effective in a group with less developed emotional and cognitive abilities. Separation of such a service from adult providers would also assist in preventing experienced drug users from influencing more naive users. Ultimately, a tiered approach would appear appropriate, since it would allow maximum utility of current services and focused development of new services. Generic services in primary health care could provide accurate screening with initial referral to youth-oriented services within existing departments. Beyond this, referral to specialist and super-specialist regional services could be employed to provide secure environments with the option of residential rehabilitation and therapeutic communities. Once engaged they may benefit from a range of possible therapies from family work and cognitive behavioural therapy to pharmacotherapy and self-help groups.

Pregnancy and breastfeeding

Maternal opioid use poses a risk to both the mother and foetus. Pregnancy can be a specific point when women try to address their opioid use problem. The management of the pregnant opioid user should follow the same guiding principles as for other opioid users; additionally, there should be close liaison between addictions and maternity services, the general practitioner and other relevant agencies (Table 4.2.3.1.8).

Women who are already on methadone maintenance treatment can remain on methadone but should be encouraged to stop illicit opioid use. For women who are not prescribed methadone, the first step is to initiate stabilization on methadone. Methadone maintenance may continue at a stable dose throughout pregnancy. During the third trimester, maternal metabolism may increase the need for methadone and so the dose may need to be increased or alternatively the daily dose could be split. Methadone increases the risk of respiratory depression in the neonate and should always be pre-considered for the delivery plan. Women prescribed opioids may also need increased pain relief during delivery. The long-term outcome in women who enter methadone treatment programmes during pregnancy is better in terms of their pregnancy, childbirth, and infant development, irrespective of continuing illicit drug use.[(36)] Methadone is not contraindicated for breast feeding.

Some women prefer to be abstinent from opioids during pregnancy. These women will often need a gradual pharmacologically assisted detoxification, which should be avoided in the first trimester, ideally undertaken in the second trimester and undertaken with caution in the third trimester. Detoxification is best undertaken within a dedicated inpatient facility, however, this may not always be possible and therefore community detoxification can be undertaken. During stabilization on methadone or detoxification, it is important to prevent the pregnant woman experiencing opioid withdrawal as this is dangerous for both mother and fetus.

Currently, there is insufficient evidence regarding the use of buprenorphine during pregnancy or breastfeeding to be able to define its safety profile. However, women well maintained on buprenorphine prior to pregnancy refusing alternative pharmacotherapy could be kept on buprenorphine following full informed consent.

Forensic

It has been estimated that up to two-thirds of people arrested have taken substances prior to arrest, whilst approximately 15–50 per cent of the prison population were previously dependent on drugs or alcohol. It is difficult to estimate exact opioid use and dependence, but approximately one-fifth of the prison population injects drugs. Access to illicit substances is not prevented by imprisonment; indeed some users may increase or start using drugs whilst imprisoned.[(37)] Improving identification of drug users before sentencing is important. In addition, identification of drug related crimes and offering court diversion schemes with drug treatment interventions can be an alternative to a custodial sentence. Prisoners will benefit from education, good primary health care, blood borne virus testing, and hepatitis vaccination. In addition, prisoners can undertake opioid detoxification or commence/continue opioid maintenance treatment whilst in prison. Release from prison is associated with extremely high risk of opioid overdose death, particularly in the first few weeks, and therefore quick access to drug services following release (or prior to release) may reduce deaths.

Accessing treatment and the range of services

Those who experience problems with opioids may present to a wide range of professionals within the health-care, social, and legal systems. The range of treatment options available from statutory and non-statutory agencies in any particular area will vary, as will the provision of either maintenance or detoxification for opioid dependents depending upon differing treatment philosophies and treatment settings.

Outcomes

Heroin dependence is a chronic relapsing condition and opioid use reduces morbidity and mortality more than any other drug use.[38] Treatment saves lives and improves psychosocial function as well as reducing risk to both the individual and the community. Outcomes are broadly comparable to those seen with other chronic medical conditions.[39] Abstinence rates following treatment vary widely, but 10 to 40 per cent of treated patients are still drug free at 6 months.[40] The majority of those who relapse following treatment do so within 3 months of discharge. Longer treatment is associated with better outcomes and greater pre-treatment severity of psychopathology is associated with worse outcomes. Long-term follow-up studies suggest that successful and lasting cessation of opioid use can be a very slow process and becomes increasingly unlikely if users continue into their late thirties.

Results from three longitudinal studies ranging from 3–5 years based in the United Kingdom, Australia and United States of America have shown that treatment leads to better outcomes against all parameters as compared to no treatment.[41,42,43] Patients who enter drug treatment are more likely to significantly reduce use of heroin and other illicit drugs and longer treatment times have been associated with better treatment outcomes. Reductions in heroin use have also been mirrored by reductions in heroin overdose rates. Therefore opioid treatment increases morbidity and mortality in opioid users.

The Australian Treatment Outcome Study (ATOS) reported that half the number of opioid overdoses occurred in the participants in treatment at 1 year as compared to the same participants prior to entering treatment. In addition this study showed that levels of psychopathology reduced, physical health improved and crime rates in this population reduced following treatment.[43] The National Treatment Outcome Research Study (NTORS) based in the UK had increased rates of abstinence, reduced heroin use and reduced injecting and sharing of injecting related equipment with both residential and community treatment.[42] Findings from the Drug Abuse Treatment Outcome Studies (DATOS) based in the USA were similar to both the UK and Australia studies.[41]

Longer term outcomes have been observed in a study following up 581 male heroin users since 1962. At the 33-year follow up, 284 subjects were dead and 242 were interviewed. Over a fifth were still using heroin and 40.5 per cent admitted to using heroin in the last year. There were high rates of health problems, mental health problems, and criminal justice system involvement. Heroin abstinence was associated with improved outcomes in all these domains. Deaths increased steadily over time with a relatively stable pattern of heroin use in the subjects.[44] A further analysis of the results assessed years of life lost through heroin use and concluded that on average, 18.3 years of potential life were lost before the age 65, which is significantly higher than that of US population.[45]

Conclusion

Opioid dependence is a chronic relapsing and remitting disorder affecting a large proportion of people throughout the world with severe physical, psychological, and social consequences. Opioid overdose and spread of blood borne viruses are major causes of morbidity and mortality. Assessment of opioid use and dependence should be systematic and confirmation of dependence is of paramount importance before initiating treatment. The prescription of substitute opioids should be managed carefully to prevent harm, diversion to others and improve safety. Management of opioid dependence can greatly improve outcomes and may be based on opioid maintenance stabilization or detoxification combined with psychosocial interventions.

Further information

Department of Health (England) and the developed administrations. Drug misuse and dependence: UK guidelines on clinical management. 1999. HMSO, London. http://www.dh.gov.uk/prod_consum_dh/groups/dh_digitalassets/@dh/@en/documents/digitalasset/dh_4078198.pdf

National Treatment Agency for Substance Misuse website for guidelines. http://www.nta.nhs.uk/

The Cochrane Library for Cochrane Systematic Reviews on Opioids. http://www3.interscience.wiley.com/cgi-bin/mrwhome/106568753/HOME

National Institute for Clinical Excellence. www.nice.org.uk/

References

1. Stahl, S.M. (2006). *Essential Psychopharmacology*, Cambridge University Press, Cambridge.
2. Simonato, M.(1996). The neurochemistry of morphine addiction in the neocortex. *Trends in Pharmacological Science*, **17**, 410–15.
3. Strang, J., Griffiths, P., Gossop, M., *et al.* (1997). Heroin in the United Kingdom: different forms, different origins, and the relationship to different routes of administration. *Drug and Alcohol Review*,**16**, 329–37.
4. Strang, J., Griffiths, P., Powis, B., *et al.(1999).* Heroin chasers and heroin injectors: differences observed in a community sample in London. *American Journal on Addictions*, **8**(2),148–60.
5. Maurer, H.H., Sauer, C., Theobald, D.S., *et al.* (2006) Toxicokinetics of drugs of abuse: current knowledge of the isoenzymes involved in the human metabolism of tetrahydrocannabinol, cocaine, heroin, morphine, and codeine. *Therapeutic Drug Monitoring,* **28**(3), 447–53.
6. Annual report on the state of the drugs problem in the European Union 2000 European Monitoring Centre for Drugs and Drug Addiction (EMCDDA). Accessed April 2007.
7. Gossop, M., Griffiths, P., Powis, B., *et al.* (1996). Frequency of non-fatal heroin overdose. *British Medical Journal*, **313**, 402.
8. United Kingdom drug situation: annual report to the European Monitoring Centre for Drugs and Drug Addiction (EMCDDA) 2005.
9. Stimson, G.V. (1995). AIDS and injecting drug use in the UK, 1987–1993: the policy response and the prevention of the epidemic. *Social Sciences and Medicine*, **41**, 699–716.
10. Fingerhood, M.I., Jasinski, D.R., Sullivan, J.T. *et al.*(1993). Prevalence of hepatitis C in a chemically dependent population. *Archives of International Medicine*, **153**, 2025–30.
11. Verthein, U., Degkwitz, P., Haasen, C., *et al.*(2005). Significance of comorbidity for the long-term course of opiate dependence. *European Addiction Resarch*, **11**(1),15–21.

12. Marsden, J., Gossop, M., Stewart, D., *et al.* (2000). Psychiatric symptoms among clients seeking treatment for drug dependence. Intake data from the National Treatment Outcome Research Study. *The British Journal of Psychiatry*, **176**,285–9.
13. Lloyd, C.(1998). Risk factors for problem drug use: identifying vulnerable groups. *Drugs: Education, Prevention and Policy*, **5**, 217–32.
14. Darke, S., Ross, J.(2002). Suicide among heroin users: rates, risk factors and methods. *Addiction*, **97**(11),1383–94.
15. Havard, A., Teesson, M., Darke, S., *et al.* (2006). Depression among heroin users: 12-Month outcomes from the Australian Treatment Outcome Study (ATOS). *Journal of Substance Abuse Treatment*, **30**(4), 355–62.
16. NICE technology appraisal guidance 114. (2007). Methadone and buprenorphine for the management of opioid dependence.
17. Mattick, R.P., Breen, C., Kimber, J., *et al.* (2003). Methadone maintenance therapy versus no opioid replacement therapy for opioid dependence. *Cochrane Database of Systematic Reviews*. Issue 2, Art. No.: CD002209. DOI: 10.1002/14651858.CD002209.
18. Faggiano, F., Vigna-Taglianti, F., Versino, E., *et al.* (2003). Methadone maintenance at different dosages for opioid dependence. *Cochrane Database of Systematic Reviews*. Issue 3, Art. No.: CD002208. DOI: 10.1002/14651858.CD002208.
19. Caplehorn, J. and Drummer, O.H. (1999). Mortality associated with New South Wales methadone programs in 1994: lives lost and saved. *Medical Journal of Australia*, **170**, 104–9.
20. Mattick, R.P., Kimber, J., Breen, C., *et al.* (2003). Buprenorphine maintenance versus placebo or methadone maintenance for opioid dependence. *Cochrane Database of Systematic Reviews*. Issue 2, Art. No.: CD002207. DOI: 10.1002/14651858.CD002207.pub2.
21. Ferri, M., Davoli, M., Perucci, C.A., *et al.* (2006). Heroin maintenance treatment for chronic heroin-dependent individuals: a Cochrane systematic review of effectiveness. *Journal of Substance Abuse Treatment*, **30**(1), 63–72.
22. Eder, H., Jagsch, R., Kraigher, D., *et al.* (2005) Comparative study of the effectiveness of slow-release morphine and methadone for opioid maintenance therapy. *Addiction*, **100**(8), 1101–9.
23. Robertson, J.R., Raab, G., Bruce, M., *et al.* (2006). Addressing the efficacy of dihydrocodeine versus methadone as an alternative maintenance treatment for opiate dependence: a randomized controlled trial. *Addiction*, **101**, 1752–9.
24. Gowing, L., Ali, R., White, J., *et al.* (2006). Buprenorphine for the management of opioid withdrawal. *Cochrane Database of Systematic Reviews*. Issue 2, Art. No.: CD002025. DOI: 10.1002/14651858. CD002025.pub3.
25. Amato, L., Davoli, M., Minozzi, S., *et al.* (2005). Methadone at tapered doses for the management of opioid withdrawal. *Cochrane Database of Systematic Reviews*. Issue 3, Art. No.: CD003409. DOI: 10.1002/14651858.CD003409.pub3.
26. Gowing, L., Farrell, M., Ali, R., *et al.* (2004). Alpha2 adrenergic agonists for the management of opioid withdrawal. *Cochrane Database of Systematic Reviews*. Issue 4, Art. No.: CD002024. DOI: 10.1002/14651858.CD002024.pub2.
27. NICE technology appraisal guidance 115 – January 2007. Naltrexone for the management of opioid dependence.
28. Marlatt, G.A., and Gordon, J.R. (ed.) (1985). *Relapse prevention: maintenance strategies in the treatment of addictive behaviour*. Guilford Press, New York.
29. Prochaska, J.O., and Di Clemente, C.C. (1986). Towards a comprehensive model of change. In *Treating addictive behaviours: process of change* (eds. W.R. Miller and N. Heather). Plenum Press, New York.
30. Miller, W., and Rollnick, S. (1991). *Motivational interviewing*. Guilford Press, New York.
31. Narcotics Anonymous webpage http://www.na.org/accessed April 2007
32. Mayet, S., Farrell, M., Ferri, M., *et al.* (2005), Psychosocial treatment for opiate abuse and dependence. *Cochrane Database of Systematic Reviews*, **25**(1).
33. Amato, L., Minozzi, S., Davoli, M., *et al.* (2004). Psychosocial and pharmacological treatments versus pharmacological treatments for opioid detoxification. *Cochrane Database of Systematic Reviews*. Issue 4, Art. No.: CD004147. DOI: 10.1002/14651858.CD004147.pub2.
34. Department of Health. (1999). Drug misuse and dependence: guidelines on clinical management. HMSO, London.
35. Strang, J., Kelleher, M., Best, D., *et al.* (2006). Emergency naloxone for heroin overdose. *British Medical Journal*, **333**(7569), 614–5.
36. Fischer, G. (2000). Treatment of opioid dependence in pregnant women. *Addiction*, **95**(8), 1141–4.
37. Stover H. (2002). Drug and HIV/AIDS services in European Prisons Bibliotheks-und Unfomationssystems der Universitat Oldenurg BJS
38. Darke, S., Degenhardt, L., Mattick, R., *et al.* (2007). *Mortality amongst illicit drug users: epidemiology, causes and intervention*. Cambridge University Press, Cambridge.
39. McLellan, A.T., Lewis, D.C., O'Brien, C.P., *et al.* (2000). Drug dependence, a chronic medical illness: implications for treatment, insurance, and outcomes evaluation. *Journal of the American Medical Association*, **284**(13), 1689–95.
40. McLellan, A.T., Alterman, A.I., Metzger, D., *et al.* (1994). Similarity of outcome predictors across opiate, cocaine and alcohol treatments: role of treatment services. *Journal of Consulting and Clinical Psychology*, **62**, 1141–58
41. Hubbard, R.L., Craddock, S.G., Anderson, J., *et al.* (2003). Overview of 5-year follow up outcomes in the drug abuse treatment outcome studies (DATOS). *Journal of Substance Abuse Treatment*, **25**(3), 125–34.
42. Gossop, M., Marsden, J., Stewart, D., *et al.* (2003) The National Treatment Outcome Research Study (NTORS): 4-5 year follow-up results. *Addiction*, **98**(3), 291–303.
43. Darke, S., Ross, J., Teesson, M., *et al.* (2007). The Australian Treatment Outcome Study (ATOS): what have we learnt about treatment for heroin dependence? *Drug and Alcohol Review*, **26**(1), 49–54.
44. Hser, Y.I., Hoffman, V., Grella, C.E., *et al.* (2001). A 33-year follow-up of narcotics addicts. *Archives of General Psychiatry*, **58**(5), 503–8.
45. Smyth, B., Hoffman, V., Fan, J., *et al.* (2007). Years of potential life lost among heroin addicts 33 years after treatment. *Preventive Medecine*. **44**(4), 369–74. Epub 2007, Feb 8.

4.2.3.2 **Disorders relating to the use of amphetamine and cocaine**

Nicholas Seivewright and Robert Fung

Introduction

Amphetamine and cocaine are classed as stimulant drugs, although the distinction between stimulants and depressants can be criticized on the grounds that the same drug may have both actions in turn. This does indeed occur with amphetamine and cocaine, but the initial desired effects are increased energy and activity, and elevation in mood. These appear to be mainly due to enhanced central transmission of dopamine and noradrenaline (norepinephrine), with a similar enhancement of serotonin playing a less certain role.

Pharmaceutical preparations of amphetamine were previously widely used for treatment of depression and obesity, with some misuse of these occurring. In the period since the 1970s of increasing recreational drug use, the powder preparation of 'street' amphetamine (commonly known as 'speed' or 'whizz') has largely displaced the pharmaceutical forms to become a common drug of misuse in many countries. The powder is typically very impure and constitutes a racemic mixture of d- and l-isomers, with the l-form being relatively inactive. A stronger street preparation is the 'base', sometimes more a moist paste, and both these forms of the drug may be swallowed (either on their own or in a drink), snorted, or injected. (For the methylated forms 'ecstasy' and 'crystal meth', see Chapter 4.2.3.5.)

The coca shrub is indigenous to countries in South America, where the leaf is chewed, and use of the derived cocaine powder has spread extensively to the United States and elsewhere. The powder may be injected, sometimes along with heroin, by polydrug users, or snorted, the image of which is sometimes linked with executive lifestyles. Cocaine has become more dangerous as usage has gradually transferred in many countries to the 'crack' form, which is made from cocaine hydrochloride powder in a simple chemical process, and is more potent in its effects and withdrawal effects. Very rapid increases in blood levels of the drug can be achieved by smoking crack, and this is the usual route, although it is injected by committed intravenous drug users.

Clinical features

The effects and withdrawal effects of amphetamine and cocaine can be considered together, as the main features are equivalent. However, amphetamine has a slower onset of action than cocaine and longer elimination half-life, while crack is the most quickly absorbed of the cocaine preparations. This is reflected not only in the generally more intense effects of cocaine than amphetamine, but in the timescales involved. Thus an amphetamine user may experience desired effects, unwanted mental effects, and withdrawal features over the course of a few days, while a crack user can report the same sequence occurring in a matter of hours or even less. The main effects and withdrawal effects of these two stimulant drugs are shown in Table 4.2.3.2.1.

The list of effects can be seen as merging from the desired to the undesired. These drugs are typically taken in situations where stimulation is the aim, with sleep and eating regarded as hindrances. Mood is elevated, but characteristically this progresses to suspicion, in which true paranoid symptoms may be experienced. This is usually recognized by the individual as indicating that the episode of use should be terminated, but if use persists symptoms may become severe, or a more confused state develop. After stopping the drugs there are typically withdrawal effects of depressed mood, hyperphagia, and hypersomnia; no consensus exists as to whether such features are best viewed as 'rebound' symptoms, a truer withdrawal syndrome, or simply users catching up on sleeping and eating after a period without either.

Table 4.2.3.2.1 Effects and withdrawal effects of amphetamine and cocaine

Effects	Withdrawal effects
Increased energy	Depression
Hyperactivity	Irritability
Euphoria	Agitation
Reduced appetite	Craving
Insomnia	Hyperphagia
Paranoid symptoms	Hypersomnia
Confusion	

Such withdrawal features have been delineated most closely in relation to cocaine. A three-stage process has long been recognized[(1)]: initially agitation, anorexia, and acute craving; second, excessive tiredness, depression, and hyperphagia; finally, a normalization of most features, but a return of craving when triggered by environmental cues. This description is from before the escalation in crack use, and depression, craving, and agitation especially are often much more severe with this form of the drug. While environmental cues are clearly relevant in precipitating the use of any drug, a powerful surge of craving on encountering situations associated with previous use appears particularly characteristic of cocaine and crack.[(2)] The three-stage description of withdrawal features suggests that this phenomenon may occur after months or even years of abstinence.

Are amphetamine and cocaine addictive?

It is commonly observed that amphetamine and cocaine are non-addictive, or cause psychological but not physical dependence. Such observations rest on a distinction in which the condition of addiction, or physical dependence, requires visible bodily withdrawal symptoms, but critics claim this is of limited meaning now that there is an understanding of the neurobiological basis of drug withdrawal states. The current classification systems do retain some distinctions between physical and psychological dependence, and the issue is largely one of definition and semantics. The credibility of the label 'non-addictive' is certainly tested by individuals who have injected amphetamine 10 or more times every day for many years, or who spend vast amounts of money using crack in a highly compulsive manner.

Classification

Table 4.2.3.2.2 shows the classification within ICD-10 and DSM-IV-TR of disorders that may relate to the use of cocaine. In both systems the same diagnoses can be applied to amphetamine, in ICD-10 within a category 'other stimulants'.

Importantly, the list of diagnoses in ICD-10 is a standard one to be used across all psychoactive substances, with the second digit of the code number simply changed according to substance, and so does not imply that all those conditions can be caused by amphetamine or cocaine. The DSM-IV-TR listing is somewhat more specific, in that the diagnoses are selected from a wider general list of conditions which can apply to the range of substances. In this way the DSM-IV-TR classification recognizes that cocaine and amphetamine can produce states of dependence and withdrawal, as well as psychosis, affective disorders, and the other conditions included.

Diagnosis

The use of amphetamine or cocaine can be detected by drug screening of a plain urine sample, in laboratory testing or with instant kits. The importance of urine testing as a relatively simple procedure to employ, in any setting, in cases where drug use is suspected must be emphasized, as it is surprisingly often neglected. The two main limitations are possible doubts about authenticity, where mouth swabs for oral mucosal transudate can be a useful

Table 4.2.3.2.2 Classification of disorders relating to cocaine in ICD-10 and DSM-IV-TR

ICD-10		DSM-IV	
F14.0	Acute intoxication	292.89	Cocaine intoxication
		292.81	Cocaine intoxication delirium
F14.1	Harmful use	305.60	Cocaine abuse
F14.2	Dependence syndrome	304.20	Cocaine dependence
F14.3	Withdrawal state	292.0	Cocaine withdrawal
F14.4	Withdrawal state with delirium		
F14.5	Psychotic disorder	292.11	Cocaine-induced psychotic disorder, with delusions
		292.12	Cocaine-induced psychotic disorder, with hallucinations
		292.84	Cocaine-induced mood disorder
		292.89	Cocaine-induced anxiety disorder
		292.89	Cocaine-induced sexual dysfunction
		292.89	Cocaine-induced sleep disorder
F14.6	Amnesic syndrome		
F14.7	Residual and late-onset psychotic disorder		

alternative, and the short time for which drugs remain detectable in urine—as little as 24 h for cocaine. By contrast drugs remain in hair from the head or other parts of the body for the whole period of growth, but this technique which gives much longer-term information is a specialized one.

Obtaining a history and compliance with sampling may be particularly problematic in psychotic states. In such conditions it is also important to recognize that detected drug use may be incidental rather than necessarily causative.

Epidemiology

In most countries, the use of illicit drugs is commonest among young males of lower socio-economic status. Stimulant use overall reflects this, although of the various drugs of misuse, cocaine powder has been exceptional in the extent of usage also by more affluent individuals.

The biggest epidemic of cocaine use outside South America has been in the United States, where it peaked in the mid-1980s.[3] Household surveys at that time estimated that approximately one-tenth of the population had used the drug; the same epidemiological method has charted the subsequent general decline in occasional use, but an increase in more dependent use of crack. Cocaine use in other countries has not generally spread as widely as was predicted from the United States experience. In Europe the population lifetime prevalence of cocaine use has remained in low single-figure percentages,[4] much of it among inner-city polydrug users, although snorting cocaine powder is seemingly increasing among young people, rather displacing the recreational use of 'ecstasy'.

Even in areas where stimulant use is common, such users tend to present relatively rarely to treatment services. Priority is generally given to opioid substitution treatment of heroin addicts, and so service statistics will nearly always underestimate stimulant problems.

Aetiology

Broadly the same familial, social, and psychological factors are relevant in the aetiology of amphetamine and cocaine misuse as in other forms of drug misuse. Approximately half of the drug misusers are deemed in studies to have an underlying personality disorder,[5] usually of the antisocial type, although the figure has sometimes been found to be lower for stimulant misusers than for those dependent on opiates. This may be partly methodological, to do with the difficulty in distinguishing true personality characteristics from behaviours inherent in the activity of highly dependent drug misuse, but is probably also a reflection of the use of stimulant drugs by a generally broader population.

Course and prognosis

Course

A far greater proportion of amphetamine and cocaine misuse than opiate misuse is recreational in nature, with few significant complications if the medical harms are avoided. It is assumed that the vast majority of those who are identified in school and teenage surveys as having used stimulants simply give them up in due course, although little systematic data is available. Complications and involvement with treatment services are more likely where there is dependent usage, and there may be psychiatric contact in episodes of psychosis. A very small proportion of amphetamine injectors progress to high-dose daily usage, while the heavy use of cocaine appears to be less sustainable and is therefore usually periodic in nature.

Other drug use

After being stimulated with amphetamine or cocaine, many individuals will use sedatives such as alcohol, benzodiazepines, or cannabis to 'come down' from their drug. Increasingly heroin is being used for this purpose, sometimes to the point of becoming dependent on the opiate and requiring substitution treatment. The use of cocaine in particular is commonly encountered as a secondary form of drug misuse in methadone patients,[6] with some individuals undoubtedly switching their preferred illicit drug from heroin to cocaine when treatment is established.

Prognosis

The drug misuse literature in general would suggest that stimulant use is more likely to progress and become problematic in individuals with associated personal or social difficulties or psychiatric disorder. Usage by individuals with severe mental illness, which often contains an element of 'self-medication' of distress even though in the long run stimulants will render symptoms worse, can be particularly entrenched.[7]

Complications

Many of the complications of amphetamine and cocaine misuse are complications of drug misuse in general, including those related to injecting. The range includes general physical decline, weight loss, dental problems, infective complications ranging from abscesses to hepatitis and infection with the human immunodeficiency virus (HIV), reduced foetal growth in pregnancy, mood disturbances, and various social problems. Complications in the following areas are somewhat more specific to stimulant misuse:

- Cardiovascular—hypertension, arrhythmias, myocardial infarction, cerebrovascular accident
- Obstetric—premature labour, placental abruption
- Psychiatric—anxiety, depression, aggressive behaviours, psychosis
- Other—perforation of nasal septum (cocaine snorting)

The cardiovascular problems relate to increased catecholamine secretion, and represent the most serious hazard of cocaine abuse.[8] With obstetric complications, it is difficult to separate the effects of drugs from other risk factors such as poor diet, smoking, or adverse social conditions, but there appears to be a particular link between stimulants and placental abruption.

There are also various psychiatric disorders that are particularly associated with amphetamine and cocaine misuse. Anxiety as a symptom is common in relation to the agitation produced by the drugs, while depression is a classic withdrawal effect. An assessment of the true clinical significance of these features therefore requires withdrawal from drugs, while in acute presentations both can be extremely distressing. Aggressive behaviour may be due to an underlying personality disorder, but it is also characteristic of withdrawal from crack cocaine when severe craving is experienced. Paranoid psychosis, sometimes indistinguishable from an acute schizophrenic episode, is the best-known complication of stimulant misuse. The earliest descriptions were of cases where symptoms quickly subsided after withdrawal of the drugs, but it is now recognized that through mechanisms which represent a kind of sensitization, symptoms which are drug-induced can persist and recur even with avoidance of substance use.[9]

Treatment

Evidence

A very large number of medications have been investigated in cocaine misuse, mainly compounds which through actions on catecholamines or serotonin could be expected to alleviate withdrawal effects. After decades of such work the evidence is very discouraging, with no medications consistently found to reduce stimulant abuse.[10] Inpatient programmes and psychological treatments basically represent modifications of those approaches used across all forms of drug misuse, although cocaine abuse appears particularly amenable to the 'contingency management' approach of providing material incentives for abstinence.[11]

Management

Faced with the limitations in treatment for these forms of drug misuse that have high morbidity and mortality, drug services have had to consider how best to achieve some benefits in terms of very practical management.[12] The factors that appear important in such provision are:

- specific outreach programmes
- harm-reduction approaches
- rapid response where necessary
- targeted use of treatments
- admission in severe cases

To engage stimulant users at all can require outreach aimed at the subcultural groups in whom usage is common. Basic harm-reduction measures must be offered, including drug information, education about health risks, advice to reduce damaging injecting practices, and the provision of clean equipment. Counselling of a supportive or more behavioural kind may be provided by various types of agency.

The periodic nature of stimulant problems means that rapid response can be important, for instance in states of acute crack withdrawal or psychiatric disturbance. Use of tranquillizers and antipsychotic medications may be necessary for some presentations, while fluoxetine appears to be increasingly favoured over other antidepressants, due to a possible anticraving effect and good acceptability. Inpatient admission can be required in cases where no long-term measure is able to make much impact between acute crises. The possibility of any substitute prescribing in stimulant misuse is highly controversial, with some services seeing a role for oral dexamphetamine in heavily dependent amphetamine users experiencing extreme problems from injecting.[13]

Drug-induced psychosis

The two aspects of management of this complication are the treatment of psychotic symptoms and the withdrawal of the drug which is thought to be causative. The latter can be very problematic other than as an inpatient, and is not guaranteed even then. In practice, ongoing low-grade psychotic states in individuals who have not completely stopped drug use are common, and treatment may have to be attempted in such circumstances. The use of antipsychotic medications does not differ significantly from that in psychoses not produced by drugs.

Prevention

The prevention of drug misuse lies largely outside the clinical domain, in the areas of education, enforcement and social improvement. A more biological development in cocaine misuse of vaccination, whereby limited exposure produces antibodies to subsequently block the drug's effects, remains experimental.

Further information

National Institute of Drug Addiction-Research Report for Cocaine Addiction: www.nida.nih.gov/ResearchReports/cocaine.html

Amphetamine Dependence: www.mentalhealth.com/dis/p20-sb02.html

Sadock, B.J. and Sadock, V.A. (2003). Kaplan and Sadock's synopsis of psychiatry; Substance-related disorders, Chap. 12. Lippincott, Williams & Wilkins, Philadelphia.

European Monitoring Centre for Drugs and Drug Addiction. (2006). *Annual report: the state of the drugs problem in Europe*. Office for Official Publications of the European Communities, Luxembourg. Chapter 4, Amphetamines, ecstasy and other psychotropic drugs, and Chapter 5, Cocaine and crack cocaine.

References

1. Gawin, F.H. and Kleber, H.D. (1986). Abstinence symptomatology and psychiatric diagnoses in cocaine abusers: clinical observations. *Archives of General Psychiatry*, **43**, 107–13.

2. van de Laar, M.C., Licht, R., Franken, I.H.A., *et al.* (2004). Event-related potentials indicate motivational relevance of cocaine use in abstinent cocaine addicts. *Psychopharmacology*, **177**, 121–9.
3. Withers, N.W., Pulvirenti, L., Koob, G.F., *et al.* (1995). Cocaine abuse and dependence. *Journal of Clinical Psychopharmacology*, **15**, 63–73.
4. European Monitoring Centre for Drugs and Drug Addiction. (2006). Cocaine and crack cocaine. In *Annual report: the state of the drugs problem in Europe*. Office for Official Publications of the European Communities, Luxembourg.
5. Grant, B.F., Stinson, F.S., Dawson, D.A., *et al.* (2004). Co-occurrence of 12-month alcohol and drug use disorders and personality disorders in the United States. *Archives of General Psychiatry*, **61**, 361–8.
6. Williamson, A., Darke, S., Ross, J., *et al.* (2006). The association between cocaine use and short-term outcomes for the treatment of heroin dependence: findings from the Australian treatment outcome study. *Drug and Alcohol Review*, **25**, 141–8.
7. Seivewright, N., Iqbal, M.Z., and Bourne, H. (2004). Treating patients with comorbidities. In *Drug treatment: what works?* (eds. P. Bean and T. Nemitz), pp. 123–41. Routledge, London.
8. Edgred, M. and Davis, G.K. (2005). Cocaine and the heart. *Postgraduate Medical Journal*, **81**, 568–71.
9. Curran, C., Byrappa, N., and McBride, A. (2004). Stimulant psychosis: systematic review. *The British Journal of Psychiatry*, **185**, 196–204.
10. de Lima, M.S., de Oliveira Soares, B.G., Alves, A., *et al.* (2002). Pharmacological treatment of cocaine dependence: a systematic review. *Addiction*, **97**, 931–49.
11. Higgins, S.T., Heil, S.H., Dantona, R., *et al.* (2007). Effects of varying the monetary value of voucher-based incentives on abstinence achieved during and following treatment among cocaine-dependent outpatients. *Addiction*, **102**, 271–81.
12. Seivewright, N., McMahon, C., and Egleston, P. (2005). Stimulant use still going strong. *Advances in Psychiatric Treatment*, **2**, 262–9.
13. Grabowski, J., Shearer, J., Merrill, J., *et al.* (2004). Agonist-like replacement pharmacotherapy for stimulant abuse dependence. *Addictive Behaviors*, **29**, 1439–64.

4.2.3.3 Disorders relating to use of PCP and hallucinogens

Henry David Abraham

PCP

Introduction

Phencyclidine (PCP, 'angel dust') is an arylcyclohexylamine dissociative anaesthetic. It was first abused in the United States in New York and San Francisco in the 1960s, but abuse declined when a broad range of adverse complications was noted.[1]

Epidemiology

While use of the unadulterated drug occurs, PCP is more frequently mixed with LSD or cannabis. The drug may be ingested or injected, but is more commonly smoked or snorted. Data suggest use in the United States and Europe. In the United States, a stable trend of 3 per cent of high school seniors have tried PCP at least once.[2] It traffics under a long and colourful list of street names. It has been suggested that any illicit smoked drug with an unrecognized street name (dust, mist, THC, embalming fluid, *inter alia*) should be considered PCP until proven otherwise.

Acute physiological effects

The drug has a delayed onset of activity when taken orally. Unlike the major hallucinogens, PCP requires doses in milligrams to be effective, a factor facilitating toxicological identification. When smoked, the onset of its main effects occurs immediately. The drug has particular affinity for the sigma opioid receptor, and non-competitively blocks the *N*-methyl-D-aspartate-type excitatory amino acid receptor. Other effects appear to be mediated indirectly by catecholamine release, cholinergic stimulation, and serotonergic receptors.

DSM-IV lists as criteria for acute PCP intoxication the following:

- agitation
- belligerence
- impaired judgement
- nystagmus
- hyperacusis
- hypertension
- tachycardia
- numbness
- ataxia
- dysarthria
- rigidity
- salivation
- seizures
- coma

It is clear from this daunting inventory that impaired judgement is likely to be present beforehand in any person intentionally choosing to abuse this drug.

Adverse effects

PCP affects not only adults, but fetuses and nursing infants.[3] Neurological consequences in infants include poor attention, hypertonia, and depressed neonatal reflexes.[4] *In vitro* studies show that PCP causes inhibited axon outgrowth, degeneration, and death in human fetal cerebral cortical neurones.[5]

In adults signs of severe PCP toxicity include:

- hyperthermia
- opisthotonus
- cardiac arrhythmia
- stroke

PCP is capable of provoking extreme muscular agitation, rhabdomyolysis and renal failure in 2.5 per cent of users.[6] DSM-IV lists psychiatric effects of PCP including intoxication, delirium, PCP-induced psychotic, mood, and anxiety disorders, and PCP abuse and dependence. A criterion for diagnosis is the emergence of the disorder within a month of drug use.

PCP delirium

Unlike acute intoxication with other hallucinogens, PCP delirium is associated with neurological disturbances. A continuum of effects is noted depending on dose.[7] Psychiatric symptoms occur early in drug use, with stupor and coma occurring later. Shortly after drug use, patients appear confused and ataxic. Analgesia in fingers and toes may be described. PCP can produce complex hallucinations resembling LSD intoxication. Differentiating the two drugs in emergencies is important, since high-potency neuroleptics, which are useful in PCP toxicity, may exacerbate LSD, while the use of benzodiazepines, helpful in acute LSD toxicity, may disinhibit an assaultive PCP patient. Unlike LSD, PCP is readily identified in routine toxicological screening of blood and urine, but such data may not be readily available. One rapid bedside technique to differentiate the two drugs is the palm sign. The examiner asks the patient to describe the names of all the colours seen in the examiner's outstretch palm. A typical LSD patient reports a vision of multiple colours and images. A PCP patient simply attacks the hand. Dexterity of the examiner is suggested. Unfocused aggression makes PCP delirium a particularly dangerous disorder. The spectrum of violence includes both suicide and homicide.[8] The technique of 'talking down' acutely toxic patients is contraindicated. Environmental stimuli should be minimized, and the patient provided with protective supervision. The use of physical restraints is relatively contraindicated because of the potential for rhabdomyolysis.

Specific treatments involve:

- intravenous naloxone to rule out narcotics overdose
- activated charcoal
- acidification of the patient's urine with vitamin C, ammonium chloride, cranberry juice
- diuresis with frusemide (furosemide, Lasix)
- antihypertensives
- high-potency neuroleptics or barbiturates

PCP has mixed agonist and antagonist effects at cholinergic receptors. Anticholinergic drugs may precipitate a synergistic reaction with PCP, worsening delirium. Thus, low-potency neuroleptics, tricyclic antidepressants, and the anticholinergic antiparkinsonian drugs should be avoided.

PCP-induced psychotic disorder

PCP delirium may evolve into a chronic PCP psychosis that is differentiated from schizophrenia only with difficulty. Alternatively, a PCP delirium may clear, only to be replaced by the insidious onset of a post-PCP psychotic disorder. Certain features of PCP psychosis, namely neurological abnormalities, dose-related severity of symptoms, and regularity of the length of illness, are not noted with other psychedelic drugs, leading to the suggestion that PCP psychosis is a toxic drug effect rather than a functional illness. Four classes of agents are reported to help PCP psychosis:

- benzodiazepines
- neuroleptics
- acetylcholinesterase inhibitors (physostigmine)
- catecholamine depleters (reserpine)

Otherwise, treatment considerations are those for PCP delirium. The long-term prognosis for this disorder appears to be poor, according to data from an 8-year follow-up of 10 patients.[9]

PCP abuse, dependence, and organic mental disorder

Rhesus monkeys will self-administer PCP in a dose-dependent way,[10] suggesting that repeated abuse in humans may be associated with psychophysiological dependence. This in turn is likely to be associated with a decline in social and occupational function characteristic of other forms of addiction. Because of its widespread neuropsychological effects, any intentional, informed use of PCP should be considered maladaptive. For the habituated patient, long-term treatment is indicated. Issues that should be addressed in the process are:

- emotional lability
- cognitive defects
- depression
- possible PCP withdrawal
- nutritional status

Many of the treatments applicable to patients addicted to the opiates, alcohol, and cocaine apply to this population. Several aspects of treating the PCP patient depart from the more conventional addiction treatments. A triad of confusion, decreased cognitive function, and assaultiveness mark an organic mental disorder associated with PCP use. Reduced cognition is a barrier to recovery that must be recognized and addressed in any prospective treatment plan. Neuropsychological assessment is helpful in this regard. Secondly, there is murine evidence that PCP is sequestered in fat and by melanin for at least 3 weeks following a single exposure.[11] Conditions associated with weight loss are likely to release long-held PCP into the blood and brain.

Hallucinogens

Introduction

Agents that alter perception and mood without disorientation typify hallucinogenic drugs. They have been known and used for millennia for purposes ranging from magical to medical. Anthropologists trace back the earliest use of hallucinogens to Paleolithic Europe, although 80 per cent of extant hallucinogenic plants are to be found in the New World. Galen (AD 130–200) wrote that it was customary to give dinner guests hemp seeds to promote the evening's proceedings. The ergot-bearing fungus *Claviceps purpurea* infected rye in tenth-century France and claimed 40 000 lives. Despite such calamities, ergot continued to be used by midwives in medieval Europe. In search of a benign ergot derivative for use in childbirth, Albert Hofmann synthesized lysergic acid diethylamide (LSD-25) in 1938, described in his classic monograph, *LSD: my problem child.*

In 1947, Stoll in Switzerland published the first experimental use of LSD in psychiatry. Intelligence agencies worldwide seized on the misnomer of LSD as an instrument of 'mind control'. Academicians including Sandison and Elkes in England, Cohen and Eisner in the United States, Leuner in Germany, and Grof in Czechoslovakia engaged in human studies. But within a decade the drug the genie was out of the bottle, as the drug moved from the hands of scientists to clinicians, clergy, curious professors, and a widening number of students on both sides of the Atlantic. Military investigators in the United States gave the drug surreptitiously to recruits. By the late 1960s LSD and cannabis led the way to a pandemic of drug abuse among the young.

Drug preparations

Hallucinogenic drugs comprise not so much a single class of compounds, but a multiple classes affecting different neuronal receptors. Hofmann and Schultes describe 11 classes of hallucinogenic compounds which can be isolated from botanicals.[12] Hallucinogens are readily available. Botanicals are easily grown. Indole and phenethylamines can be easily synthesized, especially with the rise of the Internet. Chemically pure hallucinogens are psychoactive in microgram quantities, and are easily concealed, transported and sold, accounting for their enduring role as abusable substances.

LSD is psychoactive in a single droplet of solvent. The drug is easily dissolved in an aqueous solution. Drops of the drug are placed on sugar cubes or blotting paper stamped with coloured cartoon figures to mark the drug's location. Sheets of the paper are then distributed, and the figures ingested. Dosages commonly range from 25 to 100 μg. A hallucinogenic trip can occur after 75 μg. Other hallucinogens, such as dimethyltryptamine, are injected. The serotonin-2A receptor has been shown to bind strongly to many hallucinogenic drugs, and these drugs appear to act as partial agonists.[13]

Common **botanical hallucinogens** include fungi and angiosperms (flower-bearing plants), of which approximately 100 are recognized with hallucinogenic properties. Ibogaine is derived from the root of the *Tabernanthe iboga* plant cultivated in Gabon and eaten as a rite of passage. Ayahuasca is a tea of dimethyltryptamine from the Amazon vine, *Banisteriopsis*, potentiated by beta-carbolines which inhibit monoamine oxidase. Mescaline is a predominant hallucinogen in the cactus *Lophophora williamsii*. Strips of cactus are cut from the plant, dried, and eaten. The Mexican mint, *Salvia divinorum*, contains a diterpene kappa-opioid agonist. *Salvia* is easily bought from the Internet from scores of Websites in the United States and Europe.[14]

Hallucinogenic mushrooms contain psilocybin and psilocin, which are phosphorylated hydroxylated congeners of dimethyltryptamine. Mushrooms are ingested for their effect, or brewed first and the broth consumed. Responses vary widely between individuals and occasions. The American psychologist William James reported ingesting several dozen hallucinogenic mushrooms and only experiencing headache. Shulgin has synthesized and tested 179 phenylethylamines for hallucinogenic properties. Their effects on the human brain are complex and largely unknown.

Epidemiology

Annual surveys in United States college students indicate that LSD use fell from 1995 to 2005 from a lifetime prevalence of 11.5 to 3.7 per cent. This was offset by an increase in the lifetime use of psilocybin mushrooms, from 6.5 to 10.6 per cent. This increase in the use of non-LSD hallucinogens is reflected across secondary grades and young adults between 19 and 28 as well,[1] and follows a period of rising LSD use in Germany, the United Kingdom, and the United States in the 1990s. Factors which may explain this decrease in LSD use include student reports of less availability, greater perceptions of risk, and the substitution of psilocybin and MDMA for LSD. A cross-sectional study of 904 women from 14 to 26 found that LSD users were more often Caucasian, victims of physical abuse, and suffering depression.[15]

Acute effects

The characteristic LSD trip comprises:

- autonomic arousal
- marked mydriasis
- sensory disturbances
- emotional lability

Progressive modulations of visual imagery appear to be generated both from external objects and distortions of eidetic sources. Ordinarily benign objects may take on new emotional meanings. Geometric imagery may rise and fall before one's eyes. A prevalent feeling one experiences is a sense of helplessness to control one's streaming images and emotions, hence the hippie advice of 'going with the flow'. The loss of cognitive, perceptual, and affective control for some users leads to panic, which in turn results in the so-called 'bad trip'. As these effects decline, they may be replaced with a sense of oceanic well-being or residual paranoia.

Adverse effects

Adverse reactions to hallucinogens include panic reactions associated with a bad trip, hallucinogen persisting perception disorder, and prolonged psychoses.

(a) Panic reaction

Panic may arise during the acute drug experience. It is characterized by a crescendo of rising anxiety accompanied by autonomic arousal in the context of streaming emotions and imagery. Mydriasis is greater than that seen in non-drug-induced panic. The use of an oral benzodiazepine such as diazepam 20 mg is utterly effective in stopping the panic within minutes.

(b) Hallucinogen persisting perception disorder (HPPD)

It became apparent within the first few years of experimentation with LSD that this class of drugs was capable of inducing visual disturbances days to weeks following drug exposure. Subsequent research found that these disturbances, dubbed 'flashbacks' because of their evanescent visual appearance, appeared to be an intermittent form of post-drug visual disorder that in its extreme form was experienced continually. Thus, HPPD patients are capable of describing a range of visual disturbances that fluctuate in intensity, but are observable from moment to moment (Abraham, 1983). Such imagery includes:

- geometric hallucinations
- false perceptions of movement
- afterimagery
- the perception of trails behind moving images
- pinpoint dots in the air (aeropsia)

Symptoms drawn by HPPD patients have been published on the Internet.[16] Patients also describe derealization and depersonalization. Symptoms are intensified by stimulation from:

- emergence into a dark environment
- marijuana
- amphetamines
- cocaine

- anxiety
- the stress of intercurrent illnesses

While recovery may occur over months and years following last drug use, approximately half of the patients so afflicted appear to develop a permanent alteration of the visual apparatus. Studies of psychophysics in HPPD patients reveal quantified prolongations in afterimagery.(17) Neurophysiological studies confirm cerebral disinhibition involving those regions of the cortex processing visual information.(18)

Management: Because the disorder is exacerbated by psychological and physiological conditions of arousal, benzodiazepines have been helpful for management of visual symptoms.(19) The results of these efforts are palliative at best, and complicated by the prospect of treating a drug abuser with an abusable substance. Recent case reports of treatment with sertraline, naltrexone, and clonidine are encouraging.

In addition to pharmacotherapy, HPPD patients often require supportive psychotherapy to deal with the issues of learning to cope with what may be a permanent alteration in perception. Therapy is also indicated to educate the patient, and prevent the development of common comorbid disorders in HPPD. These are:

- major depression
- panic disorder
- alcohol dependence from self-medication

(c) Psychosis

Evidence supporting the hypothesis that the use of potent hallucinogens can trigger prolonged psychotic episodes is found in multiple longitudinal, cross-sectional, and case studies (Abraham *et al.* 1996). Psychiatric patienthood appears to be a risk factor for the development of psychosis following LSD. The clinical picture of post-LSD psychosis resembles schizoaffective disorder more than it does schizophrenia, with the commonly added feature of chronic visual disturbances. Clinically such patients resemble those with good-prognosis schizophrenia, since they possess more affect than those with poor prognosis, have less thought disorder, are more socially related, and appear to have fewer signs of negative schizophrenia. Mystical preoccupations reminiscent of acute drug experiences can predominate. Visual hallucinations often are of the variety that are seen in HPPD, although in contradistinction to such patients, psychotic patients may describe delusions and auditory hallucinations as well.(20)

Management: Atypical pharmacotherapies appear to have an important role in treatment, and in selected cases are preferable to dopamine-blocking neuroleptics. Reports in the literature describe cases responding to electroconvulsive therapy, lithium, anticonvulsants, and the serotonin precursor, l-5-hydroxytryptophan. Long-term supportive psychotherapy is almost always indicated to help the patient and his family make painful adjustments to the patient's chronic disappointments in relationships and employment, frequently made all the more poignant by the illness' propensity to preserve the patient's insight as it progresses. This last factor may partially explain the apparently high risk for suicide.

Human experimentation with hallucinogens

The discovery of the effects of LSD in 1943 led to a flurry of experimental activity with the drug in humans, at its worst with dubious methodology and indifferent to the protection of human subjects. But the ability of this unique class of drugs to alter perception, cognition, and affect has prompted a new wave of research with selected hallucinogens with regulatory oversight. Studies have examined the safety of peyote in religious use(21); the psychological effects of psilocybin, dimethyltryptamine, and ketamine(22); their use as a tool in modelling the pathophysiology of psychosis,(23) and possible therapeutic uses.

Hallucinogens have been used as experimental psychoses. Vollenweider *et al.* have found increased metabolic activity in the frontal cortex of subjects on the dissociative anaesthetic ketamine,(24) and in subjects during an experimental psychosis from psilocybin, increased serotonin-2 agonist activity.(25) Finally, the study of treatment with hallucinogens for psychiatric disorders has cautiously reemerged. In a randomized trial of ketamine for depression, Zarate *et al.* found that the drug had benefits for a week following a single dose.(26)

Further information

Abraham, H.D. (1983). Visual phenomenology of the LSD flashback. *Archives of General Psychiatry*, **40**, 884–9.

Abraham, H.D., Aldridge, A.M., and Gogia, P. (1996). The psychopharmacology of hallucinogens. *Neuropsychopharmacology*, **14**, 285–98.

Hofmann, A. (1980). *LSD: my problem child.* McGraw-Hill, New York.

McCarron, M.M., Schulze, B.W., Thompson, G.A., *et al.* (1981). Acute PCP intoxication: incidence of clinical findings in 1000 cases. *Annals of Emergency Medicine*, **10**, 237–42.

References

1. McCarron, M.M., Schulze, B.W., Thompson, G.A., *et al.* (1981). Acute PCP intoxication: incidence of clinical findings in 1000 cases. *Annals of Emergency Medicine*, **10**, 237–42.
2. Johnston, L.D., O'Malley, P.M., Bachman, J.G., *et al.* (2006). *Monitoring the future national survey results on drug use, 1975–2005: secondary school students*, Vol. I (NIH Publication No. 06-5883). National Institute on Drug Abuse, Bethesda, MD.
3. Tabor, B.L., Smith-Wallace, T., and Yonekura, M.L. (1990). Perinatal outcome associated with PCP versus cocaine use. *American Journal of Drug and Alcohol Abuse*, **16**, 337–48.
4. Golden, N.L., Kuhnert, B.R., Sokol, R.J., *et al.* (1987). Neonatal manifestations of maternal PCP exposure. *Journal of Perinatal Medicine*, **15**, 185–91.
5. Mattson, M.P., Rychlik, B., and Cheng, B. (1992). Degenerative and axon outgrowth-altering effects of PCP in human fetal cerebral cortical cells. *Neuropharmacology*, **31**, 279–91.
6. Akmal, M., Valdin, J.R., McCarron, M.M., *et al.* (1981). Rhabdomyolysis with and without acute renal failure in patients with PCP intoxication. *American Journal of Nephrology*, **1**, 91–6.
7. Milhorn, H.T.J. (1991). Diagnosis and management of PCP intoxication. *American Family Physician*, **43**, 1290–302.
8. Poklis, A., Graham, M., Maginn, D., *et al.* (1990). PCP and violent deaths in St. Louis, Missouri: a survey of medical examiners' cases from 1977 through 1986. *American Journal of Drug and Alcohol Abuse*, **16**, 265–74.
9. Wright, H.H., Cole, E.A., Batey, S.R., *et al.* (1988). PCP-induced psychosis: eight-year follow-up of ten cases. *Southern Medical Journal*, **81**, 565–7.
10. Campbell, U.C., Thompson, S.S., and Carroll, M.E. (1998). Acquisition of oral PCP (PCP) self-administration in rhesus monkeys: effects of dose and an alternative non-drug reinforcer. *Psychopharmacology (Berlin)*, **137**, 132–8.
11. Misra, A.L., Pontani, R.B., and Bartolomeo, J. (1979). Persistence of PCP (PCP) and metabolites in brain and adipose tissue and implications for long-lasting behavioural effects. *Research Communications in Chemistry, Pathology, and Pharmacology*, **24**, 431–45.

12. Schultes, R. and Hofmann, A. (1980). *The botany and chemistry of hallucinogens*. Thomas, Springfield, IL.
13. Glennon, R.A., Titeler, M., and McKenney, J.D. (1984). Evidence for 5-HT2 involvement in the mechanism of action of hallucinogenic agents. *Life Sciences*, **35**, 2505–11.
14. Prisinzano, T.E. (2005). Psychopharmacology of the hallucinogenic sage *Salvia divinorum*. *Life Sciences*, **78**, 527–31.
15. Rickert, VI., Siqueira, L.M., Dale, T., *et al.* (2003). Prevalence and risk factors for LSD use among young women. *Journal of Pediatric and Adolescent Gynecology*, **16**, 67–75.
16. Abraham, H.D. (2005). at http://www.drabraham.com/html/hppd.htm
17. Abraham, H.D. and Wolf, E. (1988). Visual function in past users of LSD: psychophysical findings. *Journal of Abnormal Psychology*, **97**, 443–7.
18. Abraham, H.D. and Duffy, F.H. (1996). Stable quantitative EEG difference in post-LSD visual disorder by split-half analysis: evidence for disinhibition. *Psychiatry Research and Neuroimaging*, **67**, 173–87.
19. Lerner, A.G., Gelkopf, M., Skladman, I., *et al.* (2003). Clonazepam treatment of lysergic acid diethylamide-induced hallucinogen persisting perception disorder with anxiety features. *International Clinical Psychopharmacology*, **18**, 101–5.
20. Bowers, M.B. Jr (1977). Psychoses precipitated by psychotomimetic drugs: a follow up study. *Archives of General Psychiatry*, **34**, 832–5.
21. Halpern, J.H., Sherwood, A.R., Hudson, J.I., *et al* (2005). Psychological and cognitive effects of long-term peyote use among Native Americans. *Biological Psychiatry*, **58**, 624–31.
22. Gouzoulis-Mayfrank, E., Heekeren, K., Neukirch, A., *et al.* (2005). Psychological effects of (S)-ketamine and *N,N*-dimethyltryptamine (DMT): a double-blind, cross-over study in healthy volunteers. *Pharmacopsychiatry*, **38**, 301–11.
23. Javitt, D.C. and Zukin, S.R. (1991). Recent advances in the PCP model of schizophrenia. *The American Journal of Psychiatry*, **148**, 1301–8.
24. Vollenweider, F.X., Leenders, K.L., Scharfetter, C., *et al.* (1997). Metabolic hyperfrontality and psychopathology in the ketamine model of psychosis using positron emission tomography (PET) and [^{18}F]fluorodeoxyglucose (FDG). *European Neuropsychopharmacology*, **7**, 9–24.
25. Vollenweider, F.X., Vollenweider-Scherpenhuyzen, M.F., Babler, A., *et al.* (1998). Psilocybin induces schizophrenia-like psychosis in humans via a serotonin-2 agonist action. *Neuroreport*, **9**, 3897–902.
26. Zarate, C.A. Jr, Singh, J.B., Carlson, P.J., *et al.* (2006). A randomized trial of an *N*-methyl-D-aspartate antagonist in treatment-resistant major depression. *Archives of General Psychiatry*, **63**, 856–64.

4.2.3.4 **Misuse of benzodiazepines**

Sarah Welch and Michael Farrell

Epidemiology and patterns of use

The rise in benzodiazepine prescribing in the United Kingdom in the 1960s and 1970s was a development that followed the previous period of prescribing of barbiturates and other sedatives. Concerns about the obvious toxicity of barbiturates, and previously other sedatives, in overdose, together with knowledge of their dependence-inducing characteristics, led to their replacement with the safer benzodiazepines as the commonly prescribed anxiolytic and hypnotic drugs. Case reports of patients who escalated their dose of benzodiazepines above the recommended dose, and who experienced convulsions and confusional states on stopping them, began to appear in the 1970s.[1,2] In the mid-1970s and onward, regulatory bodies in the United Kingdom and United States began to recognize the abuse potential of benzodiazepines even in therapeutic doses. Dependence on benzodiazepines was well described in the early literature on the development of these drugs but surprisingly clinical dependence was not reported in the medical literature until the early 1980s.[3,4] Dependence on therapeutic doses of prescribed benzodiazepines is covered in Chapter 6.2.2. In this chapter we are concerned with abuse of and dependence on high doses of benzodiazepines.

The upsurge in the drug epidemic in the 1980s was associated with an increase in misuse of hypnosedatives, and in the late 1980s there was a series of reports on the intravenous use of benzodiazepines, in particular temazepam.[5,6] Because benzodiazepines are the most commonly prescribed anxiolytics and hypnotics it is not surprising to find that they are also reported to be commonly misused. However, patterns of misuse vary, from episodic use of non-prescribed medication with up to 15 per cent of young people reporting some experience with benzodiazepines, to continuous high-dose use. Since the mid-1980s there has been a substantial drop in the prescription of benzodiazepines as anxiolytic agents but use as hypnotics has remained relatively steady with the concentration of long-term use being in the elderly population. Changes in prescribing practices are likely to influence diversion of benzodiazepines to the illicit market.

Reports indicate that supra-therapeutic dose misuse and dependence is strongly associated with polydrug and alcohol abuse and dependence.[7,8] This pattern of benzodiazepine misuse and dependence is probably much less common than iatrogenic benzodiazepine dependence. However, it presents a substantial problem to many clinicians in primary care and specialist settings. In particular, high-dose misuse is likely to be associated with 'doctor shopping' and efforts to extract additional medication on top of that already prescribed. The high doses used present a particular risk because they are often used in combination with other substances such as alcohol, opiates, and stimulants. High-dose use may be intermittent in nature (in a 'binge' pattern), and not associated with dependence (in which case the initiation of a prescription may change a pattern of intermittent binge use to daily dependent use in a manner that entrenches polydrug use; see the section below on guidelines for management). Drug misusers use benzodiazepines in a non-dependent fashion for a variety of reasons. For example, benzodiazepines may be used to enhance the effect of other drugs (such as boosting the euphoria with heroin), or to alleviate unwanted effects from other drugs (to 'cushion' the 'come-down' from cocaine), or to help alleviate withdrawal symptoms when drugs such as heroin are unobtainable, or in attempts at self-detoxification from other drugs. Misuse of benzodiazepines may also arise from injudicious patterns of prescribing for the treatment of alcohol dependence, or from attempts at self-treatment for alcohol dependence. Some drug users will also develop a dependent pattern of use of benzodiazepines in their own right. Benzodiazepine dependence may be a factor contributing to poor outcome for patients who are attempting opiate detoxification.

High-dose use is associated with substantial tolerance to the sedating effects of the medication but some of the other effects may not be equivalently protected by tolerance. Thus, some individuals may consume extraordinarily high doses, and not appear sedated, but experience profound amnesia for their actions. Such effects of amnesia may also be associated with the reported high rates of risk-taking behaviour, and amnesia may be more pronounced in injecting benzodiazepine users, although there are no good data to confirm this.

The potential of different benzodiazepines for misuse and dependence

In view of the frequency of prescribing of benzodiazepine drugs, it is an important question as to whether some benzodiazepines are more likely to be misused, or to lead to dependence, than others. The similarities between different benzodiazepines are much greater than the differences. Patients may maintain that they need a specific named benzodiazepine, but there is marked cross-tolerance, and patients changed to an equivalent dose of a different benzodiazepine under double-blind conditions show almost complete cross-dependence (i.e. no difference in withdrawal symptoms from those whose medication has been unchanged).[9] However, this cross-dependence was shown for patients who were already benzodiazepine dependent. It is possible that the properties of certain benzodiazepines lead to a stronger motivation for people to desire their effects, to escalate the dose, and to persist with their use.

Factors that have been considered to influence the liability to misuse and development of dependence include the relative potency of the drug, and its elimination half-life.[10] Triazolam, a very short-acting benzodiazepine prescribed for insomnia, was withdrawn from the British market following concerns about the severity of rebound anxiety experienced even after a single dose. Triazolam is a very potent benzodiazepine that binds very readily to benzodiazepine receptors, and experience with its use suggested that it had a more euphoriant effect than other benzodiazepines, resulting in greater potential for misuse and for the development of dependence. Other benzodiazepines that have high potency and have caused concern include flunitrazepam and lorazepam. Flunitrazepam is relatively rarely prescribed in the United Kingdom, but frequently reported as one of the most common benzodiazepines misused in many European countries and in Australia. It is not marketed in the United States. Concerns about its availability on the illicit market continue.[11,12] It has attracted media attention as a drug used to facilitate 'date rape'; it is unclear why this particular benzodiazepine should have this image, although it is a potent drug. Lorazepam, also a potent benzodiazepine, is much more widely prescribed in the United Kingdom, and alprazolam is used in the United States. Some studies suggest that lorazepam and alprazolam may be associated with an earlier and more difficult withdrawal process than diazepam.[9,13] In one European study, triazolam and lorazepam were found to feature more highly among individuals dependent on high doses of benzodiazepine drugs than among those dependent on low or 'therapeutic' doses.[14] In summary, it appears that potency is a contributory factor in the abuse and dependence-inducing potential of benzodiazepine drugs. However, this picture is somewhat complicated by the fact that drugs such as lorazepam tend to have been marketed at higher equivalent doses than some other benzodiazepines. The elimination half-life influences the nature of withdrawal; if it is short, withdrawal symptoms appear more rapidly and may appear more severe, although withdrawal of more insidious onset in longer-acting benzodiazepines may be just as problematic.

As well as properties of the drugs themselves, the abuse potential of different benzodiazepines is also associated with broader prescribing patterns which affect the potential for diversion to illicit market. Diazepam and temazepam have been the most widely prescribed benzodiazepines in the United Kingdom, and are therefore the most likely to be obtained by drug users and problem drinkers. Drugs such as clonazepam which tend to be prescribed much less widely, and generally for epilepsy rather than for anxiety or insomnia, seem infrequently to raise concerns about misuse[10] but are frequently requested as the treatment of choice for those who are both epileptic and drug dependent. In other parts of Europe where flunitrazepam is more commonly prescribed, there are reports of its high levels of misuse among the illicit drug-using population.

The potential for misuse by injecting

Over time, there have been reports of misuse of various benzodiazepines by injection.[7] A number of factors have influenced this practice. These include the availability of the drug, its short-acting nature, and also the formulation of the drug. In the 1980s temazepam was marketed as a liquid-filled capsule, which enabled easy extraction of the contents to put into a syringe for injecting. The later gel formulation was also injected, by heating to liquidize the gel, resulting in very damaging injecting complications. Some medications that come in easily soluble form can also be converted into a form for injecting, such as liquid diazepam.

The injection of benzodiazepine drugs is associated with substantially more harmful drug misuse in a number of respects,[15] with increased rates of reported sharing of injecting equipment,[9,16] increased risks of overdose, and poorer general health.[8]

Evidence-base for management of benzodiazepine misuse

The literature on management of 'ordinary dose' benzodiazepine dependence, relating mainly to patients prescribed benzodiazepines for treatment of psychiatric disorders, is far more extensive and systematic than that concerning illicit drug users. At the time of writing, there are no meta-analyses or indeed well-conducted randomized controlled trials specifically addressing this problem. In practice, the applicability of the 'ordinary dose' dependence literature is affected not only by clinical differences, but also by concerns about abuse and diversion of prescribed supplies by illicit drug users. So far, no clear guidelines for management have been produced, and the management principles covered in the section below are based on expert clinical consensus statements: these involve some extrapolation from the 'ordinary dose' benzodiazepine dependence literature, and some from established evidence-based principles for management of misusers of other drugs such as opiates.[17] For example, unlike the established evidence that supervised substitute prescribing of methadone reduces injecting in intravenous heroin users, there is no clear evidence that substitute prescribing of benzodiazepines reduces injecting behaviour in injecting misusers of these drugs. Nevertheless, prescribing of oral benzodiazepines with daily supervised consumption is sometimes instituted for this group of patients, especially if they are already established in supervised treatment for concurrent intravenous heroin use (see section on concurrent opioid dependence below).

Guidelines for management of misuse of non-prescribed benzodiazepines

These are a complex group of patients to manage and in general such patients should be referred for specialist assessment.

Assessment

Assessment should attempt to confirm evidence for benzodiazepine dependence. Assessment over a number of visits should involve obtaining urine specimens to determine objectively the regularity (or intermittent nature) of benzodiazepine consumption. Part of the initial assessment process should identify underlying psychiatric disorders that may have been the trigger for a doctor initiating a prescription or for the patient obtaining drugs for the purpose of self-medication. High levels of psychiatric morbidity have been found among samples of patients with severe benzodiazepine dependence.[(18)] The commonest conditions are probably anxiety disorders for which anxiolytics have been prescribed injudiciously; however, in some instances major depressive disorders may be treated or self-medicated with benzodiazepines. Thorough assessment should explore for evidence of major depression and if identified, consideration should be given to the use of antidepressant medication combined with cognitive behavioural therapy.

Treatment

In the presence of polydrug abuse or dependence, caution needs to be exercised about initiating a prescription for benzodiazepines (see section on opioid drug users). Where dependence is established, dose titration should aim to ameliorate withdrawal symptoms rather than to match the large doses of medication that the patient reports consuming. Long-acting benzodiazepines such as diazepam are preferred (Chapter 6.2.2), and doses should rarely exceed 40 to 60 mg daily. Where large doses are prescribed these should ideally be dispensed on a daily pick-up basis from the community pharmacist. The prescribing doctor should avoid succumbing to pressure from the patient to increase the dose without a thorough dose assessment and evidence of withdrawal symptoms. Prescriptions issued on a routine 'repeat' basis should be avoided, and the patient should be informed that lost medication will not be replaced. Requests for replacement medication or additional medication should encourage the doctor to review the overall care plan and to consider reducing and stopping the benzodiazepine prescription. Virtually all benzodiazepine prescriptions should be time limited and part of a detoxification plan with gradual reduction over a clearly stated and negotiated time period. Alternatively, inpatient detoxification, perhaps with longer admissions, may be the best course of action where reduction regimens fail in the community setting. Reduction regimens with benzodiazepines are very variable and many clinicians opt for a very gradual withdrawal with small dose reduction at wide intervals. There is no evidence to indicate that such a gradual approach is any more effective than 20 to 25 per cent reductions over a shorter, more clearly defined time (such as 6 weeks). Carbamazepine can also be effective in ameliorating withdrawal symptoms and in seizure prevention, and may be used as an adjunct in withdrawal management in high-dose benzodiazepine dependence,[(19)] though drug interactions need to be considered for patients who are also prescribed opioid substitute drugs for treatment of heroin dependence (see section on concurrent benzodiazepine and opioid dependence).

Special considerations for managing concurrent benzodiazepine and alcohol dependence

There are high reported rates of alcohol dependence among the homeless, and there are substantial reports of benzodiazepine abuse and dependence in this population also. Cross-tolerance between benzodiazepines and alcohol permits individuals who are alcohol dependent to tolerate high doses of benzodiazepines. Patients may be prescribed benzodiazepines to manage alcohol withdrawal, but injudicious prescribing that is not targeted towards the management of alcohol withdrawal symptoms may result in iatrogenic benzodiazepine dependence.

The extensive research on pharmacological interventions for management of alcohol withdrawal in alcohol-dependent patients has been examined in a meta-analysis by Mayo-Smith, who subsequently produced a systematic review with treatment guidelines.[(20)] This review supports the use of benzodiazepines as the treatment of choice for managing withdrawal symptoms for patients whose symptoms are of sufficient severity to warrant medication, and is consistent with a more recent Cochrane review.[(21)] However, carbamazepine is established as an acceptable alternative to benzodiazepine drugs in treatment of alcohol withdrawal, and is effective both in reducing withdrawal symptoms and in seizure prevention.[(17)] Agents such as clomethiazole and the barbiturate phenobarbital, are less well-supported by controlled trials than benzodiazepines, and carry higher risks of adverse effects.

The potential for misuse of benzodiazepines must be considered in alcohol-dependent patients. However, this is not an adequate reason for avoiding the use of benzodiazepines in the management of withdrawal in view of their superiority in effectiveness, and possibly in potential for harmful misuse, over other treatments. Benzodiazepines with a slower onset of action such as chlordiazepoxide, appear to have less potential for misuse. The prolonged use of benzodiazepines in withdrawal is rarely necessary or helpful, and evidence for benefits of 'substitute prescribing' of benzodiazepines for alcohol users in the longer term is lacking. Use of benzodiazepines to manage phobic and anxiety disorders associated with alcohol dependence should be avoided. For alcohol-dependent patients with a history of benzodiazepine misuse, especially where the patient wishes to avoid further benzodiazepine use, management of withdrawal using carbamazepine alone should be explored.

Special considerations for managing concurrent benzodiazepine and opioid drug dependence

Currently there is no evidence base for long maintenance prescribing of benzodiazepines for those who are high-dose injecting polydrug abusers. However, this intervention has not been subject to any structured evaluation and merits further study in the face of the difficulties of managing such patients. There are two particular areas of concern in managing opioid drug users who also misuse benzodiazepines. The first is the potential for toxicity and overdose when combining illicit or prescribed opioid drugs with benzodiazepines, particularly because of the sedative and respiratory depressant effect of both. Two studies comparing the effects of benzodiazepine use in conjunction with either methadone or buprenorphine treatment have reported higher subjectively reported opioid toxicity symptoms[22] and greater peak effects on objectively assessed performance measures[23] for patients on methadone than for patients on buprenorphine. Where substitute prescribing for heroin or other opioid drug dependence is to be undertaken, the patient needs clear information about the effects of combining opioid and benzodiazepine drugs. Close supervision of prescribed medication (such as daily supervised consumption in the clinic or pharmacy) should be maintained in the early stages of treatment. As many opioid drug users use benzodiazepines somewhat erratically, for example as a substitute when heroin is not available, then stabilization on either methadone or buprenorphine as a regular dose may allow them to stop benzodiazepine use without any other intervention. Initiation of any prescribing intervention addressing benzodiazepine dependence is usually best delayed until it is clear that dependent use has continued despite well-established treatment for opioid dependence. The second area of concern is the potential poor prognosis of opioid withdrawal programmes for patients with concurrent benzodiazepine dependence. Opioid withdrawal symptoms may be more pronounced in patients with both problems, and treatment protocols may need to be adjusted to address this.[24]

Conclusion

There is a valuable role for benzodiazepines, and a need for vigilance and care in their use, as well as active recognition and management of those who are dependent. However, there is a need for greater awareness of the risks of polydrug dependence with misuse of high doses of benzodiazepines in conjunction with both alcohol dependence and opiate dependence. Caution needs to be used in assessing patients, and benzodiazepine prescribing should be restricted to those where there is clear evidence of dependence.

The risk of synergistic effects with other drugs and consequent overdose should be explained to all patients who are identified as being involved in such behaviour. Community detoxification or inpatient detoxification is the best option based on the evidence of available research and evaluation of current interventions.

Further information

Seivewright, N. (2000). *The case for other substitute drugs. Community treatment of drug misuse: more than methadone*, pp. 49–81. Cambridge University Press, Cambridge, UK.

Lingford-Hughes, A.R., Welch, S., and Nutt, D. (2004). Evidence-based guidelines for the treatment of substance misuse, addiction and comorbidity: recommendations from the British Association for Psychopharmacology. *Journal of Psychopharamacology*, **18**, 293–335.

References

1. Woody, G.E., O'Brien, C.P., and Greenstein, R. (1975). Misuse and abuse of diazepam: an increasingly common medical problem. *International Journal of Addiction*, **10**, 843–8.
2. Bliding, A. (1978). The abuse potential of benzodiazepines with special reference to oxazepam. *Acta Psychiatrica Scandinavia Supplementum*, **274**, 111–16.
3. Petursson, H. and Lader, M.H. (1981). Benzodiazepine dependence. *British Journal of Addiction*, **76**, 133–45.
4. Hallstrom, C. and Lader, M. (1981). Benzodiazepine withdrawal phenomena. *International Pharmacopsychiatry*, **16**, 235–44.
5. Farrell, M. and Strang, J. (1988). Misuse of temazepam. *British Medical Journal*, **297**, 1402.
6. Ruben, S.M. and Morrison, C.L. (1992). Temazepam misuse in a group of injecting drug users. *British Journal of Addiction*, **87**, 1387–92.
7. Strang, J., Seivewright, N., and Farrell, M. (1992). Intravenous and other novel abuses of benzodiazepines: the opening of Pandora's box? *British Journal of Addiction*, **87**, 1373–5.
8. Ross, J., Darke, S., and Hall, W. (1997). Transitions between routes of benzodiazepine administration among heroin users in Sydney. *Addiction*, **92**, 697–705.
9. Murphy, S.M. and Tyrer, P. (1991). A double-blind comparison of the effects of gradual withdrawal of lorazepam, diazepam and bromazepam in benzodiazepine dependence. *The British Journal of Psychiatry*, **158**, 511–16.
10. Tyrer, P. (1993). Pharmacological differences in the dependence potential of benzodiazepines. In *Benzodiazepine dependence* (ed. C. Hallstrom), pp. 77–90. Oxford University Press, Oxford.
11. Simmons, M.M. and Cupp, M.J. (1998). Use and abuse of flunitrazepam. *Annals of Pharmacotherapy*, **32**, 117–19.
12. Woods, J.H. and Winger, G. (1997). Abuse liability of flunitrazepam. *Journal of Clinical Psychopharmacology*, **17**(Suppl. 2), 1S–57S.
13. Rickels, K., Case, W.G., Schweizer, E.E., *et al.* (1986). Low dose dependence in chronic benzodiazepine users; a preliminary report on 119 patients. *Psychopharmacology Bulletin*, **22**, 415–17.
14. Martinez-Cano, H., Vela-Bueno, A., De Iceta, M., *et al.* (1996). Benzodiazepine types in high versus therapeutic dose dependence. *Addiction*, **91**, 1179–86.
15. Darke, S., Hall, W., Ross, M., *et al.* (1992). Benzodiazepine use and HIV risk-taking behaviour among injecting drug users. *Drug and Alcohol Dependence*, **31**, 31–6.
16. Klee, H., Faugier, J., Hayes, C., *et al.* (1990). AIDS-related risk behaviour, polydrug use and temazepam. *British Journal of Addiction*, **85**, 1125–32.
17. Lingford-Hughes, A.R., Welch, S., and Nutt, D. (2004). Evidence-based guidelines for the treatment of substance misuse, addiction and comorbidity: recommendations from the British Association for Psychopharmacology. *Journal of Psychopharamacology*, **18**, 293–335.
18. Busto, U.E., Romach, M.K., and Sellers, E.M. (1996). Multiple drug use and psychiatric comorbidity in patients admitted to the hospital with severe benzodiazepine dependence. *Journal of Clinical Psychopharmacology*, **16**, 517.
19. Denis, C., Fatseas, M., Lavie, E., *et al.* (2006). Pharmacological interventions for benzodiazepine monodependence management in outpatient settings. *Cochrane Database of Systematic Reviews*, (3), CD005194.
20. Mayo-Smith, M.F. (1997). Pharmacological management of alcohol withdrawal: a meta-analysis and evidence-based practice guideline. *The Journal of the American Medical Association*, **278**, 144–50.
21. Ntais, C., Pakos, E., Kysaz, P., *et al.* (2005). Benzodiazepines for alcohol withdrawal. *Cochrane Database of Systematic Reviews*, (3), CD005063.
22. Nielsen, S., Dietze, P., Lee, N., *et al.* (2007). Concurrent buprenorphine and benzodiazepines use and self-reported toxicity in opioid substitution treatment. *Addiction*, **102**, 616–22.
23. Lintzeris, N., Mitchell, T.B., Bond, A., *et al.* (2006). Interactions on mixing diazepam with methadone or buprenorphine in maintenance patients. *Journal of Clinical Psychopharmacology*, **26**, 274–83.
24. de Wet, C., Reed, L., Glasper, A., *et al.* (2004). Benzodiazepine co-dependence exacerbates the opiate withdrawal syndrome. *Drug and Alcohol Dependence*, **76**, 31–5.

4.2.3.5 Disorders relating to the use of ecstasy and other 'party drugs'

Adam R. Winstock and Fabrizio Schifano

Introduction

Participation in the dance music/rave scene has been associated with an ever-growing range of primarily stimulant and hallucinogenic drugs since its inception in the Balearic Islands in the mid-1980s. The last two decades have seen the globalization of the dance music scene and the gradual adoption of these and other drugs by mainstream drug using populations. Although 'Ecstasy' (**MDMA**, 3,4-methylenedioxymethamphetamine) was the archetypical dance drug inducing both stimulant and empathogenic effects, dance drug use is polydrug use with cocaine, amphetamine, nitrates, ketamine, and GHB all being common.[(1)] The use of this diverse group of drugs is now no longer confined to either young adults or the dance floor with use common for example, at house parties or other more intimate social gatherings.[(2)] Although not typically identified as dance drugs, alcohol and cannabis are of course highly prevalent among this group.

Ecstasy (3,4-methylenedioxymethamphetamine)

Background

Incorrectly termed a designer drug (a drug whose chemical structure is modified to avoid being included within a list of drugs/chemical structures prohibited by legislation), MDMA was first synthesized in 1912 by Merck Pharmaceuticals. It was never marketed and remained largely ignored until the 1950s when the United States Army explored its military potential. It was not until the late 1960s and early 1970s however that drug users on the west coast of America began to popularize its recreational use along with MDA (methylenedioxymethamphetamine).

Although MDMA may claim its place as the mother of dance drugs and possessor of the best branding in terms of name, MDMA is only one of a large number of synthetic amphetamine type drugs possessing varying degrees of stimulant, hallucinogenic, and empathogenic effects that are used within the dance scene. Characterized by its stimulant and prosocial effects the sought after experiences of disinhibition, euphoria, energy, and empathy are ideally suited to the 'dance scene' where energetic and prolonged dancing is commonplace. Indeed it may be that dancing offsets the psychomotor agitation that stimulants can induce or that MDMA-like drugs may enhance enjoyment and ability to dance to dance music. In the United Kingdom MDMA is classified as a Class B drug.

Preparations, purity, and routes of use

MDMA is most commonly taken orally though it may be snorted or injected. MDMA is most commonly sold as branded tablets ('pills'), with different tablets being identified by an imprinted logo (for example of a cartoon character, car manufacturer, or animal), but may also be found as capsules or powder. The average dose of an ecstasy tablet containing MDMA is about 70 mg (range 50–150 mg). The cost has reduced markedly over the last 20 years from £20/tablet in 1985 to as little at 50 pence/tablet when bought in bulk (typical price in the United Kingdom for a single tablet would be 2–5).[(3)]

Because of the illicit nature of MDMA production, variation in precursor availability, and the large number of possible synthetic pathways for its production, tablets sold as ecstasy may contain a wide range of substances other than MDMA. In the United Kingdom and Europe especially in the 1990s, ecstasy tablets were often found to contain substances (usually psychoactive) other than MDMA. These included analogues of MDMA, such as methylenedioxyamphetamine (**MDEA**), *N*-methyl-1-(1,3-benzodioxol-5-yl)-2-butanamine (**MBDB**), and methylenedioxyethylamphetamine (**MDEA**), or combinations of stimulants such as ephedrine or amphetamine and hallucinogens such as LSD or ketamine.[(4)] While these other psychoactive substances may be marketed as distinct substances with their own branding (e.g. 4-Bromo-2, 5-dimethoxyphenethylamine sold as 2CB and 4 MTA as 'flatliners') more commonly they and the MDMA analogues MDEA, MBDB, and MDA, which broadly share the effects of MDMA, are sold under the generic term 'ecstasy'. More recent evidence would suggest that the proportion of tablets sold as ecstasy that contains MDMA in the United Kingdom is very high, with purity levels of 80–90 per cent not being uncommon.[(5)]

Pill testing

Some users utilize various pill testing methods (such as the Marquis test which gives colorimetric result by mixing the substance with a reagent) and websites (www.EcstasyData.org) which provide the contents of different pills following more elaborate analytical methods. Although it may be the case that these approaches may have some role in getting users to consider risks and promote the uptake of harm reduction practices, it is only on very few occasions that such methods have identified potentially far riskier psychoactive contents such as paramethoxyamphetamine (PMA).[(6)] In such cases, early warning through such websites may be potentially helpful. However, even with more sophisticated analytic processes (e.g. GMS, HPLC), knowing the content of your tablet never guarantees the user a positive experience and does not guarantee that they will not experience severe adverse effects.[(4)] In addition, most ecstasy-related deaths have involved tablets containing MDMA. Most deaths have not been related to dose and would have been unpredictable from knowing the content of the tablet.[(3)]

Prevalence and patterns of ecstasy use

British population studies show that 54 per cent of 20- to 22-year-olds have been offered ecstasy at some time and 15 per cent have tried it at least once.[(7)] The prevalence of use appears higher in those associated with the dance music drug scene with over 90 per cent reporting ever use. Similar findings have been reported from Europe,[(8)] Australia,[(9)] and the United States.

The typical pattern of use in the United Kingdom and Europe is one to four tablets a night, though many users will often consume larger number of tablets during a binge session especially when holidaying in summer dance resort destinations. Regular users will use between once or twice a week to once every fortnight, though there has been increasing recognition of a minority of users who take very large numbers of tablets (20 or 30) over a single session, or with the availability of very cheap 'pills' extended periods of low-level daily use. Ecstasy, especially within the context of dance clubs is rarely taken in isolation and polydrug use is the norm, with different adjunctive substances taken at different times over the course of a night.[1] For example, alcohol is taken with ecstasy at the beginning of the night to get a stronger/better high.[10] Cocaine, amphetamines, and/or additional ecstasy tablets are taken to maintain arousal and a state of alertness (the MDMA enactogenic effects fade away in 2–4 h). Finally depressants such as cannabis, alcohol, benzodiazepines, and more rarely opiates, may be taken in the last part of the night to calm down before going home, since the untoward after-effects of ecstasy (namely irritability, insomnia, and restlessness) may persist well beyond its 'pleasurable' effects. With a chronic high dosage, ecstasy users develop tolerance and experience a decrease in the desired effects over time, which could lead to exploration of use of other stimulants and hallucinogens.[1]

Physical effects and complications

Physiologically sympathomimetic properties similar to amphetamine predominate including tachycardia, anorexia, increased respiratory rate, blood pressure, increased motor activity, tremor, mydriasis, increased temperature, and sweating. Jaw tightening (bruxism), xerostomia, teeth grinding with molar erosion, may also be seen (see Table 4.2.3.5.1). Sleep architecture modification[11] and sexual activity alteration[12,13] have also been described.

After MDMA intake a number of untoward effects may commonly occur including nausea, vomiting, diarrhoea, tachycardia, and palpitations. Pathologies less commonly seen include arrhythmias, hypertension as well as potentially life-threatening, metabolic acidosis, cerebral haemorrhages, convulsions, coma, rhabdomyoloysis, thrombocytopenia, disseminated intravascular coagulation, SIADH, acute kidney failure, acute liver failure, dehydration, and malignant hyperthermia.[14–18]

Hyperthermia although enhanced by exertional activity and poorly ventilated environments may be somewhat independent from the setting in which the drug is taken, with MDMA having thermal dysregulation effects in its own right. Dehydration is common and thirsty clubbers naturally tend to replace body fluids lost during sweating sensibly with fruit juices, other isotonic fluids or water, or less sensibly but quite commonly with alcohol. Very rarely excessive intake of hypotonic fluids, coupled with an increase in vasopressin levels, has led to the occurrence of lethal hyponatraemia.[19] Deaths as a result of SIADH are very rare but can be fatal in association with excessive hypotonic fluid consumption with MDMA potentially impairing judgement or stimulating repetitive compulsive behaviours. In normal subjects who take ecstasy and do not develop SIADH there does appears to be an increase in both ADH and oxytocin levels,[20] the latter perhaps responsible for the drug's prosocial effects. MDMA is a potentially damaging cardiac stimulant;[21] with reports suggesting long-term MDMA use may possibly lead to a fenfluramine-like valvular heart disease condition. All users of ecstasy develop a (mild, in most cases) serotonin syndrome after acute drug intake.[13,22] Unfortunately although being reported by almost half ecstasy users, Verheyden and Henry[23] found that concerns about physical health are not perceived as important as concerns about mental health.[23]

Table 4.2.3.5.1 Psychological and physical effects of MDMA

Physical	Psychological
Increase in physical and emotional energy	Relaxation/euphoria
Dilated pupils, dry mouth	Feelings of well-being
Tachycardia, hypertension, increased respiratory rate	Enhanced closeness and sociability
Increased sweating, dehydration	Heightened perceptual awareness
Increased motor activity, tremor	Disinhibition
Blurred/double vision	Increased response to touch/empathy
Anorexia, nausea, weight loss	Anxiety/panic/paranoia
Teeth grinding, jaw clenching	Agitation and restlessness

MDMA psychological effects and problems (see Table 4.2.3.5.1, adapted from Liester *et al.*[24])

Being structurally related to both amphetamine and mescaline, 'empathogens' or 'entactogens'[25] like MDMA possess both stimulant and hallucinogenic properties which allow them to be discriminated from other related substances. After MDMA ingestion, enhanced mood, increased energy, openness, heightened sensory perception, and mild perception alterations are reported[15,17] (Table 4.2.3.5.1).

MDMA is described as evoking 'an easily controlled altered state of consciousness with emotional and sensual overtones',[26] with the substance's appeal resting in its 'dramatic and consistent ability to induce in the user a profound feeling of attachment and connection'. With this in mind it is perhaps not surprising that the Los Angeles dealer who coined the street name 'ecstasy' for MDMA would have preferred the name 'empathy' but he did not feel that his typical customer would know what it meant. It was also these qualities that led to the enthusiasm of a small number of physicians and therapists in the United States to explore its use within a clinical psychotherapeutic setting and more recently led to its approval as a research agent in the treatment of PTSD.[27]

Acute psychological problems associated with MDMA use

There have been reports of acute episodes of anxiety, panic, paranoia, and rarely brief psychotic episodes following consumption of MDMA by some users. Many users of MDMA report 'midweek blues', with some individuals reporting clinically borderline levels of depression in the days following MDMA[28] which could reflect depletion of serotonin following the acute elevation that follows ingestion of MDMA. This could be seen as a parallel to the 'crash' reported after abstinence of cocaine use or as a hangover effect from all night dancing, excessive alcohol, and minimal sleep. Although depression, anxiety, and mood fluctuations attributed to ecstasy are reported to be strongly related to the number of occasions of MDMA use,[29,30] Morgan *et al.*[31] found that higher depression scores among current heavy ecstasy users, in comparison to drug-naïve and polydrug controls, were no longer significant after treating cannabis use as a covariate.

Other consequences of use

(a) Neurotoxicity and evidence for 5-HT disruption in humans (see Table 4.2.3.5.2)

Although, in humans, the relationship between MDMA intake, putative 5-HT neurotoxicity, and persistent functional consequences is somewhat controversial,[32] the average single dose size consumed by humans approaches levels found to be neurotoxic in animals.[10] Core ambient temperature and hydration status have been implicated as key factors in the development of neurotoxicity.[13]

Although Colado *et al.*[33] suggested that MDMAs ability to produce neurodegeneration of dopamine nerve endings is open to debate, MDMA is generally considered to be a selective 5-HT neurotoxin. After administration of MDMA, animals have reduced levels of 5-HT, 5-hydroxyindole acetic acid, and tryptophan hydroxylase. Abnormal 5-HT regrowth has been reported after MDMA-induced damage with a decrease in 5-HT terminal density, suggestive of a 'chemical axotomy'. Pathological investigations suggest that 5-HT nerve terminals arising from the dorsal raphe nucleus are specifically involved. Duration and magnitude of these neurotoxic effects are dose dependent and are followed by differential rates of recovery, with 5-HT damage persisting for up to a year in the rat, and dopaminergic damage for up to 3 years in the rhesus monkey. These changes appear to be species specific with primates being more sensitive to the neurotoxic damage than rodents.

Markers for 5-HT damage may be sought either by direct assessment of metabolite levels or indirectly by assessing those functions thought to be dependent on an intact 5-HT system (see Table 4.2.3.5.2). MDMA users may show reduced brain 5-HTT (serotonin transporter) levels; there might be an association between degree of MDMA exposure and degree of reduction in 5-HTT ligand binding.[34]

Further evidence for disruption of the 5-HT system comes from blunted neuroendocrine responses (cortisol and prolactin) to d-fenfluramine in former MDMA users;[13] from cognitive disturbances in former MDMA users and from PET studies showing a decrease in a structural component of 5-HT neurones.

(b) Neuropsychological impairment and psychiatric presentation of ecstasy users

MDMA users as a group demonstrate a range of cognitive deficits in comparison to alcohol users, non-drug controls, and MDMA-naïve polydrug controls, including cannabis users.[31,35] Although the issue is somewhat controversial the most consistent neuropsychological finding in former MDMA users is a deficit in verbal memory under both immediate- and delayed-recall conditions.[36] Deficits in other areas of cognitive function, such as verbal fluency, executive function, impulse control, reaction time, and processing speed have been reported as well.[31] Evidence for attentional deficits varies depending on the task employed.[37] MDMA use may be associated with longer visual scanning times, reaction times, or planning times. Interpretation of these data is somewhat complicated by the fact that MDMA users typically use other drugs which may exert independent or interactive effects on cognitive performance.[37]

MDMA intake may put users at significant risk for developing psychiatric problems,[23] although some have suggested that this may occur only in vulnerable individuals.[39] Studies suggest that ecstasy users may report both childhood emotional/physical abuse[40] and history of familial depression, anxiety, and panic attacks[41] more frequently than ecstasy-naïve controls.

Thus although fraught with confounders, especially other drug use and premorbid functioning, there does appear to be an association between MDMA use and increased rates of anxiety,[24] panic, major depressive disorder,[38] prolonged depersonalization, psychosis, flashbacks, and even craving for chocolate.

Table 4.2.3.5.2 Clinical signs of intoxication with amphetamine

Physical	Psychological	Behavioural
Elevated P, BP, temperature	Euphoria/energized	Motor hyperactivity
Increased respiratory rate	Anxious/irritable	Restless/twitching
Sweating/dehydrated	Rapid thoughts	Talkative, pressured speech
Dilated pupils	Paranoia	Aggressive
Tremor/shakiness	Perceptual disturbance	Stereotyped movements

(c) Depression and its management in ecstasy users

In the case of a patient presenting with psychological problems who has a history of MDMA use, the crucial assessment issues are the identification of any premorbid disorders, where in the cycle of use/post use they are, and the persistence of any symptoms beyond a 2–4 week period following cessation of use. As with amphetamine use, in the days after taking MDMA there is a period characterized by symptoms attributable to monoamine depletion and subsequently repletion. A period of acute 5-HT depletion due to vesicular monoamine depletion (Tuesday blues), is likely to be the most potent cause for the relative reduction in monoamine neurotransmitters. Repeated use of MDMA over several days will be associated with markedly diminished effects. Recovery is delayed further by inhibition of the rate-limiting enzyme (tyrosine hydroxylase in the case of MDMA) and the relative absence especially in chronic users, of a good source of monoamine precursors following stimulant-induced anorexia and malnutrition. It is likely that, as with other stimulant drugs, including cocaine, a period of extended but less intense withdrawal symptoms (mood, sleep) may be seen with persistent abstinence which may take weeks or months to recede and are associated with the more gradual reversal of neuroadaptive changes in dopaminergic receptor sensitivity/expression.[42]

History taking should specifically endeavour to identify any pre-existing/persistent depressive/other disorders and to ascertain the functionality of the use of MDMA and the consequences on underlying mood and functioning in days following use. Antidepressant treatments should usually not be commenced until 2–4 weeks after cessation of MDMA use in order to allow for reassessment and confirmation of any disorder. In addition, resolution of symptoms with cessation of use may also act as powerful reinforcer of continued abstinence if an individual's mood recovers. Reassessment and treatment where necessary, is important since being depressed is associated with an enhanced initial response to stimulant drugs and higher relapse risk.

In prescribing an antidepressant to a client with a previous history of MDMA use, confining prescribing to only abstinent users is recommended since their effectiveness during a period of current use would be expected to be poor both as a result of poor compliance and monoamine depletion. In addition there are at least theoretical causes for concern over potentially fatal interactions between MDMA and selective serotonin reuptake inhibitors (SSRIs) that have very rarely been reported, possibly because some SSRIs (i.e. citalopram) can inhibit the CYP2D6 enzyme.[22] The precise effects of combining SSRIs and MDMA appears to be related to whether use of the SSRI was before or after the MDMA and whether SSRI dosing is acute or chronic. For example, SSRIs given acutely after MDMA (taken by users to intensify the ecstasy effects) may theoretically increase the risk of precipitating a serotoninergic syndrome. It is probable that SSRIs and other classes of antidepressant can be used effectively in this group if a diagnosis of responsive affective/anxiety disorder is confirmed and abstinence is maintained. CBT may be useful in this group both to address their underlying drug as well as to address any coexisting anxiety/depressive disorders.

Dependence with the development of heavy regular use patterns is possible, though there are unlikely to be any specific signs or symptoms that differentiate diagnosis of management significantly from other forms of stimulant dependence.

Methamphetamine-'crystalline methamphetamine hydrochloride' ice, crystal, shabu, yaba, meth, tina

Background

Methamphetamine is one of number of synthetic amphetamine type stimulants that includes dex-amphetamine. Whilst its use has been problematic in SE Asian countries such as Thailand, Japan, and Korea for many years it is only in the last decade that it has become a significant problem in eastern Europe, America, Australia, and elsewhere. In the United Kingdom methamphetamine was reclassified as Class A drug in 2007.

Preparation, purity, and routes of use

Unlike illicit amphetamine sulphate powder (speed), methamphetamine is often of very high purity. Crystalline methamphetamine hydrochloride (known as ice-because it can resemble shards of glass) can be up to 80% pure. Base amphetamine (sometimes known as paste), is an oily, waxy intermediate product on the way the manufacture of the crystalline hydrochloride salt of methamphetamine and has a lower purity of about 40–50 per cent. Methamphetamine is a versatile drug and can be smoked, snorted, injected, and taken orally.

Mechanism of action and metabolism

Methamphetamine closely resembles amphetamine sulphate (commonly referred to as speed) in structure and mechanism of action but is considerably more potent in its sympathomimetic effects and has a longer duration of action (half-life about 12 h). Methamphetamine has both direct sympathomimetic effects secondary to disruption of vesicular storage of monoamines and inhibition of their breakdown by MAOIs and indirect actions through inhibition of central presynaptic reuptake of catecholamines.

Prevalence and patterns of use

In the United Kingdom reports of its use are becoming more common, particularly in association with the gay and dance music scene but compared to the use of cocaine in all its forms, the prevalence of methamphetamine use at present is still low.[43]

Physical effects and complications

Sympathetic arousal induced by methamphetamine produces rapid and sometimes irregular heartbeat, sweating, pupillary dilation, hypertension, dry mouth, tremor and blurred vision, and increased body heat. Occasionally, serious medical complications arise including coronary artery syndrome, seizures, and cerebral bleeds (see Table 4.2.3.5.2).

Psychological effects and complications

Acute sought after-effects are similar to those of amphetamine and include euphoria, enhanced stamina, confidence, disinhibition, reduced appetite, improved coordination, and heightened alertness and awareness.

Other consequences of use

(a) Dependence and withdrawal

Dependence may occur and is more common among heavy male users and in those who smoke or inject the drug. Although dependent users may use every day to avoid withdrawal, more typically users tend to consume a large amount of the drug (often several grams) over several days going out without sleep (a binge) before ceasing use through physical exhaustion or an exhaustion of funds. 'Crashing' refers to the period following a binge, which is characterized by fatigue, hypersomnia, hyperphagia, and low mood due to acute monoamine depletion. The crash and subsequent comedown period may last 2–7 days. If abstinence persists a longer term withdrawal period may be seen, characterized by craving, low mood, anergia, irritability, sleep, and appetite disturbance. Similar neurobiological mechanisms involving alterations in the function and activity of the monoamine neurotransmitters are responsible for the overlap between the symptoms of depression and those of stimulant withdrawal.[42,44] Typically the withdrawal gradually diminishes over 2–4 weeks though dysphoric symptoms may persist for up to 10 weeks.

(b) Withdrawal, depression, and management

The frequency of depressive symptoms is highest during the withdrawal period. As with alcohol, there are a far fewer number of people who present with depression symptoms outside of stimulant use or withdrawal. Management of withdrawal is largely supportive and with a safe, well-supported home environment. In patient admission is rarely required other than in those with severe mental or physical illness. The patient should be placed in quiet surroundings for several days and allowed to sleep and eat as much as is needed. Because a significant component of the withdrawal syndrome is probably related to neurotransmitter depletion, recovery may be delayed because of anorexia associated with amphetamine use. It may be useful in some to provide nutritional supplements or a well-balanced diet rich in monoamine precursors: phenylalanine, tyrosine, l-tryptophan for example, pumpkin seeds, chocolate, marmite, bananas. Benzodiazepines may be prescribed on a short-term basis for agitation. Some patients may become markedly despondent during withdrawal and a suicide assessment may be necessary.

Since antidepressants have no specific anti-craving effects, and the efficacy of antidepressants in reducing depression is confined to those stimulant users who are depressed, it is useful to wait until after they have stopped using for 2–4 weeks and reassess them for depressive symptoms. The advantages of waiting are improved diagnostic accuracy, avoidance of potentially unnecessary medication, and probably an improvement in compliance and efficacy. However the persistence of depressive symptoms beyond 2–4 weeks after stopping amphetamine use may suggest that there is an underlying depressive illness and this should be treated(42) since left unmanaged its presence represents a high risk for relapse. Psychosocial treatments for stimulant abuse and dependence have been found to be effective in reducing levels of use,(45) but to date, no reliably effective pharmacological treatments have been identified and there are currently no widely accepted evidence-based pharmacotherapy regimes for the treatment of psychostimulant withdrawal.(46)

(c) Stimulant-induced psychosis

The use of high doses of methamphetamine may lead to the induction of a temporary psychotic state that may be clinically indistinguishable from paranoid schizophrenia. First recognized in 1938 in association with Benzedrine nasal inhalers, it was not until Connell's classic 1958 study that the syndrome was well described. Acute transient psychotic episodes (typically characterized by suspiciousness, unusual thought content, or hallucinations) occur in about 10–15 per cent of users. Psychotic episodes are more common in dependent users, men, injectors, and smokers, polydrug users, those with past history and following a binge in association with prolonged insomnia.(47)

Characterized by persecutory delusions and hallucinations which are typically auditory but may be visual or tactile (which can be associated with secondary delusion of parasitic infestation) amphetamine-induced psychosis typically remit within few days or at most a few weeks. Little has changed in the way of management since Connell's time who recommends 'removal of the drug and appropriate sedation'. Often, patients present with high levels of hostility and violence secondary to persecutory delusions or hallucinations, and safe containment and management of the disturbed individual can require enormous levels of both physical and chemical restraint. Benzodiazepines (often required in very high doses) should be the first-line medication with antipsychotics used only where additional tranquilization is required. A diagnosis of a possible underlying or persistent psychotic disorder must be deferred until a reassessment can be made in a drug-free state. These often florid psychoses usually remit within a few days and the user returns to normal functioning, although some retain a vulnerability to such episodes.(48) Only a minority (1–15 per cent) persist beyond 1 month and many of these patients will have underlying psychiatric disorders.(47)

The prognosis is variable with those who have experienced stimulant-induced psychotic episodes being more vulnerable to future episodes (possibly through behavioural sensitization) on re-exposure to the drug often at lower levels. Recent positron emission tomography (PET) imaging studies in chronic methamphetamine users have demonstrated a reduction in dopamine transporter concentration and this reduction was significantly associated with the duration of methamphetamine use and closely related to the severity of persistent psychiatric symptoms. Moreover, the severity of psychiatric symptoms was significantly correlated with the duration of methamphetamine use. Cessation is still potentially important since there does however appear to be some recovery of dopamine transporter function with abstinence.

Gamma hydroxy butyrate, GHB, GBH, fantasy, G, liquid ecstasy, and GBL

Background

GHB is an endogenous short-chain fatty acid found in the CNS and elsewhere in the body. A putative neurotransmitter, its precise role is yet to be identified although specific binding sites have been identified in hippocampus (linked to DA neurones). Trace amounts may also be found in certain fruits such a guava. In the United Kingdom GHB is classified as Class C drug.

Like ketamine, GHB was originally developed as an anaesthetic though the high incidence of tonic clinic seizures dampened enthusiasm among surgeons for its routine use. Subsequently it found clinical utility as a sedative, a treatment for narcolepsy, as a detoxification agent (it is effective in the management of alcohol withdrawal) and as a putative muscle growth enhancer for body builders (through its effect on increasing slow wave sleep). Since the 1990s however it has become best known for its place among the smorgasbord of drugs commonly used by those involved in the dance/rave scene. It has a reputation as a cheap stimulant drug of short duration with marked aphrodisiac properties but a narrow therapeutic threshold carrying a significant risk of overdose especially in combination with alcohol.(49)

Preparation (pro drugs), purity, and routes of use

Until the late 1990s GHB and its precursors including the psychoactive pro compounds GBL (gamma butyl-lactone) and 1,4 butanediol were widely available over the Internet. Because of its relative ease of manufacture attempts at home production were common, resulting in preparations of widely varying concentrations. The resultant formulations were sometimes caustic, resulting in gastrointestinal discomfort, vomiting, aspiration, and coma.

GHB is sold most commonly as a free acid (a colourless and odourless liquid in its pure form, with a slightly salty, acidic taste) or as a sodium salt (usually a white powder). Although varying widely in concentration typically doses are sold in plastic vials holding 5–10 ml.

Mechanism of action and metabolism

GHB readily cross the BBB and acutely leads to a transient decrease followed by increase in dopamine levels (accompanied by increase in endogenous opioid release). Increases in other neurotransmitters such as GABA, Ach, and 5-HT are also seen. At higher doses it exhibits some partial GABA-b activity (epileptogenic). GHB is usually taken orally often mixed in fruit juice or alcoholic beverage. It has a very rapid onset of action with noticeable effects occurring within 15 min of administration it has a relatively short duration of action ($t_{1/2}$ 27 min) with effects peaking at 30–60 min and being over within 2–4 h, being eliminated though its breakdown to CO_2 and H_2O.

Physical effects and complications

GHB exhibits a very narrow therapeutic index and as a result of wide interpersonal variation in tolerance and significantly enhanced toxicity (depressant effects) when combined with alcohol, overdose with GHB has been reported more widely than for any other dance drug,[50,51] overdose should be suspected in someone who presents with nystagmus, ataxia, nausea, vomiting, sedation, weakness, bradycardia, hypotension, and the rapid onset of unconsciousness (quite similar to severe alcohol intoxication but without alcohol on the breath). Management should include placing the person in the recovery position, airway management and pulse oximetry. GCS scores may be very low (<7). If oxygen saturation drops or they are so unconscious that they can tolerate a Guedels airways then ventilation should be considered. Overdoses are short lived and most awake somewhat aroused and disorientation after a few hours. Other clinical presentations include agitation, anxiety, coma, amnesia, and collapse. These patients when in coma may require ventilation and typically suddenly emerge from their coma with high levels of agitation, arousal, and violence.

Although there have been press reports of GHB being commonly used as 'date rape drug', such cases are very rare and it is still the case that the most common drug used for such purposes is alcohol alone.

Psychological effects and complications

Consumption of GHB results in a dose related euphoria and stimulation which gives way to sedation at higher doses. In combination with stimulant drugs there may be an increase of precipitating a brief psychotic reaction, whilst with alcohol the risk of fatal overdose is the primary concern. There has been a single case report of Wernicke Korsakoff syndrome.

Other consequences of use

(a) Dependence and withdrawal

More recently there have been number of reports describing GHB dependence and withdrawal. The later may present as a rapid onset, prolonged alcohol withdrawal picture. Although associated with lower levels of autonomic arousal and seizure risk, patients may exhibit marked confusion, delirium, and hallucinations. Management may require doses of diazepam markedly in excess of those typically used to manage alcohol withdrawal with a waxing and waning clinical progression that may last 2 weeks.[52]

Ketamine (K, Special K, Super K, Vitamin K, Green, Mean Green, Jet)

Background

Ketamine (2-(2-chlorophenyl)-2-(methylamino)-cyclohexanone) and PCP (angel dust) are very similar drugs, the main difference being ketamine's shorter half and less problematic 'emergence phenomena'. Ketamine has a range of useful clinical applications. It is used across several areas of medicine including paediatric analgesia and anaesthesia, emergency anaesthesia, obstetrics, and battle-zones[53] and benefits from having a wide margin of safety in overdose. Ketamine is an NMDA antagonist and is almost unique as an anaesthetic in its ability to produce a 'dissociative' state, which results in higher brain structures in the brain centres being prevented from perceiving auditory, visual or painful stimuli leading to 'a lack of responsive awareness'. Overall the effect has been described as somato-aesthetic sensory blockade with amnesia and analgesia. In recent years its non-medical use as a psychedelic has become more common. In the United Kingdom ketamine is classified as Class C drug. For a recent review see Wolff and Winstock.[54]

Mechanism of action and metabolism

Ketamine has multiple actions at numerous receptor sites particularly affecting glutaminergic and monoaminergic neurotransmission. The most significant pharmacological action of ketamine is the non-competitive antagonist binding at the cation channel of the NMDA receptor and consequent interference with excitatory amino acid transmitters—glutamate and aspartate. As a research probe in the study of schizophrenia, ketamine has given increasing prominence to the role of glutamate in the aetiology of psychotic illness. Ketamine also enhances monoaminergic transmission resulting in marked sympathomimetic effects as well as modulating activity at opioid receptors, thought to be responsible for its analgesic and dysphoric effects.

Ketamine undergoes marked first-pass metabolism and is fairly ineffective when taken orally (bioavailability may be <20 per cent). However, oral consumption does result in a two-fold higher concentration of its primary metabolite norketamine compared to, for example, intramuscular dosing. Norketamine is pharmacologically active with anaesthetic potency approaching one-third that of the parent compound. Hence although the onset of effects following ingestion may be somewhat slower than by parental routes the duration of effects would almost certainly be longer. The majority of the parent drug will be eliminated from the body within 24 h, although prolonged effects due to the presence of active metabolites may occur.

Preparations, purity, and routes of use

Ketamine may be sold illicitly in a number of preparations; as crystalline powder for intranasal use (dose-100–400 mg), in liquid, tablet, powder, or capsular form (dose-350–500 mg) for ingestion. When obtained from diverted licit sources, the formulation of the drug is a solution prepared for intravenous use. This solution may be injected or swallowed, but more typically the solution is dried and taken intranasally.[54] However, this process of desiccation may reduce the purity of the crystalline residue, and is an obvious point at which, via contamination, purity may be altered. Ketamine may be adequately absorbed via the intranasal, intravenous, subcutaneous, intramuscular, and intrathecal routes, with snorting and injecting being the most common recreational routes of use. Reports of clinical use via the rectal and transdermal routes have also been described.

Prevalence and patterns of use

Far less common in the general population than MDMA, ketamine none the less has become increasingly popular among those associated with the dance scene with a prevalence of about 20 per cent being reported among clubbers. Whilst ketamine maintains a good safety record within clinical settings, the increase in its unregulated use outside such controlled environments is a cause for concern

Table 4.2.3.5.3 Ketamine, psychological and physical effects

Psychological	Physical
Rapid onset, short duration of action (1 h), wide safety margin	
Dissociative anaesthesia 'somatosensory blockade' analgesia	Dilated pupils
Perceptual distortion/hallucinations/near death	Tachycardia
Out of body experience	Hypertension
Though disorder/synaethesia	Ataxia
Emergence phenomena	Paralysis
Cognitive impairment	Sweating
Amnesia	Hypersalivation
Derealization/depersonalization	Little effect on cough reflex

with its effects being highly sensitive to age, dose, route, set, and setting (see Table 4.2.3.5.3). Outside clinical settings ketamine is most commonly snorted or injected, with typically administered doses being small fractions of a gram (an eighth). Because of its short half-life (17 min) the psychedelic effects experienced are generally short-lived with effect duration of about 1–2 h. The short duration of effect and rapid onset of action when taken by intranasal or intravenous routes often leads recreational users to administer repeated doses over the course of an evening (session) in order to maintain a desired psychoactive effect.

Physical effects and complications

Because of its fast urinary excretion (within 2 h) the ability to identify ketamine in urine screens is almost impossible and thus a level of clinical suspicion is required especially if a history of its use is not forthcoming.[55] Detection by clinical examination relies on identifying mydriasis, moderate tachycardia, elevated BP, slurred speech, blunted affect, ataxia, delirium, nystagmus (less commonly than with PCP). Tachycardia is the most common finding on physical examination. Its short half-life of 17 min (see Table 4.2.3.5.3).

Admissions to hospital are most commonly for complaints related to sympathetic over activity with chest pain, palpitations and taccycardia, nausea, vomiting, difficulty breathing, ataxia, temporary paralysis/inability to speak, blurred vision, no awareness of pain as well as derealization/depersonalization, and amnesia. Other risks associated with its use include accidents, trauma, and risky sexual behaviours. Rarely more severe complications are reported including severe agitation and rhabdomyolysis. Although relatively safe in overdose, in combination with ethanol or other CNS depressants the use of ketamine can result in death.

Clinical findings and detection

(a) Psychological effects and complications

At low doses marked elevation in mood predominate. At higher doses intense psychedelic effects commence with sensory and perceptual distortion, euphoria, and out of body and floating experiences (see Table 4.2.3.5.3). The Harvard academic, Timothy Leary, described it as 'the ultimate psychedelic journey'. Users describe entering the 'K hole' where they experience—visits to god, aliens, their birth, past lives and the 'experiences of evolution'. Some users report taking issues of set and setting into careful consideration prior to using ketamine such preparation cannot be performed if the drug is consumed unwittingly when it has been marketed under the guise of another drug such as ecstasy. Being an amnestic it may become difficult to remember the total doses consumed.

Ketamine can also produce a psychotic picture that can briefly mimic schizophrenia. Both positive and negative symptoms of schizophrenia can be transiently seen in normal users and its use can exacerbate symptoms in those with pre-existing psychotic disorders. Other adverse effects can include frightening hallucinations/out of body experiences, thought disorder, confusion, and dissociation. Such episodes tend to be short-lived, resolving in a few hours or at the most a few days. In many respects these are similar to those adverse effects seen LSD, though with ketamine they come on after a shorter period following use and recede more quickly.

Management is by supportive monitoring (cardiovascular) in a quiet low stimulation room with symptomatic treatment with benzodiazepines if needed. Unusually, the effects of benzodiazepines are inconsistent varying between compounds and dose. For instance, whilst lorazepam may reduce emotional distress, it appears to have little impact upon the psychosis or perceptual changes observed. Midazolam, on the other hand, is able to negate ketamine's effect on thought process and perceptual disorder but has little impact upon mood problems. Interestingly haloperidol also has little effect upon the psychosis associated with ketamine, suggesting a role for receptors other than D2. Chlorpromazine should be avoided (anticholinergic effects).

Other consequences of use

(a) Ketamine dependence and long-term cognitive impairment

Animal studies demonstrate the ability for intravenous ketamine to produce dependence in rat models, with disruption of operant behaviour on withdrawal. Ketamine demonstrates reinforcing efficacy in animal self-administration models and is found to be a discriminative stimuli in operant tasks. Its effects are thus readily distinguishable from other drugs and may have abuse liability. However, ketamine is somewhat unusual in its pharmacodynamics, almost acting as a partial antagonist with regard to brain reward enhancements, being stimulatory at low doses, and inhibiting brain reward centres at higher doses.

Clinically ketamine dependence has been described, with compulsive use as primary symptom. Heavy habitual use has been described by Jansen (1990), and cases of dependence have also been reported among anaesthetic staff. Although tolerance develops there are only a few case reports of a withdrawal syndrome occurring.

Longer-term follow-up studies suggest that any impairment of semantic memory may be reversible upon cessation of use but persistent deficits may be seen in episodic memory and in subjective experience with one study suggesting persistence of schizotypal and perceptual changes after cessation of use.[56]

(b) New class of drugs

Tryptamine (1H-indole-3-ethanamine) is a naturally occurring metabolite of tryptophan. It forms the parent nucleus of a wide range of hallucinogenic drugs, some entirely synthetic (LSD, *N,N*-dimethyltryptamine) but many naturally occurring in plants, fungi (psilocybin—the psychoactive component of 'magic mushrooms'), and occasionally animals. It seems unlikely that many tryptamines other than LSD and psilocybin will be used unduly in dance clubs because they possess few stimulant properties, and need to be smoked or injected because most are inactive by mouth unless taken with a monoamine oxidase inhibitor.An example of the latter is the combination of *N,N*-dimethyltryptamine (the hallucinogen) and harmine (the activator) in the hallucinogenic drink ayahuasca or caapi used in rituals by South American Indians. Drugs such a *N,N*-dimethyltryptamine may have adverse effects upon both the cardiovascular system and on temperature regulation. They may induce unpleasant hallucinogenic experiences.

As described earlier the analogues MBDB, MDEA, and MDA all share similar properties with MDMA and at times have been marketed as distinct drugs. More recently 4-Bromo-2, 5-dimethoxyphenethylamine (also known as 2C-B, Nexus) a drug with similar hallucinogenic properties as psilocybin and mescaline has become available within the dance scene in Europe. Others such a 2C-T2 (2,5-dimethoxy-4-ethylthio-β-phenethylamine) suggest that new additions to an expanding street pharmacy are unlikely to become a thing of the past any time soon. Newer drugs are likely to be less easily detected by toxicologist and may have unfamiliar or atypical clinical manifestations.

Conclusion

MDMA, methamphetamine, GHB, and ketamine are all capable of producing acute adverse psychological experiences in normal users and exacerbating symptoms in those with underlying psychological disorders. They also to varying degrees pose the risk of long-term neuropsychiatric consequences. Although dependent patterns of use are not commonly seen with this group of drugs, methamphetamines certainly can result in the very rapid development of severe dependence. Most acute presentations are typically short-lived and self-limiting and are only very rarely life-threatening. The precipitation of an underlying psychiatric disorder or an exacerbation of premorbid traits may well be one of the longer term consequences of heavy use of these drugs. In those who present with acute drug-related psychological symptoms there should be an emphasis on follow-up since in some cases the symptoms will represent the onset of a persistent independent disorder which requires treatment. Users who have experienced acute psychological problems should be encouraged to make the attribution that there may be something inherent in them that makes them susceptible to experiencing the unpleasant reactions with a drug and that they are likely to remain vulnerable to those adverse experiences. This may be difficult to accept for potentially vulnerable young people who may prefer to think that the experience was not enjoyable because the drugs were not good – 'it was a bad pill'.

Further information

www.emcdda.europa.eu
www.erowid.org
www.maps.org

References

1. Winstock, A.R., Griffiths, P., and Stewart, D. (2001). Drugs and the dance music scene: a survey of current drug use patterns among a sample of dance music enthusiasts in the UK. *Drug and Alcohol Dependence*, **64**, 9–17.
2. Hansen, D., Maycock, B., and Lower, T. (2001). 'Weddings, parties, anything', a qualitative analysis of ecstasy use in Perth, Western Australia. *International Journal of Drug Policy*, **12**, 181–99.
3. Schifano, F., Corkery, J., Deluca, P., *et al.* (2006). Ecstasy (MDMA, MDA, MDEA, MBDB) consumption, seizures, related offences, prices, dosage levels and deaths in the UK (1994–2003). *Journal of Psychopharmacology*, **20**, 456–63.
4. Winstock, A.R., Wolff, K., and Ramsey, J. (2001). Ecstasy pill testing: harm minimization gone too far? *Addiction*, **96**, 1139–48.
5. Parrott, A.C. (2004). Is ecstasy MDMA? A review of the proportion of ecstasy tablets containing MDMA, their dosage levels, and the changing perceptions of purity. *Psychopharmacology*, **173**, 234–41.
6. Byard, R.W., Gilbert, J., James, R., *et al.* (1998). Amphetamine derivative fatalities in South Australia: is 'ecstasy' the culprit? *The American Journal of Forensic Medicine and Pathology*, **19**, 261–5.
7. Webb, E., Ashton, C.H., Kelly, P., *et al.* (1996). Alcohol and drug use in UK university students. *Lancet*, **348**, 922–5.
8. Condon, J. and Smith, N. (2003). *Prevalence of drug use: key findings from the 2002/2003 British Crime Survey. 229.* Home Office, London.
9. Copeland, J., Dillon, P., and Gascoigne, M. (2006). Ecstasy and the concomitant use of pharmaceuticals. *Addictive Behaviors*, **31**, 367–70.
10. Schifano, F. (2004). A bitter pill. Overview of ecstasy (MDMA, MDA) related fatalities. *Psychopharmacology*, **173**, 242–8.
11. McCann, U.D., Eligulashvili, V., and Ricaurte, G.A. (2000). (±)3,4 Methylenedioxymethamphetamine ('Ecstasy')-induced serotonin neurotoxicity in clinical studies. *Neuropsychobiology*, **42**, 11–6.
12. Topp, L., Hando, J., Dillon, P., *et al.* (1999). Ecstasy use in Australia: patterns of use and associated harm. *Drug and Alcohol Dependence*, **55**, 105–15.
13. Parrott, A.C. (2001). Human psychopharmacology of ecstasy (MDMA): a review of 15 years of empirical research. *Human Psychopharmacology*, **16**, 557–77.
14. Schifano, F., Oyefeso, A., Corkery, J., *et al.* (2003). Death rates from ecstasy (MDMA, MDA) and polydrug use in England and Wales 1996–2002. *Human Psychopharmacology Clinical Experimental*, **18**, 519–24.
15. Tancer, M. and Johanson, C.E. (2003). Reinforcing, subjective, and physiological effects of MDMA in humans: a comparison with d-amphetamine and mCPP. *Drug and Alcohol Dependence*, **72**, 33–44.
16. de la Torre, R., Farré, M., Ortuño, J., *et al.* (2000). Non-linear pharmacokinetics of MDMA ("ecstasy") in humans. *British Journal of Clinical Pharmacology*, **49**, 104–9.
17. Harris, D.S., Baggott, M., Mendelson, J.H., *et al.* (2002). Subjective and hormonal effects of 3,4-methylenedioxymethamphetamine (MDMA) in humans. *Psychopharmacology*, **162**, 396–405.
18. Hernandez-Lopez, C., Farre, M., Roset, P.N., *et al.* (2002). 3,4- Methylenedioxymethamphetamine (ecstasy) and alcohol interactions in humans: psychomotor performance, subjective effects, and pharmacokinetics. *The Journal of Pharmacology and Experimental Therapeutics*, **300**, 236–44.
19. Budisavljevic, M.N., Stewart, L., Sahn, S.A., *et al.* (2003). Hyponatremia associated with 3,4-methylenedioxymethylamphetamine ('ecstasy') abuse. *The American Journal of the Medical Sciences*, **326**, 89–93.
20. Wolff, K., Tsapakis, E.M., Winstock, A.R., *et al.* (2006). Vasopressin and oxytocin secretion in response to the consumption of ecstasy in a clubbing population. *Journal of Psychopharmacology*, **20**, 400–10.

21. Parrott, A.C. (2007). Ecstasy versus alcohol: Tolstoy and the variations of unhappiness. *Journal of Psychopharmacology*, **21**, 3–6.
22. Liechti, M.E. and Vollenweider, F.X. (2000). The serotonin uptake inhibitor citalopram reduces acute cardiovascular and vegetative effects of 3,4 methylenedioxymethamphetamine ('ecstasy') in healthy volunteers. *Journal of Psychopharmacology*, **14**, 269–74.
23. Verheyden, S.L., Henry, J.A., and Curran, H.V. (2003). Acute, sub-acute and long-term subjective consequences of 'ecstasy' (MDMA) consumption in 430 regular users. *Human Psychopharmacology Clinical Experimental*, **18**, 507–17.
24. Liester, M.B., Grob, C.S., Bravo, G.L., *et al.* (1992). Phenomenology and sequelae of 3,4-methylenedioxymethamphetamine use. *The Journal of Nervous and Mental Disease*, **180**, 345–54.
25. Nichols, D.E. (1986). Differences between the mechanism of action of MDMA, MBDB, and the classic hallucinogens. Identificationof a new therapeutic class: entactogens. *Journal of Psychoactive Drugs*, **18**, 305–13.
26. Shulgin, A.T. and Nichols, D.E. (1978). Characteristics of 3 new psychomimetics. In *The pharmacology of hallucinogens* (eds. N.C. Stillman and N.E. Willete). Pergamon Press, Oxford.
27. Parrott, C., Buchanan, T., Scholey, A.B., *et al.* (2002). Ecstasy/MDMA attributed problems reported by novice, moderate and heavy recreational users. *Human Psychopharmacology Clinical Experimental*, **17**, 309–12.
28. Curran, H.V. and Travill, R.A. (1997). Mood and cognitive effects of ±3,4-methylenedioxymethamphetamine (MDMA, 'ecstasy'): weekend 'high' followed by mid-week low. *Addiction*, **92**, 821–31.
29. Guillot, C. and Greenway, D. (2006). Recreational ecstasy use and depression. *Journal of Psychopharmacology*, **20**, 411–6.
30. Schifano, F., Di Furia, L., Forza, C., *et al.* (1998). MDMA ('ecstasy') consumption in the context of polydrug abuse: a report on 150 patients. *Drug and Alcohol Dependence*, **52**, 85–90.
31. Morgan, M.J., McFie, L., Fleetwood, H., *et al.* (2002). Ecstasy (MDMA): are the psychological problems associated with its use reversed by prolonged abstinence? *Psychopharmacology*, **159**, 294–303.
32. Verrico, C.D., Miller, G.M., and Madras, B.K. (2007). MDMA (Ecstasy) and human dopamine, norepinephrine, and serotonin transporters: implications for MDMA-induced neurotoxicity and treatment. *Psychopharmacology*, **189**, 489–503.
33. Colado, M.I, O'Shea, E., and Green, A.R. (2004). Acute and long-term effects of MDMA on cerebral dopamine biochemistry and function. *Psychopharmacology*, **173**, 249–63.
34. Cowan, R.L. (2007). Neuroimaging research in human MDMA users: a review. *Psychopharmacology*, **189**, 539–56.
35. Roiser, J.P., Cook, L.J., Cooper, J.D., *et al.* (2005). Association of a functional polymorphism in the serotonin transporter gene with abnormal emotional processing in ecstasy users. *The American Journal of Psychiatry*, **162**, 609–12.
36. Hanson, K.L. and Luciana, M. (2004). Neurocognitive function in users of MDMA: the importance of clinically significant patterns of use. *Psychological Medicine*, **34**, 229–46.
37. Gouzoulis-Mayfrank, E., Daumann, J., Tuchtenhagen, F., *et al.* (2000). Impaired cognitive performance in drug free users of recreational ecstasy (MDMA)[see comment]. *Journal of Neurology, Neurosurgery, and Psychiatry*, **68**, 719–25.
38. McCann, U.C. and Ricaurte, G.A. (1991). Lasting neuropsychiatric sequelae of (±)3,4 methylenedioxymethamphetamine ('ecstasy') in recreational users. *Journal of Clinical Psychopharmacology*, **11**, 302–5.
39. Gerra, G., Zaimovic, A., Giucastro, G., *et al.* (1998). Serotonergic function after (+/-)3,4-methylene-dioxymethamphetamine ('Ecstasy') in humans. *International Clinical Psychopharmacology*, **13**, 1–9.
40. Singer, L.T., Linares, T.J., Ntiri, S., *et al.* (2004). Psychosocial profiles of older adolescent MDMA users. *Drug and Alcohol Dependence*, **74**, 245–52.
41. Guillot, C.R. and Berman, M.E. (2007). MDMA (Ecstasy) use and psychiatric problems. *Psychopharmacology*, **189**, 575–6.
42. Kosten, T.R., Markou, A., and Koob, G.F. (1998). Depression and stimulant dependence: neurobiology and pharmacotherapy. *The Journal of Nervous and Mental Disease*, **186**, 737–45.
43. Bolding, G., Hart, G., Sherr, L., *et al.* (2006). Use of crystal methamphetamine among gay men in London. *Addiction*, **101**, 1622–30.
44. Lambert, G., Johansson, M., Agren, H., *et al.* (2000). Reduced brain norepinephrine and dopamine release in treatment-refractory depressive illness: evidence in support of the catecholamine hypothesis of mood disorders. *Archives of General Psychiatry*, **57**, 787–93.
45. Baker, A., Lee, N.K., and Jenner, L. (eds.) (2004). *Models of intervention and care for psychostimulant users* (2nd edn).
46. Shearer, J. and Gowing, L.R. (2004). Pharmacotherapies for problematic psychostimulant use: a review of current research. *Drug and Alcohol Review*, **23**, 203–11.
47. McKetin, R., McLaren, J., Lubman, D.I., *et al.* (2006). The prevalence of psychotic symptoms among methamphetamine users. *Addiction*, **101**, 1473–8.
48. Harris, D. and Batki, S.L. (2000). Stimulant psychosis: symptom profile and acute clinical course. *The American Journal on Addictions*, **9**, 28–37.
49. Rodgers, J., Ashton, C.H., Gilvarry, E., *et al.* (2004). Liquid ecstasy: a new kid on the dance floor. *The British Journal of Psychiatry*, **184**, 104–6.
50. Degenhardt, L., Darke, S., and Dillon, P. (2003). The prevalence and correlates of gamma-hydroxybutyrate (GHB) overdose among Australian users. *Addiction*, **98**, 199–204.
51. Deveaux, M., Renet, S., Renet, V., *et al.* (2002). Utilisation de l'acide gamma-hydroxybutyrique (GHB) dans les rave-parties et pour la soumission chimique en France: mythe ou realite? *Acta Clinica Belgica—Supplementum*, (1), 37–40.
52. Galloway, G.P., Frederick, S.L., and Gonzales, M. (1997). Gamma-hydroxybutyrate: an emerging drug of abuse that causes physical dependence. *Addiction*, **92**, 89–96.
53. White, P.F., Way, W.L., and Trevor, A.J. (1982). Ketamine—its pharmacology and therapeutic uses. *Anesthesiology*, **56**, 119–36.
54. Wolff, K. and Winstock, A.R. (2006). Ketamine: from medicine to misuse. *CNS Drugs*, **20**, 199–218.
55. Lim, D.K. (2003). Ketamine associated psychedelic effects and dependence. *Singapore Medical Journal*, **44**, 31–4.
56. Curran, H.V., Rees, H., Hoare, T., *et al.* (2004). Empathy and aggression: two faces of ecstasy? A study of interpretative cognitive bias and mood change in ecstasy users. *Psychopharmacology*, **173**, 425–33.

4.2.3.6 Disorders relating to the use of volatile substances

Richard Ives

Introduction

Volatile substance abuse (**VSA**)—also known as 'solvent abuse' and 'inhalant abuse'—is the deliberate inhalation of any of a range of products (see Table 4.2.3.6.1[(1)]), to achieve intoxication. Amyl (pentyl) and isobutyl nitrites ('poppers') have different patterns of misuse, and are not discussed here.[(2)]

VSA has dose-related effects similar to those of other hypnosedatives. Small doses rapidly lead to 'drunken' behaviour similar to the

Table 4.2.3.6.1 Some products which can be abused by inhalation

Product	Major volatile components
Adhesives	
Balsa wood cement	Ethyl acetate
Contact adhesives	Butanone, hexane, toluene, and esters
Cycle tyre repair cement	Toluene, and xylenes
Woodworking adhesives	Xylenes
Polyvinylchloride (PVC) cement	Acetone, butanone, cyclohexanone, trichloroethylene
Aerosols	
Air freshener	LPG, DME, and/or fluorocarbons
Deodorants, antiperspirants	LPG, DME, and/or fluorocarbons
Fly spray	LPG, DME, and/or fluorocarbons
Hair lacquer	LPG, DME, and/or fluorocarbons
Paint sprayers	LPG, DME, and/or fluorocarbons and esters
Anaesthetics/analgesics	
Inhalational	Nitrous oxide, cyclopropane Diethyl ether, halothane, enflurane, isoflurane
Topical	FC 11, FC 12, monochloroethane
Dust removers (air brushes)	DME, FC 22
Commercial dry cleaning and degreasing agents	Dichloromethane, FC 113, methanol, 1,1,1-trichloroethane, tetrachloroethylene, toluene, trichloroethylene (now rarely carbon tetrachloride, 1,2-dichloropropane)
Domestic spot removers and dry cleaners	Dichloromethane, 1,1,1-Trichloroethane, tetrachloroethylene, trichloroethylene
Fire extinguishers	Bromochlorodifluoromethane, FC 11, FC 12
Fuel gases	
Cigarette lighter refills	LPG
'Butane'	LPG
'Propane'	Propane and butanes
Nail varnish/nail varnish remover	Acetone and esters
Paints/paint thinners	Acetone, butanone, esters, hexane, toluene, trichloroethylene, xylenes
Paint stripper	Dichloromethane, methanol, toluene
'Room odorizer'	

(Reproduced from B. Flanagan and R. Ives Volatile substance abuse, *Bulletin on Narcotics*, **XLVI**, 49–78, copyright 1994, UNODC.).

effects of alcohol, and may induce delusions and hallucinations. Some heavy misusers inhale large quantities; 6 l of adhesive weekly have been reported.

Long-term effects include listlessness, anorexia, and moodiness. The hair, breath, and clothing may smell of the substance(s) used, and empty product containers (e.g. glue cans, cigarette lighter refills, and aerosol spray cans), and bags used to inhale from, may be found.

Being readily available, volatile substances are, along with alcohol and tobacco, the first intoxicating substances some children try. However, most VSA is experimental and does not lead to the use of other psychoactive substances; problematic misusers have other difficulties in their lives.(3)

History

Inhaling substances to achieve intoxication is not new. Inhaling ether and nitrous oxide ('laughing gas'), as well as commercially available volatile products, has a long history.

Public concern is more recent. In the United States during the 1950s and 1960s there was much publicity about glue sniffing; this helped to publicize the possibilities of glue as an intoxicant.(4) Only in the 1970s did public concern about VSA emerge in the United Kingdom, to reach a peak in 1983 when there were more press cuttings on the subject than on all other drugs.(5) Public anxiety has since waned, although the problem has not disappeared.

Prevalence of VSA

VSA is a worldwide problem. For an overview, see a WHO report,(6) and a National Institute on Drug Abuse (NIDA) report.(7) The European Schools survey Project on Alcohol and other Drugs (ESPAD) report provides 2003 data from 35 European countries: lifetime experience of VSA (i.e. whether *ever* tried VSA) among 15- to 16-year-olds varied from 2 per cent (in Romania) to 22 per cent (in Greenland). In the United Kingdom (and Iceland) 12 per cent reported trying VSA—nine countries had a higher prevalence. There was little difference between boys' and girls' lifetime prevalence.(8) Although young people from all socio-economic groups experiment with volatile substances, for some among the poor and the dispossessed, VSA is the drug of choice.(9) VSA is a particular problem among people living on the street. Chronic VSA is associated with poor socio-economic conditions, with delinquency and illegal drug use,(10) disrupted families, and other social and psychological problems.(11)

VSA deaths

Even for first-time experimenters, death from VSA is an ever-present risk. Death may ensue from convulsions and coma, inhalation of vomit, or direct cardiac or central nervous system toxicity. Sudden deaths of young people should be thoroughly investigated, as VSA-related deaths can be overlooked. Post-mortem examination usually reveals little, except perhaps acute lung congestion and possibly cold-induced burns to the mouth and throat. Toxicological examination of blood and tissue specimens is used to confirm a diagnosis of VSA-related death.(12)

A long-term study in the United Kingdom identified 2152 VSA-related deaths between 1971 and 2004.(13) The death rate peaked in 1990 with 152 deaths, declining since, with 47 deaths being recorded in 2004. Under-18s make up half the deaths, although the age of death is increasing. Most are male, although the overall proportion of female deaths has risen and in the first 5 years of the new millennium females comprised 22 per cent of the deaths (Table 4.2.3.6.2). Volatile-substance-related deaths occur in all social classes in the United Kingdom. However, '... in deaths of

Table 4.2.3.6.2 VSA-related deaths in the United Kingdom—selected years

Year	1983	1985	1987	1989	1990	1993	1996	1998	1999	2000	2001	2002	2003	2004
N	82	117	115	113	152	79	78	80	75	66	63	65	53	47

Reproduced from Field-Smith, M.E., Butland, B.K., Rarnsey, J.D. and Anderson, H.R. Trends in deaths associated with abuse of volatile substances 1971–2004, copyright 2006, St. George's University of London, London.

those under 16, there was a marked difference in mortality between social classes I and V, with nearly four times as many deaths occurring in social class V . . . compared with social class I'.[14]

Health issues

Health effects of volatile substances include the following:

- A sensitization of the heart—so that cardiac arrhythmias may occur if VSA is followed by exertion or fright.
- Cooling of the throat tissues—caused by spraying substances directly into the mouth, which may causing swelling and suffocation.
- A risk of fire—especially when combined with smoking; many products are inflammable.
- Suffocation—a particular danger if large plastic bags are used.
- Most products are mixtures of chemicals, and manufacturers do not list the constituents. Changing product formulations make the dangers unpredictable.
- Using alone in an isolated place presents special hazards.
- When combined with alcohol or other drugs, the effects can be unpredictable.
- Intoxication itself has potential dangers, for example, greater recklessness, doing bizarre things in response to hallucinations, becoming unconscious, and choking on vomit.

Apart from the real risk of death, VSA rarely causes long-term damage. However, some products contain poisonous substances, such as lead in some petrol or *n*-hexane in some glues. Chronic abuse of toluene-containing products and of chlorinated solvents such as 1,1,1-trichloroethane sometimes causes damage to the liver and kidneys. Damage to the lungs, bone marrow, and nervous system is also known, but is uncommon and generally reversible. Some people are more vulnerable (genetically or otherwise) than others to certain harmful effects. However, the long-term effects of sniffing have not been thoroughly studied, and virtually all reports of chronic toxicity are case studies, so the actual morbidity from VSA is not known.

A review article looking at the possibility of cognitive impairments concluded that: 'the possibility that permanent structural brain damage, with accompanying psychiatric manifestations, results from solvent abuse remains inconclusive'.[15]

Users develop tolerance. Although no dependence syndrome exists, a few young people develop a more compulsive and long-term habit. The UK Advisory Council on the Misuse of Drugs suggested that: 'There are . . . pharmacological reasons for suspecting that persistent exposure to volatile substances might be able to induce a dependence of the so-called depressant type'.[16]

Many volatile substance misusers are also users of other drugs, both legal and illegal. Poly-drug use may potentiate the effects of individual drugs and make it difficult to assess the risks of individual substances.[17]

VSA during pregnancy is associated with increased maternal and foetal morbidity.[18] Paternal exposure to volatile substances may also have deleterious effects on their offspring.[19] But the complexities of the chemicals involved—and the complexities of people's lives—make it difficult to identify specific causes of foetal damage difficult.

Treatment of VSA-related disorders

Emergency treatment

The immediate treatment of an intoxicated person needs a calm and firm approach. The product being misused should be removed; although not if this would lead to conflict—exertion or high emotion may raise adrenaline to dangerous levels for an over-sensitized heart. Therefore, an intoxicated person should be kept calm and never chased. It is unlikely that it will be possible to have a serious conversation with an intoxicated misuser, but calming and reassuring talk may help. After 5 to 20 min without inhalation the abuser will sober up (unless alcohol or other drugs have also been used). Subsequently, medical help might be needed; a check-up may identify particular health problems.

Cessation

No special regime is necessary when stopping misusing volatile substances. Although, being lipid-soluble, the chemicals may be detectable in the body tissues for some weeks after cessation of use, they do not have any psychoactive effect. There is no clearly defined withdrawal syndrome and special detoxification regimes are unnecessary, but rest, sleep, and good food may aid recovery.

Dealing with experimental misuse

Most teenagers never even try misusing volatile substances; those who do, do so only a few times, and even those who do so more frequently do not continue for long. Experimental or the occasional misuse of volatile substances occurs mainly from curiosity or as part of peer group activity. Appropriate intervention may simply involve a warning of the dangers, plus increased supervision. Specialist treatment is not required, and may be counterproductive, entrenching an otherwise transient activity.

Dealing with dependent misuse

Biology may predispose to dependent use, but chronic VSA is connected with other problems. As group of United Kingdom professionals put it:[20]

> Persistent misuse of volatile substances is a complex behaviour . . . frequently associated with low self-esteem, family problems, isolation and psychological difficulties. These are factors that may also be associated with the problematic use of legal and illegal drugs, and indeed,

a large proportion of people who misuse volatile substances also misuse other drugs. Chronic VSA is thus intertwined with social and psychological problems and with the misuse of illegal drugs. Therefore, counselling services for young people should not be narrowly focused on volatile substances, but should be able to deal with VSA in the context of a range of problematic behaviours.

Often, these other problems need attention first, and until these are dealt with, the misuser—even while recognizing the harm—may not give up. Consequently, generic services, which can deal more effectively with these broader problems, should lead on care, supported where necessary by specialist agencies. Mental health services, as well as drugs' services, have an important role in giving this support, for example, in the treatment of psychiatric comorbidity (dual diagnosis). Specialist services can also help to identify areas for intervention; implementation should take account of social and cultural patterns of the misuser's life. Female volatile substance misusers may not readily present for treatment and can suffer additional stigmatization. Services for young people need to be specifically designed for their needs and cognizant of issues such as confidentiality and consent. Families who struggle unaided with problematic VSA by a young family member may also need help.

The Modified Social Stress Model, developed by the WHO Street Children Project, gives a framework for understanding substance use.[21] Potential for change can be assessed using Prochaska and DiClemente's 'revolving door' model of stages of change.[22] Jumper-Thurman and colleagues point out that the treatment of volatile substance misusers:[23]

> has presented a particularly difficult challenge . . . given the general lack of direction for effective treatment strategies. In addition to the physiological, neurological, and emotional challenges abusers face . . . [they] bring with them a multitude of other problems—academic, legal, social, and family issues.

Some groups (such as people living on the street, and indigenous peoples) have special problems with substance use that require different, more holistic, attention. Treatment should work 'with the grain' of the culture, rather than imposing inappropriate 'alien' treatment models. Indigenous peoples are beginning to insist that their cultures have useful perspectives and approaches that can be utilized in the treatment of people with drug and volatile substance problems.[24]

Follow-up

After-care, long-term rehabilitation, social reinsertion, relapse management, and follow-up of discharged patients are important aspects of the treatment process.

Relapse, which is common, should be treated non-judgementally; not as 'failure' but as an opportunity for learning. Support in maintaining improvements may be helpful; for example, events for ex-users of volatile substances to help them to maintain abstinence and to utilize group support.

Harm minimization

Because of the unpredictable dangers of VSA, harm minimization advice should not be routinely given. However, very entrenched misusers may benefit from careful individual guidance on minimizing the risks, such as avoiding spraying gases directly into the mouth.

Wider aspects

Chronic VSA is not an individual problem: it arises not only from individual pathology, but also from failures in social structures. Treatment, in the broadest sense, needs to help the healing of the family, the community, and to assist in making changes in society.

Measuring outcomes

Evaluation and monitoring need careful thought and planning. But treatment interventions have multiple aims and varied outcomes. Aims may alter and be adapted as the work develops, so that outcomes will be difficult to assess in relation to the original aims. Evaluation should handle this complexity: identifying 'success' requires measures beyond the simple calculation of reduction in, or abstention from, substance use.

Building evaluation in from the start, and using it to inform the intervention throughout, makes it part of the process of intervention; the reflection that monitoring and evaluation encourages can increase the effectiveness of the intervention.

Prevention

There are many different sniffable products, many possibilities for substitution of one product for another, many different chemicals involved, and insufficient information about the relative harm of various products and practices. Volatile substance misusers are generally young, and VSA-related deaths are sudden and unpredictable. All these factors make prevention difficult.

Tackling the supply of products

This can be approached in several ways:

- Product elimination—while it is not possible to eliminate all volatile substances, some products are particularly dangerous, and have satisfactory substitutes.
- Product modification—there are three possibilities (a review paper gives more details:[25])
  - changing the formulation of the product to remove the intoxicating substance. There has been great success in Australian indigenous communities through substituting petrol with unsniffable 'Opal', an unleaded fuel with low levels of aromatics[26,27]
  - adding a chemical to make the product unpalatable (experiments with the bittering agent, *Bitrex*, have been inconclusive)
  - and modifying the container to make misuse difficult.
- Warning labels—these may be helpful, although labelling draws attention to the potential for misuse. Many sniffable products in the United Kingdom carry the 'SACKI' warning, 'Solvent Abuse Can Kill Instantly'.[28]
- Education for suppliers—retailers need information and advice about a product's potential for misuse. This is difficult, as the various products are sold through many retail outlets.
- Legal controls on the sale and supply of misusable products—these exist in many countries but are difficult to enforce.

Tackling the demand for products

- Legal controls—in Japan, Singapore, and the Republic of Korea, VSA is an offence. However, this is not so in most countries because the criminalization of misusers of volatile substances is considered counterproductive.
- Information and education—this can be provided through public advertising, leaflets, helplines, in schools and informal education. Early education about volatile substances is essential; these products are in most people's homes and therefore (unlike illegal drugs) they can be accessed by very young children. Because many parents are unaware of the misuse potential of household products, information should also be targeted at parents.

All these strategies should be considered; as the Advisory Council on the Misuse of Drugs pointed out, 'good practice' will constitute a layered series of alternative or multiple strategies rather than any one master stroke.[29]

Further information

Advisory Council on the Misuse of Drugs. (1995). *Volatile substance abuse*. HMSO, London.

Skellington Orr, K. and Shewan, D. (2006). *Review of evidence relating to volatile substance abuse in Scotland*. Scottish Executive Substance Misuse Research Programme, Edinburgh (www.scotland.gov.uk/Resource/Doc/147377/0038818.pdf accessed 22-03-07).

The UK Government's. (2005). Strategy for tackling volatile substance (*Out of sight—Not out of mind. Children, young people and volatile substance abuse (VSA) A framework for VSA*) can be downloaded from http://www.dh.gov.uk/assetRoot/04/11/56/05/04115605.pdf.) (accessed 22-03-07).

Flanagan, R.J., Streete, P.J., and Ramsey, J.D. (1997). *Volatile substance abuse: practical guidelines for the analytical investigation of suspected cases and interpretation of results*. United Nations Drug Control Programme, Vienna.

Field-Smith, M.E., Butland, B.K., Ramsey, J.D., *et al.* (2006). *Trends in deaths associated with abuse of volatile substances 1971–2004*. St George's, University of London, London.

Ron, M. (1986). Volatile substance abuse: a review of possible long-term neurological, intellectual and psychiatric sequelae. *The British Journal of Psychiatry*, **148**, 235–46.

Reading list from the UK's DrugScope www.drugscope.org.uk/wip/7/PDFS/Inhalants%20and%20solvents.pdf (accessed 22-03-07).

Information on UK VSA-related deaths: www.vsareport.org

USA National Inhalants Prevention Coalition: www.inhalants.org

References

1. Flanagan, B. and Ives, R. (1994). Volatile substance abuse. *Bulletin on Narcotics*, **46**, 49–78.
2. Haverkos, H. and Dougherty, J. (eds.) (1988). *Health hazards of nitrite inhalants, NIDA Research Monograph 83*. National Institute on Drug Abuse, Rockville, MD.
3. Davies, B., Thorley, A., and O'Connor, D. (1985). Progression of addiction careers in young adult solvent misusers. *British Medical Journal*, **290**, 6482.
4. Brecher, E. (1972). How to launch a nation-wide drug menace. In *Licit and illicit drugs*, (eds. E.M. Brecher and the Editors of Consumer Report Magazine) pp. 321–34. Little, Brown, Boston, MA.
5. Ives, R. (1986). The rise and fall of the solvents panic. *Druglink*, **1**, 10–12.
6. WHO Programme on Substance Abuse. (1999). *Volatile substance abuse: a global overview*. WHO, Geneva.
7. Kozel, N., Sloboda, Z., and De La Rosa, M. (eds.) (1995). *Epidemiology of inhalant abuse: an international perspective (NIDA Research Monograph series No. 148)*. NIDA, Washington, DC.
8. Ives, R. (2006). Volatile Substance Abuse: a review of findings in ESPAD 2003. *Drugs: Education, Prevention and Policy*, **13**, 441–9.
9. Beauvais, F., Wayman, J. C., Jumper-Thurman, P., *et al.* (2004). Inhalant abuse among American Indian, Mexican American, and non-Latino white adolescents. *The American Journal of Drug and Alcohol Abuse*, **28**, 2171–87.
10. NSDUH. (2005). *Inhalant use and delinquent behaviors among young adolescents* (USA 'National Survey on Drug User and Health') (http://oas.samhsa.gov/2k5/inhale/inhale.htm (accessed 22-03-2007)).
11. Ives, R. (1999). *Volatile substance abuse: a report on survey evidence*. Health Education Authority, London.
12. Flanagan, R.J., Streete, P.J., and Ramsey, J.D. (1997). *Volatile substance abuse: practical guidelines for the analytical investigation of suspected cases and interpretation of results*. United Nations Drug Control Programme, Vienna.
13. Field-Smith, M.E., Butland, B.K., Ramsey, J.D., *et al.* (2006). *Trends in deaths associated with abuse of volatile substances 1971–2004*. St George's, University of London, London.
14. Esmail, A., Meyer, L., Pottier, A., *et al.* (1993). Deaths from volatile substance abuse in those under 18 years: results from a national epidemiological study. *Archives of Disease in Childhood*, **69**, 356–60 (see p. 358).
15. Ron, M. (1986). Volatile substance abuse: a review of possible long-term neurological, intellectual and psychiatric sequelae. *The British Journal of Psychiatry*, **148**, 235–46.
16. Advisory Council on the Misuse of Drugs. (1995). *Volatile substance abuse*, paragraph 3.11. HMSO, London.
17. Ives, R. and Ghelani, P. (2006). Polydrug use (the use of drugs in combination): a brief review. *Drugs: Education, Prevention and Policy*, **13**, 225–32.
18. Wilkin, H. and Gabow, P. (1991). Toluene abuse during pregnancy: obstetric complications and perinatal outcomes. *Obstetrics and Gynaecology*, **77**, 504–8.
19. Robaire, B. and Hales, B. (1993). Paternal exposure to chemicals before conception (editorial). *British Medical Journal*, **307**, 341–2.
20. Network VSA. (1997). *Network VSA statement about volatile substance misuse*. Network VSA, Blackburn, Lancs.
21. WHO Programme on Substance Abuse. (1997). *Street children, substance use and health: training for street educators*, p. 48. WHO, Geneva.
22. Prochaska, J. and DiClemente, C. (1986). Towards a comprehensive model of change. In *Treating addictive behaviours: processes of change* (eds. W. Miller and N. Heather), pp. 3–27. Plenum Press, New York.
23. Jumper-Thurman, P., Plested, B., and Beauvais, F. (1992). Treatment strategies for volatile substance abusers in the United States. In *Inhalant abuse: a volatile research agenda* (eds. C. Sharpe, F. Beauvais, and R. Spence), NIDA Research Monograph 129. National Institute on Drug Abuse, Rockville, MD.
24. Brady, M. (1992). *Heavy metal. The social meaning of petrol sniffing in Australia*. Aboriginal Studies Press, Canberra.
25. MacLean, S. and d'Abbs, P. (2006). Will modifying inhalants reduce volatile substance misuse? A review. *Drugs: Education, Prevention and Policy*, **13**, 423–39.
26. Shaw, G., Biven A., Gray, D., *et al.* (2004). *An evaluation of the Comgas scheme*. Australian Government Department of Health and Human Ageing, Canberra, ACT.
27. www.health.gov.au/petrolsniffingprevention (accessed 22-03-07).
28. www.bama.co.uk/educ_3.html (accessed 22-03-07).
29. Advisory Council on the Misuse of Drugs. (1995). *Volatile substance abuse*, paragraph 5.5. HMSO, London.

4.2.3.7 **The mental health effects of cannabis use**

Wayne Hall

Cannabis the drug

Cannabis products are derived from the female plant of *Cannabis sativa* and contain the psychoactive constituent delta-9-tetrahydrocannabinol (**THC**).[1] Marijuana (THC content typically 0.5–5 per cent) is prepared from the dried flowering tops and leaves of the plant. Hashish (THC content typically 2–20 per cent) consists of dried cannabis resin and compressed flowers.[1]

Cannabis is usually smoked in a 'joint', like a tobacco cigarette, or in a water pipe, often mixed with tobacco. Although marijuana and hashish may be eaten, cannabis is usually smoked because this is the most efficient way to achieve the desired effects.[2]

THC acts on a widely distributed, specific receptor in brain regions that are involved in cognition, memory, reward, pain perception, and motor coordination.[1] These receptors respond to an endogenous ligand, anandamide, which is considerably less potent and has a shorter duration of action than THC.[1]

Patterns of cannabis use

Cannabis has been tried by many young adults in Europe, the United States, and Australia.[3] Most cannabis users in these countries start in their mid to late teens and stop in their middle to late 20s.[3,4] In the United States and Australia, about 10 per cent of those who ever use cannabis become daily users, and another 20 to 30 per cent use weekly.[3] This pattern of use differs from that found in traditional cannabis-using countries, such as Egypt and India, where recreational cannabis use is uncommon and heavy cannabis use is confined to small, marginalized groups.[3]

'Heavy' cannabis use is usually defined as daily or near-daily use.[5] This pattern of use places users at the greatest risk of experiencing adverse psychological and physical consequences.[2,3] Daily cannabis users are also more likely to be regular users of alcohol and tobacco and to use amphetamines, hallucinogens, psychostimulants, sedatives, and opioids.[2,3]

Acute psychological effects of cannabis use

Cannabis produces euphoria and relaxation, perceptual alterations, impaired short-term memory and attention, and intensification of ordinary sensory experiences.[2] The most common unpleasant psychological effects are anxiety and panic reactions,[2] that are most often reported by naive users and are a common reason for discontinuing use.[2] Cannabis produces dose-related impairments in cognitive and behavioural functions that may impair ability to drive an automobile.[6]

Chronic psychological effects of cannabis use

Cannabis dependence

Animals and humans develop tolerance to the effects of THC,[1] and some heavy users experience withdrawal symptoms on the abrupt cessation of cannabis use.[7] During the 1990s there was an increase in the number of persons in the United States, Australia, and Europe seeking help to stop their cannabis use.[3]

A cannabis-dependence syndrome occurs in heavy chronic users of cannabis who report problems in controlling their cannabis use, but who continue despite experiencing adverse personal and social consequences.[8] The lifetime prevalence of cannabis abuse and dependence (as defined in DSM-IIIR) in the United States has been estimated at 4.4 per cent of adults.[9] Around 10 per cent of those who ever use cannabis will meet criteria for dependence at some point in their lives.[2,9]

It is not clear how cannabis dependence is best managed. Roffman and Stephens,[10] in summarizing the results of controlled trials of cognitive behavioural, relapse prevention and other psychological approaches to treatment, report low rates of abstinence at 12 months but substantial reductions in cannabis use and problems among those who continue to use cannabis.

Cannabis psychosis

High doses of THC have been reported to produce visual and auditory hallucinations, delusional ideas, and thought disorder in normal volunteers.[2] In traditional cannabis-using cultures, such as India, a 'cannabis psychosis' has been reported in which the symptoms are preceded by heavy cannabis use and remit after abstinence[11] but the existence of a 'cannabis psychosis' in Western cultures is still a matter for debate.[11]

Cannabis and schizophrenia

Cannabis use and schizophrenia are associated[12,13] and there is consistent evidence from a series of prospective studies in a number of different countries suggesting that cannabis use can precipitate schizophrenia in persons who are vulnerable because of a personal or family history of this disorder,[12,13] and possibly a genetic vulnerability.[14] This hypothesis is consistent with the stress-diathesis model of schizophrenia[15] and it is also biologically plausible because psychotic disorders involve disturbances in the dopamine neurotransmitter systems and cannabinoids, such as THC, increase dopamine release.[1]

Individuals with psychotic symptoms who use cannabis should be encouraged to stop or, at the very least, to reduce their frequency of use. The major challenge is in finding ways to persuade individuals with psychoses to stop doing something they enjoy and to help those who want to stop using cannabis but find it difficult to do so. Psychological interventions for cannabis dependence in individuals without psychoses produce modest rates of abstinence and many individuals with schizophrenia lack social support, may be cognitively impaired, are often unemployed, and may not comply with treatment. A recent Cochrane review[16] found no clear evidence that supported any type of substance abuse treatment in schizophrenia over standard care. The development of more effective pharmacologic and psychological methods of treatment for cannabis dependence in persons with psychoses is a research priority.

Other disorders

Cognitive impairment

Cannabis use acutely impairs cognitive functioning but long-term heavy use of cannabis does not appear to produce severe or grossly debilitating impairment of cognitive function that is comparable to the impairments found in chronic heavy alcohol drinkers.[17] There is evidence that the long-term use of cannabis produces more subtle cognitive impairment in the higher cognitive functions of memory, attention and organization, and the integration of complex information.[16] This evidence suggests that, longer the period of heavy cannabis use, the more pronounced is the cognitive impairment.[17] But it remains to be decided whether these cognitive impairments antedate cannabis use, reflect poorer learning in non-academically oriented young people, or reflect neurotoxic effects of cannabis use that can be reversed after an extended period of abstinence.[18]

An 'amotivational syndrome'

Anecdotal reports that chronic heavy cannabis use impairs motivation and social performance have been described in societies with a long history of cannabis use, such as Egypt, the Caribbean, and elsewhere.[2] A similar pattern of behaviour among young Americans who were heavy cannabis users in the early 1970s was described as an 'amotivational syndrome'.[19] Field studies of chronic heavy cannabis users in societies with a tradition of such use, for example Costa Rica and Jamaica,[2] have produced evidence that has usually been interpreted as failing to demonstrate the existence of the amotivational syndrome. Critics have argued that these studies are unconvincing because the chronic users studied have come from socially marginal groups, so that the cognitive and motivational demands of their everyday lives were insufficient to detect any impairment caused by chronic cannabis use.[2]

The status of the amotivational syndrome remains contentious. Many clinicians find the cases of 'amotivational syndrome' compelling, while many researchers are more impressed by the largely negative findings of the field and epidemiological studies. Regular cannabis users can experience a loss of ambition and impaired school and occupational performance[2] and former cannabis users report that impaired occupational performance was their reason for stopping.[2] It may be more parsimonious to explain impaired motivation as a symptom of chronic cannabis intoxication and dependence than to invent a new syndrome.[2,3]

Flashbacks

There are case reports of users experiencing cannabis 'flashbacks', i.e. symptoms of cannabis intoxication days or weeks after the individual last used cannabis.[20] Because of their rarity, and the fact that many affected individuals have also used other drugs, it is difficult to decide whether these are rare events that are coincidental with cannabis use, the effects of other drugs that are often taken together with cannabis, rare consequences of cannabis use that only occur at much higher than usual doses, experiences that require unusual forms of personal vulnerability, or the results of interactions between cannabis and other drugs.[2]

Behavioural effects in adolescence

There has been understandable societal concern about the effects of rising rates of cannabis use among adolescents on their school performance, mental health and adjustment, and their use of other more hazardous illicit drugs.[3,21]

There is a strong cross-sectional association between heavy cannabis use in adolescence and the risk of discontinuing a high-school education and experiencing job instability in young adulthood.[20,22] However, in longitudinal studies the strength of this association is reduced but not eliminated when statistical adjustments are made for the fact that heavy cannabis users have lower academic aspirations and poorer high-school performance prior to using cannabis than their peers.[22]

There is some evidence that heavy cannabis use has adverse effects upon family formation, mental health, and involvement in drug-related crime.[3] In each case, the strong associations in cross-sectional studies are more modest in longitudinal studies after statistically controlling for associations between cannabis use and other pre-existing characteristics which independently predict these adverse outcomes.[22] It remains uncertain to what degree these modest relationships represent residual confounding[22] or real relationships.

A consistent finding in the United States[23] has been the regular sequence of initiation into drug use, in which cannabis use has typically preceded involvement with 'harder' illicit drugs such as stimulants and opioids. The interpretation of this sequence of events remains controversial.[24] There is support for two hypotheses: (i) there is a selective recruitment into cannabis use of non-conforming adolescents who have a propensity to use a variety of other illicit drugs and (ii) once recruited to cannabis use, it is the social interaction with drug-using peers and greater access to illicit drug markets that increases the likelihood of using other illicit drugs.[23]

A major public health challenge will be finding effective ways of explaining the mental health risks of cannabis use to young people. In addition to a possible increased risk of psychosis, young people also need to be informed about the risks of developing dependence on cannabis, impairing their educational attainment, and possibly increasing their risk of depression.[21]

School-based drug education programmes produce small, statistically significant reductions in cannabis use but their primary effect is on knowledge rather than behaviour change and most reductions in use occur among less frequent users rather than the heavier users who are at greater risk of adverse mental health effects.[25,26]

Summary

The major adverse acute psychological effects of cannabis use are as follows:

- Anxiety, dysphoria, panic, and paranoia, especially in naive users
- Impairment of attention, memory, and psychomotor performance while intoxicated
- An increased risk of accident if an intoxicated person attempts to drive a vehicle.

The major psychological effects of daily heavy cannabis use over many years remain contested but probably include the following:[3]

- A cannabis-dependence syndrome
- Subtle forms of cognitive impairment that affect attention and memory and which persist while the user remains chronically intoxicated
- Impaired educational achievement in adolescents with a history of poor school performance, whose achievement may be limited

by the cognitive impairments produced by chronic intoxication with cannabis

- Among those who initiate cannabis use in the early teens, a higher risk of progressing to heavy cannabis and other illicit drug use, and becoming dependent on cannabis.

Further information

Some useful books

Castle, D.J. and Murray, R.M. (2004). *Marijuana and madness*. Cambridge University Press, Cambridge.

Hall, W.D. and Pacula, R.L. (2003). *Cannabis use and dependence: public health and public policy*. Cambridge University Press, Cambridge.

Iversen, L. (2000). *The science of marijuana*. Oxford University Press, Oxford.

Kandel, D.B. (2002). *Stages and pathways of drug involvement: examining the gateway hypothesis*. Cambridge University Press, New York.

Roffman, R.A. and Stephens, R.S. (2006). *Cannabis dependence: its nature, consequences and treatment*. Cambridge University Press, Cambridge.

Solowij, N. (1998). *Cannabis and cognitive functioning*. Cambridge University Press, Cambridge.

Some useful websites

Commonwealth of Australia Department of Health and Ageing. http://www.health.gov.au/internet/wcms/publishing.nsf/Content/health-pubhlth-publicat-mono.htm (A monograph reviewing the health effects of cannabis that is periodically updated)

European Monitoring Centre for Drugs and Drug Addiction. http://www.emcdda.europa.eu/ (Regularly reports data on patterns of cannabis use and cannabis related harm in Europe including treatment seeking)

National Drug and Alcohol Research Centre (Australia). http://ndarc.med.unsw.edu.au/ (This site includes research and resources on the health effects of cannabis and the treatment of cannabis dependence)

National Institute on Drug Abuse (USA). http://www.nida.nih.gov/ (Provides regular research updates on the effects of cannabis and the treatment of cannabis dependence)

Substance Abuse and Mental Health Services Administration (USA). http://www.samhsa.gov/(Provides regular updates of USA survey data on patterns of cannabis use)

Trimbos-Instituut/Netherlands Institute of Mental health and Addiction. http://www.trimbos.nl/ (A useful source for research on cannabis use and dependence in the Netherlands)

United Nations Office on Drugs and Crime (Vienna). World drug report. http://www.unodc.org/pdf/WDR_2006/wdr2006_volume1.pdf. (A very useful overview of global trends in cannabis use and the global cannabis market)

World Health Organization. http://www.who.int/substance_abuse/publications/psychoactives/en/index.html (This contains authoritative reviews of the health effects of cannabis that are periodically updated)

References

1. Adams, I.B. and Martin, B.R. (1996). Cannabis: pharmacology and toxicology in animals and humans. *Addiction*, **91**, 1585–614.
2. Hall, W.D., Degenhardt, L., and Lynskey. M.T. (2001). *The health and psychological effects of cannabis use*. Commonwealth Department of Health and Aged Care, Canberra.
3. Hall, W.D. and Pacula, R.L. (2003). *Cannabis use and dependence: public health and public policy*. Cambridge University Press, Cambridge.
4. Chen, K. and Kandel, D.B. (1995). The natural history of drug use from adolescence to the mid-thirties in a general population sample. *American Journal of Public Health*, **85**, 41–7.
5. Kandel, D.B. and Davies, M. (1992). Progression to regular marijuana involvement: phenomenology and risk factors for near-daily use. In *Vulnerability to drug abuse* (ed. M.D. Glantz), pp. 211–53. American Psychological Association, Washington, DC.
6. Ramaekers, J.G., Berghaus, G., van Laar, M., *et al.* (2004). Dose related risk of motor vehicle crashes after cannabis use. *Drug and Alcohol Dependence*, **73**, 109–19.
7. Lichtman, A.H. and Martin, B.R. (2006). Understanding the pharmacology and physiology of cannabis dependence. In *Cannabis dependence: its nature, consequences and treatment* (eds. R.A. Roffman and R.S. Stephens), pp. 37–57. Cambridge University Press, Cambridge, New York.
8. Babor, T. (2006). The diagnosis of cannabis dependence. In *Cannabis dependence: its nature, consequences and treatment* (eds. R.A. Roffman and R.S. Stephens), pp. 21–36. Cambridge University Press, Cambridge, New York.
9. Anthony, J.C., Warner, L., and Kessler, R. (1994). Comparative epidemiology of dependence on tobacco, alcohol, controlled substances and inhalants: basic findings from the National Comorbidity Survey. *Experimental and Clinical Psychopharmacology*, **2**, 244–68.
10. Roffman, R.A. and Stephens, R.S. (2006). *Cannabis dependence: its nature, consequences and treatment*. Cambridge University Press, Cambridge, New York.
11. Hall, W.D. and Degenhardt, L. (2004). Is there a specific cannabis psychosis? In *Marijuana and madness* (eds. D.J. Castle and R.M. Murray), pp. 89–100. Cambridge University Press, Cambridge.
12. Hall, W.D. and Degenhardt, L. (2006). What are the policy implications of the evidence on cannabis and psychosis? *Canadian Journal of Psychiatry. La Revue Canadienne de Psychiatrie*, **51**, 15–23.
13. Arseneault, L., Cannon, M., Witton, J., *et al.* (2004). Causal association between cannabis and psychosis: examination of the evidence. *The British Journal of Psychiatry*, **184**, 110–7.
14. Caspi, A., Moffitt, T.E., Cannon, M., *et al.* (2005). Moderation of the effect of adolescent-onset cannabis use on adult psychosis by a functional polymorphism in the catechol-*O*-methyltransferase gene: longitudinal evidence of a gene X environment interaction. *Biological Psychiatry*, **57**, 1117–27.
15. Gottesman, I.I. (1991). *Schizophrenia genesis: the origins of madness*. W.H. Freeman, New York.
16. Jeffery, D.P., Ley, A., and McLaren, S.N.S. (2004). Psychosocial treatment programmes for people with both severe mental illness and substance misuse. *The Cochrane Database of Systematic Reviews*, 2000, CD001088.
17. Solowij, N. (1998). *Cannabis and cognitive functioning*. Cambridge University Press, Cambridge.
18. Pope, H.G. Jr, Gruber, A.J., Hudson. J.I., *et al.* (2003). Early-onset cannabis use and cognitive deficits: what is the nature of the association? *Drug and Alcohol Dependence*, **69**, 303–10.
19. Cohen, S. (1982). Cannabis effects upon adolescent motivation. *Marijuana and youth: clinical observations on motivation and learning*. National Institute on Drug Abuse, Rockville, MD.
20. Edwards, G. (1983). Psychopathology of a drug experience. *The British Journal of Psychiatry*, **143**, 139–42.
21. Hall, W.D. (2006). Cannabis use and the mental health of young people. *Australian and New Zealand Journal of Psychiatry*, **40**, 105–13.
22. Macleod, J., Oakes, R., Copello, A., *et al.* (2004). Psychological and social sequelae of cannabis and other illicit drug use by young people: a systematic review of longitudinal, general population studies. *Lancet*, **363**, 1579–88.
23. Kandel, D.B. (2002). *Stages and pathways of drug involvement: examining the gateway hypothesis*. Cambridge University Press, New York.

24. Hall, W.D. and Lynskey, M. (2005). Is cannabis a gateway drug? Testing hypotheses about the relationship between cannabis use and the use of other illicit drugs. *Drug and Alcohol Review*, **24**, 39–48.
25. White, D. and Pitts, M. (1998). Educating young people about drugs: a systematic review. *Addiction*, **93**, 1475–87.
26. Tobler, N.S., Lessard, T., Marshall, D., *et al.* (1999). Effectiveness of school-based drug prevention programs for marijuana use. *School Psychology International*, **20**, 105–37

4.2.3.8 Nicotine dependence and treatment

Mª Inés López-Ibor

Introduction

Tobacco use is the single most important preventable health risk in the developed world, and an important cause of premature death worldwide.[(1)] Smoking causes a wide range of diseases, including many types of cancer, chronic obstructive pulmonary disease, coronary heart disease, stroke, peripheral vascular disease, and peptic ulcer disease.[(2)] According to the World Health Organization (WHO) smoking prevalence is estimated at around 28.6 per cent (40 per cent among males and 18.2 per cent among females),[(3)] it is therefore the most prevalent form of drug dependence in the world.

Tobacco causes around 13 500 deaths per day, currently, approximately 5 million people are killed annually by tobacco use. In the last few years the standardized death rate for lung cancer among men across the European region has fallen but it has increased in women.[(3)] By 2030, estimates based on current trends indicate that this number will increase to 10 million, with 70 per cent of deaths occurring in low- and middle-income countries.[(4)]

Tobacco remains the leading contributor to the disease burden in the majority of the developed countries. According to the WHO tobacco-related health care costs between 1 per cent and 1.1 per cent of Gross Domestic Product (GDP) in many countries.[(5,6)]

Despite the considerable efforts made to fight smoking in the last few decades, there are still substantial number of people who, in full knowledge of the health hazards, begin smoking or continue smoking. Since 2002 many countries have implemented smoke-free policies, strengthening product regulation, restrictions on smoking in public places and in work places, which for the first time are extended to bars and restaurants.[(7)]

Traditionally, experimentation with and the initiation of the smoking habit were related to issues such as rebellious adolescent behaviour, a need to affirm maturity, challenging authority, imitating idols, peer group pressure (from friends or relatives who are smokers) and associating smoking with being successful from a professional, financial, or sexual point of view. More recently, other perspectives, such as the specific personality pattern typified by the search for challenges (sensation seeking behaviour) and the characteristics of neuropsychological development, also began to be considered.[(8)]An other important issue is that smokers are much more likely than non-smokers to use or even to abuse other psychoactive drugs. Over 90 per cent of alcoholic persons smoke, drink more coffee, or take other drugs like cannabis, cocaine, or amphetamines. The reasons that smokers have such difficulty in ceasing smoking are probably similar to those of organic dependence.[(9–11)]

Cigarette smoking and nicotine dependence

Approximately one-third of those individuals who experiment with cigarettes become regular smokers.[(12)] Once dependence develops, tobacco addiction can become a chronic relapsing disorder with direct and serious medical consequences.[(13)]

Nicotine dependence explains why approximately 70 per cent of smokers who want to quit smoking do not succeed. Of these, approximately one-third succeed for only 1 day and less than 10 per cent remain abstinent for 12 months.[(13)] The definitive cessation of smoking generally occurs only after various attempts, and the relapse rate is very high, 88 per cent.[(14)] The percentage of smokers in which relapse occurs is similar in almost all social classes, even when including individuals, such as health care professionals, who are more informed about tobacco-related diseases.

On the other hand, only a portion of smokers develop such dependence. Why is it that not all smokers follow the same course? This question about smoking relates to the wider one of why only some people exposed to drugs become addicted to them.[(15)]

Why is nicotine so addictive?

The psychoactive component of tobacco is nicotine, which has its central nervous system effects by acting as agonist at the nicotine subtype of acetylcholine receptors. About 25 per cent of the nicotine inhaled when smoking a cigarette reaches the blood, and reaches the brain in about 15 s. The half-life of nicotine is about 2 h.[(13)]

Nicotine is believed to have positive reinforcing and addictive properties because it activates the dopaminergic pathway projecting from the ventral tegmental area to the cerebral cortex and the limbic system, the system that is affected by cocaine and amphetamine. In addition to activating the reward system, nicotine causes an increase in the concentrations of circulating norepinephrine and epinephrine, and increased release of vasopressin, β-endorphin, adrenocorticothropine, and cortisol.[(16)]

The development of dependence is enhanced by strong social factors that encourage smoking in some settings.[(17)]

Other central effects

The stimulatory effects of nicotine result in improved attention, learning, reaction time, and problem-solving ability. Nicotine also decreases psychological tension and lessens depressive feelings.

The effects of nicotine in the cerebral blood flow (CBF) have been studied and results suggest that short-term nicotine exposure increases the CBF without changing cerebral oxygen metabolism but that long-term nicotine exposure is associated with decrease in the CBF.[(18)]

Genetic issues

Epidemiological studies have shown that the genetic component can play a significant role in the smoking habit, being responsible for 40 per cent to 60 per cent of the variability in the risk of addiction.[(19,20)] The first studies relating genetics to smoking date from 1958[(21)] when it was suggested that there were genes that, in youth, predispose individuals to become smokers and, later, to present with lung cancer.[21]

Many twin concordance studies have indicated that genetic inheritance plays a role in smoking addiction.[22] Such studies have demonstrated a higher concordance rate in relation to smoking among monozygotic twins than among dizygotic twins, whether raised together or separately.[23,24] More recent studies with larger study samples, a better classification of phenotypes, and more sophisticated statistical models, point to a rather significant influence of the genome in determining the smoking phenotype.[25]

The most extensively studied genes of the dopaminergic pathway are those that regulate the flow of dopamine in the central nervous system. Five different dopamine receptors are known, and the genes that encode them have been cloned (DRD1, DRD2, DRD3, DRD4, and DRD5). Among those, the DRD2 receptor has been studied most widely, because of its association with other addictive behaviours, and because nicotine has a dopamine-releasing effect.[26–28]

Smoking in psychiatric patients

Nicotine has been said to provide anxiety relief, oral gratification, and self-medication of psychotic symptoms in psychiatric patients.[29] Patients with schizophrenia and severe mental illness smoke cigarettes at rates that well exceed the general population.[30] Little is known about the correlates and sequels of increased smoking severity on persons with severe mental illness. Greater smoking severity has however been associated with greater perceived stress, poorer overall subjective quality of life, and lower satisfaction with finances, health, leisure activities, and social relationships, results that may lend support to a self-medication hypothesis.[31]

Nicotine intoxication and withdrawal symptoms

The primary addictive substance in cigarette smoking is nicotine. Cigarette smoking is very efficient nicotine delivery system because nicotine is nebulized and subsequently absorbed through the extensive pulmonary lung vessels. Consequently, smoking produces high arterial nicotine concentrations.[12] These high arterial concentrations, higher than venous concentrations, deliver a bolus of 1–3 mg of nicotine rapidly to the brain, a few seconds after smoking. With nicotine receptor activation, neurotransmitters are released including dopamine, norepinephrine, serotonin, and endogenous opioids. The immediate positive reinforcing effects of smoking include a reduction in anxiety and increased alertness and concentration.[32]

Nicotine's half-life is 2 h; therefore, repeated administration is needed through the day to maintain its effects. Consequently smokers usually smoke at frequent intervals to maintain narrow range of nicotine concentration in the blood. Paradoxically, chronic administration of nicotine results in an increase in the number of nicotine receptors. This paradoxical effect is probably due to a chronic nicotine receptor desensitization and inactivation. An increased number of receptors may play a role in the withdrawal symptoms that many smokers experience with prolonged cigarette abstinence.[33]

Nicotine is a highly toxic chemical; doses of 60 mg in adults are fatal secondary to respiratory paralysis (an average cigarette has an average dose of 0.5 mg). At low doses, symptoms of toxicity are nausea, vomiting, salivation, pallor due to peripheral vasoconstriction, weakness, abdominal pain, diarrhoea, dizziness, headache, increased blood pressure, tachycardia, tremor, and cold sweats. Toxicity is also associated with inability to concentrate, confusion, and sensory disturbances. During pregnancy, smoking is associated with an increased incidence of low-weight-birth babies.[32]

DSM-IV does not have a diagnostic category for nicotine intoxication; however, it has a category for nicotine withdrawal.[34] ICD-10 does have a category for nicotine intoxication (F17.0, mental and behavioural disorders due to use of tobacco, acute intoxication).[35] Withdrawal symptoms can develop within 2 h after having smoked the last cigarette. Withdrawal symptoms include dysphoria and depressed mood, insomnia, irritability, anxiety, frustration, difficulty in concentration and increase in appetite, and weight gain. Withdrawal symptoms peak within 24–36 h after cessation and usually diminish after 1 week of abstinence but can last for much longer. Some individuals continue smoking to avoid the negative symptoms of withdrawal.[36,37]

Nicotine dependence

The cumulative findings of more than 2500 scientific papers were summarized in the *1988 Surgeons General's Report on the Health Consequences of Smoking: Nicotine Addiction*.[38] Nicotine has a pronounced effect on the major stress hormones, and the dose-related effects of nicotine on neuroendocrine responses appear to constitute a critical component of its pharmacological action. Hypothalamic corticotrophin-releasing factor (CRF) is stimulated by nicotine, and levels of hypophyseal hormones including ACTH and arginine-vasopressin are increased in a dose-related manner. At higher doses, growth hormone (GH) and prolactin are entrained, and corticosteroid levels are related to plasma nicotine levels.[15,39,40]

Treatment for tobacco dependence

Many of the adverse health effects of smoking are reversible, and smoking cessation treatments represent some of the most cost-effective of all health care interventions. Although the greatest benefit accrues from ceasing smoking when young, even quitting in middle age avoids much of the excess health care risk associated with smoking.[41–43]

In order to improve smoking cessation rates, effective behavioural and pharmacological treatments, coupled with professional counselling and advice, are required. Since smoking duration is the principal risk factor for smoking-related morbidity, the treatment goal should be early cessation and prevention of relapse.[44,45]

The health benefits are various: smoking cessation has a major and immediate health benefit for persons with or without smoking-related diseases; former smokers live longer than those who continue to smoke; smoking cessation decreases the risk of lung cancer, myocardial infarction, cerebrovascular diseases, and chronic lung diseases.[46]

Non-pharmacological treatment

Physician counselling and pharmacotherapeutic interventions for smoking cessation are among the most cost-effective clinical interventions. Several strategies can be used for smoking cessation, counselling differs according to the patient's readiness to quit. For smokers who do not intend to quit smoking, physicians should inform and sensitize them about tobacco use and cessation. For smokers ready to quit, the physician should show strong support, help set a quit date, prescribe pharmaceutical therapies for nicotine dependence, if needed.(47,48)

There is insufficient information to know which elements of behavioural support are effective or whether one approach, such as motivational interviewing or cognitive behavioural therapy, is more effective than another. There is some evidence to suggest that group support may be more effective in general than one-to-one support(49) and that it should involve multiple sessions.(50) There is also evidence that such sessions can be effective even if conducted over the telephone.(51)

Of the many web-based support packages available on the Internet, only two have been evaluated in randomized controlled trials,(52,53) these trials of tailored programmes enrolled smokers who were using nicotine replacement. Both trials showed significant benefits 10–12 weeks after the quit date.

There are a few adequate studies examining complementary therapies in smoking cessation. Meta-analysis of trials of acupuncture and hypnotherapy showed no benefit but could not exclude small effects.(54,55)

Nicotine replacement therapies

Nicotine replacement therapies (NRTs) were designed in order to enhance efficacy rates during smoking cessation by replacing some of the nicotine usually delivered by smoking. All replacement therapies have shown to have high rates of efficacy. The choice of NRT depends on patient's preference, side effects, presence of concomitant medical conditions, and a history of previous success or failure.(56,57)

(a) Nicotine gum and nicotine lozenge

Nicotine gum was the first NRT marketed for smoking cessation, contains nicotine bound to an iron resin. The nicotine is slowly released into the mouth and is absorbed through the mucosa of the mouth, only 50 per cent of the nicotine in a piece of gum is systemically absorbed and concentrations reach a maximum peak in 30 min after onset of chewing.(12) The staring dose for individuals who smoke 20 cigarettes a day should be 2 mg. The gum should not be prescribed in patients with temporo-mandibular joint disease and those with dental or oral problems. The nicotine lozenge contains nicotine bound to a prolacrilex ion-exchange resin, does not require chewing and therefore is preferable to the gum for patients with dental problems.(58)

(b) Transdermal nicotine

Transdermal nicotine, commonly known as the nicotine patch, produces a constant delivery of nicotine that is very useful for patients with poor treatment adherence. Eight weeks of treatment are generally sufficient for smoking cessation.(59)

Transdermal nicotine is available in a variety of formulations and dosing schedules (i.e. 15 mg/16 h; 7, 14, 21 mg/24 h). Peak nicotine concentrations for the various systems are reached 2–6 h after application and steady state conditions occur 2–3 days after continued patch use.(59)

(c) Nicotine nasal spray and inhaler

Nicotine nasal spray delivers nicotine through the nasal mucosa. One advantage is that it relieves tobacco cravings quickly. It is available only by prescription. One spray to each nostril constitutes a dose, approximately 1 mg nicotine. Patients should use one or two doses per hour; the nasal spray delivers nicotine rapidly, with venous nicotine peaking at 5–10 min after administration.(60) Side effects include some initial irritation of the nasal mucosa should be avoided in patients with rhinitis, nasal polyps, or sinusitis.

Nicotine vapour inhaler is used by puffing through a cartridge inhaler, and may be useful for smoking cessation in some patients because its use is similar to the smoking ritual, and it delivers nicotine rapidly. It is only available by prescription. The recommended treatment period is up to 24 weeks.(45)

Pharmacological treatments

Considering that not all smokers respond well to nicotine replacement therapies and some smokers have comorbid symptoms there has been considerable interest in non-nicotine medications to treat nicotine dependence. The observations that some antidepressant-like bupropion and other selective serotonin-reuptake inhibitors (SSRIs) are useful as a treatment for smoking cessation, led to intensive research to study dopamine, serotonin, norepinephrine, glutamate, gamma-aminobutyric acid (GABA), nicotine, cannabinoid, and opiod receptors.(61,62)

Sustained-released bupropion

The sustained-released bupropion is currently considered as a first-line treatment for cigarette smokers. The mechanism of action of this antidepressant in the treatment of nicotine dependence likely involves blockade of dopamine and norepinephrine reuptake as well as antagonism of high-affinity nicotine acetylcholine receptors.(63)

The goals of bupropion therapy for nicotine dependence are (1) cessation of smoking behaviour and (2) reduction of nicotine withdrawal symptoms. In addition, bupropion SR may delay cessation-induced weight gain.(64)

A study by Hurt *et al.*(65) established the efficacy and safety of bupropion SR for treatment of nicotine dependence, and led to its approval for this indication by the FDA in 1998. Bupropion treatment also reduces weight gain associated with smoking cessation and significantly reduced nicotine withdrawal symptoms at a dose of 150–300 mg/day. Major side effects are headache, dry mouth, nausea, vomiting, and insomnia.(65)

Nortrityline

This tricycle antidepressant appears to have efficacy rates similar to bupropion in smoking cessation.(66) The mechanism of action is thought to be related to its noradrenergic and serotoninergic reuptake blockade. Side effects are those of the typical tricyclic antidepressants and include dry mouth, blurred vision, constipation, and orthostatic hypotension. Nortryptiline has been recommended as a second-line treatment.(61,67)

Clonidine

Because clonidine appears to have some efficacy for alcohol and opioid withdrawal, it has been evaluated for the treatment of nicotine withdrawal. However, it has not proved to be as effective as other therapies. Several clinical trials used oral or transdermal clonidine in doses of 0.1–0.4 mg/day for 2–6 weeks with or without behaviour therapy. Most common side effects of clonidine are dry mouth, sedation, and constipation, postural hypotension, and depression.(61)

Selective serotonin reuptake inhibitors

The available evidence provides little support for the use of SSRIs to assist in smoking cessation, either alone or in combination with other therapies. Placebo-controlled trials of fluoxetine or paroxetine failed to show an increase in smoking cessation.[61]

Varenicline

Varenicline is a selective alpha (4) beta (2) nicotinic acetylcholine receptor partial agonist and the first non-nicotine-containing medication developed with the sole purpose of treating nicotine addiction.[68]

Varenicline seems to be more efficacious than bupropion 24 weeks after randomization to a 12-week treatment course and 1 year after randomization in an identical trial. There are no contraindications except hypersensitivity and the drug is generally well tolerated. Varenicline, which is recently approved for smoking cessation, offers an option to patients who cannot tolerate the adverse effects associated with nicotine-replacement therapy and bupropion. It is also an alternative to consider for patients with contraindications to such therapies. Varenicline is completely absorbed orally and not affected by food. Steady state is reached within 4 days of administration.[69,70]

Other pharmacological treatments

Several new therapies are emerging as possible treatment options for smoking cessation. Rimonabant, a selective cannabinoid antagonist, blocks dopamine release in the nucleus accumbens, a primary reward centre for the brain. Studies have found that Rimonabant may not only be effective as a smoking cessation aid but may also assist in the maintenance of nicotine abstinence. Rimonabant has also demonstrated a weight-loss benefit, which may be attractive to smokers concerned with weight gain associated with smoking cessation.[71–73]

Three nicotine vaccines are currently in development, each acting to sequester nicotine from the bloodstream, thereby preventing its penetration of the central nervous system. Ongoing studies will evaluate their use as established therapies for smoking cessation.[74,75]

Conclusions

Despite the reality that smoking remains the most important preventable cause of death and disability, most clinicians underperform in helping smokers quit. Nearly 70 per cent of smokers want to quit, and 42.5 per cent attempt to quit each year. The most effective smoking cessation programmes involve a combination of pharmacotherapy and behavioural and/or cognitive counselling to improve abstinence rates. Ways to counter clinicians' pessimism about cessation include the knowledge that most smokers require multiple attempts before they succeed in quitting.

Further information

Fiore, M.C., Bailey, W.C., Cohen, S.J., *et al.* (2000). *Treating tobacco use and dependence. Quick reference guide for clinicians.* U.S. Department of Health and Human Services, Rockville, MD. Public Health Service. (http://www.surgeongeneral.gov/tobacco/tobaqrg.htm)

www.tobaccofreekids.org Information on Youth Smoking

www.findhelp.com Foundation for Innovations in Nicotine Dependence

www.quitnow.org Self-help Website Support for Quitting Smoking

References

1. Peto, R., López, A.D., Boreman, J., *et al.* (1996). Mortality from smoking world wide. *British Medical Bulletin*, **52**, 12–21.
2. Collihaw, N.E. and López, A.D. (1996). *The tobacco epidemic: a public health emergency.* World Health Organization (WHO) Tobacco Alert. WHO, Geneva.
3. Esson, K.M. and Leeder, S.R. (2004). *The millennium developments goals and tobacco control.* World Health Organization Publications, Geneva.
4. Thun, M.J., Day-Lacally, C.A., Calle, E.E., *et al.* (1995). Excess mortality among cigarette smokers: changes in a 20 years interval. *American Journal of Public Health*, **85**, 1223–30.
5. Mathers, C.D. and Loncar, D. (2006). Projections of global mortality and burden of disease from 2002 to 2030. *PLoS Medicine*, **3**(11), e512.
6. Jha, P. and Chaloupka, F.J. (2000). *Tobacco control in developing countries.* Oxford University Press, Oxford, UK.
7. Davis, K.C., Nonnemaker, J.M., and Farrelly, M.C. (2007). Association between national smoking prevention campaigns and perceived smoking prevalence among youth in the United States. *The Journal of Adolescent Health*, **41**(5), 430–6. Epub 4 September 2007.
8. Fagerström, K. (2002). The epidemiology of smoking: health consequences and benefits of cessation. *Drugs*, **62**(Suppl. 2), 1–9.
9. Choquet, M., Morin, D., Hassler, C., *et al.* (2004). Are alcohol, tobacco, and cannabis use as well as polydrug use increasing in France? *Addictive Behaviours*, **29**, 607–14.
10. Riala, H., Hakko, M., Isohanni, M.R., *et al.* (2004). Teenage smoking and substance use as predictors of severe alcohol problems in late adolescence and in young adulthood. *The Journal of Adolescent Health*, **35**, 245–54.
11. Farrell, M., Howes, S., Bebbington, P., *et al.* (2001). Nicotine, alcohol and drug dependence and psychiatric comorbidity. Results of a national household survey. *The British Journal of Psychiatry*, **179**, 432–7.
12. Henningfield, J.E. (1995). Nicotine medications for smoking cessation. *The New England Journal of Medicine*, **333**, 1196–203.
13. Scelling, T.C. (1992). Addictive drugs: the cigarette experience. *Science*, **225**, 430.
14. Yudkin, P., Hey, K., Roberts, S., *et al.* (2003). Abstinence from smoking eight years after participation in randomized controlled trial of nicotine patch. *British Medical Journal*, **327**(7405), 28–9.
15. Volkow, N.D. (2005). What do we know about drug addiction? *The American Journal of Psychiatry*, **162**(8), 1401–2.
16. Brody, A.L., Mandelkern, M.A., London, E.D., *et al.* (2006). Cigarette smoking saturates brain alpha 4 beta 2 nicotinic acetylcholine receptors. *Archives of General Psychiatry*, **63**(8), 907–15.
17. Mamede, M., Ishizu, K., Ueda, M., *et al.* (2007). Temporal change in human nicotinic acetylcholine receptor after smoking cessation: 5IA SPECT study. *Journal of Nuclear Medicine*, EPub 17 October 2007.
18. Heath, A.C., Kirk, K.M., Meyer, J.M., *et al.* (1999). Genetic and social determinants of initiation and age at onset of smoking in Australian twins. *Behavior Genetics*, **29**(6), 395–407.
19. Sullivan, P.F. and Kendler, K.S. (1999). The genetic epidemiology of smoking. *Nicotine & Tobacco Research*, **1**(Suppl. 2), S51–7; discussion S69–70.
20. Batra, V., Patkar, A.A., Berrettini, W.H., *et al.* (2003). The genetic determinants of smoking. *Chest*, **123**(5), 1730–9.
21. Fisher, R.A. (1958). Cancer and smoking. *Nature*, **182**(4635), 596.
22. Berrettini, W.H. and Lerman, C.E. (2005). Pharmacotherapy and pharmacogenetics of nicotine dependence. *The American Journal Psychiatry*, **162**(8), 1441–51.
23. Tapper, A.R., McKinney, S.L., and Nashmi, R. (2004). Nicotine activation of alpha4 receptors: sufficient for reward, tolerance, and sensitization. *Science*, **306**, 1029–32.
24. True, W.R., Heath, A.C., Scherrer, J.F., *et al.* (1997). Genetic and environmental contributions to smoking. *Addiction*, **92**(10), 1277–87.

25. Munafo, M., Clark, T., Johnstone, E., *et al.* (2004). The genetic basis for smoking behavior: a systematic review and meta-analysis. *Nicotine & Tobacco Research*, **6**(4), 583–97.
26. Swan, G.E., Benowitz, N.L., Jacob, P. III, *et al.* (2004). Pharmacogenetics of nicotine metabolism in twins: methods and procedures. *Twin Research*, **7**(5), 435–48.
27. do Prado-Lima, P.A., Chatkin, J.M., Taufer, M., *et al.* (2004). Polymorphism of 5HT2A serotonin receptor gene is implicated in smoking addiction. *American Journal of Medical Genetics. Part B Neuropsychiatric Genetics*, **128**(1), 90–3.
28. Arinami, T., Ishiguro, H., and Onaivi, E.S. (2000). Polymorphisms in genes involved in neurotransmission in relation to smoking. *European Journal of Pharmacology*, **410**(2–3), 215–26.
29. Medoff, D.R., Wohlheiter, K., DiClemente, C., *et al.* (2007). Correlates of severity of smoking among persons with severe mental illness. *American Journal of Addiction*, **16**(2), 101–10.
30. Strand, J.E. and Nybäck, H. (2005). Tobacco use in schizophrenia: a study of cotinine concentrations in the saliva of patients and controls. *European Psychiatry*, **20**(1), 50–4.
31. Gershon, R.B., Hwang, S., Han, J., *et al.* (2007). Short-term naturalistic treatment outcomes in cigarette smokers with substance abuse and/or mental illness. *The Journal of Clinical Psychiatry*, **68**(6), 892–8; quiz 980–1.
32. Di Chiara, G. (2000). Role of dopamine in the behavioural actions of nicotine related to addiction. *European Journal of Pharmacology*, **393**, 295–314.
33. Dani, J.A. and De Biasi, M. (2001). Cellular mechanism of nicotine addiction. *Pharmacology, Biochemistry, and Behavior*, **70**, 439–66.
34. American Psychiatric Association. (2000). *Diagnostic and statistical manual of mental disorders* (4th edn, revised). American Psychiatric Association, Washington, DC.
35. WHO. (1992). *The ICD-10 classification of mental and behavioural disorders*, pp. 70–4. World Health Organization, Geneva.
36. Hughes, J.R. and Hatsukami, D. (1986). Signs and symptoms of tobacco withdrawal. *Archives of General Psychiatry*, **43**, 289–94.
37. Heatherton, T.F., Kozlowski, L.T., Frecker, R.C., *et al.* (1991). The Fagerström test for nicotine dependence: a revision of the Fagerström tolerance questionnaire. *British Journal of Addiction*, **86**, 1119–27.
38. Jarvis, M. (2001). Patterns of use, epidemiology, adverse effects and specific issues concerning treatment for nicotine dependence. In *Oxford textbook of psychiatry* (eds. N. Andreasen, M. Gelder, and J.J. López-Ibor), pp. 554–9.
39. Maskos, U., Molles, B.E., and Pons, S. (2005). Nicotine reinforcement and cognition restored by targeted expression of nicotinic receptors. *Nature*, **436**, 103–7.
40. Kremer, I., Bachner-Melman, R., Reshef, A., *et al.* (2005). Association of the serotonin transporter gene with smoking behavior. *The American Journal of Psychiatry*, **162**(5), 924–3028.
41. Fiore, M.C., Bailey, W.C., and Cohen, S.J. (2000). *Treating tobacco use and dependence. Quick reference guide for clinicians.* US Dept of Health and Human Services, Public Health Service, Rockville, MD.
42. Schroeder, S.A. (2005). What to do with a patient who smokes. *The Journal of the American Medical Association*, **294**(4), 482–7.
43. Law, M. and Tang, J.L. (1995). An analysis of the effectiveness of interventions intended to help people to stop smoking. *Archives of Internal Medicine*, **155**, 1993–41.
44. Lerman, C., Patterson, F., and Berrettini, W. (2005). Treating tobacco dependence: state of the science and new directions. *Journal of Clinical Oncology*, **23**(2), 311–23.
45. Ocken, C.A. and George, T.P. (2005). Tobacco. In *Clinical manual of addiction psychopharmacology*, American Psychiatric Publishing, Arlington, pp. 315–38.
46. Chatkin, J.M. (2006). The influence of genetics on nicotine dependence and the role of pharmacogenetics in treating the smoking habit. *Journal of Brasileiro de Pneumologia*, **32**(6), 573–9.
47. [No authors listed] (2000). A clinical practice guideline for treating tobacco use and dependence: a US public health service report. The tobacco use and dependence clinical practice guideline panel, staff, and consortium representatives. *The Journal of the American Medical Association*, **283**(24), 3244–54.
48. Cornuz, J. (2007). Smoking cessation interventions in clinical practice. *European Journal of Vascular Endovascular Surgery*, **34**(4), 397–404. Epub 1 August 2007.
49. McEwen, A., West, R., and McRobbie, H. (2006). Effectiveness of specialist group treatment for smoking cessation vs. one-to-one treatment in primary care. *Addictive Behaviors*, **31**, 1650–60.
50. Aveyard, P., Brown, K., Saunders, C., *et al.* (2007). Weekly versus basic smoking cessation support in primary care: a randomised controlled trial. *Thorax*, **62**(10), 892–903.
51. Stead, L.F., Perera, R., and Lancaster, T. (2006). Telephone counselling for smoking cessation. *Cochrane Database of Systematic Reviews*, (3), CD002850.
52. Strecher, V.J., Shiffman, S., and West, R. (2005). Randomized controlled trial of a web-based computer-tailored smoking cessation program as a supplement to nicotine patch therapy. *Addiction*, **100**, 682–8.
53. Swartz, L.H., Noell, J.W., Schroeder, S.W., *et al.* (2006). A randomised control study of a fully automated internet based smoking cessation programme. *Tobacco Control*, **15**, 7–12.
54. White, A.R., Rampes, H., and Campbell, J.L. (2006). Acupuncture and related interventions for smoking cessation. *Cochrane Database of Systematic Reviews*, (1), CD000009.
55. Abbot, N.C., Stead, L.F., White, A.R., *et al.* (1998). Hypnotherapy for smoking cessation. *Cochrane Database of Systematic Reviews*, (2), CD001008.
56. George, T.P. and O'Malley, S.S. (2004). Current pharmacological treatment for nicotine dependence. *Trends in Pharmacological Sciences*, **25**, 42–48.
57. Perkins, K.A., Stitzer, M., and Lerman, C. (2006). Medication screening for smoking cessation: a proposal for new methodologies. *Psychopharmacology (Berl)*, **184**(3–4), 628–36.
58. Shiffamn, S., Dresler, C.M., and Hajek, P. (2002). Efficacy of a nicotine lozenge for smoking cessation. *Archives of Internal Medicine*, **162**, 1267–76.
59. Fiore, M.C., Smith, S.S., and Jorenby, D.E. (1994). The effectiveness of the nicotine patch for smoking cessation. *The Journal of the American Medical Association*, **271**, 1940–8.
60. Shuterland, G., Sappleton, J.A., and Russell, M.A. (1992). Randomised controlled trial of nasal nicotine spray in smoking cessation. *Lancet*, **340**, 324–9.
61. Sullivan, M.A. and Covey, L.S. (2002). Nicotine dependence: the role for antidepressants and anxiolytics. *Current Opinion in Investigational Drugs*, **3**(2), 262–71.
62. Slemmer, J.E., Martin, B.R., and Damaj, M.I. (2000). Bupropion is a nicotinic antagonist. *The Journal of Pharmacology and Experimental Therapeutics*, **295**, 321–7.
63. Lerman, C., Shields, P.G., Wileyto, E.P., *et al.* (2003). Effects of dopamine transporter and receptor polymorphisms on smoking cessation in a bupropion clinical trial. *Health Psychology*, **22**(5), 541–8.
64. Gonzales, D.H., Nides, M.A., and Ferry, L.H. (2001). Bupropion SR as an aid to smoking cessation in smokers treated previously with bupropion: a randomized placebo-controlled study. *Clinical Pharmacology and Therapeutics*, **69**, 438–44.
65. Hurt, R.D., Sachs, D.P., and Glover. E.D. (1997). A comparison of sustained released bupropion and placebo for smoking cessation. *The New England Journal of Medicine*, **337**, 1195–202.
66. Hall, S.M., Humfleet, G.L., and Reus, V.I. (2002). Psychology intervention and antidepressant treatment in smoking cessation. *Archives of General Psychiatry*, **59**, 930–6.

67. Haggstram, F.M., Chatkin, J.M., Sussenbach-Vaz, E., *et al.* (2006). A controlled trial of nortriptyline, sustained-release bupropion and placebo for smoking cessation: preliminary results. *Pulmonary Pharmacology & Therapeutics*, **19**(3), 205–9.
68. Stack, N.M. (2007). Smoking cessation: an overview of treatment options with a focus on varenicline. *Pharmacotherapy*, **27**(11), 1550–7.
69. Potts, L.A. and Garwood, C.L. (2007). Varenicline: the newest agent for smoking cessation. *American Journal of Health-System Pharmacy*, **64**(13), 1381–4.
70. Tonstad, S., Tønnesen, P., Hajek, P., *et al.* (2006). For the varenicline phase 3 study group. Effect of maintenance therapy with varenicline on smoking cessation: a randomized controlled trial. *The Journal of the American Medical Association*, **296**, 64–71.
71. Garwood, C.L. and Potts, L.A. (2007). Emerging pharmacotherapy's for smoking cessation. *American Journal of Health-System Pharmacy*, **64**(16), 1693–8.
72. Fowler, J.S., Volkow, N.D., Wang, G.J., *et al.* (1996). Brain monoamine oxidase. An inhibition in cigarette smokers. *Proceedings of the National Academy of Sciences of the United States of America*, **93**(24), 14065–9.
73. Markou, A., Paterson, N.E., and Semenova, S. (2004). Role of gamma-aminobutyric acid (GABA) and metabolic glutamate receptors in nicotine reinforcement: potential pharmacotherapy for smoking cessation. *Annals of the New York Academy of Sciences*, **1025**, 491–503.
74. Dwoskin, L.P., Joyce, B.M., Zheng, G., *et al.* (2007). Discovery of a novel nicotinic receptor antagonist for the treatment of nicotine addiction: 1-(3-Picolinium)-12-triethylammonium-dodecane dibromide (TMPD). *Biochemical Pharmacology*, **74**(8), 1271–82. Epub 21 July 2007.
75. Oliver, J.L., Pashmi, G., Barnett, P., *et al.* (2007). Development of an anti-cotinine vaccine to potentiate nicotine-based smoking cessation strategies. *Vaccine*, **25**(42), 7354–62. Epub 30 August 2007.

4.2.4 Assessing need and organizing services for drug misuse problems

John Marsden, Colin Bradbury, and John Strang*

Introduction

In the present decade, there has been substantial investment in drug misuse treatment thereby expanding the workforce, the capacity of the treatment system and leading to reduced waiting times and better integration of local services. In 2006–07, an in-treatment population of approximately 200 000 individuals were recorded by the National Drug Treatment Monitoring System (NDTMS). Capture-recapture estimates suggest that there are approximately 327 000 users of opioids and/or crack cocaine.

About two-thirds of adults entering drug misuse treatment services are dependent on illicit heroin—a clinical presentation complicated by between 20 per cent to 50 per cent of admissions by concurrent dependence on cocaine and other substances such as the misuse of pharmaceutical medications (such as benzodiazepines). Cannabis is reported as the main problem drug for younger patients under 18 years of age. Overall, treatment services for clients of all ages are able to assess and provide interventions across all illicit drugs including amphetamine-type stimulants, sedative/hypnotics, cannabis, hallucinogens and volatile substances (solvents and inhalants). Hazardous and harmful alcohol use characterizes a significant, but priority group of drug misuse treatment seekers.

In 2006, a revised national drug misuse treatment effectiveness strategy stressed the need for better local partnerships to commission and organize local services and promote reintegration of treated patients into the community. A core component of the strategy was the creation of Criminal Justice Integrated Teams (CJITS) who were given the role of treatment case coordination for individuals involved in the justice system with identified drug misuse. Nevertheless, improvements to the reach, operation, and effectiveness of treatments remains a priority—particularly tackling high-risk behaviours linked to the acquisition and transmission of blood-borne infections and ensuring that all service users receive good quality assessment and care coordination.

Local coordination of treatment

Drug Action Teams (DATs) were originally set up in 1995 under a Government white paper on drug misuse. The purpose of the DAT was to co-ordinate the activity and spend of local statutary commissioning agencies who have an interest in reducing the harm caused by illicit drug use to individuals, their families, and the community. DATs and their membership typically consists of senior commissioning representatives from local Police, Health, Local Authority and Probation services. Increasingly, the Prison Service are represented following the announcement of a new Integrated Drug Treatment System for prisoners which seeks to ensure that the same appropriate and evidenced drug treatment interventions are available to individuals regardless of whether they are in prison or in the community. Under the Police Reform Act (2002), the process of combining the activity of DATs with their equivalent bodies for crime (Crime and Disorder Reduction Partnerships (CDRPs) was started. Local areas organize their activity in differing ways, but the concept of co-ordination of action between the DAT and CDRP is now universal.

DATs are charged with consulting with and involving local communities, stakeholders, treatment providers, and crucially—users and carers—in the development of their local commissioning strategies. DATs are allocated a hypothecated fund for improving capacity and quality of drug treatment services for their residents. This Pooled Treatment Budget is typically banked by a partner agency (usually the PCT) but is intended to be commissioned jointly (along with mainstream monies that partner agencies allocate for drug treatment) via the DAT Partnership structure. DAT Partnerships typically have a sub-group know as the Joint Commissioning Group (JCG) which seeks to operationalize the DAT's agreed strategy for the locality.

The National Treatment Agency for Substance Misuse (NTA) is a Special Health Authority set up in 2001 to oversee and performance manage the commissioning of effective drug treatment.

* The views expressed in this chapter are those of the authors and do not necessarily reflect the views of the National Treatment Agency. The commissioning, performance management and planning of drug treatment varies significantly across the United Kingdom. Unless stipulated to the contrary, the following text applies specifically to England.

DAT Partnerships submit a treatment plan on an annual basis which is signed off by the NTA and other regional partners and performance monitored on a quarterly basis. Since 2005–06, the NTA has issued guidance on conducting a Needs Assessment for the local population and increasingly assessment of need is being seen as the centrepiece of DAT Partnership commissioning activity. DAT Partnerships are encouraged to set up expert groups which (in combination with available local data sources of prevalence and treatment) should be used to carefully consider available information and intelligence in order to inform the local Joint Commissioning Group of assessed levels of unmet need, therefore enabling them to set and update commissioning priorities on a cyclical basis.

Types of treatment

In the UK, treatment for substance use disorders vary on several core dimensions, as follows: (a) setting (outpatient/community or inpatient/residential), modality (pharmacological or behavioural); (b) content (e.g. cognitive behavioural therapy, motivational approaches, contingency management; couples therapy); (c) goals (harm reduction, partial or complete abstinence); (d) intensity (brief interventions or intensive therapeutic contact); (e) extent of external contingency (e.g. self-referral or criminal justice mandate); and (f) type of provider (NHS, non-governmental organiztion and private/commercial). In 2002, the NTA promulgated a national service framework for drug misuse services and updated this four years later. The framework uses a practical framework to aid rational and evidence-based commissioning of drug treatment in England with services for drug misusers grouped into four broad bands, or tiers.

Tier 1 interventions

This first tier involves the provision of information, advice, screening and referral to drug users by generic medical and social care services (e.g. Accident and Emergency Departments, community retail pharmacies). It includes liaison and partnership working with specialist drug treatment services to provide specific interventions (e.g. treatment of patients with health problems caused by Hepatitis C infection).

Tier 1 services for adults are not structured drug or alcohol treatment, but can be part of the local substance misuse treatment system. These services work with a wide range of clients including drug and alcohol misusers, but their sole purpose is not drug or alcohol treatment. Tier 1 services comprise a range of interventions which are not drug-specific, but offer a variety of generic health and social care interventions. In this context, the role of Tier 1 includes the provision of their own services plus, as a minimum, screening drug misusers and referral to local drug and alcohol treatment services in Tiers 2 and 3. Tier 1 provision for drug and alcohol misusers may also include assessment, services to reduce drug-related harm, and liaison or joint working with Tiers 2 and 3 specialist drug and alcohol treatment services. Tier 1 services are crucial to providing services in conjunction with more specialized drug and alcohol services (e.g. general medical care for drug misusers in community-based or residential substance misuse treatment, or housing support and aftercare for drug misusers leaving residential care or prison).

Tier 2 interventions

The second tier describes interventions involving specific drug-related information and advice to help drug users reduce or avoid hazardous and harmful patterns of use or attain and maintain abstain harm. Services are delivered from dedicated community locations as well as outreach and may also include brief, structured psychosocial interventions, various harm minimization interventions (including syringe and needle exchange) and aftercare support. Tier 2 services may also provide triage assessment and linked referral to structured drug treatment and in this respect may operated independently or in the same setting as a Tier 3 intervention team. Tier 2 interventions for adults provide accessible drug and alcohol specialist services for a wide range of drug and alcohol misusers referred from a variety of sources, including self-referrals. This tier is defined by its low threshold to access services, and limited requirements on drug and alcohol misusers to receive services. Often drug and alcohol misusers will access drug or alcohol services through Tier 2 and progress to higher tiers. Tier 2 interventions include advice and information, drop-in services, needle exchange and motivational interviewing.

Tier 3 interventions

In terms of the volumes of people receiving treatment, this tier is at the centre of the system. It includes specialized care-planned pharmacotherapy (opioid agonist and antagonist and adjunctive medication prescribing to treat dependence) and a broad array of psychosocial interventions delivered by combined or separate teams in the community and primary care. There is an emphasis on high-quality assessment, care planning, liaison and review and regular contact with a clinical keyworker and other team members. The frequency of scheduled contact varies widely across Tier 3 services but is particularly indented to be intensive among users attending 'structured day programmes'. Tier 3 interventions for adults are provided solely for drug and alcohol misusers in structured programmes of care. Tier 3 structured services include psychotherapeutic interventions and structured counselling (e.g. cognitive behavioural therapy, motivational interventions), methadone maintenance programmes, community detoxification, or day care provided either as a drug- and alcohol-free programme or as an adjunct to methadone treatment. Community-based aftercare programmes for drug and alcohol misusers leaving residential rehabilitation or prison are also included in Tier 3 interventions. There is interest in developing behaviour therapies to treatment drug dependence on contingency management. Psychoactive substances can exert unconditioned reinforcing effects and repeated administration produce several conditioned responses. For example, voucher-based reinforcement therapy uses vouchers of increasing value for goods and services with various bonus incentives to subjects who can provide drug-free urine tests. The National Institute for Health and Clinical Excellence (NICE) has produced guidelines for the effective delivery of various psychosocial treatment interventions tailored to the needs of drug misusers, including brief motivational interventions, contingency management and behavioural couples therapy.

Tier 4 interventions

The fourth tier of the treatment system denotes specialist inpatient (and general ward) inpatient services providing stabilization and medically supervised withdrawal (detoxification), residential rehabilitation programmes (providing psychosocial and practical, vocational supports designed to maintain abstinence and promote long-term recovery) and a range of halfway houses and supportive accommodation. Some inpatient and residential programmes are directly linked. These services vary in duration from brief (<10 days), short-term (<3 months) and long-term (>3 months). Tier 4 services are highly structured interventions underpinned by assessments and close monitoring of clinical progress. Rehabilitation programmes have been pioneered and then sustained chiefly in the voluntary sector. Some adhere to or have adopted a therapeutic philosophy (e.g. 12-Step based on the Minnesota Model of addiction recovery developed in the USA) or therapeutic community model, while others operate as 'general houses'—which seek to foster responsible communal living and community reintegration. Tier 4 substance misuse interventions for adults are aimed at individuals with a high level of presenting need and usually require a higher level of commitment from drug and alcohol misusers than is required for services in lower tiers. Tier 4 services are rarely accessed directly by clients. Referral is usually from Tiers 2 or 3 services or via community care assessment.

NICE has produced guidelines for the delivery of psychosocial interventions in residential rehabilitation services and also for the organization and delivery of opioid detoxification services.

Commissioning treatment services

The national drugs strategy requires Crime and Drug Partnerships to commission services (or ensure access to) structured treatment (Tiers 3 and 4). The balance of l*f*ocal drug misuse treatment services and their detailed delivery mechanisms should be tailored to fit the needs of the local population; commissioners are encouraged to think systemically rather than focusing on putting in place individual services. Poorly defined care pathways between services and the lack of a joined-up care planned approach is clearly an unsatisfactory situation. Many individuals may require the provision of several different types of treatment service over time. It is quite common for an individual receiving treatment from one provider to receive additional welfare support and other social inclusion services which are provided by other agencies (e.g. housing support, legal advice). These supports are important elements in an effective package of care services that can evolve over the course of an individual's treatment. Together, the four tiers are meant to imply a continuum of care. Generic service providers and state agencies can refer an individual both up and down the four tiers to access appropriate treatment or support services.

Needs assessment

In the following section, we use an epidemiologically-based conceptualization of population treatment needs to discuss the organization of treatment services and methods for assessing need. Needs assessment occupies an importance place in the evidence-based planning process for the design and delivery of substance misuse services. It is the systematic collection of information about a geographically defined population and then applying this to make changes that will be beneficial to health. In the drug misuse field, there is a specific focus on two groups in the community: (a) those that are not in contact with services and treatment agencies and have unmet need; (b) those in contact with inefficient, ineffective or inappropriate health care services who have unmet need or for whom outcomes could be improved. Good needs assessment practice involves the application of epidemiological (and sometimes spatial geographical) techniques to estimate the number of people in the two groups above, clear understanding of the costs and benefits of interventions, a close collaboration with clinical services and the range of community stakeholders, and a planning and evaluation process to effect change. There is active encouragement for drug misuse partnerships and commissioners to undertake comprehensive needs assessments in the area of drug misuse with a specific target to assess the needs of young people. However, there have been few systematic quantitative and qualitative studies conducted in the drug misuse field in the UK. In fact, most studies in the mental health service field have been mainly or exclusively qualitative, relying on focus group discussion material. Multiple indicator methods and capture-recapture techniques have enabled estimates to be derived of the number of problem drug users in local areas.

Target groups

At the level of the individual patient, several headline factors may be influential in the assessment and treatment planning process: age, gender, race, and culture; pregnancy; familial pattern; quantity, frequency, and route of administration of psychoactive substances used; acute intoxication (overdose liability); extent of impairment and complications; social and occupational environmental supports and stressors—including acute housing need, training, and education. Complex cases will usually (but not always) be characterized by drug-related impairment, dependence, regular injecting, high tolerance levels and co-morbid problems across physical, psychological and personal/social functioning domains. At the population level, we identify six, non-independent groups. The prevalence of these groups and their case-mix at the local level will have ramifications for the assessment of health care needs and the planning, commissioning, delivery and monitoring of treatment services.

(a) Non-dependent, hazardous substance users

This group comprises individuals who are experiencing drug-related problems but they do not meet the criteria for dependence. This group may include large numbers of younger users who have begun to use drugs relatively recently. Because members of this group (both adults and particularly young people) are at risk of advancing their drug involvement to more serious levels they may be ideal clients for early intervention services.

(b) Drug injectors

This group comprises individuals who are injecting drugs and who may be at risk of acquiring and transmitting blood borne diseases. Community surveys suggest that less than 1:3 drug injectors share needles and syringes but 1:2 share injecting equipment (filters, spoons and flushing water). Research Individuals who inject drugs are much more likely to be dependent and experience drug-related harms. They constitute a priority group to be attracted to appropriate harm reduction and structured treatment programmes and retained in treatment as appropriate.

(c) Acutely intoxicated drug users

The specific needs of this group are identified because of the morbidity and mortality risks to health due to adverse reactions and drug overdose. This sub-group may overlap with sub-group B (the IDU). There is evidence that some two-thirds of heroin users have experienced an overdose. Risk of overdose is increased for opiates users who have also consumed other central nervous system depressants—commonly other opiates, alcohol and benzodiazepines. Preventing drug overdose and overdose mortality is a specific priority area. Acute intoxication is a discrete event although an individual's needs may advance to those associated with dependence, co-morbidity and withdrawal management and support. Most services provided to the intoxicated drug user will be found outside specialist drug or mental health services (e.g. accident and emergency departments, police custody). All services, which have contact with opiate users, should have prompt access to the injectable opiate antagonist naloxone which may be administered intravenously, intramuscularly or subcutaneously and can be life-saving in the event of an opiate overdose. There is now widespread recognition of the problem of drug dependence among the prison population and evidence from database linkage studies showing that newly released prisoners are at substantial risk of fatal overdose. In a study of 48 771 male and female sentenced prisoners in England and Wales released during 1998–2000, there were 442 recorded deaths (59 per cent drug-related) in year following release. There were 342 observed male deaths (45.8 expected in the general population) and 100 observed female deaths (8.3 expected). Drug-related male deaths were relatively more likely to involve heroin and female deaths were relatively more likely to involve benzodiazepines, cocaine and tricyclic antidepressants.

(d) Dependent drug users

This group comprise individuals who have drug-related problems and meet ICD/DSM dependence criteria. Dependence ranges in severity and is characterized by substantial impairment in the ability to control the frequency and amount used and various neuro-adaptational aspects. The majority of people presenting to specialist drug misuse services are in this group. They will require carefully planned community (and often residential treatment) together with the offer of aftercare support and access to social inclusion services to assist problems with housing, employment and training.

(e) Drug users with psychiatric co-morbidity

There is widespread concern about improving services and outcomes for people who have co-morbid psychiatric and substance use disorders. There is currently no research and clinical evidence-base for the effective management and care of patients in psychiatric inpatient units with psychoactive substance misuse co-morbidity and this is an important development area. There is some evidence that people with substance use problems and co-morbid psychiatric disorders appear to have a relatively high contact with medical services and may require more intensive treatment. However, it would appear that substance use disorders amongst people admitted for psychiatric treatment are of a less severe nature than those entering treatment for primary substance use problems. It is also important to consider and plan for the possibility that people with drug misuse and severe mental illness will not respond well or comply with traditional care plans and arrangements. In terms of client attributes, the presence of psychiatric co-morbidity in drug users entering treatment has been linked to poorer outcomes. Pre-treatment psychiatric severity has been found to be predictive of outcome and this should be taken into account when selecting appropriate treatments. The importance of providing social inclusion and reintegration services, particularly in the first three months of treatment has been advocated for community-based treatment services. However, the intensity or comprehensiveness of services *per se* is not consistently associated with improved outcome. The matrix of client attributes and treatment factors and processes has important implications for referral, assessment and client treatment-placement activities.

(f) Drug users in recovery

This group denotes individuals who have achieved a state of abstinence from their main problem drug (or all drugs), usually through successful completion of a health care treatment episode. This group may require residential rehabilitation services or community based aftercare programmes and other supports.

The process and techniques of needs assessment

Service commissioners should follow a sequence of steps to inform the needs assessment for their population requirements. The overarching goal is to produce a strategic commissioning framework which can be agreed across the health, social, and criminal justice partners. This remains an evolving area with guidance available from the NTA to assist the commissioning and implementation of work in this area. The usual steps when conducting a needs assessment are as follows:

- Allocation of resources and establishment of an agreed plan/methods.
- Prevalence estimation of target population and identification and profiling of sub-groups.
- Mapping of treatment services provided in the locality and an audit of treatment commissioning purchasing from services located outside the geographical boundary of the drug misuse partnership (e.g. Social Services purchasing of residential rehabilitation) to determine the extent to which demand is being met elsewhere.
- Audit of the demand profile of treatment services (capacity; number of episodes; estimated number in need).
- Personal interviews with key informants across commissioning, provision and advocacy sectors.
- Focus group discussions with key stakeholders (commissioners, clinicians, treatment providers, service users, carers of service users) to explore what they want from services.
- A 'gaps' analysis of current and desired profile of service provision (often qualitative exercise involving estimation of desired range of services to increase coverage for specific special groups).
- Recommendations for increasing treatment coverage, purchasing efficiency, and service effectiveness based on available evidence.
- Assessment of reactions to recommendations from strategists, commissioners, purchasers, services providers, and service users.
- Development of an implementation plan based on the identification of activities, resources, and timetables.

People in the seven sub-groups summarized above are not all the same and it is necessary to characterize each group on the basis of the severity of their problems (and extent of any complications). It is important to note that the above sub-categories are not mutually exclusive. Indeed, it is likely that an individual patient will occupy more than one category at any particular point in time (e.g. the injecting dependent heroin user with co-morbidity of HBV infection). The multiple occupation of different categories may also vary over time. In addition to these six primary groups, there is a further category which can be labelled 'at risk'. There is particular concern about segments of the younger population (see below) thought to be at risk; prevention initiatives and general educational programmes are Drug misuse services and treatment modalities.

The appraisal of the healthcare needs of the target populations and commissioning of strategic service responses should be flexible and adaptive to changing circumstances in each locality, including: variations and new trends in drugs use and consumption patterns; the geographical distribution and concentration of drug use; variations in demand for services; the changing relationship between drug use and other conditions (notably HIV infection, and blood borne viral hepatitis); changes in the organization of health services and monitoring the evidence-base for current and new treatment services.

Needs assessment activities are potentially costly activities. Intensive surveys of the resident population in most areas will be time consuming and expensive. It is quite likely that most partnerships will employ alternative (and less precise) estimation methods with which to inform the direction and success of commissioning strategies. A qualitative approach to needs assessment can be undertaken relatively quickly and can answer important questions concerning what commissioners, purchasers, service providers and service users want from treatment services and supports. Service user satisfaction surveys may be a useful means of gathering information about the extent to which a programme is perceived to have met an individual's treatment wants and needs. A range of issues has been examined including the accessibility, adequacy, content, and impact of services received. In addition to serving a simple monitoring function for treatment service providers and their commissioners, treatment satisfaction is argued to be a valuable indicator of treatment experience. Treatment satisfaction can act as a moderator of treatment outcome, since it is reasonable to assume that less satisfied clients may leave treatment prematurely or have different responses to interventions. Both users and carers should be routinely involved and consulted on service development and the setting of commissioning activities. Many DAT Partnerships (and the services they commission) now have good user/carer involvement mechanisms and guidance exists to enable the development of these mechanisms where they are still lacking.

Monitoring the impact of interventions

Drug interventions are from identical in their structure and operation, and outcome studies show that their level of effectiveness varies widely. Many service providers have been interested in monitoring their own outcomes reflecting organizational learning and quality values. The National Treatment Agency has now further developed the NDTMS as a national outcomes monitoring system. There are several benefits from collecting assessment and outcome information. Firstly, many patients perceive that a structured approach to assessment and recording outcome is a reflection of a service that is committed to providing the best care.

The feedback of information describing during-treatment changes to the patient (and his/her spouse/partner or carers) by clinical staff can be a powerful motivational influence to reinforce progress and assist in personal treatment goal setting. Secondly, clinical staff can monitor the characteristics and outcomes of their caseloads and identify areas of priority work. Thirdly, service managers can aggregate information across staff as an indicator of how well the agency is serving its patients. Fourthly, information on samples of cases of aggregate summaries across services can be provided to funding bodies and other government agencies to show the overall impact of treatment provision for a particular area.

In 2007, the NTA launched a national outcome monitoring system for substance misuse treatment services. A brief, outcome monitoring instrument—the Treatment Outcomes Profile (TOP) has been validated for this purpose. The TOP contains 30 items in four domains and is shown in Table 4.2.4.1. From these, a subset of 20 items are compiled at a national level to assess the overall effectiveness of the treatment system.

Case mix and performance analysis

Prognostic models of treatment outcome have been developed in our health care arenas with some success but the approach is in its infancy in the substance use disorders field. Essentially, a set of variables which predict a health or other outcome are identified using a statistical technique. Various methods can then be used to rank individual treatment provider's outcome performance can then be ranked against this averaged outcome. Having adjusted for

Table 4.2.4.1 The Treatment Outcomes Profile (TOP)

Domain/section	Item—in past 28 days
Substance use	Number of days used the following substances alcohol; opiates; cocaine; crack cocaine; amphetamines; cannabis; other (named) Typical quantity consumed on typical day (recorded as units, grams or amount spent) Number of days injected drugs in past 28 days Whether shared needles and syringes (direct receptive sharing); Yes/No Whether injected using a spoon, water or filter used by someone else (indirect receptive sharing; yes/no)
Crime	Days committed shop theft; days sold drugs Whether committed theft from or of vehicle (yes/no) Whether committed other property theft (yes/no) Whether committed fraud, forgery handling stolen goods (yes/no) Whether committed assault or violence (yes/no)
Health and social functioning	Had acute housing need (yes/no) Was at risk of eviction (yes/no) Number of days had paid work in past 28 days Number of days attended college or school in past 28 days Subjective rating of physical health (0 [poor] to 20 [good]) Subjective rating of psychological health (0 [poor] to 20 [good]) Subjective rating of quality of life (0 [poor] to 20 [good])

patient case mix differences, the objective is then to isolate the characteristics of very successful service providers as well as the correlates of less successful delivery of care. The results of this process can then be used to guide the development of the local treatment system.

Further information

For information on the UK drug misuse strategy and national treatment system in UK see the following websites: http://drugs.homeoffice.gov.uk/ http://www.nta.nhs.uk/

References

1. Audit Commission (2004). *Drug Misuse 2004: Reducing the Local Impact.* London:Audit Commission.
2. NTA and Department of Health (2005). *Statistics From the National Drug Treatment Monitoring System* (NDTMS), 1 April 2003, 31 March 2004. London: DH.
3.. Hay, G., Gannon, M., MacDougall, J., *et al.* (2006). Local and national estimates of the prevalence of opiate use and/or crack cocaine use (2004/05). In: *Measuring Different Aspects of Problem Drug Use: Methodological Developments* (eds. N. Singleton, R. Murray & L. Tinsley). London: Home Office. http://www.homeoffice.gov.uk/rds/pdfs06/rdsolr1606.pdf.
4. National Treatment Agency (2002). *Models of Care for Treatment of Adult Drug Misusers.* NTA, London.
5. National Treatment Agency (2006). *Models of Care for Treatment of Adult Drug Misusers:* update 2006.London: NTA.
6. Higgins, S. T., Delaney, D. D., Budney, A. J., *et al.* (1991). A behavioral approach to achieving initial cocaine abstinence. *American Journal of Psychiatry*, **148**, 1218–24.
7. Silverman, K., Chutuape, M. A., Bigelow, G. E.*et al.* (1999). Voucher-based reinforcement of cocaine abstinence in treatment-resistant methadone patients: effects of reinforcement magnitude. *Psychopharmacologia*, **146**, 128–38.
8. National Institute for Health and Clinical Excellence (2007). Drug misuse: psychosocial interventions.NICE guideline (http://guidance.nice.org.uk/CG51). Accessed on 27.07.07.
9. National Institute for Health and Clinical Excellence (2007). Drug misuse: opioid detoxification. NICE guideline (http://guidance.nice.org.uk/CG52). Accessed on 27.07.07.
10. Marsden, J., Strang, J., Lavoie, D., *et al.* (2000). Epidemiologically-based needs assessment: Drug misuse. In *Health Care NeedsAssessment: the epidemiologically based needs assessment reviews* (eds. A. Stevens, J. Raftery, and J. Mant). First Series Update. Radcliffe Medical Press, Ltd, Abington.
11. Stevens, A., and Gillam, S., (1998)/ Needs assessment: from theory to practice. *British Medical Journal*, **316**, 1448–52.
12. Hostick, T., (1995)/ Research design and methodology for a local mental health needs assessment. *Journalof Psychiatric & Mental Health Nursing*. **2**, 295–99.
13. Frischer, M., Heatlie, H., and Hickman, M., (2004). Estimating the prevalence of problematic and injecting drug use for Drug Action Team areas in England: a feasibility study using the Multiple Indicator Method. Home Office: Online Report 34/04 http://www.homeoffice.gov.uk/rds/pdfs04/rdsolr3404.pdf). Accessed 27.07.07.
14. Health Protection Agency (2005). *Shooting up: infections among injecting drug users in the United Kingdom 2004.* An update: October 2005. HPA, London.
15. Darke, S., and Zador, D., (1996). Fatal heroin 'overdose': a review. *Addiction*, **91**, 1765–72.
16. Darke, S., Ross, J., and Hall, W., (1996). Overdose among heroin users in Sydney, Australia: II. Responses to overdose. *Addiction*, **91**, 413–17.
17. Gossop, M., Griffiths, P., Powis, B., *et al.* (1996). Frequency of non-fatal heroin overdose: survey of heroin users recruited in non-clinical settings, *British Medical Journal*, 313, 402.
18. Darke, S., Ross, J., and Hall, W., (1996). Overdose amongst heroin users in Sydney: I. Prevalance and correlates of non-fatal overdose. *Addiction*, **91**, 405–11.
19. Powis, B., Strang, J., Griffiths, P., *et al.*(1999). Self-reported overdose among injecting drug users in London: Extent and nature of the problem. *Addiction*, **94**, 471–8.
20. Strang, J., Griffiths, P., Powis, B., *et al.* (1999). Which drugs cause overdose among opiate misusers? Study of personal and witnessed overdoses. *Drug and Alcohol Review*, **18**, 253–61.
21. Boys, A., Farrell, M., Bebbington, P., *et al.* (2002). Drug use and initiation in prison: results from a national prison survey in England and Wales. Addiction, **97**,1551–60.
22. Bird, S.M. and Hutchinson, S.J. (2003). Male drugs-related deaths in the fortnight after release from prison: Scotland, 1996–99. Addiction, **98**, 185–90.
23. Farrell, M., and Marsden, J. (2005). Drug-related mortality among newly released offenders 1998 to 2000. Home Office online report 40/05.
24. Johns, A., (1997). Substance misuse: a primary risk and a major problem of comorbidity. *International Review of Psychiatry*, **9**, 233–41.
25. Alterman, A.I., McLellan, T., *et al.* (1993). Do substance patients with more psychopathology receive more treatment? *Journal of Nervous and Mental Disease*, **181**, 576–82.
26. Lehman, A.F., Myers, C.P., and Corty, E. (1994). Severity of substance use disorders among psychiatric in-patients. *Journal of Nervous and Mental Disease*, **182**, 164–7.
27. McLellan, A.T., and Wisner, C. (1996). Achieving the public health potential of substance abuse treatment: implications for patient referral, treatment "matching" and outcome evaluation. In, *Drug Policy and Human Nature* (eds. W. Bickel and R. DeGrandpre), Philadelphia, PA.
28. National Treatment Agency for Substance Misuse (2007). Needs Assessment Manual. (http://www.nta.nhs.uk/publications/documents/nta_needs_assessment_manual_july_06.pdf) Accessed on 27.07.07.
29. Pascoe, G. (1983). Patient satisfaction in primary health care: a literature review and analysis. *Evaluation and Program Planning*, **6**, 185–210.
30. Marsden, J., Farrell, M., Bradbury, C., *et al.* (2007). The Treatment Outcomes Profile (TOP): A structured interview for the evaluation of substance misuse treatment. London: National Treatment Agency for Substance Misuse.

4.3

Schizophrenia and acute transient psychotic disorders

Contents

4.3.1 Schizophrenia: a conceptual history
Nancy C. Andreasen

4.3.2 Descriptive clinical features of schizophrenia
Peter F. Liddle

4.3.3 The clinical neuropsychology of schizophrenia
Philip D. Harvey and Christopher R. Bowie

4.3.4 Diagnosis, classification, and differential diagnosis of schizophrenia
Anthony S. David

4.3.5 Epidemiology of schizophrenia
Assen Jablensky

4.3.6 Aetiology

4.3.6.1 Genetic and environmental risk factors for schizophrenia
R. M. Murray and D. J. Castle

4.3.6.2 The neurobiology of schizophrenia
Paul J. Harrison

4.3.7 Course and outcome of schizophrenia and their prediction
Assen Jablensky

4.3.8 Treatment and management of schizophrenia
D. G. Cunningham Owens and E. C. Johnstone

4.3.9 Schizoaffective and schizotypal disorders
Ming T. Tsuang, William S. Stone, and Stephen V. Faraone

4.3.10 Acute and transient psychotic disorders
J. Garrabé and F.-R. Cousin

4.3.1 Schizophrenia: a conceptual history

Nancy C. Andreasen

We know that psychotic disorders have been present and publicly recognized at least since classical times because of their portrayals in literature: the madness of Medea, the frenzied behaviour in *The Bacchae*, or the paranoia of Othello. Perhaps the most 'valid' portrayal from a modern clinical perspective is the feigned madness of 'Poor Tom' in King Lear. Poor Tom is a 'bedlam beggar' who encounters Lear during the great scenes of madness, portrayed while the world itself is also in the midst of a terrible storm. Tom's speech is a classical example of schizophrenic thought disorder, but he also experiences delusions and visual hallucinations:

> Who gives anything to poor Tom? Whom the foul fiend hath led through fire and through flame, and through ford and whirlpool, o'er bog and quagmire, that hast laid knives under his pillow, and halters in his pew; set ratsbane by his porridge; made him proud of heart, to ride on a bay trotting-horse over four-inch'd bridges, to course his own shadow for a traitor. Bless thy five wits! Tom's a-cold, –O, do de, do de, do de. Bless thee from whirlwinds, star-blasting, and taking! Do poor Tom some charity, whom the foul fiend vexes. There could I have him now, –and there, –and there again, and there. (*King Lear*, III. iv. 51–60)

However, the definition and delineation of schizophrenia as a discrete disorder is a relatively recent phenomenon.

The founding fathers of the concept: Kraepelin and Bleuler

The earliest academic formulations of the concept of schizophrenia occurred in the mid-nineteenth century in the work of Bénédict-Auguste Morel and Karl Kahlbaum.[1] Morel coined the term 'démence precoce' to refer to a disorder that he observed in young people that was characterized by cognitive impairments and progressive degeneration. He did not develop the concept fully, however. Instead, under the influence of Darwinian thinking, he became preoccupied with the general concept of hereditary degeneration, which he described in disorders ranging from intellectual disability to alcoholism. This general concept was highly influential throughout the nineteenth and early twentieth century, which led to some of the earliest studies of the familiality of mental illnesses, and laid early foundations for later efforts to examine the role of genetic factors in schizophrenia. Kahlbaum's seminal contribution was an emphasis on using course of illness (as opposed to symptoms) to define discrete disorders. He objected to the concept that there was only one form of severe mental illness ('unitary psychosis' or 'einheitspsychose') and argued that various kinds of psychotic disorders could be differentiated from one another based on changing patterns of symptoms and long-term outcome. Kahlbaum identified one type as 'hebephrenia'.

Our modern concept of schizophrenia primarily derives, however, from the interaction between two great clinicians early in the twentieth century: Emil Kraepelin and Eugen Bleuler.

Although his ideas were presaged by Morel and Kahlbaum, Emil Kraepelin was clearly the first to give a detailed description of this syndrome and a compelling justification for its delineation. Kraepelin highlighted his concept of the key features of the disorder in the name that he chose for it: It was an illness that tended to begin at an early age ('praecox') and to have a relatively chronic course characterized by significant cognitive and social impairment ('dementia'). Alois Alzheimer was a member of Kraepelin's department in Munich and used the tools of neuropathology to study a similar dementia that began at a later age; examination of the brains of these individuals at post-mortem revealed a characteristic neural signature—plaques and tangles. Kraepelin began to call this disorder Alzheimer's disease and thus gave it its current name, as well as its differentiation from dementia praecox. A similar neuropathological signature was sought for dementia praecox, but it was never found, although Kraepelin hypothesized that it must be a disease involving prefrontal and temporal regions[2]:

> If it should be demonstrated that the disease attacks by preference the frontal areas of the brain, the central convolutions and the temporal lobes, this distribution would in a certain measure agree with our present views about the site of the psychic mechanisms which are principally injured by the disease. (p. 219)

Kraepelin did not select any specific clinical feature as pathognomic, but he did stress the importance of several symptoms as characteristic:

> . . . there are apparently two principal groups of disorders which characterise the malady. On the one hand we observe a *weakening of those emotional activities which permanently form the mainsprings of volition*. In connection with this, mental activity and instinct for occupation become mute. The result of this part of the morbid process is emotional dullness, failure of mental activities, loss of mastery over volition, of endeavor, and of ability for independent action.

> The second group of disorders . . . consists in the *loss of the inner unity* of the activities of intellect, emotion, and volition in themselves and among one another ... the near connection between thinking and feeling, between deliberation and emotional activity on the one hand, and practical work on the other is more or less lost. Emotions do not correspond to ideas. The patients laugh and weep without recognizable cause, without any relation to their circumstances and their experiences, smile while they narrate the tale of their attempts at suicide . . . (pp. 74–5).

Thus, for Kraepelin, what we now refer to as negative symptoms and fragmenting of thought were two key features of the disorder.

Bleuler was a near contemporary of Kraepelin. During their two long careers they maintained a dialogue between their native countries of Germany and Switzerland. Kraepelin was a thoroughgoing empiricist with a keen eye for detail, while Bleuler was primarily a high-level conceptualizer, although he clearly also had vast clinical experience. Bleuler chose to highlight fragmenting of thinking as the most fundamental feature of schizophrenia and designated it as the pathognomonic symptom. That is, he explicitly stated that this particular symptom ('loosening of associations') was present in all patients with schizophrenia and did not occur in other disorders. Because of the importance that he gave to this particular symptom, he renamed the illness after it (schizophrenia = fragmenting of mind). To this symptom, he added several others that he also considered to be of high importance. These included loss of volition, impairment in attention, ambivalence, autism, and affective blunting. He regarded these symptoms as basic or fundamental and the other symptoms observed in the disorder, such as delusions or hallucinations, as secondary or accessory. He pointed out that these accessory symptoms tended to occur in a variety of other conditions, such as manic-depressive illness, delirium, or dementia.

> Certain symptoms of schizophrenia are present in every case and in every period of the illness even though, as with every other disease symptom, they must have attained a certain degree of intensity before they can be recognized with any certainty . . . Besides the specific permanent or fundamental symptoms, we can find a host of other, more accessory manifestations such as delusions, hallucinations, or catatonic symptoms . . . As far as we know, the fundamental symptoms are characteristic of schizophrenia, while the accessory symptoms may also appear in other types of illness (p. 13).

Bleuler's conceptualization of the disorder captured the imagination of clinicians and investigators throughout the world, and the name he chose for the disorder eventually became the one that is now universally used. The prophecy of Kraepelin's tombstone came true: 'though his name will be forgotten, his work will live on'. During the much of the twentieth century, Bleuler's conceptualization and terminology prevailed. Although he drew on Kraepelinian concepts, very few people were aware of the magnitude of Kraepelin's contributions. Students of schizophrenia used Bleuler's name for the disorder and defined it in terms of 'the four A's' (associations, autism, affect, and ambivalence).

Schneiderian symptoms, psychosis, and the dominance of diagnostic criteria

The Bleulerian emphasis slowly began to change, however, beginning in the late 1960s and 1970s. This change in emphasis arose primarily from an interest in improving diagnostic precision and reliability. Because they are essentially 'all or none' phenomena, which are relatively easy to recognize and define, florid psychotic symptoms such as delusions and hallucinations were steadily given greater prominence and indeed even placed at the forefront of the definition of schizophrenia. Bleuler's secondary or accessory symptoms began to be treated as the pathognomonic symptoms.

The emphasis on florid psychotic symptoms arose because of the influence of Kurt Schneider and the interpretation of his thinking by influential British psychiatrists. Schneider was greatly influenced by the work of Karl Jaspers, who explored phenomenology and created a bridge between psychiatry and philosophy. Jaspers believed that the essence of psychosis was the experience of phenomena that were 'nonunderstandable'—i.e. symptoms that a 'normal' person could not readily imagine experiencing. Schneider, like Bleuler, wished to identify symptoms that were fundamental. He concluded that one critical component was an inability to find the boundaries between self and not-self and a loss of the sense of personal autonomy. This led him to discuss various 'first-rank' symptoms that were characterized by this loss of autonomy, such as thought insertion or delusions of being controlled by outside forces.[3–5]

Schneiderian ideas were introduced to the English-speaking world by British investigators and began to exert a powerful influence on the concept of schizophrenia. An emphasis on Schneiderian first-rank symptoms satisfied the fundamental need to find an anchor in the perplexing flux of the phenomenology of schizophrenia. Schneiderian symptoms were incorporated into the first major structured interview developed for use in the International Pilot Study of Schizophrenia, the Present State Examination (PSE).[6] From this major base, they were thereafter introduced into other standard diagnostic instruments such as the Schedule for Affective Disorders and Schizophrenia (SADS),[7] Research Diagnostic Criteria (RDC),[8] and the *Diagnostic and Statistical Manual* (*DSM-III*).[9]

The emphasis on positive symptoms, and especially Schneiderian symptoms, derived from several concerns. The first was that Bleulerian symptoms were difficult to define and rate reliably. They are often continuous with normality, while positive psychotic symptoms were clearly abnormal. In addition to concerns about reliability, work with the IPSS and the US/UK study also had indicated that in the United States the concept of schizophrenia had broadened to an excessive degree, particularly in the Northeastern parts of the United States. Thus, in the United States, there was clearly a need to narrow the concept of schizophrenia. Stressing florid psychotic symptoms, particularly Schneiderian symptoms, was a useful way to achieve this end, since it appeared that schizophrenia was often being diagnosed on the basis of mild Bleulerian symptoms. When diagnostic criteria such as the RDC and later *DSM-III* were written, these placed a substantial emphasis on positive symptoms and minimized negative symptoms.

While there have been many good consequences of this progression and of the interest in Schneider's work, there have also been problems.

From a Schneiderian perspective, Schneider's work and point of view has been oversimplified and even misunderstood. As a Jasperian phenomenologist, Schneider was in fact deeply interested in the subjective experience of schizophrenia—in understanding the internal psychological processes that troubled his patients. For him, the fundamental core of the illness was not the specific first-rank symptoms themselves, but rather the internal cognitive and emotional state that they reflected. It is somewhat ironic that he has become the symbol of objective quantification and reductionism. He himself was a complex thinker who was concerned about individual patients.

The development of diagnostic criteria for schizophrenia has also had both advantages and disadvantages. When *DSM-III* was originally developed, it was intended only as a 'provisional consensus agreement' based on clinical judgement. The criteria were created by a small group of individuals who reached a decision about what to include based on a mixture of clinical experience and research data available up to that point. The criteria were chosen to serve as a gatekeeper that would include or exclude individual cases, and they were not intended to be a full description of the illness. Unfortunately, they are now sometimes treated as a textbook of psychiatry. Further, the criteria have become reified and given a power that they originally were never intended to have.

Diagnostic criteria have substantial and undeniable advantages, they improve reliability, provide a basis for cross-centre standardization both nationally and internationally, improve clinical communication, and facilitate research. However, they may also have potential disadvantages and even abuses: they provide an oversimplified and incomplete view of the clinical picture, discourage clinical sensitivity to individual patients and comprehensive history-taking, lead students and even clinicians to believe that 'knowing the criteria is enough', reify an agreement that was only intended to be provisional, and discourage creative or innovative thinking about the psychological and neural mechanisms of schizophrenia.

The concept of positive and negative symptoms

Neither Kraepelin nor Bleuler actually used the terms 'positive symptoms' or 'negative symptoms', although the concepts are embedded in their writings. While various sources for this term can be cited,[10] one of the earliest and most prominent was Hughlings-Jackson.[11] Although Jackson's work was not published until much later, in the late nineteenth century Jackson speculated about the mechanisms that might underlie psychotic symptoms:

> Disease is said to 'cause' the symptoms of insanity. I submit that disease only produces negative mental symptoms, answering to the dissolution, and that all elaborate positive mental symptoms (illusions, hallucinations, delusions, and extravagant conduct) are the outcome of activity of nervous elements untouched by any pathological process; that they arise during activity on the lower level of evolution remaining.

Thus Jackson believed that some symptoms represented a relatively pure loss of function (negative symptoms answer to the dissolution), while positive symptoms such as delusions and hallucinations represented an exaggeration of normal function and might represent release phenomena. Jackson presented these ideas at a time when Darwinian evolutionary theories were achieving ascendance, and his concepts concerning the mechanisms that produced the various symptoms were clearly shaped by a Darwinian view that the brain is organized in hierarchical evolutionary layers. Positive symptoms represent aberrations in a primitive (perhaps limbic) substrate that is for some reason no longer monitored by higher cortical functions. Thus Jackson's concept of negative versus positive symptoms rather closely resembles those which are currently discussed. Although today most investigators do not necessarily embrace the specific mechanism that he proposed, they accept his view that they must be understood in terms of brain mechanisms, as well as his basic descriptive psychopathology.

References to positive and negative symptoms occurred sporadically during the 1970s, sometimes making clear references to Jackson's ideas and sometimes simply presenting notions about the clinical meaning of the distinction. Notable examples include the descriptions of Fish,(3) a reference to the terms by Strauss and others,(12) and Iowa work on affective blunting and on thought disorder, classifying it as positive versus negative.(13, 14)

In 1980, Crow published an influential paper describing a two syndrome hypothesis of schizophrenia using the terms 'positive' and 'negative' symptoms.(15) He proposed that schizophrenia could be divided into two different syndromes, which he referred to as Type I and Type II. Type I schizophrenia was characterized by prominent positive symptoms, an acute onset, good premorbid adjustment, a good response to treatment, intact cognition, intact brain structure, and an underlying mechanism that was neurochemical (dopaminergic) and therefore reversible. Type II schizophrenia was characterized by prominent negative symptoms, an insidious onset, poor premorbid adjustment, a poor response to treatment, impaired cognition, structural brain abnormalities (i.e. ventricular enlargement as visualized by Computerized Tomography [CT]), and an underlying mechanism that was characterized by neuronal loss and therefore irreversible. This proposal was highly generative for research in schizophrenia during the 1980s, primarily because it combined speculations about clinical presentation and about underlying neural mechanisms within a single hypothesis.

Two major problems were inherent in Crow's presentation of this hypothesis, however, which initially limited its empirical testing. One problem was its failure to specify a clear method for measuring positive and negative symptoms, and the second was its failure to indicate which of the broad array of variables associated with each of the two syndromes should be considered dependent or independent. Which symptoms of schizophrenia should be considered to be positive and which negative? Which variable—or group of variables—should be used to define the separate syndromes and test whether the hypothesized relationships were present?

Solutions to these problems were proposed by the investigative team at the University of Iowa.(16) Reliable methods for defining and differentiating positive and negative thought disorder and other negative symptoms such as affective blunting had already been developed at Iowa(13, 14) and the research group there also had a long tradition of developing diagnostic criteria. Consequently, we developed structured scales for the assessment of both positive and negative symptoms, the Scale for the Assessment of Negative Symptoms (SANS) and the Scale for the Assessment of Positive Symptoms (SAPS).(16–18) These scales were intended to provide a more comprehensive, reliable, and well-anchored set of measurements for the evaluation of psychopathology in schizophrenia than had been provided by standard instruments such as the Brief Psychiatric Rating Scale (BPRS).(19) They were subjected to rigorous assessment of their psychometric properties, including internal consistency, reliability, and validity. They were quickly translated into a variety of languages and widely used throughout the world.

In addition, a solution to the second problem was implemented by using a standard strategy in the study of psychopathology: the core clinical syndrome would be treated as the independent variable, while the various associated features would be (somewhat arbitrarily) designated as dependent. To this end, criteria were developed that could be used to classify schizophrenic patients as positive, negative, or mixed. Initial work with these criteria suggested that this strategy could be quite useful.(16, 17) As Crow hypothesized, negative patients differed from positive patients in the predicted direction: larger ventricular brain ratio (VBR), poorer premorbid adjustment, lower educational achievement, and poorer cognitive performance. Many subsequent studies continued to explore the two syndrome hypothesis, with the majority confirming at least some aspects of it. However, other problems with this hypothesis also became evident. Perhaps the most vexing for the hypothesis, and for the application of criteria to categorize patients based on clinical presentation, was the large number of patients with a mixture of positive and negative symptoms. The hypothesis had difficulty in explaining how patients who were both positive and negative could have both reversible and irreversible abnormalities, good and poor premorbid adjustment, and other counterintuitive and contradictory findings. For these reasons, most investigators have regretfully abandoned this appealingly simple and heuristic hypothesis during recent years.

However, the clinical distinction between positive and negative symptoms has remained relatively robust. The tendency to distinguish between these two classes of symptoms has become widespread, and the terms have passed into standard clinical usage. The alacrity with which the terms have been adopted suggests that they fill a useful linguistic and conceptual niche. Negative symptoms are an important component of schizophrenia, and the use of the 'positive' and 'negative' terminology gives them recognition and even equal weight. As the Bleulerian symptoms received de-emphasis because of concerns about reliability, they left a void in the descriptive lexicon. Patients were designated as having 'recovered' when their delusions and hallucinations were no longer present or prominent; yet many remained unemployed, unable to return to school, or socially isolated. What might explain this outcome if their symptoms were genuinely absent? Upon reflection, it became evident that only some of their symptoms were absent, and that a group of 'no name' symptoms were the likely explanation. If these symptoms could be named 'negative', grouped together, measured objectively and reliably, and related to outcome and treatment, an important mechanism for clinical description and communication was restored. Although the oversimplified distinction between positive and negative implied in the two syndrome hypothesis might be misleading, it was useful to recognize that some symptoms tend to get patients hospitalized and to call these 'positive' and that other symptoms tend to lead to psychosocial morbidity and to call these 'negative'. Thus the distinction at the level of symptoms (as opposed to syndromes or disease categories) is helpful descriptively.

The distinction has also persisted because standardized and reliable methods have been developed for assessing these symptoms and placing them in broad general classes. Instruments such as the SANS and SAPS have facilitated the persistence of the terminology because they have provided the tools for rating and measuring. Although tools were at hand for most positive symptoms, no scale was available at all for negative symptoms prior to the SANS. The extensive and repeated documentation of its reliability has quieted concerns that negative symptoms are too 'soft' to be assessed precisely, accurately, and objectively. Furthermore, other simpler scales, targeted primarily for use in clinical drug trials, have also been developed.[20] By the time that *DSM-IV*[21] and *ICD*-10[22] were written, the concept of positive and negative symptoms was so widely accepted that negative symptoms were included in their diagnostic criteria for the first time.

Beyond diagnostic criteria and the search for fundamental mechanisms

As the present moves towards the future, corrective readjustments are continuing to occur. Paradoxically, these often occur by returning to the past and coming back full circle to the work of Kraepelin, Bleuler, Jackson, and Schneider.

Clinically, the emphasis on negative as well as psychotic symptoms is leading to increased interest in the full range of symptoms of schizophrenia and in developing methods for treating that full range. In particular, there has been a growing interest in developing improved treatments for negative symptoms. The interest in negative symptoms has been complemented by a return to an interest in cognitive aspects of schizophrenia. Many negative symptoms are cognitive in nature—alogia (poverty of thought and speech), avolition (inability to formulate plans and pursue them), and attentional impairment. While their assessment may emphasize objective aspects of behaviour in order to achieve reliability, their underlying essence is in the domains of thought and emotion. Increasingly, therefore, investigators are returning to the original insights of Kraepelin and Bleuler that the core symptoms of schizophrenia represent a fundamental deficit in cognition and emotion.

Several prominent investigators have turned from a focus on explaining and 'localizing' the specific symptoms of schizophrenia to a search for more fundamental underlying cognitive mechanisms.[23] Examples include Frith's hypotheses concerning an inability to think in 'metarepresentations',[24] Goldman-Rakic's studies of working memory,[25] our descriptions of cognitive dysmetria Andreasen,[26] or the work of Holzman,[27] Braff,[28] Swerdlow and Geyer,[29] and Freedman[30] on information processing and attention. These cognitive models provide a general theory of the disease that is consistent with its diversity of symptoms, permit testing in human beings with a variety of convergent techniques (e.g. imaging, neurophysiology), and even permit modelling in animals. This efficient and parsimonious approach offers consider hope for the future because it facilitates the search both for improved treatments and for molecular mechanisms.

Further information

Ackerknect, E. (1959). *A short history of psychiatry*, Hafner, New York.

Zilboorg, G. (1967). *A history of medical psychology*, WW Norton, New York.

References

1. Shorter, E. (1997). *A history of psychiatry: from the era of the asylum to the age of prozac.* John Wiley & Sons, New York.
2. Kraepelin, E., Barclay, R.M., and Robertson, G.M. (1919). *Dementia praecox and paraphrenia.* E. & S. Livingstone, Edinburgh.
3. Fish, F.J. (1962). *Schizophrenia.* Williams and Wilkins, Baltimore.
4. Mellor, C.S. (1970). First rank symptoms of schizophrenia. I. The frequency in schizophrenics on admission to hospital. II. Differences between individual first rank symptoms. *The British Journal of Psychiatry*, **117**(536), 15–23.
5. Schneider, K. (1959). *Clinical psychopathology.* Grune & Stratton, New York.
6. Wing, J.K., Cooper, J.E., and Sartorius, N. (1974). *Measurement and classification of psychiatric symptoms; an instruction manual for the PSE and Catego Program.* Cambridge University Press, New York, London.
7. Endicott, J. and Spitzer, R.L. (1978). A diagnostic interview: the schedule for affective disorders and schizophrenia. *Archives of General Psychiatry*, **35**(7), 837–44.
8. Spitzer, R.L., Endicott, J., and Robins, E. (1978). Research diagnostic criteria: rationale and reliability. *Archives of General Psychiatry*, **35**(6), 773–82.
9. Association AP, Statistics CoNa. (1980). *Diagnostic and statistical manual of mental disorders* (*DSM-III*) (3rd edn). American Psychiatric Association, Washington, DC.
10. Berrios, G.E. (1985). Positive and negative symptoms and Jackson. A conceptual history. *Archives of General Psychiatry*, **42**(1), 95–7.
11. Hughlings-Jackson, J. (1931). In *Selected writings of John Hughlings Jackson* (ed. J. Taylor). Hodder & Stoughton, Ltd., London.
12. Strauss, J.S., Carpenter, W.T. Jr, and Bartko, J.J. (1974). The diagnosis and understanding of schizophrenia. Part III. Speculations on the processes that underlie schizophrenic symptoms and signs. *Schizophrenia Bulletin*, **11**, 61–9.
13. Andreasen, N.C. (1979). Thought, language, and communication disorders. I. Clinical assessment, definition of terms, and evaluation of their reliability. *Archives of General Psychiatry*, **36**(12), 1315–21.
14. Andreasen, N.C. (1979). Affective flattening and the criteria for schizophrenia. *The American Journal of Psychiatry*, **136**(7), 944–7.
15. Crow, T.J. (1980). Positive and negative schizophrenic symptoms and the role of dopamine. *The British Journal of Psychiatry*, **137**, 383–6.
16. Andreasen, N.C. and Olsen, S. (1982). Negative v positive schizophrenia. Definition and validation. *Archives of General Psychiatry*, **39**(7), 789–94.
17. Andreasen, N.C. (1982). Negative symptoms in schizophrenia. Definition and reliability. *Archives of General Psychiatry*, **39**(7), 784–8.
18. Andreasen, N.C. (1987). The diagnosis of schizophrenia. *Schizophrenia Bulletin*, **13**(1), 9–22.
19. Overall, J.E. and Gorham, D.R. (1962). The brief psychiatric rating scale. *Psychological Reports*, **10**, 799–812.
20. Kay, S.R., Fiszbein, A., and Opler, L.A. (1987). The positive and negative syndrome scale (PANSS) for schizophrenia. *Schizophrenia Bulletin*, **13**(2), 261–76.
21. American Psychiatric Association. (1994). *Diagnostic and statistical manual of mental disorders, fourth edition* (*DSM-IV*) (4th edn). American Psychiatric Press, Inc., Washington, DC.
22. World Health Organization. (1990). Chapter V, mental and behavioral disorders (including disorders of psychological development): diagnosis criteria for research. International classification of diseases, tenth edition (ICD-10). Geneva.
23. Andreasen, N.C. (1997). Linking mind and brain in the study of mental illnesses: a project for a scientific psychopathology. *Science*, **275**(5306), 1586–93.
24. Frith, C.D. (1992). The cognitive neuropsychology of schizophrenia. Lawrence Erlbaum, East Sussix.
25. Goldman-Rakic, P.S. (1994). Working memory dysfunction in schizophrenia. *The Journal of Neuropsychiatry and Clinical Neuroscience*, **6**(4), 348–57.
26. Andreasen, N.C., Nopoulos, P., O'Leary, D.S., *et al.* (1999). Defining the phenotype of schizophrenia: cognitive dysmetria and its neural mechanisms. *Biological Psychiatry*, **46**(7), 908–20.
27. Holzman, P.S., Levy, D.L., and Proctor, L.R. (1976). Smooth pursuit eye movements, attention, and schizophrenia. *Archives of General Psychiatry*, **33**(12), 1415–20.
28. Braff, D.L. (1993). Information processing and attention dysfunctions in schizophrenia. *Schizophrenia Bulletin*, **19**(2), 233–59.

29. Swerdlow, N.R. and Geyer, M.A. (1993). Clozapine and haloperidol in an animal model of sensorimotor gating deficits in schizophrenia. *Pharmacology, Biochemistry, and Behavior*, **44**(3), 741–4.
30. Freedman, R., Waldo, M., Bickford-Wimer, P., *et al.* (1991). Elementary neuronal dysfunctions in schizophrenia. *Schizophrenia Research*, **4**(2), 233–43.

4.3.2. Descriptive clinical features of schizophrenia

Peter F. Liddle

The clinical features of schizophrenia embrace a diverse range of disturbances of perception, thought, emotion, motivation, and motor activity. It is an illness in which episodes of florid disturbance are usually set against a background of sustained disability. The level of chronic disability ranges from a mild decrease in the ability to cope with stress, to a profound difficulty in initiating and organizing activity that can render patients unable to care for themselves.

Disorders of thought and perception

Delusions

Although there are no features that provide an unambiguous distinction between the delusions of schizophrenia and those of other psychotic illnesses, the delusions most typical of schizophrenia have an enigmatic character rarely seen in other disorders. In contrast to the delusions of affective psychosis, which usually have content consistent with the prevailing emotional state, in schizophrenia delusions often appear to reflect a fragmented experience of reality. This fragmentation is manifest in several ways.

- There is a lack of logical consistency between the components of the belief, or between the belief and common understanding of what is possible. For example, a patient was very distressed by the belief that he had no head and also that there was blood all over his face.
- Behaviour bears an unpredictable relationship to the delusional belief. In some instances, the patient believes he has a special role or identity, yet for the most part, lives a life that is scarcely influenced by the belief. In the words of Bleuler[1]: 'Kings, Emperors, Popes, and Redeemers engage for the most part, in quite banal work, provided they still have any energy at all for activity'.
- In the chronic phase of the illness, patients might acknowledge that a former delusion was not justified, yet in the same interview they reiterate the delusional belief. Bleuler[1] reported: 'sometimes the patients even produce thoughts which are only understandable if it is assumed that the delusions still retain some reality for these patients even though consciously they may reject them'.

The mental mechanism of schizophrenic delusions remains to be ascertained. It is not a lack of capacity for logical thought; rather it appears that certain ideas acquire an attribute that exempts them from the normal processes of validation. This phenomenon is illustrated by the historic case of Daniel Schreber,[2] a high-ranking judge from Leipzig, who suffered a late-onset schizophrenic illness. After obtaining a court order for discharge from his second hospital admission he published his memoirs[3] in a volume that includes his own account of his beliefs, and also the report prepared by the asylum director, Dr Weber, opposing his discharge. For the purpose of understanding the nature of delusions in schizophrenia, Schreber's account is of special value because we have access to his own perceptions of his condition in addition to detailed accounts by his physician. Dr Weber reported that Schreber exhibited lively interest in his social environment, a well-informed mind, and sound judgement, while nonetheless maintaining his delusional beliefs in a manner that would accept no contrary argument. Schreber himself agreed that his beliefs were unchangeable. He believed that he had a mission to redeem the world and restore humankind to its lost state of bliss. His system of delusions included the belief that he was being transformed into a voluptuous female partner of God. He considered that his beliefs belonged to a domain that was exempt from normal logic: 'I could even say with Jesus Christ: My kingdom is not of this world; my so-called delusions are concerned solely with God and the beyond'. Furthermore, he maintained total conviction in his core beliefs despite recognizing that his experiences earlier in his illness had been unrealistic. He stated:

> Having lived for months among miracles, I was inclined to take more or less everything I saw for a miracle. Accordingly, I did not know whether to take the streets of Leipzig through which I traveled as only theatre props, perhaps in the fashion in which Prince Potemkin is said to have put them up for Empress Catherine II of Russia during her travels through the desolate country, so as to give the impression of a flourishing countryside.

Thus, in the stable phase of his illness, Schreber recognized that his earlier experiences were unrealistic and that his current beliefs defied normal logic, but appeared to regard them as exempt from the need for validation. The late onset of his illness and his high level of professional achievement are unusual for an individual with schizophrenia, and raise questions about the diagnosis. However, the fact that he eventually suffered a marked deterioration in function during his third episode of illness strongly supports the diagnosis of schizophrenia.

In many instances, the delusions of schizophrenia appear to arise from an altered experience of self. The phenomena identified by the German psychiatrist, Kurt Schneider[4] as first-rank symptoms of schizophrenia (discussed in greater detail below) include several symptoms that entail an aberrant experience of ownership of one's own thought, will, action, emotion, or bodily function, which the patient attributes to alien influence. In some cases, delusions might arise from a delusional mood, i.e. an altered sense of reality in which the current circumstances acquire an indefinable transcendental quality.

Although the delusions most characteristic of schizophrenia have an incongruous quality, it is not uncommon for schizophrenic patients to have coherent delusions that are internally consistent and produce predictable behavioural responses. In particular, coherent persecutory delusions are common, and can lead to defensive actions such barricading oneself in one's room with blinds drawn. Ideas of reference and delusions of reference are also prevalent. For example, a patient might report that television programmes refer specifically to him or her. In the International Pilot Study of Schizophrenia[5] conducted by the World Health Organization, ideas of reference were reported in 70 per cent of cases, suspiciousness in 66 per cent, and delusions of persecution in 64 per cent.

Hallucinations

Hallucinations in any modality can occur, but auditory hallucinations are the most prevalent in schizophrenia. Hearing voices speaking in the third person is the most specific. This experience is listed among the Schneiderian first-rank symptoms. Sometimes the content is mundane, as in the instance when a patient of Bleuler[1] heard a voice saying 'Now she is combing her hair' while she was grooming in the morning. In other instances there is an implied criticism, as in the case reported by Schneider[4] of a woman who heard a voice saying 'Now she is eating; here she is munching again', whenever she wanted to eat.

Second-person auditory hallucinations are also common. In the International Pilot Study of Schizophrenia,[5] voices speaking to the patient were reported in 65 per cent of cases. Voices might issue commands that the patient obeys. In some instances, the patient engages in a dialogue with the voices.

During the acute phase of illness, auditory hallucinations usually have the same sensory quality as voices arising from sources in the external world. In some instances the voice is attributed to a radio-transmitter implanted in the body, especially in the teeth. In the chronic phase, the voices are often recognized as coming from within the person's own mind. Kraepelin[6] reports: 'at other times they do not appear to the patient as sense perceptions at all; they are 'voices of conscience'; 'voices which do not speak with words''. These experiences are pseudohallucinations, but nonetheless they are a significant feature in many cases.

In schizophrenia, visual hallucinations are less common than auditory hallucinations, but do occur. Somatic hallucinations are also relatively common, and often are associated with a delusional misinterpretation. For example, a young man reported sensations in his belly that he attributed to a snake, which he believed had crawled up his anus.

Schneiderian first-rank symptoms

Kurt Schneider[4] identified a set of phenomena that he considered were strongly indicative of schizophrenia in the absence of overt brain disease. These symptoms, listed in Table 4.3.2.1, have become known as first-rank symptoms. Schneider did not consider that the diagnosis could be made simply on the presence of one such symptom; on the contrary, he warned,[4] 'a psychotic phenomenon is not like a defective stone in an otherwise perfect mosaic'. Schneider did not define the phenomena precisely, and clinicians have interpreted his writings differently. Mellor[7] formulated a precise set of definitions and found that, according to these strict criteria, 72 per cent of patients with schizophrenia exhibited at least one first-rank symptom. Applying the same criteria, O'Grady[8] found that in a series of cases assessed at admission to hospital, 73 per cent of schizophrenic patients exhibited at least one first-rank symptom, while no cases of affective psychosis did. However, applying less strict criteria, O'Grady found more broadly defined first-rank symptoms in 14 per cent of patients with affective psychosis.

Table 4.3.2.1 Schneiderian first-rank symptoms

Voices commenting—a hallucinatory voice commenting on one's actions in the third person
Voices discussing or arguing—hallucinations of two or more voices discussing or arguing about oneself
Audible thought—hearing one's thoughts aloud
Thought insertion—the insertion, by an alien sources, of thoughts that are experienced as not being one's own
Thought withdrawal—the withdrawal of thoughts from one's mind by an alien agency
Thought broadcast—the experience that one's thoughts are broadcast so as to be accessible to others
Made will—the experience of one's will being controlled by an alien influence
Made acts—the experience that acts executed by one's own body are the actions of an alien agency, rather than oneself
Made affect—the experience of emotion that is not one's own, attributed to an alien influence
Somatic passivity—bodily function is controlled by an alien influence
Delusional perception—the attribution of a totally unwarranted meaning to a normal perception

Three of the first-rank symptoms (voices commenting, voices discussing, and audible thoughts) involve auditory hallucinations, while the remainder entail delusional attributions to experiences or perceptions. Although Schneider himself avoided speculating on the theoretical implications of these phenomena, it is notable that most of them involve a disorder of the sense of ownership of one's own mental or physical activity. Thought broadcast, thought withdrawal, and thought insertion reflect the experience of loss of autonomy over thought, while made will, made acts, made affect, and somatic passivity reflect loss of autonomy over action, will, affect, and bodily function.

Mellor[7] emphasizes that there are two aspects to these phenomena: the experience of loss of autonomy and the delusional attribution to alien influence. As an illustration of made acts, Mellor reports a patient who reported that his fingers moved to pick up objects 'but I don't control them ... I sit there watching them move, and they are quite independent, what they do is nothing to do with me. I am just a puppet ... I am just a puppet who is manipulated by cosmic strings'. To illustrate made affect, Mellor quotes a young woman: 'I cry, tears roll down my cheeks and I look unhappy, but inside I have a cold anger because they are using me in this way, and it is not me who is unhappy, but they are projecting unhappiness into my brain'.

Delusional perception, in which an entirely unwarranted conclusion is drawn from a normal perception, illustrates the incongruity between a delusional idea and concurrent mental activity, which is characteristic of schizophrenia. However, the way in which delusional perceptions often crystallize from a delusional mood indicates that it is not merely a matter of illogical inference; the delusional idea is more like a divine revelation. Mellor[7] gives the example of an Irishman who experienced a sense of foreboding while seated at the breakfast table in a lodging house. When another lodger innocently pushed the salt cellar towards him, he suddenly knew this meant that he must return home to greet the Pope who was visiting his family to thank them because Our Lord was to be born again to one of the women.

Disorders of the form and flow of thought

The speech of schizophrenic patients is often difficult to understand because of abnormalities of form of the underlying thought. However, the clinical assessment of thought form disorder remains a major challenge. This is due in part to the fact the essential features of formal thought disorder in schizophrenia have yet to be defined in a fully satisfactory manner. Furthermore, thought disorder is usually manifest during spontaneous speech, making it difficult to create circumstances in which the phenomena can be elicited reliably.

Bleuler[1] coined the term loosening of associations to describe the weakening of the connections between words and ideas that bind thoughts into a coherent whole. While this term is a useful label for one of the major types of disorder of the form of speech and thought, it does not encompass the entire range of such disorders. In addition to disordered connections between words and ideas, there are oddities in the use of language. One of the most comprehensive catalogues is the Thought, Language, and Communication Scale compiled by Andreasen.[9] This scale includes several items that involve different aspects of the loosening of associations:

- Derailment—wandering off the point during the free flow of conversation
- Tangentiality—answers to questions that are off the point
- Incoherence—a breakdown of the relationships between words within a sentence so that the sentence no longer makes sense
- Loss of goal—failure to reach a conclusion or achieve a point.

The Thought, Language, and Communication Scale also includes several items that refer to unusual use of language:

- Metonyms—unusual uses of words (e.g. hand-shoe instead of glove)
- Neologisms—new words invented by the patient.

The various aspects of loosening of associations and peculiarities of language use are commonly regarded as positive thought disorder. The Thought, Language, and Communication Scale also include negative thought disorders that entail impoverishment of thinking:

- Poverty of speech—a disorder of the flow of speech in which the rate of speech production is reduced
- Poverty of content—the amount of information conveyed is relatively little in proportion to the number of words uttered.

The Thought, Language, and Communication Scale has proved to be one of the most successful of recent attempts to define and quantify formal thought disorder, but it has several limitations. Most important of these is that the positive thought disorder items defined in the scale do not discriminate well between manic thought disorder and florid schizophrenic thought disorder.[10] Secondly, the scale is not sensitive to the subtle thought form disorders that occur in first-degree relatives of schizophrenic patients.

These limitations are dealt with, at least partially, in the Thought Disorder Index devised by Holzman.[11] This scale employs ratings based on thought and speech elicited by the Rorschach inkblot figures and during an assessment of IQ. Two categories of disorder, disorganization (comprising vagueness, confusion, and incoherence) and idiosyncratic verbalizations, appear to discriminate fairly well between schizophrenic and manic thought.[11] Unfortunately, this scale is too cumbersome for routine clinical use.

Positive formal thought disorder is usually a transient feature of acute episodes of illness. Nonetheless, after resolution of the acute episode there is often a subtle residual thought disorder that is manifest as vague, wandering speech, or minor idiosyncrasies of word usage or ideas. Negative formal thought disorder has a greater tendency to be persistent. Chronic poverty of speech is associated with impairment in several domains of cognition[12] including abstract reasoning. It leads to impaired social relationships,[13] although it is also influenced by the social milieu. Transient poverty of speech can occur during acute episodes of illness. At its most severe, the patient is mute.

Insight

Lack of insight is one of the defining characteristics of psychotic illness. Lack of insight entails a failure to accept that one is ill and to appreciate that symptoms are due to illness. In the International Pilot Study of Schizophrenia[5] lack of insight occurred in approximately 90 per cent of cases. Insight is often partial. In particular, even in instances in which a patient acknowledges suffering from an illness, he or she might fail to accept that psychotic symptoms such as delusions or hallucinations are a manifestation of that illness. Lack of insight is one factor that contributes to unwillingness to accept treatment. However, the clinician should be aware that other factors, including lack of appropriate education about the illness and justified fear of side-effects of treatment, can also impede the development of a therapeutic collaboration between physician and patient.

Impaired cognition

In addition to delusions and disorders of thought form, a wide range of cognitive deficits occur in schizophrenia. These are discussed in Chapter 4.3.3. This chapter focuses on the relationship between cognitive impairment and other features of the illness.

In the acute phase of the illness, attentional impairment is common and is often associated with psychomotor excitation and/or formal thought disorder. It might also reflect preoccupation with delusions and hallucinations.

During the chronic phase of illness, many schizophrenic patients exhibit persistent cognitive impairments. Longitudinal studies of individuals who subsequently develop schizophrenia reveal that the deficits are discernible during childhood, suggesting that these deficits are an aspect of the predisposition to schizophrenia. The major cognitive impairments are in the realm of executive function, working memory, and long-term memory. Executive dysfunction includes impaired ability to initiate and select self-generated mental activity. Impaired ability to form and initiate plans is associated with chronic poverty of speech, blunted affect, and lack of spontaneous activity, while impaired ability to inhibit inappropriate responses is associated with chronic formal thought disorder.[12]

Disorders of emotion

An extensive range of disorders of emotion occur in schizophrenia. Blunted affect and inappropriate affect are the most characteristic, and also tend to be the most persistent, but transient excitation, irritability, lability, and depression are also common.

Blunted affect

Blunting of affect is manifest as decreased responsiveness to emotional issues, loss of vocal inflection, and diminished facial expression. These objective signs of affective blunting are sometimes accompanied by awareness of loss of emotional tone that, paradoxically, patients find to be distressing. More commonly, there is a lack of concern and even a lack of awareness of the problem. Affective blunting is one of the hallmarks of chronic schizophrenia. Bleuler[(1)] remarked that when the affects disappear, the illness becomes chronic. While blunted affect is usually chronic, it can also be a feature of acute episodes of the illness that resolves as the acute episode resolves.

Inappropriate affect

Inappropriate or incongruous affect is the expression of affect that is inappropriate in the circumstances. At its most severe it takes the form of hollow laughter that is unrelated to any apparent stimulus.

Excitation and depression

During acute exacerbations of schizophrenia, excitation, manifest as irritability, sleeplessness, agitation, and motor overactivity, is common. Depression is also common around the time of an acute episode of schizophrenia,[(14)] and is often a feature of the prodromal phase of the illness.

Depression also occurs during the chronic phase of the illness. The cross-sectional rate is approximately 10 per cent in the chronic phase,[(15)] while in a longitudinal study, Johnson[(16)] found that 65 per cent of schizophrenic patients exhibited an episode of depression in a period of 36 months after a florid psychotic episode.

Motor disorders and catatonia

Subtle disturbance of motor co-ordination is common. Home videos of children who subsequently develop schizophrenia demonstrate that even in infancy they are noticeably more clumsy than their siblings, suggesting that disturbed motor co-ordination is an aspect of the predisposition to schizophrenia.[(17)]

Catatonia is a term embracing disorders of the initiation or organization of voluntary movement or posture. The most characteristic catatonic phenomena are:

- *Immobility*—absence of motor activity
- *Posturing*—adopting an unusual body posture
- *Waxy flexibility*—allowing an examiner to adjust one's posture, yielding like a warm candle
- *Negativism*—resisting manipulation by an examiner, with force proportional to that applied by the examiner
- *Stereotypy*—aimless repetitive motor behaviour
- *Mannerisms*—apparently purposeful actions that appear odd because they are exaggerated in form or occur out of the usual context
- *Echo phenomena*—repetition of an examiners utterances or movements
- *Excitement*—excessive motor activity, usually accompanied by excessive mental activity.

These disorders can occur not only in schizophrenia, but also in other psychiatric or neurological disorder such as bipolar mood disorder or encephalitis, or alone as a primary disorder of motility.

Kahlbaum[(18)] provided the classic description of catatonia. He emphasized not only the typical phenomena but also a characteristic time course, in which a prodromal phase dominated by melancholic symptoms evolved into a fluctuating disorder in which episodes of diminished motility typically lasting for several weeks or months, were interspersed in periods of near normal function, but with a tendency towards eventual dementia in many cases. Episodes were often accompanied by confusion and in some instances, a state of stupor. In some cases, episodes of excitation occurred as well. While Kahlbaum's emphasis on both characteristic phenomena and time course laid a foundation for the subsequent delineation of major mental illnesses at the end of the nineteenth century and in particular, for Kraepelin's delineation of schizophrenia,[(7)] it is probably best to regard catatonia as a cluster of clinical features that can occur within various different illnesses.

Two major forms are retarded catatonia, characterized by slowed or diminished activity; and excited catatonia in which the dominant feature is excessive motor activity. Many variants of catatonia differing in the relative prominence of the characteristic features; or in the associated features such as autonomic instability; or in time course, have been reported in the past 150 years. Fink and Taylor[(19)] argue on the grounds similarity of clinical features and response to treatment (with benzodiazepines and/or ECT) that the variants of catatonia share a common brain pathophysiology, though different predisposing or precipitating factors might lead to variation in clinical features and time course. The variants include malignant catatonia, in which there is a sudden onset of excitation, associated with fever and autonomic instability, leading to fatal outcome in a substantial proportion of cases. The relationship between malignant catatonia and neuroleptic malignant syndrome (NMS), which is characterized by features very similar to malignant catatonia, but is triggered by antipsychotic medication, is an issue of practical clinical importance. A careful review nine cases of NMS and 17 cases of malignant catatonia by Carroll and Taylor[(20)] failed to find differences in clinical features, supporting the conclusion that NMS is a form of catatonia.

Disorders of volition

Among the most disabling of the clinical phenomena of schizophrenia are disruptions of motivation and will. Voluntary activity can be disjointed or weakened. Disjointed volition is manifest in poorly organized ill-judged activities which appear to be prompted by impulse. For example, an artistic, intelligent young woman felt cold so she lit a fire on the carpet in her bedroom, even though she was able to appreciate that this was a dangerous thing to do.

Weakened volition results in prolonged periods of underactivity. The patient might lie in bed or sit in an armchair for hours.

Anxiety and somatoform disorders

Various forms of anxiety and somatic symptoms are common in schizophrenia. Huber[21] described a non-characteristic defect state which is dominated by anxiety and asthenia. Coenesthesia, in which the patient suffers unusual or debilitating bodily experiences that do not have an apparent somatic cause, occurs frequently.

Dimensions of psychopathology in schizophrenia

Schizophrenia is heterogeneous in its clinical presentation, suggesting that several different pathophysiological processes might contribute to the illness.

Positive and negative symptom dimensions

Positive symptoms are those that reflect the presence of an abnormal mental process, and include delusions, hallucinations, and formal thought disorder. Negative symptoms reflect the diminution or absence of a normal mental function. They include poverty of speech and blunted affect. In schizophrenia, positive symptoms tend to be transient, while negative symptoms tend to be chronic. In an influential hypothesis, Crow[22] proposed that positive symptoms arise from dopaminergic overactivity, while negative symptoms reflect structural brain abnormality. While this hypothesis is consistent with a substantial body of evidence, it does not account adequately for the complexity of the heterogeneity of the clinical features in schizophrenia.

Three dimensions of characteristic symptoms

The preponderance of evidence[12, 13, 23] from factor analysis of schizophrenic symptoms indicates that the characteristic symptoms of schizophrenia segregate into three syndromes, as shown in Table 4.3.2.2. These syndromes do not reflect separate illnesses, but different dimensions of illness, in the sense that a patient might exhibit more than one of the syndromes.

The three syndromes embrace only the characteristic symptoms that are given weight in making a diagnosis of schizophrenia. In addition, there are two affective syndromes, depression and psychomotor excitation, which are prevalent in schizophrenia,[12] despite being more characteristic of mood disorders. These affective syndromes are usually transient.

Table 4.3.2.2 Three syndromes of symptoms characteristic of schizophrenia

Reality distortion
Delusions
Hallucinations
Disorganization
Thought form disorder
Inappropriate affect
Bizarre behaviour
Psychomotor poverty (core negative symptoms)
Poverty of speech
Blunted affect
Decreased spontaneous movement

An accumulating body of evidence[12] from brain imaging studies indicates that the three characteristic syndromes are associated with three distinguishable patterns of cerebral malfunction involving the areas of association cortex and related subcortical nuclei, which serve higher mental functions. In an individual case, several of these neural systems might be involved.

Although many details of the relationships between the diverse clinical features of schizophrenia remain uncertain, a growing understanding of the neural pathways involved is beginning to provide the foundation for understanding the protean manifestations of this disorder.

Further information

Cutting, J. (2003). Descriptive psychopathology. In *Schizophrenia*, Chap. 2 (2nd edn) (eds. S.R. Hirsch and D. Weinberger), pp. 15–24. Blackwell, Oxford.

Fuller, R.L.M., Schultz, S.K., and Andreasen, N.C. (2003). The symptoms of schizophrenia. In *Schizophrenia*, Chap. 3 (2nd edn) (eds. S.R. Hirsch and D. Weinberger), pp. 25–33. Blackwell, Oxford.

References

1. Bleuler, E. (1950). *Dementia praecox or the group of schizophrenias* (trans. J. Zinkin). International Universities Press, New York.
2. Spitzer, R.L., Gibbon, M., Skodol, A.E., *et al.* (eds) (1989). *DSM-IIIR casebook*. American Psychiatric Press, Washington, DC.
3. Schreber, D.P. (1955). *Denkwurdigkeiten eines Nervenkranken (Memoirs of my nervous illness)* (trans. I. Macalpine and R. Hunter). Dawson, London.
4. Schneider, K. (1959). *Clinical psychopathology* (trans. M.W. Hamilton). Grune & Stratton, New York.
5. World Health Organization. (1973). *The international pilot study of schizophrenia*. World Health Organization, Geneva.
6. Kraepelin, E. (1919). *Dementia praecox and paraphrenia* (trans. R.M. Barclay). Facsimile edition, 1971. Kreiger, New York.
7. Mellor, C.S. (1970). First rank symptoms of schizophrenia. *The British Journal of Psychiatry*, **117**, 15–23.
8. O'Grady, J.C. (1990). The prevalence and diagnostic significance of first-rank symptoms in a random sample of acute schizophrenia in-patients. *The British Journal of Psychiatry*, **156**, 496–500.
9. Andreasen, N.C. (1979). Thought language and communication disorders. I. Clinical assessment, definition of terms and evaluation of their reliability. *Archives of General Psychiatry*, **36**, 1315–21.
10. Andreasen, N.C. (1979). Thought, language and communication disorders. II. Diagnostic significance. *Archives of General Psychiatry*, **36**, 1325–30.
11. Holzman, P.S., Shenton, M.E., and Solovay, M.R. (1986). Quality of thought disorder in differential diagnosis. *Schizophrenia Bulletin*, **12**, 360–71.
12. Liddle, P.F. (1999). The multi-dimensional phenotype of schizophrenia. In *Schizophrenia in a molecular age* (ed. C.A. Taminga), pp. 1–28. American Psychiatric Press, Washington, DC.
13. Liddle, P.F. (1987). The symptoms of chronic schizophrenia: a re-examination of the positive-negative dichotomy. *The British Journal of Psychiatry*, **151**, 145–51.
14. Siris, S.G. (1991). Diagnosis of secondary depression in schizophrenia: implications for DSMIV. *Schizophrenia Bulletin*, **17**, 75–98.
15. Barnes, T.R.E., Curson, D.A., Liddle, P.F., *et al.* (1989). The nature and prevalence of depression in chronic schizophrenic inpatients. *The British Journal of Psychiatry*, **154**, 486–91.

16. Johnson, D.A.W. (1988). The significance of depression in the prediction of relapse in chronic schizophrenia. *The British Journal of Psychiatry*, **152**, 320–3.
17. Walker, E. and Lewine, R.J. (1990). Prediction of adult-onset schizophrenia from childhood home videos of the patients. *The American Journal of Psychiatry*, **89**, 704–16.
18. Kahlbaum, K.L. (1874; translated 1973). *Die Katatonie oder das Spannungsirresein*. Verlag August Hirschwald, Berlin, 1874. Translated: Kahlbaum, K. Catatonia. Translated by Y. Levis and T. Pridon. Johns Hopkins University Press, Baltimore, 1973.
19. Fink, M. and Taylor, M.A. (2003). *Catatonia. A clinicians guide to diagnosis and treatment*. Cambridge University Press, Cambridge.
20. Carroll, B.T. and Taylor, B.E. (1997) The nondichotomy between lethal catatonia and neuroleptic malignant syndrome. *Journal of Clinical Psychopharmacology*, **17**, 235–36.
21. Huber, G., Gross, G., and Schuttler, E. (1975). A long term follow-up study of schizophrenia: psychiatric course of illness and prognosis. *Acta Psychiatrica Scandinavica*, **52**, 49–57.
22. Crow, T.J. (1980). The molecular pathology of schizophrenia: more than one disease process. *British Medical Journal*, **280**, 66–8.
23. Arndt, S., Andreasen, N.C., Flaum, M., *et al.* (1995). A longitudinal study of symptom dimensions in schizophrenia. *Archives of General Psychiatry*, **52**, 352–60.

4.3.3 The clinical neuropsychology of schizophrenia

Philip D. Harvey and Christopher R. Bowie

Introduction

Impairments in a variety of cognitive functions are found in patients with schizophrenia. These impairments affect a wide array of different cognitive abilities and are often quite severe, when compared to standards based on healthy individuals of the same age, education levels, and gender. Cognitive impairments appear to be present across the lifespan, detectable at the time of the first treatment episode, if not before, and to manifest a generally stable course over time. Although the current knowledge base regarding cognition in schizophrenia is quite broad, additional research information is constantly accruing. The main purpose of this chapter is to provide a broad overview of the domains, severity, and course of cognitive impairments in schizophrenia, with a focus on functional relevance and treatment possibilities.

History

Cognitive impairments were reported by both Emil Kraepelin and Eugen Bleuer, both of whom noted that they believed that cognitive impairments were amongst the core features of the illness. The conception of dementia praecox introduced by Kraepelin focused on the cognitive and functional deficits in the illness and likened the condition to a condition such as Alzheimer's disease with an earlier onset age. Over the first half of the twentieth century research on cognition in schizophrenia focused on a variety of different topics, including memory, attention, and language skills.(1)

Clinical neuropsychology and schizophrenia

The development of clinical neuropsychology and formalized neuropsychological (NP) tests led to a substantial increase in interest in cognition in schizophrenia. Classical NP ability domains, as well as the types of tests typically used to assess them are presented in Table 4.3.3.1. Clinical NP assessments develop an understanding of areas of relative strength and weakness, comparing current functioning following illness or injury to evidence or estimates regarding prior functioning.(2) Then a profile can be developed, contrasting better or more poorly performed ability areas. Performance across these ability areas can be converted to standard scores, considering demographic factors that influence performance such as age, education level, and sex.(3) Thus, the results of a clinical NP assessment provide a summary of relative strengths and weaknesses. Clinical NP assessment has moved away from earlier efforts to anatomically localize deficits through test performance or to distinguish 'functional' versus 'organic' impairments. The current conception of neuropsychological performance is largely based on the concept of functional neural networks, which link cortical and subcortical regions through patterns of linked activation during task performance.(4)

Table 4.3.3.1 Important cognitive ability domains and tests

Ability areas	Tests
Perceptual skills	Pattern recognition
Motor skills	Manual dexterity
Attention	
Sustained attention	Continuous performance tests
Selective attention	Resistance to distraction
Working memory	
Spatial working memory	Spatial delayed response tests
Verbal working memory	Measures of verbal memory span
Episodic memory	
Verbal memory	List learning; paragraph recall
Non-verbal memory (spatial memory)	Object learning tests
Procedural memory	Pursuit rotor; mirror writing
Long-term semantic memory	Word recognition reading
Executive functions	
Concept formation	Comprehension tests
Reasoning	Proverb interpretation
Problem-solving	Wisconsin card sort; Tower of London
Inhibition	Stroop test
Processing speed	Trail-making; digit symbol
Verbal skills	
Naming	Object naming test
Verbal fluency	Animal naming

Cognitive impairment in schizophrenia

Severity

Patients with schizophrenia demonstrate impaired performance on NP tests measuring a variety of ability areas. As shown in Table 4.3.3.2, impairments across abilities range from mild to severe.(5) Further, aspects of spared functioning are quite rare, with patients performing at levels worse than population means on nearly all domains other than reading skills, object naming, and recognition memory. These impairments are not due to poor motivation or the presence of psychosis(6); it is well understood that patients demonstrate persistent NP impairments following recovery from acute psychotic episodes and that cognitive impairments are quite stable over time.

Profile

It is important to consider that patients with schizophrenia show considerably smaller overall decline in intelligence than in some specific ability areas.(7) The majority of these impaired domains are often seen to be those that are associated with the functions of the frontal lobe. However, the notion that the whole array of cognitive impairments seen in schizophrenia could originate from a single localized lesion is implausible, as impairments in cognitive functions that are impaired individuals with medial temporal-hippocampal lesions are also quite profound in patients with schizophrenia.(8)

Table 4.3.3.2 Level of impairment in cognitive abilities in schizophrenia

	Mild	Moderate	Severe
Perceptual skills	X		
Motor skills	X		
Attention			
Sustained attention			X
Selective attention		X	
Working memory			
Spatial working memory		X	
Verbal working memory			X
Episodic memory			
Verbal learning			X
Non-verbal memory (spatial memory)		X	
Delayed recall		X	
Delayed recognition	X		
Procedural memory		X	
Long-term factual memory	X		
Executive functions		X	
Processing speed			X
Verbal skills			
Naming	X		
Verbal fluency		X	

See Heinrichs and Zakzanis(5) for a description of the methods used to evaluate these levels of impairment.

There has been considerable debate about the structure of cognitive deficits in schizophrenia. This debate has focused on whether the profile of relative deficits is generalized, with similar severity across all components, or specific.(9) Proponents of the specific profile argument often site evidence of regional brain dysfunction detected with neuroimaging procedures(10) or more extreme deficits on certain NP tests such as episodic memory.(8) There have been recent factor analytic studies that found complex solution with up to six factors(11) and other studies that found a single factor characterized all of the cognitive data in large samples.(12) It does seem that tests requiring cognitive capacity and processing speed are amongst the most poorly performed and that tests examining the ability to use information acquired prior to the onset of schizophrenia are performed best.

Onset

At the time of the first treatment for schizophrenia, either inpatient or outpatient, people who receive the diagnosis perform in a manner that is nearly as impaired as more chronic patients, with a similar profile of impairment.(13) These data support the idea that cognitive impairment is not continuously progressive over the entire course of illness.(14) It is clear, however, that cognitive impairments may also be detectable in at least some people who are destined to develop schizophrenia. In population-based studies of apparently healthy individuals being screened for induction into compulsory military service, there are clear group differences in performance between individuals who eventually develop schizophrenia and those who do not.(15) These impairments have some level of sensitivity and specificity, but are clearly not diagnostic indicators at that stage. Findings of impairments in cognition prior to the patient's meeting formal diagnostic criteria for the illness do provide additional suggestions that cognitive deficits are central features of the illness.

Cognitive decline in schizophrenia?

While the course of cognitive impairments in schizophrenia appears generally stable over the lifespan, there is a substantial minority of patients with schizophrenia who manifest considerable cognitive impairments that worsen over time. The patients who show these changes tend to be older and with a chronic course of treatment-refractory positive symptoms, often accompanied by a lifetime of institutional care.(16) Longitudinal studies have suggested that younger institutionalized patients with similarly severe positive do not show declines during similar follow-up periods,(17) suggesting that there may be age-associated vulnerability to decline. Studies from multiple research sites have found a low prevalence of neurodegenerative changes at post-mortem in older schizophrenia patients,(18) suggesting that these abnormalities cannot be fully explained by degenerative conditions. At present, there is no information on whether these changes could be due to the experience of institutionalization alone, but studies of patients who were released from chronic psychiatric care have not shown evidence of reversal of these cognitive impairments. As patients with schizophrenia have evidence of considerable reduction in their 'cognitive reserve', based on the lower levels of premorbid functioning, it would expected that a variety of risk factors could lead to cognitive changes, including subclinical neurodegenerative pathology, vascular abnormalities, or other factors which can influence cognitive impairments in older individuals.

Presence in relatives and individuals with 'spectrum' conditions

Cognitive impairments are present in the relatives of people with schizophrenia and these impairments have evidence of heritability. Longitudinal studies have suggested that some aspects of cognitive impairment, such as attentional deficits, predict the development of psychotic symptoms in high risk children with at least one schizophrenic parent.(19) Further, individuals with schizophrenia spectrum conditions such as schizotypal personality disorder (SPD) show evidence of cognitive deficits similar in profile, yet reduced in severity compared to people with schizophrenia.(20) As patients with SPD do not have a markedly increased risk for schizophrenia, some aspects of cognitive functioning may represent a stable correlate of some aspects of the predisposition to schizophrenia. While studies have been in process to identify candidate cognitive processes as potential genetically mediated intermediate phenotypes,(21) specific gene-performance correlations are not large enough in magnitude yet to demonstrate that any cognitive impairment is clearly related to specific susceptibility genes for schizophrenia.

Functional relevance

One of the reasons for the increased interest in NP impairment in schizophrenia over the past decade is the developing understanding of the functional relevance of NP impairment. In specific, NP impairment in schizophrenia is the single strongest correlate of impairments in everyday living skills, in social outcomes, and in seeking and maintaining employment or other productive activities. This realization was spurred by several high-profile reviews of the literature(22) and a developing interest in both disability reduction and the direct measurement of disability. While the correlations between impairments in individual NP ability areas and specific aspects of everyday disability are only moderate in size, correlations between composite measures of multiple NP domains and global measures of outcome are often fairly substantial, in the range of Pearson correlations of $r = 0.7$ (reflecting 50 per cent shared variance). In contrast, in similar studies, the cross-sectional correlation between the severity of psychotic (i.e. positive) symptoms is often closer to $r = 0.1$, reflecting about 1 per cent shared variance.(12) This difference in correlations is likely accentuated by the unstable and episodic nature of positive symptoms, in contrast to both functional disability and NP performance, which are both known to be quite stable over time.

Studies of the ability to perform skilled acts (i.e. independent living and social skills) in analogue situations have found that the correlation between impairment on NP tests and deficits in 'functional capacity' is greater than the correlation between NP performance and real world functional performance.(23) This difference in correlations is probably due to the fact that there are multiple factors other than ability that determine everyday outcomes. Opportunities, disability compensation, environmental support, and familial resources are all factors that could lead to discrepancies between what a person can do (i.e. their competence) and what they actually do (i.e. their everyday performance). The fact that disability, in terms of reduced competence, can be measured directly with performance-based tests is quite important, as some of these measures could actually be used in everyday clinical practice or as outcomes in treatment studies.

Treatment of cognitive impairment in schizophrenia

Although antipsychotic medications have been shown for years to be effective in reducing psychotic symptoms in about 70 per cent of patients with schizophrenia, effects on cognitive impairments are much smaller. Although cognitive impairments are apparently not worsened by conventional antipsychotic treatments, their beneficial effects are small and limited to a subset of cognitive domains. Atypical antipsychotic treatment appears to have a somewhat greater effect, suggested by meta-analyses and large-scale studies to be about 0.25 standard deviations.(24) Given the substantial magnitude of impairments in the illness, this level of improvement does not come close to normalization for most patients.

Targeted treatments aimed at cognitive functioning have come from both pharmacological and cognitive remediation domains. Most pharmacological interventions have had quite modest effects, while the results of recent cognitive remediation interventions have been more promising. At least three different interventions, using computerized interventions in randomized trials have shown both cognitive improvements and generalization of improvement to functionally relevant aspects of everyday outcome.(25) Concurrent antipsychotic treatments may be responsible for the poor outcomes of pharmacological interventions, as some of these treatments that have shown minimal benefits in patients with schizophrenia receiving antipsychotic treatments have shown beneficial effects in healthy individuals and in persons with schizotypal personality disorder. This is an issue that will require further study.

Conclusion

Cognitive impairments in schizophrenia are related to the functional disability in the illness and may produce much of the morbidity associated with the condition. These impairments are wide ranging and are found in multiple important domains, with onset at the time of, or in many cases, prior to the first episode of illness. No single focal lesion appears responsible for the array of deficits seen. Relatives of people with schizophrenia and individuals with non-psychotic schizophrenia-spectrum conditions are also affected by these cognitive deficits. Cognitive impairments have proven difficult to treat, but multiple initiatives are underway to improve treatment success. Both pharmacological and cognitive remediation interventions are being studied in detail at this time.

Further information

Resources: National Association for Research in Schizophrenia and Affective Disorders (NARSAD). Promotes research on these topics for junior to distinguished investigators.

Websites: Schizophrenia Research Forum. The ultimate resource for new developments in schizophrenia. http://www.schizophreniaforum.org/

References

1. Chapman, L.J. and Chapman, J.M. (1973). *Disordered thought in schizophrenia*. Appleton, Century, Crofts, New York.
2. Lezak, M.D., Howieson, D.B., and Loring, D.W. (2004). *Neuropsychological assessment* (4th edn). Oxford, New York.

3. Heaton, R.K., Miller, S.W., Taylor, M.J., *et al.* (2005). *Revised comprehensive norms for an expanded Halstead-Reitan Battery (HRB): demographically adjusted neuropsychological norms for African American and Caucasian adults.* Psychological Assessment Resources, Lutz, FL.
4. Braver, T.S. and Barch, D.M. (2002). A theory of cognitive control, aging cognition, and neuromodulation. *Neuroscience and Biobehavioral Reviews*, **26**, 809–17.
5. Heinrichs, R.W. and Zakzanis, K.K. (1998). Neurocognitive deficit in schizophrenia: a quantitative review of the evidence. *Neuropsychology*, **12**, 426–45.
6. Elevevag, A. and Goldberg, T.E. (2000). Cognitive impairment in schizophrenia is the core of the disorder. *Critical Reviews in Neurobiology*, **14**, 1–21.
7. Weickert, T.W., Goldberg, T.E., Gold, J.M., *et al.* (2000). Cognitive impairments in patients with schizophrenia displaying preserved and compromised intellect. *Archives of General Psychiatry*, **57**, 907–13.
8. Saykin, A.J., Gur, R.C., Gur, R.E., *et al.* (1991). Neuropsychological function in schizophrenia. Selective impairment in memory and learning. *Archives of General Psychiatry*, **48**, 618–24.
9. Dickinson, D., Iannone, V.N., Wilk, C.M., *et al.* (2004). General and specific cognitive deficits in schizophrenia. *Biological Psychiatry*, **55**, 826–33.
10. Hazlett, E.A., Buchsbaum, M.S., Jeu, L.A., *et al.* (2000). Hypofrontality in unmedicated schizophrenia patients studied with PET during performance of a serial verbal learning task. *Schizophrenia Research*, **43**, 33–46.
11. Gladsjo, J.A., McAdams, L.A., Palmer, B.W., *et al.* (2004). A six-factor model of cognition in schizophrenia and related psychotic disorders: relationships with clinical symptoms and functional capacity. *Schizophrenia Bulletin*, **30**, 739–54.
12. Keefe, R.S., Bilder, R.M., Harvey, P.D., *et al.* (2006). Baseline neurocognitive deficits in the CATIE schizophrenia trial. *Neuropsychopharmacology*, **31**, 2033–46.
13. Saykin, A.J., Shtasel, D.L., Gur, R.E., *et al.* (1994). Neuropsychological deficits in neuroleptic naive patients with first-episode schizophrenia. *Archives of General Psychiatry*, **51**, 124–31.
14. Heaton, R.K., Gladsjo, J.A., Palmer, B.W., *et al.* (2001). Stability and course of neuropsychological deficits in schizophrenia. *Archives of General Psychiatry*, **58**, 24–32.
15. Davidson, M., Reichenberg, A., Rabinowitz, J., *et al.* (1999). Behavioral and intellectual markers for schizophrenia in apparently healthy male adolescents. *The American Journal of Psychiatry*, **156**, 1328–35.
16. Harvey, P.D., Silverman, J.M., Mohs, R.C., *et al.* (1999). Cognitive decline in late-life schizophrenia: a longitudinal study of geriatric chronically hospitalized patients. *Biological Psychiatry*, **45**, 32–40.
17. Friedman, J.I., Harvey, P.D., Coleman, T., *et al.* (2001). Six-year follow-up study of cognitive and functional status across the lifespan in schizophrenia: a comparison with Alzheimer's disease and normal aging. *The American Journal of Psychiatry*, **158**, 1441–8.
18. Arnold, S.E., Gur, R.E., Shapiro, R.M., *et al.* (1995). Prospective clinicopathological studies of schizophrenia: accrual and assessment of patients. *The American Journal of Psychiatry*, **152**, 731–7.
19. Cornblatt, B.A. and Erlenmeyer-Kimling, L. (1985). Global attentional deviance as a marker of risk for schizophrenia: specificity and predictive validity. *Journal of Abnormal Psychology*, **94**, 470–86.
20. Mitropoulou, V., Harvey, P.D., Zegarelli, G., *et al.* (2005). Neuropsychological performance in schizotypal personality disorder: importance of working memory. *The American Journal of Psychiatry*, **162**, 1896–903.
21. Goldberg, T.E., Egan, M.F., Gscheidle, T., *et al.* (2003). Executive subprocesses in working memory: relationship to catechol-O-methyltransferase Val158Met genotype and schizophrenia. *Archives of General Psychiatry*, **60**, 889–96.
22. Green, M.F., Kern, R.S., Braff, D.L., and Mintz, J. (2000). Neurocognitive deficits and functional outcome in schizophrenia: are we measuring the 'right stuff?' *Schizophrenia Bulletin*, **26**, 119–36.
23. Bowie, C.R., Reichenberg, A., Patterson, T.L., *et al.* (2006). Determinants of real-world functional performance in schizophrenia subjects: correlations with cognition, functional capacity, and symptoms. *The American Journal of Psychiatry*, **163**, 418–25.
24. Harvey, P.D. and Keefe, R.S. (2001). Studies of cognitive change in patients with schizophrenia following novel antipsychotic treatment. *The American Journal of Psychiatry*, **158**, 176–84.
25. McGurk, S.R., Mueser, K.T., and Pascaris, A. (2005). Cognitive training and supported employment for persons with severe mental illness: one-year results from a randomized controlled trial. *Schizophrenia Bulletin*, **31**, 898–909.

4.3.4 Diagnosis, classification, and differential diagnosis of schizophrenia

Anthony S. David

The diagnosis of schizophrenia

Until the early 1970s, the diagnosis of schizophrenia was one of the most contentious and fraught issues in the whole of psychiatry. Since then a massive international effort has been put in motion out of which explicit diagnostic criteria emerged. Some achieved widespread and even multinational agreement, allowing the painstaking process of calculating diagnostic specificity, sensitivity, reliability, and (perhaps) validity to begin. Although criticism of the diagnosis of schizophrenia continues, mostly from outside psychiatrists, the vast majority of psychiatrists look upon the major sets of diagnostic criteria with weary acceptance, seeing them as flawed but useful and possibly 'as good as it gets' given our current state of knowledge/ignorance.

Throughout the 1970s and early 1980s there was an overabundance of criteria including the St. Louis criteria[1] and the Research Diagnostic Criteria,[2] followed by the Present State Examination (PSE-CATEGO), the ICD-9, and the DSM-III. Perhaps because of the 'cookbook' explicitness of the DSM-III or the pervasive influence of American psychiatric practice, dubbed by some 'neo-colonial', the DSM, in its fourth revision with a fifth due in 2010, is the mostly widely used. The ICD-10 is also used throughout the world, but seldom in North America.

Diagnostic criteria

The signs and symptoms of schizophrenia and related disorders are discussed in detail in Chapter 4.3.2. Also, the diagnostic process is described in general in Chapter 1.8.1. As noted, the signs and symptoms, weighted in terms of their typicality or specificity, combined with additional clinical factors such as onset, duration, social consequences, etc., are used to make a diagnosis of schizophrenia and subsequently to classify the disorder into subtypes. The DSM and ICD criteria are described below (Tables 4.3.4.1–4.3.4.3).

Table 4.3.4.1 Major diagnostic criteria for schizophrenia

	DSM-IV	ICD-10
Characteristic symptoms		
One or more for 1 month	1. Bizarre delusions	1. Thought echo/insertion/ withdrawal/broadcasting
	2. Commenting voice or voices conversing	2. Delusions of control
		3. Hallucinatory voices
		4. Persistent delusions
Or two or more	1. Delusions	1. Persistent hallucinations
	2. Hallucinations	2. Thought block/disorder
	3. Disorganized speech	3. Catatonia
	4. Grossly disorganized or catatonic behaviour	4. Negative symptoms
	5. Negative symptoms	5. Significant personality change
Time course	1 month ('significant proportion') for symptoms listed plus 6 months social/occupational disturbance	1 month (most of the time)
Exclusions	Schizoaffective disorder or brief mood disturbance	Extensive depressive/manic symptoms or diagnosis of schizoaffective disorder
	Direct effect of drugs of abuse/ medication or general medical condition	Overt brain disease; drug intoxication/withdrawal

Another group of psychotic disorders which may be distinguished on the basis of formal phenomenological properties are the delusional disorders[3, 4] formally known as paranoia (see Chapter 4.4).

Basis of classification

Atheoretical: Schneider's first-rank symptoms

These are still important for the diagnosis of schizophrenia using the ICD-10 frame of reference. They are too rare to achieve high levels of sensitivity and their specificity has been challenged. Nevertheless, first-rank symptoms perform creditably on these parameters when compared to negative symptoms.[5,6] On the other hand, the lack of aetiological and prognostic significance of first-rank symptoms has undermined the prominence claimed for them.[7,8] The negative[9] or so-called deficit syndrome[10] relates more consistently to outcome/prognosis and shows more stability over time. The constituent symptoms such as social withdrawal, apathy, lack of initiative, and self-care, have rather poor diagnostic specificity in isolation and must be distinguished from depression and parkinsonism, chronic drug dependence, and organic brain damage.

Theoretical

Attempts at a theoretical classification have been made. The first in the modern era was Crow's Type I and Type II distinction,[11]

Table 4.3.4.2 Criteria for the diagnosis of schizophrenia subtypes

Schizophrenia subtypes	DSM-IV	ICD-10
Paranoid	One or more delusions plus frequent auditory hallucinations; no prominent thought disorder, catatonia, or negative symptoms	Delusions, hallucinatory voices, hallucinations in other modalities; disturbances of affect, volition, and speech 'inconspicuous'
Disorganized DSM Hebephrenic ICD	Prominent disorganized speech behaviour and flat/inappropriate affect; no catatonia	Prominent disturbances of affect, volition, and thought; 2–3 months duration; adolescents/young adults only
Catatonic	Two of motoric immobility, excessive activity, negativism, peculiar voluntary movements, echolalia/ praxia	One or more of stupor, excitement. posturing, negativism, rigidity, waxy flexibility, automatic compliance and perserveration
Undifferentiated	Meets criteria for schizophrenia but none of the above subtypes	Meets criteria for schizophrenia but none of the above subtypes plus residual
Residual	Absence of prominent characteristic symptoms (but two or more must be present in attenuated form); continuing evidence of disturbance including negative symptoms	Prominent negative symptoms; clear-cut episode(s) in past; at least 1 year history; no dementia or depression etc.
Simple	Slowly progressive negative symptoms without other psychotic symptoms	(See schizoid personality disorder)

Table 4.3.4.3 Terminology used to describe the course of schizophrenia in the DSM-IV and ICD-10 classifications

DSM-IV	ICD-10
Continuous	Continuous
Episodic with residual symptoms	Episodic with stable deficit
Episodic with no interepisode symptoms	Episodic remittent
Single episode in partial remission	Incomplete remission
Single episode in full remission	Complete remission
Other	Other Episodic with progressive deficit

[a]Course specifiers in both DSM-IV and ICD-10 require 1 year of observation.

although it echoes older notions of 'process'-chronic and deteriorating versus 'reactive' (relapsing and remitting) typologies. The innovation was to link the distinction with proposed differences in dopamine receptor hyperactivity (Type I), associated with positive symptoms and good response to dopamine antagonist drugs, and on the other hand, to neurological damage (Type II) as evidenced by ventricular enlargement on Computerized Tomography (CT) brain scans, associated with chronicity, poor premorbid functioning, and poor response to treatment.

Building on this was the 'aetiological classification' proposed by Murray *et al.*[12] which contrasted cases with a presumed genetic aetiology and those who had other putative risk factors such as early brain damage (see Chapter 4.3.6.1). Although these attempts have served as useful stimuli for research, they have not been found to aid clinical decision-making and in fact now appear to support a blurring of diagnostic boundaries rather than a sharpening or subdivision.[13] In fact the search for 'biological markers' often called 'endophenotypes', which might validate diagnostic distinctions continues. Take for example, the presence of ventricular enlargement or cortical thinning, first detected using CT and now magnetic resonance imaging (**MRI**). Meta-analyses have confirmed that indices of 'cerebral atrophy' are strongly associated with schizophrenia but the effect sizes are small.[14] Medial temporal lobe structures are the region of most grey matter volume loss. However, there is substantial overlap between normal controls and schizophrenia cases and MRI cannot be considered a useful diagnostic test. A host of genetic markers have been identified in the last 5 years, each of small effect and some showing overlap between the major schizophrenic and affective syndromes.[15]

Positive family history remains an important finding in the psychiatric history of an individual patient. Although none of the diagnostic criteria permits the influence of family history, in clinical settings, 'odd' or withdrawn behaviour takes on a very different meaning if seen in the first-degree relative of someone with a firm schizophrenia diagnosis.

Early diagnosis?

The premorbid personality in schizophrenia is typically described as emotionally and socially detached. Such people have few friends, are often cold and aloof, and engage in solitary occupations. Their behaviour may be eccentric and they are indifferent to praise or criticism. Recent studies, including United Kingdom national cohort studies[16] and a Swedish conscript cohort study[17] indicate that children who later develop schizophrenia are more likely to have lower IQs and educational achievements than other children. They are also more likely to have interpersonal and behavioural difficulties. Parents recognize 'preschizophrenic' children as being different from their other siblings. However, such characteristics are very common in the general population so have virtually no positive predictive value.

Early diagnosis is only successful when based on psychotic symptoms. Here the diagnosis of schizophreniform psychosis (DSM-IV) and the acute schizophrenia-like psychotic disorder of the ICD-10 are relevant. The former must last for more than 1 but less than 6 months (otherwise the diagnosis is brief reactive psychosis). Hence the disorder is substantial by any common-sense definition, and unsurprisingly many cases (70 per cent) go on to develop full-blown schizophrenia, affective disorder, or schizoaffective disorder.[18] The temporal stability of the diagnosis is poor, with around 30 per cent recovering over follow-up periods averaging 16 months in one study.

New services have built up around ever earlier diagnosis with the explicit aim of secondary or even primary prevention. Criteria have been developed for the diagnosis of high-, ultra-high, or so-called 'at-risk' mental states based on transient psychotic experiences—even briefer than schizophreniform or more persistent disturbances in the sense of self ('basic symptoms') which fall short of true psychosis.[19,20] One impetus to this being the discovery that most patients when first ill endure a long duration—months or years—of untreated psychosis (DUP).

Differential diagnosis

Other psychiatric disorders

(a) Other psychoses

It could be argued that distinguishing schizophrenia from schizoaffective disorder, schizophreniform disorder, delusional disorder, etc. is an academic exercise. Despite passing enthusiasms, treatment in psychiatry is largely symptom or syndrome based.[21] Thus manic symptoms respond to antimanic agents including lithium, psychotic symptoms respond to 'neuroleptics' or first and now second-generation antipsychotic drugs (SGA), and depressive symptoms respond to antidepressants. Other 'mood-stabilizing' agents are also of value especially when combined with antipsychotics. Several SGAs are licensed for bipolar affective disorder and schizoaffective disorder although it is not clear whether they have distinct advantages over older drugs in this regard. Clozapine remains the only antipsychotic medication which is proven to be effective in at least some patients who are otherwise treatment resistant. However, it is possible that with increasing clinical experience and research more specific indications for newer agents will emerge. This will depend on the preservation of skills in history taking and the mental state examination, and a careful attitude towards making a diagnosis rather than use of sloppy catch-all labels such as 'serious mental illness' favoured by healthcare planners.

The prognostic significance of a diagnosis of schizophrenia (versus schizoaffective and affective disorders) has been discussed in Chapters 4.3.7 and 4.3.9. Although predicting outcome in individual patients is notoriously difficult because of the influence of idiosyncratic factors such as services, relationships within the family, compliance, intelligence, personality, demographics, etc., the more a disorder approaches 'typical' schizophrenia, the poorer the prognosis tends to be.

That said, schizoaffective disorder is the closest disorder, phenomenologically, to schizophrenia but combines schizophrenic symptoms with affective symptoms. The criteria are discussed in Chapter 4.3.9. Schizophreniform (DSM-IV) or acute schizophrenia-like disorders (ICD-10) differ only in terms of duration, as operationally defined (see Chapter 4.3.10). Delusional disorders (Chapter 4.4) differ from schizophrenia in being based around 'non-bizarre' delusions and few or no hallucinations. The onset and course are characteristically later and more benign respectively.

(b) Affective disorders

Typical presentations of either mania or depression usually cause few diagnostic difficulties. Overdiagnosis of schizoaffective disorder is to be resisted although the distinction from schizophrenia proper remains controversial and debatable. The guidelines given in DSM-IV attempt to exclude transient mood disturbances (<2 weeks) in people with psychosis as a basis for a schizoaffective diagnosis.

In practice reaching a diagnosis of schizophrenia in a person with evidence of one or more core symptoms of psychosis (listed under the DSM-IV and ICD-10) may be complicated for the following reasons.

(c) The presence of mood-incongruent delusions (or hallucinations)

'Congruence' is somewhat in the eye of the beholder, especially where mood may be labile or where disturbed mood is suspected but fails to follow clinical stereotypes. The clinician should try to determine if a 'grandiose' delusion is being enjoyed by the patient, and whether the content (e.g. elevated status, magical powers, material riches) is seen as justified by the patient. Similarly a delusion of depressive content (e.g. physical illness, imminent death) must be seen as undeserved or inexplicable to be deemed 'incongruent'. Auditory hallucinations may be comforting, complimentary, or, more commonly, hostile and critical. It is probably their complexity and personification which makes them 'schizophrenic' rather than their mood-incongruent content.

(d) The duration and acuteness of onset criteria

A good history may simply not be available. Symptoms may wax and wane. Partial or successful treatment may modify or curtail a potentially long episode, and onset may be complicated by the use of psychoactive drugs.

(e) Social and occupational disturbance

This is critical to the diagnosis of schizophrenia, especially the DSM-IV criteria. Here the difficulty is in distinguishing 'premorbid deficits', an illness prodrome and the illness itself. Premorbid personality factors will obscure or set in relief discontinuities in an individual's social trajectory. Objective information and informant testimony is crucial as in most of the diagnostic process. Other individual differences such as intelligence will also shape the presentation of schizophrenia. At the extreme, people with intellectual disability (learning disability) may manifest psychosis in less obvious ways (see Chapters 10.5.1 to 10.5.3). The old diagnosis of 'simple schizophrenia', retained in the ICD-10 describes 'insidious and progressive development of oddities of conduct' and the 'inability to meet the demands of society' that is, social disturbance of long duration. The progressive element distinguishes it from personality disorder although problems adjusting to changing social demands through the life cycle may give the appearance of progression in a fixed personality disorder.

Organic conditions

Differentiation of a 'primary' psychotic illness from one secondary to an organic condition may arise in essentially two situations:

- a person with a clear-cut diagnosis of a medical or neurological syndrome in which psychosis is a recognized complication (e.g. epilepsy)
- a person with a presumptive diagnosis of schizophrenia in whom significant abnormalities are detected usually following special investigation (e.g. CT brain scanning).

The list of medical conditions that could potentially give rise to psychosis is enormous. These have been the subject of extensive reviews.[22, 23] While it appears that almost any disease that causes a cerebral perturbation can give rise to psychosis, abnormalities affecting the temporal lobes and diencephalon are somewhat more likely to do this.

The time course is obviously important in this context. Chronic inflammatory lesions (e.g. sarcoidosis), degenerative disorders (e.g. presenile dementias), chronic infections (e.g. neurosyphilis, AIDS), space-occupying lesions (e.g. tumour or abscesses), metabolic disorders (e.g. hyper- or hypothyroidism and vitamin deficiencies) may mimic schizophrenia by virtue of a gradual deterioration in social functioning and self-care punctuated perhaps by odd or inexplicable behaviour and rarely hallucinations and delusions. The features of the primary disease are usually evident. Rarer conditions may be misdiagnosed, for example, Wilson's disease (hepatolenticular degeneration). This usually presents with a motor disorder with bulbar features and abnormal liver function, but personality changes and psychotic symptoms are also associated. Diagnosis is made on other associated clinical features (e.g. Kayser–Fleischer rings), copper studies, and liver biopsy. Huntington's disease is characterized by chorea and cognitive decline. Affective disorder and occasionally psychotic symptoms may occur. The main differential diagnosis is with patients with chronic psychosis and tardive dyskinesia and is usually clarified by the family history, inexorable progression, and caudate atrophy on CT or MRI. Neurosyphilis is still encountered from time to time and in the 'general paralysis of the insane' form, may present with chronic delusions (often grandiose) plus dementia. Diagnosis is by appropriate serological testing of blood and cerebrospinal fluid. Finally, metachromatic leukodystrophy, a rare inherited progressive demyelinating condition, has recently been identified as a cause of a schizophrenia-like psychosis, when onset is in childhood or early adult life.[24] Arylsulphatase-A is a diagnostic marker detectable in peripheral white blood cells.

Acute disturbances following head trauma, acute infections (viral encephalitis), cerebrovascular accidents, metabolic abnormalities (e.g. electrolyte disturbances, porphyria), or drug intoxication or withdrawal (including prescribed medication) (see below) may present with a florid psychotic picture, classically dominated by visual distortions or hallucinations and fluctuating levels of alertness, rather than the stereotyped auditory hallucinations in clear consciousness which are characteristic of schizophrenia.[25]

In practice there are few common conditions that ever give rise to real diagnostic uncertainty. The most important is **epilepsy**. It is well established that epilepsy, particularly focal (complex partial or 'temporal lobe epilepsy') can give rise to psychosis and there are inter-ictal and post-ictal patterns (see Chapter 5.3.3). A survey from a large neurology clinic showed that the incidence of schizophrenia is about nine times that of the rest of the population.[26]

Inter-ictal psychoses include the chronic schizophrenia-like psychoses described by Slater *et al.*[27] and Trimble.[28] These almost always arise in people with many years of well-established temporal lobe seizures, while the post-ictal variety occurs earlier in the life cycle but again in a person with previously diagnosed epilepsy. In post-ictal psychosis the temporal relationship to seizures, sometimes occurring in a cluster, is diagnostic, although a lucid interval is often observed. A clear history and independent description of seizures is the foundation of a diagnosis of epilepsy, with EEG confirmation. Resting EEGs show slight and subtle abnormalities in a substantial minority of patients with schizophrenia which may be accentuated by antipsychotic medication. As such, the EEG may be of limited value in differential diagnosis unless pronounced slowing or frank seizure activity is picked up (see also Chapter 5.3.3.).

(a) Symptoms

Symptoms of schizophrenic psychosis in relative isolation may give rise to diagnostic difficulties.

Auditory hallucinations may occur in alcoholic hallucinosis (see below and Chapter 4.2.2.3). Hallucinations in the context of dissociation (voices representing figures from the patient's past or embodiments of aspects of their personality) must also be distinguished from typical schizophrenic hallucinations. These are often multimodal. Pure auditory hallucinations in organic conditions including epilepsy in the absence of other psychotic features are surprisingly rare.

Certain forms of delusion suggest alternative diagnoses. Transient ill-formed but usually paranoid delusions occur in the context of confusion, memory impairment, or dementia (i.e. things going missing, strange people loitering). Delusions of misidentification are particularly associated with organic illness such as dementia or stroke.

Thought disorder may be confused with a fluent aphasia following stroke or cerebral tumours.

Personality deterioration and inappropriate or disinhibited behaviour can occur in many organic conditions in the absence of overt psychotic features. Isolated frontal lesions may cause diagnostic problems since general cognitive impairments may be absent. The widespread availability of CT and MRI in the more developed world has reduced the likelihood of such patients being misdiagnosed.

A small proportion (approximately 5 per cent) of prevalent and incident cases of schizophrenia, if investigated thoroughly, are found to have a variety of 'organic' conditions which may contribute to the illness.[29] These include metabolic abnormalities, cerebral tumours, multisystem autoimmune disease, cerebrovascular disease, etc. Some of these may be incidental; others may have precipitated the psychosis. The range of diseases counts against any specific aetiological mechanism. Similarly, the phenomenology found in such 'organic' patients is usually indistinguishable from their 'functional' counterparts.[30]

Thanks to increased application of non-invasive neuroimaging techniques to psychiatric patients, particularly those with schizophrenia, another class of organic abnormalities have been noted, namely cerebral anomalies which are often congenital. These include agenesis of the corpus callosum, cavum septum pellucidum, aqueduct stenosis, etc. Again, it is difficult to know how often such findings occur in the normal population and are asymptomatic, although the widespread use of MRI for 'minor' complaints such as mild head injury and headache is uncovering such anomalies. The examples above certainly appear to be associated with psychiatric disorders in general more than would be expected by chance. They tend to be associated with below-average IQ and other neurological problems (epilepsy in the cases of callosal agenesis).

Other factors to be taken into account in the differential diagnosis from organic conditions include the presence of a family history of schizophrenia, and abnormal premorbid personality, both of which weight aetiological judgement in favour of the functional diagnosis. This applies to the psychoses of epilepsy and those related to drug abuse especially. 'Secondary' schizophrenias also tend to have less pervasive effects on the person's personality. Treatment is again based on symptoms with the added complication that antipsychotic drugs lower the epileptic seizure threshold, and will tend to worsen extrapyramidal symptoms in patients with primary movement disorders. Treatment of the primary condition (if this has remained undiagnosed for some time) may be disappointing but should always be attempted especially in the case of chronic infections. Reversal of metabolic abnormalities, even long-standing, can lead to dramatic improvements in the mental state.

(b) Drug-induced psychoses

Many drugs of abuse and prescribed drugs can cause psychotic symptoms. The associations are also considered in Chapters 4.2.3.1 to 4.2.3.9. In the context of a differential diagnosis, drugs of abuse—in adolescents and young adults—must be considered. Chronic amphetamine psychosis may be indistinguishable from schizophrenia. The psychosis is florid and may include visual and auditory hallucinations. Phencyclidine (PCP or angel dust) is a drug of abuse in the United States and causes an acute psychosis with prominent affective symptoms as well as perceptual distortions and depersonalization. Other psychotogenic drugs include cocaine, ecstasy, and Lysergic Acid Diethylamide(LSD).

Cannabis is widely used, especially in large metropolitan areas and by certain ethnic groups (e.g. African-Caribbeans). Cannabis intoxication is more characterized by perceptual distortions and depersonalization than frank psychosis. Clinical experience suggests that cannabis has a propensity to precipitate psychotic relapse in patients with established schizophrenia and a recent meta-analysis of cohort studies concludes that cannabis use is certainly a risk factor for schizophrenia, and other psychiatric disorders.[31]

Delusions and hallucinations may occur rarely during states of alcohol intoxication but are more commonly associated with withdrawal syndromes (Chapter 4.2.2.2). Alcoholic hallucinosis is a chronic hallucinatory state of uncertain nosological status in which the patient with long-standing alcohol dependence often hears 'voices' which may be derogatory and commenting, in clear consciousness, after a lengthy withdrawal period.

(c) Prescribed medication

Again the list of agents that can cause psychotic reactions to be distinguished from schizophrenia is very long, and psychotropic drugs are particularly liable to cause psychotic reactions. Two classes of drug deserve mention because of their widespread use and relatively high incidence of major psychiatric adverse effects:

- steroids can cause a wide range of psychiatric disturbances including psychosis
- dopamine agonists used in the treatment of Parkinson's disease and some pituitary adenomas.

Frank psychosis and affective disorders may be seen. In the treatment of neurological diseases, such as Parkinson's disease, and the use of steroids for diseases of the central nervous system, there is often an interaction between the agent and the underlying condition which increases the likelihood of a drug-induced psychosis.

The diagnostic process

It used to be argued that a diagnosis of schizophrenia in itself caused disability and morbidity due to social 'labelling' and stigmatization. Evidence that this accounts for schizophrenic disability is lacking but the reality of the stigma of mental illness and negative attitudes towards 'schizophrenics' cannot be denied. This is especially delicate in the case of early intervention with people presenting without the full-blown schizophrenic syndrome since arguably, the balance of harms and benefits of diagnosis is tilted slightly away from benefit. Hence, making a diagnosis of schizophrenia should not be taken lightly. In the author's experience, very few psychiatrists spontaneously convey the diagnosis to the patient. If a patient asks whether he or she has schizophrenia, the clinician should first try to understand the motivation behind the question and the patient's knowledge and understanding of the term. Ultimately there is seldom justification in withholding the diagnosis if it is established. A schizophrenia diagnosis can be framed in a relatively positive light—this is a condition which we are now beginning to understand and for which there are effective treatments—and may lessen the burden of responsibility and blame that the patient and his or her family may carry for the disorder.

Further information

McKenna, P.J. (2007). *Schizophrenia and related syndromes* (2nd edn). Routledge, Hove, East Sussex.

The Cochrane Schizophrenia Group: http://www.update-software.com/Abstracts/SCHIZAbstractIndex.htm

References

1. Feighner, J.P., Robins, E., Guze, S., *et al.* (1972). Diagnostic criteria for use in psychiatric research. *Archives of General Psychiatry*, **26**, 57–62.
2. Spitzer, R.L., Endicott, J., and Robins, E. (1977). *Research diagnostic criteria for a selected group of functional disorders* (3rd edn). Biometrics Research Division, New York State Psychiatric Institution, New York.
3. World Health Organization. (1992). F20-F29 schizophrenia, schizotypal and delusional disorders. *The ICD-10 classification of mental and behavioural disorders. Clinical descriptions and diagnostic guidelines*, pp. 97–109. WHO, Geneva.
4. American Psychiatric Association. (1994). Schizophrenia and other psychotic disorders. *Diagnostic and statistical manual of mental disorders, DSM-IV* (2nd edn), pp. 284–306. American Psychiatric Association, Washington, DC.
5. David, A.S. and Appleby, L. (1992). Diagnostic criteria in schizophrenia: accentuate the positive. *Schizophrenia Bulletin*, **18**, 551–7.
6. Andreasen, N.C. and Flaum, M. (1991). Schizophrenia: the characteristic symptoms. *Schizophrenia Bulletin*, **17**, 27–39.
7. Wing, J.K., Cooper, J.E., and Sartorius, N. (1974). *Measurement and classification of psychiatric symptoms*. Cambridge University Press, Cambridge.
8. McGuffin, P., Farmer, A., Gottesman, I.I., *et al.* (1984). Twin concordance for operationally defined schizophrenia: confirmation of familiarity and heritability. *Archives of General Psychiatry*, **41**, 541–5.
9. Andreasen, N.C. and Olsen, S. (1982). Negative v. positive schizophrenia: definition and validation. *Archives of General Psychiatry*, **39**, 789–94.
10. Amador, X.F., Kirkpatrick, B., Buchanan, R.W., *et al.* (1999). Stability of the diagnosis of deficit syndrome in schizophrenia. *The American Journal of Psychiatry*, **156**, 637–9.
11. Crow, T.J. (1980). Molecular pathology of schizophrenia: more than one disease process? *British Medical Journal*, **280**, 1–9.
12. Murray, R.M., Lewis, S.W., and Reveley, A.M. (1985). Towards an aetiological classification of schizophrenia. *Lancet*, **i**, 1023–6.
13. Murray, R.M., Sham, P., Van Os, J., *et al.* (2004). A developmental model for similarities and dissimilarities between schizophrenia and bipolar disorder. *Schizophrenia Research*, **71**, 405–16.
14. Wright, I.C., Rabe-Hesketh, S., Woodruff, P.W.R., *et al.* (2000). Meta-analysis of regional brain volumes in schizophrenia. *The American Journal of Psychiatry*, **157**, 16–25.
15. Craddock, N., O'Donovan, M.C., and Owen, M.J. (2006). Genes for schizophrenia and bipolar disorder? Implications for psychiatric nosology. *Schizophrenia Bulletin*, **32**, 9–16.
16. Jones, P. (1997). The early origins of schizophrenia. *British Medical Bulletin*, **53**, 135–55.
17. Malmberg, A., Lewis, G., David, A., *et al.* (1998). Premorbid adjustment and personality in schizophrenia. *The British Journal of Psychiatry*, **172**, 308–13.
18. Strakowski, S.M. (1994). Diagnostic validity of schizophreniform disorder. *The American Journal of Psychiatry*, **151**, 815–24.
19. Yung, A.R., Stanford, C., Cosgrave, E., *et al.* (2006). Testing the ultra high risk (prodromal) criteria for the prediction of psychosis in a clinical sample of young people. *Schizophrenia Research*, **84**, 57–66.
20. Owens, D.G.C. and Johnstone, E.C. (2006). Precursors and prodromata of schizophrenia: findings from the Edinburgh High Risk Study and their literature context. *Psychological Medicine*, **36**, 1501–14.
21. Johnstone, E.C., Crow, T.J., Frith, C.D., *et al.* (1988). The Northwick Park 'functional' psychoses study: diagnosis and treatment response. *Lancet*, **ii**, 119–26.
22. Davison, K. and Bagley, C.R. (1969). Schizophrenia-like psychoses associated with organic disorders of the central nervous system. In *Current problems in neuropsychiatry* (ed. R.N. Herrington). British Journal of Psychiatry Special Publication No. 4. Headley Brothers, Ashford, Kent.
23. Lishman, W.A. (1997). *Organic psychiatry: the psychological consequences of cerebral disorder* (3rd edn). Blackwell Science, Oxford.
24. Hyde, T.M., Ziegler, J.C., and Weinberger, D.R. (1993). Psychiatric disturbances in metachromatic leukodystrophy. Insights into the neurobiology of psychosis. *Archives of Neurology*, **50**, 131.
25. Cutting, J. (1987). The phenomenology of acute organic psychosis: comparison with acute schizophrenia. *The British Journal of Psychiatry*, **151**, 324–32
26. Mendez, M.F., Grau, R., Doss, R.C., *et al.* (1993). Schizophrenia in epilepsy: seizure and psychosis variables. *Neurology*, **43**, 1073–7.

27. Slater, E., Beard, A.W., and Glithero, E. (1963). The schizophrenia-like psychoses of epilepsy. *The British Journal of Psychiatry*, **109**, 95–150.
28. Trimble, M.R. (1990). First-rank symptoms of Schneider. A new perspective? *The British Journal of Psychiatry*, **156**, 195–200.
29. Johnstone, E.C., Cooling, N., Frith, C.D., *et al.* (1988). Phenomenology of organic and functional psychoses and the overlap between them. *The British Journal of Psychiatry*, **153**, 770–6.
30. Johnstone, E.C., Macmillan, J.F., and Crow, T.J. (1987). The occurrence of organic disease of possible or probably aetiological significance in a population of 268 cases of first episode schizophrenia. *Psychological Medicine*, **17**, 371–9.
31. Moore, T.H.M., Zammit, S., Lingford-Hughes, A., *et al.* (2007). Cannabis use and risk of psychotic or affective mental health outcomes: a systematic review. *Lancet*, **370**, 319–28.

4.3.5 Epidemiology of schizophrenia

Assen Jablensky

Introduction

Epidemiological research into schizophrenia aims to answer four essential questions.

- What is the 'true' population frequency of the disorder in various populations and how is it distributed across the various groups within populations?
- Do the incidence, manifestations, and course of schizophrenia vary in relation to factors of the physical and social environment?
- Who is at risk and what forces determine or influence the risk of developing schizophrenia?
- Can the answers to the above questions help explain what causes the disorder and how to prevent it?

The hallmark of the epidemiological method (see Chapter 2.7) is the referral of a measure (numerator) of the occurrence of a disorder, or of any associated characteristics, to a population base (denominator), such as **person-years at risk**. The epidemiological study of diseases usually proceeds from a description of its frequency and associations (establishing rates of occurrence) to testing hypotheses about risk factors and causes by analysing ratios between rates.

Schizophrenia has been studied extensively from an epidemiological perspective since Kraepelin[(1)] introduced the concept of *dementia praecox* in 1896. In the first half of the twentieth century, epidemiological research into schizophrenia took two divergent paths. While European studies tended to focus on population distributions and genetic risks, North American researchers investigated the social ecology of the disorder. A variety of methods were explored and successfully applied by the pioneers of psychiatric epidemiology, and the contours of the epidemiological map of schizophrenia in Europe and North America were effectively laid down between the two World Wars. The early studies were carried out by dedicated researchers who often spent months or years collecting data 'door-to-door' in small communities. Close knowledge of the respondents, access to multigenerational records from the local parish registers, and the cooperation of the community resulted in studies that remain landmarks of psychiatric epidemiology (Table 4.3.5.1).

During the last several decades, the scope of epidemiological studies of schizophrenia has expanded to include populations in Asia, Africa, and South America about which little had been known previously. The World Health Organization (**WHO**) International Pilot Study of Schizophrenia and its successor, the WHO 10-country epidemiological study[(9,10)] were the first systematic investigations of the comparative incidence, clinical manifestations, and course

Table 4.3.5.1 Historical landmarks in the epidemiology of psychoses

Author	Method	Target population	Case-finding	Assessment
Koller (1895)[(2)]	The first epidemiological case-control study of psychoses	Probands with psychoses (n = 287) and non-psychiatric controls (n = 370)	Records of psychiatric hospitals and clinics	Genealogical inquiry
Luxenburger (1928)[(3)]	Twin concordance/discordance analysis; sampling design	Monozygotic and dizygotic twin pairs	Census of inpatients; search of birth registers for twin births	Emphasis on reliability of diagnosis: 'definite' and 'probable'
Brugger (1931)[(4)]	Census (door-to-door survey)	Area in Thuringia, population 37 561	Records and key informants consulted to detect 'suspected' cases	Personal examination of 'suspected' cases and of a control sample
Klemperer (1933)[(5)]	Birth cohort study	Random sample (n = 1000) from all births in Munich, 1881–90	Attempted tracing of all cohort members, 44% successfully traced	Personal examination or key informant interview (271 examined)
Ödegaard (1946)[(6)]	Cumulative national case register	Entire population of Norway	Registration of all first-admissions 1926–35 (n = 14 231)	Statistical analysis of hospital diagnoses and records
Essen-Möller *et al.* (1956);[(7)] Hagnell (1966)[(8)]	Census followed by repeated follow-up surveys	Rural community, initial population 2550 (+1013 new residents in the course of follow-up)	Complete census; tracing of migrants	Personal examination (and re-examination) of all residents

of schizophrenia in both developing and developed countries. The WHO programme was an impetus for similar studies in India, China, the Caribbean, and Australia. Two major studies of psychiatric morbidity in the United States, the Epidemiological Catchment Area project,[11] and the National Comorbidity Survey,[12] generated data on the prevalence of DSM-III/IIIR schizophrenia and related disorders in representative population samples. In the 1980s and 1990s, epidemiological studies increasingly utilized existing large databases such as cumulative case registers or birth cohorts to test hypotheses about risk factors, and began to include methods of genetic epidemiology. There is a current tendency towards integrating epidemiological approaches with other types of aetiological research in schizophrenia. This predicts an important role for epidemiology in the era of molecular biology of mental disorders.

Epidemiological methods and instruments in the study of schizophrenia

The measurement of the prevalence, incidence, and disease expectancy of schizophrenia depends critically on the sensitivity of the case-finding method (i.e. its capacity to identify all affected persons in a given population) and the availability of a diagnostic instrument or procedure that selects 'true' cases (i.e. those corresponding to an established clinical concept).

Case-finding

Case-finding designs fall into three broad groups: case detection in clinical populations, door-to-door surveys of population samples or whole communities, and birth cohort studies. Each method has its advantages and limitations.

While case-finding through the mental health services provides a relatively easy access to a substantial proportion of all persons with schizophrenia, the **cases in treatment** may not be fully representative of all individuals with the disorder. Bias related to gender, marital status, socio-economic factors, culture, or ethnicity are known to affect the probability of being in treatment at a given time in a given setting, and generalizations about schizophrenia from hospital or clinic samples are liable to error. Some of the deficiencies of case-finding through service contacts are avoided in cumulative national or regional psychiatric case registers, which cover large well-defined populations and can be linked to other population databases (e.g. birth records). This makes registers efficient research instruments in low-incidence disorders such as schizophrenia.

Surveys involve accounting for every person at risk within a defined community or a population sample in terms of either being or not being a case. Face-to-face interviews (and follow-up) of all residents in defined communities has been a feature of some high-quality research, especially in the Scandinavian countries. However, since the size of the populations surveyed in this way is limited, the number of detected cases of schizophrenia is usually too small to generate stable estimates of epidemiological parameters. Surveys of large populations involve two basic designs: a single-phase survey of a probability sample drawn from the general population, and a two-phase survey where a validated screening test is first applied to the entire population and only those scoring as screen-positive proceed to a full assessment. In the instance of schizophrenia, logistics dictates a choice between assessing large numbers less rigorously and investigating a smaller sample in greater depth. In the absence of a simple and valid screening procedure for schizophrenia, such as a biological or psychological test, the advantages of the two-phase survey may be offset by poor sensitivity or specificity of the screening device which is usually a questionnaire or checklist.

The study of **birth cohorts** at ages when their members have passed through the greater part of the period of risk for onset of schizophrenia is usually done by direct interviewing or by analysing available case register data. Well-characterized birth cohorts are among the best tools for the study of the incidence of schizophrenia and associated risk factors. However, even in settings where the population is stable and mortality and morbidity are adequately monitored, the size of birth cohorts with prospectively collected data may not be sufficient for conclusive epidemiological inferences.

All this suggests that there is no single 'gold standard' of case-finding for schizophrenia that could be applied across all possible settings, and the assets and liabilities of particular case-finding procedures need to be evaluated in the context of each study. This makes the detailed reporting of case-finding methods a mandatory prerequisite for an 'evidence-based' epidemiology of schizophrenia.

Diagnosis

Variation in diagnostic concepts and practices always explains a proportion of the variation in the results of schizophrenia studies, especially if they involve different populations or different periods. Until the 1960s, the diagnostic rules used in epidemiological research were seldom explicitly stated. In the late 1960s, the WHO International Pilot Study of Schizophrenia[10] examined diagnostic variation in schizophrenia across nine countries by comparing the diagnoses made by psychiatrists using a semi-structured clinical interview with diagnostic classification by a computer algorithm[13] utilizing the same interview data. The results demonstrated that in the majority of settings psychiatrists were using comparable diagnostic concepts in the Kraepelin–Bleuler tradition. The introduction of explicit diagnostic criteria and rules with the consecutive editions of **DSM** and the WHO's **ICD-10** improved further the reliability of diagnosis but did not resolve all diagnostic issues with implications for epidemiology. While ICD-10 and DSM-IV tend to agree well on the core cases of schizophrenia, they agree less well on the classification of atypical or milder cases. Such differences may be less important in clinical practice but they present a problem for epidemiological and genetic studies. By providing more restrictive criteria for schizophrenia, both classifications aim to identify clinically similar cases and to minimize false-positive diagnoses. This is not an unequivocal advantage for epidemiology. Applying such criteria at case-finding may result in the rejection of potential cases which fail to meet the full set of criteria at initial assessment. Therefore it is desirable to develop less restrictive screening versions of the DSM and ICD criteria for epidemiological research.

Instruments

The diagnostic instruments used in surveys which involve interviewing fall into two categories: fully structured interviews such as the Diagnostic Interview Schedule (**DIS**)(12) and the Composite International Diagnostic Interview (**CIDI**)(14) both written to match exactly the diagnostic criteria of DSM-IIIR/IV and ICD-10, and semi-structured interview schedules such as the Present State Examination (**PSE**)(13) and the Schedules for Clinical Assessment in Neuropsychiatry (**SCAN**),(15) which cover a broad range of psychopathology and elicit data that can be processed by alternative diagnostic algorithms.

The DIS/CIDI type of instrument is reliable and capable of generating standard diagnoses of common mental disorders in a single-phase survey design. Its clinical validity in schizophrenia is less certain because symptoms may not be reported accurately or impairment may be underestimated by the respondent. In contrast, the PSE/SCAN allows a greater amount of psychopathological data to be elicited in a flexible clinical interview format, but its use in epidemiological studies presupposes availability of clinically trained interviewers. While SCAN and other similar interviews are suitable as second-stage diagnostic instruments, there is still a need for a relatively simple and effective screening procedure for case-finding of schizophrenia in field surveys.

Persons, place, time: descriptive epidemiology of schizophrenia

The epidemiological description of schizophrenia draws on extensive evidence available today on its frequency, age, and sex distribution in relatively large populations or geographical areas. Less than complete information is available on variations in its epidemiological characteristics that may be found in unusual or isolated populations, or on the temporal trends in its occurrence.

Prevalence, incidence, and disease expectancy

(a) Prevalence

Prevalence provides an estimate of the number of cases per 1000 persons at risk present in a population at a given time or over a defined period. **Point prevalence** refers to the 'active' (i.e. symptomatic) cases on a given date, or within a brief census period. Since asymptomatic cases (e.g. persons in remission) will be missed in a point prevalence survey, it is useful to supplement the assessment of the present mental state with an enquiry about past episodes of the disorder to obtain a **lifetime prevalence** index. In schizophrenia, which tends to a chronic course, estimates of point and lifetime prevalence will be closer to each other than in remitting illnesses.

An overview of selected prevalence studies of schizophrenia spanning nearly seven decades is presented in Table 4.3.5.2. The studies differ in many aspects of methodology but the majority of them feature a high intensity of case-finding. Several studies are repeat surveys in which the original population was reinvestigated following an interval of 10 or more years (the resulting consecutive prevalence figures are indicated by arrows).

The majority of studies have produced point prevalence estimates in the range 2.1 to 7.0 per 1000 population at risk and lifetime prevalence of schizophrenia in the range 15.0 to 19.0 per 1000. The figures are not uniformly standardized, and should be compared with caution because of demographic differences between populations related to factors such as age-specific mortality and migration. A **systematic review** of 188 studies in 46 countries, published between 1965 and 2002,(16) estimated the median value for point prevalence at 4.6 per 1000 persons and for lifetime prevalence at 7.2 per 1000.

Certain populations and groups deviate markedly from the central tendency. Strikingly high prevalence of schizophrenia (two to three times the national or regional average) has been found in geographically and genetically **isolated populations**, including small communities in Northern Sweden and Finland, and several Western Pacific islands (see Table 4.3.5.2). At the other extreme, a virtual absence of schizophrenia and a high rate of depression have been claimed for the Hutterites of South Dakota, a Protestant sect whose members live in close-knit endogamous communities sheltered from the outside world.(33) Negative social selection for schizoid individuals who fail to adjust to the lifestyle of the majority and eventually migrate without leaving progeny has been suggested (but not definitively proven) as an explanation. Results of two surveys in Taiwan,(21) separated by 15 years, point to a falling prevalence of schizophrenia (from 2.1 to 1.4 per 1000) in the context of major socio-economic change and an overall increase in total mental morbidity in the population.

The question about the extent of true variation in the prevalence of schizophrenia across populations has no simple answer. Methodological differences among studies, related to sampling, case-finding, and diagnostic assessment are likely to account for a good deal of the observed variation. As an example, the high mean prevalence rate of DSM-III schizophrenia reported from the Epidemiologic Catchment Area study in the United States(25) is difficult to reconcile with inconsistencies, such as a 13-fold difference in the rates for age group 18–24 years across the various sites of the survey. One possible reason is that the principal diagnostic instrument of the survey (DIS), administered by lay interviewers, may produce both false-positive and false-negative diagnoses of schizophrenia in a number of cases. Similarly, computer-generated diagnoses of 'non-affective psychosis' in the National Comorbidity Survey,(12) based on a version of the CIDI administered by lay interviewers, were found to agree poorly with clinicians' diagnoses when a subsample of the respondents were re-interviewed over the telephone.(34)

Notwithstanding such caveats in the interpretation of survey findings, the prevalence rates are fairly similar in the majority of studies, though certain specific populations clearly deviate from the modal value. Even in those instances, however, the magnitude of the deviation is modest compared with the 10- to 30-fold differences in prevalence observed in other multifactorial diseases (e.g. diabetes, ischaemic heart disease, multiple sclerosis) across populations.

(b) Incidence

The incidence rate (an estimate of the annual number of first-onset cases in a defined population per 1000 persons at risk) is of greater interest for the study of risk factors than prevalence since it represents the so-called force of morbidity (the probability of disease occurrence) in a given population, and is closer in time to the action of antecedent or precipitating factors. The estimation of incidence depends critically on the ability to determine reliably the point of **onset** of the disorder. In the case of schizophrenia, the long prodromal period and the fuzzy boundary between premorbid state and onset of psychosis make this particularly difficult. In the absence of an objective biomarker of the disease, onset is usually defined as

Table 4.3.5.2 Selected prevalence studies of schizophrenia

Author	Country	Population	Method	Prevalence per 1000 population at risk
Brugger (1931)[4]	Germany	Area in Thuringia (*n* =37 561); age 10+	Census; interview of sample	2.4
Strömgren (1938)[17]; Bøjholm and Strömgren (1989)[18]	Denmark	Island population (*n* = 50 000)	Census interviews; repeat census	3.9→3.3
Böök (1953);[19] Böök *et al.* (1978)[20]	Sweden	Genetic isolate (*n* = 9000); age 15–50	Census interviews; repeat census	9.5→17.0
Essen-Möller *et al.* (1956);[7] Hagnell (1966)[8]	Sweden	Community in Southern Sweden	Census interviews; repeat census	6.7→4.5
Lin *et al.* (1989)[21]	Taiwan	Population sample	Census interviews; repeat census	2.1→1.4
Crocetti *et al.* (1971)[22]	Croatia	Sample of 9201 households	Census based on hospital records and interviews	5.9
Dube and Kumar (1972)[23]	India	Four areas in Agra (*n* = 29 468)	Census based on hospital and clinic records	2.6
Rotstein (1977)[24]	Russia	Population sample (*n* = 35 590)	Census based on hospital and clinic records	3.8
Keith *et al.* (1991)[25]	USA	Aggregated data across five ECA sites	Sample survey; interviews	7.0 (point) 15.0 (lifetime)
Jeffreys *et al.* (1997)[26]	UK	London health district (*n* = 112 127)	Census; interview of sample (*n* = 172)	5.1
Kebede *et al.* (1999)[27]	Ethiopia	25 districts of Addis Ababa (*n* = 2 228 490)	Screening by self-report questionnaire, interviews of sample (*n* = 2042)	7.0 (point) 9.0 (lifetime)
Jablensky *et al.* (2000)[28]	Australia	Four urban areas (*n* = 1 084 978)	Census, screen for psychosis; interviews of sample (*n* = 980)	3.1–5.9 (point)[a] 3.9–6.9 (period, one year)[b]
Waldo *et al.* (1999)[29]	Micronesia	Island of Kosrae Genetic isolate	Screen of hospital records, interviews	6.8 (point)
Arajärvi *et al.* (2005)[30]	Finland	Birth cohort (*n* = 14 817) Genetic isolate	Case register data; interviews of 55% of register cases	15.0 (lifetime) 19.0[c] (lifetime)
Wu *et al.* (2006)[31]	USA (California)	Medicaid/Medicare health insurance data	20% random sample of insured subjects	5.1 (period, 1 year)
Perälä *et al.* (2007)[32]	Finland	National sample (*n* = 8028)	Screen for psychosis, interviews of sample; register and case note data also used	10.0 (lifetime) 22.9[d] (lifetime)

[a]All psychoses.

[b]Schizophrenia and other non-affective psychotic disorders.

[c]Schizophrenia spectrum disorders.

[d]Non-affective psychotic disorders.

the point in time when clinical manifestations become recognizable and diagnosable according to specified criteria. The first hospital admission, which has been used as a proxy for disease onset in many studies, is not a robust indicator because of the variable time lag between the earliest appearance of symptoms and the first-admission across treatment facilities and settings. A better approximation is provided by the first-contact, i.e. the point at which any psychiatric, general medical, or alternative 'helping' agency is accessed by symptomatic individuals for the first time. A limitation common to both first-admission and first-contact studies is that they produce rates of 'treated' incidence and miss symptomatic cases that do not present for assessment or treatment. This limitation can be overcome by periodically repeated door-to-door surveys of the same population or by longitudinal cohort studies (though both are difficult to mount for reasons of cost and logistics).

Table 4.3.5.3 summarizes the essential features of 12 selected incidence studies of schizophrenia. Studies using a 'broad' definition of schizophrenia (ICD-8 or ICD-9) estimate about three-fold difference in the variation of rates, in the range from 0.17 to 0.57 per 1000 population per year, for first-admissions or first contacts. Studies using more stringent criteria, such as the Research Diagnostic Criteria (**RDC**),[121] DSM-IV, ICD-10, or **Catego S+**,[13] have reported incidence rates two to three times lower than those based on 'broad' criteria. A **systematic review** of data from some 160 studies from 33 countries, published between 1965 and 2001,[35] yielded a median value of 0.15 and mean value of 0.24 per 1000, with a five-fold range of the rates and a tendency for more recent studies to report lower rates.

Considering the methodological differences among individual studies, generalizing about the incidence of schizophrenia from pooled data may be problematic. To date, the only investigation

Table 4.3.5.3 Selected incidence studies of schizophrenia

Author	Country	Population	Method	Rate per 1000
Ödegaard (1946)[6]	Norway	Total population	First-admissions 1926–35 (n = 14 231)	0.24 (Hospital diagnoses)
Walsh (1969)[36]	Ireland	City of Dublin (n = 720 000)	First-admissions	0.57 (males, ICD-8); 0.46 (females, ICD-8)
Murphy and Raman (1971)[37]	Mauritius	Total population (n = 257 000)	First-admissions	0.24 (Africans); 0.14 (Indian Hindus); 0.09 (Indian Moslems)
Lieberman (1974)[38]	Russia	Moscow district (n = 248 000)	Follow-back of prevalent cases	0.20 (males) 0.19 (females)
Helgason (1977)[39]	Iceland	Total population	First-admissions (case register)	0.27 (ICD-8)
Lin *et al.* (1989)[21]	Taiwan	Three communities (n = 39 024)	Door-to-door survey	0.17 ('Bleulerian' criteria)
Castle *et al.* (1991)[40]	UK	London (Camberwell)	First-admissions (case register)	0.25 (ICD-9); 0.17 (RDC); 0.08 (DSM-III)
Rajkumar *et al.* (1993)[41]	India	Area in Madras (n = 43 097)	Door-to-door survey and key informants	0.41 (ICD-9)
Wig *et al.* (1993)[42]	India	A rural area (n = 1 036 868) and an urban area (n = 348 609) in Northern India	Case-to-case finding and key informants	0.38 (urban, ICD-9); 0.09 (urban, Catego S+); 0.44 (rural, ICD-9); 0.12 (rural, Catego S+)
Brewin *et al.* (1997)[43]	UK	Nottingham	Two cohorts of first contacts (1978–80 and 1992–94)	0.25→0.29 (All psychoses, ICD-10); 0.14→0.09 (ICD-10 schizophrenia)
Mahy *et al.* (1999)[44]	Barbados	Total population (n = 262 000)	First contacts; PSE interviews; Catego	(0.32 ICD-9); (0.28 Catego S+)
Bresnahan *et al.* (2000)[45]	USA (California)	Birth cohort (n = 12 094)	Case register study; cumulative risk by age 38	0.93 (males, DSM-IV) 0.35 (females, DSM-IV)

that has applied a uniform design and common research tools to generate directly comparable incidence data for different populations is the **WHO 10-country study.**[9] Incidence counts in the WHO study were based on first-in-lifetime contacts with any 'helping agency' within defined areas (including traditional healers in the developing countries) which were monitored over a 2-year period. Potential cases and key informants were interviewed by clinicians using standardized instruments, and the timing of onset was ascertained for the majority of the patients. In 86 per cent of the 1022 patients the onset of diagnostic symptoms of schizophrenia was within the year preceding the first-contact, and therefore the first-contact incidence rate was adopted as a reasonable approximation to the 'true' onset rate. Two definitions of 'caseness', differing in the degree of specificity, were used to determine incidence: a 'broad' clinical definition comprising ICD-9 schizophrenia and paranoid psychoses, and a more restrictive definition of PSE/Catego S+[13] 'nuclear' schizophrenia manifesting with Schneiderian **first-rank symptoms**. The rates for eight of the catchment areas are shown in Table 4.3.5.4.

The differences between the area rates for 'broadly' defined schizophrenia (0.16–0.42 per 1000) were significant ($p < 0.001$) but those for 'nuclear' schizophrenia were not, suggesting that the frequency of this diagnostic subgroup varies less across different populations. No differences were found between cases meeting only 'broad' ICD-9 criteria and the Catego S+ cases with regard to age at onset, or 2-year course and outcome. Therefore it is unlikely that 'nuclear' and 'broad' schizophrenia define two different clinical illnesses.

Replications of the design of the WHO 10-country study, including its research procedures and instruments, have been carried out with very similar results in India, the Caribbean, and the United Kingdom (Table 4.3.5.3).

(c) Disease expectancy (morbid risk)

This is the probability (expressed as a percentage) that an individual born into a particular population will develop the disease if he or she survives the period of risk for that disease. In the instance of schizophrenia the **period of risk** is usually defined as 15 to 54 years. If age- and sex-specific incidence rates are known, disease expectancy can be estimated directly by a summation of the age-specific rates within the period of risk. Alternatively, disease expectancy can be estimated indirectly from prevalence data.

The estimates of disease expectancy produced by a number of studies are fairly consistent across populations and over time. Excluding outliers, such as the northern Swedish isolate,[19,20] they vary about five-fold; in the WHO study, they range from 0.59 per cent (Aarhus) to 1.8 per cent (Chandigarh, rural area) for ICD-9 schizophrenia and from 0.26 per cent (Honolulu) to 0.54 per cent (Nottingham) for Catego S+ 'nuclear' schizophrenia. The frequently cited modal estimate of lifetime disease expectancy for broadly defined schizophrenia at around 1 per cent seems to be consistent with the evidence.

(d) Associations with age and sex

Schizophrenia may have its onset at any age—in childhood as well as past middle age—although the vast majority of onsets fall within the 15 to 54 years of age interval. Onsets in men peak steeply in the

Table 4.3.5.4 Incidence rates per 1000 population, age 15–54, for a 'broad' and a 'narrow' case definition of schizophrenia (WHO 10-country study)

Country	Area	'Broad' definition (ICD-9)			'Narrow' definition (CATEGO S+)		
		Male	Female	All	Male	Female	All
Denmark	Aarhus	0.18	0.13	0.16	0.09	0.05	0.07
India	Chandigarh (rural area)	0.37	0.48	0.42	0.13	0.09	0.11
	Chandigarh (urban area)	0.34	0.35	0.35	0.08	0.11	0.09
Ireland	Dublin	0.23	0.21	0.22	0.10	0.08	0.09
Japan	Nagasaki	0.23	0.18	0.20	0.11	0.09	0.10
Russia	Moscow	0.25	0.31	0.28	0.03	0.03	0.02
United Kingdom	Nottingham	0.28	0.15	0.22	0.17	0.12	0.14
United States of America	Honolulu	0.18	0.14	0.16	0.10	0.08	0.09

(Taken from Report of the international pilot study of schizophrenia, WHO 10-country study, © World Health Organization, www.who.int)

age group 20 to 24 years; thereafter the rate of inception remains more or less constant at a lower level. In women, a less prominent peak in the age group 20 to 24 years is followed by another increase in incidence in age groups older than 35. While the age-specific incidence up to the mid-thirties is significantly higher in men, the male-to-female ratio becomes inverted with age, reaching 1:1.9 for onsets after age 40 and 1:4 or even 1:6 for onsets after age 60. There seems to be no real 'point of rarity' between the symptomatology of late-onset schizophrenia and schizophrenia of an early onset.

The sex differences in mean age at onset are unlikely to be an invariant biological characteristic of schizophrenia. For example, within families carrying high-genetic risk (two or more affected members), no significant differences in age at onset have been found between male and female siblings with schizophrenia. In some populations (e.g. India and China) the male predominance in the frequency of onsets in the younger age groups is attenuated or even inverted.(46,47)

The question of whether the total lifetime risks for men and women are about the same, or different, has not been answered definitively. In the WHO 10-country study, the cumulated risks for males and females up to the of age 54 were found to be approximately equal. Scandinavian studies which followed up population cohorts into very old age (over 80) reported a higher cumulated lifetime risk in women than in men.(48)

Male–female differences have been described in relation to the premorbid history (better premorbid functioning in women), the occurrence of brain abnormalities (more frequent in men), course (a higher percentage of remitting illness episodes and shorter hospital stay in women), and outcome (higher survival rate in the community, less disability in women). However, there is no unequivocal evidence of consistent sex differences in the symptom profiles of schizophrenia, including the frequency of positive and negative symptoms. Generally, the sex differences described in schizophrenia are more likely to result from normal sexual dimorphism in brain development, as well as from gender-related social roles, rather than from sex-specific aetiological factors.

Fertility, mortality, and comorbidity

(a) Fertility

Earlier studies reported low fertility in both men and women diagnosed with schizophrenia. The mean number of children fathered by men with schizophrenia in Sweden was 0.9, and the average number of live births over the entire reproductive period of women treated for schizophrenia in Norway between 1936 and 1975 was 1.8, compared with 2.2 for the general female population.(49) Yet this phenomenon is neither universal nor consistent over time. In the WHO 10-country study,(9) the fertility of women with schizophrenia in India did not differ from that of women in the general population within the same age groups and geographic areas. Although men with schizophrenia continue to be reproductively disadvantaged, the fertility of women with schizophrenia has increased over the last decades and this trend is likely to be sustained as a result of deinstitutionalization and the greater number of people with mental disorders being able to live in the community.

(b) Mortality

Excess mortality associated with schizophrenia has been well documented by epidemiological studies on large cohorts. National case register data for Norway, 1926–1941 and 1950–1974, indicate that, while the total mortality of psychiatric patients was decreasing, the relative mortality of patients with schizophrenia remained unchanged at a level higher than twice that of the general population.(6) Similar findings have been reported from other European countries and North America, with standardized mortality ratios of 2:6 or higher for patients with schizophrenia, which corresponds to about 20 per cent reduction in life expectancy. A **meta-analysis** of 18 studies(50) estimated a crude mortality rate of 189 deaths per 10000 population per year and a 10-year survival rate of 81 per cent. Mortality among males was significantly higher than among females, and the difference was primarily due to an excess in suicides and accidents. Unnatural causes apart, the leading causes of death among schizophrenia patients are similar to those in the general population, with the exception of a significantly lower than expected cancer morbidity and mortality, especially for tobacco-related malignancies in males with schizophrenia.(51) This puzzling phenomenon has been replicated by several case register and record linkage studies(52,53) and does not appear to be an artifact. Its causes remain unknown, though protective effects of both genes and antipsychotic pharmacological agents have been proposed.

The single most common cause of death among schizophrenia patients at present is **suicide** (aggregated standardized mortality ratios 9.6 for males and 6.8 for females) which accounts for 28 per cent of the excess mortality in schizophrenia.[54] The suicide rate in schizophrenia patients is at least equal to, or may indeed be higher, than the suicide rate in major depression. In China, the relative risk of suicide in individuals with schizophrenia compared to those without has been estimated at 23.8.[47] Several risk factors, relatively specific to schizophrenia, have been suggested: being young and male, experiencing multiple relapses and remissions, comorbid substance use, awareness of the deteriorating course of the condition, and loss of faith in treatment. Data from successive patient cohorts in Denmark,[55] United Kingdom,[56] and Australia[57] suggest an alarming trend of increasing mortality in first-admission patients with schizophrenia. In the Danish study,[55] the 5-year cumulated standardized mortality ratios increased from 5.30 (males) and 2.27 (females) between 1971 and 1973 to 7.79 (males) and 4.52 (females) between 1980 and 1982. Particularly striking was the standardized mortality ratio of 16.4 for males with schizophrenia in the first year after diagnosis. In the Australian study,[57] suicide risk was highest in the first 7 days after discharge from inpatient care. These trends seem to parallel the significant reductions in the number of psychiatric beds. Whether the increases in suicide mortality are associated with the shift in the management of schizophrenia from hospital to community care remains to be established.

(c) Comorbidity: physical disease

There is significant comorbidity in schizophrenia, comprising: (i) common medical problems and diseases that affect schizophrenia patients more frequently than attributable to chance; and (ii) certain rare conditions or abnormalities which tend to co-occur with the disorder.

Physical disease is common but tends to be seriously undetected and underdiagnosed. Between 46 per cent and 80 per cent of inpatients with schizophrenia, and between 20 per cent and 43 per cent of outpatients, have been found in different surveys to have concurrent medical illnesses.[58] Persons with schizophrenia, and especially those who are homeless or injection drug users, are at increased risk for potentially life-threatening **communicable diseases**, such as HIV/AIDS, hepatitis C, and tuberculosis.[59, 60] Among the chronic non-communicable diseases, patients with schizophrenia have significantly higher than expected rates of epilepsy, diabetes, arteriosclerosis, and ischaemic heart disease.[61–63] Obesity and the concomitant **metabolic syndrome** involving insulin resistance are becoming increasingly common problems in schizophrenia patients.[64] Although a high incidence of **diabetes** in schizophrenia patients had been described long before the introduction of neuroleptic treatment, a contributing role for some of the second-generation antipsychotic agents has not been ruled out.

Some rare genetic or idiopathic disorders, such as metachromatic leucodystrophy, acute intermittent porphyria, and coeliac disease, as well as dysmorphic features such as high-steepled palate, malformed ears and other minor physical anomalies have also been reported to co-occur with schizophrenia.[65,66] On the other hand, several studies have found a lower than expected rate of rheumatoid arthritis in schizophrenia patients.[67]

(d) Comorbidity: substance abuse

Substance abuse is at present by far the most common associated health problem among patients with schizophrenia[68] and may involve any drug of abuse or a polydrug combination. It seems, however, that the addictive use of cannabis, stimulants, and nicotine is disproportionately high among schizophrenia patients and may be linked to the underlying neurobiology of the disorder.[69,70] In a nationwide sample of patients with psychotic disorders in Australia,[28] a lifetime diagnosis of comorbid drug abuse, or dependence was made in 36.3 per cent of males and 15.7 per cent of females with schizophrenia (compared to 3.1 per cent and 1.3 per cent respectively in the general population). In addition to poor prognosis of schizophrenia in patients with heavy cannabis use,[71] a **systematic review** of published data on **cannabis** exposure and the onset of schizophrenia[72] concluded that early use increased the risk of psychosis in a dose-related manner, especially in persons at high genetic risk of schizophrenia. Similarly, **stimulants** tend to exacerbate acute psychotic symptoms in over 50 per cent of schizophrenia patients.[73] The prevalence of cigarette **smoking** among schizophrenia patients is, on the average, two to three times higher than in the general population,[74] but the evidence regarding any adverse effects of nicotine use on the onset and course of schizophrenia is equivocal. A population cohort study[75] found that smoking at ages 18–20 was associated with a lower risk of schizophrenia in later life and could have a specific neuroprotective effect independent of its overall harmful impact on health.

Geographical and cultural variation

To date, no population or culture has been identified in which schizophrenic illnesses do not occur. Also, there is no strong evidence that the incidence of schizophrenia is either uniform, or varies widely across populations, provided that the populations being compared are large enough to minimize the effects of small-area variation. The evidence that specific **psychosocial** or cultural factors play an aetiological role in schizophrenia is also inconsistent.[76] However, there are well-replicated findings of variations in the course and outcome of schizophrenia across populations and cultures that involve, above all, a higher rate of symptomatic recovery and a lower rate of social deterioration in traditional rural communities. Data supporting this conclusion were provided by the WHO studies[9] which found a higher proportion of recovering or improving patients in developing countries such as India and Nigeria than in the developed countries. Sampling bias (e.g. a higher percentage of acute-onset schizophreniform illnesses of good prognosis among Third World patients) was not a likely explanation. A better outcome in the developing countries was found in patients with various modes of onset, and the initial symptoms of the disorder did not distinguish good-outcome from poor-outcome cases. What causes such differences in the prognosis of schizophrenia remains largely unknown. The follow-up in the WHO studies demonstrated that the outcome of paranoid psychoses and affective disorders was also better in the developing countries. Such a general effect on the outcome of psychiatric disorders may result from psychosocial factors, such as availability of social support networks, non-stigmatizing beliefs about mental illness, and positive expectations during the early stages of psychotic illness, as well as from unknown genetic or ecological (including nutritional) factors influencing brain development.

The disease and disability burden of schizophrenia

According to WHO estimates[77,78] no less than 25 per cent of the total 'burden of disease' in the established market economies is at present attributable to neuropsychiatric conditions. Measured as proportion of the disability-adjusted life-years (**DALYs**) lost, schizophrenia, bipolar affective disorder, and major depression together account for 10.8 per cent of the total, i.e. they inflict on most communities losses that are comparable to those due to cancer (15 per cent) and higher than the losses due to ischaemic heart disease (9 per cent).

An epidemiological perspective on risk factors and antecedents

Studies on clinical samples suggest a great variety of putative risk factors in schizophrenia. As clinical samples are rarely representative and often vulnerable to bias, epidemiological evidence helps in evaluating the significance of such conjectures. Genetic and environmental risk factors are considered further in Chapter 4.3.6.1.

Genetic risk: necessary and sufficient?

Family aggregation of schizophrenia is at present the only epidemiologically well-established risk factor for the disorder, with a relative risk for first-degree relatives of persons with schizophrenia in the range from 9 to 18. Allowing for diagnostic variation, the risk estimates generated by different studies are similar and suggest a general pattern of descending risk as the proportions of shared genes between any two individuals decrease.[79,80] Although **heritability** (commonly estimated at about 80 per cent) provides the basis for the search of specific genes and gene networks involved in schizophrenia causation, the extent to which genetic vulnerability alone is necessary and sufficient to produce the disorder remains unclear. While an environmental contribution to the aetiology of schizophrenia is highly plausible, the evidence in support of it is inferential, typically proceeding from the observation that the concordance for schizophrenia in monozygotic twins (sharing 100 per cent of their genes) is only about 50 per cent. The majority of investigators now agree that genes and environments should be studied jointly and three models of conjunction have been proposed[81]:

- The effects of predisposing genes and environmental factors are additive and increase the risk of disease in a linear fashion;
- Genes modulate the sensitivity of the brain to environmental insults;
- By fostering certain personality traits and associated behaviour, genes influence the likelihood of an individual's exposure to stressful environments.

Epidemiological research into possible environmental contributions to the causation of schizophrenia focuses on three main areas: pre- and perinatal brain damage, factors affecting neurodevelopment from infancy to late adolescence, and factors of the social and urban ecology. (See also Chapter 4.3.6.1)

Factors maintaining the incidence of schizophrenia in populations

Since the first epidemiological study on the reproduction patterns of people with psychoses,[82] reduced fertility among individuals with schizophrenia has been documented by numerous investigators. Coupled with the evidence that the lifetime risk of the disorder (about 1 per cent) is similar across populations and remains stable over time, the question about factors that sustain the incidence of schizophrenia despite a reduced **reproductive fitness**. An early hypothesis was proposed in 1964 by Huxley *et al.*[83] who argued that the high frequency of schizophrenia was evidence of 'genetic morphism' (a balanced polymorphism) whereby the low fertility of affected individuals could be compensated for by a higher than average fertility of clinically unaffected 'cryptoschizophrenic carriers' who possessed some selective advantage, e.g. resistance to shock, autoimmune disease, or infection. However, attempts to demonstrate such advantage in terms of disease resistance, adaptability to extreme environments, or ability and creativity, have been unsuccessful. Importantly, the selective advantage hypothesis assumed that schizophrenia was a single-gene disorder with low penetrance, whereas the majority of investigators today agree that schizophrenia is a **complex polygenic disorder** with incomplete or variable expression of the genotype, and widespread locus and allelic heterogeneity. The polygenic model implies that loss of susceptibility alleles resulting from the lower reproductive fitness of affected individuals would have a negligible effect on the overall gene pool in the population. The more recent hypothesis, that *de novo* germ-line mutations inherited from an ageing father[84] may be responsible for a substantial proportion of incident cases of schizophrenia, is difficult to reconcile with current knowledge that mutation rates for most human genes are within the range of 10^{-6} to 10^{-5} per generation, i.e. their contribution to the maintenance of schizophrenia in the population would be insignificant. Considering that both multiple genes and multiple exogenous factors are likely to be involved in the causation of schizophrenia, neither increased fertility in asymptomatic carriers of the risk genes, nor paternal inheritance of germ-line mutations appear to be necessary or sufficient for the persistence of the disorder.

Environmental insults during early development

(a) Season of birth

A 5 per cent to 8 per cent winter–spring excess of schizophrenic births was first described in 1929[85] and since then reported by numerous studies, mostly in the northern hemisphere (southern hemisphere data are less consistent). Though some of these studies did not have the sample size or statistical design needed to definitively prove or rule out a seasonal effect, **winter–spring births** were associated with a mild but significant increase of the relative risk for schizophrenia (RR = 1.11; CI 1.06–1.18) in a large population cohort from Denmark.[86] Thus, birth seasonality appears to be a robust finding in the epidemiology of schizophrenia,[87] though few biologically plausible and testable causal hypotheses have been advanced to explain it. One of them is the seasonally increased risk of intrauterine exposure to viral infection.

(b) Prenatal exposure to infection

In utero exposure to **influenza** has been implicated as a risk factor since a report that a significant proportion of adult schizophrenia in Helsinki was associated with presumed second-trimester *in utero* exposure to the 1957 A2 influenza epidemic.[88] Numerous studies, attempting to replicate the link between maternal influenza and schizophrenia, have since reached conflicting results, with negative findings reported from an increasing number of studies based on large population samples,[89,90] as well as studies including data on schizophrenia risk in the offspring of women with prospectively recorded influenza infection during pregnancy.[91] However, positive association between schizophrenia in the offspring and maternal infection during pregnancy has been reported for **rubella**[92] and **toxoplasmosis**[93] and the issue of prenatal infection contributing to schizophrenia risk merits further study.

(c) Pregnancy and birth complications

Maternal obstetric complications, ranging from placental abnormalities in the first trimester of pregnancy to diabetes, pre-eclampsia, perinatal hypoxia, and low birth weight, are widely regarded to be risk factors in schizophrenia. This view is supported by a number of studies of small to moderate size, typically using a case-control design and relying on maternal recall of adverse events during pregnancy.[94] Population-based studies[95,96] using prospectively recorded obstetric data tend to report conflicting or inconclusive results, with generally small effect sizes (odds ratio less than two) for any positive findings.[97] However, several birth cohort studies with long-term follow-up have found significantly increased risk of adult schizophrenia in individuals who had survived severe, mainly **hypoxic perinatal brain damage**.[98,99] Birth weight (adjusted for gestation) is another factor that may have a complex relationship with schizophrenia risk. A large cohort study in Sweden[100] found a reverse J-shaped association between **birth weight** and adult schizophrenia, with significant hazard ratios of 7.03 for males of low birth weight (<2500 g) and 3.37 for those of high birth weight (>4000 g). It remains unclear, however, if severe obstetric complications, such as perinatal hypoxia or low birth weight, are capable of raising substantially the risk of schizophrenia in the adult in the absence of increased genetic risk. Maternal schizophrenia is associated with a higher rate of pregnancy complications, including low birth weight,[101] but it is not known if the effects of genetic liability and obstetric complications on schizophrenia risk in the offspring are additive or interactive. It is also possible that genetic predisposition sensitizes the developing brain to lesions resulting from randomly occurring less severe obstetric complications. Such gaps in knowledge or inconsistencies among research findings caution against an unqualified acceptance of obstetric complication as a proven risk factor in schizophrenia. Clarification of their role remains an important priority for epidemiological research.

Further information about studies of obstetric complications and hypoxic-ischaemic damage as risk factors for schizophrenia can be found in Chapter 4.3.6.1.

Developmental antecedents of schizophrenia

(a) Brain development and neurobehavioural markers

Children at high genetic risk for schizophrenia (i.e. having parents or other first-degree relatives with the disorder) tend to show early signs of aberrant neurodevelopment, including ventricular enlargement on computerized tomography[102] and decreased activation in the prefrontal and parietal regions of the heteromodal association cortex on functional magnetic resonance imaging.[103] Such imaging studies are limited by small sample size and their results may not be generalizable. However, population-based or cohort studies, such as the National Child Development Study in the United Kingdom have demonstrated a higher incidence of abnormal **motor and speech development** before 2 years of age, and of soft neurological signs (poor motor control, coordination, and balance), non-right handedness and speech defects between ages 2–15.[104]

(b) Cognitive and neurophysiological markers

Deficits in verbal memory, sustained attention and executive functions, as well as abnormalities in event-related brain potentials and oculomotor control[105–107] are common in patients with schizophrenia and antedate the onset of clinical symptoms. They also occur in a proportion of their clinically normal biological relatives, but are rare in control subjects drawn from the general population (see Chapter 4.3.3). Their specificity to schizophrenia needs to be investigated in larger population samples. Should such **endophenotypes** be validated as biological markers of schizophrenia by epidemiological studies, the power of risk prediction at the level of the individual is likely to increase substantially.

(c) Premorbid intelligence (IQ)

In a cohort study from Sweden,[108] involving a 15-year follow-up of 109 643 men conscripted into the army at age 18 to 20, the individuals who subsequently developed schizophrenia were compared with the rest of the cohort on the performance of IQ-related tests and tasks at the time of conscription. Controlling for potential confounders, the risk of schizophrenia was found to increase linearly with the decrement of IQ. The effect was mainly attributable to poor performance on verbal tasks and tests of reasoning. Similar results have been reported from a study in Israel linking psychometric assessment data of the army draft board with the national psychiatric case register.[109]

Premorbid social impairment

Individuals who develop schizophrenia as adults are more likely to manifest difficulties in social interaction during childhood and adolescence than individuals who do not develop schizophrenia. Among children at increased genetic risk (having a parent with schizophrenia), those who develop schizophrenia as adults have been found to show poorer social competence at age 7 to 12 and more passivity and social isolation in adolescence, as compared to those who do not develop the disorder.[110] The association between early 'schizoid' traits and risk of schizophrenia is not restricted to offsprings of parents with schizophrenia. Population-based evidence of early **socialization difficulties** (school problems, social anxiety, and preference for solitary play) in children who develop schizophrenia as adults is provided by the prospective study of a national birth cohort in the United Kingdom.[104] In the Swedish conscript study,[108] poor social adjustment during childhood and adolescence was significantly more common among those who subsequently developed schizophrenia than among those who did not. It should be noted, however, that the early behavioural traits that tend to be associated with schizophrenia in adult life have low specificity and their predictive value is limited.

Further information about studies of premorbid social impairment can be found in Chapter 4.3.6.1.

The social and family environment

(a) Early rearing environment

Support for an effect of the early rearing family environment on the risk of developing schizophrenia is provided by a study of a Finnish sample of **adopted children** born to mothers with schizophrenia (a high-risk group) and a control sample of adoptees at no increased genetic risk.[111] Though the rates of adult psychosis or severe personality disorder were significantly higher in the high-risk group compared with the control group, the difference was entirely attributable to a subset of the high-risk children who grew up in dysfunctional or otherwise disturbed adoptive families—a result consistent with a gene-environment model of genetic influence on a person's sensitivity to psychosocial adversity.

(b) The urban environment

Earlier hypotheses that urban environments increase the risk of psychosis, either by contributing to causation (the breeder effect) or by attracting vulnerable individuals (the drift effect), have been revived in the light of recent epidemiological findings suggesting that urban birth is associated with a moderate but statistically significant increase in the incidence of schizophrenia, affective psychoses, and other non-affective psychoses.[112] It remains unclear whether the effect is linked to a factor operating pre- or perinatally, or a factor influencing postnatal development (see also Chapter 4.3.6.1).

(c) Social class

Since the 1930s, numerous studies in North America and Europe have consistently found that the economically disadvantaged social groups contribute disproportionately to the first-admission rate for schizophrenia. Two explanatory hypotheses, of **social causation** ('breeder') and of **social selection** ('drift'), were originally proposed.[113] According to the social causation theory, the greater socio-economic adversity characteristic of lower-class living conditions could precipitate psychosis in genetically vulnerable individuals who have a restricted capacity to cope with complex or stressful situations. In the 1960s, this theory was considered to be refuted by a single study[114] which found that the social class distribution of the fathers of schizophrenic patients did not deviate from that of the general population, and that the excess of low socio-economic status among schizophrenic patients was mainly attributable to individuals who had drifted down the occupational and social scale prior to the onset of psychosis. As a result, aetiological research in schizophrenia in recent decades has tended to ignore such 'macrosocial' variables. However, the possibility remains that social stratification, socio-economic status, and acculturation stress are contributing factors in the causation of schizophrenia.

(d) Migrants and ethnic minorities

An exceptionally high-incidence rate of schizophrenia (about 6.0 per 1000) has been found in the African–Caribbean population in the United Kingdom.[115,116] The excess morbidity is not restricted to recent immigrants and is higher in the British-born second generation of migrants. Similar findings of nearly four-fold excess over the general population rate have been reported for the Dutch Antillean and Surinamese immigrants in Holland.[117]

The causes of the phenomenon remain obscure. Incidence studies in the Caribbean do not indicate any excess morbidity in the indigenous populations from which migrants are recruited. Explanations in terms of biological risk factors have found little support.[118,122] A finding in need of replication is the significant increase of schizophrenia among the siblings of second-generation African–Caribbean schizophrenia patients compared with the incidence of schizophrenia in the siblings of white patients.[119] Such 'horizontal' increase in the morbid risk suggests that an environmental factor may be modifying the penetrance of the genetic predisposition to schizophrenia carried by a proportion of the African–Caribbean population. Psychosocial hypotheses involving acculturation stress, demoralization due to racial discrimination, and blocked opportunities for upward social mobility have been suggested but not yet definitively tested (see also Chapter 4.3.6.1).

Epidemiological issues for the next decade

The unprecedented growth of basic knowledge about the brain and the human genome opens up novel perspectives and opportunities in the study of complex disorders such as schizophrenia, which integrate concepts and tools of genetics, neuroscience, and epidemiology. Several issues with wide implications for future research are already emerging.

Is schizophrenia a single disease or a group of aetiologically distinct disorders?

Schizophrenia is characterized by extensive phenotypic variability and likely genetic heterogeneity. These two factors may be contributing disproportionately to the multitude of research findings that are inconsistent or difficult to replicate and there is increasing concern that the categorical diagnostic concept of schizophrenia may not demarcate a biologically homogeneous entity.[120] The likely existence of different **subtypes** of the disorder (Bleuler's notion of a 'group of schizophrenias') is rarely considered in genetic and other biological research into schizophrenia. Disaggregating a **complex phenotype** by identifying intermediate (endo-) phenotypes and quantitative traits as covariates has been a successful strategy in the genetic study of disorders such as type I diabetes, asthma, and dementia. While the clinical concept of schizophrenia as a broad syndrome with some internal cohesion and a characteristic course over time is well supported by current epidemiological evidence, its dissection into modular endophenotypes with specific neurocognitive and neurophysiological underpinnings is beginning to be perceived as a promising approach in schizophrenia genetics. The study of endophenotypes cutting across the conventional diagnostic boundaries may reveal unexpected patterns of associations with symptoms, personality traits or behaviours, as well as genetic polymorphisms, providing epidemiology with rich material for hypothesis testing at population level.

Molecular epidemiology of schizophrenia

Notwithstanding the difficulties accompanying the genetic dissection of complex disorders, novel methods of genetic analysis will eventually identify genomic regions, genes, and **interacting gene networks** underlying the predisposition to schizophrenia. The majority of genes involved are believed to be of small effect, although one cannot exclude the possibility that genes of moderate effects may also be found, especially in relation to the neurophysiological abnormalities associated with schizophrenia. Clarifying the function of such genes will be a complex task. Part of the solution is likely to be found in the domain of epidemiology, since establishing their population frequency and associations with a variety of phenotypic expressions is a prerequisite for understanding their causal role. Thus the molecular epidemiology of schizophrenia is likely to be the next major chapter in the search for its causes and cures.

Can schizophrenia be prevented?

The increasing investment in early diagnosis and treatment of **first episodes** of schizophrenia has raised questions whether people likely to develop schizophrenia can be reliably recognized prior to the onset of symptoms, and whether early pharmacological, cognitive, or social intervention can prevent the development of the disorder. While early diagnosis and timely treatment of symptomatic cases may improve the short- or medium-term outcome, the detection of people at risk with a view to preventative intervention is problematic. Screening young age groups in the population by using predictors such as family history of psychosis, obstetric complications, or abnormal eye tracking is likely to result in multiple false-positive and false-negative results and a generally low positive predictive value. Other candidate risk factors have not been evaluated at all epidemiologically. Problems of reliability of measurement apart, population-based screening will pose huge practical and ethical problems of having to treat a large number of individuals who do not have the disorder and missing many others who eventually will develop the disorder. From an epidemiological point of view, pre-symptomatic detection and preventative intervention in schizophrenia do not appear to be feasible for the time being.

Summary and conclusions

After nearly a century of epidemiological research, essential questions about the nature and causes of schizophrenia still await answers. Two major conclusions stand out.

- The clinical syndrome of schizophrenia is robust and can be identified in diverse populations, regardless of wide-ranging demographic, ecological, and cultural differences among them. This suggests that a common pathophysiology is likely to underlie the characteristic symptoms of schizophrenia. On balance, the evidence suggests that schizophrenia incidence and disease risk show relatively modest variation at the level of large population aggregates. However, the study of 'atypical' populations or pockets of very high or very low frequency of schizophrenia, such as in genetic isolates or minority groups, may provide **novel clues** to the aetiology and pathogenesis of disorder.
- No single environmental risk factor of major effect on the incidence of schizophrenia has yet been discovered. Further studies using large samples are required to evaluate potential risk factors, antecedents, and predictors for which the present evidence is inconclusive. Assuming that methodological pitfalls will be avoided by risk-factor epidemiology, and that multiple environmental risk factors of small to moderate effect will eventually be identified, the results will complement those of genetic research which also implicate multiple genes and networks. All this suggests that the key to understanding schizophrenia is likely to be in the unraveling of complex **gene-environment interactions**.

Further information

Susser, E., Schwartz, S., Morabia, A., and Bromet, E. (eds.) (2006). *Psychiatric epidemiology. Searching for the causes of mental disorders.* Oxford University Press, Oxford.

Murray, R.M., Jones, P.B., Susser, E., van Os, J., and Cannon, M. (eds.) (2003). *The epidemiology of schizophrenia.* Cambridge University Press.

Hirsch, S.R. and Weinberger, D.R. (eds.) (2003). *Schizophrenia* (2nd edn). Blackwell Science, Oxford.

www.schizophreniaforum.org Schizophrenia Research Forum (sponsored by NARSAD, the Mental Health Research Association, through a contract with the National Institute of Mental Health).

References

1. Kraepelin, E. (1896). *Psychiatrie. Ein Lehrbuch für Studirende und Aerzte. Barth, Leipzig* (Reprint: edition 1976 by Arno Press Inc., New York).
2. Koller, J. (1895). Beitrag zur Erblichkeitsstatistik der Geisteskrankheiten in Canton Zürich. *Archiv für Psychiatrie*, **27**, 269–94.
3. Luxenburger, H. (1928). Vorläufiger Bericht über psychiatrische Serienuntersuchungen an Zwillingen. *Zeitschrift für die gesamte Neurologie und Psychiatrie*, **116**, 297–326.
4. Brugger, C. (1931). Versuch einer Geisteskrankenzählung in Thüringen. *Zeitschrift für die gesamte Neurologie und Psychiatrie*, **133**, 252–390.
5. Klemperer, J. (1933). Zur Belastungsstatistik der Durchschnittsbevölkerung. Psychosehäufigkeit unter 1000 stichprobenmässig ausgelesenen Probanden. *Zeitschrift für die gesamte Neurologie und Psychiatrie*, **146**, 277–316.
6. Ödegaard, Ö. (1946). A statistical investigation into the incidence of mental disorders in Norway. *The Psychiatric Quarterly*, **20**, 381–401.
7. Essen-Möller, E., Larsson, H., Uddenberg, C.E., *et al.* (1956). Individual traits and morbidity in a Swedish rural population. *Acta Psychiatrica et Neurologica Scandinavica*, (Suppl. 100), 1–136.
8. Hagnell, O. (1966). *A prospective study of the incidence of mental disorder*. Svenska Bokforlaget, Lund.
9. Jablensky, A., Sartorius, N., Ernberg, G., *et al.* (1992). Schizophrenia: manifestations and course in different cultures. A World Health Organization ten-country study. *Psychological Medicine, Monograph Supplement*, **20**, 1–97.
10. World Health Organization. (1973). *The international pilot study of schizophrenia*, Vol. 1. WHO, Geneva.
11. Robins, L.N. and Regier, D.A. (eds.) (1991). *Psychiatric disorders in America. The Epidemiologic Catchment Area Study*. Free Press, New York.
12. Kessler, R.C., McGonagle, K.A., Zhao, S., *et al.* (1994). Lifetime and 12-month prevalence of DSM-IIIR psychiatric disorders in the United States. Results from the National Comorbidity Survey. *Archives of General Psychiatry*, **51**, 8–19.
13. Wing, J.K., Cooper, J.E., and Sartorius, N. (1974). The measurement and classification of psychiatric symptoms. Cambridge University Press, Cambridge.
14. Robins, L.N., Wing, J., Wittchen, H.U., *et al.* (1988). The Composite International Diagnostic Interview: an epidemiologic instrument suitable for use in conjunction with different diagnostic systems and in different cultures. *Archives of General Psychiatry*, **45**, 1069–77.
15. Wing, J.K., Babor, T., Brugha, T., *et al.* (1990). SCAN. Schedules for clinical assessment in neuropsychiatry. *Archives of General Psychiatry*, **47**, 589–93.
16. Saha, S., Chant, D., Welham, J., *et al.* (2005). A systematic review of the prevalence of schizophrenia. *PLoS Medicine*, **2**, 413–33. (www.plosmedicine.org)
17. Strömgren, E. (1938). Beiträge zur psychiatrischen Erblehre, auf Grund von Untersuchungen an einer Inselbevölkerung. *Acta Psychiatrica et Neurologica Scandinavica*, (Suppl. 19), 1–86.
18. Bøjholm, S. and Strömgren, E. (1989). Prevalence of schizophrenia on the island of Bornholm in 1935 and in 1983. *Acta Psychiatrica Scandinavica*, **79**(Suppl. 348), 157–66.
19. Böök, J.A. (1953). A genetic and neuropsychiatric investigation of a North Swedish population (with special regard to schizophrenia and mental deficiency). *Acta Genetica*, **4**, 1–100.

20. Böök, J.A., Wettenberg, L., and Modrzewska, K. (1978). Schizophrenia in a North Swedish geographical isolate, 1900–1977: epidemiology, genetics and biochemistry. *Clinical Genetics*, **14**, 373–94.
21. Lin, T.Y., Chu, H.M., Rin, H., *et al.* (1989). Effects of social change on mental disorders in Taiwan: observations based on a 15-year follow-up survey of general population in three communities. *Acta Psychiatrica Scandinavica*, **79**(Suppl. 348), 11–34.
22. Crocetti, G.J., Lemkau, P.V., Kulcar, Z., *et al.* (1971). Selected aspects of the epidemiology of psychoses in Croatia, Yugoslavia, II. The cluster sample and the results of the pilot survey. *American Journal of Epidemiology*, **94**, 126–34.
23. Dube, K.V. and Kumar, N. (1972). An epidemiological study of schizophrenia. *Journal of Biosocial Science*, **4**, 187–95.
24. Rotstein, V.G. (1977). Material from a psychiatric survey of sample groups from the adult population in several areas of the USSR. *Zhurnal Nevropatologii I Psikhiatrii*, **77**, 569–74 (in Russian).
25. Keith, S.J., Regier, D.A., and Rae, D.S. (1991). Schizophrenic disorders. In *Psychiatric disorders in America. The Epidemiologic Catchment Area Study* (eds. L.N. Robins and D.A. Regier), pp. 33–52. Free Press, New York.
26. Jeffreys, S.E., Harvey, C.A., McNaught, A.S., *et al.* (1997). The Hampstead schizophrenia survey 1991. I. Prevalence and service use comparisons in an inner London health authority, 1986–1991. *The British Journal of Psychiatry*, **170**, 301–6.
27. Kebede, D. and Alem, A. (1999). Major mental disorders in Addis Ababa, Ethiopia. I. Schizophrenia, schizoaffective and cognitive disorders. *Acta Psychiatrica Scandinavica*, **100**, 11–7.
28. Jablensky, A., McGrath, J., Herrman, H., *et al.* (2000). Psychotic disorders in urban areas: an overview of the Study on Low Prevalence Disorders. *The Australian and New Zealand Journal of Psychiatry*, **34**, 221–36.
29. Waldo, M.C. (1999). Schizophrenia in Kosrae, Micronesia: prevalence, gender ratios, and clinical symptomatology. *Schizophrenia Research*, **35**, 175–81.
30. Arajärvi, R., Suvisaari, J, Suokas, J., *et al.* (2005). Prevalence and diagnosis of schizophrenia based on register, case record and interview data in an isolated Finnish birth cohort born 1940–1969. *Social Psychiatry and Psychiatric Epidemiology*, **40**, 808–16.
31. Wu, E.Q., Shi, L., Birnbaum, H., *et al.* (2006). Annual prevalence of diagnosed schizophrenia in the USA: a claims data analysis approach. *Psychological Medicine*, **36**, 1535–40.
32. Perälä, J., Suvisaari, J., Saarni, S.I., *et al.* (2007). Lifetime prevalence of psychotic and bipolar I disorders in a general population. *Archives of General Psychiatry*, **64**, 19–28.
33. Eaton, J.W. and Weil, R.J. (1955). *Culture and mental disorder. A comparative study of the Hutterites and other populations.* Free Press, Glencoe, IL.
34. Kendler, K.S., Gallagher, T.J., Abelson, J.M., *et al.* (1996). Lifetime prevalence, demographic risk factors, and diagnostic validity of nonaffective psychosis as assessed in a US community sample. *Archives of General Psychiatry*, **53**, 1022–31.
35. McGrath, J., Saha, S., Welham, J., *et al.* (2003). A systematic review of the incidence of schizophrenia: the distribution of rates and the influence of sex, urbanicity, migrant status and methodology. *BMC Medicine*, **2**, 1–22. (www.biomedcentral.com/1741-7015/2/13)
36. Walsh, D. (1969). Mental illness in Dublin–first admissions. *The British Journal of Psychiatry*, **115**, 449–56.
37. Murphy, H.B.M. and Raman, A.C. (1971). The chronicity of schizophrenia in indigenous tropical peoples. Results of a twelve-year follow-up survey in Mauritius. *The British Journal of Psychiatry*, **118**, 489–97.
38. Lieberman, Y.I. (1974). The problem of incidence of schizophrenia: material from a clinical and epidemiological study. *Zhurnal Nevropatologii I Psikhiatrii*, **74**, 1224–32 (in Russian).
39. Helgason, L. (1977). Psychiatric services and mental illness in Iceland. *Acta Psychiatrica Scandinavica*, **53**(Suppl. 268), 1–140.
40. Castle, D., Wessely, S., Der, G., *et al.* (1991). The incidence of operationally defined schizophrenia in Camberwell, 1965–1984. *The British Journal of Psychiatry*, **159**, 790–4.
41. Rajkumar, S., Padmavati, R., Thara, R., *et al.* (1993). Incidence of schizophrenia in an urban community in Madras. *Indian Journal of Psychiatry*, **35**, 18–21.
42. Wig, N.N., Varma, V.K., Mattoo, S.K., *et al.* (1993). An incidence study of schizophrenia in India. *Indian Journal of Psychiatry*, **35**, 11–7.
43. Brewin, J., Cantwell, R., Dalkin, T., *et al.* (1997). Incidence of schizophrenia in Nottingham. *The British Journal of Psychiatry*, **171**, 140–4.
44. Mahy, G.E., Mallett, R., Leff, J., *et al.* (1999). First-contact incidence rate of schizophrenia on Barbados. *The British Journal of Psychiatry*, **175**, 28–33.
45. Bresnahan, M.A., Brown, A.S., Schaefer, C.A., *et al.* (2000). Incidence and cumulative risk of treated schizophrenia in the prenatal determinants of schizophrenia study. *Schizophrenia Bulletin*, **26**, 297–308.
46. Murthy, G.V.S., Janakiramaiah, N., Gangadhar, B.N., *et al.* (1998). Sex difference in age at onset of schizophrenia: discrepant findings from India. *Acta Psychiatrica Scandinavica*, **97**, 321–5.
47. Phillips, M.R., Yang, G., Li, S., *et al.* (2004). Suicide and the unique prevalence pattern of schizophrenia in mainland China: a retrospective observational study. *Lancet*, **364**, 1062–8.
48. Helgason, T. and Magnusson, H. (1989). The first 80 years of life. A psychiatric epidemiological study. *Acta Psychiatrica Scandinavica*, **79**(Suppl. 348), 85–94.
49. Ödegaard, Ö. (1980). Fertility of psychiatric first admissions in Norway, 1936–1975. *Acta Psychiatrica Scandinavica*, **62**, 212–20.
50. Brown, S. (1997). Excess mortality of schizophrenia. A meta-analysis. *The British Journal of Psychiatry*, **171**, 502–8.
51. Dupont, A., Jensen, O.M., Strömgren, E., *et al.* (1986). Incidence of cancer in patients diagnosed as schizophrenic in Denmark. In *Psychiatric case registers in public health* (eds. S.H. Ten Horn, R. Giel, and W. Gulbinat), pp. 229–39. Elsevier, Amsterdam.
52. Dalton, S.O., Mellemkjær, L., Thomassen, L., *et al.* (2005). Risk for cancer in a cohort of patients hospitalized for schizophrenia in Denmark, 1969–1993. *Schizophrenia Research*, **75**, 315–24.
53. Grinshpoon, A., Barchana, M., Ponizovsky, A., *et al.* (2005). Cancer in schizophrenia: is the risk higher or lower? *Schizophrenia Research*, **73**, 333–41.
54. Heilä, H. and Lönnqvist, J. (2003). The clinical epidemiology of suicide in schizophrenia. In *The epidemiology of schizophrenia* (eds. R.M. Murray, P. Jones, E. Susser, J. van Os, and M. Cannon), pp. 288–314. Cambridge University Press, Cambridge.
55. Mortensen, P.B. and Juel, K. (1993). Mortality and causes of death in first admitted schizophrenic patients. *The British Journal of Psychiatry*, **163**, 183–9.
56. Geddes, J.R. and Juszczak, E. (1995). Period trends in rate of suicide in first 28 days after discharge from psychiatric hospital in Scotland, 1968-92. *British Medical Journal*, **311**, 357–60.
57. Lawrence, D., Holman, C.D.J, Jablensky, A., *et al.* (2001). Increasing rates of suicide in Western Australian psychiatric patients: a record linkage study. *Acta Psychiatrica Scandinavica*, **104**, 443–51.
58. Jeste, D.V., Gladsjo, J.A., Lindamer, L.A., *et al.* (1996). Medical comorbidity in schizophrenia. *Schizophrenia Bulletin*, **22**, 413–30.
59. Susser, E., Valencia, E., and Conover, S. (1993). Prevalence of HIV infection among psychiatric patients in a New York City men's shelter. *American Journal of Public Health*, **83**, 568–70.
60. Martens, W.H. (2001). A review of physical and mental health in homeless persons. *Public Health Reviews*, **29**, 13–33.
61. Mortensen, P.B. (2003). Mortality and physical illness in schizophrenia. In *The epidemiology of schizophrenia* (eds. R.M. Murray, P. Jones, E. Susser, J. van Os, and M. Cannon), pp. 275–87. Cambridge University Press, Cambridge.

62. Lawrence, D.M., Holman, C.D.J., Jablensky, A.V., *et al.* (2003). Death rate from ischaemic heart disease in Western Australian psychiatric patients 1980–1998. *The British Journal of Psychiatry*, **182**, 32–6.
63. Goff, D.C., Sullivan, L.M., McEvoy, J.P., *et al.* (2005). A comparison of ten-year cardiac risk estimates in schizophrenia patients from the CATIE study and matched controls. *Schizophrenia Research*, **80**, 45–53.
64. Saari, K.M., Lindeman, S.M., Viilo, K.M., *et al.* (2005). A 4-fold risk of metabolic syndrome in patients with schizophrenia: the Northern Finland 1966 birth cohort study. *The Journal of Clinical Psychiatry*, **66**, 559–63.
65. Hyde, T.M., Ziegler, J.C., and Weinberger, D. (1992). Psychiatric disturbances in metachromatic leucodystrophy. *Archives of Neurology*, **49**, 401–6.
66. Murphy, K.C. and Owen, M.J. (1996). Minor physical anomalies and their relationship to the aetiology of schizophrenia. *The British Journal of Psychiatry*, **168**, 139–42.
67. Eaton, W.M., Hayward, C., and Ram, R. (1992). Schizophrenia and rheumatoid arthritis: a review. *Schizophrenia Research*, **6**, 181–92.
68. Murray, R.M., Grech, A., Phillips, P., *et al.* (2003). What is the relationship between substance abuse and schizophrenia? In *The epidemiology of schizophrenia* (eds. R.M. Murray, P. Jones, E. Susser, J. van Os, and M. Cannon), pp. 317–42. Cambridge University Press, Cambridge.
69. Koethe, D., Llenos, I.C., Dulay, J.R., *et al.* (2007). Expression of CB1 cannabinoid receptor in the anterior cingulate cortex in schizophrenia, bipolar disorder, and major depression. *Journal of Neural Transmission*, **114**, 1055–63.
70. Myers, C.S., Robles, O., Kakoyannis, N., *et al.* (2004). Nicotine improves delayed recognition in schizophrenic patients. *Psychopharmacology*, **174**, 334–40.
71. Henquet, C., Murray, R., Linszen, D., *et al.* (2005). The environment and schizophrenia: the role of cannabis use. *Schizophrenia Bulletin*, **31**, 608–12.
72. Semple, D.M., McIntosh, A.M., and Lawrie, S.M. (2005). Cannabis as a risk factor for psychosis: systematic review. *Journal of Psychopharmacology*, **19**, 187–94.
73. Curran, C., Byrappa, N., and McBride, A. (2004). Stimulant psychosis: systematic review. *The British Journal of Psychiatry*, **185**, 196–204.
74. De Leon, J. and Diza, F.J. (2005). A meta-analysis of worldwide studies demonstrates an association between schizophrenia and tobacco smoking behaviors. *Schizophrenia Research*, **76**, 135–57.
75. Zammitt, S., Allebeck, P., Dalman, C., *et al.* (2003). Investigating the association between cigarette smoking and schizophrenia in a cohort study. *The American Journal of Psychiatry*, **160**, 2216–21.
76. Boydell, J. and Murray, R. (2003). Urbanization, migration and risk of schizophrenia. In *The epidemiology of schizophrenia* (eds. R.M. Murray, P. Jones, E. Susser, J. van Os, and M. Cannon), pp. 49–67. Cambridge University Press, Cambridge.
77. Murray, C.J.L. and Lopez, A.D. (eds.) (1996). *The global burden of disease. A comprehensive assessment of mortality and disability from diseases, injuries, and risk factors in 1990 and projected to 2020.* Harvard School of Public Health, Cambridge, MA.
78. Jablensky, A. (2000). Epidemiology of schizophrenia: the global burden of disease and disability. *European Archives of Psychiatry and Clinical Neuroscience*, **250**, 274–85.
79. Gottesman, I.I. (1991). *Schizophrenia genesis: the origins of madness.* W.H. Freeman, New York.
80. Lichtenstein, P., Björk, C., Hultman, C.M., *et al.* (2006). Recurrence risks for schizophrenia in a Swedish National Cohort. *Psychological Medicine*, **36**, 1417–25.
81. Kendler, K.S. and Eaves, L.J. (1986). Models for the joint effect of genotype and environment on liability to psychiatric illness. *The American Journal of Psychiatry*, **143**, 279–89.
82. Essen-Möller, E. (1935). Untersuchungen über die Fruchtbarkeit gewisser Gruppen von Geisteskranken. *Acta Psychiatrica et Neurologica*, **8**, 1–314.
83. Huxley, J., Mayr, E., Osmond, H., *et al.* (1964). Schizophrenia as a genetic morphism. *Nature*, **204**, 220–1.
84. Sipos, A., Rasmussen F., Harrison, G., *et al.* (2004). Paternal age and schizophrenia: a population based cohort study. *British Medical Journal*, **330**, 147–8.
85. Tramer, M. (1929). Über die biologische Bedeutung des Geburtsmonates, insbesondere für die Psychoseerkrankung. *Schweizerischer Archiv für Neurologie und Psychiatrie*, **24**, 17–24.
86. Mortensen, P.B., Pedersen, C.B., Westergaard, T., *et al.* (1999). Effects of family history and place and season of birth on the risk of schizophrenia. *The New England Journal of Medicine*, **340**, 603–8.
87. Torrey, E.F., Miller, J., Rawlings, R., *et al.* (1997). Seasonality of births in schizophrenia and bipolar disorder: a review of the literature. *Schizophrenia Research*, **28**, 1–38.
88. Mednick, S.A., Machon, R.A., Huttunen, M.O., *et al.* (1988). Adult schizophrenia following prenatal exposure to an influenza epidemic. *Archives of General Psychiatry*, **45**, 189–92.
89. Morgan, V., Castle, D., Page, A., *et al.* (1997). Influenza epidemics and incidence of schizophrenia, affective disorders and mental retardation in Western Australia: no evidence of a major effect. *Schizophrenia Research*, **26**, 25–39.
90. Grech, A., Takei, N., and Murray, R.M. (1997). Maternal exposure to influenza and paranoid schizophrenia. *Schizophrenia Research*, **26**, 121–5.
91. Cannon, M., Cotter, D., Coffey, V.P., *et al.* (1996). Prenatal exposure to the 1957 influenza epidemic and adult schizophrenia: a follow-up study. *The British Journal of Psychiatry*, **168**, 368–71.
92. Brown, A.S., Cohen, P., Harkavy-Friedman, J., *et al.* (2001). Prenatal rubella, premorbid abnormalities, and adult schizophrenia. *Biological Psychiatry*, **49**, 473–86.
93. Brown, A.S., Schaefer, C.A., Quesenberry, C.P., *et al.* (2005). Maternal exposure to toxoplasmosis and risk of schizophrenia in the offspring. *The American Journal of Psychiatry*, **162**, 767–73.
94. Cannon, T.D. (1997). On the nature and mechanisms of obstetric influence in schizophrenia: a review and synthesis of epidemiological studies. *International Review of Psychiatry*, **9**, 387–97.
95. Done, D.J., Johnstone, E.C., Frith, C.D., *et al.* (1991). Complications of pregnancy and delivery in relation to psychosis in adult life: data from the British perinatal mortality survey sample. *British Medical Journal*, **202**, 1576–80.
96. Buka, S.L., Tsuang, M.T., and Lipsitt, L.P. (1993). Pregnancy/delivery complications and psychiatric diagnosis: a prospective study. *Archives of General Psychiatry*, **50**, 151–6.
97. Cannon, M., Jones, P.B., and Murray, R.M. (2002). Obstetric complications and schizophrenia: historical and meta-analytic review. *The American Journal of Psychiatry*, **159**, 1080–92.
98. Zornberg, G.L., Buka, S.L., and Tsuang, M.T. (2000). Hypoxic-ischemia-related fetal/neonatal complications and risk of schizophrenia and other nonaffective psychoses: a 19-year longitudinal study. *The American Journal of Psychiatry*, **157**, 196–202.
99. Cannon, T.D., Rosso, I.M., Hollister, J.M., *et al.* (2000). A prospective cohort study of genetic and perinatal influences in the etiology of schizophrenia. *Schizophrenia Bulletin*, **26**, 351–66.
100. Bennedsen, B.E., Mortensen, P.B., Olesen, A.V., *et al.* (2001). Obstetric complications in women with schizophrenia. *Schizophrenia Research*, **47**, 167–75.
101. Jablensky, A.V., Morgan, V., Zubrick, S.R., *et al.* (2005). Pregnancy, delivery, and neonatal complications in a population cohort of women with schizophrenia and major affective disorders. *The American Journal of Psychiatry*, **162**, 79–91.
102. Cannon, T.D., Mednick, S.A., Parnas, J., *et al.* (1993). Developmental brain abnormalities in the offspring of schizophrenic mothers. *Archives of General Psychiatry*, **50**, 551–64.

103. Keshavan, M.S., Diwadkar, V.A., Spencer, S.M., *et al.* (2002). A preliminary functional magnetic resonance imaging study in offspring of schizophrenic patients. *Progress in Neuro-Psychopharmacology & Biological Psychiatry*, **26**, 1143–49.
104. Leask, S.J., Done, D.J., and Crow, T.J. (2002). Adult psychosis, common childhood infections and neurological soft signs in a national birth cohort. *The British Journal of Psychiatry*, **181**, 387–92.
105. Thaden, E., Rhinewine, J.P., Lencz, T., *et al.* (2006). Early-onset schizophrenia is associated with impaired adolescent development of attentional capacity using the identical pairs continuous performance test. *Schizophrenia Research*, **81**, 157–66.
106. Winterer, G., Egan, M.F., Raedler, T., *et al.* (2003). P300 and genetic risk for schizophrenia. *Archives of General Psychiatry*, **60**, 1158–67.
107. Calkins, M.E., Curtis, C.E., Iacono, W.G., *et al.* (2004). Antisaccade performance is impaired in medically and psychiatrically healthy biological relatives of schizophrenia patients. *Schizophrenia Research*, **71**, 167–78.
108. Zammitt, S., Allebeck, P., David, A.S., *et al.* (2004). A longitudinal study of premorbid IQ score and risk of developing schizophrenia, bipolar disorder, severe depression, and other nonaffective psychoses. *Archives of General Psychiatry*, **61**, 354–60.
109. Reichenberg, A., Weiser, M., Rabinowitz, J., *et al.* (2002). A population-based cohort study of premorbid intellectual, language, and behavioral functioning in patients with schizophrenia, schizoaffective disorder, and nonpsychotic bipolar disorder. *The American Journal of Psychiatry*, **159**, 2027–35.
110. Cannon, T.D., Mednick, S.A., and Parnas, J. (1990). Antecedents of predominantly negative- and predominantly positive-symptom schizophrenia in a high-risk population. *Archives of General Psychiatry*, **47**, 622–32.
111. Wahlberg, K.E., Wynne, L.C., Oja, H., *et al.* (1997). Gene-environment interaction in vulnerability to schizophrenia: findings from the Finnish adoptive family study of schizophrenia. *The American Journal of Psychiatry*, **154**, 355–62.
112. van Os, J., Hanssen, M., Bak, M., *et al.* (2003). Do urbanicity and familial liability coparticipate in causing psychosis? *The American Journal of Psychiatry*, **160**, 477–82.
113. Mischler, E.G. and Scotch, N.A. (1983). Sociocultural factors in the epidemiology of schizophrenia; a review. *Psychiatry*, **26**, 315–51.
114. Goldberg, E.M. and Morrison, S.L. (1963). Schizophrenia and social class. *The British Journal of Psychiatry*, **109**, 785–802.
115. Bhugra, D., Leff, J., Mallett, R., *et al.* (1997). Incidence and outcomes of schizophrenia in Whites, African-Caribbeans, and Asians in London. *Psychological Medicine*, **27**, 791–8.
116. Harrison, G., Glazebrook, C., Brewin, J., *et al.* (1997). Increased incidence of psychotic disorders in migrants from the Caribbean to the United Kingdom. *Psychological Medicine*, **27**, 799–806.
117. Selten, J.P., Slaets, J.P.I., and Kahn, R.S. (1997). Schizophrenia in the Surinamese and Dutch Antilean immigrants to the Netherlands: evidence of an increased incidence. *Psychological Medicine*, **27**, 807–11.
118. Selten, J.P., Slaets, J., and Kahn, R. (1998). Prenatal exposure to influenza and schizophrenia in Surinamese and Dutch Antillean immigrants to the Netherlands. *Schizophrenia Research*, **30**, 101–3.
119. Hutchinson, G., Takei, N., Fahy, T.A., *et al.* (1996). Morbid risk of schizophrenia in first-degree relatives of White and African-Caribbean patients with psychosis. *The British Journal of Psychiatry*, **169**, 776–80.
120. Jablensky, A. (2006). Subtyping schizophrenia: implications for genetic research. *Molecular Psychiatry*, **11**, 815–36.
121. Spitzer, R.L., Endicott, J., and Robins, E. (1978). Research diagnostic criteria. Rationale and reliability. *Archives of General Psychiatry*, **35**, 773–82.
122. Hutchinson, G., Takei, N., Bhugra, D., *et al.* (1997). Increased rate of psychosis among African-Caribbeans in Britain is not due to an excess of pregnancy and birth complications. *The British Journal of Psychiatry*, **171**, 145–7.

4.3.6 Aetiology

Contents

4.3.6.1 Genetic and environmental risk factors for schizophrenia
R. M. Murray and D. J. Castle
4.3.6.2 The neurobiology of schizophrenia
Paul J. Harrison

4.3.6.1 Genetic and environmental risk factors for schizophrenia

R. M. Murray and D. J. Castle

One thing that is certain about the aetiology of schizophrenia is that there is no single cause. This might reflect the fact that the schizophrenia construct itself is heterogeneous, such that specific subtypes might in the future be found to have specific causes. But it is more useful at this stage of our knowledge to conclude that, like other disorders such as ischaemic heart disease and diabetes mellitus, schizophrenia results from the cumulative effects of a number of risk factors. These may be crudely divided into the familial-genetic and the environmental, though there are clearly interactions between the two.

Familial–genetic risk

The most powerful risk factor for schizophrenia is having a relative afflicted with the disorder. Numerous studies have shown that the lifetime risk for broadly defined schizophrenia increases from about one per cent in the general population to about 10 per cent cent in first-degree relatives of patients with schizophrenia and to close to 50 per cent in those with two parents with the disorder.(1) However, familial aggregation does not prove that a condition is genetically transmitted; to look at this issue we need to turn to adoptee and twin studies.

Adoption studies

Adoptee studies offer the opportunity of separating the effects of familiality from genetics. In the first such study of schizophrenia, Heston and Denney(2) demonstrated that five out of 47 children of mothers with schizophrenia who were adopted away within a few days of their birth, later developed schizophrenia compared with none out of 50 adoptees with no family history of schizophrenia. Similar findings were reported from the Danish-American Study of Rosenthal *et al*(3) who found that a significantly higher proportion of the adopted-away offspring of parents with schizophrenia were classified as having schizophrenia or 'borderline schizophrenia', than were control adoptees. This study originated the concept of the schizophrenia spectrum disorder, which has come to include not only frank schizophrenia but also schizophreniform disorder, as well as schizotypal and possibly paranoid personality disorder.

In an extension of the Danish-American collaboration, Kety *et al.*(4) took all adoptees in Denmark who had schizophrenia and examined their biological and adoptive relatives; unlike the earlier adoption studies this one also used operational definitions of the schizophrenia spectrum conditions. Fully 23.5 per cent of the biological first-degree relatives received a schizophrenia spectrum diagnosis compared with only 4.7 per cent of the biological relatives of normal control adoptees; the adoptive relatives of both groups of adoptees had very low rates of spectrum disorders.

Finally, Wender *et al.*[5] studied the grown-up children of normal individuals who, by mischance, had been placed with an adoptive parent who later developed schizophrenia, and found that they were at no increased risk of the disorder. Thus, adoption studies consistently indicate that the familial aggregation of schizophrenia is determined by individuals inheriting genes from someone with the disorder (or a related spectrum condition) rather than any effect of the intrafamilial culture (e.g. being brought up by a parent with schizophrenia).

Twin studies

Twin studies have come to the same conclusion. Gottesman,[1] who reviewed the literature, calculated the average probandwise concordance rate for broadly defined schizophrenia in monozygotic twins to be 46 per cent, compared with 14 per cent in dizygotic twins. This difference reflects that while monozygotic twins share all their genes, dizygotic twins share, on average, only half. Further evidence of the effect of heredity comes from the evidence that the concordance rate in 12 pairs of monozygotic twins who were reared apart was 58 per cent.[1]

The above twin studies preceded the introduction of operational definitions of schizophrenia. When studies with such definitions were carried out, the rates for both monozygotic and dizygotic twins were both lower, but the disparity between the two remained. Cardno *et al.*[6] examined 108 consecutive pairs of twins seen at the Maudsley Hospital in London, and reported probandwise concordance rates for DSM-IIIR schizophrenia of 42.6 per cent in monozygotic twins and 0 per cent in dizygotic twins.

What is the range of the clinical phenotype transmitted?

The fact that an individual can have the same genes as their co-twin with schizophrenia but have a better than evens chance of remaining non-psychotic indicates that it is not schizophrenia *per se* which is inherited but rather a susceptibility to it. Further evidence in support of this comes from a study which showed that the offspring of the identical but well co-twins of individuals with schizophrenia carry a risk of the disorder similar to that of the offspring of the affected twin.[7] Thus, the predisposition is transmitted without being expressed as schizophrenia.

As noted earlier, sometimes the predisposition may be expressed as non-psychotic spectrum disorders. In addition, family studies show that relatives of people with schizophrenia also show an increased risk of other psychotic conditions such as schizoaffective disorder, atypical and schizophreniform psychoses, and affective psychosis with mood-incongruent delusions. Thus, the clinical phenotype transmitted encompasses a range of psychotic conditions, as well as schizotypal personality disorder and paranoid personality. Within schizophrenia, researchers have asked whether different subtypes are differentially inherited. The results have in general been negative which is not surprising since clinicians know that an individual patient can appear predominantly hebephrenic on one admission and schizoaffective on another. However, there has been a consensus that paranoid schizophrenia is less familial than other types and is associated with a lower monozygotic twin concordance. Also, very late onset schizophrenia (late paraphrenia) appears to carry less genetic loading than early-onset types.

It has been repeatedly shown that schizophrenic symptoms can be summarized as three main factors: delusions and hallucinations (reality distortion), negative symptoms (psychomotor poverty), and disorganization or positive thought disorder.[8,9] Is schizotypal personality particularly closely related to one of these three core syndromes? Mata *et al.*[10] showed that schizotypal personality scores in non-psychotic relatives were significantly correlated with the presence of delusions and hallucinations in the probands; indeed, they were also correlated with premorbid schizoptypal traits in the childhood of the probands. Thus, it seems that certain families transmit schizotypal traits which manifest themselves in childhood; some family members remain schizotypal throughout life but in others this predisposition is compounded by other (genetic or environmental) factors so that the individual passes a threshold for the expression of delusions and hallucinations.

Genetic models

From the data reviewed above, we can conclude that schizophrenia cannot be explained by the inheritance of a single major gene. In any case, such simple Mendelian inheritance would be hard to square with the persistence of schizophrenia in the population. Since people with schizophrenia tend to reproduce less frequently than the rest of the population, one would have expected that a single major gene with such damaging consequences would have been selected out of the gene pool.

The evidence is compatible with oligogenic inheritance (a small number of genes involved) but most parsimonious is a polygenic model which postulates that a number of genes of small effect are involved. Support for this model comes from the fact that the risk to an individual increases with the number of affected relatives[1] and also that the monozygotic concordance rate is higher for those twins who had an early rather than late onset of psychosis.[6]

Family studies also show that the relatives of probands with an early onset have a higher morbid risk of psychosis than the relatives of late-onset patients.[11] These findings are compatible with the idea that schizophrenia is in part a developmental disorder and that some of the susceptibility genes may be involved in the control of neurodevelopment.[12]

Molecular genetic studies

Researchers have been using molecular techniques to seek the gene or genes that predispose to schizophrenia. The first technique to be used was that of linkage in which large families with several members affected with schizophrenia are studied to try and find a genetic marker that co-segregates with the disease. Two decades of linkage studies suggest that no gene can exist which increases the overall risk of schizophrenia by more than a factor of around three, and that, therefore, there are likely to be a number of susceptibility genes of small effect. This is the mode of transmission for other chronic disorders such as diabetes and hypertension, and, as with these disorders, the genetic basis of schizophrenia is beginning to be unravelled. In the past few years, findings from linkage studies have led on to detailed mapping studies of certain chromosomal regions which have in turn implicated specific genes. Those for which there is most evidence currently are neuregulin and dysbindin.

Neuregulin[13]: An association between schizophrenia and a multi marker haplotype (a pattern of DNA within a gene) of Neuregulin 1 (**NRG1**) on chromosome 8p21–22 was found in an Icelandic sample in 2002 and soon replicated in a Scottish population. Subsequently, neuregulin has been implicated in other studies although the exact haplotype has varied in the different studies.

Dysbindin: Also in 2002, Straub *et al.*[14] reported, in Irish families, association between schizophrenia and several SNPs (single nucleotide polymorphisms) and multimarker haplotypes spanning the gene encoding dystrobrevin-binding protein 1 (**DTNBP1**), or dysbindin, located at chromosome 6p22.3. Some but not all other studies have replicated this association.

Another way of identifying susceptibility genes is through the study of chromosomal rearrangements. Thus, Blackwood, *et al.*[15] reported that a large Scottish pedigree showed strong evidence for linkage between a balanced chromosomal translocation (1, 11) (q42;q14.3) (two portions of the different chromosomes swapping positions with each other) and a broad phenotype consisting of schizophrenia, bipolar disorder, and recurrent depression. This translocation caused the disruption of a gene, termed disrupted in schizophrenia 1 (**DISC1**). Subsequent studies have examined DISC1 in Finnish and US samples, and have suggested that it may be a susceptibility gene for both schizophrenia and bipolar disorder.

A third approach, that of association studies, takes a gene that is suspected of involvement in the pathogenesis of the disorder and compares the frequency of its various alleles in a series of individuals with schizophrenia as opposed to a control group without schizophrenia. One such gene is the catecholamine O-methyl transferase (**COMT**) gene which has been extensively investigated because of its role in dopamine metabolism, especially in the prefrontal cortex.[16, 17] A mis-sense mutation (incorrect unit in the genetic code) generates a valine to methionine substitution at codon 158 (Val158Met), producing an unstable enzyme with reduced degradation of dopamine. The evidence that this polymorphism is in itself a susceptibility gene is uncertain but as we shall see later, it may compound other risk factors for schizophrenia.

Neuregulin, dysbindin, and DISC 1 are the most replicated putative susceptibility genes for schizophrenia but other plausible candidate genes identified by linkage and follow-up studies such as **G72** (D–amino acid oxidase activator, DAOA), have been suggested. G72 and several of the other putative risk genes appear to carry not only an increased risk of schizophrenia but also of bipolar disorder, and are thus congruent with the results of a twin study which suggested substantial genetic overlap between the two major psychoses.

Nevertheless, none of the above genes can yet be said to be 100 per cent proven as a cause of schizophrenia since there remain inconsistencies between the specific risk alleles and haplotypes among studies. It is unlikely that there is a simple relationship between carrying one risk allele and developing schizophrenia. Rather, an individual may need to carry a number of risk genes and be exposed to several environmental risk factors. In such a dynamic multifactorial model, several genes of small effect interact with each other and with time-specific exposure to environmental risk factors contribute to both the onset and outcome of schizophrenia.

Biological abnormalities in the relatives of people with schizophrenia

Relatives have been examined for some of the biological abnormalities which are found in their kin with schizophrenia. Thus, in the Maudsley Study of families multiply affected with schizophrenia, both the members with schizophrenia and those unaffected relatives who appeared to be transmitting the liability to the disorder (so-called obligate carriers) showed larger lateral ventricles than controls.[18, 19] McDonald *et al.*[20] went on to show that such families transmit a grey matter pattern that shows deficits in frontal and temporal areas and that the greater the genetic liability, the greater the deficit.

In the same Maudsley Family Study, the non-psychotic relatives exhibited other neurophysiological abnormalities such as an excess of delayed P300 event-related potentials; their prevalence was not as high as in the patients themselves but higher than in unaffected controls.[21] Those patients who showed an excess of saccadic distractability errors tended to have relatives with the same eye-tracking abnormalities.[22] The patients with schizophrenia and their well relatives from these multiply affected families also showed more integrative neurological abnormalities than controls.[23]

These findings suggest that what is being transmitted is not genes for schizophrenia *per se* but rather genes for a variety of characteristics (e.g. schizotypal personality, enlarged lateral ventricles, grey matter deficit, delayed P300, integrative neurological abnormalities) which may increase the risk of schizophrenia or at least be markers thereof. Individuals can inherit these characteristics without being psychotic; perhaps schizophrenia only ensues when an individual inherits a number of such endophenotypic abnormalities and passes a critical threshold of risk.[24]

Advancing paternal age in non-familial schizophrenia

An interesting finding first noted over 30 years ago is that schizophrenia is commoner in those whose fathers were old at the time they were born. One of the largest studies to demonstrate this comes from Sipos *et al.*[25] who studied the risk of schizophrenia in 754 330 people born in Sweden. The overall hazard ratio for developing schizophrenia increased with each 10 year increase in paternal age. This association between paternal age and schizophrenia has been repeatedly shown to be present in those with no family history of the disorder, but not in those with a positive family history. This stronger association between paternal age and schizophrenia in people without a family history raises the possibility that accumulation of de novo mutations in paternal sperm with ageing contributes to the risk of schizophrenia.

Environmental factors

It is evident from above that genes exert a probabilistic rather than a deterministic effect on the development of schizophrenia; environmental risk factors appear to be necessary for the disease to become manifest in many, if not all, cases.[26] But what are these environmental risk factors?

Pre- and perinatal complications

More than 20 studies have shown that patients suffering from schizophrenia are more likely to have a history of pre- or perinatal complications (collectively termed obstetric complications) than are healthy subjects from the general population, patients with other psychiatric disorders, and their own healthy siblings.[27] Some of the studies which reported these findings were based upon interviews with patients' mothers asking them to recall their pregnancies; such interviews are obviously open to distortion by recall bias. However, similar findings have been reported by studies examining data collected in obstetric records at the time of birth of patients and controls.[28] Indeed a meta-analysis of large epidemiologically sophisticated studies which used contemporary records confirmed that there is modest but consistent effect of obstetric complications. [29]

Of course, it is possible that the excess obstetric complications in schizophrenia may be the consequence of some pre-existing abnormality. Since the foetus plays an active role in the normal progress of pregnancy and labour, foetal impairment induced by earlier abnormality may itself result in some perinatal complications. Also, some studies have shown that women with schizophrenia who become pregnant tend to have more obstetric complications, possibly owing to their behaviour during pregnancy, for example smoking and not attending antenatal visits.

The term 'obstetric complications' covers a broad range of obstetric events. An international study on 700 schizophrenic patients and a similar number of controls found that low birth weight, prematurity, and resuscitation at birth were particularly increased in the schizophrenic patients;[27] other complications that have been implicated include retarded foetal growth and rhesus incompatability. Thus, a common characteristic of most of the obstetric complications implicated is that they increase the risk of hypoxia.

Could hypoxic–ischaemic damage be the mechanism that increases the risk of later schizophrenia? Children who were subject to cerebral hypoxia at or before birth show an excess of abnormalities on MRI scan, of minor neurological signs, and of cognitive and behavioural problems, characteristics also found in many preschizophrenic children.[30] As one might predict, studies of monozygotic twins discordant for schizophrenia have shown that the affected twins have larger lateral ventricles and smaller hippocampi than their well co-twins;[31,32] furthermore, those twins who have been subjected to the most severe perinatal difficulties have the largest ventricles and smallest hippocampi.[33]

Similarly, Stefanis *et al.*[34] compared hippocampal volume in three groups, viz, schizophrenia patients with affected relatives but with no personal history of obstetric complications; schizophrenia patients with no affected relatives but who had a history of significant obstetric complications; and normal controls. Hippocampal volume was normal in the first schizophrenia group but reduced in the second group, implying that it is hypoxic-ischaemic damage rather than genetic predisposition alone that determines decreased hippocampal volume in schizophrenia.

Season of birth and maternal exposure to infection

Many studies have shown (in the Northern Hemisphere at least) that people born in late winter and spring are slightly more likely than expected to later develop schizophrenia. Since respiratory viral infections such as influenza tend to occur in autumn and winter, maternal infection might provide the explanation. A number of epidemiological studies have, therefore, addressed the question of whether maternal exposure to influenza during the second trimester of pregnancy is a risk factor for schizophrenia; some but not all studies have suggested that it is.[35] One study[36] reported an association between the presence of antibodies to the influenza virus in first trimester blood, but not during the other trimesters. The possibility that prenatal exposure to rubella may have a similar risk-increasing effect for schizophrenia has been raised, and a significant association has been reported with serologically-documented rubella exposure in gestation[37] Some studies have implicated other infectious agents such as herpes simplex, cytomegalovirus and toxoplasmosis, but there is as yet no consensus as to whether these findings are replicable or not.

Severe prenatal malnutrion appears to have an effect. Thus, children born following the Dutch Hunger Winter when the Nazi occupiers systematically starved the population were shown to have a higher risk of schizophrenia and this finding has recently been replicated in a Chinese population.[38,39]

Childhood risk factors

There is now a wealth of evidence attesting to the fact that a proportion of individuals who later manifest schizophrenia show abnormalities in their early development. The evidence for early developmental abnormalities in schizophrenia come from three main sorts of study:

- high-risk studies in which the offspring of parent(s) with schizophrenia are examined;
- follow-back studies where cases of schizophrenia are ascertained, and their early developmental trajectory plotted with the help of history from the individual and family, sometimes also including such evidence as school reports; and
- cohort studies, where birth cohorts are followed up prospectively, and individuals who later manifest schizophrenia are compared with the rest of the cohort in terms of their early development.

(a) High-risk studies

Studies of the offspring of mothers with schizophrenia, the so-called 'high-risk studies', show that between a quarter to a half show some deviation from normal in terms of their early development (reviewed by Davies *et al.*[40]) In the neonatal period, there is a tendency to hypotonia and decreased cuddliness; in infancy, milestones are delayed; in early childhood, there is poor motor co-ordination; and in later childhood, there are deficits in attention and information processing. Fish *et al.*[41] followed their cohort of 12 high-risk infants into adulthood. One developed schizophrenia and six showed schizotypal or paranoid personality traits; these authors coined the term 'pandysmaturation' to describe the abnormalities which included delayed motor milestones in the first two years of life.

(b) Follow-back studies

High-risk studies have been criticized on the basis that they are unrepresentative because only a minority of people who develop schizophrenia have a mother with the same illness. Therefore, a separate set of studies of representative groups of patients with schizophrenia have used maternal recall to document the early development of adults with schizophrenia. These have shown impairment of cognitive and neuromotor development and interpersonal problems. These findings are more commonly reported in males than females, and tend to be associated with an early onset of illness.[42] The findings are not specific to schizophrenia, being reported also in the early development of some children who later manifest an affective psychosis.[43]

Of course, one of the major criticisms of follow-back studies is the likelihood of recall bias. Studies that have avoided this problem include those which have accessed IQ scores assessed prior to illness onset; these have shown that premorbid IQ is, on average, lower in those, particularly males, who later manifest schizophrenia.[44, 45]

Another source of material mapping early development has been childhood home videos, which have been reviewed by researchers 'blind' to whether the individual later manifested schizophrenia.[46] In comparison with their healthy siblings, the preschizophrenic children showed higher rates of neuromotor abnormalities (predominantly left-sided) and overall poorer motor skills; the group differences were significant only at two years of age.

(c) Cohort studies

Cohort studies have overcome many of the criticisms of follow-back studies. In an investigation of the 1958 British Perinatal Mortality cohort, comprising 98 per cent of all children ($n = 15\,398$) born in the United Kingdom in a certain week in March 1958, Done *et al.*[47] compared those who later manifested schizophrenia ($n = 40$), affective psychosis ($n = 35$), and neurotic illness ($n = 79$) with each other as well as with 1 914 randomly selected individuals with no history of mental illness. At age seven years, teacher ratings showed the preschizophrenic children to have exhibited more social maladjustment than controls; the effect was most marked in boys. The preaffective children differed little from normal controls, whilst the preneurotic children (expressly girls) showed some maladjustment (over- and under-reaction) at age 11 years.

In a similar study of the 1946 British Birth Cohort, Jones *et al.*[48] determined that 30 out of 4 746 individuals had, in adulthood, developed schizophrenia. This group was more likely than the rest of the cohort to show delayed milestones and speech problems, to have a lower premorbid IQ and lower education test scores at ages 8, 11, and 15 years, and to prefer solitary play at ages 4 and 6 years. Perhaps the most influential of all the cohort studies has been the Dunedin Birth Cohort Study, which followed the development of 1 037 children through the ages of 3 to 15 years, and assessed them again at the ages of 18, 21, and 26 years.[49] This study found that poorer motor development, poorer receptive language, and a lower IQ all increased the risk of subsequently developing schizophreniform disorder by age 26 years. The Dunedin cohort additionally provided evidence that a proportion of children who develop schizophrenia are already experiencing 'quasi-psychotic' phenomena by age 11 years.[50] These phenomena include beliefs that people are reading their minds or following or spying on them, or they are already hearing voices. Children with strong evidence of quasi-psychotic symptomatology were up to 16-times more likely to develop schizophreniform disorders by the age of 26 years; making these phenomena some of the most powerful early predictors of later psychosis.

Together, such studies provide compelling evidence for a tendency of individuals with schizophrenia to show abnormalities in development which antedate the onset of illness. The findings are compatible with the notion that subtle brain abnormalities (which may be genetically or environmentally mediated, or both) underpin schizophrenia. However, it is also possible that some of the childhood risk factors are independent and act in an additive manner to set individuals on an increasingly deviant trajectory towards schizophrenia.

Social and geographic risk factors

Recent dogma about schizophrenia has held that the incidence does not vary by time or place, even though such an occurrence would have made schizophrenia unique among diseases! Now this curious belief has been disproved by a raft of studies. In particular, a systematic review by McGrath *et al.*[50] concluded that the incidence of schizophrenia shows prominent worldwide variation (up to five-fold), and that it is about 40 per cent greater in men than women.

In 1939, Faris and Dunham[52] reported that an excess of individuals with schizophrenia was found in certain deprived inner-city areas. These authors suggested that social isolation in poor deprived parts of the city could precipitate schizophrenia. However, subsequently, their results were interpreted as a consequence of social drift, i.e. the idea that individuals with this illness 'drift' down the social scale.[53] This effect was postulated to result from not only the illness itself but also its prodroma and consequences such as loss of employment and estrangement from family. A related finding is that of lack of upward social mobility in individuals with schizophrenia. For example, Hollingshead and Redlich[54] reported that individuals with schizophrenia to be less likely than expected to attain the socio-economic status of their fathers.

More recently, research has focused on the apparent excess of individuals who later manifest schizophrenia, who actually start life in a setting which appears to increase the subsequent risk of schizophrenia. Kohn[55] stated that '... in all probability, lower class families produce a disproportionate number of schizophrenics' but the evidence concerning such 'social causation' is contradictory. Thus, Turner and Wagenfeld[56] reported fathers of schizophrenia patients to be themselves over-represented in lower socio-economic groups. However, Jones *et al.*[48] did not find this.

It may be that it is not so much poverty as being born or brought up in a city which increases the risk of the disorder. For example, Lewis *et al.*[57] found that Swedish conscripts who later manifested schizophrenia were 1.65 times more likely to have been born in urban than rural areas. Similarly, Marcelis *et al.*[58] reported that birth in an urban area of Holland carried twice the risk of later schizophrenia of birth in a rural area. Similar findings have come from Denmark where those individuals born in Copenhagen appear to have twice the risk of schizophrenia of those born in rural areas.[59] It is now generally accepted that the incidence is higher amongst those brought up in urban areas, and that the larger the town, and the longer the individual has lived in the city, the greater the risk. The exact mechanisms underlying this effect remain unclear.

Immigration

Since the classic study of Odegaard in 1932,[60] many studies have reported that migrants are at increased risk of schizophrenia. A recent meta-analysis of 18 studies of migrants from different backgrounds confirmed a weighted mean relative risk for first-generation migrants of 2.7 (95 per cent CI 2.3–3.2) and for second generation migrants, 4.5 (95 per cent CI 1.5–13.1). Risk was higher for migrants from lower socio-economic countries, and for black people moving into predominantly white societies.[61]

A notable example has come from a series of studies of African-Caribbeans resident in the United Kingdom, who show a markedly higher rate of schizophrenia than do their white

British-born counterparts.[62]This is in the absence of any increased risk to Caribbeans who remain in the West Indies.[63] The increase is striking. The large and sophisticated AESOP study of three English cities demonstrated a ninefold increase in the incidence of schizophrenia among African Caribbeans, and a six-fold increase among those of African origin.[64] Boydell *et al.*[65] further demonstrated that migrants were especially vulnerable if relatively isolated in localities where their own ethnic group were in a small minority. Of particular interest is that this increased risk also pertains to British-born offspring of Caribbean migrants, discounting an explanation in terms of migration stress alone. Furthermore, there is a marked increased risk in the siblings but not the parents of this second generation;[63] this suggests an environmental effect operating particularly upon this second generation.

Initial studies sought to ascertain any evidence of developmental disadvantage such as poor maternal nutrition, poor obstetric care, and possible maternal susceptibility to novel viruses. However, these studies have shown that, if anything, African-Caribbean schizophrenic patients in England show less evidence of neurodevelopmental insult than their white counterpart patients. Other research focuses on the possibility that a paranoid reaction to social disadvantage and discrimination may be one factor. The findings relating to skin colour potentially support the notion of perceived or real discrimination being an important variable. Other work suggests that people in certain migrant communities are particularly likely to be exposed to risk-increasing factors such as childhood adversity (e.g. parental separation) and adult social exclusion.

Life events

Brown and Birley[66] reported an excess of life events in the 3 weeks preceding schizophrenic relapse. Further studies were conflicting in their findings, possibly due to methodological problems. The study of Bebbington *et al.*[67] avoided many of the methodological pitfalls, assessing life events in 97 psychotic patients (52 with schizophrenia) and general population controls. There was a significant relationship between life events and onset or relapse of schizophrenia, although it was not as strong as for depressive psychosis. One possibility is that certain types of schizophrenic patients are particularly vulnerable to relapse following adverse life events. For example, Bebbington *et al.*[67] found females to be particularly prone, whilst van Os *et al.*[9] found life events to be associated with a less severe good-outcome illness.

There is also evidence that families who exhibit high 'expressed emotion' (comprising critical comments, hostility, and/or over-involvement) can provide an environment which enhances the risk of relapse in a family member with schizophrenia. Again, cause and effect are difficult to tease apart. Thus, it is possible that patients with more severe and intractable illnesses may induce more expressed emotion in their relatives. It is clear, though, that family interventions aimed at reducing levels of expressed emotion can be effective in reducing relapse rates in the individual.

Drug abuse

Numerous studies attest to the fact that illicit substance use is more prevalent in patients with schizophrenia than in the general population; estimates of the prevalence of such comorbidity in individuals with schizophrenia range from 20 to 60 per cent, and are consistently higher than in well controls.[68]

Whether illicit substances actually cause schizophrenia has been very contentious. The most robust methodology to consider this issue is a cohort design, and a number of such studies have now investigated whether premorbid exposure to cannabis is associated with an increased later risk of schizophrenia. Arseneault *et al.*[69] reviewed these studies and concluded that cannabis could be considered a cumulative casual factor in some cases of schizophrenia, operating in consort with other predisposing factors to 'tip the scales' in some individuals who might not otherwise have manifested the disorder. This literature needs to be seen in the light of the fact that the vast majority of people who use cannabis do not develop schizophrenia, and the majority of cases of schizophrenia are not caused by cannabis; it has been estimated that the population attributable fraction for cannabis and schizophrenia is of the order of 5 per cent to 8 per cent.

Similarly, although clinical wisdom suggests that illicit substance use has a negative impact on the longitudinal course of schizophrenia, there are few methodologically sound studies in this area.[70,71] Indeed, even the finding of an excess of use, and the association of such use with a poor longitudinal course, is potentially explicable by confounding factors such as substance abuse by the patients who are more ill. On balance, though, it seems reasonable to conclude that illicit substances make the longitudinal course of illness worse, and that patients with schizophrenia should be strongly advised to seek help to cease such behaviours.

Risk factors, age of onset, and outcome

Individuals who have been exposed to certain risk factors for schizophrenia tend have an earlier onset of psychosis than those who have not. Thus, age of onset is earlier in those whose relatives show a high morbid risk of schizophrenia;[11] similarly, those twin pairs in which the schizophrenia has an early onset show the highest monozygotic concordance.[6]

Schizophrenia patients with an early age at onset of psychosis are also more likely than those with later onset to have had a history of exposure to obstetric complications,[72] while those who showed childhood deficits such as low IQ also tend to have an early onset.[45] Schizophrenia patients who abuse cannabis have also recently been shown to have an earlier onset than those who do not.

If a factor operates to increase the risk of schizophrenia and to bring on its onset, then it is logical to think that if it is still present then it will be associated with a poor outcome. Thus, a family history of schizophrenia, a history of obstetric complication, childhood low IQ, and continued drug abuse are all associated with a poor outcome. On the other hand, those patients who develop psychosis following stressful life-events tend to have a better outcome than those with no such precipitant.[9]

The risk factor model: Gene–environment interaction

Thus, one way of construing the aetiology of schizophrenia is to see individuals on a stress-vulnerability continuum in which genetic and environmental factors act in an additive manner until a threshold of liability for expression of psychosis is passed. An individual might, for instance, inherit a schizotypal personality but not develop frank psychosis unless exposed to some cerebral insult which causes cognitive impairment; the sum of the two factors could produce the psychotic illness.

Assuming such a model in which a number of genes and environmental factors of small effect act additively, then the heritability of schizophrenia can be calculated to be between 66 and 85 per cent (i.e. a high proportion of liability to the disorder is under genetic influence). However, this assumes that the various factors operate additively, and much evidence is against this assumption. Rather, it seems that there is often an interaction between genetic susceptibility and environmental effects. As van Os and Marcelis[26] point out, it seems that certain individuals exposed to an environmental risk factor have a high risk of developing schizophrenia while others with a different genotype are at low risk.

Thus, the quality of upbringing can interact with genetic predisposition. For example, the Finnish Adoption Study has shown that when the offspring of women with schizophrenia are placed in a well-adjusted family, they have a lower risk of developing a schizophrenia spectrum disorder than if they are placed in a dysfunctional family, i.e the genotype renders the individual susceptible to the adverse effect of an adverse family environment.[73] Obstetric complications also appear to interact with, and compound, a genetic liability; the offspring of parents with schizophrenia are more likely to develop increased ventricular size following obstetric complications.

Similarly, there is evidence that individuals with a family loading for schizophrenia may be more susceptible to psychosis following abuse of cannabis.[74] The latter situation may be complicated by the possibility that individuals who inherit certain personality characteristics may be more likely to take drugs such as cannabis, i.e. their genotype renders them more liable to expose themselves to a factor to which they are genetically susceptible. Caspi *et al.*[75] investigating the Dunedin birth cohort study, presented evidence of a gene by environment (G x E) interaction between a functional polymorphism in the catechol-O-methyltransferase gene (COMT) and exposure to cannabis. The enzyme COMT has an essential role in the breakdown of dopamine in the prefrontal cortex. Caspi and colleagues showed that COMT moderates the influence of adolescent cannabis use, with at least a five-fold increased risk of developing schizophreniform disorder in cannabis users homozygous for the high activity Val allele (COMT); the Met/Met status offered relative protection (OR=1.1) while risk for heterozygotes was intermediate (OR=2.5). Furthermore, there was no correlation between the COMT genotype and cannabis use, indicating that COMT genotype does not influence cannabis consumption. This appears to be a the first clear example of a specific gene x environmental interaction predisposing for schizophrenia, but it remains to be replicated.

The implications

Having identified various risk factors for schizophrenia, we can proceed to consider the theoretical possibility of reducing the prevalence of certain risk factors and thus reducing the incidence of the disorder. From the point of view of public health, rare risk factors which have a big effect are much less important than common risk factors of even small effect. Thus, although familial risk has by far the biggest effect, it makes a smaller contribution to the total incidence of the disorder than environmental effects. Therefore, if all cases with an affected first-degree relative could be prevented, we would eliminate only about 10 per cent of the total cases. However, because being born in an urban area is so common, this small effect accounts for a much greater proportion of the population attributable fraction (33 per cent), i.e. if we could bring down the incidence of schizophrenia in cities to that in the countryside, we could theoretically eliminate one-third of all cases of the disorder. Of course, we could only do this if we knew what the critical urban factors were!

The importance of the evidence that early developmental factors are involved in the aetiology of schizophrenia lies in the fact that at least some of these are preventable. For example, advances in antenatal and perinatal care have reduced the frequency, and toxicity, of some obstetric complications. Similarly, vaccination programmes have reduced exposure to some viral infections in pregnancy and childhood. There could be a link between these developments and the decreased incidence of schizophrenia which has been observed in some western countries over recent decades.[76]

Nevertheless, most babies who are exposed to even severe obstetric complications will not later suffer from schizophrenia. Thus, there is at present no sense in attempting to improve antenatal care with the aim of reducing the occurrence of schizophrenia. There is one important exception. It is indisputable that the children of schizophrenic mothers have a higher risk of the disease if they are also exposed to obstetric complications. Therefore those women with schizophrenia who conceive must have the best possible antenatal care during their pregnancy, and steps should be taken to avoid any event (e.g. prolonged labour) which might lead to hypoxic damage to the baby.

The fact that preschizophrenic children show a number of impairments raises the possibility that predisposed individuals could be identified and 'rescued' by some intervention. Unfortunately, the childhood characteristics of such children are non-specific, and their predictive value for the later manifestation of the illness is too low to be of value for any preventative intervention, i.e. many children who show such deviation from normal in terms of early development do not later manifest schizophrenia, whilst other children who later develop schizophrenia have perfectly 'normal' early development. Furthermore, any such abnormalities must be seen in the total context of development, and it should be remembered that many such abnormalities are not static, but may be evident at some stages of development and not at others.

One might think that there is as yet little that can be done systematically to reduce the incidence of schizophrenia. However, one area where prevention is possible concerns drug abuse. The evidence concerning the abuse of cannabis is clear. If the population could be persuaded to avoid heavy use of cannabis, particularly the more potent varieties, then it is likely that a small but nevertheless significant proportion of cases of schizophrenia could be avoided.

Further information

Murray R.M., Jones P.B., Susser E., *et al.* (eds.) (2003) *The Epidemiology of Schizophrenia*. Cambridge: Cambridge University Press.

Van Os J., Marcelis, M. (1998) The ecogenetics of schizophrenia: a review. *Schizophrenia Research*, **32**, 127–35.

Harrison, P.J., Owen, M.J. (2003) Genes for schizophrenia? Recent findings and their pathophysiological implications. *Lancet*, **361**, 417–419.

Jones, P., Cannon, M. (1998) The new epidemiology of schizophrenia. *Psychiatric Clinics of North America*, **21**, 1–25.

References

1. Gottesman, I.I. (1991). *Schizophrenia Genesis: The Origins of Madness*. W.H. Freeman, New York.
2. Heston, L.L. and Denney, D. (1968). Interactions between early life experience and biological factors in schizophrenia. In *The transmission of Schizophrenia* (ed. D. Rosenthal and S. Kety), pp. 363–76. Pergamon Press, Oxford.
3. Rosenthal, D., Wender, P., Kety, S., *et al.* (1971). The adopted-away offspring of schizophrenics. *American Journal of Psychiatry*, **128**, 307–11.
4. Kety, S.S. *et al.* (1994). Mental illness in the biological relatives of schizophrenic adoptees. Replication of the Copenhagen study in the rest of Denmark. *Archives of General Psychiatry*, **51**, 442–55.
5. Wender, P.H., *et al.* (1974). Cross-fostering: a research strategy for clarifying the role of genetic and experimental factors in the etiology of schizophrenia. *Archives of General Psychiatry*, **30**, 121–8.
6. Cardno, A., Marshak, J., Coid, B., *et al.* (1999). Relationships between symptom dimensions and genetic liability to psychotic disorders in the Maudsley Twin Psychosis Series. *Archives of General Psychiatry*, **56**, 162–8.
7. Gottesman, I.I. and Bertelsen, A. (1989). Confirming unexpressed genotypes for schizophrenia: risks in the offspring of Fischer's Danish identical and fraternal discordant twins. *Archives of General Psychiatry*, **46**, 867–72.
8. Liddle, P.F. (1987). Symptoms of chronic schizophrenia. *British Journal of Psychiatry*, **151**, 145–51.
9. van Os, J. *et al.* (1994). The influence of life events on the subsequent course of psychotic illness: a follow-up of the Camberwell Collaborative Psychosis study. *Psychological Medicine*, **24**, 503–13.
10. Mata, I., Sham, P., and Murray, R.M. (2003) Schizotypal personality traits in nonpsychotic relatives are associated with positive symptoms in psychotic probands. *Schizophrenia Research*, **29**, 273–83
11. Sham, P. *et al.* (1994). Age at onset, sex and familial psychiatric morbidity in schizophrenia. Report from the Camberwell Collaborative Psychosis Study. *British Journal of Psychiatry*, **165**, 466–73.
12. Jones, P. and Murray, R.M. (1991). The genetics of schizophrenia is the genetics of neurodevelopment. *British Journal of Psychiatry*, **158**, 615–23.
13. Li D, Collier D.A. and He L. (2006) *Meta-analysis shows strong positive association of the neuregulin 1 (NRG1) gene with schizophrenia.* Molecular Genetics 1995–2002.
14. Straub, R.E., *et al.* (2002). Genetic variation in the 6p22.3 gene DTNBP1, the human ortholog of the mouse dysbindin gene, is associated with schizophrenia. *American Journal of Human Genetics*. **71**, 337–48.
15. Blackwood, D.H.R., Fordyce, A., Walker, M.T., *et al.* (2001). Schizophrenia and affective disorders – cosegregation woth a translocation at chromosome 1q42 that directly disrupts brain-expressed genes: clinical and P300 findings in a family. *American Journal of Human Genetics*. **69**, 428–433.
16. Li T, Vallada H, Curtis D, *et al.* (1997). Catechol-O-methyltransferase Val158Met polymorphism: frequency analysis in Han Chinese subjects and allelic association of the low activity allele with bipolar affective disorder. *Pharmacogenetics*, **7**, 349–53.
17. Egan, M.F., *et al.* (2001). Effect of COMT Val108/158Met genotype on frontal lobe function and risk for schizophrenia. *Proceedings of the National Academy of Science, U.S.A.* **98**, 691–722.
18. Sharma, T. *et al.* (1998). Brain changes in schizophrenia: volumetric MRI study of families multiply affected with schizophrenia-the Maudsley Family Study 5. *British Journal of Psychiatry*, **173**, 132–8.
19. Sharma, T., Lancaster, E., Sigmondson, J., *et al.* (1999). Loss of cerebral asymmetry in familial schizophrenics and their relatives detected by magnetic resonance imaging. *Schizophrenia Research*, **40**, 111–20.
20. McDonald C, Bullmore E T. Sham P C, *et al.* (2004). Association of genetic risks for schizophrenia and bipolar disorder with specific and generic brain structural endophenotypes. *Archives of General Psychiatry*, **61**, 974–84
21. Frangou, S. *et al.* (1997). The Maudsley Family Study II: endogenous event-related potentials in familial schizophrenia. *Schizophrenia Research*, **23**, 45–53.
22. Crawford, T., Sharma, T., Puri, B.K., *et al.* (1998). Saccadic eye movements in families multiply affected with schizophrenia. *American Journal of Psychiatry*, **155**, 1703–10.
23. Griffiths, T.D., Sigmundsson, T., Takei, N., *et al.* (1998). Neurological abnormalities in familial and sporadic schizophrenia. *Brain*, **121**, 191–203.
24. Wickham, H. and Murray, R.M. (1997). Can biological markers identify endophenotypes predisposing to schizophrenia? *International Review of Psychiatry*, **9**, 355–64.
25. Sipos, A., Rasmussen, F., Harrison, G.T., *et al.* (2004), Paternal age and schizophrenia: a population based cohort study British Journal of Psychiatry, 329:1070.
26. van Os, J. and Marcelis, M. (1998). The ecogenetics of schizophrenia. *Schizophrenia Research*, **32**, 127–35.
27. Geddes, J.R., Verdoux, H., Takei, N., *et al.* (1999). Individual patient data meta-analysis of the association between schizophrenia and abnormalities of pregnancy and labour. *Schizophrenia Bulletin*, **25**, 413–23.
28. Hultman, C.M., Sparen, P., Takei, N., *et al.* (1999). Prenatal and perinatal risk factors for schizophrenia, affective psychosis and reactive psychosis. *British Medical Journal*, **318**, 421–5.
29. Cannon, M., Jones, P.B. and Murray, R.M. (2002). Obstetric complications and schizophrenia: historical and meta-analytic review. *American Journal of Psychiatry* **159**, 1080–92.
30. Stewart, A.L., Rifkin, L., Amess, P.N., *et al.* (1999). Brain structure, neurocognitive and behavioural function in adolescents who were born very preterm. *Lancet*, **353**, 1653–7.
31. Reveley, A.M., Reveley, M.A., Clifford, C.A., *et al.* (1982). Cerebral ventricular size in twins discordant for schizophrenia. *Lancet*, **i**, 540–1.
32. Suddath, R.L. *et al.* (1990). Anatomical abnormalities in the brains of monozygotic twins discordant for schizophrenia. *New England Journal of Medicine*, **322**, 789–94.
33. McNeill, T.F., Cantor-Graae, E., and Weinberger, D.R. (2000). Relationship of obstetric complications and differences in size of brain structures in monozygotic twin pairs discordant for schizophrenia. *American Journal of Psychiatry*, **157**, 203–12.
34. Stefanis, N., Frangou, S., Yakeley, J., *et al.* (2000). Hippocampal volume reduction in schizophrenia is secondary to pregnancy and birth complications. *Biological Psychiatry*, **46**, 697–702.
35. McGrath, J. and Murray, R.M. (1995). Risk factors for schizophrenia: from conception to birth. In *Schizophrenia* (ed. S. Hirsch and D. Weinberger), pp. 187–205. Blackwell Science, Oxford.
36. Brown, A. S., Begg, M. D., Gravenstein, S., *et al.* (2004a) Serologic evidence of prenatal influenza in the etiology of schizophrenia. *Archives of General Psychiatry*, **61**, 774–80.
37. Brown, A. S., Cohen, P., Greenwald, S. *et al.* (2000a) Nonaffective psychosis after prenatal exposure to rubella. *American Journal of Psychiatry*, **157**, 438–43.
38. Susser, E.S. and Lin, S.P. (1992). Schizophrenia after prensatal exposure to the Dutch hunger winter. *Archives of General Psychiatry*, **49**, 938–88.
39. St Clair, D., Xu, M., Wang, P., *et al.* (2005) Rates of adult schizophrenia following prenatal exposure to the Chinese famine of 1959–1961. *Journal of the American Medical Association*, **294**, 557–62.
40. Davies, N., Russell, A., Jones, P., *et al.* (1998). Which characteristics of schizophrenia predate psychosis? *Journal of Psychiatric Research*, **32**, 121–31.

41. Fish, B., Marcus, J., Hans, S.L., *et al.* (1992). Infants at risk for schizophrenia. *Archives of General Psychiatry*, **49**, 221–35.
42. Castle, D.J. and Murray, R.M. (1991). The neurodevelopmental basis of sex differences in schizophrenia. *Psychological Medicine*, **21**, 565–75.
43. Foerster, A., Lewis, S.W., Owen, M.J., *et al.*. (1991). Premorbid personality in psychosis: effects of sex and diagnosis. *British Journal of Psychiatry*, **158**, 171–6.
44. Aylward, E., Walker, E., and Bettes, B. (1984). Intelligence in schizophrenia: meta-analysis of the research. *Schizophrenia Bulletin*, **10**, 430–59.
45. Russell, A.J., Munro, J.C., Jones, P.B., *et al.*(1997). Schizophrenia and the myth of intellectual decline. *American Journal of Psychiatry*, **154**, 635–9. Letters and reply: *American Journal of Psychiatry*, **155**, 1633–7 (1998).
46. Walker, E.F., Savoie, T., and Davis, D. (1994). Neuromotor precursors of schizophrenia. *Schizophrenia Bulletin*, **20**, 441–51.
47. Done, J.D., Crow, T.J., Johnstone, E.C., *et al.* (1994). Childhood antecedents of schizophrenia and affective illness: social adjustment at ages 7 and 11. *British Medical Journal*, **309**, 699–703.
48. Jones, P.D., Rodgers, B., Murray, R.M., *et al.*(1994). Child developmental risk factors for adult schizophrenia. *Lancet*, **344**, 1398–402.
49. Cannon, M., Caspi, A., Moffitt, T.E., *et al.* (2002b). Evidence for early-childhood, pan-developmental impairment specific to schizophreniform disorder: results from a longitudinal birth cohort. *Archives of General Psychiatry*. **59**, 449–56.
50. Poulton, R., Caspi, A., Moffitt, T.E., *et al.* (2000). Children's self-reported psychotic symptoms and adult schizophreniform disorder: a 15-year longitudinal study. *Archives General of Phychiatry*, **57**, 1053–58.
51. McGrath J.J. (2006). Variations in the incidence of schizophrenia: data versus dogma. *Schizophrenia Bulletin*. **32**, 195–7.
52. Faris, R.B.L. and Dunham, H.W. (1939). *Mental disorders in urban areas. an ecological study of schizophrenia and other psychoses*. University of Chicago Press.
53. Goldberg, S.M. and Morrison, S.L. (1963). Schizophrenia and social class. *British Journal of Psychiatry*, **109**, 785–802.
54. Hollingshead, A.B. and Redlich, F.C. (1954). Schizophrenia and social structure. *American Journal of Psychiatry*, **110**, 695–701.
55. Kohn, M.L. (1975). Social class and schizophrenia: a critical review and reformulation. In *Annual review of the schizophrenic syndrome* (ed. R. Cancro). Brunner-Mazel, New York.
56. Turner, R.J. and Wagenfeld, M.O. (1967). Occupational mobility and schizophrenia: an assessment of the social causation and social selection hypothesis. *American Sociological Review*, **32**, 104–13.
57. Lewis, G., David, A., Andreasson, S., *et al.* (1992). Schizophrenia and city life. *Lancet*, **340**, 137–40.
58. Marcelis, M., Navarro-Mateu, F., Murray, R., *et al.* (1998). Urbanization and psychosis: a study of 1942–1978 birth cohorts in The Netherlands. *Psychological Medicine*, **28**, 871–9.
59. Mortensen, P.B., Pedersen, C.B., Westergaard, T., *et al.* (1999). Effects of family history and place and season of birth on risk of schizophrenia. *New England Journal of Medicine*, **340**, 603–8.
60. Odegaard, O. (1932). Emigration and insanity. *Acta Psychiatrica Scandinavica Supplementum*, **4**.
61. Cantor-Graae, E. And Selten, J-P. (2005). Schizophrenia and migration: a meta-analysis and review. *American Journal of Psychiatry*, **162**, 12–24.
62. van Os, J., Castle, J., Takei, N., *et al.* (1996). Psychotic illness in ethnic minorities: clarification from the 1991 census. *Psychological Medicine*, **26**, 203–8.
63. Hutchinson, G. *et al.* (1996). Morbid risk of psychotic illness in first degree relatives of white and African-Caribbean patients with psychosis. *British Journal of Psychiatry*, **169**, 776–80.
64. Fearon P, Kirkbride JB, Morgan C,*et al.* (2006). Incidence of schizophrenia and other psychoses in ethnic minority groups: results from the MRC AESOP Study. *Psychological Medicine*, **36**, 1541–50.
65. Boydell, J., van Os, J., McKenzie, K. (2001). Incidence of schizophrenia in ethnic minorities in London: ecological study into interactions with environment. *British Medical Journal*. **323**, 1336–8.
66. Brown, G.W. and Birley, J.L.T. (1968). Crises and life changes and the onset of schizophrenia. *Journal of Health and Social Behaviour*, **9**, 203–14.
67. Bebbington, P. *et al.* (1993). Life events and psychosis: initial results from the Camberwell Collaborative Psychosis Study. *British Journal of Psychiatry*, **162**, 72–9.
68. Meuser, K.T. *et al.* (1990). Prevalence of substance use in schizophrenia. *Schizophrenia Bulletin*, **16**, 31–56.
69. Arseneault, L., Cannon, M., Witton, J., *et al.* (2004). Cannabis as a potential causal factor in schizophrenia. In: *Marijuana and Madness* (ed. D.J. Castle and R.M. Murray), pp. 101–18. Cambridge: Cambridge University Press.
70. Turner, W.M. and Tsuang, M.T. (1990). Impact of substance use on the course and outcome of schizophrenia. *Schizophrenia Bulletin*, **16**, 87–96.
71. Grech, A. (1998). Drug abuse and psychosis in London and Malta. M.Sc. Thesis, University of London.
72. Verdoux, H. *et al.* (1997). Obstetric complications and age at onset in schizophrenia: an international collaborative meta-analysis of individual patient data. *American Journal of Psychiatry*, **154**, 1220–7.
73. Wahlberg, K.E., Wynne, L.C., Oja, H., *et al.* (1997). Gene-environment interaction in vulnerability to schizophrenia. *American Journal of Psychiatry*, **154**, 355–62.
74. McGuire, P., Jones, P., Harvey, I., *et al.* (1994). Cannabis and acute psychosis. *Schizophrenia Research*, **24**, 995–1011.
75. Caspi A, Moffitt T E, Cannon M, *et al.* (2005). Moderation of the effect of adolescent-onset cannabis use on adult psychosis by a functional polymorphism in the Catechol-O-Methayltransferase Gene: Longitudinal evidence of a gene X environment interaction. *Biological Psychiatry*, **57**, 1117–27.
76. Der, G., Gupta, S., and Murray, R.M. (1990). Is schizophrenia disappearing? Evidence from England and Wales 1952–1986. *Lancet*, **335**, 513–16.

4.3.6.2 The neurobiology of schizophrenia

Paul J. Harrison

The neurobiology of schizophrenia remains the subject of intense research activity. Here, the key issues and findings are described, divided into functional and structural aspects, and followed by a summary of the major neurobiological theories. Where possible, meta-analyses and systematic reviews are cited in preference to individual studies.

Functional neurobiology of schizophrenia

Dopamine

The dopamine hypothesis of schizophrenia has been neurochemically pre-eminent since the 1960s.[1] It proposes that the symptoms of schizophrenia result from dopaminergic overactivity, whether due to excess dopamine, or to an elevated sensitivity to it, for example because of an increased number of dopamine receptors. The hypothesis originated with two complementary observations: that effective antipsychotics were dopamine (D_2) receptor antagonists, and that dopamine-releasing agents such as amphetamine produce a paranoid psychosis.[2] It received support from various findings of increased dopamine content and higher densities of D_2 receptors in post-mortem brain studies of schizophrenia, but proved difficult to refine or refute, for two main reasons. First, predictably, antipsychotics have marked effects on the dopamine system, confounding all studies of drug-treated subjects. Second, molecular biology revealed an unexpected complexity and diversity of dopaminergic genes, increasing the number of potential sites of dysfunction and mechanisms by which it might occur. For example, soon after the D_4 subtype of dopamine receptor was cloned, there were high profile reports that the receptor was up-regulated several-fold in schizophrenia, and might also be relevant for the actions of clozapine. However, neither suggestion was confirmed by further studies, and interest in this topic has subsided.

Despite these difficulties, substantial support for the dopamine hypothesis has now emerged, attributable largely to the availability of imaging-based methods to assess the dopamine system in the brain in vivo, free of medication, and post-mortem confounds. Notably, there is now strong evidence for a pre-synaptic dopamine abnormality, with several studies showing elevated dopamine synthesis, release, and higher dopamine receptor occupancy in the striatum.[3] The findings indicate a dysregulation and hyper-responsiveness of dopaminergic neurones in schizophrenia, sometimes referred to as 'hyperdopaminergia'. These abnormalities are present in patients with acute psychosis but not in patients in remission; recent data suggest that they may also occur in subjects in the prodrome of schizophrenia, and that they are localized to the associative parts of the striatum. It is not known whether the findings are specific to schizophrenia or common to other acute psychoses, whether they also affect dopamine pathways in the cerebral cortex, and whether they apply in all subjects with schizophrenia.[4] Neither is the cause of the hyperdopaminergia understood; one hypothesis is that it is downstream of a developmental deficit in the glutamatergic projections that regulate dopamine transmission,[5] another that it involves an imbalance between phasic and tonic modes of dopamine release.[6]

In addition to the excessive dopamine function associated with acute psychosis, there is also increasing evidence that deficiencies in dopamine transmission, especially in the dorsolateral prefrontal cortex, and genetically influenced, may underlie the working memory and allied cognitive deficits that occur in the disorder.[7] The relationship between these two facets of dopaminergic involvement in schizophrenia is not understood.

Glutamate

Phencyclidine and other non-competitive antagonists of the *N*-methyl-D-aspartate (NMDA) subtype of glutamate receptor produce a psychosis closely resembling schizophrenia.[8] This has driven the hypothesis of glutamatergic dysfunction in the disorder, particularly a disturbance of NMDA receptor-mediated glutamate transmission.[9] In support, drugs that enhance NMDA receptor function (via a variety of indirect mechanisms, since direct agonists are toxic) have some beneficial effects on positive, negative, and cognitive symptoms.[10] Also, impairment of NMDA receptor function in animal models, induced by either genetic or pharmacological manipulation, produces behavioural, structural, and neurochemical findings consistent with a 'schizophrenia-like phenotype'.[11,12] There is also a range of alterations in parameters of glutamate transmission in subjects with schizophrenia, including levels of glutamate receptors and of endogenous glutamate receptor modulators such as D-serine.[9,13] Interest in the glutamate system has been heightened with the realization that many of the putative susceptibility genes for schizophrenia have effects on NMDA receptors and their pathways[14] (see below).

Other neurotransmitters

A 5-hydroxytryptamine (5-HT, serotonin) involvement in schizophrenia was suggested because the hallucinogen lysergic acid diethylamide (LSD) is a 5-HT agonist. Recently, interest has focused on the 5-HT_{2A} receptor, for several reasons.[15] There is lowered 5-HT_{2A} receptor expression in the frontal cortex in schizophrenia, and a blunted neuroendocrine response to 5-HT_2 agonists; a high affinity for the receptor may contribute to the profile of atypical compared to typical antipsychotics, and variants in the gene are weakly associated with response to clozapine, and perhaps with schizophrenia. Elevated cortical 5-HT_{1A} receptors are also a replicated finding. Explanations for 5-HT involvement in schizophrenia include the trophic role of the 5-HT system in neurodevelopment, interactions between 5-HT and dopaminergic neurones, and impaired 5-HT_{2A} receptor-mediated activation of the prefrontal cortex.

GABA, the major inhibitory transmitter in the brain, has been implicated in schizophrenia, on the basis of findings of alterations in specific markers of GABAergic neurones and their connections as well as changes in GABA receptors.[16,17] The position of these alterations in the pathogenesis of schizophrenia is not known, as is also the case for the many other neurochemical differences that have been reported, e.g. in neuropeptides, endocannabinoids, muscarinic receptors, etc.[18]

Functional neuroimaging and cerebral activity

Cerebral activity in schizophrenia has been investigated by several methods, initially using positron emission tomography to measure regional cerebral blood flow and glucose utilization, and more recently using functional magnetic resonance imaging. The studies have addressed several questions: are there differences between cases and controls at rest, or correlations between patterns of activity and clinically defined groups of subjects, or does brain activation during the performance of cognitive tasks differ in those with and without the illness?

Hypofrontality—decreased activity in the frontal lobes—has been widely studied in schizophrenia since the first report in 1974. Results have broadly supported the notion, but with several important qualifications. The current view is that, whilst hypofrontality does occur in unmedicated subjects,[19] it is not an invariable finding, and may be related to clinical state.[20] Similarly, there are few other robust baseline differences in cerebral activity or perfusion between cases and controls. Instead, the focus has shifted towards the link between regional patterns of activation with specific symptoms, or with performance during cognitive tasks. Among the former category, a well-known example is that of Liddle *et al.*[21] who found that each of the three subsyndromes of chronic schizophrenia they had identified by factor analysis was associated with a different regional profile of cerebral blood flow. A relationship between superior temporal gyrus metabolic activity and auditory hallucinations has often been reported, sometimes lateralized to the left hemisphere.[22] Many other correlations between regional patterns of (de)activation and individual symptoms have also been reported.

A number of studies have investigated regional brain activation during the performance of various neuropsychological tests. For example, the hypofrontality of schizophrenia can be seen most clearly during working memory tasks, such as the Wisconsin Card Sort Test, which require activation of the frontal lobes, and at which patients are impaired. Conversely, when groups are matched for performance, subjects with schizophrenia show increased activation of these areas compared to controls, suggesting that they are less 'efficient' in how the information is processed, and requir greater 'effort' to achieve the same result. These issues illustrate that the situation is more complex than simply hypo- (or hyper-) frontality, but rather that there is a dynamic disturbance of frontal cortex function and regulation.(23) Beyond working memory and hypofrontality, a range of other specific correlations of this kind have been reported, but the key conclusion of this research is that cerebral dysfunction in schizophrenia is better conceptualized not as reflecting a static or single focal disorder, but as arising from abnormalities in distributed circuits linking specific cortical areas and subcortical nuclei. A prominent model is that of Andreasen,(24) who proposed the concept of 'cognitive dysmetria', in which deficits in activity in a circuit involving the cerebral cortex, thalamus, and cerebellum are key, and underlie the memory difficulties of schizophrenia. The view of the disorder as one of disturbed neural connectivity affecting multiple brain regions and their integration is supported by structural imaging and neuropathological data (see below). The model also highlights two other recent research themes: first, that brain areas beyond the 'traditional' ones (e.g. prefrontal cortex, hippocampus) and their interconnections are involved in the pathophysiology of the disorder; the most notable region of this kind is the cerebellum, formerly overlooked because of the erroneous view that it is entirely involved in motor control.(25) Second, the model places the cognitive deficits of schizophrenia centre stage in its pathophysiology, a view that was neglected for many years, but has regained prominence and is now widely cepted (Refs26–28; see Chapter 4.3.3).

Electrophysiology

A number of electrophysiological indices are altered in schizophrenia, and are relevant to the understanding of its neurobiology.(29) First, evoked potentials (electrical activity in the brain measured after a brief sensory stimulus); in particular, the P300 component is reduced and delayed in response to auditory and visual stimuli, indicative of impaired sensory processing.(30) Second, there is a high rate of eye movement abnormalities in schizophrenia, especially affecting smooth pursuit tracking, suggestive of impairment in the neural pathways subserving oculomotor control.(29) There are also differences in the cortical signal to noise ratio in the electroencephalogram, suggestive of an impairment of cortical information processing,(31) and consistent with the hypothesized abnormalities in cortical neural circuitry.

Structural neurobiology of schizophrenia

Finding the neuropathology of schizophrenia has been one of the major quests of biological psychiatry for over 100 years. Indeed, Alzheimer wrote a paper on the subject in 1897, 10 years before he described the disease that bears his name. However, whilst fundamental neuropathological discoveries were made in the dementias, there was no such progress for schizophrenia. In the past 20 years or so, the situation has changed. There is now compelling evidence that there is a neuropathology of schizophrenia, in the sense that there are statistically robust structural differences in the brains of patients with the disorder compared to normal subjects, both on structural imaging and at post-mortem (Table 4.3.6.2.1). On the other hand, the details and meaning of these changes are still elusive, and they are of limited clinical utility—they are not diagnostically specific, and they are only demonstrable when groups of cases and controls are compared.

Table 4.3.6.2.1 Morphological findings in schizophrenia

Replicated positive findings
Enlarged lateral and third ventricles
Decreased brain size and weight
Decreased cortical volume, especially temporal lobes
Fewer neurones in pulvinar thalamic nucleus
Decreased synaptic markers
Replicated negative findings
No increased incidence of Alzheimer's disease
No gliosis
Selected controversial findings
Increased density of cortical neurones
Smaller neurones
Reduced density of parvalbumin-positive interneurones
Aberrant distribution of white matter neurones
Fewer glia (oligodendrocytes)
Smaller mediodorsal thalamus with fewer neurones
Hemispheric asymmetry of pathology
Decreased dendritic markers
Effects of antipsychotic drugs on brain structure

Structural neuroimaging and macroscopic findings

The landmark study of Johnstone and colleagues showed, using computerized tomography, enlargement of the lateral ventricles in schizophrenia.(32) Although similar findings had been reported by pneumoencephalography, it was this paper which stimulated the field. It has been followed by many imaging studies, mostly in the last 20 years using magnetic resonance imaging,(33) and several meta-analyses. The latter show clearly that ventricular enlargement (with an average volume increase of ~40 per cent) is a feature of schizophrenia.(34–36) Accompanying this change there are decreases in cortical and whole brain volume of ~3 per cent,(36, 37) paralleled by a similar reduction of brain weight.(38) The regional localization of volume deficits is less clear, with different studies and meta-analyses implicating the hippocampus,(39) left superior temporal gyrus and medial temporal lobe (including hippocampus),(40) other regions of cerebral cortex, and thalamus.(41) For a narrative review of structural MRI studies, see Shenton *et al.*(42)

Structural brain changes are present in first episode patients.(43) Some differences are also present in subjects before they develop psychosis,(44,45) as well as in unaffected relatives,(46) indicating that part of the structural pathology is related to risk for schizophrenia (whether genetic or otherwise). Equally, other volumetric changes develop in high-risk subjects when they develop psychosis (e.g. hippocampal volume loss), suggesting that these changes are state-related rather than trait-related.(45, 47)

Two issues regarding structural imaging in schizophrenia remain controversial. First, the extent to which changes are progressive after the onset of established illness.[48] The meta-analyses of the cross-sectional studies show no clear evidence of progression (in keeping with the stability of cognitive impairments, and the nature of the neuropathology to be described). On the other hand, several longitudinal studies do report greater shrinkage of various brain regions with time compared to control subjects, leading to pathophysiological theories related to aberrant plasticity and neurotoxicity.[49,50] The second controversy, which may be related to the first, concerns medication effects. Again, there is little consensus: there are positive and negative reports concerning effects of antipsychotics on whole or regional brain volumes, and some suggesting differential effects of typical versus atypical antipsychotics.[51]

Recent studies are using novel imaging methods to assess the status of white matter tracts in schizophrenia, to investigate hypotheses of aberrant anatomical connectivity.[52] A number of abnormalities have been demonstrated, broadly consistent with these notions,[53] although their interpretation (i.e. what is different functionally and/or anatomically) is not wholly clear.

The neuropathology is not degenerative

Despite the continuing uncertainties, the appreciation that there are structural brain changes in schizophrenia in terms of magnetic resonance imaging findings helped stimulate a new generation of morphometric and molecular post-mortem studies designed to determine the histological and cellular basis of the observations.

The most robust and important histological findings in schizophrenia are both negative.[54] Firstly, the neuropathology is not degenerative[55–57]: there are no lesions such as neurofibrillary tangles, amyloid plaques, or Lewy bodies, which would indicate the presence of any known neurodegenerative process.[56,57] Importantly, this conclusion even applies to the significant subgroup of elderly patients who develop dementia; the neuropathological basis for the dementia of schizophrenia is entirely unexplained.[56] Secondly, there is no excess of gliosis in the brains of patients with schizophrenia.[58] Gliosis, the proliferation and hypertrophy of astrocytes, is a sign of inflammation, injury, or other ongoing pathological processes. Hence the lack of gliosis is taken to denote that the disorder is likely to be neurodevelopmental in origin, affecting mechanisms involved in the normal maturation of the brain. Indeed, some recent studies suggest there is actually a decrease in the number or activity of some glial cells, an issue returned to later.

Morphometric and cytoarchitectural changes

Having ruled out these important possibilities, it has been difficult to pin down just what the histological changes are, and therefore the cellular basis for decreases in regional brain volumes. Nevertheless, the positive findings can be grouped together and viewed as broadly cytoarchitectural in nature—i.e. affecting the morphology and spatial organization of neurones and their processes (Ref.[54]; Table 4.3.6.2.1).

As a rule, the more dramatic (and well publicized) the initial finding, the less robust it has proved to be. For example, dysplasia (disorganized, misplaced, and misshapen neurones) in the entorhinal cortex was reported in 1986. Such a finding would be strongly suggestive of a prenatal developmental anomaly. However, subsequent studies have, at best, only partially replicated this observation. Similarly, a report that pyramidal neurones in the hippocampus are not aligned in their usual regular orientation, also indicative of a developmental disturbance, has not been consistently observed.

A decreased size of neurones, particularly in the hippocampus and prefrontal cortex, has been found in several studies. The size of a neurone is related to the volume of axon and dendrites, which it has to support, and also to its metabolic activity. Thus, the finding of smaller neurones in schizophrenia suggests the neurones may be receiving and making fewer, abnormal, or less-active connections. Support for this interpretation comes from studies of synaptic and dendritic markers, which have been reasonably consistent in showing decreases in the same brain areas.[59] It is unclear as to which specific populations of neurones and synapses are most affected in schizophrenia, and it may vary from one region to another; in both hippocampus and prefrontal cortex, there is evidence for involvement of excitatory (glutamatergic) pathways[60, 61] as well subtypes of inhibitory (GABAergic) ones,[16,17] especially the class of parvalbumin-positive interneurones.[17] In addition to the neuronal pathology, several recent studies show reductions in markers of oligodendrocytes and their activity.[62] This type of glial cell is intimately involved in myelination, and contributes to synaptic homeostasis, and therefore their involvement in schizophrenia is in keeping with the occurrence of synaptic as well as white matter pathology.

A further area of interest is the thalamus, specifically the pulvinar and mediodorsal nuclei. Both have been found to be smaller and to contain fewer neurones in several studies of schizophrenia; in the case of the pulvinar nucleus, the evidence is amongst the most compelling of any brain region, coming from four methodologically rigorous studies (as well as complementary findings in the imaging literature, noted above), and with no corresponding negative studies.[63] These thalamic nuclei have extensive reciprocal connections with the prefrontal and temporal association cortices, and it is assumed that there is some causal link between the changes in each thalamic nucleus and its cortical partner.

Neuropathology and medication effects

Most patients studied neuropathologically were treated in life with antipsychotic drugs, and so the findings in schizophrenia are open to the criticism that they may have been caused by antipsychotic medication.[64] However, as noted above, many imaging studies show that the pathology, at least in terms of the gross alterations summarized in Table 4.3.6.2.1, is present in first episode and medication-naïve subjects. Also, in post-mortem studies, the reported neuropathological findings rarely if ever correlate with the extent of antipsychotic exposure. In some instances it may also be that medication ameliorates the disease effects. Nevertheless, the possibility that antipsychotic drugs have neuropathological effects should not be overlooked. Firstly, typical antipsychotics produce enlargement of, and synaptic structural alterations in, the basal ganglia (caudate, putamen, globus pallidus).[64] Secondly, a recent monkey study found that chronic administration of haloperidol or olanzapine at therapeutic levels led to decreased brain volume[65] along with increased neuronal density and decreased glial density,[66] thus reproducing several of the changes reported in schizophrenia.

Neurobiological theories of schizophrenia

Schizophrenia as a neurodevelopmental disorder

The neurodevelopmental model of schizophrenia is the prevailing pathogenic hypothesis.[5,67–69] Neurobiological data form an important component of the evidence, along with epidemiological and other observations (Table 4.3.6.2.2). A specific version of the theory is that the pathology of schizophrenia originates in the second trimester *in utero*. An earlier timing is excluded since overt brain abnormalities would be seen if neurogenesis were affected, whilst the lack of gliosis has been taken to mean that the changes must have occurred prior to the third trimester when the gliotic response begins.[57] Other forms of the neurodevelopmental theory advocate abnormalities in processes such as myelination, synaptic pruning, and apoptosis, all of which continue long into post-natal life. Overall, a parsimonious view is that the neuropathological data are indicative merely of a basically developmental, as opposed to degenerative, disease process, but do not, in isolation, point to a particular mechanism or timing.

Schizophrenia as a disorder of connectivity

The functional imaging and histological data summarized above have together contributed to the emerging consensus that the pathophysiological basis of schizophrenia is one of connectivity.[24, 54, 70–72] The nature of the 'dysconnectivity' is not a simple lack, or gross mis-routing, of connections, but likely a subtle change in a more fine-grained aspect, such as the precise molecular composition, location, or activity of subpopulations of synapses.[71] Both intrinsic (local) and extrinsic (long-range) connections may be affected. The extent to which there is a structural basis to the aberrant connectivity remains uncertain,[73] but in so far as it exists, the histological basis of the syndrome is a difference in the circuitry, or 'wiring' of the brain, manifested by the cytoarchitectural differences in the morphology and organization of neurones and their synapses. If there is indeed a structural basis to the pathophysiology of the syndrome, it would help explain why many of the cardinal features are trait rather than just state abnormalities, and perhaps why individuals are vulnerable to relapse, in that a 'miswired' brain may be less able to respond rapidly, appropriately, or fully to environmental stressors.

Table 4.3.6.2.2 Evidence adduced for a neurodevelopmental basis to schizophrenia

- Usual age of onset in late adolescence and early adulthood
- Most environmental risk factors operate prenatally or in early childhood
- Neuromotor, intellectual, and behavioural differences in children many years prior to onset
- Structural brain changes and cognitive impairments present at, and prior to, onset of illness
- Nature of the neuropathological findings—lack of gliosis or neurodegeneration, plus cytoarchitectural disturbances
- Changes in expression of neurodevelopmental genes (e.g. reelin)
- Minor physical anomalies—for example, craniofacial dysmorphology and dermatoglyphics.
- Animal models—early lesions or pharmacological interventions lead to delayed 'schizophrenia-like' phenotypes

(Reprinted from P.J. Harrison, Schizophrenia susceptibility genes and neurodevelopment, *Biological Psychiatry*, **61**, 1119–20, copyright 2007, with permission from Elsevier)

For reviews and other references, see text.

Cerebral asymmetry and schizophrenia

Many neuropathological, neurochemical, neuropsychological, and electrophysiological studies of schizophrenia report lateralized abnormalities. Although there are also important negative findings, reductions in normal brain asymmetries, and a left hemisphere preference of the pathology, do seem more common than one would expect by chance.[74,75] Crow's influential theory sees a fundamental connection between schizophrenia, asymmetry, handedness, and language, causally linked to each other and to the same gene.[76] Alternatively, altered asymmetry in schizophrenia is viewed as an epiphenomenon of its developmental origins, a process which interferes with normal brain lateralization.

Susceptibility genes and neurobiology

Given its high heritability,[77] it can be assumed that genes are the major influence on the neurobiological features of schizophrenia, likely modified by the various environmental risk factors (see Chapter 4.3.6.1). The recent discovery of several probable susceptibility genes[14,78] now allows this question to be addressed more specifically, in terms of the normal functions of the genes, and how this is altered in those carrying the risk variants of the genes.

Neuregulin 1 (NRG1) is the best established susceptibility gene.[79] It encodes a family of proteins that have multiple roles in the nervous system, ranging from cell fate determination, to neuronal migration, neuronal-glial signalling, and NMDA receptor functioning.[80] As such, it is a good candidate gene for schizophrenia given the existing theories outlined above regarding aberrations in neurodevelopment, connectivity, and glutamate synaptic transmission. Equally, at present it is not clear which of these functions is actually affected in schizophrenia or explains the contribution that NRG1 plays in the disease process,[81] and determining this will not be simple. Initial data suggest an impairment of NRG1 signalling via its receptors,[82] and an alteration in the expression of one specific subtype of NRG1.[83,84]

An interaction with synaptic neurotransmission is also seen for most of the other leading susceptibility genes (Table 4.3.6.2.3), leading to the notion that this effect is a point of pathophysiological convergence of the genes.[14] Such a convergence is an attractive concept for several reasons, not least parsimony, but whilst there is some evidence to support it, it remains highly speculative. Indeed,

Table 4.3.6.2.3 Susceptibility genes and their neurobiological functions

Gene symbol	Functions include
NRG1	Multiple roles in brain development, synaptic plasticity, and glutamate signalling
DTNBP1	Glutamate release
DISC-1	Multiple roles in development, cell functioning, and synaptic signalling
PPP3CC	Critical molecule for integration of dopamine and glutamate signalling
DAOA	Affects metabolism of the NMDA receptor modulator D-serine
COMT	Regulation of dopamine function in frontal cortex

NRG1, neuregulin 1; DTNBP1, dysbindin; DISC-1, disrupted in schizophrenia-1; PPP3CC, calcineurin Aγ subunit; DAOA, D-amino acid oxidase activator COMT, catechol-*O*-methyltransferase.

Table 4.3.6.2.4 Key recent findings in the neurobiology of schizophrenia

- Elevated dopamine release and receptor occupancy during acute psychosis
- Confirmation (by meta-analysis) of structural brain changes, including in first-episode patients, and in unaffected relatives
- Exclusion of a neurodegenerative disease process
- Discovery of neuregulin and several other putative susceptibility genes, and of molecular mechanisms by which they may increase schizophrenia susceptibility

Table 4.3.6.2.5 Current key questions to be addressed in the neurobiology of schizophrenia

- Which, if any, of the neurobiological findings are clinically useful (i.e. will influence diagnosis, treatment, or prognosis)?
- What is the relationship between the dopaminergic changes, and those affecting other neurochemical systems and brain structure?
- Are there differing neurobiological substrates for the psychotic, cognitive, and negative components of schizophrenia?
- How do the genes interact with each other, and with the environmental risk factors, to produce their effects?

it will probably remain difficult to determine in detail the genetic contribution to the neurobiology of schizophrenia, given that there are many genes, each of small and complex effects.[85]

Summary

Significant progress has been made in understanding the neurobiology of schizophrenia over the past decade (Table 4.3.6.2.4). In particular, there is now good evidence for a dopaminergic dysfunction, and for structural brain changes that are present at, and in part before, the onset of illness. There is also emerging evidence for several susceptibility genes, accompanied by data suggesting mechanisms by which these genes contribute to the neurodevelopmental and other pathogenic processes that are thought to lead to schizophrenia. Whilst highlighting the progress, one must also acknowledge that much remains unknown (Table 4.3.6.2.5), and it is a moot point how and when the research advances will impact on the diagnosis, treatment, or prognosis of schizophrenia.

Further information

Lawrie, S.A., Weinberger, D.R., Johnstone, E.C. (2004). *Schizophrenia. From neuroimaging to neuroscience*. Oxford University Press, Oxford.

Schizophrenia Research Forum (www.schizophreniaforum.org)—links to all aspects of schizophrenia research, including up-to-date bibliographies, discussion forum, and a genetics database.

Weinberger, D.R. and Harrison, P.J. (2009). *Schizophrenia* (3rd edn). Wiley Blackwell, Oxford.

References

1. Matthyse, S. (1973). Antipsychotic drug actions: a clue to the neuropathology of schizophrenia? *Federation Proceedings*, **32**, 200–5.
2. Davis, K.L., Kahn, R.S., Ko, G., *et al.* (1991). Dopamine in schizophrenia: a review and reconceptualization. *The American Journal of Psychiatry*, **148**, 1474–86.
3. Laruelle, M. and Abi-Dargham, A. (1999). Dopamine as the wind of the psychotic fire: new evidence from brain imaging studies. *Journal of Psychopharmacology*, **13**, 358–71.
4. Abi-Dargham, A., Rodenhiser, J., Printz, D., *et al.* (2000). Increased baseline occupancy of D_2 receptors by dopamine in schizophrenia. *Proceedings of the National Academy of Sciences of the United States of America*, **97**, 8104–9.
5. Weinberger, D.R. (1987). Implications of normal brain development for the pathogenesis of schizophrenia. *Archives of General Psychiatry*, **44**, 660–9.
6. Grace, A.A. (1993). Cortical regulation of subcortical dopamine systems and its possible relevance to schizophrenia. *Journal of Neural Transmission*, **91**, 111–34.
7. Weinberger, D.R., Egan, M.F., Bertolino, A., *et al.* (2001). Prefrontal neurons and the genetics of schizophrenia. *Biological Psychiatry*, **50**, 825–44.
8. Javitt, D.C. and Zukin, S.R. (1991). Recent advances in the phencyclidine model of schizophrenia. *The American Journal of Psychiatry*, **148**, 1301–8.
9. Tsai, G. and Coyle, J.T. (2002). Glutamatergic mechanisms in schizophrenia. *Annual Review of Pharmacology and Toxicology* **42**, 165–79.
10. Tuominen, H.J., Tiihonen, J., and Wahlbeck, K. (2005). Glutamatergic drugs for schizophrenia: a systematic review and meta-analysis. *Schizophrenia Research*, **72**, 225–34.
11. Lipska, B.K. and Weinberger, D.R. (2000). To model a psychiatric disorder in animals: schizophrenia as a reality test. *Neuropsychopharmacology*, **23**, 223–39.
12. Tordjman, S., Drapier, D., Bonnot, O., *et al.* (2007). Animal models relevant to schizophrenia and autism: validity and limitations. *Behavioral Genetics*, **37**, 61–78.
13. Konradi, C. and Heckers, S. (2003). Molecular aspects of glutamate dysregulation: implications for schizophrenia and its treatment. *Pharmacology & Therapeutics*, **97**, 153–79.
14. Harrison, P.J. and Weinberger, D.R. (2005). Schizophrenia genes, gene expression, and neuropathology: on the matter of their convergence. *Molecular Psychiatry*, **10**, 40–68.
15. Dean, B. (2003). The cortical serotonin$_{2A}$ receptor and the pathology of schizophrenia: a likely accomplice. *Journal of Neurochemistry*, **85**, 1–13.
16. Benes, F.M. and Berretta, S. (2001). GABAergic interneurons: implications for understanding schizophrenia and bipolar disorder. *Neuropsychopharmacology*, **25**, 1–27.
17. Lewis, D.A., Hashimoto, T., and Volk, D.W. (2005). Cortical inhibitory neurons and schizophrenia. *Nature Reviews Neuroscience*, **6**, 312–24.
18. Fallon, J.H., Opole, I.O., and Potkin, S.G. (2003). The neuroanatomy of schizophrenia: circuitry and neurotransmitter systems. *Clinical Neuroscience Research*, **3**, 77–107.
19. Andreasen, N.C., O'Leary, D.S., Flaum, M., *et al.* (1997). Hypofrontality in schizophrenia: distributed dysfunctional circuits in neuroleptic-naive patients. *Lancet*, **349**, 1730–4.
20. Spence, S.A., Hirsch, S.R., Brooks, D.J., *et al.* (1998). Prefrontal cortex activity in people with schizophrenia and control subjects. Evidence from positron emission tomography for remission of 'hypofrontality' with recovery from acute schizophrenia. *The British Journal of Psychiatry*, **172**, 316–23.
21. Liddle, P.F., Friston, K.J., Frith, C.D., *et al*, (1992). Patterns of cerebral blood flow in schizophrenia. *The British Journal of Psychiatry*, **160**, 179–86.
22. Weiss, A.P. and Heckers, S. (1999). Neuroimaging of hallucinations: a review of the literature. *Psychiatry Research: Neuroimaging*, **92**, 61–74.

23. Callicott, J.H., Mattay, V.S., Verchinski, B.A., *et al.* (2003). Complexity of prefrontal cortical dysfunction in schizophrenia: more than up or down. *The American Journal of Psychiatry*, **160**, 2209–15.
24. Andreasen, N.C. (1998). A unitary model of schizophrenia: Bleuler's 'fragmented phrene' as schizencephaly. *Archives of General Psychiatry*, **56**, 781–7.
25. Picard, H., Amado, I., Mouchet-Mages, S., *et al.* (2008). The role of the cerebellum in schizophrenia: an update of clinical, cognitive, and functional evidences. *Schizophrenia Bulletin*, **34**, 155–72.
26. Aleman, A., Hijman, R., De Haan, E.H.F., *et al.* (1999). Memory impairment in schizophrenia: a meta-analysis. *The American Journal of Psychiatry*, **156**, 1358–66.
27. Green, M.F. and Neuchterlein, K.H. (1999). Should schizophrenia be treated as a neurocognitive disorder? *Schizophrenia Bulletin*, **25**, 309–19.
28. Goldberg, T.E., David, A., and Gold, J.M. (2003). Neurocognitive deficits in schizophrenia. In *Schizophrenia* (2nd edn) (eds. S.C. Hirsch and D.R. Weinberger), pp. 168–86. Blackwell, Oxford.
29. Salisbury, D.F., Krljes, S., and McCarley, R.W. (2003). Electrophysiology. In *Schizophrenia* (2nd edn) (eds. S.C. Hirsch and D.R. Weinberger), pp. 298–309. Blackwell, Oxford.
30. Bramon, E., Rabe-Hesketh, S., Sham, P., *et al.* (2004). Meta-analysis of the P300 and P50 waveforms in schizophrenia. *Schizophrenia Research*, **70**, 315–29.
31. Winterer, G. and Weinberger, D.R. (2004). Genes, dopamine and cortical signal-to-noise ratio in schizophrenia. *Trends in Neurosciences*, **27**, 683–90.
32. Johnstone, E.C., Crow, T.J., Frith, C.D., *et al.* (1976). Cerebral ventricular size and cognitive impairment in chronic schizophrenia. *Lancet*, **2**, 924–6.
33. Andreasen, N.C., Nasrallah, H.A., Dunn, V., *et al.* (1986). Structural abnormalities in the frontal system in schizophrenia. A magnetic resonance imaging study. *Archives of General Psychiatry*, **43**, 136–44.
34. Daniel, D.G., Goldberg, T.E., Gibbons, R.D., *et al.* (1991). Lack of a bimodal distribution of ventricular size in schizophrenia—a Gaussian mixture analysis of 1056 cases and controls. *Biological Psychiatry*, **30**, 887–903.
35. Lawrie, S.M. and Abukmeil, S.S. (1998). Brain abnormality in schizophrenia—a systematic and quantitative review of volumetric magnetic resonance imaging studies. *The British Journal of Psychiatry*, **172**, 110–20.
36. Wright, I.C., Rabe-Hesketh, S., Woodruff, P.W.R., *et al.* (2000). Meta-analysis of regional brain volumes in schizophrenia. *The American Journal of Psychiatry*, **157**, 16–25.
37. Ward, K.E., Friedman, L., Wise, A., *et al.* (1996). Meta-analysis of brain and cranial size in schizophrenia. *Schizophrenia Research*, **22**, 197–213.
38. Harrison, P.J., Freemantle, N., and Geddes, J.R. (2003). Meta-analysis of brain weight in schizophrenia. *Schizophrenia Research*, **64**, 25–34.
39. Nelson, M.D., Saykin, A.J., Flashman, L.A., *et al.* (1998). Hippocampal volume reduction in schizophrenia as assessed by magnetic resonance imaging—a meta-analytic study. *Archives of General Psychiatry*, **55**, 433–40.
40. Honea, R., Crow, T.J., Passingham, D., *et al.* (2005). Regional deficits in brain volume in schizophrenia: a meta-analysis of voxel-based morphometry studies. *The American Journal of Psychiatry*, **162**, 2233–45.
41. Konick, L.C. and Friedman, L. (2001). Meta-analysis of thalamic size in schizophrenia. *Biological Psychiatry*, **49**, 28–38.
42. Shenton, M.E., Dickey, C.C., Frumin, M., *et al.* (2001). A review of MRI findings in schizophrenia. *Schizophrenia Research*, **49**, 1–52.
43. Steen, R.G., Mull, C., McClure, R., *et al.* (2006). Brain volume in first-episode schizophrenia—systematic review and meta-analysis of magnetic resonance imaging studies. *The British Journal of Psychiatry*, **188**, 510–18.
44. Lawrie, S.M., Whalley, H., Kestelman, J.N., *et al.* (1999). Magnetic resonance imaging of brain in people at high risk of developing schizophrenia. *Lancet*, **353**, 30–3.
45. Pantelis, C., Velakoulis, D., McGorry, P.D., *et al.* (2003). Neuroanatomical abnormalities before and after onset of psychosis: a cross-sectional and longitudinal MRI comparison. *Lancet*, **361**, 281–8.
46. Boos, H.B.M., Aleman, A., Cahn, W., *et al.* (2007). Brain volumes in relatives of patients with schizophrenia—a meta-analysis. *Archives of General Psychiatry*, **64**, 297–304.
47. Velakoulis, D., Wood, S.J., Wong, M.T.H., *et al.* (2006). Hippocampal and amygdala volumes according to psychosis stage and diagnosis—a magnetic resonance imaging study of chronic schizophrenia, first-episode psychosis, and ultra-high-risk individuals. *Archives of General Psychiatry*, **63**, 139–49.
48. Weinberger, D.R. and McClure, R.K. (2002). Neurotoxicity, neuroplasticity, and magnetic resonance imaging morphometry—what is happening in the schizophrenic brain? *Archives of General Psychiatry*, **59**, 553–8.
49. Lieberman, J.A. (1999). Is schizophrenia a neurodegenerative disorder? A clinical and neurobiological perspective. *Biological Psychiatry*, **46**, 729–39.
50. Woods, B.T., Ward, K.E., and Johnson, E.H. (2005). Meta-analysis of the time-course of brain volume reduction in schizophrenia: implications for pathogenesis and early treatment. *Schizophrenia Research*, **73**, 221–8.
51. Lieberman, J.A., Tollefson, G.D., Charles, C., *et al.* (2005). Antipsychotic drug effects on brain morphology in first-episode psychosis. *Archives of General Psychiatry*, **62**, 361–70.
52. Davis, K.L., Stewart, D.G., Friedman, J.I., *et al.* (2003). White matter changes in schizophrenia—evidence for myelin-related dysfunction. *Archives of General Psychiatry*, **60**, 443–56.
53. Kubicki, M., McCarley, R., Westin, C.F., *et al*, (2007). A review of diffusion tensor imaging studies in schizophrenia. *Journal of Psychiatric Research*, **41**, 15–30.
54. Harrison, P.J. (1999). The neuropathology of schizophrenia. A critical review of the data and their interpretation. *Brain*, **122**, 593–624.
55. Harrison, P.J. (2003). Schizophrenia and its dementia. In *The neuropathology of dementia* (eds. M. Esiri, V. Lee, and J. Trojanowski), pp. 497–508. Cambridge University Press, Cambridge.
56. Arnold, S.E. and Trojanowski, J.Q. (1996). Cognitive impairment in elderly schizophrenia: a dementia (still) lacking distinctive histopathology. *Schizophrenia Bulletin*, **22**, 5–9.
57. Arnold, S.E., Trojanowski, J.Q., Gur, R.E., *et al.* (1998). Absence of neurodegeneration and neural injury in the cerebral cortex in a sample of elderly patients with schizophrenia. *Archives of General Psychiatry*, **55**, 225–32.
58. Roberts, G.W. and Harrison. P.J. (2000). Gliosis and its implications for the disease process. In *The neuropathology of schizophrenia* (eds. P.J. Harrison and G.W. Roberts), pp. 137–50. Oxford University Press, Oxford.
59. Eastwood, S.L. (2004). The synaptic pathology of schizophrenia: is aberrant neurodevelopment and plasticity to blame? *International Review of Neurobiology*, **59**, 47–72.
60. Lewis, D.A. and Gonzalez-Burgos, G. (2000). Intrinsic excitatory connections in the prefrontal cortex and the pathophysiology of schizophrenia. *Brain Research Bulletin*, **52**, 309–17.
61. Hof, P.R., Haroutunian, V., Copland, C., *et al.* (2002). Molecular and cellular evidence for an oligodendrocyte abnormality in schizophrenia. *Neurochemical Research*, **27**, 1193–200.
62. Harrison, P.J. and Eastwood, S.L. (2001). Neuropathological studies of synaptic connectivity in the hippocampal formation in schizophrenia. *Hippocampus*, **11**, 508–19.
63. Byne, W., Fernandes, J., Haroutunian, V., *et al.* (2007). Reduction of right medial pulvinar volume and neuron number in schizophrenia. *Schizophrenia Research*, **90**, 71–5.

64. Harrison, P.J. (1999). The neuropathological effects of antipsychotic drugs. *Schizophrenia Research*, **40**, 87–99.
65. Dorph-Petersen, K.A., Pierri, J.N., Perel, J.M., *et al.* (2005). The influence of chronic exposure to antipsychotic medications on brain size before and after tissue fixation: a comparison of haloperidol and olanzapine in macaque monkeys. *Neuropsychopharmacology*, **30**, 1649–61.
66. Konopaske, G.T., Dorph-Petersen, K.A., Pierri, J.N., *et al.* (2007). Effect of chronic exposure to antipsychotic medication on cell numbers in the parietal cortex of macaque monkeys. *Neuropsychopharmacology*, **32**, 1216–23.
67. Murray, R.M. and Lewis, S.W. (1987). Is schizophrenia a neurodevelopmental disorder. *British Medical Journal*, **295**, 681–2.
68. Weinberger, D.R. (1995). From neuropathology to neurodevelopment. *Lancet*, **346**, 552–7.
69. Lewis, D.A. and Levitt, P. (2002). Schizophrenia as a disorder of neurodevelopment. *Annual Review of Neuroscience*, **25**, 409–32.
70. McGuire, P.K. and Frith, C.D. (1996). Disordered functional connectivity in schizophrenia. *Psychological Medicine*, **26**, 663–7.
71. Frankle, W., Lerma, J., and Laruelle, M. (2003). The synaptic hypothesis of schizophrenia. *Neuron*, **39**, 205–16.
72. Stephan, K.E., Baldeweg, T., and Friston, K.J. (2006). Synaptic plasticity and dysconnection in schizophrenia. *Biological Psychiatry*,**59**, 929–93.
73. Konrad, A. and Winterer, G. (2008). Disturbed structural connectivity in schizophrenia—primary factor in pathology or epiphenomenon? *Schizophrenia Bulletin*, **34**, 72–92.
74. Holinger, D.P., Galaburda, A., and Harrison, P.J. (2000). Cerebral asymmetry. In *The neuropathology of schizophrenia* (eds. P.J. Harrison and G.W. Roberts), pp. 151–72. Oxford University Press, Oxford.
75. Sommer, I., Aleman, A., Ramsey, N., *et al.* (2001). Handedness, language lateralisation and anatomical asymmetry in schizophrenia—meta-analysis. *The British Journal of Psychiatry*, **178**, 344–51.
76. Crow, T.J. (2004). Cerebral asymmetry and the lateralization of language: core deficits in schizophrenia as pointers to the gene. *Current Opinion in Psychiatry*, **17**, 97–106.
77. Sullivan, P.F., Kendler, K.S., and Neale, M.C. (2003). Schizophrenia as a complex trait—evidence from a meta-analysis of twin studies. *Archives of General Psychiatry*, **60**, 1187–92.
78. Owen, M.J., Craddock, N., and O'Donovan, M.C. (2005). Schizophrenia: genes at last? *Trends in Genetics*, **21**, 518–25.
79. Li, D.W., Collier, D.A., and He, L. (2006). Meta-analysis shows strong positive association of the neuregulin 1 (*NRG1*) gene with schizophrenia. *Human Molecular Genetics*, **15**, 1995–2002.
80. Harrison, P.J. and Law, A.J. (2006). Neuregulin 1 and schizophrenia: genetics, gene expression, and neurobiology. *Biological Psychiatry*, **60**, 132–40.
81. Corfas, G., Roy, K., and Buxbaum, J.D. (2004). Neuregulin 1-erbB signaling and the molecular/cellular basis of schizophrenia. *Nature Neuroscience*, **7**, 575–80.
82. Hahn, C.G., Wang, H.Y., Cho, D.S., *et al.* (2006). Altered neuregulin 1-erbB4 signaling contributes to NMDA receptor hypofunction in schizophrenia. *Nature Medicine*, **12**, 824–8.
83. Law, A.J., Lipska, B.K., Weickert, C.S., *et al.* (2006). Neuregulin 1 transcripts are differentially expressed in schizophrenia and regulated by 5′ SNPs associated with the disease. *Proceedings of the National Academy of Sciences of the United States of America*, **103**, 6747–52.
84. Tan, W., Wang, Y., Gold, B., *et al.* (2007). Molecular cloning of a brain-specific, developmentally regulated neuregulin 1 (NRG1) isoform and identification of a functional promoter variant associated with schizophrenia. *The Journal of Biological Chemistry*, **282**, 24343–51.
85. Harrison, P.J. (2008). Schizophrenia genes: searching for common features, functions, and mechanisms. In *Cortical deficits in schizophrenia: from genes to function* (ed. P. O'Donnell), pp. 1–16. Springer, Norwell, MA.

4.3.7 Course and outcome of schizophrenia and their prediction

Assen Jablensky

Introduction

The course of schizophrenia is as variable as its symptoms. Systematic investigations of course of the psychoses were initiated by Kraepelin who believed that, in the absence of demonstrable brain pathology and aetiology, a common outcome into 'psychic weakness' of the clinical syndromes he grouped together as **dementia praecox** would provide a validity test for the disease entity. Later, Kraepelin revised his claim that the prognosis of dementia praecox was invariably poor and noted that 'permanent cures' had occurred in about 15 per cent of his cases.[1] Subsequent longitudinal studies have confirmed the striking variability of course as one of the salient characteristic of the 'natural history' of schizophrenia.

Methodological issues

The large number of studies on the course and outcome of schizophrenia published since the beginning of the twentieth century might suggest that the longitudinal aspects of the disorder are well established and exhaustively documented. Unfortunately, this is not the case since the methodological difficulties that accompany this type of research are complex and few studies have adequately dealt with all the major sources of error and confounding, including sample selection, definition of outcome, and diagnostic criteria used.[2,3]

The studies of the course and outcome of schizophrenia comprise statistical reports on admissions and discharges, long-term **follow-back studies** (in which the initial features of the cases and the course of the disorder are reconstructed retrospectively from admission records), and prospective investigations (in which patients are enlisted at an early stage of the disorder and followed up for a varying length of time). Each design is vulnerable to bias: admission and discharge statistics usually comprise patients at different stages of disease progression; follow-back studies rely on prevalence samples in which chronic cases tend to be over-represented; and **prospective studies**, though superior to other designs, tend to exclude patients who initially have diagnoses other than schizophrenia but are subsequently re-diagnosed as schizophrenic. The methodological issues that need to be considered in interpreting the results from longitudinal research into schizophrenia include the following.

Diagnosis

The use of either 'broad' or 'restrictive' definitions of schizophrenia may result in vastly different samples on which follow-up data are reported. Systems with an inbuilt illness duration criterion, such as **DSM-III**, **DSM-IIIR**, and **DSM-IV** which require at least 6 months of unremitting symptoms and a decline in functioning, are likely to overselect patients already developing a chronic course. The result would be a greater homogeneity of outcome at the cost of a compromised representativeness of the sample as regards the range of possible outcomes of schizophrenia. Diagnostic systems which emphasize the cross-sectional features of the disorder, such as **ICD-10** (which requires 1 month's duration of clinically characteristic symptoms) avoid this limitation, possibly at the expense of including some cases of good prognosis that may be aetiologically or pathogenetically different from poor prognosis schizophrenia. However, until aetiology is elucidated, or validating biomarkers are established, the decision as to what constitutes 'true' schizophrenia will remain arbitrary. With regard to prognostic studies, less restrictive diagnostic systems have the advantage that a broad spectrum of outcomes would be available at the end point of prospective observation, allowing for subgroups to be identified and their characteristics related to the initial manifestations of the disorder and various risk factors.

Definitions and assessment of course and outcome variables

There is no single measure of course and outcome of a complex disorder such as schizophrenia. Blanket terms such as 'recovery', 'improvement', or 'deterioration' tend to conflate substantially different aspects of the evolution of the disorder over time. Most investigators today agree that course (comprising the pathways or trajectories of the disorder) and outcome (the net balance of the clinical and functional descriptors at the end point of observation) are multivariate composites. As a minimum, three domains that need not co-vary over time should be independently assessed: symptom severity; functional impairments including cognitive deficits, and disablement in social and occupational role performance. Each one of these can be further articulated into a number of areas or dimensions. In addition, one must consider extrinsic variables such as measures of environmental and treatment-related influences on course and outcome, as well as subjective experiences commonly described as 'quality of life'. Standardized, reliable instruments (interviews, inventories, rating scales) are required for the assessment of most variables. **Operational definitions** and criteria of relapse and remission have been proposed.[4,5] It should not be forgotten, however, that some of the richest sources of information are the perceptive, in-depth clinical case studies based on personal patient contact over many years. Collectively, such single case observations can generate hypotheses for testing in epidemiologically designed studies.

Length of follow-up

The evidence from previous research suggests that very different impressions of the course and outcome of schizophrenia would be gained depending on the duration of prospective observation and the degree of control over the inclusion of patients that are comparable in terms age and length of previous illness.

Cohort attrition

In any follow-up study, a proportion of cases will be lost to observation because of death, migration, refusal of contact, or other reasons for untraceability. Since such loss of subjects is likely to correlate with particular patterns of course and outcome, it is essential to estimate its possible effect (e.g. by statistical modelling) on the interpretation of the final results, especially if cohort attrition is greater than 15–20 per cent of the original sample.

Other aspects of study design

Variation in the sources of recruitment of cases (e.g. any admission to a treatment facility or catchment area sampling), and of information regarding course and outcome variables (e.g. face-to-face interviews or collateral data from case notes or informants), can obviously influence the results of any follow-up study. In addition, subtle variations in study design, such as whether investigators assessing patients' symptoms and functioning at any point in time are 'blind' to data from previous assessments, can bias the final results. Inclusion of a comparison group (e.g. patients with other psychotic disorders) would help evaluate the extent to which any observed patterns of course and outcome are specific to schizophrenia, whereas appropriate controls drawn from the general population can provide reference points for assessing social variables, such as occupational functioning, stressful life events, or habit-related behaviour such as substance use.

Statistical analysis

Longitudinal research poses a number of specific requirements with regard to data analysis. Thus, the problem of **multiple comparisons** is likely to arise when examining the data for significant associations; time series, survival, or path analysis may be required when observations are made and recorded at successive time points in the evolution of the disorder; and methods of unconfounding are called for at each step of the analysis of longitudinal data. While no single study up to date has met all the rigorous methodological requirements, a number of studies have succeeded in controlling at least some of the sources of bias and confounding. The results from previous research are, therefore, not strictly comparable in specific detail, but are informative as regards general trends and patterns.

The 'natural history' of schizophrenia before the neuroleptic era

Since the great majority of schizophrenic patients are today receiving pharmacological treatment, current and recent studies may not reflect the 'natural' course and outcome of the disorder. Studies in urban communities in Scotland[6] and India,[7] and a study in a rural community in China[8] estimated the proportions of never hospitalized schizophrenic patients at 6.7 per cent, 28.7 per cent, and 30.6 per cent, respectively. About half of the Scottish patients had been prescribed neuroleptics by their general practitioners while the Indian and Chinese patients had been virtually untreated. In all three settings the outcomes of these interesting samples (which presumably approximate the 'natural' history of the disorder) were heterogeneous but, except for a larger proportion of Chinese patients having marked psychotic symptoms, they did not differ much from the outcomes in the treated groups. In a historical study of 70 Swedish patients with first admissions in 1925, lifetime records were retrieved and re-diagnosed in accordance with DSM-III.[9] None of these patients had received neuroleptics. The final outcome was rated as good in 33 per cent (but no patient was considered as completely recovered), as 'profoundly deteriorated' in 43 per cent, and as intermediate in 24 per cent.

A long-term perspective on the course of schizophrenia ove successive generations is provided by a meta-analysis of 320 outcome studies on schizophrenia or dementia praecox published between 1895 and 1992 and including a total of 51 800 subjects.[10]

Overall, about 40 per cent of the patients were reported as improved after an average length of follow-up 5.6 years. There was a significant increase in the rate of improvement during the period 1956–1985 compared to 1895–1955, clearly related to the introduction of neuroleptic treatment, but a secular trend towards better outcomes with every successive decade had been present for much longer. Coupled with the virtual disappearance of the most malignant or 'catastrophic' forms of schizophrenia resulting in a profound defect state after a first psychotic episode, or death ('lethal catatonia'), these observations suggest that a transition to a less deteriorating course of the disorder had occurred prior to modern pharmacological treatment. Among the factors explaining this shift one should consider improvements in general care, progressive changes in attitudes and hospital regime which occurred in a number of institutions on both sides of the Atlantic in the 1930s and 1940s, as well as heightened expectations that psychosocial measures such as psychotherapy or rehabilitation could result in a cure in some cases.

Long-term prognosis

Results of course and outcome studies published over the last six decades are shown in Table 4.3.7.1. The studies have been selected on the basis of the length of follow-up (>5 years), effective sample size (>50), and intensity of follow-up and assessment to provide a global overview of the long-term course of schizophrenia.

Although the studies differ in their design (prospective, follow-back, or retrospective), their results have much in common.

Manfred Bleuler's monograph[11] is the account of an intensive study of 208 patients first admitted in 1942–1943 and personally followed up by the author for 22 years or until death. A recent re-interpretation of Bleuler's diagnoses in terms of DSM-IIIR, DSM-IV, and ICD-10 diagnostic criteria concluded that although some 30 per cent of the original cases would today meet criteria for schizoaffective disorder, the distribution of the types of long-term course did not change significantly.[12] Another 23-year follow-up of 504 patients admitted in 1945–1959 has been completed by Ciompi,[14] and Huber *et al.*[15] interviewed 289 surviving patients in Switzerland first admitted between 1900 and 1962 (median follow-up length 36.9 years).

Notwithstanding methodological constraints which apply to these studies, their findings are a unique record of what probably represents the closest approximation to the 'natural history' of schizophrenia. In summary, they indicate the following.

- Lasting recovery ('complete cure') occurred in 15 per cent to 26 per cent of the cases; 43 per cent had either remitted or exhibited mild residual abnormalities which did not interfere with their living in the community.
- Forty-four per cent were still in hospital and severe chronic states had developed in 14 to 24 per cent.

Table 4.3.7.1 Results of selected course and outcome studies in schizophrenia, 1972–2005

Author	Country	Sample size	Length of follow-up (years)	Proportion good outcome*
Bleuler (1972)[11]	Switzerland	208	23	20% Complete remission; 33% mild defect
Tsuang *et al.* (1979)[13]	USA	186	35	46% Recovered or improved significantly
Ciompi (1980)[14]	Switzerland	289	37	20% Recovered; 43% definitely improved
Huber *et al.* (1980)[15]	Germany	502	22	26% Recovered; 31% remission with mild defect
Harding *et al.* (1987)[16]	USA	118	32	62% Recovered or improved significantly
Ogawa *et al.* (1987)[17]	Japan	140	21–27	31% Recovered; 46% improved
Shepherd *et al.* (1989)[18]	UK	107	5	22% Recovered, no relapse
Johnstone *et al.* (1990)[19]	UK	530	3–13	14% Excellent; 18.5% very good social adjustment
Carone *et al.* (1991)[20]	USA	79	5	17% Complete remission
Marneros *et al.* (1992)[21]	Germany	249	25	Full remission in 24% ('broad') or 7% ('pure') schizophrenia
Thara *et al.* (1994)[22]	India	90 (first-onset cases)	10	12% Complete recovery; 62% remission
Mason *et al.* (1995)[23]	UK	67	13	17% Complete recovery; 52% remission
Wieselgren and Lindström (1996)[24]	Sweden	120	5	30% Good outcome
Wiersma *et al.* (1998)[25]	Holland	82	15	27% Complete; 50% partial remission
Ganev *et al.* (1998)[26]	Bulgaria	60	16	32% Complete; 5% partial remission
Gureje and Bamidele (1999)[27]	Nigeria	120	13	22% Unimpaired (social outcome); 19% some impairment
Finnerty *et al.* (2002)[28]	Ireland	67 (first-onset cases)	15	35% Complete remission; 46% partial remission
Thara (2004)[29]	India	90 (first-onset cases)	20	6% Complete recovery; 15% clinically stable
Lauronen *et al.* (2005)[30]	Finland	91 (birth cohort members)	To age 31 years	4% Complete recovery; 3% partial remission

*Descriptive categories used by the authors.

- In 50 per cent to 75 per cent of the patients, a clinically stable state set in after the fifth year since onset, with no significant further deterioration.
- Remitting course with multiple episodes and full remissions characterized 22 per cent of the patients; catastrophic course (rapid onset of chronic deterioration) was observed in 1 per cent to 4 per cent.
- The 20-year suicide rate was 14 per cent to 22 per cent.

Two American studies largely concur with these findings. In the Vermont study,[16] no less than 62 per cent of the cohort had achieved significant improvement or recovery after an average length of follow-up 32 years; the corresponding proportion in the Iowa 500 study[13] was 46 per cent.

The most striking finding from the long-term follow-up studies is the high proportion of patients who recover, either completely or with mild residual abnormalities, after decades of severe illness[31] This contrasts with the ingrained image of schizophrenia as an intractable, deteriorating illness that many clinicians tend to adopt on the basis of a limited follow-up horizon and patient samples selected for unfavourable course and treatment response. It is unlikely that the high percentage of recoveries in the long-term studies could be explained by cases of affective illness or brief transient psychoses misdiagnosed as schizophrenia (the retrospective re-diagnosis of cases according to DSM-III criteria in the American studies did not alter significantly the results). Similarly unlikely would be the attribution of all the good outcomes to the antipsychotic treatment many of these patients received in the later stages of their illnesses, since comparable proportions of improvement of recovery had been reported for patients who never received neuroleptics.[32] A tentative conclusion from such follow-up research would be that schizophrenia is not an invariably chronic deteriorating disorder, and that the progression of the disease can be arrested or even reversed at any stage. The causes of such reversibility remain poorly understood, but research focusing specifically on the recovering cases will undoubtedly provide essential clues for understanding the nature of schizophrenia.

The results of longitudinal studies published in the last decade generally tend to corroborate the pattern of outcomes outlined by the earlier studies. However, several recent studies suggest a trend of worsening clinical and social outcomes in patients with schizophrenia in both developed countries[28,30] and developing countries.[27,29] A 13-year follow-up of 120 Nigerian patients[27] reported much higher rates of severe impairment in social and occupational functioning than those found in the same region of the country by follow-up studies in the 1970–1980s.

Patterns and stages of the course of schizophrenia

The marked heterogeneity of the course of schizophrenia can be reduced to a limited number of patterns into which cases tend to cluster over time. In earlier long-term follow-up studies, eight different categories of course have been described by Bleuler[11] and by Ciompi,[14] and 12 by Huber *et al.*[15] These classifications were derived from empirical observation, rather than statistical modelling, and conflated into single categories the mode of onset, longitudinal aspects such as frequency and duration of psychotic episodes, remissions, and end states. Treating these various aspects of the longitudinal profile of the illness as independent dimensions has been recommended.[19] However, the complexity of statistical modelling of the course of schizophrenia is such that the development of a classification of course that would be both useful in clinical practice and rigorous in a statistical sense may not be easy to achieve. Therefore, a heuristic compromise between these two requirements should, as a minimum, define operationally and assess separately: (i) the number and duration of discrete episodes of illness; (ii) the predominant clinical features of each episode (e.g. psychotic or affective); (iii) the number and length of remissions and their quality (presence/absence of residual negative or deficit symptoms and signs). By combining these variables, several patterns of course have been derived that have found good empirical support in international follow-up studies:

1. single psychotic episode followed by complete remission;
2. single psychotic episode followed by incomplete remission;
3. two or more psychotic episodes, with complete remissions between episodes;
4. two or more psychotic episodes, with incomplete remissions between episodes;
5. continuous (unremitting) psychotic illness.

With some modifications, these longitudinal patterns have been incorporated into ICD-10 and DSM-IV as additional descriptors.

Although the components of the course patterns, such as episode, remission, residual symptomatology, etc. may not represent 'pure' dimensions, it is desirable to restrict the definition of **pattern of course** to clinical variables only, in order to be able to examine its correlations with risk factors and predictors, such as premorbid impairments, mode of onset, or social outcomes. Assessing social functioning independently of the clinical pattern of course is critical to the study of illness-environment interactions and the causes of disablement in schizophrenia.

At present it does not seem possible to define with any precision **discrete stages** in the progression of schizophrenic illnesses by using combined clinical and pathological criteria, as in cancer or cardiovascular disease. Nevertheless, a 'softer' form of staging is feasible since there is on the whole a good agreement between the results of different studies on the general pattern of course in schizophrenia. On the basis of long-term follow-up studies, the lifetime course of schizophrenia can be articulated into a premorbid phase (from birth to the onset of psychosis), a phase of acute or positive schizophrenic symptomatology, and a residual phase.[21] Various sub-stages have been proposed to describe in finer detail the pre-onset and early psychosis period.[33,34] For most practical and research purposes, a three-stage classification of **post-onset course** has been proposed:[24]

1. an early deteriorating phase (the first 5–10 years);
2. a middle (stabilization) phase;
3. a gradual improvement phase.

This model agrees well with the empirical evidence and could be useful in the collection and summarizing of data on individual risks and prognosis.

Geographical and cultural variation

Three prospective investigations initiated by the World Health Organization (WHO): the **International Pilot Study on**

Table 4.3.7.2 Two-year course and outcome features of 1070 patients with schizophrenia in the WHO 10-country study(37)

Course and outcome descriptor	% Patients in developing countries[1] (n = 467)	% Patients in developed countries[2] (n = 603)
Remitting, complete remissions	62.7	36.8
Continuous or episodic, no complete remission	35.7	60.9
Psychotic <5% of the follow-up	18.4	18.7
Psychotic >75% of the follow-up	15.1	20.2
No complete remission during follow-up	24.1	57.2
Complete remission for >75% of the follow-up	38.3	22.3
On antipsychotic medication >75% of the follow-up	15.9	60.8
No antipsychotic medication during follow-up	5.9	2.5
Hospitalized for >75% of follow-up	0.3	2.3
Never hospitalized during follow-up	55.5	8.1
Impaired social functioning throughout follow-up	15.7	41.6
Unimpaired social functioning >75% of follow-up	42.9	31.6

[1] Colombia, India, Nigeria.

[2] Czech Republic, Denmark, Ireland, Japan, Russia, United Kingdom, United States.

Table 4.3.7.3 Long-term (15- and 25-year) outcome in patient cohorts assessed in the International Study of Schizophrenia (ISoS)

Outcome variable	Incidence cohorts (N = 1171, including 15-year follow-up of the WHO 10-country cohort)	Prevalence cohorts (N = 462, including 25-year follow-up of 373 cases from the WHO IPSS)
Recovered at follow-up (Bleuler's criteria)	48.1	53.5
Not psychotic in the past 2 years	42.8	40.8
GAF-S[1] > 60	54.0	56.7
Working most of past 2 years	56.8	73.9
GAF-D[2] > 60	50.7	60.3
SMR[3] (range)	0.00–5.71[4]	1.04–8.88[5]

[1] Global assessment of functioning—symptoms scale.

[2] Global assessment of functioning—disability scale.

[3] Standard mortality ratio.

[4] Rochester (0.00), Moscow (1.41), Chandigarh urban (1.88), Prague (2.53), Chandigarh rural (3.02), Honolulu (3.13), Nottingham (3.31), Dublin (4.10), Nagasaki (5.71).

[5] Sofia (1.04), Cali (1.31), Madras (1.90), Agra (1.86), Beijing (2.97), Prague IPSS (3.84), Mannheim (5.55), Hong Kong (5.76), Groningen (8.88).

Schizophrenia (IPSS);(35,36) the 10-country study on **Determinants of Outcome of Severe Mental Disorders**;(37) and the study on **Assessment and Reduction of Psychiatric Disability**(38,39) laid the ground for a broad-based, cross-cultural evaluation of the course and outcome of schizophrenia. These studies comprise extensive initial and follow-up information on a total of 2736 patients in 16 countries, diagnosed with schizophrenia according to strict and comparable criteria. Identical or closely similar, standardized assessment procedures and instruments were employed, ensuring a high level of comparability across the multiple sites. Results of the WHO 10-country study (pooled data on 1070 patients in all the research sites) are presented in Table 4.3.7.2.

A more recent, transcultural investigation coordinated by WHO, the **International Study of Schizophrenia** (ISoS) involving 18 research centres in 14 countries,(40,41) achieved tracing 75 per cent of cases assessed in the earlier WHO studies referred to above, as well as additional cohorts from mainland China, Hong Kong, and India. Follow-up data were collected on a total of 1633 cases (surviving or dead), and 890 patients were re-interviewed at either 15- or 25-year follow-up since their first assessment. Key findings from this landmark study are presented in Table 4.3.7.3.

The following general conclusions can be drawn from the WHO studies.

1 There is a striking heterogeneity and variability of the course and outcome of schizophrenia, both across and within populations. Patients with similar clinical and diagnostic characteristics at baseline assessment develop a spectrum of outcomes ranging from stable clinical and social recovery after a single psychotic episode to chronic unremitting psychosis and severe impairment. Long-term follow-up studies lend credibility to the conclusion that a high proportion (over 30 per cent) of patients meeting the diagnostic criteria for schizophrenia have relatively favourable outcomes.

2 The frequencies of both relapses and remissions tend to increase over time: while at 2-year follow-up of the International Pilot Study of Schizophrenia (IPSS)(35)11 per cent of the patients had experienced two or more psychotic episodes followed by complete remission, and another 18 per cent had two or more episodes followed by residual symptoms and impairments, the corresponding proportions at 5-year follow-up were 15 per cent and 33 per cent.(36) These trends are now bolstered by the findings of the International Study of Schizophrenia (ISoS)(40) which found a 48 per cent recovery rate at the 15-year follow-up and 54 per cent at the 25-year follow-up.

3 Regardless of the increasing relapse rate, the cumulative proportion of follow-up time during which patients have psychotic symptoms (as a percentage of the total follow-up time), tends to remain stable or decrease. At the end of the 5-year follow-up, 57 per cent of the patients had experienced a total of less than 9 months of active psychosis; only 22 per cent had been psychotic for 45–60 months. At 15-year and 25-year follow-up, 43 per cent and 41 per cent, respectively, have been free of active psychotic symptoms for the past 2 years.

4 The levels of social impairment assessed at 2 years changed very little during the subsequent years of follow-up. Overall, most of the observed change in the clinical state and social functioning of patients between the 2-year follow-up and the 5-year follow-up

was towards improvement rather than deterioration. This also is congruent with the findings at 15-year and 25-year follow-up.

5 While the percentage of patients with continuous, deteriorating illness was similar across the sites of the WHO studies, there were significant differences in the proportions of patients who achieved symptomatic and social recovery. In this respect, outcome was generally better in the developing countries. This unexpected finding of the first follow-up of the International Pilot Study of Schizophrenia patients,[35] who had been recruited from consecutive hospital admissions with the attendant possibilities of a selective bias, was subsequently replicated by the 10-country study which had an epidemiological design and recruited only first-contact patients from delimited populations.[37] The better course and outcome in the developing country areas could not be attributed to any particular subtype of the disorder, e.g. cases of acute onset, since it applied equally to the cases of slow, insidious onset. The main outcome difference across the study areas was in the occurrence and average length of symptom-free remissions. Remissions tended to be more frequent and to last longer in the developing countries. No single factor accounting for this difference could be identified and it is likely that complex interactions between illness and environment are involved that may include both population differences in **predisposing genes**,[42] and environmental or cultural factors, such as relative absence of an institutionalized role of 'the schizophrenic',[43] less intrafamilial **expressed emotion** towards the affected family member,[44] or better integration of the mentally ill person in the domestic economy in traditional rural communities. It should be noted, however, that the long-term WHO follow-up studies include patients whose onset of psychotic illness occurred decades ago, and that increasing social and economic stresses experienced by both rural and urban communities in many developing countries may have eroded the traditional support systems, resulting in worse outcomes, as suggested by several recent studies.

Whether the better outcome of schizophrenia in the developing countries is 'transportable' following migration to other settings, remains unclear. Data on immigrants treated for first episodes of schizophrenia in the United Kingdom suggest that while Asian patients have a lower relapse and readmission rate than British-born Whites, Afro-Caribbean's show a higher rate.[45] The marked social and family structure differences between the Asian and the Afro-Caribbean immigrant communities suggest that the likelihood of a more benign course in the new setting may depend on the degree to which the immigrant group has retained its traditional values and intra-group cohesion.

First episode psychosis

The recent focus on early detection and treatment of first episodes of psychosis, driven by theoretical considerations and clinical concerns, is supported by evidence suggesting that the course and outcome of the earliest stages of a schizophrenic illness may have a **pathoplastic effect** on its subsequent course. Specifically, the period between the first onset of psychotic symptoms and the initiation of treatment (**duration of untreated psychosis, DUP**) has been shown to correlate with increased time to remission and poor response to treatment.[46,47] Plausible clinical considerations have been proposed in support of the view that the first episode of psychosis represents a critical developmental transition that may impact the subsequent course of schizophrenia, possibly by inducing neurotoxic alterations in neural networks, thus preparing the ground for chronic illness.[48] An extension of this mode of thinking is the suggestion that a behavioural or pharmacological intervention prior to the onset of psychotic symptoms could delay or prevent the onset of schizophrenia.[49]

None of these hypotheses has been conclusively tested. However, a number of studies focusing on the **prodrome** and the earliest manifestations of psychosis have highlighted features such as a presymptomatic drop in cognitive performance and social functioning;[50] early co-occurrence of 'positive' and 'negative' symptoms;[37] as well as a general malleability of such dysfunction in response to appropriate behavioural interventions and low-dose, time-limited pharmacological treatment.[51–53] This suggests that clinical research bridging the gap between statistical investigations of risk factors or antecedents of disease and individual pathways to psychotic illness may have an important role to play in understanding and, ultimately, influencing the development and course of schizophrenia.

Prognosis of specific clinical symptoms and syndromes

Longitudinal studies suggest that the characteristic symptoms of schizophrenia tend to 'breed true', i.e. only a minority of patients are eventually reclassified into other disease categories because of a significant and lasting change in the predominant symptoms. However, the proportion of cases warranting a re-diagnosis seems to increase with the length of follow-up.

Depression in schizophrenia

In the WHO International Pilot Study of Schizophrenia,[35, 36] the proportion of patients with initial schizophrenic symptomatology who developed non-schizophrenic (mostly affective) episodes in the course of time increased from 3 per cent in the first 2 years to 17 per cent at the end of the 5-year follow-up. In contrast, subsequent episodes with schizophrenic features occurred in less than 10 per cent of the patients with an initial diagnosis of major depression. Depression is the most common non-schizophrenic syndrome co-ocurring with schizophrenia also in those patients who retain the essentially schizophrenic character of their illnesses. The proportion of patients who develop clear-cut episodes of major depression ranges from 15 per cent during a 5-year follow-up[54] to 24 per cent during a 12-year follow-up.[55] This is a much higher period prevalence than depression in the general population, which suggests that mood disorder may be an intrinsic part of the clinical spectrum of schizophrenia. Based on such data, a diagnostic rubric of **post-schizophrenic depression** has been added to the classification of schizophrenia in ICD-10.

First-rank (schneiderian) symptoms

Subjective thought disorder phenomena, such as thought broadcast or insertion, passivity ('replacement of will') experiences, and particular type of auditory hallucinations (third-person or commenting 'voices') were attributed 'first-rank' significance in the differential diagnosis between schizophrenic and affective psychoses by Kurt Schneider.[56] These symptoms are accorded special diagnostic weight in the current diagnostic criteria of both ICD-10 and DSM-IV. Although Schneider explicitly disclaimed any particular prognostic value for the first-rank symptoms, they have a strong tendency to recur in the course of schizophrenia. In the WHO 10-country study, patients with one or more first-rank symptoms on the initial examination had a three-fold increased risk of recurrence of such symptoms in subsequent episodes compared to patients with no first-rank symptoms at initial examination.[(37)]

Prognosis of schizophrenia subtypes

The evidence that each of the 'classic' subtypes of schizophrenia is associated with a characteristic pattern of course is generally weak but surprisingly good for some of the subtypes. Consistent differences have been reported between **paranoid**, **hebephrenic**, and **undifferentiated** schizophrenia (diagnosed according to DSM-III) on a long-term follow-up of 19 years.[(57)] Paranoid schizophrenia tended to have a remittent course, and to be associated with less disability, in contrast to hebephrenia which had an insidious onset and poor long-term prognosis. Undifferentiated schizophrenia occupied an intermediate position. In the WHO International Pilot Study of Schizophrenia,[(35)] four alternative groupings of the ICD-9 subtypes were tested by a discriminant function for differences with regard to six course and outcome measures. Clear discrimination was achieved between simple and hebephrenic schizophrenia grouped together, on the one hand, and the schizoaffective subtype on the other. However, the comparison of simple and hebephrenic schizophrenia with paranoid schizophrenia resulted in a considerable degree of overlap.

Better discrimination has been claimed for groups of patients diagnosed according to the criteria of Leonhard.[(58)] A 5–13 years follow-up study of 178 patients admitted with a diagnosis of schizophrenia and re-diagnosed according to the Leonhard's criteria as **systematic schizophrenia**, atypical (unsystematic) schizophrenia, **cycloid psychosis**, or **reactive psychosis**[(59)] resulted in marked outcome differences on blind assessment. While only 10 per cent of the cases in the two schizophrenia groups were judged to have 'recovered', the corresponding proportion in the cycloid and reactive psychoses group was 38 per cent. Conversely, the proportions of 'unimproved' cases were 49 per cent and 3 per cent.

The question whether good prognosis, remitting schizophrenia with an acute onset is a separate subtype that could be distinguished symptomatologically was addressed in the WHO 10-country study[(37)] by comparing 274 patients with an initial ICD-9 diagnosis of acute schizophrenic episode and 752 patients with other schizophrenia subtypes. The group of acute cases tended to be younger and had a lower male/female ratio, but was no different from the rest of the schizophrenic patients with regard to initial symptomatology. This argues against acute **schizophreniform** illness being a discrete syndrome, outside the clinical spectrum of schizophrenia.

The course and outcome data on **schizoaffective** disorders seem to support their placement within the broad category of schizophrenia. A retrospective and prospective study of 150 schizoaffective patients and 95 bipolar affective patients[(60)] established general similarities between the two groups but the schizoaffective cases were less likely to achieve a full remission and more likely to develop a residual state (in 57 per cent compared to 24 per cent in the bipolar group). An intermediate outcome between that of schizophrenia and bipolar affective disorder is a common finding in schizoaffective disorders.

Predictors of course and outcome

A wide range of variables have been explored as possible predictors of course and outcome in schizophrenia: (i) socio-demographic characteristics; (ii) features of the premorbid personality and premorbid functioning; (iii) family history of psychiatric disorder; (iv) history of past psychotic episodes and treatments; (v) substance use; (vi) characteristics of the onset; (vii) features of the initial clinical state and treatment response; and (viii) variables related to brain morphology and neurocognitive functioning. Many predictors have been independently replicated by different investigators and there is reasonable agreement on the general direction of their effects. However, definitions of both the independent (predictor) and the dependent (outcome) variable tend to vary across studies, and the statistical methods employed range from basic descriptive statistics (e.g. *x* per cent of the patients with characteristic *y* developed outcome *z*) to complex statistical models with capacity to quantify the independent contribution of individual variables to a specified outcome.

Table 4.3.7.4 lists the best predictors of the 2-year outcome in the WHO 10-country study[(37)] and Table 4.3.7.5 summarizes the findings about predictors of 15-year outcome for the subset of participants in the WHO 10-country study who were re-examined as part of the International Study of Schizophrenia.[(40)] Apart from the variable 'setting' (i.e. research centre), which is a proxy for an unspecified number of local area features ranging from population genetic background to the multiple facets of 'culture', the mode of onset of symptoms (acute versus insidious), drug abuse, and premorbid psychosocial functioning were the best predictors of the duration of psychotic episodes, achievement of remission, and social outcome at 2-year follow-up. Importantly, the total time with psychotic symptoms during the first 2 years post-onset emerged as the best predictor of 15-year outcome, highlighting the potential importance of interventions aiming to contain and minimize active psychosis during this critical stage.

Limitations of clinical prediction

The explanatory power of any predictor in schizophrenia (in terms of accounting for a proportion of the outcome variance) varies depending on sample size, setting, homogeneity of patient groups, and measurement error, but generally tends to be limited (rarely exceeding 30 per cent of the outcome variance). This suggests that no single background or premorbid characteristic of the person, and no clinical symptom or sign among the initial manifestations of the disorder, is strongly associated with its prognosis in the longer-term. Similarly to the genetic epidemiology of schizophrenia, where non-shared environmental influences account for a greater amount of variance than the shared environment, person-specific, emergent life events or changes in the mental state may have a similar or even greater impact on the outcome as the initial or premorbid predictors. Indeed, variables such as negative symptoms have been shown to gain in predictive power if they are assessed two or more years after the onset, or after the patients have received adequate treatment. The predictive capacity of other variables, for example, mode of onset, or a high index of expressed emotion, tends to become attenuated in the course of time. Thus, there is

Table 4.3.7.4 Best predictors of 2-year course and outcome in the WHO 10-country study (log-linear analysis of 1078 cases)

	Course and outcome variables			
Predictor	**Pattern of course**	**Time in psychosis**	**Remission/no remission**	**Social functioning**
Age	n.s.	n.s.	n.s.	*
Sex	*	*	**	**
Marital status	**	***	***	***
Acute versus gradual onset	***	***	***	***
Time since onset (duration of untreated psychosis)	n.s.	n.s.	**	***
First-rank symptoms at baseline	n.s.	n.s.	n.s.	n.s.
Adjustment in childhood	n.s.	n.s.	**	***
Adjustment in adolescence		***	***	***
Close friends	*	*	***	***
Street drug use	*	*	***	***
Setting (developing/ developed country)	***	n.s.	***	***

n.s., Not significant.
*Significant at $p \leq 0.05$.
**Significant at $p \leq 0.01$.
***Significant at $p \leq 0.001$.

Table 4.3.7.5 Best predictors of 15-year outcome in the WHO 10-country study (stepwise linear regression analysis of 766 cases included in ISoS)

	Course and outcome variables			
Predictor	**GAF-S[1] (centre in the analysis)**	**GAF-S (area variables in the analysis)**	**GAF-D[2] (centre in the analysis)**	**GAF-D (area variables in the analysis)**
Percentage of time psychotic (first 2 years)	*	*	*	*
Setting (centre)	*	–	*	–
Blunted affect at initial examination	–	*	–	*
National health insurance available	–	–	–	*
Street drug use	–	–	–	*
Family involvement in care	–	–	–	*

[1] Global assessment of functioning—symptoms scale.
[2] Global assessment of functioning—disability scale.
* Significant at $p \leq 0.05$.
– Not significant or not applicable.

no fixed set of predictors of the course and outcome of schizophrenia, but rather a number of prognostic indicators which allow a judgement to be made about the probability of one or another type of course over a limited time period (usually not exceeding 5 years).

Short-term predictors

There is good agreement between different studies on the factors that help predict a relapse of psychotic symptoms after a period of stabilization or remission. By and large, the best predictor of relapse in the short-term remains the withdrawal of antipsychotic medication, usually due to non-compliance.(61) Heavy cannabis use has been shown to be associated with an increased risk of relapse in a dose-response relationship.(62) Other factors, such as stressful **life events**(63) and **expressed emotion** (EE) within the family,(44) have attracted considerable interest, both as independent predictors and as modifiers of the effects of pharmacological treatment. A high expressed emotion index, assessing a key family member's emotional over-involvement with, and concomitant criticism of the patient, has been found to be a reliable short-term predictor of psychotic relapse. However a limitation of the method is that it is only applicable to situations of intensive daily interaction between a patient and a carer (typically a family member) which may not be the case for many people with schizophrenia living in hostels or marginal accommodation. Moreover, the cross-cultural validity of the expressed emotion index still remains to be established.(64)

Medium- and long-range predictors

In first-episode cases, male sex, single marital status, premorbid social withdrawal and insidious onset have been shown to be relatively robust predictors of a poor outcome in the short- to medium-term (2–5 years), while female sex, being married, having social contacts outside the home, and acute onset predict a relatively good outcome. No consistent findings have been reported for age at onset as a predictor, and the long-term follow-up studies do not lend support to the view that an early onset is always associated with a poor prognosis. Similarly, a history of psychotic illness (including schizophrenia) in a first-degree relative does not necessarily predict a worse prognosis. On the contrary, in some studies(65) patients with a high familial load were found on follow-up to have a better outcome than 'sporadic' cases with no psychotic illness among their first-degree relatives.

A consistent finding of many studies is that the clinical symptoms in either the early, or the advanced stages of schizophrenia, have limited capacity to predict future course and outcome. An exception is the modest predictive power of clear-cut negative symptoms appearing early in the course of the disorder, or when assessed under the conditions referred to above.

The **socio-cultural setting**, i.e. a developing country or a developed country, was found to be among the best predictors of 2-year and 5-year outcome in the WHO studies.(35,36) It remained a significant predictor of 15-year outcome in the International Study of Schizophrenia.[40] Exactly what factors may be underlying these marked cultural differences in the prognosis of schizophrenia remains an unresolved issue.

There is a growing interest in the predictive power of **neurocognitive functions**, such as verbal memory, working memory, processing speed, and sustained attention. Though positive results have been reported from a number of studies, the proportion of variance in outcome measures that could be explained by such factors varies from low 14 per cent[66] to as high as 60 per cent,[67] depending on sample selection, patients' age, and length of follow-up. Overall, there is increasing evidence that neurocognitive functioning at the early stages of a schizophrenic illness predicts significantly global psychosocial and occupational functioning in the medium-term. Neurocognition is therefore likely to be an increasingly important target for novel pharmacological and cognitive behavioural interventions in schizophrenia.

Recovery from schizophrenia

There is consistent evidence from longitudinal studies reviewed in this chapter that, notwithstanding the high risk of chronic disability, loss of developmental potential, and diminished quality of life associated with schizophrenia, there is a non-negligible proportion of people who meet the current diagnostic criteria for the disease but ultimately attain nearly complete recovery and a stable level of psychosocial functioning. The existence of a good outcome subgroup within schizophrenia has been known for a long time and the prevailing view is that it is not an artefact of misdiagnosis. Yet little focused research has been conducted to bring to light the characteristics and predictors of this clinical subpopulation. A retrospective study of 436 people diagnosed with schizophrenia in the United Kingdom[68] found that over a follow-up period of 6 years, 15.6 per cent had a single psychotic episode with complete remission. A 15-year prospective study of 145 patients in the United States[69] revealed that up to 25 per cent of DSM-III diagnosed schizophrenia patients had ceased on their own accord antipsychotic medication since the first 5 years of follow-up and the majority of them had remained symptom-free for the rest of follow-up. Common findings in these two studies were that the non-relapsing, high-functioning patients were characterized by a higher level of premorbid occupational achievement and social competence, were less likely to use street drugs,[68] had better insight and an internal 'locus of control'.[69] Further study of the implications of such indicators of better prognostic potential and internal resources should advance efforts to design management and treatment strategies reducing the disabling impact of the disorder.

Summary and conclusions

Studies conducted over many decades consistently demonstrate that schizophrenia presents a broad spectrum of possible outcomes and course patterns, ranging from complete or nearly complete recovery after acute episodes of psychosis to continuous, unremitting illness leading to progressive deterioration of cognitive performance and social functioning. Between these extremes, a substantial proportion of patients show an episodic course with relapses of psychotic symptoms and partial remissions during which affective and cognitive impairments become increasingly conspicuous and may progress to gross deficits. Although no less than one-third of all patients with schizophrenia have relatively benign outcomes, in the majority the illness still has a profound, lifelong impact on personal growth and development. The initial symptoms of the disorder are not strongly predictive of the pattern of course but the mode of onset (acute or insidious), the duration of illness prior to diagnosis and treatment, the presence or absence of comorbid substance use, as well as background variables such as premorbid adjustment (especially during adolescence), educational and occupational achievement, marital status, and availability of a supportive social network allow a reasonable accuracy of prediction in the short- to medium-term (2–5 years).

One of the most striking aspects of the longitudinal course of schizophrenia is the so-called 'terminal improvement'. A relatively high proportion of patients tend to improve substantially with ageing. What determines this long-term outcome is far from clear but the stereotype view of schizophrenia as an invariably progressive, deteriorating disorder does not accord well with the evidence. Similarly, a model of schizophrenia as a static **neurodevelopmental encephalopathy** decompensating post-adolescence under the influence of a variety of stressors fits only part of the spectrum of course patterns. In a significant proportion of cases, the disorder exhibits the unmistakable features of a shift-like process with acute exacerbations and remissions which may progress to severe deterioration or come to a standstill at any stage. Whether a single underlying pathophysiology can explain the variety of clinical outcomes, or several different pathological processes are at work, remains obscure. It has been suggested that the longitudinal course of schizophrenia should be seen as an open-ended, dynamic life process with multiple, interacting biological and psychosocial determinants. Obviously, such issues cannot be resolved by clinical follow-up studies alone, and require a strong involvement of neurobiological research in prospective investigations of representative samples of cases spanning the entire spectrum of course and outcomes. No such studies have been possible until recently, both because of the technical complexity of such an undertaking and because of the tendency to selectively recruit for biological investigations patients from the severe, deteriorating part of the spectrum. Overcoming such limitations will be essential to the uncovering of the mechanisms driving the 'natural history' of schizophrenia.

Further information

Hopper, K., Harrison, G., Janca, A., *et al.* (eds.) (2007). *Recovery from schizophrenia. An international perspective. A report from the WHO collaborative project the international study of schizophrenia.* Oxford University Press, New York.

References

1. Kraepelin, E. (1919). *Dementia praecox and paraphrenia.* Livingstone, Edinburgh.
2. van Os, J., Wright, P., and Murray, R.M. (1997). Follow-up studies of schizophrenia I: natural history and non-psychopathological predictors of outcome. *European Psychiatry*, **12**(Suppl. 5),327s–41s.
3. Olesen, A.V. and Mortensen, P.B. (2002). Readmission risk in schizophrenia: selection explains previous findings of a progressive course of disorder. *Psychological Medicine*, **32**, 1301–7.

4. Bebbington, P.E., Craig, T., Garety, P., *et al.* (2006). Remission and relapse in psychosis: operational definitions based on case-note data. *Psychological Medicine*, **36**, 1551–62.
5. Nuechterlein, K.H., Miklowitz, D.J., Ventura, J., *et al.* (2006). Classifying episodes in schizophrenia and bipolar disorder: criteria for relapse and remission applied to recent-onset samples. *Psychiatry Research*, **15**, 153–66.
6. Geddes, J.R. and Kendell, R.E. (1995). Schizophrenic subjects with no history of admission to hospital. *Psychological Medicine*, **25**, 859–68.
7. Padmavathi, R., Rajkumar, S., and Srinivasan, T.N. (1998). Schizophrenic patients who were never treated—a study in an Indian urban community. *Psychological Medicine*, **28**, 1113–17.
8. Ran, M., Xiang, M., Huang, M., *et al.* (2001). Natural course of schizophrenia: 2-year follow-up study in a rural Chinese community. *The British Journal of Psychiatry*, **178**, 154–8.
9. Jonsson, S.A.T. and Jonsson, H. (1992). Outcome in untreated schizophrenia: a search for symptoms and traits with prognostic meaning in patients admitted to a mental hospital in the preneuroleptic era. *Acta Psychiatrica Scandinavica*, **85**, 313–20.
10. Hegarty, J.D., Baldessarini, R.J., Tohen, M., *et al.* (1994). One hundred years of schizophrenia: a meta-analysis of the outcome literature. *The American Journal of Psychiatry*, **151**, 1409–16.
11. Bleuler, M. (1972). Die schizophrenen Geistesstörungen im Lichte langjähriger Kranken- und Familiengeschichten. G. Thieme, Stuttgart. English translation by S.M. Clemens (1978) The schizophrenic disorders. Long-term patient and family studies. Yale University Press, New Haven.
12. Modestin, J., Huber, A., Satirli, E., *et al.* (2003). Long-term course of schizophrenic illness: Bleuler's study reconsidered. *The American Journal of Psychiatry*, **160**, 2202–8.
13. Tsuang, M., Woolson, R., and Fleming, J. (1979). Long-term outcome of major psychoses. I. Schizophrenia and affective disorders compared with psychiatrically symptom-free surgical conditions. *Archives of General Psychiatry*, **36**, 1295–301.
14. Ciompi, L. (1980). Catamnestic long-term study on the course of life and aging of schizophrenics. *Schizophrenia Bulletin*, **6**, 606–18.
15. Huber, G., Gross, G., Schüttler, R., *et al.* (1980). Longitudinal studies of schizophrenic patients. *Schizophrenia Bulletin*, **6**, 592–605.
16. Harding, C., Brooks, G.W., Ashikara, T., *et al.* (1987). The Vermont longitudinal study of persons with severe mental illness. I. Methodology, study sample, and overall status 32 years later. *The American Journal of Psychiatry*, **144**, 718–26.
17. Ogawa, K., Miya, M., Watarai, A., *et al.* (1987). A long-term follow-up study of schizophrenia in Japan—with special reference to the course of social adjustment. *The British Journal of Psychiatry*, **151**, 758–65.
18. Shepherd, M., Watt, D., Falloon, I., *et al.* (1989). The natural history of schizophrenia: a five-year follow-up study of outcome and prediction in a representative sample of schizophrenics. *Psychological Medicine*, Monograph Supplement 15, 1–46, Cambridge University Press.
19. Johnstone, E.C., Macmillan, J.F., Frith, C.D., *et al.* (1990). Further investigation of the predictors of outcome following first schizophrenic episodes. *The British Journal of Psychiatry*, **157**, 182–9.
20. Carone, B.J., Harrow, M., and Westermeyer, J.F. (1991). Posthospital course and outcome in schizophrenia. *Archives of General Psychiatry*, **48**, 247–53.
21. Marneros, A., Deister, A., and Rohde, A. (1992). Comparison of long-term outcome of schizophrenic, affective and schizoaffective disorders. *The British Journal of Psychiatry*, **161**(Suppl. 18), 44–51.
22. Thara, R., Henrietta, M., Joseph, A., *et al.* (1994). Ten-year course of schizophrenia—the Madras longitudinal study. *Acta Psychiatrica Scandinavica*, **90**, 329–36.
23. Mason, P., Harrison, G., Glazebrook, C., *et al.* (1995). Characteristics of outcome in schizophrenia at 13 years. *The British Journal of Psychiatry*, **167**, 596–603.
24. Wieselgren, I.M. and Lindström, L.H. (1996). A prospective 1-5 year outcome study in first-admitted and readmitted schizophrenic patients: relationship to heredity, premorbid adjustment, duration of disease and education level at index admission and neuroleptic treatment. *Acta Psychiatrica Scandinavica*, **93**, 9–19.
25. Wiersma, D., Nienhuis, F.J., Sloof, C.J., *et al.* (1998). Natural course of schizophrenic disorders: a 15-year follow-up of a Dutch incidence cohort. *Schizophrenia Bulletin*, **24**, 75–85.
26. Ganev, K., Onchev, G., and Ivanov, P. (1998). A 16-year follow-up study of schizophrenia and related disorders in Sofia, Bulgaria. *Acta Psychiatrica Scandinavica*, **98**, 200–7.
27. Gureje, O. and Bamidele, R. (1999). Thirteen-year social outcome among Nigerian outpatients with schizophrenia. *Social Psychiatry and Psychiatric Epidemiology*, **34**, 147–51.
28. Finnerty, A., Keogh, F., O'Grady-Walsh, A., *et al.* (2002). A 15-year follow-up of schizophrenia in Ireland. *Irish Journal of Psychological Medicine*, **19**, 108–14.
29. Thara, R. (2004). Twenty-year course of schizophrenia: the Madras longitudinal study. *Canadian Journal of Psychiatry*, **49**, 564–69.
30. Lauronen, E., Koskinen, J., Veijola, J., *et al.* (2005). Recovery from schizophrenic psychoses within the northern Finland 1966 birth cohort. *The Journal of Clinical Psychiatry*, **66**, 375–83.
31. Auslander, L.A. and Jeste, D.V. (2004). Sustained remission of schizophrenia among community-dwelling older outpatients. *The American Journal of Psychiatry*, **161**, 1490–3.
32. Harrow, M. and Jobe, T.H. (2007). Factors involved in outcome and recovery in schizophrenia patients not on antipsychotic medications: a 15-year multifollow-up study. *The Journal of Nervous and Mental Disease*, **195**, 406–14.
33. Häfner, H., Maurer, K., Löffler, W., *et al.* (2003). Modeling the early course of schizophrenia. *Schizophrenia Bulletin*, **29**, 325–40.
34. McGorry, P.D., Hickie, I.B., Yung, A.R., *et al.* (2006). Clinical staging of psychiatric disorders: a heuristic framework for choosing earlier, safer and more effective interventions. *The Australian and New Zealand Journal of Psychiatry*, **40**, 616–22.
35. World Health Organization. (1979). *Schizophrenia. An international follow-up study*. Wiley, Chichester.
36. Leff, J., Sartorius, N., Jablensky, A., *et al.* (1992). The international pilot study of schizophrenia: five-year follow-up findings. *Psychological Medicine*, **22**, 131–45.
37. Jablensky, A., Sartorius, N., Ernberg, G., *et al.* (1992). Schizophrenia: manifestations, incidence and course in different cultures. A World Health Organization ten-country study. *Psychological Medicine* Monograph Supplement 20, Cambridge University Press, Cambridge.
38. Jablensky, A., Schwarz, R., and Tomov,T. (1980). WHO collaborative study of impairments and disabilities associated with schizophrenic disorders. *Acta Psychiatrica Scandinavica*, (Suppl. 285), **62**, 152–63.
39. Wiersma, D., Nienhuis, F.J., Giel, R., *et al.* (1996). Assessment of the need for care 15 years alter onset of a Dutch cohort of schizophrenic patients and an international comparison. *Social Psychiatry and Psychiatric Epidemiology*, **31**, 114–21.
40. Harrison, G., Hopper, K., Craig, T., *et al.* (2001). Recovery from psychotic illness: a 15- and 25-year international follow-up study. *The British Journal of Psychiatry*, **178**, 506–17.
41. Hopper, K., Harrison, G., Janca, A., *et al.* (eds.) (2007). *Recovery from schizophrenia. An international perspective. A report from the WHO collaborative project the international study of schizophrenia.* Oxford University Press, New York.
42. Freedman, M.L., Reich, D., Penney, K.L., *et al.* (2004). Assessing the impact of population stratification on genetic association studies. *Nature Genetics*, **36**, 388–93.
43. Waxler, N.E. (1979). Is the outcome for schizophrenia better in non-industrial societies? The case of Sri Lanka. *The Journal of Nervous and Mental Disease*, **167**, 144–58.
44. Leff, J.P., Wig, N.N., Bedi, H., *et al.* (1990) Relatives' expressed emotion and the course of schizophrenia in Chandigarh: a two-year follow-up of a first-contact sample. *The British Journal of Psychiatry*, **156**, 351–6.

45. Bhugra, D., Leff, J., Mallett, R., *et al.* (1997). Incidence and outcome of schizophrenia in Whites, African-Caribbeans and Asians in London. *Psychological Medicine*, **27**, 791–8.
46. Perkins, D., Gu, H., Boteva, K., *et al.* (2005). Relationship between duration of untreated psychosis and outcome in first-episode schizophrenia: a critical review and meta-analysis. *The American Journal of Psychiatry*, **162**, 1785–804.
47. Marshall, M., Lewis, S., Lockwood, A., *et al.* (2005). Association between duration of untreated psychosis and outcome in cohorts of first-episode patients: a systematic review. *Archives of General Psychiatry*, **62**, 975–83.
48. Lieberman, J.A. (1999). Is schizophrenia a neurodegenerative disorder? A clinical and neurobiological perspective. *Biological Psychiatry*, **46**, 729–39.
49. McGlashan, T.H. and Johannessen, J.O. (1996). Early detection and interbention with schizophrenia: rationale. *Schizophrenia Bulletin*, **22**, 201–22.
50. Johnstone, E.C., Ebmeier, K.P., Miller, P., *et al.* (2005). Predicting schizophrenia: findings from the Edinburgh High-Risk Study. *The British Journal of Psychiatry*, **186**, 18–25.
51. Szymanski, S.R., Cannon, T.D., Gallacher, F., *et al.* (1996). Course and treatment response in first-episode and chronic schizophreni a. *The American Journal of Psychiatry*, **153**, 519–25.
52. McGorry, P.D., Edwards, J., Mihalopoulos, C., *et al.* (1996). EPPIC: an evolving system of early detection and optimal management. *Schizophrenia Bulletin*, **22**, 305–26.
53. Menezes, N.M., Arenovich, T., and Zipursky, R.B. (2006). A systematic review of longitudinal outcome studies of first-episode psychosis. *Psychological Medicine*, **36**, 1349–62.
54. Sheldrick, C., Jablensky, A., Sartorius, N., *et al.* (1977). Schizophrenia succeeded by affective illness: catamnestic study and statistical enquiry. *Psychological Medicine*, **7**, 619–24.
55. Breier, A., Schreiber, J.L., Dyer, J., *et al.* (1991). National Institute of Mental Health longitudinal study of chronic schizophrenia. *Archives of General Psychiatry*, **48**, 239–46.
56. Schneider, K. (1959). *Clinical psychopathology* (trans. M.W. Hamilton). Grune & Stratton, New York.
57. Fenton, W.S. and McGlashan, T.H. (1991). Natural history of schizophrenia subtypes. I. Longitudinal study of paranoid, hebephrenic, and undifferentiated schizophrenia. *Archives of General Psychiatry*, **48**, 969–77.
58. Leonhard, K. (1999). *Classification of endogenous psychoses and their differentiated etiology* (2nd revised and enlarged edn). Springer, Wien, New York.
59. Stephens, J.H. and Astrup, C. (1963). Prognosis in 'process' and 'non-process' schizophrenia. *The American Journal of Psychiatry*, **119**, 945–53.
60. Angst, J., Felder, W., and Lohmeyer, B. (1980). Course of schizoaffective psychoses: results of a follow-up study. *Schizophrenia Bulletin*, **6**, 579–85.
61. Dencker, S.J., Malm, U., and Lepp, M. (1986). Schizophrenic relapse after drug withdrawal is predictable. *Acta Psychiatrica Scandinavica*, **73**, 181–5.
62. Linszen, D.H., Dingemans, P.M., and Lenior, M.E. (1994). Cannabis abuse and the course of recent-onset schizophrenic disorders. *Archives of General Psychiatry*, **51**, 273–9.
63. Brown, G.W. and Birley, J.L.T. (1968). Crises and life changes and the onset of schizophrenia. *Journal of Health and Social Behaviour*, **9**, 203–14.
64. López, S.R., Hipke, K.N., Polo, A.J., *et al.* (2004). Ethnicity, expressed emotion, attributions, and course of schizophrenia: family warmth matters. *Journal of Abnormal Psychology*, **113**, 428–39.
65. Johnstone, E.C., Macmillan, J.F., Frith, C.D., *et al.* (1990). Further investigation of the predictors of outcome following first schizophrenic episodes. *The British Journal of Psychiatry*, **157**, 182–9.
66. Milev, P., Ho, B.C., Arndt, S., *et al.* (2005). Predictive values of neurocognition and negative symptoms on functional outcome in schizophrenia: a longitudinal first-episode study with 7-year follow-up. *The American Journal of Psychiatry*, **162**, 495–506.
67. Evans, J.D., Heaton, R.K., Paulsen, J.S., *et al.* (2003). The relationship of neuropsychological abilities to specific domains of functional capacity in older schizophrenia patients. *Biological Psychiatry*, **53**, 422–30.
68. Rosen, K. and Garety, P. (2005). Predicting recovery from schizophrenia: a retrospective comparison of characteristics at onset of people with single and multiple episodes. *Schizophrenia Bulletin*, **31**, 1–16.
69. Harrow, M. and Jobe, T.H. (2007). Factors involved in outcome and recovery in schizophrenia patients not on antipsychotic medications: a 15-year multifollow-up study. *The Journal of Nervous and Mental Disease*, **195**, 406–14.

4.3.8 Treatment and management of schizophrenia

D. G. Cunningham Owens and E. C. Johnstone

Introduction

Historically, there was no shortage of interventions to 'treat' insanity, and later, schizophrenia. Most were palliative, barely effective and often barbaric. It was only with the development of antipsychotic drugs and evolution of trial methodology in the 1950s that a new era of care arrived.

With chronic or recurrent psychiatric disorders, 'treatment' and 'management' are not strictly synonymous. The former has a narrow, patient-specific and largely *symptom* focus, comprising traditional medical tools, especially medications, while the latter can be defined as encompassing a broader range of targets with techniques less specifically part of traditional 'medical' repertoires, including psychological, social, and behavioural interventions. In both its 'treatment' and 'management' aspects, schizophrenia has undergone a concerted therapeutic assault in the past few years but rather than introducing clarity into care, the recent literature might indicate that certainties which seemed so recently within our grasp, remain elusive.

Evidence-based medicine (EBM) has had a major impact on care recommendations for those suffering from schizophrenia. A number of national and international 'guidelines' have been published[1–3] and the Cochrane database provides reviews on a range of relevant issues. This move has been important in smoothing out variability in patient care but although influential and increasingly endorsed, the trend is not beyond criticism. Guidelines are largely derived from *efficacy* data, which may translate awkwardly to real-life *effectiveness*, while considering solely the 'bottom lines' of trials masks the qualitative problems inherent to design, execution, and analysis. Furthermore, over-adherence to guidelines diminishes the impact that *individual variability* within the patient pool makes to optimizing treatment choices while deskilling those charged with care of a complex condition where 'quality' requires greater skill than is usually credited to those who do it well.

Thus, while evidence-based guidelines can offer a *framework* for good care practices, they are *not* a substitute for a broad range of expertise in *individualized* care planning.

Evidence for efficacy

Drug treatment

Schizophrenia comprises a number of domains of disability that form useful targets for drug treatment. These include:

- 'positive' features
- 'negative' features
- cognitive ability
- affective symptomatology
- general behaviour

In addition, comprehensive treatment planning requires awareness of efficacy in:

- maintenance and
- treatment resistance

(a) 'Positive' features

In providing a scientific basis for the use of antipsychotic drugs in 'acute' schizophrenia, the NIMH/VA Collaborative Study comparing the efficacy of three phenothiazines of differing chemical type (chlorpromazine, thioridazine, trifluoperazine) cannot be bettered.[4] Although its conclusions referred specifically to *phenothiazines*, subsequent research justifies the generalization of its findings to 'antipsychotics', making this elegant study relevant still.

Five main points emerged:

1 *Antipsychotics produce a significantly greater improvement in patients with acute schizophrenic symptomatology than placebo.* This action on the positive (or 'acute') symptomatology is the *primary class action* and is beyond doubt. Reviewing the first two decades of antipsychotic use, Davis and Garver[5] found that in 86 per cent of controlled studies chlorpromazine was superior to placebo and that *all* 26 trials utilizing more than 500 mg/day reported definitely greater benefit than placebo. In this dose range *no* trials found only marginal benefits. A similar view can be drawn regarding the efficacy of licensed second-generation antipsychotics.

LEARNING POINT: The antipsychotic effect of antipsychotic drugs (or the magnitude of that effect) is *not* shared by other types of psychotropic agent such as sedatives, is not in need of further replication, and forms a valid basis for classification.

2 *Antipsychotics of (three) different chemical types do not differ in efficacy.* The conclusion that all antipsychotics have comparable 'acute' efficacy is *not* to say that clinically there is nothing to choose between them. Although sharing a primary class action, antipsychotics encompass diverse pharmacologies that in practice can overshadow the action they share in common. There are therefore many ways of viewing class members apart from the traditional subgrouping by chemical structure—e.g. clinical adverse effect profile, subdivided into *general* or *extrapyramidal* tolerability; pharmacodynamically in terms of potency, receptor-binding profile or binding characteristics ('loose' or 'tight'), etc. This is a large 'extended' family!

Table 4.3.8.1 Antipsychotic and placebo response rates in schizophrenia

	Antipsychotic	Placebo	%
Very much improved	16	1	15
Much improved	29	11	18
Improved	16	10	6
Slightly improved	31	31	0
Not improved	6	15	
Worse	2	33	

Data from NIMH Collaborative Study.[4]

LEARNING POINT: In choosing an antipsychotic drug for 'acute' treatment, tolerability not efficacy, is the key consideration.

3 *A substantial proportion of patients show limited or no response to antipsychotic drugs.* Overall, 61 per cent of those on active drug were considered 'improved' to 'very much improved'.[4] It has usually been agreed that standard drugs produce a satisfactory response in approximately 60–70 per cent of patients with 'acute' schizophrenia, while approximately 6–8 per cent do not respond at all.[6] However, if one includes placebo response rates a less favourable picture emerges, suggesting that significant benefits could be more realistically expected in approximately 40 per cent of patients (Table 4.3.8.1).

Not all those non-responders could be classified as 'treatment resistant' (this concept, now operationally defined, long post-dated the Collaborative Study), but it does mean that in the mixture of first episode and relapsed patients presenting in routine practice, expectations for 'acute' (i.e. 'positive') symptom resolution must be *realistic* and cannot necessarily be improved by increasingly aggressive drug treatments alone.

LEARNING POINT: While providing a necessary foundation for clinical improvement to *acute* psychotic symptomatology, expectations of antipsychotic drugs on this single domain must be realistic. Treatment objectives should be correspondingly broad-based.

4 *A rapid phase (over the first week) of improvement is followed by a slower, more protracted pattern of improvement (over several weeks).* This finding has recently been replicated but with a somewhat different interpretation to that traditionally adopted. In a review of placebo-controlled studies, Agid *et al.*[7] also found that standardized ratings of positive symptomatology began to decline in the first week and improvement was significantly greater in the first 2 weeks of treatment than in the subsequent two. This was interpreted as rejecting the conventional view that antipsychotic onset is delayed. In an early clinical test of the dopamine hypothesis, Johnstone *et al.*[8] compared the two isomers of flupenthixol (flupentixol), one a dopamine blocker, the other not. They found that antipsychotic efficacy between the two groups, although evident in the first week, only became *significant* in the third week, often taken as supportive of the delayed onset hypothesis. A compromise between these two viewpoints comes from other data from this study, which showed that the first week of treatment

was also a time of significant improvement in non-specific symptomatology, especially anxiety, in those exposed to the antidopaminergic isomer.[9]

LEARNING POINT: While early improvement on antipsychotics may comprise a component of primary efficacy, such early benefits should be interpreted circumspectly in treatment planning, especially dose modifications, as they may reflect *mainly* non-specific changes.

5 *Patients in placebo arms of antipsychotic drugs trials can—and do—show improvements in positive symptomatology*. This is a standard finding in clinical trials often overlooked in routine practice. Non-specific benefits that can accrue from the environment where treatment is undertaken can contribute to maximizing outcomes.

LEARNING POINT: Drug effects have a context!

Despite their limitations, antipsychotics are unquestionably *the* key element in acute treatment. In a unique study, May *et al.* compared response rates and outcomes in a large group of schizophrenic patients randomly assigned to one of five regimes: individual psychotherapy, antipsychotics, individual psychotherapy plus antipsychotics, ECT, and 'milieu' therapy (ward environment). Patients who received physical treatments did better with increased rates of discharge, reduced lengths of stay, and decreased need for additional treatments.[10] Two years after discharge, twice as many of those treated with antipsychotics as with psychotherapy were in employment, while in the 3 years post-discharge, drug-treated patients spent less time back in hospital.[11]

(b) 'Negative' features

The issue of whether antipsychotics exert *efficacy* on negative schizophrenic features rose to prominence in the 1980s as a result of the implications of Crow's Type 1/Type 2 hypothesis.[12] The inference of this is that efficacy is 'unlikely' owing to different pathophysiological substrates proposed for 'positive' and 'negative' states. Controversy has persisted, with claims that whatever the case may be for first-generation drugs, new generation antipsychotics do possess this action. Recent reviews, however, have been increasingly circumspect.[13]

One consequences of testing Crow's proposal was that 'negative' schizophrenic symptomatology came to be viewed as something ratable *cross-sectionally*. This was a radical shift for traditionally the 'defect state' was conceptualized as a set of phenomena evident mainly from *longitudinal* appraisal, relating to complex behavioural *signs* such as psychosocial and occupational functioning. This switch assumed that the varied states that can underlie 'negative' presentations can be distinguished using cross-sectional clinical means alone. This assumption has never been validated and seems to push at the limits of clinical examination.

A major confound in assessing trial data in this field is the bradykinesia of drug-related parkinsonism, a common, pervasive feature in those exposed to antipsychotics yet one whose boundaries remain poorly defined, especially for its *subjective* components.[14] Changing to drugs or doses with lower extrapyramidal liability, or improving psychotic phenomena that may underlie social withdrawal is a therapeutic action of sorts, but hardly addresses the question. Likewise, utilizing elaborate statistics (e.g. path analysis) to support efficacy for second-generation antipsychotics ignores the fact that the problem is clinical attribution, not analysis.

Table 4.3.8.2 The classification of 'negative' states in schizophrenia

Primary	Authentic schizophrenic state

Secondary	Positive symptomatology
	Depressed mood
	Extrapyramidal disorder
	  Early dysphoria
	  Bradykinesia
	Psychosocial isolation

After Carpenter et al.[29]

Carpenter and colleagues[15] raised awareness of this issue by emphasizing the varied clinical states that can present 'negatively', thereby introducing a differential diagnosis (Table 4.3.8.2). Furthermore, by emphasizing 'durability' in their definition of 'deficit' syndrome,[16] they reintroduced a longitudinal component, aligning this more with the historical concept of schizophrenic negativity. Interestingly, this group found clozapine's benefits on negative features to be confined to patients who did *not* conform to criteria for 'deficit' state.[17]

One cannot help wondering whether the quest for antipsychotic 'therapy' of negative states has been a wild goose chase, predicated on assessment that was reliable—but lacking validity. This view will be controversial, as will our conclusion that Crow's hypothesis has *not* yet been disproven—that it remains to be shown that antipsychotics as a class exert any therapeutic benefits on primary negative schizophrenic symptomatology.

(c) Cognitive ability

The importance of cognitive deficits underlying the overt symptomatology of schizophrenia is being increasingly highlighted. They comprise a valid endophenotype in predisposed individuals, general cognition suffers a decline in the shift to florid illness and specific cognitive impairments, especially in executive function and memory, may relate to structural changes in specific brain areas.[18] The pharmacological question is whether drug treatments can enhance cognitive performance and thereby promote benefits in other domains.

Evaluation of cognitive actions of antipsychotics faces major methodological problems and findings remain contradictory. Standard antipsychotics initially impair aspects of attention and motor behaviour which improve following continued exposure, though working memory and long-term recall do not appear to be fundamentally affected.[19] Paced performance tests tend to be affected while those that are untimed tend to be insensitive, perhaps reflecting subtle motor effects.[20]

While new generation drugs may be associated with marginally less cognitive impairment than standard drugs, data are inadequate for firm conclusions.[21] In the absence of consistent evidence of differential effects on a range of neuropsychological tests, it has been suggested that measurements of 'social competence' may represent a more appropriate target for study.[22]

Furthermore, in studies evaluating cognitive-enhancing agents as 'add on' therapy no consistent evidence of utility has emerged.[21,23]

(d) Non-specific symptomatology

Affective symptomatology is prominent in schizophrenia but the efficacy of antipsychotics on such features has received little attention.

Their utility in the treatment of *anxiety* and other manifestations of 'arousal' in acute episodes of illness has not been systematically addressed and rests largely on clinical wisdom.

There is however, a tradition in Continental Europe of attributing *antidepressant* actions to low-dose antipsychotics[24,25] (e.g. flupentixol, sulpiride L-enantiomer, amisulpride) when they may exert preferential actions at presynaptic (autoreceptor) dopaminergic sites. Data remain inconclusive but it is unlikely that such an action would be clinically useful, as presynaptic selectivity is lost at doses usually required for antipsychotic efficacy.

Depression is a common feature of untreated schizophrenia and resolves as positive psychotic phenomena diminish.[26] This probably does not reflect an antidepressant action but symptom covariation. Of greater concern is what was formerly referred to as the 'depressogenic' action of antipsychotics.[27] This again raises the difficulty of distinguishing between similar presentations of pathophysiologically different states. Van Putten and May described a dysphoric mood state in antipsychotic-treated patients ('akinetic depression'),[28] which resolved following administration of anticholinergic. This was most likely a subjective manifestation of bradykinesia.

(e) Behaviour

Behaviour can be variously disturbed in schizophrenia, though is seldom considered other than as part of a global assessment. While certain confrontational behaviours such as hostility, belligerence, and resistiveness do improve with antipsychotics,[29] this is usually attributed to improvement in positive symptoms. There is, however, evidence that certain types of behavioural disorder correlate with negative, not positive, features and may represent a distinct domain of disorder.[30] It seems likely that certain manifestations of behavioural disorganization represent independent dimensions of pathology with their own, predominantly negative, prognostic implications.[31]

(f) Maintenance

With mood disorders, 'relapse' (exacerbation of an ongoing episode) and 'recurrence' (emergence of a new episode) are well-defined. In schizophrenia, where full remission of acute symptomatology may not be a realistic treatment goal, the distinction is less clear. As the long-term aim is usually minimizing the likelihood of florid exacerbation in a disorder characterized by persisting symptomatology, the term 'maintenance' is preferable to 'prophylaxis'.

The efficacy of antipsychotic drugs in long-term maintenance of schizophrenic illness is beyond doubt.[32] This applies to first-episode patients and to those who have suffered multiple episodes. Nonetheless, it remains difficult to quantify the effect as published figures vary widely. Reviewing relevant trials (covering variable follow-up intervals), Janicak *et al.* concluded that on average 55 per cent of those on placebo relapsed compared to 21 per cent on active medication, providing overwhelming statistical support for the maintenance effect.[32] In qualification, maintenance studies tend to be biased towards patients who have already shown a degree of response and it is likely that the magnitude of this effect, at least over 12–24 months, is less than trial-based analyses suggest.

A crucial question for clinicians is how long maintenance medication should be continued. The evidence is clear. Relapse rates have been shown to be similar following cessation in groups maintained well for differing lengths of time, from months to years.[33] Furthermore, no difference in relapse has been found in those who responded well compared to those whose response was less good.[34] The implication is that, no matter the *duration* or the *quality* of well-being on antipsychotic maintenance, relapse is *inevitable* following discontinuation in those with an established relapsing-remitting illness pattern (i.e. two or more episodes), which comprise the majority.

Not only is relapse a characteristic inherent to these illnesses, it seems so too is *time* to relapse. Davis *et al.* showed that placebo relapses plotted over a 2-year period occurred along an exponential line, indicating a constant *rate* of relapse, calculated from pooled data at a steady 11.5 per cent per month.[35]

Thus, the clinician's position is clear—for maintenance of well-being following second or subsequent acute episodes, 'long-term' antipsychotic maintenance means 'lifelong'. Should patients decide to discontinue, past experience can offer an invaluable tool in predicting when relapse is likely.

Some patients see long-term maintenance as 'well-being' only of sorts, in which quality-of-life is unacceptably impaired. In such individuals, *targeted intervention*, where treatment is focused on prodromal relapse symptomatology, has intuitive appeal. Alas, the trial evidence does not support this as a general strategy. No controlled studies so far have found advantage in targeted intervention and in a meta-analysis, Davis *et al.* calculated 25 per cent relapse rates in those continuously treated, rising to 50 per cent in the targeted group.[36] While carefully selected individuals, who can work with family and psychiatrists, may prefer this approach, a further potential concern is that intermittent exposure to antipsychotics may increase liability to tardive dyskinesia.[14]

Intermittent treatment is, of course, a feature of poor compliance (also known as 'adherence' or 'concordance'), itself perhaps *the* major contributor to relapse. In terms of major medical events, antipsychotics have a highly favourable risk:benefit ratio but in terms of medically trivial but unpleasant, intrusive adverse effects, the risk:benefit ratio is *unfavourable*, something often overlooked. Ensuring a maximally effective *and* tolerable maintenance regime is a joint exercise, from which the doctor cannot be excused.

The evidence that depot formulations enhance compliance is strong, if largely indirect. Support comes from 'mirror image' studies, where time in hospital is compared prior to and after starting depot. Six such studies were unanimous in showing substantial reductions in time spent in the hospital after switching to depot (average reduction: 77.8 per cent).[36] There is nothing to suggest that this reflects additional *therapeutic* advantage inherent to depots, whose benefit lies simply in facilitating regular administration and objective monitoring of compliance. Long-acting injectable risperidone (not a 'depot' in the traditional sense) has so far received favourable assessment[37] but it is too early to provide head-to-head comparative data with conventionally formulated depots. Dosages are also an important consideration in maintenance, as those compatible with maximizing long-term tolerability and well-being are likely to be considerably *lower* than those necessary for acute symptom control. However, the data are insufficiently clear to provide specific guidance. Kane *et al.* showed that relapse rates were significantly higher in patients receiving fluphenazine decanoate in a dose of 1.25 to 5 mg two weekly compared to those receiving 25 mg,[38] yet Baldessarini *et al.* have calculated that in long-term treatment, half-maximal effective doses (ED50) may be as low as one-fifth to one-tenth those normally employed.[39] In the absence of specifics, general principles must suffice. Kane and colleagues also showed that while relapse was more likely on low-dose regimes, neurological tolerability and psychosocial/quality-of-life parameters were superior.(38) Gradual pursuit of the minimal effective dose is all that can be recommended. Bearing in mind the exponential pattern of relapses, with a modal point at 3–5 months,(40) 'gradual' should equate to decrements at intervals of *months*, not weeks.

(g) Treatment resistance

The limitations of antipsychotic treatment in schizophrenia have been known since the 1960s but the concept of 'treatment resistance' only sprang to prominence with publication of the US multicentre clozapine study.(41) Within an operationally defined framework of 'resistance' (failure to respond to at least two antipsychotics of different chemical type administered in adequate dose for a minimum of 8 weeks), Kane *et al.* showed that 30 per cent of those on clozapine improved, while only 4 per cent on chlorpromazine/benztropine did likewise ($P < 0.001$).(41)

This has been interpreted as proving that clozapine possesses superior *efficacy* over standard agents. While this is one interpretation, it is not the only one. In this study, a chlorpromazine: clozapine dose equivalence of 2:1 was assumed, which might have disadvantaged chlorpromazine, allowing the interpretation that clozapine's advantage lies in its unique neurological *tolerability*. However, many other studies have confirmed clozapine's edge in patients who fail to respond satisfactorily to other antipsychotics and whatever the explanation, this is *real* added benefit. It does not mean however, that clozapine is a 'miracle' drug. While 30 per cent of such patients improving is welcome, the criteria for 'improvement' here were modest and subsequent review has failed to show substantial long-term benefits in higher level functioning, such as occupational ability.(42) Overall expectations of clozapine, a potentially difficult drug to administer, and for patients to tolerate, must be realistic.

Similar benefit has been claimed for other second-generation antipsychotics. However, there is *no* conclusive evidence that such advantages can be attributed to *any* other antipsychotic agent.

Management: psychological and psychosocial interventions

While nowadays, there is no suggestion that *the* core intervention in schizophrenia should be anything but medication, the limitations of medication alone in symptomatic, relapse prevention, and satisfaction/quality-of-life terms have long prompted interest in wider forms of management. Randomized-controlled studies of psychological and psychosocial interventions are complex and expensive to undertake and hold many potential problems—sample representativeness, high drop-outs, appropriateness of controls, fidelity to the intervention, blindness, etc. As a result, there have been many fewer such studies than of drugs, though in recent years new work, evaluating especially psychological interventions, has been published.

The major types of intervention include:

- Cognitive behaviour therapy
- Psychodynamic psychotherapy
- Social skills training
- Psychoeducation
- Family interventions

It is also convenient to consider aspects of service organization here.

(a) Cognitive behaviour therapy

As striking as the decline in dynamic psychotherapies over the past two decades has been the rise of *cognitive behaviour therapy* (CBT) as a clinical and research focus across psychiatry. Especially in the UK, this has extended to advocacy in schizophrenia. With over 20 randomized-controlled trials and five meta-analysis seeming to support its use, a place in management should be beyond doubt.(43)

The fact is, however, that doubt *does* remain. A recent Cochrane review(44) found that CBT did *not* reduce relapse and readmission compared to standard care (though it did decrease the risk of staying in hospital) and while it improved mental state over the medium term, after a year these slight benefits had disappeared. Continuous measures on mental state did not demonstrate consistent effects. Compared to supportive psychotherapy, CBT had no effect on relapse and when combined with a psychoeducational approach, no significant reduction in readmission rates relative to standard care alone could be demonstrated.

While some individual studies have shown impressive results, the powerful advocacy CBT has attracted as adjunctive management in schizophrenia seems, at this stage, disproportionate to the evidence base. Studies have been built around fundamental design flaws, most notably in relation to control conditions, allowing some to conclude that CBT can be shown to work only in poorly controlled trials and not in well controlled ones.(45) Even between studies showing benefit, it is difficult to discern what the most appropriate target(s) should be and what components ought to comprise an/the ideal CBT package. A further problem, specific to assessing CBT in group contexts, is inappropriate data analysis where independence of observations is universally assumed, something group interactions violate, with a resultant increase in Type 1 errors.(46) While CBT *may* hold promise, widespread endorsement of a resource intensive management would seem premature until more and better designed work reports.

A further application of CBT techniques in psychosis has been in enhancing compliance. While *compliance therapy*,(47) combining cognitive behaviour and motivational interviewing techniques, has shown promise, it has been insufficiently evaluated to support robust recommendations. A recent Cochrane review(48) identified only one study comparing this with non-specific counselling. No significant differences were found in overall 'non-compliance' rates or in mental state measures, attitudes to treatment, global functioning, or quality of life. Although at 1 and 2 year follow-ups, average number of days in hospital was reduced, this was not statistically significant. This study did not show any effect on insight, but other work has claimed that improvements can be achieved by short, insight-focused CBT interventions, but at the expense of increasing depression,(49) an observation also reported with non-CBT approaches targeting insight.(50)

Cognitive remediation (or rehabilitation), in which the desired end-point is not symptom reduction per se but improved *global* functioning via amelioration of cognitive deficits such as impaired vigilance, attention, and planning/decision-making, has also been applied in adjunctive management. Once again, while some individual findings are encouraging, data remain inconclusive.(51)

LEARNING POINT: While present evidence does support the use of CBT led interventions in adjunctive management of schizophrenia, the research is flawed and further, *well controlled* studies are necessary to determine a precise role.

(b) Psychodynamic psychotherapy

Unlike Freud, many analysts of the early-mid twentieth century were undaunted in pursuit of psychodynamic understanding of, and management for, schizophrenia but theories were universally unsupported by evidence. When assessed against supportive psychotherapy, no advantages could be demonstrated.[3] While some modest revival of interest may be detected, especially amongst advocates of 'early intervention', a recent review provided no support for such revisionism.[52] Furthermore, May's study[10,11] offers a cautionary warning of the potential for harm.

LEARNING POINT: Insight-orientated dynamic psychotherapy has no current place in the management of schizophrenia.

(c) Social skills training

As a result of the early age of onset, relapsing nature, and persistence of many clinical features, schizophrenia can potently disrupt smooth acquisition and evolution of skills essential for developing mature interpersonal relationships, occupational competence, and independent living. *Social* (or life) *skills training* evolved in the context of resettlement programmes aimed at discharging long-stay, institutionalized patients but in various forms remain widely practised. It is based on a structured learning-orientated approach to the acquisition of skills relevant to the individual and the demands of his/her environment.

Unfortunately, social skills training is difficult to evaluate, as this has become a 'blanket term' covering a wide range of applications and targets. While some studies have focused on rehearsal of activities of daily living, others concentrate on communication and conversational skills, and although some view improvement in symptoms as the underlying goal, for others the benefit lies with cognitive ability. Blindness of assessments is a major problem, though can be easily achieved using blinded video techniques. Thus, while individual studies have found improvements in assertiveness, general social competence, and even speed of discharge, with benefits extending to a widened social network and that generalize, a recent Cochrane review failed to find conclusive evidence of benefit.[53]

Illness self-management is part of several social skills training programmes but has been singled out as the focus of specialized techniques, comprising video modelling, role-play, and specific problem-solving combined with homework. While promising results have been reported,[54,55] this intensive approach requires further evaluation.

Vocational training (or rehabilitation) is not directly dependent on social skills training but is related to it. Although the majority of schizophrenic patients end up unemployed (up to 85 per cent in the US; 73 per cent in the UK),[56] specialist vocational training remains a scarce component of long-term illness management in most services. A review[56] concluded that *supported employment* models were significantly more effective than *pre-vocational training* in facilitating competitive employment, the latter being no better than standard community care. Supported employment was also associated with higher earnings and more hours working per month. It is sobering that even in trial contexts an average of only 34 per cent of individuals in supported employment were actually employed at 18 months, the comparable figure for those who received pre-vocational training being 12 per cent.[56]

LEARNING POINT: Although intuitively sound and generally appreciated by patients and families, 'social skills training' can only be given a firm evidence base with further well controlled studies in which individual components of therapy are 'teased out' for separate evaluation and specific end-points are genuinely blindly assessed.

(d) Psychoeducation

Much of the above comprises an element of 'education' in the widest sense but programmes have been advocated in which information exchange is *the* key intention. *Psychoeducation* can be targeted on the patient to improve outcomes, enhance compliance, and increase knowledge, including on early relapse recognition, thereby contributing to a better sense of well-being. Imparting factual material is also a fundamental component of many family interventions (see below).

In general, patients appreciate sessions in which their illness is explained, reinforcing the idea that some understanding is possible in situations which may seem incomprehensible. Furthermore, explaining bizarre experiences and beliefs in *illness* terms can help de-stigmatize preconceptions they themselves may hold.

Like most psychological and social interventions advocated as adjunctive strategies for schizophrenia, 'psychoeducation' is not a single procedure with standardized delivery, something that inherently limits systematic reviewing. Nonetheless, it has a favourable review in the Cochrane Library,[57] which found that relapse and readmission rates were significantly reduced (NNT = 9) at 9 to 18 months. Beyond this however, no effect was found on insight, medication-related attitudes or overall satisfaction with services by patients or families. Thus, while data to date are consistent with some *overall* benefits from psychoeducation, those that are proven remain few.

LEARNING POINT: Psychoeducation, as a blanket concept, is attractive to patients and carers and, because it is brief and inexpensive, to service providers, but its *therapeutic* impact may be limited. Future studies must define component elements and address complexities, such as the distinction between knowledge and understanding, and the vulnerability of learned material to degeneration.

(e) Family interventions

The therapeutics of schizophrenia broadened from sufferers to families and carers with the observation that criticism and hostility from a close relative ('expressed emotion': EE) was an important determinant of relapse. As families remain the key element of support for most patients, development of positive, constructive ways of helping them provide this has rightly formed a considerable research focus over the past 30 years. With regard to EE, the consensus is that reduction reduces relapse risk when combined with maintenance medication.[58] However, this appraisal is *not* unanimous and the importance of EE reduction is in need of modern systematic review.

Family interventions have broadened to include not only educational input about the illness, its consequences and service availability, but also psychosocial interventions aimed at developing an alliance (especially important during first presentations), reducing emotional distress, boundary setting, and instillation of realistic expectations of both patient and services. This component heterogeneity again makes straight literature comparisons difficult. A recently updated Cochrane review[59] reported somewhat more equivocal findings than previously, suggesting that while family intervention *may* decrease relapse frequency, the number needed to be treated to prevent an episode of relapse (NNT) had risen from six in a previous review to eight. The authors emphasized that some negative studies may have been missed by their search, rendering even this figure tentative. There was clearer evidence of an effect in reducing hospital admission (NNT = 8) and a *likely* beneficial effect on compliance (NNT = 7). There was no effect on the tendency of individuals to drop out of care but a *likely* improvement in general social impairment and in levels of EE. The effect on suicide seemed neutral. While this may be taken as an endorsement of family interventions, the reviewers offer a salutary caution, suggesting that interested parties—clinicians, patients, policy makers—'cannot be confident on the effects of family intervention from the findings of this review'.

LEARNING POINT: Families generally welcome professional input dedicated to *them* and *their* needs at distressing times such as first diagnosis and subsequently, with realization of the implications. As a quality-of-care issue, such involvement is beyond the benefits trial evaluation can provide. However, in proposing what *works* therapeutically—and works *best*—further research is necessary to define specific elements of interventions that are not only appreciated but that contribute unequivocally to well-being of sufferers and family members.

So—using the *evidence*—what can be concluded from the above? In reviewing psychosocial management strategies advocated for those with schizophrenia and their relatives, two observations emerge. First, is a certain 'regression to the mean'—the more interventions are studied, the harder it becomes to replicate benefits enthusiastically identified early on. The second might be viewed as cynical but is worth stating nonetheless—namely, that in our quest to maximize the care of those with this fell disorder, it has been conclusively established that *drugs plus* 'something' produces better outcomes than *drugs alone*. What remains unclear is whether 'something' amounts to more than projecting high levels of professionalism and/or a common humanity or whether there is indeed a *specific* therapeutic component (or components) to any or all of these 'somethings'.

It is disappointing that after decades of research such a conclusion is still possible and future studies not only need to address the standardization of component element(s) of psychosocial management but must establish a supremacy for it/them before psychiatrists in routine practice and policy makers alike are able to invest not simply in services that others 'like' but that doctors can confidently endorse as having firm *evidence* of therapeutic benefit.

(f) Service organization

The rationale of 'community care' in promoting independence and choice is noble but its implementation has frequently been found wanting. A major thrust in community care management has been the introduction of *community mental health teams* (CMHTs), comprising a comprehensive range of disciplines that bring both collectivism to decision-making and varied expertise to service delivery. Compared to non-team care, CMHT management does promote a greater acceptance of treatment options but further advantages are hard to identify, though reductions in admission and suicides are *possible* benefits.[60]

It has long been clinical experience that not all patients with acute psychoses, including schizophrenia, require hospitalization and, although the research base (specifically in relation to schizophrenia) is slender, *home treatment* programmes have vocal advocates, partly because of the promise they hold for reduction in costly bed numbers. While patient satisfaction is usually high, early quality-of-life benefits may not be sustained and, owing to ongoing need for inpatient facilities, cost benefits may be limited long-term.[61,62] These are difficult services to organize, require intensive staffing and sophisticated multiagency working, and even then, staff morale can be hard to sustain.[63] They are highly selective in who they accept[64] and may work most effectively for those whose family units remain well-integrated and supportive,[65] such as adolescents, but doubts spanning all the potential benefits are sufficient to suggest caution in making empirically based leaps to such radical service reorganization in the absence of further data.

The policy of institutional closures that began in most developed countries in the 1960s/1970s did not result in reduced patterns of acute bed usage. In fact, *rising* admission rates caused concern that day and outpatient care alone were inadequate because of failure to maintain engagement or to meet complex needs. Case management and a variant, assertive community treatment (ACT), arose as ways of optimizing ongoing service involvement and ensuring coordination and delivery of care appropriate to individual clinical and social needs. Both aim to: maintain patients in contact with services; reduce frequency and durations of admissions; improve outcomes, especially social functioning and quality of life. Case management is essentially based on 'brokerage', where an *individual* member of the multi-disciplinary team is responsible for assessing needs, developing a care plan, arranging implementation and monitoring quality and engagement, and is also involved in an element of delivery. This is now seen as the least robust model and more complex variants have arisen. With ACT, the emphasis lies in *team* working.

Systematically reviewed, *case management* ensures that more people remain in contact with services but with the consequence of *increased* admission rates.[66] Furthermore, rather than shortening admissions, it may actually increase their duration. There is no evidence that it improves outcomes on any clinical or social variables. Compared to standard community care, patients receiving ACT are more likely to remain in contact with services, less likely to be admitted, and spend less time in hospital with other benefits in terms of accommodation, employment, and satisfaction.[67] However, mental state and social functioning are *not* improved and with overall costs accounted for, ACT is *not* less expensive. In comparison to case management, ACT has advantages in terms of reduced time in hospital but overall there are no cost benefits.[67] Few other comparisons are possible due to inadequate data.

The impression that case management should be dropped and ACT flourish[67] is somewhat oversimplified. The negative appraisal of case management as of 'questionable value' has been criticized[68] while the 'effectiveness' of ACT seems to rest on the recurrent problems of content and fidelity of delivery noted in relation to all the psychosocial interventions discussed here.

LEARNING POINT: Like drugs, organizational structures operate in a social and service development context and what applies to one patient group in one national or local environment might not reap similar benefits in another. Community-based

or otherwise, *the* weakness in the care of those with chronic, relapsing-remitting disorders like schizophrenia, characterized by autistic withdrawal and social dislocation, is failure to maintain engagement with specialist services. Any structure that fosters a proactive approach to engagement while maintaining staff morale is likely to be better appreciated and to provide better outcomes.

Treatment and management principles

The following is based on UK experience and may not translate completely across international borders where local traditions and organizational constraints may modify practice. It is only presented as an *outline* of issues to be considered and cannot provide a universal blueprint for care. As will become apparent, the authors would argue that such 'blueprints' do not best serve the interests of patients or the expertise of those implementing care.

Doctors confronted with a patient believed to be acutely psychotic must address three preliminary questions:

1 *Does the patient require admission or can they be managed as an outpatient?*

Some of the issues were aired above but from the *medical* point of view, there are a number of scenarios in which admission remains a priority (Table 4.3.8.3).

2 *Can the clinical situation be dealt with informally or are compulsory legal powers required?*

Table 4.3.8.3 Considerations in relation to admission policies in patients with acute schizophrenia

Supporting admission	Supporting non-admission
Unstable mental state Rapidly extending content Variable affect	Mental state disorder stable/slowly evolving
Imperative auditory hallucinations To harm self To harm others	Absent/no will to act
Marked affective change Suspiciousness, anger Depression	Affective change mild/amenable to reassurance
Behavioural disturbance Disorganization Dangerousness Commission Omission	Minimal behavioural disturbance/risk of harm
Cognitive disturbance Lack of insight Impaired attention/distractability Inability to comprehend advice Hopelessness/suicidal ideation	No barrier to engagement
Inadequate social support Living alone Vagrancy/neglect	Good social supports
Any (other) reason for non-compliance	Likelihood of compliance
Medical state Intercurrent physical illness Substance misuse/dependency	Physically fit
'Asylum'	Aversion to inpatient care

This will depend on the thorough *risk assessment* that must be a part of every examination. This must, of course, include the *health* risks, not solely those involving threat. The details of implementing compulsory detention for assessment and/or treatment will differ in different jurisdictions.

3 *What is the best first step in treatment?*

There is *no* single first–line drug for the treatment of acute schizophrenic episodes—nor, the authors would suggest, any first-line *type* of antipsychotic. Guidelines are fairly unanimous in recommending 'atypical' antipsychotics, especially in first episodes, and any recommendation qualifying this requires justification.

Despite its persistence, the term 'atypical' has never attained *pharmacological* credibility. It rests on a single *clinical* parameter—a perceived reduction in liability to promote extrapyramidal side-effects (EPS)—*quite specifically*, drug-induced parkinsonism. The problems surrounding a subclassification based on such a vague parameter are multiple (e.g. the boundaries of parkinsonism; inadequacies of rating schedules; discrepancies in dose equivalences between trial and comparator agents) making 'atypicality' of dubious scientific validity.[14] Carefully conducted trials, not sponsored by industry, have recently raised questions about putative advantages in EPS tolerability, even with high potency comparators such as haloperidol, when appropriate equivalence is used.[69] With quality-of-life parameters no different after up to 1 year, and no detectable patient preference,[70,71] objectively it is hard to see 'atypicality' as having any merits beyond product marketing. There is certainly little to support any *inherent* value for clinical decision-making beyond the fact that new generation drugs extend the options.

However, there is now strong *evidence* to challenge the blinkered 'algorithmic' prescribing guidelines can foster, especially in relation to 'atypical' antipsychotics. Results of the Clinical Antipsychotic Trials of Clinical Effectiveness (CATIE) study raise important issues about the tolerability profiles of different new generation compounds in relation to first-generation drugs[72] and challenge cost-effectiveness benefits.[73] These data form part of an emerging trend that, we contend, opens up once again the *full range* of antipsychotics—new and old—to consideration as treatment options.

An alternative to 'algorithmic' practice is to view guidelines as providing a *framework* only, within which *all* clinical information can be brought to bear in prescribing decisions. This approach takes its cue from drug regulation, where the appropriateness of granting a license is based on an *individual risk: benefit appraisal*. This is a *clinical* judgement, the outcome of which is dependent on *context* (e.g. not simply adverse effect burden but availability of alternatives). Patients, psychotic illnesses and drugs to treat them are each diverse, harbouring far greater differences than the few similarities they share. These diversities should be entered into the individual risk:benefit appraisal in making prescribing choices. So too should the *phase* of illness one is planning for—acute through to maintenance—as the risk:benefit appraisal may shift between these in particular individuals.

Some examples of issues for consideration in individual risk: benefit appraisals are shown in Table 4.3.8.4, but the professionalism psychiatry claims can only come from expertise in recognizing and accounting for the many varied possibilities.

Table 4.3.8.4 Individual risk:benefit appraisal in the use of antipsychotics : examples of some considerations

Presentation	Possible Strategies	Schedule
Behavioural disturbance 'positive' or 'negative' = arousal	Low potency standard (solo treatment)	'diminuendo' or 'crescendo'
Prominent non-specific affective symptomatology	Low potency standard Or New generation + benzodiazepine (potentiation)	Rapid 'crescendo' to tolerance
Marked insomnia	New generation + benzodiazepine Or low potency standard	'crescendo' to 6–8 hours nocturnal sleep + maximum of two hours in the day
High risk of psychiatric emergency	Low potency standard (+/- additional medication)	Slow 'diminuendo'
Tenuous engagement Poor past medication experiences (tolerability) Overfamiliarity with common regimes	New generation (solo treatment)	Slow 'crescendo'
Poor physical health Overweight Family history of CV disease	High potency standard	'crescendo'
Middle aged High CVS risk factors	High potency standard	Low dose regime assessed without change over protracted period
Prior or present EPS symptomatology	'loose binding' new generation (quetiapine)	Slow 'crescendo'
Established history of poor long-term engagement/ compliance	Long-acting injectable	Ultra-slow 'crescendo'

'diminuendo' = starting with higher doses and tailing down to tolerability

'crescendo' = starting with lower doses and building up to tolerability

Identifying goals and defining structure

The key to avoiding confusion and 'decision paralysis' in dealing with the complex clinical situations schizophrenia presents is to delineate the *structure* within which it is hoped to achieve a series of treatment/management *goals*. Although arbitrary, three 'phases' can be identified:

- Acute
- Post-acute
- Maintenance

The acute phase

This encompasses treatment during the maximally florid symptomatic period, corresponding to first presentation or subsequent acute exacerbations (Fig. 4.3.8.1). It is characterized by a significant shift to *illness*, though surprisingly, it remains unclear exactly what changes define this shift.

The goals include:

i) control of intrusive, non-specific symptomatology (e.g. anxiety, agitation, and especially insomnia);

ii) maximizing safety and well-being of the patient and others by containing chaotic, socially damaging behaviours;

iii) engaging the patient in therapeutic recommendations and (mental state permitting) gaining consent for treatment plans;

iv) implementing an appropriate foundation drug regime;

v) stabilizing positive symptomatology;

vi) preventing, or if unavoidable, treating psychiatric emergencies.

The risk:benefit appraisal at this early stage is driven by the first four of these, for the ultimate goal of acute phase treatment—stabilization of positive symptomatology—is, as noted, likely to be delayed. It is important not to overlook other goals that can be achieved quickly, especially those that can be held up as evidence of progress, such as improved sleep.

These goals may be achieved using a single antipsychotic, which is the *ideal*. In this regard, low potency first-generation drugs, such as chlorpromazine, have appeal because of low cost, extensive usage, wide dose flexibility and potent, if rapidly habituating, sedative properties. Flexible dose studies suggest the majority of responses will be achieved in the range of 500–600 mg/day[5] with some suggestion that first-episode patients may respond at lower doses. While low potency drugs have a justifiably admirable reputation in the treatment of presenting, acute phase symptomatology, they are not generally ideal as sole long-term treatment in view of the often intrusive effects of lingering sedation. As patients who have experienced benefit on a particular regime tend not to like changes, and such switches can be clinically problematic because of poor dose equivalence data, chlorpromazine alone is usually best reserved as an initial, short-term strategy.

High potency first-generation drugs, especially haloperidol, have also been widely used, especially in the United States, and while effective, contain a potential problem. High potency drugs are *safe* and tend to be used in higher doses than low potency ones (in one study, 4–6 times the low potency equivalent[74]). This undoubtedly follows from the fact that low potency compounds are inherently dose-limited by anti-autonomic and sedative actions. Unsurprisingly, liberal early use of high potency drugs is associated with higher rates of EPS (dystonias, akathisia, and parkinsonism).[14] Two points should be borne in mind in using high potency first-generation antipsychotics. Firstly, it has been shown in both clinical and functional imaging (PET) studies using D2 occupancy levels that usual minimum effective daily doses of haloperidol lie somewhere between 2 and 5 mg.[75,76] Secondly, even utilizing slightly higher doses, EPS need present no greater problems with haloperidol than they do with placebo or olanzapine.[69,75]

Nowadays, most clinicians tend to pursue a new generation drug as their first choice and this does have some practical advantages, not least single dosing and orodispersable formulations. However, while most new generation drugs have some sedative properties, these are clinically less prominent than with low potency first-generation compounds, so achieving early acute phase goals can be protracted. Furthermore, these drugs usually now come with defined protocols relating to starting doses and rate of increments which do not apply to older drugs. A number of guidelines address

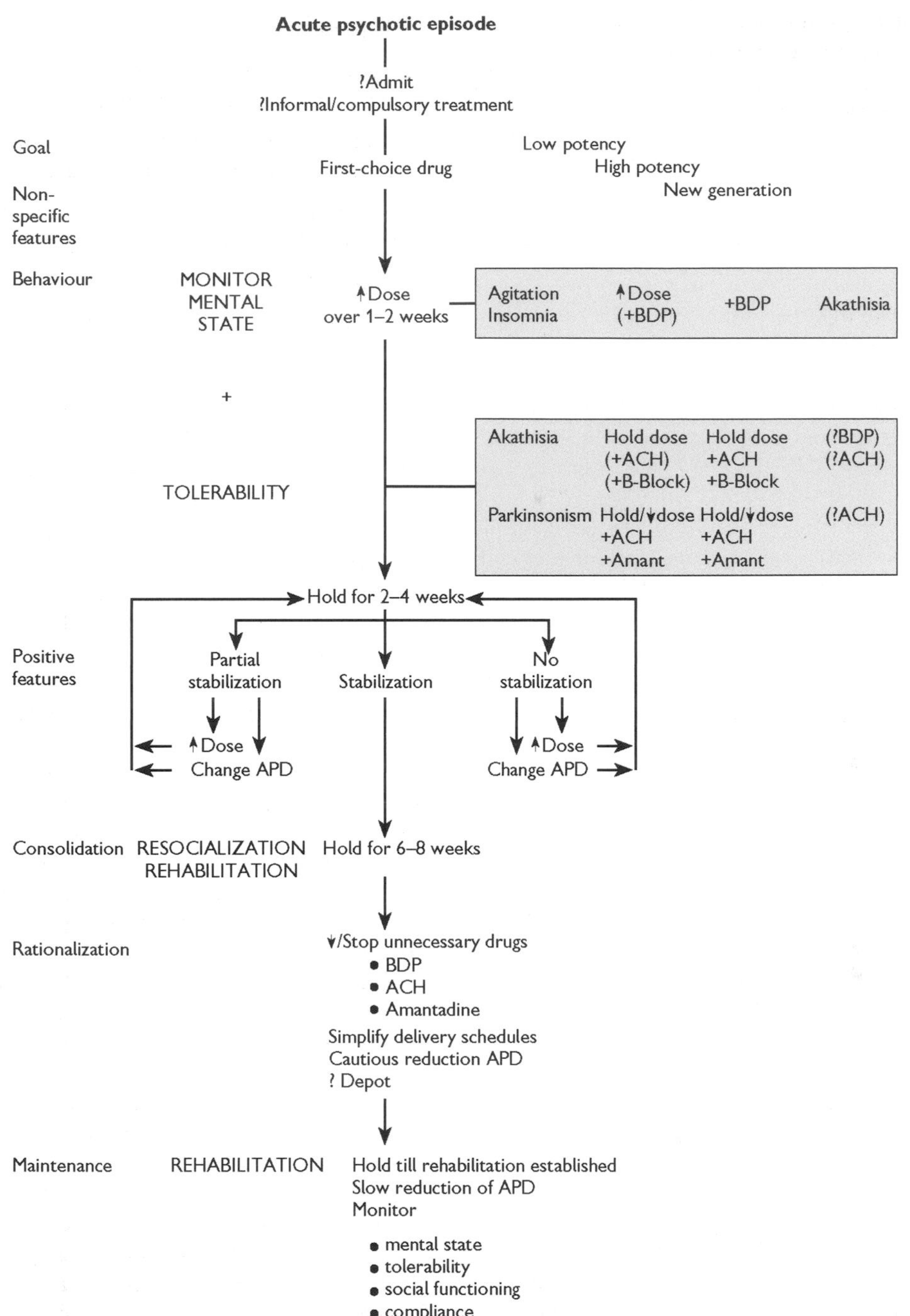

Fig. 4.3.8.1 Outline plan for treatment/ management of schizophrenia: APD, antipsychotic drug; BDP, benzodiazepine; ACH, anticholinergic; B-Block, ß-blocker; Amant, amantadine.

the potential impediment this introduces into achieving acute phase goals by recommending the adjunctive use of a sedative drug, especially benzodiazepines, to gain early control of intrusive non-specific symptomatology.[77] While this is sound, there is another, more traditional, approach—namely, the addition of a second, sedative antipsychotic.

This introduces the issue of polypharmacy, against which the literature has long (and rightly) railed. However, notwithstanding these many cautions, it might seem more logical to treat non-specific symptomatology that is *psychotically mediated* with an antipsychotic, even if one's goals are largely short-term and symptomatic, rather than to introduce a further class of medication whose benefits will not contribute to the fundamental treatment issue (see below) and may cause their own, unrelated problems, including behavioural 'dyscontrol'. Antipsychotic polypharmacy *must* be reviewed regularly, justified constantly and rationalized when possible. The real 'sin' of polypharmacy is its persistence in the treatment plan 'by default'. However, it must be acknowledged that behavioural disturbance and non-specific symptomatology may be so overwhelming that benzodiazepines may be useful in order to avoid over-rapid, excessive escalations of antipsychotic doses.

Even if not introduced as a fixed part of early treatment recommendations, prescription of additional antipsychotic on an 'as required' (or 'PRN') basis is virtually standard practice, allowing nursing staff to intervene at their discretion in the face of escalating symptomatology. This has no trial basis[78] and although a pragmatic solution to inherently unstable situations, must be utilized with discretion. Indications, maximum doses, frequencies, and modes of administration must all be written up separately and unambiguously. Such regimes should *not* be viewed merely as a means of 'keeping the peace' but should be used to inform judgements about how far short of practical requirements initial treatment recommendation fall, invaluable information to incorporate into each treatment review.

Antiparkinsonian medication should be automatically used with higher doses of high potency standard antipsychotics (=/> 10 mgms haloperiod daily or equivalent)[69]but not with lower doses or other acute phase choices.[14] While anticholinergics reduce the risk of acute EPS, only a minority will develop these to a clinically significant degree and antiparkinsonian drugs will interact with antipsychotics to interfere with their actions. These drugs have their own profile of antimuscarinic effects which can be minimized by choosing the most M1-selective compounds (e.g. biperiden, procyclidine) should be used.[14]

A further point relates to goal (iii) above. Patients are often more experienced psychopharmacologists than their doctors! In deciding treatment regimes in those with past histories, be advised by the patient. Medications in which they have confidence should always be one's first-line in treating acute relapses.

Prior to the emergence of goal (v) above, monitoring of acutely psychotic patients should be *frequent*, and preferably daily, each assessment resulting in a review and, if necessary, modification of the treatment plan. At this stage it is rarely useful to commence formal psychosocial, including educational, programmes with patients, whose cognitive difficulties will make it hard to engage meaningfully, though as part of one's ongoing dialogue, monitoring progress and addressing tolerability and compliance serves an elementary educational purpose. Likewise, one's interactions with families are best restrained to exchange of such basic information as the patient will permit (e.g. diagnosis and treatment) and to general support.

The boundary of acute phase of treatment is not rigidly defined, nor is it necessarily set by major symptomatic reversals. The ultimate aim is 'stabilization', as evidenced by the psychotic process becoming less 'active', delusions are recalled as yesterday's events, hallucinations become less preoccupying, behaviour more amenable. It may also be that sedation, previously an ally, becomes intrusive and a source of complaint.

The post-acute phase

This is characterized by the re-emergence of stability in both mental state and behaviour. The following goals should be considered:

i) consolidation of clinical improvements;

ii) rationalization of treatment regimes;

iii) resocialization.

The different domains of schizophrenic symptomatology do not all improve at the same rate and the first signs of amelioration should not be taken as evidence that the tide has turned. Global improvements need to mature into *specific* improvements in particular domains of symptomatology before this can be assumed. Practically, caution is important as over-rapid reductions in antipsychotic dosages before fundamental therapeutic changes have bedded down increases the risk of symptom exacerbation and although there is little evidence on the matter, clinical experience suggests that such very early setbacks are not only demoralizing but more difficult to stabilize, requiring higher doses for longer periods to recapture previous gains.

Nonetheless, the transition from acute to post-acute phase usually marks a pivotal point when the balance of appraisal shifts towards the increasing contribution of 'risk' to the risk:benefit assessment. Taking account of this shift is important in maximizing compliance, both short and long term. So an important step of post-acute treatment is about *gradual* change towards simplifying regimes and maximizing tolerability. The emphasis on 'gradual' is still important, as over-rapid reductions may be implemented ahead of relapse set in train by previous reductions.

In monitoring progress, two issues should be borne in mind. First, is a clear impression of the *criteria* on which 'improvement' are to be based. The traditional medical emphasis is on symptomatology, especially positive symptoms, but elimination of *all* psychotic phenomena, or development of *full* insight, may be unrealistic goals, particularly in those with established illness. Such attempts usually come at the expense of dose regimes significantly higher—and with correspondingly greater long-term risks—than are necessary for a good quality of life and maximum compliance.

Secondly, patients and families—and those who pay for care—often have unrealistic expectations of the timescale over which outcomes can be assessed in acute schizophrenic episodes. Considering both psychopathology and 'degree' of remission, Lieberman *et al.* found that the median time to 'remission' was 11 weeks, with a *mean* time of almost 37 weeks—and that, in a first-episode sample![79] Other studies have produced similar findings. Even if full 'remission' is not the goal of acute and post-acute treatment, the relatively protracted timescales over which 'benefit' is to be considered must be taken into account. There is *no* evidence that this process can be speeded up by escalating doses, which on the contrary, may prolong the situation by introducing unnecessary and intrusive adverse effects.

In this regard, it is worth introducing another concept from past studies. In the 1960s a number of authors described a phenomenon of so-called 'neuroleptic toxicity', an apparently paradoxical worsening of mental state with escalating antipsychotic doses.[80] In reviewing the dose–response literature, Baldessarini and colleagues suggested that the curvilinear relationships usually found may be explained by increasing extrapyramidal symptomatology.[39] Thus, with antipsychotic drugs, while 'less' may not necessarily be 'more', 'more is usually less'!

The post-acute phase is the time to introduce appropriate elements of wider 'management'. With the patient, this might include 'education' in a more formal sense than hitherto, tackling the nature of the condition and, most importantly, the key role of medication in its treatment, including addressing potential long-term recommendations. Regardless of one's interpretation of the literature on its specific benefits, CBT *principles* can be helpful in structuring goals and realistic pathways to attaining them and in re-instilling a sense of control and optimism. Families, too, can now more productively be brought into formal educational programmes, either singly or in groups.

The maintenance phase

The boundary between post-acute and maintenance phases is the least defined but is reached when remission—maximal improvements in all major domains of disorder—can reasonably be considered to have occurred. The major goals now are:

i) maximum well-being with minimum adverse effects;

ii) monitoring efficacy/effectiveness and tolerability;

iii) continuing or extending rehabilitation and social integration.

Attempts to reduce medication should still be cautious but, over the longer term more determined, as one seeks the *minimal effective dose*. As noted, evidence suggests that maintenance regimes can be considerably lower than those utilized for acute treatment but this aspect of long-term care is often omitted, perhaps on the basis that no one wishes to 'rock the boat'. The result is that maintenance may be facilitated by unnecessarily high doses that, in turn, may impede compliance and increase the liability to long-term adverse effects. These need not be simply neurological but may extend to wider domains of functioning. In the Northwick Park First Episodes study significantly more patients in the placebo group were found to have some clear achievement at 2-year follow-up compared to those on active antipsychotic.[(81)]

This finding referred to small numbers but raises the important question of what are the most satisfactory criteria by which to gauge long-term treatment response-domain-specific criteria or global outcomes. Whichever is selected, a second important shift occurs in the risk:benefit appraisal in this phase, the goal being the active elimination of as many components of 'risk' (i.e. side-effects) as possible.

Monitoring neurological tolerability should involve both enquiry into *subjective* adverse effects as well as examination for signs,[(14)] the most efficient being simply an assessment of the patient walking.

The most ambitious aim of maintenance comprises engagement in management geared to attaining the highest possible level of psychosocial and, where possible, occupational functioning for the patient, with carers able to exert the greatest degree of understanding and coping skills.

Depression, affecting up to 70 per cent of patients in the acute phase, tends to remit with the psychosis[(26,82)] but as many as one-third will develop depression in the maintenance phase. This *post-psychotic* (or post-schizophrenic) *depression* is likely to be as aetiologically heterogeneous as depression in other contexts but has been poorly studied including from a therapeutic perspective. Despite initial pessimism, there is evidence that such mood states respond to tricyclic antidepressants[(83)] though response is impeded in those experiencing residual or recurring psychotic symptoms on low maintenance antipsychotic regimes.[(84)]

Negative symptoms are present throughout the course of schizophrenia but are most likely to raise specific therapeutic issues during maintenance. An outline of care options is shown in Table 4.3.8.5.

Table 4.3.8.5 Outline management of 'negative' states in schizophrenia

Question	Intervention
1 Is the patient actively psychotic?	Start/increase antipsychotics Reduce levels of stimulation
If not: 2 Is there evidence of extrapyramidal side-effects?	Anticholinergics Amantadine Reduce antipsychotic doses Switch antipsychotic New generation Low ptency
If not: 3 Is there evidence of dysphoric mood?	Antidepressants Anxiolytics Reduce antipsychotics Supportive management Switch to new-generation antipsychotic
If not: 4 Has psychosis recently resolved?	Supportive management
If not: 5 Is the environment impoverished?	Resocialization Rehabilitation
If not: 6 Is the patient receiving long-term medication?	Reduce to reasonable maintenance dose Switch to new-generation antipsychotic Clozapine
Then: 7 Is the problem a 'deficit' state?	Adapt expectations to the patient's capabilities

After Carpenter *et al.* (29)

Prodromes

Some would say the above is far from comprehensive, missing *the* key element in the care of schizophrenia nowadays—prevention. In fact, they would argue, by concentrating on recommendations that only apply once the possibility of prevention has passed, we are submitting to traditional therapeutic pessimism, which is out-of-step with the optimism of the times.

Prodrome refers to features that, for any illness, characterize the difference between well-being and the state of illness evolution. The patient is not unwell as such but the journey to illness has commenced.

In schizophrenia research, 'prodrome' applies to two scenarios. The first, and perhaps most therapeutically relevant, relates to second and subsequent episodes where the clinical team may have a basis for prevention—not of the illness but of the episode (i.e. *relapses*). The universally negative trial evidence in relation to targeted intervention on early relapse symptomatology has been mentioned but this may be one of those situations in which trial *efficacy* does not translate well to *real-life* situations. Maybe the patients selected for such approaches must be 'targeted' as much as the symptomatology!

Early symptom recognition should certainly be a key part of the education of both patients and their families, a task helped by the fact that as a rule, psychotic episodes run 'true to form'. Non-specific and positive features recognized from an earlier episode can be recruited to help identify emergence of subsequent episodes. Especially sensitive, is a change in sleep pattern. As was noted, if patients have stopped maintenance medication, knowledge of the *time* to relapse following previous cessations can be useful in high lighting the 'critical period' for subsequent relapse. Such knowledge can be empowering, especially for families and carers and even though trial support is lacking, clinical experience suggests it can sometimes be useful in facilitating swift reintroduction of medication or increasing dosages from maintenance to treatment levels.

Relapse prevention through early symptom recognition is *not*, however, from where optimism currently springs. This comes from the second application of 'prodrome'—to the early phase of *illness*, not episode, development.

The '*early intervention*' movement has swelled to an influential grouping within both the research and policy arms of psychiatry. Its origins lie in a very real concern—the delay that many schizophrenic patients experience between the first signs of illness and entry into specialist care. This so-called 'duration of untreated psychosis' (DUP) is on average 1–2 years but can be longer[(85)] and has been linked to adversity of outcome, initially on the theoretical basis of some factor mediating neurotoxicity,[(86)] though this remains unsupported.

While a degree of consensus is possible on what the key elements *might* comprise, it is as yet impossible to construct a valid model of what 'early intervention' *should* comprise and thereafter to measure fidelity.[(87)] Nonetheless, its principles have been enthusiastically adopted and development of services is government policy in many countries, including the UK. This does however, remain controversial—not at the *quality-of-care* level, where the aims of improving awareness and service access are inherently sound, but at the *scientific* level, where evidence supporting improved outcomes remains weak.

Recent systematic reviews do point to modest benefits in terms of a lower symptom burden and delayed readmission in the short-intermediate term.[(88,89)] However, assessment of DUP is invariably retrospective and although it may be done with reliability, validity remains suspect. Also, the link may be confounded by, for example, some illness characteristic that mediates both delay in entering services and poor outcome, making interpretation difficult. The authors' own work with those at high risk of developing schizophrenia has pointed to the problems of attributing a 'prodromal' psychotic state solely to the emergence of what are traditionally considered 'psychotic' symptoms and to the non-specific nature of those symptoms that do seem to point to a later formal diagnosis.[(90)]

The precise delineation of pathway(s) to illness remains to be refined to a degree that provides meaningful positive predictive values, thereby avoiding the awkward issue of unnecessary and potentially risky interventions in those whose 'operationally defined normality' is merely different, not necessarily prepsychotic. Continued investment in 'early intervention' services must for the present be driven more by quality-of-care considerations than an evidential base.

Psychiatric emergencies

In dealing with acutely ill psychotic patients, one must always bear in mind the 'unpredictability factor' and the *potential* for aggressive or violent outbursts during acute symptomatic 'shifts'. Risk assessment of dangerousness is an imprecise science but should be incorporated into all routine clinical assessments during acute phase treatment—and conclusions *documented*. Caution should be exercised with patients who are profoundly suspicious, verbally aggressive, resistant to engagement, whose presentation does not allow for comprehensive mental state examination, whose clinical condition is complicated by substance misuse and especially, those who have a past history of assaultive or threatening behaviour.

Principles of wider management are crucial in *avoiding* emergency situations including the quality of the (ward) environment, staff:patient ratios, etc., but even with high levels of vigilance, pre-emptive plans and good quality management, emergency situations may still occur and must be dealt with decisively.

An outline plan relating to emergency situations is shown in Fig. 4.3.8.2.

Poor response and treatment resistance

Where a patient has not responded satisfactorily to an adequate dose (600–800 mg/day chlorpromazine or its equivalent) of antipsychotic for an adequate period of time (at least 6–8 weeks) they might be considered a 'poor responder' but not yet 'treatment resistant'. Several strategies have been suggested in this situation.

Antipsychotics

Conventionally, the first approach is to modify the antipsychotic regime by:

1 increasing first-choice drug to a high-dose schedule (up to 1000 mg chlorpromazine or its equivalent) for 6–8 weeks;

2 changing to a drug of different chemical type in standard dose ranges for 6–8 weeks. (Current research would suggest this should include changes between not just old and new drugs, but in the other direction too);

3 increasing the dose of the second-choice drug to a high-dose schedule for 6–8 weeks.

As far as the literature is concerned, it is only when at least one, and preferably two, of these steps have failed that the illness should be considered 'treatment resistant'.[(41)]

Despite adoption in routine practice, there is little evidence that such manoeuvrings are of themselves effective. More *time* may still be the crucial factor. There is some evidence that in those switching from a new generation drug, slightly better results may be achieved with risperidone and olanzapine than quetiapine or ziprazidone,[(91)] though this might be saying simply that, when tolerated, relatively high potency compounds do better than relatively low potency ones.

In clinical practice, especially when external pressures and a sense of therapeutic confusion have clouded therapeutic goals, antipsychotic doses can escalate 'by default'. The issue of 'neuroleptic toxicity' has been mentioned and where high-dose regimes cannot be specifically *justified*, it is worth *reducing* to average or low doses and assessing response. Furthermore, patients showing poor response may benefit from addition of a *depot*, even when compliance is not in doubt, possible advantages perhaps relating to adverse pharmacokinetic parameters, such as poor absorption or enhanced metabolism with complex or high-dose oral regimes.

IMPENDING EMERGENCY

Non-drug intervention	Drug intervention
• Talking down • Distraction • Seclusion	Antipsychotic (with sedative properties) orally e.g. chlorpromazine 50 – 100mgs (liquid/tabs) haloperidol 5 – 10mgms Low-distribution benzodiazepine e.g. lorazepam 1 – 2mgms

Review 30 –60 minutes
If no response – repeat
Or
If no response or no initial co-operation

• Talking down • Distraction • Seclusion • Monitor physically	(Sedative) antipsychotic IM e.g. haloperidol 5-10mgs olanzapine 10mgms chlorpromazine 50-100mgms (with care in frail elderly or drug naïve) Low-distribution benzodiazepine e.g. lorazepam 1-2mgms

Revise treatment plan – start/increase baseline antipsychotic
Review 30 –60 minutes
If no response – repeat (with higher dose ranges, vital signs permitting)
Revise treatment plan

ESTABLISHED EMERGENCY

Non-drug intervention	Drug intervention
• Seclusion • Talking down • Monitor vital signs	sedative antipsychotic IM (as above) in adequate dose ± Low distribution benzodiazepine as above, administered separately (depending on severity of incident) Or zuclopentixol acetate (Acuphase) IM * High potency antipsychotic IV e.g. haloperidol 5 – 10mgms

Review 30 – 60 minutes
Revise treatment plan
Repeat if necessary (vital signs permitting)

* should be used with care in the frail or drug naïve

Fig. 4.3.8.2 Outline plan for treatment/management of psychiatric emergencies.

Adjunctive medications

Simplifying any complexities that may have entered into treatment is a useful strategy when response is poor, such as reducing or stopping anticholinergics or other drugs, such as antidepressants, where possible. For kinetic (and possibly dynamic) reasons, such drugs may be acting against the primary therapeutic aim.

While a number of other drugs have been recommended for adjunctive treatment of suboptimally responding schizophrenia, there is inadequate evidence to support any of them.

Lithium, independent of its actions on mood, is not 'antipsychotic'[92] but has been recommended for patients with schizoaffective disorders. The evidence is inconclusive and its use is best considered empirical in those with prominent affective symptoms.[93] There is some evidence of a more rapid improvement in symptoms with *valproate* augmentation but any benefits seem to be transient.[94] This is more than can be said for *carbamazepine*, whose widespread adjunctive use comes with no supporting evidence, though such studies that have been done have been small.[95] A recent Cochrane review of the role of *lamotrigine* did provide tentative support from small, poor quality studies, suggesting that PANSS total and positive and negative subscale scores significantly decline on lamotrigine compared to placebo.[96] Further work is required before clear recommendations can be made.

At one time, *benzodiazepines* were advocated in both the sole and adjunctive treatment of schizophrenia, usually in high doses

(~100 mg/day diazepam). Benefits beyond simple sedation have been hard to find and systematic reviews highlight a small number of small, supporting studies.(97) While, as noted, benzodiazepines are widely used for treating psychotically mediated acute behavioural disturbance, such evidence as there is suggests little difference between them and antipsychotics.(97)

Finally, it is worth remembering that the theory behind the introduction of ECT, however flawed, related to *schizophrenia* and there is some evidence to support its use in this condition, especially when rapid global improvement is required and when antipsychotic response has been limited.(98) However, as in depression, its benefits are usually short-lived and do not substitute for an effective long-term medication strategy.

When the patient satisfies criteria for 'treatment resistance', the evidence is, as noted, overwhelming that *clozapine* is better than any other drug regime.(41) There is *no* evidence that any other antipsychotic, old or new, shares its edge and in this regard, clozapine remains a *unique* compound.

Of the psychosocial interventions, only CBT has been suggested as possibly helpful in modifying symptoms and improving outcomes in those with 'treatment resistance'(99) though further work is required to confirm these tentative findings.

Concluding remarks

The above might be interpreted as inferring that nothing much has changed in the treatment and management of schizophrenia, which remains a somewhat pessimistic, even unrewarding, area of therapeutic endeavour: one that is regressing far less moving on. This is far from our experience and the opposite of the impression we wish to create.

Certainly, as far as drug treatments are concerned, no single agent or type of agent now seems more satisfactory across the board than any other, but the challenge to 'atypicality' as a valid subgrouping of antipsychotics does not limit options—rather it *broadens* them, restoring to the treatment repertoire the wide range of choices that is the key to individualized care planning. With psychosocial interventions, there does remain more work to be done in *proving* absolute efficacy and/or effectiveness and the relative place of each, but in service development and care planning, risk:benefit appraisal is sophisticated enough to encompass what has qualitative *value* as well as what is quantitatively *proven*.

As in all branches of medicine where chronic and relapsing disease is encountered, restoring order on chaos, fostering engagement and lighting a way forward when none may be obvious are for the highest levels of skill, in which evidence-based practice can provide the direction but not yet the specific path. We are fortunate in now having available to us the greatest *ever* range of interventions to bring to the care of those who suffer from this most complex and fell disorder. None is comprehensive, all have limitations, but if we wish to provide quality care, care that accounts for the multifarious manifestations patients present, it is our duty to apply not only the experience of others but of ourselves too.

There is no 'quick fix' in gaining competence in the treatment and management of schizophrenia—and, as yet, no curative 'holy grail' either. But there is, more than ever, the opportunity for clinicians to demonstrate *real* expertise in moulding the range of therapeutics now at our disposal. If that is not reason for medical optimism, what is!

Further information

There is at present a sense of 'flux' in care recommendations for those who suffer from schizophrenia and the authors would recommend that some of the articles below should be *read* as opposed to just 'referred to'. Both the American(2) and the Australian(3) guidelines are good examples of present trends in this approach, though illustrate the slight differences of emphasis that even 'evidence' permits. The CATIE study(72) is seminal and mandatory reading for all those involved in treatment planning (the background to this is presented in *Schizophrenia Bulletin* (2003, vol. 29(1))—the CUtLASS study likewise.(71) Both mark a change from simply efficacy-based studies to pragmatic, 'everyday' designs that is likely to intensify. For a background to the importance of absolute doses of standard comparator drugs in efficacy trials and dose equivalence issues, the studies of Rosenheck *et al.*(69) and Strakowski *et al.*(70) are informative, as is that of Baldessarini *et al.*(74) from an earlier period. Crow's original paper on the Type 1/Type 2 dichotomy(12) is historically important (in the 1980s/1990s, the most cited source of research-testable hypotheses in psychiatry) and helpful in understanding what was being proposed and the limitations of subsequent efforts to disprove it.

The authors would contend that behind much of the confusion in the clinical psychopharmacology of the antipsychotic drugs in recent years lurks the long shadow of parkinsonism. This, rather than tardive dyskinesia, has always been the extrapyramidal side-effects issue, partly because of its pervasive presence but also because of its wide and ill-defined boundaries. Those wishing to familiarize themselves with more than just the basics are referred to the book by Owens,(14) one of the few texts to specifically present drug-induced parkinsonism in both its subjective and objective components for primarily a psychiatric audience.

Finally, all practicing psychiatrists nowadays should be familiar with the address of the Cochrane Library (www.thecochranelibrary.com) and its Database of Systematic Reviews and should feel comfortable referring to it themselves, not just second-hand. It presents quality syntheses of complex material of relevance to many key areas of psychiatric practice.

References

1. National Institute for Clinical Excellence. (2002). *Schizophrenia: core interventions in the treatment and management of schizophrenia in primary and secondary care*. NICE, London.
2. Lehman, A.F., Lieberman, J.A., Dixon, L.B., *et al.* (2004). Practice guideline for the treatment of patients with schizophrenia (2nd edn). *The American Journal of Psychiatry*, **161**(Suppl. 2), 1–56.
3. McGorry, P. (2005). Royal Australian and New Zealand College of Psychiatrists clinical practice guidelines for the treatment of schizophrenia and related disorders. *The Australian and New Zealand Journal of Psychiatry*, **39**, 1–30.
4. Cole, J.O. and the NIMH Psychopharmacology Service Center Collaborative Study Group. (1964). Phenothiazine treatment in acute schizophrenia. *Archives of General Psychiatry*, **10**, 246–61.
5. Davis, J.M. and Garver, D.L. (1978). Neuroleptics—clinical use in psychiatry. In *Handbook of psychopharmacology* (eds. L.L. Iversen, S. Iversen, and S. Snyder), pp. 129–64. Plenum Press, New York.
6. Tuma, A.H. and May, P.R.A. (1979). And if it doesn't work, what next? A study of treatment failures in schizophrenia. *The Journal of Nervous and Mental Disease*, **167**, 566–71.

7. Agid, O., Kapur, S., Arenovich, T., *et al.* (2003). Delayed-onset hypothesis of antipsychotic action: a hypothesis tested and rejected. *Archives of General Psychiatry*, **60**, 1228–35.
8. Johnstone, E.C., Crow, T.J., Frith, C.D., *et al.* (1978). Mechanism of the antipsychotic effect in the treatment of acute schizophrenia. *Lancet*, **i**, 848–51.
9. Johnstone, E.C. (1979). The clinical implications of dopamine receptor blockade in acute schizophrenia. In *Proceedings of an international symposium on neuroleptics and schizophrenia* (ed. J.M. Simister), pp. 21–8. Lundbeck, Luton.
10. May, P.R.A., Tuma, A.H., Yale, C., *et al.* (1976). Schizophrenia: a follow-up study of the results of five forms of treatment. II. Hospital stay over two to five years. *Archives of General Psychiatry*, **33**, 481–6.
11. May, P.R.A., Tuma, A.H., Yale, C., *et al.* (1981). Schizophrenia: a follow-up study of the results of five forms of treatment. *Archives of General Psychiatry*, **38**, 776–84.
12. Crow, T.J. (1980). Molecular pathology of schizophrenia: more than one disease process. *British Medical Journal*, **280**, 66–8.
13. Erhart, S.M., Marder, S.R., and Carpenter, W.T. (2006). Treatment of schizophrenia negative symptoms: future prospects. *Schizophrenia Bulletin*, **32**, 234–371.
14. Cunningham Owens, D.G. (1999). *A guide to the extrapyramidal side-effects of antipsychotic drugs*. Cambridge University Press, Cambridge.
15. Carpenter, W.T., Heinrichs, D.W., and Alphs, L.D. (1985). Treatment of negative symptoms. *Schizophrenia Bulletin*, **11**, 440–52.
16. Carpenter, W.T., Heinrichs, D.W., and Wagman, A.M.I. (1988). Deficit and non-deficit forms of schizophrenia: the concept. *The American Journal of Psychiatry*, **145**, 578–83.
17. Breier, A., Buchanan, R.W., Kirkpatrick, B., *et al.* (1994). Effects of clozapine on positive and negative symptoms in outpatients with schizophrenia. *The American Journal of Psychiatry*, **151**, 20–6.
18. Owens, D.G.C. and Johnstone, E.C. (2006). Precursors and prodromata of schizophrenia: findings from the Edinburgh high risk study and their literature context. *Psychological Medicine*, **36**, 1501–14.
19. King, D.J. (1990). The effects of neuroleptics on cognitive and psychomotor function. *The British Journal of Psychiatry*, **157**, 799–811.
20. King, D.J. (1994). Psychomotor impairment and cognitive disturbances induced by neuroleptics. *Acta Psychiatrica Scandinavica*, **89**(Suppl. 380), 53–8.
21. Harvey, P.D. and McClure, M.M. (2006). Pharmacological approaches to the management of cognitive dysfunction in schizophrenia. *Drugs*, **66**, 1465–73.
22. Harvey, P.D., Patterson, T.L., Potter, L.S., *et al.* (2006). Improvement in social competence with short-term atypical antipsychotic treatment: a randomised, double-blind comparison of quetiapine versus risperidone for social competence, social cognition, and neuropsychological functioning. *The American Journal of Psychiatry*, **163**, 1918–25.
23. Ferreri, F., Agbokou, C., and Gauthier, S. (2006). Cognitive dysfunctions in schizophrenia: potential benefits of cholinesterase inhibitor adjunctive therapy. *Journal of Psychiatry & Neuroscience*, **31**, 369–76.
24. Salminen, J.K., Lehtonen, V., Allonen, H., *et al.* (1980). Sulpiride in depression: plasma levels and effects. *Current Therapeutic Research*, **27**, 109–15.
25. Margakis, B.P. (1990). A double-blind comparison of oral amitriptyline and low-dose intramuscular flupenthixol decanoate in depressive illness. *Current medical Research and Opinion*, **12**, 51–7.
26. Knights, A. and Hirsch, S.R. (1981). 'Revealed' depression and drug treatment for schizophrenia. *Archives of General Psychiatry*, **38**, 806–11.
27. de Alarcon, R. and Carney, M.W.P. (1969). Severe depressive mood changes following slow-release intramuscular fluphenazine injection. *British Medical Journal*, **3**, 564–7.
28. Van Putten, T. and May, P.R.A. (1978). 'Akinetic depression' in schizophrenia. *Archives of General Psychiatry*, **35**, 1101–7.
29. Klein, D. and Davis, J.M. (1969). *Diagnosis and drug treatment of psychiatric disorders*. Williams and Wilkins, Baltimore, MD.
30. Owens, D.G.C. and Johnstone, E.C. (1980). The disabilities of chronic schizophrenia: their nature and factors contributing to their development. *The British Journal of Psychiatry*, **136**, 384–95.
31. Miller, P.M., Johnstone, E.C., Lang, F.H., *et al.* (2000). Differences between patients with schizophrenia within and without a high security psychiatric hospital. *Acta Psychiatrica Scandinavica*, **102**, 12–18.
32. Janicak, P.G., Davis, J.M., Preskorn, S., *et al.* (1993). *Principles and practice of psychopharmacology*. Williams and Wilkins, Baltimore, MD.
33. Johnson, D.A.W. (1979). Further observations on the duration of depot neuroleptic maintenance therapy in schizophrenia. *The British Journal of Psychiatry*, **135**, 524–30.
34. Morgan, R. and Cheadle, J. (1974). Maintenance treatment of chronic schizophrenia with neuroleptic drugs. *Acta Psychiatrica Scandinavica*, **50**, 78–85.
35. Davis, J.M., Shaffer, C.B., Killan, G.A., *et al.* (1980). Important issues in the drug treatment of schizophrenia. *Schizophrenia Bulletin*, **6**, 70–87.
36. Davis, J.M., Metalon, L., Watanabe, M., *et al.* (1993). Depot antipsychotic drugs: place in therapy. *Drugs*, **47**, 741–73.
37. Kane, J.M., Eerdekens, M., Lindenmayer, J.-P., *et al.* (2003). Long-acting injectable risperidone: efficacy and safety of the first long-acting atypical antipsychotic. *The American Journal of Psychiatry*, **160**, 1125–32.
38. Kane, J.M., Rifkin, A., Woerner, M., *et al.* (1983). Low dose neuroleptic treatment of outpatient schizophrenics. *Archives of General Psychiatry*, **40**, 893–6.
39. Baldessarini, R.J., Cohen, B.M., and Teicher, M.H. (1990). Pharmacological treatment. In *Schizophrenia—treatment of acute episodes* (eds. S.T. Levy and P.T. Ninan), pp. 61–118. American Psychiatric Press, Washington, DC.
40. Hirsch, S.R. (1986). Clinical treatment of schizophrenia. In *The psychopharmacology and treatment of schizophrenia* (eds. P.B. Bradley and S.R. Hirsch), pp. 286–339. Oxford University Press, Oxford.
41. Kane, J.M., Honigfeld, G., Singer, J., Meltzer, H.Y., and the Clozaril Collaborative Study Group. (1988). Clozapine for the treatment-resistant schizophrenic: a double-blind comparison with chlorpromazine. *Archives of General Psychiatry*, **45**, 789–96.
42. Wahlbeck, K., Cheine, M.V., and Essali, A. (1999). Clozapine versus typical neuroleptic medication for schizophrenia. *Cochrane Database of Systematic Reviews*, Issue 4. Art. No.: CD000059. DOI: 10.1002/14651858.CD000059.
43. Kingdon, D. (2006). Psychological and social interventions for schizophrenia: robust evidence supports a wide range, including cognitive therapy. *British Medical Journal*, **333**, 212–13.
44. Jones, C., Cormac, I., Silveira de Mota Neto, J.I., *et al.* (2004). Cognitive behaviour therapy for schizophrenia. *Cochrane Database of Systematic Reviews*, Issue 4. Art. No.: CD000524. DOI: 10.1002/14651858.CD000524.pub2.
45. McKenna, P.J. (2006). Cognitive behaviour therapy is not effective. *British Medical Journal*, **333**, 353.
46. Baldwin, S.A., Murray, D.M., and Shadish, W.R. (2005). Empirically supported treatments or type 1 errors? Problems with the analysis of data from group-administered treatments. *Journal of Consulting and Clinical Psychology*, **73**, 924–35.
47. Kemp, R., Kirov, G., Everitt, B., *et al.* (1998). Randomised controlled trial of compliance therapy: 18 month follow-up. *The British Journal of Psychiatry*, **172**, 413–19.
48. McIntosh, A.M., Conlon, L., Lawrie, S.M., *et al.* (2006). Compliance therapy for schizophrenia. *Cochrane Database of Systematic Reviews*, Issue 3. Art. No.: CD003442. DOI: 10.1002/14651858.CD003442.pub2.
49. Rathod, S., Kingdon, D., Smith, P., and Turkington, D. (2005). Insight into schizophrenia: the effects of cognitive behavioural therapy on the components of insight and association with sociodemographics—data on a previously published randomised controlled trial. *Schizophrenia Research*, **74**, 211–19.

50. Carrol, A., Fattah, S., Clyde, Z., *et al.* (1999). Correlates of insight and change in schizophrenia. *Schizophrenia Research*, **35**, 247–53.
51. Hayes, R.L. and McGrath, J.J. (2000). Cognitive rehabilitation for people with schizophrenia and related conditions. *Cochrane Database for Systematic Reviews*, (3), CD000968. DOI: 10.1002/14651858.CD000968.
52. Malmberg, L. and Fenton, M. (2001). Individual psychodynamic psychotherapy and psychoanalysis for schizophrenia and severe mental illness. *Cochrane Database of Systematic Reviews*, Issue 3. Art. No.: CD001360. DOI: 10.1002/14651858.CD001360.
53. Robertson, L., Connaughton, J., and Nicol, M. (1998). Life skills programmes for chronic mental illnesses. *Cochrane Database of Systematic Reviews*, Issue 3. Art. No.: CD000381. DOI: 10.1002/14651858.CD000381.
54. Eckman, T.A., Wirshing, W.C., Marder, S.R., *et al.* (1992). Technique for training schizophrenic patients in illness self-management: a controlled trial. *The American Journal of Psychiatry*, **149**, 1549–55.
55. Linszen, D., Dingemans, P., Van der Does, J.W., *et al.* (1996). Treatment, expressed emotion and relapse in recent onset schizophrenic disorders. *Psychological Medicine*, **26**, 333–42.
56. Crowther, R., Marshall, M., Bond, G., *et al.* (2001). Vocational rehabilitation for people with severe mental illness. *Cochrane Database of Systematic Reviews*, Issue 2. Art. No.: CD003080; DOI: 10.1002/14651858.CD003080.
57. Pekkala, E. and Merinder, L. (2002). Psychoeducation for schizophrenia. *Cochrane Database of Systematic Reviews*, Issue 2. Art. No.: CD002831.DOI: 10.1002/14651858.CD002831.
58. Leff, J., Kuipers, L., Berkowitz, R., *et al.* (1982). A controlled trial of social intervention in the families of schizophrenic patients. *The British Journal of Psychiatry*, **141**, 121–34.
59. Pharoah, F., Mari, J., Rathbone, J., *et al.* (2006). Family intervention for schizophrenia. *Cochrane Database of Systematic Reviews*, Issue 4. Art. No. CD000088. DOI: 10.1002/14651858.CD000088.pub2.
60. Tyrer, P., Coid, J., Simmonds, S., *et al.* (1998). Community mental health teams (CHMTs) for people with severe mental illnesses and disordered personality. *Cochrane Database of Systematic Reviews*, Issue 4. Art. No. CD000270. DOI: 10.1002/14651858. CD000270.
61. Marks, I.M., Connolly, J., Muijen, M., *et al.* (1994). Home-based versus hospital-based care for people with serious mental illness. *The British Journal of Psychiatry*, **164**, 179–94.
62. Grawe, R.W., Falloon, I.R.H., Widen, J.H., *et al.* (2006). Two years of continued early treatment for recent-onset schizophrenia: a randomised controlled study. *Acta Psychiatrica Scandinavica*, **114**, 328–36.
63. Audini, B., Marks, I.M., Lawrence, R.E., Connolly, J., and Watts, V. (1994). Home-based versus out-patient/in-patient care for people with serious mental illness. Phase II of a controlled study. *The British Journal of Psychiatry*, **164**, 204–10.
64. Harrison, J., Alam, N., and Marshall, J. (2001). Home or away: which patients are suitable for a psychiatric home treatment service. *Psychiatric Bulletin*, **25**, 310–13.
65. Fitzgerald, P. and Kulkarni, J. (1998). Home-oriented management programme for people with early psychosis. *The British Journal of Psychiatry*, **172**(Suppl. 33), 39–44.
66. Marshall, M., Gray, A., Lockwood, A., *et al.* (1998). Case management for people with severe mental disorders. *Cochrane Database of Systemic Reviews*, Issue 2. Art. No.: CD000050. DOI: 10.1002/14651858.CD000050.
67. Marshall, M. and Lockwood, A. (1998). Assertive community treatment for people with severe mental disorders. *Cochrane Database of Systematic Reviews*, Issue 2. Art. No.: CD001089. DOI: 10.1002/14651858.CD001089.
68. Rosen, A. and Teesson, M. (2001). Does case management work? The evidence and the abuse of evidence-based medicine. *The Australian and New Zealand Journal of Psychiatry*, **35**, 731–46.
69. Rosenheck, R.A., Perlick, D., Bingham, S., *et al.* (2003). Effectiveness and cost of olanzapine and haloperidol in the treatment of schizophrenia: a randomised controlled trial. *The Journal of the American Medical Association*, **290**, 2693–702.
70. Strakowski, S.M., Johnson, J.L., DelBello, M.P., *et al.* (2005). Quality of life during treatment with haloperidol or olanzapine in the year following a first psychotic episode. *Schizophrenia Research*, **78**, 161–9.
71. Jones, P.B., Barnes, T.R.E., Davis, L., et al. (2006). Randomised controlled trial of the effect on quality of life of second-vs-first generation antipsychotic drugs in schizophrenia: Cost Utility of the Latest Antipsychotic Drugs in Schizophrenia Study (CUtLASS 1). *Archives of General Psychiatry*, **63**, 1079–87.
72. Lieberman, J.A., Stroup, T.S., McEvoy, J.P., *et al.* (2005). Effectiveness of antipsychotic drugs in patients with chronic schizophrenia. *The New England Journal of Medicine*, **353**, 1209–23.
73. Rosenheck, R.A., Leslie, D.L., Sindelar, J., *et al.* (2006). Cost-effectiveness of second-generation antipsychotics and perphenazine in a randomised trial of treatment for chronic schizophrenia. *The American Journal of Psychiatry*, **163**, 2080–9.
74. Baldessarini, R.J., Katz, B., and Cotton, P. (1984). Dissimilar dosing with high-potency and low-potency neuroleptics. *The American Journal of Psychiatry*, **141**, 748–52.
75. Oosthuizen, P., Emsley, R.A., Turner, J., *et al.* (2001). Determining the optimal dose of haloperidol in first-episode psychosis. *Journal of Psychopharmacology*, **15**, 251–5.
76. Kapur, S., Zipursky, R., Roy, P., *et al.* (1997). The relationship between D2 receptor occupancy and plasma levels on low dose oral haloperidol: a PET study. *Psychopharmacology*, **131**, 148–52.
77. Taylor, D., Kerwin, R., and Paton, C. (eds.) (2005). *The Maudsley 2005–2006 prescribing guidelines*. Taylor and Francis, London.
78. Whicher, E., Morrison, M., and Douglas-Hall, P. (2002). 'As required' medication regimes for seriously mentally ill people in hospital. *Cochrane Database of Systemic Reviews*, Issue 1. Art. No.: CD003441. DOI: 10.1002/14651858. CD003441.
79. Lieberman, J., Jody, D., Geisler, S., *et al.* (1993). Time course and biologic correlates of treatment response in first-episode schizophrenia. *Archives of General Psychiatry*, **50**, 369–76.
80. Bishop, M.P., Gallant, D.M., and Sykes, T.F. (1965). Extrapyramidal side effects and therapeutic response. *Archives of General Psychiatry*, **13**, 155–61.
81. Johnstone, E.C., Macmillan, F.J., Frith, C.D., *et al.* (1990). Further investigations of the predictors of outcome following first schizophrenic episodes. *The British Journal of Psychiatry*, **157**, 182–9.
82. Birchwood, M., Iqbal, Z., Chadwick, P., *et al.* (2000). Cognitive approach to depression and suicidal thinking in psychosis. I. Ontogeny of post-psychotic depression. *The British Journal of Psychiatry*, **177**, 516–21.
83. Siris, S.H., Morgan, V., Fagerstrom, R., *et al.* (1987). Adjunctive imipramine in the treatment of post-psychotic depression: a con trolled study. *Archives of General Psychiatry*, **44**, 533–9.
84. Siris, S.H., Pollack, S., Bermanzohn, P., *et al.* (2000). Adjunctive imipramine for a broader group of post-psychotic depressions in schizophrenia. *Schizophrenia Research*, **44**, 187–92.
85. McGlashan, T.H. (1999). Duration of untreated psychosis in first episode schizophrenia: marker or determinant of course. *Biological Psychiatry*, **46**, 899–907.
86. Lieberman, J.A. (1999). Is schizophrenia a neurodegenerative disorder? A clinical and neurobiological perspective. *Biological Psychiatry*, **46**, 729–39.
87. Marshall, M., Lockwood, A., Lewis, S., *et al.* (2004). Essential elements of an early intervention service for psychosis: the opinions of expert clinicians. *BMC Psychiatry*, **4**.
88. Marshall, M., Lewis, S., Lockwood, A., *et al.* (2005). Association between duration of untreated psychosis and outcome in cohorts of first-episode patients: a systematic review. *Archives of General Psychiatry*, **62**, 975–83.

89. Perkins, D.O., Gu, H., Boteva, K., *et al.* (2005). Relationship between duration of untreated psychosis and outcome in first-episode schizophrenia: a critical review and meta-analysis. *The American Journal of Psychiatry*, **162**, 1785–804.
90. Owens, D.G.C., Miller, P., Lawrie, S.M., *et al.* (2005). Pathogenesis of schizophrenia: a psychopathological perspective. *The British Journal of Psychiatry*, **186**, 386–93.
91. Stroup, T.S., Lieberman, J.A., McEvoy, J.P., *et al.* (2006). Effectiveness of olanzapine, quetiapine, risperidone and ziprasidone in patients with chronic schizophrenia following discontinuation of a previous atypical antipsychotic. *The American Journal of Psychiatry*, **163**, 611–22.
92. Johnstone, E.C., Crow, T.J., Frith, C.D., *et al.* (1988). The Northwick Park 'functional' psychosis study: diagnosis and treatment response. *Lancet*, **ii**, 119–26.
93. Leucht, S., McGrath, J., and Kissling, W. (2003). Lithium for schizophrenia. *Cochrane Database of Systematic Reviews*, Issue 3. Art. No.: CD003834. DOI: 10.1002/14651858.CD003834.
94. Basan, A. and Leucht, S. (2003). Valproate for schizophrenia. *Cochrane Database of Systematic Reviews*, Issue 3. Art. No.: CD004028. DOI: 10.1002/14651858.CD004028.pub2.
95. Leucht, S., McGrath, J., White, P., *et al.* (2002). Carbamazepine for schizophrenia and schizoaffective psychoses. *Cochrane Database of Systematic Reviews*, Issue 3. Art. No.: CD001258. DOI: 10.1002/14651858.CD001258.
96. Premkumar, T.S. and Pick, J. (2006). Lamotrigine for schizophrenia. *Cochrane Database of Systematic Reviews*, Issue 4. Art. No.: CD005962. DOI: 10.1002/14651858.CD005962.pub2.
97. Volz, A., Khorsand, V., Gillies, D., *et al.* (2007). Benzodiazepines for schizophrenia. *Cochrane Database of Systematic Reviews*, Issue 1. Art. No.: CD006391. DOI: 10.1002/14651858.CD006391.
98. Tharyan, P. and Adams, C.E. (2005). Electroconvulsive therapy for schizophrenia. *Cochrane Database of Systematic Reviews*, Issue 2. Art. No.: CD000076. DOI: 10.1002/14651858.CD000076.pub2.
99. Pilling, S., Bebbington, P., Kuipers, E., *et al.* (2002). Psychological treatments in schizophrenia. I. Meta-analysis of family intervention and cognitive behaviour therapy. *Psychological Medicine*, **32**, 763–82.

4.3.9 Schizoaffective and schizotypal disorders

Ming T. Tsuang, William S. Stone, and Stephen V. Faraone

Introduction

This chapter focuses on two disorders in the schizophrenia 'spectrum': schizoaffective disorder and schizotypal personality disorder. The emphasis includes the clinical features, classification, diagnosis, epidemiology, aetiology, course, prognosis, and possibilities for prevention for each disorder. Some aspects will be underscored to reflect controversial issues, such as the heterogeneity apparent in each condition. Such issues relate to the accurate classification of the disorders, which is important for at least two reasons. First, it is essential to develop reliable and valid diagnostic criteria in order to study the aetiology of the disorders and then utilize that knowledge to develop rational and testable intervention strategies. Heterogeneity adds variance to the process that reduces both the reliability of diagnosis and also the statistical power of experimental designs to detect intervention/treatment effects. Second, the development of newer generations of psychopharmacological treatments holds the promise of matching more appropriate and efficacious medications with specific syndromes or types of symptoms. This trend underscores the importance of differential diagnosis in determining what treatment a patient will receive. Heterogeneity within a diagnostic category complicates achievement of this goal. Another area to be emphasized involves the goal of early interventions, in addition to palliative treatments for these disorders. In contrast, other areas such as the genetic aetiology of schizoaffective disorder and schizotypal personality disorder, and treatments for schizoaffective disorder, will receive less emphasis here, to avoid redundancies with other chapters in this volume. Each disorder will be considered separately, starting with a review of schizoaffective disorder, the more severe of the two spectrum conditions.

Schizoaffective disorder

Clinical features

Schizoaffective disorder afflicts patients having schizophrenic and affective symptoms. Either they have affective symptoms of sufficient severity and chronicity to exclude an uncomplicated diagnosis of schizophrenia, or they show features of schizophrenia that are sufficient to exclude an uncomplicated diagnosis of an affective disorder.[(1)] These types of symptoms may or may not occur simultaneously, which underscores the importance of viewing the course of the illness longitudinally in addition to its cross-sectional presentation. Symptom clusters that are primarily affective or primarily schizophrenic predominate at different times.

Compared to patients with schizophrenia, patients with schizoaffective disorder often (though not always) demonstrate relatively high levels of premorbid function,[(2,3)] but nevertheless show significant premorbid weaknesses in multiple cognitive and clinical functions.[(4)] Patients with schizoaffective disorder also tend to show more identifiable precipitating events. The nature of the precipitating stressor may vary widely; for example it may be physical (e.g. recently giving birth or experiencing a head injury) or interpersonal (e.g. change in an important relationship). The clinical course of the disorder is often characterized by a periodic, rapid onset of symptoms that shows a relatively high degree of remission after several weeks or months. As Vaillant pointed out in the 1960s, many of these patients 'recover' completely after an episode, and resume their lives at premorbid levels of function.[(5)] As will be noted further below, the clinical features of some cases of schizoaffective disorder mainly resemble those of schizophrenia, while the features of other cases are more similar to those of bipolar disorder. Regardless of the subtype or variant of the disorder, however, the mortality rate is of special concern. Rates of death due mainly to suicide or accident show elevations in this disorder that are similar to those observed in schizophrenia and in major affective disorders.[(6)]

In general, schizoaffective disorder is more common in females than in males.[(3)] The age of onset varies, but tends to be younger than that of unipolar or bipolar disorder. Tsuang *et al.* found the median age of onset for schizoaffective disorder was 29 years, which was significantly lower than groups with bipolar or unipolar affective disorder, but similar to a group with schizophrenia.

Marneros *et al.*[2] also reported that a median age of onset of 29 years for schizoaffective disorder was lower than the median age for groups with affective disorders (35 years), but reported that it was higher than a group with schizophrenia (24 years). In contrast, Reichenberg *et al.*[4] reported no differences in the age of first hospitalization between patients with schizophrenia, schizoaffective disorder, or non-psychotic bipolar disorder. These differences between studies reflect differences in both the diagnostic criteria employed, and the heterogeneity of the disorder.

Classification

The classification of schizoaffective disorder has always been controversial. Kraepelin reported in 1919 that patients with both affective and schizophrenic symptoms complicated the differential diagnosis due to the 'mingling of morbid symptoms of both psychoses'. Kasanin first employed the term 'acute schizophrenic psychoses' in 1933 to describe a group of patients who experienced a rapid onset of emotional turmoil and psychotic symptoms, but who recovered after several weeks or months.[3] In other words, the symptoms appeared similar to schizophrenia during periods of exacerbation, but unlike schizophrenia, they showed a greater tendency to remit between episodes. These features sparked an ongoing debate by the 1960s about the proper classification of schizoaffective disorder. Much of this discussion involved the following proposals:

1 It was a type of schizophrenia (e.g. 'remitting schizophrenia');

2 It was a type of affective disorder;

3 It was a unique disorder that was separate from both schizophrenia and bipolar disorder;

4 It reflected an arbitrary categorization of clinical symptoms that masked a continuum of pathology between schizophrenia and affective illness;

5 It contained a heterogeneous collection of 'interforms' between schizophrenia and affective disorder (i.e. symptoms of both disorders).

The last possibility is not mutually exclusive of the first four; for example, one or more variants of schizoaffective disorder may be related closely to schizophrenia, while another may be related more closely to an affective disorder.

The puzzle has yet to be solved. Family and outcome studies provide useful ways of assessing the relative merits of each of the possibilities outlined above. These approaches are informative and will be reviewed below, although interpretations of such studies are complicated at times by the use of different diagnostic criteria across investigations.

(a) Family studies

Family studies provide an important tool for assessing the relationship between disorders. They are a type of genetic study that assumes that related disorders will co-aggregate more frequently among biologically related individuals than they would in the general population. Thus, a disorder is more likely to be in the schizophrenia spectrum if it occurs more frequently among the relatives of schizophrenic patients, compared with suitable controls. Similarly, a disorder is more likely to be in the affective spectrum if it occurs more frequently among the relatives of patients with affective disorders. Evidence for the inclusion of schizoaffective disorder in the schizophrenia spectrum is discussed in greater detail elsewhere (see Chapter 4.3.6.1). Only representative findings pertinent to the present discussion about the classification of schizoaffective disorder will be summarized here.

Bertelsen and Gottesman[7] summarized a series of seven family studies published between 1979 and 1993, using structured diagnostic criteria. Analyses of risk to the development of schizophrenia, schizoaffective disorder, and affective disorder in the first-degree relatives of patients with schizoaffective disorder, were included. In all seven studies, the relatives showed a higher risk of developing an affective disorder than of developing schizoaffective disorder. In five of the seven studies the risks of developing schizophrenia was equal to or greater than the risk of developing schizoaffective disorder. Thus, the relatives of schizoaffective patients showed generally higher risks of developing disorders other than the one with which they were diagnosed. These findings were consistent with a heterogeneous view of schizoaffective disorder, in which individual cases represented subtypes of either schizophrenia or of affective disorder. The findings were also consistent with the possibility that schizoaffective disorder represents a chance collection of 'interforms' between schizophrenia and affective disorder.

These findings were not consistent with the view that schizoaffective disorder represented a continuum between the other two disorders, because in that case, the rate of schizoaffective disorder in first-degree relatives would have been higher, compared with the rates at which these relatives developed schizophrenia or affective disorder. The findings were also inconsistent with the possibility that schizoaffective disorder represented a unique disorder that was independent of either schizophrenia or an affective disorder. In that case, the first-degree relatives of patients with schizoaffective disorder should show relatively high rates of schizoaffective disorder itself, but relatively low rates of the other disorders. In the series of studies reviewed by Bertelsen and Gottesman,[7] the morbid risk for schizoaffective disorder itself ranged from 1.8 to 6.1 per cent in first-degree relatives of patients with schizoaffective disorder, which was still higher than the rate observed in the general population (see the section on epidemiology below). These results, taken together with the higher risks for both schizophrenia and affective disorder, suggest that schizoaffective disorder is a heterogeneous condition. Recent reviews of family studies, including those that considered depressed (i.e. unipolar) and bipolar subtypes, have also underscored both the heterogeneity of schizoaffective disorder, and the controversial nature of its classification.[8,9]

(b) Outcome studies

A majority of outcome studies show that schizoaffective disorder has a better course than schizophrenia, but a poorer course than affective disorder.[10–12] For example, Tsuang and colleagues reviewed 10 outcome studies reported between 1963 and 1987 that assessed patients with either schizoaffective disorder or schizophrenia.[10] Global, marital, social, occupational, hospital course, and symptom dimensions of outcome were measured. In each category, patients with schizophrenia showed poorer outcomes. In contrast, their review of 11 outcome studies comparing schizoaffective disorder with affective disorder showed that affective disorder was associated with equal or better outcomes on almost all dimensions. Thus, despite differences in methodology and diagnostic criteria, schizoaffective disorder was frequently associated with clinical outcomes that were intermediate between those associated with schizophrenia and those related to affective disorder.

Other researchers reported similar findings. Kendler *et al.*, for example, showed intermediate levels of clinical impairment for schizoaffective disorder in an epidemiological family study.[13] Marneros *et al.* reported on outcomes as part of the Cologne Longitudinal study, using modified DSM-III-R diagnoses.[14] The outcomes were measured by symptoms in five dimensions (psychotic symptoms, reduction of energetic potential, qualitative and quantitative disturbances of affect, and other disturbances of behaviour) that persisted for at least 3 years. Consistent with the pattern described thus far, poor outcomes in the schizoaffective group occurred at a rate (49.5 per cent of the sample) that was intermediate between those observed in the schizophrenic (93.2 per cent) and affective groups (35.8 per cent), and differed significantly from both of them. In a more recent study, Jäger *et al.* studied 241 patients at the time of their first hospitalization, and then again 15 years later.[15] Similar to these other examples, schizoaffective subjects presented a clinical picture that was less impaired than the one shown by schizophrenic subjects, but more impaired than the one shown by affective subjects.

While these studies show schizoaffective disorder to have intermediate outcomes generally, there are categories in which it resembles schizophrenia or affective disorder more closely. For example, Samson *et al.*[10] and Reinares *et al.*[12] noted that outcomes for schizoaffective disorder were equivalent to those for affective disorder in several dimensions. Marneros *et al.*, showed that 70 per cent of a schizoaffective group was rated as good or excellent on a measure of social adjustment, which did not differ significantly from 84 per cent of an affective group who received the same rating.[12] Both groups differed significantly from a schizophrenic group, however, in which only 44 per cent of the group demonstrated good or excellent outcomes. Moreover, the schizoaffective and affective disorder groups did not differ on a rating scale of psychological impairments (e.g. body language, affect display, conversation skills, and cooperation), although both were rated as significantly less impaired than the schizophrenic group.

Other studies, however, such as Kendler *et al.*[13] reported similarities between some types of psychotic symptoms in schizoaffective disorder and schizophrenia, including the severity of delusions and positive thought disorder, and the frequency of hallucinations. Each of these groups showed higher levels of these symptoms than an affective disorders group. Hizdon *et al.* showed recently that individuals with schizoaffective disorder did not differ from individuals with schizophrenia on basic cognitive measures of executive function, memory, and processing speed, although the schizoaffective group did perform better on measures of social cognition.[16] Reichenberg *et al.* showed that individuals with schizophrenia and schizoaffective disorder who were assessed premorbidly performed similar to each other but lower than individuals who later developed non-psychotic bipolar disorder, on tests of non-verbal and verbal intellectual function, and on tests of basic reading and reading comprehension.[4]

These overall differences in outcome serve to validate the classification of schizoaffective disorder as a separate syndrome further. Its heterogeneity, however, raises the issue of whether such intermediate outcomes might reflect the mean of a combination of mainly good and mainly poor outcomes. This in turn leads to the question of whether schizoaffective disorder can be subtyped in a useful and valid manner. If so, are better and worse outcomes associated with different variants of the syndrome?

Vaillant suggested in the 1960s that prognostic indicators, including a good premorbid level of adjustment, the presence of precipitating factors, an acute onset, confusion, the presence of affective symptoms, and a familial history of affective disorder (or the absence of a schizophrenic history), could predict remission in approximately 80 per cent of cases of 'remitting schizophrenia'.[17] The inclusion of affective symptoms and a positive family history for affective illness on the list contributed (later) to hypotheses that variants of schizoaffective disorder were related to affective illness and to better outcomes. In contrast, variants associated more with schizophrenic symptoms or family history were associated more with schizophrenia and with relatively poor outcomes.[18]

There have been a variety of attempts to subtype schizoaffective disorders, based on whether affective or schizophrenic symptoms predominate. The validity of many of these attempts, however, is inconclusive. Bertelsen and Gottesman noted, for example, that at best, relatives of individuals with affective type schizoaffective disorder, or schizophrenic type schizoaffective disorder, showed only trends towards higher rates of affective disorder or schizophrenia, respectively.[7] Similarly, Kendler *et al.* did not detect different rates of schizophrenia or affective illness in first-degree relatives of patients with schizoaffective disorder when the patients were subtyped into bipolar and depressive subgroups.[13] Moreover, the subtypes did not predict differences in outcomes.

Conversely, a latent class analysis of psychotic patients from the Roscommon study showed that most cases of DSM-III-R schizoaffective disorder were categorized in either a bipolar schizomania class ($n = 19$), or in a schizodepression class ($n = 13$), rather than in schizophrenia ($n = 1$), major depression ($n = 0$), schizophreniform ($n = 3$), or hebephrenia ($n = 3$) classes.[19] Moreover, Reinares *et al.* reviewed evidence showing that bipolar and depressive subtypes differed from each other in ways consistent with differences between bipolar and unipolar affective disorders.[12] For example, the bipolar schizoaffective subtype was associated with more total episodes, more episodes with shorter periods and cycles, and higher frequency of cycles. Higher numbers of cycles were associated with poorer long-term outcomes. Taken together, these studies show at least some recent support for the subtyping of schizoaffective disorder into mainly affective and mainly schizophrenic variants.

Other factors associated with poor outcomes include poor inter-episode recoveries,[13] persistent psychotic symptoms in the absence of affective features, poor premorbid social adjustment, chronicity, a higher number of schizophrenia-like symptoms,[20] and the presence of schizoaffective mixed states.[12]

Diagnosis and differential diagnosis

The DSM-IV diagnosis of schizoaffective disorder[1] is listed in the category of 'schizophrenia and other psychotic disorders'. The major feature of the disorder is that, in addition to meeting the clinical criteria for schizophrenia (criterion A), an individual must also experience a major depressive, manic, or mixed episode concurrently. In addition, in the same period of illness, a patient must experience symptoms of psychosis (hallucinations and/or delusions) for a period of at least 2 weeks, in the absence of mood-related symptoms (criterion B). Nevertheless, affective symptoms must comprise a substantial portion of total duration of the illness (criterion C), and symptoms may not be attributable to either substance use or to a major medical condition (criterion D). Two subtypes of the disorder, including bipolar type and depressive type, may be diagnosed.

The criteria for schizoaffective disorder in ICD-10 are similar to those in DSM-IV. The essential requirement is that prominent symptoms of affective disorder and prominent symptoms of schizophrenia are present together for at least 2 weeks. Depressive, manic, and mixed subtypes are recognized.

The differential diagnosis includes, most prominently, either schizophrenia or affective disorder, which may be differentiated in part by consideration of the longitudinal criteria (criteria B and C), in addition to the cross-sectional criteria (criterion A). The presence of conditions relating to general medication and substance use should also be considered in the differential diagnosis.

Epidemiology

The epidemiological status of schizoaffective disorder is somewhat uncertain compared with schizophrenia, largely because of dilemmas related to the diagnosis and classification of the disorder. To help in the standardization of data from different studies, representative incidence and prevalence estimates will be emphasized from recent investigations that utilized research diagnostic, DSM-III-R or DSM-IV criteria.

(a) Incidence

Earlier studies showed that new cases of 'schizomanic' patients (i.e. manic patients who also demonstrated schizophrenic or paranoid symptoms) numbered approximately 1.7 per 100 000 per year.[(20)] This was less than the 4 per 100 000 per year shown by 'schizodepressive' patients. The number of schizoaffective cases in this study exceeded the number of manic patients, and made up half of the number of schizophrenic cases. Since then, Tien and Eaton analysed data from the Epidemiologic Catchment Area study for three non-overlapping groups with psychotic symptoms.[(21)] One of these groups comprised individuals with 'psychotic affective syndrome', which was similar to schizoaffective disorder except that most members of the group (59 per cent) demonstrated psychotic symptoms only in conjunction with a mood disturbance (essentially DSM-III-R mood disturbance with psychotic symptoms). The incidence of this disorder was 1.7 per 1000 per year, which was approximately equal to the rate for schizophrenia (2.0 per 1000 per year). Even if the 59 per cent of the group who met the criteria for a mood disorder with psychotic features was excluded, the remaining 41 per cent would still comprise a higher incidence rate than that detected by earlier studies. Differences in sampling procedures (treated versus non-treated samples) may have contributed to the differences observed in the rates. More importantly, however, these studies showed that schizoaffective disorder occurred at 50 to 85 per cent of the rate of schizophrenia, thus confirming that patients with this disorder comprise a clinically significant population. One current but long-standing issue involves questions about the temporal stability of incidence rates in schizophrenia-related disorders, as reflected by reports of both increases and decreases.

(b) Prevalence

Until recently, prevalence estimates for schizoaffective disorder relied mainly on samples that were treated in clinics or other psychiatric settings. Because a variety of factors influence the decision to enter and remain in treatment, the estimates varied substantially. For example, Okasha reviewed studies that reported rates varying between 2 and 29 per cent.[(8)] A recent epidemiological study in Finland using 8028 people who were at least 30 years old showed a lifetime prevalence rate of 0.32 per cent for schizoaffective disorder (compared to 0.87 per cent for schizophrenia), which accounted for 10.5 per cent of all psychotic disorders.[(22)] This is a lower estimate than many earlier studies reported, and likely results from a combination of factors (including a narrowing of diagnostic criteria, and increased utilization of multiple sources of information such as case notes and registers, in addition to interview data) that together have improved diagnostic accuracy. Prevalence estimates of putative schizoaffective subtypes remain subject to the same inconsistencies of diagnosis and selection factors that affect schizoaffective disorder itself. Not surprisingly, there is little consensus about whether manic or schizophrenic subtypes predominate (see also Tsuang *et al.*[(20)]).

(c) Review of evidence

Treatments for schizoaffective disorder are the same as those for schizophrenia and affective disorders alone. As the nature and efficacy of those treatments are discussed elsewhere, they will not be considered here. Rather, this section will focus on management issues related to the need to treat symptoms of both disorders simultaneously, or sequentially.

Management

The authors have found it useful to consider psychopharmacological treatment in terms of putative subtypes, including affective type schizoaffective disorder and schizophrenic type schizoaffective disorder.

Treatment of schizoaffective disorder, affective subtype, will include antipsychotic medication (e.g. clozapine, risperidone quetiapine, ziprasidone, or olanzepine), particularly if psychotic symptoms are present. In addition, antidepressants, mood stabilizers (e.g. lithium), or anticonvulsants (e.g. valproate or carbamazepine) may be useful with this group. It will be necessary in such cases to weigh the potential risks of such medications, such as elevated toxicity, against the potential benefits.

In schizoaffective disorder, schizophrenic subtype, combination treatments may also be more effective than a single treatment. We find, however, that antipsychotic treatments alone may be more efficient in many cases. This is particularly true if affective symptoms (i.e. depression) are largely secondary to the experience of having a psychotic condition, and its attendant interpersonal, social, and financial difficulties. In these cases, remediation of the psychotic symptoms may also have the effect of easing the affective problems. For other cases, which include more of a treatment-refractory depression, antipsychotic medication may be augmented with lithium (or another mood stabilizer) or antidepressant medication. Moreover, electroconvulsive therapy may reduce mortality rates in schizoaffective patients.

The authors note that it may be difficult at times to distinguish the affective subtype from the schizophrenic subtype, especially in the presence of florid psychotic symptoms. In these cases, treatment decisions may rest on the presenting symptoms of the patient. Treatment during intermorbid periods is in part dependent on the presence or absence of psychotic symptoms. As noted above, psychotic episodes in this period are associated with relatively poorer outcomes, and are likely to require chronic antipsychotic therapy.

Schizotypal personality disorder

Clinical features

Like schizoaffective disorder, schizotypal personality disorder is a complex and chronic condition that includes some, but not all, of the features of schizoaffective disorder and schizophrenia. Most notably, persistent psychosis is not part of the syndrome, although mild forms of thought disorder may occur, such as magical thinking or ideas of reference (as opposed to delusions of reference, which indicate psychosis). Moreover, brief episodes of psychosis may occur in times of stress, but will not persist.

Schizotypal patients show pervasive deficits in social and interpersonal traits. They often demonstrate aloofness, poor eye contact, affective constriction, and suspiciousness. Consequently, close interpersonal relationships are either avoided, or cause discomfort and anxiety. These individuals usually have few friends. Not surprisingly, schizotypal patients are often deficient in accurately sensing social cues or affective signals from others. Although they can interact with people when necessary, they often prefer not to, and do not become more comfortable in social situations with time.

Schizotypal patients may also show magical thinking, ideas of reference, unusual perceptions (e.g. sensing the presence of another person, or that people are talking about them), and/or perceptual illusions (e.g. often perceiving a dimly lit lamp-post as a person). Both their social deficits and these cognitive–perceptual problems contribute to an overall impression of oddness. However, this feature may occur independently of other clinical symptoms,[(23)] and manifest itself in odd speech or unusual appearance. The oddness or eccentricities evident in these patients are often ego syntonic (i.e. they are not experienced as problems). Moreover, schizotypal patients show deficits in attention, long-term verbal memory, and executive functions. These deficits are qualitatively similar to those seen in schizophrenia (and schizoaffective disorder), but like many other clinical manifestations of this disorder, they are quantitatively milder.

Like schizophrenia, schizotypal personality disorder is often evident by early adulthood, but schizotypal traits may be evident in late childhood or adolescence. Once it appears, the disorder tends to show a chronic course, but one that includes periodic exacerbations and attenuations of symptoms. A recent study that followed individuals with schizotypal personality disorder for 2 years showed that paranoid thoughts and unusual perceptual experiences were among the most stable and least malleable DSM-IV symptoms, while the most changeable were odd behaviours and restricted affect.[(24)] The former symptoms were thus more trait-like, and the latter were more intermittent. Consistent with these findings, the same group also showed that in the course of 2 years (with treatment), 61 per cent of schizotypal patients no longer met DSM-IV diagnostic criteria for the disorder.[(25)] With a more stringent definition of improvement (12 months with two or less symptoms meeting criteria), the rate of remission dropped to 23 per cent. These studies show that both the severity and the expression of the disorder vary over time and probably, as a function of treatment.

Classification

In contrast to the controversy surrounding the classification of schizoaffective disorder, family, twin, and adoption studies clearly support the view that schizotypal personality disorder is best classified in the schizophrenia spectrum.[(26)] Nevertheless, it is a complex and chronic disorder that in all likelihood, is also heterogeneous. Kendler pointed out that this heterogeneity was at least partly related to the two primary methods used to study the disorder.[(27)] One of these involves the 'clinical method', which identifies patients with mild forms of schizophrenic or psychotic-like symptoms. This type of patient, for example, is often characterized by relatively high levels of positive psychiatric symptoms (e.g. magical thinking and perceptual distortions).

In contrast, the 'family research method' identifies relatives of patients with schizophrenia who have subtle, schizophrenia-like symptoms. Features associated more with familial than with clinical schizotypal personality disorder include a predominance of negative symptoms (e.g. social withdrawal and impairment, and higher levels of anxiety and poor rapport), cognitive impairments (e.g. impaired language comprehension, eye-tracking, and attentional dysfunctions), and elevated rates of schizophrenia and related disorders in family members.[(26)] Thaker *et al.* reported that familial and clinical schizotypal personality disorders were similar on measures of physical or social anhedonia,[(28)] and that some neuropsychological deficits were also associated with both groups.[(26)]

The concept of familial schizotypal disorder is particularly important because it may share a common genetic basis with schizophrenia. Paul Meehl first proposed the term 'schizotaxia' to describe the genetic vulnerability to schizophrenia, and suggested that individuals with schizotaxia would eventually develop either schizotypal personality disorder or schizophrenia, depending on the protection or liability afforded by environmental circumstances. As the concept evolved, Meehl reformulated it to allow for the possibility that some people with schizotaxia would develop neither schizophrenia nor schizotypal personality disorder. In fact, evidence now shows that the clinical symptoms observed in many non-psychotic, first-degree relatives of people with schizophrenia are similar to those observed in familial schizotypal personality disorder.[(26)] Psychiatric features in such relatives frequently include an aggregation of negative symptoms that are qualitatively similar to, but milder than, those often cited in schizophrenia.[(29)] Positive symptoms, however, are usually less evident in these relatives than they are in schizophrenia or in schizotypal personality disorder. Neuropsychological impairments in biological relatives of people with schizophrenia are also qualitatively similar to, but milder than, those seen in people with schizophrenia.[(26)] In particular, these neuropsychological deficits frequently include problems in working memory/attention, long-term verbal memory, and concept formation/abstraction.

Faraone *et al.* recently suggested a reformulation of Meehl's concept of schizotaxia that focuses on these features of negative symptoms and neuropsychological deficits.[(26)] Unlike schizotypal personality disorder, which occurs in less than 10 per cent of the adult relatives of patients diagnosed with schizophrenia, the basic symptoms of schizotaxia occur in 20 to 50 per cent of adult relatives, suggesting further that the genetic liability to schizophrenia does not lead inevitably to schizophrenia, schizotypal personality disorder, or schizoid personality disorder.

Diagnosis and differential diagnosis

The DSM-IV criteria for schizotypal personality disorder include a 'pervasive pattern of social deficits' and 'cognitive or perceptual distortions' and behavioural 'eccentricities' (criterion A).[1] At least five of nine specific symptoms (e.g. ideas of reference, constricted affect, odd behaviour, or appearance) must be present to satisfy this criterion. These symptoms must occur by early adulthood. They must not occur exclusively during the course of four other conditions, including schizophrenia, a mood disorder with psychotic features, any other psychotic disorder, or a pervasive developmental disorder (criterion B).

The differential diagnosis includes a variety of other disorders. A key difference between schizotypal personality disorder and schizophrenia, a psychotic mood disorder, or another psychotic condition involves the transient nature of psychotic symptoms in schizotypal personality disorder. It may be distinguished from developmental communication disorders by a lack of compensatory means (e.g. gestures) of communicating, and it may be distinguished from autistic or Asperger's disorders by the relatively greater deficits in social awareness and frequent presence of stereotyped behaviours in those syndromes. Schizotypal personality disorder may be confused with several other personality disorders, but can be distinguished from them. In particular, it differs from schizoid personality disorder by its pattern of cognitive–perceptual distortions, and by the odd appearance or behaviour shown frequently by schizotypal patients. The pattern of schizotypal symptoms also differs from that manifested in borderline personality disorder, although there are similarities between these conditions. Schizotypal personality disorder differs from borderline personality disorder, however, in that psychotic-like symptoms and social isolation are more likely to persist in the absence of affective turmoil, and schizotypal individuals are less likely to display the impulsive and manipulative traits that are often associated with borderline personality disorder.

Epidemiology

(a) Incidence

To the authors' knowledge, there continue to be no published incidence studies for schizotypal personality disorder.

(b) Prevalence

A review by Lyons showed that prevalence rates for schizotypal personality disorder in non-clinical samples ranged from 0.7 to 5.1 per cent, with a median near 3.0 per cent.[30] Higher rates occurred in clinical samples—2.0 to 64.0 per cent, with a median of 17.5 per cent. More recently, Torgersen *et al.* reported a rate of 0.6 per cent for DSM-III-R in a community sample, which is lower than the rates in studies reviewed by Lyons.[31] Similar to recent prevalence rates reported for schizoaffective disorder (described above), more recent studies have tended to show lower rates than earlier studies. In contrast to non-clinical samples, the prevalence of schizotypal personality disorder among the relatives of schizophrenic individuals is as high as 10 per cent.[32]

Treatment

(a) Review of evidence

There is, unfortunately, a dearth of outcome studies involving psychotherapy, psychosocial, or psychopharmacological treatments for schizotypal personality disorder. Older published studies often show methodological limitations (e.g. small samples, subjects with mixed diagnoses, inadequate controls, and problems with internal validity), or provide outcome data on only limited aspects of the disorder. Despite these caveats, it is clear that few treatment gains are evident in earlier studies. This is particularly true of studies that utilized psychodynamically oriented psychotherapy, either alone or in combination with other treatments (e.g. group therapy or art therapy) as the primary treatment modality.[33] Recent evidence for the efficacy of psychotherapy for personality disorders is more promising, but is limited mainly to other personality disorders.[34]

Several earlier studies investigated the usefulness of medications in treating schizotypal personality disorder, although they typically employed small numbers of subjects, combined samples of schizotypal and borderline personality disorders, and showed little clinical improvement.[33] Typical antipsychotic drugs, in particular, were proposed to reduce positive symptoms or depressed mood in times of acute stress, but the high incidence of adverse side effects discouraged their widespread use at other times, including the more chronic stable (i.e. non-crisis) phases of the disorder. Other types of medication, including fluoxetine, have shown generally non-specific effects of treatment.

Hymowitz *et al.* administered a low dose of haloperidol, a first-generation antipsychotic medication, to 17 outpatients with DSM-III diagnoses of schizotypal personality disorder, for 6 weeks.[35] The initial dose of 2.0 mg was intended to rise to 12.0 mg, but side effects prevented increases beyond a mean dose of 3.6 mg. Even with lower doses, 50 per cent of the sample withdrew from the study because of side effects. The 17 subjects who completed 2 weeks of the protocol improved somewhat in ratings of ideas of reference, odd communications, social isolation, and overall functioning.

More recently, Koenigsberg *et al.* employed a double-blind protocol to administer low doses of risperidone (0.25 mg/day—2.0 mg/day), a second-generation antipsychotic medication, to 25 patients with DSM-IV schizotypal personality disorder, for 9 weeks.[36] Compared to a placebo control group, patients who received risperidone demonstrated significant reductions in positive and negative symptoms, with no difference in dropout rates between groups. These findings are encouraging and consistent with evidence described above that schizotypal symptoms are amenable to change.[24,25] Hopefully, findings like this will stimulate additional research into pharmacological treatments for this disorder.

Management

Patients with schizotypal personality disorder often view their worlds as odd and threatening places and may require extended courses of treatment. Although trust and rapport with the therapist are often difficult to establish in schizotypal personality disorder, the therapeutic relationship may be used to mitigate the marked deficits in interpersonal relationships that characterize this syndrome.[37] The frequent occurrence of paranoia and suspiciousness, together with social aloofness and constricted affect, may make exploratory psychotherapeutic approaches less effective than supportive cognitive behavioural therapies. In fact, these patients may only seek treatment to alleviate circumscribed problems, like anxiety or somatic complaints. Approaches that emphasize concrete, interim goals, and stipulate explicit means of attaining them, thus have the best chances of success. Because individuals with this disorder are vulnerable to decompensation during times of stress and may experience transient episodes of psychosis, they may also benefit from techniques to facilitate stress reduction (e.g. relaxation techniques, exercise, yoga, and meditation). Fortunately, some people with schizotypal features are likely to seek treatment in times of stress.[38] In the short-term, brief courses of antipsychotic treatment may be useful if symptoms of psychosis appear.

Cognitive problems are also frequently amenable to concrete goal-oriented approaches to treatment. Patients benefit from understanding their cognitive strengths and weaknesses because it helps them confront and cope with long-standing difficulties in their lives. For example, problems in attention, verbal memory, or organizational skills contribute to failures in educational, occupational, and social endeavours, while reinforcing negative self-images and increasing performance anxiety. Knowledge of circumscribed cognitive problems allows patients to reframe their difficulties in a more positive manner, and facilitate selection of realistic personal, educational, and occupational goals. Moreover, specific cognitive deficits are often subject to partial remediation. For example, standard procedures will attenuate deficits in the acquisition, organization, and retrieval of new information (e.g. writing information down in a 'memory notebook', using appointment books or planners, and rehearsing new information, among others). In some instances, the documentation of specific cognitive deficits (e.g. attention) can lead to academic accommodations in school (e.g. more time to take exams), which will help individuals function closer to their intellectual potentials.

Possibilities for prevention

At present, most early intervention programmes involve secondary prevention, which includes the early identification and treatment of clinical (usually psychotic or psychotic-like) symptoms. While intervention is necessary to alleviate clinical symptoms at any point during the disorder, it is particularly important early on because it might alter the course of the illness. Patients treated with antipsychotic medication during their first or second hospital admission, for example, show better outcomes than those who are not treated until later in the course of their disorders.

Primary prevention, which involves treatment before the disorder manifests itself clinically, is not yet available for schizoaffective disorder, schizotypal personality disorder, or other disorders in the schizophrenia spectrum. To develop such treatments, it will be necessary to predict who is most likely to develop a disorder. There are a few encouraging approaches, including ongoing 'high-risk' studies that follow the offspring of schizophrenic parents longitudinally.[39] Such studies help to identify traits early in life that predict which individuals are most likely to experience emergent clinical symptoms in adulthood. This type of study is particularly important because it can facilitate the formation of homogeneous high-risk groups, which in turn can facilitate the development of focused prevention strategies.

With our current knowledge, it is difficult to justify preventive treatments—especially medication—for people without symptoms. The authors have argued elsewhere, however, that if people in high-risk groups (like first-degree biological relatives of patients with schizophrenia) show clinically meaningful symptoms that can be organized into valid liability syndromes, then intervention attempts may become appropriate.[26] The authors proposed this course of action for people with 'schizotaxia', and suggested preliminary research guidelines.[40]

Eventually, prevention will be a primary therapeutic approach for the treatment of disorders in the schizophrenia spectrum. While primary prevention has yet to occur, the authors are optimistic that high risk studies, progress in secondary prevention, and progress in discovering the genetic aetiology of the schizophrenia spectrum, will facilitate primary prevention strategies eventually.

Further information

Raine, A. (2006). Schizotypal personality: neurodevelopmental and psychosocial trajectories. *Annual Review of Clinical Psychology*, **2**, 291–326.

Evans, J.D., Heaton, R.K., Paulsen, J.S., McAdams, L.A., Heaton, S.C., and Jeste, D.V. (1999). Schizoaffective disorder: a form of schizophrenia or affective disorder? *The Journal of Clinical Psychiatry*, **60**, 874–82.

Tsuang, M.T., Stone, W.S., and Lyons, M.J. (2007). Toward prevention of schizophrenia: early detection and intervention. In *Recognition and prevention of major mental and substance abuse disorders* (eds. M.T. Tsuang, W.S. Stone, and M.J. Lyons), pp. 213–37. American Psychiatric Publishing, Inc, Washington DC.

References

1. American Psychiatric Association. (1994). *Diagnostic and statistical manual of mental disorders (DSM-IV)*. American Psychiatric Association, Washington, DC.
2. Marneros, A., Deister, A., and Rohde, A. (1990). Sociodemographic and premorbid features of schizophrenic, schizoaffective and affective psychoses. In *Affective and schizoaffective disorders* (eds. A. Marneros and M.T. Tsuang), pp. 130–45. Springer-Verlag, Berlin.
3. Tsuang, M.T., Simpson, S.J.C., and Fleming, J.A. (1986). Diagnostic criteria for subtyping schizoaffective disorder. In *Schizoaffective psychoses* (eds. A. Marneros and M.T. Tsuang), pp. 50–62. Springer-Verlag, Berlin.
4. Reichenberg, A., Weiser, M., Rabinowitz, J., *et al.* (2002). A population-based cohort study of premorbid intellectual, language and behavioral functioning in patients with schizophrenia, schizoaffective disorder, and nonpsychotic bipolar disorder. *The American Journal of Psychiatry*, **159**, 2027–35.
5. Vaillant, G. (1962). The prediction of recovery in schizophrenia. *The Journal of Nervous and Mental Disease*, **135**, 534–43.
6. Simpson, J. (1988). Mortality studies in schizophrenia. In *Nosology, epidemiology and genetics of schizophrenia*, Vol. 3 (eds. M.T. Tsuang and J.C. Simpson), pp. 245–73. Oxford, Elsevier Science Publishers B.V., Amsterdam, New York.
7. Bertelsen, A. and Gottesman, I.I. (1995). Schizoaffective psychoses: genetical clues to classification. *American Journal of Medical Genetics (Neuropsychiatric Genetics)*, **60**, 7–11.
8. Okasha, A. (2007). The concept of schizoaffective disorder: utility versus validity and reliability—a transcultural perspective. In *The overlap of affective and schizophrenic spectra* (eds. A. Marneros and A.H. Akiskal), pp. 104–32. Cambridge University Press, Cambridge.
9. Coryell, W. (2007). Phenomenological approaches to the schizoaffective spectrum. In *The overlap of affective and schizophrenic spectra* (eds. A. Marneros and A.H. Akiskal), pp. 133–44. Cambridge University Press, Cambridge.

10. Samson, J.A., Simpson, J.C., and Tsuang, M.T. (1988). Outcome of schizoaffective disorders. *Schizophrenia Bulletin*, **14**, 543–54.
11. Angst, J. (1986). The course of schizoaffective disorders. In *Schizoaffective psychoses* (eds. A. Marneros and M.T. Tsuang), pp. 63–93. Springer-Verlag, Berlin.
12. Reinares, M., Vieta, E., Benabarre, A., *et al.* (2007). Clinical course of schizoaffective disorders. In *The overlap of affective and schizophrenic spectra* (eds. A. Marneros and A.H. Akiskal), pp. 145–55. Cambridge University Press, Cambridge.
13. Kendler, K.S., McGuire, M., Gruenberg, A.M., *et al.* (1995). Examining the validity of DSM-III-R schizoaffective disorder and its putative subtypes in the Roscommon Family Study. *The American Journal of Psychiatry*, **152**, 755–64.
14. Marneros, A., Rohde, A., and Deister, A. (1998). Frequency and phenomenology of persisting alterations in affective, schizoaffective and schizophrenia disorders: a comparison. *Psychopathology*, **31**, 23–8.
15. Jager, M., Bottlender, R., Strauss, A., *et al.* (2004). Fifteen-year follow-up of ICD-schizoaffective disorders compared to schizophrenia and affective disorders. *Acta Psychiatrica Scandinavica*, **109**, 30–7.
16. Fiszdon, J.M., Richardson, R., Greig, T., *et al.* (2007). A comparison of basic and social cognition between schizophrenia and schizoaffective disorder. *Schizophrenia Research*, **91**, 117–21.
17. Vaillant, G. (1964). Prospective prediciton of schizophrenic remission. *Archives of General Psychiatry*, **11**, 509–18.
18. Levitt, J.J. and Tsuang, M.T. (1988). The heterogeneity of schizoaffective disorder: implications for treatment. *The American Journal of Psychiatry*, **145**, 926–36.
19. Kendler, K.S., Karkowski, L.M., and Walsh, D. (1998). The structure of psychosis: latent class analysis of probands from the Roscommon family study. *Archives of General Psychiatry*, **55**, 492–9.
20. Tsuang, M.T., Levitt, J.J., and Simpson, J.C. (1995). Schizoaffective disorder. In *Schizophrenia* (eds. S.R. Hirsch and D.R. Weinberger). Blackwell Scientific, Oxford.
21. Tien, A.Y. and Eaton, W.W. (1992). Psychopathologic precursors and sociodemographic risk factors for the schizophrenia syndrome. *Archives of General Psychiatry*, **49**, 37–46.
22. Perala, J., Suvisaari, J., Saarni, S.I., *et al.* (2007). Lifetime prevalence of psychotic and bipolar I disorders in a general population. *Archives of General Psychiatry*, **64**, 19–28.
23. Battaglia, M., Cavallini, M.C., Macciardi, F., *et al.* (1997). The structure of DSM-III-R schizotypal personality disorder diagnosed by direct interviews. *Schizophrenia Bulletin*, **23**, 83–92.
24. McGlashan, T.H., Grilo, C.M., Sanislow, C.A., *et al.* (2005). Two-year prevalence and stability of individual DSM-IV criteria for schizotypal, borderline, avoidant, and obsessive-compulsive personality disorders: toward a hybrid model of axis II disorders. *The American Journal of Psychiatry*, **162**, 883–9.
25. Grilo, C.M., Sanislow, C.A., Gunderson, J.G., *et al.* (2004). Two-year stability and change of schizotypal, borderline, avoidant and obsessive-compulsive personality disorders. *Journal of Consulting and Clinical Psychology*, **72**, 767–75.
26. Faraone, S.V., Green, A.I., Seidman, L.J., *et al.* (2001). Schizotaxia: clinical implications and new directions for research. *Schizophrenia Bulletin*, **27**, 1–18.
27. Kendler, K.S. (1985). Diagnostic approaches to schizotypal personality disorder: a historical perspective. *Schizophrenia Bulletin*, **11**, 538–53.
28. Thaker, G., Moran, M., Adami, H., *et al.* (1993). Psychosis proneness scales in schizophrenia spectrum personality disorders: familial vs. nonfamilial samples. *Psychiatry Research*, **46**, 47–57.
29. Tsuang, M.T., Gilbertson, M.W., and Faraone, S.V. (1991). Genetic transmission of negative and positive symptoms in the biological relatives of schizophrenics. In *Positive vs. negative schizophrenia* (eds. A. Marneros, M.T. Tsuang, and N. Andreasen), pp. 265–91. Springer-Verlag, New York.
30. Torgersen, S., Kringlen, E., and Cramer, V. (2001). The prevalence of personality disorders in a community sample. *Archives of General Psychiatry*, **58**, 590–6.
31. Lyons, M.J. (1995). Epidemiology of personality disorders. In *Textbook in psychiatric epidemiology* (eds. M.T. Tsuang, M. Tohen, and G.E. Zahner), pp. 407–36. Wiley-Liss, New York.
32. Battaglia, M. and Torgersen, S. (1996). Schizotypal disorder: at the crossroads of genetics and nosology. *Acta Psychiatrica Scandinavica*, **94**, 303–10.
33. Tsuang, M.T., Stone, W.S., and Faraone, S.V. (1998). Overview for treatment for schizotypal and schizoid personality disorders: present and future. *NOOS Aggiornamenti in Psichiatria*, **4**, 201–15.
34. Verheul, R. and Herbrink, M. (2007). The efficacy of various modalities of psychotherapy for personality disorders: a systematic review of the evidence and clinical recommendations. *International Review of Psychiatry*, **19**, 25–38.
35. Hymowitz, P., Frances, A., Jacobsberg, L.B., *et al.* (1986). Neuroleptic treatment of schizotypal personality disorders. *Comprehensive Psychiatry*, **27**, 267–71.
36. Koenigsberg, H.W., Reynolds, D., Goodman, M., *et al.* (2003). Risperidone in the treatment of schizotypal personality disorder. *The Journal of Clinical Psychiatry*, **64**, 628–34.
37. Bender, S. (2005). The therapeutic alliance in the treatment of personality disorders. *Journal of Psychiatric Practice*, **11**, 73–87.
38. Poreh, A. and Whitman, D. (1993). MMPI-2 schizophrenia spectrum profiles among schizotypal college students and college students who seek psychological treatment. *Psychological Reports*, **73**, 987–94.
39. Stone, W.S., Faraone, S.V., Seidman, L.J., *et al.* (2005). Searching for the liability to schizophrenia: concepts and methods underlying genetic high-risk studies of adolescents. *Journal of Child and Adolescent Psychopharmacology*, **15**, 403–17.
40. Tsuang, M.T., Stone, W.S., Seidman, L.J., *et al.* (1999). Treatment of nonpsychotic relatives of patients with schizophrenia: four case studies. *Biological Psychiatry*, **41**, 1412–18.

4.3.10 Acute and transient psychotic disorders

J. Garrabé and F.-R. Cousin

Historic introduction

Acute and transient psychotic episodes have been described since the end of the nineteenth century. Descriptions have varied from one country to another, so that the exact nosology has not yet been established. The links between acute psychoses (generally defined as having brief obvious psychotic symptomatology) and chronic psychoses (schizophrenic psychoses and psychoses with persistent delusions) are still under discussion.

For instance, Sections F20 and F21 in ICD-10[(1)] are devoted to 'Schizophrenia, schizotypal and delusional disorders'. A specific diagnostic category named 'Acute and transient psychotic disorders' is included, distinct from Schizophrenia (F20), Schizotypal disorder (F21), Persistent delusional disorder (F22), Induced delusional disorder (also called *folie à deux*) (F24), and Schizoaffective disorder (F25).

In this textbook, the acute and transient psychotic disorders (Chapter 4.3.10) appear in the section dedicated to schizophrenia, which also includes schizotypal disorders and schizoaffective disorders (Chapter 4.3.9). However, this section is clearly distinguished from the chapter in which the persistent delusional disorders are discussed (Chapter 4.4). These taxonomic divergences are justified more by the history of acute psychoses than by scientific findings.

In the nineteenth century, German psychiatrists had already described *akute primäre Verruckheit*,[2] termed *paranoia acuta* by Karl Westphal. In 1876 (published in 1878), Westphal used this term to describe an acute form of paranoia with an outburst of perceptual hallucinations, consisting mostly of hallucinatory voices and delusions, with clouding of consciousness. In 1890, Meynert repeated the clinical description but named the condition amentia.[3] Sigmund Freud chose this type of acute delusion with hallucinations for his psychoanalytic conception of psychosis.[4]

In the sixth edition of his textbook, published in 1899, Kraepelin[5] included all the paranoias under dementia praecox, and in the eighth edition (1908–1915) he combined manic and melancholic periodic disorders in a single group, leaving acute psychosis with no place between these two diagnostic categories.

In 1911, Bleuler[6] replaced the single disease dementia praecox by the concept of a group of schizophrenias of various clinical forms. He noticed that schizophrenia often began with an acute excitatory episode lasting from a few hours to a few years. He described a wide variation of outcome of acute forms of psychosis, but he separated acute schizophrenias from simple schizophrenia as he believed that acute forms do not necessarily end in deterioration.

In 1916, based on Karl Jaspers' psychopathology, the Danish psychiatrist Wimmer[7] described psychogenic psychosis as a reactive psychosis arising after psychosocial trauma. Mayer-Gross,[8] who proposed an organic aetiology for schizophrenia, described 'oneiroid states' consisting of acute psychotic symptomatology with no other specific organic features.

In 1961, Leonhard[9] used Kleist's concept of marginal psychosis (*Randpsychosen*) to develop his description of 'cycloid psychoses' as endogenous psychoses separate from schizophrenic psychoses and from manic and melancholic psychoses. These cycloid psychoses tend to have a benign and periodic course.

Earlier (1933), Kasanin[10] had described 'acute schizoaffective psychoses', raising questions about the links between schizophrenic and affective diseases.

Langfeldt[11] suggested that observation for 5 years was required to be able to distinguish schizophrenia and what he called schizophreniform psychosis. This long-term observation is a reminder of the Bleulerian concept of acute schizophrenias which could last for several years. Epidemiological studies have led to the presence in modern classifications of a group of acute schizophreniform psychoses under the rubric 'Schizophreniform disorder' (DSM-IV Section 295.40) or 'Acute psychotic disorder schizophrenic-like' (ICD-10 Section F23.2).

In France, the concept of *bouffée délirante* led naturally to a specific class of acute psychoses. In 1895, Magnan[12] and his disciple Legrain[13] described *bouffée délirante* or *délire d'emblée* (immediate delusion) within the polymorphic delusions of the chronic insane. This concept is based on Morel's theory of degeneration, commonly accepted in the nineteenth century. The question of whether there is a susceptibility or a predisposition to the occurrence of an acute psychosis remains unanswered.[14]

In 1954, Ey[15,16] described the development of the concept of *bouffées délirantes* and of acute psychoses with hallucinations from the time of Magnan to a symposium devoted to the clinical subdivision of schizophrenic psychoses held at the First World Congress of Psychiatry in 1950, where the various ideas were discussed by Langfeldt, Karl Leonhard, and Aubrey Lewis (Table 4.3.10.1).

Table 4.3.10.1 Historical development of the terminology of acute and transient psychotic disorders

Historic term	Current terminology
1876 Westphal *Akute primäre Verruckheit* *Paranoia acuta*	F23.3 Other acute predominantly delusional psychotic disorder
1890 Meynert Amentia	
1895 Magnan and Legrain *Bouffées délirantes*	F23.0 Acute polymorphic psychotic disorder without symptoms of schizophrenia
1899 Kraepelin Dementia praecox	F20.0 Schizophrenia
1909–1913 Kraepelin Paranoia	F22.0 Persistent delusional disorder
1911 Bleuler Acute-onset forms of schizophrenia	F23.1 Acute polymorphic psychotic disorder with symptoms of schizophrenia F23.2 Acute schizophrenia-like psychotic disorder
1916 Wimmer Psychogenic psychosis	F23.3 Other acute predominantly psychotic disorder
1924 Mayer-Gross *Oneroide Erlebnisform*	F23.3 Acute schizophrenia-like psychotic disorder
1933 Kasanin Acute schizoaffective psychoses	F25 Schizoaffective disorders
1939 Langfeldt Schizophreniform states	F23.2 Acute schizophrenia-like psychotic disorder
1954 Ey *Bouffées délirantes et psychoses hallucinatoires aigues*	F23.0 Acute polymorphic psychotic disorder without symptoms of schizophrenia
1961 Leonhard Cycloid psychoses	F23.0 Acute polymorphic psychotic disorder without symptoms of schizophrenia

Clinical description: psychopathology

The heterogeneous group of acute and transient psychotic disorders are characterized by three typical features, listed below in descending order of priority:

- suddenness of onset (within 2 weeks or less);
- presence of typical syndromes with polymorphic (changing and variable) or schizophrenic symptoms;
- presence of associated acute stress (stressful events such as bereavement, job loss, psychological trauma, etc.).

The onset of the disorder is manifested by an obvious change to an abnormal psychotic state. This is considered to be abrupt when it occurs within 48 h or less. Abrupt onset often indicates a better outcome. Full recovery occurs within 3 months and often in a shorter time (a few days or weeks). However, a small number of patients develop persistent and disabling states.

The general (G) criteria for these acute disorders in DCR-10 (Diagnostic Criteria Research of ICD) are as follows.

G1 There is acute onset of delusions, hallucinations, incomprehensible or incoherent speech, or any combination of these. The time interval between the first appearance of any psychotic symptoms and the presentation of the fully developed disorder should not exceed 2 weeks.

G2 If transient states of perplexity, misidentification, or impairment of attention and concentration are present, they do not fulfil the criteria for organically caused clouding of consciousness as specified for F05, criterion A.

G3 The disorder does not satisfy the symptomatic criteria for manic episode (F30), depressive episode (F32), or recurrent depressive disorder (F33).

G4 There is insufficient evidence of recent psychoactive substance use to satisfy the criteria for intoxication (F1x.0), harmful use (F1x.1), dependence (F1x.2), or withdrawal states (F1x.3 and F1x.4). The continued moderate and largely unchanged use of alcohol or drugs in the amounts or with the frequency to which the individual is accustomed does not necessarily exclude the use of F23; this must be decided by clinical judgement and the requirements of the research project in question.

G5 There must be no organic mental disorder (F00–F09) or serious metabolic disturbances affecting the central nervous system (this does not include childbirth). (This is the most commonly used exclusion clause.)

A fifth character should be used to specify whether the acute onset of the disorder is associated with acute stress (occurring 2 weeks or less before evidence of first psychotic symptoms):

- F23.x0 without associated acute stress and
- F23.x1 with associated acute stress.

For research purposes it is recommended that change of the disorder from a non-psychotic to a clearly psychotic state is further specified as either abrupt (onset within 48 h) or acute (onset in more than 48 h but less than 2 weeks).

Six categories of acute psychoses are presented in ICD-10, and we shall discuss them in order.

F23.0 acute polymorphic psychotic disorder without symptoms of schizophrenia

The diagnostic criteria are based on the classical symptoms of the true *bouffée délirante* described by Magnan and Legrain.

(a) Suddenness of onset

Bouffée délirante occurs over a period of a few hours or days, usually to young adults and often women in their 30s. The onset of the delirious episode is 'like a thunderbolt in a serene sky'. This aphorism from Legrain has the same meaning as the French classical expression *délire d'emblée* (immediate delusion).

Although premonitory symptoms, such as increasing perplexity and anxiety, may occur, the delusions start suddenly and are always accompanied by a break-up in the individual psychic life. If the onset is preceded by a stressful or traumatic event, such as resettlement or acculturation, this may take place some months previously and the outburst of the delirious episode is delayed. The fifth code character of category F23 is used to specify whether acute stress is associated with the onset of the disorder (e.g. F23.00 has no associated acute stress).

(b) Polymorphic psychotic symptoms

The delusional themes are varied and include grandeur, persecution, influence, possession, body transformation (depersonalization), derealization, or world alteration; these themes change with time and may combine. Other symptoms are also varied, including hallucinations, illusions, interpretations, and intuitions.

(c) The emotional state

As a consequence of the delusions the patient experiences mood change and emotional turmoil (happiness, ecstasy, anxiety, irritability). However, the criteria for manic episode, depressive episode, schizoaffective disorder, and schizophrenia are not satisfied.

Consciousness fluctuates with the delirious convictions and changes of emotion. There is a specific disorientation with respect to time and place—the passage of time (*temps vécu* according to Eugène Minkowski) and 'temporality' (*Sein und Zeit* according to Ludwig Binswanger) are disturbed. This disorientation, described by Karl Jaspers as a 'first delirious experience' (*Erlebnisse*), has to be understood as a dream-like state.

Ey[15,16] differentiated the acute psychoses in terms of the specific alteration in the perception of time rather than their transient course. According to Jacksonian ideas, the acute psychoses are the expression of a destructuring of consciousness to levels related to each acute psychosis.

(d) The duration of the delirious experience

In ICD-10, the criterion of a duration of less than a month distinguishes other categories from schizophrenia (F20) and manic or depressive episodes (F30 and F32).

(e) Short recovery time

In most cases recovery from the acute psychotic disorder occurs within a few weeks or months. However, long-term prognosis is difficult because of the risk of relapse into either a repeated episode or a more chronic disease. If resolution of the symptoms has not occurred after 3 months, the diagnosis should be changed to persistent delusional disorder (F22) or non-organic psychotic disorder (F28).

(f) Suggested criteria

Pull *et al.*[17] have suggested the following empirical criteria for *bouffée délirante*.

- Abrupt or acute onset, with no previous psychiatric disorder except other similar episodes.
- Absence of chronicity: the active stages disappear completely in a few weeks or months. Relapses can occur, but there is no psychiatric disorder between consecutive episodes.
- Specific symptoms: delusions and/or any type of hallucination, depersonalization and/or derealization with or without confusion, and affective disturbance manifesting as depression or euphoria. The symptoms change from day to day and even from hour to hour.
- There is insufficient evidence for organic mental disorder, alcoholism, or drug addiction. The exclusion clauses are less restrictive in ICD-10, since a moderate, continued, and unchanged use of alcohol or drugs in habituated individuals does not exclude the diagnosis.

- The true acute psychotic disorder occurs without any associated psychosocial stress factor. When psychosocial stress factors are found, there is only a temporal link with the so-called 'reactive' acute psychosis.

(g) Long-term evolution

Bleuler[6] described one-third of cases of acute schizophrenic psychoses as single episode, one-third as recurrent episodes with repetition of the same acute and transient psychoses (either manic or depressive), and one-third following a course which developed as schizophrenia.

Between 1976 and 1989, Metzger and Weiber[18] studied 885 cases of acute psychoses. Using the criteria of Pull *et al.*[17] they found group 303 cases of genuine *bouffée délirante* (two-thirds female, one-third male, average age of 32 years). They followed the course of 191 cases (over an average period of 6.2 years): 34 per cent did not relapse, 24 per cent had recurrent and transient episodes, 34 per cent developed schizophrenia, and over 7 per cent developed a periodic affective disorder (manic and depressive states). The relapse or chronic course rate was higher in the group without triggering factors ($n = 92$) than in the group with triggering factors ($n = 99$). The difference between true *bouffée délirante* (no triggering factors) and other acute and transient psychotic disorders raises questions about their pathogenesis.

In the first 2 years, it is essential to distinguish *bouffée délirante* from schizophrenia[19] and other acute psychoses.[20] Follow-up during this period must be very careful.

F23.1 acute polymorphic disorder with symptoms of schizophrenia (*bouffée délirante* or cycloid psychosis with symptoms of schizophrenia)

This diagnostic category combines the symptoms of acute polymorphic psychotic disorder with some typical symptoms of schizophrenia (F20) present for most of the time. However, the schizophrenic symptoms are not precisely listed. F23.1 can be a provisional diagnosis, which is changed to schizophrenia if the criteria of F20 persist more than a month.

Acute polymorphic disorder with symptoms of schizophrenia satisfies the general criteria for acute and transient psychotic disorders:

- acute onset of less than 2 weeks
- polymorphic delusions and hallucinations or perceptual disturbances leading to incomprehensible or incoherent speech
- clouding of consciousness with impairment of attention or concentration, disorientation, perplexity, etc.
- emotional turmoil and affective symptoms (depressed mood, euphoria, anxiety, irritability) without the symptomatic criteria for manic–depressive or recurrent depressive disorders
- rapid changes of the type and intensity of symptoms
- no evidence of causation by organic or psychoactive substances.

It is also associated with some schizophrenic symptoms which are present most of the time:

- mental automatism (thought echo, insertion, withdrawal, or broadcasting)
- control, influence, passivity referred to body movements, thoughts, actions, or sensations
- hallucinations with commentary
- catatonic behaviour
- negative symptoms.

The ICD-10 clinical criteria give no information about psychotic or schizophrenic symptoms or about the action of antipsychotic drugs on these symptoms.

Leonhard[9] described cycloid psychosis as an episode with clouding of consciousness and a marked alteration of thinking. Many authors have reported follow-up studies of cycloid psychoses,[21–23] which confirm the better prognosis of cycloid psychoses than of schizophrenias and schizoaffective disorders.

F23.2 acute schizophrenia-like psychotic disorder (schizophreniform psychosis)

This acute psychotic disorder lasts for less than a month and is mostly schizophrenic. The polymorphic psychotic symptoms are stable (no rapid changes, no emotional turmoil or confusion), sometimes with emotional instability.

The duration criterion is the most important. This category is a provisional diagnosis and appears to include such disparate descriptions as oneirophrenia (oneiroid states or *Erlebnisform*[8]), schizophrenic reaction (DSM.IV 298.8, Brief reactive psychoses), and schizophreniform psychosis.[11] In ICD-10, if the first episode lasts for more than a month, it has to be considered as an acute onset of schizophrenia.

The Scandinavian psychiatric school[24] justify the retention of this category because of the very good and rapid recovery, and have tried to determine factors in the personal and family history predicting the onset of schizophrenia.

Schizophreniform disorder remains in DSM-IV (295.40) because the evidence linking it to typical schizophrenia remains unclear, but the duration criterion is less restrictive (up to 6 months). Features suggesting a good prognosis are onset within 4 weeks, confusion at the height of the psychotic episode, previously good social and occupational functioning, and absence of blunted or flat affect.

F23.3 other acute predominantly delusional psychotic disorders

The main clinical features of this category are delusions and hallucinations. The foreground delusions are mostly persecutory (delusions that the person or close relatives are being malevolently treated or are under external influence, with thought disturbances); auditory hallucinations are present in the background. Despite their stability, these psychotic features do not meet the criteria for schizophrenia (F20).

As for F23.0, the duration of this acute predominantly delusional psychotic episode must be less than 3 months. If the persecutory delusions persist for more than 3 months, the diagnosis changes to persistent delusional disorders (F22). This development from F23.3 to F22 is reminiscent of the classical *paranoia acuta*. Thus, both paranoid reaction and psychogenic paranoid psychosis are included in F23.3. Paranoid reaction must be distinguished from induced delusional disorder or *folie à deux* (F24), in which the delusions of the 'dominated' patient disappear when the two people are separated (see Chapter 4.4).

If the background auditory hallucinations persist for more than 3 months, the diagnosis is changed to other non-organic psychotic disorders (F28). This diagnostic category is defined by exclusion: the persistent hallucinatory disorder does not meet the criteria for schizophrenia (F20), persistent delusional disorders (F22), acute and transient psychotic disorders (F23), psychotic types of manic episode (F30.2), or severe depressive episode (F32.3). F28 also corresponds to chronic hallucinatory psychosis, as explicitly noted in ICD 10.

F23.8 other acute and transient psychotic disorders

This category includes any other acute and transient psychotic disorders with no evidence of organic cause that are not classifiable under previous F23 categories, such as ephemeral delusions or hallucinations and undifferentiated excitement.

F23.9 acute and transient psychotic disorder unspecified

Brief psychotic disorder (298.8) is defined in DSM-IV as an episode of acute and transient psychotic disorders (delusions and hallucinations with disorganized speech and behaviour) which lasts at least a day but less than a month with eventual full return to previous level of functioning. If the symptoms occur after stressful events in the person's life, brief psychotic disorder with marked stressor(s) has to be specified. If the symptoms occur within 4 weeks post-partum, brief psychotic disorder with post-partum onset has to be specified.

Cultural variants

Other forms of acute psychoses have been observed in both traditional and developing countries, with high prevalence in Asia, Africa, and Latin America. These brief psychotic episodes are culture-bound syndromes, often with immediate precipitating stress or life events.[25] There is disorganized behaviour, delusions, thought disorders, confusion, and mood disorders, usually with full recovery and no relapse in a 1-year follow-up.

The culture-specific disorders[26] and their potentially related syndromes are often acute and transient. The status of these culture-reactive disorders is controversial and needs more clinical and epidemiological research. The mode of assignment to categories in ICD-10 does not suggest category F23.

Appendix I of DSM-IV (Outline for cultural formulation and glossary of culture-bound syndromes) lists 25 syndromes, with a glossary mostly using the local terms (seven in Hispanic languages, five in English, and one in French). *Bouffée délirante*, described only in West Africa and Haiti, is defined as episodes resembling brief psychotic disorder and classified in F23.0. Messich and Lin[25] have suggested that the whole group of culture-bound syndromes should be classified as acute and transient psychotic disorders, although this is justified only for a very few such as *amok* (dissociative episode with persecutory ideas and aggressive behaviour from Malaysia), *shin-byung* (Korean dissociation and possession), and spell (trance state in southern United States).

ICD-10 includes the two Malaysian syndromes *koro* and *latah* as well as *dhat* (India) in F48.8, Other specified neurotic disorders.

International follow-up studies have shown that cultural factors can influence the course and prognosis of acute psychotic disorders. In 1979, the World Health Organization compared the course of schizophrenia (295), psychotic depression, mania, and other psychoses in different cultures, using the ICD-9 criteria for the diagnoses. The outcome for the schizophrenic group was better in emerging countries than in the industrialized world. These results probably explain the individualization of category F23 in ICD-10.

Some authors[27] have suggested that short-lived psychotic episodes are expressions of overcharged mechanisms of defence, or of individual psychological fragility. The brief psychosis is an understandable development of the psychic life of the subject and has a cathartic effect.

Culturally related syndromes are discussed further in Chapter 4.16.

Treatment

Short-term treatment

Acute psychotic syndromes require early hospitalization in either an inpatient psychiatric unit or a crisis centre. These syndromes are to be considered as psychiatric emergencies. The decision to admit to hospital is taken in order to make a careful physical and mental examination clinical evaluation, to separate the patient from his or her environment, to provide a reassuring setting, and to prevent any suicidal or aggressive tendencies.[28]

The goals are to prevent auto or heteroagressivity (suicidal potential, affective symptoms, agitation, aggressive behaviour, command hallucinations, etc.), to reduce the acute psychotic symptoms, to suppress the causal factors and to establish an early therapeutic alliance with the patient and his family. Antipsychotic drugs medications are prescribed.[29] Some clinicians wait for a day or two before starting neuroleptic therapy in order to eliminate an organic cause (a general medical condition or substance abuse disorder can be present with acute and transient psychoticsymptoms) and prescribe benzodiazepines rather than neuroleptics. More often, however, antipsychotic treatment starts immediately after physical, electrophysical, radiological assessments, and laboratory tests (CBC, blood electrolytes, cholesterol, triglycerides, toxicology screen, etc.) to evaluate health status.

The choice of antipsychotic medication depends on the clinician's experience and the clinical features. Second-generation antipsychotic medications (amisulpride, aripiprazole, olanzapine, quetiapine, risperidone, ziprasidone) are commonly prescribed as first-line treatment; clozapine is reserved to schizophrenia with high suicidal potential or to resistant schizophrenia. First-generation antipsychotic medications (chlorpromazine, haloperidol, etc.) are second choice or adjunctive medications.

In cases of major anxiety or agitated behaviour, short-acting sedative drugs neuroleptics such as first-generation antipsychotics chlorpromazine (100–500 mg/day), (loxapine: 50–300 mg/day), with or without benzodiazepines (lorazepam) can be prescribed or levomepromazine (25–300 mg/day) are chosen, or zuclopenthixol acetate (100–300 mg every 3 days by intramuscular injection) is used as a short-acting depot antipsychotic. Parenteral administration (standard intramuscular administration) may be required if the patient refuses oral medication, or if a rapid effect is required because the patient is seriously uncooperative or is too dangerously disturbed.

Predominance of delusions and hallucinations indicates a high-potency antipsychotic agent as haloperidol (5–15 mg/day) or flupenthixol (80–200 mg/day).

Benzodiazepines may be given to potentiate the action of the neuroleptics. Alprazolam (0.5–4 mg/day), clorazepate (50–200 mg/day), and lorazepam (2–5 mg/day) produce rapid sedation in acutely psychotic patients if they are used with a neuroleptic. Some clinicians prefer the combination of two neuroleptics (haloperidol–levomepromazine, haloperidol–cyamemazine).

New compounds with fewer adverse effects can be used (amisulpride, 800–1200 mg/day; olanzapine, 5–20 mg/day; quetiapine, 75–500 mg/day; risperidone, 2–10 mg/day).

In culture-bound syndromes the prescription of antidepressants is often recommended as primary treatment.

The dosage may be adjusted from low doses and gradually increased, or adjusted to the standard dose after a first loading dose. Frequent monitoring to assess drug response and adverse effects (extrapyramidal side-effects, orthostatic hypotension, anticholinergic effects, and temperature dysregulation) is essential, and corrections and prophylactic prescriptions (e.g. antiparkinsonian medications) may be necessary.

Sociotherapy (occupational or intensive) and psychotherapy (reality–adaptive–supportive) are indicated depending on the state of the patient and his environment, with individual, family, or rehabilitation care.

Continuation treatment

The effectiveness of psychopharmacotherapy is usually manifested in the first 6 weeks, with improved sleep, regression of agitation, recovery from anxiety and delusion, and finally disappearance of the psychotic features. When there is no recovery or improvement either another antipsychotic drug should be used or the dosage of the first increased. Worsening of the symptoms, serious side-effects, or a poor response to pharmacotherapy may lead to the main indications for electroconvulsive therapy.

If mood disorders or cyclic episodes occur, treatment with antidepressants, mood stabilizers (lithium or valproate), or an anticonvulsant drug (carbamazepine) may be indicated. Care must be taken to distinguish between a post-neuroleptic depression and the development of a (schizo)affective disorder.

Prevention of recurrence

The possibility that psychotic symptoms may re-emerge has to be borne in mind during the first 2 years of follow-up. Low-dosage pharmacotherapy must be maintained for 1 or 2 years after recovery. During this long-term follow-up, periodic assessment and effective clinical care with social and psychological therapy are essential.

Advice about management

Patients are often hospitalized under constraint because they do not acknowledge the disorder. The initial non-compliance leads to the frequent use of first-generation antipsychotic medications classic intramuscular neuroleptics. After remission recovery, a switch to a second-generation antipsychotic medication newer antipsychotic drug, which is better tolerated, helps to ensure the acceptance of long-term treatment when the psychotic symptoms have disappeared.

In general, psychotherapy and psychosocial care are more effective in an outpatient setting after symptomatic remission recovery has started. A good relationship between patient and psychiatrist together with collaboration with the family practitioner and social workers improve the long-term prognosis. If resources allow, psychotherapy by a trained practitioner, behavioural therapy, or family therapy may be combined with a low-dose pharmacotherapy.[30]

Further information

There are no substantial sources of information in the English language. The following will be of use to those who read French or Spanish. Others should seek further information using an information retrieval system such as Medline.

Weibel, H. and Metzger, J.Y. (2007). Psychoses délirantes aiguës. *Encyclopédie Médico—chirurgicale. Psychiatrie*, 37–230 A 1O 15 p. 142 ref.

Segarra, E.R., Eguiliz, U.I., and Gutierrez, F. (2007). Trastorno esquizofreniforme y trastorno esquizoafectivo. 158 ref. in *Trastornos psicoticos (457–592)* Coordinador M. Roca Benassar. Fundacion española de Psiquiatria y Salud mental. Barcelona: Ars medica.

References

1. World Health Organization. (1992). *International statistical classification of diseases and related health problems,* 10th revision. WHO, Geneva.
2. Bercherie, P. (1980). L'école d'Illenau. In *Les fondements de la clinique* (ed. Le Seuil), pp. 119–28. Ornicar, Paris.
3. Meynert, T. (1890). *Klinische vorlesungen über psychiatrie auf wissenschaftlichen grundlagen*. Braumüller, Vienna.
4. Freud, S. (1917). Metapsychologie Ergänzung Zurtraumlehre. In *Gesammelte werke*. Internationales Psychoanalytischer Verlag, Leipzig, 1947.
5. Kraepelin, E. (1899). *Psychiatrie* (6th edn). Barth, Leipzig.
6. Bleuler, E. (1911). Dementia praecox oder Gruppe der Schizophrenien. In *Aschaffenburg Handbuch des Psychiatrie*. Deuticke, Leipzig.
7. Wimmer, A. (1916). Psykogene sindssygdomsformer. In St. Hans Hospital, Jubilee Publication. Gad, Copenhagen.
8. Mayer-Gross, W. (1924). Selbschilderungen der Verwirrtheit (Die oneroïde Erlebnisform). Stringler, Berlin.
9. Leonhard, K. (1961). Cycloid psychoses: endogenous psychoses which are either schizophrenic or manic-depressive. *Journal of Nervous and Mental Diseases*, **107**, 633–48.
10. Kasanin, J. (1933). The acute schizo-affective psychoses. *American Journal of Psychiatry*, **13**, 97–126.
11. Langfeldt, G. (1939). *The schizophreniform states*. Oxford University Press, London.
12. Magnan, V. (1893). *Leçons cliniques sur les maladies mentales*. Bataille, Paris.
13. Legrain, M. (1895). *Du délire des dégénérés*. Progrés Medical, Paris.
14. Samuel-Lajeunesse, B. and Heim, A. (1994). Psychoses délirantes aigues. In *Encyclopedie de medecin et de chirurgie*, 37 230, A10. Editions Techniques, Paris.
15. Ey, H. (1954). Bouffées délirantes et psychoses hallucinatoires aigues. In *Etudes psychiatriques*, Vol. III. Desclée de Brower, Paris.
16. Ey, H. (1955). Psychoses délirantes aigues (bouffées délirantes aigues, psychoses hallucinatoires aigues, états oniroïdes). In *Encyclopedie de medecin et de chirurgie*, 37 230, A10, pp. 1–6. Editions Techniques, Paris.
17. Pull, C.B., Pull, M.C., and Pichot, P. (1987). Des critères empiriques français pour les psychoses. II-Consensus des psychiatres français et définitions provisoires. *Encéphale*, **13**, 53–7.
18. Metzger, J.-Y. and Weibel, H. (1991). Les bouffées délirantes. *Congrès de psychiatrie et de neurologie de langue française*. Masson, Paris.
19. World Health Organization. (1979). *Schizophrenia: an international follow-up study*. Wiley, Chichester.
20. Guilloux, J. (1987). Psychoses délirantes aigues. Statut nosologique et evolution. *Revue Française de Psychiatrie*, **5**, 9–13.

21. Perris, L. (1974). A study of cycloid psychoses. *Acta Psychiatrica Scandinavica*, **253**(Suppl.), 1–75.
22. Brockington, I.F., Perris, L., Kendell, R.E., *et al.* (1982). The course and outcome of cycloid psychoses. *Psychiatry in Medicine*, **12**, 97–105.
23. Barcia, D. (1998). *Psicosis cicloides (psicosis marginales, bouffées délirantes)*. Triacastela, Madrid.
24. Strömgren, E. (1963). Schizophreniform psychosis. *Acta Psychiatrica Scandinavica*, **41**, 483–9.
25. Messich, J. and Lin, K.M. (1995). Acute and transient psychotic disorders and culture-bound syndromes. In *Comprehensive textbook of psychiatry* (eds. H. Kaplan and B. Sadock) (6th edn), Vol. 1, pp. 1049–57. Williams and Wilkins, Baltimore, MD.
26. World Health Organization. (1993). *The ICD-10 classification of mental and behavioural disorders-diagnostic criteria for research, Annex 2*. World Health Organization, Geneva.
27. Cousin, F.R. and Vanelle, J.M. (1987). Défense et illustration du concept de bouffée délirante aiguë. *Information Psychiatrique*, **63**, 315–21.
28. American Psychiatric Association (2004). Practice guideline for the treatment of patients with schizophrenia. *Supplement to the American Journal of Psychiatry*, **161**.
29. Janicak, P., Davis, J., Preskorn, S., *et al.* (1997). Management of acute psychosis. In *Principles and practice of psychopharmacotherapy* (eds. P.G. Janicak, J.M. Davis, S.H. Preskorn, and F.J. Ayd) (2nd edn), pp. 110–39. Williams and Wilkins, Baltimore, MD.
30. Rochet, T., Daléry, J., and De Villard, R. (1995). Troubles psychotiques aigus et transitoires. In *Thérapeutique psychiatrique* (eds. J.L. Senon, D. Sechter, and D. Richard), pp. 797–803. Hermann, Paris.

4.4

Persistent delusional symptoms and disorders

Alistair Munro

Introduction

Delusional disorder (DSM-IV 297.1 and ICD-10 F22)[1,2] is a psychotic illness with some superficial resemblances to schizophrenia from which, however, it is quite distinct. It presents with a stable and well-defined delusional system, which is typically 'encapsulated' within a personality, which retains many normal aspects, unlike the situation in schizophrenia in which there is widespread personality disorganization in addition to the psychotic features. Nevertheless, although many normal aspects of the personality are preserved, the individual's way of life becomes progressively distorted by the intensity and intrusiveness of the delusional beliefs. Hallucinations may be present but are not usually prominent. This is a chronic disorder, probably lifelong in most instances, which retains an unjustified reputation for being untreatable. Because of the nature of their delusions, many patients are unwilling to accept that they have a mental disorder or that they require psychiatric treatment but, if they can be persuaded to cooperate and accept appropriate medication, the condition can be shown to respond to treatment in a remarkably high proportion of cases.

Delusional disorder used to be known as 'paranoia', and the terms are virtually synonymous. Paranoia and its related disorders were regarded as an important group of psychiatric illnesses until the early part of the twentieth century. Then, because of changing diagnostic and classificatory approaches, especially a tendency to overdiagnose schizophrenia, the diagnosis of paranoia all but disappeared from standard classificatory systems. In 1987, paranoia was again officially recognized by DSM-IIIR but was renamed delusional (paranoid) disorder—since simplified to delusional disorder. It is the only officially acknowledged member of the old group of paranoid illnesses appearing in DSM-IV and ICD-10.

Although the diagnosis of paranoia all but ceased for many years, the illness and its sufferers did not disappear. When the phenomena of the disorder came to attention the patient was either labelled as schizophrenic or else a specific feature of the delusional phenomenology was seized upon and spurious diagnoses were described. Thus we have a multiplicity of apparently disparate diagnoses such as de Clérambault's syndrome (delusional erotomania), the Othello syndrome (delusional jealousy), querulant paranoia (a form of persecutory delusional disorder), monosymptomatic hypochondriacal psychosis (delusional disorder with somatic preoccupations), and many others. The result has been an extraordinarily scattered literature with cases recorded in a variety of medical and non-medical sources, but very few in psychiatric journals until recently. Since DSM-IIIR there has been a serious attempt to resolve the confusion and to diagnose paranoia/delusional disorder by its own intrinsic features, but many problems still bedevil the nomenclature.

Jaspers, in discussing paranoia, said: 'Why are the paranoics as defined by Kraepelin so rare, yet when they do occur they are so typical?' This remains true because there are striking similarities from case to case and the illness' features clearly distinguish it from other psychoses, yet many psychiatrists continue to label it erroneously.

DSM-IV and ICD-10 provide criteria to differentiate delusional disorder as an illness *sui generis* and these are now widely accepted. This section adopts that official approach but with two caveats. The first is that the descriptions are bald and not very helpful to the clinician who has not actually seen cases of the disorder. The second is that the category of delusional disorder (persistent delusional disorders in ICD-10) may well be overrestrictive as it stands. However, some well-respected authorities take a somewhat different approach, regarding 'delusional disorders' as all psychiatric illnesses with delusions and then subcategorizing according to the underlying syndrome, which might be severe mood disorder, schizophrenia, actual delusional disorder, etc. Therefore the reader of any text must be aware of a particular author's criteria for diagnosis in this area.

Emil Kraepelin (1856–1926) clearly described paranoia and included it in a continuum of illnesses with delusional features, especially paraphrenia and paranoid schizophrenia. This so-called 'paranoid spectrum' will be briefly alluded to later. Paranoid schizophrenia continues to be a widely used diagnosis but usually in the context of schizophrenia. Paraphrenia is not officially acknowledged in DSM-IV or ICD-10 but cases fitting its traditional description are quite commonly seen in practice. The present author regards it as a significant entity and the reader is encouraged to become familiar with descriptions to be found elsewhere.

At present, 'delusional disorder' is both an illness category and essentially the only syndrome contained within that category. In recent years, another diagnosis—delusional misidentification syndrome (**DMIS**)—has come into increasing prominence. Originally described in 1923 by Capgras and Reboul-Lachaux[3] as an illness in which the individual is delusionally convinced that someone familiar in the environment has been replaced by an almost exact double, this 'Capgras syndrome' led a rather marginal existence in the literature for many years. Lately, however, there have been considerably more case-reports of better quality and clinical subtypes have been established. Most importantly, sound psychological and neuropathological work has increasingly shown significant cerebral pathologies in a high proportion of sufferers.

DMIS is not currently recognized by DSM or ICD but in many respects it resembles delusional disorder and should certainly be included in an expanded category of that disorder.

Finally, there is an important phenomenon which is found in association with all illnesses with delusions, especially delusional disorder. This is named 'shared psychotic disorder' in DSM-IV and 'induced delusional disorder' in ICD-10, but is often still referred to by its long-established name *folie à deux*. Here, the primary patient has a bona fide delusional illness and a secondary patient has come to accept the delusional beliefs as true. The secondary patient is usually a highly impressionable individual living in prolonged close contact with the other; he or she is not truly deluded, but retains the beliefs tenaciously as long as the intimate relationship is maintained. A less common variety is when two people each have genuine delusional disorders and, through close proximity, come to share identical abnormal beliefs. *Folie à deux* is not uncommon and, as will be explained later, there are very practical reasons why the clinician should be aware of its possible presence and the ways in which it may influence management of the case.

The paranoid spectrum[4]

Since Kraepelin's time there has been a tacit acceptance by many psychiatrists of a spectrum simplified as:

delusional disorder—paraphrenia—paranoid schizophrenia.

Somewhat anecdotally, the literature suggests that approximately 10 per cent of cases of delusional disorder or paraphrenia will deteriorate to schizophrenia though, in general, most cases of delusional disorder remain diagnostically stable in the long term. Several reports have indicated that, as one moves to the delusional disorder end, a family history of schizophrenia becomes progressively less common. The risk for schizophrenia in the close family of a case of delusional disorder appears to be much the same as in the general public. In paranoid schizophrenia the family history of schizophrenia is approximately half as common as in other schizophrenias and profound disintegration of personality is less frequent.

When dealing with cases in this general area the clinician should bear in mind the concept of a paranoid spectrum. This, plus knowledge of constituent illnesses, will make it easier to distinguish delusional disorder from superficially similar conditions, a matter of considerable importance when considering treatment and prognosis.

Problems of nomenclature

Although English-speaking psychiatrists (and most members of the public) use the word 'paranoid' to mean 'persecutory', strictly speaking it just means 'delusional'. In many writings on 'paranoia' and 'paranoid' disorders, authors do not make it clear whether delusions are present or not in their cases.

Unfortunately, with the passage of time, the term 'paranoid' has come to be used so loosely that it has lost any meaningful clinical connotation. Paranoia should now be regarded as an historical usage, pretty well synonymous with delusional disorder.

The word 'paranoid' is still used in the official diagnoses of paranoid schizophrenia and paranoid personality disorder. The former is acceptable because the illness has delusions as a prominent feature, but it is quite illogical in describing a personality disorder, which cannot have delusions. Since it is unlikely that the personality disorder will be renamed soon, the reader should be aware of such pitfalls in our psychiatric terminology and consequently the need for ultra-careful case-descriptions.

Although the **form** of delusional disorder is remarkably characteristic, the delusional **contents** and the ways in which cases come to attention are extremely varied, and this has led to an extraordinarily complex history. The core description, that of paranoia, gradually crystallized in the latter half of the nineteenth century and was definitively delineated by Kraepelin, who recognized subtypes with delusional contents of grandiosity, persecution, erotomania, and jealousy, and also allowed for the possibility of a hypochondriacal content. He clearly differentiated paranoia from *dementia praecox* (i.e. schizophrenia). Kraepelin later doubted whether hallucinations could be present: in fact, non-prominent hallucinations are now acceptable and in every other respect Kraepelin's century-old definition of paranoia still largely serves to describe present-day delusional disorder.[5]

Subsequently, Kraepelin[5] introduced the concept of paraphrenia, an illness similar to paranoid schizophrenia but with significantly better preservation of affect and of personality. As already mentioned, he regarded paranoia, paraphrenia, and paranoid schizophrenia as a relatively discrete group of illnesses, later referred to as the paranoid spectrum.

It was later found that a minority of cases of paranoia and paraphrenia eventually deteriorated to schizophrenia and this somewhat illogically led to these diagnoses being progressively ignored. Despite this, speculation on the nature of delusions continued, most notably by Jaspers (1883–1969),[6] Kretschmer (1888–1964),[7] and Freud (1856–1939) and his followers. These speculations contributed a good deal to the descriptive phenomenology of delusions but whereas we know a good deal about delusional contents, we understand little about the origin of delusions or of delusional illnesses, or the reasons for their unique features.[8] Unfortunately, as much of the writing on delusions appeared when most psychoses, and certainly paranoia, had no effective treatments, writers usually dwelt on the untreatability of paranoia, a pessimistic view that persists but is no longer warranted.

From the 1970s onwards, interest in paranoia reappeared and a more optimistic view of treatment emerged. Since its renaissance as delusional disorder in DSM-IIIR in 1987, paranoia has again become a respectable diagnosis. Not only that, it has subsumed several quasi-disorders which were undoubtedly delusional but which had been described superficially on the strength of their delusional content alone. Several of these have already been noted (see p. 281).

Nowadays the clinical description of delusional disorder is well established, but adequate case series are rare and scientific investigations are in their infancy, except in the case of the diagnosis which still remains officially unrecognized, delusional misidentification syndrome, in which underlying brain abnormalities are commonly demonstrable. The separateness of delusional disorder from schizophrenia is beyond doubt, but its relationship to the other constituents of the paranoid spectrum still has to be determined. Delusional disorder is no longer regarded as rare, but many years of neglect have left many psychiatrists sadly unaware of its characteristic features.

Delusions: clinical aspects

A delusion may be defined very loosely as a mistaken idea which is held unshakably by the patient and which cannot be corrected. As will be seen, this is not a satisfactory definition, although it may be a useful starting point for clinical recognition of a delusional process. This brief exposition is concerned to facilitate clinical recognition and not to dwell on psychopathological theories, which are dealt with in detail elsewhere in this book.

It is a widely held opinion that delusions are qualitatively different from normal ideas or beliefs and have an all-or-nothing aspect. The DSM-IV definition initially seems to accept this viewpoint, stating that a delusion is 'A false belief based on an incorrect inference about external reality that is firmly sustained despite what almost everyone else believes and despite what constitutes incontrovertible and obvious proof or evidence to the contrary. The belief is not one ordinarily accepted by other members of the person's culture or subculture'. But the definition goes on to say that it is often difficult to distinguish between a delusion and an overvalued idea (in which there is an unreasonable belief or idea but not held with such pathological certitude as in a delusion), and that 'Delusional conviction occurs on a continuum' from normal to abnormal. These two statements markedly lessen the initial description of the absolute nature of the delusional wrongness.

The definition of delusion by Mullen[9] based on the earlier description by Jaspers is widely quoted and its implications are largely accepted by DSM-IV and ICD-10. He characterizes delusions as follows:

1 They are held with absolute conviction.
2 The individual experiences the delusional belief as self-evident and regards it as of great personal significance.
3 The delusion cannot be changed by an appeal to reason or by contrary experience.
4 The content of delusions is unlikely and often fantastic.
5 The false belief is not shared by others from a similar socio-economic group.

Clinicians widely employ the terminology on delusions introduced by Jaspers, for example when they use terms such as 'primary' and 'secondary' delusions, 'delusional mood' (*Wahnstimmung*), and 'delusional memory'. These concepts are of some descriptive and possibly heuristic value, but they do not prove particularly helpful in distinguishing delusions from overvalued ideas in individual cases, nor in deciding whether a particular delusional phenomenon is specific to a given mental disorder.

In a sense, all delusions are secondary in that they are the product of a pathological process in the brain which, in most cases, we can only guess at. It is sometimes useful to differentiate clinically between the 'primary' or 'autochthonous' delusion, which appears fully fledged and relatively suddenly, and the 'secondary' delusion, which is a further development within the delusional system and may sometimes seem to be the individual's way of rationalizing his delusional beliefs although, of course, the rationalization must necessarily be filtered through a mind already thought-disordered and affected by delusions. For example, the initial belief may be that the police are watching him night and day; the secondary delusion 'explains' that this is because he has secret information about aliens which the authorities do not wish divulged. The better organized the delusions, the more convincing are the 'explanations', even to outsiders.

Not all primary delusions arise suddenly and, in fact, it must be presumed that in most cases the suddenness is more apparent than real. Almost certainly, unless the delusion is the result of an acute brain dysfunction such as may follow a head injury or delirium, there is a lead-up process, which may be accompanied by the aforementioned *Wahnstimmung*, a mood state compounded of anxiety, perplexity, and a sense of impending crisis. When the delusion crystallizes, the delusional mood often disperses and is replaced by a sense of revelation and of certainty. It seems likely that this phenomenon occurs in a proportion of delusional disorder patients and it often happens that, at the moment of revelation, some coincidental but irrelevant circumstance is picked upon to explain the appearance of the new belief. For example, a media event, a thunderstorm, a chance telephone call, etc., may thereafter be, in the patient's mind, the 'cause'.

While we regard delusions as one of the most characteristic elements of all the psychotic illnesses and a sine qua non in the diagnosis of delusional disorder, clear-cut description, and delineation have proved elusive despite many years of study and experiment.[10] In fact, it would seem that none of the characteristics of delusion which we traditionally accept stand up completely to scientific scrutiny. In particular, nowadays the so-called bizarreness of a delusion has been shown to have little or no distinguishing value.[11]

Much of the classical work on delusions was done in pretreatment times when the chronic condition was readily available for study in institutions. In the present era our aim is to diagnose psychotic disorders as early as possible, sometimes even before frank delusions are evident, and to begin treatment at once. Neuroleptics rapidly interfere with many psychopathological processes; they certainly suppress delusions, although not necessarily permanently. Of course this makes ongoing experimental observations of delusions, especially of the acute variety, all but impossible in clinical circumstances. Psychiatrists find themselves in the paradoxical situation of diagnosing illness because of the presence of delusions whose scientific validity is largely unsubstantiated, and then causing these to disappear before they can be verified properly. Nevertheless, until we have more objective means of making diagnoses it remains essential that, as far as we can, we recognize delusions when they occur and separate them from other abnormal psychopathological appearances.

How can a clinician deal with this? Firstly it seems inescapable that he or she be both experienced and insightful. Given these qualities, it often does seem possible to have an informed sense of whether a belief is true or false and, if the latter, whether it is being held with delusional intensity. A key element in the decision is a comparison between the patient's current beliefs and those he habitually held, and here a corroborative account from an informed outside source is usually necessary.

The observer's educated suspicion that a delusion is present is the starting point, but it is evident that that suspicion has to be aroused by the context of the apparently delusional idea because, no matter how isolated it appears to be, it nearly always occurs in the setting of a mental disorder whose other features may indicate a specific psychiatric diagnosis. Illogically, instead of recognizing the delusion and using it to make a definite diagnosis, we develop the conviction that we are dealing with a probable psychosis and thereafter judge all the patient's utterances in light of that. While he may indeed be experiencing delusions, it is essential that we do not automatically assume that anything the psychotic individual says has of necessity to be of a delusional nature.

We must accept that we cannot be absolute in our recognition of a delusion. In addition to the illness context we base our estimate on a series of nuances, no one of which is pathognomonic but an accumulation of which becomes increasingly convincing. The abnormalities to be sought are as follows:

1 An idea or belief is expressed with unusual persistence or force.

2 As far as we can tell, the idea is not typical of the individual's previously prevailing thinking and is not shared by his or her social community.

3 The idea appears to exert an undue influence on the person's life and consequently the way of life is altered to an extraordinary degree.

4 Despite the significance to the patient of the belief, he or she often displays secretiveness or resentment when questioned about it.

5 The individual tends to be humourless and oversensitive about the belief.

6 There is a quality of 'centrality'; no matter how strange the belief or its consequences, the patient rarely questions that incredible things are happening to him or her. For example, why should a perfectly ordinary harmless person be singled out for constant surveillance by the security agencies? But this is simply accepted.

7 Attempts to contradict the belief are likely to arouse an inappropriately strong emotional reaction, often with irritability and hostility and with a superciliousness that may be a form of grandiosity.

8 On reflection the belief appears unlikely to the observer, but at the time of history-taking the vehemence of its expression may temporarily disguise its improbability.

9 The patient is so emotionally overinvested in the idea that it swamps other elements in the psyche, and many everyday activities are neglected.

10 If the delusion is acted out, uncharacteristic behaviours, sometimes involving violence, will occur which may be partly understood in terms of the abnormal belief.

11 Others who know the patient well will usually observe that his or her thinking and behaviour are alien, unless *folie à deux* is present when, paradoxically, the other person's denials of abnormality are themselves possible confirmation of the presence of delusion.

12 An odd feature of delusions is that, no matter how strongly they are held, when the patient is given the opportunity to obtain real proof he or she persistently evades accepting the opportunity.

13 One must always look for the features which frequently accompany delusions, especially suspiciousness, hauteur, grandiosity, evasiveness, and eccentric or threatening behaviour, as well as evidence of thought disorder, mood change, and hallucinations.

Particular features of delusions in delusional disorder

In addition to any of the above, in delusional disorder we find several other elements, which are of importance in leading to the diagnosis:

1 The delusional system is stable and is expressed or defended with intense affect and with highly rehearsed arguments. The form of logic used by the patient is very consistent but the propositions are based on false premises. Since the individual is so focused on his beliefs and is so self-assured, he often succeeds in making the enquirer feel inept.

2 The delusional system is markedly 'encapsulated', so that the beliefs therein and their accompanying symptoms are to a considerable extent separated from the rest of the personality which retains a good deal of normal function. However, the compelling force of the delusions often overshadows these normal aspects and this is increasingly so with advancing chronicity of the illness, when the tendency to express and act out the delusions may well increase.

3 When the individual is preoccupied with the delusional system there is strong emotional and physiological arousal, but when he or she is engaged on neutral topics, the arousal abates and an ordinary conversation can take place. Switching between normal and abnormal 'modes', sometimes very rapidly, is virtually pathognomonic of delusional disorder.

4 Because of the encapsulation of the delusions and the normal–abnormal switch just described, the patient may have phases of relative normality interspersed with psychotic periods. The switch can occur spontaneously or as a result of external provocation; the two are difficult to disentangle because the hypervigilant individual may perceive provocation in almost anything. Since it is a chronic illness the symptoms never remit, but if they are temporarily in the background the patient may converse and function almost normally and may have sufficient quasi-insight to keep the delusions concealed for the moment. Total denial of mental abnormality and resistance to psychiatric referral are almost universal in cases of delusional disorder and lead to severe underestimation of the illness's frequency.

5 As a result of the features just described, many delusional disorder patients can continue to exist in society, sometimes with very abnormal but harmless beliefs but in other instances with highly malignant delusions, which they may or may not act out.

6 As will be repeatedly emphasized, delusional disorder must be diagnosed on the **form** of the illness and the content of the delusion is not used to make the primary diagnosis. On the other hand, the particular content is employed to categorize into subgroups, as will shortly be described.

Delusional disorders: clinical features

Official diagnostic criteria

The DSM-IV and ICD-10 criteria are shown in Tables 4.4.1 and 4.4.2, respectively.

As will be seen, the DSM-IV and ICD-10 descriptions are very similar in overall outline but with a number of rather striking minor differences. The following specific items should be noted:

1 DSM-IV uses the term 'non-bizarre' delusions; this criterion has been shown to have little or no validity.[11]

2 DSM-IV allows the presence of tactile and olfactory hallucinations, while ICD-10 mentions only auditory hallucinations; in practice most modalities may be represented but the important point is that they are relatively non-prominent and usually parallel to the content of the delusion(s).

3 DSM-IV says that delusions should have been present for 1 month and ICD-10 insists on 3 months. Both are guesses, but ICD-10 is probably right to err on the side of caution and it provides category F22.8 as a temporary niche until the definitive diagnosis emerges.

4 Both classifications exclude delusional illnesses due to organic brain disorder, medical illnesses, medication effects, or psychoactive substance abuse. In essence this is correct, especially in an illness of acute onset. However, as will be noted later, an apparently typical delusional disorder may arise as a long-term complication of any of these factors.

5 DSM-IV and ICD-10 agree emphatically that delusional disorder is not schizophrenia and DSM-IV notes that general functioning is not impaired. Both say that mood disturbance may accompany the delusional illness but is not a cause of it.

6 The list of subtypes according to delusional content is similar in both classifications, although ICD-10 adds self-referential and litigious themes.

Table 4.4.1 DSM-IV delusional disorder (297.1)

Principal features

(a) Non-bizarre delusions of at least 1 month's duration

(b) Criterion A for schizophrenia has never been met, although tactile and olfactory hallucinations may be acceptable if they are related to the delusional theme

(c) Apart from the impact of the delusion(s) or its consequences, functioning is not markedly impaired and behaviour is not obviously odd or bizarre

(d) Concurrent mood episodes, if present, are brief relative to the duration of the delusional disorder

(e) The disturbance is not the direct outcome of a drug or medication or of a medical disorder

Subtypes

Erotomanic
Grandiose
Jealous
Persecutory
Somatic
Mixed (allowing for the presence of more than one of the foregoing)
Unspecified or other

Table 4.4.2 ICD-10 persistent delusional disorders

Delusional disorder (F22.0)

Principal features

(a) A delusion or set of related delusions, other than those described as typically schizophrenic, must be present; the most common are persecutory, grandiose, hypochondriacal, jealous, or erotic

(b) The delusion(s) must be present for at least 3 months

(c) The general criteria for schizophrenia are not fulfilled

(d) There are no persistent hallucinations, but there may be transitory or occasional auditory hallucinations that are not speaking in the third person or making a running commentary

(e) Depressive symptoms or episodes may be intermittently present, but the delusional symptoms must persist at times when there is no disturbance of mood

(f) There must be no evidence of primary or secondary organic mental disorder or of a psychotic disorder due to psychoactive substance use

Subtypes

Persecutory
Litigious
Self-referential
Grandiose
Hypochondriacal
Jealous
Erotomanic

Other persistent delusional disorders (F22.8)

This is a residual category for persistent disorders with delusions that do not fully meet the criteria for delusional disorder or schizophrenia. Illnesses with prominent delusions accompanied by persistent hallucinatory voices or by psychotic symptoms insufficient to satisfy the criteria for schizophrenia are included here. A delusional disorder of less than 3 months' duration is coded under Acute and Transient Psychotic Disorders (F23) until proven otherwise.

7 Neither classification specifies that the essence of delusional disorder is a highly organized delusional system, largely encapsulated from normal aspects of the personality, although DSM-IV hints at this when it comments that functioning is not markedly impaired and behaviour is not obviously odd or bizarre. Neither comments that the patient can demonstrate alternating 'normal' and 'delusional' modes.

8 The ICD-10 category of 'other persistent delusional disorders' is vaguely described and is largely a catch-all heading or, as mentioned above, a temporary holding station. However, it could conceivably be used for the time being to subsume the unofficial delusional disorder diagnoses of paraphrenia and delusional misidentification syndrome.

9 Overall, DSM-IV and ICD-10 give rather laconic descriptions of delusional disorder and it will be necessary to flesh them out with relevant clinical details. This will be done after the next section on aetiological considerations.

General aetiological considerations in delusional disorders

It must be stressed that knowledge of aetiology in delusional disorder is scanty and highly speculative, largely because so little modern research has been conducted. What follows is an outline, and certain other factors will be noted when we come to consider some of the illness.

(a) Genetic factors

Changes in definitions of paranoia/delusional disorder over the years and the frequent confusion with schizophrenia make most studies all but impossible to interpret. Conclusions are inferential rather than evidence based. However, it seems well established[12] that delusional disorder and paranoid schizophrenia are less directly inherited than other forms of schizophrenia, and that there is little or no evidence of a genetic link between delusional disorder and schizophrenia.

There may be genetic links with certain severe personality disorders, especially of the paranoid and schizoid varieties, but these are difficult to substantiate. There does seem to be an excess of such disorders in relatives and premorbidly in delusional disorder patients themselves. It is suggested that paranoid and schizoid traits are particularly liable to lead to social isolation and aggravation of delusional tendencies.[13,14]

(b) Organic brain factors

Recent evidence from the study of delusional misidentification syndrome (see later) indicates that delusions of a very specific type may arise in association with certain well-defined brain insults. There are strong hints, but much less supportive evidence, to suggest that organic brain factors may also be important in cases of delusional disorder. For example, head injury may lead to the development of marked paranoid symptoms, and there is a long-established association between chronic alcoholism and pathological jealousy.[15] Old age itself may be linked to the onset of symptoms typical of delusional disorder, and early evidence of brain changes, especially in subcortical areas, is starting to appear in studies of various kinds of senile 'paranoid' illness.[16–18] Amphetamine and cocaine abuse[19] can induce delusional illness, as can therapeutic drugs, including L-dopa and methyldopa,[20] at times. Delusional illness induced by the brain effects of AIDS infection has been documented.[21]

Gorman and Cummings[22] have proposed that delusional illnesses of organic origin have underlying features in common, particularly temporal lobe or limbic involvement and an excess of dopamine activity in certain areas of the brain.

If organic factors predominate in a particular case, delusions must be seen as a secondary feature of an organic brain disorder. However, if the organic factors are subtle and of long duration, the clinical appearances may be those of a quite typical delusional disorder which, interestingly, may well respond to neuroleptic treatment as effectively as idiopathic cases. (In fact, 'idiopathic' may simply denote organicity at a more subtle level.) It is very possible that organic brain factors are much more common than we suspect in delusional disorder, especially in young males who have previously abused alcohol or drugs or have suffered a head injury in the past, and in older patients (more commonly female) who suffer from effects of an ageing brain.[23,24]

(c) Interplay with mood factors

We have already seen that DSM-IV and ICD-10 agree that mood symptoms may accompany delusional disorder but not cause it. Delusional and mood disorders are separate illnesses with their own natural histories and responses to treatment, yet there is a complex relationship between them, as is also the case with mood disorder and schizophrenia. For example, it is well documented that some cases of apparently typical mood illness, unipolar or bipolar, can progress to delusional disorder or schizophrenia over time. Conversely, cases which appear to be delusional disorder but with an episodic course may prove to be bipolar illness. There are a number of anecdotal reports of delusional disorder responding to antidepressant treatment, and it is more than likely that these represent a failure to recognize the true nature of a mood disorder associated with delusions.

Both depressive disorder and mania may be complicated by delusions. On the other hand, mood symptoms, especially dysphoria with anxiety, are a common complication of delusional disorder, while individuals with the grandiose subtype may show elation, which mimics mania but is far more sustained. In recovering delusional disorder, one may see postpsychotic depression of varying degrees of severity and this is described later. Suicide is not unknown in delusional disorder but its frequency is undetermined.

In many delusional disorder patients the illness is profoundly isolating and sets them at odds with the rest of the society, which often generates suspiciousness, dejection, anxiety, and agitation in the individual. It seems that a vicious circle results whereby the delusion induces distress and physiological overarousal which, in turn, reinforces the strength of the delusion and progressively diminishes reality input.

(d) Psychodynamic theories of causation

The psychodynamic literature continues to discuss aspects of 'paranoia' but often fails to differentiate clearly between trait, symptom, personality disorder, and psychotic illness. Most of the emphasis is on the persecutory aspect of paranoia, with only occasional references to other types of delusional content. Since psychotherapists rarely treat psychotic patients, their experience of delusional phenomena must actually be rare and their knowledge of the features correspondingly scanty. Their theoretical bias is to interpret the origins of paranoia in terms of psychological maldevelopment, ignoring the increasing weight of evidence that faulty brain mechanisms are involved. One must read the psychoanalytic literature on this particular topic with an ultracritical attitude, since it usually fails to provide adequate illness definitions or clear case reports and generates explanatory theories which are unjustifiably presented as proven facts.

(e) Conclusions regarding aetiology

No systematic research on paranoia took place for more than half a century and modern investigations into delusional disorder are only beginning to appear. Therefore it is premature to propose specific aetiological theories. However, a gathering weight of evidence does suggest a localized and relatively circumscribed brain disorder associated with the possible influence of abnormal neurotransmitter activity, probably involving dopamine overactivity. Whatever the original basis of delusional disorder, it certainly seems that provocative influences such as head injury, alcohol abuse, and ill effects of drugs may play a part, whereas speculation about psychological causations suggest that this is at most a secondary influence. There is an urgent need for the study of extended case series utilizing modern neurophysiological and neuropsychological investigative methods.

Delusional disorder: general features and introduction to the subtypes

We have already outlined the diagnostic criteria for delusional disorder in DSM-IV and ICD-10 and have amplified these with descriptions of many of the clinical phenomena associated with the illness. It has been emphasized that this is a stable and readily recognizable disorder, provided that the clinician is informed of the essential criteria and has dealt with at least several cases to familiarize him- or herself with its very characteristic 'feel'. With this experience it becomes much more possible to delve under the prominent symptoms related to delusional content and to discern the underlying form of the illness. However, it is the predominant delusional content in an individual case, and the symptoms and behaviours related to this, which decide how a patient will present for assessment. Therefore we shall consider the main subtypes in some detail. It cannot be stressed enough that these are not separate types of illness, but variants on a single psychopathological theme.

All cases of delusional disorder occur in clear consciousness and have a stable and persistent delusional system which is relatively encapsulated. Since much of the personality remains remarkably intact, a considerable degree of social functioning is retained in many cases. The patient experiences a heightened sense of self-reference within the delusional context and ordinary events take on unusual significance. He or she clings to the delusion with fervid intensity and spurns any suggestion that a mental illness is present. Outside the delusional system the patient shows quite normal thinking, affect, and behaviour, but there is a marked tendency for gradual pushing to one side of these normal aspects. The retention of such a degree of normality makes the illness totally different from schizophrenia.

Earlier it has been indicated that the DSM-IV criterion of non-bizarreness is unhelpful, although in all cases of delusional disorder the delusions are relatively well structured, coherent, and consistent, and the logic would often be acceptable if it weren't that its basic premises are irrational. Many affected individuals can maintain overtly normal activities, at least in public, but increasing pressure of the delusion tends to cause corresponding responses in behaviour; these may be channelled socially, as in hypochondriacally deluded patients who utilize medical resources, albeit excessively, or antisocially, as in the aggression of the jealously deluded individual. Mood abnormalities are common as a response to the effects of the illness.

Hallucinations do occur in some cases and may affect any modality, but they are often difficult to assess and to differentiate from delusional misinterpretations and illusions. Widespread persistent hallucinations in more than one sensory sphere should make one cautious about the diagnosis of delusional disorder.

The illness appears to affect men and women approximately equally, but it is not clear if this is true of all subtypes. Despite older assertions that the illness is restricted to the middle-aged and elderly, the age of onset can actually be from late adolescence to extreme old age, with male patients appearing on average to experience earlier initiation. Some patients behave in an eccentric or fanatical fashion and, as a group, delusional disorder sufferers are excessively likely to be unmarried, divorced, or widowed, probably reflecting restriction of affective responses and some isolative tendencies. Despite this, the condition can be compatible with marriage and continued employment. The premorbid personality is usually described as asocial and there may indeed be an excess of long-standing schizoid and paranoid personality disorders. However, when a patient makes a good recovery there may be little evidence of this, and it is possible that in some cases a 'personality disorder' is actually the prolonged and insidious prodrome of the illness.

Onset may be gradual or acute. In the latter the patient often identifies a precipitating stressor, which is difficult to confirm (e.g. the person who has a delusion of skin infestation may attribute it to a single insect bite many years previously). While most individuals are secretive about their abnormal beliefs or express them by such means as physical complaints or legal processes, a certain number actually utilize them, perhaps within the context of an extreme religious sect or by becoming an excessively insistent agitator on some social issue. Disinhibited and overtly aggressive behaviour seems more likely to occur in males, at times leading to clashes with the authorities.

In all cases of delusional disorder, no matter what the nature of the delusional theme, the investigator should look for the relatively unique feature of the illness—the patient's ability to move between normal and delusional modes of thinking. In the former there is relatively calm mood, reasonable rapport, and appropriate emotional responses, whereas in the latter there is overalerting, suspiciousness, and the sense that the person is being remorselessly driven by the delusional beliefs. This situation is difficult for the inexperienced observer to comprehend, since it is inconceivable to most people that someone who can appear perfectly rational at one moment can almost instantaneously change to a possessed irrational being—and then back again just as quickly. In a sense the same patient is both sane and insane, and when in the latter mode may be ultrapersuasive about the acceptability of his or her beliefs. One may imagine the plight of a lawyer faced with a client who has committed some uncharacteristically outrageous act as a result of a delusion, who can then discuss his case with apparent insight and logic, and even genuine remorse, but who nevertheless remains totally self-justifying. As a corollary, the client will usually deny the possibility of mental illness and often refuses to cooperate with psychiatric assessment. He may also refuse to cooperate with the legal process, to his knowing detriment.

Delusional disorder, when it was known as paranoia, often had a bad reputation because patients were regarded as angry, suspicious, accusatory, and potentially violent. Some undoubtedly are, but as we consider the various subtypes nowadays we realize that many sufferers, perhaps the majority, lead lives of internalized despair in progressively isolated circumstances. Anger and suspiciousness are often secondary, at least in part, to the perceived neglect of their overwhelming concerns. The illness is chronic and self-reinforcing, and it is likely that only a minority of cases are recognized or helped. Psychiatry does not have an impressive record of helpfulness towards this group of patients.

The subtypes of delusional disorder

As previously noted, DSM-IV recognizes five main subtypes based on the predominant delusional themes: the erotomanic, grandiose, jealous, persecutory and somatic, plus mixed and unspecified types. ICD-10 also recognizes these subtypes, and adds litigious and self-referential categories. Here, the litigious variety is included within the persecutory group and self-referential cases are not given separate status since self-reference is, in reality, a feature of the illness as a whole and prominent in all cases.

When delusional disorder was resurrected in DSM-IIIR, single delusional themes were emphasized, but the mixed category in DSM-IV accepts the reality that, for example, a hypochondriacal individual can also feel persecuted and an erotomanic patient can be extremely grandiose. Also, we shall find that there are considerable individual variations within the overall themes, so that in the somatic subtype there are cases involving different body systems. Yet the range of major themes does not appear to be all that wide and we have no explanation for this relative restriction in their number. The 'unspecified' category in DSM-IV allows us to accommodate any case whose delusional theme is unusual and leaves a door open to the discovery of other themes in the future.

In presenting the subtypes, relatively more attention will be given to the somatic form. This should not be taken as an indication that this is the most common variant; rather, it happens to be the one which has been best documented in the recent psychiatric literature. Other types of delusional presentation are much more often described in non-psychiatric and non-medical sources, where the fundamental nature of the illness may be overlooked, and so we are only beginning to correlate such descriptions with modern findings on delusional disorder.

Delusional disorder: persecutory and litigious subtypes

In most people's minds the persecutory type of delusional disorder is the archetype of 'paranoia' and it is usually assumed that it is the most common variety. Therefore it is surprising to find that the literature, while full of speculation, is very lacking in good descriptions of the phenomenology of the illness and, apart from unreliable psychoanalytic theory, says relatively little about persecutory delusions themselves.

Clinical features

By definition the illness is a chronic psychotic disorder with a well-systematized delusional system and with relative sparing of the surrounding personality. The persecutory threats may be perceived simply as coming from 'them', but can elaborate to descriptions of the most labyrinthine plots involving a variety of known and unknown adversaries. The beliefs are extremely stable and usually increase in complexity with the passage of time. There is heightened awareness and misinterpretation of neutral environmental cues and, not unnaturally suspiciousness, extreme anxiety, and irritability are present. Elements of grandiosity are not uncommon, with the individual accepting that he or she is the centre of focused and malignant attention that would be inexplicable to the normal person. As the illness progresses there is a tendency to involve an increasing number of people in the persecutory system, not uncommonly relatives, physicians, law-enforcement agencies, aspects of government, and others.

As with other subtypes of delusional disorder, many individuals are able to conceal their increasingly insistent delusions for some time, but because of fear of harm they are likely to isolate themselves more and more. If they live alone they may come to be regarded as eccentrics, but if they remain in contact with society the suspicion and anger must eventually become evident, so that interactions with family, social agencies, or the authorities become increasingly confrontational.[24] Despite the reputation of 'paranoia' for violence, only a small proportion of these individuals resort to threat or assault, but with those who do the danger may be profound as the individual is without reservation in his beliefs and will act as though genuinely under severe provocation. Disinhibition may at times be engendered by alcohol or drug use, which makes such situations even more volatile.

Even in a long-standing illness, islands of normal functioning remain; despite this there is little or no insight and the patient resists any psychological explanation for his beliefs. He usually refuses to see a psychiatrist voluntarily; many patients of this kind are encountered in a forensic setting only after an outburst of unacceptable behaviour and are minimally cooperative.[25]

Litigious variety of the persecutory subtype (querulous paranoia)[26,27]

In some individuals with delusional disorder there is a profound and persistent sense of having been wronged in some way, and these people endlessly and repetitively seek redress, sometimes personally but often through the legal system. In a proportion of cases there may initially have been a genuine grievance and there may also have been unsatisfactory recompense, but the subsequent pursuit of 'justice' becomes never-ending and also becomes self-reinforcing because no satisfactory resolution is possible.

This group may not be large but it generates considerable media publicity. Reports of cases naturally tend to be in the literature of the legal profession, the law-enforcement agencies, and, to some extent, forensic psychiatry, but rarely from general psychiatry. Because the individual appears relatively high functioning apart from his delusional beliefs, the complaintive behaviour may be regarded as mere eccentricity for a long time. As in many cases of delusional disorder, the immediate complaint and behaviour may seem coherent and not unreasonable but over time their ongoing, never-ending, and extraordinarily demanding quality begin to raise the suspicion of severe underlying psychopathology. Even then, unless the person begins to be perceived as a threat, little may be done and prolonged harassment of officialdom and the legal system may be tolerated for surprisingly long periods. In some national communities (e.g. Germany and the Scandinavian countries) there are legal provisions to stop 'barratry' or unreasonable use of the law by declaring an individual a querulous litigant.

Goldstein[28] has described three typical ways in which 'litigious paranoia' presents. The first is the 'hypercompetent defendant' who knows and uses the letter of the law up to and beyond its limits but pays no heed to its spirit. The second is the 'paranoid party in a divorce proceeding' who is often consumed with jealousy and pursues vendettas against the ex-spouse, the lawyers on both sides, and even the judge. The third is the 'paranoid complaining witness' who endlessly initiates litigation despite repeated adverse judgements. All such individuals pursue their grievances in a driven manner, see conspiracy in every corner, and are often quite unscrupulous in their single-mindedness, blatantly bending facts to fit with their beliefs. Since they hold the delusional belief with total conviction, they can accept no counterargument or contrary facts. In the past, persistent litigation was virtually a preserve of the rich, but many modern societies provide a variety of avenues for complaintiveness and will even support complaint procedures, and so abnormally litigious behaviour appears to be on the increase.[29]

Diagnosis of the persecutory subtype

All the features of a delusional disorder as previously described are present. In this subtype, wariness, irritability, suspiciousness, and threatening behaviour are especially prominent, and both impulsive and planned violence may occur. Gaining confidence is extremely difficult, but if this succeeds, the more normal aspects of the individual's personality may become apparent and one may also perceive how chronically anxious and overalerted he or she is.

Differential diagnosis

The illness must be distinguished especially from the following:

- paranoid schizophrenia
- paranoid and antisocial personality disorders
- substance-related disorders
- organic brain disorders, including early dementia and some epileptic disorders
- obsessive-compulsive disorder.

Epidemiology

Virtually nothing is known of the frequency and distribution of persecutory delusional disorder. As with other subtypes it occurs in both sexes, but male cases are probably overreported because of a readier tendency to violence and antisocial acts. The literature is biased by the reporting of the most overt cases, often in the news media or through the courts. It is open to speculation how many cases avoid diagnosis; as noted, relatively few come to the clinical attention of psychiatrists other than in forensic work.

Course and prognosis

Delusional disorder is very chronic, and it is presumed that cases of the persecutory subtype are as likely as others to be lifelong and to show increasing psychopathology with the passage of time. In a proportion of cases there is always a risk of violence and illegal behaviour. Since cooperation with assessment and treatment is usually minimal, the overall figures for prognosis must be bad, but we have no reliable data to confirm this.

Forensic complications[30,31]

If someone with a generalized psychotic disorder like schizophrenia becomes sufficiently disorganized, functioning in the community becomes impossible. In contrast, many delusional disorder patients retain a sufficient grasp of reality to continue existing in society, sometimes indefinitely. However, this does not imply that their illness is quiescent. Intellectual ability, capacity for reasoning, and the form of thought remain relatively intact, but the delusional process worsens. They retain the ability to brood on their beliefs so that normal thought processes and delusions interweave, as do normal and abnormal behaviours. Anger may express itself explosively, but some individuals carry out violent actions in a very calculated way, believing that a just vengeance is being exacted. Afterwards there may be real regret and a clear awareness of a wrong having been committed against society, but the actions are seen as justifiable and necessary. The patient is usually aware that by societal standards his deed is legally and morally wrong, but that awareness resides within the normal non-delusional aspect of his mental functioning. Within the confines of the delusional system, the person unswervingly believes that it was obligatory for him to behave as he did.

In such cases, the judge and jury are placed in a quandary, made worse by the individual's frequent arrogance (related to grandiosity), self-justification, and ambivalent expression of regret. The ability to acknowledge the wrongness of one's action in general terms and even to show remorse for it, while also asserting that it was necessary to carry it out, may well be regarded as indicating wilfulness or hypocrisy. Then, paradoxically, culpability may be determined by the content of the delusion, although this has minor relevance to the disinhibition of behaviour. Thus, as Goldstein has pointed out, if the person felt threatened because of a delusional belief and reacted, as he genuinely perceived, in self-defence, his degree of blame may be adjudged to be low. But if he were equally deluded and carefully plotted revenge, this might be seen as highly culpable. Such a distinction cannot be defended logically either in the clinical situation or at law.

Delusional disorder defies any definition of insanity in black or white terms; it is both black and white. Because few psychiatrists, even in the forensic field, are familiar with its detailed characteristics, psychiatry has had limited success in educating the legal profession about the subtleties of the illness or the conundrum that delusions can induce such abnormal behaviour in an individual who superficially appears rational and for significant periods of time is effectively sane even though the illness is always lurking there.

Treatment of the persecutory subtype

Treatment is discussed later in this chapter in the section on overall treatment aspects.

Delusional disorder: somatic subtype (monosymptomatic hypochondriacal psychosis)

Modern society, especially in developed countries, is preoccupied with health concerns. While much of this is positive, there is no doubt that many people worry excessively about health matters and a proportion of these show pathological self-concern. This can shade into hypochondriasis, in which there is a persistent conviction of illness in the absence of objective evidence, with misinterpretation of bodily sensations as disease and with inability to accept reassurances. In many cases the individual shows some degree of body image disturbance, sometimes of extreme degree.[32] Usually we think of hypochondriasis as referring to physical complaints, but nowadays it seems that an increasing number of people are also liable to complain of psychological disorder.

Hypochondriasis is common and may be a personality trait, but it can also be an accompaniment to many psychiatric illnesses, both delusional and non-delusional. It is the presenting feature of the somatic subtype of delusional disorder and in different patients we see many varieties of alteration of body image expressed in delusional terms. Certain themes of delusional content tend to predominate and this has meant an unfortunate proliferation of descriptive names scattered across a fragmented literature, leading to many difficulties in conceptualizing the subtype and in separating it from other psychiatric disorders with prominent hypochondriasis. As with all subtypes of delusional disorder, the clinician must bear in mind the advice already given that, for the diagnosis of delusional disorder, it is the characteristic form of the illness, which is of prime importance, not the content of the delusional beliefs. The hypochondriasis in delusional disorder may superficially resemble that of somatoform disorder, psychotic depression, or obsessive-compulsive disorder, but careful investigation will reveal an illness very different from these.

Clinical features

We shall consider the manifestations of the somatic subtype under four major theme areas:

1 delusions involving the skin;

2 delusions of ugliness or misshapenness (dysmorphic delusions);

3 delusions of body odour or halitosis;

4 miscellaneous.

(a) Delusions involving the skin[33]

In the delusion of skin infestation, the patient insists that he has organisms, usually insects, crawling over the surface of the skin and sometimes burrowing into the skin or under the nails. In most instances he cannot see the creatures, but sometimes there may be graphic descriptions. This may represent a visual hallucination but more usually seems to be a vivid ideational projection.

The delusion of parasites burrowing deeply under the skin is often attributed to worm-like parasites, and internal body sensations or the rippling of small superficial muscles are misinterpreted as evidence of their activities. Sometimes the patient believes that the worms have spread throughout the body or intermittently migrate from place to place.

In the delusion of discrete foreign bodies under the skin or nails, these bodies are occasionally described as inanimate, but generally the patient says they are seed-like or believes that they are parasite eggs. In some individuals this is associated with an irresistible urge to pick, and multiple deep excoriations may result. Such people are sometimes labelled as having 'neurotic excoriations' or factitious disorder, but in fact the picking behaviour is delusionally motivated and is an irresistible urge to stem the invasion of the parasites.

Chronic cutaneous dysaesthesia[34] is an unremitting burning sensation of the skin or mucosae, sometimes generalized but at other times largely confined to complaints of glossodynia or vulvodynia. A minority of these patients appear to have a delusional disorder.

A subgroup of patients with trichotillomania and onychotillomania[35] have delusional illnesses, and the hair-pulling or nail-picking may be part of the attempt to rid themselves of parasites.

In all the above presentations, the delusion and its associated behaviours typically occur in the setting of many well-retained personality features and the patient can often make very clear-cut and apparently rational complaints, convincing the many physicians they attend, at least for a time, that actual physical disease is present. However, no somatic treatment works and the complaining becomes increasingly shrill and unreasonable. The sufferer cannot be persuaded that infestation is not present and often becomes very angry at the perceived incompetence of the dermatologists he has visited.

Usually the story of the infestation is presented in great detail, perhaps involving an original event such as an insect bite. 'Proof' is presented by displaying skin lesions, deformed nails, bald patches, etc. The 'matchbox' or 'pill-bottle' sign, in which the patient produces a small container in which 'insect corpses' or 'eggs' are kept, is typical; the contents nearly always turn out to be dried mucus, skin scrapings, or pieces of lint. Often, there is incessant cleaning of self and surroundings, and repeated demands may be made to local authorities or pest-control agencies for disinfestation of the home. At times bizarre and even dangerous self-treatment is resorted to, such as applying boiling water or corrosive substances to the skin. The more normal part of the psyche is dominated by shame or fear of passing on the infestation, so that progressive social isolation tends to occur, with attendance on doctors as virtually the only outside activity.

(b) Dysmorphic delusions

'Dysmorphophobia', an old term which implies a morbid fear of being deformed, is still sometimes employed to describe cases in this category but should be abandoned since it has been so loosely used to denote both delusional and non-delusional complaints as well as a variety of very different illnesses.[36] In the present context we are considering only cases typical of delusional disorder, which present with a false belief of ugliness or deformity. In some instances there may indeed be some minor deformity, but the complaining and demand for alleviation are out of all proportion and expressed with delusional intensity.

A specific feature is often singled out by the complainer, such as an overlong nose, prominent ears, over-large or undersized breasts, dissatisfaction with the appearance of the genitalia, a skin blemish, or some other. However, in other cases the total body is perceived as abnormal, and there is evidence that a small group of apparent cases of anorexia nervosa and bulimia nervosa may have an underlying delusional disorder.

Many of the patients with dysmorphic delusions go from surgeon to surgeon demanding cosmetic procedures and usually being refused, but if the surgeon does not perceive the illogicality of the complaint an operation may take place. While some successes have been reported, the general consensus is that most cases need psychiatric rather than surgical intervention and unnecessary operations may seriously worsen the mental disorder in the long term.

It is sometimes very difficult to distinguish cases of delusional disorder of somatic subtype from severe somatization disorder, and claims have been made that there is a continuum between these illnesses.[37] The evidence for this is minimal and a diagnostic distinction is essential since treatments of the two disorders are very different.

(c) Delusion of smell or of halitosis[38]

In this category it is often very difficult to distinguish between delusions and hallucinations of smell or taste. The term 'olfactory reference syndrome' is often used to describe olfactory delusions, but in fact it should properly only refer to hallucinatory experiences. Sometimes the deluded patient will say that he or she has not actually experienced the odour, which is usually unpleasant, but 'knows' that it is present because of remarks made by others or their avoidant behaviour. In other cases the stench is described graphically and consistently (like 'burning rubber' or 'faeces') and here a hallucination may be present. There may be no explanation, or else the smell may be attributed to escaping flatus, abnormal sweat secretion, or sinus or dental problems leading to halitosis etc. As is typical, an unending and escalating search for a physical cure occurs.

(d) Miscellaneous delusional contents

Presumably there is an almost infinite possibility of different themes, but in practice their numbers are somewhat limited. The following have been described.

(i) Dental

Although his dentition is satisfactory, the patient insists that his dental bite is abnormal and obtains repeated corrective treatments from successive dentists, none of which works. This has been termed the 'phantom bite syndrome', and may sometimes be associated with complaints of facial pain for which no physical basis is apparent. There may also be delusional complaints of deformity of the jaw or abnormality of the temporomandibular joint.

(ii) Delusion of transmitting non-sexual diseases

Some patients may be convinced that they are causing illnesses in others (e.g. tuberculosis), and they will cite as evidence, for example, that everyone starts coughing when they enter a room.

(iii) Delusion of sexually transmitted disease[39]

Hypochondriasis is, of course, rampant around the topic of sexually transmitted disease. A subgroup of delusional disorder patients develop the conviction that they have venereal disease, often when there is no evidence of risk-taking behaviour having occurred. In the past syphilis was probably the greatest fear, but nowadays it is usually AIDS. Repeated tests showing negative serology have no reassuring effect. Interestingly, a few cases of actual AIDS have been described in which a delusional illness with hypochondriasis has emerged, usually due to direct effects of the virus on the brain.

Differential diagnosis of delusional disorder: somatic subtype

First, the presence of a significant physical disorder must be excluded (although it is possible for a physical illness and delusional disorder to coexist). The illness must be distinguished from the following:

- paranoid schizophrenia
- substance-related disorders (e.g. itching related to alcohol-related liver failure, cocaine abuse, etc.)
- organic brain disorders
- severe depressive disorder with hypochondriacal delusions
- somatoform disorders, especially body dysmorphic disorder
- obsessive-compulsive disorder
- factitious disorder

Epidemiology

Cases usually present in medical and surgical practices and much less often in a psychiatric context. We have no idea of the frequency because non-psychiatrists make a variety of diagnoses, often untranslatable in psychiatric terms. However, the somatic subtype of delusional disorder is certainly not uncommon, and this is increasingly being revealed as consultation–liaison psychiatry develops.

These cases make a strong impression on physicians and surgeons because of their insistence and unreasonable demands. To date, dermatologists have been most aware of the nature of the delusional complaining and, in some cases, have learned to treat the deluded patients satisfactorily with appropriate medication. Infectious and tropical disease specialists also have an awareness, as do gastroenterologists and some dentists, and they are gradually referring more cases for psychiatric help. Plastic and cosmetic surgeons see a considerable number of cases with dysmorphic delusions, but it is still rather uncommon for them to seek psychiatric consultations. Since the patient with delusional disorder generally refuses to visit a psychiatrist willingly, it is often necessary for us to consult on the other specialists' territory in order to offer practical help and to obtain a better idea of the illness's frequency.

From what we know, the somatic subtype affects both sexes approximately equally and the age of onset may be from late adolescence to extreme old age. The illness is more common in the unmarried, divorced, and widowed.

Course and prognosis

Typically the illness is long term with a tendency to worsen with time. Some patients eventually lapse into a rather apathetic state, and some attempt or commit suicide in chronic despair, but the majority continue to move from doctor to doctor demanding treatment on their own deluded terms.

Treatment of the somatic subtype

Treatment is discussed later in this chapter in the section on overall treatment approaches.

Delusional disorder: jealousy subtype[40]

This is sometimes known as the Othello syndrome, but the term is not recommended as it lacks specificity.

The phenomenon of jealousy

Jealousy can arise in various contexts, but here we shall deal with sexual jealousy. This is a virtually universal human emotion, especially when a rival is attempting to lure away someone's sexual partner. Males and females are equally prone to jealousy but may express it differently; Mullen and Martin[41]suggest that men are mainly concerned with losing the partner whereas women worry about the effect of infidelity on the ongoing relationship.

Broadly there are three levels of jealousy. Normal jealousy is understandable in terms of the situation and the individual's perception of it, and its expression can range from pique to severe rage. How it is expressed is largely related to temperament; some people habitually vent anger with slight provocation and others usually bottle up their feelings. On the whole, men tend to act out their jealous anger more physically.

Neurotic jealousy occurs where the mood and its mode of expression are relatively normal but owing to non-psychotic psychiatric illness, including personality disorder, the reaction is impulsive and excessive. Although the individual is reacting to an overvalued idea rather than a delusion, this type of jealousy can be irrational and quite persistent, and may be expressed dangerously.

Psychotic jealousy, as in delusional disorder, is characterized by a fixed delusional belief which cannot be swayed by reasoned argument or presentation of contrary evidence. This is the most alarming type since there is no dissuasion and there is an inexorability about the way that the individual accuses, controls, and even stalks the victim. Since the accusations are usually untrue, the latter is bewildered by them, but occasions do arise when a partner actually has been unfaithful and it is then very difficult for the observer to know at first how much of the jealousy is justified and how much is delusional. Eventually the savageness and unreasonableness of the accusations reveal themselves as undoubtedly abnormal, but meanwhile a frightened partner will have suffered enormous abuse and possibly repeated assault.

When does jealousy become pathological?

Jealousy, which appears justifiable is regarded as normal, although perhaps not laudable, and it will usually be accepted by society if its manifestations are not antisocial. Nowadays we increasingly disapprove of jealous violence, whether provoked or not, but in some communities there is still acknowledgement of the *crime passionel*, the crime committed out of jealous love. However, this is an excuse extended only to males, and the jealous woman who commits assault or murder is usually treated more harshly.

Cobb[42] proposed the following as clinical features of pathological jealousy, whether it be neurotic or psychotic.

1 The jealous thinking and behaviour are unreasonable in expression and intensity.

2 The jealous individual is convinced of the partner's guilt but the evidence is dubious to others.

3 A recognizable psychiatric illness is present which could plausibly be associated with abnormal jealousy.

4 In a proportion of cases, the jealous person has habitual personality characteristics of jealousy, suspiciousness, and overpossessiveness.

5 The jealousy persists unduly and reinforces itself.

6 Pathological jealousy is usually focused on one specific person.

In neurotic jealousy, which in some ways resembles obsessive-compulsive disorder, there is high self-awareness of the emotion and sometimes of its irrationality. In delusional jealousy the person is totally at one with the belief, which has come to occupy much of his or her time. Counterargument or contrary evidence is rejected, yet in delusional disorder the individual may be so high functioning that he or she is totally convincing to outsiders and may even be able to brainwash the innocent victim into admission of guilt, a form of *folie à deux*.

The impact of pathological jealousy

Delusional jealousy is anguishing to the sufferer and even more so to the sexual partner who is accused of infidelity. The latter is subjected to escalating emotional abuse, and indignation, protest, and proof of innocence are unavailing. Physical violence, especially by males, is common[43] and in a proportion of cases finally ends in homicide, sometimes followed by the suicide of the perpetrator.[44] Subjected to prolonged threat, many victims are too terrified to speak up, and some become housebound in a vain attempt to prevent accusations of philandering. From time to time the situation reveals itself when the desperate partner attempts suicide and talks to a helping professional when recovering.

Clinical features

The person's belief in the other's infidelity is absolute and brooks no contradiction. There is much associated irritability, despondency, and, in some cases, aggressiveness. An ever-increasing proportion of time is spent searching for spurious 'proofs', and 'clues' are pounced upon and misinterpreted; for example, an innocent stain is declared to be semen. The victim is put through endless interrogations and is kept under constant surveillance.

Paradoxically, when the jealous individual is questioned closely about his or her specific charges, details prove vague, there is dismissiveness, and there are self-justifying repetitive assertions. Evidence is always about to be produced but rarely materializes. Strangely too, the jealous person often avoids taking the action, which might provide definite proof of guilt or innocence, and this passivity in the midst of intensiveness may be evidence of some volitional defect.

As noted, delusional jealousy is more commonly reported in men, but this is probably an artefact due to their greater likelihood of violence. Also, there is a link between chronic alcohol abuse, as well as amphetamine and cocaine abuse, and delusions of jealousy, and it is known that these substance abuses are more common in males.

Epidemiology

The overall prevalence of abnormal jealousy and the specific prevalence of the delusional disorder subtype are unknown and, because of fear on the part of the victim, both are invariably underreported. Both heterosexual and homosexual cases occur, and family patterns of jealous behaviour have been described, but there is little evidence of direct inheritance.

Course and prognosis

The condition may appear gradually or suddenly, but even when the onset seems rapid there may have been a previous period of rumination and perplexity of varying duration. When the delusion crystallizes the perplexity vanishes and the patient is then totally sure of his belief.

Delusional jealousy is typical in being chronic and often lifelong. Without treatment the prognosis is poor and the danger to the victim is ever present. Most patients refuse psychiatric help and unfortunately may only receive it after incarceration for a violent crime.

Differential diagnosis

The illness must be distinguished from the following:

- actual marital or sexual problems, including spousal infidelity
- mental handicap, where a simple-minded person may develop a 'crush' and be unable to understand that the other person does not reciprocate, or else enters into a sexual relationship and cannot cope with the partner's motives and behaviours
- schizophrenia, especially of the paranoid type
- major mood disorder with delusions, either depressive or manic
- personality disorder, especially of the paranoid, antisocial, borderline, histrionic, and narcissistic types
- obsessive-compulsive disorder

- substance abuse (which may complicate any of the other differential diagnoses)
- organic brain disorders, including dementias and some epileptic disorders
- sexual dysfunction may lead to fears that a normal partner is seeking satisfaction elsewhere

It should be noted that an important part of the diagnostic process, an accurate collateral history, may be impossible to obtain in cases of delusional jealousy because of the victim's fears.

Forensic complications

In cases of identified physical abuse in a relationship one possibility that must always be considered is delusional disorder of jealous type. Severe assault and even murder are not uncommon, and the physician has a duty to warn and protect the partner if these dangers seem real, perhaps divulging confidential information if necessary. Of course the patient denies that his beliefs are unjustified and may present his case more convincingly than the terrified victim can. If involuntary committal is necessary it may be very difficult to sustain, partly because of the individual's ability to maintain a pseudonormal facade and often because he or she threatens litigation.

Occasionally, cases of stalking, usually of females by deluded males, are jealousy related and the victim is nearly always well aware of the stalker's identity in these instances.

Treatment

This will be discussed when considering the overall treatment approach to delusional disorder. If successful treatment can be achieved, the couple may require considerable psychotherapy and counselling to re-establish a trusting and fear-free relationship.

Delusional disorder: erotomanic subtype[45–48]

In erotomania the individual has strong erotic feelings towards another person and has the persistent, unfounded belief that this other person is deeply in love with him or her. The belief is usually delusional, though a small number of non-delusional cases have been reported. Occasionally the imagined lover does not actually exist, but more often he or she is a real person who is unaware of the situation. The phenomenon is often referred to as de Clérambault's syndrome, but this usage is obsolete and can be misleading since it is used to describe erotomanic manifestations in a number of different mental illnesses.

In the older literature it was claimed that erotomanic delusions were largely confined to women, especially isolated and frustrated elderly spinsters, but more and more cases of male erotomania are being reported nowadays.[49] In both sexes the majority of cases described involve heterosexual emotions, but homosexual erotomania is now well documented in both males and females.

Clinical features

The patient yearns for another person and has the unshakeable belief that these feelings are reciprocated. The person is often socially unattainable, may be of higher social status, and can be a celebrity. There has rarely been close contact and the love object will usually be unaware of the situation, but despite this the patient believes that the other initiated the imagined relationship, often with covert signals or utterances. Many patients experience strong erotic, even orgasmic, feelings, but some insist that the 'relationship' is platonic and that the other person is maintaining a non-sexual attitude of watchful protectiveness.

In many instances the patient makes no attempt to get in touch with the love object, perhaps writing letters or buying gifts but not sending them. When given a chance to make actual contact he or she will frequently avoid doing so and will make spurious excuses such as not wanting to offend the other person's spouse. In those cases where the patient does attempt contact, false reasons are presented to explain the almost inevitable rejection that results.

Since this is erotomania in the setting of delusional disorder, the illness will have the typical form of a tightly knit delusional system with preservation of relatively normal personality features and with greater or lesser ability to continue functioning in society. There is often enough insight or inhibition present for the patient to keep the delusional beliefs concealed. However, at times he or she may be profoundly angered by being 'inexplicably' rejected and may act this out, occasionally dangerously. This is more likely to occur in males.

The onset of erotomania can be gradual or apparently sudden. Hallucinations are sometimes present but are not prominent, although the patient may be encouraged by 'hearing' the other person express passionate feelings. Occasionally, the presence of tactile hallucinations leads the patient to believe that a lover has paid a visit during the night (sometimes picturesquely referred to as the 'incubus syndrome').

Diagnosis and differential diagnosis

Many covert examples necessarily go unrecognized and so there is a bias towards diagnosis of cases with some sort of acting out behaviour. Otherwise the most common situation is one where the patient, after years of silent suffering, becomes unhappy enough to be treated for depression and then, during sympathetic history-taking, lets the delusional belief slip out. There is often much accompanying anguish and perhaps anger, and of course the beliefs are regarded as indisputable. Obviously, if the patient has been very secretive, a confirmatory history may be impossible to obtain. In married patients the spouse may be totally unaware of delusions which have lasted for years.

The following disorders may be associated with secondary erotomanic features:

- Schizophrenia, especially paranoid, in which the erotomania coexists with other delusions, florid hallucinations, and more widespread thought disorder.
- Major mood disorder, in depressive or manic phases.
- Organic brain disorders, including epilepsy, post-head-injury states, following long-term substance abuse, senile dementia, and possibly as a side effect of steroid treatment.
- Mental handicap, in which misunderstanding occurs regarding another's feelings or intentions. However, we must remember that the mentally handicapped are liable to sexual abuse and we must not unthinkingly dismiss sexually laden remarks that they may make about other individuals. Conversely, we must also remember that mental handicap can coexist with psychotic disorders and delusional expressions.

- Delusional misidentification syndrome has occasionally been described with erotomanic features.
- Non-delusional erotomanic beliefs may emerge in unstable individuals, sometimes complicating transference in the course of psychotherapy. If associated with histrionic traits there may be florid acting out, but the beliefs do not have the qualities of a delusion.

Epidemiology

Nothing is known of the frequency of erotomania in general, or of the erotomanic subtype of delusional disorder. As will be noted below, the more dangerous aspects of the illness are proving to be not uncommon.

Course and prognosis

Without treatment this is a chronic illness, which is likely to worsen gradually over time.

Forensic complications[50]

Males who irrationally act out their erotomanic delusions are usually diagnosed as schizophrenic but some prove to have delusional disorder. Often the overt behaviour is in the nature of harassment, but even without violence the individual's persistent intrusiveness and incorrigibility can be thoroughly alarming to the victim, who is bewildered by the situation and by the other's accusations of duplicity.[51]

Severely aggressive behaviour can lead to assault, kidnapping, and even murder, sometimes of the love object but at other times of an acquaintance who is viewed as a rival. A manifestation, which has gained much recent publicity is that of victim stalking, and in a considerable number of cases the victim has no idea who is carrying out the stalking.

While women are generally less prone to aggressive acting out of their delusions, they may sometimes demonstrate their false beliefs in devastating ways. For example, a deluded woman may claim publicly that a physician, counsellor, or teacher has demonstrated strong erotic feelings towards her. This belief may be the result of a delusional memory. If she has an undeteriorated personality, is coherent, totally believes her own story, and presents it with typical vehemence and persistence, it may be virtually impossible to persuade the public and the authorities that the accusations are totally false. Any professional person dealing with deluded patients must be aware of abnormal transference emotions that may arise in the patient during treatment, usually of a heterosexual nature but sometimes homosexual. Great circumspection is then required and the therapist must immediately seek collegial (and possibly legal) help.

Treatment

Treatment is discussed later in the section on overall treatment of delusional disorder.

Delusional disorder: grandiose subtype[23]

This is the least well-described variant of delusional disorder, not surprisingly in view of its nature. An individual who is habitually elated, even exalted, and who may believe himself or herself rich or powerful is unlikely to seek help, especially psychiatric help. If he or she remains sufficiently high functioning to remain in the community, the delusions may be undetected; indeed some people capitalize on their beliefs by belonging to fringe organizations, apocalyptic religious groups, or doomsday sects. Sometimes these groups develop malignant qualities, especially under a deluded but charismatic leader, and one cannot minimize the dangerous qualities of the forceful megalomaniac whose grandiosity is alloyed with persecutory anger. Like-minded and impressionable people are readily drawn in and a kind of mass shared psychotic disorder may result; comparisons with Nazi Germany are not inapt.

Clinical features

This disorder often only becomes apparent over time and with observation. The few cases that we identify tend to fall into two categories. The first are those whose state of bliss is so profound that they totally neglect self-care. The rest are usually seen in custody after they have committed an offence under delusional influence. The characteristic underlying features of a delusional disorder have already been well described.

Differential diagnosis

The illness must be distinguished from the following.

- Mania, in which grandiosity is associated with euphoria, overactivity, and, at times, irritability and suspiciousness. As the mood is often volatile and/or phasic, so the grandiose features are unstable.
- Schizophrenia in which there is marked incongruity between ecstatic affect and relative thought poverty.
- Organic brain disorders, especially affecting the prefrontal cerebral lobes, which cause labile mood, disinhibited behaviour, and some degree of cognitive deficit. Cerebral syphilis (general paralysis of the insane) used to be the best-known exemplar.
- Antisocial personality disorder in which the individual feels above the law and may express grandiose ideas and behaviours. In these cases one finds evidence of lifelong impulsivity, lack of remorsefulness, and usually a long history of delinquency.

Epidemiology

We have virtually no information. The illness can occur in either sex and apparently at any age from adolescence onwards. It may appear gradually or suddenly.

Course and prognosis

As far as we know, the grandiose subtype is as chronic and unremitting as the other subtypes of delusional disorder. For many years the presence of grandiosity in any psychiatric disorder has been regarded as a bad prognostic factor. In delusional disorder this may be so, because a grandiose delusional system is particularly likely to be associated with spurning of treatment. Even if treatment begins to be effective, the abandoning of highly pleasurable beliefs may not be welcomed by some patients.

There may be forensic complications if grandiose delusions are acted out.

Treatment

This is discussed later when considering the overall treatment of delusional disorder.

Delusional disorder: mixed and unspecified subtypes

There is little to be added regarding these categories. In DSM-IV it is accepted that more than one delusional theme can exist side by side so that, provided that the form of the illness is that of delusional disorder, it is acceptable to have combined themes of, for example, hypochondriasis and persecution, persecution and grandiosity, erotomania and jealousy, etc.

The unspecified type is a residual category and again the illness must have the form of a delusional disorder, but the delusional content is one other than those specifically listed. No reliable data exist on either the mixed or the unspecified subtypes.

Other disorders with persistent delusions

As mentioned previously, ICD-10 has a category for 'other persistent delusional disorders' (F22.8), but this is too loosely worded to delineate any coherent clinical entity. Paraphrenia, as has been noted before (p. 283) is regarded by some, including the present author, to be a candidate for inclusion in an expanded category of delusional disorders but currently is not receiving official notice. Therefore, the only condition we shall consider here is delusional misidentification syndrome.

Delusional misidentification syndromes (DMIS)[52]

The abilities to recognize individual faces and to discriminate between different faces are fundamental human processes and normally we are extraordinarily adept at them. Changes in a familiar facial appearance can be unsettling and even frightening, in both children and adults. A great deal of sophisticated neurophysiological and neuropsychological investigation has been carried out on normal and abnormal face-recognition processes.

A number of clearly defined neurological disorders are associated with very specific abnormalities of face recognition.[53] Here we shall emphasize those cases in which a delusion of misidentification is the principal symptom of the disorder and in which the form or structure of the illness is in many ways similar to that of delusional disorder. These are the delusional misidentification syndromes. However, it is important to note that superficially similar presentations may occur as secondary features in cases of schizophrenia, severe mood disorder, or dementia, and in these we refer to a misidentification phenomenon rather than syndrome.

(a) Clinical features

There are four main variants of DMIS:

1 the Capgras syndrome, in which the individual falsely perceives that someone in his environment, usually a close relative or friend, has been replaced by an almost exact double

2 the Frégoli syndrome, where the patient believes that one or more individuals have altered their appearances to resemble familiar people, usually to persecute or defraud him or her

3 intermetamorphosis, in which the patient believes that people around have exchanged identities so that A becomes B, B becomes C, and so on

4 the syndrome of subjective doubles, where the patient is convinced that exact doubles of him- or herself exist, a kind of *Doppelgänger* phenomenon

Additional alternative forms have been described and sometimes features of more than one variant occur in an individual case, especially in the subjective doubles phenomenon.

Although the patient is convinced of the deception, he is often aware that something is wrong and that the replacements are subtly incorrect. Many sufferers are extremely distressed and frightened and fear impending harm. In some cases, they may become enraged and attack the 'impostor' with considerable violence. Their belief is of delusional intensity and they usually cannot be dissuaded by argument or by demonstration of contrary proof.

It is of particular interest that the misidentification is not indiscriminate but involves a limited number of usually familiar people. In some cases, substitution also involves places and objects. An admixture of depersonalization and derealization is not unusual, especially in the earlier stages.

(b) Classification

Delusional misidentification syndromes have not been included in DSM-IV or ICD-10, though if misidentification occurs in the setting of a psychotic illness like schizophrenia it is regarded as a feature of that illness. However, if it is the principal aspect of a psychosis it should be regarded as a disorder *sui generis*. In those cases where there is a discrete delusional system occurring in clear consciousness and within a relatively intact personality, it would seem logical to assign it as a new subcategory within Delusional Disorder (DSM-IV) or Persistent Delusional Disorders (ICD-10). In cases where organic brain disease is prominent, the proper assignment would be to Mental Disorders due to a General Medical Condition (DSM-IV) or Organic, Including Symptomatic, Mental Disorders (ICD-10).

(c) Diagnosis and differential diagnosis

The diagnosis is based on recognition of the delusional nature of the belief, the accompanying agitation, and uncharacteristic behaviours, possibly including violent attacks on others. A full neurological investigation is mandatory.

Differential diagnosis includes:

- Schizophrenia
- delusional disorder, persecutory subtype
- major mood disorder with delusions
- organic brain disorder
- substance abuse disorders.

(d) Epidemiology

The frequency of DMIS is unknown but an increasing number of cases are being reported. The disorder occurs in both sexes and across a wide age range, but particularly in the middle-aged and elderly.

(e) Aetiology

When DMIS was first recognized, attempts were made to explain its symptoms on psychodynamic grounds. Such theories have been almost totally undermined of late by the increasing recognition of significant brain pathology in a high proportion of cases.

Nowadays we have many reports on brain dysfunction in DMIS[18,54,55] but large case series are lacking. There is some consensus that abnormalities of the right cerebral hemisphere, especially temporoparietal, are especially likely to be present but are not inevitable, and lesions in other cerebral locations have been found. The lesions can be regarded as causal of specific abnormalities of face recognition, a function mediated especially in the right hemisphere. Also, there appears to be dissociation of sensory information from its normal affective accompaniment and failure of suppression of inappropriately repetitive behaviours (also a right-sided function). These last two features are very typical of delusional disorders in general.

We know little of the biological substrate of delusional symptoms, but one proposal is that there may be a dysfunction of the limbic–basal ganglia mechanisms, with particular emphasis on dopamine overactivity. In DMIS there seems to be a breakdown in integration of information between the right parietotemporal cortex, the limbic system, and certain basal ganglia, resulting in the specific misidentification, associated with inappropriate emotion and inability to suppress abnormal thoughts and behaviours. Very tentatively it is possible to postulate a complex brain mechanism which normally integrates sensory and affective impulses and downregulates repetitive behaviour, and whose malfunction results in delusional beliefs, altered judgement, overintense mood, and inability to change or develop insight. The particular delusional content might be determined by the specific site within the mechanism at which the brain dysfunction occurred.[(56)]

Although the above is simply an attempt at a paradigm, it is also a model with potential for the study of delusional and concomitant phenomena by modern neurobiological investigative methods. It also allows us to conjecture about the general similarities and specific differences between DMIS and delusional disorder.

(f) Course and prognosis

Although DMIS may appear insidiously, it not infrequently appears relatively suddenly in a previously normal individual, presumably related to the underlying cerebral pathology. Where brain damage is substantial, the prognosis is that of the brain disease. If the brain dysfunction is more subtle and does not remit, the delusional symptoms may become chronic. Forensic complications may occur if the patient becomes violent,[(47)] and a small number of murders by patients have been reported in DMIS.

(g) Treatment

Acute treatment may involve sedation and antipsychotic medication. Ongoing treatment is by maintenance doses of an antipsychotic with possible addition of an anticonvulsant. Psychological counselling may be beneficial as the patient improves.

Folie à deux: a phenomenon which may accompany illnesses with delusions[(57,58)]

This phenomenon is listed as a psychiatric disorder in DSM-IV (Shared Psychotic Disorder, 297.3) and in ICD-10 (Induced Delusional Disorder, F24) but there is a conceptual difficulty in regarding it as a psychotic illness in its own right, as will be discussed shortly.

Folie à deux is a venerable term used to describe a situation in which mental symptoms, usually but not invariably delusions, are communicated from a psychiatrically ill individual (the 'primary patient') to another individual (the 'secondary patient') who accepts them as truth. As noted, DSM-IV and ICD-10 refer to this by different names and there have been several confusing changes of official terminology over the years. The older name, which is used as an alternative by DSM-IV, is well known to most psychiatrists and is used here by preference. However, *à deux* may sometimes be a misnomer since several people can be involved, and then we read of *folie à trois*, *folie à plusieurs*, *folie à ménage*, etc.

Taking the dyad as the classical situation, the two people are usually closely associated, especially husband–wife, siblings, or parent–child, and often live in social isolation. The content of the shared belief depends on the predominant delusion(s) of the primary patient and can include convictions of persecution, delusional parasitosis, belief in having a child who does not exist, misidentification delusions, and many others. There have been descriptions of shared persecutory and apocalyptic beliefs in quasi-religions and cults led by a charismatic leader with gullible followers. In many shared delusional examples there is a sense of antagonism from 'them' who may be defined or who may be what Cameron[(59)] referred to as the 'paranoid pseudocommunity', the hovering 'they' who carry out oppression which is evident to the sufferers but not to normal others.

Once thought rare, *folie à deux* has been increasingly described in the literature. Milder cases may not be recognized and, also, many delusional people strive to avoid psychiatric referral; collusion between primary and secondary patient in this has been noted. The physician should be aware of *folie à deux* and never overlook it.

'Shared psychotic' and 'induced delusional' both imply that two members of the dyad are psychotic. In delusional disorder the primary patient is psychotic but the recipient of the beliefs usually is not. Most often, the latter is highly impressionable and dependent and adopts the false beliefs because of their intense and unceasing transmission by the primary patient. Social isolation, accentuated by induced mistrust of 'them', discourages adequate reality testing. Thus one can say that the content of the secondary patient's false belief derives from psychotic thinking, but he or she is not usually psychotic.

Nearly all cases of *folie à deux* are reported in association with schizophrenia, delusional disorder, severe depressive disorder with delusions, or early dementia, but it is probable that the condition also sometimes coexists with non-psychotic illnesses such as obsessive-compulsive disorder, somatoform disorder, and histrionic–dissociative personality disorder, in which the beliefs are intensely held and communicated but are not delusional. This makes the DSM-IV and ICD-10 terms even less appropriate.

Subtypes

In practice, the great majority of cases are of the type described, sometimes known as *folie imposée* because the belief is impressed on the secondary patient.

However, one occasionally sees an alternative presentation, the so-called *folie simultanée*, in which two predisposed people develop illnesses with delusions and through long and over-close association come to share identical false beliefs. This is said to be likelier when there is a genetic link (for example two unmarried siblings) or when older people have lived together in considerable isolation for many years.

Classification

Folie à deux is included with schizophrenia and other psychotic disorders in DSM-IV and with schizophrenia, schizotypal, and delusional disorders in ICD-10, and is regarded as a separate psychotic illness. It would be better to treat it as an important clinical phenomenon, which may be associated with other identifiable mental disorders. However, rather than encourage pedantic argument, it is best to alert the clinician to its existence, its frequency, and, as will be seen, its importance.

Diagnosis

The phenomenon is recognized by the identical nature of the two individuals' false beliefs, their gross affective investment in these, and their refusal to accept alternatives even when overwhelming proof is presented. Careful history-taking will usually readily distinguish the primary from the secondary patient, but this can sometimes prove difficult. In the much less common *folie simultanée*, the distinction is largely irrelevant.

Epidemiology

This is unknown except that, by definition, it will occur most in association with an illness characterized by delusional beliefs or severely overvalued ideas, especially under isolated conditions, and it is by no means rare. It is extremely important for the clinician to be on the lookout for it. He or she may be convinced that a patient is expressing delusional ideas but be thoroughly perplexed when an apparently rational relative unswervingly supports these. This can lead to serious mismanagement of the case. Conversely, recognition of *folie à deux* may solve a baffling diagnostic problem and result in appropriate care for both individuals.

Aetiology

Folie à deux appears to arise from a combination of the following:

1 innate impressionability and marked dependence on the primary patient

2 personality traits such as suggestibility, low initiative, poor reality testing, etc. in the secondary patient

3 in some cases, low intelligence in the secondary patient

4 the intensity of the abnormal beliefs expressed by the primary patient

5 the length of time over which the abnormal beliefs have been imposed

6 the degree of social isolation

Treatment

In *folie imposée* the logical approach is to identify the primary patient and treat his or her mental disorder adequately. It may also be helpful to separate the two individuals for a time, for example by hospitalizing the primary patient. With both people, every attempt must be made to reduce social isolation and to reintroduce them to reality. If the primary patient's delusions improve with treatment, the secondary patient's beliefs usually also improve. It is rarely appropriate to treat the secondary patient with antipsychotic medication, although this is sometimes mistakenly done.

In *folie simultanée*, both patients require neuroleptic treatment.

Theoretically, treatment is straightforward but in practice it can be problematic. For example, the primary patient with delusional disorder often resists psychiatric help, and subterfuge and resistance by both individuals is common. In group situations, for example a cult, this resistance is likely to be widespread and intense, and will be justified by the participants in terms of religious, social and legal rights, which they claim are being suppressed. The propagators should be separated from the recipients as much as possible, and the treatment team has to expend much time and diplomacy in gaining some confidence and a degree of cooperation. Direct challenge of the beliefs in any shared delusional situation is usually totally counterproductive.

Mass suicide is a reported outcome of shared delusions in some cult situations and any danger of this must be countered with great urgency.[60]

Treatment of delusional disorder

There are special aspects to the treatment of delusional disorder, which need emphasis, especially since many clinicians are unfamiliar with them. The first is that we must realize that delusional disorder is indeed treatable, despite frequent pessimistic statements to the contrary. In fact, the greatest difficulty is not treatment responsiveness, but persuading the patient that he needs psychiatric help because his delusions militate against this. With careful diagnosis and an approach that encourages the patient to cooperate, delusional disorder can respond to treatment, which in all cases will primarily be by neuroleptics.

General aspects of the treatment of delusions[61]

We usually aim to treat the illness of which the delusion is a part, but there is good evidence that delusions themselves, as well as hallucinations, can be considerably modified by a psychological approach. In severe psychotic illnesses the initiation of psychological treatment usually has to follow the initial controlling of serious symptoms with medications or, on occasion, electroconvulsive therapy. Thereafter, a cognitive behavioural approach or, to a much lesser extent, conventional psychotherapy can help the individual to reduce preoccupation with false beliefs, become less isolated, and reorientate towards reality.[62,63] But there is no good evidence that psychological methods by themselves can completely eliminate established delusions.

Since many illnesses are associated with delusions we have to tailor the psychopharmacological approach to suit each particular condition. In delusional disorder, the schizophrenias, and schizoaffective disorder, neuroleptics are the mainstay, with antidepressants, mood stabilizers, and electroconvulsive therapy sometimes playing subsidiary roles.

The rate of symptom response to treatment in a psychotic disorder is not uniform. For example, hallucinations often resolve quite quickly, but delusions can be much more persistent. Despite vigorous treatment they can last for many months and, in some patients, never fully remit. If the patient continues to be deluded, non-compliance with treatment is likely to be present, especially in delusional disorder where the individual is often expert at concealing his or her lack of cooperation. At present it appears that all the subtypes of delusional disorder are potentially responsive to treatment. If treatment fails, always consider non-compliance before abandoning the current approach.

Treatment approaches

Since so many delusional disorder patients actively resist seeing a psychiatrist, it is best to see them in a non-psychiatric setting if possible, for example in the office of the referring specialist or family physician. The psychiatrist who treats cases of delusional disorder needs much patience and tact, and it is common to spend one or more sessions first gaining the individual's confidence and finally persuading him to give a psychotropic medication a trial. Many of them argue vehemently and with well-organized pseudologic against the premise that they are mentally ill and use all kinds of sophistry to deny the need for a neuroleptic, but a calm and persistent approach will gain cooperation in a good proportion of cases.

Whatever neuroleptic is prescribed it is essential to begin with the lowest effective dose. This dose is only raised if required and then very gradually to avoid side effects which are guaranteed to prompt withdrawal from treatment. The patient should be seen at least once a week as an outpatient in the initial stages. Inpatient treatment is not often indicated, although forensic cases will nearly always be seen in an institutional setting.

With a positive treatment response it is not unusual to see minor improvements in a few days, such as reduced agitation, a slight increase in well-being, improved sleep, and a little less preoccupation with the delusion. On average it is about 2 weeks before the delusional system is significantly ameliorated, but in some patients this may take 6 weeks or more.

Quite often if this degree of improvement occurs the patient decides that there is no further need of treatment and stops it. Within days or weeks there is an inevitable return of the delusion with its accompanying agitation and preoccupation. It is then that the psychiatrist must be available to encourage resumption of medication. Although at this stage the patient still believes in his delusions, the experience of improvement followed by relapse makes a deep impression and, given trust in the therapist, often leads to long-term cooperation.

It is striking that good recovery is often relatively rapid and can be surprisingly complete, even when the illness has been present for many years. Some patients return to a considerable degree of intrapsychic, interpersonal, and occupational functioning, with little evidence of the personality disorder that is supposed to be so prevalent in delusional disorder. Also, many patients require surprisingly little counselling or psychotherapy in resuming a reasonable life, although these should always be available if required. Such results suggest that this profound illness may be due to a relatively circumscribed brain abnormality and also that, in some cases at least, a very insidious onset may cause initial symptoms, which mimic personality disorder.

In most cases, treatment has to be continued for an indefinite period since delusional disorder is potentially a lifelong illness. Naturally the drug dosage should be the lowest, which keeps symptoms under control and this maintenance dose is often very low indeed. Perhaps up to one-third of patients can eventually be weaned successfully from medication, but we have no means of predicting who these will be, so that any reduction in effective treatment must be carried out with extreme caution. Sadly, a proportion of relapses are due to injudicious withdrawal of treatment by a physician and we must assume the need for treatment to be permanent unless proved otherwise. It is interesting that successfully treated patients, whether on maintenance drugs or not, keep a lookout for subsequent recurrences themselves and may report that tension-inducing circumstances provoke some reappearance of symptoms. Such patients may then request to have their medication resumed or increased.

There is no necessary correlation between acquired insight into the desirability of taking one's medication and true insight into the illness itself. Many patients never fully accept the psychotic nature of their experience, but as long as they are benefiting from treatment and are functioning reasonably there is nothing to be gained from challenging them on this. If, despite treatment, the delusions remain intrusive, cognitive behavioural therapy and counselling should be available,[62,63] but intrusive psychotherapy must be avoided.

Overall, the best-attested treatment results refer to the somatic subtype, with smaller literatures on the erotomanic, jealousy, and persecutory subtypes, and virtually nothing on the grandiose form. A wide variety of neuroleptics have been reported, but for a considerable time pimozide, a diphenylbutylpiperidine, was the drug of first choice.[64] Recently a study by Manschrek and colleagues[65] has apparently shown that some of the newer atypical antipsychotics can produce comparable results. Antidepressants and benzodiazepines are ineffective as first-line treatments and monoamine oxidase inhibitor antidepressants are absolutely contraindicated.

Currently, the best estimate of treatment outcomes is that, if the diagnosis is correct, the patient compliant, and the treatment adequate, recovery (defined as 'return to full function with total or near-remission of symptoms') occurs in approximately 50 per cent of all patients, and a further 30 per cent will show significant but less complete improvement. An unknown, but considerable, proportion of those who show no improvement can be assumed to have been non-compliant. Although mostly based on non-blind trials, these figures are culled from a worldwide literature, which does show considerable consistency.

Recognition and treatment of postpsychotic depression

Ten per cent or more of delusional disorder patients whose illness responds to neuroleptics experience significant degrees of mood disorder during recovery, sometimes very severe depression with suicidal risks.[66] This has also been noted in recovering schizophrenics. Various explanations have been proposed such as a medication side effect or perhaps the achievement of painful insight. The most likely reason is neurochemical, due to rapid changes in neurotransmitter balance.

If the neuroleptic is withdrawn, the depression tends to improve but the delusions return. Therefore the proper approach is to continue with the minimum effective dose of neuroleptic and to add an antidepressant drug in an effective dose. Occasionally, in extremely severe cases, electroconvulsive therapy is required. Subsequently the neuroleptic is continued but, in most instances, the antidepressant can be gradually reduced.

All cases of delusional disorder should be monitored for the possible emergence of mood symptoms during recovery and treatment immediately instituted if necessary. If suicidal symptoms appear, inpatient admission is highly recommended.

Conclusions

Paranoia/delusional disorder is unique in psychiatry in that it is virtually a newly discovered illness, yet much of the fundamental descriptive work was done a century or more ago. This long hiatus means that most practitioners have little knowledge or experience of the disorder, and the few who are aware of it usually only see a small part of the fabric. The dermatologist treats a case of delusional parasitosis, the cosmetic surgeon has an impossible patient wth a dysmorphic delusion, the lawyer does not know what to do with a totally unreasonable litigant, the police officer has to deal with a jealous murderer or an erotomanic stalker, and the personnel officer has an employee who is convinced his fellow workers are persecuting him, etc. How can we draw all this scattered material together and add it to the psychiatric literature to make a whole cloth? The answer is largely by consciousness raising and education.

Kendler, an authority in this field, has said, 'The paranoid disorders may be the third great group of functional psychoses, along with affective disorder and schizophrenia'.[(67)] If he is correct, it is imperative that we hone our diagnostic and treatment skills in order to improve the help we might offer to delusional disorder sufferers and to facilitate research which is so badly needed.

Further information

Bhugra, D. and Munro, A. (eds.) (1997). *Troublesome disguises: underdiagnosed psychiatric syndromes*. Blackwell Science, Oxford.

Cash, T.F. and Pruzinsky, T. (eds.) (1990). *Body images: development, deviance and change*. Guilford Press, New York.

Freeman, D., Bentall, R., and Garety, P. (2008) *Persecutory delusions: assessment, theory and treatment*. Oxford University Press, Oxford.

Garety, P.A. and Hemsley, D.R. (1994). *Delusions: investigations into the psychology of delusional reasoning*. Maudsley Monograph No. 36. Oxford University Press, Oxford.

Manschrek, T.C. (ed.) (1992). Delusional disorders. *Psychiatric Annals*, **22**, 225–85.

Munro, A. (1999). *Delusional disorder*. Cambridge University Press, Cambridge.

Sedler, M.J. (ed.) (1995). Delusional disorders. *Psychiatric Clinics of North America*, **18**, 199–425.

Sharma, V.P. (1991). *Insame jealousy*. Mind Publications, Cleveland, TN.

References

1. American Psychiatric Association. (1994). *Diagnostic and statistical manual of mental disorders* (4th edn). American Psychiatric Association, Washington, DC.
2. World Health Organization. (1992). *International statistical classification of diseases and related health problems*, 10th revision. WHO, Geneva.
3. Capgras, J. and Reboul-Lachaux, J. (1923). L'illusion des 'sosies' dans un délire systématisé chronique. *Bulletin de la Societé Clinique de Médecine Mentale*, **2**, 6–16.
4. Munro, A. (1997). Paraphrenia. In *Troublesome disguises: underdiagnosed psychiatric syndromes* (eds. D. Bhugra and A. Munro), pp. 91–111. Blackwell Science, Oxford.
5. Kraepelin, E. (1896). *Lehrbuch der Psychiatrie* (5th edn). Barth, Leipzig.
6. Jaspers, K. (1963). *General psychopathology* (7th edn) (trans. J. Hoenig and M. Hamilton). Manchester University Press, Manchester.
7. Kretschmer, E. (1927). *Der sensitiver Beziehungswahn* (2nd edn). Springer, Berlin.
8. Garety, P.A. and Hemsley, D.R. (1994). *Delusions: investigations into the psychology of delusional reasoning*. Maudsley Monograph No. 36. Oxford University Press, Oxford.
9. Mullen, P. (1979). Phenomenology of disordered mental function. In *Essentials of postgraduate psychiatry* (eds. P. Hill, R. Murray, and G. Thorley), pp. 25–54. Academic Press, London.
10. Butler, R.W. and Braff, D.L. (1991). Delusions: a review and integration. *Schizophrenia Bulletin*, **17**, 633–47.
11. Flaum, M., Arndt, S., and Andreasen, N.C. (1991). The reliability of 'bizarre' delusions. *Comprehensive Psychiatry*, **32**, 59–65.
12. Farmer, A.E., McGuffin, P., and Gottesman, I.I. (1987). Searching for the split in schizophrenia: a twin study perspective. *Psychiatric Research*, **13**, 109–18.
13. Kendler, K.S. and Gruenberg, A.M. (1982). Genetic relationship between paranoid personality disorder and the 'schizophrenic spectrum' disorders. *The American Journal of Psychiatry*, **139**, 1185–7.
14. Kendler, K.S. (1987). Paranoid disorders in DSM III, a critical review. In *Diagnosis and classification in psychiatry* (ed. G.L. Tischler), pp. 57–83. Cambridge University Press, Cambridge.
15. Michael, A., Mirza, S., Mirza, K.A.H., *et al.* (1995). Morbid jealousy in alcoholism. *The British Journal of Psychiatry*, **167**, 668–72.
16. Feinstein, A. and Ron, M.A. (1990). Psychosis associated with demonstrable brain disease. *Psychological Medicine*, **20**, 793–803.
17. Almeida, O.P., Howard, R., Förstl, H., *et al.* (1992). Late paraphrenia: a review. *International Journal of Geriatric Psychiatry*, **7**, 543–8.
18. Flint, A.J., Rifat, S.L., and Eastwood, M.R. (1991). Late-onset paranoia: distinct from paraphrenia? *International Journal of Geriatric Psychiatry*, **6**, 103–9.
19. Connell, P.H. (1958). *Amphetamine psychosis*. Maudsley Monograph No. 5. Chapman & Hall, London.
20. Morimotom, K., Miyatake, R., and Nakamura, M., (2002). Delusional disorder: molecular genetic evidence for dopamine psychosis. *Neuropsychopharmacology*, **26**, 794–801.
21. Reilly, T.M. and Batchelor, D.H. (1991). Monosymptomatic hypochondriacal psychosis and AIDS (letter). *The American Journal of Psychiatry*, **148**, 815.
22. Gorman, D.G. and Cummings, J.L. (1990). Organic delusional syndrome. *Seminars in Neurology*, **10**, 229–38.
23. Munro, A. (1988). Delusional (paranoid) disorder: etiologic and taxonomic considerations. The possible significance of organic brain factor in etiology of delusional disorders. *Canadian Journal of Psychiatry*, **33**, 171–4.
24. Munro, A. (1998). *Delusional disorder*. Cambridge University Press, Cambridge.
25. Kennedy, H.G., Kemp, L.I., and Dyer, D.E. (1992). Fear and anger in delusional (paranoid) disorder: the association with violence. *The British Journal of Psychiatry*, **160**, 488–92.
26. Ungvari, G.S. and Hollokoi, R.I.M. (1993). Successful treatment of litigious paranoia with pimozide. *Canadian Journal of Psychiatry*, **38**, 4–8.
27. Rowlands, M.W.D. (1988). Psychiatric and legal aspects of persistent litigation. *The British Journal of Psychiatry*, **153**, 317–23.
28. Goldstein, R.L. (1987). Litigious paranoids and the legal system: the role of the forensic psychiatrist. *Journal of Forensic Sciences California*, **32**, 1009–15.
29. Freckelton, I. (1988). Querulent paranoia and the vexatious complainant. *International Journal of Law and Psychiatry*, **11**, 127–43.
30. Reavis, D.J. (1995). *Ashes of Waco: an investigation*. Simon & Schuster, New York.
31. Weightman, J.M. (1984). *Making sense of the Jonestown suicides: a sociological history of the people's temple*. Edwin Mellen Press, Lewiston, NY.
32. Pruzinsky, T. (1990). Psychopathology of body experience: expanded perspectives. In *Body images: development, deviance and change* (eds. T.F. Cash and T. Pruzinsky), pp. 170–89. Guilford Press, New York.

33. Van Moffaert, M. (1992). Psychodermatology: an overview. *Psychotherapy and Psychosomatics*, **58**, 125–36.
34. Koblenzer, C.S. and Bostrom, P. (1994). Chronic cutaneous dysesthesia syndrome: a psychotic phenomenon or a depressive symptom? *Journal of the American Academy of Dermatology*, **30**, 370–4.
35. Stein, D.J. and Hollander, E. (1992). Low-dose pimozide augmentation of serotonin reuptake blockers in the treatment of trichotillomania. *The Journal of Clinical Psychiatry*, **53**, 123–6.
36. Munro, A. and Stewart, M. (1991). Body dysmorphic disorder and the DSM-IV: the demise of dysmorphophobia. *Canadian Journal of Psychiatry*, **36**, 91–6.
37. McElroy, S.L., Phillips, K.A., Keck, P.E., *et al.* (1993). Body dysmorphic disorder: does it have a psychotic subtype? *The Journal of Clinical Psychiatry*, **54**, 389–95.
38. Malasi, T.H., El-Hilu, S.R., Mirza, I.A., *et al.* (1990). Olfactory delusional syndrome with various aetiologies. *The British Journal of Psychiatry*, **156**, 256–60.
39. Bhanji, S. and Mahony, J.D.H. (1978). The value of a psychiatric service within the venereal disease clinic. *British Journal of Venereal Disease*, **54**, 266–8.
40. Crowe, R.R., Clarkson, C., Tsai, M., *et al.* (1988). Delusional disorder: jealous and nonjealous types. *European Archives of Psychiatric and Neurological Science*, **237**, 179–83.
41. Mullen, P.E. and Martin, J. (1994). Jealousy: a community study. *The British Journal of Psychiatry*, **164**, 35–43.
42. Cobb, J. (1984). Morbid jealousy. In *Contemporary psychiatry* (ed. S. Crown), pp. 68–79. Butterworths, London.
43. Mowat, R.R. (1966). *Morbid jealousy and murder*. Tavistock Publications, London.
44. Fishbain, D.B. (1986). Suicide pacts and homicide. *The American Journal of Psychiatry*, **143**, 1319–20.
45. Gillett, T., Eminson, S.R., and Hassanyeh, F. (1990). Primary and secondary erotomania: clinical characteristics and follow-up. *Acta Psychiatrica Scandinavica*, **82**, 65–9.
46. Segal, J.H. (1989). Erotomania revisited: from Kraepelin to DSM-IIIR. *The American Journal of Psychiatry*, **146**, 1261–6.
47. Silva, J.A., Leong, G.B., Weinstock, R., *et al.* (1994). Delusional misidentification syndromes and dangerousness. *Psychopathology*, **27**, 215–19.
48. Raschka, L.B. (1979). The incubus syndrome, a variant of erotomania. *Canadian Journal of Psychiatry*, **24**, 549–53.
49. Goldstein, R.L. (1987). More forensic romances: de Clérambault's syndrome in men. *Bulletin of the American Academy of Psychiatry and the Law*, **15**, 267–74.
50. Purcell, R., Pathé, M., and Mullen, P.E. (2005). Association between stalking victimisation and psychiatric morbidity in a random community sample. *The British Journal of Psychiatry*, **187**, 416–20.
51. Pathé, M. and Mullen, P.E. (1997). The impact of stalkers on their victims. *The British Journal of Psychiatry*, **170**, 12–17.
52. Ellis, H.D. and Young, A.W. (1990). Accounting for delusional misidentifications. *The British Journal of Psychiatry*, **157**, 239–48.
53. Weinstein, E.A. (1994). The classification of delusional misidentification syndromes. *Psychopathology*, **27**, 130–5.
54. Cummings, J.L. (1985). Organic delusions: phenomenology, anatomical correlations, and review. *The British Journal of Psychiatry*, **142**, 184–97.
55. Förstl, H., Burns, A., Jacoby, R., *et al.* (1991). Neuroanatomical correlates of clinical misidentification and misperception in the senile dementia of the Alzheimer type. *The Journal of Clinical Psychiatry*, **52**, 268–71.
56. McAllister, T.W. (1992). Neuropsychiatric aspects of delusions. *Psychiatric Annals*, **22**, 269–77.
57. Arnone, D., Patel, A., and Giles, M.Y.T. (2006). The nosological significance of folie à deux: a review of the literature. *Annals of General Psychiatry*, **5**, 11–22.
58. Silveira, J.M. and Seeman, M.V. (1995). Shared psychotic disorder: a critical review of the literature. *Canadian Journal of Psychiatry*, **40**, 389–95.
59. Cameron, N. (1959). The paranoid pseudocommunity revisited. *American Journal of Sociology*, **65**, 57–61.
60. Myers, P.L. (1988). Paranoid pseudocommunity beliefs in a sect milieu. *Social Psychiatry and Psychiatric Epidemiology*, **23**, 252–5.
61. Fennig, S., Fochtmann, L.J., and Bromet, E.J. (2005). Delusional and shared psychotic disorder. In *Comprehensive textbook of psychiatry* (8th edn) (eds. H.J. Kaplan and B.J. Saddock), pp. 1525–33.
62. Kingdon, D., Turkington, D., and John, C. (1994). Cognitive behaviour therapy of schizophrenia. *The British Journal of Psychiatry*, **164**, 581–7.
63. Silva, S.P., Kim, C.K., Hofmannn, S.G., *et al.* (2003). To believe or not to believe: cognitive and psychodynamic approaches to delusional disorder. *Harvard Review of Psychiatry*, **11**, 20–9.
64. Munro, A. and Mok, H. (1995) An overview of treatment in paranoia/delusional disorder. *Canadian Journal of Psychiatry*, **40**, 616-22
65. Manschrek, T.C. and Khan, N.L. (2006). Recent advances in the treatment of delusional disorder. *Canadian Journal of Psychiatry*, **51**, 114–19.
66. Mandel, M.R., Severe, J.B., Schooler, N.R., *et al.* (1982). Development and prediction of postpsychotic depression in neuroleptic-treated schizophrenics. *Archives of General Psychiatry*, **39**, 197–203.
67. Kendler, K.S. (1982). Demography of paranoid psychosis (delusional disorder): a review and comparison with schizophrenia and affective illness. *Archives of General Psychiatry*, **39**, 890–902.

4.5

Mood disorders

Contents

4.5.1 Introduction to mood disorders
John R. Geddes

4.5.2 Clinical features of mood disorders and mania
Per Bech

4.5.3 Diagnosis, classification, and differential diagnosis of the mood disorders
Gordon Parker

4.5.4 Epidemiology of mood disorders
Peter R. Joyce

4.5.5 Genetic aetiology of mood disorders
Pierre Oswald, Daniel Souery, and Julien Mendlewicz

4.5.6 Neurobiological aetiology of mood disorders
Guy Goodwin

4.5.7 Course and prognosis of mood disorders
Jules Angst

4.5.8 Treatment of mood disorders
E. S. Paykel and J. Scott

4.5.9 Dysthymia, cyclothymia, and hyperthymia
Hagop S. Akiskal

4.5.1 Introduction to mood disorders

John R. Geddes

Mood and disorders of mood

The concept of mood is difficult to define. In psychiatry, it has come to mean a pervasive emotional tone varying along an axis from happiness to sadness—and perhaps anxiety. The boundaries between normal and abnormal mood are equally difficult to define. Nonetheless, there is usually no doubt about the most extreme manifestations of low mood, **depression**, or elevated mood, **mania**.

Early history

Descriptions of variations in mood which go beyond normal limits and are associated with functional impairment are present in the oldest writings of mankind.[1] The ancient Greeks identified that mood disorders were diseases of the body, rather than the effects of supernatural spirits and identified the link between elevation of mood and states of despondency or depression. The Hippocratics also identified that mental disorders were located in the brain. This insight was lost for 2000 years under the influence of Galen's humoral theory which held that melancholia was due to an excess of black bile and mania due to an excess of yellow bile. During this period, attempts to put forward empirical theories in both Western and Eastern civilizations often fell foul of increasingly dominant religious dogma.

Development of modern psychiatric nosology

In Europe, during the Enlightenment of the seventeenth and eighteenth centuries, reason and empiricism once again emerged. In *Anatomy of Melancholy*, published in 1632, Richard Burton provides a comprehensive review of previous writings on mood disorder.[2] Burton, who writes with the penetrating insight of someone with extensive personal experience of mood disorder, clearly makes the link between mood elevation and enhanced creativity, cycling with periods of low mood, when all pleasure is lost:

> When I go musing all alone
> Thinking of divers things fore-known.
> When I build castles in the air,
> Void of sorrow and void of fear,
> Pleasing myself with phantasms sweet,
> Methinks the time runs very fleet.
> All my joys to this are folly,
> Naught so sweet as melancholy.
> When I lie waking all alone,

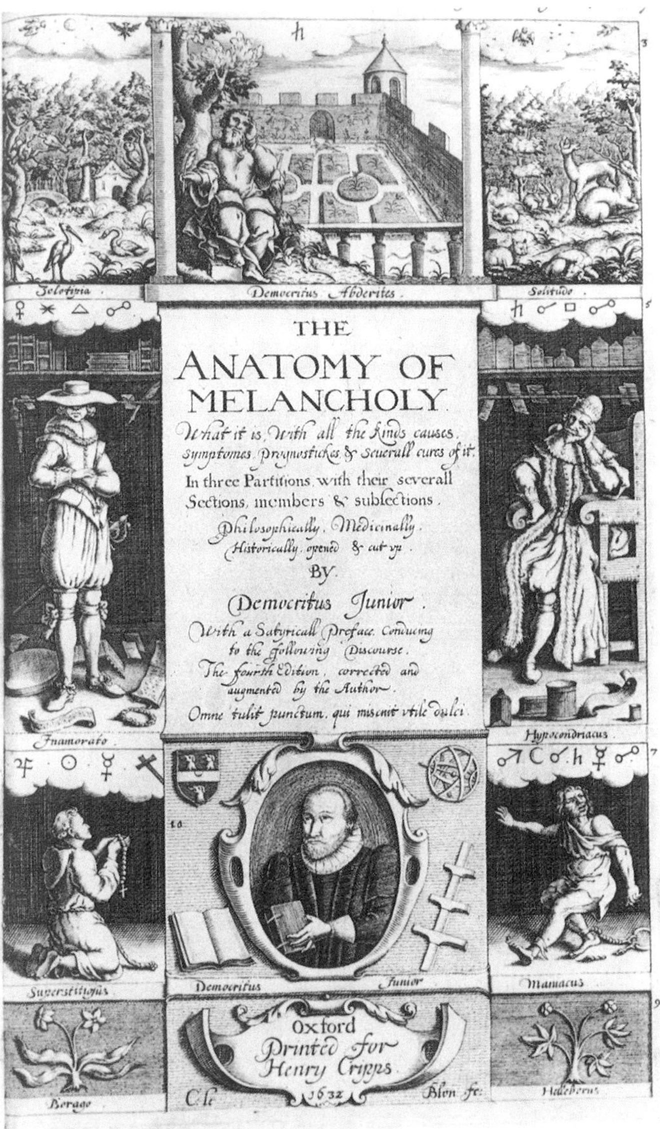

Fig. 4.5.1.1 Frontispiece to Burton's *Anatomy of Melancholy.*

Recounting what I have ill done,
My thoughts on me then tyrannise,
Fear and sorrow me surprise,
Whether I tarry still or go,
Methinks the time moves very slow.
All my griefs to this are jolly,
Naught so mad as melancholy.

(extract from The Author's Abstract of Melancholy, *Anatomy of Melancholy*)

Burton's work is an erudite and comprehensive review of the work on mood disorders until the early seventeenth century, although of course not systematic in the modern sense. Following Burton, Thomas Willis (1621–1675), Sedleian Professor of Natural Philosophy at Oxford University, perhaps better known for his description of the eponymous circle of Willis, is now recognized as one of the first to (re)localize psychiatric disorders within specific body organs, primarily the brain, rather than due to the circulation of bodily humours. In *Cerebri anatomi* (1664) Willis writes[3]:

> Melancholy is a complicated distemper of the brain and heart. For as melancholick people talk idly, it proceeds from the vice or fault of the brain and the inordination of the animal spirits dwelling in it, but as they become very sad and fearful, this is deservedly attributed to the passion of the heart. But we cannot here yield to what some physicians affirm, that melancholy doth arise from a melancholick humour. Melancholy being a long time protracted, passes oftentimes into stupidity, or foolishness, and sometimes into madness.

This identification of the physical brain as the location of the involved pathological processes initiated the modernist project of the scientific study of serious mood disorder, using contemporarily available scientific methods to generate insights into diagnosis, aetiology, course, and treatment. The first steps in this project were diagnosis and classification. Modern psychiatric diagnostic systems can be traced to post-Enlightenment Europe—in particular, France. The development of the mental hospital system throughout Europe provided the populations of patients for the early psychiatrists to study, as they created and refined diagnostic systems. In 1854, Esquirol described *la folie circulaire* which remains a recognizably modern description of bipolar disorder.[4] Despite this, the prevalent view throughout the nineteenth century was that manic and depressive states were separate entities. At the turn of the twentieth century, Kraepelin distinguished *dementia praecox* from *manic-depressive insanity*[5] Kraepelin emphasized the episodic course of the latter, the relatively benign prognosis and the family history of mood disorder.

Expanding the scope of mood disorder and recognition of diagnostic heterogeneity

In the twentieth century, diagnostic systems that had derived from the populations of large mental hospitals were challenged by the recognition that mental disorders were widespread in milder forms in the general population. Under the influence of Freud, Bleuler expanded Kraepelin's original concept of dementia praecox to include some of the less severe forms that he identified in the general population and renamed the disorder *schizophrenia* to reflect his views of the fundamental psychology of the psychosis.[6] A similar process to this occurred with the mood disorders, eventually leading to the recognition that milder, albeit still severe enough to cause impairment of function, forms of depression, and anxiety were the commonest forms of mental disorder in the general population. Indeed, after the World Health Organization and World Bank's Global Burden of Disease study in the 1990s, it became clear that unipolar depression was the among the most important causes of disability worldwide.[7] With the expansion in the scope of mood disorders, it was recognized that there is also heterogeneity in the way in which mood disorders manifest themselves. There was debate about existence of subtypes of depression, often based on the severity of symptoms and hypothesized links to an underlying brain process. For example, Gillespie's *reactive depression* in which the depressive disorder develops in response to external circumstances and remains subject to influence by external influences during its course, can be contrasted with *endogenous* and *melancholic* subtypes which were held to arise from a primary neurobiological abnormality.

The distinction between unipolar and bipolar disorders

Despite having some descriptive clinical utility, most postulated depressive subgroups have remained of uncertain status. The distinction between unipolar and bipolar disorders, however, has become accepted and is included in modern diagnostic systems. Initially, during the twentieth century, diagnostic systems continued to maintain the Kraepelinian approach to mood disorder with *manic-depressive insanity* including both severe mania and depression.—i.e. illnesses that were characterized only by depressive episodes and illnesses which included both poles.

The school of Kleist and Leonhard identified the heterogeneous nature of patients with manic-depressive illness—some had both manic and depressive episodes while others had only depressions. They coined the terms bipolar and unipolar to describe these two forms. Carl Perris and Jules Angst later provided some empirical validation for the separation on the basis of family history.[8,9]

Modern diagnostic systems—the birth of diagnostic criteria

Under the influence of psychoanalytic thought, psychiatric diagnoses had become very vague and unreliable by the 1960s—particularly in the United States where psychoanalysis was particularly influential. Following the observation that schizophrenia was more prevalent in the United States than in United Kingdom, the US–UK Diagnostic project showed conclusively that the apparent differences appeared to be due to the differences in diagnostic practice rather than true differences in prevalence.[10] The US–UK Diagnostic project highlighted the unacceptable reliability of psychiatric diagnoses which fuelled the arguments of critics of psychiatry. It was recognized that more reliable diagnostic systems were required which were explicitly based on evidence of validity. The defining feature of these systems was the use of explicit diagnostic criteria and, historically, the most important of these was the third edition of the Diagnostic and Statistical Manual of the American Psychiatric Association.[11]

International classification systems were based on compromise between national views rather than evidence and were therefore slower to change. The ninth edition of the World Health Organization's International Classification of diseases retained the concept 'Manic-Depressive Illness' which included both unipolar and bipolar disorders. However, the distinction was finally made in the 10th edition in 1993.[12]

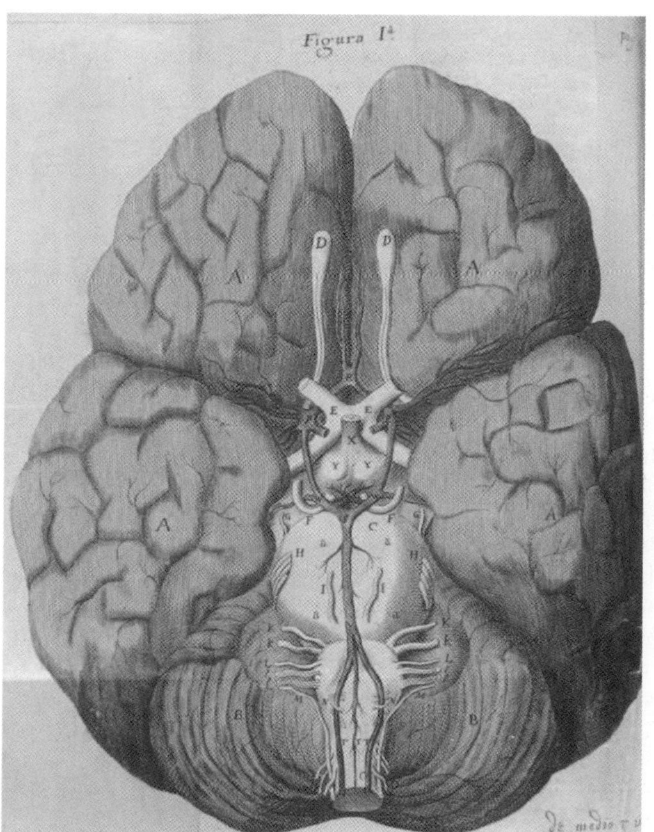

Fig. 4.5.1.2 Illustration by Christopher Wren from *Cerebi anatome* by Thomas Willis.

Refining the concept—subgroups of unipolar and bipolar disorder

As well as the fundamental Kraepelinian distinction between mood disorders and schizophrenia and the subsequent distinction between unipolar and bipolar mood disorders, there have been several attempts to subclassify mood disorders.

Unipolar disorder

A crucial distinction has been made between *endogenous* and *reactive* forms of unipolar depressive disorder (see above). Current classifications do not emphasize the distinction because it is now recognized that both typical endogenous and reactive clinical pictures can be related to external stressors. Nonetheless, the concept of a melancholic subtype remains.

Bipolar disorder

As more is known about the epidemiology of bipolar disorder, it has become apparent that some people do not experience manic episodes, but nonetheless do experience episodes of mood elevation that are clearly noticeable to themselves and others (hypomania)- as well as depressive episodes. To accommodate these heterogeneous clinical pictures, bipolar disorder has been divided into bipolar disorder, type 1 (mania ± depression) and bipolar disorder, type 2 (hypomania + depression). A focus of intense current research is the concept of bipolar spectrum disorder—in other words, the recognition that there is probably a continuum of mood phenomena from normal mood through to extreme mania.

Future developments in the classification of mood disorders

We can expect more changes in the diagnostic classification as knowledge continues to accrue. Our current classifications remain entirely descriptive, based on cross-sectional clinical symptoms and longitudinal course. As such, the classifications have been therapeutically useful—we now have increasing evidence for the diagnosis-specific effects of treatments. In the future, as out knowledge of the basic neurobiology of mood disorder increases, incremental or fundamental changes may be required.

Further information

Goodwin, F.K. and Jamison, K.R. (2007). *Manic-depressive illness: bipolar disorders and recurrent depression* (2nd revised edn). Oxford University Press, USA.

References

1. Goodwin, F.K. and Jamison, K.R. (1990). *Manic depressive illness.* Oxford University Press, New York.
2. Burton, R (1632). *Anatomy of Melancholy.* http://onlinebooks.library.upenn.edu/webbin/gutbook/lookup?num=10800
3. Willis, T. (1664). *Cerebri anatome: cui accessit nervorum descriptio et usus.* J. Martyn & J. Allestry, London.
4. Esquirol, J.E.D. (1838). *Des maladies mentales.* Balliere, Paris.
5. Kraepelin, E. (1896). *Lehrbuch der psychiatrie* (5th edn). Barth, Leipzig.
6. Bleuler, E. (1950). *Dementia praecox or the group of schizophrenias.* International Universities Press, New York.
7. Murray, C.J. and Lopez, A.D. (1997). Global mortality, disability, and the contribution of risk factors: global burden of disease study. *Lancet*, **349**, 1436–42.
8. Perris, C.A. (1966b). Study of bipolar (manic-depressive) and unipolar recurrent depressive psychoses I. Genetic investigation. *Acta Psychiatrica Scandinavica*, **42**(Suppl. 194), 15–44.
9. Angst, J. (1966). *Zur Ätiologie und Nosologie endogener depressiver Psychosen.* Springer, Berlin.
10. Cooper, J.E., Kendell, R.E., Gurland, B.J., *et al.* (1972). *Psychiatric diagnoses in New York and London.* Maudsley Monograph No. 20. Oxford University Press, London.
11. American Psychiatric Association. (1980). *Diagnostic and statistical manual of mental disorders* (3rd edn DSM-III). APA, Washington, DC.
12. World Health Organization. (1992). *The ICD-10 classification of mental and behavioural disorders.* World Health Organization, Geneva.

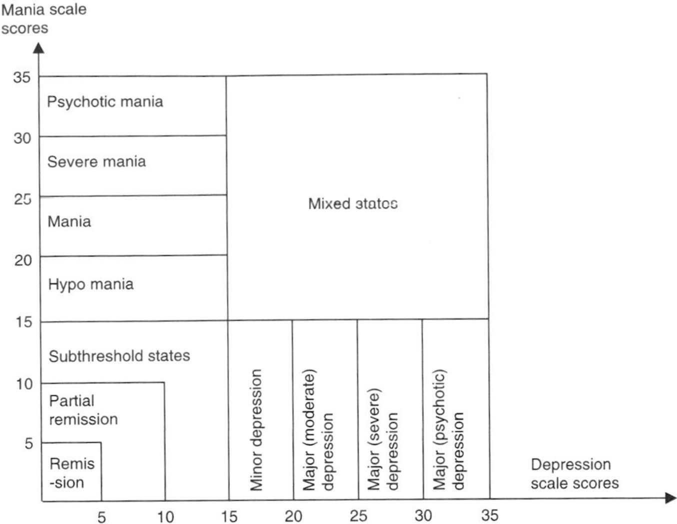

Fig. 4.5.2.1 Patient state fluctuations within the spectrum of mood states from the subthreshold states over minor mood states (hypomania or minor depression) to major states (mania/psychotic mania or major depression without or with psychotic symptoms) and to the mixed states.

4.5.2 Clinical features of mood disorders and mania

Per Bech

Introduction

The clinical features of mood disorders are dimensional, i.e. distributed according to their severity.[1] The categorical approach as manifested in the DSM-IV or ICD-10 does not, however, preclude dimensional descriptions, because in DSM-IV as well as in ICD-10 the categories or diagnoses are essentially defined by minimum and maximum cut-off scores on the symptomatic states.

Fig. 4.5.2.1 shows a coordinate system in which the ordinate represents the dimension of manic states and the abscissa the dimension of depressive states. The cut-off scores refer to the standardization of the isometric rating scales for mania and depression.[1–3] Jamison[4] has argued that the term 'bipolar' perpetuates the notion that: '... depression exists rather tidily segregated in its own pole, while mania clusters off neatly and discretely on another. This polarisation of two clinical states flies in the face of everything that we know about the fluctuating nature of manic-depressive illness . . . and it minimises the importance of mixed manic-depressive states'. William James referred to the stream of consciousness to emphasize its continuity in contrast to its conception as a series of discrete states. However, William James actually confessed that during his own depressive episodes, his mood states,[5] to a large extent, blocked his own stream of consciousness.[6] In the perspective outlined by Jamison,[4] polarity in the clinical world is not two opposites that contradict each other by a logical relationship of juxtaposition. Polarity should rather, as shown in Figs. 4.5.2.1 and 4.5.2.2, be considered at a level of psychological intercorrelations in which clinical mania and depression exist by virtue of each other involving both negative and positive correlations.

The symptom rating scales shown in Fig. 4.5.2.1 measure the severity of mania, depression, or mixed states and have a time frame of 3 days. Clinically, this is the minimum for the measurement of the spectrum of mood states ranging from subthreshold states to states of psychotic severity.

Ultrashort states of mood swings are often seen without any reference to mood disorders. In one of Henry James' masterpieces, The Ambassadors, his autobiographical hero has a tendency towards being introverted in the morning, while in the afternoon and evening he is more extraverted, like a man ' . . . who, elately finding in his pocket more money than usual . . . ', though without spending a lot. This 24-h 'cyclothymia' between introversion and extraversion displays too mild a symptomatology to be part of a 'bipolar' disorder and might be referred to as a temperamental neuroticism. Thus, Eysenck's original questionnaire for measuring neuroticism included items of being moody without any apparent reason or being inclined to having frequent ups and downs in mood.[7] Neuroticism now seems to include subclinical, temperamental, low, negative affectivity (worrying, gloomy, dysphoric, and hostile).

Fig. 4.5.2.2 shows another coordinate system in which the ordinate is representing the dimension of mania severity and the abscissa the dimension of depression severity, but covering the lifelong correlation of the courses of manic and depressive episodes,

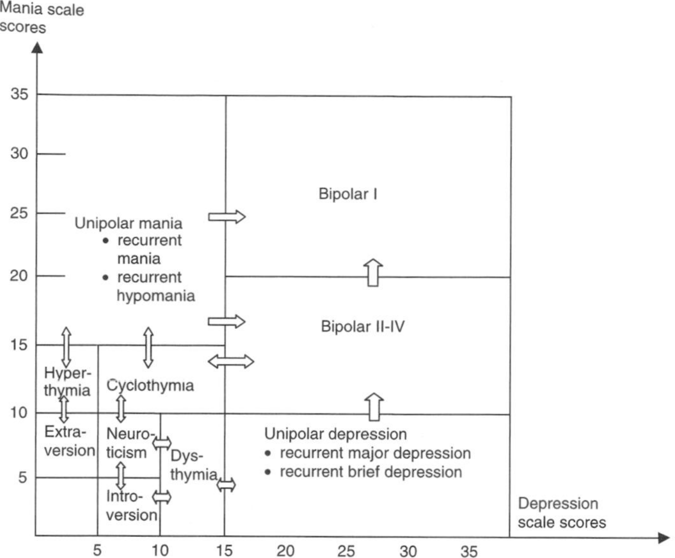

Fig. 4.5.2.2 Patient state lifetime fluctuations within the spectrum of mood polarity syndromes or disorders from the temperamental neuroticism over minor disorders (dysthymia or cyclothymia) to major unipolar disorders (hypomania/mania or brief/major depression) and to the various bipolar disorders.

i.e. the longitudinal diagnosis of mood polarity disorders. While a unipolar course of manic episodes without any depressive episodes is very rare,[8] the course of unipolar depressive episodes without manic episodes is much more frequent. Angst[9] has criticized the DSM-IV definitions of depressive episode disorders (a duration of at least 2 weeks) and of manic episode disorder (a duration of at least 1 week). Thus, Angst has shown that these episode duration criteria are not only too narrow (not sensitive enough), but they also lack empirical evidence (not validated). The spectrum of mood polarity as shown in Fig. 4.5.2.2 is an attempt to refer to the DSM-IV definitions, though modified with reference to Angst.[9] The mood polarity disorder as shown in Fig. 4.5.2.2 is defined by the highest score a given patient has obtained in the coordinate system at any time. Unipolar depression, however, with a score of 10 or less on the mania scale, as shown in Fig. 4.5.2.2, remains a lifelong uncertain diagnosis. Thus, Angst[9] has demonstrated a persistent risk of 1–2 per cent per year of a diagnostic change from unipolar to bipolar disorder.

The dimensional approach has been valid also in regard to personality disorder. As discussed by Angst,[9] only around 15 per cent of the general population seem to report no lifelong personality disorders, and he therefore calls these persons 'supernaturals'. Thus, nearly everyone has some kind of personality disorder, and within the spectrum of mood personality disorders, extraversion, introversion, neuroticism, hyperthymia, dysthymia, and cyclothymia are to be considered subthreshold disorders as shown in Fig. 4.5.2.2.

It has recently been argued that when taking into account both the subthreshold levels of symptoms and the short states of 2–3 days' duration rather than the whole DSM-IV episodes, there appears to be a linear correlation between mania and depression in the course of illness in many patients with mood disorders.[10]

The depressive episode: duration and severity

Table 4.5.2.1 shows the DSM-IV and ICD-10 depressive symptoms for the diagnosis of major depression, which to a large extent covers the rating scale dimension in Fig. 4.5.2.1. Thus, the individual symptoms should be present most of the day and nearly every day during an episode. Kendler and Gardner[11] have shown that the risk of developing a new major depressive episode (i.e. of a duration of 14 days or more) is as high for patients with major depressive symptoms lasting from 5 to 13 days as for patients with symptoms lasting from 14 to 59 days.

The study by Kendler and Gardner[11] has also demonstrated that patients with a subthreshold quantity of depressive symptoms (i.e. just below five out of the nine DSM-IV symptoms listed in Table 4.5.2.1 or minor depression in Fig. 4.5.2.1) had the same risk of developing a new major depressive episode as patients fulfilling the symptomatic criteria of major depression. It has been shown that approximately 50 per cent of the patients fulfilling the ICD-10 category of mild depression also fulfil the criteria for DSM-IV major depression.

To illustrate how a major depressive episode often develops on a continuum of depressive symptoms from the first prodromes of decreased positive well-being (introversion) to the major depressive episode, a layman's description is shown in Box 4.5.2.1. These autobiographical notes of the late William Styron (1925–2006) describe his first episode of depression at the age of 60.[12] As indicated, the symptom of anxiety (not included in DSM-IV or ICD-10) is a very important symptom of major depression from its very onset. When suicidal impulses developed, he was admitted to Yale New Hospital.

Table 4.5.2.1 Depression symptoms as included in DSM-IV and ICD-10

	Symptoms of depression	DSM-IV	ICD-10
1	Depressed mood most of the day, nearly every day	+	+
2	Markedly diminished interest or pleasure in all, or almost all, activities most of the day, nearly every day	+	+
3	Loss of energy or fatigue nearly every day	+	+
4	Loss of confidence or self-esteem	–	+
5	Unreasonable feelings of self-reproach or excessive or inappropriate guilt, nearly every day	+	+
6	Recurrent thoughts of death or suicide, or any suicidal behaviour	+	+
7	Diminished ability to think or concentrate, or indecisiveness, nearly every day	+	+
8	Psychomotor agitation or retardation nearly every day	+	+
9	Insomnia or hypersomnia nearly every day	+	+
10	Change in appetite (decrease or increase with corresponding weight change)	+	+

+ indicates that the symptom is included; – indicates that the symptom is not included.

Box 4.5.2.1 The stages from decreased positive well-being through mild depression to major depression without psychotic features

- The shadows of nightfall seemed more sober, my mornings were less buoyant, walks in the woods became less zestful, and there was a moment during my working hours when a kind of panic and anxiety overtook me, just for a few minutes, accompanied by a visceral queasiness . . .
- . . . As the disorder gradually took full passion of my system, I began to conceive that my mind itself was like one of those outmoded small-town telephone exchanges, being gradually inundated by flood-waters.
- . . . I particularly remember the lamentable near disappearance of my voice . . . The libido also made an early exit . . . food, like everything else within the scope of sensation, was utterly without savor.
- . . . My few hours of sleep were usually terminated at three or four in the morning, when I started up into yawning darkness . . . I'm fairly certain that it was during one of these insomnia trances that there came over me the knowledge that this condition would cost me my life, if it continued on such a course . . . I had not conceived precisely how my end would come. In short, I was still keeping the idea of suicide at bay . . . What I had begun to discover is that the grey drizzle of horror, induced by depression, takes on the quality of physical pain . . .

(from W. Styron (1990), *Darkness visible. A memoir of madness*, Random House, New York.)

Major depression with or without melancholia

Negative beliefs such as 'loss of self-esteem' or 'inappropriate guilt' are among the most specific core symptoms of major depression. Inappropriate guilt can be experienced as a punishment for past misdeeds (prior to the current episode of depression). The prevailing element of negative beliefs is a sense of loss which is associated with lower self-esteem experienced retrospectively. The symptom which discriminates best between anxiety states and major depressive disorder is guilt.

However, also states of anxiety with worrying and panic are important symptoms of depression. Anxiety is among the core items of the Hamilton Depression Scale.(13) Patients suffering from subthreshold depression experience less anxiety than patients with major depression. Another important symptom of depression included in the depression dimension of Fig. 4.5.2.1, but not in Table 4.5.2.1, is emotional and social withdrawal. Within the flux between mania and depression, this is probably another specific symptom (the emotionally intrusive behaviour in mania is its opposite pole).

Both in DSM-IV and ICD-10, major depressive states can be further specified as melancholic or somatic syndromes. In earlier descriptions (including Freud's 'Mourning and melancholia'), endogenous or somatic depression is distinguished from psychogenic or reactive depression by 'early morning awakening' and 'depression regularly worse in the morning'. These two signs are the only features of somatic or melancholic depression not included in the list of symptoms in Table 4.5.2.1. Strictly speaking, diurnal variation of symptoms is not a symptom itself, but rather a description of the fluctuation. The most 'somatic' symptom in Table 4.5.2.1 is change in body weight (Styron had lost 20 to 25 pounds over a period of 6 weeks, when the illness developed into a major depression).(14)

Styron's depression (Box 4.5.2.1) included the somatic feature of early morning awakening and suicidal thoughts. The latter are not just a consequence of the other symptoms. Styron described how during depression he could still keep '...the idea of suicide at bay...'. At a later stage (not shown in Box 4.5.2.1), just before he was admitted to hospital, Styron tried to write a suicide letter. Suicidal thoughts were often present late at night, when anxiety symptoms had lifted.

Measurements of social behaviour and subjective distress have shown that acute major depression is one of the most disabling and distressing of medical disorders.(6) The constant mental pain and the suicidal symptoms seriously affect quality of life. The suicidal risk in major depression is especially high when psychomotor retardation is improving in the course of treatment. The treating physician or the relatives typically observe improvement in the depressive symptoms before the patient does, because psychomotor retardation improves before mood state or hopelessness do. The risk is especially high in socially isolated people. Major depression has the highest risk of suicide of all mental disorders, and all patients with major depression should be assessed for the risk of suicide. It has been shown that patients with unipolar depression have higher suicide rates than patients with bipolar I and bipolar II disorders. However, concerning the core items of severe depressive states, no differences in the intensity of symptoms have been seen between unipolar and bipolar patients.

Major depression with psychotic features

According to DSM-IV or ICD-10, the term 'psychotic depression' is not synonymous with endogenous or melancholic depression. This agrees with Hamilton(13) who used the term 'psychosis' to refer to the severity of symptoms. As stated by Hamilton:(13) '. . . a schizophrenic patient, who has delusions is not necessarily worse than one who has not, but a depressive patient who has is much worse . . .'.

Recurrent depression

Recurrent major depression

After a single episode of major depression, around 85 per cent of patients experience recurrent episodes. While the first episode of major depression is often provoked by a negative life event such as loss of job, retirement, marital separation or divorce, subsequent episodes are often unprecipitated (but positive life events can also provoke depression). Depressive episodes typically increase in frequency and duration as they return.(3)

Recurrent brief depression

The symptoms of recurrent brief depression, first described by Angst, are similar to those of major depression (Table 4.5.2.1) with regard to both number and severity. Recurrent brief depression is a state of major depression lasting 2–3 days. Its diagnosis has not been adopted fully in DSM-IV, but it is included in ICD-10. It should be distinguished from recurrent suicidal behaviour, for example in patients with borderline personality disorder.

Seasonal depression

Seasonal depression is seen most frequently in winter, and less frequently in summer. In DSM-IV, seasonal depression has been adopted as a specifier (rather than a diagnostic category) which can be applied not only to recurrent depression but also to bipolar disorder. The seasonal episodes (e.g. winter depression) have to outnumber any non-seasonal depressive episodes in the same patient. In ICD-10 only seasonal depression is briefly mentioned, but only in an annex for disorders under consideration.

According to DSM-IV, the symptoms of seasonal depression are similar to those of major depression. However, it has been shown that the symptoms differ from those of major depression, with hypersomnia, overeating, carbohydrate craving, and weight gain (often referred to as atypical depression).

Atypical depression

DSM-IV atypical depression has a specifier which can be applied both to major depression and to bipolar I and bipolar II, but also to dysthymia. The core item is mood reactivity (i.e. the mood brightens in response to actual or potential positive events), while the associated symptoms are hypersomnia, overeating, and weight gain, leaden feelings in arms or legs, and interpersonal rejection sensitivity. It has been shown that mood reactivity is more often seen in bipolar II disorders than in unipolar depression disorders.

The manic episode: duration and severity

Table 4.5.2.2 shows the symptoms of mania according to DSM-IV and ICD-10, which to a large extent covers the rating scale dimension in Fig. 4.5.2.1. The episode criteria for hypomania and mania are shorter than those for major depression. For hypomania, the symptoms should have lasted at least 4 days, and it has been suggested to accept as little as 2 days (e.g. for states of hypomania).[15] In DSM-IV, but not in ICD-10, the category bipolar II disorder has been adopted (Fig. 4.5.2.2), referring to patients with a major depressive episode, who previously have experienced episodes of hypomania. It has been shown that patients with cyclothymia have the same risk of developing bipolar II depression as patients with hypomania. It has been proposed to extend the bipolar spectrum to include a category of bipolar III to refer to depressed patients who have developed hypomania episodes during treatment with antidepressant medication,[16] while bipolar IV refers to depressed patients having a substance-induced hypomania.

Patient-reported questionnaires have recently been published to identify previous episodes of hypomania in depressed patients. It has been shown that the Hypomania Checklist[17] is superior to the Mood Disorder Questionnaire in identifying patients with bipolar II disorder.

The problem with self-reported questionnaires to measure manic symptoms is that many patients do not perceive their hypomanic symptoms as pathological. They may describe themselves as 'normal' or their response pattern may show that they play 'the manic game'.

Studies with clinician-rated mania scales have shown that the various symptoms in Table 4.5.2.2, when quantified, can be rank-ordered in one single dimension of severity, analogously to the depressive symptoms in Table 4.5.2.1. This is illustrated by Box 4.5.2.2, which lists the three stages of mania from the longitudinal study by Carlson and Goodwin[18] on hospitalized patients in the untreated stage of their illness.

Table 4.5.2.2 Manic symptoms as included in DSM-IV and ICD-10

	Symptoms of mania	DSM-IV	ICD-10
1A	Elevated mood	+	+
1B	Irritable mood	+	+
2	Increased self-esteem or grandiosity	+	+
3	Decreased need for sleep	+	+
4	Increased talkativeness	+	+
5	Flight of ideas	+	+
6	Distractibility	+	+
7A	Increased social activities or contacts	+	+
7B	Psychomotor agitation	+	+
8	Risk taking behaviour	+	+
9	Increased sexual activities	–	+

+ indicates that the symptom is included; – indicates that the symptom is not included.

Hypomania

Hypomania can be the first stage of a spiralling upswing of mood (Box 4.5.2.2). According to DSM-IV, hypomania is more in concordance with the following description by Jamison[4] than with Box 4.5.2.2: '... When you're high it's tremendous. The ideas and feelings are fast and frequent ... Shyness goes, the right words and gestures are suddenly there, the power to captivate others a felt certainty ... Sensuality is pervasive and the desire to seduce and be seduced irresistible'. The shyness or introversion seen in mild depression or dysthymia contrast with the lack of shyness and extraversion seen in the hypomanic patient.

As described in Box 4.5.2.2, the dysphoric or irritable mood is often a core symptom of hypomania, which in the next stage of mania develops further, to cooperation difficulties and impulsive hostility. Although hypomania might cause hyperactiveness in social functioning,[15] the more or less hidden hostility often causes marked impairment in the hypomanic individual's ability to pursue some necessary task or to maintain an acceptable contact with family members. In this respect, therefore, dysphoric hypomania may cause as much clinically significant impairment in social functioning as cyclothymia.

Mania without psychotic features

In mania, the elevated spirit seen in hypomania is often mixed with irritability and hostility. Jamison[4] has described the change: 'Humor and absorption on friends' faces are replaced by fear and concern. Everything previously (in the hypomanic state) moving with the grain is now against—you are irritable, angry, frightened, uncontrollable ...'.

Box 4.5.2.2 The three stages of the acute manic episode as observed in untreated inpatients

- **Hypomania**

  Increased well-being and/or irritable mood, more busy, pressured speech, makes more telephone calls, seductive

- **Mania**

  Nearly always pleasant and cheerful. Occasionally losing insight and cooperation, impulsive, angry, very hyperactive, less sleep, more pressure of speech, makes repeated telephone calls, racing thoughts, more expansive, some grandiosity

- **Mania with psychotic features**

  Emotionally labile, can be very angry, very intrusive. Uncooperative, severely agitated, no sleep, very talkative, loud, flight of thoughts, grandiosity, religious delusions 'hearing God', sexually very preoccupied

(modified from G.A. Carlson and F.K. Goodwin (1973), The stages of mania. A longitudinal analysis of the manic episode, *Archives of General Psychiatry*, **28**, 221–8.)

The psychomotor symptoms of mania are restlessness and less need for sleep. There is pressure of speech; the patient talks more and in a louder voice. There is intrusive behaviour, arguments, and attempts to dominate others. Expansiveness is manifested as increased self-esteem; for example, the patient clearly overestimates his or her own capacities or hints at unusual abilities. Jamison[4] has described how in periods of mania she did not worry about money: 'The money will come from somewhere; I am entitled; God will provide. Credit cards are disastrous, personal cheques even worse . . . mania is a natural extension of the economy . . . So I bought precious stones, elegant and unnecessary furniture, three watches within an hour (in the Rolex rather than Timex class) . . .'.

To be diagnosed as a manic episode, the disorder should last at least a week. The criteria for mania are elevated or clearly irritable mood, and at least three of the symptoms listed in Table 4.5.2.2. These symptoms should be severe enough to cause marked impairment of occupational functioning. Hospital admission is often needed to prevent the patient from harming him/herself or others.

The psychomotor restlessness and the pressured speech in the dysphoric hypomanic state present a clinical picture of agitated depression, i.e. a mixed state (Fig. 4.5.2.1). The taste for talking is observed more frequently in females than in males, but otherwise no significant differences are seen between males and females in the manic dimension (Fig. 4.5.2.1).

Mania with psychotic features

Psychotic states of mania are characterized by greater pressure of speech, more open hostility, severe agitation, no need for sleep, flight of thoughts, severe distractibility, and grandiose delusions. In younger people, psychotic mania is often misdiagnosed as schizophrenia.

In hospital, the increased social contact of manic patients is clearly different from the emotional bluntness of schizophrenics. The intrusive behaviour seen in severe mania is of an extremely dominating and manipulative nature, out of context with the setting. Hamilton found this to be one of the most important mania symptoms. Secondary persecutory delusions often develop. The expansive religious delusion 'hearing God' should be differentiated from the schizophrenic patient's religious hallucinations.

Both DSM-IV and ICD-10 differentiate between mood-congruent psychotic symptoms (such as grandiose delusions of religion and voices supporting the patient's superhuman powers) and mood-incongruent psychotic symptoms (which are often the secondary delusions of persecution mentioned above).

Mixed states

The mixture of manic and depressive symptoms is the essential feature of mixed states (Fig. 4.5.2.1). It is not necessarily a bipolar course of symptoms, but the mixture of depressive and manic symptoms nearly every day. DSM-IV requires that the duration of a mixed episode should be at least 1 week; ICD-10 requires at least 2 weeks.

Kraepelin described transitory moods of depression in acute manic states. Transitory moods of depression have been recorded in manic patients by use of a rating scale administered by the nursing staff. Such short-lived states of 'depression' in patients with acute mania should be referred to as 'microdepressions' and not mixed episodes. Winokur described 'microdepressions' very clearly:

> . . . If one allows a manic patient to talk, one will note that he shows fleeting episodes of depression embedded within mania (microdepressions). He may be talking in grandiose and extravagant fashion and then suddenly for 30 seconds breaks down to give an account of something he feels guilty about . . . His eyes will fill with tears but in 15 to 30 seconds he will be back to talking in his expansive fashion.

Rapid cycling

DSM-IV has a specifier for rapid cycling, which refers to patients with bipolar I or bipolar II disorders, who have experienced at least four episodes during the previous 12 months. The episode has to be demarcated by partial or full remission for at least 2 months or a switch to an episode of opposite polarity.

Conclusion

The clinical spectrum of the states of depression and mania has been described in Fig. 4.5.2.1 by the symptomatic dimensions of severity as validated by clinician-rated scales. Thus, symptom severity is a key issue of the spectrum of mood states.

The spectrum of mood polarity disorders covering the longitudinal diagnosis of manic and depressive episodes is shown in Fig. 4.5.2.2. Recent research has demonstrated how important it is to recognize subthreshold states of mania and depression, as they can have a major impact on both social functioning and quality of life, since many patients with mood disorders spend much time in subthreshold disorders, i.e. cyclothymia, dysthymia, or neuroticism.

While the severity spectrum of the states of mania and depression has been accepted as evidence-based, we still lack a validation of the mood polarity spectrum in long-term follow-up studies.

Acknowledgement

I wish to thank Jules Angst and Rasmus W. Licht for their valuable comments and suggestions during the revision of this chapter.

Further information

The greatest resource book for research is Goodwin, F.K. and Jamison, K.R. (2007). *Manic depressive illness* (2nd edn). Oxford University Press, Oxford.

Other sources for further information are:

Marneros, A. and Goodwin, F.K. (eds.) (2005). *Bipolar disorders: mixed states, rapid cycling and atypical forms*. Cambridge University Press, Cambridge.

Stein, D.J., Kupfer, D.J., and Schatzberg, A.F. (eds.) (2006). *Textbook of mood disorders*. American Psychiatric publishing, Washington, DC.

Ghaemi, S.N. (2003). *The concepts of psychiatry. A pluralistic approach to the mind and mental illness*. Johns Hopkins University Press, Baltimore.

References

1. Bech, P. (1993). *Rating scales for psychopathology, health status and quality of life*. Springer Verlag, Berlin.
2. Bech, P. (2005). The Bech-Rafaelsen Mania and Melancholia Scales in clinical trials: a 25-year review of their use as outcome measure in bipolar and unipolar patients. In *Focus on bipolar disorder research* (ed. M.C. Brown), pp. 131–51. Nova Science Publishers, Hauppauge, New York.
3. Goodwin, F.K. and Jamison, K.R. (2007). *Manic-depressive illness* (2nd edn). Oxford University Press, New York.
4. Jamison, K.R. (1995). *An unquiet mind. A memoir of moods and madness*. Knopf, New York.
5. James, W. (1890). *Principles of psychology*. Holt, New York.
6. Bech, P. (1998). *Quality of life in the psychiatric patient*. Mosby-Wolfe, London.
7. Eysenck, H.J. (1958). A short questionnaire for the measurement of two dimensions of personality. *Journal of Applied Psychology*, **42**, 14–17.
8. Klerman, G.L. (1981). The spectrum of mania. *Comprehensive Psychiatry*, **22**, 11–20.
9. Angst, J. (2007). The bipolar spectrum. *The British Journal of Psychiatry*, **190**, 81–6.
10. Cassano, G.B., Rucci, P., Frank, E., *et al*. (2004). The mood spectrum in unipolar and bipolar disorder: arguments for a unitary approach. *The American Journal of Psychiatry*, **161**, 1264–9.
11. Kendler, K.S. and Gardner, C.O. (1998). Boundaries of major depression: an evaluation of DSM-IV criteria. *The American Journal of Psychiatry*, **155**, 172–7.
12. Styron, W. (1990). *Darkness visible. A memoir of madness*. Random House, New York.
13. Hamilton, M. (1960). A rating scale for depression. *Journal of Neurology, Neurosurgery, and Psychiatry*, **23**, 56–62.
14. West, J.L.W (1998). *William Styron. A life*. Random House, New York.
15. Benazzi, F. (2007). Bipolar disorder—focus on bipolar II disorder and mixed depression. *Lancet*, **369**, 935–45.
16. Klein, D.N., Shankman, S.A., and McFarland, B.R. (2006). Classification of mood disorders. In *Textbook of mood disorders* (eds. D.J. Stein, D.J. Kupfer, and A.F. Schatzberg), pp. 17–32. American Psychiatric Publishing Inc., Washington, DC.
17. Angst, J., Adolfsson, R., Benazzi, F., *et al*. (2005). The HCL-32: towards a self-assessment tool. *Journal of Affective Disorders*, **88**, 217–33.
18. Carlson, G.A. and Goodwin, F.K. (1973). The stages of mania. A longitudinal analysis of the manic episode. *Archives of General Psychiatry*, **28**, 221–8.

4.5.3 Diagnosis, classification, and differential diagnosis of the mood disorders

Gordon Parker

Introduction

Varying expressions of mood disorders make for difficulties in definition, diagnosis, and classification. DSMIV and ICD10 formal classifications with decision rules (see Chapter 1.9) provide a structure but their underlying models may or may not be valid. This chapter therefore considers how mood disorders can be variably conceptualized and structured—an issue of intrinsic importance but also influencing identification of causes and management. Some definitional and boundary issues are first detailed prior to considering sub-typing and differential diagnostic issues.

Definitions

(a) Depression

The term *depression* is extremely broad, variably defining an affect, mood states, disorders, or syndromes—as well as disease states. A depressed 'affect' usually occurs in response to a specific situation and is defined as a transient and non-substantive state of feeling 'depressed', 'sad', or 'blue'.

A *depressed mood* is more pervasive, more likely to be experienced as unusual or atypical, associated with negative ideation (e.g. hopelessness, helplessness, pessimism about the future), and may influence behaviour. Its quintessential construct is lowering of the individual's intrinsic level of self-esteem, with the extent of self-esteem lowering roughly equating to the severity of the mood state. Experienced by most people, it generally lasts only minutes to days in non-clinical situations.

A *depressive condition* (be it a disorder, syndrome, or disease) is generally distinguished by a longer duration, more clinical (and more pathological) features, and distinct social impairment. A duration criterion ensures that a transient depressed mood state does not alone establish psychiatric 'case' status, with a minimum duration of 2 weeks capturing most conditions other than the so-called 'adjustment disorders'. Additional clinical features (detailed shortly) inform us about severity (e.g. 'major' and 'minor' depressive disorders) and sub-typing, while the social impairment criterion further cleaves 'normal' mood states from clinical depressive conditions.

At times, depressive conditions are described as *primary or secondary*, a distinction necessarily imprecise. We comfortably concede 'secondary depression' when depression emerges during the course of a substantive psychiatric condition (e.g. schizophrenia) or medical condition, or following certain aetiologically defined triggers (e.g. substance abuse). However, as depression is commonly contributed to by other psychiatric disorders (e.g. severe anxiety states) and primary psychosocial factors, it might be logical to also call these 'secondary' depressive disorders, and yet this rarely occurs. The term 'secondary depression' therefore generally imputes a substantive primary condition with depression as a clear-cut consequence.

(b) Bipolar/unipolar depression specifics

Turning from cross-sectional to longitudinal definition, the course specifier 'bipolar' is applied to those having had at least one manic or hypomanic episode, whether preceded or not by a depressive episode. Originally, Leonhard[1] introduced the concept of 'monopolar' (or 'unipolar') depression to distinguish those who had episodes of the melancholic sub-type of depression, but no manic episode. Regrettably, the term 'unipolar' depression is now used to define a residual (i.e. non-bipolar) category, so heterogeneous as to be of limited meaning and utility.

(c) Mania/hypomania

As described in Chapter 4.5.2, such conditions are the converse of depression and fundamentally represent hedonistic, high energy states. Here self-esteem is almost invariably increased, the mood generally infectious, the individual energized or 'wired', disinhibited, with creativity and religiosity often enhanced, while psychotic features may be present.

Distinguishing 'hypomania' and 'mania' is imprecise in the formal classificatory systems, as noted shortly. To some theorists, the presence of psychotic features determines manic (as against hypomanic) status. Others subscribe to a dimensional model. For example, Goodwin and Jamison[2] suggest that hypomania and mania differ little in mood components, but that cognition, perception, and behaviour differ in severity and manifestation.

(d) Bipolar categories

In recent years, bipolar disorder has been principally subcategorized into bipolar I and bipolar II expressions, with 'manic' and 'hypomanic' episodes, respectively, defining the 'highs'. The term 'bipolar III' refers to a manic or hypomanic 'switch' on exposure to—or cessation of—an antidepressant drug and may reflect a pure drug effect and/or a vulnerability to switching in those with a latent bipolar condition. Numerous other bipolar categories (e.g. IV, V, and VI) have been proposed in the last few decades.[3] Many describe a 'hyperthymic' bipolar type (where the individual tends to be frequently cheerful, overly talkative, extroverted, self-assured, and full of ideas). Whether this is merely an exuberant personality style or a mild or sub-clinical expression of bipolar disorder remains to be clarified. The growth in bipolar sub-types has led to the dimensional concept of a 'bipolar spectrum'.

(e) 'Mixed states'

Here the individual with a bipolar disorder shows depressive features during a manic episode or manic features during a depressive episode. While sometimes used to describe the transition from one polar mood disturbance to another, it more commonly refers to the coterminous presence of manic and depressive features. Clinically, such patients more tend to report perturbing agitation rather than elevated mood in conjunction with depressive symptoms.

Depressive disorders: contrasting models

Unitary or binary?

The extended debate as to whether the depressive disorders are best conceptualized as comprising one or more distinct disorders warrants overview. The 'unitarian' model presupposes one depressive disorder, varying essentially by severity. The strict 'binarian' view postulated two separate types (i.e. 'endogenous'/'psychotic' versus 'neurotic'/'reactive'). There were a number of ascriptions to the 'endogenous' (now termed 'melancholic') type. Firstly, as indicated by its naming, its determinants weighted genetic and other biological factors rather than exogenous psychosocial factors. Secondly, that it had a distinctive pattern of ('endogeneity') symptoms and signs—noted shortly. Thirdly, that it showed a preferential response to physical treatments (e.g. antidepressant drugs and ECT) and less responsivity to psychotherapy. By contrast, the second 'neurotic' or 'reactive' depressive type was viewed as more reflecting depression emerging as an interaction of a predisposing personality style and precipitating life-event stressors.

The debate was strongly influenced by Lewis's clinical study[4] finding no clear demarcation between depressive types, examined both cross-sectionally and longitudinally, thus delivering support to the unitarian view. The introduction of multivariate statistical approaches led to the debate being reactivated in the 1960s, with the so-called Newcastle School arguing strongly that their analyses supported a binary view. In a representative paper, Kiloh and Garside[5] used a factor-analytic strategy to argue for separate 'endogenous' and 'neurotic' depressive conditions. However, factor analysis is not ideal for developing a typology, in that it produces dimensions (here of symptoms) rather than groupings of patients. Subsequently, more appropriate strategies have been used, such as cluster analysis[6] and latent class analysis,[7] and with those studies providing some support for separate classes. Critics suggest, however, that such classes or subgroups could still be determined by severity or, even if sub-types can be identified, question whether sub-classification has any management importance.[8–10]

This latter challenge is fundamental, taking us to the heart of any consideration of the diagnosis and classification of the depressive disorders. To the unitarians, as depression essentially varies only by degree, treatment choices (e.g. electroconvulsive therapy (ECT), antidepressant drugs, psychotherapy, or cognitive behavioural therapy) are commonly decided on the basis of severity. The opposing argument—for conceding sub-types—was well put by Kendell,[11] who drew on historical analogies. For example, he noted that distinguishing between cardiac and renal forms of 'dropsy' allowed prediction of those who would respond to digitalis.

Thus, if there are valid depressive sub-types, the contribution of putative psychosocial and biological risk factors may vary across each, and exert differential responses to differing treatment modalities. If the sub-typing model is valid, forcing homogeneity by creating dimensionally based categories such as 'major depression' will ensure muddied results. As noted by Hickie,[12] numerous studies of patients with DSM-defined 'major depression' have failed to demonstrate any coherent pattern of neurobiological changes, replicate key biological correlates, and demonstrate any specific pattern of treatment response outside inpatient treatment settings.

Approaches in the classificatory systems

How then have the official classificatory systems addressed such a substantive issue? In developing the DSM-III system,[13] the working group was required to make a decision on the competing unitarian or binarian models. While the binarians were at the door, they had, until then, failed to prove their case and the DSM-III committee chose a compromise. Thus, DSM-III depression classification was predicated on an initial dimensional component (i.e. 'major' versus 'minor' disorders). If criteria for a major disorder were met, second-order and more categorical decisions about the presence of melancholia or psychotic depression were specified. This model proved unsatisfactory for melancholia. For example, Zimmerman and colleagues[14] noted that the DSM-III melancholia criteria set, unlike the definition provided in the predecessor (DSM-II), 'did not predict treatment response'. Thus, the DSM-III-R[15] criteria set for melancholia was revised to include complete recovery after previous episodes, previous good response to somatic treatments, and no significant personality disturbance, to overcome the lack of predictive validity by building into the definition some of the 'givens' held by many clinicians about melancholia. However, the criteria set for melancholia developed for DSM-IV returned essentially to the DSM-III set, with limitations considered below. The contrasting system, ICD-10, is essentially based on a stricter dimensional or unitarian view of the depressive disorders—comprising 'severe', 'moderate', and 'mild' disorders.

During the extended debate as to whether a categorical and more 'biological' type of depression exists—it was variably termed 'endogenous', 'endogenomorphic', 'autonomous', and 'melancholic' depression. The last is probably preferable as numerous studies have quantified few or no differences in the likelihood of those with 'endogenous' and 'non-endogenous' depression reporting antecedent life events, so arguing against any term weighting 'internal' or 'external' causes.

Whether psychotic (or delusional) depression is a 'severe' form of melancholia or a separate entity also remains problematic. DSM-III had a category 'major depression with psychotic features' for use when delusions or hallucinations are present or when there is 'depressive stupor (the individual is mute and unresponsive)', thus viewing 'psychotic depression' as a sub-type of the generic 'major depression' category rather than a sub-type of melancholia. While 'depressive stupor' may be a useful marker or proxy for the condition, this criterion was not retained in DSM-III-R or DSM-IV, but is included in ICD-10. Two points argue for psychotic depression as a distinct entity: the presence of psychotic features, and its poor response to antidepressant medication alone and to neuroleptic medication alone in comparison to high responsiveness to their combination.[16]

A strict interpretation of the 'binary' view would place the non-psychotic, non-melancholic depressive conditions in a pure second class. However, rather than view this as a pure 'type', this class is best regarded as a heterogeneous residue category (i.e. non-melancholic depression), with its heterogeneity expressed widely—across aetiological factors, clinical expression, and natural and treated history.

Classification of affective mood disorders

Formal classification—depressive disorders

Both ICD-10 and DSM-IV have multiple conditions and specifiers. The ICD-10 system allows mild and moderate depressive episodes (with or without a 'somatic syndrome' conceptualized as reflecting 'melancholic' features), and severe depressive episode (with or without psychotic symptoms). There are separate codes for a similar set of 'recurrent' disorders, while several 'persistent' mood disorders (including cyclothymia and dysthymia) and residual conditions are listed. DSM-IV has two principal 'stem' disorders (major depressive episode and dysthymia), with the first having a number of optional specifiers including 'with' melancholic, catatonic, psychotic, or atypical features, as well as including disorders showing longitudinal patterns of rapid cycling or a seasonal pattern. Both systems have categories for affective disorders secondary to organic disease, while DSM-IV includes mood disorders due to a general medical condition or substance use, or occurring in the post-partum period. Both classificatory systems include adjustment disorders with depression.

Formal classifications are therefore built principally on severity, features of current episode, patterns of disorder expression over time, as well as persistence and recurrence. Few diagnoses are consistent across the ICD-10 and DSM-IV systems and, while each provides definitions that allow a 'shared language' to be used by clinicians and researchers, the extent to which their severity-weighted groupings capture 'meaningful' depressive sub-types remains problematic.

For example, and as detailed elsewhere,[17] 'major depression' has come to be viewed as an entity, sufficient in and of itself for testing antidepressant therapies and to generate treatment recommendations. Limitations to such a model become apparent if we consider the analogy of 'major breathlessness', which could be a transient consequence of acute exercise, or reflect quite differing pathological processes (e.g. asthma, pneumonia, or a pulmonary embolus) benefiting from quite differing treatment approaches. Thus, a diagnosis of 'major depression' or 'clinical depression' is, in reality, a first-level domain diagnosis, and benefiting from secondary specification. The latter tends to proceed on the basis of severity, but alternative and more categorical models have long been proposed as considered elsewhere in this chapter.

Formal classification—bipolar disorders

The DSM-IV definition effectively requires an initial or previous manic episode for bipolar I disorder, while bipolar II disorder requires hypomanic episodes and one or more previous episode of major depression.

To meet DSM-IV diagnostic status, manic episodes must have lasted 7 days and hypomanic episodes 4 days. Both ICD-10 and DSM-IV have course specifiers for bipolar disorder containing 10 and 4 subgroups, respectively. In addition to the number of subgroups, differences include a greater emphasis on distinguishing bipolar I and II in DSM-IV, and cyclothymia being listed as a 'bipolar disorder' in DSM-IV as against being a 'persistent' mood disorder overlapping with a personality style in ICD-10. Distinguishing 'hypomania' and 'mania' is regrettably imprecise in the formal classificatory systems. Both DSM-IV[18] and ICD-10[19] disallow a diagnosis of hypomania if psychotic features are present but, conversely, do not require psychotic features for a diagnosis of mania. DSM-IV lists essentially similar clinical criteria (and criteria number cut-off) for hypomanic and manic episodes, but distinguishes mania by the presence of marked impairment in social functioning (risking subjective judgement), requirement for hospitalization (which is logically more a consequence than a defining criterion although it may have some proxy value), and the presence of psychotic features in a manic episode. As noted earlier, ICD-10 views hypomania as 'an intermediate state without delusions, hallucinations, or complete disruption of normal activities'.

Thus, formal 'cleavage' between bipolar I and II (and constituent manic and hypomanic states) is largely dimensional in relation to clinical features and with some logical fallacies. Further, duration criteria (i.e. at least 7 days for mania and at least 4 days for hypomania in DSM-IV) do not appear sustainable. In recent years there have been many studies[20] indicating that clinical definition of bipolar disorder is not dependent on the duration of the highs, and that imposing DSM-IV duration criteria for both mania and hypomania may exclude a significant percentage of those with true bipolar disorder.

A sub-typing model for classifying depression

As detailed earlier, there are intrinsic difficulties in classifying depression according to any single model when it is a term encompassing normal mood states through to possibly categorical diseases, and when any imposition of a severity-based model raises problems about how to differentiate meaningful groups (e.g. 'cases' from 'non-cases'). A personal mixed model is now detailed for consideration—one shaped by clinical experience and supported by research findings. It is described in line with the 'reasoning steps' that a clinician might employ in assessing a potential depressive disorder.

(a) Step 1: Is a depressive disorder present?

For all the depressive disorders, the first building block generally requires evidence of a depressed mood (although some with a melancholic or psychotic depression may deny 'depression'). Useful questions include the following: 'Do you feel depressed'?, 'Has there been any change in your self-esteem or from the way you generally value yourself'?, and 'Are you being more self-critical or harder on yourself than usual'?

The next clinical priority is to determine if the depression is sufficiently severe as to warrant 'case' status, and here the DSM-IV criteria for a major depressive episode have common acceptance in terms of representative symptoms and duration criteria. That criteria set lists the following:

- four mood items (depressed mood, loss of interest or pleasure, feelings of worthlessness or inappropriate guilt, recurrent thoughts of death, and suicidal ideation)
- weight changes
- sleep disturbance
- fatigue
- impaired concentration
- psychomotor disturbance

A positive diagnosis requires five or more of the nine, evidence of functional impairment, and a minimum duration of 2 weeks.

(b) Step 2: If a depressive disorder is present, what sub-type?

If 'caseness' criteria are met, the next decision should be to determine the diagnostic sub-type. We favour a three-class hierarchical model (i.e. respectively psychotic, melancholic, and a heterogeneous non-melancholic class)—hierarchical in the sense that those in the two highest classes have class-specific features as well as possessing features of the subordinate classes. Clinical assessment then allows a sequencing process to diagnosis.

In essence: does this individual have a melancholic or non-melancholic depression; are there psychotic features indicative of a psychotic depression? That sequence will now be detailed. The left half of Fig. 4.5.3.1 details the so-called 'structural model'. A shared mood disorder component is present and varying in severity across the three principal sub-types. However, sub-type distinction proceeds on the basis of two class-specific components—psychomotor disturbance and psychotic features.

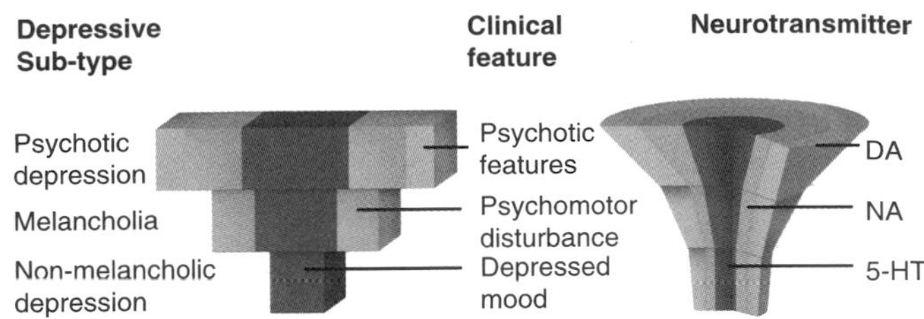

Fig. 4.5.3.1 The structural and functional model of three depressive classes. DA = dopamine; NA = noradrenalin; 5-HT = serotonin.

(c) Step 3: Differentiating melancholic and non-melancholic depression

In DSM-IV, the 'melancholic features specifier' requires, in addition to a base diagnosis of major depression, either one of two A criteria and three (or more) of six B criteria, with most of the latter comprising so-called 'endogeneity symptoms'. However, some such DSM criteria have limitations. Firstly, criterion A (loss of pleasure and/or lack of mood reactivity) is generally met by both 'melancholic' and 'non-melancholic' patients. Secondly, some criterion B features are vague. For example, 'distinct quality' is defined as a mood different to that experienced after 'the death of a loved one', and is a negative definition (akin to defining 'psychiatry' as 'not cardiology'). A second, 'excessive or inappropriate guilt', is a concatenated descriptor, subsuming the excessive expression of normal guilt, as well as guilt held at an overvalued or delusional level. Others are non-specific (e.g. early morning wakening, significant anorexia, or weight loss), being common in other psychiatric conditions (e.g. anxiety disorders) as well as in other expressions of depression. Further, as DSM-IV-defined major depression and melancholia share several similar features (e.g. anhedonia, psychomotor disturbance, weight loss), even those two conditions are poorly cleaved.

Features of melancholia: Any improvement on DSM-IV distinction of melancholia would benefit from identification of features specific to—or distinctly over-represented in—melancholia. Nelson and Charney[21] undertook a review of 33 studies using multivariate statistical approaches to identify melancholic or 'endogeneity symptoms'. They found no support for appetite/weight loss and insomnia, little support for early morning wakening and 'distinct quality', but some support for a severely depressed and non-reactive mood, loss of interest in pleasurable activities (or anhedonia), and psychotic features. The most strongly associated feature was psychomotor change (with retardation more consistently associated than agitation). When Rush and Weissenburger[22] examined nine diagnostic systems for diagnosing melancholia or endogenous depression, the only common criterion in all nine was psychomotor retardation (with psychomotor agitation included in six). Our research[23] has established that the specificity of psychomotor disturbance to 'melancholia' is dependent on measuring it as a sign, with that diagnostic weighting more recently detailed and endorsed by others.[24] Thus, and returning to a hierarchical model, differentiation between the non-melancholic and melancholic disorders (on the basis of clinical features) appears assisted principally by the specific feature of behaviourally evident psychomotor disturbance. As measured by the sign-based CORE system,[23] psychomotor disturbance is reflected along three dimensions—impaired cognitive processing and motor retardation and agitation, although components are not mutually exclusive. For example, those with significant agitation may have it present for much of the time or, and more commonly, have a base of retardation with intermittent epochs of agitation.

In younger individuals with true melancholia, overt psychomotor disturbance is less distinctive, although they still tend to report distinct concentration problems. In addition to such 'signs', symptoms seemingly over-represented in melancholia include: distinct anergia often preventing the individual from getting out of bed to bathe; anergia and mood distinctly worse in the morning (i.e. diurnal variation); and an anhedonic and non-reactive mood.

The non-melancholic disorders have no specific features—apart from some (e.g. mood reactivity) that are the converse of their expression in melancholic disorder (i.e. non-reactive mood). Thus, these conditions are effectively diagnosed by excluding the two higher order conditions of melancholic and psychotic depression.

(d) Step 4: Implications of the distinction

Classification should never be sterile. It should at least provide us with a lexicon and, ideally, inform us about management nuances. We suggest that there are important treatment implications associated with distinguishing melancholic and non-melancholic disorder. The right half of Fig. 4.5.3.1 offers a 'functional model' that operates in parallel with the 'structural model'. As detailed,[25] it assumes that if there is any neurotransmitter perturbation underpinning the non-melancholic disorders, then it is principally serotonergic in origin, shaping the hypothesis that there is no advantage in proceeding beyond a narrow-action Selective Serotonin Reuptake Inhibitor (SSRI) antidepressant. It further assumes a greater noradrenergic contribution (and possibly dopaminergic contribution) to melancholia, and shapes the hypothesis that broad-action antidepressants will overall be more effective than SSRI antidepressants—and any psychotherapy—for melancholic depression. Both hypotheses have been supported in a number of trials and naturalistic studies[26] arguing the importance of distinguishing the melancholic sub-type.

(e) Step 5: Distinguishing psychotic depression

In psychotic (or delusional) depression, the central mood component is generally even more severe than in melancholic depression but many will deny or minimize a depressed mood. A number of 'endogeneity symptoms' are also frequently more severe (particularly non-reactive mood, anhedonia, and constipation). One frequent feature in melancholic depression (i.e. diurnal variation of mood) is, however, rarely present at episode nadir, as the patient is more likely to be persistently depressed across the days. Observable psychomotor disturbance is present and generally distinctly more severe than in melancholic depression. In some, the combination of the cognitive processing problems and motor change (retardation in particular) can give the impression of a dementing process, and provides an example of 'pseudodementia'.

The key class-specific feature, however, is the presence of psychotic features. Delusions are almost invariably present while hallucinations (auditory most commonly) are present in 10 to 20 per cent. DSM-IV subdivides delusions and hallucinations as 'mood congruent' (where themes of guilt, disease, death, nihilism, and personal inadequacy dominate) and 'mood incongruent' (where psychotic features appear independent of the depressive theme and might include persecutory themes, delusions of control, as well as thought insertion and thought broadcasting) states. It is important to emphasize that mood-incongruent states are common and do not, by themselves, necessarily challenge a diagnosis of delusional depression or argue for a schizophrenic illness of necessity.

A significant percentage (approximately one-third) of patients with psychotic depression develop constipation. In many it is a primary feature (not merely a side-effect of psychotropic medication), and may serve as a nidus of delusional interpretation (e.g. the depressed patient who believes that their bowels have turned to concrete, or that they have a bowel cancer).

When psychomotor disturbance is extremely severe, it may not be possible for psychotic features to be elicited, particularly if the patient is mute. Many patients are diffident about revealing psychotic material, and here indirect questions can often be useful. In particular, pursuing the presence of 'guilt' can assist, with guilt here defined as a sense of self-blame and not merely self-criticism, together with a sense of remorse for wrong acts or omissions that are independent of any concern about potential evaluation by others. In psychotic depression, the guilt is more likely to be held at the level of an overvalued idea or at a formally delusional level. If direct inquiry does not elicit delusional material, then asking 'Do you feel any sense that you deserve to be punished'? can help elicit previously unexpressed psychotic material.

Our 'functional model' (Fig. 4.5.3.1) argues that there is likely to be a greater dopaminergic (than noradrenergic and serotonergic) contribution to psychotic depression, a hypothesis supported by meta-analyses[16,27] quantifying this condition as showing a 25 per cent response to an antidepressant alone, 33 per cent to an antipsychotic alone, and 80 per cent to their combination and to ECT.

(f) Step 6: If a non-melancholic depressive disorder, can this class be sub-typed?

There is no generally accepted sub-typing system for this residual group, and where symptoms reflecting the lower order mood construct dominate the clinical picture. In the absence of any class-specific features, any categorical sub-typing model is unlikely to be valid, and dimensional models more appropriate. But what are the salient constructs for dimensionalizing? DSM-IV and ICD-10 proceed largely on a severity dimension for the mood disorder (e.g. 'major' and 'minor') but also on patterns of recurrence and persistence, all appropriate candidate dimensions.

Historically, terms such as 'neurotic depression' and 'reactive depression' were used, with the former emphasizing a pre-morbid style of neuroticism and high anxiety, and the latter defining depression developing largely in response to life-event stressors. This suggests another set of candidate constructs, dimensionalizing both personality and severity of stress components—and modelling their interaction.

Several earlier studies argued for some clinical utility emerging from such a model. Thus, an early factor-analytic study[28] suggested both a 'hostile' type (evidenced by irritability as well as anxiety) and an 'anxious-tense' type. Blashfield and Morey[29] reviewed 11 cluster analytic studies suggesting separate 'hostile' and 'anxious' depressive subgroups. In an extensive review of the then published studies, Roth and Barnes[30] suggested three principal subgroups, with depression associated with a personality disorder, in addition to 'hostile' and 'anxious' depression.

While such 'hostile' and 'anxious' subgroups have been identified for a lengthy period, clear and consistent descriptions are lacking. Grinker *et al.*[31] described those with 'hostile' depression as unappreciative, actively angry, provocative, and making excessive demands of—and complaints about—their therapists, suggesting a personality disorder contribution. The second ('anxiety') subgroup is variably interpreted as defining either those with an anxious personality or temperament, or the presence of significant coterminous anxiety symptoms when primarily depressed.

The model we favour is one that respects historical description (i.e. 'reactive' versus 'neurotic') but develops the 'personality' contribution beyond the simple diagnostic allocation of 'neurotic depression'.

Terms such as 'reactive depression' or 'situational depression' (or as used in DSM-IV and ICD-10, 'adjustment disorder') concede that some individuals develop a non-melancholic depressive disorder largely or purely as a consequence of a stressful life event, which may produce, trigger, and/or maintain depressive episodes. In an empirical study,[32] the authors were unable to establish clinical, family history, and even life-event stress differences between those with 'situational' and 'non-situational' major depression. Our research[33] indicated that for the acute reactive 'disorders', the impact emerged less from the severity of the stressor and more from its perceived 'meaning' or 'salience'. We suggested a cognitive 'lock and key model', whereby individuals may be predisposed by perturbing developmental events such as a highly judgemental parent (creating 'locks'). In adult life, exposure to a mirroring situation (e.g. a judgemental boss) might act as a 'key' for precipitating a 'reactive' depression. For more chronic 'situational depression' scenarios, here we presume that the stressor is a chronic one and/or that the stressor induces a 'learned helplessness' mind set in the individual, where they believe that it does not matter what they do or attempt to do—there will be no impact on outcome—and they develop a sense of 'powerlessness' along with depressive symptoms.

A spectrum model

In modelling non-melancholic disorders reflecting a personality contribution, we suggest the utility of a 'spectrum' model, a term variably used but which argues for a continuum between temperament/personality style and symptom states,[34] or some level of inter-dependency. This spectrum model views certain biological factors as shaping temperament and personality style—which then shape surface marker symptoms during a non-melancholic depressive episode. An earlier research report[35] identified those presenting with an 'irritable/hostile' depression as being more likely to have a cluster B personality and to report 'acting out' behaviours when stressed (i.e. demonstrating a 'short fuse' response to stress). By contrast, those with an 'anxious depressive' spectrum disorder appeared more likely to internalize anxiety. They tended to have shown shyness and behavioural inhibition in childhood, to have high rates of lifetime anxiety disorders, score high on trait anxiety, view themselves as 'worriers', 'nervy', or 'tense', and to rate as having a cluster C personality style. When stressed, they were somewhat more likely to 'act in' by becoming quiet, retiring to their room, crying, and 'stewing'. Thus, anxiety was evident both in the temperament pattern and in the prominent symptom profile when depressed—demonstrating the 'spectrum'. The suggested profile of these spectrum disorders is not only important for clinical consideration, but in facilitating research into possible neurobiological determinants and to consider any treatment specificity. For example, Blashfield and Morey[36] reviewed studies indicating that 'anxious depressives respond well to major and minor tranquillizers but not to tricyclics, while hostile depressives show little improvement with conventional drug therapies'. Further, Fava *et al.*[37] reported that anxious depressives were more likely to be responders to a selective serotonin reuptake inhibitor (SSRI) than other depressive expressions (including 'hostile depression').

We have more recently pursued the 'spectrum model' for non-melancholic disorders beyond the two candidate groupings (i.e. hostile/irritable and anxious depressive) considered above. Both clinical observation and literature review indicated eight predisposing personality styles[38] but an application study[39] suggested that the spectrum model could be supported up to a six-factor personality model. The latter spectrum model is now detailed.

Those who scored high on the personality measure of 'anxious worrying' were, when depressed, indecisive, and self-blaming, as well as feeling anxious and tense. Those high on the 'irritability/snappiness' personality dimension were likely, when depressed, to be irritable and impulsive. Rather similar personality dimensions of 'personal reserve' and 'social avoidance' identified some differential coping responses apart from a shared social withdrawal response, with the former avoiding others and losing interest in people, while those high on social avoidance reported avoiding pleasurable activities. Those high in 'perfectionism' were more likely to focus on trying to solve the problem and to seek distraction. The sixth personality style benefits from more detailed consideration as it informs us about the nature of 'atypical depression', a condition which—while listed in DSM-IV and held to show a specific response to monoamine oxidase inhibitor antidepressant drugs—has been quite variably interpreted over time.[40] In that review, we argued for the primacy of the personality style of 'rejection sensitivity'. In our spectrum study,[39] those high on 'rejection sensitivity' were distinctly more likely to report some of its characteristic features (e.g. food cravings, hypersomnia), but also a set of cognitive extensions of their personality style (e.g. a tendency to feel abandoned, rejected, and put down) as well as distinct self-consolatory strategies (e.g. spending money, seeking support, and even crying).

While such a spectrum model is not a categorical one (in circumscribing 'pure' depressive conditions) nor sufficiently consistent in expression to deserve endophenotypic status, such 'fuzzy set' patterning may have clinical implications in terms of assisting a richer diagnostic formulation and in providing therapies that address any predisposing personality style, rather than merely treat the surface marker of non-melancholic 'depression'. Much research will be required to determine if candidate expressions show any differential response to contrasting antidepressant strategies, necessary to ensure that classification has clinical utility.

A sub-typing model for classifying bipolar disorders

As considered earlier, the formal official classificatory systems fail to provide pristine cleavage between bipolar I and bipolar II disorders. We briefly describe a model that supports an historical approach to this issue (by preserving the definition of mania—and bipolar I status—to those who have had psychotic features during a 'high') and which links the bipolar disorders with psychotic and melancholic depression.

The 'isomer model' illustrated in Fig. 4.5.3.2 builds on studies suggesting that 'bipolar depressive episodes' are highly likely to be psychotic or melancholic in type, albeit with some differences in that individuals not infrequently report 'atypical features' of hypersomnia and food cravings rather than more characteristic melancholic features of insomnia and appetite loss. The model was further shaped by findings derived in one clinical sample.[41] Firstly, bipolar patients who had experienced a psychotic 'high' had a 50 per cent chance of having a depressive episode with psychotic features. Secondly, of the bipolar patients who had never been psychotic during a high, none had experienced psychotic features.

The 'isomer model' therefore posits two contrasting 'mirror image states'. Those with bipolar states oscillate across parameters of energy and mood (elevated in highs, depressed in lows). More specifically, individuals with bipolar II disorder oscillate between non-psychotic depression and hypomania—never experiencing psychotic depression or psychotic mania. By contrast, those with bipolar I disorder have had psychotic manic episodes (by definition) and, when depressed, are at increased risk of having psychotic episodes.

The advantage to the model is that it respects and formalizes the historical view of regarding the presence or absence of psychotic features during a high as distinguishing mania and hypomania (and respective bipolar I and II disorders). Further, it suggests that aetiological studies might well focus on pursuing the nature of two oscillators—one of mood and energy, and one of psychotic features. Thirdly, it offers a template for pursuing management options for the two differing bipolar disorders. Currently, there are many treatment guidelines for managing bipolar I—but only informal templates for managing bipolar II disorder[42]—and it may be unwise to extrapolate such bipolar I guidelines for managing bipolar II disorder.

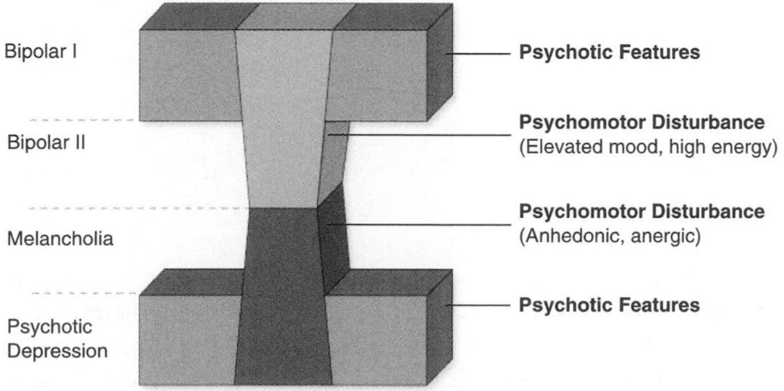

Fig. 4.5.3.2 The isomer model for conceptualizing bipolar I and bipolar II conditions. (Reproduced from Parker *et al.*[41])

Differential diagnosis and ascertainment difficulties

Depression

The three key features of lowered self-esteem, increased self-criticism, and a depressed mood distinguish depression phenomenologically from states such as grief or bereavement—where there is a distinct sense of 'loss' of something valued, but no primary 'loss' of self-esteem. They also assist phenomenological differentiation from anxiety, where the individual is more likely to report a sense of insecurity, fear, apprehension, worry, panic, or of 'going mad'. Subsequent questioning of clinical symptoms and observation should clarify if a clinical syndrome exists, its diagnostic sub-type and—from a longitudinal perspective—whether the individual has a unipolar or bipolar course.

At the practical level, such a definitional approach may fail in certain groups. A percentage of those with psychotic or melancholic depression appear more emotionally blunted and 'flat' rather than depressed. They may deny depression, self-blame and worthlessness, and instead note a lack of feeling (or vitality), sluggishness, enervation, or emphasize physical states, such as anergia. Less commonly, they may evidence 'corporization' by Schneider,[43] with reports of pain or physical sensations in the head, chest, or stomach. As noted earlier, others may have such profound psychomotor disturbance that they do not respond to questioning and appear as if they have a dementia (here a so-called 'pseudodementia'). In such instances, pursuit of proxy items (severe psychomotor disturbance, pathological guilt, overvalued ideas) may assist. If unsuccessful, the diagnosis may require corroborative reports and clinical observation, as well as certain investigations (e.g. CT or MRI scans, single-photon emission CT scans, EEG) to exclude a dementia. In a percentage of the elderly, however, a depressive episode and dementia may coexist (particularly a vascular dementia), and reflect a shared aetiological process.

Secondly, there are some patients and certain cultures where psychological issues are either denied or expressed somatically, although careful and directed questioning about central depressive descriptors will usually clarify the possibility. If unsuccessful, diagnostic clarification may require corroborative reports and clinical observation.

Thirdly, it is commonly difficult to define 'clinical depression' in those with a medical illness. Here, general depression criteria sets risk false-positive diagnoses by including certain features which may be secondary to the medical illness (e.g. fatigue, insomnia, anorexia) rather than reflecting depression *per se*. Common corrective strategies include the 'aetiological approach', where only symptoms viewed as independent of the medical condition are counted, the 'exclusive approach', eliminating potentially confounded items such as anorexia, the 'inclusive approach', where all symptoms are counted irrespective of their origin, and the 'substitutive approach', excluding features that could be due to the medical illness and substituting features such as social withdrawal and crying.

In some cases where depression has been established, the salient clinical difficulty is in determining whether depression is or is not the primary disorder in those with concomitant major medical problems, excessive alcohol intake, organic central nervous system disease, and certain psychiatric conditions (e.g. anxiety states, depressive personality disorder). Clinical judgement is generally required with two alternate logical approaches: either weighting the disorders hierarchically or sequentially. The hierarchical approach assumes that the more severe disorder is the primary one, while the sequential approach weights the antecedent condition (e.g. organic disorder, schizophrenia, anxiety). Acceptance of one approach does not logically bind the clinician to any therapeutic consequence (such as necessarily treating only the more severe or primary condition).

Mania/hypomania

The differential diagnoses for manic states essentially include other psychotic conditions (e.g. schizophrenia, drug-induced psychosis) and, rarely, a primary organic state. While cross-sectional dissection of the phenomenology can be helpful, there is wisdom in also weighting the longitudinal course. Thus, those with manic states are more likely to describe complete restoration of function between episodes (of mania and/or depression), while this is less likely for those with schizophrenia. Definitive distinction is not always possible, and a diagnosis of 'schizoaffective' disorder may then be appropriate. In severe mania, an 'organic' picture may be suggested, and require exclusion of a dementia or delirium.

The differential diagnosis of hypomanic states is often quite difficult. Questioned about having 'highs' often elicits defensive response from those with true states, while some depressed people will present a remission to a euthymic state as a 'high'. Highly creative people may affirm many hypomanic descriptors when possessed by the muse (e.g. less need for sleep, feeling creative, and overconfident, being enthused and energized), as may those with a distinctly extroverted or cyclothymic personality when stimulated. Some patients with a cluster B personality style (especially of the borderline type) may also describe mood states that approximate to hypomania. Clarification is probably best assisted by a sequence of strategies, including asking the individual about times when, neither depressed nor feeling normal, they have states of feeling overly 'energetic and wired', that they have an appropriate number of concomitant criterion features during such highs, that there was a 'trend break' where 'highs' became a new phenomenon (most commonly mid-adolescence or later), and that—during their highs—any usual level of anxiety melts away, and by interviewing a corroborative witness.

Conclusions

Current formal classificatory systems list a large number of mood disorders, with criteria designed to assist diagnostic reliability. Most reflect attempts to create classes on the basis of severity-weighted dimensional models. Terms such as 'major depression' and 'unipolar depression'—as well as 'bipolar spectrum disorder'—have achieved acceptance in recent years, for such diagnoses are easily made (and easily reified), but the limitations inherent to their heterogeneity should not be ignored. Until the dissonance between the formal classifications and clinician-derived models has been resolved, practitioners should proceed by recognizing the advantages and limitations to competing approaches. A functional classificatory system should have clinical utility, going beyond mere description and informing the clinician about treatment differentiation.

Further information

Parker, G. and Manicavasagar, V. (2005). *Modelling and managing the depressive disorders. A clinical guide*. Cambridge University Press, Cambridge.

Parker, G. (2007). *Modelling and managing bipolar II disorder: a clinical guide*. Cambridge University Press, Cambridge (in press).

http://www.blackdoginstitute.org.au

References

1. Leonhard, K. (1957). *The classification of endogenous psychoses* (trans. R. Berman). Irvington, New York.
2. Goodwin, F.K. and Jamison, K.R. (1990). *Manic-depressive illness*. Oxford University Press, New York.
3. Phelps, J. (2008). The bipolar spectrum. In *Modelling and managing bipolar II disorder. A clinical guide* (ed. G. Parker), pp. 15–45, Cambridge University Press, Cambridge.
4. Lewis, A. (1934). Melancholia: a clinical survey of depressive states. *Journal of Mental Science*, **80**, 277–378.
5. Kiloh, L.G. and Garside, R.F. (1963). The independence of neurotic depression and endogenous depression. *The British Journal of Psychiatry*, **109**, 451–63.
6. Paykel, E.S. (1971). Classification of depressed patients: a cluster analysis derived grouping. *The British Journal of Psychiatry*, **118**, 275–88.
7. Parker, G., Hadzi-Pavlovic, P., Mitchell, P., *et al*. (1994). Defining melancholia: properties of a refined sign-based measure. *The British Journal of Psychiatry*, **164**, 316–26.
8. Parker, G. (2006). The DSM classification of depressive disorders: debating its utility. *Canadian Journal of Psychiatry*, **51**, 871–3.
9. Parker, G. (2006). Through a glass darkly: the disutility of the DSM nosology of depressive disorders. *Canadian Journal of Psychiatry*, **51**, 879–86.
10. Goldney, R.D. (2006). The utility of the DSM nosology of mood disorders. *Canadian Journal of Psychiatry*, **51**, 874–7.
11. Kendell, R.E. (1989). Clinical validity. In *The validity of psychiatric diagnosis* (eds. L.N. Robins and J.E. Barrett), pp. 305–23. Raven Press, New York.
12. Hickie, I. (1996). Issues in classification: III. Utilising behavioural constructs in melancholia research. In *Melancholia: a disorder of movement and mood. A phenomenological and neurobiological review* (eds. G. Parker and D. Hadzi-Pavlovic), pp. 38–56. Cambridge University Press, New York.
13. American Psychiatric Association. (1980). *Diagnostic and statistical manual of mental disorders* (3rd edn). American Psychiatric Association, Washington, DC.
14. Zimmerman, M., Black, D.W., and Coryell, W. (1989). Diagnostic criteria for melancholia. The comparative validity of DSM-III and DSM-III-R. *Archives of General Psychiatry*, **46**, 361–8.
15. American Psychiatric Association. (1987). *Diagnostic and statistical manual of mental disorders* (3rd edn). American Psychiatric Association, Washington, DC.
16. Spiker, D.G., Weiss J.C., Dealy, R.S., *et al*. (1985). The pharmacological treatment of delusional depression. *The American Journal of Psychiatry*, **142**, 430–5.
17. Parker, G. (2005). Beyond major depression. *Psychological Medicine*, **35**, 467–74.
18. American Psychiatric Association. (1994). *Diagnostic and statistical manual of mental disorders* (4th edn). American Psychiatric Association, Washington, DC.
19. World Health Organization. (1992). *The ICD-10 classification of mental and behavioural disorders—clinical descriptions and diagnostic guidelines*. World Health Organization, Geneva.

20. Parker, G. (2008). Defining and measuring bipolar II disorder. In *Modelling and measuring bipolar II disorder. A clinical guide.* Cambridge University Press, Cambridge, 46–60.
21. Nelson, J.C. and Charney, D.S. (1981). The symptoms of major depressive illness. *The American Journal of Psychiatry*, **138**, 1–13.
22. Rush, A.J. and Weissenburger, J.E. (1994). Melancholic symptom features and DSM-IV. *The American Journal of Psychiatry*, **151**, 489–98.
23. Parker, G. and Hadzi-Pavlovic, D. (1996). *Melancholia: a disorder of movement and mood. A phenomenological and neurobiological review.* Cambridge University Press, New York.
24. Taylor, M.A. and Fink, M. (2003). Catatonia in psychiatric classification: a home of its own. *The American Journal of Psychiatry*, **160**, 1233–41.
25. Malhi, G., Parker, G., and Greenwood, J. (2005). Structural and functional models of depression: from sub-types to substrates. *Acta Psychiatrica Scandinavica*, **111**, 94–105.
26. Parker, G. (2007). Defining melancholia: the primacy of psychomotor disturbance. *Acta Psychiatrica Scandinavica*, **115**(Suppl. 433), 21–30.
27. Parker, G., Roy, K., Hadzi-Pavlovic, D., *et al.* (1992). Psychotic (delusional) depression: a meta-analysis of physical treatments. *Journal of Affective Disorders*, **24**, 17–24.
28. Overall, J.E., Hollister, C.E., Johnson, M., *et al.* (1966). Nosology of depression and differential response to drugs. *The Journal of the American Medical Association*, **195**, 946–8.
29. Blashfield, R.K., and Morey, L.C. (1979). The classification of depression through cluster analysis. *Comprehensive Psychiatry*, **20**, 516–27.
30. Roth, M. and Barnes, T.R.E. (1981). The classification of affective disorders: a synthesis of old and new concepts. *Comprehensive Psychiatry*, **22**, 54–77.
31. Grinker, R.R., Miller, J., Sabshin, M., *et al.* (1961). *The phenomena of depressions.* Harper and Row, New York.
32. Hirschfeld, R.M.A., Klerman, G.L., Andreasen, N.C., *et al.* (1985). Situational major depressive disorder. *Archives of General Psychiatry*, **42**, 1109–14.
33. Parker, G., Gladstone, G., Roussos, J., *et al.* (1998). Qualitative and quantitative analyses of a 'lock' and 'key' hypothesis of depression. *Psychological Medicine*, **28**, 1263–73.
34. Cassano, G.B., Michelini, S., Shear, M.K., *et al.* (1997). The panic–agoraphobic spectrum: a descriptive approach to the assessment and treatment of subtle symptoms. *The American Journal of Psychiatry*, **154**(Suppl.), 27–38.
35. Parker, G., Hadzi-Pavlovic, D., Roussos, J., *et al.* (1998). Non-melancholic depression: the contribution of personality, anxiety and life events to subclassification. *Psychological Medicine*, **28**, 1209–19.
36. Blashfield, R.K., and Morey, L.C. (1979). The classification of depression through cluster analysis. *Comprehensive Psychiatry*, **20**, 516–27.
37. Fava, M., Uebelacker, L.A., Alpert, J.E., *et al.* (1997). Major depressive subtypes and treatment response. *Biological Psychiatry*, **42**, 568–76.
38. Parker, G., Manicavasagar, V., Crawford, J., *et al.* (2006). Assessing personality traits associated with depression: the utility of a tiered model. *Psychological Medicine*, **36**, 1131–9.
39. Parker, G. and Crawford, J. (2007). A spectrum model for depressive conditions: extrapolation of the atypical depression prototype. *Journal of Affective Disorders*, **103**, 155–163.
40. Parker, G., Roy, K., Mitchell, P., *et al.* (2002). Atypical depression: a reappraisal. *The American Journal of Psychiatry*, **159**, 1470–9.
41. Parker, G., Hadzi-Pavlovic, D., and Tully, L. (2006). Distinguishing bipolar and unipolar disorders: an isomer model. *Journal of affective Disorders*, **96**, 67–73.
42. Parker, G. (2008). *Modelling and managing bipolar II disorder. A clinical guide.* Cambridge University Press, Cambridge.
43. Schneider, K. (1920). The stratification of emotional life and the structure of the depressive states. *Zentrallblat für Neurologie, Psychiatrie*, **59**, 281.

4.5.4 Epidemiology of mood disorders

Peter R. Joyce

The Global Burden of Disease, which is a comprehensive assessment of mortality and disability from diseases and injuries in 1990 and projected to 2020, highlights the importance of mood disorders for the world. Using the measure of disability-adjusted life years, it was determined that unipolar major depression was the fourth leading cause of disease burden in the world. It was also projected that, in the year 2020, unipolar major depression would be the second leading cause of disease burden in the world. Disability-adjusted life years is based on both mortality and disability. If one looks at disability alone, then unipolar major depression was the leading cause of disability in the world in 1990, and bipolar disorder was the sixth leading cause. Across the world, 10.7 per cent of disability can be attributed to unipolar major depression and, in developed countries, unipolar major depression contributes to nearly 20 per cent of disease burden in women aged from 15 to 44 years.[1]

The mood disorders have received considerable attention in psychiatric epidemiology over the last 25 years. These received particular attention in the five-site United States National Institutes of Mental Health Epidemiologic Catchment Area Study (**ECA**), as well as in the epidemiological studies in other countries around the world that used the ECA methodology. Mood disorders also received particular attention in the National Comorbidity Survey (**NCS**) in the United States, in the National Psychiatric Morbidity Survey of Great Britain, and most recently in the World Mental Health Survey (**WMH**) across many countries. Thus, there is substantial data from around the world on the epidemiology of these disorders. In addition, many of the population-based twin registries, such as in Virginia (USA), have also paid particular interest to mood disorders and have the additional advantage of being able to consider genetic as well as environmental risk factors.

Bipolar disorders

Diagnostic issues

While classical bipolar disorder with episodes of euphoric mania interspersed with episodes of depression is one of the clearest clinical syndromes in psychiatry, the boundaries of bipolar disorder remain contested. As case definition is central to epidemiology, all the contested boundaries of bipolar disorder could influence prevalence rates and our understanding of risk factors. Some of the major boundary issues for bipolar disorder include the overlap of bipolar disorder with psychotic features, with schizoaffective disorder and schizophrenia, and the overlap of bipolar disorder with unipolar major depression when patients who present primarily with depression have brief or mild episodes of hypomania. There is also an overlap of bipolar disorder with apparent personality disorder, especially Cluster B personality disorders such as borderline and narcissism, and the issue of when hyperthymic personality merges into bipolar disorder.[2,3] When bipolar disorder is comorbid with substance abuse there are also important diagnostic issues.

Another important issue in determining caseness of bipolar disorder for epidemiological surveys is symptom pattern and duration. A number of the diagnostic instruments for assessing bipolarity in population surveys limit the questions on mania to a type of symptom profile characterized by euphoria, grandiosity, increased energy, and decreased sleep. Whether the commonly used epidemiology interviews adequately detect those individuals who have manic episodes characterized by irritability, anger, and activation is very debatable. The other key diagnostic issue is what criteria are used to categorize the minimum duration for hypomania; is four days too long, is even two days too long? Furthermore, as insight is sometimes impaired in hypomania and mania, and as these are low prevalence disorders, the accuracy of case detection of bipolar disorders in populations remains an issue for further research.[4]

Prevalence

Population studies such as the ECA, and its related cross-national studies, and the NCS reported that the lifetime prevalence of bipolar disorder varies from 0.3 to 1.5 per cent. The NCS data include only bipolar I data, while the ECA includes bipolar I and bipolar II disorder.[4,5] In all studies, the six-month prevalence is not much lower than the lifetime prevalence of bipolar disorder. These findings reflect the high degree of chronicity and/or recurrence associated with bipolar disorder. Broader definitions of mania/hypomania have resulted in lifetime prevalence rates increasing to about 4 per cent.[6]

In these population studies, the mean age of onset of bipolar disorder has varied from 17 to 27 years. However, as age of onset is not normally distributed, the mean is a slightly misleading variable; in clinical samples, while the mean age of onset may be in the twenties, the most common age of onset are the teenage years.

In bipolar disorder, the prevalence in males and females is similar. This is in contrast to the reasonably consistent female excess found in major depression.

Comorbidity

In the NCS, all identified bipolar I individuals suffered from at least one, and often up to three or more, comorbid disorders. The most common comorbid disorders included the full range of anxiety disorders, alcohol and drug dependence, and conduct disorder or other antisocial behaviours.

Alcohol and drug abuse and/or dependence are commonly comorbid with bipolar disorder. Old studies found that binge drinking was especially common in bipolar individuals and that this binge pattern of drinking was more associated with manic episodes than with depressive episodes. Clinical studies find that bipolar patients with comorbid substance dependence are less compliant with prescribed mood stabilizers and have more frequent hospital readmissions. Stimulant abuse/dependence rates are especially increased in bipolar disorder.

Individuals with bipolar disorder have the full range of anxiety disorders, including phobias, panic disorder, and obsessive–compulsive disorder. Perhaps surprisingly, comorbid rates of these anxiety disorders tend to be higher in bipolar disorder than in major depression.

Another area of high comorbidity with bipolar disorder is that of childhood conduct disorder and attention deficit disorder. One of the issues in understanding this high rate of comorbidity is whether childhood conduct disorder and/or childhood attention-deficit disorder are sometimes the first manifestations or precursors of bipolar disorder. Certainly, if the pattern of conduct-disorder symptoms or attention-deficit symptoms is episodic rather than consistent over time, the issue becomes whether these are not early manifestations of bipolar disorder rather than truly independent comorbid conditions. The other key diagnostic controversy in this area is the status of juvenile or childhood bipolar disorder.

Use of health services

In the ECA study, 39 per cent of those with bipolar I or bipolar II disorders received outpatient psychiatric treatment within 1 year and about 10 per cent would receive inpatient treatment within a 6-month period. In the NCS study, 45 per cent of those with bipolar disorder had received psychiatric treatment in the previous 12 months; although 93 per cent reported lifetime treatment for their bipolar disorder. However, both of these studies suggest that more than half the individuals with bipolar disorder are not currently in psychiatric treatment and, given the high morbidity and mortality associated with bipolar disorder, this is of major concern.[4]

Risk factors for bipolar disorders

In considering the risk factors for bipolar disorder, it is useful to separate risk factors into those that are risk factors for lifetime vulnerability (for example genetic factors) and those that are risk factors for the onset of an episode of depression or mania (for example, life events). Thus, in determining risk factors for lifetime vulnerability, genetic factors constitute the largest single risk factor. However, if one is considering who is vulnerable to an episode of mania over the next six months, genetic factors will play a relatively smaller part and predictions may be best based on other factors such as past history, childbirth, being treated for depression with antidepressant medication, and the approach of spring or summer. Genetic risk factors are discussed further in Chapter 4.5.5.

Although organic factors, such as some type of central nervous system damage, are unusual risk factors in young adults, in late-onset bipolar disorder (age of onset more than 50 years) organic disease of the central nervous system is an increasing factor for the development of mania. In younger adults, AIDS and head injury are two important aetiological factors in a limited number of cases of bipolar disorder.

Risk factors for manic episodes in people with bipolar disorder

A range of other biological factors are particularly relevant risk factors to the onset of episodes of illness, but they may contribute a relatively small part to lifetime vulnerability. Many women have their first episode of depression or mania in the postpartum period. While a limited number of women may have manic episodes limited to the postpartum period, postpartum episodes of mania are more commonly part of a long-term bipolar disorder and these women will have episodes both precipitated by childbirth and at other times in their life. Indeed, in the postpartum period, having a history of bipolar disorder is one of the strongest risk factors for the development of a postpartum psychosis.

There is substantial evidence that seasonal patterns influence the onset of manic and depressive episodes. There are consistent findings of an excess of manic episodes in late spring and early summer. To date, however, the nature of the environmental factors that influence this late spring, early summer peak of manic episodes is less clear.

There is also substantial evidence that disruptions of normal biological rhythms may precipitate the onset of manic or depressive episodes. This has been documented in relation to international travel involving east–west or west–east travel with disruption of circadian rhythms. Disruption of circadian rhythms through shift-work or other factors, which disrupt the normal sleep cycles, may also be important triggers to the onset of episodes of mania. These findings have led to the development of a social rhythm metric, as an adjunct to interpersonal psychotherapy (interpersonal social rhythms therapy) as a treatment for individuals with bipolar disorder.

Adverse life events have been well documented to be precipitants of manic episodes, as well as depression. It appears that life events are more likely prior to the first or second episode of mania and are less likely later in the course of illness. The critical factor in life events triggering mania may be whether there is associated sleep disruption, rather than the 'psychological' meaning of the event.

Depressive disorders

Diagnostic issues

A key issue for the epidemiology of depressive disorders is defining the boundaries of major depression and dysthymia. Depressive symptoms in the community are common, and defining both the symptom count and the duration at which depressive symptoms count as part of a clinical disorder is arbitrary. When Kendler and Gardner[7] examined the boundaries of major depression as defined by DSM-IV in a population-based twin sample of women, they found that, if a twin had four or fewer depressive symptoms, syndromes composed of symptoms involving no or minimal impairment, and episodes lasting less than 14 days, then the individual's co-twin was still at an increased risk of major depression. Kendler and Gardner concluded that they could find no empirical support for the DSM-IV requirement of duration for two weeks, five symptoms, or clinically significant impairment. These authors suggested that major depression, as articulated by DSM-IV, may be a diagnostic convention imposed on a continuum of depressive symptoms of varying severity and duration. Wainwright *et al.*,[8] using data from the National Psychiatric Morbidity Survey of Great Britain, have also suggested that research should move beyond a binary decision of case versus non-case, and utilize a probablistic measure of psychiatric case status, replacing the arbitrary threshold with a smooth transition. This type of approach allows the benefits of syndrome diagnosis to be retained, while not falling into the dilemma of an arbitrary threshold that lacks validity.

Provided that one accepts the arbitrary definition of major depression, then determining the rates of current depressive disorders is not especially problematic. However, there are major methodological issues involved in determining whether an individual has ever had a lifetime episode of major depression. Lifetime prevalence rates vary from 4.4 per cent in the United States ECA study, to 17.1 per cent in the NCS, and to over 30 per cent in Kendler's Virginia twin sample of women. In part, subjects in the community may forget or fail to report past episodes of major depression (recall bias), and the manner in which the questions are asked may importantly influence lifetime rates of depression. In the Diagnostic Interview Schedule, which was used in the ECA, respondents were asked about lifetime symptoms, a lifetime diagnosis was made, and then recency of the lifetime diagnosis was determined. More recent diagnostic interview schedules, such as the Composite International Diagnostic Interview, first ask about current depressive symptoms and then, having 'primed' individuals about depressive symptoms, go on to enquire about past depressive episodes. Interviews that follow the schedule of 'priming' before asking about past episodes appear to obtain considerably higher rates of lifetime major depression. Determining lifetime rates of depression with greater precision is an important task, as the vulnerability to depression conferred by risk factors such as genetic factors and childhood experiences may be wrongly estimated if lifetime rates of major depression are imprecise. For instance, when Kendler *et al.*[9] examined the heritability of major depression and corrected for the moderate reliability of a lifetime diagnosis of major depression, the heritability estimate increased from 40 per cent to over 70 per cent. As concluded by Kendler, major depression is not a disorder of high reliability and moderate heritability, but is a diagnosis of moderate reliability and high heritability.

DSM-IV allows major depression to be further subclassified into subtypes, such as melancholia, atypical, psychotic, and by severity and recurrence. Most of the traditional epidemiology studies have tended to ignore the issue of subtyping major depression. Recently, however, the issue of the atypical depression subtype has received particular attention in the study of the Virginia twins and in the NCS. In both these studies, latent class analysis suggests that atypical depression is a distinct subtype with several distinctive features, such as higher rates of parental alcohol- and drug-use disorders, higher interpersonal dependency, and higher rates of conduct disorder. If risk factors for atypical depression are, in part, distinct from risk factors for other subtypes of major depression, then for epidemiology to contribute to an understanding of aetiology it will be important to undertake further work on depressive subtypes.[10]

Prevalence

In the ECA, the six-month prevalence of major depression across five sites was 2.2 per 100. In ECA equivalent studies the six-month prevalence rate ranged up to 5.3 per 100. In the NCS, the 1-month prevalence of a major depressive episode was 6.1 per 100.[11] In the National Psychiatric Morbidity Surveys of Great Britain, the one-week rate of a depressive episode was 2.1 per 100.[12] Together, these studies would suggest that the current rate of major depression is in the realm of two to five per cent.

The estimates of the lifetime rate of major depression are much more variable. The lowest rate reported is 4.4 per 100 from the ECA study, while, in the study of Virginia twins, the lifetime rate of major depression is over 30 per cent. It is reasonable to believe that the true lifetime rate of major depression is probably in the realm of 10 to 20 per 100, but caution should be exercised in expressing lifetime rates of depression with undue precision.

These rates of major depression may also be lower if the rate of bipolar disorder is higher. Isolated clinical studies have found that one in two, not one in ten, individuals presenting with depressive disorders have features of bipolar spectrum disorders. If these figures are correct, then this would presumably lower the rates of major depression, but would correspondingly increase the rates of bipolar disorders.

Over the past decade, one of the controversial findings in the epidemiology of major depression has been whether the rates of depression are increasing, and whether it is occurring at a younger age. Despite methodological concerns about the reliability of lifetime major depression, studies across countries have reasonably consistently documented an increasing rate of major depression with an earlier age of onset.[(13)] As mood disorders are the single largest risk factor for suicide, it is also of note that, in most Western countries, the rate of suicide, especially in young adults, increased considerably from the 1970s to 1990s, although the suicide rate is now declining in many countries. This could, however, reflect better recognition and treatment of depression.

Risk factors

(a) Genetics

There is now substantial evidence that genetic factors are of major importance as risk factors for vulnerability to major depression. While traditional estimates have put the heritability at about 40 per cent, when Kendler *et al.*[(9)] allowed for the moderate reliability of the diagnosis of major depression, the heritability estimate increased to 70 per cent. Of greater interest is that the genes for major depression do not appear to be unique for depression, but overlap with the genes for anxiety and the genes for neuroticism.[(14, 15)] The greater prevalence of depression in women may be due to the strong association of anxiety and neuroticism with depression, and that the higher rates of anxiety and neuroticism in women lead to higher rates of depression.

(b) Gender

One of the most consistent findings in the epidemiology of major depression is that the ratio of women to men is approximately 2:1. This increased rate of major depression in women arises during puberty, as in childhood there is a slightly higher prevalence of depression in boys than girls. The timing of this transition in rates by gender is related to biological puberty rather than just to age.

(c) Childhood experiences

Early theorizing suggested that the loss of a parent in childhood increased the later risk for major depression; although many studies have examined this issue, they have inconsistently found it to be a risk factor for adult depression. However, studies that examine the nature of child–parent attachment using a measure such as the Parental Bonding Instrument have consistently found that a lack of parental care is associated with increased rates of depression.[(16)] More recently, childhood sexual abuse has been established as a risk factor for adult major depression.

However, cumulative childhood disadvantage almost certainly poses a greater risk to later depression than any single childhood variable in isolation. Thus, if studies only look at single childhood risk factors, they may miss the full impact of global childhood adversity. The converse of childhood risk factors is childhood resilience, and it is probable that one good relationship with an adult and high intelligence in the child may, in part, protect from other adversities.

(d) Personality

There has been a long history of interest in the likelihood that people with certain personality traits are more vulnerable to depression than others. It is likely that those individuals who are unduly anxious, impulsive, and obsessional may have increased rates of later major depression. The best data exists for neuroticism, which emerges as a clear risk factor for the later development of depressive and anxiety disorders. However, as already mentioned, the same genes seem to contribute to the development of neuroticism and to later anxiety and depressive disorders.

(e) Social environment

There has been considerable interest in the role of marital status as a risk factor for major depression. For men, it appears clear that married men have the lowest rate of depression, while separated or divorced men have the highest rates of major depression. In women, the association is slightly less clear, but in the ECA study the same findings applied for women as for men. Understanding the nature of the association between marital status and rates of depression is more problematic. If personality is a risk factor for depression, then the same traits could interfere with the ability to marry or to stay married. There is little doubt that depression sometimes contributes to marital maladjustment and separation or divorce. Finally, the stresses associated with divorce and separation could increase the likelihood of an episode of depression occurring.

In the classic and influential work of George Brown on working-class women, having three or more children, a lack of paid employment, and the lack of a confident were risk factors for the development of an episode of depression. Subsequent studies have inconsistently replicated the risk factors of having children or lack of paid employment, but have supported the finding that the lack of a confident increases the risk of depression.

It is well established that adverse life events, particularly those characterized by loss, increases the risk of an episode of major depression. Interestingly, however, the life events which may constitute the greatest risk may be 'dependent' rather than 'independent' life events. The increased vulnerability to an episode appears to last for a period of two to three months following such an event.

Early thinking about depression suggested that there would be those depressions that occurred for largely biological reasons and those precipitated by adverse life events; however, it is now clear that such a dichotomous view is incorrect. Kendler *et al.*[(17)] showed that there is a significant genotype by environment interaction in the prediction of onset of major depression. They proposed that genetic factors influence the risk of onset of depression, in part, by increasing the sensitivity of individuals to the depression-inducing effects of stressful life events.

(f) Physical illness

Having a chronic or severe physical illness is associated with an increased risk for depression. The mechanisms behind this increased risk may vary depending upon the physical disorder. In disorders such as Parkinson's disease, it is possible that there are shared neurotransmitter abnormalities between Parkinson's disease and depression. In post-stroke depression, there is good evidence that the location of the lesion, at least in part, contributes to the rate of depression, which suggests a neuroanatomical/neurotransmitter connection between the physical illness and the likelihood of depression. For non-central nervous system disorders, such as acute myocardial infarction, diabetes, and cancers, the mechanism for this association is less clear. However, at least in the case of patients with cancer, most do not suffer from major depression and, if they do, the key risk factors are family history and a past history of depression. This suggests that the stress associated with a serious or chronic physical illness may act by bringing out an individual's lifetime vulnerability to depression.

An integrated aetiological model

The ultimate purpose of studying risk factors for depressive disorders is to contribute to the development of an integrated aetiological model. The most promising research in this area has been performed by Kendler and colleagues on twins from the Virginia Twin Register.[18] In this study, both female–female and male–male twin pairs of known zygosity have been assessed on a series of occasions at longer than one-year intervals. A range of predictor variables; including genetic factors, parental warmth, childhood parental loss, childhood disorders, lifetime traumas, neuroticism, self esteem, social support, past depressive episodes, recent difficulties, and recent stressful life events have been examined to see how they contributed prospectively to the development of an episode of major depression over the next 12 months. In considering the results from this study, it is important to bear in mind the limitations of this landmark study, especially the fact that they were predicting the onset of an episode over 12 months and not predicting lifetime episodes. However, despite these caveats, Kendler and colleagues developed a model that predicted over 50 per cent of the variance in the liability to develop major depression in the next twelve months. The strongest predictors to depression were as follows:

- stressful life events
- genetic factors
- previous history of major depression
- neuroticism

It is of note that some of the risk factors exerted these effects directly, while other effects were largely indirect. Thus, 60 per cent of the effect of genetic factors on liability to depression was direct, but the remaining 40 per cent was indirect and largely mediated by past episodes of depression, stressful life events, and neuroticism. Variables such as perceived parental warmth had no direct effect on liability to develop an episode of major depression, but did impact upon neuroticism, a history of a past depressive episode, recent difficulties, and lifetime traumas.The most comparable prospective studies looking at risk factors for the development of major depression have been undertaken during the postpartum period, which is a time of increased risk of depression. In this special case, the most consistent risk factors are family history and a past history of depression, and there is lesser support for a lack of social support, neuroticism, and complications during childbirth.

As one of the key tasks of epidemiology is to contribute to an understanding of aetiology, models that integrate risk factors are important strategies for further research. They provide clinicians with predictive power, and can also guide intervention studies to prevent the onset of episodes of depression.

Comorbidity

One of the important contributions of epidemiology to the study of mood disorders over the past twenty five years has been the recognition of the extent to which depression and other psychiatric disorders are often comorbid. In both the ECA study and NCS, over two-thirds of all individuals identified as having an episode of major depression also met the criteria for one or more other psychiatric disorders. Not surprisingly, the most common comorbid disorders are anxiety disorders and substance-abuse disorders. In the NCS, the anxiety disorders with the highest odds ratios indicating comorbidity were generalized anxiety disorder, panic disorder, and post-traumatic stress disorder. It is also important to note that for most anxiety disorders, with the exception of panic disorder, the anxiety disorder usually predates the onset of the depressive disorder.[19] This is of considerable importance, as the risk factors for pure major depression differed from the risk factors for comorbid major depression. Furthermore, the cohort effects of increasing rates of major depression were largely attributable to increasing rates of comorbid major depression, rather than to increasing rates of pure major depression. These results raise important issues for prevention, as it may well be that targeting young people with anxiety disorders and could be a major step to the prevention of the development of later major depressive disorders.

The second key area of comorbidity with major depression is with alcohol dependence. Data from the Virginia Twin Register suggest that part of this comorbidity is due to shared genetic factors, although there is also a smaller common environmental risk factor to both disorders.

Another area of considerable comorbidity with major depression is the personality disorders. The comorbidity between major depression and these disorders is receiving considerable attention in clinical samples but, to date, there are only limited data in epidemiological samples on the importance of these patterns of comorbidity.

Use of health services

One of the major challenges for psychiatry presented by epidemiological studies of depression has been the consistent finding that the majority of cases of depression in the community are not recognized, diagnosed, nor treated. In the ECA study, it was found that 65 to 70 per cent of people with depression had visited a health professional in the last 6 months, but only 15 to 20 per cent had had a visit for a mental health reason and only about 10 per cent had seen a mental health specialist. Ormel *et al.*[20] found that patients with depression who present with largely somatic rather than psychological symptoms are extremely unlikely to be recognized by general practitioners. Even if major depression is recognized in the primary care setting, it is often not adequately treated.[21]

References

1. Murray, C.J.L. and Lopez, A.D. (1996). *The global burden of disease and global health statistics.* Harvard University Press, Boston, MA.
2. Akiskal, H.S. (2003). Validating 'hard' and 'soft' phenotypes within the bipolar spectrum: Continuity or discontinuity? *Journal of Affective Disorders*, **73**, 1–5.

3. Blacker, D. and Tsuang, M.T. (1992). Contested boundaries of bipolar disorder and the limits of categorical diagnosis in psychiatry. *American Journal of Psychiatry,* **149**, 1473–83.
4. Kessler, R.C., Rubinow, D.R., Holmes, C., *et al.* (1997). The epidemiology of DSM-III-R bipolar I disorder in a general population survey. *Psychological Medicine,* **27**, 1079–89.
5. Weissman, M.M., Bland, R.C., Canino, G.J., *et al.* (1996). Cross national epidemiology of major depression and bipolar disorder. *Journal of the American Medical Association,* **276**, 293–9.
6. Angst, J. (1998). The emerging epidemiology of hypomania and bipolar II disorder. *Journal of Affective Disorders,* **50**, 143–51.
7. Kendler, K.S. and Gardner, C.O. (1998). Boundaries of major depression: an evaluation of DSM-IV criteria. *American Journal of Psychiatry,* **155**, 172–7.
8. Wainwright, N.W.J., Surtees, P.G., and Gilks, W.R. (1997). Diagnostic boundaries, reasoning and depressive disorder, I. Development of a probabilistic morbidity model for public health psychiatry. *Psychological Medicine,* **27**, 835–45.
9. Kendler, K.S., Neale, M.C., Kessler, R.C., *et al.* (1993). The lifetime history of major depression in women. Reliability of diagnosis and heritability. *Archives of General Psychiatry,* **50**, 863–70.
10. Sullivan, P.F., Prescott, C.A. and Kendler, K.S. (2002). The subtypes of major depression in a twin registry. *Journal of Affective Disorders,* **68**, 273–84.
11. Blazer, D.G., Kessler, R.C., McGonagle, K.A., *et al.* (1994). The prevalence and distribution of major depression in a national community sample: the National Comorbidity Survey. *American Journal of Psychiatry,* **151**, 979–86.
12. Jenkins, R., Lewis, G., Bebbington, P., *et al.* (1997). The National Psychiatric Morbidity Surveys of Great Britain—initial findings from the household survey. *Psychological Medicine,* **27**, 775–89.
13. Cross National Collaborative Group (1992). The changing rate of major depression. Cross national comparisons. *Journal of the American Medical Association,* **268**, 3098–105.
14. Kendler, K.S., Neale, M.C., Kessler, R.C., *et al.* (1992). Major depression and generalized anxiety disorder. Same genes (partly) different environment. *Archives of General Psychiatry,* **49**, 716–22.
15. Andrews, G., Stewart, G., Allen, R., *et al.* (1990). The genetics of six neurotic disorders: a twin study. *Journal of Affective Disorders,* **19**, 23–9.
16. Parker, G. (1983). Parental 'affectionless control' as an antecedent to adult depression. A risk factor delineated. *Archives of General Psychiatry,* **40**, 956–60.
17. Kendler, K.S. and Karkowski-Shuman, L. (1997). Stressful life events and genetic liability to major depression: genetic control of exposure to the environment? *Psychological Medicine,* **27**, 539–47.
18. Kendler, K.S., Gardner, C.O. and Prescott, C.A. (2002). Toward a comprehensive developmental model for major depression in women. *American Journal of Psychiatry,* **159**, 1133–45.
19. Kessler, R.C., Nelson, C.B., McGonagle, K.A., *et al.* (1996). Comorbidity of DSM-III-R major depressive disorder in the general population: results from the US National Comorbidity Survey. *British Journal of Psychiatry,* **168**, 17–30.
20. Ormel, J., Koeter, M.W.J., Van den Brink, W., *et al.* (1991). Recognition, management and course of anxiety and depression in general practice. *Archives of General Psychiatry,* **48**, 700–6.
21. Schulberg, H., Block, H.R., Madonia, M.J., *et al.* (1996). Treating major depression in primary care practice, eight-month clinical outcomes. *Archives of General Psychiatry,* **53**, 913–19.

4.5.5 Genetic aetiology of mood disorders

Pierre Oswald, Daniel Souery, and Julien Mendlewicz

Introduction

Advances towards the understanding of the etiological mechanisms involved in mood disorders provide interesting yet diverse hypotheses and promising models. In this context, molecular genetics has now been widely incorporated into genetic epidemiological research in psychiatry. Affective disorders and, in particular, bipolar affective disorder (BPAD) have been examined in many molecular genetic studies which have covered a large part of the genome, specific hypotheses such as mutations have also been studied. Most recent studies indicate that several chromosomal regions may be involved in the aetiology of BPAD. Other studies have reported the presence of anticipation in BPAD and in unipolar affective disorder (UPAD).[1–3] In parallel to these new developments in molecular genetics, the classical genetic epidemiology, represented by twin, adoption and family studies, provided additional evidence in favour of the genetic hypothesis in mood disorders. Moreover, these methods have been improved through models to test the gene-environment interactions.

In addition to genetic approaches, psychiatric research has focused on the role of psychosocial factors in the emergence of mood disorders. In this approach, psychosocial factors refer to the patient's social life context as well as to personality dimensions. Abnormalities in the social behavior such as impairment in social relationships have been observed during episode of affective disorders, and implicated in the etiology of affective disorders. Further, gender and socio-economic status also emerged as having a possible impact on the development of affective disorders. Finally, the onset and outcome of affective disorders could also be explained by interactions between the social life context and the individual's temperament and personality. The importance of temperament and personality characteristics in the etiology of depression has been emphasized in various theories, although disagreement exists with regard to terminology and the etiology.

While significant advances have been done in these two major fields of research, it appears that integrative models, taking into account the interactions between biological (genetic) factors and social (psychosocial environment) variables offer the most reliable way to approach the complex mechanisms involved in the etiology and outcome of mood disorders. This chapter will review some of the most promising genetic and psychosocial hypotheses in mood disorders that can be integrated in interactive models.

Genetic epidemiology of mood disorders

The various strategies available to investigate genetic risk factors in psychiatric disorders belong to the wider discipline of genetic epidemiology. This combines both epidemiological and genetic investigations and has the primary objective of identifying the genetic and non-genetic (environmental) causes of a disease. Genetic epidemiological data in affective disorders has come mostly from family, twin, adoption and segregation (within families) studies. Family, twin and adoption studies are the mainstay in establishing the genetic basis of affective disorders. These methods firstly demonstrated that genetic factors are involved in the aetiology of these disorders.[4] Twin and adoption data may also be used to investigate the relative contributions of genetic and environmental factors to the aetiology of a disease.[5] The exact contribution of these factors is not yet firmly understood for affective disorders but some studies provide contributing findings. The study of adoptees who are separated from their biological parents has consistently favoured the gene-environment hypothesis in the aetiology of diverse psychiatric disorders.[6] In adoption studies, both UPAD and BPAD have been described to be more frequent in biological relatives of the adopted subject, suffering from affective disorders than in adopted relatives.[7]

The diagnostic validation and the structure of the genetic and environmental risk factors in mood disorders are also approached in twin studies.[8] From the landmark study of Rosanoff *et al.* in 1934 to more recent works from Mc Guffin *et al.*[9] and Kieseppa *et al.*,[10] concordance rates for BPAD are higher in monozygotic twins (20–100 per cent) than in dizygotic twins (0–38 per cent).

Molecular genetics in affective disorders

The rapid advance in molecular genetic techniques over the last decade has generated a large database of DNA markers across the whole human genome and has enabled chromosomal regions throughout almost the entire genome to be studied in affective disorders. These studies have been performed mainly using linkage and association methodologies. Current linkage and association methods investigate heritable factors at a molecular genetic level, and enable genes to be mapped.[11] These approaches are mostly applied to BPAD, which is considered to be the 'core' phenotype in affective disorders. Linkage analysis tests the hypothesis that a linkage relationship exists between a known genetic marker and a trait which is known to be genetically determined but has not yet been mapped on a chromosome.[12] Two genetic loci are linked if they are located closely together on a chromosome. In linkage analysis, the distance between a marker locus and the gene under investigation is used for gene mapping. This method was originally designed to explore a major single genetic transmission and to evaluate the extent of co-segregation between genetic markers and the phenotype investigated in pedigrees. The major problems which linkage methodology face when applied to affective disorders are the complex aetiology and inheritance patterns. More than one locus are probably involved in susceptibility to these disorders, and the exact mode of transmission is not known. Mis-specification of the genetic parameters of the phenotype may lead to errors in linkage studies.[12] Furthermore, the linkage approach fails to detect minor gene effects which contribute to genetic susceptibility to the disorder.[13] More recently, genome-wide linkage studies have been performed on samples of families with multiply affected members.[14]

The association method offers an alternative strategy of studying genetic factors involved in complex diseases in which the mode of transmission is not known.[15] The association strategy does not require genetic parameters to be known (non-parametric method). The purpose of association studies is to compare frequencies of genetic marker alleles in patient and control populations in order to detect linkage disequilibrium. Linkage disequilibrium between the disease locus and the marker tested is defined as a level of concordance between the two loci which is higher than would be expected by chance. The major reason for this is their proximity on a chromosome. The major advantage of association studies is that they can detect genes with minor effects other than a single major locus (SML). The major limitation of this approach is that spurious associations between a genetic marker and a disorder may result from variations in allele frequency between cases and controls observed if the two populations are ethnically different (population stratification). It is important in this case to compare populations which are homogenous in their ethnic background. A further major difficulty in association studies is the interpretation of the precise meaning of the association observed.[16] The result may be interpreted as linkage disequilibrium between the disease locus and the associated marker allele(s). Alternatively, the associated marker may be interpreted as a susceptibility factor which is directly involved in the disease. The candidate gene approach in association studies is a useful method to investigate linkage between markers and diseases. A candidate gene refers to a region of the chromosome which is potentially implicated in the aetiology of the disorder concerned. The possibility of false positive results must be taken into account, as a very large number of candidate genes now exist. The probability that each of these genes is involved in the aetiology of the disorder is relatively low.

Linkage studies in affective disorders (See[17] for review)

From more than two decades of linkage studies, it seems that several chromosomal locations have been associated with affective disorders, sometimes with conflicting results. Mendlewicz *et al*[18] first reported possible genetic linkage between manic depression and coagulation Factor IX (F9) at Xq27 in 11 pedigrees. Another region of interest seems to be the chromosome 18 where the pericentromeric region was suggested to carry susceptibility genes. The chromosome 11 has been thoroughly investigated in AD but showed contradictory results. Chromosomes 4, 6, and 10 were also investigated with conflicting and/or unreplicated results. Darier's disease (keratosis follicularis), a rare autosomal dominant skin disorder associated with increased prevalence of epilepsy and mental retardation, whose gene was mapped on chromosome 12 (12q23–24.1), was found to cosegregate with BPAD in one pedigree. This result was replicated in several family studies. Genome-wide linkage analyses provide an accurate tool to study regions of interest. In BPAD, early positive and promising results were contradicted by further analyses. This fact is not surprising, since these studies were performed on small samples sizes, insufficient to replicate modest linkage signals.[19] Meta-analyses were thus performed on BPAD to increase the power to detect modest linkage signals.[14] Bipolar loci with evidence of linkage were found on the following arms: 4p, 6p, 6q, 9p, 10q, 12q, 13 q, 14q, 17q, 18p–q, 21q, 22q.[14,20] McQueen *et al.*[21] found susceptibility loci on chromosomes 6q and 8q by using a combined analysis of eleven linkage studies. A recent study from Schumacher *et al.*,[22] in four European samples, confirmed previously reported loci, 4q31 and 6q24, and provided evidence for a new linkage locus, 1p35-36.

Candidate genes in affective disorders

Serotonin markers

Dysfunction of the serotoninergic system has long been suspected in major depression and related disorders. Depression can successfully be treated with selective drugs which target serotonin receptors. The serotonin transporter may also be involved in susceptibility to affective disorders and in the response to treatment with these drugs. Most recent replication studies did not support these initial positive findings. This has been the case for 5HTT.(17) The tryptophan hydroxylase (TPH1) gene, which codes for the rate limiting enzyme of serotonin metabolism, is also an important candidate gene for affective disorders and suicidal behavior. Bellivier *et al*(23) reported a significant association between genotypes at this marker and BPAD, no association was found with suicidal behaviour. In a previous study in depressed patients suicidal behaviour has been associated with one variant of this gene.(24) The tryptophan hydroxylase isoform (TPH2) showed an association between BPAD and suicidality.(25)

Other candidate genes

Among other pathways, DRD2, DRD3, DRD4 and DAT1 were largely studied and replicated. Unfortunately, results remain conflicting. Recent studies have implicated neurotrophic factors in the underlying disease processes of affective disorders. Brain-derived neurotrophic factor (BDNF), the most abundant of the neurotrophins in the brain, enhances the growth and maintenance of several neuronal systems, serves as a neurotransmitter modulator, and participates in plasticity mechanisms such as long-term potentiation and learning.(26) Although promising, BDNF did not confirm its role in the pathophysiology of affective disorders.(27,28) Several new candidate genes from the well-known molecular cascades have been tested: PIK3C3 in the intracellular signalling pathway; PCDH11Y, a proto-cadherin and GSK3β, a target molecule of lithium. Finally, studies of circadian rhythm-related genes showed promising results in BPAD, such as ARNTL.(29,30)

Anticipation and expanded trinucleotide repeat sequences

Anticipation implies that a disease occurs at a progressively earlier age of onset and with increased severity in successive generations. This may explain the non-Mendelian pattern of inheritance observed in some inherited diseases. Anticipation has been found to correlate with specific mutations in these syndromes: expanded trinucleotide repeat sequences. An expanded repeat sequence is unstable and may increase in size between family members, leading to increased disease severity of the disorder.

Anticipation has been described in BPAD and in UPAD.(1,3) One study highlighted an association between Cysteine-Alanine-Glycine (CAG) trinucleotide repeats and BPAD illness in Swedish and Belgian patients with affective disorder.(31) CAG repeats have been detected by the Repeat Expansion Detection method (RED-method). This hypothesis has also been tested in a family sample of two-generation pairs with BPAD.(32) A significant increase in CAG repeats between parents and offspring generations was observed however, when the phenotype increased in severity, i.e. changed from major depression, single episode or unipolar recurrent depression to BPAD. This is the first evidence of genetic anticipation in BPAD families and should be followed by the identification of loci within the genome containing triplet repeats. CTG 18.1 on chromosome 18q21.1 and ERDA 1 on chromosome 17q21.3 are two repeat loci recently identified but were not found to be associated with BPAD.(33) A newly identified CTG/CAG repeat was found to be associated with BPAD.(34)

Phenotype definition

Facing the heterogeneity of results, it has been hypothesized that genetic factors could explain some symptoms or clinical features of the syndromes, such as severity of the disease, age at onset or gender predominance. Early-onset, and more specifically pediatric-onset, BD has been suggested to have its own pattern of genetic susceptibility factors. Family studies have consistently found a higher rate of BD among the relatives of early-onset BD patients than in relatives of later-onset cases.(35) Among the most recent studies, Faraone *et al.*(36) found, in a genome-wide scan, 3 regions of interest that may influence age at onset of mania in BPAD. Geller *et al.*(37) found an association between BDNF and BPAD with early-onset. Massat *et al.*(38) provided evidence for the influence of HTR2C in early-onset BPAD

More specific neurophysiologic, neuroimaging, neurocognitive, or neurochemical trait measures might identify homogeneous groups of patients. These 'traits' are called 'endophenotypes' and are believed to represent the genetic liability of the disorder among non-affected subjects.(39) Endophenotypes in BD are difficult to define. Circadian rythms, stress reactivity and appetite regulation have been proposed. Bipolar patients are also suggested to show inappropriate emotional responsiveness. Using emotional facial stimuli, depressed BD patients show impaired recognition of happy and sad facial expressions.(40) These findings confirm a particular pattern of characteristics in BD, and suggest that genetic factors may explain these characteristics, rather than the whole clinical picture.

Shared genetic predisposition between BPAD and schizophrenia

If BPAD and schizophrenia (SCZ) are distinguishable, they may share some characteristics. Indeed, family studies show partial overlap in familial susceptibility for these two conditions.(41) Evidence for linkage of both BPAD and SCZ were found on 18p11, 13q32, 10p14, 22q11–13 and 6p22.2.(42–44) More interestingly, two genes showed promising results in molecular genetic studies in these two conditions. From the first report from Hattori *et al.*,(45) G72, found on 13q34 and encoding d-amino acide oxidase activator (DAOA), was found to be associated with delusion or psychosis, rather than with the entire bipolar or schizophrenic clinical pictures.(46) Although robust, these results were confirmed in a recent meta-analysis from Detera-Wadleigh *et al.*(47) Largely distributed in neurones, DISC1 (Disrupted in Schizophrenia 1) interacts with many proteins and is related to several neuronal functions. Thomson *et al.*(48) found a robust association between DISC1 and BPAD, but this result needs confirmation. Theses cases of shared genetic predisposition emphasizes the need, in future classification systems such as DSM-V, to focus on classification that may more closely represent expression of underlying biologic systems.(49)

Pharmacogenetics

One of the main difficulties in clinical practice is the inability to know *a priori* which psychotropic drug will be best suited for each case. Therefore, several groups worldwide try to overcome that obstacle by searching genetic markers that might be predictive of treatment response.

BPAD

The first studies on the relationship between response to lithium and family history have been published in the 1970s, supporting an association between a family history of BPAD and satisfactory response to treatment. Mendlewicz *et al.*(50) first reported a study of 36 patients through a double blind study of lithium prophylaxis. They found that 66 per cent of the responders to lithium had at least one first-degree relative with BPAD, and that only 2–1 per cent of the lithium nonresponders had a first-degree relative with BPAD. Lipp *et al.*(51) first reported an association between DRD2 and non-response to lithium. Several studies have followed (See(52) for review). Positive results were found in TPH and 5HTT.(53,54)

UPAD

Previous studies of an association between poor antidepressant response in depressive patients and 5HTT were largely replicated and could be considered as a robust finding (see(55) for exhaustive review and discussion). Among more recent findings, GNB3 (beta3 subunit of G protein) and DAT1 were found to be associated with treatment response. Binder *et al.*(56) found an association between FKBP5, which plays an important role in the glucocorticoid receptor function, and rapid response to antidepressant. Interestingly, this group of patients was characterized by a high rate of relapses. Finally, the large STAR*D (Sequenced Treatment Alternatives to Relieve Depression) project provided recent promising data for HTR2A 5HTT and GRIK4, which codes for the kainic acid-type glutamate receptor KA1 and treatment response.(57–59)

Psychosocial factors in affective disorders

Impairment in social relationships, dysfunctional cognition, gender, economic status, and temperament has been suggested as involved in the emergence of mood disorders. However, empirical studies on psychosocial factors of patients with affective disorders examine psychosocial features assessed after recovery from or/and at the time of episodes of affective disorders. These retrospective studies might not be able to distinguish between premorbid psychosocial patterns and those which result from previous episodes of illness. Further, longitudinal studies focusing on the role of psychosociological factors have involved predictions of recurrence or exacerbation of symptomatology in previously affected people, but not regarding the onset of the diseases. Thus, the demonstration of temporal antecedence to the initial onset of affective disorder is extremely difficult.(60) Thus, the conclusions in terms of etiological psychosocial factor are limited.

Impairment in social and familial relationships

Difficulties in social functioning are concomitant to depressive disorders.(61) The concept of social support has been widely used to predict general health and more specifically psychiatric symptoms.(62) Previous research revealed that the degree of integration in a social network, or structural support, have a direct positive effect on well-being, reducing negative outcomes in both high and low stress life events. Among depressed individuals, dysfunction in social activities has been found to persist long time after remission from the depressive episode.(63) The social dysfunctioning concerns more specifically marital relationships, parental, and familial relationships.

The relationship between marital disturbance and affective disorders has received increased attention over the past decades. First, descriptive studies have suggested that marital conflict correlates highly with concomitant depression,(64) and marital therapy has been found to be effective in reducing the symptoms of depression, alone as well as in combination with pharmacotherapy. Further, previous research found dysfunctional patterns of communication in couples with a depressed spouse.(65, 66) The lack of a confiding and intimate relationship leaves individuals vulnerable to depression.(67, 68) Finally, marital distress may also exacerbate difficulties experienced in extramarital relationships,(69) thereby increasing introverted behavior and social isolation. In similar manner, the absence of a marital partner may hasten the onset of depression among vulnerable individuals.(70)

The parental relationships seem also to have a great impact in the course of affective disorders. A variety of authors have emphasized the importance of the quality of early experiences with parents in the development of adult depression. Beck first, explicitly attributes the development of negative cognition and negative schemata of self to critical, disapproving parents.(71)

Dysfunctional cognition

According to the helplessness model of depression(73) vulnerability to depression derives from a habitual style of explaining the causes of life events, known as attributional style. A large body of research found that individuals suffering of depression think more negatively than healthy individuals. Specifically, depressed patients have a tendency to make internal, stable, and global causal attributions for negative events, and to a lesser extent, the attribution of positive outcomes to external, specific, and unstable causes. In other words, depressed patients have a low self-esteem.(74,75) Thus, when thinking about the self, past, current and future circumstances, depressed patients emphasize the negative, and this process is likely to contribute to the perpetuation of their depressed mood.

Gender

Evidence for sex differences in responses to depression comes from a large number of studies. Women are consistently reported to have greater prevalence of affective disorders than men.(76,77) First, women may experience two important periods, known to be associated with higher rates of depression: pregnancy and post-partum. The prevalence of major or minor depression among pregnant women ranges from 7 per cent to 26 per cent.(78) Depression during pregnancy is a strong predictor of postpartum depression. The prevalence of postpartum depression ranges from 10 per cent to 15 per cent in the first year after childbirth.(79) Besides these two specific conditions, the reasons for this sex difference are unclear, and are as likely to be social as biological.

Divergences in the number and quality of social and occupational roles have been proposed to explain the greater prevalence of affective disorders among women. In the context of marital relationship, previous research has indicated that for men, marriage confers a protection against illness, while it appears to be associated with higher rates of depression for women.[80] There has been some evidence that within the marriage the traditional female role is limiting, restricting, which may lead to depression.[81,82] For example, the role of child caretaker has consistently been shown to be associated with both high levels of stress and a higher incidence of depression for women.[83]Women are found to have more depressive symptoms when there are young children in the home, and this tends to increase in an almost linear fashion according to the number of children in the household.[84] Further, since women who are employed outside the home also tend to be responsible for household chores,[85] the notion that differentiation in occupational roles could partially explain the prevalence of depression for women is supported.

Socio-economic status

Many studies have reported that low socio-economic status is associated with high prevalence of mood disorders.[86] Since a long time, in social psychiatry, the 'social causation' and 'social selection' hypotheses have been formulated to explain the role of the low socio-economic status in the disease. The causation hypothesis suggests that the stress associated with low social position, that is exposure to adversity and lack of resource to cope with difficulty, may contribute to the development of the affective disorder[87] while the social selection hypothesis argued that genetically predisposed persons drift down to or fail to rise out of such positions.[88,89] Thus, the social selection hypothesis emphasizes the genetic interpretation of cause, while social causation hypothesis focuses on the etiologic role of the environment. Few longitudinal data sets are available to test the causal hypothesis. Nevertheless, there is evidence that disadvantaged socio-economic status, poverty, or education and occupation can be considered as risk factors for mood disorders.[90,91] Nevertheless, Bruce and Hoff found that the effect of poverty is substantially reduced when controlling for degree of isolation from friends and family, suggesting that social isolation mediates some of the relationships between economic status and mood disorders.[92]

In summary, a positive relationship has been found between socio-economic status and vulnerability to affective disorders, with higher rates of vulnerability found among individuals with lower educational and social achievement levels.

Temperament and behaviour

Temperament has been defined in terms of differences in the adaptative systems, that is differences in reactivity and self-regulation to the social context.[93–95]

The model of temperament developed by Eysenck approaches temperament in terms of cortical arousal.[96] Eysenck suggested that individuals differ in their basic arousability and therefore, in their optimal level of stimulation. These physiological differences give rise to the primary personality dimension of introversion-extraversion. Introverts are said to possess relatively reactive reticular systems, and thus to attain their optimal level of cortical arousal at relatively low level of stimulation. As a result of their low optimal arousal level, introverts are expected to prefer and seek out mild forms of stimulation and to avoid more intense and novel forms of stimulation. In contrast, extraverts are said to possess relatively unreactive reticular systems, to have correspondingly high optimal levels of cortical arousal, and to therefore, approach more intense and novel forms of stimulation.

The differences between the Cloninger's model and other models are that Cloninger assumes relationships between biogenic amine neurotransmitters (norepinephrine, serotonin, and dopamine) and personality dimensions. Specifically, Cloninger defined temperament dimensions in terms of individuals' differences in associative learning in response to novelty, danger or punishment, and reward. Further, he hypothesized a positive correlation between serotoninergic activity and harm avoidance, dopaminergic activity and novelty seeking, and finally between noradrenergic activity and reward dependence. According to this author, these aspects of personality denote traits that are usually considered temperament factors because they are heritable, manifest early in life, and apparently involved in learning. The possible tridimensional combinations of extreme (high or low) variants on these basic stimulus response characteristics correspond closely to the traditional descriptions of personality disorders. The specific relationship between temperament and mood disorder is not yet understood satisfactorily. Studies have been done regarding the Tridimensional Personality Questionaire (TPQ) scores in relation to mood disorder, the data available suggest that depressed patients have elevated harm avoidance scores.[97–100]

The possible role of candidate genes has been investigated in personality. Association between a personality trait (Novelty Seeking) and the 7 repeat allele in the locus for Dopamine receptor D4 gene (DRD4) has been observed in a group of 124 unrelated Israeli normal subjects.[101] Novelty Seeking was assessed from the Tridimensional Personality Questionnaire (TPQ).[102] An association was also observed between similar personality traits and long alleles of DRD4 gene in 315 subjects, mostly male siblings from United States.[103] This last study utilized the NEO Personality Inventory (NEO-PI-R)[104] from which TPQ Novelty-Seeking scores can be estimated. More recent studies also suggest a pattern of influence on temperamental dimension exerted by serotonergic and dopaminergic genes.[105] They studies, even not definitive, suggest that the contribution of these polymorphisms to the clinical presentation of mood disorders could be mediated by an influence on personality differences.

The gene-environment hypothesis

The availability of molecular genetic findings in affective disorders offers new directions in this research field. It is now possible to consider the gene-environment hypotheses using the DNA as the genetic liability variable. In primate models, early experiences of maternal separation were found to confer increased risk of depression during adult age.[106] Barr *et al.* found that infant rhesus monkeys showing a specific polymorphism in 5HTT were more likely to engage in rough play than were individuals without this polymorphism.[107] In humans, a landmark study demonstrated that a functional polymorphism in the promoter region of 5HTT gene moderated the influence of stressful life events on depression and suicidal behaviour.[108] This study was replicated with conflicting results using different methodologies.[109–112] However, these results support the notion that a combination of genetic predisposition and specific life events may interact to facilitate the development of affective disorders.

Conclusion

The complexity and heterogeneity of affective disorders is a major limitation for gene-environment studies.This could be attributed to their non-Mendelian mode of inheritance. BPAD and UPAD are, in fact, phenotypes which do not appear to exhibit classic Mendelian recessive or dominant inheritance involving a single major locus. The presence of both environmental as well as genetic factors and phenotypic diversity also represent important problems when dealing with these diseases. After the era of enthusiasm due to first results from linkage and association studies, the lack of replication and the identification of potential methodological biases led to a period of pessimism. However, recent technological advances allow for the analysis of hundreds of components in a biological system simultaneously. Gene expression micro-arrays may analyse the expression of hundreds of genes in a specific tissue. More specifically, micro-array technologies measure levels of messenger ribonucleic acid (mRNA), an intermediate product between gene and protein.[113] The levels of these 'transcripts' are compared between a population suffering from a specific disease and control subjects. The analysis of mRNA transcripts, instead of DNA regions, may provide additional information on genetic regulation processes of illness. Ultimately, the understanding of neurobiological processes underlying affective disorders may help developing therapeutic and prevention strategies.

Further information

Serretti, A. and Mandelli, L. (2008). The genetics of bipolar disorder: genome 'hot regions', genes, new potential candidates and future directions. *Mol Psychiatry*, **13**, 742–71

The Wellcome Trust Case Control Consortium http://www.wtccc.org.uk

References

1. McInnis, M.G., McMahon, F.J., Chase, G.A. *et al.* (1993). Anticipation in bipolar affective disorder. *American Journal of Human Genetics*, **53**, 385–90.
2. Nylander, P.-O, Engstrom, C., Chotai, J., *et al.* (1994). Anticipation in Swedish Families with Bipolar Affective Disorder. *Journal of Medical Genetics*, **9**, 686–89.
3. Engström, C., Johansson, E.L., Langström, M., *et al.* (1995). Anticipation in unipolar affective disorder. *Journal of Affective Disorder*, **35**, 31–40.
4. Mendlewicz, J. (1994) The search for a manic depressive gene: from classical to molecular genetics. *Progress in Brain Research*, **100**, 225–59.
5. Vieland, V.J., Susser, E. and Weissman, M.M. (1995) Genetic epidemiology in psychiatric research. In *Genetics of Mental Disorders Part I: Theoretical aspects. Baillière's Clinical Psychiatry, International Practice and Research* (eds. G.N. Papadimitriou and J. Mendlezicz), pp. 19–46. Vol. 1, No 1, Bailliere Tindall, London.
6. Cadoret, R.J., Winokur, G., Lengbehn, D., *et al.* (1996) Depression spectrum disease, I: the role of gene-environment interaction. *American Journal of Psychiatry*, **153**, 892–9.
7. Mendlewicz, J., Rainer, J.D. (1977). Adoption study supporting genetic transmission in manic--depressive illness. *Nature*, **268**(5618), 327–9.
8. Kendler, K.S., Eaves, L.J., Walters, E.E. *et al.* (1996) The identification and validation of distinct depressive syndromes in a population-based sample of female twins. *Archives General of Psychiatry*, **53**, 391–9.
9. McGuffin, P., Rijsdijk, F., Andrew, M., (2003). The heritability of bipolar affective disorder and the genetic relationship to unipolar depression. *Archives General of Psychiatry*, **60**(5), 497–502.
10. Kieseppä, T., Partonen, T., Haukka, J., *et al.* (2004). High concordance of bipolar I disorder in a nationwide sample of twins. *American Journal of Psychiatry*, **161**(10), 1814–21.
11. Weiss, K.M. (1993) Genetic variation and human disease: principles and evolutionary approaches. Cambridge University Press, Cambridge, pp.117-148.
12. Ott, J. (1991) Analysis of human genetic linkage (2nd edn.). Johns Hopkins University Press, Baltimore.
13. Propping, P., Nothen, M.M., Fimmers, R. *et al.* (1993). Linkage versus association studies in complex diseases. *Pychiatric Genetics*, **3**, 136–9.
14. Maier, W., Zobel, A., Rietschel, M,. (2003). Genetics of schizophrenia and affective disorders. *Pharmacopsychiatry*, **36** (Suppl 3), S195–202.
15. Hodge, S.E. (1993) Linkage analysis versus association analysis: distinguishing between two models that explain disease-marker associations. *American Journal of Medical Genetics*, **53**, 367–84.
16. Hodge, S.E. (1994) What association analysis can and cannot tell us about the genetics of complex disease. *American Journal of Medical Genetics*, **54**, 318–23.
17. Oswald, P., Souery, D., Mendlewicz, J. (2003). Molecular genetics of affective disorders. *International Journal of Neuropsychopharmacol*, **6**(2), 155–69.
18. Mendlewicz, J., Simon, P., Sevy, S., *et al.* (1987). Polymorphic DNA marker on chromosome and manicdepression. *Lancet*, **1**, 1230–2.
19. Suarez, B.K. and Hampe, C.L. (1994). Linkage and association. *American Journal of Human Genetics*, **54**(3), 554–9
20. Green, E.K., Raybould, R., Macgregor, S., *et al.* (2005). Operation of the schizophrenia susceptibility gene, neuregulin 1, across traditional diagnostic boundaries to increase risk for bipolar disorder. *Archives General of Psychiatry*, **62**(6), 642–8.
21. McQueen, M.B., Devlin, B., Faraone, S.V., *et al.* (2005). Combined analysis from eleven linkage studies of bipolar disorder provides strong evidence of susceptibility loci on chromosomes 6q and 8q. *American Journal of Human Genetics*, **77**(4), 582–95
22. Schumacher, J., Kaneva, R., Jamra, R.A., *et al.* (2005). Genomewide scan and fi ne-mapping linkage studies in four European samples with bipolar affective disorder suggest a new susceptibility locus on chromosome 1p35–p36 and provides further evidence of loci on chromosome 4q31 and 6q24. *American Journal of Human Genetics*, **77**(6), 1102–11.
23. Bellivier, F., Leboyer, M., Courtet, P., *et al.* (1998) Association between the tryptophan hydroxylase gene and manic-depressive illness. *Archives of General Psychiatry*, **55**, 33–7.
24. Mann, J.J., Malone, K.M., Nielsen, D.A., *et al.* (1997) Possible association of a polymorphism of the tryptophan hydroxylase gene with suicidal behavior in depressed patients. *American Journal of Psychiatry*, **154**, 1451–3.
25. De Luca, V., Mueller, D.J., Tharmalingam, S., *et al.* (2004). Analysis of the novel TPH2 gene in bipolar disorder and suicidality. *Molecular Psychiatry*, **9**(10), 896–7.
26. Murer, M.G., Yan, Q., Raisman-Vozari R Brain-derived neurotrophic factor in the control human brain, and in Alzheimer's disease and Parkinson's disease. *Progress in Neurobiology*, **63**(1), 71–124.
27. Oswald, P., Del-Favero, J., Massat, I., *et al.* (2004). Non-replication of the brain-derived neurotrophic factor (BDNF) association in bipolar affective disorder: a Belgian patient-control study. *American Journal of Medical Genetics. Part B, Neuropsychiatric Genetics*, **129**(1), 34–5.
28. Schumacher, J., Jamra, R.A., Becker, T., *et al.* (2005). Evidence for a relationship between genetic variants at the brain-derived neurotrophic

factor (BDNF) locus and major depression. *Biological Psychiatry*, **58**(4), 307–14.

29. Nievergelt, C.M., Kripke, D.F., Barrett, T.B., (2006). Suggestive evidence for association of the circadian genes PERIOD3 and ARNTL with bipolar disorder. *American Journal of Medical Genetics. Part B, Neuropsychiatric Genetics,* **141**(3), 234–41.
30. Mansour, H.A., Wood, J., Logue, T., *et al.* (2006). Association study of eight circadian genes with bipolar I disorder, schizoaffective disorder and schizophrenia. *Genes, Brain, and Behavior*, **5**(2), 150–7.
31. Lindblad, K., Nylander, PO., De bruyn, A., *et al.* (1995) Expansion of trinucleotide CAG repeats detected in Bipolar Affective Disorder by the RED-(rapid expansion detection) method. *Neurobiology of disease*, **2,** 55–62.
32. Mendlewicz, J., Lipp, O., Souery, D. *et al.* (1997) Possible maternal genomic imprinting on expended trinucleotide CAG repeats in bipolar affective disorder. *Biological Psychiatry*, **42**, 1115–22.
33. Mendlewicz, J., Souery, D., Del-Favero, J., *et al.* (2004). Expanded RED products and loci containing CAG/ CTG repeats on chromosome 17 (ERDA1) and chromosome 18 (CTG18.1) in trans-generational pairs with bipolar affective disorder. *American Journal of Medical Genetics. Part B, Neuropsychiatric Genetics,* **128**(1), 71–5.
34. Tsutsumi, T., Holmes, S.E., McInnis, M.G., *et al.* (2004). Novel CAG/ CTG repeat expansion mutations do not contribute to the genetic risk for most cases of bipolar disorder or schizophrenia. *American Journal of Medical Genetics. Part B, Neuropsychiatric Genetics,* **124**(1), 15–9.
35. Faraone, S.V., Glatt, S.J., Tsuang, M.T. (2003). The genetics of pediatric-onset bipolar disorder. *Biological Psychiatry*, **53**, 970–7.
36. Faraone, S.V., Glatt, S.J., Su, J., *et al.* (2004). Three potential susceptibility loci shown by a genome-wide scan for regions infl uencing the age at onset of mania. *American Journal of Psychiatry*, **161**(4), 625–30.
37. Geller, B., Badner, J.A., Tillman, R., *et al.* (2004). Linkage disequilibrium of the brain-derived neurotrophic factor Val66Met polymorphism in children with a prepubertal and early adolescent bipolar disorder phenotype. *American Journal of Psychiatry*, **161**(9), 1698–700.
38. Massat, I., Lerer, B., Souery, D., *et al.* (2007). HTR2C (cys23ser) polymorphism infl uences early onset in bipolar patients in a large European multicenter association study. *Molecular Psychiatry*, **12**(9), 797–8.
39. Leboyer, M., Bellivier, F., Nosten-Bertrand, M., *et al.* (1998). Psychiatric genetics: search for phenotypes. *Trends in Neurosciences*, **21**, 102–5.
40. Rubinow, D.R. and Post, R.M. (1992). Impaired recognition of affect in facial expression in depressed patients. Biological Psychiatry, **31**, 947–53.
41. Berrettini, W. (2003). Evidence for shared susceptibility in bipolar disorder and schizophrenia. *American Journal of Medical Genetics. Part C, Seminars in Medical Genetics*, **123**(1), 59–64.
42. Berrettini, W. (2000). Susceptibility loci for bipolar disorder: overlap with inherited vulnerability to schizophrenia. *Biological Psychiatry*, **47**(3), 245–51.
43. Walss-Bass, C., Escamilla, M.A., Raventos, H., *et al.* (2005). Evidence of genetic overlap of schizophrenia and bipolar disorder: linkage disequilibrium analysis of chromosome 18 in the Costa Rican population. *American Journal of Medical Genetics. Part B, Neuropsychiatric Genetics*, **139**(1), 54–60.
44. Schulze, T.G., Buervenich, S., Badner, J.A., *et al.* (2004). Loci on chromosomes 6q and 6p interact to increase susceptibility to bipolar affective disorder in the national institute of mental health genetics initiative pedigrees. *Biological Psychiatry*, **56**(1), 18–23.
45. Hattori, E., Liu, C., Badner, J.A., *et al.* (2003). Polymorphisms at the G72/G30 gene locus, on 13q33, are associated with bipolar disorder in two independent pedigree series. *American Journal of Human Genetics*, **72**(5), 1131–40.
46. Chen, Y.S., Akula, N., Detera-Wadleigh, S.D., *et al.* (2004). Findings in an independent sample support an association between bipolar affective disorder and the G72/G30 locus on chromosome 13q33. *Molecular Psychiatry,* **9**(1), 87–92.
47. Detera-Wadleigh, S.D. and McMahon, F.J. (2006). G72/G30 in schizophrenia and bipolar disorder: review and meta-analysis. *Biological Psychiatry*, **60**(2), 106-14.
48. Thomson, P.A., Wray, N.R., Millar, J.K., *et al.* (2005). Association between the TRAX/ DISC locus and both bipolar disorder and schizophrenia in the Scottish population. *Molecular Psychiatry*, **10**(7), 657–8, 616.
49. Merikangas, K.R. and Risch, N. (2003). Will the genomics revolution revolutionize psychiatry? *American Journal of Psychiatry*, **160**(4), 625–35.
50. Mendlewicz, J., Fieve, R.R. and Stallone, F. (1973). Relationship between the effectiveness of lithium therapy and family history. *American Journal of Psychiatry,* **130**, 1011–13.
51. Lipp, O., Mahieu, B., Souery, D., *et al.* (1997). Molecular genetics of bipolar disorders: Implication for psychotropic drugs. *European Neuropsychopharmacology*, **7**(suppl 2), 112–3.
52. Oswald, P., Souery, D. and Mendlewicz, J. (2006). Pharmacogenetics of bipolar disorders. In *Psychopharmacogenetics* (eds. P. Gorwood and M. Hamon), pp. 75–100, Springer, USA.
53. Serretti, A., Lilli, R., Lorenzi, C., *et al.* (1999). tryptophan hydroxylase gene and response to lithium in mood disorders. *Psychiatry Research*, **33**, 371–7.
54. Serretti, A., Lilli, R., Mandelli, L., *et al.* (2001). Serotonin transporter gene associated with lithium prophylaxis in mood disorders. *Pharmacogenomics Journal*, **1**(1), 71–7.
55. Serretti, A. and Artioli, P. (2004). From molecular biology to pharmacogenetics: a review of the literature on antidepressant treatment and suggestions of possible candidate genes. *Psychopharmacology (Berl)*, **174**(4), 490–503.
56. Binder, E.B., Salyakina, D., Lichtner, P., *et al.* (2004). Polymorphisms in FKBP5 are associated with increased recurrence of depressive episodes and rapid response to antidepressant treatment. Nature Genetics, **36**(12), 1319–25.
57. McMahon, F.J., Buervenich, S., Charney, D., *et al.* (2006). Variation in the gene encoding the serotonin 2A receptor is associated with outcome of antidepressant treatment. *American Journal of Human Genetics*, **78**(5), 804–14.
58. Hu, X.Z., Rush, A.J., Charney, D., *et al.* (2007). Association between a functional serotonin transporter promoter polymorphism and citalopram treatment in adult outpatients with major depression. *Archive General of Psychiatry*, **64**(7), 783–92.
59. Paddock, S., Laje, G., Charney, D., *et al.* (2007). Association of GRIK4 with outcome of antidepressant treatment in the STAR*D cohort. *American Journal of Psychiatry*, **164**(8), 1181–8.
60. Depue, R.A. and Monroe, S.M. (1986). Conceptualization and measurement of human disorder in life stress research: the problem of chronic disturbance. *Psychological Bulletin,* **99**, 36–51.
61. Hirschfeld, R.M.A, Klerman, G.L., Clayton, P.J., *et al.* (1983). Assessing personality: Effects of the depressive state on trait measurement. *American Journal of Psychiatry,* **140**, 695–9.
62. Kendler, K.S. (1997) Social support: a genetic epidemiologic analysis. *American Journal of Psychiatry,* **154**, 1398–404.
63. Shapira, B. *et al.* (1999). Social adjustment and self-esteem in remitted patients with unipolar and bipolar affective disorder: a case-control study. *Comprehensive Psychiatry,* **40**, 24–30.
64. Crowther, J.H. (1985). The relationship between depression and marital maladjustment: A descriptive study. *Journal of nervous and mental disease,* **173**, 227–31.
65. Kahn, J., Coyne, J.C., and Margolin, C. (1985). Depression and marital disagreement: The social construction of despair. *Journal of social and Personal Relationships,* **2**, 447–61.

66. Biglan, A., Hops, H., Sherman, L., *et al.* (1985). Problem-solving interactions of depressed women and their husbands. *Behavior Therapy*, **16**, 431–51.
67. Brown, G.W. and Prudo, R. (1981). Psychiatric disorder in a rural and urban population: 1. Etiology of depression. *Psychological medicine*, **11**, 581–99.
68. Costello, C.G. (1982). Social factors associated with depression: A retrospective community study. *Psychological Medicine*, **12**, 329–39.
69. Coyne, J.C., and DeLongis, A. (1986). Going beyond social support: The role of social relationships in adaptation. *Journal of Consulting and Clinical Psychology*, **54**, 454–60.
70. Brown, G.W., and Harris T. (1978). *Social origin of depression*. London: Free Press.
71. Beck, A.T. (1967). *Depression: Clinical, experimental, and theoretical aspects*. Harper & Row, New York.
72. Peterson, C. and Seligman, M.E.P. (1984). Causal explanations as a risk factor for depression: Theory and evidence. *Psychological Review*, **91**, 347–74.
73. Peterson, C. and Seligman, M.E.P. (1984). Causal explanations as a risk factor for depression: Theory and evidence. *Psychological Review*, **91**, 347–74.
74. Tracy, A., Bauwens, F., Martin, F., *et al.* (1992). Attributional style and depression: a controlled comparison of remitted unipolar and bipolar patients. *British Journal of Clinical Psychology*, **31**, 83–4.
75. Pardoen, D., Bauwens, F., Tracy, A., (1993). Self-esteem in recovered bipolar and unipolar out-patients. *British Journal of Psychiatry*, **163**, 755–62.
76. Bebbington, P.E., *et al.* (1998) The infl uence of age and sex on the prevalence of depressive conditions: report from the National Survey of Psychiatric Morbidity. *Psychological Medicine*, **28**, 9–19.
77. Kroenke, K., and Spitzer, R.L. (1998). Gender differences in the reporting of physical and somatoform symptoms. *Psychosomatic Medicine*, **60**, 150–5.
78. Hobfoll, S.E., Ritter, C., Lavin, J., *et al.* (1995). Depression prevalence and incidence among inner-city pregnant and postpartum women. *Journal of Consulting and Clinical Psychology*, **63**(3), 445–53.
79. Afifi, M. (2007).Gender differences in mental health. *Singapore Medical Journal*, **48**(5), 385–91.
80. Weissman, M.M. (1987). Advances in psychiatric epidemiology: Rates and risks for major depression. *American Journal of Public Health*, **77**, 445–51.
81. Gove, W.R., and Tudor, J.F. (1973). Adult sex roles and mental illness. *American Journal of Sociology*, **78**, 1308–14.
82. Ramsey, E.R. (1974). Boredom: the most prevalent american disease. *Harpers*, **249**, 12–22.
83. Thoits, P.A. (1986). Multiple identities: Examining gender and marital status differences in distress. *American Sociological Review*, **51**, 259–72.
84. Radloff, L.S. (1975). Sex differences in depression: The effects of occupation and marital status. *Sex Roles*, **1**, 249–65.
85. Rosenfield S. (1992). The costs of sharing: wives' employment and husbands' mental health. *Journal of Health and Social Behavior*, **33**, 213–25.
86. Dohrenwend, B.P., *et al.* (1992). Sosioeconomic status and psychiatric disorders: the causation-selection issue. *Science*, **255**, 946–52.
87. Faris, R.E.L., and Dunham, W. (1939). *Mental disorders in urban areas*. University of Chicago Press, Chicago.
88. Jarvis, E. (1971). Insanity and idiosy in Massachusetts: report of the commission of Lunacy, 1855. Harvard University Press, Cambridge.
89. Odegaard, O. (1956). The incidence of psychoses in various occupations. *International Journal of Social Psychiatry*, **2**, 85–104.
90. Bruce, M.L., Takeuchi, D.T., and Leaf, P.J. (1991). Poverty and psychiatric status: Longitudinal evidence from the New Haven Epidemiologic Catchment Area Study. *Archives of General Psychiatry*, **48**, 470–4.
91. Gallo, J.J., Royall, D.R., and Anthony, J.C. (1993). Risk factors for the onset of depression in middle age and later life. *Social Psychiatry Psychiatr Epidemiology*, **28**, 101–8.
92. Bruce, M.L., and Hoff, R.A. (1994). Social and physical health risk factors for fi rst-onset major depressive disorder in a community sample. *Social Psychiatry and Psychiatric Epidemiology*, **29**, 165–71.
93. Cloninger, C.R., Svrakic, D.M., and Przybeck, T.R. (1993). A psychobiological model of temperament and character. *Archives of General Psychiatry*, **50**, 975–90.
94. Derryberry, D., and Rothbart M.K. (1984). Emotion, attention, and temperament. In *Emotion, Cognition, & Behavior* (eds. C.E. Izard, J. Kagan, and R.B. Zajonc), pp 133–66. Cambridge University Press, New York.
95. Derryberry, D, and Rothbart, M.K. (1997). Reactive and effortful processes in the organization of temperament. *Developmental Psychopathology*, **9**, 633–52.
96. Eysenck, H.J. (ed.) (1981). *A model of personality*. Springer- Verlag, New York.
97. Joffe, R.T., Bagby, R.M., Levitt, A.J., *et al.* (1993). The Tridimensional Personality Questionnaire in major depression. *American Journal Psychiatry*, **150**, 959–60.
98. Kleifield, E.I., Sunday, S., Hurt, S., *et al.* (1994). The effects of depression and treatment on the Tridimensional Personality Questionnaire. *Biological Psychiatry*, **36**, 68–70.
99. Nelsen, M.R., and Dunner, D.L. (1995). Clinical and differential diagnostic aspects of treatment-resistant depression. *Journal of Psychiatry Research*, **29**, 43–50.
100. Chien, A.J., and Dunner, D.L. (1996). The Tridimensional Personality Questionnaire in depression: state versus trait issues. *Journal of Psychiatry Research*, **30**, 21–7.
101. Ebstein, R.P., Novick, O., Umansky, R., *et al.* (1996) Dopamine D4 receptor (D4DR) exon III polymorphism associated with the human personality trait of Novelty-Seeking. *Nature Genetics*, **12**, 78–80.
102. Cloninger, C.R. (1987) A systematic method for clinical description and classifi cation of personality variants. *Archives of General Psychiatry*, **44**, 573–88.
103. Benjamin, J., Li, L., Paterson, C., *et al.* (1996). Population and familial association between the D4 dopamine receptor gene and measures of Novelty-Seeking. *Nature Genetics*, **12**, 81–4.
104. Costa, P.T.J and McCrae, R.R. (1992). In Revised NEO Personality Inventory (NEOPI-R) and NEO Five Inventory (NEO-FFI) professional manual. *Psychological Assessment Ressources*, Odessa, FL.
105. Serretti, A., Mandelli, L., Lorenzi, C., *et al.* (2006). Temperament and character in mood disorders: influence of DRD4, SERTPR, TPH and MAO-A polymorphisms. *Neuropsychobiology*, **53**(1), 9–16.
106. Lesch, K.P., Bengel, D., Heils, A. *et al.* (1996). Association of anxiety-related traits with a polymorphism in the serotonin transporter gene regulatory region. *Science*, **274**, 1527–31.
107. Barr, C.S., Newman, T.K., Schwandt, M., *et al.* (2004). Sexual dichotomy of an interaction between early adversity and the serotonin transporter gene promoter variant in rhesus macaques. *Proceedings of the National Academy of Sciences of the United States of America*, **101**(33), 12358–63.
108. Caspi, A., Sugden, K., Moffitt, T.E., *et al.* (2003). Influence of life stress on depression: moderation by a polymorphism in the 5-HTT gene. *Science*, **301**(5631), 386–9.
109. Eley, T.C., Sugden, K., Corsico, A., *et al.* (2004). Gene-environment interaction analysis of serotonin system markers with adolescent depression. *Molecular Psychiatry*, **9**(10), 908–15.
110. Kaufman, J., Yang, B.Z., Douglas-Palumberi, H., *et al.* (2004). Social supports and serotonin transporter gene moderate depression in maltreated children. *Proceedings of the National Academy of Sciences of the United States of America*, **101**(49), 17316–21.

111. Grabe, H.J., Lange, M., Wolff, B., *et al.* (2005). Mental and physical distress is modulated by a polymorphism in the 5-HT transporter gene interacting with social stressors and chronic disease burden. *Molecular Psychiatry*, **10**(2), 220–4.
112. Wilhelm, K., Mitchell, P.B., Niven, H., *et al.* (2006). Life events, fi rst depression onset and the serotonin transporter gene. *British Journal of Psychiatry*, **188,** 210–5.
113. Konradi, C. (2005). Gene expression microarray studies in polygenic psychiatric disorders: applications and data analysis. *Brain Research. Brain Research Reviews*, **50**(1), 142–55.

4.5.6 Neurobiological aetiology of mood disorders

Guy Goodwin

Introduction

Neurobiology provides an explanation of behaviour or experience at the level, either of systems of neurones or individual cells. The current era of progress is driven by contemporary cognitive neuroscience and a rapid evolution in the platform technologies of imaging and genetics. These will allow us to improve our accounts of the functional anatomy of the component elements of mood and its disorder, their functional neurochemistry and, in all probability, give meaning to what a cellular account of depressive illness may eventually describe. This chapter will offer a partial and personal view of these developments to date.

There are now authoritative models of causation in mood disorder, established from well designed, large-scale twin studies (see Chapter 4.5.5). These inform the classical formulation of mood disorder as requiring a vulnerability, a precipitating factor or factors, and maintaining factors which prevent spontaneous recovery. Neurobiology will be addressed under these headings.

Vulnerability to mood disorder

The key vulnerability factors appear to be genes, temperament (also in substantial part genetic), and early adversity. There has been limited work on the neurobiology of these risk factors, as opposed to the vast effort to understand the depressed phenotype. However, for potential prevention either of onset or relapse, such factors appear more logical targets for current research effort and will be covered first. Success in depression would parallel that seen in moving the management of heart disease from the acute episode of infarction to the treatment of metabolic risk factors.

(a) Genetics

Neurobiology has informed the genetic search for candidate genes, starting with the human serotonin transporter (SERT) gene (see Chapter 4.5.5). There has been a terrific proliferation of possible genetic effects deriving from neurobiological theories designed either to explain elements of the actions of psychotropic drugs, the depressed phenotype or from animal experiments. The latter are limited by the validity of animal models of depression per se. Some of the former will be noticed below.

Genes making small contributions to the risk of psychiatric disorder are emerging from direct analysis of the genome (see Chapter 2.4.2). Consistent findings must inform biological investigations in future. At this point it is uncertain whether insights will come from studying variation in individual genes, as has often been assumed, or from a much more complex understanding of cellular function regulated only in part by genetic variation. On the latter assumption the role of genetic hits is to direct attention to processes which may go wrong in the relevant disease. For mood disorder, these seem likely to be developmental or related to stress regulation.

(b) Temperament

The way in which genes may regulate the expression of vulnerability traits is suggested by animal studies. For example, when animals are selected for differences in emotional behaviour they also show different hypothalamic–pituitary–adrenal (HPA) axis function. Specifically, Roman high- and low-avoidance rats differentially acquire a two-way active avoidance response in a shuttle box. High-avoidance animals show greater prolactin and HPA axis responsivity to stress compared with low-avoidance animals. However, young Roman strain rats show identical HPA axis reactivity, although prolactin responses and behaviour are different.[1] In other words, reactivity to the environment may share a measure of common genetic control across physiological and behavioural domains, but HPA abnormality per se develops secondary to emotional experience, or at least is magnified by it.

In human studies, neuroticism is an old psychological construct often criticized as reflecting an average or habitual mood state rather than a truly independent risk. We have studied extremes of the dimension (high and low N) in young subjects before the onset of depression and in older groups who may or may not have experienced depressive episodes. Interestingly, high neuroticism with or without a history of depression is associated with increased awakening cortisol[2] in mature subjects, but not in subjects under 20 years of age, echoing the rodent finding. Thus, N has a purely biological consequence that develops with emotional experience, but is independent of depression per se.

What the neuroticism construct has also lacked hitherto has been a plausible psychological dimension. Cognitive bias relevant to the onset of depression can be detected in young high N subjects. In emotional categorization and memory tasks, high N volunteers were faster to classify dislikeable self-referent personality characteristics and produced fewer positive memory intrusions. They also had a higher threshold for identifying happy faces. This suggests the hypothesis that risk for depression is largely manifest as reduced positive processing of emotional information[3]; increased negative processing appears to develop only after the actual experience of depression. Neural biases underlying this behaviour are even more readily detected.[4] Our hypothesis is that high neuroticism is not just an habitual low mood but is **biologically** founded in negative biases in attention, processing, and memory for emotional material. Indeed, there is now genetic evidence favouring a common genetic locus in human beings and rodent.[5] How emotional bias translates into either low-level symptoms or a full mood episode will be of great interest. Furthermore, depressive episodes per se appear to have an impact on brain function, and increase the risk of further relapse (see below).

(c) Early adverse experience

Adverse childhood experience was identified in genetically uncontrolled studies as a risk factor predisposing women to subsequent depression (Chapter 4.5.5) and has been confirmed in genetically informative designs.[6] In a clinical context, such developmental or social effects are usually viewed as separable from biology. Indeed, their very existence is usually taken to validate a 'social' approach to psychiatry. From a more unified point of view, however, one would predict measurable neurobiological consequences. In fact, such effects have proved to be more profound than most biologists anticipated.

Variations in maternal care produce individual differences in neuroendocrine responses to stress in rats. The offspring of mothers that exhibited more licking and grooming of pups during the first 10 days after birth showed, in adult life, reduced plasma ACTH and corticosterone responses to acute stress.[7] In addition, there was increased hippocampal glucocorticoid-receptor messenger RNA (**mRNA**) expression, enhanced glucocorticoid feedback sensitivity, and decreased levels of hypothalamic corticotrophin-releasing hormone (**CRH**) mRNA. Greater early maternal attention also substantially reduced subsequent behavioural fearfulness in response to novelty, increased benzodiazepine receptor density in the amygdala and locus coeruleus, increased α_2-adrenoreceptor density in the locus coeruleus, and decreased CRH receptor density in the locus coeruleus. Thus, maternal care serves to programme behavioural responses to stress in the offspring by altering the development of the neural systems that mediate fearfulness.

When BALB/cByJ mice were raised by an attentive C57BL/6ByJ dam, their excessive stress-elicited HPA activity was reduced, as were their behavioural impairments. However, cross-fostering the more resilient C57BL/6ByJ mice to an inattentive BALB/cByJ dam failed to elicit behavioural disturbances. In other words, vulnerable offspring may have their problems exacerbated by maternal behaviour, while early-life manipulations may have less obvious effects in relatively hardy animals.[8] Whether separation or stress paradigms in rodents can be taken as precise models of the mechanisms underlying the risk of mood disorder or other psychiatric problems cannot yet be decided, but their general relevance to the human case seems obvious. At present, data in human subjects is limited but findings that relate to the better characterized animal models are emerging.[9]

In fact, epidemiological data have linked increased risks of cardiovascular, metabolic, neuroendocrine, and psychiatric disorders in adulthood with an adverse *foetal* environment as well. Glucocorticoid excess may be the mechanism.[10] Low-birth-weight babies have higher plasma cortisol levels throughout adult life, which suggests a permanent change in HPA function. Whether such effects and later effects of environmental stress in childhood can in part mediate co-morbidity between a range of psychiatric and physical disorders is of growing contemporary interest. It is unclear how, over- or underactivity in stress regulation contributes to psychiatric disorder: both appear to be implicated since awakening cortisol responses may be blunted in subjects with early adversity[9] or enhanced in at risk neurotic individuals.

Gene–environment interaction is the likely basis of the neurobiology of mood disorder. In general terms this must be correct. Either the genetic/biological or the environmental factors could be targets for prevention. Whether the genetic mechanisms can be brought into sufficient focus to allow specific new pathways to be identified remains the major current challenge. It is often assumed that mediating characteristics or the endophenotype may have a simpler genetic architecture than the disease itself: unfortunately, the evidence so far gives reason for caution. This debate is currently very polarized between optimists (see Chapter 2.5.3 by Meyer-Lindenberg & Goldberg) and pessimists (see Chapter 2.4.2 by Flint). The genetic and developmental routes into distal common pathways regulating stress responses may be very numerous. Disorders that are both common and very variable in expression, such as depression, may turn out to have little specificity that is worth talking about. Every illness may be an ensemble of many specific factors, none of which is individually going to lead to a more focused treatment or a better prediction of treatment response.

Precipitating factors: the neurobiology of life events

Like early adversity, the role of life events in depression has been affirmed in genetically controlled studies. Life events are relevant to almost all first episodes of depression, but are less significant in its recurrence. The biology of life events is subsumed in the biology of stress, at best a clumsy term. In human studies it will be always difficult to isolate the critical ingredients of a particular psychological stress from the individual differences that stressed individuals bring to their experience. There have been few recent contributions to the field of direct relevance to depression.[11] However, a key clinical feature of the illness course in depression is the association of life events most strongly with first episodes of depression. Subsequent episodes appear to need a less substantial environmental trigger, as if the patient becomes sensitized.[12] Patients with a strong family history may effectively be presensitized. Accordingly the effect of life events and the brain changes that occur with repeated or chronic illness is of great relevance to prevention and reduction of the risk of future episodes.

Maintaining factors: biological studies of the depressed state

In the majority of biological studies of affective disorder, patients have been studied when ill and compared with normal controls. Over the years, this kind of design has produced a range of positive findings, usually of modest effect. It remains true to say that no biological changes have ever been found that distinguish between depressed patients and controls better than does the clinical assessment of the patients. What is also curious, and not a little tantalizing, is the impression that some symptoms may, in part, represent biological adaptations directed to put things right. Thus, on the one hand, there may be consistent effects upon hormone secretion or sleep that represent phenomena of illness. On the other, deliberate changes in hormone status or sleep deprivation may modify the state of depression. Depression is also so common in its less severe forms, that it is tempting to see it as a biologically adaptive mechanism in response to loss or social defeat. Informative animal analogues might be expected to exist, but theoretical comparisons with other biological models such as early separation in primates or hibernation in bears are limited by the species gap.[13]

However, what makes depression the clinical burden it is, remains its tendency to persist and sometimes become chronic. The biological factors contributing to this are still poorly understood, but they would provide an obvious target for novel drug development. In general it is not yet obvious which symptoms of acute depression are related to this key biology and which are either irrelevant or even adaptive. If there is now a consistent interest, it has been stimulated by the gradual acceptance that some cells divide to produce neurones in the mature brain, especially in the hippocampus. It is very tempting to suppose that the plastic effects maintaining the unwanted brain state in depression may be related to neurogenesis or its failure, which is a beautiful hypothesis requiring confirmation by direct evidence.

(a) The depressed state: functional anatomy

Perfusion or metabolic imaging can indirectly detect changes in neuronal activity (see Chapters 2.3.6 and 2.3.8). Signals can be well localized, but their meaning is ambiguous. They may reflect either reversible changes in function or a semi-permanent loss of neuronal connectivity. Reductions in function in anterior brain structures have been typical in major depression. Hypoperfusion tends to be greatest in frontal, temporal, and parietal areas and most extensive in older patients; high Hamilton scores tend to be associated with reduced perfusion.[14] Reductions in frontal areas may be more likely in patients with impoverished mental states. Thus, neuropsychological testing in major depression shows evidence of slowing in motor and cognitive domains, with additional prominent effects on mnemonic function that are most marked in the elderly. These effects are correlated with reduced frontal perfusion in the elderly. In younger patients, there may actually be increased perfusion in the frontal and cingulate cortex. Metabolic increases in the cingulate gyrus have been associated with a good treatment response.[15] Highly localizing findings have been unusual, however. The only exceptions have been within-subject changes on recovery in the mesial frontal cortex and perhaps the basal ganglia.[14]

There has been a dramatic expansion of imaging studies of emotional processing in normal volunteers, now usually with fMRI (see Chapters 2.3.8 and 2.5.4). It is well summarized by meta-analysis of over 300 such emotion induction and cognitive task. Emotion induction resulted in inferior medial activation and cognitive tasks resulted in dorsolateral activation.[16] However, the broad spread of precise loci of activation means that localization within the frontal lobes has proceeded little further. It may explain the diffuse reports typical of the depression literature. Nevertheless, a focus on limbic activity has led to quite specific, quasi-neurological hypotheses about connectivity in frontal areas and to treatment innovation: deep brain stimulation adjacent to subgenual cingulated cortex (Brodmann area 25).[17] How effective, and how localized this treatment effect really is, will be an important challenge to the field. However, it underlines that 'functional imaging' of brain perfusion primarily informs anatomy.

Isotope-based imaging of receptor occupation could more plausibly offer mechanistic understanding of psychiatric disorder. In depression, it has progressed with the availability of suitably informative ligands. However, the field generally tends to employ small sample sizes, and fundamental advances are difficult to identify. Single-photon emission tomography (**SPET or SPECT**) with the dopamine $D_{2/3}$ ligand [123I]IBZM showed increased binding in the striatum.[18] There were significant correlations between IBZM binding in the left and right striatum and measures of reaction time and verbal fluency, but not of mood as such. This finding has been confirmed with a PET ligand.[19] Increased $D_{2/3}$ binding in the striatum probably reflects a reduced dopamine function, whether due to a reduced release or secondary upregulation of receptors. Binding to the 5-HT1a receptor appears to be reduced in unipolar depression, an effect also present in recovered atients.[20]

In recent years, new SPET and PET ligands for the serotonin and dopamine transporter have become available (see Chapter 2.3.6 by Grasby). For the serotonin transporter in acute depression, the story is not consistent.[21,22] Binding to the dopamine transporter appears to correlate with depressive symptoms in healthy volunteers.[23] Hence trait effects may confound state effects and vice versa. Isotope-based imaging has been slow to develop a wide choice or availability of ligands, hence its role has been largely to follow rather than stimulate new ideas. Its specificity does mean that it can critically test hypotheses about specific receptors.

Such ligands have not yet made an impact on treatment strategies, as dopamine receptor ligands have for the antipsychotics. However, there are interesting preliminary conclusions: for example, drugs that bind to the serotonin transporter appear to saturate the site at therapeutic doses and increase the availability of dopamine reuptake sites.[24]

In summary, functional imaging has served to implicate frontal and limbic rather than posterior brain areas, in broad confirmation of anatomical conclusions derived from observing the effects of lesions or brain stimulation. Relevant neuropsychological challenges are now being incorporated into imaging protocols and we have the first example of an imaging-led treatment innovation—deep brain stimulation. Finally, 'functional' abnormalities may importantly predict structural abnormality in depression.

(b) Neuroendocrine challenge tests

Secretion of hormones in the anterior pituitary is under control, both direct and indirect, of central neuronal cell bodies that may project relatively widely within the brain. The secretion of a given hormone in response to specific precursors or agonists for individual neurotransmitter receptors has been proposed as a way of testing the security of such connections. Hormone secretion provides a bioassay of the system of interest. There is a measure of consensus about the findings in major depression, which, indeed, forms the most consistent basis for our understanding of disturbed neurotransmission in depression. However, the approach no longer leads the neurobiology, and merits consideration instead, in the more specific context of neuroendocrine function (see Chapter 2.3.3). The main findings are described below.

Neuroendocrine drug challenge suggests attenuated serotonergic function and increased cholinergic function in depression. Reduced responses to adrenergic and dopaminergic challenge also suggest impaired neurotransmission. Interpretation of tests with agonists is always difficult, because blunting may occur in an overactive system that has been downregulated. In addition, if the secretion of the assay hormone itself is actually directly affected by the state of depression, interpretation in terms of specific neurotransmitter abnormalities may be misleading. This is a particular problem for ACTH/cortisol responses (see below). In fact, enthusiasm for neuroendocrine surrogate markers of monoamine transmission within the brain has probably diminished in recent years, but the paradigm of drug challenge nevertheless remains interesting. We must assay brain responses of the monoamine projections more centrally involved in mood regulation.

(c) Hypercortisolaemia

About half of all patients with major depression have a raised cortisol output, which tends to return to normal on recovery. It is most consistently associated with an 'endogenous' pattern of illness (see Chapter 4.5.3). While cortisol is always regarded as a 'stress' hormone, and is secreted in response to various types of acute stress, the stresses that commonly result in long-term hypercortisolaemia are poorly understood. The idea that there is a relatively specific link between chronic high cortisol levels and mood disorder is notably persistent. In major depression there is peripheral hypertrophy of the adrenal glands, measurable in MRI body scans, and an enhanced response to corticotrophin. The MRI change, like the hypercortisolaemia itself, reverses on recovery.[25]

Suppression of cortisol secretion occurs normally via glucocorticoid receptor-mediated inhibitory feedback to the hypothalamus; it is readily produced by dexamethasone, which is a potent exogenous glucocorticoid (the dexamethasone suppression test (**DST**)). For example, Non-suppression of endogenous cortisol after dexamethasone occurs in Cushing's disease. It implies either reduced feedback and/or enhanced central drive to release cortisol. It was initially observed that the 1-mg DST showed high specificity (96 per cent) and sensitivity (67 per cent) as a putative diagnostic test for melancholia.[26] At this point of time the result attracted intense interest, but has since proved difficult to generalize. The high specificity established against normal controls was less against other patient groups. Thus, DST non-suppression has not been accepted as a diagnostic test. This failed effort to give medical respectability to psychiatric diagnosis came to devalue what remains an important observation. Non-suppression usually reflects hypercortisolaemia, which is itself a robust phenomenon of mood disorder that requires explanation like any other core biological symptom. Other symptoms that we identify as part of the depressive syndrome lend themselves less easily to investigation. The DST also has potential clinical uses beyond diagnosis. DST non-suppression predicts a low placebo response rate to drug treatment,[27] and hypercortisolaemia predicts a low rate of clinical response to psychological intervention.[28]

It remains unclear whether cortisol contributes to the clinical state of depression by a direct action on the brain. Exogenous cortisol administration is associated with affective symptoms, and chronic excessive cortisol secretion commonly appears to produce depressive symptoms in Cushing's disease. An HPA axis programmed to hypersecrete cortisol under stress could be a pathogenic mechanism explaining why depression or mania develops. This view has provoked efforts to treat mood disorder by inhibition of cortisol synthesis with metyrapone or blocking the post-synaptic receptors. The effects of such manipulations appear primarily, and unexpectedly, to influence cognitive function more than mood per se. Thus the anti-glucocorticoid, mifepristone improved spatial working memory in bipolar depression[29] and the anti-mineralocorticoid, spironolactone significantly impaired selective attention and delayed recall of visuospatial memory in healthy volunteers without effects on CCK-induced panic anxiety.[30]

There is a final twist: when depressed patients are given large doses of cortisol they tend to show acute mood enhancement[31] and oral dexamethasone has been reported to elevate mood in major depression, especially in hypersecretors.[32] This leads to the converse hypothesis that an HPA axis appropriately adapted to chronic stress early in development might be unable to mount a normal effective response to acute stress later in life. Cortisol may then be seen as a euphoriant (or antidepressant), and hypercortisolaemia as an antidepressant response of the stress-regulating mechanisms of the brain. Based on this view, all cortisol levels seen in depression may be set inappropriately low for the ongoing stress, however high or low they are compared with the normal range.

Whether one supposes cortisol levels to be set too high or too low in depression, it remains inconvenient that either a suppression or an augmentation of steroid effect seems, initially at least, to elevate mood. A way out of this complication may lie in cortisol's action on two receptors in the brain (the glucocorticoid and mineralocorticoid receptors) that may have opposite actions. However, we still need better-controlled replicated data on the effects of steroid manipulations, both in at-risk subjects and in major depression. It is also possible that peripheral cortisol levels are largely irrelevant to the brain and that receptor regulation may critically modulate their central action: one challenging hypothesis is that antidepressants work through changing receptor disposition.[33]

An increased cortisol production is associated with an increased release of hypothalamic β-endorphin and probably a pulsatile increase in ACTH. The paraventricular nucleus of the hypothalamus represents the highest level of dedicated neurones in the HPA axis. The neurosecretory cells of the paraventricular nucleus release the peptides CRH and AVP into the portal hypophyseal blood. These hormones in turn stimulate the release of ACTH from the anterior pituitary. Major depression is characterized by a blunted ACTH response to CRH, an elevated level of CRH in the cerebrospinal fluid, and increased numbers of neurones expressing CRH mRNA in the paraventricular nucleus of the hypothalamus post-mortem.[34] CRH is not confined to the paraventricular nucleus, but is expressed in a variety of other central nuclei whence it can produce anxiogenic behavioural effects. CRH receptors, which exist in two forms, are widely distributed in the hypothalamus and cortex. A related peptide, urocortin, has a similar pharmacology. Knocking out the CRH-1 receptor gene in mice impaired the HPA stress response and reduced anxiety-like behaviour. Non-peptide antagonists of CRH action, and of other peptide hormones implicated in stress responses have been taken very seriously as putative anxiolytics or antidepressants.[35] If effective, they will be among the first of a new generation of truly novel treatments based on peptide neurotransmission. The failure to see new compounds of this general kind by now is disappointing, and in the case of a neurokinin antagonist, aprepitant, there has been a high profile failure in major depression.[36]

(d) Thyroid abnormalities

In unselected major depression, thyroid hormone levels are usually normal, but there may be abnormalities of the thyrotropin (thyroid-stimulating hormone) response to thyrotropin-releasing hormone. The thyrotropin response is blunted in a significant number of patients, but this effect is poorly understood and has few accepted clinical associations. In contrast, a subgroup of patients may show an enhanced thyrotropin response with normal thyroid hormone levels (referred to as grade II hypothyroidism). These associations and the use of thyroid hormones in treatment suggest that there is more to be learned in this area (see Chapter 4.5.8).

(e) Sleep disturbance

Sleep is often disturbed in depression but in a variety of ways. Early-morning waking is the most typical in endogenous or melancholic depression, with the sleep patterns in such patients being similar to those seen in patients with mania. Trouble getting to sleep, frequent awakenings, and unsatisfactorily prolonged sleep are also commonly seen in depression. Like other biological manifestations of the disorder, the extent to which sleep is simply a consequence of the state of depression or a contribution to its biology is uncertain. Patients with severe depression or mania may respond to sleep deprivation with a transient elevation in mood. It implies that the sleep–wake cycle is directly involved with mood regulation and its disorder.

In severe depression (melancholia) the typical effects are a reduction in the total length of slow-wave sleep and a shortened latency in the appearance of rapid eye movement (**REM**) or dreaming sleep.[37] The cholinergic projections from the hindbrain may be REM-ON cells, while serotonergic and noradrenergic cells may be REM-OFF cells. The disturbed sleep of depression could be due to an increased cholinergic and/or a decreased serotonergic/noradrenergic drive; simplistic though it sounds, the experimental evidence is supportive. Depressed patients challenged with a cholinergic agonist in the second non-REM period enter REM significantly faster than psychiatric and normal control subjects. The reduced sensitivity of the noradrenergic system is suggested because clonidine fails to suppress REM in depressed patients compared with controls.[38] Tryptophan depletion (to attenuate 5-HT function) partially mimics the changes seen in depression in recovered patients.[39]

Sleep tends to recover on recovery from depression, and the tricyclic antidepressants in particular suppress REM sleep. However, sleep disturbance may be an early predictor of relapse, and disturbed sleep parameters predict a poor response to cognitive behaviour therapy.[40] Indeed, depressed patients may have inherently weak slow-wave sleep processes because unaffected subjects with a family history of depression show reduced slow-wave sleep and increased REM density in the first sleep cycle[41].

Interest in sleep as a fundamental key to understanding mood disorder has waned in the last two decades. However, its neurobiology is increasingly well understood, and its time may come again.

(f) Monoamine metabolite turnover

The earliest studies to investigate the actions of tricyclic antidepressants highlighted their actions on the turnover of the monoamine metabolites in animal brain. The 'monoamine theory of depression' proposed the reduced functioning of monoamine transmission in depression. Therefore it was natural to seek relevant measures of monoamine chemistry in the cerebrospinal fluid of patients and controls. The study of what became irreverently known as 'neural urine' and indeed of urine itself, since peripheral measures of monoamine turnover are also potentially relevant, virtually defined a decade of biological psychiatry in the 1970s and 1980s. Drugs had similar effects on neurotransmitter turnover as seen in animal studies, demonstrating that the human techniques were sufficiently sensitive. Indeed the monoamine theory is, at its best, a theory about drug action because the monoamine and metabolite changes produced by illness in patients have proved remarkably unconvincing.[42] The findings for the noradrenaline metabolite MHPG and the 5-HT metabolite 5-hydroxyindoleacetic acid were negative. The dopamine metabolite homovanillic acid did show the predicted decrease, but only significantly in women. There were trends to modest increases in all the major metabolites in mania. Although disappointing, cerebrospinal fluid studies could never reflect the activities of smaller groups of neurones localized in areas critical for the modulation of mood. Such a focus is only possible in isotope imaging (PET or SPET) or better post-mortem studies of the brain.

(g) Tryptophan depletion

The most convincing evidence that 5-HT is intimately involved in mood disorder has come from depletion of tryptophan, the amino acid precursor of 5-HT. The level of tryptophan in both peripheral blood and the brain can be driven to very low levels by a short-term low-protein diet and subsequent loading with large neutral amino acids. These compete with tryptophan for access to the brain amino acid transporter and also increase its peripheral metabolism, which results in the reduced synthesis and release of 5-HT. Initial observations appeared to bear primarily on the mechanism of drug action. Thus, patients who had recovered from major depression while taking a serotonin-selective reuptake inhibitor experienced a clear-cut return of severe symptoms lasting for several hours after tryptophan depletion. This finding has now been critically extended to patients with a history of recurrent major depression who were euthymic but not taking any medication.[43] Prominent objective symptoms of retardation and cognitive distortion returned in a stereotyped and severe way, reflecting previous symptoms. The effects on mood in patients who have had a previous episode of depression are qualitatively different from the more minor changes seen in normal female controls or even subjects with a strong family history. This may imply the formation of a form of neurobiological template, which increases the vulnerability to subsequent relapse or recurrence. The immediacy of the link between neurotransmitter function and symptoms may be the reason why patients with recurrent major depression need long-term treatment with antidepressant drugs to remain well.

(h) Does mood disorder have a functional neuropathology?

Severe mood disorder is virtually defined by its frequent recurrence or its chronicity. The first episodes of severe depression occur more frequently with increasing age and tend to be more refractory to treatment. Severe mood disorder is associated with ventricular enlargement and sulcal prominence.[44] Late-onset depression is characterized by pronounced impairments in most areas of cognitive function, in particular executive function and processing speed and is increasingly regarded as having a quasi-neurological quality. Indeed, there is an increased rate of white matter lesions, perhaps related to vascular disease, in older patients.[44] The relationship between cognitive deficits and underlying neuropathological changes requires further examination. Elderly patients with early-onset depression demonstrate greater preservation of executive functioning and processing speed, which may reflect partially distinct disease processes possibly mediated by different neuropathological mechanisms.[45] The key hypothesis must be that it is the particular pattern of functional disruption resulting from any cellular pathology that increases the risk of depression. It may be reasonable to describe such a change as a functional neuropathology.

In younger patients, the issue is whether depression per se leads to a functional neuropathology. In patients with unusual refractoriness and chronicity, MRI scanning again suggested reduced grey matter parameters, most significantly in the left hippocampus but also more diffusely in the left parietal and frontal association cortices. Left hippocampal grey matter density was correlated with measures of verbal memory, supporting the functional significance of the imaging changes. In contrast, patients with severe illnesses fully responsive to treatment showed no differences from controls. Any finding in the chronic group could predate the onset of depression, or be the result of the illness process or its treatment. It is fashionable to attribute structural changes in depression to hypercortisolaemia, but in this study that was not the explanation.[46] A failure of BDNF, related neurogenesis or loss of synaptic plasticity is also a possibility. Reduced hippocampal volume is a relatively consistent finding in many studies of modest size which have also implicated inter-linked structures in basal ganglia and thalamus.[47]

Rather surprisingly, a correlation between lifetime duration of illness and memory performance was also seen in a very large outpatient sample studied after recovery from a discrete episode.[48] It favours a toxic link between the burden of depression and cognition, which has implications for public health. It also means that the mechanisms associated with very severe depression are also relevant in less severe ambulant forms.

Post-mortem studies of the brain in mood disorder have been rare and are limited by tissue availability. Such studies in elderly depression have greater potential validity than the much more numerous investigations of schizophrenia. The Stanley Neuropathology consortium has made samples of tissue widely available from small but well-characterized patient series. In the hippocampus, the most consistent findings are of reduced GABA function and abnormal measures of synaptic density or neuronal plasticity.[49] Such studies have seldom focused on other 'candidate regions' such as the inferior frontal or cingulate cortex or amygdale.[50] Several studies suggest a particular involvement of glial cells.[51] Since glia support the energy requirements of neurones, and their deficient function could account for aspects of the imaging abnormalities found in these disorders: elevated levels of glucocorticoids acting on glia could change their function, or glial changes could represent responses to primary neuronal withdrawal (see also Chapter 2.3.5).

Post-mortem studies can also address the neurochemistry, perhaps more directly and completely than other methods. Normal ageing is accompanied by a decline in a variety of indices of monoamine function including presynaptic markers of 5-HT innervation. In a small series of depressed suicides, there were 54 per cent fewer neurones in the dorsal raphe nucleus expressing SERT mRNA compared with controls.[52] Whether a reduced serotonergic innervation is the critical change that increases the vulnerability to mood disorder of patients with advancing years is not yet established. If so, the potential for MDMA to have long-term effects in heavy users is real and worrying.[53]

In suicide, post-mortem findings have broadly paralleled those in depression, with an important emphasis on 5-HT metabolism and neurotransmission (see Chapter 4.15.3). Whether 5-HT neurotransmission, perhaps like that involving the other monoamines, represents a functional domain implicated independently in a variety of psychiatric syndromes and behaviours remains to be well established.

Conclusions

Mood disorder has an important neurobiological basis. This stretches from a vulnerability, which seems to be attributable to polymorphism in genes critical to stress regulation, through the impact that early experience has on the subsequent programming of the brain for stress responses, to the final responsiveness when encountering particular personal adversity in later life. Biological studies have highlighted the role of key brain areas within the limbic system such as the cingulate cortex and amygdala. We are still a long way from understanding, with any precision, the critical connections and cellular mechanisms, but the function of monoamine neurones generally, and of serotonergic projections in particular, is closely associated with mood regulation. Peptide neurotransmitters have long seemed likely to play a central role in stress regulation, but their potential as targets for antidepressant drug action are yet to be fulfilled. Finally, observations in the most chronic illnesses and in the elderly with depression have highlighted the possibility of a functional neuropathology underlying severe mood disorder. Depression seems to be critically related to the evolving story around neurogenesis in the brain. It is perhaps appropriate that its resolution will require fundamental advances in brain science: psychiatry has always posed, or anyway implied, the most demanding of scientific questions: how does the brain work?

Further information

American College of Neuropsychopharmacology: 5th Generation of progress. Available at: http://www.acnp.org/Default.aspx?Page=5thGenerationChapters

References

1. Castanon, N., Perez-Diaz, F., and Mormede, P. (1995). Genetic analysis of the relationships between behavioral and neuroendocrine traits in Roman high and low avoidance rat lines. *Behavior Genetics*, **25**(4), 371–84.
2. Portella, M.J., Harmer, C.J., Flint, J., *et al.* (2005). Enhanced early morning salivary cortisol in neuroticism. *The American Journal of Psychiatry*, **162**(4), 807–9.
3. Chan, S.W.Y., Goodwin, G.M., and Harmer, C.J. (2007). Highly neurotic never-depressed students have negative biases in information processing. *Psychological Medicine*, **37**, 1281–92.
4. Chan, S.W.Y., Norbury, R., Goodwin, G.M., *et al.* (2008). Risk for depression is associated with exaggerated neural responses to fearful facial expressions of emotion. *British Journal of Psychiatry* (in Press).
5. Fullerton, J., Cubin, M., Tiwari, H., *et al.* (2003). Linkage analysis of extremely discordant and concordant sibling pairs identifies quantitative-trait loci that influence variation in the human personality trait neuroticism. *American Journal of Human Genetics*, **72**(4), 879–90.
6. Kendler, K.S., Kuhn, J.W., and Prescott, C.A. (2004). Childhood sexual abuse, stressful life events and risk for major depression in women. *Psychological Medicine*, **34**(8), 1475–82.
7. Liu, D., Diorio, J., Tannenbaum, B., *et al.* (1997). Maternal care, hippocampal glucocorticoid receptors, and hypothalamic–pituitary–adrenal responses to stress. *Science*, **277**(5332), 1659–62.
8. Caldji, C., Tannenbaum, B., Sharma, S., *et al.* (1998). Maternal care during infancy regulates the development of neural systems mediating the expression of fearfulness in the rat. *Proceedings of the National Academy of Sciences of the United States of America*, **95**(9), 5335–40.
9. Heim, C., Plotsky, P.M., and Nemeroff, C.B. (2004). Importance of studying the contributions of early adverse experience to neurobiological findings in depression. *Neuropsychopharmacology*, **29**(4), 641–8.
10. Seckl, J.R. and Meaney, M.J. (2006). Glucocorticoid 'programming' and PTSD risk. *Annals of the New York Academy of Sciences*, **1071**, 351–78.
11. Biondi, M. and Picardi, A. (1999). Psychological stress and neuroendocrine function in humans: the last two decades of research. *Psychotherapy and Psychosomatics*, **68**(3), 114–50.

12. Kendler, K.S., Thornton, L.M., and Gardner, C.O. (2000). Stressful life events and previous episodes in the etiology of major depression in women: an evaluation of the 'kindling' hypothesis. *The American Journal of Psychiatry*, **157**(8), 1243–51.
13. Tsiouris, J.A. (2005). Metabolic depression in hibernation and major depression: an explanatory theory and an animal model of depression. *Medical Hypotheses*, **65**(5), 829–40.
14. Goodwin, G.M. (1997). Neuropsychological and neuroimaging evidence for the involvement of the frontal lobes in depression. *Journal of Psychopharmacology*, **11**(2), 115–22.
15. Mayberg, H.S., Brannan, S.K., Mahurin, R.K., *et al.* (1997). Cingulate function in depression: a potential predictor of treatment response. *Neuroreport*, **8**(4), 1057–61.
16. Steele, J.D. and Lawrie, S.M. (2004). Segregation of cognitive and emotional function in the prefrontal cortex: a stereotactic meta-analysis. *Neuroimage*, **21**(3), 868–75.
17. Mayberg, H.S., Lozano, A.M., Voon, V., *et al.* (2005). Deep brain stimulation for treatment-resistant depression. *Neuron*, **45**(5), 651–60.
18. Shah, P.J., Ogilvie, A.D., Goodwin, G.M., *et al.* (1997). Clinical and psychometric correlates of dopamine D-2 binding in depression. *Psychological Medicine*, **27**(6), 1247–56.
19. Meyer, J.H., McNeely, H.E., Sagrati, S., *et al.* (2006). Elevated putamen D-2 receptor binding potential in major depression with motor retardation: an [C-11] raclopride positron emission tomography study. *The American Journal of Psychiatry*, **163**(9), 1594–602.
20. Bhagwagar, Z., Rabiner, E.A., Sargent, P.A., *et al.* (2004). Persistent reduction in brain serotonin(1A) receptor binding in recovered depressed men measured by positron emission tomography with [C-11]WAY-100635. *Molecular Psychiatry*, **9**(4), 386–92.
21. Meyer, J.H. (2007). Imaging the serotonin transporter during major depressive disorder and antidepressant treatment. *Journal of Psychiatry & Neuroscience*, **32**(2), 86–102.
22. Staley, J.K., Sanacora, G., Tamagnan, G., *et al.* (2006). Sex differences in diencephalon serotonin transporter availability in major depression. *Biological Psychiatry*, **59**(1), 40–7.
23. Newberg, A., Amsterdam, J., and Shults, J. (2007). Dopamine transporter density may be associated with the depressed affect in healthy subjects. *Nuclear Medicine Communications*, **28**(1), 3–6.
24. Shang, Y.L., Gibbs, M.A., Marek, G.J., *et al.* (2007). Displacement of serotonin and dopamine transporters by venlafaxine extended release capsule at steady state—a [I-123]2 beta-carbomethoxy-3 beta-(4-iodophenyl)-tropone single photon emission computed tomography imaging study. *Journal of Clinical Psychopharmacology*, **27**(1), 71–5.
25. Rubin, R.T., Phillips, J.J., Sadow, T.F., *et al.* (1995). Adrenal gland volume in major depression: increase during the depressive episode and decrease with successful treatment. *Archives of General Psychiatry*, **52**(3), 213–18.
26. Carroll, B.J., Feinberg, M., Greden, J.F., *et al.* (1981). A specific laboratory test for the diagnosis of melancholia. Standardization, validation, and clinical utility. *Archives of General Psychiatry*, **38**(1), 15–22.
27. Ribeiro, S.C.M., Tandon, R., Grunhaus, L., *et al.* (1993). The DST as a predictor of outcome in depression: a meta-analysis. *The American Journal of Psychiatry*, **150**(11), 1618–29.
28. Thase, M.E., Dube, S., Bowler, K., *et al.* (1996). Hypothalamic–pituitary–adrenocortical activity and response to cognitive behavior therapy in unmedicated, hospitalized depressed patients. *The American Journal of Psychiatry*, **153**, 886–91.
29. Young, A.H., Gallagher, P., Watson, S., *et al.* (2004). Improvements in neurocognitive function and mood following adjunctive treatment with mifepristone (RU-486) in bipolar disorder. *Neuropsychopharmacology*, **29**(8), 1538–45.
30. Otte, C., Moritz, S., Yassouridis, A., *et al.* (2007). Blockade of the mineralocorticoid receptor in healthy men: effects on experimentally induced panic symptoms, stress hormones, and cognition. *Neuropsychopharmacology*, **32**(1), 232–8.
31. Goodwin, G.M., Muir, W.J., Seckl, J.R., *et al.* (1992). The effects of cortisol infusion upon hormone secretion from the anterior pituitary and subjective mood in depressive illness and in controls. *Journal of Affective Disorders*, **26**(2), 73–83.
32. Dinan, T.G., Lavelle, E., Cooney, J., *et al.* (1997). Dexamethasone augmentation in treatment-resistant depression. *Acta Psychiatrica Scandinavica*, **95**(1), 58–61.
33. Pariante, C.M., Thomas, S.A., Lovestone, S., *et al.* (2004). Do antidepressants regulate how cortisol affects the brain? *Psychoneuroendocrinology*, **29**(4), 423–47.
34. Mitchell, A.J. (1998). The role of corticotropin releasing factor in depressive illness: a critical review. *Neuroscience and Biobehavioral Reviews*, **22**(5), 635–51.
35. Nemeroff, C.B. and Vale, W.W. (2005). The neurobiology of depression: inroads to treatment and new drug discovery. *Journal of Clinical Psychiatry*, **66**, 5–13.
36. Keller, M., Montgomery, S., Ball, W., *et al.* (2006). Lack of efficacy of the substance P (neurokinin(1) receptor) antagonist aprepitant in the treatment of major depressive disorder. *Biological Psychiatry*, **59**(3), 216–23.
37. Berger, M. and Riemann, D. (1993). REM sleep in depression—an overview. *Journal of Sleep Research*, **2**(4), 211–23.
38. Schittecatte, M., Garcia Valentin, J., Charles, G., *et al.* (1995). Efficacy of the 'clonidine REM suppression test (CREST)' to separate patients with major depression from controls; a comparison with three currently proposed biological markers of depression. *Journal of Affective Disorders*, **33**(3), 151–7.
39. Moore, P., Gillin, J.C., Bhatti, T., *et al.* (1998). Rapid tryptophan depletion, sleep electroencephalogram, and mood in men with remitted depression on serotonin reuptake inhibitors. *Archives of General Psychiatry*, **55**(6), 534–9.
40. Thase, M.E., Simons, A.D., and Reynolds, C.F. III. (1993). Psychobiological correlates of poor response to cognitive behavior therapy: potential indications for antidepressant pharmacotherapy. *Psychopharmacology Bulletin*, **29**(2), 293–301.
41. Lauer, C.J., Schreiber, W., Holsboer, F., *et al.* (1995). In quest of identifying vulnerability markers for psychiatric disorders by all-night polysomnography. *Archives of General Psychiatry*, **52**(2), 145–53.
42. Schatzberg, A.F., Samson, J.A., Bloomingdale, K.L., *et al.* (1989). Toward a biochemical classification of depressive disorders. X.Urinary catecholamines, their metabolites, and D-type scores in subgroups of depressive disorders. *Archives of General Psychiatry*, **46**(3), 260–8.
43. Smith, K.A., Fairburn, C.G., and Cowen, P.J. (1997). Relapse of depression after rapid depletion of tryptophan. *Lancet*, **349**(9056), 915–19.
44. Videbech, P. (1997). MRI findings in patients with affective disorder: a meta-analysis. *Acta Psychiatrica Scandinavica*, **96**(3), 157–68.
45. Herrmann, L.L., Goodwin, G.M., and Ebmeier, K.P. (2007). The cognitive neuropsychology of depression in the elderly. *Psychological Medicine*, **37**, 1693–702.
46. Shah, P.J., Ebmeier, K.P., Glabus, M.F., *et al.* (1998). Cortical grey matter reductions associated with treatment-resistant chronic unipolar depression: controlled magnetic resonance imaging study. *The British Journal of Psychiatry*, **72**(172), 527–32.
47. Sheline, Y.I. (2003). Neuroimaging studies of mood disorder effects on the brain. *Biological Psychiatry*, **54**(3), 338–52.
48. Gorwood, P., Corruble, E., Falissard, B., *et al.* (2008). Toxic effects of depression on brain function: impairment of delayed recall reflects the cumulative length of the depressive disorder in a large sample of depressed out-patients. *American Journal of Psychiatry*, **165**, 731–9.
49. Knable, M.B., Barci, B.M., Webster, M.J., *et al.* (2004). Molecular abnormalities of the hippocampus in severe psychiatric illness: postmortem findings from the Stanley neuropathology consortium. *Molecular Psychiatry*, **9**(6), 609–20.

50. Harrison, P.J. (2002). The neuropathology of primary mood disorder. *Brain*, **125**, 1428–49.
51. Cotter, D.R., Pariante, C.M., and Everall, I.P. (2001). Glial cell abnormalities in major psychiatric disorders: the evidence and implications. *Brain Research Bulletin*, **55**(5), 585–95.
52. Arango, V., Underwood, M.D., Boldrini, M., *et al.* (2001). Serotonin 1A receptors, serotonin transporter binding and serotonin transporter mRNA expression in the brainstem of depressed suicide victims. *Neuropsychopharmacology*, **25**(6), 892–903.
53. Green, A.R. and Goodwin, G.M. (1996). Ecstasy and neurodegeneration. *British Medical Journal*, **312**(7045), 1493–4.

4.5.7 Course and prognosis of mood disorders

Jules Angst

The importance of course

Ever since Kahlbaum's monograph 1863[1] the course and outcome of mental disorders have played important roles as criteria and validators of psychiatric classification. The prognosis is fundamental for doctor and patient when deciding whether to start long-term prophylactic medication and, at a later stage, whether to stop a successful long-term treatment. Course is a crucial factor in estimating the social consequences, costs, suicide risk, and mortality associated with mood disorders.

The description of course includes the age of onset, episode length, recurrence of episodes, residual symptoms between episodes and outcome (remission, chronicity, death). These aspects are covered in this chapter.

Stability of the diagnoses of mood disorders

Mood disorders can be roughly sub-classified into unipolar mania, bipolar disorder, and unipolar depression.[2] The three groups differ significantly as regards family history, personality, course and outcome, including mortality. Unipolar mania has not yet been studied extensively, and for this reason will not be dealt with here.

Distinguishing between bipolar disorder and unipolar depressive disorder is hampered by the fact that the diagnosis of unipolar depression is always uncertain. Many depressives are hidden bipolar patients: a long-term follow-up study over 27 years showed a constant rate of diagnostic change from depression to hypomania of 1.25 per cent per year of follow-up. As a consequence of this diagnostic instability, the exact ratio of bipolar to unipolar depressive subjects in the population is unknown; modern estimates range from 1:5 to 1:1. The discussion of bipolar disorder has therefore to take account of its unipolar counterpart.

Bipolar disorder

Onset

In patients admitted to hospital between 1913 and 1940 and not treated by electroconvulsive therapy or modern psychotropic drugs, bipolar disorder clearly manifested earlier than unipolar depression; this finding is confirmed by modern community studies. In most patients bipolar disorder begins during adolescence but in some cases may already manifest in childhood. Unfortunately pediatric psychiatry cannot yet provide prospective data from large representative community studies on the onset and course of bipolar disorder starting in childhood or adolescence.

In the offspring of bipolar parents social functioning up to the age of 18 develops normally before the onset of their illness.

Bipolar disorders usually begin as depression, and it takes a further 5 years on average until the first manic syndrome manifests.[3] There may be unspecific prodromal symptoms in the form of mood lability, vegetative lability, somatization, or being hyper-alert or easily excited; there may also be discrete cognitive impairment present before the onset of the affective disorder.[4] After the onset of the disorder social functioning often begins to be impaired.

The first depressive and manic manifestations are commonly mild, brief, or uncharacteristic, and are often only diagnosed in retrospect after years.

Prospective epidemiological studies in adolescents and young adults found the onset of bipolar disorder to occur in the teens (with means and medians around 15 years or later), whereas studies of hospitalized patients date its onset in retrospect in the early 20s or in the 30s.

Bipolar-I illness manifests earlier than bipolar-II and psychotic bipolar disorder. Late-onset bipolar disorder is extremely rare but does occur and may be associated with specific neuropathology. An early age of onset of the disorder, usually manifesting as depression, is correlated with suicidality, comorbid substance-use disorder and a rapid cycling course.

A two-peak distribution of the age of onset has sometimes been described for both bipolar disorder and depression in men and women, with no specific association in women between the second peak and the menopause.

Duration of episodes

Most episodes are short, but 10 to 20 per cent become chronic (lasting more than 2 years); the distribution of episode length is log normal, and therefore percentiles and not averages should be used as parameters. Using data collected a century ago on the natural length of episodes of mania and bipolar disorder, mainly among hospitalized patients, it is possible to compute a median length of 4 to 6 months for mania and 5 to 6 months for bipolar disorder. These figures do not differ from those obtained today despite a wide range of antimanic and antidepressant treatments. Among hospitalized bipolar patients episode length (median) was 4.2 months; 25 per cent of bipolar episodes lasted more than 7.3 months.

About 20 to 30 per cent of episodes are *biphasic* (mania with subsequent switch into depression, or depression with subsequent, switch into hypomania/mania); such high switch rates were already observed before the introduction of electroconvulsive therapy and antidepressants. An effective treatment does not induce a switch but increases (compared to placebos) the rates of responders; and the response is a precondition for the natural switch.

Recurrence of episodes

Recurrence is typical of mood disorders. It can be described by the number of episodes, the length of intervals (measured from remission to the onset of a new episode), and the length of cycles (measured from the beginning of one episode to the beginning of the next). In prospective studies, time to the onset of a new episode is frequently used as a parameter for survival analyses and frailty analyses of recurrence.

In both bipolar disorder and unipolar depression the time from the first to the second episode is on average much longer than from the second to the third episode and so on. This progressive shortening of cycles and free intervals then levels off and fluctuates around a certain (but still variable) individual limit. Most published data on interval length or cycle length are methodologically flawed because they have not been corrected for the number of episodes/cycles observed. Nonetheless, multiple episodes obviously follow each other in more rapid succession than a few episodes distributed over a lifetime. Statistically, a normal distribution of cycle length can be obtained by log *n* transformation. Even after taking episode numbers into account, there is a clear intra-individual trend to a progressive shortening of cycle length, as demonstrated by frailty analyses[5] dimming the prognosis for both bipolar disorder and unipolar depression. Initial cycle length tends to be shorter in late-onset than in early-onset mood disorders, increasing the risk of recurrence in the elderly.

Precipitating events play an important role in the onset of the first few affective episodes; thereafter recurrence seems to become gradually autonomous with stressful events contributing little or nothing to the process. Stressors may not only precipitate episodes but also increase a pre-existent vulnerability, sensitizing the individual and thereby making him or her more vulnerable to further episodes (kindling effect). In bipolar illness there is no difference in the quality or quantity of stressors precipitating depressive and manic episodes; a legacy or the loss of a relative can induce depression or mania. The sensitivity to stressors has also a genetic component.

Over a patient's lifetime his condition continuously fluctuates on a dimension of severity, which ranges from psychotic, via major and minor syndromes (cyclothymic and minor bipolar disorders), cyclothymic temperament within the norm, symptomatic to symptom-free.

The NIMH Collaborative Depression Study with annual assessments of outpatients over an average of 13 years, demonstrated that bipolar-II patients spent slightly more time with symptoms/syndromes (33 per cent) than bipolar-I patients (27 per cent). In both subtypes of bipolar disorders depressive periods were three times more common than manic periods[6] but bipolar-I patients suffered more from psychotic features. In a 25-year follow-up study of hospitalized mood disorder patients, manic and depressive episodes were about equally present in bipolar-I patients, whereas in bipolar-II patients the course was dominated by depression.

Daily assessments of the course by the life-chart methodology over more than 3 years confirmed that bipolar outpatients spent a three-fold greater amount of time in depression than hypomania. But it was also shown that bipolar-I patients spent significantly more time in hypomania than their bipolar-II counterparts but an equal time in depression; in more than half the time the patients were euthymic.

Over lifetime bipolar patients experience twice as many episodes as unipolar depressives, a difference which is not explained by the manifestation of manic episodes in addition to depression. The total number of episodes observed depends on the length of observation. In a 22- to 26-year follow-up study, bipolar patients experienced a median of 10 episodes, but depressive patients only four. A family history of mood disorders increases recurrence. The proportion of mania to depression remains fairly stable across multiple episodes, but over their lifetime patients spend more time in depression than in mania.

Outcome

(a) Incomplete remission of episodes

Remission after bipolar episodes is frequently incomplete in terms of symptomatic and functional recovery. Residual symptoms are common in patients in both psychiatric and general practice settings and bipolar subjects identified in community studies. Residual depressive symptoms are more impairing than hypomanic symptoms, which may even enhance functioning.[7] The chronic residual symptoms are mainly depressed mood, anxiety, and somatic disturbances, such as insomnia, hypersomnia, headaches, neurasthenic complaints, reduced libido, and gastrointestinal symptoms. Functional recovery was found to develop later than symptomatic recovery. Short-term outcome is less favourable in patients with agitation, rapid cycling, poor premorbid functioning, comorbidity with anxiety disorders, social phobia, substance use, OCD, obesity, personality disorders, sexual trauma, abuse, and behaviour disorders in childhood.[8] Manic versus mixed episodes do not differ in outcome after 1 year.

(b) Long-term course and outcome

The long-term course and outcome of bipolar disorders is characterized by high recurrence rates, frequent residual symptoms between episodes; compared to depression they carry a higher risk of suicide attempts but lower risk of suicides.

Bipolar disorder has a poorer outcome than depression and there is no burn-out with age. After a follow-up of 22 to 26 years, definitive recovery (at least 5 years with good social adaptation) was found in 25 per cent of 186 depressive subjects, whereas the figure was only 16 per cent of the 220 bipolar patients; a chronic course lasting at least 2 years without remission was present in 12 to 14 per cent of depressive and bipolar patients. A chronic course is associated with early life adversity, including sexual and physical abuse.

Comorbidity with alcoholism, a factor known to correlate with poorer outcome and increased mortality, was found in 30 per cent of the bipolar patients. Modern treatment has improved the outcome of mood disorders by reducing chronicity and rehospitalization.

Recurrence (number of hospital admissions) may increase the risk of dementia.

Mortality

Mortality is expressed by the standardized mortality ratio (**SMR**) in comparison with the normal population (SMR = 1.0). Data on hospitalized psychiatric patients in Sweden[9] give an overall SMR for bipolar men of 2.5 and for women 2.7. The high mortality is a consequence not only of suicides (SMR = 15.0 for males and 22.4 for females) but of most other causes of death (excluding cancer): infections, endocrine, cardiovascular, cerebrovascular, respiratory and gastrointestinal disorders, homicides, accidents, traffic accidents and secondary substance-use disorders (mainly alcohol use disorder), etc. This is true for both men and women.

Consequences for treatment

Incomplete recovery and high recurrence are the main problems in the treatment of bipolar disorders. In the treatment of an acute episode the primary goals are full recovery and the prevention of relapses. The length of treatment of an acute episode depends on its estimated spontaneous duration, which may be derived from earlier episodes. In case of doubt, 6-months' maintenance treatment after recovery is the rule. Long-term prophylaxis should be maintained lifelong.

Most time is spent in depression, therefore a combination of a mood stabilizer with an antidepressant is often indicated. The same is true for the long-term medication of the disorder, where combined treatments are the rule.

Special attention should be given to suicidal bipolar patients, who should preferably be treated with drugs shown to be antisuicidal (lithium or clozapine combined often with antidepressants). A lifelong study demonstrated a three- to five-fold reduction of suicides. Comorbidity with alcohol use disorder increased the mortality but not the suicide rate.

Major depressive disorder (MDD)

Onset

Unlike bipolar disorder, depression may start at any time of life and has therefore a later mean age of onset. In the United Kingdom a mean age of onset of 33 years was found in hospitalized patients. In a large United States study of outpatients the mean was 29.4 years, but in 53 per cent of cases the onset was before the age of 21. The distribution of the age of onset is bimodal, with peaks in the 30s and 50s.

Prospective data suggest that MDD very often begins as subthreshold depression; this is especially true for late-onset cases, where the full MDD episodes also tend to last longer and to become chronic more often. Age of onset and earlier episodes assessed in retrospect are subject to dramatically false recall.

There is no true dichotomy between early-onset and late-onset depression but a continuous distribution accompanied by a systematic decrease in genetic vulnerability (morbid risk among first-degree relatives) and an increase in precipitation by environmental factors. The correlation of age of onset with the genetic component was found in both patient and community samples. Childhood traumata create a vulnerability which promotes earlier onset and higher comorbidity.

Duration of episodes

The length of depressive episodes is log normally distributed; therefore simple mean values are meaningless. Compared to bipolar disorder, episodes of depressive disorders last about 1 month longer (median duration of 5.4 months); and about 18 to 25 per cent of patients develop chronic depression with a minimum duration of 2 years. In the general population, among whom there are many untreated cases of depression, episodes were found to be shorter; the 25th, 50th, and 75th percentiles were 4, 8, and 16 weeks respectively for recurrent episodes.

Chronicity is clearly correlated with age and persistent cognitive deficits; it is common in the elderly but relatively rare in adolescents. As is in bipolar disorder chronicity is associated with early life adversity, including sexual and physical abuse.

Recurrence of episodes

Major depression is recurrent in about 85 per cent of cases; compared to bipolar disorders, however, depressive patients experience only half as many episodes over their lifetime. The cycle length (time from the start of an episode to the start of a subsequent episode) is consequently longer than in bipolar disorders. There is also a systematic shortening of cycle length with the increasing number of episodes, as shown by frailty analyses. The precipitation of episodes by life events—frequent initially—decreases as the number of episodes grows; the periodicity becomes increasingly autonomous. A twin study suggests that undesirable life events play a significant role in the recurrence of depression in women with a low genetic risk.

In a recent large representative record study in Denmark (N = 20 350 first admissions) unipolar depressives had strikingly lower recurrence rates (hospitalizations) than bipolars, the rates for both correlating with the number of previous episodes.[10] The authors concluded: 'The course of severe unipolar and bipolar disorder seems to be progressive in nature despite the effect of treatment and irrespective of gender, age and type of disorder'. Risk factors for recurrence are previous recurrence, long duration of episodes, late onset, age, severity, and incomplete remission.

Residual symptoms represent a strong risk factor for further recurrence; a survival analysis by Paykel *et al.*[11] found a three-fold higher risk of recurrence (76 per cent) in patients with residual symptoms than in those without (25 per cent). This sub-threshold depressive morbidity is clinically relevant and a clear risk factor for future recurrence and suicidality, especially in the elderly.

Outcome

In long-term follow-up studies, 43 to 52 per cent of depressed outpatients became symptom-free between their episodes, and the other half continued to suffer from dynamically fluctuating residual syndromes or symptoms. The corresponding cross-sectional status may be diagnosed as dysthymia, recurrent brief depression, minor depression, residual syndromes and symptoms, or as full recovery. Initial severity and comorbidity are positively correlated with poor outcome in terms of poorer functioning and incomplete remission. In a British study residual symptoms of major depression, defined by a score of eight or more on the 17-item Hamilton Depression scale, were found in 32 per cent of 60 patients 12 to 15 months after remission.[11] In a large cross-cultural study ($N = 968$) conducted over 9 months, between 25 and 48 per cent of cases experienced complete remission,[12] rates which also depended on the severity of the depression and comorbidity. Severe residual symptoms correlate with long-term morbidity, impaired social functioning at work and in relationships and suicidal behaviour, especially in the elderly, amongst whom remission is present in only about one third of cases.

Recent evidence from a 30-month prospective community-based cohort study of 75-year-old subjects suggests that a history of depression may increase the risk of senile dementia,[13] which is compatible with findings from Denmark that recurrence (number of hospital admissions) increases the risk of dementia.[14]

Mortality

Unipolar depressives have twice the mortality risk of the general population. The SMR (standardized mortality ratio) for suicide is

21 for males and 27 for females;[9] these figures are higher than those for bipolar disorder. Many other causes of death are also more common among unipolar depressives than in the general population but to a lesser extent than among bipolar patients.

The frequently quoted suicide rate of 12 to 19 per cent is only valid for selected hospitalized patient samples, which, by definition, include many suicidal patients. In community and outpatient samples, suicides account for a considerably smaller percentage of deaths; but long-term data is not available yet.

A lifelong follow-up study showed a suicide-preventive effect of administering low-dose antidepressant medication to severe unipolar depressives.

Course of other subtypes of mood disorders

Dysthymia

Subjects with a depressive personality disorder are especially prone to develop dysthymia. Dysthymia is by definition a chronic form of depression; nevertheless dysthymic patients have a similar outcome to major depressives: in outpatients the 5-year recovery rate was 53 per cent. Dysthymia is highly comorbid with other psychiatric disorders, especially with major depression (which it may precede or follow), so worsening the prognosis.

Minor depression

In the general population the recurrence rates of minor depression are comparable to those of major depression, a fact confirmed by survival analyses.[15] A diagnostic change from minor to major depression, or the reverse, is frequent during the course of mood disorders. Minor depression increases about five-fold the risk for the development of major depression. Primary minor depression, like depressive symptoms in general, is a significant risk factor for major depression. It can also represent a residual state of major depression and is a strong risk factor for further recurrence.

Among the elderly minor depression is common as a residual state. Both minor and major depression should be considered seriously as a target for preventive intervention and treatment; full recovery should be the goal.[15]

Seasonal affective disorder

Many patients experience depressive episodes mainly in autumn and winter; mania tends to occur more often in summer. Seasonal affective disorder (SAD) remained seasonal in 70 per cent of 43 cases followed up over 2 to 5 years and in 42 per cent over 8.8 years.[16] The diagnostic stability of SAD was fairly good (26 to 57 per cent). A large number of patients developed seasonal subthreshold (subsyndromal) depression, whereas full remission was present in only 15 to 20 per cent.

Rapid cycling mood disorder

There is no generally accepted definition of rapid cycling; it is usually defined by the occurrence of at least four episodes per year, counting arbitrarily a biphasic episode as two episodes. Rapid cycling occurs almost exclusively in bipolar disorder; it is more frequent in females and in the bipolar-II subtype. Rapid cycling often manifests at an early age and increases the risk of suicide attempts but does not appear to represent a final course pattern of bipolar disorder: it is often a transient, non-familial manifestation of the disorder. In a prospective follow-up conducted over approximately 3 years the diagnosis was stable in about half the cases and the other half became simply recurrent (non-rapid cycling); in a control group 10 per cent of the non-rapid-cycling patients converted to rapid cycling.[17] Studies on the long-term prognosis are inconclusive.

Consequences for treatment

Antidepressant treatment can shorten the time to recovery. Therapeutic decisions on the length of acute treatment will depend on the length of the individual's previous episodes and on the average episode length observed in follow-up studies. The length of affective episodes has probably not changed in 100 years. Antidepressants cannot shorten the episodes but can minimize the symptoms. Treatment should be maintained for the full duration of episodes, which are frequently masked, otherwise relapses must be expected. Full symptomatic and functional remission to the premorbid level should be the goal of treatment.

As with acute treatment, the choice of a long-term prophylactic medication should take into consideration the previous individual course of the disorder plus the general scientific knowledge of course and prognosis, and keep in mind the increased mortality, especially the high suicide risk associated with depression. Recurrence is also a feature of mild cases, but in contrast to severe cases the suicide mortality is probably low.

Over a patient's lifetime, each new recurrence is associated with a new risk of suicide and requires long-term prophylaxis with lithium, combined with low-dose antidepressants. This is especially necessary in the presence of suicidality in the previous or in the family history. If further studies confirm that the recurrence of affective episodes increases the risk of dementia, such a long-term prophylaxis may become even more important.

Conclusions

Bipolar disorder and depression are serious illnesses responsible for most suicides in the population and are recurrent lifelong in most cases. The remission between episodes is often incomplete, increasing the risk of recurrence. Compared to depression bipolar disorder is twice as recurrent and complicated by higher comorbidity with multiple somatic and psychiatric disorders, especially with substance-use disorder which shortens life expectancy even more. Most patients spend about half their lifetime in good health but the other half in largely depressive mood states fluctuating on the broad severity spectrum. Sub-diagnostic morbidity has been recognized as clinically very relevant and in need of permanent treatment. Great progress in the study of continuous fluctuations has been made by the introduction of the life-chart methodology and by computer-assisted daily assessments, methods which hold further promise.[18] Treatment should focus on all manifestations of the illness, including minor morbidity, in order to achieve full recovery to the premorbid level of functioning; in a long-term perspective the primary goal remains the prevention of recurrence, secondary substance-use disorders and suicides.

Future studies should also try to reduce the dementia associated with affective disorders.[13,19,20]

Acknowledgement

I wish to thank Per Bech for his valuable comments and suggestions during the revision of this chapter.

Further information

Goodwin, F.K. and Jamison, K.R. (2007). *Manic-depressive illness* (2nd edn). Oxford University Press, New York.

Maj, M., Akiskal, H.S., Lopez-Ibor, J.J., *et al.* (eds.) (2002). *Bipolar disorder.* John Wiley & Sons, Chichester.

Marneros, A. (ed.) (2004). *Das Neue Handbuch der Bipolaren und Depressiven Erkrankungen.* Georg Thieme, Stuttgart.

References

1. Kahlbaum, K. (1863). *Die Gruppirung der psychischen Krankheiten und die Eintheilung der Seelenstörungen.* A.W. Kafemann, Danzig.
2. Angst, J. (2007). The bipolar spectrum. *The British Journal of Psychiatry*, **190**, 189–91.
3. Hillegers, M.H.J., Reichart, C.G., Wals, M., *et al.* (2005). Five-year prospective outcome of psychopathology in the adolescent offspring of bipolar parents. *Bipolar Disorders*, **7**, 344–50.
4. Christensen, M.V., Kyvik, K.O., and Kessing, L.V. (2006). Cognitive function in unaffected twins discordant for affective disorder. *Psychological Medicine*, **36**, 1119–29.
5. Kessing, L.V., Hansen, M.G., Andersen, P.K., *et al.* (2004). The predictive effect of episodes on the risk of recurrence in depressive and bipolar disorders—a life-long perspective. *Acta Psychiatrica Scandinavica*, **109**, 339–44.
6. Judd, L.L., Schettler, P.J., Akiskal, H.S., *et al.* (2003). Long-term symptomatic status of bipolar I vs. bipolar II disorders. *International Journal of Neuropsychopharmacology*, **6**, 127–37.
7. Judd, L.L., Akiskal, H.S., Schettler, P.J., *et al.* (2005). Psychosocial disability in the course of bipolar I and II disorders. A prospective, comparative, longitudinal study. *Archives of General Psychiatry*, **62**, 1322–30.
8. Paykel, E.S. (1998). Remission and residual symptomatology in major depression. *Psychopathology*, **31**, 5–14.
9. Ösby, U., Brandt, L., Correia, N., *et al.* (2001). Excess mortality in bipolar and unipolar disorder in Sweden. *Archives of General Psychiatry*, **58**, 844–50.
10. Kessing, L.V., Andersen, P.K., Mortensen, P.B., *et al.* (1998). Recurrence in affective disorder. I. Case register study. *The British Journal of Psychiatry*, **172**, 23–8.
11. Paykel, E.S., Ramana, R., Cooper, Z., *et al.* (1995). Residual symptoms after partial remission: an important outcome in depression. *Psychological Medicine*, **25**, 1171–80.
12. De Almeida Fleck, M.P., Simon, G., Herrman, H., *et al.* (2005). Major depression and its correlates in primary care settings in six countries. 9-month follow-up study. *The British Journal of Psychiatry*, **186**, 41–7.
13. Fischer, P., Zehetmeyer, S., Jungwirth, S., *et al.* (in press). Risk factors for Alzheimer dementia in a community-based birth-cohort at age 75. *Dementia and Geriatic Cognitive Disorders.*
14. Andersen, K., Lolk, A., Kragh-Sorensen, P., *et al.* (2005). Depression and the risk of Alzheimer disease. *Epidemiology*, **16**, 233–8.
15. Kessler, R.C., Zhao, S., Blazer, D.G., *et al.* (1997). Prevalence, correlates, and course of minor depression and major depression in the National Comorbidity Survey. *Journal of Affective Disorders*, **45**, 19–30.
16. Schwartz, P.J., Brown, C., Wehr, T.A., *et al.* (1996). Winter-seasonal affective disorder: a follow-up study of the first 59 patients of the NIMH seasonal studies program. *The American Journal of Psychiatry*, **153**, 1028–36.
17. Bauer, M.S., Calabrese, J., Dunner, D.L., *et al.* (1994). Multisite data reanalysis of the validity of rapid cycling as a course modifier for bipolar disorder in DSM-IV. *The American Journal of Psychiatry*, **151**, 506–15.
18. Bauer, M., Grof, P., Rasgon, N., *et al.* (2006). Self-reported data from patients with bipolar disorder: impact on minimum episode length for hypomania. *Journal of Affective Disorders*, **96**, 101–5.
19. Angst, J., Gamma, A., Gerber-Werder, R., *et al.* (2007). Does long-term medication with lithium prevent or attenuate dementia in bipolar and depressed patients? *International Journal of Psychiatry in Clinical Practice*, **11**, 2–8.
20. Kessing, L.V. and Andersen, P.K. (2007). Does the risk of developing dementia increase with the number of episodes in patients with depressive disorder and in patients with bipolar disorder? *Journal of Neurology, Neurosurgery, and Psychiatry*, **75**, 1662–6.

4.5.8 Treatment of mood disorders

E. S. Paykel and J. Scott

Evidence

Medication and physical treatments

(a) Acute treatments for depression

(i) Antidepressants: general issues

The first modern antidepressants became available in the late 1950s, coinciding with introduction of randomized controlled trials in psychiatry. Tightening of licensing requirements has ensured good efficacy for new antidepressants. Overall efficacy and speed of response of most antidepressants are similar. In addition to meta-analyses of specific antidepressant classes, there have been meta-analyses confirming efficacy in specific patient groups or disorder subtypes, including dysthymia[1] and the elderly.[2]

There are moderate, but not very large, effect sizes. About 30 per cent more subjects respond well on antidepressants than on placebo, partly because good response is often seen in placebo groups, probably not due to the placebo but to spontaneous improvement and non-specific treatment effects such as those of seeing a helping figure, supportive psychotherapy, and hospitalization. Non-specific outcome tends to be worse among severely ill patients, but here also antidepressants may be less effective. Placebo-controlled trials are still mandated by regulatory authorities for new antidepressants, since comparisons between active drugs have high risk of type 2 error.

Table 4.5.8.1 lists the principal antidepressants and recommended doses, omitting minority drugs limited to a small number of countries. Some of the antidepressants listed are not available in all countries. Recommended doses depend partly on national authorities and readers should check the situation in their own country.

(ii) Reuptake inhibitors

Tricyclic antidepressants. In addition to the tricyclics listed in Table 4.5.8.1, maprotiline and amoxapine are available in some countries. There have been many older efficacy reviews, with

Table 4.5.8.1 Antidepressant medications*

Drug	Usual dose range (mg/day)**
Reuptake inhibitors	
Tricyclics	
Amitriptyline	75–300
Clomipramine	75–300
Desipramine	75–300
Dosulepin (dothiepin)	75–225
Doxepin	75–150
Imipramine	75–300
Lofepramine	70–210
Nortriptyline	75–150
Proptriptyline	15–60
Trimipramine	75–300
Serotonin and noradrenaline reuptake inhibitors (SNRIs)	
Duloxetine	60
Venlafaxine	75–375 (check)
Selective serotonin reuptake inhibitors (SSRIs)	
Citalopram	20–60
Escitalopram	10–20
Fluoxetine	20–80
Fluvoxamine	50–300
Paroxetine	20–60
Sertraline	50–200
Selective noradrenaline reuptake inhibitor (NARI)	
Reboxetine	4–12
Monoamine oxidase inhibitors	
Irreversible monoamine oxidase inhibitors	
Isocarboxazid	30–60
Phenelzine	45–90
Tranylcypromine	20–30
Reversible monoamine oxidase inhibitor (RIMA)	
Moclobemide	300–600
Others	
Bupropion	200–450
Mianserin	30–90
Mirtazepine	15–45
Trazodone	150–600

*This list is not fully comprehensive because of new developments and national differences.

**Official dose recommendations vary between countries and should always be checked.

further studies accumulating as tricyclics have been included in placebo-controlled trials of new antidepressants.

Earlier views that tricyclics were more effective in endogenous and psychotic depressives have not been confirmed and effects extend across a broad spectrum of depressives, extending more widely into anxiety disorders, panic disorder, and obsessive-compulsive disorder. Tricyclic use has lessened in recent years in favour of antidepressants with fewer side effects.

Serotonin and noradrenaline reuptake inhibitors (SNRIs). Selective SNRIs share the proposed therapeutic mechanisms of tricyclics but with fewer and different side effects, including the serotoninergic effect of nausea, and for venlafaxine at high dose, risk of blood pressure elevation and cardiac arrhythmia, with toxicity in overdose. There is good efficacy evidence for venlafaxine, with possible superiority over SSRIs,(3) and emerging evidence for duloxetine.(4) A further SNRI in some countries is milnacipran.

Selective serotonin reuptake inhibitors (SSRIs). Meta-analyses of SSRIs(5) show efficacy comparable with tricyclics, but lower rates of side effects and discontinuation. There is conflicting evidence as to whether SSRIs are less effective than tricyclics and SNRIs in severe depression. SSRIs and clomipramine, the most serotoninergic tricyclic, are more effective than noradrenergic tricyclics in obsessive-compulsive disorder.

There have been vigorous debates regarding effects of antidepressants, particularly SSRIs, on suicidal behaviour, with many studies.(6) Actual suicide does not appear to be increased and may be reduced. There is some evidence that suicidal feelings and attempts may be increased in the early weeks after starting, particularly for SSRIs, with development of tension or agitation, and in children and adolescents. On the other hand SSRIs and other newer antidepressants are considerably safer in overdose than tricyclics and SNRI. Warnings were issued by regulatory authorities in the United States and the United Kingdom when the evidence started to emerge. Most strongly the findings argue for careful clinical surveillance of patients prescribed antidepressants, particularly in the early phases of treatment when risk of suicidality has long been recognized as increased. This is in any case important in depressed patients.

Noradrenaline reuptake inhibitors. Only one newer selective NARI is available, reboxetine. It is clearly superior to placebo.(7)

(iii) Monoamine oxidase inhibitors (MAOIs)

Irreversible MAOIs. There are few MAOIs available, reflecting hypertensive and other interactions and limited use. The older MAOIs bind irreversibly to the enzyme, and new enzyme needs to be synthesized over 1–2 weeks to reverse the effect. Controlled trials(8) show superiority to placebo in depression, and in anxiety disorders. Often high doses are necessary and the hydrazine MAOIs, phenelzine, and isocarboxazid, show better clinical response in slow acetylators. Tranylcypromine has additional stimulant effects, and has been viewed as more effective but with more risk of interactions.

From the late 1950s, there were suggestions of particular efficacy in atypical depression, variously regarded as non-endogenous depression, anxiety disorder with depression, or as a pattern of reversed vegetative symptoms with increased appetite, increased sleep, evening worsening, reactivity, and other features, a meaning currently predominant in the United States. Evidence is not strong, but comparative trials of phenelzine and tricyclics point to better effects than tricyclics with anxiety disorders and reversed vegetative symptoms.(8) On the other hand MAOIs are mostly used as second-line drugs by psychiatrists, where other antidepressants have failed, irrespective of clinical picture.

Reversible competitive inhibitors. The reversible MAO-A selective drug moclobemide can dissociate from the enzyme and be displaced by substances with higher affinity, including tyramine. It shows superiority to placebo,(9) but not at doses below 450 mg daily, and evidence is best for 600 mg. Many clinicians view moclobemide as less effective than older MAOIs.

(iv) Other antidepressants

Bupropion. Bupropion is relatively stimulant and is epileptogenic. It is licenced for depression in the United States, and in some other countries as an aid to smoking cessation.

Mianserin. Mianserin, an older drug which blocks alpha-2 autoreceptors, is sedative in side effects and carries a definite although low risk of agranulocytosis.

Mirtazepine. Mirtazepine blocks alpha-2, 5HT2, and 5HT3 receptors. It has been shown superior to placebo and is also a sedative.[10]

Trazodone. Trazodone, an older drug is relatively sedative carries a risk of priapism in males.

New classes of antidepressants, not yet licenced, are continually being sought.[11] Agomelatine, an agonist at melatonin MT1 and MT2 receptors and a 5HT2C antagonist has shown evidence of efficacy. Efforts have been made to develop drugs, which inhibit cortisol secretion. Development pathways for new antidepressants are long and failures due to weak treatment effects or major adverse effects are common.

(b) Electroconvulsive therapy (ECT)

ECT, the earliest of modern treatments, is still the most effective in severe depression. In a meta-analysis.[12] It has been found more effective than simulated ECT in blind trials, and more effective than pharmacotherapy. Bilateral ECT appears more effective than unilateral but this may not be true at adequate stimulus intensity. Best effects occur in psychotic depression with delusions or psychomotor retardation. There is also some evidence, which is not conclusive, that ECT may benefit mania.

Other physical treatments

(a) Bright light

Bright light, reviewed in Chapter 6.2.10.2 is the established treatment for seasonal affective disorder. Several studies in non-seasonal depressions as adjunctive treatment have suggested some benefit, although the effect may not be sustained.[13]

(b) Repetitive transcranial magnetic stimulation (TMS)

TMS is reviewed in Chapter 6.2.10.3. There is clear evidence of superiority of left prefrontal TMS compared with sham therapy but the degree of benefit appears weak. There is still uncertainty regarding optimal stimulation parameters. At present the evidence is not sufficient for widespread use of TMS in clinical practice.

(c) Vagus nerve stimulation

Stimulation of afferent left cervical vagus nerve fibres by a stimulator implanted in the chest wall is approved by regulatory authorities in a number of countries for resistant epilepsy and in the United States for resistant depression. Controlled evidence is still limited.[14]

(d) Deep brain stimulation

Chronic stimulation of white matter tracts adjacent to the subgenual cingulate region by implanted electrodes has been reported to produce striking remission in a small number of patients with resistant depression, associated with marked reduction in local cerebral blood flow.[15] Further experience is still needed.

Longer-term treatment

(a) Continuation treatment

In recent years, it has become apparent from follow-up studies that the long-term outcome of depression is still often problematic. It is customary to distinguish between relapse, or early symptom return, and later recurrence of a new episode.[16] In parallel, drug treatment after the acute episode has been divided into earlier continuation treatment, to prevent relapse, and longer-term maintenance treatment to prevent recurrence.

There have been many controlled trials of continuation treatment on active drug for 6 to 8 months after the acute episode against withdrawal to placebo, showing substantial benefit from continuation.[17] A fluoxetine study with staged withdrawal showed benefit of continuation for 24 and 38 weeks, but not 62 weeks, suggesting that routine continuation should be for 9–12 months rather than 6 months.[18] A controlled trial of early lithium withdrawal after augmentation showed very high relapse rate indicating a need for lithium continuation[19] and there is evidence for continuation drugs after ECT.

(b) Maintenance treatment

Longer-term studies in unipolar depression have shown clear benefit from maintenance antidepressants,[17] although recurrence rates in drug-treated patients may be high.

Withdrawal reactions requiring temporary restarting can occur if antidepressants are stopped abruptly, particularly after high doses for long periods, with malaise, coryza-like symptoms, vomiting, and diarrhoea. This may occur with a variety of antidepressants including SSRIs, tricyclics, and SNRIs.

Trials of lithium in maintenance treatment of severe recurrent unipolar depressives also show benefit over placebo.[20] Comparative efficacy against antidepressants is not clear.

(c) Acute treatments for bipolar disorder

In the treatment of bipolar depression there is a good evidence for efficacy of antidepressants.[21] The major risks are precipitation of mania and rapid cycling, which appear to occur more with tricyclics and venlafaxine than with other antidepressants, suggesting the preferential use of SSRIs, MAOIs, or ECT and covering with lithium. Lamotrigine has also been found effective.[22] For lithium alone as an antidepressant the evidence is less clear-cut.

In the treatment of acute mania, lithium has been extensively reviewed and the evidence is good.[23] Anticonvulsants have been increasingly evaluated, with good controlled trial evidence in mania for valproate and carbamazepine, but not lamotrigine or other anticonvulsants.[22] There is also controlled trial evidence for antipsychotics, both older and newer.[24] Available trials do not clearly point to choice of treatment.

(d) Maintenance treatment of bipolar disorder

Controlled trials of maintenance lithium against placebo in bipolar disorder show clear reduction of recurrences, particularly of mania, with weaker effects on depression.[25] There is also reduction of suicide in mood disorder more generally.

There are high rates of early recurrence, particularly of mania, when lithium is discontinued after long-term use, particularly if discontinuation is rapid.[26] This mandates slow withdrawal in practice. One study.[27] has indicated greater benefit on residual symptoms for doses producing blood levels 0.8 to 1.0 mmol/l than for 0.4 to 0.6 mmol/l. This is important since follow-up studies of bipolar patients show that subsyndromal symptoms are common.

There have been fewer long-term studies of anticonvulsants.[22] For valproate evidence is suggestive rather than conclusive. For lamotrigine two controlled trials have confirmed prophylaxis of bipolar depression. Although carbamazepine has been used for longer, evidence from placebo-controlled trials is mainly for acute treatment of mania.

Several manufacturer-sponsored trials have indicated prophylactic effects of olanzapine in maintenance. Older antipsychotics have long been used as adjunctive treatment in bipolar maintenance.

Psychological treatments

There is high public demand for psychotherapies. Guidelines are less well developed and less robustly based than for pharmacotherapy. The concept of empirically supported psychotherapies (EST) assists definition of the evidence base.[28]

(a) Acute treatment of depression

(i) Psychological treatments: general issues

The therapy models can broadly be divided into 'process-orientated' therapies such as psychodynamic or supportive–expressive therapies, and 'outcome-orientated' therapies, such as cognitive behaviour therapies (CBT) and interpersonal therapy (IPT), which primarily focus on symptom reduction. The latter EST are protocol or guideline driven, with a manual describing the therapy in detail. In large-scale randomized controlled treatment trials (RCTs) they have been found superior to pill or psychological placebo-controlled treatments or efficacious as antidepressants or other established treatments.[28] The EST are usually brief (12–20 sessions), delivered by a trained therapist, establishing a working alliance and using an individualized case formulation to focus on specific 'here and now' problems, encouraging between session 'homework' tasks to enable development of new coping skills.

(ii) Meta-analyses

The two best-evaluated therapies are CBT (including behaviour therapies) and IPT, with many meta-analyses of a large number of RCTs. There are fewer studies of dynamic therapies. Early outcome studies and resultant meta-analyses were hampered by use of 'completer' samples rather than 'intent-to-treat' analyses, but found specific psychological therapies, particularly CBT, more effective than other verbal therapies or waiting-list controls. A meta-analysis of 29 carefully selected controlled trials,[29] using intent to treat analyses, found efficacies of individual CBT (response rate, 50 per cent), behavioural therapy (55 per cent), and IPT (52 per cent) in the treatment of the acute episode were not significantly different to pharmacotherapy (58 per cent). Brief dynamic psychotherapies, mainly group therapies, were less effective (35 per cent) and only marginally superior to waiting-list controls (30 per cent). CBT was less effective in a group format, behavioural therapy was equally effective, and IPT was more beneficial when a significant other took part in therapy.

A recent meta-analysis[30] found CBT and IPT equally effective in reducing depressive symptoms in heterogeneous groups of patients with depressive symptoms and syndromes, and both were superior to counselling, other therapies or control treatments in primary care. When compared in meta-analyses to an active treatment, however, CBT and IPT show only equivalent efficacy or marginal superiority. Almost all RCTs of psychological therapies have been in outpatient depressives, not above moderate severity and comparisons with pharmacotherapy do not represent severe or inpatient disorder.

(iii) Cognitive therapy

Earlier CBT studies suggested it was effective over a range of severity and endogenicity. However, in the three-centre NIMH study,[31] which sought to overcome earlier methodological flaws, a secondary analysis found CBT less effective than pharmacotherapy in the more severe disorders within the outpatient range studied. Another study found that individuals with mild or moderately severe depression did equally well with either 8 or 16 sessions, but those with severe depression showed better response with 16 sessions. A large RCT in subjects with severe major depressive disorder[32] found no difference overall between antidepressants and CBT, but also significantly greater effects for antidepressants at the trial centre where the CBT therapists were less experienced.

(iv) IPT

IPT Has been found effective in moderate numbers of RCTs, in a variety of situations, including combination studies with antidepressants and some situations where medication as a first-line treatment for depression is not easily feasible (pregnancy, postpartum, adolescence, and in a developing country).[33] The NIMH study[31] is the only one that has compared IPT with a pill-placebo control. Interpersonal therapy was nearest to the effectiveness of imipramine but a little weaker, and IPT was more beneficial than CBT in patients with more severe outpatient depression.

(v) Other psychotherapies

Fewer acute controlled trials of other therapies have been published. Two large-scale RCTs of individual behavioural therapy found respectively greater efficacy than insight-orientated therapy, which disappeared by 3 months follow-up, and no differences from several other treatments.

The only published RCTs on marital therapy mainly draw on behavioural approaches with behavioural marital therapy or CBT both more effective than waiting-list controls in one study and an advantage for behavioural marital therapy over CBT one study of depressed individuals with marital discord. Couples therapy was more effective than pharmacotherapy in a study of depressed patients living with a critical partner. An RCT of family therapy in inpatients with affective disorder[34] found benefit on role function for female patients on discharge, and for bipolars but not unipolars on follow-up.

Counselling is often offered alone or in combination with medication, particularly in primary care or non-specialist mental health settings. Recent meta-analyses[30] suggest limited benefits, with superiority over treatment as usual or waiting-list control conditions lost beyond about 3 months. Individuals who are socially isolated and lack a confidante may particularly benefit.

(vi) Combined psychotherapy and pharmacotherapy

Data on whether combination of psychotherapy and pharmacotherapy bestows additional benefit over either treatment alone are not conclusive, but some studies suggest a small advantage at the level of severity usually studied, both for CBT and for IPT. However, in a meta-analysis of eight outcome studies, neither CBT, behavioural therapy, nor IPT added to antidepressants were any more effective than pharmacotherapy alone.(35)

In a large RCT of antidepressant and cognitive behavioural analysis system of psychotherapy (CBASP) given alone, or in combination for major depressive episode persisting for longer than 1 year(36) the group receiving the combined treatment had significantly greater overall reduction in depressive symptoms and attainment of remission as compared with single therapies.

In other studies, treatment with an antidepressant alone or in combination with IPT has been found more effective than IPT alone in dysthymics, and greater benefit of combined treatment has been reported in an RCT of group CBT and medication. These studies indicated that combined treatments improved quality of life over and above individual treatments. There is also some evidence that social adjustment is particularly benefited by IPT.

(b) Longer-term psychological treatment

(i) Continuation and maintenance trials

Psychological treatments are more expensive than antidepressants, but the balance could change if they reduced relapse rates.(37) Naturalistic follow-ups suggest this, but are hard to interpret because the original RCTs were not designed or powered to evaluate long-term outcome.

The use of continuation and maintenance psychotherapy is a relatively new concept. The key maintenance trial for IPT(38) assigned subjects with recurrent depression to imipramine, placebo, or monthly IPT with or without medication. There was a highly significant effect for antidepressants on recurrence rates and a modest effect (at the end of year 1 and year 3) for IPT. The first study of IPT, by its originators 15 years earlier, did not find it reduced relapse, compared with antidepressant continuation.

Five longer-term RCTs have now shown relapse and recurrence reduction with CBT.(37) Three of these, in individuals in remission using mindfulness or other techniques have only found benefit in subjects with a previous history of repeated episodes.

At least 20 per cent of people with an initial episode of major depressive disorder do not recover within 2 years, and those with residual depressive symptoms have a high risk of relapse. In a RCT(39) in 158 subjects with persistent residual depressive symptoms following major depression assigned to antidepressant continuation or antidepressant plus CBT, at 18-month follow-up relapse rates in the CBT plus antidepressant group were reduced by 45–50 per cent compared with the control group. Relapse prevention persisted for 3.5 years. Similar findings have been obtained in three small RCTs.(40)

(c) Bipolar disorder

Until very recently, research in psychological treatments for bipolar disorder was limited. Prior to 1995 a number of small studies, few of them randomized trials, suggested that adherence to medication was improved.(41) More recently good RCTs have been completed. The earlier of these found some benefit from psychological treatments in preventing relapse, with a hint that the briefer interventions are more effective in preventing mania than depression. A meta-analysis of relapse rates(42) found an odds ratio (OR) for relapse in the intervention as compared to the control group of 0.31. Three recent large efficacy trials used CBT, family therapy, or group psycho-education, respectively. A separate meta-analysis of these(42) found a similar odds ratio for relapse, with more benefit for depressive than manic/hypomanic relapses.

The MRC multicentre RCT in the United Kingdom(43) was one of the few pragmatic effectiveness trials, with over 250 subjects randomized to CBT plus usual psychiatric treatment or usual treatment alone. Over 50 per cent of the sample had a recurrence by 18 months, with no overall significant differences between groups, but a significant interaction with number of previous episodes such that CBT was significantly more effective than treatment as usual in subjects with fewer than 12 previous episodes, but less effective in those with more episodes.

One variant of IPT has been evaluated in a large RCT, interpersonal and social rhythm therapy (IPSRT), which includes an approach to stabilize social rhythms.(44) It was found to reduce bipolar relapse rates more than did IPT. The full advantages and disadvantages of different forms of psychotherapy for bipolar disorders are yet entirely clear, but further evidence is expected to emerge soon.

Management

Treatment of unipolar disorder

(a) General aspects: where to manage

The goals of depression treatment are to alleviate acute symptoms, to restore psychosocial functioning, and to prevent relapse and recurrence. Crucial decisions are the selection of an intervention and treatment setting. These involve four key issues: severity of the disorder including risk of self-harm, availability of treatments (specific antidepressants, trained therapists), patient preference, and nature of any associated difficulties. Recent guidelines include those of the UK National Institute for Health and Clinical Excellence(45) and of CANMAT.(46)

(b) Treatment setting

Very severe depression with definite suicidal risk is best managed in inpatient facilities to allow careful monitoring. With less suicidal risk and good social support severe cases can be managed with intensive community support, partial hospitalization, day care, or combined outpatient and home-based care. Moderate or mild depression should be managed in outpatient settings, unless treatment is complicated by severe physical illness, or non-response requires more detailed assessment.

(c) Primary or secondary care

Worldwide, most depressed patients are treated in primary care or general medical settings. Cases are referred to specialist mental health services because the disorder is more severe, chronic, treatment resistant, or because other difficulties, such as alcohol misuse or marital problems, complicate the clinical picture.

(d) Medication or psychological therapy

Although severe depression may respond to psychotherapy alone, recovery is slower than with drugs or ECT. Psychotherapy may be used in addition, rather than alone. In milder depressions, choice depends partly on patient preference and availability of psychotherapies, although when major depression criteria are reached antidepressants should preferably not be withheld. In the complex situations requiring specialist referral it is often necessary to use combinations of drugs and psychosocial approaches. Although physical and psychological treatments are described separately in this section, treatment rarely involves only prescribing, but education and support of patient and family are important aspects of any clinical management.

Medication

(a) When to treat

The most important indications for use of medication are severity and persistence. A severity threshold has been shown a little below major depression at which tricyclic antidepressants start to show superiority over placebo.(47) SSRIs may show benefit in minor depression.(48) Antidepressants are also superior to placebo in dysthymia. In mild depressive episodes highly reactive to major stress, and in acute grief, prognosis for spontaneous resolution is often good, and medication may be delayed, provided that improvement is occurring. Impairment of function and suicidal feelings are other indications to treat. Recent guidelines recommend use in depression of moderate severity, major depression, or ICD-10 depressive episode.

(b) What antidepressant to choose

Since SSRIs are comparatively free of side effects and are not costly if out of patent, they are generally recommended as first choice antidepressants. Where there is a previous history of response to a specific drug or class, the best first choice is that antidepressant.

With few exceptions, symptom pattern is not a good guide to treatment. Effects of antidepressants extend widely across the spectrum of depression and in to anxiety disorders. The place of SSRIs in very severe depression is still debated. MAOIs or SSRIs or are a reasonable first choice in atypical depression. With comorbid obsessive-compulsive disorder the SSRIs, SNRIs, or clomipramine are preferable to noradrenergic antidepressants. Light therapy is indicated for seasonal affective disorder, alone or with antidepressant.

(c) How to use an antidepressant

There is a delay in clinical antidepressant effects of 1 to 3 weeks or longer, although some improvement may be seen earlier. An antidepressant needs to be continued for a minimum duration of 6 weeks at adequate or high dose before being regarded as ineffective.

Since side effects often occur more in the early weeks, with later tolerance, build-up of dose over 2 to 3 weeks is useful. For fluoxetine, the exceptionally long half-life of the active metabolite means that blood levels build-up for some weeks, even on a standard dose. Standard dosage regimes fail to allow for the considerable interindividual variability in pharmacokinetic mechanisms that occurs. Low doses are usually ineffective. Where response is not occurring and there are only minor side effects doses should be increased towards maximum, except in the elderly, who are vulnerable to poor elimination and to side effects.

Dose division during the day can be based on pharmacology. Half-lives of most antidepressants, combined with delay in therapeutic effects, mean that one dose per day may be adequate, but for most, two doses per day are better and three doses may be useful for some patients. Moclobemide, which is easily displaced from MAO and metabolized, should be given in three doses daily. For sedative antidepressants, administration of two-thirds of the dose at night may avoid hypnotics. Doses at bedtime of the more stimulant antidepressants, including SSRIs and older MAOIs, should be avoided.

Common side effects of SSRIs and SNRIs are nausea, and other gastrointestinal disturbances, insomnia, and sometimes tension and restlessness. Blood pressure should be monitored with high dose venlafaxine and it should not be used with hypertension or risk of ventricular arrhythmias. Common side effects of tricyclics clinically are sedation and anticholinergic side effects of dry mouth, blurred near vision, urinary retention, orthostatic hypotension, and confusion in the elderly. Dose-limiting side effects of MAOIs are hypotension, insomnia, and ankle oedema and tyramine containing foods and interacting drugs must be avoided.

(d) What to use if the first choice does not work

The evidence base for second choice of antidepressant after poor response to the first is weak. The large non-blind partially randomized STAR*D study,(49) has shown few differences between different choices after weak first response to citalopram.

The major pragmatic options are switch to a different antidepressant or combination. Switch should be to an antidepressant of a different class, or to a broad action SNRI. If this is not adequate, lithium augmentation is the best-supported change. Where depression is severe ECT is an alternative second choice.

(e) What to use in special situations

(i) Suicidal risk

Major suicidal risk requires consideration of lethality of particular antidepressants in overdose. Tricyclics and SNRIs should be avoided. SSRIs and most other newer antidepressants are comparatively safe in overdose, with careful monitoring for increased risk early in treatment.

(ii) Psychotic depression

Evidence as to choice of antidepressant is weak, but suggests SNRIs or tricyclics, rather than SSRIs. Combination with an antipsychotic may be useful, but antipsychotics are not adequate alone.(50) ECT is an alternative.

(iii) Medical illness

Antidepressant treatment with medical disorders is often difficult, because of toxicity due to illness, high blood levels from impaired metabolism, side effects, and drug interactions. Cardiac problems indicate use of an SSRI or other newer non-tricyclic non-SNRI antidepressant, and treatment after myocardial infarction may enhance survival. MAOIs lower blood pressure as a dose-related effect and should be avoided.

Concomitant epilepsy may be controlled by adjustment of anticonvulsant dose. Tricyclics and bupropion are epileptogenic and should be avoided. Epileptic potential is usually less with newer antidepressants but is often not clear, and the only antidepressants established not to be epileptogenic are older MAOIs.

(iv) The elderly

The elderly are particularly liable to side effects. SSRIs and newer antidepressants are preferable to tricyclics.

(v) Children

Antidepressants are not first choice treatments for depression in children and adolescents, for whom psychological therapy is preferable. Where the depression is not improving and is severe, an antidepressant may be needed. Tricyclics are not effective.[51] There is more evidence for SSRIs, best for fluoxetine,[52] but the risk-benefit ratio is argued. For adolescents combination of SSRIs with CBT may be useful. The risk of increased suicidality early in treatment mandates careful observation. The FDA issued an Advisory in 2004 but not a contraindication.

(vi) Pregnancy and lactation

Tricyclics have been used in pregnancy for many years and do not carry risk of foetal malformation. For SSRIs the current evidence is contradictory and for some newer drugs evidence is lacking. Lithium and anticonvulsants carry some risk of foetal malformation and are contraindicated in the early months of pregnancy. Psychotropic drugs used at the time of delivery may produce complications of anaesthesia and foetal sedation and if possible should be withdrawn temporarily. Most psychotropic drugs appear in breast milk in small quantities. Breast feeding should be discussed with the patient.

Electroconvulsive therapy

Use of ECT varies internationally. Many psychiatrists use it as a first choice treatment in severe depression with psychomotor retardation or mood-congruent depressive delusions, or where an antidepressant has failed, and for moderately severe depressions which have not responded to one or two courses of antidepressant.

The UK National Institute for Clinical Excellence has recommended use only to achieve rapid improvement where a trial of other treatment has failed or the condition is potentially life threatening, in severe depression, catatonia, and prolonged or severe mania.[53] Detailed recommendations on how ECT should be administered also can be consulted.[54]

Non-response and resistant depression

Controlled trials of treatments for depressives who do not respond to first or second treatments are limited. There is good evidence for lithium augmentation of antidepressants[55] and limited evidence for potentiation by triiodothyronine (T3).[56] A variety of other augmenters have been tried including tryptophan, pindolol, buspirone, and combinations of antidepressants such as SSRI-bupropion, SNRI-mirtazepine, tricyclic-MAOI, with weak evidence.

We therefore depend on clinical experience.[57] If there is still limited response after several antidepressant treatments, a systematic approach to resistant depression should be adopted:

1 Reassess the situation thoroughly, with full history, assessment, and laboratory investigation of thyroid function to ask the following questions: (a) Is the diagnosis correct? Wrong diagnosis is in practice unusual. (b) Are there perpetuating factors in personality, family environment, or the social setting? Commonly, where depression has been long-term, secondary role loss (including work), and family adaptations to a non-functioning member mean there are no roles or relationships for the patient to return to and remission cannot occur, or is transient, unless psychotherapy, family therapy, and rehabilitation are employed to change the situation. (c) Is hypothyroidism impairing response? This may develop as a result of earlier use of lithium.

2 Consider previous treatment. Failure to use high or maximal doses of antidepressants when response is not occurring can lead to apparently resistant depression.

3 Employ drug and other physical treatments.

4 As remission occurs, introduce psychotherapeutic, cognitive, and rehabilitative interventions.

The treatment decisions depend on what has been used before. Start with the most promising antidepressant suggested by the history and push to a very high dose. If there is no good clue venlafaxine may be useful, with monitoring of blood pressure for elevation as high doses are reached.

The next intervention is augmentation. Lithium is easiest and best. Blood levels required for augmentation are not established. If response occurs, the lithium should be continued for some months, although not as long as antidepressant. Care should be taken to monitor for a serotonin syndrome (excitability, restlessness, temperature elevation), with serotoninergic antidepressants.

T3 may produce fewer side effects than lithium but evidence is weaker and care must be exercised if there are cardiac problems. L-tryptophan may potentiate MAOIs and the more serotoninergic uptake inhibitors. Its effect is weak, but may be combined with lithium. Pindolol, which blocks 5-HT_{1A} autoreceptors, can accelerate speed of antidepressant response but increased amount of response is less clear.

At one time tricyclic-MAOI combinations were often used and occasionally still have a place, combined with lithium. SSRIs, SNRIs, and clomipramine risk of serotonin syndrome and are contraindicated. Doses should be increased gradually. More ordinarily 1 to 2 weeks should intervene between stopping an older MAOI and starting a reuptake inhibitor.

When vigorous medication regimens have still not produced a response, it is often helpful to add bilateral ECT to maximal drug therapy, even when ECT alone has not previously helped. The practical places for vagus nerve stimulation and deep brain stimulation are not yet clear. In intractable severe chronic depression, psychosurgery still has an occasional place, followed by active rehabilitation.

Longer-term treatment

(a) Continuation treatment: a routine

Continuation antidepressant for 9–12 months should be routine following response to acute treatment. Antidepressant or lithium are also advisable after ECT. The continuation dose should initially be the same as the acute treatment dose. After 2 to 3 months this may be reduced if side effects are a problem, but only by a small amount, to avoid symptom return.

Before the antidepressant is withdrawn the patient should also be completely free of residual symptoms for at least 4 months. These symptoms or history of previous relapse or recurrence suggest longer continuation. Withdrawal should then be carried out slowly, over 2 to 3 months, to minimize the risk of relapse, and of withdrawal symptoms.

In some patients, after withdrawal, or achievement of a low dose, depressive symptoms return. Full dose should be resumed, followed by continuation for a further period of 9 months to a year. Some of these patients relapse again on later drug withdrawal, and long-term maintenance should then be considered.

(b) Maintenance treatment

Longer-term maintenance is indicated where there have been several recurrences, such as two episodes in the last 2 years, or three episodes in 5 years.[16,45] This also depends on the severity of episodes, their potential impact on personal life, family life, and career, and the patient's preferences. Discussion is required, to reach a joint decision.

For most unipolar depressives the maintenance treatment choice will be whichever antidepressant has been effective and well tolerated. Where antidepressants have not been fully effective, lithium or combination are required. Antidepressant doses should be the same or a little lower than those needed for acute treatment in the particular patient. The length of maintenance is harder to specify, and it depends on the history. Two to three years will be a minimum, longer where remission has been difficult to achieve or recent episodes more frequent, 5 years or more where risk is greater, and indefinite or lifelong where two or three attempts to withdraw have been followed by another episode within a year.[16] Withdrawal of antidepressants, lithium, or other drugs after long-term maintenance should always be gradual. Where withdrawal is followed soon after by a recurrence, longer-term maintenance is indicated, and where this sequence has been repeated, lifelong treatment.

Psychological treatments

The psychological management of acute depression ranges across basic clinical management, psychoeducation for the individual and partner or family, supportive psychotherapy, to formal psychotherapy.

(a) Clinical management

Clinical management is a key component of the care of all individuals with depression regardless of the specific treatment. It includes education about the nature of the disorder, its polarity, course and prognosis, treatment options, their advantages and disadvantages, delay in benefits, probable side effects and how to manage these, and planned length of treatment. This dialogue can help build a strong treatment alliance, overcome misconceptions such as fears of addiction to antidepressants, and improve medication adherence. Involving 'significant others' also in some sessions facilitates information and engagement in the treatment process, clarifies what aspects of care are the clinician's responsibility, and can help reduce tension in interpersonal relationships resulting from the patient's depression. For many depressed individuals the reduction in symptoms from this basic approach and medication restores the previous level of functioning. They are again able to use their coping skills to resolve personal problems and no other form of psychological input is needed.

(b) When to use psychological therapies

If additional strategies are needed, a number of factors should guide their choice, including treatment setting, severity, chronicity, complexity, patient preferences, and availability of therapists. Most management approaches are multifaceted and in a dynamic state so the divisions below, structured by severity of depression, although useful may be somewhat artificial.

(i) Mild depression

For individuals with milder depression, usually treated in primary care, psychological approaches can be used alone as alternatives to medication, and there is little advantage in combined treatment. Many patients express their own treatment preferences. Some primary care physicians offer extended treatment sessions for depression, but many utilize counsellors. A course of counselling, lasting 8–10 sessions, is particularly useful to patients who lack a confidante. Benefits appear in the first 3 months, but there is no evidence of longer-term benefits compared to other treatments or 'watchful waiting'[45] (regular appointments with a clinician offering monitoring and support without medication or other interventions).

The next option may be CBT or IPT. There are no robust predictors of differential response to these as opposed to medication so choice often depends on availability of a suitable therapist. Difficulties in timely access have led to development of computerized CBT and of self-help approaches. The individual is offered a computer version of therapy or a written manual to guide self-therapy (bibliotherapy), with possible 1–3 sessions from a therapist to explain the process and overcome hitches. In other circumstances, including management of depressed pregnant women, telephone versions of IPT have been developed. There is not yet consensus on the efficacy of these alternatives but a trial may be used in mild depression.

(ii) Moderate depression

Formal psychotherapy may be offered to individuals with moderate depression as the only treatment, or preferably combined with medication. Usually this comprises 15–20 sessions of individual therapy, but since more than 20 per cent of couples report marital discord in association with depression, marital or family approaches should also be considered. Psychological treatments may also be required where medical conditions or needed medications contraindicate antidepressants, or the patient refuses medication. Other important considerations include previous coping skills, premorbid stressors requiring problem-solving approaches, ability to articulate emotions and difficulties. If there are doubts regarding suitability, referral may be offered for assessment. Patient preference for therapy does not imply benefit, and dropout rates are about similar to those for medication. Also consider whether needs can be met through a time-limited input or if longer-term support is preferable through day services or a community support worker. Therapists adherence to the therapy model, their level of expertise and skill and the provision of regular and adequate supervision to the practitioner are other factors and may account for some 30 per cent of the variance in patient's improvement.[58]

(iii) Severe depression or complex presentations

Research evidence suggests that CBT or IPT may be used alone in severe depression if delivered by an expert therapist. However improvement is slower than with antidepressants and in practice these are usually combined with medication, which is commenced first. In severe depressions it may be difficult for an individual to concentrate until the mental state has been stabilized by medication. Patients who fail to respond adequately to antidepressants alone require reassessment. In many instances medication has improved the vegetative symptoms of depression, but the individual manifests psychological vulnerabilities, such as Axis II comorbidity or long-standing, low self-esteem, or social stressors, acting as maintenance factors and amenable to therapy. The evidence suggests that IPT or CBT are the most useful therapies to combine with antidepressants in unipolar disorders, but the more severe or complex the case, the more important therapist factors become.[58] More severe or chronic disorders also require more prolonged therapy.

Continuation and maintenance therapy

Some patients may benefit from regular but less frequent sessions of continuation or maintenance CBT or IPT to prevent relapse, with about eight additional sessions over the course of a year, to explore whether the techniques learnt in therapy are being used well and to identify potential triggers of relapse or recurrence. It is unrealistic to offer this to all those who receive an acute course of IPT or CBT, but it may be considered for those at high risk of relapse or recurrence due to residual symptoms, history of highly recurrent episodes, ongoing severe psychosocial stressors, refusal to take continuation medications. A full course of CBT may also be offered now, rather than during the acute illness, if remission is partial with residual symptoms.

Treatment of bipolar disorder

Recent guidelines on treatment of bipolar disorder, providing supporting evidence, include those from the UK National Institute for Health and Clinical Excellence,[59] the CANMAT consensus statement,[60] and the APA Practice Guideline.[61]

(a) Treating acute mania

Most mood stabilizers and antipsychotics have acute antimanic effects, but lithium or valproate are the drugs of first choice. Since response may take 7 to 14 days, an antipsychotic is also often required, with effects within days in controlling the acute manic symptoms. The older antipsychotic, haloperidol should not be used with lithium due to risk of neurotoxicity syndrome. Benzodiazepines such as lorazepam and clonazepam may also be used temporarily to treat hyperactivity, insomnia, and agitation. The loss of insight, impaired judgement, hyperactivity, and disinhibited behaviour of manic patients often mean that hospitalization is required to ensure patient safety and commence treatment. For severe mania, ECT may occasionally be used.

(b) Treating bipolar depression

Treatment of bipolar depression is in principle similar to unipolar, but with mood stabilizer cover. If severity indicates antidepressant use, an SSRI, bupropion, or MAOI should be used, but not a tricyclic or SNRI, because of higher risk of mania and cycling. A mood stabilizer should be used in addition. Lamotrigine may produce benefit alone. If cycling occurs in spite of this, an antipsychotic may be added, and the antidepressant cautiously reduced. ECT may be indicated, as in unipolar depression, and does not appear to lead to rapid cycling.

(c) Continuation and maintenance treatment for bipolar disorder

Continuation treatment is needed after acute bipolar episodes, using the single medication or combination that has been used in acute treatment. Bipolar disorder is more recurrent than unipolar disorder, and mania can have catastrophic effects on personal life. The threshold for maintenance treatment is therefore lower and it should be used for 1 to 2 years following a first episode of mania and longer after bipolar recurrences.

Choice of mood stabilizer includes an increasingly wide range. Probably lithium is still the first choice, in the absence of major side effects. Doses should achieve blood levels 12 h after the last dose of 0.4 to 0.8 mmol/l, but sometimes higher levels are needed to prevent recurrences, and to reduce residual symptoms. After some months blood levels are often very stable and only require occasional monitoring. Advice needs to be given on circumstances, which may disturb levels such as dehydration, gastrointestinal upset, travel, hot climates. Thyroid function should be monitored for hypothyroidism every 6 to 12 months.

Poor or partial responses are not uncommon, and valproate is a first choice alternative. Lamotrigine may be helpful where depression is a main feature. In treatment-resistant cases, two mood stabilizers may be required, particularly lithium and valproate. Antipsychotics, particularly olanzapine, may also be added or substituted if response is poor.

Antidepressants can often be withdrawn slowly after mood stabilizers are well established, but may be necessary to prevent chronic or recurrent depression. Antidepressants should not usually be used alone for maintenance in view of the risk of mania. A few patients require multiple combinations of mood stabilizers, an antipsychotic, and an antidepressant.

Length of maintenance treatment varies, from a few years, to lifelong where several recurrences have followed withdrawal. Withdrawal of lithium should always be slow, over 3 to 6 months, to avoid rebound mania. It is best to do the same for the anticonvulsants.

(d) Rapid cycling

Treatment of established rapid cycling may be difficult. It is important to avoid a cycling alternation of antidepressant and antimanic medication, following too late after mood changes. The patient should be established on mood stabilizers, usually in high dose and often more than one in combination. Antipsychotic may be added. Antidepressants are better avoided but may be needed in addition, used cautiously and with slow dose increase and an effort to establish a constant dose. Thyroid function should be checked initially and regularly.

(e) Pregnancy

Management in pregnancy is complicated by the risk of foetal malformations with lithium and anticonvulsants. These should be withdrawn for the first trimester. Antipsychotics and antidepressants may be used if necessary. Olanzapine may be appropriate but safety of newer antipsychotics and antidepressants is less well established than for older ones. In later pregnancy lithium and anticonvulsant mood stabilizers may need to be reinstituted. Medication should be withdrawn at the time of delivery to avoid effects on the foetus, but started again as soon as possible thereafter, as risks of relapse are increased postpartum.

Psychological treatments

(a) Acute treatment of mania

Psychotherapy has not been evaluated in manic patients and the evidence for benefit in bipolar disorders is for relapse reduction when delivered during euthymia. Access to therapy in most countries is limited and it is important to use clinical management, supportive therapy, and psychoeducational sessions as part of general treatment. Use should be made of systematic care packages to address psychosocial problems, to facilitate recognition of early warning symptoms of relapse, and to implement self-monitoring and self-management strategies.[59] Support should also include education about the disorder and treatment options, and help in adjusting to the diagnosis and should, if possible, include the patient's 'significant others'. About six sessions of family therapy may have beneficial effects extending beyond discharge.

Therapy with individuals with bipolar disorders can be challenging, requiring skilled and experienced therapists who also understand aetiology and pharmacology. There is a trend towards more cost-efficient group approaches, which allow individuals to observe the strengths and weaknesses of coping strategies employed by peers. However, a key study of group psychoeducation found benefits only with a structured group with a coherent treatment plan and not with unstructured groups without expert professional leadership.

The therapies currently found effective to treat acute bipolar depressive episodes or to reduce the risk of future relapse in RCTs do not differ markedly in either their overall efficacy or their core content. They incorporate four key components: psychoeducation and adjustment to the disorder, lifestyle regularity and 'harm reduction' (reducing substance misuse), enhancing medication adherence, and developing self-management skills to reduce the risk of relapse by recognizing potential triggers or prodromal signs or symptoms.

There are no consistent predictors of therapy response. There is some consensus that patients with Axis I or II comorbidity, particularly substance misuse or borderline personality disorder will benefit from an extended course of therapy. Likewise, where there have been many previous episodes of bipolar disorder, patients are unlikely to be able to assimilate and implement all the problem-solving and coping strategies being offered, in a time-limited therapy. Even where therapy does not clearly reduce relapse, many recipients value the opportunity to discuss their problems in detail, reporting improved quality of life and social functioning. Clinically, if the goal is relapse prevention, it may be appropriate to particularly target for therapy those individuals at an earlier stage of their 'bipolar career', whom evidence suggests may benefit more.[(43)]

Longer-term treatment of bipolar disorders

Supportive or other psychological therapies may extend over considerable periods of time. People with affective disorders also form 15 to 20 per cent of the long-stay patient populations of United Kingdom and United States mental hospitals. Rehabilitation techniques, as applied to schizophrenia and other severe mental disorders, are important for instilling hope and developing day-to-day living skills in people with chronic or recurrent affective disorders. Lastly, individuals with chronic health problems are at high risk of non-adherence with medication. There is an important role for psychotherapy in enhancing the acceptance of long-term medication[(23,62)] and there is emerging evidence that psychological interventions targeted directly or indirectly at enhancing medication adherence can have a beneficial impact on outcome in bipolar disorders.

Further information

Beck, A.T. (2005). The current state of cognitive therapy: a 40-year retrospective. *Archives of General Psychiatry*, **62**, 953–9.

Canadian Psychiatric Association and the CANMAT Depression Work Group. (2001). Clinical practice guidelines for the treatment of depressive disorders. *Canadian Journal of Psychiatry*, **46**(Suppl. 1), 5S–90S.

NICE. (2004). *Depression. Management of depression in primary and secondary care.* NICE Clinical Guideline 23 National Institute for Clinical Excellence, London.

NICE. (2006). *Bipolar disorder. The management of bipolar disorder in adults, children and adolescents, in primary and secondary care.* NICE Clinical Guideline 38 National Institute for Health and Clinical Excellence, London.

Stein, D.J., Lerer, B., and Stahl, M. (2005). *Evidence based psychopharmacology*. Cambridge University Press, Cambridge.

Weissman, M.M., Markowitz, J.C., and Klerman, G.L. (2000). *Comprehensive guide to interpersonal psychotherapy.* Basic Books, New York.

References

1. De Lima, M.S., Hotopf, M., and Wessely, S. (1999). The efficacy of drug treatments for dysthymia: a systematic review and meta-analysis. *Psychological Medicine*, **29**, 1273–89.
2. Wilson, K., Mottram, P., Sivanranthan, A., *et al.* (2001). Antidepressants versus placebo for the depressed elderly. *Cochrane Database of Systematic Reviews*, (1). CD000561. DOl: 1O.1002/14651858.CD000561.
3. Smith, D., Dempster, C., Glanville, J., *et al.* (2002). Efficacy and tolerability of venlafaxine compared with selective serotonin reuptake inhibitors and other antidepressants: a meta-analysis. *The British Journal of Psychiatry*, **180**, 396–404.
4. Hudson, L.L., Wohlreich, M.M., Kajdasz, D.K., *et al.* (2005). Safety and tolerability of duloxetine in the treatment of major depressive disorder: analysis of pooled data from eight placebo-controlled clinical trials. *Human Psychopharmacology*, **20**, 327–41.
5. MacGillivray, S., Arroll, B., Hatcher, S., *et al.* (2003). Efficacy and tolerability of selective serotonin reuptake inhibitors compared with tricyclic antidepressants in depression treated in primary care: systematic review and meta-analysis. *British Medical Journal*, **326**, 1014.
6. Goldney, R.D. (2006). Suicide and antidepressants: what is the evidence? *The Australian and New Zealand Journal of Psychiatry*, **40**, 381–5.
7. Schatzberg, A.F. (2000). Clinical efficacy of reboxetine in major depression. *The Journal of Clinical Psychiatry*, **61**(Suppl. 10), 31–8.
8. Paykel, E.S. (1990). Monoamine oxidase inhibitors: when should they be used. In *Dilemmas and difficulties in the management of psychiatric patients* (eds. K. Hawton and P. Cowen), pp. 17–30. Oxford University Press, Oxford.
9. Paykel, E.S. (1995). Clinical efficacy of reversible and selective inhibitors of monoamine oxidase A in major depression. *Acta Psychiatrica Scandinavica*, **91**(Suppl. 386), 22–7.
10. Anttila, S.A. and Leinonen, E.V. (2001). A review of the pharmacological and clinical profile of mirtazapine. *CNS Drug Reviews*, **7**, 249–64.
11. Norman, T.R. (2006). Prospects for the treatment of depression. *The Australian and New Zealand Journal of Psychiatry*, **40**, 394–401.
12. The UK ECT Review Group. (2003). Efficacy and safety of electroconvulsive therapy in depressive disorders: a systematic review and meta-analysis. *Lancet*, **361**, 799–808.
13. Tuunainen, A., Kripke, D.F., and Endo, T. (2004). Light therapy for non-seasonal depression. *Cochrane Database of Systematic Reviews*, (2). CD004050. DOl: 1O.1002/14651858.CD004050.pub2.
14. Nemeroff, C.B., Mayberg, H.S., Krahl, S.E., *et al.* (2006). VNS therapy in treatment-resistant depression: clinical evidence and putative neurobiological mechanisms. *Neuropsychopharmacology*, **31**, 1345–55.
15. Mayberg, H.S., Lozano, A.M., Voon, V., *et al.* (2005). Deep brain stimulation for treatment-resistant depression. *Neuron*, **45**, 651–60.
16. Paykel, E.S. (2001). Continuation and maintenance therapy in depression. *British Medical Bulletin*, **57**, 145–59.
17. Geddes, J.R., Carney, S.M., Davies, C., *et al.* (2003). Relapse prevention with antidepressant drug treatment in depressive disorders: a systematic review. *Lancet*, **361**, 653–61.
18. Reimherr, F.W., Amsterdam, I.D., Quitkin, F.M., *et al.* (1998). Optimal length of continuation therapy in depression: a prospective assessment during long-term fluoxetine treatment. *The American Journal of Psychiatry*, **155**, 1247–53.

19. Bauer, M., Bschor, T., Kunz, D., *et al.* (2000). Double-blind, placebo-controlled trial of the use of lithium to augment antidepressant medication in continuation treatment of unipolar major depression. *The American Journal of Psychiatry*, **157**, 1429–35.
20. Cipriani, A., Smith, K., Burgess, S., *et al.* (2006). Lithium versus antidepressants in the long-term treatment of urupolar affective disorder. *Cochrane Database of Systematic Reviews*, (4). CD003492. DOl: 10.1002/14651858. CD003492. pub2.
21. Gijsman, H.J., Geddes, J.R., Rendell, J.M., *et al.* (2004). Antidepressants for bipolar depression: a systematic review of randomized, controlled trials. *The American Journal of Psychiatry*, **161**, 1537–47.
22. Bowden, C.L. and Karren, N.U. (2006). Anticonvulsants in bipolar disorder. *The Australian and New Zealand Journal of Psychiatry*, **40**, 386–93.
23. Goodwin, F.K. and Jamison, K.R. (2007). *Manic depressive illness. Bipolar Disorders and Recurrent Depression* (2nd edition). Oxford University Press, New York.
24. Jones, R.M., Thompson, C., and Bitter, I. (2006). A systematic review of the efficacy and safety of second generation antipsychotics in the treatment of mania. *European Psychiatry*, **21**, 1–9.
25. Geddes, J.R., Burgess, S., Hawton, K., *et al.* (2004). Long-term lithium therapy for bipolar disorder: systematic review and meta-analysis of randomized controlled trials. *The American Journal of Psychiatry*, **161**, 217–22.
26. Baldessarini, R.J., Tondo, L., Floris, G., *et al.* (1997). Reduced morbidity after gradual discontinuation of lithium treatment for bipolar I and II disorders: a replication study. *The American Journal of Psychiatry*, **154**, 551–3.
27. Keller, M.B., Lavori, P.W., Kane, I.M., *et al.* (1992). Subsyndromal symptoms in bipolar disorder: a comparison of standard andlow serum levels of lithium. *Archives of General Psychiatry*, **49**, 371–6.
28. Chambless, D.L. and Hollon, S.D. (1998). Defining empirically supported therapies. *Journal of Consulting and Clinical Psychology*, **66**, 7–18.
29. Agency for Health Care Policy and Research. (1993). Depression Guideline Panel. *Depression in primary care: treatment of major depression*, Vol. **2**. Clinical Practice Guideline Number 5. USDHHS, Public Health Service, Rockville, MD.
30. Churchill, R., Hunot, V., Comey, R., *et al.* (2001). A systematic review of controlled trials of the effectiveness and cost-effectiveness of brief psychological therapies in depression. *Health Technology Assessment*, **5**, No 35. Southampton: HTA.
31. Elkin, I., Shea, M., Watkins, J., *et al.* (1992). National Institute of Mental Health treatment of depression collaborative treatment programme. *Archives of General Psychiatry*, **46**, 971–82.
32. DeRubeis, R., Hollon, S., Amsterdam, J., *et al.* (2005). Cognitive therapy v medication in the treatment of moderate to severe depression. *Archives of General Psychiatry*, **62**, 409–16.
33. Weissman, M. (2007). Recent non-medication trials of interpersonal psychotherapy for depression. *International Journal of Neuropsychopharmacology*, **10**, 117–22.
34. Clarkin, J, Glick, I, Haas, G., *et al.* (1990). A randomized clinical trial of inpatient family intervention: results for affective disorder. *Journal of Affective Disorder*, **18**, 17–28.
35. Depression Guideline Panel. (1993). *Clinical practice guideline No 5: depression in primary care. Treatment of major depression*, Vol 2, pp. 71–123. US Department of Health and Human Services, AHCPR Publications, Rockville, MD.
36. Keller, M.B., McCullough, J.P., Klein, D.N., *et al.* (2000). A comparison of nefazodone, the cognitive behavioral-analysis system of psychotherapy, and their combination for the treatment of chronic depression. *The New England Journal of Medicine*, **342**, 1462–70.
37. Paykel, E.S. (2007). Cognitive therapy in relapse prevention in depression. *The International Journal of Neuropsychopharmacology*, **10**, 131–6.
38. Frank, E., Kupfer, D., Perel, J., *et al.* (1990). Three year outcomes for maintenance therapies in recurrent depressions. *Archives of General Psychiatry*, **47**, 1093–9.
39. Paykel, E.S., Scott, J., Cornwall, P.L., *et al.* (2005). Duration of relapse prevention after cognitive therapy in residual depression: a follow-up of controlled trial. *Psychological Medicine*, **35**, 59–68.
40. Fava, G.A., Ruini, C., Rafanelli, C., *et al.* (2004). Six-year outcome of cognitive behavior therapy for prevention of recurrent depression. *The American Journal of Psychiatry*, **161**, 1872–6.
41. Scott, J. and Gutierrez, M.J. (2004). The current status of psychological treatments for bipolar disorders: a systematic review of relapse prevention. *Bipolar Disorders*, **6**, 498–503.
42. Scott, J., Colom, F., and Vieta, E. (2006). A meta-analysis of relapse rates with adjunctive psychological therapies compared to usual psychiatric treatment for bipolar disorders. *The International Journal of Neuropsychopharmacology*, **9**, 1–7.
43. Scott, J., Paykel, E., Morriss, R., *et al.* (2006). Cognitive behavioural therapy for severe and recurrent bipolar disorders: randomised controlled trial. *The British Journal of Psychiatry*, **188**, 313–20.
44. Frank, E., Kupfer, D.J., Thase, M.E., *et al.* (2005). Two-year outcomes for interpersonal and social rhythm therapy in individuals with bipolar I disorder. *Archives of General Psychiatry*, **62**, 996–1004.
45. NICE. (2004). *Depression. Management of depression in primary and secondary care.* NICE Clinical Guideline 23 National Institute for Clinical Excellence, London.
46. Canadian Psychiatric Association and Canadian Network for Mood and Anxiety Treatments (CANMAT). (2001). Clinical guidelines for the treatment of depressive disorders. *Canadian Journal of Psychiatry*, **46**(Suppl. 1), 5S–90S.
47. Paykel, E.S., Hollyman, J.A., Freeling, P., *et al.* (1988). Predictors of therapeutic benefit from amitriptyline in mild depression: a general practice placebo-controlled trial. *Journal of Affective Disorders*, **14**, 83–95.
48. Judd, L.L., Rapaport, M.H., Yonkers, K.A., *et al.* (2004). Randomized, placebo-controlled trial of fluoxetine for acute treatment of minor depressive disorder. *The American Journal of Psychiatry*,**161**, 1864–71.
49. Valenstein, M. (2006). Keeping our eyes on STAR*D. *The American Journal of Psychiatry*, **163**, 1484–6.
50. Wijkstra, J., Lijmer, J., Balk, F.J., *et al.* (2006). Pharmacological treatment for unipolar psychotic depression: systematic review and meta-analysis. *The British Journal of Psychiatry*, **188**, 410–5.
51. Hazell, P., O'Connell, D., Heathcote, D., *et al.* (2002). Tricyclic drugs for depression in children and adolescents. *Cochrane Database of Systematic* Reviews, (2). CD002317. DOl: 1O.1002/14651858. CD002317.
52. Whittington, C.J., Kendall, T., Fonagy, P., *et al.* (2004). Selective serotonin reuptake inhibitors in childhood depression: systematic review of published versus unpublished data. *Lancet*, **363**, 1341–5.
53. NICE. (2003). *Guidance on the use of electroconvulsive therapy*. Technology Appraisal 59 National Institute for Clinical Excellence, London.
54. Royal College of Psychiatrists. (1995). *Council report CR39: the ECT handbook. The second report of the Royal College of Psychiatrists special committee on ECT*. Royal College of Psychiatrists, London.
55. Bauer, M. and Dopfmer, S. (1999). Lithium augmentation in treatment-resistant depression: meta-analysis of placebo-controlled studies. *Journal of Clinical Psychopharmacology*, **19**, 427–34.
56. Aronson, R., Offman, H.J., Joffe, R.T., *et al.* (1996). Triiodothyronine augmentation in the treatment of refractory depression. A meta-analysis. *Archives of General Psychiatry*, **53**, 842–8.
57. Kennedy, N. and Paykel, E.S. (2004). Treatment and response in refractory depression: results from a specialist affective disorders service. *Journal of Affective Disorders*, **81**, 49–53.
58. Roth, T. and Fonagy, P. (1996). *What works for whom?* pp. 57–103. Guilford Press, London.
59. NICE. (2006). *Bipolar disorder. The management of bipolar disorder in adult: children and adolescents, in primary and secondary care.* NICE Clinical Guideline 38 National Institute for Health and Clinical Excellence, London.

60. Yatham, L.N., Kennedy, S.H., O'Donovan, C., *et al.* (2005). Canadian network for mood and anxiety treatments. Canadian Network for Mood and Anxiety Treatments (CANMAT) guidelines for the management of patients with bipolar disorder: consensus and controversies. *Bipolar Disorders*, **7**(Suppl. 3), 5–69.
61. American Psychiatric Association. (2002). *Practice guideline for the treatment of patients with bipolar disorder* (2nd edn). American Psychiatric Press, Washington.
62. Tacchi, M.J. and Scott, J. (2005). *Medication adherence in schizophrenia and bipolar disorders*, p. 110. John Wiley & Sons, London.

4.5.9 Dysthymia, cyclothymia, and hyperthymia

Hagop S. Akiskal

Subthreshold affective conditions, personality, and temperament

Long before psychiatry moved to the outpatient arena in the latter part of the twentieth century, psychiatrists had observed milder mood disturbances among the kin of patients hospitalized for endogenous or psychotic depressions or mania. Some were described as sullen, morose, or otherwise moody, without discrete episodes; others reported self-limited episodes, but often went untreated. With the advent of modern treatments, practitioners are being increasingly consulted by patients presenting with attenuated affective disturbances. Although the relationship of these ambulatory mood states and more classical severe affective disorders has not been resolved, there is emerging sleep electroencephalography (**EEG**) and familial-genetic evidence[1–3] that a continuum exists between them. Along the same lines, studies conducted in the United States and Germany[4,5] into what were once described as 'neurotic' depressions have revealed a progression to more endogenous, psychotic, or bipolar switching. For these and related reasons, current official classification systems such as the ICD-10 and DSM-IV, have dropped the neurotic-endogenous dichotomy. Sceptics would perhaps argue that the new categorization of depressive disorders into dysthymic and major subtypes is not much of an improvement. Nonetheless, the new terminology has drawn attention to a large universe of human suffering that had been neglected in the past, and the conceptualization of dysthymia as a variant of mood disorder has had a far-reaching impact on diagnostic and therapeutic habits of clinicians worldwide.[6] The emerging concept of the bipolar spectrum, which does include manic, cyclic depressive (bipolar II), cyclothymic, hyperthymic and related conditions, is beginning to have a similar impact on practice.[7]

The subthreshold mood disorders are not only in continuum with more pathological mood states, but they also provide a bridge with normal affective conditions. In this context, temperament, as a construct encompassing affective personalities, is currently enjoying a renaissance as one of the possible substrates for the origin of mood disorders. Temperament classically refers to an adaptive mixture of traits which, in the extreme, can lead to illness or modify the expression of superimposed affective states. The subthreshold conditions covered in this chapter represent the extreme expressions of these temperaments. A new self-administered instrument, the TEMPS-A,[8] now validated in 10 language versions, is being used internationally to measure the classical constructs of depressive, cyclothymic, hyperthymic, and irritable, as well as anxious temperaments.

In the current literature, various terms such as 'minor affective states', 'intermittent depression', 'hysteroid dysphoria', and 'atypical depression' are often used for subthreshold disorders.[9] These terms are avoided here, because in contemporary practice these conditions are at least as 'typical' as major mood disorders: their impact on the sufferer is not time-limited, nor minor, and involves more than a state of demoralization and moral foible. The following passage from Sir Aubrey Lewis[10] is *à propos*:

> . . . Severe emotional upsets ordinarily tend to subside, but mild emotional states . . . tend to persist, as it were, autonomously. Hence the paradox that a gross blatant psychosis may do less damage in the long run than some meager neurotic incubus: a dramatic attack of mania or melancholia, with delusions, wasting, hallucinations, wild excitement may have far less effect on the course of man's life than some deceptively mild affective illness which goes on so long that it becomes inveterate. The former comes as a catastrophe and when it has passed the patient takes up his life again . . . while with the latter he may never get rid of his burden.

It is a curious fact that most subthreshold affective conditions, while symptomatologically attenuated, tend to pursue a chronic course. This raises the question, partially addressed in this chapter, whether these conditions in their trait expressions might serve some useful function, even as they burden the individual with cares and instability which could predispose to full-blown affective disease. By their very chronicity, these subaffective conditions pose difficult conceptual and clinical questions about their differentiation from personality disorders.[11] Sceptics might argue that subthreshold affective conditions are nothing more than personality disorders and/or expressions of 'neuroticism'. Actually, a close examination of the Eysenck personality inventory, which ranges over a large terrain of depressiveness, anxiousness, emotionality, and mood lability among others, reveals low-grade intermittent affective symptomatology.[12] And at least one genetic investigation has reported that neuroticism and major depression in women share substantial genetic underpinnings.[13] Nonetheless, clinicians have always preferred categorical constructs, because neuroticism and related personality constructs do not do justice to the rich clinical phenomenology of disorders within the subaffective realm. I finally wish to point out that terms like 'neurotic', 'psychopathic', or 'personality disorder' used as epithets to describe a person have pejorative connotations. They tend to describe what is negative about someone, whereas 'temperament' refers to the optimum mixture of both liabilities and assets regarding a human being, thereby rendering therapeutic work possible with relatively little countertransference. This is particularly relevant when we consider the distinct possibility that the many dysthymic and cyclothymic individuals might otherwise be labeled 'borderline.'[11]

The dysthymic spectrum

History

The term 'dysthymia' (meaning 'bad mood') originated in classical Greek and is still in current use in that country with the same connotation.

In the Hippocratic School, it was considered as part of the broader concept of melancholia (meaning 'black bile'). A temperament predisposed to melancholia was also delineated, and referred to individuals who were lethargic, brooding, and insecure. It was not until the early nineteenth century that dysthymia was reintroduced into medicine by the German physicians, Stark and Fleming to describe depressions in inpatients that pursued a chronic course.[14] Eventually, dysthymia came to subsume all mood disorders. The major residue of dysthymia in the latter sense in Europe today is the French rubric of *les dysthymies*, as a synonym for *troubles de l'humeur*; the DSM-IV or ICD-10 'dysthymic disorder' in that country is translated as *le trouble dysthymique*.

The more direct lineage of our current usage of the term dysthymia is to be found in the latter part of the nineteenth century in the work of Kraepelin, who delineated the depressive disposition as one of the constitutional foundations of affective episodes. The condition often began early in life, such that by adolescence many showed an increased sensitivity to life's sorrows and disappointments: they were tormented by guilt, had little confidence in their abilities, and suffered from low energy. As they grew into adulthood, they experienced 'life with its activity [as] a burden which they habitually [bore] with dutiful self-denial without being compensated by the pleasures of existence'. In some, these temperamental peculiarities were so marked that they could be considered 'morbid without the appearance of more severe, delimited attacks . . .' (clearly foreshadowing the modern concept of trait dysthymia). In other cases, recurrent melancholia arose from this substrate without definite boundaries (again anticipating the concept of 'double-depression').

Subsequently, Kurt Schneider in his opus *Psychopathic Personalities* devoted considerable space to a depressive type whose entire existence was entrenched in suffering. Building on this rich phenomenological tradition, our research in Memphis[15] helped in operationalizing the core characteristics of such patients encountered in contemporary practice: gloomy, sombre, and incapable of having fun; brooding, self-critical, and guilt-prone; lack of confidence, low self-esteem, preoccupation with failure; pessimistic, easily discouraged; easy to tire, sluggish, and bound to routine; non-assertive, self-denying, and devoted; shy and sensitive. These traits have excellent internal consistency and discriminatory ability.[16] Similar concepts have also appeared in the Japanese literature,[17] with particular emphasis on self-critical attitudes, persistence in work habits, and devotion to others. Finally, the French construct of *la depression constitutionelle*[18] has emphasized the lethargic aspects with a sense of inadequacy. A self-rated scale in all of these languages[8] now can assist in reliable and valid assessment of depressive temperament traits.

The classical tenet in psychiatry has been that affectively ill patients recover from their acute episodes with relatively little symptomatic residua and dysfunction. Community psychiatry, which has given renewed visibility to the temperamentally expressed low-grade fluctuating depressive disorders, has challenged this classic view. With the advent of DSM-III, such patients are now officially designated as 'dysthymic.' In the ICD-10 classification, the low-grade depressive baseline is considered the main pathology; only an occasional superimposed depressive episode is permitted, provided that it is mild. In DSM-IV, at least two patterns have been described: pure dysthymia uncomplicated by major depression and a more prevalent pattern of dysthymia complicated by major depressive episodes that could be even moderate or severe in intensity (and which has been dubbed 'double depression').

The mystery of this incapacitating depressive subtype—long recognized, but only recently sanctioned in official diagnostic manuals—is that, in their habitual condition, sufferers lack the classical 'objective' or 'major' signs of acute clinical depression, such as profound changes in psychomotor and vegetative functions. Instead, patients consult their doctors for more fluctuating complaints consisting of gloominess, lethargy, self-doubt, and lack of *joie de vivre*; they typically work hard, but do not enjoy their work; if married, they are deadlocked in bitter and unhappy marriages which lead neither to reconciliation nor separation; for them, their entire existence is a burden: they are satisfied with nothing, complain of everything, and brood about the uselessness of existence. As a result, in the past those who could afford it were condemned to the couch for what often proved to be interminable analysis. The legitimization of dysthymia as a clinically significant variant of affective disorder in both the United States and WHO classifications has helped the cause of more cost-effective treatments.

To sum up, for nearly 2500 years physicians have described individuals with a low-grade chronic depressive profile marked by gloominess, pessimism, low enjoyment of life, relatively low drive, yet endowed with self-critical attitudes and suffering for others.[19] This constellation is as much a virtue as it is a disposition to melancholy, and many dysthymic patients presenting clinically have various admixtures of major depression. This is compatible with a spectrum-concept of depressive illness, which defines various degrees of severity.

Clinical picture and diagnostic considerations[20]*

Diagnostic criteria for dysthymia in both DSM-IV and ICD-10 stipulate a two-year duration of low-grade depressive symptoms, exclusive of such indicators of severity as suicidality and psychomotor disturbances. Dysthymia is distinguished from chronic major depressive disorder by the fact that it is not a sequel to well-defined major depressive episodes. Instead, patients often complain that they have always been depressed. Most are of early onset (less than 20 years). A late-onset subtype first manifesting after the age of 50 is much less prevalent and has not been well characterized clinically, but it has been identified largely through studies in the community.

At their best, dysthymic individuals invest whatever energy they have in work, leaving none for leisure or social activities. According to Tellenbach, such dedication to work represents overcompensation against depressive disorganization. Kretschmer had earlier suggested that such persons were the 'backbone of society,' devoting their lives to jobs that require dependability and great attention to detail. These features represent the obsessoid facet of dysthymia. Such individuals may seek outpatient counseling and psychotherapy for what some clinicians might consider 'existential depression': individuals who complain that their life lacks lustre, joy, and meaning. Others present clinically because of an intensification of their gloom to the level of clinical depression; history of lifelong low-

* Unless otherwise specified, in the remainder of this chapter, references to concepts, historical developments, and research covering dysthymia and cyclothymia through the year 2000 can be found in this centenary review of Kraepelinian psychiatry.[20]

grade depressive symptoms would distinguish them from episodic major depressive patients.

The proverbial dysthymic patient will often complain of having been 'depressed since birth'. In the eloquent words of Kurt Schneider, "they view themselves as belonging to an 'aristocracy of suffering". These hyperbolic descriptions of suffering in the absence of more objective signs of depression earn such patients the label of 'characterological depression'. The description is further reinforced by the fluctuating depressive picture that merges imperceptibly with the patient's habitual self, leading to the customary clinical uncertainty as to whether dysthymic disorder belongs to the affective or personality disorder domains.

At their worst, patients with low-grade depression having an intermittent course can present such instability in their life, including suicidal crises, that some clinicians would entertain the diagnosis of borderline personality disorder. This is not consistent with the classic picture of dysthymia arising from a temperamental type with more mature ego structure described above. Depressives with unstable (that is to say, 'borderline') personality structure more often belong to the irritable cyclothymic–bipolar II spectrum.

The greatest overlap of dysthymia is with major depressive disorder, but differs from it in that symptoms tend to outnumber signs (more subjective than objective depression). Thus, marked disturbances in appetite and libido are uncharacteristic, and psychomotor agitation or retardation is not observed. Nonetheless, subtle 'endogenous' features are not uncommonly reported: inertia, lethargy, and anhedonia that are characteristically worse in the morning. Because many patients with dysthymia presenting clinically fluctuate in and out of a major depression, the core DSM-IV criteria for dysthymia tend to emphasize vegetative dysfunction, whereas the alternative criterion B for dysthymia in a DSM-IV appendix lists cognitive symptoms; although the latter appear more characteristic of trait dysthymia, the DSM-IV field trial could not demonstrate their specificity for dysthymia.

A Milan-San Diego collaboration of a large sample from community and primary-care medical settings revealed that negative mood (by definition), along with low energy, poor concentration, low self-esteem, sleep and appetite disturbance, and hopelessness (in descending order) were the most common symptoms of dysthymia. These data suggest that the cognitive and somatic symptoms are not easily separable in practice. None the less, this study did raise the possibility that factors could be discerned along two different axes: 'negative affectivity' and 'lassitude with poor concentration'. In our experience, patients loading on the latter factor often complain of hypersomnia and may exhibit subtle bipolar signs; alternatively, they might have some link to the poorly defined constructs of neurasthenia, chronic fatigue syndrome, and fibromyalgia. In terms of differential diagnosis, patients with chronic fatigue syndrome present with disabling fatigue and, typically, deny depressive symptoms; patients with fibromyalgia complain of pain; by contrast, the typical patient with dysthymia cannot stop relating to the physician his or her litany of depressive symptoms. Polysomnography, though not yet definitive, may shed some light on differentiating fibromyalgia from dysthymia proper.

Although dysthymic disorder represents a more restricted concept than does its parent, neurotic depression, it is still quite heterogeneous. Anxiety is not a necessary part of its clinical picture, yet dysthymia is sometimes diagnosed in patients with anxiety and neurotic disorders. That clinical situation is perhaps to be regarded as a secondary or 'anxious dysthymia' or, as some British authors seem to prefer, as part of a 'general neurotic syndrome' (an implicit partial return to the now defunct concept of neurotic depression).

Table 4.5.9.1 The core characteristics of dysthymia

Long-standing subthreshold depression of a fluctuating or persistent nature
Gloomy and joyless disposition
Brooding about the past and guilt prone
Low drive and lethargy
Low self-esteem and preoccupation with failure
Identifies suffering as part of the habitual self

Summarized from Akiskal.[19]

The clinical picture of dysthymic disorder that emerges from the foregoing descriptions is quite varied, with many who fluctuate in and out of major depression, whereas in others the pathology is woven into the habitual self. Prospective follow-up supports a continuum between temperament, dysthymia and major depression. These considerations suggest that a clinically satisfactory operationalization of dysthymia must include both symptoms and trait characteristics (Table 4.5.9.1). The following vignette illustrates this more prototypical form of dysthymic suffering.

Case Study: This 37-year-old never-married male teacher presented with the complaint that he was 'tired of living' and was considering 'ending it all'. He said that much of his life had been 'wasted', he had never known any joy, and that all human existence for him was a 'tragic mistake of God'. He was known to be a dedicated and talented teacher, but he felt all his efforts had been 'useless and in vain'. He said he probably was 'born depressed', because he had not known any happiness and that the only utility he could have for mankind was 'to serve as a specimen to be researched—to shed light on human misery'. Although he conceded that some women found him interesting, even intellectually stimulating, he said he could not enjoy physical intimacy, that even orgasm lacked passion; nonetheless, he masturbated frequently, fantasizing about married female teachers—only to feel guilty. We could not document any major affective episodes. He stated that he had always functioned at a 'mediocre level' (which was at variance with the good feedback students had given him year after year); but did admit he 'appreciated work, because there was nothing else to do'. He denied alcohol and drug habits. There had never been any periods of hypomania, but one of his maternal aunts had been treated for a 'cyclical depression' and was apparently doing well on lithium. The patient's mother was a sombre serious work-oriented woman who had raised three children and had done voluntary work for the church, but had no depressive complaints. His father had died from a coronary attack, but his side of the family was otherwise unremarkable.

Although both DSM-IV and ICD-10 omit suicidal preoccupations in their diagnostic criteria for dysthymia, as testified by the above case, this is what often brings patients to clinical attention.

Course[20]

An insidious onset of depression dating back to late childhood or the teens, preceding any superimposed major depressive episodes by years, even decades, is the most typical developmental

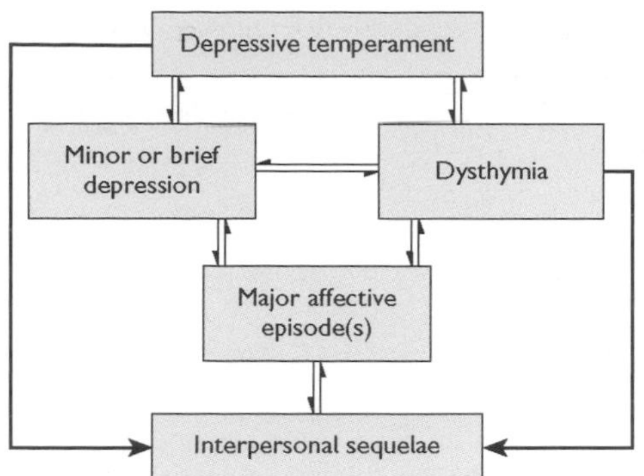

Fig. 4.5.9.1 Diagram to show putative relationships within a broad depressive spectrum.

background of dysthymic disorder. A return to the low-grade depressive pattern is the rule following recovery from superimposed major depressive episodes, if any, hence the designation 'double depression'.

Few studies have studied the phenomenology of dysthymia in childhood. DSM-IV does not seem to distinguish between childhood and adult dysthymia, yet current clinical experience indicates that the main symptoms in childhood dysthymia include irritability, low self esteem, fatigue, low mood, guilt, poor concentration, anhedonia, and hopelessness; as in adults, comorbid anxiety disorders were prevalent; suicidality was more common in adolescents. These findings should be useful in dysthymic children in future studies. A long-term prospective Pittsburgh study of prepubertal children has revealed an episodic course of dysthymia with remissions and exacerbations, and eventual complication by major depressive episodes, as well as hypomanic, manic, or mixed episodes postpubertally. Persons with dysthymic disorder presenting clinically as adults tend to pursue a chronic 'unipolar' course, which may or may not be complicated by major depression: they rarely develop spontaneous hypomania or mania. However, when treated with antidepressants, some adult patients with dysthymia may experience brief hypomanic switches that typically disappear when the antidepressant dose is decreased. Although ICD-10 and DSM-IV would not 'allow' the occurrence of such switches in dysthymia, systematic clinical observation have verified their occurrence in between 10 and 30 per cent of dysthymic patients. In that special dysthymic subgroup, the family histories are typically positive for bipolar disorder. Such patients, often conforming to the double depressive pattern, represent a clinical bridge between major depressive disorder and bipolar II.

A 12-year NIMH prospective study has shown that patients with major depressive disorder spent 44 per cent of their course in low-grade depression (versus 15 per cent of time in major depressive episodes). This suggests that major depression, dysthymia, or otherwise subsyndromal depression constitute somewhat artificial conventions on the threshold and duration of depressive illness, representing alternative manifestations of the same diathesis. In this context, residual intermorbid depressive symptoms have been confirmed as being strongly predictive of a rapid relapse into a new major depressive episode. Various 'major' and 'minor' depressive conditions described in DSM-IV and its appendix must not be viewed as distinct depressive subtypes, but part of a symptomatic continuum. Fig. 4.5.9.1 shows a diagram of these putative relationships within a broad depressive spectrum.

Epidemiology[20]

From 1966 to 1980, *Index Medicus* listed no more than 10 articles on chronic depressions. Since 1980, when dysthymia was first introduced in DSM-III, at least 500 articles have appeared on chronic depression, mostly on dysthymia. This phenomenal growth in research interest parallels the increasing public health significance of this disorder. It is estimated that 3–5 per cent of the world population is suffering from dysthymia. Like major depressive disorders, dysthymia is twice as common in women as in men. Because of its chronicity, dysthymia is among the most prevalent psychiatric conditions in clinical practice. Dysthymia is more disabling, as far as quality of life in social and personal areas, work, and leisure, than depression in the setting of a severe anxiety disorder like agoraphobia. Celibacy is also common in early-onset dysthymia, but not for long; modern successful treatments often lead to a change in marital status!

UCLA research in primary care has focused on depressive symptoms falling short of the major depressive threshold, as far as symptom intensity is concerned, as well as falling short of the two year duration criterion for dysthymia. Despite its chronicity, 50 per cent of people remain unrecognized by general practitioners. Despite the low-grade nature of their depressive complaints, these patients report high degrees of morbidity and impairment in a variety of health domains and quality of life, including 'bed days' (namely, the number of days per year they stayed ill in bed). Actually, these impairments are generally more pronounced than those of patients with a variety of medical conditions, such as hypertension, diabetes, arthritis, and chronic lung disease; only coronary artery disease exceeded the disability of low-grade depression in several domains. Stroke has recently been added on this list.

In light of the foregoing developments, both the World Psychiatric Association[21] and the World Health Organization[22] have developed programmes to address the challenges of educating general practitioners in the proper recognition and treatment of dysthymia.

Aetiological considerations[20]

Some sensitivity to suffering, a cardinal feature of the depressive temperament, represents an important attribute in a species like ours, where caring for young and sick individuals is necessary for survival. This temperament, historically the *Anlage* of dysthymia, in the extreme often leads to clinical depression. The constitutional viewpoint, while dominant in the early part of the twentieth century, gradually disappeared from psychiatric thinking. One reason was that Kurt Schneider preferred to conceptualize such conditions as 'psychopathy', by which he meant abnormal personality development. Independently, Freud's disciples took this one step further and, eventually in outpatients, all milder depressions with a tendency to chronicity came to be considered as the expressions of a character neurosis. In support for this position, these authors could point to the long-standing nature of the interpersonal difficulties in the lives of these individuals. When, and if, antidepressants were prescribed, they were given in homeopathic doses; worse, many patients received stimulants or benzodiazepines rather than genuine antidepressants. Failure to respond to these incorrectly chosen pharmaceutical agents seemed to further reinforce the notion of a 'character' defect.

Several lines of observation during the latter part of the 20th century have challenged the concept of 'character neurosis' as an explanation for low-grade depression, and thereby forced a return to the more classical European concept of temperament with its biological underpinnings. First, in a 1980 Memphis study of rapid eye movement (REM) latency (normally 90 min, measured from sleep onset to the first REM period) conducted in 'depressive characters' who were not in a state of major depression, we reported that REM latency was less than 60 min, and REM was redistributed to the early part of the night (which was the reverse of what we observed in chronic anxious patients). Moreover, a family history for major affective illness (including bipolar) was significantly high in short-REM latency patients. (The reverse was true for those with familial alcoholism and sociopathy.) The sleep findings were so reminiscent of those seen in major affective illness that we were compelled to give our patients systematic open trials with desipramine and nortriptyline (the best-tolerated secondary amine tricyclics in those days) or lithium carbonate if antidepressants failed (based on the observation of familial bipolar disorder in some). Nearly 40 per cent remitted, of whom one out of three developed brief hypomania. The sleep findings have been replicated in other laboratories. Furthermore, a Hungarian study has shown that patients with dysthymia experience transient lifting of their mood with sleep deprivation. Other studies have shown high rates of affective illness in a systematic familial investigation of dysthymic probands. There also exist dysthymic patients whose lifelong suffering and discontent appear, in retrospect, a legacy of an unsatisfactory childhood marked by deprivation or abuse at the hands of alcoholic and/or sociopathic parents or step-parents. Although it is clinically attractive to invoke the notion of 'learned helplessness' secondary to such inescapable childhood traumata, an alternative hypothesis is that the helplessness of these individuals might develop secondary to an inherited diathesis which biases these children's early experiences in a dysphoric direction.

As for neuroendocrine markers, thyroid-releasing hormone-thyroid-stimulating hormone challenge and electrodermal activity similar to those with major depressive disorders are the main findings; by contrast, dexamethasone suppression and catecholamine metabolism are essentially unaltered in dysthymia. These observations, along with the REM latency findings, suggest that dysthymia represents trait depression. Coupled with the family history data, this traitness can be postulated to be of constitutional origin. Certainly, the occurrence of major affective episodes in the long-term course of dysthymia, in both community and clinical samples, is in line with this position. It is, therefore, of great theoretical and practical significance that shortened REM latency has been reported in the offspring of the affectively ill. More recently a variety of other biological findings have been reported in dysthymia, further strengthening the link with major depression: low testosterone and adrenal-gonadal steroid levels,[24] neuro-immune abnormalities,[25] effects of prenatal maternal dysthymia on foetal growth,[26] as well as small genual corpus callosum volume[27] and enlarged amygdalar volume.[28] Coupled with s-allele polymorphism of the serotonin transmitter,[29,30] that subthreshold depression, however defined, is not a 'neurotic' phenomenon in the traditional psychodynamic sense of the term, but part of the spectrum of depressive illness! Table 4.5.9.2 summarizes the foregoing links between dysthymia and major depressive disorder, and which support its inclusion within the family of mood disorders.

Table 4.5.9.2 Evidence for considering dysthymia as a variant of major depressive disorder

Familial affective loading
Phase advance of rapid eye-movement sleep
Diurnality of inertia, gloominess, and anhedonia
Thyroid-releasing hormone-thyroid-stimulating hormone challenge test abnormalities
Low testosterone
Lowered interlukin-1-beta production
Amydalar enlargement
s-allele in serotonin transporter gene
Prospective course complicated by recurrent major depressive episodes
Positive response to selected thymoleptics
Treatment-emergent hypomania

Updated from Akiskal.[19]

There are also exist medical and neurological factors that may contribute to dysthymic symptom formation. Actually, joint medical-neurological and non-affective psychiatric disease is often contributory to extreme refractoriness among the chronic depressive states of these patients. Such patients are at risk for suicide, especially those with epilepsy or progressive degenerative neurological disease. Interestingly, living with a medically disabled spouse or family member, too, can be associated with some chronicity of depression.

The emergence of pathogenetic understanding, as outlined above, is all the more impressive, given the controversies on the very nature of dysthymia and its legitimacy as a nosological entity.[31]

Treatment[20]

The trait nature of dysthymia can be further observed in the fact that dysthymia often pursues an unrelenting course towards chronicity. Thus, spontaneous recovery has been shown to occur in no more than 13 per cent of subjects in the community over 1 year. In outpatient clinics, the outcome is somewhat better, but this is probably due to the treatment received and a longer follow-up.

Most classes of antidepressants have been shown to be effective in dysthymia in double-blind studies (Table 4.5.9.3). The rationale for using classic antidepressants such as tricyclic compounds in our mood clinic was our observation of shortened REM latency in

Table 4.5.9.3 Major controlled pharmacological trials in dysthymia worldwide*

Reference	Country	Medication
Vallejo *et al.* (1987)	Spain	Phenelzine versus imipramine
Kocsis *et al.* (1987)	USA	Imipramine versus placebo
Stewart *et al.* (1989)	USA	Phenelzine versus placebo
Thase *et al.* (1996)	USA	Sertraline versus imipramine
Vanelle *et al.* (1998)	France	Fluoxetine versus placebo
Lecrubier *et al.* (1996)	France	Amisulpride versus placebo
Versiani *et al.* (1997)	Brazil	Moclobemide versus imipramine

*Summarized from references[19,20]

dysthymic subjects in our sleep laboratory. Irreversible monoamine oxidase inhibitors such as phenalzine were used because of the belief that non-classical depressions respond preferentially to this class of drugs; the same can be said for the reversible inhibitors of type A monoamine oxidase. Amisulpride was tried, because it reverses 'negative' symptoms in schizophrenia and, by analogy, it was hypothesized that the low motivation and lethargy seen in some patients with dysthymia reflected a shared underlying dimensional transnosological pathology. The selective serotonin re-uptake inhibitors (SSRIs) were used empirically, because of good tolerance compared with the tricyclic antidepressants, and later it was suggested that improvement in dysthymia correlates with normalization of serotonergic indices. The foregoing trials, conducted in different countries during the past 12 years represent the most eloquent evidence for the increasing worldwide acceptance of the concept of dysthymia as a clinically significant variant of affective disorder.[21,22]

The treatment of dysthymia should continue in most cases for 2 years or more. Tricyclic antidepressants have too many side-effects in clinically effective doses (desipramine equivalent of 150 mg or more per day). Given dietary and medication prohibitions, monoamine oxidase inhibitors are also not practical as first-line drugs. Overall good tolerance in long-term use, despite sexual side-effects, has made the SSRIs first-line intervention treatment for dysthymia; given that many people with dysthymia are young individuals who should be eager to form families, their acceptance of long-term SSRI use is an indication that the alleviation of the depressive suffering of dysthymia is genuine and far outweighs the sexual dysfunction. However, 75 to 150 mg bupropion-SR can be taken in the morning on the desired day of sexual union, but preferably no more than once a week. Moclobemide also spares sexual function, but seems more effective in anxious and milder cases of dysthymia. Amisulpride, which rarely causes amenorrhoea and/or galactorrhoea, is otherwise well tolerated in dysthymia in the more lethargic forms of the illness seen in general medical practice.

The dosage of nearly all antidepressants in dysthymia is in the full range for that recommended for major depression (20–40 mg for fluoxetine). In the case of amisulpride, the dosage is low (25–50 mg), because at this dosage the drug is a dopamine agonist, believed to be the necessary ingredient for its mechanism of action in dysthymia. Both dysthymia and double depression respond equally well, and the duration of underlying dysthymia does not seem to matter. The main difference in treatment for these two course patterns is that dysthymia need not be treated for a lifetime, but double depression should probably be treated indefinitely. Women seem to have a preferentially better response to SSRIs, which have the added benefit of treating the premenstrual accentuation of dysthymic symptoms. Borderline thyroid function (e.g. a high baseline thyroid-stimulating hormone level) preferentially occurs in women with dysthymia, so that these women would benefit from thyroid augmentation (levothyroxine 175 mg/day) of the antidepressant. In those patients who oversleep in the morning, terminal sleep deprivation and/or morning phototherapy represent useful adjuncts to antidepressants. Although there are no controlled studies in children, our clinical experience indicates that SSRIs often prove effective in this population, with the appropriate dosage reduction for body-weight. In adults, concurrent personality disturbances (for instance, obsessoid, avoidant, dependent, and hostile features) do not compromise therapeutic responses. Indeed, more often than not, such personality disturbances recede with the successful alleviation of dysthymic suffering; social function improves in tandem. (However, extremely hostile patients, who may meet symptomatological criteria for 'dysthymia' but whose irritable dysphoria more appropriately belongs to the cyclothymic domain, are best managed with mood-stabilizing anticonvulsants, for example divalproex 600 to 1200 mg/day.)

In a Memphis study, we have shown that, with the judicious use of the foregoing modalities in private practice, three out of four patients with dysthymia engulfed in gloom for much of their lives had sustained remissions for five or more years. Depressive episodes *and* suicidal preoccupation and/or crises were prevented, in tandem with the alleviation of the dysthymia. Approximately 15 per cent experienced 'overcorrection' of their dysthymia in the direction of mild hypomania; this is particularly likely in the presence of inhibited-social phobic traits as part of dysthymia, and when the family history is bipolar. The hypomania is typically short-lived, and tends to disappear when the antidepressant dose is reduced; in some cases, it is necessary to provide lithium (600–900 mg/day) or valproate augmentation (500–750 mg/day). The question has been raised whether selective serotonin-reuptake inhibitors, in particular fluoxetine, change the personality in a hyperthymic direction. In our experience, most observed changes are compatible with adaptive behaviour that emerge as a result of alleviation of depressive suffering; the more distinctly protracted hypomanic changes nearly always require familial bipolar diathesis. It is, nonetheless, true that with SSRIs we have entered an era of 'dimensional psychopharmacology', whereby the clinician could dose the patient to a desired end from a functional standpoint. Many become care-less rather than careless. The present author has also encountered some patients treated with SSRIs who view a life without cares as negative; in such cases, one should opt for very low doses and a more gradual lifting of the dysthymia, and help the patient adjust to a new self-image of normalcy.

As for psychotherapy, there is little credible evidence for its efficacy as monotherapy in the treatment of dysthymia. Actually, some female mental health experts have argued that exploration of one's mental inadequacies, in the 'passive' psychoanalytical situation, is particularly negative for women; the more 'active' cognitive behavioural approaches, which encourage thinking, and behaviours reinforcing for the individual, are preferable. Many clinicians profitably use the latter strategy along with pharmacotherapy to boost the self-esteem of the patient. In a more practical vein, there are clinical management strategies that are specifically useful for both the patients and their clinicians (Table 4.5.9.4).

Table 4.5.9.4 Psychotherapeutic principles in dysthymia*

Provide a believable dose of optimism
Optimize compliance to pharmacotherapy
Limit destructive expression of negative feelings
Address accumulated conflicts
Combat postdepressive resignation and inertia
Provide support for patient and significant others
Be aware of countertransference feelings
Consult experts with extensive experience in treating chronic depression
Gradually mobilize patient's skills and resources

*Updated from Akiskal.[6]

It is particularly important for the clinician not to be submerged by the negative thinking of the patient, and it is even more crucial for the therapist to recognize that a relative lack of progress can generate feelings of 'impotence' and countertransference; periodic consultation with more experienced clinicians in the treatment of chronic depression would be desirable.

Interpersonal psychotherapy has been used in medication failures. This is best viewed as a more practical abbreviation of psychodynamic psychotherapy, with a strong emphasis on support and encouragement for patients with dysthymia who seek help at a time of loss or role transition in their lives. Knowledge of the interpersonal context of depression is obviously important in formulating how the clinician would stage the psychological recovery process from dysthymia. Nonetheless, there are some suggestions that SSRIs often lead to improved coping behaviour, even without formal psychotherapy. Indeed, Canadian studies have shown that a successful response to SSRIs is often associated with decreased emotion-focused coping and decreased perception of daily hassles, as well as alleviation of the sense of loneliness one experiences in chronic depression.

No matter what the active ingredients in antidysthymic treatments, there is little doubt that for the first time in the history of psychiatry we have potent practical treatments to alleviate a major source of chronic human suffering, including what were once deemed depressive characterological attributes inseparable from the habitual self. Helping patients attain a new homeostasis of the self is an art unparalleled in the history of medical science. In our view, it does not constitute what Kraemer has erroneously labeled 'cosmetic psychopharmacology'.[32]

Prevention opportunities[20]

Community subjects with pure dysthymia have been found in two prospective studies to be at risk for major depressive episodes. Because dysthymia often makes its first appearance in juvenile years, identifying the disorder at this early stage represents a special opportunity for prevention in child psychiatry and paediatrics. 'Pure' dysthymia, even without major depression, responds better to pharmacotherapy better than to placebo in 8 out of 9 social domains. St. John's Wort, on the other hand, does not appear to be effective in dysthymia![33]

In still another group of patients, low-grade chronic depressive developments occur in the setting of disabling systematic medical and neurological disorders, and are best categorized as 'secondary dysthymias'. For instance, poliomyelitis may not only lead to deformities in musculoskeletal structures in children, but could permanently scar the sufferer's sense of enjoyment, fulfillment, and outlook of life. Likewise, low-grade chronic depressive development often complicates neurodegenerative cerebrovascular disease later in life. In both situations, psychological factors might be operative, yet the contribution of specific cerebral lesions to the subthreshold mood disturbance may be substantial. This group as a whole is not well captured by the conventional depressive categories in ICD-10 and DSM-IV. In these subacute dysthymic-like conditions, the affective state is often disabling, yet symptomatologically less severe than major depression; it is low grade, yet not as chronic as dysthymia. 'Minor depression' would not capture the clinical significance of their condition. Indeed, there is emerging data that treating these subacute dysthymias may improve the prognosis of the underlying neurological disorder.[22]

In concluding this review of the legitimacy of dysthymia from clinical, biologic and therapeutic standpoints, it is relevant to point out that dysthymia—properly defined—may well serve as a behavioral endophenotype for depressive illness.[34] Such a conceptualization highlights its potential as a target for preventing strategies for major depressive illness.

Cyclothymic disorder and labile-irritable variants[20]

History

Kraepelin included the cyclothymic disposition as one of the temperamental foundations from which manic-depressive illness arose. Kretschmer went one step further and proposed that this constitution represented the core characteristic of the illness: some patients were more likely to oscillate in a sad direction, while others would more readily resonate with cheerful situations; these were merely viewed as variations in the cyclothymic oscillation between these two extremes. Kurt Schneider, who did not endorse the concept of 'temperament', instead referred to 'labile psychopaths' whose moods constantly changed in a dysphoric direction, and who bore no relationship to patients with manic depression. To confuse matters further, Schneider used the term 'cyclothymia' as a synonym for all manic depressive illness, from the mildest to the most severe psychotic forms. Today, 'cyclothymia' is still sometimes used in this broader sense in Germanophone psychiatry. But in much of the rest of the world, cyclothymia (short for 'cyclothymic disorder') is reserved for a form of extreme temperament related to bipolar disorder.

Cyclothymia, which in ICD-9 and DSM-II was subsumed under the affective personalities, was first introduced into DSM-III and DSM-IV and subsequently into ICD-10 as a form of attenuated chronic mood disorder. The diagnosis is not commonly made in clinical practice, because it is almost always seen when a patient presents with major depressive episodes, warranting the designation of 'bipolar II'. Indeed, Hecker used cyclothymia as a synonym for what today we call bipolar II; his short monograph has recently been translated into English.[35] Nonetheless, systematic clinical and familial validation studies conducted in Memphis[36,37] have shown that the construct of cyclothymic temperament is of great theoretical, psychometric and practical significance as one of the possible substrates for major mood disorders. Moreover, it could shed light on social and occupational maladjustment and/or addictive behaviours that could otherwise be misattributed to personality disorder.

Clinical features and diagnostic considerations[20]

By definition, individuals with cyclothymia report short cycles of depression and hypomania that fail to meet the sustained duration criterion for major affective syndromes. At various times, they exhibit the entire range of manifestations required for the diagnosis of depression and hypomania, but only from a few days at a time up to 1 week, rarely longer. These cycles follow each other in an irregular fashion, often changing abruptly from one mood to another, with only rare interposition of 'even' periods. The unpredictability of mood swings is a major source of distress for cyclothymes, as they do not know from moment to moment, how they will feel. As one patient put it, 'my moods swing like a

Table 4.5.9.5 Discriminatory biphasic characteristics of cyclothymic disorder*

Lethargy alternating with eutonia
Shaky self-esteem alternating between low self-confidence and overconfidence
Decreased verbal output alternating with talkativeness
Mental confusion alternating with sharpened thinking
Introverted self-absorption alternating with uninhibited people-seeking

*Summarized from Akiskal *et al.*(36,37)

pendulum, from one extreme to another'. The rapid mood shifts, which undermine the patients' sense of self, may lead to the misleading diagnostic label of borderline personality. But unlike a personality disorder, the mood changes in cyclothymes have a circadian component. One patient described it as follows: 'I would go to bed in a cheerful mood and wake up down in the dumps'. This observation is in line with NIMH psychophysiological data on mood-switching occurring out of the rapid eye movement sleep phase, as reported in more typical cases of manic depression.

The mood swings of cyclothymes are biphasic: eutonia versus anergic periods; people-seeking versus self-absorption; sharpened thinking versus mental paralysis. Table 4.5.9.5 provides an empirically tested set of criteria. In addition, the following presentations characterize their roller-coaster biography.

Irritable periods. At one time or another, labile angry or irritable moods are observed in virtually all these patients. Cyclothymes, unlike patients with epilepsy, are aware of their 'fits of anger', which lead to considerable personal and social embarrassment after they subside. The patients often feel 'on edge, restless, and aimlessly driven'; family and friends report that during these periods patients seem inconsiderate and hostile toward people around them. The contribution of alcohol and sedative-hypnotic drugs to these moods cannot be denied, but the moods often occur in the absence of drugs. Electroencephalography typically reveals no seizure or subseizure activity. The interpersonal costs of such unpredictable interpersonal explosiveness can be quite damaging. One of our patients reported frequent periods where he would start unprovoked fights with very close friends, only to shift into periods of prolonged 'soul-searching, guilt, shame, and embarrassment'. In other patients, outbursts of anger are 'reactive' to minor interpersonal disputes—but once in full force, they are like emotional avalanches with the distinct potential to destroy relationships. Should they dominate the clinical picture, especially among young women who hurt themselves in response to interpersonal contexts, the problematic diagnosis of borderline personality disorder is often invoked (more so in North America than elsewhere). Although controversial, contemporary research suggests that many 'borderline' patients represent a severe labile-irritable variant of cyclothymia on the border of manic-depressive psychosis.(38) On the other hand, bizarre episodes of self-harm with features of post-traumatic stress are uncharacteristic of cyclothymia, and suggest other diagnoses.

Romantic–conjugal failure. It is easy to understand how individuals with mercurial moods would charm others when in an expansive people-seeking mode, and rapidly alienate them when dysphoric. In effect, the life of many of these patients is a tempestuous chain of intense but brief romantic liaisons, often with a series of unsuitable partners. Some rationalize their behaviour on the grounds that their spouse or partner is 'too conservative in sex, too unimaginative, too unaware of the intensity' needed to stimulate them. As expected, frequent marital separations, divorces, and remarriage to the same person occur.

Financial extravagance. One patient in our case series reported going to bars and buying people drinks because he wanted everybody to feel like him. Another patient intermittently showered his lovers with expensive jewellery. In general, however, the extravagance of the cyclothymic group reflects gregariousness and tends to occur on a smaller scale compared to the psychotic manner in which manic patients bring financial ruin to themselves and their families.

Uneven school and work record. Repeated and unpredictable shifts in work and study habits occur in most people with cyclothymia, giving rise to a dilettante biography. Although some do better during their 'high' periods—for example, one car salesman would sell cars only 'when up'—for others, the occasional 'even' periods were more conducive to meaningful work. It is sometimes unappreciated by clinicians inexperienced with bipolarity that the hypomanic period can be one of disorganized and unpatterned busyness that could easily lead to a serious drop in net productivity. For instance, one insurance salesman related that he was less successful when 'high', because he tended to enter into unproductive arguments with his clients. When 'down', productivity obviously abates, although two creative individuals in our case series—one inclined poetically, the other towards painting—produced their better work when coming out of mini-depressions.

Alcohol and drug abuse. An alternating pattern of the use of 'uppers' and 'downers' occurs in at least 50 per cent of patients. We have clinically evaluated at least five cyclothymes who 'sold dope' to maintain their habit: two went to prison. These and other observations suggest that a proportion of substance-abusing, especially stimulant-abusing, patients might be suffering from subtle or cryptic forms of bipolar disorder. The bipolar nature of mood swings in alcohol- or substance-abusing individuals can be documented by demonstrating mood swings well past the period of detoxification; in some cases, escalating mood instability makes its first appearance following abrupt drug or alcohol withdrawal. The DSM-IV criteria for drug-induced or drug withdrawal-induced mood disorder are, in our opinion, biased against the diagnosis of otherwise treatable bipolar spectrum disorders. New evidence suggests that the temperamental disorder might serve as the anlage for self-enhancement or augmentation with cocaine, other stimulants and heroin.(39,40) These features might raise differential diagnostic questions from adult attention deficit hyperactivity disorder (ADHD). The social warmth observed among most people with cyclothymia distinguishes them from ADHD. Also, elation and inflated self-confidence, which occur periodically in cyclothymia, are uncharacteristic of ADHD; the moodiness in the latter is largely depressive in nature. Finally, antidepressants and stimulants typically worsen the moods in cyclothymia; they treat ADHD. In rare cases, however, cyclothymia and ADHD can coexist.

Course patterns

In cyclothymia, hypomania and mini-depression alternate with each other from adolescence. For instance, the optimistic, overconfident, people-seeking phase can give way to self-absorption, self-doubt, pessimism, and a sense of futility, emptiness, and suicidal ideation. More commonly, depressive periods dominate the clinical picture, interspersed by 'even', 'irritable', and occasional hypomanic periods. Indeed, most people with cyclothymia who present clinically do so because of depression. These depressions are typically short-lived, yet unrelenting in their cyclic course, creating much interpersonal havoc for the patient. The following vignette illustrates the cardinal clinical features of cyclothymia that has not yet progressed to major depression.

Case Study: This 24-year-old songwriter presented with the chief complaint of 'depression so bad that I become totally dysfunctional—I cannot even get out of bed'. Since her mid-teens she had experienced periods lasting from a few days up to a week, during which she would withdraw into herself, losing confidence and interest, feeling drained of energy, and crying when approached by anybody. These periods were particularly prevalent during the autumn and winter months, but they did not coincide with the premenstrual phase. All she needed sometimes was restful sleep to 'feel alive again'; at other times, she would have little sleep, and would wake up 'wired', 'ready to go', 'open to experience all the joy waiting for me out there'; she would exude confidence, 'sensuality and sexual aroma'. These occurred less frequently than the 'down' periods and usually lasted for 1 to 3 days, but were not associated with creative spurts. The latter came as she was descending from 'highs' into a more 'mellow depression'. Her success in music had been sporadic, paralleling the sporadic nature of her 'muses' that visited her on the descending limb of 'hypomania merging with tears'. However, the major toll of her mood swings had been in her personal life, the intensity of her moods had driven away most men she had loved, of whom she had lost count. She described periods of such intense sexual arousal, that sometimes she would go to bed 'with anybody, including women of all ages, shapes, and description'. But, she added: 'I am not a lesbian—oral love is just one way of relating to these women—why not?' She had also experimented with drugs, such as stimulants, which had made her moodiness worse. More recently, she had been prescribed at least two SSRIs, which after a period of 'success' for a few months, had made her depressive swings more frequent and lower in amplitude, leading to the present consultation in our clinic.

As documented in this case, sexual excesses with both sexes are often readily admitted by patients. Winter accentuation or clustering of depressive periods, as exemplified here, is not uncommon in cyclothymia. We also would like to point out the special relationship of the moods to artistic productivity which occur in up to 8 per cent of cyclothymic depressions.(41) The 4-day threshold for hypomania in the official diagnostic manuals is too conservative; as shown in this case, most patients with cyclothymia (and bipolar II disorder) report a threshold of 1 to 3 days (though on occasion, one would observe a hypomanic duration of 1 week or longer). It is also noteworthy that the episodes are short-lived and do not reach the duration threshold for rapid cycling. Sometimes, the term 'ultra rapid cycling' is used for these patients, but we prefer to reserve this for extremely severe cases who require hospitalization. The short cycle length in cyclothymia is, in part, a selection artifact: the universe of patients with bipolar disorder is composed of an extreme variety of overlapping patterns.

The relationship of a cyclothymic temperament to the bipolar spectrum is more complex than that of dysthymia to major depressive disorder. Although cyclothymia can be observed in some patients with full-blown manic-depressive illness (bipolar I with severe or hospitalized mania), it is more commonly associated with the bipolar II pattern (of recurrent major depression with self-limited hypomanias). In a recent French national study of patients with major depression, 88 per cent of those with a cyclothymic disposition belonged to the bipolar II subtype. (Mania, by contrast, has been reported to more likely represent either an extension of hyperthymic traits, or a reversal from a depressive temperamental baseline.)

One-third of patients with cyclothymia studied by us on a prospective basis, progressed to spontaneous affective episodes with more protracted hypomanias and clinical (major) depression.(36,37) Thus, 6 per cent of the original cyclothymic cohort could be reclassified as bipolar I, and 30 per cent as bipolar II. The tendency to switch to hypomania was further augmented by the administration of antidepressants. A larger National Institute of Mental Health study of patients with major depression who switched to bipolar II during a prospective observation period of up to 11 years, found that a temperamental mix of 'mood-labile', 'energetic-active', and 'daydreaming' traits (reminiscent of Kretschmer's concept of the cyclothymic temperament were the most specific predictors of such outcome. Actually such temperamental factors predict who among the offspring of bipolar probands will progress during prospective course to clinical episodes.(42) New data further indicate that cyclothymia might be one of the pathways to suicidality among adolescents.(42)

The foregoing clinical and course characteristics suggest that a cyclothymic temperament leading to major depressive recurrences represents a distinct longitudinal pattern of 'cyclothymic depression', and which appears to capture the core features of bipolar II disorder in contemporary clinical practice. Because hypomanic episodes cannot be easily ascertained by history, assessing cyclothymia in clinically depressed patients represents a more sensitive and specific approach to the diagnosis of bipolar II.

Epidemiology

An excess of interpersonal difficulties and psychiatric consultations distinguish people with cyclothymia in the community from controls; excessive use patterns of stimulants, caffeine, nicotine, and alcohol, have also been well documented. Explosive traits, probably representing the irritable component of cyclothymia, have been reported to be prevalent in the community in a British study. More recently, we found that 6.3 per cent of a national cohort of 1010 Italian students between the ages of 14 and 26 years of age scored above two standard deviations for cyclothymia; this was more prevalent in females, with a ratio of 3:2. Overall, the foregoing data testify to the fact that a cyclothymic and/or labile disposition can be accurately measured, is prevalent, and represents a population at risk for affective disorders. Table 4.5.9.6 summarizes the rates in different populations.

Aetiological aspects

The flamboyant behaviour and the restless pursuit of romantic opportunities in cyclothymia suggest the hypothesis that its

Table 4.5.9.6 Prevalence of cyclothymic and related mood-labile temperaments[20]*

Reference	Population (Country)	Rate (%)
Akiskal *et al.* (1977)	Mental health centre (USA)	10
Weissman and Myers (1978)	Community (USA)	4
Depue *et al.* (1981)	College students (USA)	6
Casey and Tyrer (1986)	Community (UK)	6
Wicki and Angst (1991)	Community (Zurich)	4
Placidi *et al.* (1988)	14–26-year old students (Italy)	6

*These data derive from interview-based studies. For more recent psychometric data based on cyclothymic and a broader range of sub-bipolar temperaments in a self-reported format can be found in a new monograph.[8]

constituent traits may have evolved as a mechanism in sexual selection.[23] Even their creative bent—in poetry, music, painting, or fashion design—may have evolved to subserve such a mechanism. Cyclothymic traits appear to lie on a polygenic continuum between excessive temperament and manic depression. Indeed, clinically identified cyclothymes have patterns of familial affective illness, as one would expect for a *forme fruste* disorder.

Cyclothymia has also been observed in the offspring of manic-depressive probands, with onset in the postpubertal period. Finally, family studies of patients with a bipolar disorder have revealed an excess of cyclothymia. Hypothetically, this temperament might represent one of, if not the most important, inherited trait diathesis for bipolar disorder. For instance, moody-temperamental individuals are over-represented in the 'discordant' monozygotic co-twins of Danish manic-depressives. Alternatively, and in a more theoretical vein, manic-depressive illness might be the genetic reservoir for the desirable cyclothymic traits in the population at large.[23,44] In line with these data and considerations, cyclothymia can be considered a behavioral endophenotype for bipolar disorder.[45] This is supported by recent findings from both Europe and the United States which have shown that it is present in the clinically well relatives of bipolar probands. Cyclothymia might also share familial-genetic relationship with alcohol and substance use,[40] bulimic,[46] panic,[47] obsessive-compulsive[48] as well as atypical depressive and borderline conditions.[49]

Clinical management

The proper pharmacological treatment for cyclothymic excesses is low doses of lithium (600–900 mg/day) or valproate (500–750 mg/day). These are based on open systematic studies.[50] There is some data from a controlled trial with lithium about the prevention of depression in cyclothymic individuals. Similarly controlled data exist for a related construct—'labile personality'. Generally speaking, patients with cyclothymia object to the 'overcontrol' that may come from mood stabilizers, and this is particularly the case with lithium. Lamotrigine is also being used on clinical grounds in the unstable dysthymic-cyclothymic spectrum. In those with 'borderline' features, lamotrigine is particularly promising.

Patients should be taught how to live with the extremes of their temperamental inclinations, and to seek professions where they determine the hours that they work. Marriage to a work-oriented or a rich older spouse might sustain them for a while, but eventually interpersonal friction and sexual jealousy terminate such marriages. The artistically inclined among them should be encouraged to live in those parts of a city inhabited by artists and other intellectuals, where temperamental excesses are better tolerated. ltimately, the decision to use mood stabilizers in such individuals should balance any benefits from decreased mood instability against the social and creative spurts that the cyclothymic disposition can bring to them. Their clinical management represents a challenging task for the psychiatrist who is willing to learn about the lifestyle of these individuals, not prejudging them by the more mundane norms of society. But the psychiatrist should also be there to help them during the multiple crises of their lives. Low-dose sedating neuroleptics, both classical (e.g. thioridazine 50 mg at bedtime) and atypical (e.g. quetiapine 25–50 mg at bedtime) may temporarily help to diffuse such crises. It is only when a clinician has earned therapeutic alliance with a patient that the latter will permit limit-setting on his or her extravagant or outrageous behaviour. Parents might also benefit from some counselling, because the dilettante life of their children is often a source of great sorrow for them. Rarely, parents or spouses are rewarded by great artistic or intellectual achievement, which does not necessarily reduce the pain that the volatile cyclothymes bring to their loved ones.

Kurt Schneider admonished the kin of labile individuals (who might approximate the contemporary concept of borderline personality disorder) 'on their bad days . . . to keep out of their way as far as possible'. Cyclothymes with some insight into their own temperament would give the same advice to their loved ones. A cautious trial of anticonvulsants will often prove effective in those distressed enough by their behaviour to comply with such treatment.

Prevention

The offspring of patients with bipolar disorder who exhibit a cyclothymic level of temperamental dysregulation represent a logical population for prevention studies. This is a challenge for the 21st century. Presumably molecular genetic testing will one day identify those moody individuals who carry the genes for bipolar disorder. At present, it would be useful to conservatively follow-up the cyclothymic offspring of people with bipolar disorders and provide them with psychoeducation about the necessity of avoiding stimulants and sleep deprivation. It may not be entirely possible to prohibit the use of occasional alcohol consumption, but benzodiazepines should not be used. It is also imperative, should they get depressed, to protect them from the indiscriminate prescription of antidepressants.

Mood-labile female prisoners, commonly given the diagnosis of antisocial or borderline personality disorder, may represent affective variants with irritable cyclothymic features. Formal studies are needed in prison populations, to assess more precisely the rates of preventable cryptic bipolarity among female and male offenders.

It is finally worthwhile to mention that affective temperaments with irritable, cyclothymic and irritable-hyperthymic traits might predispose to HIV infection. The public health dimensions of this question deserve further research focus.

The hyperthymic temperament[38]*

History and description

Although well described by classical German psychiatrists (e.g. Schneider), the hyperthymic type appears neither in DSM-IV nor in ICD-10. A lifelong disposition, hyperthymia must be distinguished from short-lived hypomanic episodes. Alternatively, this disposition can be characterized as trait hypomania. It derives from the ancient Graeco-Roman sanguine temperament, believed to represent the optimal mixture of behavioural traits. They are full of zest, fun-loving, and prone to lechery: their habitual disposition is one of buoyant action-orientation, extraverted people-seeking, overconfidence, and swift thinking. Typically short sleepers, they possess boundless energy to invest in sundry causes and projects, which often earn them leadership positions in the various professions and politics, yet their carefree attitudes and propensity for risk-taking can bring them to the brink of ruin; this is particularly true for their finances and sexual life, which can be marred by scandal. A hyperthymic lifestyle is so reinforcing that some resort to 'augmenting' it with stimulants such as amphetamines or cocaine. In brief, while a hyperthymic temperament *per se* does not constitute affective pathology—indeed, it represents a constellation of adaptive traits—in excess it could lead to undesirable complications. The latter will be our main focus here.

Epidemiology

The foregoing considerations partly explain why such a temperament has received scant research attention in the community. Extrapolating from studies on intermittent hypomania in the community, if strictly limited to hypomania with early onset and persistent course, the prevalence of hyperthymic temperament can be estimated to be slightly under 1 per cent. On the other hand, the traits that constitute the hyperthymic profile are so desirable that normal individuals tend to endorse them; in a recent Pisa-San Diego collaboration[16] involving 1010 students aged between 14 and 26, of whom 8.2 per cent met the full criteria for hyperthymic temperament, all participants scored between the first and second positive standard deviation. The TEMPS-A tends to validate these findings in Lebanon,[51] Argentina[52] and Hungary.[53] More work needs to be done on the psychometric standardization of this temperamental construct; on the other hand, all studies are consistent in showing marked male predominance.

Diagnostic aspects

On the positive side, hyperthymic individuals are enterprising, ambitious, and driven, often achieving considerable social and vocational prominence. Abuse of stimulants is not so much an attempt to ward off depression and fatigue as an effort to enhance their already high-level drive and, sometimes, to further curtail their already reduced need for sleep. Hyperthymic individuals typically marry three or more times. Others, without entering into legally sanctioned matrimony, form three or more families in different cities; these men are capable of maintaining such relationships for long periods, testifying to their financial and personal resourcefulness, as well as their generosity towards their lovers and the offspring from such unions. Unlike the antisocial psychopath who is predatory on others and neglects or abuses his women and children, these men care for their loved ones. But obviously, the 'arrangement' involving women of different generations is complex, and a fertile soil for jealousy, drama, scandal, and tragedy. Nonetheless, it is not uncommon to see more than three or four women crying profusely and expressing their common grief at the funerals of these men!

Although individuals with hyperthymia optimally enjoy the advantage of their reduced need for sleep (giving more time and energy to invest in work and pleasure), some present clinically because of insomnia. Thus, in a predominantly male sample of executives presenting to a sleep centre,[54] habitual sleep need was 4 to 5 h; however, they had been intermittently bothered by 'nervous energy' and difficulty falling asleep. Now, in late middle age, alcohol was no longer an effective hypnotic. Although they vigorously denied depressive and other mental symptoms—indeed, they had extremely low scores on self-rated depression—spouses or lovers provided collateral information about brief irritable-depressive dips, especially in the morning and, in some cases, more protracted 'fatigue states' of days to weeks during which the subject would vegetate. Despite these depressive dips, these patients were distinguished from the constantly shifting moods of cyclothymic patients by the fact that the depressions arose from a baseline of trait hypomania of a more or less stable course. Our most current diagnostic guidelines for a hyperthymic temperament consist of the following traits on a habitual basis since at least early adulthood: cheerful, overoptimistic, or exuberant; extraverted and people-seeking, often to the point of being overinvolved or meddlesome; overtalkative, eloquent, and jocular; uninhibited, stimulus-seeking, and sexually-driven; vigorous, full of plans, improvident; overconfident, self-assured, and boastful attitudes that may reach grandiose proportions.

A systematic retrospective review of the case records of people with manic depression, whose course was dominated by manic episodes, was recently undertaken in Munich, yielding attributes overlapping with our proposed list: active, vivid, extraverted, verbally aggressive, self-assured, strong willed, engaged in self-employed professions, risk-taking, sensation-seeking, breaking social norms, spendthrift, and generous. The fact that at least 10 per cent of patients with major depression in an Italian study could be characterized as premorbidly hyperthymic, suggests that this temperament has relevance to both major affective poles. This is an important diagnostic consideration, because rather than being considered narcissistic depressions, these should be recognized as a soft bipolar variant.

Aetiological aspects

It is of interest that Gardner's ethological analysis[55] of what constitutes 'leadership' led to a description that overlaps with a hyperthymic profile: cheerfulness, joking, irrepressible infectious quality, unusual warmth, expansive, strong sense of confidence in one's abilities, scheming, robust, tireless, pushy, and meddlesome. Hypothetically, this temperament evolved in primates whose social life required leadership to better face challenges to the group from within and without.

In a sleep electroencephalography study,[54] REM latency was found to be shortened; similar findings have been reported on the sleep of manic patients, thereby supporting the notion of a trait-state continuum at the neurophysiological level. (Although counter-intuitive, this neurophysiological marker appears to be shared between the depressive and hyperthymic poles.) Finally, family

* Unless otherwise specified, this review article contains most of the references to the concepts, history, and research on the hyperthymic type.

history for frank bipolar disorder characterizes many such individuals. The foregoing data, albeit limited, suggest that hyperthymic traits share several key biological underpinnings of affective disorder.

Course and treatment

Little is known about the natural course of the hyperthymic temperament, except what can be reconstructed retrospectively from biographical and clinical studies. Given their overoptimistic and self-assured style of thinking, these individuals feel perfectly fit in all areas of functioning and thus have no need to consult a psychiatrist. They do so only when forced by loved ones. There are no systematic treatment studies on hyperthymia. Anecdotally,[50] low doses of anticonvulsants such as valproate (e.g. 500–750 mg/day) can be useful in reducing drivenness, when deemed appropriate on clinical grounds, such as in the presence of cardiovascular disease, or when enormous sexual appetite places them at risk for social scandals and, in some cases, exposure to HIV infection.[56] Stimulant-abusing subjects with hyperthymia can be detoxified with valproate, carbamazepine, or gabapentin. Clinically depressed subjects with a hyperthymic temperament often respond poorly to antidepressants. In our opinion, the efficacy of lithium augmentation in resistant depression is partly based on the high prevalence of hyperthymia in resistant populations; it would be wise to keep the dose of lithium in augmentation in such individuals to a lower to middle range (i.e. 600–900 mg/day).

People with hyperthymia are action-oriented, and are not inclined to any type of self-examination. Furthermore, their hypertrophied sense of denial makes them poor candidates for psychotherapy. The physician must, nonetheless, attempt psychoeducation about the harm that can come to them and their loved ones because of their temperamental excesses. Alcohol consumption, which is common in these individuals, should not be abruptly interrupted because of the risk of the switch to a suicidal depression. If detoxification is necessary for health reasons, admission to a suitable inpatient facility should be arranged. The occasion might be profitably used for whatever counselling is deemed appropriate for life and health situations confronting them at the time.

Therapeutic and preventive aspects

In clinical practice, hyperthymic individuals are likely to be confused with narcissistic or antisocial types. Otherwise, they rarely present to psychiatrists, except as the premorbid adjustment of manic-depressive illness. Hyperthymic individuals are often the driving force of society in economic and political life and unless they are involved in scandals or suicidal behavior, rarely come to the attention of clinicians. In the rare circumstances they seek psychiatric advice, it is due to exasperated pressure from loved ones; even then, they tend to dictate rather than follow treatment recommendations. Their sense of entitlement derives in part from the fact these individuals have considerable leadership talent and often bequeath large sums of endowments for research, museums and other community projects. Some are performing artists. Others are famed for their erotic life in the tabloid and popular press. Rare biological investigations have been conducted on hyperthymia involving fascinating neurophysiologic and endophenotype studies.[57,58] The preventive potential of such investigations for manic-depressive illness remains uncertain at this time.

Further information

Akiskal, H.S., Akiskal, K.K. (eds.) (2005). TEMPS: Temperament Evaluation of Memphis, Pisa, Paris and San Diego. Special Issue, *Journal of Affective Disorders*, **85**, 1–242.

References

1. Akiskal, H.S., Judd, L.L., Gillin, J.C., *et al.* (1997). Subthreshold depressions: clinical and polysomnographic validation of dysthymic, residual and masked forms. *Journal of Affective Disorders*, **45**, 53–63.
2. Meier, W., Lichterman, D., Minges, J., *et al.* (1992). The risk of minor depression in families of probands with major depression: sex differences and familiality. *European Archives of Psychiatry and Clinical Neuroscience*, **242**, 89–92.
3. Kendler, K.S., Neale, M.C., and Kessler, R.C. (1992). A population-based twin study of major depression in women: the impact of varying definitions of illness. *Archives of General Psychiatry*, **49**, 257–66.
4. Akiskal, H.S., Bitar, A.H., Puzantian, V.R., *et al.* (1978). The nosological status of neurotic depression: a prospective three-to-four year examination in light of the primary-secondary and unipolar-bipolar dichotomies. *Archives of General Psychiatry*, **35**, 756–66.
5. Bronisch, T., Wittchen, H.-U., Krieg, C., *et al.* (1985). Depressive neurosis: a long-term prospective and retrospective follow-up study of former inpatients. *Acta Psychiatrica Scandinavica*, **71**, 237–48.
6. Akiskal, H.S. and Cassano, G.B. (ed.) (1997). *Dysthymia and the spectrum of chronic depressions*. Guilford Press, New York.
7. Akiskal, H.S., Akiskal, K.K., Lancrenon, S., *et al.* (2006). Validating the bipolar spectrum in the French National EPIDEP Study: Overview of the phenomenology and relative prevalence of its clinical prototypes. *Journal of Affective Disorders*, **96**, 197–205.
8. Akiskal, H.S. and Akiskal, K.K., (eds.) (2005). TEMPS: Temperament Evaluation of Memphis, Pisa, Paris and San Diego. Special Issue, *Journal of Affective Disorders*, **50**, 1–242.
9. Akiskal, H.S. and Weise, R.E. (1992). The clinical spectrum of so-called 'minor' depressions. *American Journal of Psychotherapy*, **46**, 9–22.
10. Lewis, A. (1936). Melancholia: a prognostic study. *Journal of Mental Science*, **82**, 488–558.
11. Akiskal, H.S. (1981). Subaffective disorders: dysthymic, cyclothymic and bipolar II disorders in the 'borderline' realm. *Psychiatric Clinics of North America*, **4**, 25–46.
12. Snaith, R.P. (1991). Measurement in psychiatry. *British Journal of Psychiatry*, **159**, 78–82.
13. Kendler, K.S., Neale, M.C., Kessler, R.C., *et al.* (1993). A longitudinal twin study of personality and major depression in women. *Archives of General Psychiatry*, **50**, 853–62.
14. Brieger, P. and Marneros, A. (1997). Dysthymia and cyclothymia: historical origins and contemporary development. *Journal of Affective Disorders*, **45**, 117–26.
15. Akiskal, H.S. (1983). Dysthymic disorder: psychopathology of proposed chronic depressive subtypes. *American Journal of Psychiatry*, **140**, 11–20.
16. Placidi, G.F., Signoretta, S., Liguori, A., *et al.* (1998). The Semi-Structured Affective Temperament Interview (TEMPS-I): reliability and psychometric properties in 1010 14–26 year students. *Journal of Affective Disorders*, **47**, 1–10.
17. Kasahara, Y. (1991). The practical diagnosis of depression in Japan. In *The diagnosis of depression* (eds. J.P. Feighner and W.F. Boyer), pp. 163–75. Wiley, Chichester.
18. Montassut, M. (1938). *La dépression constitutionnelle: l'ancienne neurasthénie dans ses rapports avec la médecine générale; clinique biologie, thérapeutique*. Masson, Paris.

19. Akiskal, H.S. (1996). Dysthymia as a temperamental variant of affective disorder. *European Psychiatry*, **11** (Supplement), 117s–22s.
20. Akiskal, H.S. (2001). Dysthymia and cyclothymia in psychiatric practice a century after Kraepelin. *Journal of Affective Disorders*, **62**, 17–31.
21. The WPA Dysthymia Working Group (1995). Dysthymia in clinical practice. *British Journal of Psychiatry*, **166**, 174–83.
22. Licinio, J., Prilpko, I., and Bolis, C.L. (eds.) (1997). Dysthymia in neurological disorders. In *Proceedings of the WHO Meeting*. World Health Organization, Geneva.
23. Akiskal, K., Akiskal, H.S. (2005). The theoretical underpinnings of affective temperaments: implications for evolutionary foundations of bipolarity and human nature. *Journal of Affective Disorders*, **85**, 231–9.
24. Markianos, M., Tripodianakis, J., Sarantidis, D., *et al.* (2006). Plasma testosterone and dehydroepiandrosterone sulfate in male and female patients with dysthymic disorder. *Journal of Affective Disorders*, **101**, 255–8.
25. Brambilla, F., Monteleone, P., Maj, M. (2004). Interleukin-1beta and tumor necrosis factor-alpha in children with major depressive disorder or dysthymia. *Journal of Affective Disorders*, **78**, 273–7.
26. Field, T., Diego, M.A., Hernandez-Reif, M., *et al.* (2008). Prenatal dysthymia versus major depression effects on maternal cortisol and fetal growth. *Depressive Anxiety*, **22**, in press.
27. Lyoo, I.K., Kwon, J.S., Lee, S.J., *et al.* (2002). Decrease in genus of the corpus callosum in medication-Naïve, early-onset dysthymia and depressive personality disorder. *Biological Psychiatry*, **52**, 1134–43.
28. Tebartz van Elst, L., Woermann, F.G., Lemieus, L., *et al.* (1999). Amygdala enlargement in dysthymia—a volumetric study of patients with temporal lobe epilepsy. *Biological Psychiatry*, **46**, 1614–23.
29. Oliveira, J.R., Carvalho, D.R., Pontual, D., *et al.* (2000). Analysis of the serotonin transporter polymorphism (5-HTTLPR) in Brazilian patients affected by dysthymia, major depression and bipolar disorder. *Molecular Psychiatry*, **5**, 348–9.
30. Gonda, X., Zsombok, T., Rihmer, Z., *et al.* (2006). The 5HTTLPR polymorphism of the serotonin transporter gene is associated with affective temperaments as measured by TEMPS-A. *Journal of Affective Disorders*, **91**, 125–31.
31. Burton, S.W. and Akiskal, H.S. (ed.) (1993). Dysthymic disorder. Gaskell and Royal College of Psychiatrists, London.
32. Kraemer, P.D. (1993). *Listening to Prozac*. Viking Press, New York.
33. Randlov, C., Mehlsen, J., Thomsen, C.F., *et al.* (2006). The efficacy of St. John's Wort in patients with minor depressive symptoms or dysthymia—a double-blind placebo-controlled study. *Phytomedicine*, **13**, 215–21.
34. Niculescu, A.B., Akiskal, H.S. (2001). Proposed endophenotypes of dysthymia: evolutionary, clinical and pharmacogenomic considerations. *Molecular Psychiatry*, **6**, 363–6.
35. Koukopoulos, A. (2003). Ewald Hecker's description of cyclothymia as a cyclical mood disorder: its relevance to the modern concept of bipolar II. *Journal of Affective Disorders*, **73**, 199–205.
36. Akiskal, H.S., Djenderedjian, A.H., Rosenthal, R.H., *et al.* (1977). Cyclothymic disorder: validating criteria for inclusion in the bipolar affective group. *American Journal of Psychiatry*, **134**, 1227–33.
37. Akiskal, H.S., Khani, M.K., and Scott-Strauss, A. (1979). Cyclothymic temperamental disorders. *Psychiatric Clinics of North America*, **2**, 527–54.
38. Akiskal, H.S. (1992). Delineating irritable-choleric and hyperthymic temperaments as variants of cyclothymia. *Journal of Personality Disorders*, **6**, 326–42.
39. Maremmani I, Perugi G, Pacini M, *et al.* (2007). Toward a unitary perspective on the bipolar spectrum and substance abuse: opiate addiction as a paradigm. *Journal of Affective Disorders*, **93**, 1–12.
40. Merikangas, K.R., Herrell, R., Swendsen, J., *et al.* (2008). Specificity of bipolar spectrum conditions in the comorbidity of mood and substance use disorders: results from the Zurich cohort study *Archives of General Psychiatry*, **65**, 47–52.
41. Akiskal, H.S. and Akiskal, K. (1988). Re-assessing the prevalence of bipolar disorders: Clinical significance and artistic creativity. [Psychiatric et Psychologic] *European Psychiatry*, **3**, 29s–36s.
42. Akiskal, H.S., Downs, J., Jordan, P., *et al.* (1985). Affective disorders in the referred children and younger siblings of manic-depressives: Mode of onset and prospective course. *Archives of General Psychiatry*, **42**, 996–1003.
43. Kochman, F.J., Hantouche, E.G., Ferrari, P., *et al.* (2005). Cyclothymic temperament as a prospective predictor of bipolarity and suicidality in children and adolescents with major depressive disorder. *Journal of Affective Disorders*, **85**,181–9.
44. Akiskal H.S., Akiskal, K.K. (2007) In search of Aristotle. *Journal of Affective Disorders*, **100**, 1–6.
45. Evans, L., Akiskal, H.S., Greenwood, T.A., *et al.* (2008). Suggestive linkage of a chromosomal locus on 18p11 to cyclothymic temperament in bipolar disorder families. *American Journal of Medical Genetics B Neuropsychiatric Genetics*, in press.
46. Perugi, G., Toni, C., Passino, M.C., *et al.* (2006). Bulimia nervosa in atypical depression: the mediating role of cyclothymic temperament. *Journal of Affective Disorders*, **82**, 91–7.
47. Akiskal, H.S., Akiskal, K.K., Perugi, G., *et al.* (2006). Bipolar II and anxious reactive 'comorbidity': toward better phenotypic characterization suitable for genotyping. *Journal of Affective Disorders*, **96**, 239–47.
48. Hantouche, E.G., Angst, J., Demonfaucon, *et al.* (2003). Cyclothymic OCD: a distinct form? *Journal of Affective Disorders*, **75**, 1–10.
49. Perugi, G., Toni, C., Travierso, M.C., *et al.* (2003). The role of cyclothymia in atypical depression: toward a data-based reconceptualization of the borderline-bipolar II connection. *Journal of Affective Disorders*, **73**, 87–98.
50. Akiskl, H.S. (1977). Chronic disturbances of temperament. *Bibliotheca Psychiatrica (Basel)*, **167**, 29–32.
51. Karam, E.G., Mneimneh, Z., Salamoun, M., *et al.* (2005). Psychometric properties of the Lebanese-Arabic TEMPS-A: a national epidemiologic study. *Journal of Affective Disorders*, **87**, 169–183.
52. Vázquez, G.H., Nasetta, S., Mercado, B., *et al.* (2007). Validation of the Temps-A Buenos Aires: Spanish psychometric validation of affective temperaments in a population study of Argentina. *Journal of Affective Disorders*, **100**, 23–9.
53. Rózsa, S., Rihmer, Z., Gonda, X., *et al.* (2007). A study of affective temperaments in Hungary: Internal consistency and concurrent validity of the TEMPS-A against the TCI and NEO PI-R. *Journal of Affective Disorders*, in press.
54. Akiskal, H. (1984). Characterologic manifestations of affective disorders: toward a new conceptualization. *Integrative Psychiatry*, **2**, 83–8.
55. Gardner, R. Jr. (1982). Mechanisms in manic-depressive disorder: an evolutionary model. *Archives of General Psychiatry*, **39**, 1436–41.
56. Moore, D., Atkinson, J.H., Gonzalez, B.A., *et al.* (2005). Temperament and risky behaviors: A pathway to HIV? *Journal of Affective Disorders*, **85**, 191–200.
57. Hensch, T., Herold, U., Brocke, B. (2007). An electrophysiological endophenotype of hypomanic and hyperthymic personality. *Journal of Affective Disorders*, **101**, 13–26.
58. Chiaroni, P., Hantouche, E.G., Gouvernet, *et al.* (2004). [Hyperthymic and depressive temperaments study in controls, as a function of their familial loading for mood disorders.] *Encephale*, **30**, 509–15.

4.6

Stress-related and adjustment disorders

Contents

4.6.1 Acute stress reactions
Anke Ehlers, Allison G. Harvey, and Richard A. Bryant

4.6.2 Post-traumatic stress disorder
Anke Ehlers

4.6.3 Recovered memories and false memories
Chris R. Brewin

4.6.4 Adjustment disorders
James J. Strain, Kimberly Klipstein, and Jeffrey Newcorm

4.6.5 Bereavement
Beverley Raphael, Sally Wooding, and Julie Dunsmore

4.6.1 Acute stress reactions

Anke Ehlers, Allison G. Harvey, and Richard A. Bryant

Introduction

Exceptionally stressful life events can cause severe psychological symptoms, including anxiety, feelings of derealization and depersonalization, and hyperarousal. In one of the first studies to comprehensively document acute reactions to extreme stress, Lindemann[1] observed that the symptoms reported by survivors of the Coconut Grove Fire included avoidance, re-experiencing scenes from the fire, reports of derealization, and the experience of anxiety when exposed to reminders of the event. Similarly, acute responses reported by soldiers who fought in the First and Second World Wars included re-experiencing symptoms and dissociative responses such as numbing, amnesia, and depersonalization.[2]

The *International Classification of Diseases* has recognized acute stress reactions since 1948 (ICD-6).[3] In the most recent edition (ICD-10),[4] early reactions to exceptionally stressful life events are diagnosed as acute stress reaction, one of the diagnoses in the section headed 'reactions to severe stress, and adjustment disorders'.

In contrast, the *Diagnostic and Statistical Manual of Mental Disorders* did not formally recognize that exceptionally stressful life events are a sufficient cause of psychological symptoms until 1980 when its third edition (DSM-III)[5] introduced the diagnosis of post-traumatic stress disorder (**PTSD**). DSM-III did not stipulate a duration for the symptoms, but the revised third version (DSM-III-R)[6] required that the symptoms of PTSD must be present for more than 1 month after the traumatic event. This stipulation precluded the inclusion of acutely traumatized individuals who instead were diagnosed with adjustment disorder.[7] In 1994 the fourth edition of DSM (DSM-IV)[8] formally recognized acute trauma reactions by introducing the new diagnosis of acute stress disorder into the anxiety disorders section.

The diagnoses of acute stress reactions in ICD-10 and of acute stress disorder in DSM-IV have similarities in that they are caused by extreme stress and have some overlap in symptom patterns. They can be considered as two separate points on a continuum from transient to more enduring symptoms. However, there are also differences in the underlying concepts, as we will discuss in this chapter.

Clinical features

Acute stress reactions, as defined in ICD-10, are transient reactions to exceptional physical and/or mental stress. There is an initial stage of a 'daze', including narrowing of attention, inability to comprehend stimuli, and disorientation. This is followed by a rapidly changing picture of symptoms that may include withdrawal from the surrounding situation, flight reactions, panic anxiety, and autonomic hyperarousal, depression, anger, or despair. Symptoms usually begin to diminish after 24 to 48 h and should be minimal after about 3 days.

In contrast, acute stress disorder, as defined in DSM-IV, is only diagnosed if the psychological symptoms persist for more than 2 days. Dissociative symptoms dominate the disorder. Dissociation refers to a disruption of the usually integrated feelings of consciousness, memory, identity, or perception of the environment. Symptoms include a subjective sense of numbing or detachment, reduced awareness of surroundings, derealization, depersonalization, or dissociative amnesia. In addition, patients with acute stress disorder experience symptoms that are typical of PTSD, namely re-experiencing aspects of the event, avoidance of reminders of the event, and hyperarousal symptoms. Acute stress disorder is seen in DSM-IV as a precursor of PTSD. If the re-experiencing, avoidance, and hyperarousal symptoms persist for more than 4 weeks, PTSD is diagnosed.

Classification

ICD-10 classifies acute stress reactions (F43.0) among the reactions to severe stress and adjustment disorders (F43) that are primarily caused by stressful events. DSM-IV classifies acute stress disorder (308.3) among the anxiety disorders, like PTSD (see also Chapter 4.6.2).

Diagnosis and differential diagnosis

The main diagnostic criteria for acute stress reactions (ICD-10) and acute stress disorder (DSM-IV) are compared in Table 4.6.1.1.

Stressor criterion

Both ICD-10 and DSM-IV require that acute stress responses must occur in the immediate aftermath of an exceptionally stressful event. ICD-10 uses a broad concept of what qualifies as an 'exceptional mental or physical stressor'. This includes stressors that would be regarded as traumatic (e.g. rape, criminal assault, natural catastrophe) as well as unusually sudden changes in the social position and/or network of the individual (e.g. domestic fire or multiple bereavement). In contrast, DSM-IV uses a narrow definition of stressors that lead to acute stress disorder, which is identical to the stressor criterion of PTSD. It requires (i) that the traumatic event must have involved actual or threatened death or serious injury, or a threat to the physical integrity of self or others, and (ii) that the person's response to the traumatic event must have involved intense fear, helplessness, or horror (or disorganized or agitated behaviour in children) (see Chapter 4.6.2 for the rationale underlying this definition).

Symptom patterns

As shown in Table 4.6.1.1, the diagnostic criteria for acute stress reactions (ICD-10) and acute stress disorder (DSM-IV) overlap, in that they include symptoms of dissociation, anxiety, and hyperarousal. DSM-IV puts a much greater emphasis on dissociation, requiring a minimum of three of the dissociative symptoms specified in Table 4.6.1.1 (Criterion B). According to ICD-10, any combination of a minimum of four symptoms of generalized anxiety disorder (specified in Criterion C, Table 4.6.1.1) would be sufficient to establish the diagnosis of acute stress reaction. In addition, DSM-IV, but not ICD-10, requires the individual to have at least one re-experiencing symptom, to show marked avoidance of reminders of the trauma, and to experience significant distress or impairment of functioning.

In contrast to DSM-IV, ICD-10 distinguishes between mild, moderate, and severe forms of acute stress reactions on the basis

Table 4.6.1.1 Comparison of the criteria for acute stress reaction (ICD-10) and acute stress disorder (DSM-IV)

	Acute stress reaction (ICD-10 research diagnostic criteria)	Acute stress disorder (DSM-IV)
Stressor	Exposure to exceptional mental or physical stress	(1) Exposure to event involving actual or threatened death or serious injury to self or others (2) Experience of fear, helplessness, or horror
Symptoms	*Criterion C: Symptoms of generalized anxiety disorder (at least 4 symptoms)* Palpitations, sweating, trembling, dry mouth, difficulty breathing, choking, chest pain, nausea, dizziness, derealization or depersonalization, fear of losing control, fear of dying, hot flushes, numbness or tingling, muscle tension, restlessness, keyed up, difficulty swallowing, exaggerated startle response, difficulty concentrating, irritability, difficulty getting to sleep *Criterion C: Additional symptoms to determine severity* Social withdrawal, narrowed attention, disorientation, aggression, hopelessness, overactivity, excessive grief	*Criterion B: Dissociation (at least 3 symptoms)* Numbing, reduced awareness, derealization, depersonalization, dissociative amnesia *Criterion C: Re-experiencing* (at least one *symptom)* Recurrent images, thoughts, dreams, illusions, flashbacks, reliving, distress on exposure *Criterion D: Marked avoidance* Avoidance of thoughts, feelings, conversations, activities, places, people associated with the trauma *Criterion E: Marked anxiety or increased arousal* Difficulty sleeping, irritability, poor concentration, hypervigilance, exaggerated startle response, motor restlessness *Criterion F: Clinically significant distress or impairment in functioning*
Time from trauma	Onset within 1 h	Onset within 4 weeks; lasts for at least 2 days
Time course	Transient; symptoms begin to diminish within 48 h	May result in post-traumatic stress disorder
Relationship to post-traumatic stress disorder	Alternative diagnosis	Precursor
Diagnostic group	Reactions to severe stress	Anxiety disorder
Exclusion criteria	No other concurrent (within last 3 months) mental or behavioural disorder, except for generalized anxiety disorder or personality disorder	(1) Not due to effects of a substance or general medical condition (2) Not better accounted for by brief psychotic disorder (3) Not merely exacerbation of pre-existing Axis I or Axis II disorder

of additional symptoms (Criterion C, additional symptoms, Table 4.6.1.1) such as social withdrawal, hopelessness, or excessive grief. A mild severity is stipulated when none of these symptoms are present, moderate when two are reported, and severe when four are reported or when there is dissociative stupor.

Time course of symptoms

The two diagnoses cover distinct periods on a continuum from transient to more persistent symptoms. Specifically, to meet the criteria for an acute stress reaction (ICD-10), symptoms must be manifest within 1 h of the stressor (Criterion B) and begin to diminish after no more than 8 h for a transient stressor and after no more than 48 h for an enduring stressor (Criterion D).

The diagnostic criteria for acute stress disorder (DSM-IV) require that the disturbance must last for a minimum of 2 days and a maximum of 4 weeks post-trauma, after which a diagnosis of PTSD can be considered.

Assessment instruments

There are two recognized clinician-administered and two self-report measures of acute stress disorder (DSM-IV) available. As yet, there are no established standardized assessment instruments for transient acute stress reactions (ICD-10).

(a) Acute stress disorder interview

This structured clinical interview establishes the presence or absence of 19 symptoms of acute stress disorder.[9] The sum of the symptoms scored as being present indicates acute stress disorder severity. This measure has very good internal consistency ($r = 0.90$), and, with clinician-based diagnoses as the criterion, very good sensitivity (91 per cent) and specificity (93 per cent). Test–retest reliability is strong ($r = 0.88$).

(b) Structured clinical interview for DSM-IV (SCID[10])

The SCID interview indexes the presence, absence, or subthreshold presence of each acute stress disorder symptom specified in DSM-IV. An advantage of employing this interview is that it provides a comprehensive assessment of the differential diagnoses and comorbid disorders that can be present in trauma populations.

(c) Stanford acute stress reaction questionnaire[11]

This self-report inventory asks patients to rate the frequency of a range of dissociative, intrusive, somatic anxiety, hyperarousal, attention disturbance, and sleep disturbance symptoms. The questionnaire has very good internal consistency (Cronbach's alpha = 0.90 and 0.91 for dissociative and anxiety symptoms, respectively) and concurrent validity with scores on the Impact of Event Scale ($r = 0.52$ to 0.69).[12,13] It can be employed as a measure of the severity of symptoms, but does not allow the diagnosis of acute stress disorder to be established as it has not yet been validated against clinician diagnoses.

(d) Acute stress disorder scale[14]

This self-report scale is scored on a 5-point scale that reflects degree of severity of 19 acute stress disorder symptoms. The Acute Stress Disorder Scale possesses good sensitivity (95 per cent) and specificity (83 per cent) relative to the Acute Stress Disorder Interview. Test–retest reliability with a re-administration interval of 2 to 7 days is strong ($r = 0.94$).[14]

Differential diagnoses

Both ICD-10 and DSM-IV require that the symptoms are not merely an exacerbation of a pre-existing disorder. In addition, a number of alternative diagnoses need to be considered.

(a) Post-traumatic stress disorder

In ICD-10, PTSD is conceptualized as an alternative diagnosis of acute stress reactions. The definitions of acute stress reaction and PTSD differ in terms of the stressor criterion (exceptionally stressful life event versus exceptionally threatening or catastrophic event), the time course (symptoms start to diminish within 48 h versus no time limit), and symptom pattern (PTSD, but not acute stress reaction, includes involuntary re-experiencing the traumatic event).

In DSM-IV, acute stress disorder can be distinguished from PTSD by the time-frame covered by the diagnoses. Acute stress disorder refers to the period from 2 days to 1 month post-trauma, after which a diagnosis of PTSD can be considered. The primary difference between the symptom criteria for acute stress disorder and PTSD in DSM-IV is the former's emphasis on dissociative reactions.

(b) Adjustment disorder

This diagnosis covers a wide range of emotional or behavioural symptoms indicative of distress, which are judged to be out of proportion to the stressor experienced. This broad coverage can be contrasted with (i) the specific set of symptoms described by the acute stress disorder and acute stress reaction criteria, and (ii) the stipulation that the stressor involves both a threat to life and a subjective response of fear for the acute stress disorder and an exceptional stressor in the case of acute stress reaction.

(c) Brain injury

A number of acute stress disorder symptoms overlap with symptoms of brain injury including reduced awareness, depersonalization, derealization, irritability, and concentration difficulties.[15] While results from neuropsychological and neurological investigations may assist in the differential diagnosis, there appear to be a group of individuals with a mild head injury for whom there are no known tools to differentiate whether the disturbance is due to brain injury or acute stress disorder, or whether both are present.

(d) Brief psychotic disorder

When there is one or more psychotic symptoms present after experiencing an extreme stressor, the brief psychotic disorder diagnosis should be considered.

(e) Dissociative disorders

Given the emphasis on dissociative symptoms in acute stress disorder, it needs to be distinguished from dissociative amnesia and depersonalization disorder. The criteria for these diagnoses stipulate that if the amnesia or depersonalization can be accounted for by acute stress disorder then a dissociative disorder cannot be diagnosed (see Chapter 5.2.4).

Epidemiology

Incidence

There is little research into what proportion of people develop acute stress reactions to severe stress. In a study of accident survivors, 14 per cent experienced a response pattern characterized by derealization, and a further 17 per cent exhibited strong anxiety or dysphoria.[16]

Estimates of the incidence of acute stress disorder range from about 14 per cent in motor vehicle accident survivors to 33 per cent in witnesses of a mass shooting.[17] Given the variable procedures and assessment tools employed across studies, it is difficult to determine whether the different rates of acute stress disorder detected are attributable to differences in method or in the type of trauma.

Comorbidity

Data on comorbidity are sparse. Given the similarities between acute stress disorder and PTSD it is likely that the conditions found to be comorbid with PTSD, in particular depression and substance abuse, will be applicable to acute stress disorder (see Chapter 4.6.2).

Aetiology

Both psychological and biological theories have attempted to explain the symptoms of acute stress disorder. They overlap largely with theories of PTSD (see Chapter 4.6.2). Given that acute stress reaction describes a transient disturbance, there are no specific theories of acute stress reactions as defined in ICD-10.

Psychological theories

The psychological mechanism that has received the most attention in relation to acute stress disorder is dissociation, as reflected in the DSM-IV criteria. It has been argued that dissociation minimizes the adverse emotional consequences of trauma by restricting awareness of the experience to avoid overwhelming fear and loss of control.[13] Dissociation is thought to prevent recovery because it prevents the integration of the traumatic experience into existing schemas[18] and it prevents the full activation of the trauma memory which is thought to be necessary for its modification.[19] In line with these hypotheses, dissociation during or immediately after a traumatic event predicts PTSD.[20] In contrast, an alternate view posits that dissociation at the time of trauma may serve a protective function because it may limit the encoding of aversive experiences and this may assist adaptation.[21] Consistent with this view, there is evidence that persisting dissociation (which is a form of cognitive avoidance) is more predictive of PTSD than dissociation that occurs at the time of trauma.[22,23]

Psychological theories of acute stress disorder and PTSD focus on the personal meaning of the trauma and its consequences, and characteristics of the trauma memory. Several hypotheses about the problems in memory that are responsible for the characteristic re-experiencing symptoms (i.e. unwanted memories of aspects of the trauma that occur in response to a wide range of stimuli) have been suggested (see also Chapter 4.6.2). Foa and colleagues[24,25] suggested that PTSD is characterized by a pathological network in memory that is particularly large and easily triggered. It contains many stimulus propositions that are erroneously linked to danger, causing fear responses to harmless stimuli that are associated with the traumatic event in memory. Brewin *et al.*[26] postulated that two different representations of the trauma are formed in memory. The first, termed verbally accessible memory, contains the conscious recollection of the trauma. The second memory representation, termed situationally accessible memory, comprises sensory, physiological, and motor aspects of the trauma in the form of codes that enable the re-experiencing of the original experience. Ehlers and Clark[27] suggested three memory processes to explain that a wide range of stimuli can trigger vivid memories and strong emotional responses, which are experienced as if the traumatic event was happening at present. First, trauma memory is thought to be inadequately linked to its context in memory, which leads to poor inhibition of stimulus-driven retrieval. Two other basic memory processes, perceptual priming and associative learning, are thought to further enhance the chances of stimulus-driven retrieval of memories. Consistent with these psychological theories, there is evidence that chronic PTSD is predicted by impaired access to autobiographical memories[28] and the perceived 'nowness' of trauma memories.[29] There is also evidence that maladaptive appraisals such as 'I am inadequate', 'My reactions since the trauma mean I am losing my mind', or 'I have permanently changed for the worse' in the acute phase after trauma exposure predict chronic PTSD.[30,31]

Psychological models also concur that successful adaptation to trauma involves integration of corrective information, and any strategies that minimize this process will contribute to subsequent PTSD. Excessive use of such avoidant strategies (e.g. trying not to think about the trauma, efforts to push intrusive memories out of one's mind, ruminating about how the trauma could have been avoided) prevent recovery.[24–27] There is preliminary empirical evidence supporting this hypothesis.[30–33]

Biological theories

Biological models have focused on fear conditioning and progressive neural sensitization in the weeks after trauma.[34] Specifically, when a traumatic event (unconditioned stimulus) occurs, people typically respond with fear (unconditioned response). It is argued that the strong fear elicited by the trauma will lead to strong associative conditioning between the fear and the stimuli surrounding the trauma. As reminders of the trauma occur (conditioned stimuli), people then respond with fear reactions (conditioned response). It has been hypothesized that extreme sympathetic arousal at the time of a traumatic event may result in the release of stress neurochemicals (including norepinephrine and epinephrine) into the cortex, mediating an overconsolidation of trauma memories. It is possible that sensitization occurs as a result of repetitive activation by trauma reminders and re-experiencing symptoms, elevating sensitivity of limbic networks, and that as time progresses these responses become increasingly conditioned to trauma-related stimuli.[35] In support of these proposals, there is evidence that people who eventually develop PTSD display elevated resting heart rates in the initial week after trauma.[36] There is also evidence that most people with acute stress disorder suffer panic attacks during the traumatic experience, and most of these people continue to suffer ongoing panic attacks in the subsequent month.[37]

Course and prognosis

Time course of symptoms

Whereas the ICD-10 criteria define an acute stress reaction as a disorder that remits within a few days, DSM-IV conceptualizes acute stress disorder as a marker of those vulnerable to the development of PTSD. Evidence relating to these different assumptions was sparse at the time the diagnoses were established. One explicit goal of the acute stress disorder diagnosis is to identify people who will develop PTSD. This goal is difficult to achieve because most people who initially display acute stress reactions adapt in the following 3 months.[38] Across 12 studies that have assessed the relationship between acute stress disorder and PTSD, most studies have found that whereas most people with acute stress disorder do develop PTSD, the acute stress disorder diagnosis does not capture the majority of people who develop PTSD.[38] It appears that the requirement for dissociative symptoms in the acute phase to be present results in a failure to identify many people who are high risk for PTSD development. It is important to note that similar patterns have been noted in prospective studies of children after trauma.[39–41] Across studies, people who have more severe symptoms of PTSD in the weeks following trauma have a poorer prognosis than those with less severe symptoms.[42,43]

Predictors of acute stress disorder

Little is known about predictors of acute stress reactions. A history of psychiatric disorder, depressive and dissociative symptoms prior to the traumatic event, and previous trauma predict acute stress disorder.[22,44,45]

Treatment

Psychological treatments

(a) Debriefing

Critical incident stress debriefing is a widely practised intervention that has the goal of promoting adaptation to traumatic events. Debriefing is generally conducted in a group within 24 to 72 h of the trauma. However, these parameters have been modified to permit more flexible interventions. Mitchell[46] proposes that debriefing comprises seven phases:

1 an initial outline of the purpose and benefits of debriefing;

2 the fact phase, in which participants relate what happened to them;

3 a thought phase, in which participants relate their initial thoughts after the critical incident;

4 a feeling phase, which requires participants to focus on the worst aspects of the incident and engage in their emotional reactions to the incident;

5 an assessment phase, in which participants are trained to note their physical, cognitive, emotional, and behavioural symptoms;

6 an education phase, which provides information about stress responses and ways to manage them;

7 the re-entry phase, in which the information given is summarized and referral information offered.

These phases may take 1 to 5 h, and are usually coordinated by a trained mental health professional.

Anecdotal evidence and clinical reports attest to the efficacy of debriefing. However, despite its widespread use, few controlled trials have been conducted. These have mainly focused on single session individual debriefing. A Cochrane review of 15 randomized controlled studies of psychological debriefing[47] found that although participants usually found the intervention useful, debriefing did not prevent the onset of PTSD nor reduce psychological distress compared to control. The two studies with the longest follow-up actually found that the debriefing group had a worse long-term outcome than the control group.[48–50] These results suggest that single session individual debriefing is not effective.[47]

In line with these results on individual debriefing, the first two non-randomized controlled studies of the efficacy of group debriefing found that the intervention had no beneficial effects on post-trauma symptoms.[51,52] One of the studies found negative effects of the intervention after 18 months.[52] A large trial of 1050 soldiers on a peacekeeping mission found no differences on all outcomes between a full programme of critical incident stress debriefing, stress education, and no intervention.[53]

(b) Cognitive behaviour therapy

Cognitive behavioural interventions are effective in treating PTSD (see Chapter 4.6.2). The results of randomized controlled studies of rape victims and road traffic accident survivors suggest that a brief five-session version of this treatment is effective in acute stress disorder and prevents the development of chronic post-trauma reactions.[54–58] Treatment involved the following:

1 education about trauma reactions;

2 progressive muscle relaxation;

3 prolonged exposure;

4 cognitive restructuring of fear-related beliefs;

5 graded *in vivo* exposure.

Cognitive behaviour therapy was found to be superior to other psychological therapies such as non-directive therapy or relaxation in preventing chronic PTSD.[59,60]

Psychopharmacological treatment

Little is known about which pharmacological interventions are effective in acute stress reactions/disorder. Preliminary studies report the utility of tricyclic antidepressants, but no or even harmful effects of benzodiazepines.[59–61] Research on PTSD suggests that selective serotonin reuptake inhibitors are, to date, the best pharmacological treatment for persistent reactions to traumatic stress (see Chapter 4.6.2).

There is growing interest in pharmacological interventions in the acute phase following the trauma that may prevent the development of PTSD symptoms.[62] A pilot study attempted to prevent PTSD by administering propranolol (a β-adrenergic blocker) within 6 h of trauma exposure.[63] This approach is based on evidence that propranolol abolishes the epinephrine enhancement of fear conditioning.[64] Although propranolol did not result in reduced PTSD relative to a placebo condition, patients receiving propranolol displayed less reactivity to trauma reminders 3 months later. This outcome accords with an uncontrolled study that found that propranolol administered immediately after trauma resulted in reduced PTSD 3 months later.[65] These preliminary data suggest that propranolol administration shortly after trauma exposure may limit fear conditioning that may contribute to subsequent PTSD development. Two other pilot studies found that high doses of hydrocortisol given to medical patients in an intensive care environment had a beneficial effect on subsequent PTSD symptoms.[62,66] One possible pathway of action is that cortisol contains strong epinephrine responses during stress, and may thus indirectly influence the strength of fear conditioning.[62] However, these experimental studies are as yet too preliminary to suggest clinical application.[60]

Information and self-help booklets

Several studies have evaluated the effectiveness of information or self-help booklets as early interventions after trauma. They consistently found that such interventions are ineffective and do not decrease the risk of chronic PTSD symptoms, although patients report that they find the booklets helpful.(67,68)

Advice about management

As acute stress reactions (ICD-10) are transient, and trials showed that early psychological debriefing is not effective in reducing future symptoms, psychological interventions that focus on recounting the traumatic event and ventilation of feelings are not indicated in the initial days after trauma exposure.(59,60) Instead, clinicians should focus on ensuring trauma survivors' safety and security, providing support and practical assistance, and encouraging them to actively use their social support.(59,60) Although drug treatments are not recommended as a preventative intervention following traumatic exposure,(60) clinicians may consider short-term hypnotic medication or longer term use of antidepressants for the management of significant sleep disturbance in the acute phase after trauma.(59,61) Furthermore, patients may find information about common reactions to trauma and their course, and practical advice about issues such as hospital procedures, police questioning, insurance claims, legal procedures, and media pressure to tell one's story helpful. Clinicians should offer follow-up appointments and monitor trauma survivors for the development of PTSD.(59)

An important clinical task is the early identification of those trauma survivors who are likely to develop chronic and disabling post-trauma symptoms.(47,59) If symptoms persist for 2 weeks or longer, treatment may be indicated. However, patients with low symptom severity at 2 weeks have a good chance of recovering without intervention, and clinicians may want to initially monitor symptom progression for a month to determine whether the patient is recovering naturally.(59) A number of short symptom screening questionnaires have been developed that may provide useful predictive information for this purpose in the future, but still await cross-validation in other samples.(69)

For trauma survivors with more severe acute stress disorder symptoms, a course of cognitive behavioural treatment should be considered.(59,60) This form of intervention is typically not provided within 2 weeks of trauma exposure. If the patient is offered cognitive behavioural treatment, therapists need to be aware that avoidance is a hallmark symptom of acute stress disorder and may reduce the likelihood that an individual will attend treatment sessions regularly. Flexible treatment procedures (e.g. initial contacts by telephone, scheduling sessions around the patient's preferences) and discussions about the ambivalence towards treatment may be helpful. Therapists need to be knowledgeable about the conditions surrounding the traumatic event and be sensitive to the particular socio-cultural background of the patient, which will affect the personal meaning of the event. Other forms of psychological treatment that do not address traumatic memories (such as relaxation or non-directive therapy) should not be routinely offered.(59)

The lack of randomized controlled trials suggests that pharmacological treatment cannot be considered a front-line treatment for acute stress disorder,(59,60) but research on PTSD suggests that selective serotonin reuptake inhibitors and other antidepressants may be helpful (see Chapter 4.6.2).

Possibilities for prevention

Identifying highly symptomatic individuals with acute stress disorder and providing a cognitive behavioural intervention from 2 weeks post-trauma onwards may reduce the risk of chronic PTSD. Additional preventive methods have been explored that prepare individuals 'at risk' (e.g. emergency services and military personnel) for experiencing trauma so as to enhance their coping strategies and reduce the risk of them developing longer-term symptomatology. For those individuals at high risk of experiencing a trauma, providing them with training to remain calm, evaluate the situation objectively,(70) to not identify with victims, to utilize social supports, and to express emotional reactions(71) have all been found to be associated with better coping after the trauma. However, evidence remains preliminary and it remains unclear whether they affect the risk of PTSD.

Further information

McNally, R.J., Bryant, R.A., and Ehlers, A. (2003). Does early psychological intervention promote recovery from posttraumatic stress? *Psychological Science in the Public Interest*, **4**, 45–79.

National Institute of Clinical Excellence. (2005). *Clinical guideline 26: post-traumatic stress disorder: The management of PTSD in adults and children in primary and secondary care.* http://guidance.nice.org.uk/CG26

National Center for Posttraumatic Stress Disorder. http://www.ncptsd.va.gov/ncmain/providers/ and PILOTS database http://www.ncptsd.va.gov/ncmain/publications/pilots/

Australian Centre for Posttraumatic Mental Health. (2007). *Australian guidelines for the treatment of acute stress disorder and posttraumatic stress disorder.* http://www.acpmh.unimelb.edu.au/Resources/guidelines/ACMPH_PractionerGuideForASDandPTSD.pdf

References

1. Lindemann, E. (1944). Symptomatology and management of acute grief. *The American Journal of Psychiatry*, **101**, 141–8.
2. Sargent, W. and Slater, E. (1941). Amnesic syndromes in war. *Proceedings of the Royal Society for Social Medicine*, **34**, 757–74.
3. World Health Organization. (1948). *International statistical classification of diseases, injuries, and causes of death* (6th revision). World Health Organization, Geneva.
4. World Health Organization. (1992). *The ICD-10 classification of mental and behavioural disorder: diagnostic criteria for research* (10th revision). World Health Organization, Geneva.
5. American Psychiatric Association. (1980). *Diagnostic and statistical manual of mental disorders* (3rd edn). American Psychiatric Association, Washington, DC.
6. American Psychiatric Association. (1989). *Diagnostic and statistical manual of mental disorders* (3rd edn, revised). American Psychiatric Association, Washington, DC.
7. Pincus, H.A., Frances, A., Davis, W.W., *et al.* (1992). DSM-IV and new diagnostic categories: holding the line on proliferation. *The American Journal of Psychiatry*, **149**, 112–17.
8. American Psychiatric Association. (1994). *Diagnostic and statistical manual of mental disorders* (4th edn). American Psychiatric Association, Washington, DC.
9. Bryant, R.A., Harvey, A.G., Dang, S., *et al.* (1998). Assessing acute stress disorder: psychometric properties of a structured clinical interview. *Psychological Assessment*, **10**, 215–20.
10. First, M.B., Spitzer, R.L., Gibbon, M., *et al.* (1995). *Structured clinical interview for DSM-IV Axis I disorders-patient version (SCID-I/P, Version 2.0)*. Biometrics Research Department of the New York State Psychiatric Institute, New York.

11. Cardeña, E., Classen, C., and Spiegel, D. (1991). *Stanford acute stress reaction questionnaire*. Stanford University Medical School, Stanford, CA.
12. Koopman, C., Classen, C., and Spiegel, D. (1994). Predictors of post-traumatic stress symptoms among survivors of the Oakland/Berkeley, Calif. firestorm. *The American Journal of Psychiatry*, **151**, 888–94.
13. Spiegel, D. (1991). Dissociation and trauma. In *American psychiatric press review of psychiatry*, Vol. 10 (eds. A. Tasman and S.M. Goldfinger), pp. 261–75. American Psychiatric Press, Washington, DC.
14. Bryant, R.A., Moulds, M., and Guthrie, R. (2000). Acute Stress Disorder Scale: a self-report measure of acute stress disorder. *Psychological Assessment*, **12**, 61–8.
15. Harvey, A.G. and Bryant, R.A. (1998). Acute stress disorder following mild traumatic brain injury. *The Journal of Nervous and Mental Disease*, **186**, 333–7.
16. Schnyder, U. and Malt, U.F. (1998). Acute stress response patterns to accidental injuries. *Journal of Psychosomatic Research*, **45**, 419–24.
17. Harvey, A.G. and Bryant, R.A. (2002). Acute stress disorder: a synthesis and critique. *Psychological Bulletin*, **128**, 886–902.
18. Koopman, C., Classen, C., Cardena, E., *et al.* (1995). When disaster strikes, acute stress disorder may follow. *Journal of Traumatic Stress*, **8**, 29–46.
19. Foa, E.B. and Hearst-Ikeda, D. (1996). Emotional dissociation in response to trauma: an information-processing approach. In *Handbook of dissociation: theoretical and clinical perspectives* (eds. L.K. Michelson and W.J. Ray), pp. 207–22. Plenum Press, New York.
20. Ozer, E.J., Best, S., Lipzey, T.L., *et al.* (2003). Predictors of posttraumatic stress disorder and symptoms in adults: a meta-analysis. *Psychological Bulletin*, **129**, 52–73.
21. Bryant, R.B. (2007). Does dissociation further our understanding of PTSD? *Journal of Anxiety Disorders*, **21**, 183–91.
22. Murray, J., Ehlers, A., and Mayou, R.A. (2002). Dissociation and posttraumatic stress disorder: two prospective studies of road traffic accident victims. *The British Journal of Psychiatry*, **180**, 363–8.
23. Briere, J., Scott, C., and Weathers, F. (2005). Peritraumatic and persistent dissociation in the presumed etiology of PTSD. *The American Journal of Psychiatry*, **162**, 2295–301.
24. Foa, E.B. and Riggs, D.S. (1993). Post-traumatic stress disorder in rape victims. In *Annual review of psychiatry*, Vol. 12 (eds. J. Oldham, M.B. Riba, and A. Tasman), pp. 273–303. American Psychiatric Association, Washington, DC.
25. Foa, E.B., Steketee, G., and Rothbaum, B.O. (1989). Behavioral/cognitive conceptualizations of post-traumatic stress disorder. *Behavior Therapy*, **20**, 155–76.
26. Brewin, C.R., Dalgleish, T., and Joseph, S. (1996). A dual representation theory of post-traumatic stress disorder. *Psychological Review*, **103**, 670–86.
27. Ehlers, A. and Clark, D.M. (2000). A cognitive model of post-traumatic stress disorder. *Behaviour Research and Therapy*, **38**, 319–45.
28. Harvey, A.G., Bryant, R.A., and Dang, S.T. (1998). Autobiographical memory in acute stress disorder. *Journal of Consulting and Clinical Psychology*, **66**, 500–6.
29. Michael, T., Ehlers, A., Halligan, S., *et al.* (2005). Unwanted memories of assault: what intrusion characteristics predict PTSD? *Behaviour Research and Therapy*, **43**, 613–28.
30. Ehring, T., Ehlers, A., and Glucksman, E. (in press). Do cognitive models help in predicting posttraumatic stress disorder, phobia and depression after trauma? *Journal of Consulting and Clinical Psychology*.
31. Kleim, B., Ehlers, A., and Glucksman, E. (2007). Prediction of chronic posttraumatic stress disorder after assault. *Psychological Medicine*, **37**, 1457–68.
32. Ehlers, A., Mayou, R.A., and Bryant, B. (1998). Psychological predictors of chronic post-traumatic stress disorder after motor vehicle accidents. *Journal of Abnormal Psychology*, **107**, 508–19.
33. Harvey, A.G. and Bryant, R.A. (1998). The effect of attempted thought suppression in acute stress disorder. *Behaviour Research and Therapy*, **36**, 583–90.
34. Charney, D.S., Deutch, A.Y., Krystal, J.H., *et al.* (1993). Psychobiologic mechanisms of posttraumatic stress disorder. *Archives of General Psychiatry*, **50**, 294–305.
35. Post, R.M., Weiss, S.R.B., and Smith, M.A. (1995). Sensitization and kindling: implications for the evolving neural substrates of post-traumatic stress disorder. In *Neurobiological and clinical consequences of stress: from normal adaptation to post-traumatic stress disorder* (eds. M.J. Friedman, D.S. Charney, and A.Y. Deutch), pp. 203–24. Lippincott Williams and Wilkins, Philadelphia, PA.
36. Bryant, R.A. (2006). Longitudinal psychophysiological studies of heart rate: mediating effects and implications for treatment. *Annals of the New York Academy of Sciences*, **107**, 19–26.
37. Nixon, R. and Bryant, R.A. (2003). Peritraumatic and persistent panic attacks in acute stress disorder. *Behaviour Research and Therapy*, **41**, 1237–42.
38. Bryant, R.A. (2003). Early predictors of posttraumatic stress disorder. *Biological Psychiatry*, **53**, 789–95.
39. Kassam-Adams, N. and Winston, F.K. (2004). Predicting child PTSD: the relationship between acute stress disorder and PTSD in injured children. *Journal of the American Academy of Child and Adolescent Psychiatry*, **43**, 403–11.
40. Meiser-Stedman, R., Yule, W., Smith, P., *et al.* (2005). Acute stress disorder and posttraumatic stress disorder in children and adolescents involved in assaults or motor vehicle accidents. *The American Journal of Psychiatry*, **162**, 1381–3.
41. Bryant, R.A., Salmon, K., Sinclair, E., *et al.* (2007). The relationship between acute stress disorder and posttraumatic stress disorder in injured children. *Journal of Traumatic Stress*, **20**, 1075–9.
42. Rothbaum, B.O., Foa, E.B., Riggs, D.S., *et al.* (1992). A prospective examination of post-traumatic stress disorder in rape victims. *Journal of Traumatic Stress*, **5**, 455–75.
43. Blanchard, E.B., Hickling, E.J., Barton, K.A., *et al.* (1996). One-year prospective follow-up of motor vehicle accident victims. *Behaviour Research and Therapy*, **34**, 775–86.
44. Barton, K.A., Blanchard, E.B., and Hickling, E.J. (1996). Antecedents and consequences of acute stress disorder among motor vehicle accident victims. *Behaviour Research and Therapy*, **34**, 805–13.
45. Harvey, A.G. and Bryant, R.A. (1999). Predictors of acute stress following motor vehicle accidents. *Journal of Traumatic Stress*, **12**, 519–26.
46. Mitchell, J. (1983). When disaster strikes. The critical incident stress debriefing process. *Journal of Emergency Medical Services*, **8**, 36–9.
47. Rose, S., Bisson, J., Churchill, R., *et al.* (2002). Psychological debriefing for preventing posttraumatic stress disorder (PTSD). *Cochrane Database of Systematic Reviews*, (2), CD000560, DOI: 10.1002/14651858.CD000560.
48. Bisson, J.I., Jenkins, P.L., Alexander, J., *et al.* (1997). Randomised controlled trial of psychological debriefing for victims of acute burn trauma. *The British Journal of Psychiatry*, **171**, 78–81.
49. Hobbs, M., Mayou, R., Harrison, B., *et al.* (1996). A randomised controlled trial of psychological debriefing for victims of road traffic accidents. *British Medical Journal*, **7**, 1438–9.
50. Mayou, R.A., Ehlers, A., and Hobbs, M. A (2002) three year follow-up of a randomised controlled trial of psychological debriefing for road traffic accident victims. *The British Journal of Psychiatry*, **176**, 589–93.
51. Kenardy, J.A., Webster, R.A., Lewin, T.J., *et al.* (1996). Stress debriefing and patterns of recovery following a natural disaster. *Journal of Traumatic Stress*, **9**, 37–49.
52. Carlier, I.V.E., Lamberts, R.D., van Uchelen, A.J., *et al.* (1998). Disaster-related post-traumatic stress in police officers: a field study of the impact of debriefing. *Stress Medicine*, **14**, 143–8.

53. Litz, B. (2004). Cited in Rose, S., Bisson, J., Churchill, R., and Wessely, S. (2002). Psychological debriefing for preventing posttraumatic stress disorder (PTSD) (Review). *Cochrane Database of Systematic Reviews*, (2), CD000560, DOI: 10.1002/14651858. CD000560, p. 8.
54. Bryant, R.A., Harvey, A.G., Dang, S.T., *et al.* (1998). Treatment of acute stress disorder: a comparison of cognitive behaviour therapy and supportive counselling. *Journal of Consulting and Clinical Psychology*, **66**, 862–6.
55. Bryant, R.A., Sackville, T., Dang, S.T., *et al.* (1999). Treating acute stress disorder: an evaluation of cognitive behavior therapy and counseling techniques. *The American Journal of Psychiatry*, **156**, 1780–6.
56. Bryant, R.A., Moulds, M.L., Guthrie, R., *et al.* (2003). Treating acute stress disorder after mild brain injury. *The American Journal of Psychiatry*, **160**, 585–7.
57. Bryant, R.A., Moulds, M.L., Guthrie, R.M., *et al.* (2005). The additive benefit of hypnosis and cognitive behavior therapy in treating acute stress disorder. *Journal of Consulting and Clinical Psychology*, **73**, 334–40.
58. Bisson, J.I., Shepherd, J.P., Joy, D., *et al.* (2004). Early cognitive behavioural therapy for post-traumatic stress symptoms after physical injury. *The British Journal of Psychiatry*, **184**, 63–9.
59. National Institute of Clinical Excellence. (2005). *Clinical guideline 26: post-traumatic stress disorder: the management of PTSD in adults and children in primary and secondary care.* http://guidance.nice.org.uk/CG26
60. Australian Centre for Posttraumatic Mental Health. (2007). *Australian guidelines for the treatment of acute stress disorder and posttraumatic stress disorder.* http://www.acpmh.unimelb.edu.au/Resources/guidelines/ACMPH_PractionerGuideForASDandPTSD.pdf
61. Davidson, J.R.T. (2006). Pharmacologic treatment of acute and chronic stress following trauma. *The Journal of Clinical Psychiatry*, **67**(Suppl. 2), 34–9.
62. Pitman, R.K. and Delahanty, D.L. (2005). Conceptually driven pharmacologic approaches to acute trauma. *CNS Spectrums*, **10**, 99–106.
63. Pitman, R.K., Sanders, K.M., Zusman, R.M., *et al.* (2002). Pilot study of secondary prevention of posttraumatic stress disorder with propranolol. *Biological Psychiatry*, **51**, 189–92.
64. Cahill, L., Prins, B., Weber, M., *et al.* (1994). Beta-adrenergic activation and memory for emotional events. *Nature*, **371**, 702–4.
65. Vaiva, G., Ducrocq, F., Jezequel, K., *et al.* (2003). Immediate treatment with propranolol decreases posttraumatic stress disorder two months after trauma. *Biological Psychiatry*, **54**, 947–9.
66. Schelling, G., Kilger, E., and Roozendaal, B. (2004). Stress doses of hydrocortisone, traumatic stress, and symptoms of posttraumatic stress disorder in patients after cardiac surgery: a randomized trial. *Biological Psychiatry*, **55**, 627–33.
67. Ehlers, A., Clark, D.M., Hackmann, A., *et al.* (2003). A randomized controlled trial of cognitive therapy, self-help booklet, and repeated assessment as early interventions for PTSD. *Archives of General Psychiatry*, **60**, 1024–32.
68. Turpin, G., Downs, M., and Mason, S. (1994). Effectiveness of providing self-help information following acute traumatic injury: randomised controlled trial. *The British Journal of Psychiatry*, **187**, 76–82.
69. Brewin, C.R. (2005). Systematic review of screening instruments for adults at risk of PTSD. *Journal of Traumatic Stress*, **18**, 53–62.
70. Hytten, K. (1989). Helicopter crash in water: effects of simulator escape training. *Acta Psychiatrica Scandinavica*, **80**(Suppl. 355), 73–8.
71. Fullerton, C.S., McCarroll, J.E., Ursano, R.J., *et al.* (1992). Psychological responses of rescue workers: fire fighters and trauma. *The American Journal of Orthopsychiatry*, **62**, 371–8.

4.6.2 **Post-traumatic stress disorder**

Anke Ehlers

Introduction

Clinicians have long noted that traumatic events can lead to severe psychological disturbance. At the end of the nineteenth and the beginning of the twentieth centuries, railway disasters, the World Wars, and the Holocaust prompted systematic descriptions of the symptoms associated with traumatic stress reactions. These include the spontaneous re-experiencing of aspects of the traumatic events, startle responses, irritability, impairment in concentration and memory, disturbed sleep, distressing dreams, depression, phobias, guilt, psychic numbing, and multiple somatic symptoms. A variety of labels were used to describe these reactions including 'fright neurosis', 'combat/war neurosis', 'shell shock', 'survivor syndrome', and 'nuclearism'.[1–3]

Whether the traumatic event can be considered a major cause of these psychological symptoms, has been the subject of considerable debate. Charcot, Janet, Freud, and Breuer suggested that hysterical symptoms were caused by psychological trauma, but their views were not widely accepted. The dominant view was that a traumatic event in itself was not a sufficient cause of post-trauma symptoms, and experts searched for other causes. Many suspected an organic cause. For example, damage to the spinal cord was suggested as the cause of the 'railway spine syndrome', microsections of exploded bombs entering the brain as the cause of 'shell shock', and starvation and brain damage as causes of the chronic psychological difficulties of concentration camp survivors. Others doubted the validity of the symptom reports and suggested that malingering and compensation-seeking ('compensation neurosis') was the major cause in most cases. Finally, the psychological symptoms were attributed to pre-existing psychological dysfunction. The predominant view was that reactions to traumatic events are transient, and that therefore only people with unstable personalities, pre-existing neurotic conflicts, or mental illness would develop chronic symptoms.[1–3]

It was the recognition of the long-standing psychological problems of many war veterans, especially Vietnam veterans, that changed this view and convinced clinicians and researchers that even people with sound personalities can develop clinically significant psychological symptoms if they are exposed to horrific stressors. This prompted the introduction of post-traumatic stress disorder (PTSD) as a diagnostic category in DSM-III.[4] It was thus recognized that traumatic events such as combat, rape, man-made, or natural disasters give rise to a characteristic pattern of psychological symptoms. The diagnostic criteria specified the experience of a traumatic event as a necessary condition for the diagnosis. ICD-10[5] emphasized the causal role of traumatic stressors in producing psychological dysfunction even more clearly, in that a specific group of disorders, 'reaction to severe stress, and adjustment disorders', was created. These disorders are 'thought to arise always as a direct consequence of the acute severe stress or continued trauma. The stressful event . . . is the primary and overriding causal factor, and the disorder would not have occurred without its impact'.

What makes a stressor traumatic?

In everyday language, many upsetting situations are described as 'traumatic', for example, divorce, loss of job, or failing an examination. However, a field study designed to establish what kinds of stressors lead to the characteristic symptoms of PTSD, showed that only 0.4 per cent of a community sample developed the characteristic symptoms of PTSD in response to such 'low magnitude' stressors.[6] Thus, in diagnosing PTSD, it appeared necessary to employ a strict definition of what constitutes a traumatic stressor.

Few people would contest that horrific events such as rape or bombings are traumatic. In an attempt to capture the essence of these stressors, the authors of DSM-IIIR required a traumatic stressor to be 'outside the range of usual human experience' and that it 'would be markedly distressing to almost anyone'.[7] However, epidemiological studies showed that stressors that can lead to PTSD are actually quite common, for example road traffic accidents[8] or sexual assault.[9] Thus, the DSM-IIIR definition appeared too restrictive.

ICD-10 uses a broader definition and characterizes traumatic stressors by their exceptional severity and the distress they would cause for the average person 'a stressful event or situation . . . of an exceptionally threatening or catastrophic nature, which is likely to cause pervasive distress in almost anyone'.[5] Thus, the ICD-10 diagnosis refers to a common sense understanding of which situations are likely to be extremely distressing.

In contrast, the authors of DSM-IV[10] attempted a specific definition. On the basis of research findings that threat to life or physical integrity during the event is one of the most consistent predictors of PTSD,[11] DSM-IV requires that the person 'experienced, witnessed, or was confronted with an event or events that involved actual or threatened death or serious injury, or a threat to the physical integrity of self or others'. The authors of DSM-IV made a further important step, in that they moved away from a purely situational definition and included the person's subjective response to the situation as an additional criterion, requiring that the 'person's response involved intense fear, helplessness, or horror' (or disorganized or agitated behaviour in the case of children).[10] The latter criterion takes into account that there is a large inter-individual variability in the psychological response to the same situation.

The stressor criterion of DSM-IV is still under debate. Recent research suggests that both components of the definition may require extension. First, it may be necessary to include further possible emotional responses to traumatic stressors. There is accumulating evidence that emotional numbing during traumatic events is predictive of PTSD.[12] Furthermore, it has been established that perpetrators of violent crime sometimes develop PTSD. Witnessing or participating in war-related crimes such as torturing or killing prisoners of war and civilians and mutilation of corpses is more closely linked to PTSD in Vietnam veterans than the threat of death associated with combat.[13] The psychological state of the perpetrators during the events that later lead to PTSD has not been studied in detail, but it isdoubtful that they would meet the current DSM-IV definition. Feelings of shame or guilt that were experienced at the time or subsequently, may be predictive of PTSD in this group.[14]

Second, the emphasis on threat to life or physical integrity may omit important dimensions of subgroups of traumatic events. The threat to the perception of oneself as an autonomous human being may be a relevant dimension of traumatic events that involve intentional harm by other people.[15] Mental defeat, the perceived loss of all autonomy, was related to PTSD in political prisoners and assault victims,[15,16] independent of other indicators of trauma severity including threat to life and perceived helplessness.

Clinical features

The most characteristic symptoms of PTSD are the re-experiencing symptoms. Patients involuntarily re-experience aspects of the traumatic event in a very vivid and distressing way. This includes: flashbacks in which the person acts or feels as if the event were recurring; nightmares; and intrusive images or other sensory impressions from the event. For example, a woman who was assaulted kept seeing the eyes of the perpetrator looking through the letterbox before he broke into her house, and a man involved in a severe car crash at night kept hearing the sound of the impact. Despite these vivid memory fragments, intentional recall of the event is often disorganized, and some patients have amnesia for parts of the event (see also Chapter 4.6.3).

Reminders of the trauma arouse intense distress and/or physiological reactions and are consequently avoided, including conversations about the event. Patients try to push memories of the event out of their mind and avoid thinking about the event in detail, particularly about its worst moments. On the other hand, many ruminate excessively about questions that prevent them from coming to terms with the event, for example about why the event happened to them, about how it could have been prevented, or about how they could take revenge.

The patients' emotional state ranges from intense fear, anger, sadness, guilt, or shame to emotional numbness. They often describe feeling detached from other people and give up previously significant activities. Various symptoms of hyperarousal include hypervigilance, exaggerated startle responses, irritability, difficulty concentrating, and sleep problems.

Classification

ICD-10[5] classifies PTSD (F43.1) among the reactions to severe stress and adjustment disorders (F43) that are primarily caused by stressful events. DSM-IV[10] classifies PTSD (309.81) among the anxiety disorders because symptom patterns, psychophysiological responses, family studies, and the efficacy of exposure treatment and serotonergic drugs suggested a relationship with other anxiety disorders. However, some of the symptoms would also suggest a relationship with dissociative disorders (e.g. amnesia) or depression (e.g. loss of interest).[17,18]

Diagnosis and differential diagnosis

Diagnostic criteria in ICD-10 and DSM-IV

Table 4.6.2.1 compares the diagnostic criteria of ICD-10 and DSM-IV.[10] ICD-10 research diagnostic criteria,[19] as well as diagnostic guidelines,[5] are included. The diagnostic systems agree on the core symptoms of PTSD (re-experiencing, avoidance, emotional numbing, and hyperarousal), but differ in the weight assigned to them. DSM-IV criteria are stricter.

Table 4.6.2.1 Diagnostic criteria for PTSD in ICD-10 and DSM-IV

ICD-10 diagnostic guidelines	ICD-10 research diagnostic criteria	DSM-IV criteria
Stressor criterion		
1 Event or situation of exceptionally threatening or catastrophic nature	(a) 1 Event or situation of exceptionally threatening or catastrophic nature	(a) 1 The person experienced, witnessed,or was confronted with an event or events that involved actual or threatened death or serious injury, or a threat to the physical integrity of self or others
2 Likely to cause pervasive distress in almost anyone	2 Likely to cause pervasive distress in almost anyone	2 The person's response involved intense fear, helplessness, or horror (or disorganized or agitated behaviour in children)
Symptom criteria		
Necessary symptom	*Necessary symptoms*	*Necessary symptoms*
1 Repetitive intrusive recollection or re-enactment of the event in memories, daytime imagery, or dreams	(b) Persistent remembering or 'reliving' of the stressor in intrusive 'flashbacks', vivid memories, or recurring dreams, and in experiencing distress when exposed to circumstances resembling or associated with the stressor	(b) The traumatic event is persistently re-experienced in one (or more) of the following ways 1 Recurrent and intrusive distressing recollections of the event, including images, thoughts, or perceptions (or repetitive play in which the themes or aspects of the trauma are expressed in children)
Other typical symptoms 2 Sense of 'numbness' and emotional blunting, detachment from others, unresponsiveness to surroundings, anhedonia 3 Avoidance of activities and situations reminiscent of trauma *Common symptoms* 4 Autonomic hyperarousal with insomnia 5 Anxiety and depression	(c) Actual or preferred avoidance of circumstances resembling or associated with the stressor which was not present before exposure to the stressor (d) 1 Inability to recall, either partially or completely, some important aspects or the period of exposure to the stressor *or*	2 Recurrent distressing dreams of the event (or frightening dreams without recognizable content in children) 3 Acting or feeling as if the traumatic event were recurring (or trauma-specific re-enactment in children) 4 Intense psychological distress at exposure to internal or external cues that symbolize or resemble an aspect of the traumatic event 5 Physiological reactivity at exposure to internal or external cues that symbolize or resemble an aspect of the traumatic event
Rare symptoms 6 Dramatic acute bursts of fear, panic, or aggression triggered by reminders	2 Persistent symptoms of increased psychological sensitivity and arousal (not present before exposure to stressor), shown by any two of the following (a) Difficulty in falling or staying asleep (b) Irritability or outbursts of anger (c) Difficulty in concentrating (d) Hypervigilance (e) Exaggerated startle response	(c) Persistent avoidance of stimuli associated with the trauma and numbing of general responsiveness (not present before trauma), as indicated by three (or more) of the following 1 Efforts to avoid thoughts, feelings, or conversations associated with the trauma 2 Efforts to avoid activities, places, or people that arouse recollections of the trauma 3 Inability to recall an important aspect of the trauma 4 Markedly diminished interest or participation in significant activities 5 Feeling of detachment or estrangement from others 6 Restricted range of affect 7 Sense of foreshortened future (d) Persistent symptoms of increased arousal (not present before the trauma), as indicated by two (or more) of the following 1 Difficulty falling or staying asleep 2 Irritability or outbursts of anger 3 Difficulty concentrating 4 Hypervigilance 5 Exaggerated startle response
Time frame		
Symptoms should usually arise within 6 months of the traumatic event	Symptoms should usually arise within 6 months of the traumatic event	Symptoms present for at least 1 month
Disability criterion		
N/A	N/A	The disturbance causes clinically significant distress or impairment in social, occupational, or other important areas of functioning

(continued)

Table 4.6.2.1 (Continued) Diagnostic criteria for PTSD in ICD-10 and DSM-IV

ICD-10 diagnostic guidelines	ICD-10 research diagnostic criteria	DSM-IV criteria
Differential diagnoses		
1 Acute stress reaction F43.0 (immediate reaction in the first 3 days after event) 2 Enduring personality change after a catastrophic experience F62.0 (present for at least 2 years, only after extreme and prolonged stress) 3 Adjustment disorder (less severe stressor or different symptom pattern) 4 Other anxiety or depressive disorders (absence of traumatic stressor or symptoms precedes stressor)	Same as ICD-10 diagnostic guidelines	1 Acute stress disorder (duration of up to 4 weeks) 2 Adjustment disorder (less severe stressor or different symptom pattern) 3 Mood disorder or other anxiety disorder (symptoms of avoidance, numbing, or hyperarousal present before exposure to the stressor) 4 Other disorders with intrusive thoughts or perceptual disturbances (e.g. obsessive–compulsive disorder, schizophrenia, other psychotic disorders, substance-induced disorders)

- DSM-IV puts a stronger emphasis on the avoidance/numbing cluster of symptoms by requiring a minimum of three of these symptoms.
- DSM-IV states two additional criteria that are not included in ICD-10, namely a minimum symptom duration of 1 month and significant distress or impaired functioning.

A large-scale study[20] found a prevalence of ICD-10 PTSD of 6.9 per cent, and a prevalence of DSM-IV PTSD of 3 per cent.

Differential diagnoses

Differential diagnoses are summarized in Table 4.6.2.1. Distinguishing features include the following:

- the type of stressor (adjustment disorders, enduring personality change)
- the symptom pattern (adjustment disorders, enduring personality change)
- the duration of the symptoms (acute stress disorder, acute stress reaction)
- the question of whether the avoidance, numbing, and hyperarousal symptoms were present before the traumatic event occurred (other anxiety or depressive disorders)
- the nature of the intrusive cognitions and perceptual disturbances (obsessive-compulsive disorder, psychotic symptoms, substance-induced symptoms).

Prolonged repeated trauma, such as captivity or repeated childhood sexual abuse, may lead to a more complex pattern of symptoms, 'complex PTSD', that is characterized by somatization, dissociation, affect dysregulation, poor impulse control, self-destructive behaviour, and pathological patterns of relationships.[21] It was debated whether to include a category 'disorders of extreme stress not otherwise specified' (DESNOS) into DSM-IV to accommodate these cases, but the decision was not to include it.[17] In ICD-10, the diagnosis 'enduring personality changes after catastrophic experience' covers such long-standing consequences of enduring trauma.

Furthermore, it is currently being debated whether an additional diagnostic category 'traumatic grief' should be included into the psychiatric classification systems.[22]

Ongoing research on symptom criteria

Some research has questioned the symptom clusters of DSM-IV. In particular, it may be preferable to assess the emotional numbing symptoms separately from the avoidance symptoms, because these symptoms do not load on the same factor in factor analyses and may have different underlying mechanisms. Furthermore, it may be preferable to include severity criteria for the symptoms rather than relying on counting the presence of symptoms.[23]

Assessment instruments

Several semi-structured interviews assess the DSM-IV criteria for PTSD. The most commonly used diagnostic interviews are the Structured Clinical Interview for DSM-IV (SCID)[24] and the Clinician Administered PTSD scale (CAPS).[25]

The most widely used self-report measure of PTSD symptoms used to be the Impact of Event scale.[26] The original scale contained two scales, an intrusion and an avoidance scale. It has been expanded to include an additional hyperarousal scale (IES-R).[27] The IES-R does not cover all the symptoms of PTSD specified in DSM-IV. This is why new measures that are modelled on the DSM-IV criteria are now commonly used in research studies, for example the Post-traumatic Stress Diagnostic scale (PDS)[28] or the PTSD Checklist (PCL).[29]

Epidemiology

The available epidemiological data so far stem mainly from large-scale studies in industrialized societies such as the United States or Australia. It remains to be investigated whether these data replicate in other countries. One has to bear in mind that the society and natural environment set conditions for exposure to traumatic events. For example, in the last decades, people in developing countries have had a much greater exposure to war and natural disasters than people in industrialized western societies.[30]

How common are traumatic events in the population?

Traumatic events are common. In a large representative United States' sample, Kessler *et al.*[31] found that 60.7 per cent of the men and 51.2 per cent of the women had experienced at least one traumatic event meeting DSM-IIIR criteria in their lifetime. The most common types of trauma were witnessing someone being killed or severely injured, accidents, and being involved in a fire, flood, or natural disaster. Using DSM-IV criteria, Stein *et al.*[32] found a lifetime exposure to serious traumatic events of 81.3 per cent for men, and 74.2 per cent for women. Sudden death of a loved person was one of the most frequent traumatic stressors (DSM-IV criteria).[33]

What types of trauma are associated with high PTSD rates?

PTSD rates depend on the type of traumatic event. Rape was associated with the highest PTSD rates in several studies. For example, 65 per cent of the men and 46 per cent of the women who had been raped met PTSD criteria in the Kessler *et al.*[31] study. Other traumatic events associated with high PTSD rates included combat exposure, childhood neglect and physical abuse, sexual molestation; and for women only, physical attack and being threatened with a weapon, kidnapped, or held hostage. Accidents, witnessing death or injury, and fire or natural disasters were associated with relatively low-lifetime PTSD rates of less than 10 per cent.[31] Other research has shown high PTSD rates for torture victims,[34] survivors of the Holocaust,[35] and prisoners of war.[36] The emphasis in DSM-IV on threat to life or physical integrity has led to increasing awareness that medical illness and treatment (e.g. waking up during anaesthesia) can lead to PTSD.[37]

What proportion of people develop PTSD in response to a traumatic stressor?

Kessler *et al.*[31] found that the risk of developing PTSD after a traumatic event is 8.1 per cent for men, and 20.4 per cent for women. For young urban populations, higher risks have been reported; Breslau *et al.* found an overall risk of 23.6 per cent[38]; 13 per cent for men and 30.2 per cent for women.[39]

The figures reported in these studies may be influenced by two types of biases that have opposite effects on probability estimates. First, Breslau *et al.*[33] have pointed out that previous studies overestimated the PTSD-risk imposed by traumatic events because participants reported on the worst trauma that they had experienced. When assessment focused on the symptoms induced by a traumatic event that was randomly selected from the ones that a person had experienced, the conditional risk of PTSD following exposure to trauma was found to be 9.2 per cent, using DSM-IV criteria.

Second, the retrospective methodology used in the epidemiological studies may have led to underestimation of PTSD rates due to selective recall. For example, the prevalence of PTSD 3 months after road traffic accidents was found to be around 20 per cent in prospective longitudinal studies,[40,41] whereas the retrospective studies found prevalences below 10 per cent.

How prevalent is PTSD in the population?

Kessler *et al.*[31] estimated that the lifetime prevalence of PTSD is 7.8 per cent, using DSM-IIIR criteria. Women had a higher prevalence than men (10.4 versus 5.0 per cent). This was due to both a greater exposure to high-impact trauma (rape, sexual molestation, childhood neglect, and childhood physical abuse) and a greater likelihood of developing PTSD when exposed to a traumatic event. Other studies using DSM-IIIR criteria have yielded similarly high prevalence rates.[9,39] Estimates for the 12-month prevalence range between 1.3 per cent in an Australian study[42] and 3.6 per cent in an US study.[43] A study using DSM-IV criteria and found a past-month PTSD prevalence of 2.7 per cent for women and 1.2 per cent for men.[32]

Earlier studies using DSM-III criteria had reported lower lifetime prevalences of about 1 per cent. Besides differences in procedures and sampling methods, the low PTSD prevalence in these earlier studies may be due to the use of an interview schedule with low sensitivity in detecting PTSD.[44] In particular, the early interviews asked global questions about the occurrence of traumatic events and lacked the repeated probing for specific events or event categories that seems to be necessary in eliciting relevant experiences.

Partial PTSD

Several studies have found substantial levels of distress and disability for traumatized people who met some, but not all, of the PTSD criteria specified in DSM-IV.[32] These people may be at greater risk of developing the full PTSD syndrome than people with fewer symptoms.[40,41]

Comorbidity of PTSD with other disorders and symptoms

PTSD shows a substantial comorbidity with affective disorders, other anxiety disorders, substance-use disorders, and somatization. In the study by Kessler *et al.*,[31] 88.3 per cent of the men and 78.1 per cent of the women with PTSD had comorbid psychiatric diagnoses. Studies of veterans with PTSD have also indicated an enhanced level of problems in family and marital adjustment and violent behaviour,[45] and heavy smoking.[46] Furthermore, reports of poor health and increased rates of various diseases, in particular infectious and nervous system diseases, are associated with PTSD.[47]

Is PTSD primary or secondary to the comorbid diagnoses? There is, as yet, little research into this question. The retrospective accounts obtained by Kessler *et al.*[31] suggested that PTSD was primary to comorbid affective or substance-use disorders in the majority of cases, and PTSD was primary to comorbid anxiety disorders in about half of the cases. Similarly, Breslau *et al.*[39] found that PTSD increased the risks for first-onset major depression and alcohol-use disorder. Conversely, pre-existing major depression also increased vulnerability to the PTSD-inducing effects of traumatic events and risk for exposure to traumatic events. A prospective study confirmed that PTSD increased the risk of subsequent pain, conversion symptoms, and somatization symptoms.[48]

Most of the comorbidity research has concentrated on the nature of the relationship between PTSD and alcohol or drug abuse. The majority of studies found that PTSD precedes the development of alcohol-abuse problems. There are probably several mechanisms for this relationship. In the short-term, alcohol is used to self-medicate the symptoms of PTSD, but paradoxically intoxication and withdrawal symptoms may intensify the symptoms in the long-term.[49]

Summary of main findings from epidemiological studies

- The majority of people will experience at least one traumatic event in their lifetime.
- In assessing PTSD history, interviewers should probe for specific events.
- Assault, in particular sexual assault, and combat have a higher impact than accidents and disasters.[31,32]
- If the frequency and impact of traumatic events are considered together, sudden unexpected death of a loved one[33] and road traffic accidents[8] can be considered important causes of PTSD in western industrialized societies.
- Men tend to experience more traumatic events than women, but women experience higher impact events.[31,32]
- Women are at least twice as likely as men to develop PTSD in response to a traumatic event. This enhanced risk is not explained by differences in the type of traumatic event. The estimated lifetime prevalence for women is approximately 10 to 12 per cent, and for men 5 to 6 per cent.[9,31,38,39]
- Comorbid depression and substance-use disorders appear to be secondary to PTSD in the majority of cases.

Aetiology

There is no single accepted theory of PTSD. Theoretical explanations have focused on psychological and biological mechanisms that are not mutually exclusive.

Psychological processes

(a) Fear conditioning

Mowrer's two-factor conditioning theory of phobias has been applied to PTSD.[50–52] It is suggested that through classical (Pavlovian) conditioning, stimuli that were present at the time of the trauma (unconditioned stimulus) become associated with fear and arousal responses. Subsequently, the conditioned stimuli trigger similar (conditioned) responses when presented on their own. Through stimulus generalization and higher-order conditioning, a wide variety of stimuli become triggers of distress in the aftermath of trauma. Quite naturally, the person will try to avoid the conditioned stimuli and the associated distress. The avoidance behaviour is negatively reinforced (operant or instrumental conditioning) because it leads to a reduction in psychological and physical discomfort. In the long-term, however, avoidance prevents extinction of the conditioned fear responses to reminders of the traumatic event, and thus maintains the problem.

(b) Personal meanings of the traumatic event and its aftermath

The persistence of PTSD symptoms has been explained by individual differences in the appraisal of the traumatic event: that is to say, in what personal meaning it has for them.[53–55] Some people are able to see the trauma as a time-limited terrible experience that does not necessarily have negative global implications for their view of themselves, the world or the future. These people are likely to recover quickly. Individuals with persistent PTSD are characterized by *excessively* negative appraisals of the event that go beyond what everyone would find horrific about the event. The nature of predominant emotional responses in PTSD depends on the particular appraisals; for example, appraisals concerning danger lead to fear ('Nowhere is safe'), appraisals concerning others violating personal rules lead to anger ('Others have not treated me fairly'), appraisals concerning responsibility for the traumatic event lead to guilt or shame ('It was my fault', 'I did something despicable'), and appraisals concerning loss lead to sadness ('My life will never be the same again').[55] Such appraisals distinguish between traumatized individuals with and without PTSD, and predict chronic PTSD.[16,56]

Negative appraisals involved in maintaining PTSD do not only concern the traumatic event itself, but also its sequelae such as the initial PTSD symptoms or responses of other people in the aftermath of the traumatic event.[55,57,58] In line with this hypothesis, negative interpretations of intrusive recollections (e.g. 'I am going mad') after road traffic accidents were one of the most important predictors of PTSD at 1 year after the event.[41] Perceived negative responses from other people in the aftermath of trauma predicted PTSD in studies of assault and torture victims.[15,16]

(c) Nature of trauma memories

What exactly distinguishes trauma memories from other memories and what explains the distressing re-experiencing symptoms in PTSD is still under debate.[59,60] Phenomenological observations show that although a wide range of stimuli can trigger unwanted intrusive memories of parts of the traumatic event, people with PTSD show relatively poor intentional recall of details such as the order of events and their recall appears disjointed.[60] Several theories have been put forward to explain re-experiencing symptoms. Foa and colleagues[53,58] explain re-experiencing as spreading activation in a pathological network in memory. This network is thought to be particularly large and easily triggered. It contains many stimulus propositions that are erroneously linked to danger, causing fear responses to harmless stimuli associated with the traumatic event in memory. In addition, the person's reactions during the trauma are linked to the belief that the self is incompetent. Activation of components of the trauma memory (for instance, by confrontation to a reminder, by similar bodily sensations, or by thinking about the event) will activate the whole network, including the emotional responses that the person had during the traumatic event.

Brewin and colleagues[61] have proposed that the symptoms of PTSD can only be explained if one assumes several levels of representation of the traumatic event, namely a verbally accessible memory and a memory that is triggered by situation-specific cues. PTSD is thought to be characterized by easily accessible situationally specific memories that lead to re-experiencing symptoms.

Ehlers and Clark [55] suggested that re-experiencing results from three memory processes, namely, (i) poor inhibition of stimulus-driven retrieval of parts of the trauma memory (re-experiencing) due to insufficient elaboration of the trauma memory (insufficient links to other information that would give the worst moments of the trauma a context such as 'I survived the event' or 'I complied with the requests of the perpetrator because he had threatened me with a knife'), (ii) strong perceptual priming (low perceptual threshold for stimuli with similar sensory characteristics as those present during the trauma), and (iii) strong associations among stimuli present at the time of the event (e.g. footsteps behind me associated with feeling knife in my back) and between stimuli and emotional responses (e.g. pressure on back associated with fear of death).

(d) Behaviours that maintain PTSD symptoms

Whereas many people will recover from initial PTSD symptoms, some do not get better. This has led researchers to specify possible maintaining behaviours. These include avoidance of reminders, suppression of thoughts and memories connected to the event, rumination, safety behaviours, dissociation, and the use of alcohol or drugs.(57) Ehlers and Clark(55) suggested that these behaviours and cognitive strategies maintain PTSD in three ways. First, some behaviours directly lead to increases in symptoms; for example, thought suppression leads to paradoxical increases in intrusion frequency. Second, other behaviours prevent changes in the problematic appraisals; for example, constantly checking one's rear mirror (a safety behaviour) after a car accident prevents change in the appraisal that another accident will happen if one does not check the mirror. Third, other behaviours prevent elaboration of the trauma memory and its link to other experiences. For example, avoiding thinking about the event may prevent people from incorporating the fact that they did not die into the worst moments of the trauma memory, and they thus continue to re-experience the fear of dying they originally experienced during the event. Several studies have found that avoidance, safety behaviours, thought suppression, and rumination predict maintenance of PTSD.(16,41)

Some of the cognitive processes that maintain PTSD symptoms are not intentional. Patients with PTSD have an unintentional attentional bias to stimuli that are reminiscent of the traumatic event.(6) Involuntary selective attention to reminders may be one of the reasons why these patients have frequent re-experiencing symptoms. Rumination is often described by the patient as unintentional. In particular, patients have problems stopping ruminating once they have started. Rumination may represent a cognitive habit that started as an intentional strategy employed to solve problems and that became more automatic with time.

Biological processes

A number of biological factors have been linked to PTSD symptoms. They have the effect that they make people with PTSD hyper-responsive to stressful stimuli, especially stimuli that are reminiscent of the trauma.(62)

(a) Chronic stress reaction

Patients with PTSD show several abnormalities that are consistent with a chronic stress reaction or an enhanced reactivity to minor stressors. There is evidence for an enhanced secretion of adrenaline (epinephrine) and noradrenaline (norepinephrine) to stress.(63) In psychophysiological studies, patients with PTSD showed enhanced startle responses and higher baseline heart rates and blood pressure than traumatized controls without PTSD. However, these responses may, in part, reflect anticipatory anxiety related to the expectation of trauma cues. Patients with PTSD exhibit greater physiological reactivity to trauma cues (e.g. sounds, pictures, or script-driven imagery) than control subjects without PTSD.(6)

(b) Hypothalamic-pituitary-adrenal axis abnormalities

Patients with PTSD show a different pattern of hypothalamic-pituitary-adrenal response than patients with major depression.(63) Like depressed patients, patients with PTSD hypersecrete corticotrophin-releasing factor (CRF). However, they show *lower* levels of cortisol compared to normal controls, traumatized individuals without current PTSD and depressed patients. When given a low dose of dexamethasone, PTSD patients exhibit *hyper*-suppression of cortisol. Some, but not all findings, suggest that the hypothalamic-pituitary-adrenal axis in PTSD may characterized by enhanced negative feedback.(64) Overall, the hypothalamic-pituitary-adrenal axis in PTSD appears to be set to produce large responses to further stressors.

(c) Hypothalamic-pituitary-thyroid axis

Studies suggest increased hypothalamic-pituitary-thyroid axis activity in PTSD.(63) Patients with PTSD showed increased levels of thyroid hormones, and an exaggerated thyrotropin-stimulating hormone (TSH) response to the standard TSH stimulation test.

(d) Neuroendocrinological abnormalities

Several neurotransmitter systems appear to be dysregulated in PTSD.(63,65) Research suggests exaggerated noradrenergic activity in PTSD in response to stressors.(65) People with PTSD have fewer plaletet α_2-adrenergic receptors, which has been interpreted as a response to chronic elevation of circulating catecholamines. Yohimbine (which blocks α_2-receptors) provokes flashbacks and panic attacks in a substantial subgroup of PTSD patients.(65)

There is also evidence for the involvement of the serotonergic system in PTSD.(63,65) Findings suggest decreased serotonin activity, including decreased serum concentrations, decreased sensitivity of platelet serotonin uptake sites, and blunted prolactin response to D-fenfluramine (indicative of central serotonin hypo-activity). Serotonin-reuptake inhibitors have therapeutic effects in PTSD.

Endogenous opiates have been suspected to mediate the symptoms of emotional numbing and amnesia. In the animal model, uncontrollable stress leads to the secretion of endogenous opiates that induce analgesia. There is some evidence for decreased baseline levels, but increased post-stimulation levels of ß-endorphin.(63)

The dopaminergic and γ-aminobutyric acid (GABA) systems have also been implicated in PTSD, but the evidence for these hypotheses is sparse at this stage.(63)

(e) Neuroimaging

Structural magnetic resonance imaging studies tend to show a reduced hippocampal volume in adults with PTSD, in particular in those with severe and very chronic PTSD, but not in children.(66) Disturbances of hippocampal function may lead to deficits in explicit memory and the appreciation of safe contexts. This line of research was prompted by animal studies showing that high levels of cortisol seen during stress are associated with damage to the hippocampus.(67) However, there is evidence from a study of monozygotic twins that the hippocampal volume of the *unexposed* twins correlated with the PTSD severity of the exposed twins. Thus, small hippocampal volume may be a vulnerability factor for PTSD, an effect of severe or chronic stress, or both. Preliminary evidence suggests that successful long-term treatment with paroxetine increases hippocampal volume in patients with PTSD.(67)

Functional neuroimaging studies have found differences between people with and without PTSD in neurocircuits that are involved in fear conditioning (amygdalae, medial prefrontal cortex, hippocampus). When exposed to trauma reminders or other anxiety cues,(68) people with PTSD tend to show heightened responsivity of the amygdala and diminished responsivity in the medial prefrontal cortex. The latter plays a role in extinguishing fear reactions, as animal studies established that conditioned fear responses could only be extinguished if the cortex was intact.[69] Recent studies suggest different patterns of responses to trauma reminders for people with PTSD who show high arousal to trauma reminders (involving mainly the anterior cingulate, medial prefrontal cortex, and thalamus) versus those with dissociative reactions (involving mainly the parietal, occipital, and temporal cortex).[70]

(f) Animal models of PTSD

There are biological and psychological parallels between the animal model of inescapable shock and exposure to a traumatic event. The uncontrollability of an aversive event seems to make it particularly traumatic.[71] Inescapable shock leads to changes in the noradrenergic system, the HPA axis, and endogenous opiates that parallel findings in PTSD patients.[51]

However, these effects are usually only observed after repeated exposure to inescapable shock, whereas one traumatic event can be sufficient in inducing PTSD. This is why some authors have suggested that the animal model of kindling or behavioural sensitization is more appropriate in explaining PTSD. Kindling refers to a process whereby intermittent subconvulsive electrical stimulation of the limbic system eventually has the effect that the animal will respond with a seizure to a stimulus that previously was subthreshold. Post *et al.*[72] have suggested that the repeated re-experiencing of the traumatic event may constitute a kindling process, to the effect that PTSD symptoms become more easily triggered with time. Similarly, previous exposure to stressors may sensitize people to respond with PTSD symptoms to a traumatic event.

Animal models suggest that the massive secretion of neurohormones at the time of the trauma, in particular noradrenaline and vasopressin, leads to overconsolidation (long-term potentiation) of the trauma memory. This would have the effect that the conditioned fear responses are particularly difficult to extinguish and that stimuli that resemble those present during trauma are particularly likely to trigger intrusive memories, distress, and/or the corresponding physiological responses.[62]

(g) Genetic factors

Twin studies have found a higher concordance of PTSD among monozygotic than dizygotic twins. There is also an increased prevalence of psychiatric disorders, especially anxiety disorders, affective disorders, sociopathy, and/or substance abuse, among family members of people with PTSD.[73] A study found a higher proportion of the 5-HTTLPR s/s genotype in PTSD compared to controls.[74]

Course and prognosis

Time course of symptoms

For the vast majority of PTSD cases, symptoms begin immediately after the traumatic event. Delayed onset is found in a minority (11 per cent or less) of the cases.[6]

Prospective longitudinal studies suggest that a large proportion of people who initially develop PTSD after trauma will recover on their own. However, between one-third and 50 per cent of those who develop PTSD after a traumatic event will not recover for many years.[31,75] Long-term outcome depends on initial symptom severity and the experience of further traumatic events. People with high initial PTSD severity are more likely to remain symptomatic at follow-up than those with low initial symptom severity.[41,75]

Factors that influence the risk of developing PTSD

Meta-analyses[11,76] have identified several reliable predictors of PTSD. The results are summarized in Table 4.6.2.2. Overall, peri-traumatic factors such as perceived life threat and dissociation during the trauma and post-trauma factors such as low social support appear more predictive of PTSD than pre-trauma variables.

(a) Demographic and pre-trauma variables

Women have consistently shown to have a greater risk of developing PTSD than men, but the mechanisms remain unclear.[11,31,67,76,77] Similarly, it is as yet unclear why people with lower intelligence or education,[76] people with lower socioeconomic status,[76] and people from ethnic minorities[78] have an elevated PTSD risk. Other risk factors include previous trauma, childhood adversity, a personal or family history of anxiety or depression,[76] and neuroticism.[38]

(b) Stressor variables

PTSD risk depends on the severity of the stressor. Prolonged and repeated trauma, exposure to the grotesque aftermath of violence, events that involve intentional harm by another person and abusive violence, and events that involve harm to children are particularly likely to lead to PTSD.[79,80]

Injury severity is only a weak predictor of PTSD. Long-term health problems and loss of function may play a greater role in maintaining PTSD.[41,79] There are some reports that unconsciousness during a traumatic event may decrease the risk of PTSD,[81]

Table 4.6.2.2 Risk factors for post-traumatic stress disorder

	Weighted average effect size *r*
Demographic variables	
Female sex	0.13[76]
Race (minority status)	0.05[76]
Younger age	0.06[76]
Low socio-economic status	0.14[76]
Cognitive ability	
Low education	0.10[76]
Low intelligence	0.18[76]
Psychiatric and trauma history	
Psychiatric history	0.11[76]–0.17[11]
Family psychiatric history	0.13[76]–0.17[11]
Prior trauma	0.12[76]–0.17[11]
Childhood abuse	0.14[76]
Other adverse childhood	0.19[76]
Peri-traumatic factors	
Trauma severity	0.23[76]
Perceived life threat	0.26[11]
Peri-traumatic emotions	0.26[11]
Peri-traumatic dissociation	0.35[11]
Post-trauma factors	
Low social support	0.28[11]–0.40[76]
Further life stress	0.32[76]

(Modified from meta-analyses by Brewin *et al.* (2000) and Ozer *et al.* (2003))

but other studies have found small associations in the opposite direction.[41]

(c) Psychological responses during trauma

PTSD risk depends on the degree of psychological distress the traumatic event caused. The psychological impact of the trauma depends on the perceived threat to life,[11,76] the perceived loss of control (helplessness),[82] and the perceived threat to one's autonomy (mental defeat).[15,16] Among the psychological responses predicting PTSD are feelings of anger, guilt, or shame[83] and dissociation and numbing.[11]

Factors affecting recovery from trauma

(a) Recovery environment

Recovery is facilitated by social support, [11,76] and hindered by perceived negative responses from other people.[15,16] Further stressful or traumatic life events impede recovery from PTSD.[76] This includes the stress caused by long-lasting negative effects of the event on health and personal appearance, financial difficulties, disruptions in everyday life, and ongoing litigation.[41,81,84]

(b) Psychological processes

Excessively negative appraisals of the traumatic event impede recovery (e.g. 'Nowhere is safe', 'I cannot trust anyone', 'I am inadequate').[16,56] If individuals interpret their initial PTSD symptoms as signs that they are going mad or losing control, or as signs of a permanent change for the worse, they are less likely to recover.[16,41]

If individuals engage in behaviours or cognitive coping styles that prevent them from 'working through' and accepting the trauma, they are less likely to recover. Such maladaptive behaviours include avoidance, not talking about the experience, safety behaviours, denial, thought suppression, and rumination.[16,41,80,85]

Treatment of PTSD

Meta-analyses of randomized controlled trials have identified several effective psychological and pharmacological treatments for PTSD.[86–88]

Psychological treatments

Psychological treatments lead, on average, to large improvements in PTSD symptoms. The mean effect size (Cohen's d statistic) for the difference between the pre- and post-treatment scores was $d = 1.43$ across 26 studies of psychological treatments.[86] (An effect size $d = 1$ means that the treatment led to improvement by one standard deviation). In interpreting the effect sizes of treatments, one has to bear in mind that pill-placebo or waiting list conditions also lead to some improvement. Mean effect sizes for these conditions were $d = 0.77$ and $d = 0.75$ for observer-rated PTSD symptoms, and $d = 0.51$ and $d = 0.44$ for self-rated PTSD symptoms in 61 treatment-outcome trials.[88]

Not all psychological treatments are equally effective in treating PTSD. According to the meta-analyses, trauma-focused treatments are more effective than other treatments.[86,87] Trauma-focused cognitive behaviour therapy (CBT) and eye movement desensitization and reprocessing (EMDR) were superior to stress management and other therapies such as supportive therapy or hypnotherapy.[87] On average, 67 per cent of patients who complete the trauma-focused treatments (and 56 per cent of those who enter these treatments; intent-to-treat analysis) no longer met diagnostic criteria for PTSD.[86] For supportive therapy, the corresponding recovery rates were 39 per cent among treatment completers and 36 per cent in intent-to-treat analyses.[86] On the basis of these results, recent United Kingdom and Australian treatment guidelines recommend trauma-focused CBT and EMDR as the treatments of choice for PTSD.[89,90] Both treatments address the patient's troubling memories of the traumatic events and the personal meaning of the event and its consequences.

(a) Trauma-focused psychological treatments

(i) Cognitive behavioural therapy (CBT)

All effective CBT programmes for PTSD include an element of psycho-education about common reactions to trauma that normalizes the PTSD sufferer's symptoms, and a rationale for the interventions. Trauma-focused CBT programmes for PTSD include either exposure or cognitive therapy, or a combination of these interventions. Some also include elements of stress management training such as breathing training.

Exposure. Exposure treatment for PTSD comprises two components.[58] In imaginal exposure, patients are systematically exposed to the memory of the trauma. A commonly used procedure is imaginal reliving,[58] where patients relive the traumatic event in their imagination, including their thoughts and feelings at the time. This is repeated until the reliving no longer evokes high levels of distress. Writing a trauma narrative can also be used as a method of exposure to the trauma memory.[54] In vivo exposure[58] involves confronting (safe) situations that patients avoid because they remind them of the trauma (e.g. going to the site of the traumatic event, driving again after a road traffic accident). Exposure is repeated until the patient no longer responds with high levels of distress. The effects of exposure were originally explained as an effect of habituation, but there are probably several mechanisms for its efficacy.[55,58] For example, patients realize that exposure does not lead to a feared outcome (for example, going to the site of an accident will not mean that another accident will happen; thinking about the trauma will not make them go mad) and thus helps in correcting dysfunctional beliefs about danger of the world and the meaning of PTSD symptoms. Second, the repeated exposure helps patients to create an organized memory and facilitates the distinction that intrusive thoughts and images are memories rather than something happening right now.

Whereas exposure treatment is effective in the majority of cases, a minority of patients become worse.[91] In particular, exposure treatment does not appear suitable for patients whose traumatic memories are about being perpetrators rather than victims.[92] It may also have limits in treating survivors of complex and prolonged traumatic events such as torture, war, or captivity.[93]

Cognitive therapy. Cognitive therapy for anxiety disorders focuses on the identification and modification of misinterpretations that lead the patient to overestimate threat. In PTSD, the perceived threat stems from interpretations of the trauma and its aftermath.[54,55] For example, people with PTSD may feel strong guilt or shame related to the trauma: a rape victim may blame herself for the rape; a war veteran may feel it was his fault that his best friend was killed. Others overestimate the current danger they are encountering in everyday life. An accident survivor may become convinced that he is at great risk of having a further trauma.

Others may take the intrusive re-experiencing symptoms as a sign that they are about to go crazy. By discussing the evidence for and against the interpretations, and by testing out the predictions derived from the interpretations with the help of the therapist, the patient arrives at more adaptive conclusions. The patient is encouraged to drop behaviours and cognitive strategies that prevent a disconfirmation of the negative interpretations, e.g. excessive precautions to prevent further trauma or excessive rumination about what one could have done differently during the event. Recent studies have shown that cognitive therapy is effective on its own, without additional exposure treatment.(91,94) However, when verbal challenging of dysfunctional beliefs was used as an additional procedure after a session of imaginal exposure, it did not lead to additional treatment gains.(94) However, cognitive therapy may help reduce the amount of exposure necessary to achieve large treatment effects.(95,96)

(ii) Eye-movement desensitization and reprocessing (EMDR)

Like trauma-focused CBT, EMDR(97) aims to help patients process their traumatic memory and think more positively about their experience. It involves inducing a series of rapid and rhythmic eye movements while the patient focuses on a trauma-related image and related negative emotions, sensations, and thoughts. Patients are instructed to visually track the therapist's fingers as they move back and forth in front of the patient's eyes for sets of about 20 s. After each set, the patient discusses the images and emotions they experienced during the eye movements with the therapist. This process is repeated, and includes focusing on different memories that come up in connection with the trauma. Once distress to the target image is reduced, patients are instructed to focus on the image while rehearsing a positive thought connected to the image. The mechanism of treatment is not yet understood. Several empirical studies have suggested that the eye movements may not be necessary in producing the therapeutic effects observed with EMDR.(98)

(iii) Other psychological treatments

Most other psychological treatments have a small evidence-base. In general, non-trauma focused treatments were shown to be less effective than trauma-focused treatments in randomized controlled trials.(86,87)

Stress management (stress inoculation). The goal of this treatment is to teach the patient a set of skills that will help them cope with stress. Examples include relaxation training, training in slow abdominal breathing, thought stopping of unwanted thoughts, assertiveness training, and training in positive thinking. Stress management is more effective than supportive psychotherapy, but given on its own less effective than trauma-focused treatments.(87)

Psychodynamic therapy. Several different forms of psychodynamic treatments for PTSD have been described.(99) The focus lies on resolving unconscious conflicts provoked by the stressful event by making it conscious in tolerable doses. This is thought to help the patient reengage normal mechanisms of adaptation. The goal of treatment is to understand the meaning of the stressful event in the context of the individual's personality, attitudes, and early experiences. The psychological meaning of the event is explored by a range of methods such as 'sifting and sorting through wishes, fantasies, fears, and defences stirred up by the event'.(99) Treatment strategies include exploratory insight-oriented, supportive, or directive activity. It may also include working with transference, but with the therapist using a less strict technique than that used in psychoanalysis. To date there is only one controlled study of psychodynamic therapy, and the effect size observed in that study is below those observed with trauma-focused CBT or EMDR.(88)

Hypnotherapy. The patient is given instructions to induce a state of highly focused attention, a reduced awareness of peripheral stimuli, and a heightened suggestibility. The goal of this treatment is to enhance control over trauma-related emotional distress and hyperarousal symptoms and to facilitate the recollection of details of the traumatic event. To date there is only one controlled study of hypnotherapy, and the effect size observed in that study is below those observed with trauma-focused CBT or EMDR.(88) Shalev *et al.*(93) raised concerns about the use of hypnotherapy in the treatment of PTSD as it may induce dissociative states.

Supportive therapy. Supportive therapy is primarily non-directive and non-advisory. Through a supportive therapeutic relationship, clients are encouraged to explore their thoughts, feelings, and behaviour to reach clearer self-understanding; and to find and use their strengths so that they cope more effectively with their lives by making appropriate decisions, or by taking relevant action. Supportive therapy is less effective than trauma-focused psychological treatments.(86,87)

Pharmacological treatments

Although recent guidelines(89,90) recommend trauma-focused psychological treatments as the first line treatments for PTSD, they also acknowledge a role for medication. A Cochrane review(100) found an advantage of medication over placebo with response rates of 59.1 and 38.5 per cent, respectively. Indications for medication according to recent guidelines include patient choice, severe ongoing threat, the patient is too depressed or unstable to engage in psychological treatment, and failure to respond to psychological treatment.

(a) Selective serotonin-reuptake inhibitors (SSRIs)

Among the pharmacological treatments, the SSRIs have been most widely studied and are recommended as the first line medication choice for PTSD according to expert consensus(90,101) and a recent Cochrane review.(100) Paroxetine has received the most consistent support for its efficacy.(89,100) SSRIs reduce alcohol consumption; a relevant finding given the high comorbidity of PTSD with substance abuse or dependency.(102)

(b) Monoamine oxidase inhibitors (MAOIs)

There is some evidence that phenelzine is effective in PTSD,(89,100) particularly in reducing re-experiencing symptoms and insomnia.(102) Thus, phenelzine may be considered as one of the treatment options for PTSD by mental health specialists,(89) taking into consideration the risks and necessary dietary restrictions.

(c) Other antidepressants

There is some evidence for the efficacy of tricyclic antidepressants, particularly amitriptyline, in the treatment of PTSD.(89,100) They may be considered as a treatment option for PTSD by mental health specialists.(89,90) Mirtazepine, a noradrenergic and specific serotonergic antidepressant, has shown promise in initial trials and has been recommended as one of the treatment options for PTSD.(89,90)

(d) Benzodiazepines

Benzodiazepines do not appear to be effective in the treatment of PTSD. They do not affect the re-experiencing, avoidance, and numbing symptoms, although they may show some effects on insomnia, irritability, and general anxiety and arousal symptoms.[102]

Advice on management

Diagnosing PTSD

When assessing whether a patient has experienced a trauma, it is important to ask about specific examples of traumatic events. Patients may initially feel too overwhelmed or ashamed to report details of their traumatic experience, and may find it easier to reply to factual questions with 'yes' or 'no' answers. In diagnosing PTSD, clinicians need to ascertain that the patient involuntarily re-experiences parts of the event. In addition, patients will need to have some symptoms of hyperarousal, avoidance, and emotional numbing. Self-report instruments such as the Post-traumatic Stress Diagnostic scale[28] or semi-structured interviews such as the Clinician Administered PTSD scale[25] are useful in assessing the pattern and severity of symptoms. Clinicians should ask about the impact of the symptoms (e.g. distress, restrictions, effect on family and work) on the patient's life. The DSM-IV criterion of a minimum of three avoidance or numbing symptoms appears too strict for clinical purposes. It does not appear justified to withhold treatment if the patient is disabled by the PTSD symptoms but fails to meet this criterion.

Is PTSD the main problem?

As PTSD is often comorbid with other disorders, clinicians need to ascertain whether PTSD is the main problem for which the patient presently needs help at present. The time course of the onset of the comorbid disorders and changes in the severity of symptoms provide useful information. It is also helpful to ask patients whether they believe that they would need professional help for their other problems if the PTSD symptoms are resolved. In cases of comorbid depression, the PTSD should usually be treated first (as comorbid depression improves with successful PTSD treatment), unless the depression is so severe that the patient cannot engage in treatment. In contrast, significant substance dependence usually needs to be addressed before treating the PTSD.[89]

Assessments need to include a risk assessment. If there is a high risk of suicide or harm to others, clinicians will need to concentrate on managing the risk first.[89]

Clinicians will also need to establish whether there is any serious ongoing threat or health, social, and financial problems that may need to be addressed before the patient can engage in psychological treatment.[89]

(a) Choice of treatment

Patients should be informed about effective treatments for PTSD. Information material for patients and carers is available.[103] Trauma-focused psychological treatments are the best treatment option for PTSD to date, given the strong evidence for their effectiveness,[89,90] their established long-term effectiveness,[88] and the lower dropout rates compared to medication. Meta-analyses report that, across studies, 14–21 per cent of the patients can be expected to dropout of psychological treatments,[86,88] compared to 31–36 per cent for medication.[88,100] The advantage of SSRIs and other medications compared to psychological treatments is that they are more readily available.

(i) Psychological treatment

Trauma-focused psychological treatments usually last between 8 and 12 sessions (longer for patients with multiple traumas and comorbid personality disorders). When the trauma is discussed in the session, 90 min should be allowed for the session.[89,90] The treatments require a good therapeutic alliance.[90] Depending on the nature of the trauma and comorbid problems, additional sessions for establishing trust and emotional stabilization may be needed before the trauma-focused treatment commences.[89,90]

(ii) Pharmacological treatment

Clinicians should discuss the benefits and possible side effects of the prescribed medication with the patient, and address common concerns, such as fears of addiction. Patients also need to be informed that the medication needs to be discontinued gradually. Most antidepressants recommended for the use in PTSD need to be discontinued over at least 4 weeks.[89] The risk of self-harm needs to be considered when prescribing antidepressants. Those with high risk should be seen at least weekly until the risk is no longer considered significant.[89,90] Patients receiving SSRIs need to be monitored for akathisia, suicidal ideation, and increased anxiety and agitation. Patients receiving phenelzine require careful monitoring (including blood pressure measurement) and advice about interactions with other medicines and food.[89]

(b) Special problems in the management of PTSD patients

Avoidance is one of the main symptoms of PTSD, and it can thus take years for the patient to seek help for this condition. It is important for clinicians to bear in mind that even those who seek help may find it hard to talk about the traumatic experience, and may show signs of avoidance such as irregular attendance or failure to disclose the worst moments of the trauma initially. Therapeutic techniques to deal with this problem include empathy, gradual encouragement, and giving the patient control over the timing and mode of working through the experience (e.g. writing, talking into a tape recorder, reliving with the support of the therapist).

One of the requirements for change is that the patient feels safe. Therapists therefore have to make sure that they establish a good relationship with the patient, and that the therapeutic setting or their behaviour does not remind the patient of the traumatic event. Sometimes support in changing living circumstances may be necessary if they prevent the patient from being safe (e.g. moving house if assaulted by a neighbour).

Patients with PTSD often suffer from poor sleep and concentration, and find it painful to face reminders of the trauma. For these reasons, they have difficulty in dealing with the aftermath of traumatic events such as legal procedures and continuing treatment for physical injuries, including the long delays that this usually involves. Such ongoing stressors impede recovery, and patients may therefore benefit from problem-solving and practical advice.

Further information

National Institute of Clinical Excellence. (2005). Clinical guideline 26: post-traumatic stress disorder: the management of PTSD in adults and children in primary and secondary care. http://guidance.nice.org.uk/CG26

National Center for Posttraumatic Stress Disorder. http://www.ncptsd.va.gov/ncmain/providers/ and PILOTS database http://www.ncptsd.va.gov/ncmain/publications/pilots/

Nemeroof, C.B., Bremner, J.D., Foa, E.B., *et al.* (2006). Posttraumatic stress disorder: a state-of-the art review. *Journal of Psychiatric Research*, **40**, 1–21.

Taylor, S. (2006). *Clinician's guide to treating PTSD: a cognitive-behavioral approach*. Guilford Press, New York.

References

1. Gersons, B.P.R. and Carlier, I.V.E. (1992). Post-traumatic stress disorder: the history of a recent concept. *The British Journal of Psychiatry*, **161**, 742–8.
2. Kinzie, J.D. and Goetz, R.R. (1996). A century of controversy surrounding post-traumatic stress-spectrum syndromes: the impact of DSM-III and DSM-IV. *Journal of Traumatic Stress*, **9**, 159–79.
3. Van der Kolk, B.A., Weisaeth, L., and Van der Hart, O. (1996). History of trauma in psychiatry. In *Traumatic stress* (eds. B.A. van der Kolk, A.C. McFarlane, and L. Weisaeth), pp. 47–74. Guilford Press, New York.
4. American Psychiatric Association. (1980). *Diagnostic and statistical manual of mental disorders* (3rd edn). American Psychiatric Association, Washington, DC.
5. World Health Organization. (1992). *International statistical classification of diseases and related health problems*, 10th revision. WHO, Geneva.
6. McNally, R.J. (2000). Post-traumatic stress disorder. In *Oxford textbook of psychopathology* (eds. T. Millon, P.H. Blaney, and R.D. Davis). Oxford University Press, Oxford.
7. American Psychiatric Association. (1987). *Diagnostic and statistical manual of mental disorders* (3rd edn revised). American Psychiatric Association, Washington, DC.
8. Norris, F.H. (1992). Epidemiology of trauma: frequency and impact of different potentially traumatic events on different demographic groups. *Journal of Consulting and Clinical Psychology*, **60**, 409–18.
9. Resnick, H.S., Kilpatrick, D.G., Dansky, B.S., *et al.* (1993). Prevalence of civilian trauma and post-traumatic stress disorder in a representative national sample of women. *Journal of Consulting and Clinical Psychology*, **61**, 984–91.
10. American Psychiatric Association. (1994). *Diagnostic and statistical manual of mental disorders* (4th edn). American Psychiatric Association, Washington, DC.
11. Ozer, E.J., Best, S., Lipzey, T.L., *et al.* (2003). Predictors of posttraumatic stress disorder and symptoms in adults: a meta-analysis. *Psychological Bulletin*, **129**, 52–73.
12. Roemer, L., Orsillo, S.M., Borkovec, T.D., *et al.* (1998). Emotional response at the time of a potentially traumatizing event and PTSD symptomatology: a preliminary retrospective analysis of the DSM-IV criterion A-2. *Journal of Behaviour Therapy and Experimental Psychiatry*, **29**, 123–30.
13. Yehuda, R., Southwick, S.M., and Giller, E.L. (1992). Exposure to atrocities and severity of chronic post-traumatic stress disorder in Vietnam combat veterans. *The American Journal of Psychiatry*, **149**, 333–6.
14. Evans, C., Ehlers, A., Mezey, G., *et al.* (2007). Intrusive memories in perpetrators of violent crime: emotions and cognitions. *Journal of Consulting and Clinical Psychology*, **75**, 134–44.
15. Ehlers, A., Maercker, A., and Boos, A. (2000). PTSD following political imprisonment: the role of mental defeat, alienation, and perceived permanent change. *Journal of Abnormal Psychology*, **109**, 45–55.
16. Dunmore, E., Clark, D.M., and Ehlers, A. (2001). A prospective study of the role of cognitive factors in persistent posttraumatic stress disorder after physical or sexual assault. *Behaviour Research and Therapy*, **39**, 1063–84.
17. Brett, E.A. (1996). The classification of post-traumatic stress disorder. In *Traumatic stress* (eds. B.A. van der Kolk, A.C. McFarlane, and L. Weisaeth), pp. 117–28. Guilford Press, New York.
18. Davidson, J.R.T. and Foa, E.B. (1991). Diagnostic issues in post-traumatic stress disorder: consideration for the DSM-IV and beyond. *Journal of Abnormal Psychology*, **100**, 346–55.
19. World Health Organization. (1993). *The ICD-10 classification of mental and behavioural disorders: diagnostic criteria for research*. World Health Organization, Geneva.
20. Andrews, G., Slade, T., and Peters, L. (1999). Classification in psychiatry: ICD-10 versus DSM-IV. *The British Journal of Psychiatry*, **174**, 3–5.
21. Herman, J.L. (1992). Complex PTSD: a syndrome in survivors of prolonged and repeated trauma. *Journal of Traumatic Stress*, **5**, 377–91.
22. Prigerson, H.G., Shear, M.K., Jacobs, S.C., *et al.* (1999). Consensus criteria for traumatic grief: a preliminary empirical test. *The British Journal of Psychiatry*, **174**, 67–73.
23. Foa, E.B., Riggs, D.S., and Gershuny, B.S. (1995). Arousal, numbing, and intrusion: symptom structure of PTSD following assault. *The American Journal of Psychiatry*, **152**, 116–20.
24. First, M.B., Spitzer, R.L., Gibbon, M., *et al.* (1995). *Structured clinical interview for DSM-IV Axis I disorders-patient version (SCID-I/P, Version 2.0)*. Biometrics Research Department of the New York State Psychiatric Institute, New York.
25. Blake, D.D., Weathers, F.W., Nagy, L.M., *et al.* (1995). The development of a clinician-administered PTSD scale. *Journal of Traumatic Stress*, **8**, 75–90.
26. Horowitz, M.J., Wilner, N., and Alvarez, W. (1979). Impact of Event Scale: a measure of subjective stress. *Psychosomatic Medicine*, **41**, 209–18.
27. Weiss, D.S. and Marmar, C. R. (1997). The impact of Event Scale-revised. In *Assessing psychological trauma and PTSD* (eds. J.P Wilson and T.M. Keane), pp. 399–411. Guilford Press, New York.
28. Foa, E.B., Cashman, L., Jaycox, L., *et al.* (1997). The validation of a self-report measure of post-traumatic stress disorder: the post-traumatic diagnostic scale. *Psychological Assessment*, **9**, 445–51.
29. Weathers, F.W., Huska, J.A., and Keane, T.M. (1991). *The PTSD Checklist—Civilian version (PCL-C) for DSM-IV*. National Center for PTSD—Behavioral Science Division, Boston. http://www.oqp.med.va.gov/cpg/PTSD/PTSD_cpg/content/appendices/appendixC.htm
30. McFarlane, A.C. and de Girolamo, G. (1996). The nature of traumatic stressors and the epidemiology of post-traumatic reactions. In *Traumatic stress* (eds. B.A. van der Kolk, A.C. McFarlane, and L. Weisaeth), pp. 129–54. Guilford Press, New York.
31. Kessler, R.C., Sonnega, A., Bromet. E., *et al.* (1995). Post-traumatic stress disorder in the National Comorbidity Survey. *Archives of General Psychiatry*, **52**, 1048–60.
32. Stein, M.B., Walker, J.R., Hazen, A.L., *et al.* (1997). Full and partial post-traumatic stress disorder: findings from a community survey. *The American Journal of Psychiatry*, **154**, 1114–19.
33. Breslau, N., Kessler, R.C., Chilcoat, H.D., *et al.* (1998). Trauma and post-traumatic stress disorder in the community. *Archives of General Psychiatry*, **55**, 626.
34. Maercker, A. and Schützwohl, M. (1997). Longterm effects of political imprisonment: a group comparison study. *Social Psychiatry and Psychiatric Epidemiology*, **32**, 435–42.
35. Kuch, K. and Cox, B.J. (1992). Symptoms of PTSD in 124 survivors of the Holocaust. *The American Journal of Psychiatry*, **149**, 337–40.
36. Engdahl, B.E., Dikel, T.N., Eberly, R., *et al.* (1997). Post-traumatic stress disorder in a community group of former prisoners of war: a normative response to severe trauma. *The American Journal of Psychiatry*, **154**, 1576–81.
37. Mayou, R.A. and Smith, K.A. (1997). Post traumatic symptoms following medical illness and treatment. *Journal of Psychosomatic Research*, **43**, 121–3.

38. Breslau, N., Davis, G.C., Andreski, P., *et al.* (1991). Traumatic events and post-traumatic stress disorder in an urban population of young adults. *Archives of General Psychiatry*, **48**, 216–22.
39. Breslau, N., Davis, G.C., Andreski, P., *et al.* (1997). Sex differences in post-traumatic stress disorder. *Archives of General Psychiatry*, **54**, 1044–8.
40. Blanchard, E.B. and Hickling, E.J. (1997). *After the crash. Assessment and treatment of motor vehicle survivors*. American Psychological Association, Washington, DC.
41. Ehlers, A., Mayou, R.A., and Bryant, B. (1998). Psychological predictors of chronic post-traumatic stress disorder after motor vehicle accidents. *Journal of Abnormal Psychology*, **107**, 508–19.
42. Creamer, M., Burgess, P., and McFarlane, A.C. (2001). Post-traumatic stress disorder: findings from the Australian National Survey of Mental Health and Well-being. *Psychological Medicine*, **31**, 1237–47.
43. Narrow, W.E., Rae, D.S., Robins, L.N., *et al.* (2002). Revised prevalence estimates of mental disorders in the United States: using a clinical significance criterion to reconcile 2 surveys' estimates. *Archives of General Psychiatry*, **59**, 115–23.
44. Solomon, S.D. and Davidson, J.R.T. (1997). Trauma: prevalence, impairment, service use, and cost. *The Journal of Clinical Psychiatry*, **58**, 5–11.
45. Jordan, B.K., Marmar, C.R., Fairbank, J.A., *et al.* (1992). Problems in families of male Vietnam veterans with post-traumatic stress disorder. *Journal of Consulting and Clinical Psychology*, **60**, 916–26.
46. Beckham, J.C., Kirby, A.C., Feldman, M.E., *et al.* (1997). Prevalence and correlates of heavy smoking in Vietnam veterans with chronic post-traumatic stress disorder. *Addictive Behaviors*, **22**, 637–47.
47. Schnurr, P. and Green, B.L. (eds.) (2004). *Trauma and health. Physical consequences of exposure to extreme stress*. American Psychological Association, Washington, DC.
48. Andreski, P., Chilcoat, H., and Breslau, N. (1998). Post-traumatic stress disorder and somatization symptoms: a prospective study. *Psychiatry Research*, **79**, 131–8.
49. Stewart, S.H. (1996). Alcohol abuse in individuals exposed to trauma: a critical review. *Psychological Bulletin*, **120**, 83–112.
50. Mowrer, O.H. (1939). A stimulus-response analysis of anxiety and its role as a reinforcing agent. *Psychological Review*, **46**, 553–65.
51. Charney, D., Deutch, A.Y., Krystal, J.H., *et al.* (1993). Psychobiological mechanisms of post-traumatic stress disorder. *Archives of General Psychiatry*, **50**, 294–305.
52. Keane, T.M., Zimering, R.T., and Caddell, J.M. (1985). A behavioral formulation of post-traumatic stress disorder. *Behavior Therapy*, **8**, 9–12.
53. Foa, E.B. and Riggs, D.S. (1993). Post-traumatic stress disorder in rape victims. In *Annual review of psychiatry*, Vol. 12 (eds. J. Oldham, M.B. Riba, and A. Tasman), pp. 273–303. American Psychiatric Association, Washington, DC.
54. Resick, P.A. and Schnicke, M.K. (1993). *Cognitive processing therapy for rape victims*. Sage, Newbury Park, CA.
55. Ehlers, A. and Clark, D.M. (in press). A cognitive model of persistent PTSD. *Behaviour Research and Therapy*.
56. Foa, E.B., Ehlers, A., Clark, D.M., *et al.* (1999). The post-traumatic cognitions inventory (PTCI): development and validation. *Psychological Assessment*, **11**, 303–14.
57. Ehlers, A. and Steil, R. (1995). Maintenance of intrusive memories in post-traumatic stress disorder: a cognitive approach. *Behavioural and Cognitive Psychotherapy*, **23**, 217–49.
58. Foa, E.B. and Rothbaum, B.O. (1998). *Treating the trauma of rape. Cognitive-behavior therapy for PTSD*. Guilford Press, New York.
59. McNally, R.J. (2003). *Remembering trauma*. Harvard University Press, Cambridge, MA.
60. Ehlers, A., Hackmann, A. and Michael, T. (2004). Intrusive reexperiencing in posttraumatic stress disorder: phenomenology, theory, and therapy. *Memory*, **12**, 403–15.
61. Brewin, C.R., Dalgleish, T., and Joseph, S. (1996). A dual representation theory of post-traumatic stress disorder. *Psychological Review*, **103**, 670–86.
62. Van der Kolk, B.A. (1996). The body keeps the score. Approaches to the psychobiology of post-traumatic stress disorder. In *Traumatic stress* (eds. B.A. van der Kolk, A.C. McFarlane, and L. Weisaeth), pp. 214–41. Guilford Press, New York.
63. Newport, D.J. and Nemoroff, C.B. (2000). Neurobiology of posttraumatic stress disorder. *Cognitive Neuroscience*, **10**, 211–8.
64. Kloet, C.S., Vermetten, E., Geuze, E., *et al.* (2006). Assessment of HPA-axis function in posttraumatic stress disorder: pharmacological and non-pharmacological challenge tests, a review. *Journal of Psychiatric Research*, **40**, 550–67.
65. Southwick, S.M., Rasmusson, A., Barron, J., *et al.* (2005). Neurobiological and neurocognitive alterations in PTSD. In *Neuropsychoology of PTSD: biological, cognitive and clinical perspectives* (eds. J. Vaterling and C. Brewin), pp. 27–58. Guilford Press, New York.
66. Karl, A., Schaefer, M., Malta, L.S., *et al.* (2006). A meta-analysis of structural brain abnormalities in PTSD. *Neuroscience and Biobehavioral Reviews*, **30**, 1004–31.
67. Nemeroof, C.B., Bremner, J.D., Foa, E.B., *et al.* (2006). Posttraumatic stress disorder: a state-of-the art review. *Journal of Psychiatric Research*, **40**, 1–21.
68. Shin, L.M., Rauch, S.L., and Pitman, R.K. (2006). Amygdala, medial prefrontal cortex, and hippocampal function in PTSD. *Annals of the New York Academy of Science*, **1071**, 67–79.
69. LeDoux, J.E. (1992). Emotion as memory: anatomical systems underlying indelible memory traces. In *Handbook of emotion and memory* (ed. S.A. Christianson), pp. 269–88. Erlbaum, Hillsdale, NJ.
70. Lanius, R.A., Bluhm, R., Lanius, U., *et al.* (2006). A review of neuroimaging studies in PTSD: heterogeneity of response to symptom provocation. *Journal of Psychiatric Research*, **40**, 709–29.
71. Foa, E.B., Zinbarg, R., and Rothbaum, B.O. (1992). Uncontrollability and unpredictability in post-traumatic stress disorder: an animal model. *Psychological Bulletin*, **112**, 218–38.
72. Post, R.M., Weiss, S.R.B., and Smith, M.A. (1995). Sensitization and kindling: implications for the evolving neural substrates of post-traumatic stress disorder. In *Neurobiological and clinical consequences of stress: from normal adaptation to post-traumatic stress disorder* (eds. M.J. Friedman, D.S. Charney, and A.Y. Deutch), pp. 203–24. Lippincott-Raven, Philadelphia, PA.
73. Connor, K.M. and Davidson, J.R.T. (1997). Familial risk factors in post-traumatic stress disorder. *Annals of the New York Academy of Sciences*, **821**, 35–51.
74. Lee, H.J., Lee, M.S., Kang, R.H., *et al.* (2005). Influence of the serotonin transporter promoter gene polymorphism on susceptibility to posttraumatic stress disorder. *Depression and Anxiety*, **21**, 135–9.
75. Perkonigg, A., Pfister, H., Stein, M.B., *et al.* (2005). Longitudinal course of posttraumatic stress disorder symptoms in a community sample of adolescents and young adults. *The American Journal of Psychiatry*, **162**, 1320–7.
76. Brewin, C.R., Andrews, B., and Valentine, J.D. (2000). Meta-analysis of risk factors for posttraumatic stress disorder in trauma-exposed adults. *Journal of Consulting and Clinical Psychology*, **68**, 748–66.
77. Olff, M., Langeland, W., Draijer, N., *et al.* (2007). Gender differences in posttraumatic stress disorder. *Psychological Bulletin*, **133**, 183–204.
78. Frueh, B.C., Brady, K.L., and Dearellano, M.A. (1998). Racial differences in combat-related PTSD: empirical findings and conceptual issues. *Clinical Psychology Review*, **18**, 287–305.
79. Green, B.L. (1994). Psychosocial research in traumatic stress: an update. *Journal of Traumatic Stress*, **7**, 341–62.
80. Clohessy, S. and Ehlers, A. (1999). PTSD symptoms, response to intrusive memories, and coping in ambulance service workers. *The British Journal of Clinical Psychology*, **38**, 251–66.

81. Mayou, R.A., Bryant, B., and Duthie, R. (1993). Psychiatric consequences of road traffic accidents. *British Medical Journal*, **307**, 647–51.
82. Baum, A., Cohen, L., and Hall, M. (1993). Control and intrusive memories as possible determinants of chronic stress. *Psychosomatic Medicine*, **55**, 274–86.
83. Andrews, B., Brewin, C.R., Rose, S., *et al.* (2000). Predicting PTSD in victims of violent crime. The role of shame, anger, and childhood abuse. *Journal of Abnormal Psychology*, **109**, 69–73.
84. Carr, J.V., Lewin, T.J., Webster, R.A., *et al.* (1997). Psychosocial sequelae of the 1989 Newcastle earthquake. II. Exposure and morbidity profiles during the first 2 years post-disaster. *Psychological Medicine*, **27**, 167–78.
85. Joseph, S., Dalgleish, T., Williams, R., *et al.* (1997). Attitudes towards emotional expression and post-traumatic stress in survivors of the Herald of Free Enterprise disaster. *The British Journal of Clinical Psychology*, **36**, 133–8.
86. Bradley, R., Greene, J., Russ, E., *et al.* (2005). A multidimensional meta-analysis of psychotherapy for PTSD. *The American Journal of Psychiatry*, **162**, 214–7.
87. Bisson, J., Ehlers, A., Matthews, R., *et al.* (2007). Systematic review and meta-analysis of psychological treatments for post-traumatic stress disorder. *The British Journal of Psychiatry*, **190**, 97–104.
88. Van Etten, M.L. and Taylor, S. (1998). Comparative efficacy of treatments for post-traumatic stress disorder: a meta-analysis. *Clinical Psychology and Psychotherapy*, **5**, 126–44.
89. National Institute of Clinical Excellence. (2005). Clinical guideline 26: post-traumatic stress disorder: The management of PTSD in adults and children in primary and secondary care. http://guidance.nice.org.uk/CG26
90. Australian Centre for Posttraumatic Mental Health. Australian Guidelines for the treatment of acute stress disorder and posttraumatic stress disorder. http://www.acpmh.unimelb.edu.au/Resources/guidelines/ACMPH_PractionerGuideForASDandPTSD.pdf
91. Tarrier, N., Pilgrim, H., Sommerfield, C., *et al.* (1999). A randomised trial of cognitive therapy and imaginal exposure in the treatment of chronic post traumatic stress disorder. *Journal of Consulting and Clinical Psychology*, **67**, 13–9.
92. Foa, E.B. and Meadows, E.A. (1997). Psychosocial treatments for post-traumatic stress disorder: a critical review. *Annual Review of Psychology*, **48**, 449–80.
93. Shalev, A.Y., Bonne, O., and Eth, S. (1996). Treatment of post-traumatic stress disorder: a review. *Psychosomatic Medicine*, **58**, 165–82.
94. Marks, I.M., Lovell, K., Norshirvani, H., *et al.* (1998). Treatment of post-traumatic stress disorder by exposure and/or cognitive restructuring. *Archives of General Psychiatry*, **55**, 317–25.
95. Ehlers, A., Clark, D.M., Hackmann, A., *et al.* (2003). A randomized controlled trial of cognitive therapy, self-help booklet, and repeated assessment as early interventions for PTSD. *Archives of General Psychiatry*, **60**, 1024–32.
96. Ehlers, A., Clark, D.M., Hackmann, A., *et al.* (2005). Cognitive therapy for PTSD: development and evaluation. *Behaviour Research and Therapy*, **43**, 413–31.
97. Shapiro, F. (1995). *Eye movement desensitization and reprocessing: basic principles, protocols, and procedures*. Guilford Press, New York.
98. Davidson, P.R. and Parker, K.C.H. (2001). Eye movement desensitization and reprocessing (EMDR): a meta-analysis. *Journal of Consulting and Clinical Psychology*, **69**, 305–16.
99. Kudler, H.S., Blank, A., and Krupnick, J.L. (2000). Psychodynamic therapy. In *Effective treatments for PTSD: practice guidelines from the international society for traumatic stress studies* (eds. E.B. Foa, T.M. Keane, and M.J. Friedman), pp. 176–98 and pp. 339–41. Guilford Press, New York.
100. Stein, D.J., Ipser, J.C., and Seedat, S. (2007). Pharmacotherapy for posttraumatic stress disorder (PTSD). *The Cochrane Database of Systematic Reviews. The Cochrane Library*, **2**.
101. Foa, E.B., Davidson, J.R.T., and Frances, A. (1999). The expert consensus guideline series. Treatment of post traumatic stress disorder. *The Journal of Clinical Psychiatry*, **60**(Suppl. 16).
102. Friedman, M.J. (1998). Current and future drug treatment for post-traumatic stress disorder. *Psychiatric Annals*, **28**, 461–8.
103. National Institute for Clinical Excellence. (2005). *Posttraumatic stress disorder (PTSD): the treatment of PTSD in adults and children*. Information about NICE Clinical Guidelines 26. http://guidance.nice.org.uk/CG26

4.6.3 Recovered memories and false memories

Chris R. Brewin

Clinicians working with survivors of traumatic experiences have frequently noted the existence of memory loss with no obvious physical cause and the recovery of additional memories during clinical sessions. Indeed, amnesia is described in diagnostic manuals as a feature of post-traumatic stress disorder, although its presence is not necessary for this diagnosis. In the majority of these cases, people forget details of the traumatic event or events, or forget how they reacted at the time, although they remember that the event happened. They typically report that they have endeavoured not to think about the event, but have never forgotten that it occurred. Controversy is centred on memories of traumatic events, particularly concerning child abuse, that appear to be recovered after a long period of time in which there was complete forgetting that they had ever happened. It has sometimes been suggested that many, if not all, of these apparent recovered memories are the product of inappropriate therapeutic suggestion. This argument has been promulgated in particular by the False Memory Syndrome Foundation in the United States, by its counterpart, the British False Memory Society, and by their scientific advisors.

The 'false memory' position

Loftus[(1)] suggested that at least some of the memories of child sexual abuse recovered in therapy after apparent total amnesia may not be veridical, but may be false memories encouraged or 'implanted' by therapists who have prematurely decided that the patient is an abuse victim and who use inappropriate therapeutic techniques to persuade him or her to recover corresponding 'memories'. The false memory societies have claimed that there are many cases known to them in which previously happy families have been disrupted by accusations of abuse that were only triggered when an adult child entered therapy. Particular scepticism has been levelled at reports of repeated abuse, all of which has apparently been forgotten, and it has been claimed that such reports are contradicted by what is known scientifically about memory. Reports of 'repressed' memories of childhood abuse are generally regarded as clinical speculations and the psychoanalytical concept of repression as one that has no credible scientific support.

Several reviewers claim that there is no empirical support for repression or dissociative amnesia in trauma victims.[2–4]

Lindsay and Read[5] have marshalled evidence to suggest that the creation of false memories within therapy is a possibility that must be taken seriously. For example, they review experimental studies conducted with non-clinical subjects concerning the fallibility and malleability of memory, and note the potential for inaccurate recall involved in techniques such as hypnosis. Experiments have demonstrated that people are sometimes confused about whether a recent event in the laboratory actually happened, or whether they only imagined it happening. Other experiments have repeatedly succeeded in implanting apparent childhood memories of single non-abusive events in approximately 25 to 30 per cent of subjects, particularly in those who score highly on measures of hypnotizability or suggestibility.[6] Further evidence comes from individuals who claim to remember impossible events such as being kidnapped by aliens.[4]

Critics have argued that these experiments are a long way from being evidence that therapists could implant false memories of child abuse, and even the experimental studies have shown that successful suggestion depends on the plausibility of the event subjects are asked to believe in. Nevertheless, although no one has performed experiments in an attempt to implant the notion that abuse occurred, it is reasonable to argue that some patients may be highly suggestible and inclined to go along with the beliefs of therapists who may be their only source of support. If their therapist was convinced that abuse had occurred, put overt or covert pressure on their patient to 'remember' this abuse, and was insufficiently alert to the unreliability of memory, there would be a greatly increased risk of false memories occurring.

In conclusion, the recently developed 'false memory' position goes beyond previous concerns of a general nature about errors in memory, and specifically identifies a process whereby errors arise after a person has been subjected to repeated suggestive influences that the explanation for their symptoms lies in forgotten child sexual abuse. These influences are usually thought to occur in therapy, although it has been proposed that exposure to certain books or broadcast media may have the same effect. This position relies partly on information from the false memory societies about their members, and partly on experimental evidence from non-traumatic procedures in the laboratory. There has been little independent scrutiny of the data from members of false memory societies, and many of their claims, for example that parents have been falsely accused, that accusations only follow entry into therapy, or that there is a 'false memory syndrome', are anecdotal and have not been empirically verified.[7]

Evidence for genuine 'recovered memories'

Over 20 longitudinal and retrospective studies have now found that a substantial proportion of people reporting child sexual abuse (somewhere between 20 and 60 per cent) report periods in their lives (often lasting for several years) when they could not remember that the abuse had taken place.[8,9] Although the rates vary between studies, broadly similar findings have been obtained by clinical psychologists, psychiatrists, and cognitive psychologists in both clinical and community samples. As has been pointed out by critics of these studies, this evidence supports the forgetting of trauma, but does not yet have much to say about the mechanism (for example 'repression') by which it occurs. Thus it would be true to say that while there is evidence for forgetting, there is little evidence for 'repression' as such.

Three main factors support the argument that these apparently forgotten memories are not necessarily false.

1. Surveys have also found recovered memories of other traumatic experiences such as witnessing accidents, experiencing medical procedures, and physical abuse in childhood.[10] It is unclear how these could have been brought about by suggestion.
2. A number of studies have found that apparent recovered memories occur prior to any therapy, and in the absence of any obvious prolonged suggestive influence.[11] Again, it is unclear how these could have been brought about by suggestion.
3. Surveys of psychologists and therapists found that approximately 40 per cent of those with apparent recovered memories reported corroborative evidence for the content of the memories, such as abusers' confessions, testimony from other victims, and court records. Although the quality of this corroboration has been criticized, it seems unlikely that all these cases can be summarily dismissed. There are also substantial numbers of case studies reporting more detailed corroborative evidence for apparent recovered memories, some of this evidence of reasonably high quality.[10–12]

The quality of the research evidence supporting genuine recovered memories is mixed, and almost all the studies can be argued to have some flaws, but taken together the evidence for genuine memories of major traumatic events is far more extensive than the evidence for false memories of such events. Moreover, these observations need not, as has sometimes been claimed, contradict what we know about memory. Cognitive psychology recognizes that ordinary memory relies as much for its efficiency on the ability to inhibit unwanted material as on the ability to gain rapid access to relevant material. Experimental studies clearly demonstrate the inhibition of memory retrieval and the existence of a subgroup of individuals with poor memories for negative experiences.[11]

The intimate neuroanatomical connections between brain circuits involved in emotion and those involved in memory provide a good reason for believing that memory may not behave in the same way under conditions of extreme real-world stress as it does in ordinary laboratory experiments. Whereas high levels of arousal often make events more difficult to forget, it has been argued by several well-known neuroscientists that extraordinarily high levels of catecholamines or other neuropeptides at the time of the trauma, perhaps in combination with a failure to release sufficient cortisol, may produce amnesia. More specifically, it has been suggested that extreme stress produces at the same time both enhanced fear conditioning and impaired autobiographical memory.[13] Much of the evidence is indirect and not yet compelling, but it illustrates that claims concerning recovered memories of trauma need not violate current knowledge concerning the cognitive psychology and neurobiology of memory.

Why the debate?

From a purely scientific point of view, it should be evident that the quality of the available evidence is insufficient to justify any extreme position at present. The questions are extremely difficult to study empirically, and there has been little new research since the 1990s to suggest that this state of affairs is likely to change. However, scientific considerations have sometimes been secondary to the passionate advocacy practised by parents who claim to be falsely accused, and by accusers who claim that their memories of abuse are being ignored. Psychiatrists and psychologists have in the past become caught up in the debate and in some cases abandoned any pretence at neutrality. In the face of these compelling and intensely painful personal concerns, the quality of much of the argument became debased. Thus, supposedly scientific contributions on both sides of this debate questioned the motives and integrity of people with whom they disagreed and attempted to disparage opponents' professional abilities. Some of these same authors made exclusive claims for the scientific legitimacy of their own perspective, subjecting opposing data to fierce scrutiny while being relatively uncritical of studies that supported their point of view. Much of the literature was obfuscatory and confusing. Logical errors abounded, seen for example in the conclusion that because a memory has been recovered in therapy, the practitioner must have been using 'recovered memory therapy'.

A good example of the debate in action is the article by Pope *et al.*[4] on the evidence for dissociative amnesia in trauma victims and the commentary that followed it.[14] These articles demonstrate how widely differing conclusions can be drawn from the same set of studies, depending on the way terms are defined, on assumptions about what evidence should be given the most weight, and on the rigour with which alternative explanations are evaluated.

An emerging scientific and professional consensus

What should be clear by now is that extreme views, claiming that either false memories or genuine recovered memories are rare or impossible, cannot be supported by the available data. Nevertheless, the dispute continues about whether traumatic events, and particularly repeated traumas, can be forgotten and then remembered with essential accuracy. In my view it is safe to conclude from the evidence reviewed that the hypothesized implantation of false memories by practitioners cannot account for more than a subset of recovered memories (and at present it is entirely unclear how large or small this subset might be). False memories may certainly arise in other circumstances, but as yet there is little pertinent evidence. On the other hand, there is a great deal of plausible evidence supporting the existence of genuine recovered memories.

Most commentators, including some members of the advisory boards of false memory societies,[6] now accept that traumatic events can be forgotten and then remembered. Cognitive psychologists Lindsay and Read[5] summed it up well: 'In our reading, scientific evidence has clear implications . . . memories recovered via suggestive memory work by people who initially denied any such history should be viewed with scepticism, but there are few grounds to doubt spontaneously recovered memories of common forms of child sexual abuse or recovered memories of details of never-forgotten abuse. Between these extremes lies a grey area within which the implications of existing scientific evidence are less clear and experts are likely to disagree'. Similarly, the consensus view among independent commentators, repeated in the 1995 report of the British Psychological Society's Working Party on Recovered Memories and the 1995 interim statement of the American Psychological Association's Working Group on Investigation of Memories of Childhood Abuse, is that memories may be recovered from total amnesia and they may sometimes be essentially accurate. Equally, such 'memories' may sometimes be inaccurate in whole or in part.

In practical terms, the debate has had two major effects. First, proponents of 'recovered memory therapy' are now almost impossible to find within the ranks of leading psychiatrists and psychologists. Despite the small amount of empirical support, there is widespread agreement that situations in which there is sustained suggestive influence, such as therapy, do have the potential to induce false memories. Active attempts to recover suspected forgotten memories may sometimes be appropriate in unusual or extreme cases, but both the client and the therapist must be aware of the risk of false memories. Techniques such as hypnosis and guided imagery should not be used without safeguards against potential suggestive influence. Second, good practice now requires both the therapist and the client to adopt a critical attitude towards any apparent memory that is recovered after a period of amnesia, whether or not this is within a therapeutic context, and not to assume that it necessarily corresponds to a true event. Even highly vivid traumatic memories (sometimes known as 'flashbacks') may be misleading or inaccurate in some cases. Clinical guidelines are now available to help the practitioner avoid the twin perils of uncritically accepting false memories as true or summarily dismissing genuine recovered memories.[9,15]

Further information

Brewin, C.R. (2003). *Posttraumatic stress disorder: malady or myth?* Yale University Press, New Haven, CT (see Chapters 7 and 8).

Davies, G.M. and Dalgleish, T. (eds.) (2001). *Recovered memories: seeking the middle ground.* Wiley, Chichester.

References

1. Loftus, E.F. (1993). The reality of repressed memories. *The American Psychologist*, **48**, 518–37.
2. Pope, H.G. and Hudson, J.I. (1995). Can memories of childhood abuse be repressed? *Psychological Medicine*, **25**, 121–6.
3. Pope, H.G., Hudson, J.I., Bodkin, J.A., *et al.* (1997). Can trauma victims develop 'dissociative amnesia'? the evidence of prospective studies. *The British Journal of Psychiatry*, **172**, 210–15.
4. McNally, R.J. (2003). *Remembering trauma.* Harvard University Press, Cambridge, Mass.
5. Lindsay, D.S. and Read, J.D. (1995). 'Memory work' and recovered memories of childhood sexual abuse: scientific evidence and public, professional and personal issues. *Psychology, Public Policy and the Law*, **1**, 846–908.
6. Wright, D., Ost, J., and French, C.C. (2006). Recovered and false memories. *The Psychologist*, **19**, 352–5.
7. Pope, K.S. (1996). Memory, abuse and science: questioning claims about the False Memory Syndrome epidemic. *The American Psychologist*, **51**, 957–74.
8. Gleaves, D.H., Smith, S.M., Butler, L.D., *et al.* (2004). False and recovered memories in the laboratory and clinic: a review of experimental and clinical evidence. *Clinical Psychology: Science and Practice*, **11**, 3–28.
9. Mollon, P. (1998). *Remembering trauma: a psychotherapist's guide to memory and illusion.* Wiley, Chichester.

10. Andrews, B., Brewin, C.R., Ochera, J., *et al.* (1999). The characteristics, context, and consequences of memory recovery among adults in therapy. *The British Journal of Psychiatry*, **175**, 141–6.
11. Brewin, C.R. (2003). *Posttraumatic stress disorder: malady or myth?* Yale University Press, New Haven, Conn.
12. Cheit, R. (2005). *The recovered memory project.* Internet posting http://www.brown.edu/Departments/Taubman_Center/Recovmem/Archive.html
13. Elzinga, B.M. and Bremner, J.D. (2002). Are the neural substrates of memory the final common pathway in posttraumatic stress disorder (PTSD)? *Journal of Affective Disorders*, **70**, 1–17.
14. Brewin, C.R. (1998). Commentary: questionable validity of 'dissociative amnesia' in trauma victims. *The British Journal of Psychiatry*, **172**, 216–17.
15. Pope, K.S. and Brown, L.S. (1996). *Recovered memories of abuse: assessment, therapy, forensics.* American Psychological Association, Washington, DC.

4.6.4 Adjustment disorders

James J. Strain, Kimberly Klipstein, and Jeffrey Newcorm

Introduction

The psychiatric diagnoses that arise between normal behaviour and major psychiatric morbidities constitute the problematic subthreshold disorders. These subthreshold entities are also juxtaposed between problem-level diagnoses and more clearly defined disorders. Adjustment disorder (AD) would 'trump' problem-level disorders, but would be 'trumped' by a specific diagnosis even if it were in the NOS category. The subthreshold disorders present major taxonomical and diagnostic dilemmas in that they are often poorly defined, overlap with other diagnostic groupings, and have indefinite symptomatology. It is therefore not surprising that issues of reliability and validity prevail. One of the most commonly employed subthreshold diagnosis that has undergone a major evolution since 1952 is AD (Table 4.6.4.1). The advantage of the indefiniteness of these subthreshold disorders is that they permit the classification of early or prodromal states when the clinical picture is vague and indistinct, and yet the morbid state is in excess of that expected in a normal reaction and this morbidity needs to be identified and often treated. Therefore, AD has an essential place in the psychiatric taxonomy.

Many questions prevail with regard to the concept of the AD diagnosis: (1) the role of stressors and the place of specific stressors; (2) the importance of age; (3) the role of concurrent medical morbidity, for example comorbidity of Axis I and/or Axis III disorders; (4) the lack of specificity of the diagnostic criteria; (5) the absence of a symptom checklist; (6) uncertainty as to optimal treatment protocols; and (7) undocumented prognosis or outcomes. Research data regarding these questions will be examined.

The DSM was conceptually designed with an atheoretical framework to encourage psychiatric diagnoses to be derived on phenomenological grounds with an avowed dismissal of pathogenesis or aetiology as diagnostic imperatives. In frank contradiction to this atheoretical conceptual framework, the stress-induced disorders require the inclusion of an aetiological significance to a life event—a stressor—and the need to relate the stressor's effect on the patient in clinical terms. However, the stress-related disorders are unique in that they are psychiatric diagnoses with a known aetiology—the stressor—and thus aetiology is essential for the diagnosis. Four other diagnostic categories also invoke aetiology in their diagnostic criteria: (1) organic mental disorders (aetiology-physical abnormality); (2) substance abuse disorders (aetiology-ingestion of substances); (3) post-traumatic; and (4) acute stress disorders

Table 4.6.4.1 DSM-IV Evolution of the diagnosis for adjustment disorder

(a) The development of emotional or behavioural symptoms in response to an identifiable psychosocial stressor(s), which occurs within 3 months of the onset of the stressor(s)

(b) These symptoms or behaviours are clinically significant as evidenced by either of the following

1 Marked distress that is in excess of what would be expected from exposure to the stressor

2 Significant impairment in social or occupational (academic) functioning

(c) The stress-related disturbance does not meet the criteria for any specific Axis I disorder and is not merely an exacerbation of a pre-existing Axis I or Axis II disorder

(d) The symptoms do not represent bereavement

(e) Once the stressor (or its consequences) has terminated, the symptoms do not persist for more than an additional 6 moths

Specify if:

Acute: if the disturbance lasts less than 6 months.

Persistent/chronic: if the disturbance lasts for 6 months or longer

AD is a stress-related phenomenon in which the stressor precipitates maladaptation and symptoms that are time limited until either the stressor is diminished or eliminated, or a new state of adaptation to the stressor occurs (Table 4.6.4.2). At the same time that AD was evolving, other stress-related disorders, for example, post-traumatic stress disorder and acute stress disorder were described. (Acute stress disorder was formulated by Spiegel during the development of the DSM-IV.[1,2]) Acute stress reactions could result from involvement in a natural disaster such as a flood, or an avalanche, or a cataclysmic personal event, for example, loss of a body part (aetiology-an identifiable stressor).

The diagnosis of AD also requires a careful titration of the timing of the stressor in relation to the adverse psychological sequelae that ensue. Maladaptation and disturbance of mood should occur within 3 months of the patient experiencing the stressor. Until the DSM-IV criteria, the ADs were regarded as transitory diagnoses that should not exceed 6 months in duration. Thereafter, that diagnostic appellation could not be employed and had to be changed to a major psychiatric disorder or discontinued.

Definition and history

With the opportunity in 1994 to develop another evolutionary step of the DSM, i.e. DSM-IV,[3] the authors were asked to re-examine the subthreshold diagnostic category of AD with the goal of

Table 4.6.4.2 ICD-10 definition of adjustment disorder

(a) Onset of symptoms must occur within 1 month of exposure to an identifiable psychosocial stressor, not of an unusual or catastrophic type

(b) The individual manifests symptoms or behavioural disturbances of the types found in any of the affective disorders (except for delusions and hallucinations), any disorders in F40–F48 (neurotic, stress-related, and somatoform disorders) and conduct disorders, but the criteria for an individual disorder are not fulfilled. Symptoms may be variable in both form and severity

The predominant feature of the symptoms may be further specified by use of a fifth character:

Brief depressive reaction
Prolonged depressive reaction
Mixed anxiety and depressive reaction
With predominant disturbance of other emotions
With predominant disturbance of conduct
With mixed disturbance of emotions and conduct
With other specified predominant symptoms

(c) Except in prolonged depressive reaction, the symptoms do not persist for more than 6 months after the cessation of the stress or its consequences. However, this should not prevent a provisional diagnosis being made if this criterion is not yet fulfilled

improving its acknowledged 'shortcomings'. The research included: review of the literature, reanalysis of existing studies of AD and their data sets, and examination of field studies (e.g. minor depression, minor anxiety) to observe if there was sufficient differentiation among these minor disorders from the ADs (e.g. how often was a stressor identified in those patients assigned the diagnosis; minor depression or minor anxiety?). From these three sources and consultations, modifications for DSM-IV and their rationale were formulated based on the best evidence extant.

Changes in the criteria for adjustment disorder in DSM-IV

The review of the literature, the reanalysis of the Western Psychiatric Institute and Clinic data (University of Pittsburgh), and consultations with experts supported the following changes in DSM-IV.

1 Enhance the understanding of the language.

2 Describe the timing of the reaction to reflect the duration of the AD: **acute** (less than 6 months) or **chronic** (6 months or greater).

3 Allow for the continuation of the stressor for an indefinite period; psychological reactions to chronic stress states (e.g. chronic arthritis, HIV, abuse by an alcoholic spouse) do not necessarily terminate at 6 months, nor do they necessarily lead to a major psychiatric disorder.

4 Eliminate the subtypes of mixed emotional features, work (or academic) inhibition, withdrawal, and physical complaints (as they were rarely employed by diagnosticians).

Although it might be argued that ADs could be placed in a new category of 'stress response syndromes', the literature and research reports did not support such a taxonomical organization. Another possibility was that AD could be eliminated altogether, with the advantage of maintaining the atheoretical approach of the DSM conceptual framework, and substitute in its place the appropriate minor or NOS categories as established by the accompanying mood states or behaviours. However, these solutions do not seem appropriate with recent findings that demonstrate AD to be a valid and frequently employed diagnosis.(4) AD was diagnosed in over 60 per cent of burned inpatients,(5) over 20 per cent of patients in early stages of multiple sclerosis,(6) and over 40 per cent of poststroke patients.(7) Furthermore, evaluations of patients in a psychiatric walk-in clinic showed a significant difference in the symptom profile of those assigned AD and the other diagnosis, including minor diagnoses.(8) (The McArthur field trials on the prospective assessment of minor depressive and anxiety disorders which collected data on the occurrence of stressors immediately preceding the outbreak of symptoms are important databases that need further study to establish whether stress per se is a distinguishing characteristic between AD and the other minor mood disorders.)

Problems with the adjustment disorder diagnosis

(a) The symptom profile

Critics of the AD diagnosis argue that the symptom complex is too subjective or 'depends structurally on clinical judgement' as opposed to sound, operational criteria.(9,10) Because of the lack of any quantitative behavioural or operational criteria, the problem of reliability and validity are obvious. Criterion reference was evaluated by Aoki *et al.*(11) who reported that three psychological tests, Zung's Self-Rating Anxiety Scale,(12) Zung's Self-Rating Depression Scale,(13) and the Profile of Mood States,(14) were useful tools for the diagnosis of AD in physical rehabilitation patients. While these measures succeeded in reliably differentiating AD patients from normal patients, they were not able to distinguish them from patients with major depression or post-traumatic stress disorders. Thus, the construct of AD is designed as a means for classifying psychiatric conditions having a symptom profile that is at the time of its application insufficient to meet the more specifically operationalized criteria for the major syndromes but is:

1 clinically significant and deemed to be in excess of a normal reaction to the stressor in question;

2 associated with impaired vocational or interpersonal functioning;

3 not solely the result of a psychosocial problem (V Code) requiring medical attention (e.g. non-compliance, phase of life problem, etc.).

However, field studies are being performed(15) to assess whether a reliable checklist from an elaborate list of symptoms associated with AD can be constructed (Table 4.6.4.3). (The V Codes—a problem level of diagnoses—are understandably devoid of a symptom-based diagnostic schema.)

Table 4.6.4.3 DSM-IV subtypes of adjustment disorders

Adjustment disorder with depressed mood
Adjustment disorder with anxious mood
Adjustment disorder with mixed anxiety and depressed mood
Adjustment disorder with disturbance of conduct
Adjustment disorder with mixed disturbance of emotions and conduct
Adjustment disorder unspecified

(b) The meaning of 'maladaptive'

The imprecision of the diagnostic criteria for AD is immediately apparent in the DSM-IV description of this disorder as a maladaptive reaction to an identifiable psychosocial stressor, or stressors that occurs within 3 months after onset of the stressor. It is assumed that the disturbance will remit soon after the stressor ceases or, if the stressor persists, when a new level of adaptation is achieved.[1] In addition to the problem of no symptom checklist, difficulties are inherent within each of these diagnostic elements.

First, with regard to the 'maladaptive reaction', it is unclear how this concept can or should be operationalized. Is the assessment of maladaptation subjective or objective? Who makes the decision—a third party, a mental health professional, the patients themselves, or an admixture of these? Is this decision 'culture bound'? Succinctly when does an individual cross the threshold into 'patienthood', and who will make the decision? Powell and McCone (2004) make this point in their case report of the treatment of a patient with AD secondary to the stressors of the 11 September terrorist attacks. Since there has never before been a large-scale terrorist attack in United States, how are clinicians to know what a 'normal' response to such an event would be?[16]

(c) The stressor

Most recently, in the DSM-IV text revision (DSM-IV-TR; American Psychiatric Association, 2000),[17] the term psychosocial stressor was changed to the broader concept of stressor. Emotional reactions to physical stress, such as the Chernobyl reactor incident[18] or cardiac surgery[19] are well documented in literature and suggest that psychosocial stressor as a criterion is too restrictive. Moreover, the concept of 'psychosocial' versus 'physical' stressors has led to confusion.[20]

Obviously, the stressor and its effect are central to the AD diagnosis. The second major confound emanates from the fact that the DSM-IV presents no criteria or 'guidelines' to quantify stressors or to assess their effect or meaning for a particular individual at a given time. Furthermore, the assessment of stress is not linked by an algorithm to Axis IV—a statement of stress—during the previous year and so internal consistency or reinforcement within the diagnostic lexicon is not mandated (D. Schafer, personal communication, 1990). Mezzich *et al.*[8] attempted to classify and quantify the psychosocial stressors in 13 specific domains: health, bereavement, love and marriage, parental, family stressors for children and adolescents, other familial relationships, other relationships outside the family, work, school, financial, legal, housing, and miscellaneous. Such specificity has not been defined in DSM-IV and the construct is vague and generic with minimal opportunity to achieve quantification. Despland *et al.*[21] observed that the type of stressor may indeed be of help in diagnosing AD. His study demonstrated that AD with depressed mood and mixed mood was associated with more marital problems than major depressive disorders. AD with anxiety could be distinguished from the major anxiety disorders by the quantity of family and marital problems.

(d) The time course

The time course and chronicity of both stressors and their consequent symptoms were left vague in DSM-IIIR and were not consistent with the clinical situation. The modifications introduced in DSM-IV, which differentiate between *acute* and *chronic* forms of AD, solved the problem of the 6-month limitation of the AD diagnosis in DSM-IIIR and is more in keeping with what is observed in the clinical situation. This change was validated by Despland *et al.*[21] who observed that 16 per cent of patients with AD required treatment longer than 1 year—the mean exceeded the prior limitation of 6 months.

Other problems of definition

Even serious symptomatology (e.g. suicidal behaviour) that is not regarded as part of a major mental disorder requires treatment and a 'diagnosis' under which it can be placed, for example a V Code, 'Phase of Life Problem', AD, acute stress response, etc. De Leo *et al.*[22,23] reported on AD and suicidality. Recent life events, which would constitute an acute stress, were commonly found to correlate with suicidal behaviour in a patient cohort which included those with AD.[24] Spalletta *et al.*[25] observed the assessment of suicidal behaviour to be an important tool in the differentiation among major depression, dysthymia, and AD. AD patients were found to be among the most common recipients of a deliberate self-harm diagnosis, with the majority involving self-poisoning.[26] Thus deliberate self-harm is more common in AD patients,[26] while the percentage of suicidal behaviour was found to be higher in AD patients with depressed mood.[25]

The AD DSM-IV Work Group suggested that suicide and deliberate self-harm could be subtypes of AD. However, there were concerns that patients with other diagnoses, for example major affective disorder, borderline personality disorder, etc. and suicide behaviour, would be assigned the AD diagnosis since there was a specific placement for suicidal ideation and behaviour and that would be a predominant reason to use AD. The final decision was to place the problem of suicidal symptomatology without a psychiatric diagnosis in the DSM-IV F Code section for other problems 'that may be a focus of clinical attention'. Obviously a subthreshold diagnosis, AD, does not necessarily imply the presence of subthreshold symptomatology!

Recognizing some of the limitations of the diagnosis including the aforementioned lack of specificity of symptoms and the lack of clarity of the role of the stressor, the authors of a recent article proposed adding an additional 'A-Criterion' to the DSM IV diagnosis of AD. They studied 328 young conscripts diagnosed by DSM IV with AD secondary to non-combat military stress. The diagnosis was closely associated with undisturbed psychosocial function outside of military life but with marked symptoms within military life.[9] Thus, location-specific stress was associated with location-specific symptoms, a phenomenon that the authors found helpful in distinguishing AD from other psychiatric diagnoses. Whether or not this finding would be consistent in non-military populations requires further evaluation.

'Splitting' and 'lumping' continue, for example, the subthreshold diagnosis of mixed anxiety-depressive disorder is a new category included in the DSM-IV. This disorder is very similar to AD with mixed mood; a boundary between the two is difficult to demarcate. The main difference between the two diagnoses was the chronicity of the mixed anxiety-depressive disorder (as was noted in the mixed anxiety-depression field trial).[27] The change in criterion C for AD—allowing a chronic or recurrent disturbance—confounds the differentiation of these two subthreshold diagnoses. This uncertainty is further complicated by the question of treatment. Is this an anxiety accompanied by depression, which should be treated with anxiolytics, such as benzodiazepines, or is this a depression accompanied by anxiety, which should be treated with an antidepressant, such as a selective serotonin reuptake inhibitor (SSRI)? Furthermore, it is commonly viewed that the majority of patients with AD should be treated with psychotherapy or counselling as the initial approach.

Another potential mood disorder, subsyndromal symptomatic depression (**SSD**), has been suggested.[28] It joins AD in the grey area of subthreshold diagnoses. However, there are two critical differences between SSD and AD: SSD employs a symptom checklist, and is not associated with a stressor. By definition, SSD is the simultaneous presence of any two or more symptoms of depression, persistent for most or all of the time for a duratio of at least 2 weeks, associated with social dysfunction, and occurring in patients who do not meet the criteria for minor depression (which also requires two symptoms), major depression, and/or dysthymia.[28] In some cases, the SSD diagnosis is the same as the DSM-IV diagnosis for minor depression, termed by the authors 'SSD with mood disturbance', and has to be documented as such. In other cases, the disorder is 'SSD without mood disturbance'.

In a recent study, Casey *et al.* (2006) examined variables that might distinguish AD from other depressive episodes. The patients were screened for depression severity with the Beck Depression Inventory (BDI) and then interviewed with the Schedule for Clinical Assessment in Neuropsychiatry (SCAN) which includes questions assessing the presence of AD. The authors were unable to find any independent variables that distinguished AD from other depressive episodes, including the severity of the BDI score at the outset.[29] Maercker *et al.* conceptualize AD as a stress response syndrome in which intrusions, avoidance of reminders, and failure to adapt are the central processes and symptoms.[30]

Age and medical comorbidity

In contrast with DSM-IIIR, DSM-IV has tried to accommodate the presence of comorbid medical illness. DSM-IIIR was regarded as 'medical illness and age unfair' (i.e. inadequate consideration of age and/or medical illness) (L. George, personal communication, 1981).[31] To enhance reliability and validity, there will need to be a psychiatric taxonomy that takes into account medical illness and symptomatology and developmental epochs (e.g. children and adolescents, adults, 'young' elderly, and 'old' elderly). (Actually, the original DSM did divide the AD by developmental epochs.) It is clear from the Western Psychiatric Institute studies that the symptom profile for children and adolescents is very different from that for adults with regard to the entire spectrum of diagnoses. With regard to age, recent studies report AD patients to be significantly younger compared with those with major psychiatric diagnosis.[21,32] Zarb's study[33] suggests that in cognitively impaired elderly, using individual items of the Geriatric Depression Scale, AD could be differentiated from major depression. In addition, Despland *et al.*[21] showed that patients labelled AD with depressive or mixed symptoms included more women: a sex ratio resembling that seen in major depression or dysthymia. The future evolution of the DSM needs to consider the effect of developmental epochs, gender, and medical comorbidity on symptom profiles in the various diagnostic categories.

Grassi *et al.*[34] investigated psychosomatic symptoms in patients with AD in a hospital setting in order to further characterize the diagnosis of AD in the medically ill. Results showed a considerable overlap between AD and abnormal illness behaviour including health anxiety, somatization, conversion symptoms, and demoralization among others. Only 13 out of 100 AD patients interviewed did not present with psychosomatic symptoms.

Epidemiology

The Epidemiologic Catchment Area Study (ECA) did not include AD in its historic survey of patients in the population of five major settings in the United States. Most studies are of smaller or more discrete samples and have the problem of generalization. Andreasen and Wasek[35] reported that 5 per cent of an inpatient and outpatient sample at the university hospital and clinics in Iowa were labelled as having AD. Fabrega *et al.*[36] reported that 2.3 per cent of a sample of patients presenting to a walk-in clinic (diagnostic and evaluation centre) met criteria for AD, with no other diagnoses on Axis I or Axis II; when patients with other Axis I diagnoses (i.e. Axis I and II comorbidities) were included, 20 per cent had the diagnosis of AD. In general hospital inpatient psychiatric consultation populations, AD was diagnosed as 21.5 per cent, 18.5 per cent, and 11.5 per cent, respectively.[37–39] D. Schafer (personal communication, 1990) noted that up to 70 per cent of children in the psychiatric setting may be given the diagnosis of AD in a variety of mental health care environments. Faulstich *et al.*[40] reported the prevalence of AD for adolescent psychiatric inpatients. Andreasen and Wasek,[35] utilizing a chart review, reported that more adolescents than adults experienced acting out and behavioural symptoms, but adults had significantly more depressive symptomatology (87.2 per cent versus 63.8 per cent). Anxiety symptoms were frequent at all ages.

Mezzich and coworkers[8] evaluated 64 symptoms currently present in three cohorts: subjects with specific diagnoses, those with AD, and those who were not ill. Vegetative, substance use, and characterological symptoms were greatest in the specific diagnosis group, intermediate in the AD group, and least in the group with non illness. The symptoms of mood and affect, general appearance, behaviour, disturbance in speech and thought pattern, and cognitive functioning had a similar distribution. The AD group was significantly different from the non-illness group with regard to more 'depressed mood' and 'low self-esteem' ($p \leq 0.0001$). The AD and non-illness groups had minimal pathology of thought content and perception. A positive response on the suicide indicators was obtained in 29 per cent of AD compared with 9 per cent of the non-illness group. The three cohorts did not differ on the frequency of Axis III disorders.

Associated features of adjustment disorder

Andreasen and Wasek[35] observed that in their AD cohorts 21.6 per cent of the adolescents' fathers and 11.8 per cent of the adults' fathers had problems with alcohol. Greenberg *et al.*[41] report more substance abuse in adults with diagnosed AD compared with all those with other diagnoses. Breslow *et al.*[42] comparing patients with AD and other psychiatric diagnoses, observed that alcohol or substance use/abuse did not help to differentiate between diagnostic groups. Thus, currently the higher rate of substance use does not serve as an incontrovertible predictive factor for the diagnosis of an AD diagnosis.

Aetiology—the role of stress

(a) Nature of the stressor

Andreasen and Wasek[35] described the differences between the chronicity of stressors found in adolescents compared with those in adults: present for a year or more, 59 per cent and 35 per cent; present for 3 months or less, 9 per cent and 39 per cent. Fabrega *et al.*[36] reported that their AD group had greater registration of stressors compared with other diagnoses and the non-illness cohorts. Compared with other diagnoses and the non-illness patients, AD was over-represented in the 'higher stress category'. In their consultation cohort, Popkin *et al.*[37] found that in 68.6 per cent of the cases the medical illness itself was judged to be the primary psychosocial stressor. Snyder and Strain[39] observed that stressors as assessed on Axis IV were significantly higher ($p = 0.0001$) for consultation patients with AD than for patients with other diagnostic disorders.

(b) Modifiers of stress

Stress has been described as the aetiological agent for AD. Vulnerability to stress is another risk factor. Diverse variables and modifiers are involved regarding who will experience AD following a stress. Cohen[43] argues as follows:

1 acute stresses are different from chronic stresses in both psychological and physiological terms;

2 the meaning of the stress is affected by 'modifiers' (e.g. ego strengths, support systems, prior mastery);

3 manifest and latent meanings of the stressor(s) may be associated with differential impact (e.g. loss of job may be a relief or a catastrophe).

An objectively overwhelming stress may have little impact on one individual, whereas a minor stress could be regarded as cataclysmic by another. A recent minor stress superimposed on a previous underlying (major) stress that has no observable effect on its own may have a significant additive impact (i.e. concatenation of events) (B. Hamburg, personal communication, 1990). Despland *et al.*[21] reported that stressors were present on Axis IV in 100 per cent of those assigned AD with depressed mood, while it was present in 83 per cent of those with major depression, 80 per cent of those with dysthymia, and 67 per cent of those with non-specific depression, which emphasizes the importance of stressors in the AD diagnosis.

Clinical features

Nine different types of AD are listed in DSM-IV.[1] As in DSM-III, AD is classified in DSM-IIIR according to the predominant symptom picture. In DSM-IV, AD has been reduced to six types that, again, are classified according to their clinical features:

1 AD with depressed mood;

2 AD with anxious mood;

3 AD with mixed anxiety and depressed mood;

4 AD with disturbance of conduct;

5 AD with mixed disturbance of emotions and conduct; and

6 AD not otherwise specified.

In their study, Despland *et al.*[21] suggested reducing the subtypes even further, demonstrating identical profiles for AD with depressed mood and AD with mixed mood, and proposing assimilation of mixed mood into the depressed mood category. Fifty-seven per cent of their sample was represented by these two groups; the remainder was accounted for by AD with 'anxiety' and 'other' categories.

Treatment

(a) Evidence regarding treatment

In terms of randomized controlled trials (RCTs), a search of the Cochrane Database revealed only two RCTs on psychotherapeutic treatment of AD. Gonzales-Jaimes and Turnbull-Plaza (2002) showed that 'mirror psychotherapy' for patients suffering from AD with depressed mood secondary to a myocardial infarction was both an efficient and effective treatment. Mirror therapy is described as a type of therapy with psychocorporal, cognitive, and neurolinguistic components with a holistic focus. As part of the treatment, a mirror is used to encourage patient acceptance of his/her physical condition that resulted from past self-care behaviours. In this study, mirror therapy was compared to two other treatments, Gestalt psychotherapy or medical conversation in addition to a control group. Depressive symptoms improved in all treatment groups compared with the control group, but mirror therapy appeared significantly more effective than the other treatments in decreasing symptoms of AD at post-test evaluation.[44]

In a second RCT, an 'activating intervention' was carried out for the treatment of AD which had resulted in occupational dysfunction. A total of 192 employees were randomized to receive either the intervention or care as usual.[45] The intervention consisted of an individual cognitive behavioural approach to a graded activity, similar to stress inoculation training. Goals of treatment emphasized the acquisition of coping skills and the regaining of control. The treatment proved to be effective in decreasing sick leave duration and shortening long-term absenteeism when compared to the control group; both intervention and control groups, however, showed similar amounts of symptom reduction. This study formed the basis for the Dutch Practice Guidelines for the treatment of AD in primary and occupational health care.[46] These guidelines were prepared by a team of 21 occupational health physicians and one psychologist and subsequently reviewed and tested by 15 experts, including several psychiatrists and psychologists and 21 practicing occupational health physicians.

Though no other RCTs involving the psychotherapeutic treatment of pure cohorts of patients with AD could be found, many RCTs exist that studied an array of depressive and anxiety disorders and that included AD in their cohorts. For example, a recent trial comparing brief dynamic therapy (BDT) with brief supportive therapy (BSP) in patients with minor depressive disorders, including AD, was found in the Cochrane Database. Though both therapies proved efficacious in reducing symptoms, BDT was more effective as demonstrated in a 6 months follow-up.[47]

Another therapeutic modality, eye movement desensitization and reprocessing (EMDR) has been recently studied in patients with AD.[48] EMDR, a psychotherapeutic technique shown to be effective in the treatment of post-traumatic stress disorder, was carried out on nine patients suffering from AD. Results showed significant improvement in patients with anxious or mixed features but not in those with depressed mood. Additionally, those with ongoing stressors did not show improvement.

Hameed *et al.* in a retrospective chart review sought to determine if there was a difference in antidepressant efficacy in the treatment of major depressive disorder versus AD in a primary care setting. Patients had been prescribed mostly SSRIs. DSM-IV symptoms, Patient Health Questionnaire-9 (PHQ-9) depression rating scale scores, and functional disability reports were systematically used to assess patients' response. Results showed that neither depressed, nor AD patients demonstrated a difference in clinical response to any particular antidepressant. Patients with a diagnosis of AD, however, were twice as likely to respond to standard antidepressant treatment as depressed patients. This study suggests that antidepressants are very effective in treating depression in the primary care setting and may be even more effective in the treatment for AD with depressed mood.(49)

In another recent double-blind RCT, the efficacies of etifoxine, a non-benzodiazepine anxiolytic drug, and lorazepam, a benzodiazepine, were compared in the treatment of AD with anxiety in a primary care setting.(50) Efficacy was evaluated on days 7 and 28 using the Hamilton Rating Scale for Anxiety (HAM-A). The two drugs were found to be equivalent in anxiolytic efficacy on day 28. However, more etifoxine recipients responded to the treatment. Moreover, 1 week after stopping treatment, fewer patients taking etifoxine experienced rebound anxiety, compared to those given lorazepam.(50)

Management

(a) Psychotherapy and counselling

Though brief therapeutic interventions are usually all that are needed, ongoing stressors or enduring character pathology that may make a patient vulnerable to stress intolerance may signal the need for lengthier treatments.(51)

Treatment of AD initially focuses on psychotherapeutic and counselling interventions to reduce the stressor, enhance the capacity to cope with a stressor that cannot be reduced or removed, and establish a system of support to maximize adaptation. The patient needs to be made aware of the significant dysfunction that the stressor has caused and consider strategies to manage the disability. Some stressors, for example taking on more responsibility than can be managed by the individual or putting oneself at risk (e.g. unprotected sex with an unknown partner), can be avoided or minimized. Other stressors may elicit an overreaction on the part of the patient (e.g. abandonment by a lover). The patient may attempt suicide or become reclusive, damaging his or her source of income. In this situation, the therapist would assist the patient to verbalize his or her disappointed feelings and rage rather than behaving destructively. The role of verbalization in minimizing the discomfort of the stressor and enhancing coping cannot be overestimated. It is necessary to clarify and interpret the meaning/reality of the stressor for the patient. For example, if a mastectomy has devastated a patient's feelings about her body and herself, it is mandatory to articulate that the patient is still a woman, capable of having a fulfilling relationship, including a sexual one and that recurrence of the cancer may not occur. Without the correction of distortions, the patient's pernicious fantasies—'all is lost'—may occur as sequelae to the stressor (i.e. the mastectomy) and intensify incapacitation at work and/or sex, as well as contribute to a profound disturbance of mood.

Counselling, psychotherapies, crisis intervention, family therapy, and group treatment are utilized to encourage the verbalization of fears, anxiety, rage, helplessness, and hopelessness to the stressors imposed upon a patient. As mentioned above, the goal of treatment is to expose the concerns and conflicts that the patient is experiencing, identify means to reduce the stressor(s), enhance the patient's coping skills, clarify the patient's perspective on the adversity, and enable the establishment of supporting relationships. The primary treatment for AD is talking.

(b) Psychopharmacotherapy

Should drugs be used in the treatment of AD? The pharmacological studies are not conclusive. The diagnostic dilemmas of the AD present sufficient difficulty in and of themselves.(52–54) It would be preferred that cautious psychotropic drug administration be employed, to avoid subjecting the patient to the risk of unfavourable medical drug-psychotrophic drug interaction(s). Psychotrophic drug treatment will not be necessary if the condition resolves. If it evolves into a major psychiatric illness then drug treatment needs to be actively entertained. And, for a refractory AD treatment with psychopharmacological agents should be considered. Small doses of antidepressants and anxiolytics may sometimes be appropriate for AD patients when dysphoria remains profound despite several sessions of psychological treatment.

Although formal psychotherapy is presently the treatment of choice, psychotherapy combined with benzodiazapines are utilized, especially for patients with severe life stress(es) and an unrelenting anxious component. Tricyclic antidepressants or buspirone were recommended in place of benzodiazapines for AD patients with current or past excessive alcohol use because of their greater risk of dependence.(55) The use of antidepressants may assist some patients if their maladaptation is debilitating and the accompanying mood is pervasive, especially if a trial of psychotherapy has been shown to be ineffective.

Adults and adolescents

Andreasen and Hoenk(56) report that the long-term outcome of AD has a good prognosis for adults, but that a majority of adolescents eventually have major psychiatric disorders. Follow-up at 5 years after original diagnosis of AD revealed that 71 per cent of adults were completely well, 8 per cent had an intervening problem, and 21 per cent had developed a major depressive disorder or alcoholism. However, in adolescents at 5-year follow-up, only 44 per cent were without a psychiatric diagnosis, 13 per cent had an intervening psychiatric illness, and 43 per cent went on to develop major psychiatric morbidity (e.g. schizophrenia, schizoaffective disorders, major depression, bipolar disorder, substance abuse, and personality disorders). In contrast with the adults, the chronicity of the illness and the presence of behavioural symptoms in the adolescents were the strongest predictors for major psychopathology 5 years after the initial AD diagnosis. The number and type of symptoms were less useful than the length of treatment and chronicity of symptoms as predictors of future outcome.

As Chess and Thomas(57) have reported, it is important to note that AD with disturbance of conduct, regardless of age, has a more guarded outcome. In agreement with the findings of Andreasen and Wasek,(35) Chess and Thomas(57) emphasize that:

> a significant number [of AD adolescents] did not improve or even grew worse in adolescence and early adult life. It was not possible to predict the developmental course of the disorder in the early period after its first identification. Hence, we would suggest active appropriate

therapeutic intervention in all cases but especially adolescents [and adequate follow-up].

Spalletta *et al.*[25] report that suicidal behaviour and deliberate self-harm are important predictors in the diagnosis of AD. As mentioned before, these are obviously not subthreshold symptoms; they can lead to the most dire consequence—death. This outcome, when reached, can be neither corrected nor resolved. These behaviours mandate immediate and protective interventions. The diagnosis of AD may suggest that the patient has minor symptomatology. Such erroneous assessment may be life-threatening. There needs to be a definite split from viewing a diagnosis as subthreshold, and therefore assuming the attendant symptoms to be subthreshold. It is similar to labelling a patient with hypochondriasis, which in some settings can influence a more casual physical assessment, when such a patient could have serious physical morbidity concomitant with their hypochondriacal Axis I pathology.

Although most studies do point to a more benign prognosis for the AD, it is important to realize that the risk of serious morbidity and mortality still exists. Several recent studies investigating the association between suicide and AD underscore the importance of monitoring patients closely for suicidality, especially in younger populations. Portzky *et al.* conducted psychological autopsies on adolescents with AD who had committed suicide and found that suicidal thinking in these patients was brief and evolved rapidly without warning.[60] A slightly different profile was found in two other studies that looked at suicide attempters with a diagnosis of AD. These patients were more likely to have poor overall psychosocial functioning, prior psychiatric treatment, personality disorders, substance abuse histories and a current 'mixed' symptom profile of depressed mood and behavioural disturbances.[61,62] A study of the neurochemical variables of AD patients of all ages who had attempted suicide revealed biologic correlates consistent with the more major psychiatric disorders. Attempters were found to have lower platelet MAO activity, higher MHPG activity, and higher cortisol levels than controls. Though these findings differ from the lower MHPG and cortisol levels found in patients with major depression and suicidality, they are similar to findings in other major stress-related conditions.[63]

As mentioned earlier, the diagnosis of an AD may be in the early phase of an evolving disorder that has not yet developed to the extent that full-blown symptoms are evident to reach threshold for a major psychiatric disorder. If a patient continues to worsen, becomes more symptomatic, and does not respond to treatment, it is critical to review the diagnosis for the presence of a major disorder.

A recent report by Jones *et al.* (2002) looked at 10 years of readmission data for various psychiatric diagnoses including the AD. They found that admission diagnosis was a significant predictor of readmission and that AD had the lowest readmission rates.[58] Furthermore, initial psychological recovery from an AD may in large part be attributable to removal of the stressor. This was found to be the case in prisoners who developed AD after being placed in solitary confinement and whose symptoms resolved shortly after their release.[59]

The domains of diagnostic rigour and clinical utility seem at odds for AD. Studies that employ reliable and valid instruments (e.g. depression or anxiety rating scales, stress assessments, length of disability, treatment outcome, family patterns, etc.) would enhance more exact specification of the parameters of the AD diagnosis. Identification of the time course, remission or evolution to another diagnosis, and the evaluation of stressors (characteristics, duration, and the nature of adaptation to stress) would enhance the understanding of the aetiology, mechanisms, and mediators of a stress-response illness.

Studies with adequate symptom checklists rated independently from the establishment of the diagnosis would clarify the threshold between major and minor depression and anxiety, as well as guide an entry threshold to employ the AD diagnosis. Although the upper threshold is established by the specified criteria for major syndromes, the entry threshold between an AD and problem-level diagnoses and normality is undesignated with operational criteria. The careful examination of associated demographic and treatment outcome variables would also enable clinicians to describe more specifically the boundaries among subthreshold diagnoses, problem-level diagnosis, and normal behaviour. Associated features such as family history, biological correlates, treatment response, long-term course, and so forth, are all critical to establishing the validity of a diagnosis. The theory and practice of medicine have demonstrated the need for a comprehensive multidimensional formulation of all these physiological and functional variables to describe an illness and develop the most appropriate working diagnosis.

Subthreshold syndromes can encompass significant psychopathology that must not only be identified but treated (e.g. suicidal ideation/behaviour). Cross-sectionally, AD may appear to be the incipient phase of an emerging major syndrome. Consequently, AD, despite its questionable reliability and validity, serves an important diagnostic function in the practice of psychiatry. Problem- and subthreshold-level diagnoses are critical to the function of any medical discipline. Because this may be the initial phase, or a mild form, of a dysfunction that is not yet fully developed, there is a need to describe the relationship of this incipient state to other potential diagnoses. This lack of specificity and questionable reliability and validity are the hallmark of interface disorders and subthreshold phenomena, whether they are in diabetes mellitus, hypertension, or depression.

As mentioned earlier, the characteristics of a mental disorder vary over the life cycle, and this is clearly illustrated by the AD. Certain developmental epochs may be associated with a particular symptom profile, as seen with acute myocardial infarction or appendicitis. The effect of the stressor may vary, and the assessment of functioning must be 'measured' according to the demands of the developmental stage (e.g. school [adolescents], work [adults], self-care and maintenance [elderly]). The symptom characteristics and functional assessment of other diagnoses may also vary along the developmental schema from birth to senescence; illnesses such as major depressive disorders, organic mental disorders, sexual dysfunctions, and eating disorders need to be 'recast' in another hierarchy to incorporate the stage of the life cycle extant at the time of the assessment, and symptom profiles adjusted accordingly. The normal variations across developmental epochs would make AD and the other psychiatric disorders more reliable and valid across the life cycle. Similarly, there needs to be a consideration of a possible concomitant state of medical illness. The result would be a taxonomy tempered by the vicissitudes of development and medical illness.

A taxonomy which considers the development epoch and the presence of medical illness would be more useful to child psychiatrists, paediatricians, geriatricians, geriatric psychiatrists, and primary care specialists, who are often convinced that a patient does not conform with today's psychiatry lexicon. A significant number of their patients remain at the problem level of diagnoses with their somatic complaints as well. It is not uncommon for a fever of unknown origin to not be diagnosed, or for a chest pain to remain unspecified. It is the art of medicine that makes it a profession, and a most difficult one, at the interface of medicine and psychiatry, or at the interface of normality and pathology. Freud[(64)] has emphasized the difficulty of understanding normality and pathology in her assessments of childhood. This important advice would obtain across the life cycle and be an important challenge to the developers of the subthreshold diagnoses (e.g. AD) and the future evolution of the DSM.

Further information

Grassi, L., Mangelli, L., Fava, G.A., *et al.* (2007). Psychosomatic characterization of adjustment disorders in the medical setting; some suggestions for DSM-V. *Journal of Affective Disorders*, **101**, 251–4.

Kumana, H., Ida, I., Oshima, A., *et al.* (2007). Brain metabolic changes associated with predisposition to onset of major depressive disorder and adjustment disorder in cancer patients—a preliminary PET study. *Journal of Psychiatric Research*, **41**, 591–9.

Casey, P., Maracy, M., Kelly, B.D., *et al.* (2006). Can adjustment disorder and depressive episode be distinguished? Results from ODIN. *Journal of Affective Disorders*, **92**, 291–7.

Bruinvels, D.J., Rebergen, D.S., Nieuwenhuijsen, K., *et al.* (2007). *Return to work interventions for adjustment disorders. Cochrane database of systematic reviews: protocols*, Issue 1. John Wiley & Sons, Chichester, UK.

References

1. American Psychiatric Association. (1994). *Diagnostic and statistical manual of mental disorders* (4th edn). American Psychiatric Association, Washington, DC.
2. Spiegel, D. (1994). *DSM-IV options book*. American Psychiatric Association, Washington, DC.
3. American Psychiatric Association. (1980). *Diagnostic and statistical manual of mental disorders* (3rd edn). American Psychiatric Association, Washington, DC.
4. Kovacs, M., Ho, V., and Pollock, M.H. (1995). Criterion and predictive validity of the diagnosis of adjustment disorder: a prospective study of youths with new-onset insulin-dependent diabetes mellitus. *The American Journal of Psychiatry*, **152**, 523–8.
5. Perez-Jimenez, J.P., Gomez-Bajo, G.J., Lopez-Catillo, J.J., *et al.* (1994). Psychiatric consultation and post-traumatic stress disorder in burned patients. *Burns*, **20**, 532–6.
6. Sullivan, M.J., Winshenker, B., and Mikail, S. (1995). Screening for major depression in the early stages of multiple sclerosis. *The Canadian Journal of Neurological Science*, **22**, 228–31.
7. Shima, S., Kitagawa, Y., Kitamura, T., *et al.* (1994). Poststroke depression. *General Hospital Psychiatry*, **16**, 286–9.
8. Mezzich, J.E., Dow, J.T., Rich, C.L., *et al.* (1981). Developing an efficient clinical information system for a comprehensive psychiatric institute. II. Initial evaluation form. *Behavioral Research Methods and Instrumentation*, **13**, 464–78.
9. Bonelli, R.M. and Bugram, R. (2000). Additional A-criterion for adjustment disorders. *Canadian Journal of Psychiatry*, **45**, 763.
10. Casey, P. (2001). Adult adjustment disorder: a review of its current diagnostic status. *Journal of Psychiatric Practice*, **7**, 32–40.
11. Aoki, T., Hosaka, T., and Ishida, A. (1995). Psychiatric evaluation of physical rehabilitation patients. *General Hospital Psychiatry*, **17**, 440–3.
12. Zung, W. (1971). A rating instrument for anxiety disorders. *Psychosomatics*, **12**, 371–9.
13. Zung, W. (1965). A self-rating depression scale. *Archives of General Psychiatry*, **12**, 63–70.
14. McNair, D.M., Lorr, M., and Doppelman, L.F. (eds.) (1971). *Manual for the profile of mood states*. Educational and Industrial Testing Service, San Diego, CA.
15. Strain, J.J., Newcorn, J., Mezzich, J., *et al.* (1998). Adjustment disorder: the McArthur reanalysis. In *DSM-IV source book*, Vol. 4, pp. 404–24. American Psychiatric Association, Washington, DC.
16. Powell, S. and McCone, D. (2004). Treatment of adjustment disorder with anxiety: a September 11, 2001, case study with a 1-year follow up. *Cognitive and Behavioral Practice*, **11**, 331–6.
17. American Psychiatric Association. (2000). *Diagnostic and statistical manual of mental disorders* (4th edn, text revision). American Psychiatric Association, Washington, DC.
18. Havenaar, J.M., Van den Brink, W., Van den Bout, J., *et al.* (1996). Mental health problems in the Gomel region (Belarus): an analysis of risk factors in an area affected by the Chernobyl disaster. *Psychological Medicine*, **26**, 845–55.
19. Oxman, T.E., Barrett, J.E., Freeman, D.H., *et al.* (1994). Frequency and correlates of adjustment disorder related to cardiac surgery in older patients. *Psychosomatics*, **35**, 557–68.
20. Leigh, H. (1993). Physical factors affecting psychiatric condition: a proposal for DSM-IV. *General Hospital Psychiatry*, **15**, 155–9.
21. Despland, J.N., Monod, L., and Ferrero, F. (1995). Clinical relevance of adjustment disorder in DSM-III-R and DSM-IV. *Comprehensive Psychiatry*, **36**, 456–60.
22. De Leo, D., Pellegrini, C., and Serraiotto, L. (1986). Adjustment disorders and suicidality. *Psychology Reports*, **59**, 355–8.
23. De Leo, D., Pellegrini, C., Serraiotto, L., *et al.* (1986). Assessment of severity of suicide attempts: a trial with the dexamethasone suppression test and two rating scales. *Psychopathology*, **19**, 186–91.
24. Isometsa, E., Heikkinen, M., Henriksson, M., *et al.* (1996). Suicide in non-major depressions. *Journal of Affective Disorders*, **36**, 117–27.
25. Spalletta, G., Troisi, A., Saracco, H., *et al.* (1996). Symptom profile: axis II comorbidity and suicidal behaviour in young males with DSM-III-R depressive illnesses. *Journal of Affective Disorders*, **39**, 141–8.
26. Vlachos, I.O., Bouras, N., Watson, J.P., *et al.* (1994). Deliberate self-harm referrals. *European Journal of Psychiatry*, **8**, 25–8.
27. Zinbarg, R.E., Barlow, D.H., Liebowitz, M., *et al.* (1994). The DSM-IV field trial for mixed anxiety-depression. *The American Journal of Psychiatry*, **151**, 1153–62.
28. Judd, L.L., Rapaport, M.H., Paulus, M.P., *et al.* (1994). Subsyndromal symptomatic depression: a new mood disorder? *The Journal of Clinical Psychiatry*, **55**(4 Suppl), 18–28.
29. Casey, P., Maracy, M., Kelly, B.D., *et al.* (2006). Can adjustment disorder and depressive episode be distinguished? *Journal of Affective Disorders*, **92**, 291–7.
30. Maercker, A., Einsle, F., and Kollner, V. (2006). Adjustment disorders as stress response syndromes: a new diagnostic concept and its exploration in a medical sample. *Psychopathology*, **627**.
31. Strain, J.J. (1981). Diagnostic considerations in the medical setting. *The Psychiatric Clinics of North America*, **4**, 287–300.
32. Mok, H. and Walter, C. (1995). Brief psychiatric hospitalization: preliminary experience with an urban sort-stay unit. *Canadian Journal of Psychiatry*, **40**, 415–17.
33. Zarb, J. (1996). Correlates of depression in cognitively impaired hospitalized elderly referred for neuropsychological assessment. *Journal of Clinical and Experimental Neuropsychology*, **18**, 713–23.

34. Grassi, L., Gritti, P., Rigatelli, M., *et al.* (2000). Psychosocial problems secondary to cancer: an Italian multicenter survey of consultation-liaison psychiatry in oncology. Italian Consultation-Liaison Group. *European Journal of Cancer*, **36**, 579–85.
35. Andreasen, N.C. and Wasek, P. (1980). Adjustment disorders in adolescents and adults. *Archives of General Psychiatry*, **37**, 1166–70.
36. Fabrega, H. Jr, Mezzich, J.E., and Mezzich, A.C. (1987). Adjustment disorder as a marginal or transitional illness category in DSM-III. *Archives of General Psychiatry*, **44**, 567–72.
37. Popkin, M.K., Callies, A.L., Colón, E.A., *et al.* (1990). Adjustment disorders in medically ill patients referred for consultation in a university hospital. *Psychosomatics*, **31**, 410–14.
38. Foster, P. and Oxman, T. (1994). A descriptive study of adjustment disorder diagnoses in general hospital patients. *Irish Journal of Psychological Medicine*, **11**, 153–7.
39. Snyder, S. and Strain, J.J. (1989). Differentiation of major depression and adjustment disorder with depressed mood in the medical setting. *General Hospital Psychiatry*, **12**, 159–65.
40. Faulstich, M.E., Moore, J.R., Carey, M.P., *et al.* (1986). Prevalence of DSM-III conduct and adjustment disorders for adolescent psychiatric inpatients. *Adolescence*, **21**, 333–7.
41. Greenberg, W.M., Rosenfeld, D.N., and Ortega, E.A. (1995). Adjustment disorder as an admission diagnosis. *The American Journal of Psychiatry*, **152**, 459–61.
42. Breslow, R.E., Klinger, B.I., and Erickson, B.J. (1996). Acute intoxication and substance abuse among patients presenting to a psychiatric emergency service. *General Hospital Psychiatry*, **18**, 183–91.
43. Cohen, F. (1981). Stress and bodily illness. *The Psychiatric Clinics of North America*, **4**, 269–86.
44. Gonzales-Jaimes, E.I. and Turnbull-Plaza, B. (2003). Selection of psychotherapeutic treatment for adjustment disorder with depressive mood due to acute myocardial infarction. *Archives of Medical Research*, **34**, 298–304.
45. van der Klink, J.J., Blonk, R.W., Schene, A.H., *et al.* (2003). Reducing long term sickness absence by an activating intervention in adjustment disorders: a cluster randomized controlled design. *Occupational and Environmental Medicine*, **60**, 429–37.
46. van der Klink, J.J.L. and van Dijk, F.J.H. (2003). Dutch practice guidelines for managing adjustment disorders in occupational and primary health care. *Scandinavian Journal of Work, Environment & Health*, **29**, 478–87.
47. Maina, G., Forner, F., and Bogetto, F. (2005). Randomized controlled trial comparing brief dynamic and supportive therapy with waiting list condition in minor depressive disorders. *Psychotherapy and Psychosomatics*, **74**, 43–50.
48. Mihelich, M.L. (2000). Eye movement desensitization and reprocessing treatment of adjustment disorder. *Dissertation Abstracts International*, **61**, 1091.
49. Hameed, U., Schwartz, T.L., Malhotra, K., *et al.* (2005). Antidepressant treatment in the primary care office: outcomes for adjustment disorder versus major depression. *Annals of Clinical Psychiatry*, **17**, 77–81.
50. Nguyen, N., Fakra, E., Pradel, V., *et al.* (2006). Efficacy of etifoxine compared to lorazepam monotherapy in the treatment of patients with adjustment disorders with anxiety: a double-blind controlled study in general practice. *Human Psychopharmacology*, **21**, 139–49.
51. Newcorn, J.H., Strain, J.J., and Mezzich, J.E. (2000). Adjustment disorders. In *Comprehensive Textbook of Psychiatry* (7th edn) (eds. B. Saddock and V. Saddock). Lippincott Williams and Wilkins, Philadelphia, PA.
52. Hosaka, T., Aoki, T., and Ichikawa, Y. (1994). Emotional states of patients with hematological malignancies: preliminary study. *Japanese Journal of Clinical Oncology*, **24**, 186–90.
53. Oxman, T.E., Barrett, J.E., Freeman, D.H., *et al.* (1994). Frequency and correlates of adjustment disorder relates to cardiac surgery in older patients. *Psychosomatics*, **35**, 557–68.
54. Hugo, F.J., Halland, A.M., Spangenberg, J.J., *et al.* (1996). DSM-III-R classification of psychiatric symptoms in systemic lupus erythematosus. *Psychosomatics*, **37**, 262–9.
55. Uhlenhuth, E.H., Balter, M.B., Ban, T.A., *et al.* (1995). International study of expert judgment on therapeutic use of benzodiazepines and other psychotherapeutic medications. III. Clinical features affecting experts' therapeutic recommendations in anxiety disorders. *Psychopharmacology Bulletin*, **31**, 289–96.
56. Andreasen, N.C. and Hoenk, P.R. (1982). The predictive value of adjustment disorders: a follow-up study. *The American Journal of Psychiatry*, **139**, 584–90.
57. Chess, S. and Thomas, A. (1984). *Origins and evolution of behavior disorders: from infancy to early adult life*. Brunner-Mazel, New York.
58. Jones, R., Yates, W.R., and Zhou, M.D. (2002). Readmission rates for adjustment disorders: comparison with other mood disorders. *Journal of Affective Disorders*, **71**, 199–203.
59. Andersen, H.S., Sestoft, D., Lillebaek, T., *et al.* (2000). A longitudinal study of prisoners on remand: psychiatric prevalence, incidence and psychopathology in solitary vs. non-solitary confinement. *Acta Psychiatrica Scandinavica*, **102**, 19–25.
60. Portzky, G., Audenaert, K., and van Heeringen, K. (2005). Adjustment disorder and the course of the suicidal process in adolescents. *Journal of Affective Disorders*, **87**, 265–70.
61. Pelkonen, M., Marttunen, M., *et al.* (2005). Suicidality in adjustment disorder, clinical characteristics of adolescent outpatients. *European Child & Adolescent Psychiatry*, **14**, 174–80.
62. Kryzhanovskaya, L. and Canterbury, R. (2001). Suicidal behavior in patients with adjustment disorders. *Crisis*, **22**, 125–31.
63. Tripodianakis, J., Markianos, M., Sarantidis, D., *et al.* (2000). Neurochemical variables in subjects with adjustment disorder after suicide attempts. *European Psychiatry*, **15**, 190–5.
64. Freud, A. (1968). *Normality and pathology: assessment of childhood*. International Universities Press, New York.

4.6.5 Bereavement

Beverley Raphael, Sally Wooding, and Julie Dunsmore

Bereavement is the complex set reactions that occurs with the death of a loved one: the emotions of grief with yearning, angry protest, and sadness; the cognitive processes of understanding and making meaning of the finality and nature of death; and the social, cultural, spiritual, and religious contexts of adaptation. Grief may also result from other losses such as health, home, country, and safe worlds. There have been investigations into potential neurobiological substrates, without, as yet consensus about the explanatory model.

In 'Mourning and Melancholia', Freud[1] described the psychological processes of mourning which involved the gradual relinquishment of bonds with the deceased, and how mourning differed from melancholia. Lindemann[2] described the 'Symptomatology and Management of Acute Grief' in his classic paper on his experiences assessing and treating the survivors of a nightclub fire. Engel[3] asked 'Is Grief a Disease?', and concluded in the negative.

Bowlby's work on attachment, separation, and loss[4–6] has been the most influential in informing research and clinical practice, with many studies of both adults and children utilizing such concepts. Early research focused chiefly on bereavement following the death of a spouse, describing normal, high risk, and pathological patterns of grief.[7–9] There is also a number of excellent reviews of theory and research, including those of Stroebe's group.[10,11]

Phenomenology of 'normal grief'

Common phenomena of the grief experience of adults, identified through many research studies,[12–14] relate to similar domains influenced by developmental trajectories, through childhood and adolescence. Adult studies indicate consistent patterns: numbness, disbelief; yearning, angry protest, and 'searching' behaviours representing separation distress; and sadness with reviewing of memories of the lost relationship, with a range of associated emotions; progressive acceptance of the death and changed circumstances, sometimes referred to as resolution.

Bonanno[14] has shown that resilient trajectories, defined by low overall distress, are common. Other transient phenomena described by clinicians working with bereaved people[15] include: identificatory symptoms, reflecting the deceased's illness; a sense of the deceased's ongoing at presence, at times as though seeing the face, hearing the voice, or feeling the touch of the dead person. 'Yearning' is considered to be the most pathognomic of these grief phenomena, which usually settle over the first year, but may continue, triggered by anniversaries, or specific memories. Older people who have had a long relationship with a spouse may continue this relationship in their minds for the comfort of 'talking' with the person, and a need for the ongoing closeness.[16]

Recent research[17] has modelled sequential peaks of the reactive phenomena: disbelief, yearning, anger, and depression, which bereaved people more usually describe as sadness. Grief may be a precipitant of depression in those with pre-existing or bereavement-related vulnerabilities and the differentiation of normal and more pathological forms of grief from depression is important clinically.[15,18] Intense grief and the peaks of distress identified above do not usually continue beyond the first 4–6 months.[12,13] Continuing 'acute' grief beyond this time suggests the possibility of pathological response, as do other risk indicators, although some phenomena may continue intermittently for many years. Comparative studies have demonstrated that the intensity of adult grief is likely to be greatest for the death of a child, then spouse, or partner, then parent.[12,19]

Neurobiology of bereavement

Recent research has examined the neurobiology of grief through studies using functional magnetic resonance imaging of grief[20] and brain activity in womºen grieving the break-up of a romantic relationship.[21] Workers have attempted to develop a theoretical model based on a wide range of relevant data, encompassing a 'neurobiopsychosocial' framework for sadness and loss.[22] Stress hormones[23] and psychoimmune function is a further area of research. A comprehensive model integrating the relevant research findings is yet to be established.

Risk and protective factors influencing course and outcome

Pre-existing vulnerabilities that may influence the course and outcome have been reviewed alongside other risk factors.[24] These include personality vulnerabilities related to relationship styles such as avoidant and insecure attachments. Genetic factors do not appear to have been directly studied, but it is likely that the short allele of the serotonin gene promoter polymorphism of 5HTTLPR which influences response to adversity may contribute, through gene–environment interactions.[25] Prior loss and adverse experiences may add vulnerability, for instance multiple losses faced by indigenous peoples, with loss of culture, land, and loved ones, with multiple premature deaths and separations.[26] Separation anxiety in childhood, as well as pre-existing psychiatric disorder, family psychiatric disorder, and substance abuse may add to vulnerability. Successful negotiation of earlier losses, mature defence styles, and optimism may be protective.

The nature of the lost relationship has been identified in a number of studies as being a significant factor.[15,27] The special relationship between parent and child is associated with greater vulnerabilities, including increased risk of psychiatric hospitalization and even death by suicide. Patterns of distress differ by gender with stillbirth, neonatal deaths, and sudden infant death syndromes, perhaps suggesting different attachment patterns.[28] The death of an adolescent child is not infrequently by accident, suicide, or risk-taking with illicit drugs, bringing the extra complexities of adaptation for the grieving parents.

A great deal of research has explored the grief associated with the death of a partner or spouse both young and old. High levels of dependence and ambivalence have been shown to complicate grief and to be associated with more difficult bereavement,[15,27] and prolonged or complicated grief may be more likely.

Family members may have different relationships with the deceased, and thus varying patterns and trajectories of grief, which may cloud the recognition of children's and others needs.

Adults' loss of an older parent appears to be the least distressing, although there is still sadness plus the recognition of one's own mortality. Here, as at any age, intense fantasies of reunion with the deceased may indicate risk of suicide, especially for older widowed men.

Circumstances of the death may influence outcome. When dying is *prolonged*, as in the later stages of a terminal illness, the dying person may experience grief over his or her own life, and the loved ones who will be lost to him, alongside the anticipatory grieving of family members. While palliative care systems may provide bereavement programmes, families have complex dynamics, and may require family focused interventions.[29]

Sudden unexpected deaths bring an extra level of emotional shock,[30] especially if also untimely as with children's death. When violent death occurs, as with homicide or the mass violence of terrorism or war, those bereaved may experience a complex mixture of traumatic stress reactions and grief reactions, sometimes called traumatic grief.[31] The specific issues facing those bereaved by violent deaths of loved ones have been reported in a recent volume by Rynearson,[32] which deals with homicide, terrorism, and other violent deaths. The prolonged and difficult grief in such circumstances is highlighted by findings from September 11, Oklahoma, and Bali bombings.

When people are *missing*, believed dead, the uncertainty, other stressors including complex legal and evidentiary processes (e.g. Disaster Victim Identification requirements), may lead to alternating hope and dread. When there are no remains, it will be more difficult for those bereaved to accept the reality of the death.

Seeing and 'saying goodbye' to the dead person, have been shown to help those bereaved in disasters. If remains are much disfigured, as with burns, it is important that those bereaved are supported in their choice about this.

Social support, particularly the perceptions of the supportiveness of family and social network are likely to be protective and assist the bereaved psychologically,[33] while perceptions of unhelpfulness may be associated with more negative outcomes.[9] Cultural requirements for social support may differ, as may the delineation of the period of mourning, the roles of the bereaved, and associated spiritual and religious needs.[34]

Multiple other adversities may occur, either coincidentally or as a consequence of the circumstances and the loss of the person, for instance financial difficulties, loss of resources, changed status, loss of meaning and identity, or other profound stressors of illness, injury, or other bereavements. Such additional stressors may increase vulnerability.[15]

In terms of Prolonged Grief Disorder (previously known as complicated grief disorder, and initially traumatic grief) Prigerson *et al.*[35] have carried out extensive research to refine this syndrome. Bringing together the views of international researchers, they have developed consensus criteria for a distinct psychiatric disorder to be considered for inclusion in DSM-V. This definition requires that the reaction to loss encompasses one of three symptoms of separation distress (e.g. yearning) and a minimum of five from a total of nine other symptoms, experienced at least daily, to a distressing or disruptive level. These include: shock; emotional numbing; avoidance of the reality of the loss; difficulty accepting the loss; feelings of meaninglessness; difficulty moving on with life; bitterness over the loss; mistrust; and a diminished sense of self. Such symptoms would need to last at least 6 months, and be associated with significant levels of functional impairment. These findings fit well with earlier research identifying more chronic patterns of grief.[12,13]

Physical and mental health consequences of bereavement

A recent valuable review[36] outlines the evidence of increased *mortality* for bereaved spouses, particularly males which is most pronounced in the first 6 months, and includes a range of conditions such as heart disease, leading to death from 'a broken heart'. It is also more pronounced for those younger. Death of a child is associated with even greater mortality risk, particularly for mothers. Suicide is one of the heightened risks, especially for mothers and older males.

Physical health impairments are also found,[36] with a variety of physical symptoms as well as greater use of medical services, and medications. Further research is needed to clarify the nature of any increased rate of specific diseases. Changed health behaviours, the impact of loss of a health supporting partner, functional or social changes, or shared environments of risk may contribute.

With regard to *mental health* there may be an increased level of anxiety and depressive symptoms. There may be a heightened risk for some bereaved individuals for exacerbations of pre-existing conditions, or the precipitation of new illnesses, including Post-Traumatic Stress Disorder when there is a violent death.[32] Other anxiety disorders, major depression, substance use disorder, and bipolar disorder may be precipitated by bereavement. Complicated or prolonged grief disorder may also represent a psychiatric consequence.[35]

Assessment and management

Most bereaved people do not require counselling so assessment must be a basis for intervention. Assessment should be simple, synchronous with need, and do no harm, addressing the death and its circumstances, the relationship, and the bereaved's experience since, including social support.[31] A more structured format, potentially including grief measures,[37] can clarify the presence of PTSD, Depression or Prolonged Grief, or other health needs, including physical health changes or problems, establishing the basis for intervention.

Initial management of acutely bereaved persons requires empathic, compassionate support; and responding to any acute needs in ways that are protective of their mental health, recognizing the 'roller-coaster' of emotions that may occur, and facilitating natural resilience. Concepts of Psychological First Aid are also valuable in the immediate period after the death.[38] Dealing with concerns about the deceased's suffering, and support to view the dead person's remains should the bereaved choose to, are likely to be helpful.

Most evidence-based interventions focus on psychotherapeutic methods, ranging from preventive counselling of those with demonstrated heightened risk[39] to self-help guided interventions,[40] interpersonal psychotherapy modifications for traumatic grief,[41] integrated cognitive behaviour therapy models,[42] or psychodynamically informed models[43] and web-based treatments.[44] Counselling models[45] and psychoeducation have also focused on those bereaved through specific deaths such as those of infants.[46] Other models deal with grief work and tasks,[47] as well as specific treatment for morbidity of complicated grief[48] and depressive or anxiety disorders including the use of pharmacotherapy for such conditions when indicated.[49] Rynearson's[32] work with 'restorative retelling' following violent deaths emphasizes the narrative story which is central to much bereavement counselling and testimony.

A practical approach to assessment and counselling may be initiated with some gentle queries, such as 'Can you tell me a little about your loss?', 'What happened with 'John's' death?', 'Can you tell me about 'John' and your relationship?', 'What's been happening since?'

If there is: intense continuing distress; circumstances of death which are untimely or traumatic; a complex relationship with the deceased; disruption of family functioning which is impacting on the needs of children; inadequacies of social support; 'unresolved' earlier losses; multiple additional stressors, the bereaved may be at heightened risk of adverse outcomes. Preventive counselling, which facilitates grieving, is attuned to the bereaved person's readiness, vulnerabilities, and strengths, and helps them to tell the story of their experiences and the person they have lost, is likely to improve outcomes.[39]

If assessment indicates that psychiatric disorders have arisen, for instance depression, post-traumatic stress disorder, anxiety, or substance use disorders, these conditions should be managed appropriately alongside counselling for the bereavement should this be required. The use of antidepressants or other medication is not indicated for bereavement itself but may be appropriate for such complications.[49] Monitoring for suicide risk should accompany clinical management.

Prolonged or complicated grief may benefit from cognitive behaviour therapy interventions, as well as relevant rehabilitation. Those who are both traumatized and bereaved may need the traumatic stress issues, to be dealt with first, and facilitation of grieving following this.[43]

There is a need for more comprehensive research and evaluation of prevention, early intervention and treatment modalities, and their appropriate provision, to individuals, families, or groups.[50] Culturally appropriate models of support and intervention also need to be further developed. Many bereaved people present first within primary care settings, and to their general practitioners who will need the skills and knowledge to deal with their distress, assess their needs, counsel them as appropriate, and refer when necessary.

Much support also comes from community and non-government agencies including bereavement focused groups for specific losses or for grief generally, and from specialized services in public or private mental health sectors.

Telling the bereaved person how to grieve, that they should 'forget about the past', that 'time heals all', is usually perceived as unhelpful. Treating grief as a disease, for example antidepressant medication for normal sadness, is seen by many bereaved people as interfering with their capacity to grieve for their loved one.

Counselling bereaved people requires hopeful, compassionate psychotherapeutic intervention which recognizes the human suffering involved, validates the person's strengths, and respects their spiritual needs. Loss is a central issue for all of us, both our fears of it, and its reality. Counselling requires those involved to recognize their own sensitivities in this regard, and to assist the 'journey' of those affected in dealing with their loss. Most people grieve, remember with love those whom they have lost, and continue to love, and love anew.

Further information

Kellehear, A. (2007). *A social history of dying*. Cambridge University Press, Cambridge.

http://www.childhoodgrief.org.au/

References

1. Freud, S. (1915). Mourning and melancholia. In *Sigmund Freud: collected papers*, (ed. Strachey, J.) Vol. 4. Basic Books, New York.
2. Lindemann, E. (1944). Symptomatology and management of acute grief. *The American Journal of Psychiatry*, **101**, 141–8.
3. Engel, G.L. (1961). Is grief a disease? *Psychosomatic Medicine*, **23**, 18–22.
4. Bowlby, J. (1969). *Attachment and loss, Vol. 1. Attachment*. Hogarth, London.
5. Bowlby, J. (1973). *Attachment and loss. Vol. 2. Separation, anxiety and anger*. Hogarth, London.
6. Bowlby, J. (1980). *Attachment and loss. Vol. 3. Loss: sadness and depression*. Hogarth, London.
7. Parkes, C.M. (1996). *Bereavement: studies of grief in adult life* (3rd edn). Routledge, London.
8. Maddison, D.C. and Walker, W.L. (1967). Factors affecting the outcome of conjugal bereavement. *The British Journal of Psychiatry*, **113**, 1057–67.
9. Jacobs, S. (1993). *Pathologic grief: maladaptation to loss*. American Psychiatric Press, Washington, DC.
10. Stroebe, M.S., Hansson, R.O., Stroebe, W., *et al.* (eds.) (2001). *Handbook of bereavement research: consequences, coping, and care*. American Psychological Association, Washington, DC.
11. Stroebe, M.S., Hansson, R.O., Stroebe, W., *et al.* (eds.) (2007). *Handbook of bereavement research and practice: 21st century perspectives*. American Psychological Association Press, Washington, DC.
12. Middleton, W., Raphael, B., Burnett, P., *et al.* (1998). A longitudinal study comparing bereavement phenomena in recently bereaved spouses, adult children and parents. *The Australian and New Zealand Journal of Psychiatry*, **32**, 235–41.
13. Byrne, G.J. and Raphael, B. (1994). A longitudinal study of bereavement phenomena in recently widowed elderly men. *Psychological Medicine*, **24**, 411–21.
14. Bonanno, G.A., Wortman, C.B., Lehman, D.R., *et al.* (2002). Resilience to loss and chronic grief: a prospective study from preloss to 18-months postloss. *Journal of Personality and Social Psychology*, **83**, 1150–64.
15. Raphael, B. (1983). *The anatomy of bereavement: a handbook for the caring professions*. Basic Books, New York.
16. Moss, M.S., Moss, S.Z., and Hansson, R.O. (2001). Bereavement and old age. In *Handbook of bereavement research: consequences, coping, and care* (eds. M.S. Stroebe, R.O. Hansson, W. Stroebe, and H. Schut). American Psychological Association, Washington, DC.
17. Maciejewski, P.K., Zhang, B., Block, S.D., *et al.* (2007). An empirical examination of the stage theory of grief. *The Journal of the American Medical Association*, **297**, 716–23.
18. Prigerson, H.G., Bierhals, A.J., Kasl, S.V., *et al.* (1996). Complicated grief as a distinct disorder from bereavement-related depression and anxiety: a replication study. *The American Journal of Psychiatry*, **153**, 84–6.
19. Sanders, C.M. (1980). A comparison of adult bereavement in the death of a spouse, child, and parent. *Omega*, **10**, 303–22.
20. Gündel, H., O'Connor, M., Littrell, L., *et al.* (2003). Functional neuroanatomy of grief: an fMRI study. *The American Journal of Psychiatry*, **160**, 1946–53.
21. Najib, A., Lorberbaum, J., Kose, S., *et al.* (2004). Regional brain activity in women grieving a romantic relationship break up. *The American Journal of Psychiatry*, **161**, 2245–56.
22. Freed, P.J. and Mann, J.J. (2007). Sadness and loss: toward a neurobiopsychosocial model. *The American Journal of Psychiatry*, **164**, 28–34.
23. McCleery, J.M., Bhagwagar, Z., Smith, K.A., *et al.* (2000). Modelling a loss event: effect of imagined bereavement on the hypothalamic-pituitary-adrenal axis. *Psychological Medicine*, **30**, 219–23.
24. Stroebe, M., Folkman, S., Hansson, R.O., *et al.* (2006). The prediction of bereavement outcome: development of an integrative risk factor framework. *Social Science & Medicine*, **63**, 2446–51.
25. Kaufman, J., Yang, B.-Z., Douglas-Palumberi, H., *et al.* (2004). Social supports and serotonin transporter gene moderate depression in maltreated children. *Proceedings of the National Academy of Sciences of the United States of America*, **101**, 17316–21.
26. Raphael, B., Swan, P., and Martinek, N. (1998). Intergeneration aspects of trauma for Australian aboriginal people. In *An international handbook of multigenerational legacies of trauma* (ed. Y. Danieli), pp. 327–39. Plenum Press, New York.
27. Parkes, C.M. (2006). *Love and loss: the root of grief and its complications*. Routledge, Hove, UK.
28. Vance, J.C., Boyle, F.M., Najman, J.M., *et al.* (2002). Couple distress after sudden infant or perinatal death: a 30-month follow-up. *Journal of Paediatrics and Child Health*, **38**, 368–72.
29. Kissane, D.W., McKenzie, M., Bloch, S., *et al.* (2006). Family focused grief therapy: a randomized controlled trial in palliative care and bereavement. *The American Journal Psychiatry*, **163**, 1208–18.
30. Lundin, T. (1984). Morbidity following sudden and unexpected bereavement. *The British Journal of Psychiatry*, **144**, 84–8.
31. Raphael, B., Martinek, N., and Wooding, S. (2004). Assessing loss, psychological trauma and traumatic bereavement. In *Assessing psychological trauma and PTSD* (2nd edn). The Guilford Press, New York.

32. Rynearson, E.K. (ed.) (2006). *Violent death: resilience and intervention beyond the crisis*. Routledge Psychosocial Stress Series, Taylor & Francis, New York.
33. Vanderwerker, L.C. and Prigerson, H.G. (2004). Social support and technological connectedness as protective factors in bereavement. *Journal of Loss and Trauma*, **9**, 45–57.
34. Parkes, C.M., Laungani, P., and Young, B. (1997). *Death and bereavement across cultures*. Routledge, London.
35. Prigerson, H., Horowitz, M.J., Selby, C.J., *et al.* (manuscript submitted for publication). Field trial of consensus criteria for prolonged grief disorder proposed for DSM-V. *Archives of General Psychiatry*.
36. Stroebe, M., Schut, H., and Stroebe, W. (2007). The physical and mental health consequences of bereavement: a review. Seminar for *Lancet*, **8**, 1960–73.
37. Neimeyer, R.A. and Hogan, N.S. (2001). Quantitative or qualitative? Measurement issues in the study of grief. In *Handbook of bereavement research: consequences, coping, and care* (eds. M.S. Strobe, R.O. Hansson, W. Stroebe, and H. Schut), pp. 89–118. American Psychological Association, Washington, DC.
38. National Center for PTSD Psychological First Aid Manual http://www.ncptsd.va.gov/ncmain/ncdocs/manuals/nc_manual_psyfirstaid.html
39. Raphael, B. (1977). Preventive intervention with the recently bereaved. *Archives of General Psychiatry*, **34**, 1450–4.
40. Vachon, M.L.S., Lyall, W.A.L., Rogers, J., *et al.* (1980). A controlled study of self-help interventions for widows. *The American Journal of Psychiatry*, **137**, 1380–4.
41. Shear, K., Frank, E., Houck, P.R., *et al.* (2005). Treatment of complicated grief: a randomized controlled trial. *The Journal of the American Medical Association*, **293**, 2601–8.
42. Shear, K. and Frank, E. (2006). Treatment of complicated grief: integrating cognitive–behavioral methods with other treatment approaches. In *Cognitive behavioural therapies for trauma* (eds. V. Follette and J. Ruzek), pp. 290–320. Guilford Press, New York.
43. Raphael, B., Dunsmore, J., and Wooding, S. (2004). Early mental health interventions for traumatic loss in adults. In *Early intervention for trauma and traumatic loss* (ed. B. Litz), pp. 147–78. Guilford Press, New York.
44. Wagner, B., Knaevelsrud, C., and Maercker, A. (2006). Internet-based cognitive–behaviorial therapy (INTERAPY) for complicated grief: a randomized controlled trial. *Death Studies*, **30**, 429–53.
45. Rando, T.A. (1993). *The treatment of complicated mourning*. Research Press, Champaign, IL.
46. Murray, J.A., Terry, D.J., Vance, J.C., *et al.* (2000). Effects of a program of intervention on parental distress following infant death. *Death Studies*, **24**, 275–305.
47. Worden, J.W. (1991). *Grief counselling and grief therapy*. Springer Publishing Company, New York.
48. Boelen, P.A. (2005). *Complicated grief: assessment, theory, and treatment*. Ipskamp, Enscede/Amsterdam.
49. Raphael, B., Dobson, M., and Minkov, C. (2001). Psychotherapeutic and pharmacological intervention for bereaved people chapter in *Handbook of bereavement research: consequences, coping, and care* (eds. M.S. Stroebe, R.O. Hansson, W. Stroebe, and H. Schut). American Psychological Association, Washington, DC.
50. Schut, H., Stroebe, M.S., Van Den Bout, J., *et al.* (2001). The efficacy of bereavement interventions: determining who benefits. In *Handbook of bereavement research: consequences, coping, and care* (eds. M.S. Stroebe, R.O. Hansson, W. Stroebe, and H. Schut). American Psychological Association, Washington, DC.

4.7

Anxiety disorders

Contents

4.7.1 Generalized anxiety disorders
Stella Bitran, David H. Barlow, and David A. Spiegel

4.7.2 Social anxiety disorder and specific phobias
Michelle A. Blackmore, Brigette A. Erwin, Richard G. Heimberg, Leanne Magee, and David M. Fresco

4.7.3 Panic disorder and agoraphobia
James C. Ballenger

4.7.1 Generalized anxiety disorders

Stella Bitran, David H. Barlow, and David A. Spiegel

Anxious apprehension and overconcern are common to many anxiety and mood disorders. Prior to 1980 in the American DSM diagnostic system, and 1992 in the international ICD system, individuals who experienced those symptoms in the absence of a realistic focus of concern were classified as having an 'anxiety neurosis' (DSM-II) or 'anxiety state' (ICD-9). In DSM-III, panic disorder was split off from that classification, and the residual category was renamed generalized anxiety disorder (**GAD**). A similar nomenclature was adopted in ICD-10.

Since its inception, GAD as a nosological entity has been troubled by problems of poor reliability and high comorbidity.[1] Those concerns have prompted several revisions of the DSM criteria and also have raised more basic questions regarding the validity of GAD as a disorder distinct from other anxiety and mood states. The question of what is the nature of GAD is still being debated and it remains one of the least reliably diagnosed anxiety or mood disorders.[2] This diagnostic unreliability has led to various suggestions for revisions to the diagnostic criteria and criticisms of the current definition of GAD.

Clinical features

Individuals with GAD experience persistent anxiety and worry that is out of proportion to actual events or circumstances. Typically, the anxiety and worry involve minor or everyday matters, such as work, finances, relationships, the health or safety of loved ones, and routine tasks. Often, the focus of worry shifts from one concern to another. Although people with GAD do not always consider their worries to be unrealistic or excessive, they do find them difficult to control. Consequently, the worries often interfere with concentration and performance.

Associated with the anxiety and worry, individuals with GAD have a variety of cognitive and somatic symptoms, including trembling, feeling shaky, aching in the back and shoulders, tension headaches, chest tightness, restlessness, exaggerated startle, irritability, insomnia, fatigue, dry mouth, sweating, urinary frequency, trouble swallowing, nausea, and diarrhoea. In addition, GAD may be accompanied by other conditions typically associated with stress, such as irritable bowel syndrome or atypical chest pain.

Classification

Diagnosis

(a) DSM criteria

In DSM-III, GAD was essentially a residual category for individuals with somatic symptoms of anxiety who did not meet diagnostic criteria for another, more specific, anxiety disorder. Diagnosis required the presence, for at least a month, of symptoms from three of four symptom clusters: motor tension, autonomic hyperactivity, apprehensive expectation, and vigilance and scanning. Unfortunately, clinicians had difficulty applying those criteria. In addition, its diagnosis depended on the application of the criteria for other diagnoses since GAD was not diagnosed if another anxiety disorder was present.

In DSM-III-R, apprehensive expectation was removed from the diagnostic symptom clusters, was redefined as unrealistic or excessive anxiety and worry about two or more life circumstances, and was made the essential feature of GAD. In addition, the duration criterion was changed from 1 to 6 months, and the hierarchical exclusion rule was dropped, allowing GAD to be diagnosed in addition to other disorders.

Table 4.7.1.1 DSM-IV inclusion criteria for GAD

(a) Excessive anxiety and worry, occurring more days than not for at least 6 months, about a number of events or activities
(b) The person finds it difficult to control the worry
(c) The anxiety and worry are accompanied by at least three of the following six symptoms (one in children): restlessness or feeling keyed up or on edge; being easily fatigued; difficulty concentrating or mind going blank; irritability; muscle tension; sleep disturbance
(d) The anxiety, worry or physical symptoms cause significant distress or functional impairment

(American Psychiatric Association (2000), *Diagnostic and statistical manual of mental disorders* (4th edn, text revision). APA, Washington, DC)

Despite those changes, the diagnostic reliability of GAD remained essentially unchanged.(1) Investigations revealed that the new worry criterion was problematic. Interviewers commonly disagreed as to whether two distinct spheres of worry were present, whether the worry was unrealistic or excessive, or whether the focus of the worry could be construed to be part of the symptomatology of another disorder. Moreover, studies indicated that patients with GAD did not differ substantially from control subjects in the content of their worries.(3,4) The main difference between patients and controls was that the former experienced their worrying to be uncontrollable while the latter did not.

Based on those and other findings, the GAD criteria were revised again in DSM-IV. The 'unrealistic' descriptor and the requirement for anxiety or worry to involve at least two spheres of life circumstances were deleted, and a new criterion was added that the worry must be experienced as difficult to control. In addition, the associated symptom criterion was modified to require only three of six symptoms from the previous motor tension and vigilance and scanning clusters (Table 4.7.1.1). For additional information about the evolution of the DSM criteria for GAD, see Barlow or Wincze.(5)

(b) ICD-10 criteria

Like DSM-IV, ICD-10 requires a period of 6 months of generalized anxiety and worry accompanied by certain somatic symptoms (Table 4.7.1.2). The 6 months of 'prominent' tension and worry needs to be accompanied by at least 4 of 22 associated symptoms. The ICD-10 differs from DSM-IV in that it does not require that worry be 'uncontrollable', that the symptoms of GAD occur exclusively outside the context of a mood disorder, or that they meet a 'clinical significance' criterion.

(c) Differential diagnosis

Everyone experiences anxiety and worry sometimes, and some people describe themselves as born worriers. GAD differs from these non-pathological anxiety experiences in that it is both persistent and severe enough to cause significant distress or interference. Typically also, the worries are more pervasive and difficult to control than normal worries and are associated with physical symptoms of anxiety and tension.

A number of general medical conditions can present with signs and symptoms resembling GAD (Table 4.7.1.3). In addition, substances such as caffeine, alcohol, other drugs of abuse, toxins, and some medications (Table 4.7.1.4) can cause anxiety-like

Table 4.7.1.2 ICD-10 inclusion criteria for GAD

(a) At least 6 months of prominent tension, worry, and feelings of apprehension about everyday events and problems
(b) At least four of the following 22 symptoms must be present, at least one of which must be from the autonomic arousal cluster
Autonomic arousal symptoms: palpitations or pounding heart or accelerated heart rate; sweating; trembling or shaking; dry mouth (not due to medication or dehydration)
Symptoms involving the chest and abdomen: difficulty in breathing; feeling of choking; chest pain or discomfort; nausea or abdominal distress
Symptoms involving mental state: feeling dizzy, unsteady, faint or lightheaded; derealization or depersonalization; fear of losing control, 'going crazy', or passing out; fear of dying
General symptoms: hot flushes or cold chills; numbness or tingling sensations
Symptoms of tension: muscle tension or aches and pains; restlessness and inability to relax; feeling keyed up, or on edge, or mentally tense; a sensation of a lump in the throat, or difficulty in swallowing
Other non-specific symptoms: exaggerated response to minor surprises or being startled; difficulty in concentrating, or mind 'going blank' because of worrying or anxiety; persistent irritability; difficulty getting to sleep because of worrying

(World Health Organization (2004), *International statistical classification of diseases and health related problems* (2nd edn). WHO, Geneva, Switzerland)

Table 4.7.1.3 General medical conditions that can cause symptoms resembling anxiety

Cardiac conditions: arrhythmias, coronary insufficiency, mitral valve prolapse, heart failure
Endocrine conditions: hyperthyroidism, hypoparathyroidism, hypoglycaemia
Neurological conditions: temporal lobe epilepsy, vestibular nerve disease
Respiratory conditions: asthma, hypoxia, hyperventilation, obstructive lung disease, pulmonary embolism
Other conditions: porphyria, carcinoid tumour, systemic lupus erythemacosus, pellagra

Table 4.7.1.4 Medications that can cause symptoms resembling anxiety

Psychotropics: antidepressants, neuroleptics (akathisia), sedative hypnotics (withdrawal syndrome), disulfiram
Respiratory drugs: B-adrenergic stimulants, bronchodilators
Cardiovascular drugs: antiarrhythmics, antihypertensives
Neurological disorder medications: anticonvulsants, anticholinergic agents, L-dopa
Anaesthetic drugs: pre-anaesthetics, general anaesthetics (post-anaesthetic syndrome)
Other drugs: thyroid hormone, antibiotics, non-steroidal anti-inflammatory drugs, anticancer drugs

symptoms either as a direct effect or as part of a withdrawal syndrome. These causes may be established on the basis of a medical and substance use history, physical examination, or laboratory tests.

GAD is distinguished from other psychiatric disorders, in part, by the focus of the anxiety and worry, which is not limited to a feature of another disorder. For example, the worry is not only about the possible occurrence or implications of panic attacks (as in panic disorder), or about negative evaluations by others (social phobia), gaining weight (anorexia nervosa), or having a serious illness (hypochondriasis). In obsessive–compulsive disorder, the anxiety and worry are associated with intrusive thoughts, images, or impulses that are distressing.

Generalized anxiety commonly occurs in depression, and GAD and depression also share associated symptoms such as sleep disturbance, fatigue, restlessness, and poor concentration. When the associated symptoms could fit with either disorder, the distinction is made on the basis of the presence and time course of depressed mood relative to anxiety. In DSM-IV, GAD is not diagnosed if its features occur exclusively during a mood disorder.

(d) Epidemiology

Prevalence estimates of GAD vary considerably with the diagnostic criteria used. One large-scale study found a 12-month prevalence rate of 2.07 per cent and a lifetime prevalence rate to be 4.1 per cent.[6] Socio-demographic factors associated with increased risk for GAD included being female, middle-aged, and with low income. However, being African American, Asian, or Hispanic was associated with a decreased risk.[7]

The National Comorbidity Study Replication (NCS-R), which used DSM-IV criteria and included structured interviews of over 9000 individuals in the United States, found a 12-month prevalence of GAD of 3.1 per cent and a lifetime prevalence rate at 5.7 per cent.[8,9] Lifetime prevalence rates were lowest among 18- to 29-year-olds (4.1 per cent) and those 60 or older (3.65 per cent), with the highest rates found among 45- to 59-year-olds (7.7 per cent).

(e) Comorbidity

GAD usually coexists with other anxiety and mood disorders. One large-scale study found that 68 per cent of individuals with a principal diagnosis of GAD met criteria for another Axis I disorder (Table 4.7.1.5).[10] The most frequently comorbid disorders were MDD, social phobia, or panic disorder with or without agoraphobia. Ninety-two per cent of individuals from this study with a principal diagnosis of GAD met criteria for another lifetime disorder, with 64 per cent meeting criteria for MDD. Similarly, in the major epidemiological surveys, nearly two-thirds of individuals with GAD had additional DSM Axis I diagnoses.[11] Most common among these were specific (21–59 per cent) and social (16–59 per cent) phobias, followed by panic disorder (3–27 per cent) and depression (8–39 per cent). In addition, GAD was found to be approximately twice as common among women as men. There is less information about the prevalence of personality disorders among patients with GAD.

Table 4.7.1.5 Prevalence of comorbid disorders in 279 patients with GAD

Any additional lifetime disorder	96%
Any anxiety/mood	94%
Any anxiety disorder	85%
Any mood disorder	74%
Anxiety disorders	
Panic disorder with/or without agoraphobia	47%
Social phobia	46%
Specific phobia	22%
Mood disorders	
Major depressive disorder	67%
Dysthymia	11%

(f) Is GAD a valid disorder?

The findings of only fair diagnostic reliability and high comorbidity for GAD have been interpreted as indicating poor discriminant validity of the disorder, suggesting that differentiating GAD from other anxiety and mood disorders may be artifactual. In considering those arguments, it is important to distinguish the diagnostic criteria sets specified in the DSM and ICD classification systems from the clinical syndromes they are intended to identify. Low discriminant validity for a disorder may be due to problems with the former rather than the latter. To establish the construct validity of a syndrome, one must demonstrate that it has a consistent set of features, the pattern of which separates it from other related syndromes. One approach to doing that is to compare the profiles of patients with different diagnoses across various illness dimensions.

In one such study, data from patients who took part in the DSM-IV mixed anxiety-depression field trial were examined.[12] Using factor analyses of patients' scores on 73 items from the Hamilton anxiety and depression rating scales, four clusters were identified that corresponded to the dimensions of anxiety, depression, physiological arousal, and general negative affect (containing items that loaded on both the anxiety and depression factors). Patients with a principal diagnosis of GAD had a unique profile (high on negative affect and anxiety, low on physiological arousal and depression) that distinguished them from individuals with panic disorder, major depression, anxiety or depressive disorder not otherwise specified, or no mental disorder.

A subsequent study, using an anxiety clinic sample and an expanded array of measures, yielded similar results.[13] In this case, five primary factors (corresponding to panic, agoraphobia, social anxiety, obsessions/compulsions, and general anxiety) and a higher order factor (negative affect) were identified. Again, patients with GAD had a unique factor profile.

The findings from the preceding studies were replicated and extended in an independent sample of patients.[14] As in the earlier studies, GAD was found to be distinct from other anxiety syndromes and depression, although it had the highest degree of overlap with other syndromes, especially depression. In addition, GAD was strongly associated with the non-specific dimension of negative affect, which is common to anxiety and depression. The authors suggest that GAD may represent a 'basic emotional disorder', because it consists of features that are present to varying degrees in all anxiety and mood disorders.

Finally, all three of the preceding studies (and a variety of others, e.g. Barlow *et al.*[15] support the differentiation of symptoms of autonomic arousal, which are characteristic of panic attacks, from somatic symptoms related to central nervous system tension, which form the DSM-IV-associated symptom cluster of GAD.

(g) Aetiology

Findings from genetics, neurobiology, and psychology infer a multifactorial aetiology for GAD, which has been organized into a triple vulnerabilities model.[16,17] This model suggests that anxiety disorders result from the combination of a generalized biological vulnerability, a general psychological vulnerability, and a specific psychological vulnerability.

(i) Generalized biological vulnerability

Genetic contributions. Several studies investigating genetic vulnerabilities for mental disorders have supported the notion that a shared vulnerability underlies anxiety disorders.[18] It was shown through a meta-analysis of genetic epidemiological studies that many anxiety disorders (including GAD, panic disorder, phobias, and OCD) aggregate in families and that genetics has the most influence when examining familial risk.[19] In a family study that used DSM-III criteria, GAD (but not other anxiety disorders) was five times more prevalent (19.5 per cent versus 3.5 per cent) among first-degree relatives of patients with GAD than among relatives of controls.[20] However, two twin studies using the same criteria found concordance rates for GAD were no higher among monozygotic than dizygotic twins.[21] Two subsequent studies that used DSM-III-R criteria found a shared heritability for GAD and mood disorders.[22] At present, it appears that genetic factors play a modest role in the aetiology of GAD, and one that is more closely related to vulnerability for depression than for other anxiety disorders.

Neurobiological mechanisms. A variety of neuroanatomical, neurochemical, neuroendocrine, and neurophysiological systems have been implicated in the pathogenesis of anxiety states. Much of this information has come from animal models and research on the effects of stress. Studies of neurobiological functioning in humans with GAD are limited. Some of the physical systems that may be involved in the emotion of anxiety are summarized below. Additional information may be found in reviews by Davidson,[23] and Gray and McNaughton.[24]

The noradrenergic nervous system. Noradrenergic pathway (the **locus coeruleus-noradrenaline-sympathetic nervous system**) have long been associated with fear and arousal and play an important role in the body's response to threat. However, their role in persistent anxiety states is not clear. Resting catecholamine levels in patients with GAD appear to be normal. On the other hand, GAD patients exhibit subnormal responses to both stimulation[25] and blockade[26] of α_2-adrenergic receptors and a reduced density of α_2-receptors in platelets.[27] Those findings could reflect downregulation of the α_2-receptors due to initially high levels of noradrenaline (norepinephrine).

Consistent with those neurochemical findings, somatic measures of autonomic nervous system function (e.g. skin conductance, respiratory rate, heart-rate variability, blood pressure) in patients with GAD tend to show normal resting values with blunted and sometimes prolonged responses to stressful stimuli.[27] Psychophysiological studies have found that worry is associated with restricted sympathetic arousal and low vagal tone.[27] In contrast, it has been shown that compared to controls, individuals with GAD show greater muscle tension at baseline in response to psychological challenge.[28] In addition, structural analyses suggest that GAD, unlike other anxiety disorders, is not associated with autonomic hyperarousal when levels of negative affect are held constant.[14] These findings indicate diminished autonomic nervous system responsiveness in individuals with GAD.

The hypothalamic-pituitary-adrenal axis. The **hypothalamic-pituitary-adrenal axis** and its end-product, cortisol, are also involved in reactions to stress. Activity in the hypothalamic-pituitary-adrenal axis is subject to a variety of influences. Primary control is by means of hypothalamic secretion of corticotrophin-releasing factor, which stimulates pituitary secretion of ACTH, which in turn stimulates adrenal secretion of cortisol. Circulating cortisol, and analogues such as dexamethasone, exert inhibitory feedback at the level of the pituitary gland and apparently also by means of receptors on the hippocampus.

In rats, chronic exposure to stress or exogenous steroids results in a reduction of corticosteroid receptors in the hippocampus and a consequent decrease in feedback inhibition by cortisol.[29] These animals exhibit reduced dexamethasone suppression of cortisol secretion and greater or more prolonged adrenocortical responses to stress. Reduced dexamethasone suppression also has been observed in approximately one-third of patients with DSM-III-diagnosed GAD.[30] This reduction in the normal regulatory control of cortisol secretion may be one mechanism through which chronic or repeated stress can lead to persistent anxiety.

The amygdala and the bed nucleus of the stria terminalis. LeDoux[31] and others have demonstrated the central role played by the **amygdala** in the mediation of fear reactions. The amygdala is thought to be responsible for the detection of potential threats to the organism and the mobilization of a range of defensive responses (Fig. 4.7.1.1). Through connections with the hypothalamus, it can activate the sympathetic nervous system and hypothalamic-pituitary-adrenal axis. Through efferent fibres to the central grey area of the midbrain, it can mediate behavioural defence responses such as the fight-or-flight response and behavioural 'freezing'. Through connections to the nucleus reticularis pontis caudalis, it can enhance the defensive startle reflex.

A structural magnetic resonance imaging (MRI) study of children and adolescents found that those individuals with GAD had increased total and right amygdala volume compared to non-anxious controls.[32] In addition, abnormalities in fear circuitry, especially hyperactivation in the right amygdala, have been found in adolescents with GAD.[33]

The extent to which these pathways are involved in the neurobiology of anxiety (as opposed to fear) is unclear. However, a structure

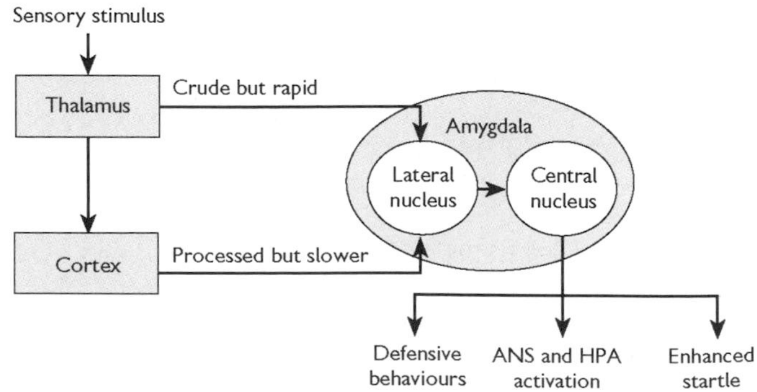

Fig 4.7.1.1 Fear pathways (based on descriptions by LeDoux[31] and Davis[34]). ANS, autonomic nervous system; HPA, hypothalamic-pituitary-adrenal axis.

closely related to the amygdala, the bed nucleus of the stria terminalis, may be involved in this emotion. The bed nucleus resembles the amygdala in its neurotransmitter content, cell morphology, and hypothalamic and brainstem connections and, like the amygdala, it exerts a modulating effect on the startle reflex.[34] Studies of this latter effect implicate it in the experience of anxiety.

Administration of corticotrophin-releasing factor into the cerebral ventricles of rats produces a state of generalized arousal resembling anxiety. Under those conditions, the startle reflex also is enhanced. Exposing rats to bright light for 5 to 20 min has similar effects. These effects are not blocked by damage to amygdala but are by lesions to the bed nucleus of the stria terminalis and by treatment with benzodiazepines or buspirone. Conversely, infusion of corticotrophin-releasing factor directly into the bed nucleus of the stria terminalis, but not the amygdala, produces a rapid increase in startle. Based on these observations, Davis[34] has suggested that the stria terminalis may play a role in anxiety analogous to that of the amygdala in fear reactions and, further, that prolonged or repeated stimulation of the stria terminalis by corticotrophin-releasing factor during periods of stress might lead to sustained activation and thus to persistent anxiety. A recent study has confirmed the differential association of these structures with fear and anxiety, respectively.[35]

The septohippocampal system (behavioural inhibition system). The bed nucleus of the stria terminalis is part of the larger septohippocampal system.[36] In 1982, based on data from several lines of research, Gray hypothesized that the septohippocampal system, together with the Papez circuit (a neural loop connecting the subicular area in the hippocampal formation to the mammillary bodies, anterior thalamus, cingulate cortex, and back to the subiculum), is responsible for mediating the emotion of anxiety as well as the major effects of anxiolytic drugs.[36] Gray called this network the **behavioural inhibition system**, because he believed that, when activated, it interrupts ongoing behaviour and redirects the organism's attention to signs of possible danger.

According to Gray's model,[24,36] the behavioural inhibition system receives information about the environment from the sensory cortex via the temporal lobe and hippocampal formation. The system checks the information for consistency with predictions, which are updated continuously by the Papez circuit based on preceding information and stored patterns, as well as for consistency with the immediate goals of the organism. When a mismatch is found, or if a predicted event is aversive, the outputs of the behavioural inhibition system are activated, resulting in a constellation of emotional and behavioural effects consistent with anxiety (Fig. 4.7.1.2).

The activation of the behavioural inhibition system appears to be moderated by ascending noradrenergic and serotonergic projections to the septohippocampal complex, providing a possible mechanism for the anxiolytic actions of some drugs. The amygdala also provides inputs to the behavioural inhibition system and may relay its outputs to the hypothalamus and autonomic nervous system, thereby mediating anxious arousal. Sustained activation of the behavioural inhibition system might therefore account for many of the features of GAD.

The benzodiazepine-γ-aminobutyric acid system. The powerful anxiolytic and sedative effects of benzodiazepines are believed to be mediated by benzodiazepine recognition sites located on γ-aminobutyric acid (**GABA**) type A receptor complexes in the central nervous system. When bound to those complexes,

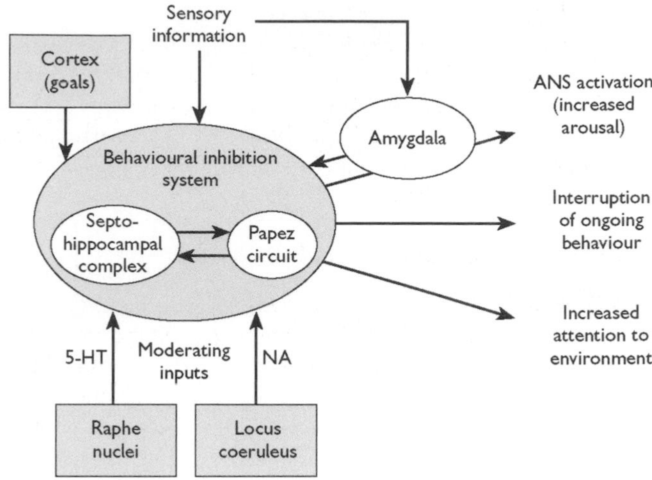

Fig 4.7.1.2 Behavioural inhibition system (based on descriptions by Gray and McNaughton[24]). ANS, autonomic nervous system; 5-HT, serotonin; NA, noradrenaline.

benzodiazepines allosterically modulate the GABA receptors to enhance the normal inhibitory effects of GABA on neurotransmission. Activation of **central benzodiazepine-GABA receptor complexes** also suppresses hypothalamic-pituitary-adrenal axis activity and, consequently, cortisol levels.

In addition to these central receptor complexes, benzodiazepine recognition sites of a different type are present widely in cells outside the central nervous system. These so-called **peripheral benzodiazepine receptors** are believed to be instrumental in controlling the synthesis of regulatory steroids. Their role in the anxiolytic actions of benzodiazepines is unknown; although they bind some drugs (e.g. diazepam), they have low affinity for others (e.g. clonazepam). Interestingly, peripheral benzodiazepine receptors are decreased in blood cells of individuals with untreated GAD but return to normal levels after successful treatment with benzodiazepines. Their numbers also vary in response to stress, being elevated following acute stressors and reduced during chronic stress.

A possible explanation for those changes has been suggested by Rocca *et al.*[37] The investigators note that peripheral benzodiazepine receptors in brain glial cells control the production of neurosteroids that act as modulators of $GABA_A$ receptor sensitivity. Their effect on GABA functioning appears to be opposite to that of clinically effective benzodiazepines, that is, they 'decrease' rather than increase the inhibitory effects of GABA. It is hypothesized that an endogenous ligand of these glial cell receptors (possibly diazepam-binding inhibitor) is released during stress, initiating the cycle of events depicted in Fig. 4.7.1.3.

The immediate effect of these events would be to enhance the stress-induced release of cortisol. However, prolonged cortisol excess is hypothesized to downregulate peripheral benzodiazepine receptors, resulting in the reduced receptor densities found in GAD. Administration of a clinically effective benzodiazepine drug would interrupt the proposed pathway at the point of the central GABA receptor, lowering cortisol levels and restoring synthesis of peripheral benzodiazepine receptors.

Other neurotransmitter systems. Individuals with GAD have been reported to have reduced serotonin levels in the cerebral spinal fluid[35] and decreased platelet binding of paroxetine, a selective serotonin reuptake inhibitor.[38] In addition, drugs that affect

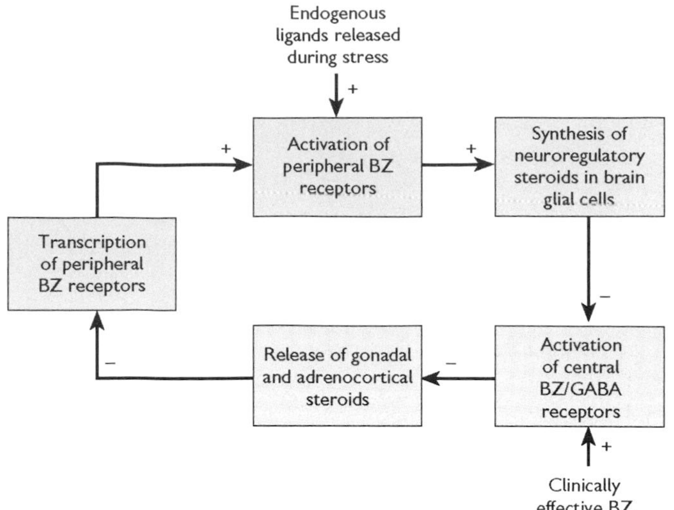

Fig 4.7.1.3 Possible involvement of peripheral benzodiazepine receptors in acute and chronic stress reactions (based on descriptions by Rocca *et al.*[37]). BZ, benzodiazepine.

serotonergic transmission (e.g. buspirone and venlafaxine) are effective in the treatment of GAD. These findings suggest that serotonin regulation may be abnormal in GAD.

Cholecystokinin neuropeptides (CCK-4 and CCK-8S) have been implicated in the genesis of arousal and fear responses.[40] It is unclear how those effects are mediated; however, cholecystokinin interacts with several neurotransmitters and systems believed to be involved in anxiety responses, including the noradrenergic nervous system, the hypothalamic-pituitary-adrenal axis, the benzodiazepine-GABA system, and serotonin.

(ii) Generalized psychological vulnerability

A diminished sense of control. Early experiences of uncontrollability may serve as a psychological vulnerability for emotional disorders.[16] Individuals in clinical populations, including people diagnosed with anxiety disorders, sexual dysfunctions, and depression, often perceive themselves as having little control over their experiences.[41,42] Patients with GAD are more likely than controls to perceive a lack of control over threatening events and to regard ambiguous information as threatening.[43] This perceived lack of control may result from a variety of events, including trauma and insecure attachment to primary caregivers.[44] In patients with GAD, worry may be an ineffective attempt to assert control on uncertain future events. Intolerance of uncertainty, a construct related to perceived lack of control, has emerged as an important variable in the study of anxiety disorders.[45] Defined as the inability to accept that future negative events may occur, intolerance of uncertainty has been associated with symptoms of several anxiety disorders, but is greater in individuals with GAD than in patients from a mixed anxiety disorder sample.[41]

Parenting. There is an extensive literature on the influences of early environmental factors on the development of anxiety and other negative emotions in children (for an integrative review, see Chorpita and Barlow[46]). Attachment theory holds that parents or other consistent caregivers serve an important function in a child's development by providing a protective and secure base from which the child can operate. Disruption of this base is hypothesized to lead initially to anxious apprehension and dependency and, if the disruption is severe, subsequently to withdrawal and depression.

An important aspect of a healthy parent–child relationship is its ability to foster in the child a sense of control over events. According to Chorpita and Barlow,[46] an individual who lacks sufficient early experiences of control may develop a general perception of personal inefficacy, which may predispose him or her to chronic negative emotional states such as GAD. Two aspects of parenting appear to be important in providing a child with opportunities to experience control: responsiveness to the child's efforts at engagement and encouragement of the child to explore and manipulate the environment. A parenting style characterized by excessive control of the child's environment (overprotection) coupled with a lack of warmth and responsiveness toward the child would deprive the child of such opportunities and thus, theoretically, could contribute to the development of anxiety.

Consistent with this theory, mothers of anxious preschool children were found to be more critical and intrusive and less responsive to their children than mothers of non-anxious children.[47] In addition, adults who rated their parenting as more protective and less caring had higher trait anxiety scores than other individuals surveyed. A similar pattern was found to distinguish patients meeting DSM-III-R criteria for GAD or panic disorder from controls.[48] One hypothesis is that the relationship of these early parenting experiences to the subsequent development of anxiety (or depression) is mediated by the early formation of cognitive vulnerability best described as a sense of uncontrollability regarding future events in one's life (Fig. 4.7.1.4).[46]

Specific psychological vulnerability. Data from twin studies suggest that environmental influences contribute more to the variance in aetiology of GAD than heredity.[19] In addition, the triple vulnerability model of the aetiology of anxiety disorders suggests that psychological and biological vulnerabilities interact with

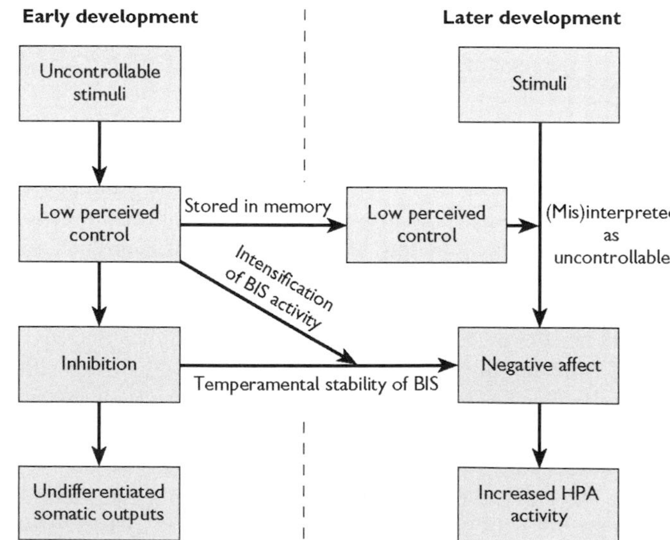

Fig 4.7.1.4 Model of the development of vulnerability for anxiety and depression. BIS, behavioural inhibition system[24]; HPA, hypothalamic-pituitary-adrenal axis (Copyright © 1998 by the American Psychological Association. Reproduced with permission. Chorpita, B.F. and Barlow, D.H. The Development of anxiety: the role of control in the early environment, *Psychological Bulletin*, **124**, 3–2. The use of APA information does not imply endorsement by APA).

environmental factors (i.e. stressful life events), to produce anxiety symptoms that reach a clinical level.[16,17] Several environmental factors have been implicated.

Stressful life events. Several studies have found an association between stressful or traumatic life events and GAD. The natures of the stressors that precede the onset of GAD remain unclear. However, in one study, 52 per cent of individuals diagnosed with GAD reported experiencing at least one past traumatic event (i.e. an event that would meet for Criterion A of the DSM-IV definition of PTSD), compared to only 21 per cent of non-anxious controls. It was unclear in this study if the events occurred prior to the onset of the GAD.[49] In addition, a variety of stressors have been associated with increased risk of GAD, including early parental death,[50] rape or combat,[51] and chronically dysfunctional marital and family relationships.[52]

Course and prognosis. Although there is evidence to the contrary, GAD has often been considered a chronic and disabling condition. The Harvard/Brown Anxiety Research Program study provides information on the course and impact of GAD among patients treated naturalistically over a 3-year period.[53] The mean age at onset of GAD was 21 years (range 2–61 years), and the average duration of illness at initial evaluation was 20 years. Excluding patients with comorbid panic disorder, one-third of subjects had never married and another 17 per cent were separated, widowed, or divorced. Unemployment was higher than average, and 37 per cent of subjects had received public financial assistance. Despite the fact that more than 80 per cent of patients received treatment during the study period, remission from GAD was uncommon (15 per cent at 1 year, 27 per cent by 3 years). Among patients with comorbid psychiatric disorders, the proportions achieving remission from GAD and coexisting anxiety disorders were only 8 per cent and 17 per cent at 1 and 3 years, respectively.

However, there is evidence that the perception of GAD as a chronic, unremitting condition may not be completely correct. A longitudinal study of individuals with GAD found that many (46 per cent of women and 56 per cent of men) experienced episodes of full remission and that the periods with no symptoms last longer in women.[54]

Treatment

(a) Pharmacotherapy

Several pharmacological agents have been shown to be effective for the treatment of GAD (for a review, see Davidson[23]). Chief among these are the benzodiazepines, azapirones, and antidepressants. Evidence shows that several types of medications may be effective for at least short-term relief of anxiety, however, many are not effective in the long term unless taken indefinitely.[55]

(i) Benzodiazepines

Benzodiazepines have for decades been prescribed for short-term relief of anxiety.[55] Although, evidence demonstrates that these drugs can be effective in relieving anxiety for a short period, there is little or no evidence that they work over a long period. However, compared with other agents used to treat anxiety disorders, they are safe, fast-acting, and have relatively few side-effects. All currently available benzodiazepines probably are efficacious for GAD. Approximately two-thirds of patients experience moderate to marked improvement, with effects being evident within the first 1 or 2 weeks of treatment.[56]

Benzodiazepines appear to be more effective for the somatic symptoms of GAD than for psychic symptoms such as apprehensive worry and irritability, possibly because of their sedative and myorelaxant properties. In some studies, irritability actually has increased during treatment with benzodiazepines. Consequently, these drugs may be better for patients whose complaints are more somatic than psychic, whereas other agents may be better when the reverse is true.

(ii) Azapirones

In recent years, azapirone drugs have become a popular alternative to benzodiazepines for the treatment of GAD. These drugs lack the sedative and muscle relaxant properties of the benzodiazepines as well as their ability to potentiate the effects of alcohol. However, improvement is somewhat slower (2–4 weeks) than with benzodiazepines. The most widely used of these agents is buspirone, whose efficacy and safety have been demonstrated in several well-controlled trials (see Rickels[57] for a review) and became, in 1996, the only non-benzodiazepine approved by the U.S. Food and Drug Administration for the treatment of GAD.[58] It is as effective as benzodiazepines for general anxiety and may reduce some of the associated features of GAD as well, including depression and agitation. Buspirone also does not seem to be associated with as much dependence and withdrawal as found with the benzodiazepines.[55] Ipsapirone, an azapirone with somewhat greater affinity and selectivity for the 5-hydroxytryptamine-1A receptor and fewer side-effects than buspirone also appears to be effective.[59] Other drugs in this class include gepirone, tandospirone, and flesinoxan.

(iii) Antidepressants

Both imipramine and trazodone have been superior to placebo for the treatment of GAD in controlled trials. In one trial, the two drugs were comparable to each other and to diazepam in reducing anxiety after the first 2 weeks of treatment.[56] In another study, imipramine was as effective as chlordiazepoxide overall and produced greater reductions in associated depression. In addition, nefazodone, an agent related to trazodone but less sedating, was effective for GAD in a small open trial.[60]

Many studies have examined the use of newer antidepressants, including selective reuptake inhibitors (SSRIs) and serotonin and norepinephrine reuptake inhibitors (SRNIs), in the treatment of GAD and have had favourable results. One placebo-controlled study of the SSRI paroxetine found that 62 per cent and 68 per cent of patients receiving 20 and 40 mg of paroxetine had significant reduction in symptoms, compared to only 46 per cent in the placebo group.[61] In addition, due to results from several large, placebo-controlled trials, venlafaxine was the first antidepressant approved by the Federal Drug Administration for the treatment of GAD.[62,63]

(b) Psychosocial treatment

Early psychological treatments for GAD consisted mostly of non-specific interventions such as supportive psychotherapy, relaxation training, and biofeedback. In general, those treatments were not very effective. However, cognitive behavioural treatment (CBT) has been found in several randomized controlled trials to be associated with clinically significant improvement. Cognitive behavioural treatment consists of psychoeducation about the nature of anxiety, symptom monitoring, relaxation training, exposure (imaginal and *in vivo*), and cognitive restructuring. Psychoeducation is a common CBT component in which the nature of anxiety is discussed in order to normalize the patient's experience. It also serves to teach patients to differentiate between adaptive and maladaptive anxiety. Symptom monitoring allows records of mood and anxiety to be recorded and allows patients to learn to observe their symptoms. Progressive muscle relaxation (PMR) is a common technique used to teach patients relaxation strategies to use in anxiety-provoking situations. Exposures are tailored to the nature of GAD and are either *in vivo* or imaginal and are often combined with rehearsal of coping skills (i.e. PMR) until anxiety subsides. Cognitive restructuring targets distorted cognitions and information-processing biases associated with GAD. Strategies to challenge catastrophizing or overestimating the probability of a negative event are often employed during this component of treatment. CBT is typically administered in a dozen or so sessions, and can be conducted in group or individual formats. In controlled trials, cognitive behavioural treatments have been more effective than no treatment or a psychological or drug placebo treatment and at least as effective as benzodiazepines (for a review, see Barlow *et al.*).[64] Attrition is low (10–15 per cent), and reductions in anxiety average about 50 per cent, with gains being maintained at follow-up. Currently, the most successful treatments combine relaxation training with cognitive interventions focused on making the worry process more controllable.

Consistent with the findings of individual studies, meta-analyses for GAD have found that CBT is more efficacious than control conditions, resulting in medium to large effect sizes when compared to pill or psychological placebo.[65] However, in studies directly comparing CBT with pharmacotherapy (most often benzodiazepines), there was no difference in effect sizes between the two treatments. Currently, neither mode of treatment has been shown to be consistently superior to the other.

Recent developments in psychosocial treatments for GAD have integrated acceptance and mindfulness approaches into traditional CBT.[66] These treatments are based on the notion that individuals' attempts to control their internal experience often backfire, resulting in increased anxiety. Components to these treatments may include experiential exercises, mindfulness training, identification of overriding values, and encouragement towards taking action in ways that are consistent with these values.[66] Further exploration with controlled trials needs to be conducted to examine the efficacy of these newer approaches with cognitive behavioural treatments.

(c) Combined pharmacotherapy and psychotherapy

Although common in clinical practice, little is known about the effects of combining pharmacotherapy and psychotherapy for GAD. In the only published study to date, Power *et al.*[67] compared cognitive behavioural therapy, diazepam, a pill placebo, cognitive behavioural therapy plus diazepam, and cognitive behavioural therapy plus a pill placebo in a sample of DSM-III-diagnosed GAD patients. At post-treatment and follow-up, patients in all three cognitive behavioural therapy conditions were more improved than those who received diazepam or placebo alone. Although the cognitive behavioural therapy groups did not differ significantly from each other on any measure, the cognitive behavioural therapy plus diazepam group improved earliest and had the largest percentage of patients achieving a criterion of clinically significant change on all measures. Unfortunately, the use of DSM-III criteria in this study makes its relevance to GAD as it is currently defined uncertain. In addition, the cognitive behavioural therapy used was briefer (seven sessions) and less specific than the currently recommended forms.

(d) Effect of comorbidity on treatment outcome and vice versa

Many treatment trials investigating GAD have excluded patients with comorbid Axis I disorders. A review of 48 GAD studies published between 1980 and 1991 found that only eight reported including patients with other psychiatric disorders.[68] When comorbid disorders have been permitted, their effect on treatment outcome generally has not been evaluated. In the Harvard-Brown Anxiety Research Program study, the presence of a comorbid psychiatric disorder reduced response rates at 1 and 3 years by nearly 50 per cent. In addition, it has been found that concurrent personality disorders impair outcome of treatment for GAD. In one study improvement was comparable among treatment completers with or without Axis II disorders, but attrition was greater in the former (44 per cent) than the latter (19 per cent) group.[69]

The high rates of comorbidity associated with GAD have important implications for treatment. Higher rates of comorbidity are associated with lower rates of remission and greater likelihood of relapse over 12-year follow-up.[70] On the other hand, successful treatment of GAD in patients with comorbid disorders often reduces the severity of the other disorders as well. Borkovec *et al.*[68] examined the effect of various psychosocial treatments for GAD on coexisting anxiety and mood disorders (except panic disorder or severe depression, which were excluded from the study). Across treatments, patients whose GAD improved exhibited reductions as well in other anxiety disorders (mostly social and simple phobia) and dysthymia. Only 4 of 13 successfully treated patients who had additional disorders at pre-treatment continued to have them at post-treatment.

Clinical management

Many anxious patients do not meet diagnostic criteria for GAD. These patients often respond to conservative measures. If the symptoms are minor or are related to a situational stressor, brief psychotherapy and support is the treatment of first choice. In one study, patients who initially reported physical or minor emotional complaints responded better to counselling than to diazepam, even when counselling was limited to only 3 h.[72] Often, an explanation of the relationship of physical symptoms to stress is reassuring to patients and can interrupt a spiral of symptoms leading to anxiety and worry about health, leading to increased symptoms, and so on. Simple behavioural interventions such as relaxation training for patients with prominent muscle tension or breathing exercises for those with dyspnoea or hyperventilation may be helpful as well.

For patients with marked adrenergic symptoms or insomnia, the temporary (a few days to a few weeks) use of a benzodiazepine may be helpful as an adjunct to psychotherapy. In some cases, a hypnotic drug alone is sufficient. In general, as-needed use of benzodiazepines should be discouraged, because it is more likely than scheduled use to foster reliance on drugs as the principal means of coping with anxiety. For the same reason, the drug dose should be kept as low as possible and should be tapered as therapy proceeds.

For patients meeting diagnostic criteria for GAD, treatment with an empirically validated form of psychosocial therapy for GAD is strongly recommended. Such treatments are available in manualized form with accompanying patient workbooks.[55]

When medication treatment is preferred, a trial of buspirone is a good initial choice. Exceptions are patients with comorbid panic disorder or marked adrenergic symptoms, for which benzodiazepines may be better if they are not contraindicated (see below). The typical starting dose of buspirone is 15 mg/day in divided doses (5 mg thrice daily or 7.5 mg twice a day), which is increased by 5 mg/day every few days to a target dose of 30 mg/day. If the response is insufficient after 2 to 4 weeks at that amount, or if the patient is experiencing significant depressive symptoms, the dose may be advanced gradually to a maximum of 60 mg/day. Improvement may continue for up to 3 months.

It is important to inform patients of the typical side-effects and response time of buspirone. Patients who have taken benzodiazepines previously may expect prompt relief and sedative side-effects from the medication and may become discouraged when these are absent. When switching from a benzodiazepine to buspirone, it may be helpful to continue the benzodiazepine during the first month of buspirone therapy before initiating a gradual taper. Remember that buspirone will not prevent benzodiazepine withdrawal symptoms.

Failing a course of buspirone, or in patients with comorbid major depression, trials of antidepressant medications (e.g. imipramine, venlafaxine, trazodone) would be a reasonable second choice. Venlafaxine may be effective at doses as low as 75 mg/day (the usual starting dose). Because of its short metabolic half-life, the extended release form is preferred, which allows once per day dosing and thus may improve compliance. The dose typically is advanced by 75 mg/day every 2 weeks to a maximum of 225 mg/day. Dosing for other antidepressants is the same as for the treatment of depression.

Because of the risk of dependence and (uncommonly) abuse, long-term use of benzodiazepines generally is reserved for patients who do not respond sufficiently to other options. Relative contraindications include a need to be alert (e.g. drivers and machinery operators), a personal or family history of alcoholism or drug abuse, and prominent aggressiveness or irritability. Generally, longer half-life benzodiazepines (e.g. diazepam, clonazepam), which can be taken once or twice daily, are preferred. A typical starting dose is 5 to 10 mg/day of diazepam or equivalent, which is advanced every few days to a maximum of 40 mg/day.

In instances where pharmacotherapy is the primary treatment, responders should be continued on medication for at least 6 months before a gradual drug taper is attempted. Even so, a substantial proportion will relapse after drug discontinuance and will require further treatment. Discontinuing pharmacotherapy in the context of effective psychosocial treatment may improve success rates.

Conclusions

Based on current knowledge, GAD seems to be the exaggerated expression of the human potential to apprehensively anticipate and prepare for future misfortune. As such, it may represent a 'basic' disorder, a better understanding of which may shed light on other anxiety and mood disorders. Although the definition of GAD has been revised considerably since being given status of a full disorder in DSM-III-R, much more information needs to be gathered regarding psychosocial treatments for GAD. In addition, due to its poor diagnostic reliability, many revisions to the diagnostic criteria of GAD have been suggested. Despite the progress in elucidating the nature of GAD, further research needs to be conducted to continue to enhance our understanding and development of effective and generalizable treatments.

Further information

Barlow, D.H. (1987). The classification of anxiety disorders. In *Diagnoses and classification in psychiatry: a critical appraisal of DSM-III* (ed. G.L. Tischler), pp. 223–42. Cambridge University Press, New York.

Brown, T.A., Barlow, D.H., and Liebowitz, M.R. (1994). The empirical basis of generalized anxiety disorder. *The American Journal of Psychiatry*, **151**, 1272–80.

Kessler, R.C., McGonagle, K.A., Zhao, S., *et al.* (1994). Lifetime and 12-month prevalence of DSM-III-R psychiatric disorders in the United States: results from the National Comorbidity Survey. *Archives of General Psychiatry*, **51**, 8–19.

Barlow, D.H., Chorpita, B.F., and Turovsky, J. (1996). Fear, panic, anxiety, and disorders of emotion. In *Nebraska symposium on motivation. Perspectives on anxiety, panic, and fear*, Vol. 43 (ed. D.A. Hope), pp. 251–328. University of Nebraska Press, Lincoln, NE.

Barlow, D.H. (2000). Unraveling the mysteries of anxiety and its disorders from the perspective of emotion theory. *The American Psychologist*, **55**, 1247–63.

Suarez, L., Bennett, S.M., Goldstein, C.M., *et al.* (2008). Understanding anxiety disorders from a "triple vulnerability" framework. In *Handbook of anxiety and the anxiety disorders* (eds. M.M. Antony and M.B. Stein). Oxford University Press, New York.

LeDoux, J. (1996). *The emotional brain: the mysterious underpinnings of emotional life*. Simon and Schuster, New York.

Craske, M.G. and Barlow, D.H. (2006). *Mastery of your anxiety and worry* (2nd edn). Oxford University Press, New York.

Barlow, D.H., Allen, L.B., and Basden, S.L. (2007). Psychosocial treatments for panic disorders, phobias, and generalized anxiety disorder. In *A guide to treatments that work* (3rd edn) (ed. P.E. Nathan and J.M. Gorman), Oxford University Press, New York.

References

1. DiNardo, P.A., Moras, K., Barlow, D.H., *et al.* (1993). Reliability of DSM-III-R anxiety disorder categories: using the Anxiety Disorders Interview Schedule-Revised (ADIS-R). *Archives of General Psychiatry*, **50**, 251–6.
2. Brown, T.A., DiNardo, P.A., Lehman C.L., *et al.* (2001). Reliability of DSM-IV anxiety and mood disorders: implications for classification of emotional disorders. *Journal of Abnormal Psychology*, **110**, 49–58.
3. Abel, J.W. and Borkovec, T.D. (1995). Generalizability of DSM-III-R GAD to proposed DSM-IV criteria and cross validation of proposed changes. *Journal of Anxiety Disorders*, **9**, 303–15.
4. Craske, M.G., Rapee, R.M., Jackel, L., *et al.* (1989). Qualitative dimensions of worry in DSM-III-R generalized anxiety disorder subjects and nonanxious controls. *Behavior Research and Therapy*, **27**, 189–98.
5. Barlow, D.H. and Wincze, J. (1998). DSM-IV and beyond: what is generalized anxiety disorder? *Acta Psychiatrica Scandinavica*, **98** (Suppl. 393), 23–9.
6. Grant, B.F., Stinson, F.S., Dawson, D.A., *et al.* (2004). Prevalence and co-occurrence of substance abuse disorders and independent mood and anxiety disorders. *Archives of General Psychiatry*, **61**, 807–16.
7. Grant, B.F., Hasin, D.S., Stinson, F.S., *et al.* (2005). Prevalence, correlates, co-morbidity, and comparative disability of DSM-IV

generalized anxiety disorder in the US: results from the National Epidemiologic Survey on Alcohol and Related Conditions. *Psychological Medicine*, **35**, 1747–59.
8. Kessler, R.C., Berglund, P., Demler, O., *et al.* (2005). Lifetime prevalence and age-of-onset distributions of DSM-IV disorders in the National Comorbidity Survey Replication. *Archives of General Psychiatry*, **62**, 593–602.
9. Kessler, R.C., Chiu, W.T., Demler, O., *et al.* (2005). Prevalence, severity, comorbidity of 12-month DSM-IV disorders in the National Comorbidity Survey Replication. *Archives of General Psychiatry*, **62**, 617–27.
10. Brown, T.A., Campbell, L.A., Lehman, C.L., *et al.* (2001). Current and lifetime comorbidity of the DSM-IV anxiety and mood disorders in a large clinical sample. *Journal of Abnormal Psychology*, **110**, 585–99.
11. Wittchen, H.-U., Zhao, S., Kessler, R.C., *et al.* (1994). DSM-III-R generalized anxiety disorder in the National Comorbidity Survey. *Archives of General Psychiatry*, **51**, 355–64.
12. Zinbarg, R.E., Barlow, D.H., Liebowitz, M., *et al.* (1994). The DSM-IV field trial for mixed anxiety-depression. *American Journal of Psychiatry*, **151**, 1153–62.
13. Zinbarg, R. and Barlow, D.H. (1996). Structure of anxiety and the anxiety disorders: a hierarchial model. *Journal of Abnormal Psychology*, **105**, 181–93.
14. Brown, T.A., Chorpita, B.F., and Barlow, D.H. (1998). Structural relationships among dimensions of the DSM-IV anxiety and mood disorders and dimensions of negative affect, positive affect, and autonomic arousal. *Journal of Abnormal Psychology*, **107**, 179–92.
15. Barlow, D.H., Chorpita, B.F., and Turovsky, J. (1996). Fear, panic, anxiety, and disorders of emotion. In *Nebraska Symposium on Motivation.* Vol. 43, *Perspectives on anxiety, panic, and fear* (ed. D.A. Hope), pp. 251–328. University of Nebraska Press, Lincoln, NE.
16. Barlow, D.H., (2002). *Anxiety and its disorders* (2nd edn). Guilford Press, New York.
17. Suarez, L., Bennett, S.M., Goldstein, C.M., *et al.* (2008). Understanding anxiety disorders from a "triple vulnerability" framework. In *Handbook of anxiety and the anxiety disorders* (eds. M.M. Antony and M.B. Stein). Oxford University Press, New York.
18. Hettema, J.M., Prescott, C.A., Myers, J.M., *et al.* (2005). The structure of genetic and environmental risk factors for anxiety disorders in men and women. *Archives of General Psychiatry*, **62**, 182–8.
19. Hettema, J.M., Neale, M.C., and Kendler, K.S. (2001). A review and meta-analysis of the genetic epidemiology of anxiety disorders. *Archives of General Psychiatry*, **158**, 1568–78.
20. Noyes, R., Clarkson, C., Crowe, R.R., *et al.* (1987). A family study of generalized anxiety. *The American Journal of Psychiatry*, **144**, 1019–24.
21. Andrews, G., Stewart, S., Allen, R., *et al.* (1990). The genetics of six neurotic disorders: a twin study. *Journal of Affective Disorders*, **19**, 23–9.
22. Kendler, K.S., Neale, M.C., Kessler, R.C., *et al.* (1992). Major depression and generalized anxiety disorder: same genes, (partly) different environments? *Archives of General Psychiatry*, **49**, 716–22.
23. Davidson R.T. (2001). Pharmacotherapy of generalized anxiety disorder. *The Journal of Clinical Psychiatry*, **62**(Suppl. 11), 46–50.
24. Gray, J.A. and McNaughton, N. (1996). The neuropsychology of anxiety: a reprise. In *Nebraska symposium on motivation. Perspectives on anxiety, panic, and fear*, Vol. 43 (ed. D.A. Hope), pp. 61–134. University of Nebraska Press, Lincoln, NE.
25. Charney, D.S., Woods, S.W., Heninger, G.R., *et al.* (1989). Noradrenergic function in generalized anxiety disorder: effects of yohimbine in healthy subjects and patients with generalized anxiety disorder. *Psychiatry Research*, **27**, 173–82.
26. Abelson, J.L., Glitz, D., Cameron, O.G., *et al.* (1991). Blunted growth hormone response to clonidine in patients with generalized anxiety disorder. *Archives of General Psychiatry*, **48**, 157–62.
27. Cameron, O.G., Smith, C.B., Lee, M.A., *et al.* (1990). Adrenergic status in anxiety disorders: platelet alpha two-adrenergic receptor binding, blood pressure, pulse, and plasma catecholamines in panic and generalized anxiety disorder patients and in normal subjects. *Biological Psychiatry*, **28**, 3–20.
28. Hazlett, R.L., McLeod, D.R., and Hoehn-Saric, R. (1994). Muscle tension in generalized anxiety disorder: elevated muscle tonus or agitated movement? *Psychophysiology*, **31**, 189–95.
29. Sapolsky, R.M. (2007). Stress, stress-related disease, and emotional regulation. In *Handbook of emotional regulation* (ed. J.J. Gross). Guilford Press, New York.
30. Tiller, J.W.G., Biddle, N., Maguire, K.P., *et al.* (1988). The dexamethasone suppression test and plasma dexamethasone in generalized anxiety disorder. *Biological Psychiatry*, **23**, 261–70.
31. LeDoux, J. (1998). Fear and the brain: where have we been, and where are we going? *Biological Psychiatry*, **44**, 1229–38.
32. DeBellis, M.D., Casey, B.J., Dahl, R.E., *et al.* (2000). A pilot study of amygdala volumes in pediatric generalized anxiety disorder. *Biological Psychiatry*, **48**, 51–7.
33. McClure, E.B., Monk, C.S., Nelson, E.E., *et al.* (2007). Abnormal attentional modulation of fear circuit function in pediatric generalized anxiety disorder. *Archives of General Psychiatry*, **64**, 97–106.
34. Davis, M. (1998). Are different parts of the extended amygdala involved in fear versus anxiety? *Biological Psychiatry*, **44**, 1239–47.
35. Waddell, J., Morris, R.W., and Bouton, M.E. (2006). Effect of bed nucleus of the stria terminalis lesions on conditioned anxiety: aversive conditioning with long-duration conditional stimuli and reinstatement of extinguished fear. *Behavioral Neuroscience*, **120**, 324–36.
36. Gray, J.A. (1982). *The neuropsychology of anxiety*. Oxford University Press, New York.
37. Rocca, P., Beoni, A.M., Eva, C., *et al.* (1998). Peripheral benzodiazepine receptor messenger RNA is decreased in lymphocytes of generalized anxiety disorder patients. *Biological Psychiatry*, **43**, 767–73.
38. Brewerton, T.D., Lydiard, R.B., Johnson, M.R., *et al.* (1995). CSF serotonin: diagnostic and seasonal differences. In *New research abstracts of the 148th meeting of the American Psychiatric Association*, Abstract NR385:151. American Psychiatric Press, Washington, DC.
39. Iny, L.J., Pecknold, J., Suranyi-Cadotte, B.E., *et al.* (1994). Studies of neurochemical link between depression, anxiety, and stress from [^{3}H]imipramine and [^{3}H]paroxetine binding on human platelets. *Biological Psychiatry*, **36**, 281–91.
40. Bradwejn, J., Koszycki, D., Couetoux du Tertre, A., *et al.* (1992). The cholecystokinin hypothesis of panic and anxiety disorders: a review. *Journal of Psychopharmacology*, **6**, 345–51.
41. Ladouceur, R., Dugas, M.J., Freeston, M.H., *et al.* (1999) Specificity of generalized anxiety disorder symptoms and processes. *Behavior Therapy*, **30**, 191–207.
42. Weisberg, R.B., Brown, T.A., Wincze, J., *et al.* (2001). Causal attributions and male sexual arousal: the impact of attributions for a bogus erectile difficulty on sexual arousal, cognitions, and affect. *Journal of Abnormal Psychology*, **110**, 324–34.
43. Rapee, R.M. (1991). Generalized anxiety disorder: a review of clinical features and theoretical concepts. *Clinical Psychology Review*, **11**, 419–40.
44. Borkovec, T.D. (1994). The nature, functions, and origins of worry. In *Worrying: perspectives on theory, assessment, and treatment* (eds. G.C.L. Davey and F. Tallis). Wiley, New York.
45. Dugas, M.J., Gagnon, F., Ladouceur, R., *et al.* (1998) Generalized anxiety disorder: a preliminary test of a conceptual model. *Behavior Research Therapy*, **36**, 215–26.
46. Chorpita, B.F. and Barlow, D.H. (1998). The development of anxiety: the role of control in the early environment. *Psychological Bulletin*, **124**, 3–21.

47. Dumas, J.E., LaFreniere, P.J., and Serketich, W.J. (1995). 'Balance of power': a transactional analysis of control in mother-child dyads involving socially competent, aggressive, and anxious children. *Journal of Abnormal Psychology*, **104**, 104–13.
48. Silove, D., Parker, G., Hadzi-Pavlovic, D., *et al.* (1991). Parental representations of patients with panic disorder and generalized anxiety disorder. *The British Journal of Psychiatry*, **159**, 835–41.
49. Roemer, L., Molina, S., Litz., B.T., *et al.* (1996). Preliminary investigation of the role of previous exposure to potentially traumatizing events in generalized anxiety disorder. *Depression and Anxiety*, **4**, 134–8.
50. Torgersen, S. (1986). Childhood and family characteristics in panic and generalized anxiety disorders. *The American Journal of Psychiatry*, **143**, 630–2.
51. Steketee, G. and Foa, E.B. (1987). Rape victims: post traumatic stress responses and their treatment: a review of the literature. *Journal of Anxiety Disorders*, **1**, 69–86.
52. Ben-Noun, L. (1998). Generalized anxiety disorder in dysfunctional families. *Journal of Behavior Therapy and Experimental Psychiatry*, **29**, 115–22.
53. Yonkers, K.A., Warshaw, M.G., Massion, A.O., *et al.* (1996). Phenomenology and course of generalised anxiety disorder. *The British Journal of Psychiatry*, **168**, 308–13.
54. Yonkers, K.A., Bruce, S.E., Dyck, I.R., *et al.* (2003). Chronicity, relapse, and illness-course of panic disorder, social phobia, and generalized anxiety disorder: findings in men and women from 8 years of follow-up. *Depression and Anxiety*, **17**, 173–9.
55. Craske, M.G. and Barlow, D.H. (2006). *Mastery of your anxiety and worry* (2nd edn). Oxford University Press, New York.
56. Rickels, K., Downing, R., Schweizer, E., *et al.* (1993). Antidepressants for the treatment of generalized anxiety disorder: a placebo-controlled comparison of imipramine, trazodone, and diazepam. *Archives of General Psychiatry*, **50**, 884–95.
57. Rickels, K. (1990). Buspirone in clinical practice. *The Journal of Clinical Psychiatry*, **51**(Suppl. 9), 51–4.
58. Apter, J.T. and Allen, L.A. (1999). Buspirone: future directions. *Journal of Clinical Psychopharmacology*, **19**, 86–93.
59. Cutler, N.R., Sramek, J.J., Keppel-Hesselink, J.M., *et al.* (1993). A double-blind, placebo-controlled study comparing the efficacy and safety of ipsapirone versus lorazepam in patients with generalized anxiety disorder: a prospective multicenter trial. *Journal of Clinical Psychopharmacology*, **13**, 429–37.
60. Hedges, D.W., Reimherr, F.W., Strong, R.E., *et al.* (1996). An open trial of nefazodone in adult patients with generalized anxiety disorder. *Psychopharmacology Bulletin*, **32**, 671–6.
61. Rickels, K., Zanielli, R., McCafferty, J., *et al.* (2003). Paroxetine treatment of generalized anxiety disorder: a double-blind, placebo-controlled study. *The American Journal of Psychiatry*, **160**, 749–56.
62. Sheehan, D.V. (1999). Venlafaxine extended release (XR) in the treatment of generalized anxiety disorder. *The Journal of Clinical Psychiatry*, **60**(Suppl. 22), 23–8.
63. Davidson, J.R., DuPont, R.L., Hedges, D., *et al.* (1999). Efficacy, safety, and tolerability of venlafaxine extended release and buspirone in outpatients with generalized anxiety disorder. *The Journal of Clinical Psychiatry*, **60**, 528–35.
64. Barlow, D.H., Allen, L.B., and Basden, S.L. (2007). Psychosocial treatments for panic disorders, phobias, and generalized anxiety disorder. In *A guide to treatments that work* (3rd edn) (ed. P.E. Nathan and J.M. Gorman). Oxford University Press, New York.
65. Mitte, K. (2005). Meta-analysis of cognitive-behavioral treatments for generalized anxiety disorder: A comparison with pharmacotherapy. *Psychological Assessment*, **4**, 224–7.
66. Orsillo, S.M., Roemer, L., and Barlow, D.H. (2003). Integrating acceptance and mindfulness into existing cognitive-behavioral treatments for GAD. *Cognitive and Behavioral Practice*, **10**, 222–30.
67. Power, K.G., Simpson, R.J., Swanson, V., *et al.* (1990). A controlled comparison of cognitive-behaviour therapy, diazepam, and placebo, alone and in combination, for the treatment of generalized anxiety disorder. *Journal of Anxiety Disorders*, **4**, 267–92.
68. Swinson, R.P., Cox, B.J., and Fergus, K.D. (1993). Diagnostic criteria in generalized anxiety disorder treatment studies. *Journal of Clinical Psychopharmacology*, **13**, 455.
69. Sanderson, W.C., Beck, A.T., and McGinn, L.K. (1994). Cognitive therapy for generalized anxiety disorder: significance of comorbid personality disorders. *Journal of Cognitive Psychotherapy*, **8**, 13–18.
70. Bruce, S.E., Yonkers, K.A., Otto, M.W., *et al.* (2005). Influence of psychiatric comorbidity on recovery and recurrence in generalized anxiety disorder, social phobia, and panic disorder: a 12-year prospective study. *The American Journal of Psychiatry*, **162**, 1179–87.
71. Borkovec, T.D., Abel, J.L., and Newman, H. (1995). Effects of psychotherapy on comorbid conditions in generalized anxiety disorder. *Journal of Consulting and Clinical Psychology*, **63**, 479–83.
72. Boulenger, J., Fournier, M., Rosales, D., *et al.* (1997). Mixed anxiety and depression: from theory to practice. *The Journal of Clinical Psychiatry*, **58**(Suppl. 8), 27–34.

4.7.2 Social anxiety disorder and specific phobias

Michelle A. Blackmore, Brigette A. Erwin, Richard G. Heimberg, Leanne Magee, and David M. Fresco

Introduction

As our classification systems have been refined, we have come to view social anxiety disorder (social phobia) and specific phobias as distinct disorders, with divergent patterns of prevalence, aetiology, and course. Moreover, treatments for these disorders have become increasingly sophisticated. This chapter presents an overview of the current state of the field with regard to social anxiety disorder and specific phobias.

Social anxiety disorder

In the first and second editions of the *Diagnostic and Statistical Manual of Mental Disorders* (**DSM**),[1,2] all phobias were grouped together. However, in 1966 Marks and Gelder[3] observed that various phobias had different ages of onset and symptom presentations, providing the initial impetus for the inclusion of *social phobia* as a distinct disorder in DSM-III.[4] At first, research into the nature and treatment of social phobia lagged behind that of other anxiety disorders, leading to its description in 1985 as the neglected anxiety disorder.[5] Over the past two decades, however, attention to the conceptualization, definition, and classification of social phobia has increased dramatically. To acknowledge the significant impairment now known to be associated with social phobia and its differentiation from specific phobia, the alternative (and increasingly utilized) label, *social anxiety disorder*, was added in DSM-IV.[6]

Clinical presentation

Anxiety in situations involving potential evaluation by others (e.g. job interviews, public speaking engagements, first dates) falls within the realm of 'normal' social anxiety. For individuals with social anxiety disorder, however, situations such as these are typically associated with incapacitating levels of anxiety and a desire for escape or avoidance. Socially anxious individuals are often self-critical and perfectionistic and go to great lengths to avoid the negative evaluation of others that they may perceive as epidemic. Commonly, persons with social anxiety disorder experience somatic symptoms such as blushing, trembling, dry mouth, or perspiring, which they believe will be noticed by others and provide further evidence of their incompetence. Children may manifest their anxiety differently than adults; they may cry, throw tantrums, freeze, shrink from interactions with strangers, and they may not acknowledge that their fears are irrational.[6] By leaving anxiety-provoking situations (escape) or foregoing them entirely (avoidance), individuals with social anxiety disorder may reduce or prevent the immediate experience of anxiety, but this behaviour reinforces beliefs in their inadequacies and serves to maintain anxiety in the absence of objective threat.[7,8]

Functional impairment

Individuals with social anxiety disorder experience significant impairment in social, educational, and occupational functioning.[5,9] They are less likely to marry and are more likely to divorce than those without the disorder.[10] They also have fewer friends and more trouble getting along with the friends they have than persons without the disorder.[11] Individuals with social anxiety disorder assessed in a primary care setting reported missing an average of 3 days of work and having an average of 6 days of reduced productivity in the last month because of their emotional problems.[12] Comparatively, mentally healthy individuals reported less than 1 day of lost work and reduced productivity combined. Unemployment, underemployment (working at a level below the individual's abilities), and financial dependency are also characteristic of individuals with social anxiety disorder.[10]

Classification

(a) DSM and ICD

Whereas the DSM is widely used in North America, the *International Classification of Mental and Behavioural Disorders* (**ICD**) is commonly used in other parts of the world. Social anxiety disorder, termed social phobia in ICD-10,[13] first appeared in ICD-10 12 years after its appearance in DSM-III. The ICD-10 criteria for social phobia are less detailed and more circumscribed than those in DSM-IV. Specifically, DSM-IV requires excessive fear of humiliation or embarrassment in social or performance situations, anxiety provoked by exposure to feared situations, recognition that the fear is excessive, avoidance of situations or endurance with distress, and significant distress or impairment. Further, the fear and avoidance cannot be better accounted for by another psychiatric disorder, a general medical condition, or the effects of a substance. The ICD-10, in contrast, requires only that the symptoms be representative of anxiety and not another psychiatric disorder, that the anxiety occurs in relation to social situations, and that avoidance of anxiety-provoking situations be present. Because most published research on social anxiety disorder relies on DSM rather than ICD criteria, this chapter will do so also.

(b) Diagnostic issues

Individuals presenting for treatment of social anxiety disorder endorse multiple fears and significant impairment. The *generalized* subtype is specified when 'most social situations' are feared, whereas the *non-generalized* subtype describes persons who fear a more limited set of social situations. Individuals with generalized and non-generalized social anxiety disorder differ on several dimensions, including symptom severity, functional impairment, and physiological symptoms when exposed to feared situations.[14] Conclusive differences between subtypes in course and response to treatment remain to be demonstrated.[15,16]

Like social anxiety disorder, avoidant personality disorder is regarded as an extreme fear of negative evaluation, leading researchers to view the two conditions on a continuum that is artificially divided at the boundary between Axes I and II. Many investigators conclude that the co-occurrence of generalized social anxiety disorder and avoidant personality disorder represent persons with the most severe social anxiety and the poorest global functioning.[17]

Social anxiety may also develop as a result of medical conditions, such as becoming excessively anxious or avoiding social situations because of obesity, acne, benign essential tremor, stuttering, or the disability associated with Parkinson's disease. These conditions are not considered exemplars of social anxiety disorder because anxiety developed secondary to the medical condition. Rather, they are assigned to the category 'anxiety disorder not otherwise specified'. However, persons who experience secondary social anxiety are often responsive to pharmacological or cognitive behavioural treatments with demonstrated efficacy for social anxiety disorder.[18]

(c) Comorbidity and differential diagnosis

Approximately 81 per cent of persons with primary social anxiety disorder meet criteria for at least one other lifetime psychiatric disorder.[19] Social anxiety disorder most commonly co-occurs with other anxiety disorders,[20] although comorbid diagnoses of depression and alcohol use disorders are also common. Differential diagnosis is complicated by the fact that certain Axis I disorders both resemble and co-occur with social anxiety disorder.

(d) Social anxiety disorder versus panic disorder with agoraphobia (PDA)

PDA can be differentiated from social anxiety disorder in several ways. Although many individuals with social anxiety disorder experience panic attacks, the attacks occur in anticipation of negative evaluation by others. For persons with panic disorder, panic attacks are often unexpected, may not be associated with specific cognitions, and can be nocturnal.[5] Persons with social anxiety disorder are more likely to experience blushing and muscle twitches, whereas individuals with PDA are more likely to experience symptoms such as blurred vision, headaches, chest pain, ringing in the ears, and fear that they will die or go crazy.[21] The age of onset for social anxiety disorder tends to be earlier than that for PDA.[22] Individuals presenting for social anxiety disorder treatment either show an equal gender distribution or are slightly more likely to be male,[23] whereas those presenting for PDA treatment are substantially more likely to be female.[21] Finally, persons with social anxiety disorder report feeling more comfortable when alone, whereas persons with PDA may feel more at ease in the presence of others.[22]

(e) Social anxiety disorder versus generalized anxiety disorder (GAD)

Individuals with GAD endorse higher levels of social anxiety than other persons with non-social anxiety disorders.[23] Although individuals with either social anxiety disorder or GAD may devote excessive amounts of time to worrying and ruminating, the focus of worry in social anxiety disorder is on fear of evaluation in social or performance situations, whereas the hallmark feature of worry in GAD is heightened focus on possible catastrophic consequences across several domains of life. Persons with social anxiety disorder are more likely to experience sweating, flushing, and breathing problems; those with GAD more commonly experience headaches, insomnia, and fear of dying.[24]

(f) Social anxiety disorder versus depression

Social anxiety disorder and depression may have withdrawal from social situations in common.[21] In differentiating between the two disorders, one must consider the reason for this withdrawal. Persons with depression withdraw because they fail to experience pleasure or lack the energy for social engagement. Individuals with social anxiety disorder fear the negative evaluation they believe to be associated with such situations. Persons with depression may be indifferent about engaging in social situations, whereas individuals with social anxiety disorder often have a strong desire to affiliate with others that is hampered by anxiety.

Epidemiology

(a) Prevalence

The National Comorbidity Survey Replication (**NCS-R**) reported a lifetime prevalence rate of 12.1 per cent[25] and a 12-month prevalence rate of 6.8 per cent[20] for social anxiety disorder. NCS-R lifetime prevalence rates render social anxiety disorder the fourth most common psychiatric disorder behind major depression (16.6 per cent), alcohol abuse (13.2 per cent), and specific phobia (12.5 per cent).

(b) Age at onset/age of treatment seeking

Social anxiety disorder often begins early in life. Mean age of onset for the disorder ranges from 13 to 20 years old, although patients often report having experienced symptoms for as long as they can remember.[26] Despite early onset, persons with social anxiety disorder often do not seek treatment for approximately 16 years after onset,[27] and many never do.[28]

(c) Gender differences

Although men and women with social anxiety disorder who seek treatment do so in relatively equal numbers,[23] epidemiological studies suggest that women are more likely than men to have the disorder.[19,25] In a clinical sample, women reported fear of more social situations and scored higher on several social anxiety disorder assessment measures.[29] Thus, although women are more likely to experience social anxiety, men are more likely to seek treatment and may do so when troubled with less severe symptoms. It may be that social anxiety disorder impairs the expected role functioning of men to a greater extent that it does for women.[29]

Aetiology of social anxiety disorder

Genetic factors appear to contribute to the emergence of social anxiety disorder. Higher rates of social anxiety disorder have been found in relatives of individuals with the disorder compared to relatives of persons without the disorder.[30] Further, rates of social anxiety disorder in first-degree relatives of probands with the generalized subtype are higher than in relatives of probands with the non-generalized subtype or with no psychiatric history.[31] Kendler *et al.*[32] report concordance rates for social anxiety disorder among monozygotic twins (24.4 per cent) to be greater than the rates for dizygotic twins (15.3 per cent). A study conducted with the same cohort 8 years later found the heritability of social anxiety disorder to be approximately 50 per cent in female twins[33] and 25 per cent in male twins.[34]

Neurobiological factors may also be associated with social anxiety disorder. Imaging studies of individuals with social anxiety disorder have demonstrated increased activity in regions associated with fear and anxiety (i.e. prefrontal cortex, amygdala, hippocampus) during anxiety-provoking tasks.[35] Given the efficacy of serotonin reuptake inhibitors and monoamine oxidase inhibitors in treating social anxiety disorder,[36] dysregulation of the serotonin[37] and dopamine[38] systems have been investigated as potential correlates of the disorder.

Several studies also suggest the importance of parental influences and significant life events in the development of social anxiety disorder. Persons with social anxiety recall observing their mothers act more fearful and avoidant of social interactions[39] and describe their parents as overprotective.[40] Stressful social and performance situations early in life (e.g. public ridicule, being bullied, mind going blank during a presentation) are also commonly reported by persons with social anxiety disorder.[41]

Course of social anxiety disorder

Social anxiety disorder is chronic and unlikely to remit without treatment. The disorder persists throughout adulthood[42] and its course is unrelated to gender, age of onset, duration of illness, level of functioning at intake, lifetime history of anxiety disorders, or current comorbidity of anxiety or depressive disorders.[42,43] Two conditions related to social anxiety disorder emerge in childhood and are relatively stable into adulthood—shyness and behavioural inhibition. Individuals who had been shy as children exhibited overall lower levels of functioning when assessed 30 years later.[44] Similarly, children described as behaviourally inhibited, or having the tendency to withdraw from novel people, settings, or objects, have demonstrated increased risk for the development of social anxiety disorder in adolescence.[45] Behavioural inhibition was also more prevalent in children of individuals with anxiety disorders and remained relatively stable for over 7 years in children initially assessed between the ages of 21 to 31 months.[46] These findings suggest that extreme shyness and behavioural inhibition may be early manifestations of social anxiety disorder.

Empirically evaluated treatments

(a) Cognitive behavioural interventions

Cognitive behavioural treatments have been subjected to the most thorough evaluation in the empirical literature. Treatments that utilize exposure alone or combined with cognitive restructuring have received the greatest empirical support and are the focus of our review. Because of space limitations, other cognitive behavioural treatments, such as social skills training and applied relaxation, will not be reviewed, and the reader is referred to other sources.[47]

(b) Exposure

Exposure requires individuals to imagine (imaginal exposure) or directly confront (*in vivo* exposure) feared stimuli. Research examining the efficacy of imaginal exposure for social anxiety disorder is limited; however, *in vivo* exposure has repeatedly demonstrated short- and long-term efficacy in therapist-directed and self-directed formats.[47] Exposure requires patients to progressively confront anxiety-provoking situations beginning with situations that elicit moderate fear. Patients turn to the next most feared situation after repeated and prolonged exposure to the previous situation no longer elicits a distressing level of fear. Individuals with social anxiety disorder treated with exposure alone experienced greater improvement than individuals receiving relaxation training,[48] pill placebo,[49] or delayed treatment.[50]

(c) Exposure combined with cognitive restructuring

Contemporary cognitive behavioural models of social anxiety disorder propose that anxiety is largely maintained by dysfunctional beliefs and information-processing biases, and that successful treatment will be associated with modification of cognition.[7,8] Accordingly, exposure is typically combined with techniques designed to modify dysfunctional thinking patterns.[51,52]

Cognitive restructuring is an intervention based on the theory that one's thoughts about a situation, not the situation itself, generate anxiety.[53] The intervention is designed to help patients challenge maladaptive beliefs by identifying irrational thoughts, evaluating the dysfunction inherent in these thoughts, and deriving rational alternatives to these thoughts. By engaging in this process and utilizing alternative thoughts during exposure to feared situations, patients acquire new, adaptive learning that competes with their previously-learned maladaptive views, and, in turn, lessens the anxiety they experience.[54]

Efficacy for the combination of cognitive restructuring and exposure has been demonstrated in comparison to wait-list control conditions,[55,56] pill placebo,[57] and psychological placebo conditions.[57,58] Several studies demonstrate equivalent outcomes for exposure alone and exposure plus cognitive restructuring, whereas others indicate the combination shows superior efficacy and additional gains at follow-up.[47] In one meta-analysis,[59] only the combination of exposure and cognitive restructuring was superior to placebo treatments, but this difference has not been reliably demonstrated.[60] Nevertheless, patients treated with exposure alone tend to show deterioration of gains after treatment, suggesting durability of gains may be enhanced with the addition of cognitive restructuring techniques.

(d) Cognitive behavioural group therapy (CBGT)

CBGT, originally developed by Heimberg and Becker,[51] is one of the most thoroughly examined cognitive behavioural treatments for social anxiety disorder. It integrates cognitive techniques and exposure and is typically conducted in 12 weekly, 2.5 h sessions, with approximately six patients and two therapists. In sessions 1–2, patients receive psychoeducation, rationale and instructions for exposure, training in cognitive restructuring, and homework assignments. Thereafter, therapists lead patients through individualized exposures preceded and followed by therapist-directed cognitive restructuring exercises. For homework, patients practice cognitive restructuring before and after exposure to real-life anxiety-provoking situations.

One study evaluating the efficacy of CBGT compared it to educational-supportive group therapy (ES), a credible placebo treatment consisting of lectures, discussions, and social support. Seventy-five per cent of CBGT patients made significant improvement compared to 40 per cent of ES patients.[58] At follow-up (4.5–6.25 years), CBGT produced durable treatment gains.[61] A comparison of CBGT to the monoamine oxidase inhibitor phenelzine, pill placebo, and ES demonstrated equivalent response and attrition rates after 12 weeks of treatment for CBGT and phenelzine, both of which were superior to placebo and ES.[57] Although the phenelzine group evidenced superior improvement on a subset of measures after 12 weeks, CBGT demonstrated more durable treatment gains, with only 17 per cent relapse compared to 50 per cent relapse in the phenelzine group after a 6-month maintenance phase and 6-month follow-up phase.[62] An intensive version of CBGT, based on a hybrid of the treatment approaches developed by Heimberg and by Clark, involving 2 weeks of daily treatment sessions separated by 1 week of homework assignments, also proved superior to a wait-list control.[63]

(e) Individual cognitive behavioural therapy

Group CBT may not always be feasible, particularly in clinical settings where it may be difficult to obtain an adequate number of patients to form a group. However, CBGT has been adapted to an individual format and proven superior to a wait-list control (Heimberg, unpublished observations). Clark[52] also developed a cognitively-focused individual treatment for social anxiety disorder that has demonstrated substantial efficacy. The treatment instructs patients on how to shift their attention externally (rather than on the self) and to reduce reliance on safety behaviours. Video feedback and exposure to feared situations aimed at restructuring distorted cognitions are also incorporated.

Individual cognitive therapy demonstrated superior efficacy to wait-list control, with clinically significant gains observed in 76 per cent of patients receiving cognitive therapy, compared to 38 per cent of patients receiving an applied relaxation treatment and 0 per cent of patients in the wait-list control group.[64] Cognitive therapy was also more efficacious than fluoxetine plus self-exposure instructions and placebo plus self-exposure instructions, with gains maintained at 1-year follow-up.[65] Although meta-analytic studies suggest that individual and group CBT are similar in efficacy,[60] individual cognitive therapy was superior to a group therapy based on Clark's model on several measures.[66] Similarly, individual cognitive therapy proved superior to a 3-week intensive group therapy based on Clark's model and treatment with psychiatrist-selected SSRIs.[67]

Pharmacotherapy

The efficacy of selective serotonin uptake inhibitors (**SSRI**s), serotonin–norepinephrine reuptake inhibitor venlafaxine (**SNRI**s), benzodiazepines, reversible and irreversible monoamine oxidase inhibitors (**MAOI**s), ß-adrenergic blockers, buspirone, gabapentin, and pregabalin have been evaluated in placebo-controlled studies. To date, most controlled trials have included patients with generalized social anxiety disorder, so it is unclear if similar efficacy would be observed among patients with the non-generalized subtype of the disorder.

(a) Selective serotonin reuptake inhibitors and venlafaxine

The SSRIs (e.g. paroxetine, sertraline, fluoxetine, fluvoxamine, and escitalopram) and the SNRI venlafaxine are regarded as first-line medication treatments for generalized social anxiety disorder, given demonstrated efficacy in placebo-controlled trials for the disorder as well as for other anxiety and affective disorders. Further, potential adverse side effects of SSRIs (e.g. sweating, sexual dysfunction) pose a lower risk than potential adverse side effects of the MAOIs (e.g. high blood pressure, seizure) or benzodiazepines (e.g. dependence, overdose).

The SSRIs have demonstrated superior efficacy to placebo as well as CBT in the short-term,[68] with the possible exception of fluoxetine.[65,69] There have been few direct comparisons of the various SSRIs or SNRIs. One study comparing escitalopram (5, 10, 20 mg), paroxetine (20 mg), and placebo, demonstrated superior efficacy for 5 mg and 20 mg of escitalopram and 20 mg of paroxetine compared to placebo at week 12.[70] At week 24, all doses of escitalopram proved superior to placebo and 20 mg of escitalopram proved superior to paroxetine on a subset of social anxiety measures. The SNRI venlafaxine produced results comparable to paroxetine, including superior efficacy relative to placebo.[71]

A fixed-dose trial of paroxetine showed 20 mg/day to be an efficacious and safe dose for the treatment of social anxiety disorder, with superior efficacy to placebo.[72] In a flexible-dose trial, paroxetine proved more efficacious than placebo after 8–12 weeks of treatment, with 55 per cent of paroxetine patients compared to 24 per cent of placebo patients identified as much or very much improved.[73] A double-blind discontinuation study demonstrated a 14 per cent relapse rate in the paroxetine group compared to a 39 per cent relapse rate in the placebo group at week 24.[74]

Van Ameringen and colleagues[75] found sertraline to be more efficacious than placebo, and a 20-week double-blind discontinuation trial demonstrated significantly lower relapse rates for patients continuing on sertraline than patients switched to placebo (4 per cent versus 36 per cent, respectively).[76] A study of fluvoxamine demonstrated superior outcome, beginning at week 8, for patients receiving fluoxamine (20 mg mean daily dose) than patients receiving placebo.[77]

Fluoxetine has yielded less promising results and is the only SSRI to date that has failed to separate from placebo in controlled trials.[65,69] However, in one study fluoxetine evidenced superior efficacy to placebo, although no differences were found between fluoxetine, CBGT, or their combination.[78]

(b) Benzodiazepines

Research suggests benzodiazapines have performed better than MAOIs and CBT in the short-term[68] and offer rapid onset of effect, good tolerability, and minimal side effects (e.g. sedation, withdrawal effects with abrupt discontinuation). However, benzodiazepines are contraindicated in the presence of substance abuse and lack efficacy for comorbid mood disorders. Clonazepam was shown to be efficacious for social anxiety disorder (2–4 mg/day), with patients showing improvement after 6 weeks of treatment and superior response rates compared to placebo patients at week 10.[79] Clonazepam also produced equivalent gains to CBGT after 12 weeks of treatment.[80] One study of alprazolam demonstrated that the medication was no more efficacious than placebo.[81]

(c) Monoamine oxidase inhibitors

MAOIs have demonstrated efficacy in the treatment of social anxiety disorder[36] similar to that of SSRIs. However, MAOI therapy requires strict dietary restrictions as ingesting foods rich in tyramine (e.g. most aged cheeses, red wine, beer) can increase the risk of rapidly escalating blood pressure. MAOIs are also associated with more adverse side effects (e.g. hypotension, sedation, weight gain, sexual dysfunction) than SSRIs. However, MAOI therapy (usually 45–90 mg/day) is justified when other treatments with more benign side effect profiles prove ineffective.

As discussed earlier, phenelzine proved superior to placebo and demonstrated equivalent response rates to CBGT after 12 weeks of treatment,[57], although CBGT evidenced more durable treatment gains.[62] Liebowitz and colleagues[82] found that after 8 weeks of acute treatment and 8 weeks of maintenance, phenelzine produced results superior to those of placebo and the ß-adreneregic blocker atenolol. Versiani and colleagues[83] found patients who received phenelzine endorsed significantly greater reductions in social anxiety than placebo patients at 8 weeks. In a comparison of phenelzine, alprazolam, CBGT, and placebo with instructions for self-exposure,[81] all groups produced relatively equivalent response. However, phenelzine demonstrated maintenance of gains at a 2-month follow-up, whereas alprazolam did not.

(d) Reversible inhibitors of monoamine oxidase

Moclobemide and brofaramine have been evaluated for the treatment of social anxiety disorder and offer fewer side effects and dietary restrictions than MAOIs. However, moclobemide has shown modest efficacy in controlled trials and is less efficacious than the SSRIs and MAOIs.[36] Although brofaramine was found to be efficacious for social anxiety, it was never marketed.

(e) ß-adreneregic blockers

ß-adreneregic blockers (e.g. atenolol) have failed to surpass placebo in controlled trials.[49] Propranolol appears to be efficacious on an as-needed basis (10–40 mg) for anxiety related to performance situations.

(f) Buspirone

Buspirone appears no more efficacious than placebo at low dosages.[84] One study demonstrated greater efficacy of buspirone in doses greater than or equal to 45 mg/day or when used as an augmentation to an SSRI.[85]

(g) Gabapentin and pregabalin

A single study shows some efficacy of high doses of the anticonvulsant gabapentin (maximum of 3600 mg/day) in the treatment of social anxiety disorder relative to placebo.[86] Pregabalin was also superior to placebo in one study,[87] but a high dose was required as well.

(h) Other agents

D-cycloserine, a partial adrenergic agonist associated with the facilitation of learning and memory consolidation, appears to enhance the efficacy of exposure. Several animal trials demonstrated enhanced fear extinction when d-cycloserine was administered prior to and after exposure trials.[88] Similar results were shown when individuals receiving d-cycloserine 1 h prior to exposure demonstrated significantly less social anxiety posttreatment than those receiving placebo.[89]

Integrating pharmacotherapy and cognitive behavioural interventions

Several studies have examined the utility of combining pharmacotherapy with cognitive behavioural interventions. Blomhoff and colleagues(90) compared sertraline and pill placebo alone and in combination with physician-directed exposure or general medical care, which included non-directive encouragement. After 12 weeks, all active treatments surpassed pill placebo and non-directive encouragement, with sertraline and exposure proving equally efficacious. Only sertraline alone or in combination with exposure proved superior to placebo at 24 weeks. However, only patients who received exposure alone demonstrated further improvement at 1-year follow-up, whereas patients receiving sertraline with or without exposure showed some degree of deterioration.(91)

Preliminary data from a study comparing CBGT, phenelzine, their combination, and pill placebo, suggests phenelzine plus CBGT may be more likely to surpass placebo than either treatment alone.(92) A similar study by Davidson and colleagues(78) found no advantage in combining fluoxetine and CBGT. Preliminary data suggests the combination of d-cycloserine with exposure may enhance the efficacy of exposure treatment.(89)

Evidence for the utility of the combination of these treatments is mixed. To summarize, different studies suggest that combining some medication treatments with CBT is no more efficacious than either treatment alone;(78) combining medication with CBT may diminish the efficacy of CBT;(91) and combining treatments may show only modest benefits over the administration of either alone.(92) The hypothesis that sequential treatments might capitalize on rapid medication response for faster symptom relief and cognitive behavioural treatment for superior relapse protection needs evaluation. Cognitive behavioural treatments may be utilized to help patients discontinue medical regimens after initial drug response.

Management of social anxiety disorder

(a) Treatment selection

Given the chronic nature of social anxiety disorder, CBT offers more enduring treatment gains compared to medication and lacks the adverse side effects. When considering cognitive behavioural interventions, it is important to assess the patient's ability and willingness to endure exposure to anxiety-provoking situations, as exposure necessitates short-term increases in anxiety over and above what the individual may typically experience. Additionally, it is helpful to assess level of compliance with previous therapy experiences (e.g. homework compliance). Managing a patient's treatment expectancy may further improve outcome as individuals reporting higher expectancy regarding the efficacy of treatment have demonstrated greater improvement and maintenance of treatment gains.(93)

Medication may be a preferred choice for individuals requiring rapid response, CBT non-responders, those with a preference for medication, or those with severe social anxiety disorder and/or comorbid depression. When selecting medication treatment, it is important to consider possible side effects, the patient's physical health, and prior medication compliance. Benzodiazepines offer rapid onset of effect, particularly beneficial for short-term performance situations, but their use may be contraindicated among patients with a history of alcohol or substance abuse. Given these concerns and their more benign side effect profile, SSRIs and venlafaxine are best regarded as the first-line medications, with the benzodiazepines and MAOIs held in reserve for non-responding patients. To date, we know little of the appropriate duration of medication treatments in social anxiety disorder, although two studies evidenced significant relapse rates upon discontinuation of SSRIs after a total treatment period of 36–40 weeks.(74,76)

(b) Other issues in management

Comorbid conditions should also be considered when treating social anxiety disorder with cognitive behavioural or pharmacological treatments. Comorbid anxiety disorders do not appear to degrade a patient's response to CBT; however, patients with comorbid mood disorders may present with more severe social anxiety symptoms and, although they improve at a similar rate, require extended treatment.(94) In general, if any comorbid condition prevents the patient from engaging in exposure exercises, taking medications in the prescribed manner, or complying with any other therapeutic activities, it may be necessary to treat the comorbid condition before the social anxiety disorder. In other cases, a comorbid condition might become the focus after social anxiety disorder treatment. Patients who abuse substances to 'treat' their social anxieties are often reticent to give up their substances before other coping strategies are made available. Ultimately, the management of comorbid conditions in individuals with social anxiety disorder depends on the analysis of the relationships between the disorders and varies from case to case.

(c) Prevention

Few studies to date have specifically examined ways of preventing social anxiety disorder; however, evidence for familial aggregation and environmental influence is strong. Parents may reinforce anxious children for making avoidant choices.(95) Thus, it is important to consider including parents of socially anxious children in treatment to provide parents with strategies to help their child manage the social anxiety. Parents with social anxiety disorder may also benefit from treatment themselves.

Since social anxiety disorder has an early age of onset, treatment of children and adolescents should help prevent social anxiety from becoming a chronic condition. Prevention programmes have been integrated into school settings to teach children and parents coping skills (e.g. cognitive restructuring, relaxation) and instruct them on the proper conduct of exposures. Individuals in the intervention group have shown significant improvement compared to non-intervention controls.(96) Similar prevention programmes have targeted at-risk youth and resulted in decreased anxiety symptoms and lower rates of anxiety disorders compared to control groups.(97)

Informational Websites

- http://www.adaa.org/GettingHelp/AnxietyDisorders/SocialPhobia.asp (Anxiety Disorders Association of America)
- http://www.nimh.nih.gov/HealthInformation/socialphobiamenu.cfm (National Institute of Mental Health)

Specific phobia

Clinical features and functional impairment

The hallmark feature of specific phobia, prior to DSM-IV called simple phobia, is a 'marked and persistent fear that is excessive or unreasonable, cued by the presence or anticipation of a specific object or situation' (6, p. 405). Commonly feared/avoided objects include animals, aspects of nature, or blood. Many individuals endorse some fear of these stimuli; however, in specific phobia, fear and avoidance cause significant interference with one's normal routine, career, academic pursuits, or social activities. Some individuals with specific phobias maintain a relatively normal routine by pursuing a lifestyle that minimizes exposure to the phobic stimulus. Often, specific phobias accompany a more impairing primary disorder that is the stimulus for seeking treatment.[98]

Classification

(a) DSM and ICD

Criteria for specific phobia are similar between DSM-IV and ICD-10. Both view fear as arising from exposure to a specific object or situation, which leads to acute autonomic and psychological symptoms of anxiety. However, ICD-10 does not stipulate that anxiety may be cued by the anticipation of the feared object or situation. Our review of specific phobia follows DSM conventions.

(b) Specific phobia subtypes

DSM-IV classifies specific phobias into five subtypes:

- animal
- natural environment
- blood-injection-injury
- situational
- other (e.g. dental/medical procedures, choking, etc.).

With the exception of blood-injection-injury phobias, exposure to the phobic stimulus evokes intense anxiety that may meet criteria for a situationally-bound panic attack. Additionally, there is extreme apprehension and desire to escape or avoid the phobic stimulus.[99] By contrast, individuals with blood-injection-injury phobias exhibit a biphasic anxiety reaction (vasovagal syncope) characterized by initial, short-lived sympathetic arousal, followed by parasympathetic arousal that may result in fainting.[100] The subjective experiences of these individuals tend to be characterized by disgust and repulsion rather than pure apprehension.[99]

(c) Comorbidity

The vast majority (83.4 per cent) of individuals with specific phobia experience at least one other lifetime psychiatric disorder.[19] In the original National Comorbidity Survey, individuals with specific phobia were 5 times more likely to have at least one additional disorder than individuals who had never met criteria for a phobic disorder. In most cases, the onset of the specific phobia preceded the onset of the other disorder.

Epidemiology

(a) Prevalence

The NCS-R reported a lifetime prevalence rate of 12.5 per cent[25] and a 12-month prevalence rate of 8.7 per cent for specific phobia.[20] One study found situational/environmental phobias to be the most common (13.2 per cent), followed by animal phobias (7.9 per cent) and blood-injection-injury phobias (3.0 per cent).[101]

(b) Age at onset/age of treatment seeking

Age at onset of specific phobia tends to be earlier than other anxiety disorders[19,102] and varies as a function of phobia subtype. For example, animal phobias onset earliest (age 7), followed by blood-injection-injury phobias (age 8), and most situational phobias (early 20s).[103] Individuals with phobic disorders often do not seek treatment for 20 years after onset.[27]

(c) Gender distribution

Women receive diagnoses of specific phobia more often than men. Lifetime rates for specific phobia in the NCS-R were 15.7 per cent for women but only 6.7 per cent for men.[25] In one study, women reported higher rates of animal and situational/environmental phobias, but rates of blood-injection-injury phobia did not differ.[101]

Aetiology of specific phobia

There is considerable evidence for familial/genetic transmission of specific phobia.[32,104] In one study, 31 per cent of first-degree relatives of persons with specific phobia also met criteria for specific phobia.[104] Rates of specific phobia were higher among first-degree relatives of persons with specific phobia and no other anxiety disorder than among first-degree relatives of persons who were never mentally ill.[105] In the Virginia Twin Study,[32] concordance rates for animal phobia were 25.9 and 11.0 per cent among monozygotic and dizygotic twins, respectively. Concordance rates for situational phobia were similar in monozygotic and dizygotic twins. Moreover, children classified as behaviourally inhibited have shown higher risk for the development of multiple specific phobias.[106]

Classical conditioning theory[107] holds that phobias are learned through the association of negative experience with an object or situation. However, individuals with more previous non-traumatic experiences with the object or situation are less likely to develop a phobia upon a negative encounter than those with less prior experience when traumatized. Two-factor learning theory[108] introduced avoidance as a critical component to the maintenance of anxiety. That is, responses of avoidance or escape are learned and serve to decrease the discomfort arising from exposure to conditioned stimuli. Repeated negative reinforcement of avoidance behaviour (i.e. reduction of arousal on removal of oneself from proximity to the phobic object or situation) maintains the fear and makes it resistant to extinction.

Some conditioning theorists assert that feared stimuli are not randomly determined; rather, humans have inherited a predisposition to fear specific stimuli through natural selection. Marks'[109] 'preparedness' theory maintains that commonly feared objects are those that historically threatened the survival of the individual or the species. In this model, phobias are viewed as instances of 'prepared learning', which is selective, easily acquired, difficult to extinguish, and non-cognitive.[110] However, a large number of studies also suggest that phobias may be acquired via observational and informational learning (e.g. hearing that the situation is dangerous).

Course of specific phobia

Individuals with specific phobias acquire their fear(s) early in life, and the disorder tends to be chronic or recurrent without treatment.[111] Often individuals with specific phobias adapt their lifestyle to avoid contact with the feared stimuli, such that only persons with the most severe specific phobias seek treatment. Events that commonly precipitate treatment seeking include a change in lifestyle that increases exposure to the feared stimulus (e.g. change in occupation that requires frequent air travel) or the experience of a panic attack in anticipation or in the presence of the feared stimulus.

Empirically evaluated treatments

(a) Cognitive behavioural interventions

(i) Exposure

Prolonged and repeated *in vivo* exposure to feared stimuli is by far the most studied and efficacious intervention for specific phobia[(112)] and should be considered the first-line treatment. Although *in vivo* exposure is generally believed to be more efficacious than imaginal exposure for specific phobia, some studies found *in vivo* and imaginal exposure techniques to be similarly efficacious.[(113)] Modelling in the form of observing another patient receive treatment has been shown to enhance the effects of exposure and to increase the speed at which positive outcomes are attained.[(114)] Multiple exposures sessions are considered more efficacious than one session, although some studies report positive outcomes for one-session treatments.[(115)] Further, one-session group *in vivo* exposure treatment has produced gains similar to those of one-session individual *in vivo* exposure treatment.[(115)] Variations in spacing of exposure sessions (e.g. 10 daily versus 10 weekly) have shown equivalent outcomes.[(116)] Finally, therapist-directed treatments have generally been more efficacious than self-directed treatments,[(117)] with gains enduring up to 8 years.[(114)] When possible, exposures should be conducted in a variety of settings to enhance generalization outside the therapeutic setting.[(54)]

In vivo exposure situations can sometimes be difficult to arrange and imaginal exposure may not achieve the reality or intensity needed to elicit an anxiety response. In such instances, virtual reality exposure (**VRE**), in which feared situations are presented in three dimensional simulations, may greatly enhance the efficacy of exposures. The salience of virtual environments can be augmented by instructing patients to touch real objects (e.g. toy spiders) which correspond with the virtual environment. Recent case studies demonstrated the efficacy of VRE either alone[(118,119)] or in combination with anxiety management training.[(120)] In a controlled trial for fear of flying, VRE training showed equivalent gains to *in vivo* exposure at 6 and 12-month follow-up[(121)]. Another study indicated that VRE produced superior gains to an attention placebo therapy, although gains were not maintained at 6-month follow-up.[(122)] D-cycloserine in combination with VRE has also shown enhanced treatment efficacy over VRE with placebo.[(123)]

(b) Applied relaxation and applied tension

Applied relaxation combines focused attention on different muscle groups while tensing and relaxing muscles,[(124)] with instruction to practice these skills first in non-anxiety-provoking situations and then in anxiety-provoking situations.[(125)] Although research is limited, applied relaxation has demonstrated efficacy,[(126)] especially among patients with higher levels of physiological reactivity than behavioural avoidance. *Applied tension*, designed specifically for blood-injection-injury phobia to treat parasympathetic arousal, requires the patient to tense different muscle groups in the presence of phobic stimuli to elevate blood pressure. Persons with phobias for blood, wounds, and injuries responded equally well to applied tension, applied relaxation, or their combination[(127)] Individuals treated with applied tension also evidenced greater treatment gains posttreatment and at 1-year follow-up than those treated with *in vivo* exposure alone.[(128)] In one dismantling study, individuals treated with applied tension and tension only (without the exposure component) evidenced equivalent gains and maintained superior outcomes at posttreatment and 1-year follow-up compared to patients who received *in vivo* exposure.[(129)]

(c) Cognitive restructuring

Phobia-specific irrational thoughts may contribute to the development of the phobia, maintain avoidance behaviour, and contribute to physiological symptoms.[(130)] When combined with exposure to feared stimuli, cognitive restructuring has proven efficacious,[(131)] although there are relatively few studies of cognitively-oriented treatments for specific phobia.

Pharmacotherapy

Drug treatments for specific phobia have consistently been shown to be less efficacious than behavioural treatments and may hinder maintenance of treatment gains. ß-Adrenergic blockers reduce some symptoms of sympathetic arousal during exposure to feared stimuli but fail to decrease subjective fear.[(132)] Although benzodiazepines (e.g. diazepam) may facilitate approach to feared stimuli, they may also reduce the efficacy of behaviour therapies by inhibiting the experience of anxiety during exposure.[(133)] Recent studies suggest d-cycloserine may facilitate exposure and extinction to specific feared stimuli. In a study of acrophobia patients, d-cycloserine was administered prior to exposure sessions and proved superior to placebo in reducing anxiety symptoms.[(123)]

Management of specific phobia

(a) Treatment selection

Exposure is clearly the treatment of choice for specific phobia, although facing feared stimuli may be particularly challenging for some patients, and their willingness and ability to participate in exposures should be assessed prior to treatment. Tailoring treatment to individual response patterns may improve outcome. For instance, patients with heightened physiological reactivity may respond preferentially to applied relaxation, whereas patients showing avoidance behaviour may respond better to *in vivo* exposure.[(126)] Further, individuals who experience anxiety primarily in the form of anxious thoughts may respond better to cognitive techniques.[(134)]

For patients unwilling or unable to engage in cognitive behavioural interventions, medication may be an appropriate alternative. However, it is first important to educate patients about the possibility of dependence with regular use and the side effects of high doses (e.g. sedation). If the patient is participating in exposure therapy, it is also necessary to explain that medication may interfere with the efficacy of exposure treatment.

(b) Prevention

Children with specific phobia were included in the Queensland Early Intervention and Prevention of Anxiety Project, but no other preventive efforts have been mounted. It is tempting to speculate that children could be 'inoculated' against a variety of the more common specific phobias by systematic exposure to potentially feared objects or situations.

Further information

http://www.adaa.org/GettingHelp/AnxietyDisorders/SpecificPhobia.asp (Anxiety Disorders Association of America)

http://www.mentalhealthamerica.net/go/phobias (Mental Health America)

References

1. American Psychiatric Association. (1952). *Diagnostic and statistical manual of mental disorders* (1st edn). American Psychiatric Press, Washington, DC.
2. American Psychiatric Association. (1968). *Diagnostic and statistical manual of mental disorders* (2nd edn). American Psychiatric Press, Washington, DC.
3. Marks, I.M. and Gelder, M.G. (1966). Different ages of onset in varieties of social phobia. *The American Journal of Psychiatry*, **123**, 218–21.
4. American Psychiatric Association. (1980). *Diagnostic and statistical manual of mental disorders* (3rd edn). American Psychiatric Press, Washington, DC.
5. Liebowitz, M.R., Gorman, J.M., Fyer, A.J., *et al.* (1985). Social phobia: review of a neglected anxiety disorder. *Archives of General Psychiatry*, **42**, 729–36.
6. American Psychiatric Association. (1994). *Diagnostic and statistical manual of mental disorders* (4th edn). American Psychiatric Press, Washington, DC.
7. Rapee, R.M. and Heimberg, R.G. (1997). A cognitive-behavioral model of anxiety in social phobia. *Behaviour Research and Therapy*, **35**, 741–56.
8. Clark, D.M. and Wells, A. (1995). A cognitive model of social phobia. In *Social phobia: diagnosis, assessment, and treatment* (eds. R.G. Heimberg, M.R. Liebowitz, D.A. Hope, and F.R. Schneier), pp. 69–93. Guilford Press, New York.
9. Schneier, F.R., Heckelman, L.R., Garfinkel, R., *et al.* (1994). Functional impairment in social phobia. *The Journal of Clinical Psychiatry*, **55**, 322–31.
10. Wittchen, H., Fuetsch, M., Sonntag, H., *et al.* (1999). Disability and quality of life in pure and comorbid social phobia: findings from a controlled study. *European Psychiatry*, **14**, 118–31.
11. Whisman, M., Sheldon, C., and Goering, P. (2000). Psychiatric disorders and dissatisfaction with social relationships: does type of relationship matter? *Journal of Abnormal Psychology*, **109**, 803–8.
12. Stein, M., McQuaid, J., Laffaye, C., *et al.* (1999). Social phobia in the primary medical care setting. *Journal of Family Practice*, **49**, 514–9.
13. World Health Organization. (1992). The ICD-10 classification of mental and behavioural disorders: clinical description and diagnostic guidelines. World Health Organization, Geneva.
14. Heimberg, R.G., Hope, D.A., Dodge, C.S., *et al.* (1990). DSM-III-R subtypes of social phobia: comparison of generalized social phobics and public speaking phobics. *The Journal of Nervous and Mental Disease*, **173**, 172–9.
15. Heimberg, R.G., Holt, C.S., Schneier, F.R., *et al.* (1993). The issue of subtypes in the diagnosis of social phobia. *Journal of Anxiety Disorders*, **7**, 249–69.
16. Vriends, N., Becker, E.S., Meyer, A., *et al.* (2007). Subtypes of social phobia: are they of any use? *Journal of Anxiety Disorders*, **21**, 59–75.
17. Heimberg, R.G. (1996). Social phobia, avoidant personality disorder and the multiaxial conceptualization of interpersonal anxiety. In *Trends in cognitive and behavioural therapies*, Vol. 1 (ed. P. Salkovskis), pp. 43–61. John Wiley & Sons, Chichester, England.
18. Schneier, F.R., Liebowitz, M.R., Beidel, D.C., *et al.* (1998). MacArthur data reanalysis for *DSM-IV*: social phobia. In *DSM-IV sourcebook*, Vol. 4 (eds. T.A. Widiger, A.H. Frances, H.A. Pincus, R. Ross, M.J. First, W. Davis, and M. Kline), pp. 307–28. American Psychiatric Press, Washington, DC.
19. Magee, W.J., Eaton, W.W., Wittchen, H.U., *et al.* (1996). Agoraphobia, simple phobia, and social phobia in the National Comorbidity Survey. *Archives of General Psychiatry*, **53**, 159–68.
20. Kessler, R.C., Chiu, W.T., Demler, O., *et al.* (2005). Prevalence, severity, and comorbidity of 12-month DSM-IV disorders in the National Comorbidity Survey Replication. *Archives of General Psychiatry*, **62**, 617–27.
21. Heckelman, L.R. and Schneier, F.R. (1995). Diagnostic issues. In *Social phobia: diagnosis, assessment, and treatment* (eds. R.G. Heimberg, M.R. Liebowitz, D.A. Hope, and F.R. Schneier), pp. 3–20. Guilford Press, New York.
22. Mannuzza, S., Fyer, A.J., Liebowitz, M.R., *et al.* (1990). Delineating the boundary of social phobia: its relationship to panic disorder and agoraphobia. *Journal of Anxiety Disorders*, **4**, 41–59.
23. Rapee, R.M., Sanderson, W.C., and Barlow, D.H. (1988). Social phobia features across the DSM-III-R anxiety disorders. *Journal of Psychopathology and Behavioral Assessment*, **10**, 287–99.
24. Reich, J., Noyes, R., and Yates, W. (1988). Anxiety symptoms distinguishing social phobia from panic and generalized anxiety disorders. *The Journal of Nervous and Mental Disease*, **176**, 510–3.
25. Kessler, R.C., Berglund, P.D., Demler, O., *et al.* (2005). Lifetime prevalence and age-of-onset distributions of DSM-IV disorders in the National Comorbidity Survey Replication. *Archives of General Psychiatry*, **62**, 593–602.
26. Hazen, A.L. and Stein, M.B. (1995). Clinical phenomenology and comorbidity. In *Social phobia: clinical and research perspectives* (ed. M.B. Stein), pp. 3–41. American Psychiatric Press, Washington, DC.
27. Wang, P.S., Berglund, P., Olfson, M., *et al.* (2005). Failure and delay in initial treatment contact after first onset of mental disorders in the National Comorbidity Survey Replication. *Archives of General Psychiatry*, **62**, 603–13.
28. Olfson, M., Guardino, M., Struening, E., *et al.* (2000). Barriers to treatment of social anxiety. *The American Journal of Psychiatry*, **157**, 521–7.
29. Turk, C.L., Heimberg, R.G., Orsillo, S.M., *et al.* (1998). An investigation of gender differences in social phobia. *Journal of Anxiety Disorders*, **12**, 209–23.
30. Tillfors, M. (2004). Why do some individuals develop social phobia? A review with emphasis on the neurobiological influences. *Nordic Journal of Psychiatry*, **58**, 267–76.
31. Stein, M.B., Chartier, M.J., Hazen, A.L., *et al.* (1998). A direct-interview family study of generalized social phobia. *The American Journal of Psychiatry*, **155**, 90–7.
32. Kendler, K.S., Neale, M.C., Kessler, R.C., *et al.* (1992). The genetic epidemiology of phobias in women: the interrelationship of agoraphobia, social phobia, situational phobia, and simple phobia. *Archives of General Psychiatry*, **49**, 273–81.
33. Kendler, K.S., Karkowski, L.M., and Prescott, C.A. (1999). Fears and phobias: reliability and heritability. *Psychological Medicine*, **29**, 539–53.
34. Kendler, K.S., Myers, J., Prescott, C.A., *et al.* (2001). The genetic epidemiology of irrational fears and phobias in men. *Archives of General Psychiatry*, **58**, 257–65.
35. Stein, M.B., Goldin, P.R., Sareen, J., *et al.* (2002). Increased amygdala activation to angry and contemptuous faces in generalized social phobia. *Archives of General Psychiatry*, **59**, 1027–34.
36. Blanco, C., Schneier, F.R., Schmidt, A., *et al.* (2003). Pharmacological treatment of social anxiety disorder: a meta-analysis. *Depression and Anxiety*, **18**, 29–40.
37. Stein, D.J. and Stahl, S. (2000). Serotonin and anxiety: current models. *International Clinical Psychopharmacology*, **15**(Suppl. 2), S1–6.
38. Schneier, F.R., Liebowitz, M.R., Abi-Dargham, A., *et al.* (2000). Low dopamine D2 receptor binding potential in social phobia. *The American Journal of Psychiatry*, **157**, 457–9.
39. Bruch, M.A., Heimberg, R.G., Berger, P., *et al.* (1989). Social phobia and perceptions of early parental and personal characteristics. *Anxiety Research*, **2**, 57–65.

40. Lieb, R., Wittchen, H.U., Hofler, M., *et al.* (2000). Parental psychopathology, parenting styles, and the risk of social phobia in offspring. *Archives of General Psychiatry*, **57**, 859–66.
41. Erwin, B.A., Heimberg, R.G., Marx, B.P., *et al.* (2006). Traumatic and socially stressful life events among persons with social anxiety disorder. *Journal of Anxiety Disorders*, **20**, 896–914.
42. Reich, J., Goldenberg, I., Vasile, R., *et al.* (1994). A prospective follow-along study of the course of social phobia. *Psychiatry Research*, **54**, 249–58.
43. Reich, J., Goldenberg, I., Goisman, R., *et al.* (1994). A prospective, follow-along study of the course of social phobia: II. testing for basic predictors of course. *The Journal of Nervous and Mental Disease*, **182**, 297–301.
44. Caspi, A., Edler, G.H., and Bem, D.J. (1988). Moving away from the world: life-course patterns of shy children. *Developmental Psychology*, **24**, 824–31.
45. Schwartz, C.E., Snidman, N., and Kagan, J. (1999). Adolescent social anxiety as an outcome of inhibited temperament in childhood. *Journal of the American Academy of Child and Adolescent Psychiatry*, **38**, 1008–15.
46. Rosenbaum, J.F., Biederman, J., Hirshfeld, D.R., *et al.* (1991). Behavioral inhibition in childhood: a possible precursor to panic disorder or social phobia. *The Journal of Clinical Psychiatry*, **52**(Suppl.), 5–9.
47. Rodebaugh, T.L., Holaway, R.M., and Heimberg, R.G. (2004). The treatment of social anxiety disorder. *Clinical Psychology Review*, **24**, 883–908.
48. Al-Kubaisy, T., Marks, I.M., Logsdail, S., *et al.* (1992). Role of exposure homework in phobia reduction: a controlled study. *Behavior Therapy*, **23**, 599–621.
49. Turner, S.M., Beidel, D.C., and Jacob, R.G, (1994). Social phobia: a comparison of behavior therapy and atenolol. *Journal of Consulting and Clinical Psychology*, **62**, 350–8.
50. Newman, M.G., Hofmann, S.G., Trabert, W., *et al.* (1994). Does behavioral treatment of social phobia lead to cognitive changes? *Behavior Therapy*, **25**, 503–17.
51. Heimberg, R.G. and Becker, R.E. (2002). Cognitive-behavioral group therapy for social phobia: basic mechanisms and clinical strategies. Guilford Press, New York.
52. Clark, D.M. (2001). A cognitive perspective on social phobia. In *International handbook of social anxiety: concepts, research and interventions relating to the self and shyness* (eds. W.R. Crozier and L.E. Alden LE), pp. 405–30. John Wiley & Sons, Chichester, United Kingdom.
53. Beck, A.T. and Emery, G. (1985). *Anxiety disorders and phobias: a cognitive perspective*. Basic Books, New York.
54. Bouton, M.E. (2002). Context, ambiguity, and unlearning: sources of relapse after behavioral extinction. *Biological Psychiatry*, **52**, 976–86.
55. Hope, D.A., Heimberg, R.G., and Bruch, M.A. (1995). Dismantling cognitive-behavioral group therapy for social phobia. *Behaviour Research and Therapy*, **33**, 637–50.
56. Butler, G., Cullington, A., Munby, M., *et al.* (1984). Exposure and anxiety management in the treatment of social phobia. *Journal of Consulting and Clinical Psychology*, **52**, 642–50.
57. Heimberg, R.G., Liebowitz, M.R., Hope, D.A., *et al.* (1998). Cognitive-behavioral group therapy versus phenelzine in social phobia: 12-week outcome. *Archives of General Psychiatry*, **55**, 1133–41.
58. Heimberg, R.G., Dodge, C.S., Hope, D.A., *et al.* (1990). Cognitive behavioral group treatment for social phobia: comparison with a credible placebo control. *Cognitive Therapy and Research*, **14**, 1–23.
59. Taylor, S. (1996). Meta-analysis of cognitive-behavioral treatments for social phobia. *Journal of Behavior Therapy and Experimental Psychiatry*, **27**, 1–9.
60. Gould, R.A., Buckminster, S., Pollack, M.H., *et al.* (1997). Cognitive-behavioral and pharmacological treatment for social phobia: a meta-analysis. *Clinical Psychology: Science and Practice*, **4**, 291–306.
61. Heimberg, R.G., Salzman, D.G., Holt, C.S., *et al.* (1993). Cognitive-behavioral group treatment for social phobia: effectiveness at five-year followup. *Cognitive Therapy and Research*, **17**, 325–39.
62. Liebowitz, M.R., Heimberg, R.G., Schneier, F.R., *et al.* (1999). Cognitive-behavioral group therapy versus phenelzine in social phobia: long-term outcome. *Depression and Anxiety*, **10**, 89–98.
63. Mörtberg, E., Karlsson, A., Fyring, C., *et al.* (2006). Intensive cognitive-behavioral group treatment (CBGT) of social phobia: a randomized controlled study. *Journal of Anxiety Disorders*, **20**, 646–60.
64. Clark, D.M., Ehlers, A., Hackmann, A., *et al.* (2006). Cognitive therapy versus exposure and applied relaxation in social phobia: a randomized controlled trial. *Journal of Consulting and Clinical Psychology*, **74**, 568–78.
65. Clark, D.M., Ehlers, A., McManus, F., *et al.* (2003). Cognitive therapy vs fluoxetine in generalized social phobia: a randomized placebo controlled trial. *Journal of Consulting and Clinical Psychology*, **71**, 1058–67.
66. Stangier, U., Heidenreich, T., Peitz, M., *et al.* (2003). Cognitive therapy for social phobia: individual versus group treatment. *Behaviour Research and Therapy*, **41**, 991–1007.
67. Mörtberg, E., Clark, D.M., Sundin, Ö., *et al.* (2007). Intensive group cognitive treatment and individual cognitive therapy vs treatment as usual in social phobia: a randomized controlled trial. *Acta Psychiatrica Scandinavica*, **115**, 142–54.
68. Fedoroff, I.C. and Taylor, S. (2001). Psychological and pharmacological treatments for social anxiety disorder: a meta-analysis. *Journal of Clinical Psychopharmacology*, **21**, 311–24.
69. Kobak, K.A., Greist, J.H., Jefferson, J.W., *et al.* (2002). Fluoxetine in social phobia: a double-blind, placebo-controlled pilot study. *Journal of Clinical Psychopharmacology*, **22**, 257–62.
70. Lader, M., Stender, K., Burger, V., *et al.* (2004). The efficacy and tolerability of escitalopram in the short-and long-term treatment of social anxiety disorder: a randomised, double blind, placebo-controlled, fixed-dose study. *Depression and Anxiety*, **19**, 241–48.
71. Liebowitz, M.R., Gelenberg, A.J., and Munjack, D, (2005). Venlafaxine extended release vs placebo and paroxetine in social anxiety disorder. *Archives of General Psychiatry*, **62**, 190–8.
72. Liebowitz, M.R., Stein, M.B., Tancer, M., *et al.* (2002). A randomized, double-blind, fixed-dose comparison of paroxetine and placebo in the treatment of generalized social anxiety disorder. *The Journal of Clinical Psychiatry*, **63**, 66–74.
73. Stein, M.B., Liebowitz, M.R., Lydiard, R.B., *et al.* (1998). Paroxetine treatment of generalized social phobia (social anxiety disorder): a randomized controlled trial. *The Journal of the American Medical Association*, **280**, 708–13.
74. Stein, D.J., Versiani, M., Hair, T., *et al.* (2002). Efficacy of paroxetine for relapse prevention in social anxiety disorder: a 24-week study. *Archives of General Psychiatry*, **59**, 1111–18.
75. Van Ameringen, M.A., Lane, K.M., Walker, J.R., *et al.* (2001). Sertraline treatment for generalized social phobia: a 20-week, double-blind, placebo controlled study. *The American Journal of Psychiatry*, **158**, 275–81.
76. Walker, J.R., van Ameringen, M.A., Swinson, R., *et al.* (2000). Prevention of relapse in generalized social phobia: results of a 24-week study in responders to 20 weeks of sertraline treatment. *Journal of Clinical Psychopharmacology*, **20**, 636–44.
77. Stein, M.B., Fyer, A.J., Davidson, J.R.T., *et al.* (1999). Fluvoxamine treatment of social phobia (social anxiety disorder): a double-blind, placebo-controlled study. *The American Journal of Psychiatry*, **156**, 756–60.
78. Davidson, J.R., Foa, E.B., Huppert, J.D., *et al.* (2004). Fluoxetine, comprehensive cognitive behavioral therapy, and placebo in generalized social phobia. *Archives of General Psychiatry*, **61**, 1005–13.
79. Davidson, J.R.T., Potts, N., Richichi, E., *et al.* (1993). Treatment of social phobia with clonazepam and placebo. *Journal of Clinical Psychopharmacology*, **13**, 423–8.

80. Otto, M.W., Pollack, M.H., Gould, R.A., *et al.* (2000). A comparison of the efficacy of clonazepam and cognitive-behavioral group therapy for the treatment of social phobia. *Journal of Anxiety Disorders*, **14**, 345–58.
81. Gelernter, C.S., Uhde, T.W., Cimbolic, P., *et al.* (1991). Cognitive-behavioral and pharmacological treatments of social phobia: a controlled study. *Archives of General Psychiatry*, **48**, 938–45.
82. Liebowitz, M.R., Schneier, F.R., Campeas, R., *et al.* (1992). Phenelzine vs atenolol in social phobia: a placebo-controlled comparison. *Archives of General Psychiatry*, **49**, 290–300.
83. Versiani, M., Nardi, A.E., Mundim, F.D., *et al.* (1992). Pharmacotherapy of social phobia: a controlled study with moclobemide and phenelzine. *The British Journal of Psychiatry*, **161**, 353–60.
84. Clark, D.B. and Agras, W.S. (1991). The assessment and treatment of performance anxiety in musicians. *The American Journal of Psychiatry*, **148**, 598–605.
85. Schneier, F.R., Saoud, J., Campeas, R., *et al.* (1993). Buspirone in social phobia. *Journal of Clinical Psychopharmacology*, **13**, 251–6.
86. Pande, A.C., Davidson, J.R.T., Jefferson, J.W., *et al.* (1999). Treatment of social phobia with gabapentin: a placebo-controlled study. *Journal of Clinical Psychopharmacology*, **19**, 341–8.
87. Feltner, D.E., Pollack, M.H., Davidson, J.R.T., *et al.* (2000). A placebo-controlled, double-blind study of pregabalin treatment of social phobia: outcome and predictors of response. *European Neuropsychopharmacology*, **10**, 345–55.
88. Walker, D.L., Ressler, K.J., Lu, K.T., *et al.* (2002). Facilitation of conditioned fear extinction by systemic administration or intra-amygdala infusions of d-cycloserine as assessed with fear-potentiated startle in rats. *The Journal of Neuroscience*, **22**, 2343–51.
89. Hofmann, S.G., Meuret, A.E., Smits, J.A.J., *et al.* (2006). Augmentation of exposure therapy with d-cycloserine for social anxiety disorder. *Archives of General Psychiatry*, **63**, 298–304.
90. Blomhoff, S., Haug, T.T., Hellstrøm, K., *et al.* (2001). Randomized controlled general practice trial of setraline, exposure therapy, and combined treatment in generalized social phobia. *The British Journal of Psychiatry*, **179**, 23–30.
91. Haug, T.T., Blomhoff, S., Hellstrøm, K., *et al.* (2003). Exposure therapy and sertraline in social phobia: 1-year follow-up of a randomized controlled trial. *The British Journal of Psychiatry*, **182**, 312–8.
92. Heimberg, R.G. (2002). Cognitive behavioral therapy for social anxiety disorder: current status and future directions. *Biological Psychiatry*, **51**, 101–8.
93. Safren, S.A., Heimberg, R.G., and Juster, H.R. (1997). Clients' expectancies and their relationship to pretreatment symptomatology and outcome of cognitive-behavioral group treatment for social phobia. *Journal of Consulting and Clinical Psychology*, **65**, 694–8.
94. Erwin, B.A., Heimberg, R.G., Juster, H., *et al.* (2002). Comorbid anxiety and mood disorders among persons with social anxiety disorder. *Behaviour Research and Therapy*, **40**, 19–35.
95. Barrett, P.M., Rapee, R.M., Dadds, M.R., *et al.* (1996). Family enhancement of cognitive style in anxious and aggressive children. *Journal of Abnormal Child Psychology*, **24**, 187–203.
96. Barrett, P. and Turner, C. (2001). Prevention of anxiety symptoms in primary school children: preliminary results from a universal school-based trial. *The British Journal of Clinical Psychology*, **40**, 399–410.
97. Dadds, M.R., Holland, D.E., Laurens, K.R., *et al.* (1999). Early intervention and prevention of anxiety disorders in children: results at 2-year follow-up. *Journal of Consulting and Clinical Psychology*, **67**,145–50.
98. Barlow, D.H., DiNardo, P.A., Vermilyea, B.B., *et al.* (1986). Co-morbidity and depression among the anxiety disorders: issues in diagnosis and classification. *The Journal of Nervous and Mental Disease*, **174**, 63–72.
99. Merckelbach, H., de Jong, P.J., Muris, P., *et al.* (1996). The etiology of specific phobias: a review. *Clinical Psychology Review*, **16**, 337–61.
100. Thyer, B.A., Himle, J., and Curtis, G.C. (1985). Blood-injury-illness phobia: a review. *Journal of Clinical Psychology*, **41**, 451–9.
101. Fredrikson, M., Annas, P., Fischer, H., *et al.* (1996). Gender and age differences in the prevalence of specific fears and phobias. *Behaviour Research and Therapy*, **34**, 33–9.
102. Scheibe, G. and Albus, M. (1992). Age at onset, precipitating events, sex distribution, and co-occurrence of anxiety disorders. *Psychopathology*, **25**, 11–8.
103. Öst, L.G. and Treffers, P.D.A. (2001). Onset, course, and outcome for anxiety disorders in children. In *Anxiety disorders in children and adolescents: research, assessment and intervention* (eds. W.K. Silverman and P.D.A. Treffers), pp. 293–312. Cambridge University Press, Cambridge.
104. Fyer, A.J., Mannuzza, S., Chapman, T.F., *et al.* (1995). Specificity in familial aggregation of phobic disorders. *Archives of General Psychiatry*, **52**, 564–73.
105. Fyer, A.J., Mannuzza, S., Gallops, M.S., *et al.* (1990). Familial transmission of simple phobias and fears: a preliminary report. *Archives of General Psychiatry*, **47**, 252–6.
106. Biederman, J., Rosenbaum, J.F., Hirshfeld, D.R., *et al.* (1990). Psychiatric correlates of behavioral inhibition in young children of parents with and without psychiatric disorders. *Archives of General Psychiatry*, **47**, 21–6.
107. Pavlov, I. (1927). *Conditioned reflexes*. Oxford University Press, London.
108. Mowrer, O.H. (1939). Stimulus response theory of anxiety. *Psychological Review*, **46**, 553–65.
109. Marks, I.M. (1969). *Fears and phobias*. Academic Press, New York.
110. Seligman, M.E. (1971). Phobias and preparedness. *Behavior Therapy*, **2**, 307–20.
111. Boyd, J.H., Rae, D.S., Thompson, J.W., *et al.* (1990). Phobia: prevalence and risk factors. *Social Psychiatry and Psychiatric Epidemiology*, **25**, 314–23.
112. Marks, I.M. (1987). Fears, phobias, and rituals: panic, anxiety, and their disorders. Oxford University Press, London.
113. Hecker, J.E. (1990). Emotional processing in the treatment of simple phobia: a comparison of imaginal and in vivo exposure. *Behavioural Psychotherapy*, **18**, 21–34.
114. Gotestam, K.G. and Berntzen, D. (1997). Use of the modeling effect in one-session exposure. *Scandinavian Journal of Behaviour Therapy*, **26**, 97–101.
115. Öst, L.G. (1996). One-session group treatment of spider phobia. *Behaviour Research and Therapy*, **34**, 707–15.
116. Chambless, D.L. (1990). Spacing of exposure sessions in treatment of agoraphobia and simple phobia. *Behavior Therapy*, **21**, 217–29.
117. Öst, L.G., Salkovskis, P.M., and Hellstrom, K. (1991). One-session therapist-directed exposure vs self-exposure in the treatment of spider phobia. *Behavior Therapy*, **22**, 407–22.
118. Carlin, A.S., Hoffman, H.G., and Weghorst, S. (1997). Virtual reality and tactile augmentation in the treatment of spider phobia: a case report. *Behaviour Research and Therapy*, **35**, 153–8.
119. North, M.M., North, S.M., and Coble, J.R. (1997). Virtual reality therapy for fear of flying. *The American Journal of Psychiatry*, **154**, 130.
120. Rothbaum, B.O., Hodges, L., Watson, B.A., *et al.* (1996). Virtual reality exposure therapy in the treatment of fear of flying: a case report. *Behaviour Research and Therapy*, **34**, 477–81.
121. Rothbaum, B.O., Hodges, L., Anderson, P.L., *et al.* (2002). Twelve-month follow-up of virtual reality and standard exposure therapies for the fear of flying. *Journal of Consulting and Clinical Psychology*, **70**, 428–32.
122. Maltby, N., Kirsch, I., Mayers, M., *et al.* (2002). Virtual reality exposure therapy for the treatment of fear of flying: a controlled investigation. *Journal of Consulting and Clinical Psychology*, **70**, 1112–8.
123. Ressler, K.J., Rothbaum, B.O., Tannenbaum, L., *et al.* (2004). Cognitive enhancers as adjuncts to psychotherapy: use of d-cycloserine in phobic individuals to facilitate extinction of fear. *Archives of General Psychiatry*, **61**, 1136–44.

124. Bernstein, D.A., Borkovec, T.D., and Hazlett-Stevens, H. (2000). *New directions in progressive relaxation training: a guidebook for helping professionals*. Prager/Greenwood, Westport, CT.
125. Öst, L.G. (1987). Applied relaxation: description of a coping technique and review of controlled studies. *Behaviour Research and Therapy*, **25**, 397–409.
126. Öst, L.G., Johansson, J., and Jerremalm, A. (1982). Individual response patterns and the effects of different behavioral methods in the treatment of claustrophobia. *Behaviour Research and Therapy*, **20**, 445–60.
127. Öst, L.G., Sterner, U., and Fellenius, J. (1989). Applied tension, applied relaxation, and the combination in the treatment of blood phobia. *Behaviour Research and Therapy*, **27**, 109–21.
128. Öst, L.G., Fellenius, J., and Sterner, U. (1991). Applied tension, exposure *in vivo*, and tension-only in the treatment of blood phobia. *Behaviour Research and Therapy*, **29**, 561–74.
129. Hellstrøm, K., Fellenius, J., and Öst. L.G. (1996). One versus five sessions of applied tension in the treatment of blood phobia. *Behaviour Research and Therapy*, **34**, 101–12.
130. Thorpe, S.J. and Salkovskis, P.M. (1995). Phobia beliefs: do cognitive factors play a role in specific phobias? *Behavior Research and Therapy*, **33**, 805–16.
131. Greco, T.S. (1989). A cognitive-behavioral approach to fear of flying: a practitioner's guide. *Phobia Practice and Research Journal*, **2**, 3–15.
132. Campos, P.E., Solyom, L., and Koelink, A. (1984). The effects of timolol maleate on subjective and physiological components of air travel phobia. *Canadian Journal of Psychiatry*, **29**, 570–4.
133. Sartory, G. (1983). Benzodiazepines and behavioral treatment of phobic anxiety. *Behavioural Psychotherapy*, **11**, 204–17.
134. Norton, G.R. and Johnson, W.E. (1983). A comparison of two relaxation procedures for reducing cognitive and somatic anxiety. *Journal of Behavior Therapy and Experimental Psychiatry*, **14**, 209–14.

4.7.3 Panic disorder and agoraphobia

James C. Ballenger

Introduction

Panic disorder draws its name from the Greek god Pan, god of flocks. Pan was known for suddenly frightening animals and humans 'out of the blue'. The spontaneous 'out of the blue' character of panic attacks is the principal identifying characteristic of panic disorder and central to its recognition and diagnosis.

We know the syndrome that we currently call panic disorder with and without agoraphobia has probably existed since the beginning of recorded history. Hippocrates presented cases of obvious phobic avoidance around 400 BC.[1] One of the first modern descriptions was by Benedikt around 1870, describing individuals who developed sudden anxiety and dizziness in public places.[2]

Certainly, our current modern ideas of panic disorder evolved essentially simultaneously in the United States and Europe in the early to mid-1960s. Donald Klein in the United States described in 1964 the panic syndrome and reported that it was responsive to imipramine.[3] Isaac Marks in the United Kingdom also described panic attacks and agoraphobic avoidance, and treating the syndrome effectively with behaviour therapy.[4]

Until the last several decades, panic disorder and agoraphobia were actually thought to be rare syndromes. It is now clear that individuals with these difficulties are anything but rare. In fact, panic disorder is one of the most common presenting problems in individuals seeking mental health treatment and the fifth most common problem seen in primary care settings.[5] It was thought to be a mild problem, but we now know that it is associated with significant dysfunction. The disability in social, occupational, and family life is in fact comparable to major depression.

Although there are differences in the understandings of panic disorder and its treatments across the world, this chapter will review the current understanding about panic disorder, its characteristics, diagnosis, aetiology, and treatments.

Clinical features

One of the earliest and most accurate descriptions of panic attacks was provided by Charles Darwin in 1872 as he described his own episodes:

> The heartbeats quickly and violently so that it palpitates and knocks against the ribs . . . the skin instantly becomes pale as during incipient faintness . . . under a sense of great fear . . . in connection with the disturbed action of the heart, the breathing is hurried . . . one of the best marked symptoms is the trembling of all the muscles of the body.[6]

The most characteristic type of panic attack is the spontaneous 'out of the blue' episode of extreme anxiety. Other 'situational panic attacks' occur immediately upon exposure, or in anticipation of exposure to particular situations, usually where panic attacks have occurred previously. Some individuals have panic attacks in certain situations some of the time, but not always, and these are labelled 'situationally predisposed panic attacks'.

Panic attacks also occur in other anxiety syndromes and are more or less the same in whatever syndrome where they occur. However, spontaneous panic attacks in panic disorder tend to have more dizziness, paraesthesia, shaking, chest pain, and fears of going mad. Shortness of breath is more common in panic attacks in agoraphobia. Certainly blushing is particularly characteristic of panic attacks in social phobia.

The symptoms of panic attacks in order of their frequency include palpitations, pounding heart, tachycardia, sweating, trembling or shaking, shortness of breath or smothering, feeling of choking, chest pain or discomfort, nausea or abdominal distress, feeling dizzy, unsteady, lightheaded or faint, derealization or depersonalization, fear of losing control or going mad, fear of dying, paraesthesia, and chills or hot flushes.

Panic attacks by definition generally involve four or more of the above symptoms to meet diagnostic criteria for panic disorder in the DSM-IV. The anxiety is crescendo in nature, building to a peak in 10 min in most cases. Panic attacks usually last for several minutes, but in some patients they can last for hours. The frequency and severity of panic attacks varies greatly between individuals and, at times, in individuals. Some have only one to three panic attacks per year, whereas others may have multiple panic attacks each day. Some individuals have bursts of panic attacks and then an absence of all attacks for a period of time. Across a large panic disorder clinical trial, the typical patient described one to two panic attacks per week.[7]

Panic attacks with fewer than four symptoms have been labelled 'limited-symptom attacks' or 'little panic attacks', and most individuals with panic disorder have these, as well as panic attacks with four or more symptoms. The threshold of four symptoms was chosen for DSM-IV because individuals with panic attacks with four symptoms or more had more disability than patients with one- to three-symptom attacks. This threshold is clearly arbitrary, and patients having panic attacks with fewer symptoms do have significant morbidity.

Panic attacks are extremely frightening and patients develop an essentially logical fear of having more panic attacks. Patients develop worry and anxiety about the possibility of panic attacks recurring. This anxiety between attacks has been called 'anticipatory anxiety' and can be almost constant, and characteristically increases prior to exposure to situations previously associated with panic attacks (e.g. having to shop in the supermarket where a panic attack has occurred).

A significant number of people with panic attacks go on to develop fear and avoidance of situations associated with previous panic attacks. They also fear situations where escape would be difficult or embarrassing, or where help might not be available. Most patients mistakenly believe they become incapacitated and incapable of taking care of themselves during a panic attack and therefore, many go on to develop avoidance of a variety of situations where they could not easily get help. Factor analytical studies demonstrate that there are clusters of situations associated with avoidance. These typically include public transportation (e.g. buses, trains, planes), riding in or driving a car, especially on heavily travelled roads, crowds (e.g. the cinema, a football match, large shopping centres), shopping (especially in supermarkets), particularly where one must stand in queues, and bridges, tunnels, elevators, and other enclosed spaces.[8] In the event of a panic attack, people often have an overwhelming need to escape or return to a place of safety such as home. Therefore they fear situations where escape is difficult or impossible, e.g. airplanes, traffic jams on a bridge, dental appointments, etc. On closer examination, it is clear that patients do not actually fear the situation itself but rather reason 'what if' the panic feelings occur while in that situation. This has led to the syndrome being called the 'what if' syndrome, emphasizing that there is actually a 'fear of the fear'.[9]

Patients tend to avoid such situations or force themselves to endure them in distress or take a companion along 'to help'. Others limit their travel to short distances from home or take longer routes where they perceive help would be available (e.g. police, doctors' offices, fire stations, etc).

Some patients develop agoraphobic avoidance following their first attack, some only after frequent and severe attacks, and some never develop agoraphobic avoidance. In community samples, one-third to half of patients who meet criteria for panic disorder also has significant agoraphobic avoidance. The rate is higher (75 per cent) in most clinical samples. A minority (5 per cent) ultimately become unable to leave their homes and are housebound.

Many patients have panic attacks that awaken them from sleep (nocturnal panic attacks), as well as during the day. These are in fact quite common and the majority of panic disorder patients experience them. These occur during slow wave sleep early in sleep. These panic attacks are essentially identical to traditional panic attacks that occur during the day. There is a group of patients who have what are called non-fearful panic attacks. These involve the sudden onset of physiological symptoms without the cognitive components of fear or anxiety. These primarily are medical patients, usually cardiac, who might have episodes of sudden tachycardia and palpitations but no fear.[10]

Classification

The earliest modern accounts of what is almost certainly the panic disorder syndrome began appearing in the mid-1900s. There were accounts beginning in 1866 of paroxysmal anxiety episodes that did not use the term 'panic attack'. During the American Civil War, patients were diagnosed with 'irritable heart syndrome' or 'Da Costa syndrome' (1871) with clear descriptions of what we now know as panic disorder. Westphal in Germany in 1872 clearly described patients having panic attacks and agoraphobic avoidance of wide open spaces.[11] Again, in the First World War (1918) the syndrome 'neurocirculatory asthenia' was described which had most of the features of panic disorder.

It was, in fact, Freud in Case IV of Katharina, published in 1895, who set the background for the modern classification of panic disorder. However, it was the Feighner criteria published in the United States in 1972 that give the first formal diagnostic recognition to the syndrome.[12] The Research Diagnostic Criteria (RDC) which followed in 1978 first split panic disorder away from what we now call generalized anxiety disorder (GAD). In the RDC, panic disorder had panic attacks while GAD did not. These diagnoses were made part of the DSM-III diagnostic scheme in 1980.

It was the conceptualization of panic disorder by Donald Klein in 1964 in the United States that led to the predominant view of the syndrome, certainly in the United States.[13] Klein argued that panic attacks were the core of the syndrome, and the remaining clinical phenomena were consequences of the panic attacks. He conceptualized that anticipatory anxiety was the fear of the possible recurrence of panic attacks, and similarly that agoraphobia was the subsequent fear and avoidance of situations where panic attacks had occurred. The bringing together of these three phenomena into one concept was accepted in the DSM-IIIR, and more recently in the DSM-IV in the United States.[14]

The biological findings that typical panic attacks could be elicited in panic disorder patients with infusions of lactate, doses of caffeine, or breathing 35 per cent CO_2 supported this conceptualization of the syndrome as primarily centered around panic attacks. This hypothesis was further supported by epidemiological findings of essentially the same illness around the world.

However, this idea remains controversial across the different sides of the Atlantic. The American DSM-IIIR and DSM-IV diagnostic schema continue to utilize the idea that panic attacks are pre-eminent and created two diagnoses: panic disorder and panic disorder with agoraphobia. In Europe and in the ICD-10, agoraphobia is conceptualized as dominant over panic attacks. Therefore, when agoraphobia and panic attacks are both present, the diagnosis is conceptualized as a phobia and that condition is diagnosed as agoraphobia with panic attacks. Beyond this theoretical debate is the clinical question whether the treatment should be aimed first at panic attacks (in the United States concept) or at agoraphobic avoidance, for example with exposure therapy (in the European schema).

(a) Diagnosis

The most recently revised diagnostic schema for this syndrome is the DSM-IV. Changes from the DSM-IIIR were made based on two principles:

1 any new empirical data that required changes be made;

2 an attempt to make the DSM-IV and ICD-10 more compatible.

For the diagnoses of panic disorder and agoraphobia, an attempt was also made to more nearly describe the prototypic patient and to move away from the pseudoquantification of using number of panic attacks per week.(14)

The DSM-IV clarified that panic attacks occurred in multiple syndromes including social phobia, obsessive–compulsive disorder, depression, and others. However, DSM-IV utilized the distinction that only in panic disorder were there recurrent spontaneous panic attacks not bound to any particular situation. The diagnosis of panic disorder has several requirements including the following:

- Recurrent, unexpected panic attacks (situational panic attacks could also occur but there would need to be at least two unexpected panic attacks by history).
- Panic attacks needed to be followed by at least 1 month of persistent anxiety about potential recurrence of further panic attacks, implications of these attacks (e.g. going mad, something wrong medically), or a significant behavioural change because of these attacks. This was necessary because some patients had panic attacks and completely changed their lives but denied that they were worried about experiencing more panic attacks or the implications of the panic attacks.(14)

The agoraphobia criteria remained largely unchanged, but it was made more clear that the diagnosis was based on persistent fear and avoidance of certain clusters of situations and listed the most common.

The controversial diagnosis of agoraphobia without a history of panic disorder was retained until further clarification is obtained through research. Our current understanding is that these patients generally have never fully met criteria for panic disorder because their panic-like symptoms have not met the diagnostic criterion requiring four full symptoms for a panic attack. Available research suggests that these patients are otherwise very much like typical patients with panic disorder and agoraphobia. Some patients actually have only one or two symptoms (e.g. fear of loss of bladder or bowel control or only tachycardia).

Perhaps the most difficult diagnostic issue is the frequent comorbidity. The Epidemiologic Catchment Area study documented that approximately 50 per cent of panic disorder patients over their lifetime have another anxiety disorder.(15)

In actuality, depression is more commonly comorbid with panic disorder than even agoraphobia and suggests a close relationship between these syndromes. Comorbid depression ranged from 22.5 to 68.2 per cent in various samples. Lifetime rates vary from 35 to 91 per cent.(16) Although approximately half the patients developed panic disorder and depression at essentially the same time, one-quarter develop depression before panic disorder and one-quarter panic disorder before depression.(17) Surprisingly, bipolar illness has been reported to be as high as 20.8 per cent.

Easily one-third of panic disorder patients abuse alcohol. The percentage in clinical samples is much higher with 13 to 43 per cent of panic disorder patients also meeting criteria for alcoholism.(18)

(b) Differential diagnosis

It is particularly important to determine whether agoraphobic avoidance is present, because its treatment usually requires some sort of exposure therapy. Patients will often not volunteer that they are avoiding certain situations out of embarrassment. As mentioned earlier, depression and panic disorder often occur together and again patients often do not describe the other syndrome, but rather describe the syndrome which is most painful to them at that time. However, proper recognition of comorbid depression is especially important because of the marked increase (four-fold) in suicide attempts in patients with panic disorder and depression.

The difference between panic disorder and GAD depends on whether patients have panic attacks and whether they have multiple, unrealistic, and excessive worries about most aspects of life, not just panic attacks. These worries in GAD often concern money, health, children, work problems, etc. The differential with social phobia centres on whether the anxiety is confined entirely towards social situations where the individual fears embarrassment and humiliation. Specific phobias involve panic attacks, but they occur in very specific situations (e.g. high places, thunderstorms) or in the presence of specific objects (e.g. animals, snakes). The post-traumatic stress disorder patient may have many panic-like symptoms, but their illness begins quite specifically after a traumatic experience and anxiety is associated with reminders of that trauma. Finally, obsessive–compulsive disorder can involve panic attacks but only in the specific context of obsessional concerns (e.g. contamination, etc.). In these patients, panic attacks are also dwarfed in importance by typical obsessions and compulsions/rituals concerning contamination, symmetry, bad events, etc.

(c) Medical conditions

Panic-like symptoms do occur in various medical conditions (hyperthyroidism, phaeochromocytoma, hyperparathyroidism, seizures, cardiac arrhythmias, especially supraventricular tachycardia, inner ear difficulties, chronic obstructive pulmonary disease, use of marijuana, withdrawal from drugs of abuse, and over the counter drugs containing caffeine or pseudoephedrine) (Table 4.7.3.1). Also, the typical panic disorder patient does report a large number of physical symptoms and usually to a non-psychiatric physician.

As mentioned, there are medical conditions that can mimic panic disorder (Table 4.7.3.1). There is also evidence that there are slightly increased rates of certain illnesses, for example hyperthyroidism (11–13 per cent) and perhaps mitral valve prolapse. However, these are uncommon in panic disorder patients. Most experts recommend a relatively conservative diagnostic medical work-up. Generally, the most valuable part of a medical examination is a careful history with follow-up of any strongly suggested possibilities, supplemented by a few laboratory tests (complete blood count, thyroid function tests, metabolic screen, and ECG, especially if the patient is over 40 years of age).

(d) Panic disorder in the general medical setting

Conservative estimates of panic disorder in primary care have ranged from 3 to 8 per cent with at least 50 per cent going unrecognized.(19) The average panic disorder patient in general medicine

Table 4.7.3.1 Medical conditions that produce panic-like symptoms

Endocrine	*Respiratory*
Hyperthyroidism	Chronic obstructive
Hypoparathyroidism	pulmonary disease
Hypoglycaemia	Asthma
Phaeochromacytoma	*Substance-induced*
Carcinoid syndrome	Caffeine
Cushing's disease	Cocaine
Cardiovascular	Marijuana
Arrhythmias (supraventricular)	Theophylline
Atypical chest pain	Amphetamines
Mitral valve prolapse	Steroids
Neurological	Alcohol/sedative
Seizures	withdrawal
Vestibular disease	*Haematological*
	Anaemia

takes 10 years or more for a correct diagnosis to be made with an escalation of the use of health care services over this period. In general, the presence of panic disorder leads to a three-fold increase in utilization of general medical services.

The percentage of panic disorder patients is also markedly higher in certain medical groups. These include the very prevalent but most difficult to diagnose patients with vague symptoms such as fatigue, back pain, headache, dizziness, chest pain, etc.[20] or multiple symptoms (more than five).[21]

In a classic study of unrecognized panic disorder patients who were referred for a psychiatric consultation from primary care, 39 per cent had cardiovascular symptoms, 33 per cent gastrointestinal symptoms, and 44 per cent neurological.[22] It is now clear that 16 to 25 per cent of patients presenting to the emergency room with chest pain have panic disorder. Fully 25 per cent of cardiology practice involves panic disorder, usually unrecognized with 80 per cent of patients with chest pain and normal angiograms ultimately diagnosed with panic disorder. We could also increase our yield of recognizing panic disorder patients in certain procedure-oriented situations. For instance, 28 per cent of patients referred for Holter monitoring for palpitations have panic disorder, as do 66 per cent of patients undergoing a work-up to rule out phaeochromocytoma.[23] Also, 44 per cent of irritable bowel syndrome and 15 per cent of patients with headache symptoms seeing a physician have panic disorder, and these are both very prevalent disorders.

Recent studies document that treatment of panic disorder in the medical setting when diagnosed there is most cost-effective.

(e) Comment

A recent large study sponsored by the World Health Organization (WHO) studied primary care patients in 14 different countries.[19] Of patients in that study who had a single panic attack in the previous month, 99 per cent had an anxiety disorder or depression, or a subthreshold anxiety disorder or depressive disorder. The occurrence of a single panic attack also predicted the onset of panic disorder in two-thirds of the patients studied in the next year, a four-fold increase in depression (51 per cent) in the next year, and marked increases in alcoholism, social phobia, and obsessive–compulsive disorder. It would appear that the occurrence of even a single panic attack may well represent the 'tip of the iceberg' and should serve as a signal for increased scrutiny for anxiety and depressive syndromes. This has been recently replicated in a large ($N = 3021$) European sample.[24]

Epidemiology

Surveys largely utilizing DSM diagnoses have found wide agreement and generally equal prevalence's of panic disorder across many countries.[16,25] Utilizing specific criteria for panic attacks, prevalence for panic attacks has generally averaged 7 to 9 per cent of the population (range 1.8–22.7 per cent). However, if criteria for panic attacks are liberalized somewhat ('fearful spells') in terms of the number of times and severity, the prevalence doubles.

There is a striking uniformity worldwide for the observed prevalence of panic disorder. In 10 community studies involving over 40 000 subjects, the majority of studies found lifetime prevalence rates for panic disorder averaging 1.5 to 3.7 per cent, with a yearly prevalence of around 1 and 1.1 per cent of panic disorder with agoraphobia (lifetime).[25] In clinical samples there is greater variability. In the previously mentioned WHO survey of 14 countries, the prevalence for panic disorder in primary care ranged from a low of 1.4 per cent to a high of 16.5 per cent for panic attacks and 0 to 3.5 per cent for panic disorder itself.[19] The average was 1.1 per cent (currently) and 3.5 per cent (lifetime), which is surprisingly similar to the community samples. As mentioned, rates are much higher in specialized medical clinics and range from 15 per cent in dizziness clinics, to 16 to 65 per cent in cardiology practices, to 35 per cent in hyperventilation clinics, etc.

Risk factors

Panic disorder has been uniformly observed to be at least two times more prevalent in females than males.[25] The Epidemiologic Catchment Area study demonstrated a prevalence of 3:2. In clinical samples it is generally 3:1. The onset of panic disorder appears to fall into two peaks. The first occurs in the early to mid-twenties (15–24 years old) with a second peak at 45–54 years of age. The onset of panic disorder after the age of 65 is rare (0.1 per cent).

The highest rates of panic disorder and agoraphobia occur in widowed, divorced, or separated individuals living in cities. Limited education, early parental loss, and physical or sexual abuse are also risk factors. Agoraphobia is clearly more prevalent in females, and females make up three-quarters of the sample with extensive avoidance. Males tend to have longer duration of illness but less agoraphobia and depression, and less frequent help seeking. Perhaps the greater necessity to perform in the workplace retards avoidance in males.

Aetiology

Genetic predisposition

Certainly the preponderance of evidence suggests there is a genetic contribution to the predisposition to develop panic attacks and agoraphobia. There are increased rates of panic disorder in first-degree relatives ranging from 2- to 20-fold with the median seven- to eight-fold. Overall, studies suggest that another affected relative can be found 25 to 50 per cent of the time, two times as often in female relatives. The increased familial aggregation is specific for panic disorder. These findings are certainly consistent with a modest genetic transmission with relatively high specificity.

Although twin studies are limited, Torgersen[26] did find increased concordance in monozygotic twins (31 versus 0 per cent). In the largest sample of interviewed female twins, a several-fold increase was again found (23.9 versus 10.9 per cent).[27] Skre *et al.*[28] found a two-fold increase of panic disorder in monozygotic twins, while other studies fail to find an increased incidence.

Overall, evidence from family and twin studies suggests that panic disorder involves modest inheritability of around 30 to 40 per cent. The best model suggests 50 per cent genetic and 50 per cent environmental influences. Recent linkage studies to confirm these hypotheses have been contradictory (e.g. with angiotensin, brain-derived neurotropic factor) but do suggest that single-gene transmission is unlikely. However, research is active in this area with positive replicated linkages with chromosomes 13q, 22q, 7p, and 9q31. Identified candidate genes include the ADOR2A, 10832/T, CCK genes, and genes coding for the 5HT1A, 5HT2A, and COMT genes and there is evidence of a link to the corticotrophin releasing hormone gene.[29] This leaves the possibilities of either heterogeneity across families and/or a polygenic inheritance.[30]

Several converging lines do link childhood anxiety with adult anxiety, consistent with a genetic predisposition. This is particularly true for separation anxiety in children. Kagan *et al.*[31] have prescribed that 10 per cent of Caucasian children are born with heightened anxiety which they call behavioural inhibition. Behavioural inhibition is higher in children of anxiety-disordered parents, and there are high rates of anxiety disorders in children of adults with panic disorder. As behaviourally inhibited children have matured, they have been found to show higher rates of anxiety and phobic disorders.[32] Currently, this is probably the best model of an inherited anxiety predisposition. A variant of this type model proposes that there is an aethological factor involving an evolutionarily determined vulnerability to unfamiliar territory. This might explain why the seemingly inherited anxiety is to specific situations. This is also consistent with the high rate of precipitating events prior to the onset of clinical difficulties. In this model an evolutionarily/genetically determined vulnerability would be clinically 'activated' by critical stressors.

Precipitating events have been reported in 60 to 96 per cent of cases. These have often centred on separation or loss, relationship difficulties, taking on new responsibility, and physiological stressors (e.g. childbirth, surgery, hyperthyroidism).[33] This is certainly consistent with a diathesis/vulnerability model with the illness being precipitated in a predisposed individual in adulthood.

There are also many studies suggesting that traumatic early events may figure in the vulnerability leading to panic disorder. The majority of children in some studies have experienced early parental separation. A traumatic event in childhood has been retrospectively reported in at least two-thirds of individuals, a three-fold increase.[34] The most common adult disorder following sexual abuse before the age of five is in fact a 44 per cent incidence of agoraphobia.[35]

There is some evidence in a prospective study involving over 3000 individuals that dependent personality traits were later associated with the development of anxiety disorders. There are also retrospective data that adult panic disorder patients describe their parents as being overly protective and less caring. It is difficult to separate the effects on individuals of the anxiety disorders themselves which create dependent behaviour, or overprotectiveness in the parents producing dependent personality traits.

Biological models

(a) Noradrenaline

There is considerable evidence implicating the brain noradrenaline (norepinephrine) brain systems and panic disorder. The noradrenergic agents yohimbine and isoproterenol stimulate panic attacks in panic disorder patients, suggesting a possible subsensitivity of pre-synaptic alpha 2 inhibitory adrenoreceptors. Both these drugs increase the firing rate of the locus ceruleus, generally thought to be part of the brain anxiety circuit. It is also true that most effective medications in the treatment of panic disorder in fact decrease locus ceruleus firing rate and most panicogenic stimuli increase the locus ceruleus firing rate.

(b) Serotonin (5HT)

Findings with 5HT brain systems in panic disorder are contradictory, probably because of the different 5HT circuits and receptors in different areas of the brain. Most investigators believe, however, that an increase in 5HT transmission decreases panic disorder perhaps because 5HT neurones in ventrolateral periaqueductal grey appear to inhibit sympathoexcitation and the fight or flight response in the rat.[36] The principal human evidence for 5HT being central in panic is that the selective serotonin reuptake inhibitors are effective and that they increase 5HT transmission after long-term use. Also, rapid depletion of 5HT has been shown to result in an increase in panic responses to flumazenil. Whether this increased neurotramsmission in fact leads to downregulation of a supersensitive post-synaptic receptor is one logical possibility, but is as yet unproven. These theories received recent support from PET scan studies demonstrating reductions in brain 5HT1A receptors[37] and 5HT transporter binding.[38]

(c) γ-Aminobutyric acid

The γ-aminobutyric acid (GABA) system is almost certainly involved in panic disorder with perhaps the strongest evidence being that benzodiazepine agonists such as alprazolam and clonazepam are clearly effective treatments for panic disorder. Also GABA antagonists such as flumezanil have panicogenic effects in panic disorder patients, and reverse benzodiazepine agonists such as β-carbolines can cause panic attacks. There is an impaired GABA neuronal response to benzodiazepines (BZs) on brain magnetic spectroscopy and decreased GABA levels in the cingulate and basal ganglia, also on magnetic spectroscopy. Also, positron emission tomography data have demonstrated decreased benzodiazepine binding in the inferior brain areas, including the inferior parieto-temporo-occipital areas.

(d) Cholecystokinin–pentagastrin

Cholecystokinin is clearly involved in anxiety in animals. Also, panic disorder patients develop panic attacks in a dose-dependent fashion with administration of pentagastrin. However, cholecystokinin antagonists have not yet been shown to be effective in humans.

Recent genetic studies implicate CCK gene polymorphisms in panic disorder.

(e) Brain imaging

The explosion of brain imaging data demonstrating a brain circuit for fear and anxiety involving the extended amygdala circuit (amygdala, hippocampus, periaqueductal grey, locus coeruleus, thalamus, cingulate, and orbitofrontal areas) has lead to the hypotheses that it is this circuit which is abnormally active in panic disorder.[39]

(f) Psychological factors

Many critics disagree with the importance of biological findings in panic disorder, principally, various European workers and the cognitive theorists. They argue that panic attacks are not 'biological' and that a phobic attitude is required, and/or certain temperamental factors. Others attempt an integrated model utilizing both findings of biological differences and psychological factors of temperament and child-rearing practices.

Course and prognosis

There is limited evidence with appropriate population-based samples to clearly delineate the course of panic disorder. Available evidence suggests that panic disorder is a stable but chronic condition once criteria for the disorder are met. Most patients seeking treatment have experienced chronic, frequently chronically worsening, illness generally for 10 to 15 years prior to diagnosis.[7] However, other evidence does suggest that there is heterogeneity in terms of course.

As previously mentioned, the Klein model suggests that spontaneous panic attacks are the first manifestation of the illness, followed by anticipatory anxiety, and agoraphobia in some individuals. However, for most panic disorder patients examined closely, a panic attack is rarely the first symptom. In some studies, over 90 per cent of patients have had mild phobic or hypochondriacal, milder symptoms prior to the onset of their first panic attack.

The first panic attack is usually in a 'phobogenic' situation such as a public place, street, store, public transportation, crowd, elevator, tunnel, bridge, or open space. As mentioned, these are often preceded by stressful life events.

The earliest studies indicated low-recovery rates with chronic waxing and waning in most patients. Some individuals have outbreaks of symptomatology with less difficulty in between, but the majority of untreated individuals seem to have a more or less continuous symptom picture which ranges from mild to severe.

Recovery rates vary from 25 to 75 per cent for 1 to 2 years follow-up. Over a 5-year follow-up, only 10 to 12 per cent had fully recovered in one study and 30 per cent in another. The most common picture is about 50 per cent of patients are neither well nor very sick with mild symptoms most of the time.[40] After diagnosis and some sort of treatment, functional recovery occurs in the majority of patients.[41]

In acute pharmacological trials, 50 to 70 per cent of patients have excellent acute responses with another 20 per cent having a moderate response. With behavioural therapy, again the majority of patients recover and in some trials over 75 per cent of patients are much improved 1 to 9 years following therapy, with an average decrease in symptoms of 50 per cent.[42]

Poor responses were most consistently associated with initial high symptom severity and high agoraphobic avoidance at baseline. Poor response is also associated with low socio-economic status, less education, longer duration, limited social networks, death of a parent, divorce or unmarried status, and personality disorders.

Treatment

Introduction

Multiple effective treatments have been developed since the early 1960s and include both psychological and pharmacological treatments. Both exposure-based treatments and imipramine were shown to be effective in treating panic disorder and agoraphobia in the early 1960s.[3,4,43] Psychological-based treatments have moved increasingly towards cognitive behavioural therapy with efficacy roughly comparable to pharmacological treatments.

Imipramine and monoamine oxidase inhibitors (MAOIs) were the first medications shown to effectively treat panic disorder in the 1960s.[3,44] The high-potency benzodiazepines (alprazolam and clonazepam) were also shown to be effective in the 1980s.[7] Most now agree that the selective serotonin reuptake inhibitors (SSRIs) are the medication of first choice.[45–47]

Factors that influence the choice of initial treatment include patient preference and past history of treatment response, costs, and often availability. Medication treatment is usually easier to obtain but does involve significant costs and side effects. Although many patients prefer psychological treatments, as many as 10–30 per cent refuse treatments that involve exposure to frightening situations or resist the time and effort required. Where available, CBT can be more cost-effective than medications.

CBT has been modified in various ways to try to make it more easily available. This has included delivery in groups by computer or telephone or in shorter amounts or in a high intensity strategy with multiple hours of therapy over just a few days. All of these approaches show promise. There is clear evidence that bibliotherapy with and without phone contacts is also effective.

Eye movement desensitization and reprocessing (EMDR) was developed for treatment of post-traumatic stress disorder. The evidence available suggests that it is not effective in panic disorder.

Panic disorder can have an onset prior to adolescence, and it does occur frequently during adolescence. Although empirical data are very limited, it is generally assumed that treatments effective in adults are also effective in children. (see American Academy of Child and Adolescent Psychiatry's *Practice Parameters for the Assessment and Treatment of Children and Adolescents with Anxiety Disorders*.[48]

Medication treatments

(a) Selection of initial pharmacotherapy

Evidence indicates that medication from five classes—the SSRIs, SNRIs, benzodiazepines, tricyclics (TCAs), and monoamine oxidase inhibitors (MAOIs) are all roughly equal in their efficacy and therefore the choice of initial therapy should be made on other factors such as tolerability, cost, prior treatments, etc. (see Table 4.7.3.2). For patients with a history or concurrent depression (usually 25 per cent), the antidepressants would be preferable to the benzodiazepines. The antidepressants generally take 4 to 6 weeks to become effective, whereas the benzodiazepines begin working within the first week. There is evidence that adding benzodiazepines to the antidepressants speeds the therapeutic response.

Table 4.7.3.2 Advantages and disadvantages of various antipanic agents

	Advantages	Disadvantages
SSRIs	Well-tolerated antidepressant Safe in overdose Little weight gain Once-daily dosing	Initial activation Nausea, headache, asthenia, insomnia initially Sexual side effects
SNRIs	Very similar to SSRIs	*Hypertension*
Benzodiazepines	Rapid efficacy Reduce anticipatory anxiety Well tolerated No initial activation Safe in overdose	Sedation Some memory problems Withdrawal Abuse potential Rare sexual dysfunction
Tricyclic antidepressants	Single daily dose Less expensive Long experience Antidepressant	Initial activation Anticholinergic side effects Weight gain Orthostatic hypotension Dangerous in overdose Sexual dysfunction
MAOIs	More effective (against comorbid depression)? Antidepressant	Dietary restrictions Hypertensive crises (rare) Initial activation, insomnia Onset delayed Anticholinergic side effects Orthostatic hypotension Dangerous in overdose

A hyperstimulation reaction has been observed to all of the antidepressants and has lead to the widespread use of very low doses initially with gradual escalation. Benzodiazepines do not appear to produce the initial hyperstimulation response and are therefore preferred by many patients. However, difficulties with tapering and discontinuing benzodiazepines are the principal negative consideration for their use.

(b) Selective serotonin reuptake inhibitors (SSRIs)

In the United States, there are now six SSRIs available and three have FDA approval for panic disorder (fluoxetine, sertraline, and paroxetine—IR and CR formulations). There is no scientific or even clinical evidence to suggest significant differences in efficacy between the SSRIs in this indication. However, there are differences in side effects, principally, weight gain and discontinuation symptoms, different potential drug interactions, and availability of generic formulations.[49]

Initial jitteriness or increased anxiety are observed with the SSRIs. Therefore, treatment is often begun with the lowest doses available (see Table 4.7.3.3). Some patients do respond at lower doses, although most require higher doses (again see Table 4.7.3.3). The reason the SSRIs are generally regarded as the first choice for pharmacotherapy include their better tolerability and absence of anticholinnergic effects, compared to the TCAs. Patients often have mild difficulties with nausea, insomnia, headache. Certainly, the most problematic side effect is sexual dysfunction in both men and women, most frequently delay in orgasm. There are rare reports of extrapyramidal side effects and gastrointestinal bleeding. Discontinued too rapidly, withdrawal symptoms of headache, irritability, dizziness, can appear in the first 1 to 5 days after withdrawal, and generally clear within 1 to 2 weeks. These can generally be avoided by taper over 1 to 3 weeks.

(c) SNRIs

The SNRI venlafaxine has recently been demonstrated in large multicenter trials to be effective in the range of 75 to 225 mg/day. The side effect profile was similar in severity and symptomatology to the SSRIs, although a small number may develop sustained hypertension. There is some evidence that venlafaxine can result in higher rates of death from overdose than the SSRIs.

(d) Tricyclics (TCAs)

The first trial demonstrating that imipramine was significantly better than placebo was published in 1964[3] and was followed by multiple controlled trials demonstrating its effectiveness. There is also a significant number demonstrating effectiveness of clomipramine and some even demonstrating greater efficacy than imipramine.[50,51] Some data are supportive of desipramine and nortriptyline. Consistent problems with poorer tolerability compared to the SSRIs has lead to the TCAs being used only infrequently.

(e) Benzodiazepines (BZs)

The most widely studied and utilized benzodiazepine has been alprazolam. The largest trial was the Cross National Collaborative

Table 4.7.3.3 Medication doses in treatment of panic disorder

	Starting dose mg/day	Therapeutic range mg/day
SSRIs		
Paroxetine	10–12.5 CR	10–40*
Fluoxetine	2.5–10	10–20
Sertraline	25	50–200**
Fluovoxamine	50	100–300
Citalopram	10	20–30***
Escitalopram	5	5–10
SNRIs		
Venlafaxine	37.5	75–225
TCAs		
Imipramine	10	50–200
Clomipramine	25	25–150
BZs	TID or QID	Acute total daily dose
Alprazolam	0.25–0.5	2–10†
Clonazepam	0.25–0.5	1–4
Lorazepam	0.5	1–7
Diazepam	5	5–40
MAOIs	BID	
Phenelzine	15	15–45 (or 90)
Tranylcypromine	10	10–40 (or 70)

*40 mg demonstrated as target dose in RCT.

**All doses equivalent in one trial 50, 100, 200.

***In one trial, 20–30 was more effective than 40–60 mg/day.

†Mean dose 5.4 mg/day in largest trial.

Panic study involving more than 1000 patients and 11 trials, the majority of which were double-blind.[7] Alprazolam was effective against all of the symptoms of panic disorder, was comparable to imipramine and better tolerated. A sustained release form of alprazolam which can be taken once-daily is currently available. This formulation's long half-life appears to have solved the inter-dose rebound symptoms and 'clock watching' which was problematic with the immediate release form.

Clonazepam has also been demonstrated to be effective and is FDA approved for panic disorder in the United States.[52] Diazepam and lorazepam have also been shown to be clinically effective. Although generally well tolerated, the benzodiazepines principal side effects include sedation, occasional ataxia, slurred speech, and small increases in memory complaints. The largest concern and controversy has been with the possibility of dependency and the possibility of recreational abuse. However, the *American Psychiatric Association Task Force on Benzodiazepine Dependence, Toxicity and Abuse*, based on multiple large trials stated 'there are no data to suggest that long-term therapeutic use of benzodiazepines by patients commonly leads to dose escalation or to recreational use'.[53] Doses in long-term treatment are either similar to short-term or lower. Discontinuation symptomatology is perhaps the largest problem with the benzodiazepines. Panic patients have more difficulty discontinuing benzodiazepines than patients with generalized anxiety disorder. Symptoms are often seen during taper and are greatest during the last part of taper and the first week after taper. It is inconclusive whether these symptoms represent withdrawal, rebound or relapse, or the combination. However, it is clear that abrupt discontinuation results in greater symptomatology than a gradual taper. Most experts suggest a taper over several months (2–4 months).[54] Gradual taper and personality issues (more symptoms with a higher anxiety sensitivity and avoidance) are more critical than half-life of the medication.

Daily doses of alprazolam have varied from 2 to 10 mg. Greater efficacy is generally seen with higher doses, and the largest trial averaged 5.4 mg/day[7] (see Table 4.7.3.3).

Doses of clonazepam are often 50 per cent or less than doses with alprazolam.[52] Some clinicians prefer clonazepam over alprazolam because its longer half-life allows it to be used less frequently each day.[52] However the recent availability of an extended release once daily alprazolam (alprazolam ER) has perhaps reversed that issue. Although the BZs are generally safe in overdose, there is recent evidence that alprazolam is associated with more morbidity than the other BZs. There are studies demonstrating that lorazepam is effective averaging 7 mg/day and 5 to 40 mg/day is effective in diazepam trials (Table 4.7.3.3). The most important aspects of benzodiazepine treatments are the rapid response and increased tolerability and perhaps the greater reduction in everyday anticipatory anxiety (Table 4.7.3.2). Certainly, the largest drawbacks are in general the lack of efficacy against depression and difficulties with the tapering and discontinuation of treatment.

(f) Monoamine oxidase inhibitors (MAOIs)

Many experienced clinicians feel the MAO inhibitors may be the most effective medication class in treatment of panic disorder. However, there is only one scientifically rigorous trial supporting its use.[44] Further, concerns about its safety and the requirement of a tyramine diet limit their use. Modern studies aimed at developing reversible inhibitors of the MAOI enzyme that could eliminate the dietary restrictions have unfortunately been disappointing. The MAOI-B inhibitor selegiline has recently been made available in the United States but there are no known studies of its use in panic disorder.

Patients must also avoid sympathomimetic agents frequently found in decongestants, the antibiotic linezolid, meperidine, fentanyl, and tramadol, serotonergic agents like fenfluramine and the migraine triptan medications. Other significant side effects include weight gain, sexual dysfunctions, postual hypotension, anticholinergic side effects, and sleepiness.

(g) Other antidepressants

There are two uncontrolled trials of buproprion and buproprion SR in panic disorder, one positive and one negative. Mirtazepine has limited evidence supporting its use, as does inositol. Reboxetine has positive and negative evidence, as does with buspirone.

(h) Other agents

Although there is no evidence that conventional antipsychotic medications are effective, there is growing clinical use of the atypical antipsychotics, particularly in treatment resistant patients. There are single trials suggesting the anticonvulsants valproate and levetiracetam may be effective.

(i) Antihypertensives

Although widely used by non-psychiatric physicians in panic patients, the evidence suggests that propranolol, although it does reduce heart rate, is ineffective in treating panic disorder.

(j) Second-line medication treatments

There is limited scientific evidence to guide the clinician in the choice of the second course of treatment if the first is ineffective. Clinically, if the patient has experienced some benefit from the first medication, most clinicians would either add a benzodiazepine or CBT (which has been shown to work in SSRI failures). If the first treatment is completely ineffective, certainly switching treatment to a different SSRI or a different class of medications would be reasonable. If the second-line treatment is also ineffective, there is preliminary evidence that use of the atypical antipsychotics, olanzapine, or resperidone might be appropriate in severe non-responsive patients, and the other atypicals are also likely to work.

(k) Length of treatment

If patients do respond to an antidepressant, continuing treatment for 6 months or longer generally results in continued improvement and a decreased risk for relapse and recurrence, especially if symptoms remit.[55] Response is generally retained as long as medications are maintained. Most studies, clinical experience, and consensus opinion suggests continuation of effective medications for 12 to 18 months or longer.

(l) Discontinuing treatment after an effective response

Although antidepressants can be tapered over 10 days, clinical evidence recommends a much slower taper involving weeks to months. With benzodiazepines, it appears critical to taper even more slowly. Discontinuation symptoms are common but are significantly minimized if taper is accomplished over 2 to 4 months.[56] CBT has been demonstrated to be helpful in decreasing discontinuation difficulties when focused on the sensations, bodily symptoms, and catastrophic misinterpretations that are often seen.

Psychological treatments

(a) Psychodynamic psychotherapy

Although psychodynamic psychotherapy remains a popular treatment for all psychiatric disorders including panic disorder, there has been very little research demonstrating its efficacy in panic disorder. There is one large case-report study of patients with panic disorder reporting that most patients did respond well. One trial compared clomipramine with clomipramine plus 15 weekly sessions of brief dynamic psychotherapy. Patients in both groups responded well with 75 per cent of the patients in the clomipramine group being panic free and all of the patients in the combination group.

In an extension of this work, an emotion-focused treatment for panic disorder has been developed which explores typical fears of being abandoned or trapped as stimuli for panic attacks. This often involves a 12-session acute treatment with six sessions of monthly maintenance in which patients are encouraged to identify, reflect upon, and attempt to change problematic feelings and their responses. A specific form of dynamic psychotherapy 'panic-focused psychodynamic psychotherapy' which is generally applied in 3-month increments, was recently shown to be effective in a RCT.[(57)†]

Behavioural treatments

(a) Exposure treatments

Behavioural treatments which utilize *in vivo* exposure to phobic situations have been the mainstay of the behavioural treatments of panic disorder. They are based on the theory and evidence that patients who enter a feared situation experience habituation of their anxiety whether they are exposed slowly or suddenly and extensively (flooding). The critical nature of exposure for improvement was made clear in one study in which patients being treated with imipramine received no improvement from imipramine when given anti-exposure instruments.[(58)] However, they significantly improved if it were simply suggested that they re-expose themselves to their previously phobic situations when ready. Exposure treatment is consistently associated with long-lasting continuation of acute improvements even without formal follow-up treatment.[(59)]

Studies have compared use of exposure therapy to cognitive behavioural therapy, and have found them to be essentially equal in efficacy.[(60)] At this point, exposure has become an integral part of most CBT protocols.

(b) Cognitive behavioural therapy (see Chapter 6.3.2.1)

Cognitive behavioural therapy of panic disorder evolved from early work of Aaron Beck, but has been applied to panic disorder primarily by Barlow and colleagues working in the United States[(42,61)] and by Clark in the United Kingdom (see Chapter 6.3.2.1).

CBT for panic disorder usually begins with education (e.g. symptoms are part of body's fear response and aren't dangerous) about panic and the cognitive model of panic attacks, use of diaries for self-monitoring of symptoms, cognitive restructuring, habituation to fearful cues including internal cues (e.g. dizziness, tachycardia, etc.) and external situations (e.g. public places, elevators, etc.), anxiety management techniques (e.g. diaphragmatic breathing), and education to prevent relapse. Although evidence suggests that breathing retraining is not an essential component of effective CBT, it is widely utilized as an anxiety management technique.

The most informative trial to date was a multicentre (N 312) 11-week acute trial with a 6-month follow-up for responders and a 6-month follow-up after discontinuation of treatment.[(62)] This trial compared imipramine to cognitive behavioural therapy, their combination, and placebo. Improvement in all the active treatment cells was approximately equal at the end of the acute trial and significantly greater than placebo on most measures. This was also true at the 6-month follow-up. Interestingly, responders to imipramine had a more robust response than responders to cognitive behavioural therapy alone. The combination of imipramine plus cognitive behavioural therapy was significantly better than CBT or imipramine treatment alone at the 6-month point where all treatments were still present. However, at follow-up 6 months after treatment, none of the treatment cells were statistically different from placebo. There are many well-controlled trials demonstrating that CBT delivered in various forms and formats is effective. Its effects are robust, and at least comparable to medications.[(62–64)] Benefits are generally long-lasting, with or without booster sessions in follow-ups to 5 years.[(63,65)] CBT delivered in a group format is also effective.

Continuation/maintenance treatments

There are now a series of studies utilizing antidepressants or benzodiazepines as maintenance treatment for 6 and 12 months for panic disorder and agoraphobia. In most trials, treatment gains from acute treatment are almost always maintained, and generally are extended while the medication is continued. In a 12-month trial comparing clomipramine and placebo, the clomipramine group continued to improve and tolerated the medication well. Placebo patients who were switched to active medication matched the good responses of the clomipramine group.

In a 6-month continuation study of alprazolam patients following an 8-week initial trial, the group maintained their efficacy with a dose at the end of the 8-week trial of 5.1 ± 2.3 mg/day. This decreased to 4.7 ± 2.1 mg/day at week 32 and subsequent follow-up 1 to 2 years later found most patients' doses had drifted down to 1 to 2 mg/day.

In the large follow-up to the Phase II Cross-National Panic Trial, there was a 32-week double-blind comparison of alprazolam, imipramine, and placebo in 181 patients. Again, efficacy was maintained with both medications with no escalation of dose. Patients on both active treatments generally extended their improvement, although the placebo patients tended to lose some efficacy and certainly had a higher drop-out rate. A long-term extension continued paroxetine, clomipramine, and placebo in 176 patients following an acute trial. During the 1-year extension, both the paroxetine and clomipramine patients continued to improve and again, placebo patients tended to lose some of their initial response.

As evidence has accumulated of the high relapse rate with discontinuation of effective medication treatments for panic disorder, longer-term treatment, generally 6 to 18 months, has become routine. Although not well documented, perhaps one of the more important issues is that it appears that patients not only continue to improve for the first 6 months but that improvements continue to be extended the longer patients are on treatment, perhaps even throughout the first 2 years of treatment.

Prevention of recurrence

Available evidence remains inconclusive about the percentage of patients who will relapse if effective pharmacotherapy of panic disorder is discontinued. Early estimates suggested that most patients relapse. It remained the prevailing opinion that 35 to 85 per cent of patients relapse after antidepressants or benzodiazepines were discontinued. However, one trial reported almost no relapse after discontinuation of clomipramine patients, perhaps because they used a gradual taper.

The early trial by Zitrin *et al.* reported only 26 per cent relapse.(65) In a modern trial comparing imipramine and cognitive behavioural therapy, the imipramine relapse rate was 40 per cent. One of the most carefully performed relapse prevention trials followed a fixed-dose study of paroxetine. After acute treatment, patients were re-randomized in double-blind fashion to receive either paroxetine at their prior dose, or to placebo for an additional 3 months of treatment. Interestingly, only 30 per cent of the patients randomized to placebo relapsed, compared with 5 per cent relapse if paroxetine was continued.(47) The relapse rate after medication discontinuation in a recent trial was only 14 per cent. Although these studies certainly need replication, it suggests that the relapse rate may be lower than previously estimated if patients are slowly tapered and carefully followed.

There is one small study that suggests that the relapse rate is lower if treatment is longer. Mavissikalian followed a small group of patients who responded to imipramine, discontinuing some after 6 months of treatment and the other group after 18 months of treatment.(66) In these patients, there was an 80 per cent relapse rate in the 6-month treatment group, but only 20 per cent in the 18-month treatment group. This suggestive finding is consistent with clinical experience but certainly needs replication; however, it is certainly supportive of the general recommendation of continued treatment for 12 to 18 months if effective.

There is certainly a strong suggestion that rapid taper of benzodiazepines produces significant withdrawal symptoms which probably stimulates relapse.

Management

The suggestions for management in this section are based on evidence of the empirically based treatments in panic disorder and agoraphobia, much of which has been reviewed above. However, as in treatment of all patients, there are suggestions that also involve the 'art' of treating these patients which have evolved, but have not been empirically studied or confirmed.

Management of the uncomplicated patient

As reviewed above, it appears clear that the average patient with panic disorder can be treated with a variety of medications or exposure-based and/or cognitive behavioural treatments designed for panic disorder with approximately equal efficacy. There are some patients who have strong feelings or prejudices for or against both medication and cognitive behavioural treatments. Given that situation, as well as the lack of any clear reason to choose one treatment over the other, ethical practice would dictate offering patients a choice of treatment. There is also some evidence that patients will respond better to the treatment they 'believe in'. Unfortunately, the types of treatments are not equally available in all settings or all countries. Psychiatrists tend to use medication treatment with education, exposure, and cognitive based work of a less systematic nature than psychologists and other non-physician caregivers. Although many behaviourally and cognitively oriented psychologists do affiliate with psychiatrists and other physicians to provide medications, for many this ease of combination treatment is not readily available.

As mentioned, most psychiatrists utilize one of the medications mentioned above, supplemented by clear educational efforts with the patient and pertinent family members. This generally includes use of some written material which the patient and spouse read and discuss with the psychiatrist. (see Appendix for suggestions) Education is also a critical part of the initial treatment of patients in exposure-based treatments and cognitive behavioural therapy. These educational efforts are almost always very helpful and in the more mildly symptomatic patients may suffice. Certainly a central issue to increase the therapeutic alliance is to make clear that the therapist does understand that panic attacks involve marked 'real' physical symptoms which are extremely frightening, even though they are not dangerous and are short-lived generally.

For the patient who will be prescribed medication, it is most reasonable to offer a discussion of which medications might be appropriate, and the pros and cons of each. As outlined in Table 4.7.3.2, each medication is different, and depending upon the individual patient's needs and previous experience, any of the classes of medications might be appropriate. As mentioned, current opinion would suggest that the medication of first choice, would probably be an SSRI. In a recent meta-analysis of all the effective medications utilized in the treatment of panic disorder, the SSRIs were shown to be more effective than the other classes.(67) Coupled with their greater tolerability, lack of weight gain, and safety in overdose, they would appear to be the logical first choice.

For clinical and other practical issues, all patients should be told initially that whatever medication is the initial treatment, there are multiple other effective medications. It is important to emphasize that there is little way of knowing which specific medication is most appropriate for which patient and that the initial choice may not be effective, but subsequent choices are likely to be effective.

There are few data to direct the choice of the medications beyond those favouring the SSRIs mentioned above (see Table 4.7.3.2). There is only one trial documenting a difference in patient type leading to a choice of medication. In the large cross-national comparison of imipramine, alprazolam, and placebo, patients with predominantly respiratory symptoms responded better to imipramine.(68) Similarly, patients with a predominantly cardiovascular symptom picture responded better to alprazolam than imipramine. Otherwise, there are no data suggesting a particular medication for a specific patient beyond the various advantages and disadvantages listed in Table 4.7.3.2.

Once medication is chosen, it is prudent to begin at the lowest dose possible (see Table 4.7.3.3). This beginning low dose also extends to the benzodiazepines but is less critical since they are not associated with an initial hyperstimulation reaction. This is one of the reasons why benzodiazepines are easier to utilize and usually more popular with patients who somehow realize that from previous experience or feedback from other patients that they are not associated with an initial worsening of symptoms and are better tolerated overall. At a practical level, management of the worries about the initial hyperstimulation reaction is one of the most important issues in the psychopharmacological management of panic disorder patients. If handled incorrectly, this issue can lead to a drop-out rate that reaches 25 to 50 per cent. With proper reassurance and close follow-up of patients, this drop-out rate can be reduced to almost zero. Patients need to be told that hyperstimulation can occur in one-third of patients but is transient and not dangerous. Because of the inherent anxiety and even phobia about taking medications, this reassurance is not usually sufficient and patients need to be invited to contact the treating physician with any anxiety or questions they might have about taking medications coupled with a quick response to their concerns.

After initial tolerance of medication is established, the dose can be raised over several weeks to a target level. Obviously, if a patient does not show a response at lower doses, the medication should be raised to maximum doses (Table 4.7.3.3).

It is important for the patient and physician alike to keep in mind that effectiveness of medications often requires a significant amount of time. The antidepressants as a class routinely take 2 to 6 weeks and with certain medications and patients as much as 6 to 12 weeks before significant effectiveness is established. This is less an issue with benzodiazepines, where initial effectiveness is generally seen in the first week or two, but there too the appropriate doses must be obtained, which often takes several weeks. Higher doses of all medicines are needed to reduce agoraphobic avoidance.

As mentioned, if agoraphobic patients do not gradually re-expose themselves to situations they fear, their avoidance fears will not be decreased. This exposure to their actual phobic situations can be accomplished in many ways. Some patients are capable of gradually re-exposing themselves after they understand the principles of exposure and the need to remain in the situation until their fears diminish. They may need help in establishing a hierarchy of their fears, although it is not actually necessary that they in fact do work-up the hierarchy in a gradually increasing fashion from 'least feared' to 'most feared'. However, it is often easier for most patients to conceptualize and accomplish it in this fashion.

Many therapists develop a hierarchical list and then monitor the patient's progress on a regular basis. Use of a standard scale which monitors the various symptom domains can be very helpful, such as *The Panic Disorder Severity scale* (PDSS).[69] There is evidence that the exposure must be regular, and extensive, often on a daily basis. Also, encouragement from the therapist and partner have both been shown to be important. Some patients can re-enter their phobic situations better if supported by their partner, or other phobics from a support group. If they are particularly afraid, an *in vivo* therapist (often recovered phobics) can be very helpful. The critical issues appear to be approaching their fears in a consistent and systematic basis in the real phobic situations accompanied by encouragement and support.

In a similar fashion, many psychiatrists combine principles of cognitive behavioural therapy without embarking on a formal cognitive behavioural therapy programme. Certainly, this should always involve education about the illness and its treatments. Other elements of identification and challenge of catastrophic thinking are widely applied by psychiatrists, but in a less systematic fashion than in formal cognitive behavioural therapy protocols.

It is important that from the beginning most patients be told that if medication treatment is effective, the expectation is to continue the medication for 12 to 18 months. An important issue to negotiate with the patient is how, when, and if effective pharmacotherapy should be tapered and discontinued.[70] Most evidence and experience suggests that patients be continued long enough to receive maximum benefit from medication treatment. In that context, patients should have experienced symptomatic and functional recovery to a maximum extent possible before discontinuation is considered. Patients should have regained a sense of confidence and control of their symptoms and lives. This might be conceptualized as a 'period of normal living' after attainment of symptomatic control before consideration is given to discontinuing an effective treatment. Relapse rates after such a remission are lower. Because the principal danger of discontinuation is relapse, the time should be carefully chosen. This should be a time when potential disruption from discontinuation symptoms and/or relapse would be least problematic.

There are strong suggestions in the literature, some of which is reviewed above, that all medications, and certainly the benzodiazepines, should be tapered very slowly, probably over 2 to 6 months, if possible.[54] This is both to minimize withdrawal symptoms which are especially frightening to panic patients and to observe for relapse symptoms as medications are slowly tapered.

The strongest reasons for discontinuing effective pharmacotherapy are the problematic side effects and expense.[70] Because this is a syndrome frequently seen in young women, the most important reason may be the wish to conceive a child or the onset of pregnancy. Certainly, routine practice is to try to taper and discontinue all medications before or during pregnancy, but sometimes this is not possible. There are now a series of women who have delivered normal children after having tried unsuccessfully to discontinue medication during pregnancy.

Many patients want to manage their own symptoms without the use of medications, and this is also a reasonable reason to taper and discontinue medications, if strongly felt by the patient.[70] The therapist should explore, however, unreasonable prejudices against the use of medications stimulated by reading, television shows, relatives, or even well-meaning physicians. Most in the field now believe that panic disorder and agoraphobia are conditions similar to hypertension and diabetes in the sense that most patients do not like the thought that they are ill and resist compliance with medication treatment. However, treatment is beneficial and not harmful, and patients often need encouragement and education in order to agree to a programme where they continue medications rather than press to discontinue them.

If medications are discontinued, the patient should be followed closely, at least by telephone, for difficulties that could include withdrawal symptoms, especially with benzodiazepines, or incipient relapse. If relapse does occur, evidence suggests that patients will respond to reinstitution of the same medication treatment regimen. If symptoms and/or functional disability associated with relapse are problematic, patients should be offered retreatment with the same medication or offered other effective non-medication treatments.

Psychological treatments

Management of patients with predominantly psychological treatments also begins with the use of educational materials, as is frequently the case with medication treatment of panic disorder. Almost all psychological treatments involve some sort of exposure-based treatment. In some, this is the predominant modality with considerable variation on how exposure to feared situations is accomplished. Although some initial exposure therapy in particularly frightened patients may be accomplished in imagination prior to *in vivo* exposure, most exposure treatments are usually attempted *in vivo* from the outset. Most treatments have been shown to be effective if they involve *in vivo* exposure. Gradual exposure is the norm, although some programmes use very rapid exposures often called 'flooding', which involves exposure to multiple phobic situations rapidly over several days. Most programmes involve therapist-assisted exposure, sometimes utilizing professional *in vivo* therapists or volunteers who accompany phobics into their feared situations. Partners of patients are often enlisted as assistants, and there is some evidence that this more effective than non-partner exposure aides.

Most exposure-based treatments involve frequent, often daily practices involving several hours. Often the critical issue is adequate support of the patient to accomplish this much exposure 'homework', as well as encouragement and praise.

Almost anything that can help the patient accomplish the actual exposure appears to be useful and helpful. For instance, manuals and computer programs, as well as telephone-based supervision and encouragement have been shown to be effective. Although many therapists utilize relaxation techniques, applied relaxation has been the most widely utilized and effective. Many therapists also employ breathing retraining, encouraging people who hyperventilate to slow their breathing by utilizing their diaphragm. Although both have been shown to be effective and are widely utilized, other studies suggest they are not essential components of treatment, and their use does vary. Although use of benzodiazepines do decrease patient anxiety about exposure, evidence suggests that the benzodiazepines interfere with the cognitive benefits and habituation effects of exposure.

Cognitive restructuring involves the patient and therapist identifying the so-called 'automatic thoughts' they have with and after each panic attack. These are the misinterpretations that patients make about what these symptoms mean. For instance, the patient and therapist together identify that these symptoms often trigger thoughts that they are very ill, having a heart attack, or perhaps even dying. Over several sessions, these are identified and it is made clear to the patient the power these thoughts have to frighten them. At that point a number of strategies can be tried to try to correct these cognitions. Some involve attempts to compute the actual probability of the catastrophic consequences that patients fear. Others involve 'decatastrophizing' in which the ultimate consequences that patients fear are exposed, and generally can then be disavowed by the patient as extremely unrealistic. Patients can be taught to correct these thoughts or substitute more positive self-statements in their place. These skills are then worked on as 'homework', including actual exposure in which negative thoughts are identified and challenged *in vivo*.

The other usual aspect of cognitive behavioural therapy for panic disorder is interoceptive exposure, in which physical symptoms that frighten patients are identified and then they are taught to habituate to those symptoms and challenge the negative cognitions that arise with them. This can easily be accomplished in an office setting. For instance, if the patients are afraid of dizzy feelings, they can be spun in a chair. If they have fears of fast heartbeat, they can run up the stairs and challenge the negative cognitions that arise.

Both exposure-based treatments and cognitive behavioural therapy often are delivered in an 8- to 16-week treatment format, with varying frequencies of follow-up and attempts are underway to shorten these treatments. There is evidence that patients failing to respond to CBT often respond to subsequent medication treatment.

Treatment of comorbid patients

Treatment of the panic disorder patient comorbid with substance abuse is probably the most difficult challenge. In general, the substance abuse problem tends to be predominant even if it were temporally secondary to panic disorder symptoms. Therefore, treatment of substance abuse generally has to be initiated and completed first, although as soon as possible treatment of panic disorder needs be initiated.

Treatment of comorbid social phobia, obsessive–compulsive disorder, or GAD has recently been made somewhat simpler with the demonstration that the SSRIs are effective in these other conditions as well. Although not yet empirically demonstrated, it is reasonable to expect that an SSRI would effectively treat the panic disorder as well as the other comorbid anxiety disorders. This is an important area for future research. Behavioural treatments specific to obsessive–compulsive disorder and to social phobia may well be needed in addition to medication treatment.

The most common comorbidity is with depression and again one of the advantages of antidepressants is probable dual treatment of panic disorder and depression.[71] Perhaps the most important management issue is recognition that comorbid depression carries with it a marked increase in suicide risk. As mentioned, there is some evidence that depressed panic disorder patients respond better to MAOIs.

Resistance to treatment

There are relatively few systematic data about treatment options for patients resistant to initial medication or to exposure- or cognitive behavioural-based treatments. Generally, however, most patients can be tried on another medication, often with success. If they are on medicine and have not tried exposure or cognitive behavioural therapy that should definitely be added. The converse is also true. Non-response can often be traced to inadequate doses or blood levels of the medication or an inadequate length of trial. Comorbid psychiatric and particularly comorbid medical conditions need to be ruled out. Apparent resistance is often related to concomitant personality disorders or failure of agoraphobics to actually attempt exposure treatments. True resistance to one medication is sometimes overcome by a switch to another medication or to two medications at a time. If the combination of an antidepressant and benzodiazepine has not been tried, that is often the first attempted combination. In highly resistant patients, sometimes a combination of tricyclic and SSRI antidepressants or an atypical antipsychotic can be utilized.

Pregnancy

Panic disorder occurs disproportionately in young women making the issue of pregnancy a critical one. The course of panic disorder through pregnancy is highly variable. Use of SSRIs may be associated with low birth weight and a higher rate of spontaneous abortions, cardiac abnormalities, pulmonary hypertension, and withdrawal symptoms in the newborn if used late in pregnancy.

In general however, increases in congenital abnormalities have not been observed with the SSRIs. Whether benzodiazepines are associated with major malformations like cleft palate is unclear. Use of benzodiazepines near delivery is associated with sedation in the newborn. Also, both antidepressants and benzodiazepines are secreted in breast milk. For all these concerns, CBT is strongly recommended for pregnant women and should be considered in women planning pregnancy.

Ethical issues

The principal ethical issues concern the availability of treatment. Because the two types of effective treatments (medications and exposure or cognitive behavioural therapy) are not widely or equally distributed in all practices or locations, sometimes caregivers face a difficult ethical choice of having only one type of treatment available. In these instances, patients should be informed of the limitations and participate in the choices made.

Most of the treatment experience and certainly the empirical evidence has been in Caucasian patients. We do know that symptoms are different across ethnic groups and that response is often less positive in non-Caucasian groups. Treatments need to be tested and developed for all ethnic and national groups as part of the ethical development of the field.

Possibilities for prevention

The best evidence now suggests that panic disorder is often preceded by an anxiety pattern in childhood. In Kagan's model of behaviourally inhibited children, there is certainly a tendency for the pattern to persist throughout life, but some children appear to lose this trait during their development. This may well be related to parental child-rearing practices in which children are encouraged to face issues they fear rather than be withdrawn and fearful. Research is needed to explore whether different parental rearing practices or educational efforts or early treatment with these children can reduce later development of anxiety disorders. If so, these efforts at the public health and school level need to developed.

The other major preventable aetiological consideration for panic disorder and agoraphobia has been the evidence of negative traumatic events occurring in the childhood of adults with panic disorder. Preventative efforts need to be aimed at these issues through public education and education of caregivers of children. Also, one of the intervention goals in helping a traumatized child should be to prevent future development of anxiety disorders and other problems.

Further information

Barlow, D.H. and Craske, M.G. (2000). *Mastery of your anxiety and panic (MAP-3): client workbook for anxiety and panic* (3rd edn). Oxford University Press, New York.

Barlow, D.H. and Crawke, M.G. (2000). *Mastery of your anxiety and panic (MAP-3): client workbook for agoraphobia* (3rd edn). Oxford University Press, New York.

Pollard, C.A. and Zuercher-White, E. (2003). *The agoraphobia workbook: a comprehensive program to end your fear of symptom attacks.* New Harbinger, Oakland, CA.

Wilson, R.R. (2003). *Facing panic: self help for people with panic attacks.* Anxiety Disorders Association of America, Silver Spring, MD.

Zuercher-White, E. (1999). *Overcoming panic disorder and agoraphobia: client manual.* New Harbinger Publication, Oakland, CA.

Bourne, E.J. (2005). *The anxiety and phobia workbook* (4th edn). New Harbinger Publications, Oakland, CA.

Brantley, J. and Kabat-Zinn, J. (2003). *Calming your anxious mind.* New Harbinger, Oakland, CA.

Foa, E.B. and Andrews, L.W. (2006). *If your adolescent has an anxiety disorder: an essential resource for parents.* Oxford University Press, New York.

Marks, I.M. (2002). *Living with fear: understanding and coping with anxiety* (2nd edn). McGraw-Hill, New York.

Anxiety Disorders Association of America, 3730 Georgia Ave., Suite 600, Silver Spring, MD 20910, www.adaa.org

References

1. Hippocrates (1870). *On epidemics V.* Section 82 (trans. S. Farrar). Cadel, London.
2. Benedikt, M. (1870). Uber Platzschwindel. *Allgemeine Wiener Medizinische Zeitung*, **15**, 488.
3. Klein, D.F. (1964). Delineation of two drug responsive anxiety syndromes. *Psychopharmacology*, **5**, 397–408.
4. Marks, I.M. (1969). *Fears and phobias.* Heinemann, London.
5. Klerman, G.L., Weissman, M., Ovellete, R., *et al.* (1991). Panic attacks in the community: social morbidity and health care utilization. *The Journal of the American Medical Association*, **265**, 742–6.
6. Noyes, R., Jr. and Barloon, T.J. (1997). Charles Darwin and panic disorder. *The Journal of the American Medical Association*, **277**, 138–41.
7. Ballenger, J.C., Burrows, G.D., Dupont, R.L., *et al.* (1988). Aprazolam in panic disorder and agoraphobia: results from a multicenter trial. I. Efficacy in short-term treatment. *Archives of General Psychiatry*, **455**, 413–22.
8. Burns, L.E. and Thorpe, G.L. (1977). The epidemiology of fears and phobias with particular reference to the national survey of agoraphobics. *The Journal of International Medical Research*, **5**, 1–7.
9. Goldstein, A.J. and Chambless, D.L. (1978). A reanalysis of agoraphobia. *Behavior Therapy*, **9**, 47–59.
10. Beitman, B.D., Kushner, M.G., Lamerti, J.W., *et al.* (1990). Panic disorder without fear in patients with angiographically normal coronary arteries. *The Journal of Nervous and Mental Disease*, **178**, 307–12.
11. Westphal, C. (1872). Agoraphobie, eine neuropahtische Erscheinung. *Archiv für Psychiatrie und Nervenkrankheiten*, **3**, 138–61.
12. Feighner, J.P., Robins, E., Guze, S.B., *et al.* (1972). Diagnostic criteria for use in psychiatric research. *Archives of General Psychiatry*, **38**, 57–63.
13. Klein, D.F. (1964). Delineation of two drug responsive anxiety syndromes. *Psychopharmacology*, **5**, 397–408.
14. Ballenger, J.C. and Fyer, A.J. (1993). Examining criteria for panic disorder. *Hospital & Community Psychiatry*, **44**, 226–8.
15. Weissman, M.M. (1990). Epidemiology of panic disorder and agoraphobia. In *Frontiers of clinical neuroscience. Clinical aspects of panic disorder*, Vol. 9 (ed. J.C. Ballenger), pp. 57–65. Wiley-Liss, New York.
16. Weissman, M.M., Bland, R.C., Canino, G.J., *et al.* (1997). The cross-national epidemiology of panic disorder. *Archives of General Psychiatry*, **54**, 305–9.
17. Lépine, J.P., Wittchen, H.U., Essau, C.A., and participants of the WHO-ADAMHA CIDI Field Trials. (1993). Lifetime and current comorbidity of anxiety and affective disorders: results from the International WHO-ADAMHA CIDI Field Trials. *International Journal of Methods in Psychiatric Research*, **3**, 67–77.
18. Lydiard, R.B. and Brady, K. (1993). Association of anxiety and alcoholism. *The Psychiatric Quarterly*, **64**, 135–49.

19. Sartorius, N., Uestuen, B., Costa e Silva, J.A., *et al.* (1993). An international study of psychological problems in primary care: preliminary report from the World Health Organization collaborative project on psychological problems in general health care. *Archives of General Psychiatry*, **50**, 819–24.
20. Kroenke, K. and Mangelsdorff, A.D. (1989). Common symptoms in ambulatory care: incidence, evaluation, therapy and outcome. *The American Journal of Medicine*, **86**, 262–6.
21. Simon, G.E. and Von Korff, M. (1991). Somatization and psychiatric disorder in the Epidemiologic Catchment Area study. *The American Journal of Psychiatry*, **148**, 1494–500.
22. Katon, W. (1984). Panic disorder and somatization. Review of 55 cases. *The American Journal of Medicine*, **77**, 101–8.
23. Ballenger, J.C. (1998). Panic disorder in primary care and general medicine. In *Panic disorder and its treatment* (eds. J. Rosenbaum and M. Pollack), pp. 1–36. Dekker, New York.
24. Goodwin, R.D., Lieb, R., Hoefler, M., *et al.* (2004). Panic attack as a risk factor for severe psychopathology. *The American Journal of Psychiatry*, **161**, 2207–14.
25. Kessler, R.C., Chiu, W.T., Jim, R., *et al.* (2006). The epidemiology of panic attacks, panic disorder, and agoraphobia in the national comorbidity survery replication. *Archives of General Psychiatry*, **63**, 415–24.
26. Torgersen, S. (1983). Genetic factors in anxiety disorders. *Archives of General Psychiatry*, **40**, 1085–90.
27. Kendler, K.S., Neale, M.C., Kessler, R.C., *et al.* (1993). Panic disorder in women: a population-based twin study. *Psychological Medicine*, **40**, 397–406.
28. Skre, I., Onstad, S., Torgersen, S., *et al.* (1993). A twin study of DSM-III-R anxiety disorders. *Acta Psychiatrica Scandinavica*, **88**, 85–92.
29. Arnold, P.D., Zai, G., and Richter, M.A. (2004). Genetics of anxiety disorders. *Current Psychiatry Reports*, **6**, 243–54.
30. Roy-Byrne, P.P., Craske, M.G., and Stein, M.G. (2006). Panic disorder. *Lancet*, **368**, 1023–32.
31. Kagan, J., Reznick, J.S., Clarke, C., *et al.* (1984). Behavioral inhibition to the unfamiliar. *Child Development*, **55**, 2212–25.
32. Rosenbaum, J.F., Biederman, J., Gersten, M., *et al.* (1988). Behavioral inhibition in children of parents with panic disorder and agoraphobia: a controlled study. *Archives of General Psychiatry*, **45**, 463–70.
33. Scocco, P., Barbieri, I., and Frank, E. (2007). Interpersonal problem areas and onset of panic disorder. *Psychopathology*, **40**, 8–13.
34. Laraia, M.T., Stuart, G.W., Frye, L., *et al.* (1994). Childhood environment of women with panic disorder and agoraphobia. *Journal of Anxiety Disorders*, **8**, 1–17.
35. Saunders, B.E., Villeponteaux, L.A., Lipovsky, J.A., *et al.* (1992). Child sexual assault as a risk factor for mental disorders among women: a community survey. *Journal of Interpersonal Violence*, **7**, 189–204.
36. Johnson, P.L., Lightman, S.L., and Lowry, C.A. (2004). A functional subset of sertonergic neurons in the rat ventrolateral periaqueductal gray implicated in the inhibition of sympathoexcitation and panic. *Annals of the New York Academy of Sciences*, **1018**, 58–64.
37. Neumeister, A., Bain, E., Nugent, A.C., *et al.* (2004). Reduced serotonin type 1_A receptor binding in panic disorder. *The Journal of Neuroscience*, **24**, 589–91.
38. Maron, E., Kuikka, J.T., Shlik, J., *et al.* (2004). Reduced brain serotonin transporter binding in patients with panic disorder. *Psychiatry Research*, **132**, 173–81.
39. Bremner, J.D. (2004). Brain imaging in anxiety disorders. *Expert Review of Neurotherapeutics*, **4**, 275–84.
40. Katschnig, H., Amering, M., Stolk, J.M., *et al.* (1996). Predictors of quality of life in a long-term followup study in panic disorder patients after a clinical drug trial. *Psychopharmacology Bulletin*, **32**, 149–55.
41. Mavissakalian, M.R. and Prien, R.F. (eds.) (1996). *Long-term treatments of anxiety disorders*. American Psychiatric Press, Washington, DC.
42. Landon, T.M. and Barlow, D.H. (2004). Cognitive-behavioral treatment for panic disorder: current status. *Journal of Psychiatric Practice*, **10**, 211–26.
43. Marks, I.M. (1987). *Fears, phobias, and rituals.* Oxford University Press, New York.
44. Sheehan, D., Ballenger, J.C., and Jacobsen, G. (1980). Treatment of endogenous anxiety with phobic hysterical and hypochondriacal symptoms. *Archives of General Psychiatry*, **37**, 51–9.
45. Jobson, K.O. and Poter, W.Z. (1995). International psychopharmacology algorithim project report. *Psychopharmacology Bulletin*, **31**, 457–507.
46. Ballenger, J.C., Davidson, J.R., Lécrubier, Y., *et al.* (1998). Consensus statement on panic disorder from the International Consensus Group on depression and anxiety. *The Journal of Clinical Psychiatry*, **59**, 47–54.
47. Ballenger, J. (1999). Selective serotonin reuptake inhibitors (SSRIs) in panic disorder. In *Panic disorder: clinical diagnosis, management and mechanisms* (eds. D. Nutt, J. Ballenger, and J.P. Lépine), pp. 159–78. Dunitz, London.
48. Connolly, S.D., Bernstein, G.A., and Work Group on Quality Issues (2007). Practice parameters for the assessment and treatment of children and adolescents with anxiety disorders. *Journal of the American Academy of Child and Adolescent Psychiatry*, **46**(2), 267–83.
49. Fava, M. (2006). Prospective studies of adverse events related to antidepressant discontinuation. *The Journal of Clinical Psychiatry*, **67**(Suppl. 4), 14–21.
50. Cassano, G.B., Petracci, A., Perugi, G., *et al.* (1998). Clomipramine for panic disorder. I. The first 10 weeks of a long-term comparison with imipramine. *Journal of Affective Disorders*, **14**, 123–7.
51. Modigh, L., Westberg, P., and Eriksson, E. (1992). Superiority of clomipramine over imipramine in the treatment of panic disorder: a placebo-controlled trial. *Journal of Clinical Psychopharmacology*, **51**, 53–8.
52. Herman, J.B., Rosenbaum, J.F., and Brotman, A.W. (1987). The alprazolam to clonazepam switch for the treatment of panic disorder. *Journal of Clinical Psychopharmacology*, **7**, 175–8.
53. American Psychiatric Association. (1990). Benzodiazepines dependence, toxicity, and abuse: a task force report of the American Psychiatric Association. APA, Washington, DC.
54. Dupont, R.L., Swinson, R.P., Ballenger, J.C., *et al.* (1992). Discontinuation of alprazolam after long-term treatment of panic-related disorders. *Journal of Clinical Psychopharmacology*, **12**, 352–4.
55. Lecrubier, Y. and Judge, R. (1997). Long-term evaluation of paroxetine, clomipramine and placebo in panic disorder. Collaborative Paroxetine Panic Study Investigators. *Acta Psychiatrica Scandinavica*, **95**, 153–60.
56. Ballenger, J.C., Pecknold, J., Rickels, K., *et al.* (1993). Medication discontinuation in panic disorder. *The Journal of Clinical Psychiatry*, **54**, 15–21.
57. Milrod, B., Leon, A.C., Busch, F., *et al.* (2007). A randomized controlled clinical trial of psychoanalyltic psychotherapy for panic disorder. *The American Journal of Psychiatry*, **164**, 265–72.
58. Mavissakalian, M. (1990). Sequential combination of imipramine and behavioral instructions in the treatment of panic disorder with agoraphobia. *Archives of General Psychiatry*, **46**, 127–31.
59. Fava, G.A., Rafanelli, C., Grandi, S., *et al.* (2001). Long-term outcome of panic disorder with agoraphobia treated by exposure. *Psychological Medicine*, **31**, 891–8.
60. Ost, L.G., Thulin, U., and Tamnero, J. (2004). Cognitive behavior therapy vs. exposure *in vivo* in the treatment of panic disorder with agoraphobia (corrected from agrophobia). *Behaviour Research and Therapy*, **42**, 1105–27.
61. Barlow, D.H., Craske, M.G., Cerny, J.A., *et al.* (1989). Behavioral treatment of panic disorder. *Behavior Therapy*, **20**, 261–82.

62. Barlow, D.H., Gorman, J.M., Shear, M., *et al.* (2000). Cognitive-behavioral therapy, imipramine, or their combination for panic disorder: a randomized controlled trial. *The Journal of the American Medical Association*. **283**, 2529–36.
63. Craske, M.G., Brown, T.A., and Barlow, D.H. (1991). Behavioral treatment of panic disorder: a two-year follow-up. *Behavior Therapy*, **22**, 289–304.
64. Butler, A.C., Chapman, J.E., Forman, E.M., *et al.* (2006). The empirical status of cognitive-behavioral therapy: a review of meta-analyses. *Clinical Psychology Review*, **26**, 17–31.
65. Zitrin, C.M., Klein, D.F, Woerner, M.G., *et al.* (1983). Treatment of phobias. I. Comparison of imipramine hydrochloride and placebo. *Archives of General Psychiatry*, **46**, 127–31.
66. Mavissakalian, M. (1990). Sequential combination of imipramine and behavioral instructions in the treatment of panic disorder with agoraphobia. *Archives of General Psychiatry*, **46**, 127–31.
67. Boyer, W. (1995). Serotonin uptake inhibitors are superior to imipramine and alprazolam in alleviating panic attacks: a meta-analysis. *International Clinical Psychopharmacology*, **10**, 45–9.
68. Briggs, A.C., Stretch, D.D., and Brandon, S. (1993). Subtyping of panic disorder by symptom profile. *The British Journal of Psychiatry*, **163**, 201–9.
69. Shear, M.K., Brown, T.A., Barlow, D.H., *et al.* (1997). Multicenter collaborative panic disorder severity scale. *The American Journal of Psychiatry*, **154**, 1571–5.
70. Ballenger, J.C. (1992). Medication discontinuation in panic disorder. *The Journal of Clinical Psychiatry*, **53**, 26–31.
71. Ballenger, J.C. (1988). Comorbidity of panic and depression: implications for clinical management. *International Journal of Clinical Psychopharmacology*, **13**(Suppl. 4), S13–17.

4.8

Obsessive–compulsive disorder

Joseph Zohar, Leah Fostick, and Elizabeth Juven-Wetzler

Introduction

Obsessive–compulsive disorder (OCD) is a common, chronic, and disabling disorder marked by obsessions and/or compulsions that are egodystonic and cause significant distress to the patients and their families. During the last 25 years, there has been a resurgence of studies into various aspects of OCD, including epidemiological, pathophysiological, and pharmacological investigations. With the progress in finding effective treatments for OCD, different algorithms for the management of these patients have been developed. The progress in OCD includes advanced methodologies of imaging studies (both before and after treatment), along with insight into the neurological aspects of OCD and OCD-related conditions, leading to selective treatments.

Up to the early 1980s, OCD was considered a rather rare, treatment-refractory, and chronic condition of psychological origin. Dynamic psychotherapy was of little benefit and several pharmacological treatments were attempted without much success.(1) Since then, several researchers have reported that the prevalence of OCD is around 2 per cent in the general population.(2,3) In addition, numerous studies have reported on the efficacy of various serotonin reuptake inhibitors, and consequently an understanding of the biological basis of OCD has begun to unfold.

The observation that clomipramine, a tricyclic antidepressant with a serotonergic profile, is effective in treating symptoms of OCD(4,5) has increased interest in OCD in general and in the relationship between serotonin and OCD in particular. Substantial evidence currently suggests that OCD is almost unique among psychiatric disorders, as only serotonergic medications appear to be effective in this disorder.(6) For example, non-serotonergic drugs, such as desipramine, a potent antidepressant and antipanic agent, are entirely ineffective in OCD.(7–9) This specific response to serotonergic drugs has paved the way for further research on the role of serotonin in the pathogenesis of OCD in particular, and in OCD-related disorders in general.

Epidemiology

The lifetime prevalence of OCD in the general population is between 2 and 3 per cent (i.e. it is more prevalent than schizophrenia).(2,10) This rate has been confirmed across different cultures.(3) The prevalence of OCD among children and adolescents appears to be as high as among adults.(11) However, Nelson and Rice(12) and Stein *et al.*(13) have suggested that the diagnosis of OCD by the Diagnostic Interview Schedule administered by lay people leads to overdiagnosis, and so have proposed lower prevalence rates of 1 to 2 per cent.

Men and women are equally likely to be affected, although some reports have suggested a slight female predominance.(3) During adolescence, boys are more commonly affected than girls. The mean age of onset is about 20 years of age. Single people are more commonly affected, probably representing the difficulty for people with OCD to maintain a relationship.

Patients with OCD are commonly afflicted by other mental disorders; for instance, the lifetime prevalence for a major depressive episode in these patients is around 67 per cent.(3,14) Other common comorbid psychiatric diagnoses include alcohol-use disorders, social phobia, specific phobia, panic disorder, eating disorders, and post-traumatic stress disorder (PTSD).(15) The comorbidity with schizophrenia and with tic disorders raises interesting pathophysiological and therapeutic implications. The rate of tic disorders approaches 40 per cent in juvenile OCD, and there is an increase in the prevalence of Tourette's syndrome among the relatives of OCD patients.(16)

The relationship between OCD and obsessive–compulsive personality disorder (OCPD) has been a focus of debate. Although prospective research is lacking, it appears that OCPD is not a prominent risk factor for developing OCD, as the prevalence of OCPD among patients with OCD is not far from its prevalence in other psychiatric disorders.

Clinical features and diagnosis

The diagnosis of OCD according to DSM-IV criteria is based on the presence of either obsessions or compulsions, which cause marked distress, are time-consuming (more than an hour per day), or significantly interfere with the person's normal routine and social and occupational activities. It stipulates that, at some point during the course of the disorder, but not necessarily during the current episode, the person has recognized that the obsessions or compulsions are excessive or unreasonable. However, if the patient does not recognize for most of the time during the current episode that the obsessions and compulsions are excessive or unreasonable, the diagnosis is OCD with poor insight.

If another Axis I disorder is present, it is mandatory that the content of the obsessions or compulsions is not restricted to it (e.g. a preoccupation with food or weight in eating disorders, or guilt feelings in the presence of a major depressive episode). The disturbance should not be due to the direct effects of a substance (e.g. of a drug abuse or a medication) or a general medical condition.

The obsessions are recurrent, intrusive, and distressing thoughts, images, or impulses, whereas the compulsions are repetitive, seemingly purposeful, behaviours that a person feels driven to perform. Obsessions are usually unpleasant and increase a person's anxiety, whereas carrying out compulsions reduces anxiety. Resistance to carrying out a compulsion results in increased anxiety. The patient usually realizes that the obsessions are irrational and experiences both the obsession and the compulsion as egodystonic.

Patients with both obsessions and compulsions constitute at least 75 per cent of the affected patients, with most patients presenting with multiple obsessions and compulsions. The symptoms may shift, for example a patient who had washing rituals during childhood may present with checking rituals as an adult.

OCD can express itself in many different symptoms, but the classical presentations include washing, checking, aggressive, religious, or sexual obsessions, and ordering, counting, hoarding, and symmetry compulsions. Dimensional approaches have been used to analyze these characteristic subtypes, and present the different symptoms in an innovative way.[17]

The most common pattern is an obsession with dirt or germs, followed by washing or avoiding presumably contaminated objects (doorknobs, electrical switches, newspapers, people's hands, telephones). Because it is hard to avoid the feared object is (e.g. faeces, urine, dust, or germs), patients wash their hands excessively and sometimes avoid leaving home because of their fear of germs. A second common pattern is an obsession of doubt, followed by a compulsion of checking. The person checks whether the oven is turned off or the front and back doors are closed—the checking may involve many trips back home to recheck what had already been checked. In OCD, the checking, instead of resolving uncertainty, often contributes to even greater doubt, which leads to further checking. The patients exhibit obsessional self-doubt, and feel guilty for having committed some damage (for instance, a fear of hurting someone while driving, leading to driving back over the same spot again and again). Other patterns include hoarding and religious obsessions. More recently, a dimensional approach to OCD has been launched by Leckman and colleagues, stating four symptom dimension of OCD: obsessions/checking, symmetry/ordering, contamination/cleaning, and hoarding.[17,18] Another pattern of OCD involves intrusive obsessional thoughts without a compulsion. Such obsessions are usually repetitious thoughts of some sexual or aggressive act that is reprehensible to the patient. Still another pattern is the need for symmetry or precision, which leads to a compulsion of slowness. Patients can take hours to eat a meal or shave, in an attempt to do things 'just right'. Unlike other patients with OCD, these patients usually do not resist their symptoms.

The gap between the knowledge that the symptoms are irrational on one hand and the overwhelming urge to perform them on the other hand contributes to the immense suffering associated with OCD.

OCD and schizophrenia

About 25 per cent of patients with chronic schizophrenia may also present with OCD symptoms (range 5 to 45 per cent)[19]; and 15 per cent of the patients with schizophrenia may fully qualify for the diagnosis of OCD. As in OCD, the OC symptoms in these patients will not necessarily surface unless specific questions are asked. Many patients with schizophrenia can distinguish the egodystonic, obsessive–compulsive symptoms, perceived as coming from within, from the egosyntonic delusions perceived as introduced from the outside. Follow-up studies demonstrate a diagnostic stability over the years, and it seems that the presence of OCD in schizophrenia predicts a poor prognosis.[19] Several studies among patients with schizophrenia and OCD reported an improvement in OCD symptomatology after the addition of serotonin reuptake inhibitors.[19]

The poor prognosis of patients with schizophrenia and OCD, preliminary data regarding their response to the unique combination of antipsychotic and anti-obsessive medications, along with the high prevalence of this presentation has led several researchers to suggest that a 'schizo-obsessive' category may be of value.[20]

Differential diagnosis

Personal distress and functional impairment, which are required for the diagnosis, differentiate OCD from ordinary or mildly excessive worries, thoughts, and habits. The medical differential diagnosis includes tic disorders (especially Tourette's syndrome), temporal-lobe epilepsy, trauma, and postencephalitic complications.

Psychiatric diagnoses that should be ruled out include depressive disorder, schizophrenia, OCPD, PTSD, phobias, delusions, hypochondriasis, and paraphilias. OCD can usually be differentiated from schizophrenia by the absence of other schizophrenic symptoms and by the patients' insight into their disorder. Moreover, patients with OCD usually attempt to resist the obsessions. OCPD does not have the degree of functional impairment characteristic of OCD and it is egosyntonic.

Phobias are distinguished by the absence of a relationship between the obsessive thoughts and the compulsions. The fears in OCD usually involve harm to others rather than harm to oneself. In addition, in OCD, when patients are 'phobic' they are usually afraid of an unavoidable stimulus (for instance, viruses, germs, or dirt) as opposed to the classic phobic objects like tunnels, bridges, or crowds.

Major depressive disorder (MDD) can sometimes be associated with obsessive ideas, but patients with OCD usually fail to meet all the criteria of MDD. Other psychiatric diagnoses closely related to OCD are hypochondriasis, body dysmorphic disorder, and trichotillomania. As these patients have repetitive worries or behaviours, although they are focal, they are still related to the 'OCD Spectrum'.

Course and prognosis

Many patients with OCD may have an onset of symptoms after a stressful event (e.g. pregnancy, a loss, or a sexual problem). Owing to the secretive nature of the disorder, there is often a delay of 5 to 10 years before patients come to psychiatric attention. However, the delay may shorten due to increased public awareness to the disorder through articles, books, and movies. The course of OCD is usually long, but variable; some patients experience a fluctuating course, while others experience a chronic course.[21]

About 20 to 30 per cent of the patients show a significant improvement in their symptoms, and 40 to 50 per cent a moderate improvement. The remaining 20 to 40 per cent become chronic or their symptoms worsen.

OCD patients are prone to depression and sometimes even to suicide. A poor prognosis is indicated by yielding (rather than resisting) to compulsions, a early onset, male gender, tic related forms of OCD with associated to hoarding/symmetry compulsions, the need for hospitalization, psychotic features, a coexisting major depressive disorder, delusional beliefs, the presence of overvalued ideas (i.e. some acceptance of the obsessions and compulsions), and the presence of personality disorder (especially schizotypal personality disorder).[22–24] A good prognosis is indicated by good social and occupational adjustment and less avoidance.[21] The obsessional content does not seem to be related to the prognosis, except for hoarding, which is usually considered to have a less favourable outcome.

Aetiology

Neurotransmitters

Many clinical trials of various serotonergic drugs lend support to the hypothesis that a dysregulation of serotonin is involved in the beneficial therapeutic effect in OCD. However, this does not necessarily reflect on pathogenesis. Abnormality of the serotonergic system, and particularly the hypersensitivity of postsynaptic 5-HT receptors, constitutes the leading hypothesis for the underlying pathophysiology of OCD.[7,25–38] However, a potential role for dopamine has been emerging as well.[39]

Clinical studies have assayed cerebrospinal levels of serotonin metabolites (e.g. 5-hydroxyindoleacetic acid [5-HIAA] a 5-HT metabolite that serves as an index of 5-HT turnover)[25,26] and affinities of imipramine and paroxetine[40] binding sites on platelets show that it binds to serotonin reuptake sites,[27–30] in some studies of OCD patients. A study supporting the relationship between a decreased function of the serotonergic system and a positive response to selective serotonin reuptake inhibitors (SSRIs), demonstrated normalization of the number of platelet 5-HT transporters following treatment with different SSRIs.[31] In an earlier study, patients who responded to clomipramine had higher pretreatment levels of 5-HIAA than the non-responders.[25] Moreover, the clinical improvement was positively correlated with a decrease in the concentration of 5-HIAA in cerebrospinal fluid.[25]

Another approach is to examine peripheral measures of serotonergic and noradrenergic function in patients with OCD. In one study, clinical improvement during clomipramine therapy closely correlated with pretreatment platelet serotonin concentration and monoamine oxidase activity, as well as with the decrease in both measures during clomipramine administration.[32] Moreover, only the plasma levels of clomipramine (a potent 5-HT reuptake inhibitor), but not the plasma levels of its primary metabolite, desmethyl clomipramine (which has noradrenergic properties), correlated significantly with an improvement in OCD symptoms. These findings suggest that the effects of anti-obsessive medications, clomipramine in this study, on serotonin function are pertinent to the anti-obsessional action observed.

Additional support for the importance of serotonin in the therapeutic response to serotonin reuptake inhibitors (SRIs) in OCD came from a study by Benkelfat *et al.*[38] in which the investigators administered the serotonin receptor antagonist metergoline and placebo to 10 patients with OCD in a double-blind crossover study. Patients receiving clomipramine on a long-term basis responded with greater anxiety to a 4-day administration of metergoline when compared with the placebo phase of the study.

Additional evidence for disturbances of the serotonergic system in OCD was provided by challenge studies. Challenges with L-tryptophan,[33] *m*-chlorophenylpiperazine (mCPP),[7,34] sumatriptan (a 5-HT1D agonist[6]), ipsapirone (a 5-HT1A receptor ligand[35]), and MK-212 (a 5-HT1A and 5-HT2C agonist[36]), among others, were used to evaluate whether they worsen obsessive–compulsive symptoms or whether they elicit different physiological responses (thermal or neuroendocrine) in patients with OCD compared with controls. Only two compounds (*m*-chlorophenylpiperazine and sumatriptan) have shown behavioural hypersensitivity and neuroendocrine hyposensitivity to be characteristic of serotonergic challenges in patients with OCD. These studies may have the potential to pinpoint the receptor subtype involved in OCD, raising the possibility that 5-HT_{1B} (but not 5-HT_{1A}) could be involved in OCD.[37]

Dopamine

The most compelling evidence for dopaminergic involvement in OCD comes from the abundance of OCD symptoms in basal ganglia disorders, such as Tourette's syndrome, Sydenham's chorea, and postencephalitic parkinsonism. The therapeutic benefits obtained with the coadministration of dopamine blockers and SRIs in a subset of patients with both OCD and tic disorder[41] has also suggested a role for dopamine dysfunction. A study evaluating levels of platelet sulphotransferase, an enzyme involved in the catabolism of catecholamines (providing a marker of presynaptic dopamine function), reported a decreased level of platelet [^{3}H]imipramine binding and a parallel increase in the level of sulphotransferase activity in OCD compared with controls. This provides further support for the hypothesis of reduced 5-HT activity and increased dopamine transmission in OCD.[28,39]

Immune factors

Study of autoimmune factors has been prompted by the association of OCD and the autoimmune disease of the basal ganglia, Sydenham's chorea. This complication of rheumatic fever is accompanied by obsessive–compulsive symptoms in over 70 per cent of cases[42]: 10 out of 11 children had antibodies directed against the caudate.[42] These children had a history of obsessive–compulsive symptoms, which started prior to the onset of the chorea, reached a peak in line with the motor symptoms, and declined with their resolution. This is consistent with the hypothesis of basal ganglia dysfunction in OCD.

Antibodies against two peptides of the basal ganglia have also been found.[43] A strong connection was reported between OCD/Tourette's syndrome and the B-cell antibody D8/17, which is another antibrain antibody.[44] The specificity of these antibodies to OCD, as well as the generalizability of these rare cases, is as yet unclear.

Brain imaging studies

The use of positron emission tomography has demonstrated the presence of increased activity (i.e. metabolism and blood flow) in the frontal lobes, the basal ganglia (especially the caudate nucleus), and the cingulum of patients with OCD.[45] Pharmacological and behavioural treatments reportedly reverse those abnormalities.[46] The data from functional imaging studies are consistent with the data from structural brain imaging studies. Both CT and magnetic resonance imaging studies have found decreased sizes of caudate bilaterally. Both functional and structural imaging procedures are also consistent with the observation that neurological procedures involving the cingulum are sometimes effective in the treatment of patients with OCD.

Overall, the brain imaging research suggests a role for the prefrontal cortex-basal ganglia thalamic circuitry. Dysfunction of these circuits can be explored by neuropsychological testing and recording evoked potentials. Indeed, a study of patients with OCD demonstrated that they are slower in performing tasks involving frontocortical systems, suggesting alterations at this level.[47] An evoked potential study showed enhanced processing negativity in the frontal cortex consistent with the prefrontal hyperactivity shown in brain imaging studies.[48] Moreover, the reflection of behavioural challenge on brain activity (brain responsivity) may be a potential tool for predicting a response to successful intervention with SSRI.[49]

Genetics

A significantly higher concordance rate was found for monozygotic twins than for dizygotic twins.[50] Of the first-degree relatives of patients with childhood-onset OCD, 35 per cent are also afflicted with the disorder.[51] Although this high rate is possibly related to the early-onset subtype, it nevertheless suggests a genetic component in OCD. Genetic research has yet to find abnormalities at the 5-HT transporter gene level. A study exploring the polymorphism of the promoter region of the gene for the 5-HT transporter failed to identify any differences between patients with OCD and controls.[52] However, several studies found polymorphism of $5HT_{1B\beta}$ in OCD,[53,54] hence providing further support for the $5HT_{1B}$ involvement in OCD.

Other biological data

Sleep electroencephalography and neuroendocrine studies have found abnormalities similar to those seen in depression, such as decreased rapid eye movement latency, non-suppression on the dexamethasone suppression test, and decreased growth hormone secretion with clonidine infusions.[55,56]

Behavioural factors

According to the learning theory, obsessions can be considered conditioned stimuli. When a relatively neutral stimulus is coupled with an anxiety-provoking stimulus, through conditioning, it will produce anxiety even when presented alone. In this regards, even the thought of the anxiety-provoking stimulus can cause anxiety, similarly to Pavlov's dog, which salivated even before he actually had food. Consequently, avoidant behaviour is being adopted in order to avoid the anxiety-provoking stimulus and any other stimuli, which remind it. The compulsions are learnt as a way to reduce anxiety. Once producing a relief of the anxiety, the relief serves as reinforce to the compulsion, which are then being repeated by the patient. Through the process of conditioning, reward and reinforcement, rituals, and avoidant strategies are become fixed.

Psychological factors

The dynamic aspects of OCD were first described by Sigmund Freud, who coined the term 'obsessional neurosis'. The disorder was thought to result from a regression from the Oedipal phase to the anal phase, with its characteristic ambivalence. The coexistence of hatred and love towards the same person leaves the patient paralyzed with doubt and indecision. Freud originally suggested that obsessive symptoms result from unconscious impulses of an aggressive or sexual nature. These impulses cause extreme anxiety, which is avoided by the defence mechanisms. One of the striking features of patients with OCD is the degree to which they are preoccupied with aggression or cleanliness (anal phase), either overtly in the content of their symptoms or in the underlying associations.

Freud described three major psychological defence mechanisms that are important in OCD: isolation, undoing, and reaction formation. According to the psychoanalytical formulation, OCD develops when these defences fail to contain the anxiety. Isolation is the separation of the idea and the affect that it arouses. Undoing is a secondary defence to combat the impulse and quit the anxiety that its imminent eruption into consciousness arouses. Undoing is a compulsive act, performed to prevent or undo the results that the patient irrationally anticipates from a frightening obsessional thought or impulse. Reaction formation is related to the production of character traits rather than symptom formation (characteristic of the above defences). The trait seems highly exaggerated and inappropriate (i.e. the switch of anger and hate into exaggerated love and dedication).

Summary

The efficacy of the SRIs for OCD, together with the lack of efficacy of adrenergic antidepressants, has suggested that serotonin is involved in the pathophysiology of OCD. This relationship was validated by research on serotonergic markers in OCD and by the challenge paradigm.[6] Which type of serotonergic receptor is involved in the pathogenesis and/or the mechanism of action of anti-obsessional drugs, is still unclear. However, the possible role of $5HT_{1B}$ has emerged. Further studies are crucial for elucidating the role of serotonin and other neurotransmitters (i.e. dopamine) in the pathophysiology and management of OCD.

The pharmacological treatment of OCD

Since the early 1980s, several potent SRIs have been studied extensively in OCD. Aggregate statistics for all SRIs suggest that 70 per cent of treatment-naive patients will improve at least moderately.[57]

Efficacy of serotonergic versus adrenergic antidepressants

Whilst anecdotal reports have suggested that clinical benefit can be obtained with a range of reuptake blockers, effectiveness has only been demonstrated consistently for the SRIs. Several studies have directly compared clomipramine with other antidepressants with a consistent finding: antidepressant drugs that are less potent SRIs than clomipramine are generally ineffective in OCD.[7–9,25]

In the late 1960s, clomipramine was the first reported effective medication for OCD.[4,5] Since then, numerous placebo-controlled studies have clearly shown clomipramine's effectiveness, and this has been confirmed in a United States multicentre controlled trial ($n = 520$).[58] In this study, after 10 weeks of treatment, 58 per cent of patients treated with clomipramine rated themselves much or very much improved versus 3 per cent of placebo-treated patients.

Besides the SRI clomipramine, the newer non-tricyclic SSRIs, such as fluoxetine, fluvoxamine, paroxetine, sertraline, citalopram, and escitalopram are gaining acceptance as effective alternatives for the treatment of OCD in controlled studies. Actually, they were found to be as effective as clomipramine.[59–62] Since SSRIs are less toxic in case of overdose, and as they have less cholinergic side-effects, they are considered as a first-line treatment for OCD.

(a) Onset of treatment response

It has been suggested that a relatively long period, up to 8 or even 12 weeks, is needed before one can consider a serotonin reuptake inhibitor to be ineffective. Several months' treatment is often needed to achieve a maximum response.

(b) Long-term treatment

Most patients relapse after prematurely discontinuing treatment, but, as stated above, it may take many months for a maximum response to be seen. Pato *et al.*[63] reported that 16 out of 18 patients with OCD relapsed within 7 weeks after stopping clomipramine, although some had been treated for more than a year (mean, 10.7 months). All patients regained the therapeutic effects when clomipramine was reintroduced. Leonard *et al.*[9] examined the effect of clomipramine substitution during a long-term clomipramine treatment in 26 children and adolescents with OCD (mean duration of treatment was 17 months). Half the patients were blindly assigned to 2 months of desipramine treatment, and then clomipramine was reintroduced. Almost 90 per cent relapsed during the 2 months' substitution period compared with only 18 per cent of those kept on clomipramine throughout the study. Therefore, it seems advisable that patients with OCD should be maintained on anti-obsessive medications for a long period, and certainly for more than a year before a very gradual attempt is made to discontinue the treatment.

The maintenance dose needed in OCD is also unclear. In a study that examined this issue, Mundo *et al.*[64] investigated the effect of dose reduction in patients previously treated successfully with fluoxetine. Patients were randomized to receive the same drug dosage or to receive a reduced dose. It appears that 'the dose that makes you well keeps you well'; i.e. that medium to high doses of SRIs are required.

(c) Drug dosage

Higher doses of SSRIs have been used in the treatment of OCD as compared to treatment of depression. Two fixed-dose studies using fluoxetine and one pan-European study with paroxetine have found some advantage with using higher doses, and those effects were found with citalopram and escitalopram studies.[6,37,62,65–67] A theoretical basis for this clinical finding, which is related to the 'stickiness' of the $5HT_{1B}$ receptor has been reported.[67,68]

Comparative studies of clomipramine versus SSRIs

The introduction of SSRIs has raised the question regarding the comparative efficacy of clomipramine versus that of the SSRIs. SSRIs are important alternatives to clomipramine, since their range of side-effects is different (absence of anticholinergic side-effects, sedation, safety with overdose, etc.). Although SSRIs may be associated with sexual side-effects, headaches, and appetite disturbances, these side-effects are usually less troublesome as compared to clomipramine's side-effects.

Fluoxetine was compared with clomipramine in 11 patients with OCD in a 10-week crossover study.[69] Although no significant differences were noted regarding clinical efficacy, the proportion of fluoxetine non-responders who later responded to clomipramine tended to be higher compared with the clomipramine non-responders who were switched to fluoxetine. However, patients reported significantly fewer side-effects while on fluoxetine. Freeman *et al.*[70] compared the efficacy of fluvoxamine and clomipramine in a multicentre randomized double-blind parallel-group comparison in 66 patients. Both drugs were equally effective and well tolerated, but fluvoxamine produced fewer anticholinergic side-effects and caused less sexual dysfunction than clomipramine, but more reports of headache and insomnia.

Paroxetine was of comparable efficacy to clomipramine and both were significantly more effective than placebo in a multinational double-blind placebo-controlled parallel group study of 399 patients with OCD.[71] Bisserbe *et al.*[72] reported that sertraline (50–200 mg/day) was significantly more effective than clomipramine (50–200 mg/day) in a double-blind study ($n = 160$).

Other pharmacological approaches and neurosurgery

Considered as one of the anxiety disorders according to DSM-IV (but not according to the ICD-10), it is not surprising that anxiolytics have been suggested for the treatment of patients with OCD. Thus, clonazepam has been reported as efficient in several uncontrolled studies and case series, and even in a small double-blind randomized multiple crossover study. However, since OCD is a chronic disorder, the long-term use of anxiolytics raises questions of dependency.

Despite reports in open studies regarding the efficacy of trazodone, buspirone, and lithium, results from double-blind studies proved negative. Adding drugs that affect dopamine function, especially the atypical antipsychotics (i.e. risperidone or quetiapine), to SRI therapy in patients with treatment-resistant OCD, may result in improvement for patients with a personal or family history of tics.[53] A combination of SSRI and small doses of high potent dopamine blocker (haloperidol or pimozide) was found to be useful for both the tics and the OC symptoms.[73]

Neurosurgery and Deep Brain Stimulation (DBS) have been reported to be effective in some patients with OCD. Neurosurgery involves procedures that disconnect the outflow pathways originating from the orbitofrontal cortex. Cingulotomy can help some intractable patients, but although the immediate results may be striking, the long-term prognosis is more reserved.[74] As for DBS, initial reports are optimistic[75] but as the total number of patients who underwent this procedure is very small, its efficacy needs to be further elucidated.

Summary of drug treatment for OCD

The first-line treatment consists of either an SSRI or clomipramine. Any one of the six SSRIs (fluoxetine, fluvoxamine, paroxetine, sertraline, citalopram, escitalopram) in current use constitutes an effective and safe choice, but choosing which SSRI depends on the drug's pharmacokinetic profile, as well as the physician's familiarity with the drug. The dose should be higher than that used for treating depression (e.g. 40–60 mg of fluoxetine) and the trial should last at least 12 weeks. If clomipramine is chosen, cardiovascular problems and closed-angle glaucoma should first be ruled out. Doses of 200 to 300 mg of clomipramine are needed, but titration should last for 1 to 3 weeks and the optimal dose should be continued for at least 12 weeks before determining a lack of response.

If the patient cannot tolerate the first drug (an SSRI) or did not respond, a trial of another SSRI or CMI is advised or augmentation (i.e. risperidone) is recommended.

The third stage in non-responders, and in cases of only a partial response, includes small doses of antipsychotics (especially in Tourette's syndrome), or the addition of lithium or trazodone, buspirone, or tryptophan. The fourth stage consists of atypical neuroleptics, thyroid supplementation, clonidine, a monoamine oxidase inhibitor, and intravenous clomipramine. In truly severe and resistant cases, neurosurgery or DBS could be tried.

Psychological approaches

The effect of a psychodynamic approach in OCD is limited, whereas modern interventions like cognitive and behavioural therapy show promising results.(76) Behavioural therapy was found to be effective in OCD,(76,77) and some data indicate that the beneficial effects of behavioural therapy may be longer lasting.(78) About two-thirds of patients with moderately severe rituals can be expected to improve substantially, but not completely. A combination of behavioural therapy and pharmacotherapy may constitute the optimal treatment for OCD. Recently, two neuroimaging studies found that patients with OCD who are successfully treated with behavioural therapy show changes in cerebral metabolism similar to those produced by successful treatment with SRIs.(47,79)

Behavioural therapy can be conducted in in- and outpatient settings. The principal behavioural approaches in OCD are exposure for obsessions and response prevention for rituals (see Chapter 6.3.2.1). Desensitization, thought stopping, flooding, implosion therapy, and aversion conditioning have also been used in patients with OCD. In behavioural therapy the patient must collaborate and perform assignments. In a study of 18 patients with OCD, those who received exposure and response prevention therapy showed significant improvement, whereas patients on a general anxiety management intervention (control) showed no improvement from baseline.(80) Direct comparisons of behavioural therapy and pharmacotherapy are few and are limited by methodological issues.

In thought stopping, the patient (or initially the therapist) shouts 'stop' or applies an aversive stimulus to counteract the obsessional preoccupation. The patient may also imagine a stop sign with a police officer nearby or another image that evokes inhibition at the same time that he or she recognizes the presence of the obsession. Another technique is to 'postpone' the thought until a specified time (e.g. an hour later) and not to think about it until then.

Psychological factors might be of considerable benefit in understanding what precipitates exacerbations of the disorder and in treating various forms of resistances to treatment, such as non-compliance to medications or to homework assignments. It is important to remember that the symptoms may have important psychological meanings that make patients reluctant to give them up.

In the absence of controlled studies of insight-oriented psychotherapy for OCD, the anecdotal reports reporting lasting change do not allow generalizations to be made regarding efficacy. Also, the efficacy of medications in producing quick improvement has rendered slow and long-term psychotherapy out of favour.

Supportive psychotherapy has a non-specific place in managing patients with OCD, and may help patients improve their functioning and adjustment. The management plan should also include attention to the family members through the provision of emotional support, reassurance, explanation, and advice on how to manage and respond to the patient. Family therapy may reduce marital discord and build a treatment alliance, as well as helping in the resistance to compulsions. Group therapy is useful as a support system for some patients.

Summary

The treatment of OCD was characterized by pessimism until 25 years ago when effective treatments including behavioural therapy and the serotonin reuptake inhibitors were developed. Although introduced for OCD in 1967, it was only in the 1980s that double-blind studies confirmed the efficacy of clomipramine, an SRI. This was followed by the introduction of the selective serotonin reuptake inhibitors, which also proved effective for OCD. The anti-obsessive activity of these drugs was found to be independent from the drugs' antidepressant effect, as established by their efficacy both in depressed and non-depressed patients. Overall, serotonergic therapies have provided a better outlook for these patients and have contributed to our understanding of the pathophysiology of OCD.(6,7) Previously thought to be a rare and untreatable disorder, OCD is now recognized as common, and there is good reason to expect that patients with OCD will benefit substantially from potent SRIs and behaviour therapy.

Many patients with OCD do not seek treatment and the disease tends to be chronic. There is about a 10-year lag between the onset of symptoms and the seeking of professional help due to feelings of embarrassment. Further delay ensues until the diagnosis and correct treatment are given.(81) Census data suggest that over $8 billion are spent in the United States each year on the management of OCD, one-fifth of that spent on cardiac disease.(82) Because patients with OCD often attempt to conceal their symptoms, it is incumbent on clinicians to screen for OCD in every mental status examination, since appropriate treatment can result in improved quality of life, reduced OCD chronicity, and a decrease in cost to the individual and society.

Further information

Kasper, S., Zohar, J., and Stein, D.J. (2002). *Decision making in psychopharmacology*. Martin Dunitz, London.

Montgomery, S. and Zohar, J. (1999). *Obsessive compulsive disorder*. Martin Dunitz, London.

Zohar, J., Hollander, E., Stein, D.J., and Westenberg, H.G. (2007). The Cape Town consensus group. From obsessive-compulsive spectrum to obsessive-compulsive disorders: the Cape Town consensus statement. *CNS Spectrums*, **12**(2 Suppl. 3).

http://www.ocfoundation.org

References

1. Salzman, L. and Thaler, F.H. (1981). Obsessive compulsive disorder: a review of the literature. *The American Journal of Psychiatry*, **138**, 286–96.

2. Robins, L.N., Helzer, J.E., Weissman, M.M., *et al.* (1984). Lifetime prevalence of specific psychiatric disorders in three sites. *Archives of General Psychiatry*, **41**, 949–58.
3. Weissman, M.M., Bland, R.C., Canino, G.J., *et al.* (1994). The cross national epidemiology of obsessive compulsive disorder. *The Journal of Clinical Psychiatry*, **55**, (Suppl. 3), 5–10.
4. Renynghe de Voxrie, G.V. (1968). Anafranil (G34586) in obsessive compulsive neurosis. *Archives Belges de Neurologie*, **68**, 787–92.
5. Fernandez-Cordoba, E. and Lopez-Ibor, A.J. (1967). La monoclorimipramina en enfermos psiquiatricos resistenses a otros tratamientos. *Actas Lusoespañolas de Neurologia, Psiquiatria y Ciencias Afines*, **26**, 119–47.
6. Dolberg, O.T., Iancu, I., Sasson, Y., *et al.* (1996). The pathogenesis and treatment of obsessive-compulsive disorder. *Clinical Neuropharmacology*, **19**, 129–47.
7. Zohar, J. and Insel, T. (1987). Obsessive-compulsive disorder: psychobiological approaches to diagnosis, treatment, and pathophysiology. *Biological Psychiatry*, **22**, 667–87.
8. Goodman, W.K., Price, L.H., Delgado, P.L., *et al.* (1990). Specificity of serotonin reuptake inhibitors in the treatment of obsessive compulsive disorder: comparison of fluvoxamine and desipramine. *Archives of General Psychiatry*, **47**, 577–85.
9. Leonard, H., Swedo, S.E., Lenane, M.C., *et al.* (1991). A double-blind desipramine substitution during long-term clomipramine treatment in children and adolescents with obsessive-compulsive disorder. *Archives of General Psychiatry*, **48**, 922–7.
10. Karno, M., Golding, J.M., Sorenson, S.B., *et al.* (1988). The epidemiology of obsessive-compulsive disorder in five US communities. *Archives of General Psychiatry*, **45**, 1094–9.
11. Flament, M.F., Whitaker, A., Rapoport, J.L., *et al.* (1988). Obsessive compulsive disorder in adolescence: an epidemiological study. *Journal of the American Academy of Child and Adolescent Psychiatry*, **27**, 764–71.
12. Nelson, E. and Rice, J. (1997). Stability of diagnosis of obsessive compulsive disorder in the epidemiologic catchment area study. *The American Journal of Psychiatry*, **154**, 826–31.
13. Stein, M.B., Forde, D.R., Anderson, G., *et al.* (1997). Obsessive compulsive disorder in the community: an epidemiologic survey with clinical reappraisal. *The American Journal of Psychiatry*, **154**, 1120–6.
14. Rasmussen, S.A. and Eisen, J.L. (1992). Epidemiology and clinical features of obsessive-compulsive disorder. In *Obsessive compulsive disorders. Theory and management* (eds. M.A. Jenike, L. Baer, and W.E. Minichiello), pp. 10–27. Year Book, Chicago, IL.
15. Sasson, Y., Dekel, S., Chopra, M., *et al.* (2005). Posttraumatic obsessive compulsive disorder—a case series. *Psychiatry Research*, **135**, 145–52.
16. Pauls, D. (1992). The genetics of OCD and Gilles de la Tourette's syndrome. *The Psychiatric Clinics of North America*, **15**, 759–66.
17. Mataix-Cols, D., Rosario-Campos, M.C., and Leckman, J.F. (2005). A multidimensional model of obsessive-compulsive disorder. *The American Journal of Psychiatry*, **162**, 228–38.
18. Leckman, J.F., Grice, D.E., Boardman, J., *et al.* (1997). Symptoms of obsessive-compulsive disorder. *The American Journal of Psychiatry*, **154**, 911–17.
19. Berman, I., Sapers, B.L., Chang, H.H.J., *et al.* (1995). Treatment of obsessive-compulsive symptoms in schizophrenic patients with clomipramine. *Journal of Clinical Psychopharmacology*, **15**, 206–10.
20. Zohar, J. (1997). Is there room for a new diagnostic subtype—the schizo-obsessive subtype? *CNS Spectrums*, **2**, 49–50.
21. Ravizza, L., Maina, G., and Bogetto, F. (1997). Episodic and chronic OCD. *Depression and Anxiety*, **6**, 154–8.
22. Mataix-Cols, D., Wooderson, S., Lawrence, N., *et al.* (2004). Distinct neural correlates of washing, checking, and hoarding symptom dimensions in obsessive-compulsive disorder. *Archives of General Psychiatry*, **61**, 564–76.
23. Mataix-Cols, D. (2006). Deconstructing obsessive-compulsive disorder: a multidimensional perspective. *Current Opinion in Psychiatry*, **19**, 84–9.
24. Iraqi, Z., El Yazaji, M., Hjiej, H., *et al.* (2005). Obsessive and compulsive symptoms in schizophrenia. Presented in the XIII WPA congress, Cairo-Egypt.
25. Thoren, P., Asberg, M., Gronholm, B., *et al.* (1980). Clomipramine treatment of obsessive compulsive disorder. II. Biochemical aspects. *Archives of General Psychiatry*, **27**, 1289–94.
26. Insel, T.R., Mueller, E.A., Alterman, I., *et al.* (1985). Obsessive compulsive disorder and serotonin: is there a connection? *Biological Psychiatry*, **20**, 1174–88.
27. Weizman, A., Carmi, M., Hermesh, H., *et al.* (1986). High affinity imipramine binding and serotonin uptake in platelets of eight adolescent and ten adult obsessive-compulsive patients. *The American Journal of Psychiatry*, **143**, 335–9.
28. Marazziti, D., Hollander, E., Lensi, P., *et al.* (1992). Peripheral markers of serotonin and dopamine function in obsessive-compulsive disorder. *Psychiatry Research*, **42**, 41–51.
29. Vitiello, B., Shimon, H., Behar, D., *et al.* (1991). Platelet imipramine binding and serotonin uptake in obsessive-compulsive patients. *Acta Psychiatrica Scandinavica*, **84**, 29–32.
30. Kim, S.W., Dysken, M.W., Pandey, G.N., *et al.* (1991). Platelet 3H-imipramine binding sites in obsessive compulsive behavior. *Biological Psychiatry*, **30**, 467–74.
31. Marazziti, D., Pfanner, C., Palego, L., *et al.* (1997). Changes in platelet markers of obsessive compulsive patients during a double-blind trial of fluvoxamine versus clomipramine. *Pharmacopsychiatry*, **30**, 245–9.
32. Flament, M.F., Rapoport, J.L., Murphy, D.L., *et al.* (1987). Biochemical changes during clomipramine treatment of childhood obsessive-compulsive disorder. *Archives of General Psychiatry*, **44**, 219–25.
33. Charney, D.S., Goodman, W.K., Price, L.H., *et al.* (1988). Serotonin function in obsessive-compulsive disorder: a comparison of the effects of tryptophan and *m*-chlorophenylpiperazine in patients and healthy subjects. *Archives of General Psychiatry*, **45**, 177–85.
34. Hollander, E., DeCaria, C.M., Nitescu, A., *et al.* (1992). Serotonergic function in obsessive-compulsive disorder: behavioral and neuroendocrine responses to oral *m*-chlorophenylpiperazine and fenfluramine in patients and healthy volunteers. *Archives of General Psychiatry*, **49**, 21–8.
35. Lesch, K.P., Hoh, A., Disselkamp-Tietze, J., *et al.* (1991). 5-Hydroxytryptamine 1A receptor responsivity in obsessive compulsive disorder. Comparison of patients and controls. *Archives of General Psychiatry*, **48**, 540–7.
36. Bastani, B., Nash, J.F., and Meltzer, H.Y. (1990). Prolactin and cortisol responses to MK-212, a serotonin agonist, in obsessive-compulsive disorder. *Archives of General Psychiatry*, **47**, 833–9.
37. Sasson, Y. and Zohar, J. (1996). New developments in obsessive-compulsive disorder research: implications for clinical management. *International Clinical Psychopharmacology*, **11**(Suppl. 5), 3–12.
38. Benkelfat, C., Murphy, D.L., Zohar, J., *et al.* (1989). Clomipramine in obsessive compulsive disorder: further evidence for a serotonergic mechanism of action. *Archives of General Psychiatry*, **46**, 23–8.
39. Denys, D., Zohar, J., and Westenberg, H.G. (2004). The role of dopamine in obsessive-compulsive disorder: preclinical and clinical evidence. *The Journal of Clinical Psychiatry*, **65**(Suppl. 14), 11–7.
40. Marazziti, D., Dell'Osso, L., Presta, S., *et al.* (1999). Platelet [3H]paroxetine binding in patients with OCD-related disorders. *Psychiatry Research*, **89**, 223–8.

41. McDougle, C.J., Goodman, W.K., Leckman, J.F., *et al.* (1994). Haloperidol addition in fluvoxamine-refractory obsessive-compulsive disorder. A double-blind, placebo-controlled study in patients with and without tics. *Archives of General Psychiatry*, **51**, 302–8.
42. Swedo, S.E., Leonard, H.L., and Kiessling, L.S. (1994). Speculations on antineuronal antibody-mediated neuropsychiatric disorders of childhood. *Pediatrics*, **93**, 323–6.
43. Roy, B.F., Benkelphat, C., Hill, J.L., *et al.* (1994). Serum antibody for somatostatin, 14 and prodynorphin 209–240 in patients with obsessive-compulsive disorder, schizophrenia, Alzheimer's disease, multiple sclerosis and advanced HIV infection. *Biological Psychiatry*, **35**, 335–44.
44. Swedo, S.E., Leonard, H.L., Mittelman, B.B., *et al.* (1997). Identification of children with pediatric autoimmune neuropsychiatric disorders associated with streptococcal infections by a marker associated with rheumatic fever. *The American Journal of Psychiatry*, **154**, 110–12.
45. Rauch, S.L. (1998). Neuroimaging in OCD: clinical implications. *CNS Spectrum*, **3**, (Suppl. 1), 26–9.
46. Baxter, L.R. Jr, Schwartz, J.M., Bergman, K.S., *et al.* (1992). Caudate glucose metabolic rate changes with both drug and behaviour therapy for OCD. *Archives of General Psychiatry*, **49**, 681–9.
47. Galderisi, S., Mucci, A., and Catapano, F. (1995). Neuropsychological slowness in obsessive-compulsive patients: is it confined to tests involving the fronto-subcortical systems? *The British Journal of Psychiatry*, **167**, 394–8.
48. Towey, J.P., Tenke, C.E., Bruder, G.E., *et al.* (1994). Brain event-related potential correlates of over focused attention in obsessive-compulsive disorder. *Psychophysiology*, **31**, 535–43.
49. Hendler, T., Lustig, M., Goshen, E., *et al.* (2003). Brain reactivity to specific symptom provocation indicates prospective therapeutic outcome in OCD. *Psychiatry research*, **124**, 87–103.
50. Rasmussen, S.A. and Tsuang, M.T. (1986). Clinical characteristics and family history in DSM-III obsessive-compulsive disorder. *The American Journal of Psychiatry*, **143**, 317–22.
51. Lenane, M.C., Swedo, S.E., Leonard, H., *et al.* (1990). Psychiatric disorders in first degree relatives of children and adolescents with obsessive-compulsive disorder. *Journal of the American Academy of Child and Adolescent Psychiatry*, **29**, 407–12.
52. Billet, E.A., Richter, M.A., King, N., *et al.* (1997). Obsessive compulsive disorder, response to serotonin reuptake inhibitors and the serotonin transporter gene. *Molecular Psychiatry*, **2**, 403–6.
53. Mundo, E., Richter, M.A., Zai, G., *et al.* (2002). 5HT1Dbeta receptor gene implicated in the pathogenesis of obsessive-compulsive disorder: further evidence from a family-based association study. *Molecular Psychiatry*, **7**, 805–9.
54. Camarena, B., Aguilar, A., Loyzaga, C., *et al.* (2004). A family-based association study of the 5-HT-1Dbeta receptor gene in obsessive-compulsive disorder. *The International Journal of Neuropsychopharmacology*, **7**, 49–53.
55. Insel, T.R., Gillin, J.C., Moore, A., *et al.* (1982). The sleep of patients with OCD. *Archives of General Psychiatry*, **39**, 1372–7.
56. Insel, T.R., Kalin, N.H., Guttmacher, L.B., *et al.* (1982). The dexamethasone suppression test in patients with primary OCD. *Psychiatry Research*, **6**, 153–8.
57. Rasmussen, S.A., Eisen, J.L., and Pato, M.T. (1993). Current issues in the pharmacological management of obsessive-compulsive disorder. *The Journal of Clinical Psychiatry*, **54**, 4s–9s.
58. Clomipramine Collaborative Study Group. (1991). Clomipramine in the treatment of patients with obsessive-compulsive disorder. *Archives of General Psychiatry*, **48**, 730–8.
59. Geller, D.A., Biederman, J., Stewart, S.E., *et al.* (2003). Which SSRI? A meta-analysis of pharmacotherapy trials in pediatric obsessive-compulsive disorder. *The American Journal of Psychiatry*, **160**, 1919–28.
60. Greist, J.H., Bandelow, B., Hollander, E., *et al.* (2003). World council of anxiety. WCA recommendations for the long-term treatment of obsessive-compulsive disorder in adults. *CNS Spectrums*, **8**, 7–16.
61. Kasper, S., Zohar, J., and Stein, D.J. (2002). *Decision making in psychopharmacology*. Martin Dunitz, London.
62. Blier, P., Habib, R., and Flament, M.F. (2006). Pharmacotherapies in the management of obsessive-compulsive disorder. *Canadian Journal of Psychiatry*, **51**, 417–30.
63. Pato, M.T., Zohar-Kadouch, R., Zohar, J., *et al.* (1988). Return of symptoms after discontinuation of clomipramine in patients with obsessive compulsive disorder. *The American Journal of Psychiatry*, **145**, 1521–5.
64. Mundo, E., Barregi, S.R., Pirola, R., *et al.* (1997). Long-term pharmacotherapy of obsessive-compulsive disorder: a double-blind controlled study. *Journal of Clinical Psychopharmacology*, **17**, 4–10.
65. March, J.S., Frances, A., Carpenter, D., *et al.* (1997). The expert consensus guideline series: treatment of obsessive-compulsive disorder. *The Journal of Clinical Psychiatry*, **58**(Suppl. 4), 1–72
66. Montgomery, S.A., Kasper, S., Stein, D.J., *et al.* (2001). Citalopram 20 mg, 40 mg and 60 mg are all effective and well tolerated compared with placebo in obsessive-compulsive disorder. *International Clinical Psychopharmacology*, **16**, 75–86.
67. El Mansari, M. and Blier, P. (2006). Mechanisms of action of current and potential pharmacotherapies of obsessive-compulsive disorder. *Progress in Neuro-Psychopharmacology & Biological Psychiatry*, **30**, 362–73.
68. Blier, P. and Szabo, S.T. (2005). Potential mechanisms of action of atypical antipsychotic medications in treatment-resistant depression and anxiety. *The Journal of Clinical Psychiatry*, **66**(Suppl. 8), 30–40.
69. Pigott, T.A., Pato, M.T., Bernstein, S.E., *et al.* (1990). Controlled comparisons of clomipramine and fluoxetine in the treatment of obsessive-compulsive disorder: behavioral and biological results. *Archives of General Psychiatry*, **47**, 926–32.
70. Freeman, C.P.L., Trimble, M.R., Deakin, J.F.W., *et al.* (1994). Fluvoxamine versus clomipramine in the treatment of obsessive compulsive disorder: a multi-center, randomized, double-blind, parallel group comparison. *The Journal of Clinical Psychiatry*, **55**, 301–5.
71. Zohar, J. and Judge, R. (1996). Paroxetine versus clomipramine in the treatment of obsessive-compulsive disorder. *The British Journal of Psychiatry*, **169**, 468–74.
72. Bisserbe, J.C., Lane, R.M., Flament, M.F., *et al.* (1997). A double-blind comparison of sertraline and clomipramine in outpatients with obsessive-compulsive disorder. *European Psychiatry*, **153**, 1450–4.
73. McDougle, J., Goodman, W.K., Price, L.H., *et al.* (1990). Neuroleptic addition in fluvoxamine-refractory obsessive-compulsive disorder. *The American Journal of Psychiatry*, **147**, 652–4.
74. Jenike, M.A., Baer, L., Ballantine, T., *et al.* (1991). Cingulotomy for refractory obsessive-compulsive disorder. *Archives of General Psychiatry*, **48**, 548–55.
75. Greenberg, B.D., Malone, D.A., Friehs, G.M., *et al.* (2006). Three-year outcomes in deep brain stimulation for highly resistant obsessive-compulsive disorder. *Neuropsychopharmacology*. **31**, 2384–93.
76. Van Balkom, A.J.L.M., De Haan, E., Van Oppen, P., *et al.* (1998). Cognitive and behavioral therapies alone versus in combination with fluvoxamine in the treatment of obsessive compulsive disorder. *The Journal of Nervous and Mental Disease*, **186**, 492–9.
77. Marks, I.M., Hodgson, R., Rachman, S., *et al.* (1975). Treatment of chronic obsessive-compulsive neurosis *in vivo* exposure: a 2-year follow-up and issues in treatment. *The British Journal of Psychiatry*, **127**, 349–64.

78. Greist, J.H. (1996). New developments in behaviour therapy for obsessive-compulsive disorder. *International Clinical Psychopharmacology*, **11**(Suppl.), 63–73.
79. Schwartz, J.M., Stoessel, P.W., Baxter, L.R. Jr., *et al.* (1996). Systematic changes in cerebral glucose metabolic rate after successful behavior modification treatment of OCD. *Archives of General Psychiatry*, **53**, 109–13.
80. Lindsay, M., Craig, R., and Andrews, G. (1997). Controlled trial of exposure and response prevention in obsessive-compulsive disorder. *The British Journal of Psychiatry*, **171**, 135–9.
81. Hollander, E. (1997). Obsessive compulsive disorder: the hidden epidemic. *The Journal of Clinical Psychiatry*, **12**(Suppl.), 3–6.
82. DuPont, R.L., Rice, D.P., Shiraki, S., *et al.* (1995). Economic costs of obsessive compulsive disorder. *Medical Interface*, **8**, 102–9.

4.9

Depersonalization disorder

Nick Medford, Mauricio Sierra, and Anthony S. David

Introduction

Depersonalization, a term coined by Dugas in 1898,[1] is defined in DSM-IV as 'an alteration in the experience of self so that one feels detached from and as if one is an outside observer of one's outside mental processes or body'. Brief, self-limiting experiences of depersonalization commonly occur in healthy people in the context of fatigue, intense stress, or during/after intoxication with alcohol or illicit drugs. However, some people experience chronic depersonalization of a disturbing intensity, causing significant distress and impacting on quality-of-life and daily functioning. This may occur as a **primary depersonalization disorder (DPD)**, or in the context of other psychiatric or neurological conditions. In this chapter, we consider the primary disorder, although some sections are also relevant to secondary depersonalization.

The depersonalization experience is one of feeling strangely altered and unreal, in a way that sufferers often find very hard to convey. It is often accompanied by the related phenomenon of **derealization**, in which the person's surroundings are experienced as somehow remote and lacking immediacy and vibrancy, as if the world itself has become oddly unreal. Patients with persistent depersonalization and derealization often use the analogy of feeling as if they are on the set of a play or film, where nothing is real and they are acting out a role rather than living a real life.

Clinical features

The diagnosis requires the presence of persistent, distressing depersonalization and/or derealization, occurring in clear consciousness, and not due to another disorder or substance. Some patients find it impossible to divide their symptoms into depersonalization and derealization, seeing them as essentially two ways of describing the same experience. Nevertheless, one may encounter patients who describe one without the other. 'Pure' derealization is, however, uncommon.

In addition, there are a number of other symptoms that occur with sufficient frequency to be considered as part of the depersonalization syndrome, although their presence is not essential for making the diagnosis. These are as follows:

Desomatization—a loss or diminution of bodily sensation, sometimes accompanied by a feeling of disembodiment.

De-affectualization—a loss or diminution of emotional reactivity-the feeling that life has somehow been drained of emotional content, or that the sufferer feels little emotion in response to people or events that would normally be expected to elicit an emotional response. This may have significance for intimate relationships. It should be noted that de-affectualization is not usually accompanied by blunted affect of the type commonly seen in schizophrenia.

De-ideation—a feeling of mental emptiness which may cause difficulty in concentrating, a distorted experience of time, and a sense of detachment from memories. Often accompanied by a feeling of 'stuffiness in the head' or 'as if my brain has turned to cotton wool'.

While 'depersonalization' and 'derealization' are well-established in the psychiatric lexicon, the three terms listed above are not widely used or discussed. However, a recent analysis of symptoms reported by patients with DPD gave strong support to the idea that the condition should be considered as a syndrome, with symptoms occurring in domains corresponding to the terms used above.[2]

Classification

In DSM-IV, DPD is classified as a dissociative disorder, while in ICD-10 it falls under the vague heading of 'other neurotic disorders', and is not linked to any other category of disorder.

It has been argued that DPD is not truly a dissociative disorder, as dissociation is generally characterized by a lack of subjective awareness of change, whereas in DPD the experience of feeling changed is central. However, this apparent contradiction can be resolved if dissociation is conceptualized as a category incorporating both types of phenomenon.[3]

Diagnosis and differential diagnosis

The diagnosis should be established by a careful clinical assessment. Because DPD remains a somewhat obscure disorder, patients with this condition may have had unproductive consultations with other professionals and formed the impression that their symptoms are baffling, perhaps even unique. Being given the correct diagnosis and the opportunity to discuss it in depth with an informed psychiatrist may come as a great relief. The reassurance derived from this may in itself have a powerful therapeutic effect.

Where there are other psychiatric symptoms (e.g. anxiety, panic attacks, depressive features), the distinction between primary and secondary depersonalization may be difficult. The best way to approach this is simply to establish what the dominant symptoms are at the time of presentation. In a patient with a history of panic disorder who has developed severe unremitting depersonalization, and now has very infrequent panic attacks, the most pragmatic approach is to diagnose DPD. The fact that the panic symptoms preceded the onset of DPD is less important than the fact that it is now the DPD symptoms that dominate the clinical picture.

This issue aside, the main psychiatric differential hinges on the possibility that when patients describe feeling altered or unreal, they are articulating delusional beliefs. It is important to establish that patients have no psychotic symptoms; in particular, that they do not literally believe themselves to be unreal or dead, as this is suggestive of psychotic depression and the Cotard delusion, rather than DPD.

Depersonalization can also occur in neurological disorders, principally temporal lobe epilepsy and migraine.[4] Here the history is usually of brief, stereotyped episodes, with associated features that should provide sufficient clues to the underlying diagnosis.

Epidemiology

Until recently, DPD was considered rare, but contemporary epidemiological work suggests that it affects 1–2 per cent of the general adult population,[5] with a gender ratio of 1:1.

Symptom surveys suggest that depersonalization is perhaps the third commonest symptom (after anxiety and low mood) in psychiatric populations. It should be noted that these studies do not distinguish between primary and secondary depersonalization.

Aetiology

Various factors have been implicated in the genesis and maintenance of the condition. Biological and psychological issues are considered separately here, but should not be seen as mutually exclusive.

Psychological factors: Many patients with primary DPD have concurrent anxiety or mood symptoms, or a previous history of anxiety and/or panic attacks. The clinical impression is often that feelings of detachment and unreality have arisen as a defence against feeling anxious and threatened—a way of keeping a stressful world at a safer psychological distance. There is sometimes a history of DPD symptoms first occurring in the context of some particularly stressful event or period. Often, however, specific precipitants are not identifiable.

Once DPD develops, further anxiety may follow—patients may worry that, for example, the peculiar feeling of unreality is a sign that they are on the verge of mental breakdown. These concerns often manifest as obsessional rumination and self-monitoring, characterized by a compulsive checking of the inner state and a comparison of this state with some idealized standard of normality. This further anxiety can lead to reinforcement and perpetuation of depersonalization and derealization, so that symptoms feed each other in a 'vicious circle'.

Biological factors: There is objective biological evidence relating to the loss of emotional reactivity that patients with DPD commonly report. Patients with DPD show attenuated skin conductance responses to emotional stimuli,[6] while fMRI work suggests that the brain's emotional response circuitry is inhibited in DPD.[7,8]

Some 10–20 per cent of patients with DPD describe symptoms beginning during or after an episode of illicit drug use, cannabis being the drug most commonly implicated. Many illicit drugs are known to cause depersonalization phenomena acutely, but it is unclear how any drug might produce chronic symptoms persisting long after the drug is cleared from the system. It seems likely that the initial symptoms are due to the drug, but become chronic and unremitting through the kind of "vicious circle" outlined above.[9]

Course and prognosis

Two large case series[10,11] suggest that age of onset is usually in late adolescence or early adulthood, although up to a third of patients describe symptoms originating in childhood. Onset may be sudden or gradual, and symptoms thereafter may be episodic or continuous. Patients often report little or no fluctuation in symptom nature or severity, although with close questioning it is often possible to establish that certain factors (e.g. stress, fatigue) worsen the symptoms.

Symptoms are often unremitting for many years. In the largest case series to date,[10] patients had been symptomatic for a mean of 13.9 years at the time of initial presentation to a specialist DPD clinic. This striking statistic may, in part, reflect the widespread lack of familiarity with the condition and consequent delays in diagnosis.

While there is little available data on which to base predictions about prognosis, symptoms that have been continuous for many years tend to be more refractory than those of more recent origin.

Evaluation of treatments

Until recently, the treatment literature consisted of small case series or single case reports, but a few larger studies have now been performed. Key findings are:

Pharmacological treatments

Lamotrigine: Despite encouraging results from a pilot study, a placebo-controlled crossover trial did not show evidence of efficacy. However, in a larger, more recent open-label study of lamotrigine-antidepressant combination therapy, significant improvements were seen in a majority of patients.[12]

Opioid antagonists: Transient reductions in symptoms have been reported in response to naloxone infusion, and a recent open-label study of oral naltrexone showed some evidence of efficacy.[13]

Clomipramine: One small open-label study, results inconclusive.[14]

There remains a paucity of data from rigorous controlled trials. To date, the only large double-blind randomised controlled trial is a study of *fluoxetine*, which found no evidence of efficacy.[15]

Psychological treatments

Despite a number of reports of successful treatment with a range of psychotherapeutic techniques, the only treatment trial is an open study of cognitive behavioural therapy (CBT), which showed significant clinical benefits.[16]

Management

It will be appreciated from the above that there is insufficient evidence on which to base definitive treatment guidelines, and as yet no drugs are licensed for the treatment of DPD in the UK. Current treatment strategies are based on encouraging results from exploratory studies, rather than on any overwhelming weight of evidence, and this limitation should not be concealed from patients.

The combination of lamotrigine (up to 500 mg per day) and an SSRI (usually citalopram or escitalopram) is often used as first-line treatment (see Medford *et al.* in Further Reading below). An alternative is clonazepam (0.5–4 mg per day).There have been no clinical trials of clonazepam in DPD, but many patients find it helpful, particularly when there is co-morbid anxiety. The risk of dependency must be carefully weighed against possible clinical benefits.

Naltrexone (see above) may also have a role, while clomipramine may be helpful when obsessional ruminations are prominent. There is anecdotal evidence to support the use of bupropion in treatment-refractory cases.

CBT may be beneficial, either alone or in combination with pharmacotherapy. Depersonalization experiences do not readily lend themselves to a cognitive behavioural analysis, but CBT techniques may be helpful in addressing associated anxieties, ruminations, and avoidance behaviours, and use of CBT should be considered whenever any of these features are prominent.

The use of standardized rating scales can assist in diagnosis and monitoring response to treatment. The Cambridge Depersonalization Scale[(17)] is particularly recommended.

In secondary depersonalization, it is usually appropriate to simply pursue conventional treatment of the primary condition, but if depersonalization becomes severe and disabling it may be necessary to treat it more specifically. Treatment of depersonalization in the context of substance misuse is particularly difficult: since most drugs of abuse can cause or exacerbate the symptoms, there is generally little point in attempting specific treatment unless abstinence has been established.

Further information

Mayer-Gross, W. (1935). On depersonalization. *British Journal of Medical Psychology*, **15**, 103–22. Classic early monograph, still of relevance.

Medford, N., Sierra, M., Baker, D., *et al.* (2005). Understanding and treating depersonalisation disorder. *Advances in Psychiatric Treatment*, **11**, 92–100. Conceptual and clinical overview by clinicians from the UK's only specialized DPD clinic.

Schilder, P. (1950). The Image and Appearance of the Human Body. New York: International Universities Press. Contains a fascinating psychodynamic account of DPD.

Simeon, D. andAbugel, J. (2006). Feeling Unreal: Depersonalization Disorder and the Loss of the Self. Oxford University Press, USA. Readable and informative book on the disorder.

References

1. Sierra, M. and Berrios, G.E. (1996) Un cas de depersonnalisation, by L.Dugas. Translation and introduction. *History of Psychiatry*, **7**, 451–61.
2. Sierra, M., Baker, D., Medford, N., *et al.* (2005). Unpacking the depersonalization syndrome: an exploratory factor analysis on the Cambridge Depersonalization Scale. *Psychological Medicine*, **35**, 1523–32.
3. Holmes, E.A., Brown, R.J., Mansell, W., *et al.* (2005). Are there two qualitatively distinct forms of dissociation? A review and some clinical implications. *Clinical Psychology Review*, **25**, 1–23.
4. Lambert, M.V., Sierra, M., Phillips, M.L., *et al.* (2002). The spectrum of organic depersonalisation: a review plus four new cases. *Journal of Neuropsychiatry and Clinical Neurosciences*, **14**, 141–54.
5. Hunter, E.C.M., Sierra, M. and David, A.S. (2004). The epidemiology of depersonalization and derealisation: a systematic review. *Social Psychiatry Psychiatric Epidemiology*, **39**, 9–18.
6. Sierra, M., Senior, C., Dalton, J., *et al.* (2002). Autonomic response in depersonalization disorder. *Archives of General Psychiatry*, **59**, 833–38.
7. Phillips, M., Medford, N., Senior, C., *et al.* (2001). Depersonalization disorder: thinking without feeling. *Psychiatry Res Neuroimaging*, **108**, 145–60.
8. Medford, N., Phillips, M., Brierley, B., *et al.* (2006) Emotional memory in depersonalization disorder. *Psychiatry Res Neuroimaging*, **148**, 93–102.
9. Medford, N., Baker, D., Hunter, E., *et al.* (2003). Depersonalization following illicit drug use: a controlled analysis of 40 cases. *Addiction*, **12**, 1731–6.
10. Baker, D., Hunter, E., Lawrence, E., *et al.* (2003). Depersonalization disorder: clinical features of 204 cases. *British Journal of Psychiatry*, **182**, 428–33.
11. Simeon, D., Knutelska, M., Nelson, D., *et al.* (2003). Feeling unreal: a depersonalization disorder update of 117 cases. *Journal of Clinical Psychology*, **64**, 990–7.
12. Sierra, M., Baker, D., Medford, N., *et al.* (2006). Lamotrigine as an add-on treatment for depersonalization disorder: a retrospective study of 32 cases. *Clinical Neuropharmacology*, **29**, 253–8.
13. Simeon, D. and Knutelska, M. (2005). An open trial of naltrexone in the treatment of depersonalization disorder. *Journal of Clinical Psychopharmacology*, **25**, 267–270.
14. Simeon, D., Stein, D.J., Hollander, E. (1998). Treatment of depersonalization disorder with clomipramine. *Biological Psychiatry*, **44**, 302–03.
15. Simeon, D., Guralnik, O., Schmeidler, J., *et al.* (2004). Fluoxetine therapy in depersonalization disorder: randomized controlled trial. *British Journal of Psychiatry*, **185**, 31–6.
16. Hunter, E., Baker, D., Phillips, M., *et al.* (2005). Cognitive-behaviour therapy for depersonalisation disorder: an open study. *Behaviour Research and Therapy*, **43**, 1121–30.
17. Sierra, M.and Berrios, G.E. (2000). The Cambridge Depersonalization Scale: a new instrument for the measurement of depersonalization. *Psychiatry Research*, **93**, 153–64.

4.10

Disorders of eating

Contents

4.10.1 Anorexia nervosa
Gerald Russell

4.10.2 Bulimia nervosa
Christopher G. Fairburn, Zafra Cooper, and Rebecca Murphy

4.10.1 Anorexia nervosa

Gerald Russell

Introduction: history of ideas

Two different approaches may be discerned in the conceptualization of anorexia nervosa.

1 The medicoclinical approach defines the illness in terms of its clinical manifestations; the main landmarks were the descriptions by William Gull in 1874[1] and Charles Lasègue in 1873.[2]

2 The sociocultural approach is unlike the more empirical clinical approach and takes causation into account by viewing the illness as a response to prevailing social and cultural systems. This was well argued by the social historian Joan Jacobs Brumberg who considers anorexia nervosa simply as a control of appetite in women responding to widely differing forces which may change during historical times.[3]

There is a strong argument for accepting the original descriptions by Gull and Lasègue as containing the essence of anorexia nervosa. They both recognized a disorder associated with severe emaciation and loss of menstrual periods, inexplicable in terms of recognized physical causes of wasting. They were both extremely cautious about the nature of the mental disorder. Gull spoke of a morbid mental state or 'mental perversity', and adopted the more general term anorexia 'nervosa' which has persisted until today. Lasègue also referred to 'mental perversity' but was bold enough to call the condition 'anorexie hystérique, faute de mieux'.

It is probably best to seek a balance between the diagnostic rectitude of the medicoclinical approach and the malleability of anorexia nervosa in different sociocultural settings. Looking back in historical times, it may well be that the self-starvation and asceticism of St Catherine of Siena corresponded to modern anorexia nervosa.[4] In more recent times the preoccupations of the patients have altered so that their disturbed experience with their own body[5] or their 'morbid fear of fatness'[6] has become one of the diagnostic criteria. Yet this concern with body size was not remarked upon by Gull or Lasègue. This is an argument for concluding that at least the psychological content, and perhaps also the form, of anorexia nervosa are changeable in response to historical times and sociocultural influences.

Epidemiology

Screening instruments

The most commonly used screening test in the detection of anorexia nervosa is the Eating Attitudes Test (**EAT**).[7] Doubt has, however, been expressed about the predictive value of the EAT in the very populations where its use was introduced, as only a small percentage of the EAT-screened positive scores will have an actual eating disorder. Thus, the EAT has limited usefulness in surveys for detecting anorexia nervosa unless it is supplemented by detailed clinical assessments. There is also a risk of failing to detect cases of anorexia nervosa as it was found that patients currently receiving active treatment were among the non-respondents, presumably because they wished to conceal their disorder.[8]

Populations surveyed

(a) General population surveys

These are often impracticable when the aim is to detect anorexia nervosa, a relatively uncommon disorder.

(b) Surveys of primary care populations

A useful compromise is that of surveying populations of patients who consult their general practitioners. A Netherlands study was successful because a large population was surveyed (over 150 000) and the general practitioners themselves, after suitable training, were responsible for making the diagnoses.[9,10]

(c) Populations thought to be more at risk

Surveys of ballet and modelling students were conducted because it was thought likely that there would be a high prevalence of anorexia nervosa among them as a result of pressures exerted to sustain a slim figure in keeping with their professional image.[11,12]

Populations of adolescent schoolgirls have also been surveyed as their susceptibility might be raised by virtue of their age, sex, and the frequency of dieting among the school population.[13] The most thorough survey of 15-year-old schoolchildren was that conducted in Göteborg, Sweden.[14]

(d) Surveys based on case registers and hospital records

Data have been obtained on patients referred to inpatient and outpatient psychiatric services, or with the addition of patients who had consulted paediatricians, general medical services, or gynaecologists.[15,16]

Results of epidemiological surveys

(a) Incidence of anorexia nervosa

The studies which counted only hospitalized patients tended to yield low estimates of the annual incidence of anorexia nervosa expressed per 100 000 population (e.g. 0.45 in Sweden[15]). Estimates based on case registers of psychiatric patients similarly yielded fairly low incidence rates (e.g. 0.64 in Monroe County, New York[15]). The incidence found in community-based studies was by far the highest (7.7 in The Netherlands[10] and 8.2 in Rochester, Minnesota[17]), presumably because they included the less severe cases.

(b) Prevalence of anorexia nervosa in vulnerable populations

A high prevalence rate was found among Canadian ballet students (6.5 per cent) and modelling students (7 per cent).[11] A similar survey in an English ballet school also showed a high prevalence of 'possible' cases of anorexia nervosa (7.0 per cent).[12]

Surveys among schoolgirls have shown a fairly wide variation in prevalence rates, ranging from 0 per cent to 1.1 per cent. In the English studies a consistent difference in prevalence rate was found between private schools (1 per cent) and state schools (0–0.2 per cent).[13] This social class distinction was not so definite in the Swedish study where the overall prevalence of 0.84 per cent of schoolgirls, up to and including 15 years of age, represents a high rate for anorexia nervosa.[14]

(c) Age and sex

Epidemiological surveys have confirmed clinical opinion that anorexia nervosa commences most frequently in the young, especially within a few years of puberty. The peak age of onset is 18 years.[13] The illness is less common before puberty, but in a series of patients admitted to a children's hospital the age of onset ranged from 7.75 to 14.33 years.[18] A prevalence of 2.0 per cent in females aged 18 to 25 was found in a community survey in Padua, Italy.[19]

A marked predominance of females over males is usually reported in surveys, for example 92 per cent in North-east Scotland[15] and 90 per cent among the children in Göteborg.[14] On the other hand a community survey in the province of Ontario gave rise to a more balanced female to male ratio (2:1) when cases of partial anorexia nervosa were included.[20]

(d) Social class and socio-economic status

The view has been widely held that anorexia nervosa occurs predominantly in patients with middle-class backgrounds, since Fenwick's classical observation that anorexia nervosa 'is much more common in wealthier classes of society than amongst those who have to procure their bread by daily labour'.[15]

Epidemiological surveys aimed at wider populations leave the question of social class distribution somewhat equivocal. Whereas a high percentage of combined social classes 1 and 2 (Registrar General's categories) were found in clinical studies,[21] a high social class predominance was not found in studies utilizing case registers.[15] On the other hand, the schoolgirl studies mentioned above tended to confirm a high social class predominance.

Has the incidence of anorexia nervosa increased since the 1950s?

From the 1970s experienced clinicians have expressed their view that anorexia nervosa had increased in frequency. This view gained support from surveys repeated on the same population after intervals of 10 years or more in Sweden, Scotland, Switzerland, and Monroe County, New York.[15] Most investigations found a clear trend for an increased incidence over time although it appears that a plateau was reached in the 1980s.[16] In the most thorough study, from Rochester, Minnesota[17] the increase was confined to female patients aged 15 to 24 years. There were similar findings from the Netherlands with a rise from 56.4 to 109.2 per 100 000 among 15- to 19-year-old females from 1985–1989 to 1995–1999.[10] Although there is support for an increased incidence of anorexia nervosa, there remain dissenting voices.

It is better to pose a different question which renders any controversy unnecessary. We should ask instead whether there has been an increase in the incidence of eating disorders including anorexia nervosa. This is especially relevant in view of the fact that bulimia nervosa is a variant of anorexia nervosa.[22] There is strong evidence that bulimia nervosa is a new disorder and has not simply appeared because of improved medical recognition.[23] Moreover, the incidence of bulimia nervosa has risen sharply at least until the mid 1990s, so that it is now about double that of anorexia nervosa[24] (see also Chapter 4.10.2). In conclusion, it is clear that since the 1960s there has been a significant increase in eating disorders, of which the two clearest syndromes are anorexia nervosa and bulimia nervosa.

Aetiology

Aetiological concepts

According to one robust opinion, it is essential to pursue the search for a specific and necessary cause of anorexia nervosa because the currently popular 'multifactorial' approach has little explanatory power. Accordingly the failure to identify a necessary causal element is regrettable. Many of the factors within a wide range of psychological, social, and physical causes so far studied may therefore only be relevant in predisposing to anorexia nervosa, whose causes still elude clarification'.[25]

The multidimensional approach to anorexia nervosa

It is precisely because we do not know the fundamental (necessary) cause of anorexia nervosa that recourse has to be had to a multi-

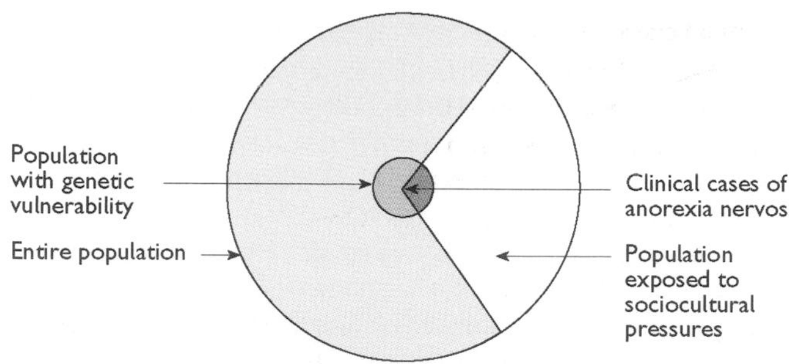

Fig. 4.10.1.1 Diagrammatic illustration of the way that genetic predisposition interacts with sociocultural pressures to cause anorexia nervosa.

dimensional approach, faute de mieux. Although it has its limitations, a multidimensional approach permits one to consider a range of possible causal factors which not only act in an additive manner but may combine in a specific way to bring about the illness: 'It is the interaction and timing of these phenomena in a given individual which are necessary for the person to become ill'.[26]

It is useful to provide a simple model of the way that two broad sets of factors may interact and augment each other (Fig. 4.10.1.1). The outer circle represents the entire population in a developed 'westernized' country. Within the circle there is a large sector representing females within an age range of 10 to 50 years who experience prevailing social pressures to acquire a slender body shape through dieting. Evidently only a small proportion of these women develop the illness. It is likely that for anorexia nervosa to develop it is also necessary to possess a genetic predisposition, represented by the small inner circle. The intersection of the inner circle and the large sector produces a small sector of females who have the genetic predisposition and also experience sociocultural pressures to lose weight, interacting to cause clinical anorexia nervosa.

Causal factors may not only interact as explained above, but they can also influence the content of the illness, its 'colouring', and its form. This modelling function is described by the term 'pathoplastic' which was introduced by Birnbaum.[27] Pathoplastic features are to be distinguished from the more fundamental causes of psychiatric illness, but they do exert a predisposing tendency as well as a modelling role.

Sociocultural causes

(a) The cult of thinness

The pathoplastic sociocultural causes of eating disorders have been subsumed under the term 'the modern cult of thinness' prevalent in westernized societies.[15] Vulnerable patients are likely to respond to this pressure by experimenting with weight-reducing diets which carry a degree of risk, and anorexia nervosa is arguably but an extension of determined dieting.[28]

It is proposed that the cult of thinness is responsible for the increase in the incidence of eating disorders since the 1950s. The social pressures which lead to dietary restraint include the publication of books and magazines advising weight-reducing diets, the fashion industry which caters mainly for the slimmer figure, television attaching sexual allure and professional success to the possession of a svelte figure, and the emphasis on physical fitness and athleticism.[3]

(b) Changes in the psychopathology of anorexia nervosa

At the beginning of this chapter it was pointed out that the psychological content and the form of anorexia nervosa have changed over historical time and in response to sociocultural influences. Whereas Gull and Lasègue spoke only of 'anorexia nervosa' and 'anorexie hystérique' respectively, more recent descriptions of the psychopathology of anorexia nervosa have stressed a disturbed experience of one's own body,[5] a weight 'phobia',[29] or a morbid dread of fatness.[6] It is precisely the modern anorectic's dread of fatness that is most in keeping with today's cult of thinness. It is arguable therefore that modern societal pressures have determined the patients' preoccupations and contributed to their food avoidance. These beliefs are held obstinately and amount to overvalued ideas.

(c) Anorexia nervosa as a culture-bound syndrome

The proposition that anorexia nervosa is a culture-bound syndrome has much support.[30,31] An intense fear of becoming obese is as culture bound as the disorder koro (a fear of shrinkage of the genitals) in Malaysia and South China.

A culture-bound syndrome may be defined as a collection of signs and symptoms which is not to be found universally in human populations, but is restricted to a particular culture or group of cultures. Implicit is the view that culture factors play an important role in the genesis of the symptom cluster . . . [30]

Anorexia nervosa meets these criteria, first because it is limited to westernized or industrialized nations, and secondly because it is clear that the psychosocial pressures on women to become thin constitute a powerful cultural force leading to anorexia nervosa.

In order to allow for exceptions to the rule, when anorexia nervosa occurs in non-westernized countries, the illness may be understood as arising from cultures undergoing rapid cultural change.[31] Anorexia nervosa is thus a 'culture-change syndrome', explaining its increased incidence in Japan and Israel. Anorexia nervosa remains rare in Asia (particularly India), the Middle East (with the exception of Israel), and generally in poorly developed countries.

Young female immigrants who move to a new culture may suffer from an increased prevalence of eating disorders. For example, children with anorexia nervosa were found among Asian families living in Britain. This was linked with an exposure to a conflicting set of sociocultural norms in comparison with their parents and grandparents.[32]

Adverse life events

Anorexia nervosa may be precipitated by adverse life events. Early clinical studies depended solely on the patient's reports of an adverse life event preceding the onset of the illness. These varied widely in severity and included the death of grandparents, a father's remarriage, a severe physical illness, stress or failure of school examinations, or being teased about being overweight.[21]

Recent studies have relied on more objective measurements of adverse life events and comparisons with control groups. In one such study,[33] life events rated included the death of a close relative, a poor relationship with parents, or an unhappy marriage. Fairly severe life events and lasting difficulties were found in the majority of patients with a late onset (after 25 years), whereas they were only found in a minority of patients with an early onset.

Anorexia nervosa can also be precipitated by sexual experiences and conflicts. In a series of 31 adolescent and young women it was observed that in 14 first sexual intercourse had occurred before the illness.[34] Sexual problems were seen by 13 patients as major precipitants of their illness; 10 of them had experienced intercourse. The authors concluded that a specific aetiological role of sexual factors seemed unlikely, but there might be a direct relationship between the onset of eating difficulties and concurrent sexual problems.

In a series of 15 patients, anorexia nervosa developed during pregnancy or, more often, during the post-natal period when it was accompanied by depression.[35] Risk factors included ambivalence about motherhood, a large weight gain during the pregnancy, physical complications during pregnancy, post-natal depression, and past psychiatric illness.

Childhood sexual abuse

Since it was reported that a high proportion of patients in a treatment programme for anorexia nervosa gave histories of sexual abuse in childhood, it has been supposed that this trauma would be a contributory causal factor.[36] It would be better if this history could be corroborated, but for obvious reasons it is often difficult to do so. Hence this subject raises unusual difficulties in judging the reliability of the data. Child sexual abuse is also discussed in the chapter on bulimia nervosa (Chapter 4.10.2).

In a careful study of childhood sexual experiences reported by women with anorexia nervosa, the authors classified the events according to the seriousness of the sexual act in childhood and concentrated on sexual experiences with someone at least 5 years older.[37] They found surprisingly high rates (about one-third) of adverse sexual experiences in women with eating disorders, and, unlike other investigators, they did not find that the frequency of these reports was less in anorexia nervosa than bulimia nervosa. They concluded that it was plausible that childhood sexual contact with an adult may in some cases contribute to a later eating disorder.

The complexity of this subject has been increased by a study on the relationship between sexual abuse, disordered personality, and eating disorders.[38] The authors found that 30 per cent of patients referred to an eating disorders clinic gave a history of childhood sexual abuse. In addition, they found that 52 per cent of their patients had a personality disorder. A significantly higher proportion of women with a personality disorder had a history of childhood sexual abuse, compared with those without a personality disorder. Surprisingly they still concluded that in patients with eating disorders it was not possible to show a clear causal link between child sexual abuse and personality disorder.

In a review of the subject a number of hypotheses were examined on the relationship between childhood sexual abuse and eating disorders.[39] One hypothesis is that child sexual abuse is more common in bulimia nervosa than in anorexia nervosa. The authors had to concede that the findings remain inconclusive. They also examined the question of whether child sexual abuse is a specific risk factor for eating disorders. They concluded that this was not the case, as the rates of child sexual abuse in eating disorder patients were similar to or less than those in various other psychiatric comparison groups. Finally, they found strong evidence that patients with eating disorders reporting child sexual abuse were more likely to show general psychiatric symptoms including depression, alcohol problems, or suicidal gestures, as well as an association with personality disorders.

Family factors

Two influential groups of family therapists (Minuchin at the Philadelphia Child Guidance Clinic and Selvini Palazzoli in Milan) have devised family models to explain the genesis of anorexia nervosa.

Minuchin *et al.* identified faulty patterns of interaction between members of the anorexic patient's family; they in turn were thought to lead to the child's attempt to solve the family problems by starving herself:[40] 'The sick child plays an important role in the family's pattern of conflict avoidance, and this role is an important source of reinforcement for his symptoms'. Five main characteristics of family interaction were identified as detrimental to the function of the family: enmeshment (a tight web of family relationships with the members appearing to read each other's minds), overprotectiveness, rigidity, involvement of the sick child in parental conflicts, lack of resolution of conflicts.

Selvini Palazzoli[41] also identified abnormal patterns of communication within these families and in addition described abnormal relationships between the family members. She assumed that anorexia nervosa amounted to a logical adjustment to an illogical interpersonal system.

Bruch[42] described girls who developed anorexia nervosa as 'good girls', who previously had a profound desire to please their families to the point of becoming unaware of their own needs. The frequency of broken families in anorexia nervosa is thought to be fairly low. Anorexic families have been found to be closer: the patients more often perceived themselves as having happy relationships within the family.

It remains uncertain whether these abnormal interactions are to blame for the illness or develop as a response by parents faced with a starving child. Careful therapists take pains to reassure parents at the commencement of family therapy: '. . . we always find it useful to spend some time discussing the nature of the illness, stressing in particular that we do not see the family as the origin of the problem'.[43]

Personality disorders

A sizeable proportion of patients (30 per cent[15] and 32 per cent[21]) were said to have had a 'normal' personality during childhood before their illness. Nevertheless there is general agreement of a close relationship between obsessional personalities and the later development of anorexia nervosa. In fact Janet, who carefully described obsessions and psychasthenia, was dubious about the validity of the diagnostic concept of anorexia nervosa. He thought that the patient's fear of fatness was an elaborate obsessional idea.[44]

In a study of patients admitted for treatment they were classified into anorexia nervosa, bulimia nervosa, or a combination of the two disorders.[45] Personality disorders were identified through the Structured Clinical Interview for DSM-IIIR personality disorders (SCID-II). Seventy-two per cent of the patients met the criteria for at least one personality disorder. Anorectics were found to have a high rate of obsessive–compulsive personality disorder.

There have been attempts to disentangle the features of premorbid personality and illness in order to clarify the personality characteristics predisposing to anorexia nervosa. Women who had recovered from restricting anorexia nervosa were tested at an 8- to 10-year follow-up, using a number of self-report instruments.[46] They were compared with two control groups: normal women and the sisters of the recovered anorexic patients. The women who had recovered rated higher on risk avoidance and conforming to authority. They also showed a greater degree of self-control and impulse control, and less enterprise and spontaneity.

Biomedical factors and pathogenesis

(a) Historical notes

Since the early part of the twentieth century a recurring theme has been the possibility that anorexia nervosa is primarily caused by an endocrine or cerebral disturbance. From 1916 there was much preoccupation with the concept of Simmonds' cachexia,[47] the assumed result of latent disease of the pituitary gland. There was diagnostic confusion between anorexia nervosa and hypopituitarism, which was only clarified much later when it became known that in true hypopituitarism weight loss and emaciation are uncommon. Hormonal deficits indicative of impaired pituitary function are indeed common in anorexia nervosa, but are merely a secondary manifestation of prolonged malnutrition.

Interest in the neuroendocrinology of anorexia nervosa led to the formulation of the hypothalamic model.[6,48] From the beginning the model was aimed at explaining pathogenesis rather than aetiology; it was not considered an alternative to the psychological origin for anorexia nervosa, but a means of explaining a constellation of disturbed neural mechanisms, as follows:

1 a disordered regulation of food intake;

2 a neuroendocrine disorder affecting mainly the hypothalamic-anterior pituitary-gonadal axis;

3 a disturbance in the regulation of body temperature.

It was known that these functions all reside within the complex of hypothalamic physiology. A 'feeding centre' had been described in the lateral hypothalamus because bilateral lesions there induced self-starvation and death in rats.[49] Over the years it has become clearer that many of the disturbances could be attributed to the patients' malnutrition, as demonstrated by experimental studies in healthy young women who were asked to follow a weight-reducing diet. It was found that ovarian function is extremely sensitive to even small restrictions of caloric intake which often lead to impaired menstrual function.[50]

(b) Cerebral lesions and disturbances

Interest in the hypothalamic model was fuelled early on by clinical reports of patients diagnosed as suffering from anorexia nervosa who were later found to have cerebral lesions, especially tumours of the hypothalamus. More recently, occult intracranial tumours have been detected, masquerading as anorexia nervosa in young children.[51]

Neuroimaging studies in anorexia nervosa have led to findings suggestive of an atrophy of the brain. CT has disclosed a widening of the cerebral sulci and less frequently an enlargement of the ventricles.[52] The outer cerebrospinal fluid spaces were enlarged markedly in 36 per cent of the patients. When the CT examination was repeated after weight gain 3 months later, the widening of the sulci had disappeared in 42 per cent of the patients who had previously shown this finding. In other patients, however, the widening remained unaltered for 1 year after body weight had returned to normal.

Functional neuroimaging techniques have also been applied to research in anorexia nervosa. Regional cerebral blood flow was measured in three series of children.[53] In the majority of the children there was an above-critical difference in the regional cerebral blood flow most often between the temporal lobes but sometimes affecting other brain regions. Hypoperfusion was found on the left side in about two-thirds of the children. Follow-up scans were undertaken in children after they had returned to normal weight; the reduced regional cerebral blood flow in the temporal lobe persisted on the same side as the initial scan. The authors found that there was a significant association between reduced blood flow and impaired visuospatial ability, impaired complex visual memory, and enhanced information processing.

(c) Genetic causes

As with general psychiatric disorders, genetic and environmental factors are no longer viewed as opposing causes of anorexia nervosa, but rather as interacting with one another. Thus there may be groups of genes that determine risk of the illness and specific environmental situations that elicit or prevent the expression of these genes. There is evidence for a family aggregation of anorexia nervosa. This does not necessarily mean that the origin of the disorder is genetic because environmental factors common to the family must also be considered. In a series of 387 first-degree relatives of 97 probands with anorexia nervosa, it was found that the illness occurred in 4.1 per cent of the first-degree relatives of the anorexic probands, whereas no case was found among relatives of the controls who were probands with a primary major affective disorder, or with various non-affective disorders.[54] The authors concluded that anorexia nervosa was familial with intergenerational transmission. It was roughly eight times more common in female first-degree relatives of anorexic probands than in the general population. The absence in the relatives of probands with major affective disorder indicated the specificity in the risk of transmission of anorexia nervosa and the absence of shared familial liability with affective disorders.

The strongest argument favouring a part-genetic causation of anorexia nervosa is derived from the classical method of comparing the concordance rate of the illness in monozygotic and dyzygotic twins. Underlying the method of twin studies is the supposition that the environment for MZ twins and DZ twins is the same, or at least it does not differ in such a way as to cause greater concordance for MZ twins. Although it is known that the environments shared by MZ twins are more often similar than those shared by DZ twins, these similarities are thought not to be of aetiological relevance to anorexia nervosa.[55] The first sizeable series of twins came from the Maudsley Hospital and St George's Hospital in London and showed higher concordance rate for MZ than for DZ twins.[56] Since then the findings have been replicated and the analysis of the twin data has suggested that the liability can be broken down into three sources of variability:

a^2 Additive genetic effects	88 per cent
c^2 Common environmental effects, found to be	0
e^2 Individual-specific environmental effects.[55]	12 per cent

The individual-specific environmental effects are those which contribute to differences between the members of the twin pair. This would happen if only one member of the twin pair had suffered from an adverse effect. It is perhaps surprising that the unique environmental effects contribute to the disorder but not the twins' common environment.

Bulik has found the concept of heritability and its estimation prone to misinterpretation. There is not just one heritability estimate because this statistic varies across the population sampled and the time of the study. One estimate of heritability of anorexia nervosa gave it as 0.74 in 17-year-old female twins.[55]

It remains uncertain how the genetic vulnerability to anorexia nervosa expresses itself in terms of the pathogenesis of this disorder. One view is that this vulnerability confers instability of the homeostatic mechanisms, which normally ensure the restoration of weight after a period of weight loss. This hypothesis would explain why in western societies, where dieting behaviour is common, those who are genetically vulnerable would be more likely to develop anorexia nervosa.[57] It has also been found that MZ twins have a higher correlation for the trait of 'body dissatisfaction' than DZ twins.[55]

(d) Neurotransmitters

Since the early 1970s, the hypothalamic model of anorexia nervosa has been transformed from a consideration of anatomical 'centres' to 'systems' involving neurotransmitters. Much evidence has been presented to show that a wide range of neurotransmitters modulate feeding behaviour, and it was only a small conceptual step to suggest that some were involved in the pathophysiology of eating disorders. At first the neurotransmitters considered were mainly the monoamine systems-noradrenaline (norepinephrine), dopamine, and serotonin. In addition, opioids, the peptide cholecystokinin, and the hormones corticotrophin-releasing factor and vasopressin have also been thought to play a part in the pathogenesis of eating disorders. During recent years the main interest has been focused on the role of serotonin (5-hydroxytryptamine, 5-HT) in the control of natural appetite, especially those aspects concerning the phenomenon of satiety, mediated through a range of processes called the 'satiety cascade'.[58] There is now strong evidence that pharmacological activation of serotonin leads to an inhibition of food consumption. It was also postulated that a defect in serotonin metabolism confers a vulnerability to the development of an eating disorder.[59]

A boost to the concept of altered serotonin activity in anorexia nervosa has come from research showing that these patients while still underweight had significant reductions in cerebrospinal fluid 5-hydroxyindoleacetic acid (**5-HIAA**). The levels became normal when the patients were retested 2 months after they reached their target weight.[60] In order to test whether these findings were secondary to malnutrition, the researchers resorted to the ingenious step of studying patients after 'recovery' when they had reached normal weight. They found elevated levels of cerebrospinal fluid 5-HIAA, possibly indicating increased serotonin activity contributing to the abnormal eating behaviour which often persists in patients who have otherwise recovered.[61] The arguments against this simple model of enhanced serotonin activity as a vulnerability trait in anorexia nervosa should be briefly presented. Serotonin function was again assessed in long-term weight-restored anorectics.[62] The investigators used a dynamic neuroendocrine challenge with d-fenfluramine as a specific probe of serotonin function, which mediates the release of prolactin. If there were any persistent abnormality in serotonin function, the response to this challenge test should differ from that in normal controls. In fact, the rise in prolactin levels was very similar in former patients and normal controls. Accordingly, this study failed to support the notion of increased central serotonin function as a vulnerability trait in anorexia nervosa.[62]

Clinical features: classical anorexia nervosa (postpubertal)

The illness usually occurs in girls within a few years of the menarche so that the most common age of onset is between 14 and 18. Sometimes the onset is later in a woman who has married and had children.

By the time the patient has been referred for psychiatric treatment she is likely to have reduced her food intake and lost weight over the course of several months, and her menstrual periods will have ceased. A regular feature of the illness is its concealment and the avoidance of treatment. Even after having lost 5 to 10 kg in weight and missed several periods, the patient's opening remark is often 'there is nothing wrong with me, my parents are unduly worried'. It is only when the clinician asks direct questions that she will admit to insomnia, irritability, sensitivity to cold, and a withdrawal from contacts with her friends, including her boyfriend if she has one.

Because of this denial, it is important to enquire from a close relative, as well as the patient, about the most relevant behavioural changes.

History

History of food intake. A **food intake history** is obtained by asking the patient to recall what she has eaten on the previous day, commencing with breakfast, which is often missed. An avoidance of carbohydrate and fat-containing foods is the rule. What remains is an often stereotyped selection of vegetables and fruit. 'Diet' drinks and unsweetened fruit juice are preferred, although some patients are partial to black coffee. It is the mother who will indicate that her daughter finds ways of avoiding meals, preferring to prepare her own food and withdrawing into her bedroom to eat it.

Weight history. The patient is usually willing to provide an accurate **weight history**. She may try to conceal her optimum weight before her decision to 'diet', but she is likely to be objective about her current weight, if only to express pride in the degree of 'self-control' she has exerted. The clinician then has an opportunity to enquire into her 'desired' weight by simply asking what weight she would be willing to return to. Her answer will betray a determination to maintain a suboptimal weight.

History of exercising. A **history of exercising** should be taken. Again, the patient is likely to conceal the fact that she walks long distances to school or to work rather than use public transport. She may also cycle vigorously or attend aerobic classes. A parent may report that his or her daughter is running on the spot or performing press-ups in the privacy of her bedroom, judging from the noise that can be heard. The amount of exercising may be grossly excessive, with the patient indulging in brisk walks or jogging even in the presence of painful knees or ankles due to soft tissue injuries.

Additional harmful behaviours, which should be enquired into include self-induced vomiting, purgative abuse, and self-injury. Vomiting and purgative abuse are similar to the behaviours that occur in bulimia nervosa (see Chapter 4.10.2). In anorexia nervosa they may occur without the prelude of overeating and the patient's motive is simply to accelerate weight loss. The laxative abuse is often at the end of the day. The favourite laxatives in the United Kingdom are Senokot and Dulcolax, and the patient is likely to take them in increasing quantities to achieve the wanted effect as tolerance develops. Self-injury should also be enquired into, and the skin of the wrists and forearms inspected for scratches or cuts with sharp instruments.

Menstrual history. The patient may not volunteer that her periods ceased soon after commencing the weight-reducing diet. On the other hand she may admit that she is relieved that her periods have stopped as she found them to be a nuisance or unpleasant.

(a) The patient's mental state

(i) Specific psychopathology

Several near-synonyms have been used to describe the specific attitude detectable in the patient who systematically avoids fatness: a 'disturbance of body image',[5] a 'weight phobia',[29] or a 'fear of fatness'.[6] Magersucht, or seeking after thinness, was a term applied in the older German literature. The patient will express a sensitivity about certain parts of her body, especially her stomach, thighs, and hips. Not only is she likely to assert that fatness makes her unattractive, but she may add that it is a shameful condition betraying greed and social failure. These distorted attitudes generally amount to overvalued ideas rather than delusions. Occasionally, however, a patient may be frankly deluded, such as one young woman who believed that her low weight was due to thin bones and that fatness was still evident on the surface of her body.

Studies have demonstrated that wasted patients, when asked to estimate their body size, see themselves as wider and fatter than they actually are.[63] Since these early observations, numerous perceptual studies have been undertaken and the conclusion drawn that anorexic patients overestimate their body width more often than normal controls. These distorted attitudes are often associated with a negative affect, so that the disturbance might be viewed as one of 'body disparagement'.[64]

The patient's dread of fatness is so common that it is pathognomonic of anorexia nervosa. There are, however, exceptions. Sometimes a patient may simply deny these faulty attitudes. Another exception is the occurrence of anorexia nervosa in eastern countries where thinness is not generally admired (e.g. Hong Kong and India). The imposition of fear of fatness as a diagnostic criterion on patients from a different culture, where slimness is not valued, amounts to a failure to understand the illness in the context of its culture.[65] An appropriate solution, proposed by Blake Woodside[66] is to accept diagnostic criteria where the psychopathology includes culture-specific symptoms which will differ for western, Chinese, and Indian ethnic groups.

(ii) Denial

Denial in anorexia nervosa is sometimes included within diagnostic criteria of the disorder, for example DSM-IV. Vandereycken[67] has written a scholarly treatize on the subject. He has pointed out that the term 'denial' is used with apparently simplicity in clinical practice, but this stands in contrast to its intriguing complexity. It is a multi-layered concept, which is difficult to measure. Denial is not a static condition but fluctuates over time. A crucial element in its assessment is the inherent conflict of perception between the patient and the clinician. The patient carries out distortions by omissions, concealments, or misrepresentations. She often denies hunger and fatigue and appears not to accept that she is thin. She shows a lack of concern for the physical and psychosocial sequelae of being underweight and may even deny the danger of her condition.

Vandereycken has proposed two categories of denial:

1 Unintentional denial (e.g. the patient's way to improve her self-esteem and preserve her sense of identity).

2 A deliberate denial including the pretence of being healthy and avoiding the treatment others want her to accept. Strong denial is often accompanied by the avoidance of treatment, but the refusal of help is not entirely due to the patient's lack of recognition of her problems.

(iii) Depression

Depression of varying severity, including a major depressive disorder, is common. The patients express guilt after eating, adding that they do not deserve food. A high rate of depression (42 per cent) was found at presentation in one study[21] and the lifetime history of depression in follow-up studies may be as high as 68 per cent.

(iv) Obsessive–compulsive features

The patients frequently eat in a ritualistic way, for example restricting their food intake to a narrow range of foods which experience tells them are 'safe' because they will not lead to weight gain. There is often a compulsive need to count the daily caloric intake. One patient rejected prescribed vitamin tablets in case they contained 'calories'. The frequency of obsessive–compulsive disorder in anorexia nervosa was found to be 22 per cent in a clinical series.[21] In studies using structured clinical interviews the frequency ranged from 25 to 70 per cent.

(v) Neuropsychological deficits

These deficits are seldom detected clinically, and an emaciated patient may pursue studies and obtain surprisingly good examination marks. On the other hand, neuropsychological testing has revealed deficits in attention, and impairment of memory and visuospatial function.[59]

(b) The endocrine disorder

(i) The impairment of hypothalamic-pituitary-gonadal function

Amenorrhoea is an early symptom of anorexia nervosa and in a minority of patients may even precede the onset of weight loss. Amenorrhoea is an almost necessary criterion for the diagnosis of anorexia nervosa. An exception is when a patient takes a contraceptive pill, which replaces the hormonal deficit and may lead her to say she still has her periods.

Generally, when the patient is undernourished, levels of gonadotrophins and oestrogens in the blood are found to be low or undetectable. Not only do malnourished patients show low blood levels of luteinizing hormone and follicle-stimulating hormone, but the secretion patterns of these pituitary hormones regress to a phase of earlier development. For example, severely wasted patients display an infantile luteinizing hormone secretory pattern with a lack of major fluctuations over the course of 24 h. With some degree of weight gain a pubertal secretory pattern appears, consisting first of a sleep-dependent increase of luteinizing hormone at night, and later displaying more frequent fluctuations.[68]

When a patient is still malnourished the ultrasound pelvic examination will reveal that ovarian volume is much smaller than in normal women.(69) Three stages can be discerned in the appearance of the ovaries as the patient gains weight:

1 small amorphous ovaries;

2 multifollicular ovaries (with cysts 3–9 mm in diameter);

3 dominant follicle (10 mm or more in diameter).

At the same time there is a corresponding return of hormonal secretion; follicle-stimulating hormone appears first, followed by luteinizing hormone and finally oestradiol which leads to enlargement of the uterus.(70)

These abnormalities signify that the patient is infertile and remains so until endocrine function recovers. Pregnancy occasionally occurs as the patient is still underweight and improving but before the appearance of the first menstrual period.(71) The pregnancy carries a risk of poor foetal growth during the first trimester, albeit with some 'catch-up' growth during the neonatal period.(72) Occasionally an underweight anorexic patient may seek treatment at an infertility clinic. Treatment with gonadotrophin-releasing hormone may restore fertility, but this practice has been severely criticized.(73)

(ii) Hypothalamic-pituitary-adrenal and hypothalamic-pituitary-thyroid axes

The emaciated anorexic patient shows an increased 24-h plasma cortisol level which returns to normal with a minimal increase in weight, as it is the nutritional intake that is critical.(74)

Reduced tri-iodothyronine (T_3) levels are linked to a reduction in energy expenditure during starvation and are adaptive in nature, so that treatment with L-thyroxin is not appropriate in anorexia nervosa.(68)

(c) Weight loss and malnutrition

(i) Body weight

The severity of weight loss may be recorded as follows:

1 As a percentage of an 'average' body weight to be found in tables for normal populations according to age and height (e.g. the *Metropolitan Life Insurance Tables*).

2 As a percentage drop from the patient's 'healthy' weight before the onset of her illness.

3 Using the Quetelet body mass index

$$\text{BMI} = \frac{\text{weight (kg)}}{(\text{height (m)})^2}$$

A BMI between 20 and 25 is regarded as healthy. A BMI of 14 or less indicates a need for hospitalization. A BMI between 10 and 12 represents the lower limit of human survival.

(ii) Physical examination

Wasting is variable but may be extremely severe, resulting in a skull-like appearance of the head, stick-like limbs, and flat breasts, buttocks, and abdomen. The hands and feet feel cold and readily turn blue in winter. The skin is dry with an excess of downy hair (lanugo) covering the cheeks, the nape of the neck, the forearms, and the legs. Heartbeat is slow (50–60 beats/min) and the blood pressure is low (e.g. 90/60 mmHg) with orthostatic lability. During the routine physical examination muscle power should be tested to detect proximal myopathy, as explained below.

Differential diagnosis of classical anorexia nervosa

The diagnosis of anorexia nervosa is usually straightforward, especially as the modern diagnostic criteria are objective. Wasting diseases such as inflammatory bowel disease (Crohn's disease or ulcerative colitis), thyrotoxicosis, and diabetes mellitus may sometimes be mistaken for anorexia nervosa, but they can be identified through specific investigations. Occasionally there is an interaction between such a medical illness and anorexia nervosa, when a patient wishes to perpetuate the weight loss caused by the former. Rarely, anorexia nervosa may be mimicked by a cerebral tumour altering the function of the hypothalamus.

In older patients there may be diagnostic difficulty with a major depressive or schizophrenic illness. The weight loss in a severe depressive illness results from loss of appetite and the patient's belief that she does not deserve food. A schizophrenic patient may avoid food because of paranoid delusions of being poisoned.

Complications of malnutrition

The complications, which are part of the illness, such as amenorrhoea due to failure of the hypothalamic-pituitary-gonadal axis, have already been discussed. The range of medical complications has been extensively reviewed,(74) with recommendations for the investigations needed on presentation of the patient.

(a) Fluid and electrolyte disturbances and cardiovascular complications

Patients who induce vomiting, abuse laxatives, or take diuretics are likely to experience dehydration and various electrolyte disturbances.

(i) Self-induced vomiting

Loss of gastric acid leads to a metabolic alkalosis and hypokalaemia. A low serum level of potassium may lead to cardiac conduction defects and arrhythmias, skeletal muscle weakness, and renal tubular dysfunction.

(ii) Laxative abuse

The abuse of laxatives is likely to cause dehydration, metabolic acidosis, hyponatraemia, and hypokalaemia.

(iii) The use of diuretics

The use of diuretics such as the thiazide group gives rise to low serum sodium levels which in turn cause fatigue and general weakness. A level below 120 mmol/l may lead to coma. The patient often justifies the use of a diuretic as a treatment for swollen ankles or even 'bloating' of the stomach, which she misinterprets as being due to fluid retention.

(iv) Impaired renal function

This may be caused by different mechanisms: pre-renal failure due to dehydration or hypokalaemic nephropathy.

(b) Peripheral oedema

Fluid retention leading to oedema occurs frequently in patients with anorexia nervosa. It is important to distinguish between 'benign' oedema, which often occurs during the course of effective refeeding, and oedema from other causes, which may have serious consequences.

(i) 'Benign' oedema

'Benign' oedema may occur during inpatient treatment. If the patient accepts a high-caloric intake, fluid retention is the rule as shown by a steep upward rise in the weight curve.

(ii) *Famine oedema*

If oedema is detected when the patient first presents clinically, or if it develops without a preceding improvement in food intake, the underlying mechanisms should be carefully investigated in order to avoid the risks of congestive cardiac failure and pulmonary oedema. By the time peripheral oedema is detectable, the amount of fluid retained in the body contributes several kilograms to the patient's weight, thereby concealing the true loss of weight. It is a misconception that peripheral oedema is usually due to a lowering of plasma albumen, as this is not necessarily so in anorexia nervosa. Therefore the clinician must look for other reasons.

1 A fall in interstitial fluid pressure has been proposed whereby water seeps from the blood into the interstitial spaces[75] whereas the total exchangeable sodium is likely to remain within the normal range.

2 'Rebound' oedema following hyponatraemia due to abuse of laxatives or diuretics.

3 Wet beri–beri: vitamin deficiency in anorexia nervosa is uncommon because many patients continue to eat vegetables and fruit. Nevertheless a lack of vitamin B_1 (thiamine) may occur in patients who eat a stereotyped diet, and Wernicke's encephalopathy may follow.[76] It may also lead to congestive cardiac failure with severe oedema from a nutritional cardiomyopathy, precipitated by refeeding without thiamine.

4 Congestive heart failure and pulmonary oedema may occur as a result of general undernutrition leading to a decreased cardiac mass, cardiac output, and volume. **Death may be caused by an injudicious intravenous infusion of fluids.**

(c) Metabolic disturbances

(i) *Hypoglycaemia*

Severe hypoglycaemia with plasma glucose levels as low as 1.0 mmol/l is recognized as a cause of death. Hypoglycaemia may go unrecognized, as a lack of sympathetic nervous response may mask the classical symptoms and signs.

(ii) *Hypercarotenaemia*

This is a benign condition causing an orange–yellow colouration of the skin of the palms, soles, forearms, and the region of the nose. It is partly due to the consumption of large amounts of foods rich in carotenoids, especially carrots, tomatoes, and the green outer leaves of vegetables.

(d) Myopathy

Weakness of specific muscle groups is common and is due to severe protein-energy malnutrition. There is a 'proximal' myopathy, affecting the musculature of the pelvic girdle and the shoulder girdle. The patient first notices an increasing difficulty in climbing stairs. Weakness may also affect the muscles of the head and neck and the face. When the patient is asked to rise from a sitting position, she will tend to push herself up using her hands and arms. She also has difficulty in rising unaided from a squatting position.[78]

There are no characteristic abnormalities in blood chemistry, although creatine kinase and liver enzymes may be elevated and the activity of the enzyme carnosinase may be reduced. Myopathic changes are consistently present in muscle biopsy specimens. Histology reveals the 'chequerboard' distribution of muscle fibres with a selective type 2 fibre atrophy. Electron microscopy reveals the presence of strikingly abundant glycogen granules between the myofibrils and under the sarcolemma.[78]

The detection of myopathy is a clear indication for the patient's admission to hospital and a refeeding programme. After a weight gain of a few kilograms her muscle strength will begin to return and a complete recovery is the rule.

(e) Osteoporosis

A high proportion of patients with anorexia nervosa risk developing osteoporosis and consequent pathological fractures. Significant reduction in bone mineral density of the femoral neck was found in all 20 patients with anorexia nervosa of 6 years or more duration.[79] The favourite method of measuring bone density in the lumbar spine and hip is by dual-energy X-ray absorptiometry. A measurement for all patients with anorexia nervosa of 2 years duration or more is recommended.[74, 79] It is difficult to disentangle the harmful effect of the nutritional deficiency itself from the associated oestrogen deficiency. The pathogenesis of osteoporosis in anorexia nervosa differs from that in postmenopausal women. In anorexia nervosa the nutritional deficiency (including a lack of calcium and vitamin D) leads to a low rate of the recycling of bone through bone formation and resorption, but the balance is disturbed with a relative increase in bone resorption.

The evidence favours the likelihood of improvement of bone density with nutritional recovery and resumption of menstruation.[79] There is much uncertainty about the best treatment. Although patients are often automatically prescribed oestrogen replacement, the only controlled trial undertaken so far indicated that oestrogen was only effective in severely underweight anorexic patients.[81] Indeed, it has been argued that oestrogen replacement could be harmful in some patients (children with premenarchal onset) and unnecessary in others with an illness of less than 3 years duration.[82] Instead the emphasis should be on encouraging weight gain, with the possible addition of calcium and vitamin D. Older patients with a poor prognosis (e.g. who have been ill over 10 years) might benefit from oestrogen replacement. There is little evidence for the use of other medication such as biphosphonates.

(f) Disturbed temperature regulation

Disturbances in the control of temperature are evident from clinical observations; the patients frequently complain of feeling cold, and in the winter they have cold and blue extremities and suffer from chilblains. In the severely malnourished patient hypothermia may be a cause of death. Severe malnutrition is accompanied by a low central body temperature, presumably because of a low metabolic rate. Ingestion of a high-calorie meal can cause a significant increase in the central body temperature[83] with complaints of heat in the periphery and sweating after food.

(g) Haematological changes

Anorexic patients may develop a significantly lowered haemoglobin level and a reduced haematocrit and white cell count, with a relative decrease in neutrophil leucocytes and an increase in lymphocytes.[84] The anaemia is usually moderate and is normocytic normochromic in type. The mechanism is that of starvation-induced bone marrow hypoplasia. Only occasionally is there an iron deficiency. The anaemia gradually becomes corrected with weight gain. A low platelet count in the blood has also been observed and there may be an associated thrombocytopenic purpura.

(h) Complications arising during rapid refeeding

(i) Acute dilatation of the stomach

This complication has been described in anorexia nervosa during the course of refeeding.[85] The patient develops copious vomiting, upper abdominal pain, distension of the upper abdomen, and rapid dehydration. Treatment is by continuous gastric aspiration, and this complication is one of the rare indications for intravenous infusions of glucose and saline. Gastric dilation is best prevented by avoiding a food intake above 1500 cal daily during the first week of refeeding.

(ii) Hypophosphataemia

When the illness has been protracted and has led to severe emaciation, the body stores of phosphate become depleted. The fall in serum phosphate is aggravated during refeeding, especially parenteral feeding.[86] Levels of phosphate may fall as low as 0.2 mmol/l. Clinical features are cardiac irregularities with a prolonged QT interval, impairment of consciousness, and delirium. Treatment is with oral phosphates rather than by intravenous administration.

Anorexic mothers as parents

A patient who is improving may conceive despite having a suboptimal weight and still not menstruating.[71] A mother may also develop the illness after having borne children. In a series of eight mothers, 9 out of 13 of their children suffered from food deprivation, identified by reductions in weight for age and in height for age as shown on Tanner–Whitehouse charts.[87] The anorexic mothers had no intention of abusing the children and indeed were affectionate towards them. **They simply extended their abnormal concern with body size to their own children**. They adopted different ways to ration their children's food intake according to their age. They might prolong breast feeding, dilute the bottle feeds, reduce the amount of food available in the home, confine eating to meal times, forbid the consumption of sweets, and prevent others giving them food. An important part of the management is to anticipate the risk to any children and conduct tactful enquiries. A whole-family approach should be adopted, focusing on the children's needs for food. The children should be followed up to ensure that they gain weight and catch-up growth is established.[87]

Clinical features: anorexia nervosa of early onset (premenarchal)

It would be too arbitrary to define an early onset by age limits such as an onset from 8 to 16 years. A more meaningful frame of reference is the onset in relation to the stage of puberty reached by the child.[88] Because puberty is a complex developmental process spanning 2 to 3 years, it is best to name as 'premenarchal' the illness which commences some time after the first signs of puberty and before its completion as shown by the first menstrual period. In true prepubertal anorexia nervosa the illness begins even earlier, before the very first signs of puberty. Postpubertal anorexia nervosa is when the illness commences after menstruation has been established.

There is much similarity between the clinical features of an illness of early onset and one which is postpubertal. However, there are two important differences. The first is the potential for the illness to interfere with the child's pubertal development. The second is the heart-rendering impact on the child's family. It follows that the management of the family is of supreme importance, and the clinician should be prepared for parental reactions, which may detract from a rational plan of treatment.

The clinical presentation is variable. Often there are precipitating events such as a family bereavement or a physical illness leading to weight loss. The onset is likely to be insidious,[18] with the parents noticing nothing amiss except for non-specific features. Symptoms of depression and irritability are common.[14,77] Some children cannot describe feelings of depression, but tearfulness may be obvious. They withdraw from friends and may refuse to go to school. Others express ideas of being underserving of love or food. Increasingly these youngsters have been found to injure themselves, especially by scratching with their nails or cutting the skin of the wrists and forearms with sharp objects, and occasionally by knocking and bruising the head. In a severe depression the child may say she hears voices calling her 'bad', but further questioning indicates that these are not true hallucinations but vivid expressions of her own thoughts. Another common presentation is with bodily symptoms, especially headaches, abdominal discomfort, and a wide range of gastrointestinal symptoms, which inevitably elicit physical investigations.

At some stage, however, the parents observe that their child is avoiding food and is reluctant to eat at normal meal times. She resorts to deviousness and secrecy. The omission of school meals often goes undetected. Eventually it is noticed that she has become thinner and may have lost a great deal of weight. Resistance is met when attempts are made to reverse the loss of weight. Even a young child may become preoccupied with the caloric values of foods and adopt additional methods of inducing weight loss. The child is likely to exercise excessively—jogging, walking, or cycling long distances. An attempt to reduce the excess activity may lead to solitary exercising in the bedroom, including press-ups or running on the spot. Other patients may induce vomiting or take laxatives even after small meals, but overeating typical of bulimia nervosa is rare in young children.[77]

(a) Weight loss

Because of the early onset while the child should still be growing in stature, there is a failure to gain the weight, which normally accompanies the growth spurt. Later there occurs an actual loss of weight and, because the child has not yet reached her optimum weight, a very low weight indeed may result—25 kg or even less. Symptoms of malnutrition ensue including tiredness, constipation, and sensitivity to cold with cold extremities.

(b) The psychological disorder

Even younger children are likely to disclose that they are fearful of becoming fat, a disturbance similar to the overvalued idea held by older patients. A minority of patients will disclose their reluctance to develop personal, sexual, or social maturity, in a manner, which fits into Crisp's model (see p. 796 of this chapter). A few may express reluctance to have menstrual periods. A girl may say she is indifferent whether she menstruates or not, but would like to develop breasts like other girls in her class. The reluctance to 'grow up' may be expressed in social terms, with the patient saying that she could not imagine herself ever leaving home or her mother. On the other hand most girls are keen to reach a normal stature.

Severe depression was found in 69 per cent of youngsters in the Göteborg study.[14] In the same series one-third of the patients had an obsessive–compulsive personality disorder, and 8 per cent developed hand-washing and other compulsions.

(c) Physical examination

Physical examination will reveal a varying degree of wasting, affecting the limbs, the abdomen, the buttocks, and the facial appearance. The extremities are blue and cold, and ischaemic changes may lead to gangrene affecting the toes. Other physical changes are similar to those in the adult, with the addition of a delay in puberty.

(d) Delay or arrest of puberty

The illness may adversely affect pubertal development depending on its time of onset. If the onset is truly prepubertal the child will not yet have shown the first signs of puberty, such as the appearance of pubic hair and breast buds. When the illness begins during the course of puberty these early signs may have appeared, but the breasts will show early growth only (Tanner stages 1 or 2), and the child will not yet have menstruated. The effects on pubertal development can be divided into those affecting growth in stature, breast development, and menstrual function.[88]

(i) Growth in stature

Growth in stature may have become arrested. In a series of 20 patients with a premenarchal onset, only two of them had reached the 50th centile in height. With successful treatment and weight gain, catch-up growth of 2 to 5 cm may be achieved, but only in patients aged 17 or less.[88]

(ii) Breast development

Breast development: in the same series only six patients had normal breasts and as many as 10 had infantile breasts. After prolonged weight gain, eight of the 14 patients showed a considerable response in breast growth.[88]

(iii) Menstrual function

Menstrual function: Primary amenorrhoea is the rule. In the series already referred to only four of the 20 patients had menstruated by the age of 16 years. A further three began their periods between 16 and 18 years of age, and four at ages ranging from 18 to 25. The remaining patients had prolonged amenorrhoea.

The above series consisted of selected patients in whom pubertal delay was severe, whereas marked pubertal delay has seldom been reported in other series in which only delayed menstruation has been remarked upon.

A young boy who develops anorexia nervosa is also likely to become preoccupied with fatness and accordingly avoids food in order to lose weight. The endocrine disorder in the male similarly consists of a disturbance of the hypothalamic-pituitary-gonadal axis. With a prepubertal onset, the penis and scrotum remain infantile, there is only a scanty growth of pubic and facial hair, and the voice may not break.

Special investigations

Pelvic ultrasound monitoring of the ovaries and uterus is a useful method of ascertaining regression and recovery in children with anorexia nervosa.[89] On first testing, and in the presence of low weight and amenorrhoea, ovarian volume and uterine volume were found to be reduced in comparison with normal pubertal girls. In the latter the normal range of ovarian volume is 3.95 ± 1.7 cm^3 and uterine volume is 14.8 ± 7.6 cm^3. On retesting the patients 18 months after the first scan those who were menstruating showed significantly larger ovarian and uterine volumes than those with amenorrhoea. The authors concluded that for ovarian and uterine maturity to occur it is necessary to achieve a mean weight of 48 kg and a mean weight-to-height ratio of 96.5 per cent. They found that pelvic ultrasound scanning helped to motivate the children to accept a higher body weight.

Differential diagnosis of early-onset anorexia nervosa

Frequent bodily complaints, loss of weight, and abnormalities of growth lead these children to be referred to paediatricians for special investigations. It has been proposed that young anorexic boys should be investigated by means of neuroimaging, so as not to miss occult intracranial tumours.[32] The diagnosis of anorexia nervosa should be distinguished from atypical eating disorders in childhood.[77]

Pervasive refusal syndrome is characterized by a child refusing to eat, drink, walk, talk, or take care of herself. Anxiety, phobic responses, and depression are also present.

Selective eating is the term applied to a child who restricts food intake to two or three different foods, such as biscuits, crisps, or potatoes, but usually remains in good health.

Food avoidance emotional disorder. this condition is one in which food avoidance is attributable to an emotional disturbance in the absence of a dread of fatness, a necessary criterion for the diagnosis of anorexia nervosa.

Food fads and food refusal. they are usually intermittent and physical health is not compromised.

Classification

ICD-10[80] (including patients with premenarchal onset[88])

1 Body weight is maintained at least 15 per cent below that expected for health. Prepubertal children may fail to gain the weight expected during the growth spurt. Weight loss is caused by avoidance of 'fattening' foods, possibly with the addition of self-induced vomiting, purgative abuse, excessive exercise, or the use of appetite suppressants.

2 The patient holds the overvalued idea of a dread of fatness and keeps her weight below a self-imposed threshold.

3 There is an endocrine failure manifest in women as amenorrhoea and in men as a loss of sexual interest and potency.

4 If the onset is premenarchal, the sequence of pubertal events is delayed: growth is arrested; in girls the breasts do not develop and there is a primary amenorrhoea; in boys the genitals remain juvenile.

DSM-IV[90]

1 Refusal to maintain body weight above the minimally normal weight for age and height (e.g. weight less than 85 per cent of that expected).

2 Intense fear of gaining weight or becoming fat, even though underweight.

3 Disturbance in the way in which one's body weight or shape is experienced.

4 In postmenarchal females, there is amenorrhoea of at least three menstrual cycles.

DSM-IV subdivides anorexia nervosa as follows.

1 Restricting type, without regular binge-eating or 'purging' behaviour (in the United States this term includes self-induced vomiting and the misuse of diuretics as well as laxatives).

2 Binge-eating/purging type.

Anorexia nervosa in males

The reduced frequency of anorexia nervosa in the male might lead one to surmise that the disorder is likely to differ between the sexes in its aetiology, clinical manifestations, and prognosis. Yet, there are remarkable similarities between the sexes as regards the age of onset and the specific features of the psychopathology.[91–93] For example, the male patients tended to select a diet which was low in fattening foods and resorted to subterfuges to dispose of food, such as self-induced vomiting and purging, and strenuous exercising. They expressed a fear of fatness and considered themselves overweight, even when they were thin.

Of course there are fundamental biological differences which inevitably alter the manifestations of the endocrine disorder in the male and, to a lesser extent, the nutritional disorder. Testicular function, as gauged by the urinary output of testosterone, is disturbed in male patients when they are emaciated. Refeeding leads to a partial correction of this abnormality.[91] The body composition of the mature male differs from that in the female; he has a lower reserve of adipose tissue so that protein depletion occurs more rapidly when he loses weight.

The relative resistance of the male against developing anorexia nervosa remains a mystery. It is even unclear whether the sex difference is likely to be due to biomedical factors or psychosocial differences. It has been suggested that young females often become preoccupied with 'fatness' because of its reproductive, biological, and social significance, whereas young males are more concerned with their musculature and its significance for strength, dominance, and masculinity.[92] These differences are linked with the frequency of dieting among adolescent girls and its rarity in boys.[94]

In a series of male patients with 'primary' anorexia nervosa most of the patients reported problems with sexuality.[95] Sexual anxieties had been present with respect to heterosexual as well as homosexual behaviour. One quarter admitted homosexual tendencies. Almost all were relieved by the loss of libido following weight loss. The authors concluded that males with atypical gender role behaviour had an increased risk of developing anorexia nervosa in adolescence.

There are only a few follow-up studies of anorexia nervosa in males. In one impressive study, 27 patients were followed up for a minimum of 2 years and a mean of 8 years.[96] Expressed in terms of the Morgan–Russell categories of general outcome, a good outcome was found in 44 per cent, an intermediate outcome in 26 per cent, a poor outcome in 30 per cent, and no deaths. Only a few predictors of outcome were identified: disturbed relationships with a parent in childhood led to a poor outcome, and the occurrence of previous sexual activity was associated with a good outcome. The outcome in males was remarkably similar to that in females.[94]

Course and prognosis

The natural outcome is defined as the long-term results of the illness or disease process. The clinical prognosis is the difficult task of forecasting the future course and final outcome of the illness in an individual patient.

Outcomes from follow-up studies in anorexia nervosa

There have been comprehensive appraisals of follow-up studies in anorexia nervosa[97] which have put forward criteria for the near-perfect follow-up study, which in practice are seldom fully met. Among these criteria are precision in the diagnostic features, the use of standardized interviews, 100 per cent success in tracing the patients, and a sufficiently long follow-up to determine eventual outcome. An arbitrary interval of at least 4 years was previously set[21] and most recent studies have adhered to this recommendation. Several groups of investigators have adopted measures of outcome based on the Morgan–Russell scales.[98] Their use gives rise to three possible categories of general outcome based on body weight and menstrual function: 'good', 'medium', and 'poor'.

In a review comparing three British studies and one Swedish study,[99] each with a mean follow-up of 5 to 6 years, it was found that the patients treated in Bristol had a better outcome than those treated at the Maudsley Hospital in London. The explanation is one of selection bias already mentioned: the Maudsley patients had all required inpatient treatment, whereas in the Bristol series the majority were outpatients. The third British study, from St George's Hospital, London, showed a quality of outcome intermediate between the other two.

The Swedish study was extended by two later follow-ups at 15 and 33 years. On the one hand, the percentage of good outcomes gradually increased and the percentage of poor outcomes diminished. On the other hand, the death rates increased with time; after 33 years the total mortality from anorexia nervosa or suicide was 18 per cent. Slow recovery was the rule: only 29 per cent of patients recovered in less than 3 years of illness, another 35 per cent within 3 to 6 years, and the remainder took much longer with recovery after 12 years being rare.[99] The Maudsley series of patients was also extended to a mean follow-up of 20 years. There was a reduction in the percentage of patients with a poor outcome, but an increase in the mortality rate close to that of the Swedish study.[100]

Prognostic predictors of outcome

In the long-term Maudsley study a poorer outcome was predicted by an older age of onset, a longer duration of illness, the presence of neurotic traits in childhood, personality problems, and the occurrence of relationship difficulties within the family.[100]

Comparison of mortality rates

In a review of 42 studies the aggregate annual mortality rate from anorexia nervosa was found to reach 0.56 per cent on average.[101] Complications of anorexia nervosa accounted for 54 per cent of deaths, suicide for 27 per cent, and other causes for 19 per cent.

A fair measure of consistency has been found in different parts of the world, especially when allowance is made for selection biases: in Denmark 0.5 per cent per annum (younger patients), in Sweden 0.75 per cent per annum, in the United States 0.66 per cent per annum, and in the United Kingdom 0.75 per cent per annum.(100)

Follow-up studies in early-onset anorexia nervosa

In a series of 60 patients in Berlin with a mean age of onset of 14.7, followed up for at least 4 years, recovery occurred in 68 per cent of patients but there was a 6.6 per cent mortality over a mean of 4.8 years,(102) a higher rate than was found in the Danish study already mentioned. A study of teenage-onset anorexia nervosa had the advantage of community screening and the use of a comparison group. At a 10-year follow-up the outcome was good in 43 per cent, intermediate in 29 per cent and poor in 20 per cent. There were no deaths. Strikingly there was a poor psychosocial outcome in half the anorexic patients with high dependence on state benefits.(103)

Conclusions

Theander(104) has provided good advice and useful definitions:

> Clinical experience has repeatedly shown that patients with anorexia nervosa can recover after a period of illness amounting to more than 10 years.

A distinction should be made between a 'chronic' illness and a long-standing illness. The word 'chronic' should be restricted to a continuous illness of more than 15 years' duration because up to then the patient is still capable of a full recovery. The term 'protracted' is preferable for an illness of prolonged duration but not as long as 15 years.

Treatment: review of evidence

In this review the evidence underpinning treatments for anorexia nervosa will be presented. Whenever possible the clinician should use a treatment whose efficacy has been established, but he will seldom be able to confine himself to such treatments. For example, in the case of the severely malnourished patient who presents as an emergency an admission to the specialized eating disorder unit may be the first necessary step, even though it has sometimes been argued that the evidence underpinning inpatient treatment is limited. In the majority of patients presenting with only moderate weight loss it is possible to select a treatment with a higher level of evidence for its efficacy. Such a treatment is family therapy, the treatment of choice in an adolescent patient.

Some cautionary words are called for on the subject of evidence-based psychiatry. For anorexia nervosa, there is no truly specific treatment in the sense of effecting a long-term 'cure'. The choice of treatment should be determined by the needs of the patient at the time when she presents for treatment and will vary according to the severity of the illness and the stage it has reached. It is wise to take into account the patient's age, her maturity, and her personality. A given treatment may be indicated for a short period only at the end of which the therapeutic aims need to be reviewed. Such a selective approach has sometimes been called the 'stepped care' approach but this concept can be misleading. The steps may not be in the same direction. They may go down as well as up. For example, a patient may be in urgent need of refeeding and if she makes good progress the next stage would consist of consolidating her improvement. If she is unfortunate, however, earlier priorities will reassert themselves.

A tendency to decry the benefits of treatment in anorexia nervosa first appeared in the early 1990s, and in more recent years cries of despair have become ever shriller. To some extent this is a side effect of the treatment evaluation industry which has unintentionally caused confusion between the usefulness of treatments on the one hand and the solid scientific evidence for their efficacy on the other. In an ideal world the two would be the same. In an illness such as anorexia nervosa they often are not, as will be illustrated further on.

A key member of the treatment evaluation industry in the United Kingdom is **the National Institute for Clinical Excellence** (NICE).(105) NICE has developed a hierarchy for the strength of the evidence underpinning various treatments, as described in Chapter 1.10. I is the strongest level of evidence, followed by Ia, IIa, IIb, III, and IV, the last being the lowest level. Anorexia nervosa is an area of care, which particularly requires Clinical Practice guidelines because of substantial dangers to life and physical health and some clinical uncertainties. So far NICE has failed to provide the required 'statements to assist practitioner decisions about appropriate health care for specific clinical circumstances'. NICE has not recognized the solid evidence favouring family therapy in adolescents (according it only Grade B in an ill-defined set of Grades A, B, and C for clinical guidelines). Family therapy should be regraded as A. NICE has also failed to identify the specific value of a specialized eating disorder service in patients with a risk to physical health and life. This should have been graded at least as B, or as (I) using the system of clinical recommendations described in Chapter 1.10. The correction of severe malnutrition requires a specialized eating disorder service rather than the involvement of a physician and medical unit (proposed by NICE) whose treatment is usually restricted to tube-feeding. NICE has also failed to recognize the value of other treatments, according them only a Grade C, implying there have been no good clinical studies.

The randomized controlled trial (RCT) has been idealized as the 'gold standard' for the level of evidence. The absence of such evidence for a given treatment does *not* signify that this treatment lacks efficacy. Some colleagues write and speak as if treatments other than those confirmed by RCT are not worthy of consideration. In truth they may well be effective, but the evidence for this is hard to come by. An effect of concentrating on RCTs and ignoring sound clinical evidence, is the conclusion reached by one authority that evidence-based treatment of anorexia nervosa is 'barely' possible. This is to ignore the fact that there are essential treatments for which evaluation by RCT has not yet been possible, because of insuperable ethical obstacles or limited patient compliance.

RCTs are particularly problematic in the assessment of treatments for patients with anorexia nervosa. For example, the NICE guidelines do not mention the role of a specialized eating disorder service, although there are oblique references to 'professionals with specialist experience of eating disorders' and 'a place for inpatient management'. Specialized eating disorder units (EDUs) long ago graduated to providing a broad service not confined to inpatient treatment but including daycare and outpatient treatment. It is important to evaluate the benefits of a specialist eating disorder service, and this is not mentioned in the NICE Guidelines. There has been only one study randomizing low weight patients to inpatient or outpatient treatments,(96) as the difficulties are obvious.

A balanced view needs to be taken towards the role of RCTs in the evaluation of treatments in anorexia nervosa. There has recently been a swing of the pendulum in the reverse direction. Some researchers have reached the surprising conclusion that RCTs in anorexia nervosa are so difficult that they should be considered as 'premature' in view of their cost and the failure of some of hem.(106)

An important reason why researchers may fail to complete a satisfactory RCT is the patient's behaviour in the course of the trial. The anorexic patient's resistance to treatment may extend to sabotaging the basic requirements of the treatment trial itself, e.g. compliance with the treatment and the follow-up assessments. These problems are difficult to eliminate entirely. Nevertheless RCTs are still possible if the researchers are assiduous in following-up their patients. Evaluators of research trials should see that the perfect trial in anorexia nervosa is a contradiction in terms. The pessimists favouring the abandonment of RCTs should remember that new ideas can emerge unexpectedly during the course of a trial, thus pointing the researcher towards fresh treatment approaches capable of being retested at a later date.

In the remainder of this section levels of evidence for the efficacy of treatments will be discussed, even when they are not considered by NICE.

Family therapy

Family therapy is the main treatment to have been carefully evaluated in anorexia nervosa, having now been tested in a number of randomized controlled trials. Any one of these trials has its imperfections, but taken as a body of evolving evidence, family therapy should be seen as the method of choice for treating anorexic patients with an early age of onset. Some of these trials will be summarized in order to illustrate ethical and technical difficulties, as well as the strength of the evidence.

(a) The first controlled trial of family therapy

The ***first controlled trial of family therapy*** was begun at the Maudsley Hospital in the early 1980s on a series of 57 patients.(107) The principles of the family therapy have been incorporated in the Maudsley model, which has been adopted by researchers in the United States who have reached broadly similar conclusions.(108) One assumption of the Maudsley model of family therapy is that the family is ineffective in helping the patient eliminate her symptoms and might indeed contribute to their maintenance, because family life has become so organized around a potentially life-threatening problem. It is considered essential to correct the patient's starvation by assisting the parents to take control of their child's eating until her weight has returned to normal.

The first Maudsley trial had to overcome ethical objections to a randomized allocation bearing in mind the severity of the illness. Risks were minimized by first ensuring that the patients' weight loss had been corrected during an admission to an eating disorders unit. Family therapy itself commenced on discharge and aimed at the prevention of relapse. The outpatient family therapy was administered for 1 year and the patients were assessed on the completion of 1 year's treatment and 5 years later.

The 57 anorexic patients were subdivided into three groups according to recognized prognostic criteria. This showed that the benefits of family therapy were confined to one of the three subgroups, namely patients with the age of onset less than 19 years and a duration of illness less than 3 years.

Patients in each subgroup were randomly allocated to family therapy or the control treatment which consisted of a supportive and problem-centred individual therapy. Most important in assessing progress was body weight. The Morgan-Russell scales were utilized to obtain categories of general outcome and measures of adjustment along five dimensions: nutritional status, menstrual function, mental state, psychosexual adjustment and socio-economic status, as well as their mean, the 'average outcome score'.

(i) Group 1: early age of onset (short history)

A tendency for the patients to lose weight on discharge from hospital was reversed more readily in patients in receipt of family therapy. The superiority of family therapy was demonstrated by a higher weight at the end of 1 year's treatment (Fig. 4.10.1.2). Family therapy was also demonstrated to be more beneficial on the Morgan-Russell scales in terms of more good outcome categories and a higher average outcome score.

(ii) Group 2: patients with late age of onset

In this group the effect of the two therapies was reversed (Fig. 4.10.1.3). Individual therapy appeared to result in a greater weight gain than family therapy but significant only at a 6-months follow-up.

It was concluded that family therapy was more effective than individual therapy in patients whose illness began before the age of 19 years and had lasted less than 3 years.

(b) Beneficial components of family therapy in adolescents: the second Maudsley RCT(109)

The finding that family therapy is effective in younger patients with anorexia nervosa has led to a search for the effective components of this therapy. Many family therapists consider that it is important to understand the way the family functions. Others, however, prefer a symptom oriented approach with an emphasis on helping the parents to manage their child's problem.(43) The relative importance of these two components of family therapy has been investigated by comparing conjoint family therapy with separated family therapy.(109) In conjoint family therapy (CFT) the whole family is seen together in the treatment sessions. In separated family therapy (SFT) the parents are seen together and the same therapist also sees

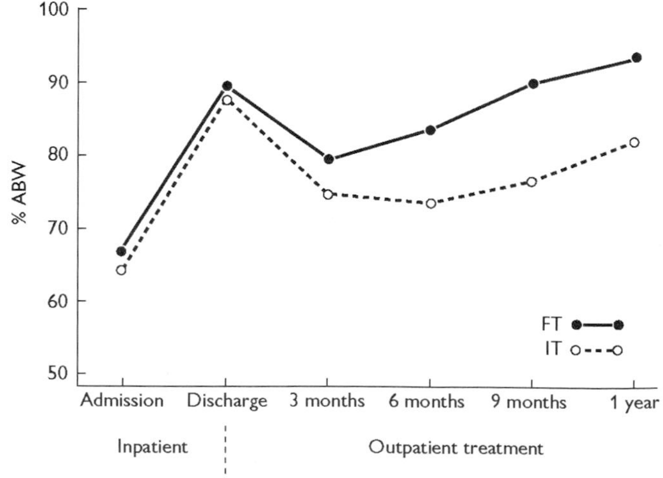

Fig. 4.10.1.2 Group of patients whose illness had an early onset and was of short duration. FT, family therapy; IT, individual therapy; ABW, average body weight.

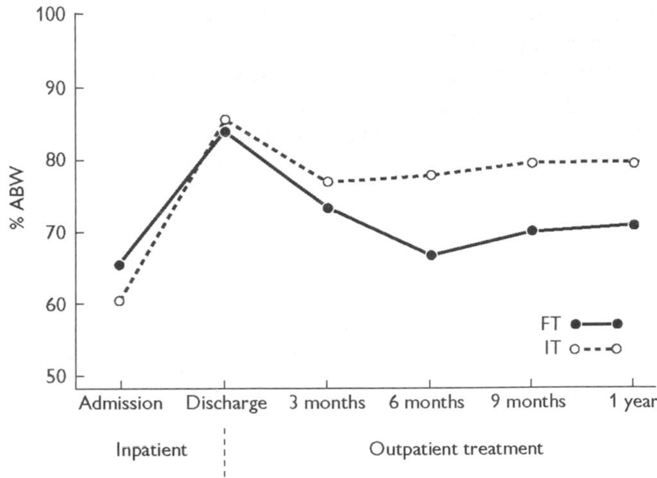

Fig. 4.10.1.3 Group of patients with relatively late onset of anorexia nervosa. FT, family therapy; IT, individual therapy; ABW, average body weight.

the patient separately for therapy and support. In CFT it is possible to observe and interpret family transactions, whereas this is not possible in SFT. The two treatments share the therapeutic advice for the parents to sustain a united approach aimed at improving their child's eating pattern.

The RCT was between CFT and SFT, given for 1 year on an outpatient basis. Forty adolescent patients were enrolled, most of them severely underweight (mean BMI 15.4).

In the course of the year the benefits of CFT and SFT were similar with considerable gains in weight (mean 8.2 kg) and marked improvements in the Morgan/Russell average outcome scores. Significant differences in the patients' responses to CFT and SFT were only obtained when treatment outcome was analysed separately in patients of high and low expressed emotion (EE) families. The patients within the high EE group allocated to SFT reached a significantly higher weight at follow-up (99.9 per cent ABW) than those in the CFT group (85.8 per cent ABW).

(c) RCT undertaken in Stanford, USA(108)

This trial was also on adolescent patients, this time comparing two courses of family therapy: one lasting for 6 months (10 sessions) and the other for 1 year (20 sessions). The aim of the study was to ascertain whether the duration of the family therapy exerted a critical effect on outcome.

The therapy was given according to the Maudsley Model, but the US study had a number of advantages, including a larger patient population (86 adolescents) and hence a greater statistical power. The therapy was given by therapists trained on a manual-based form of family therapy.

In comparison with the 2000 Maudsley Study(109) the patients were not so ill, (mean BMI 17.1). The principal measures of outcome were body weight and the eating disorder examination (EDE). There were no statistically significant differences between the two treatments.

The authors concluded that the short-term course of family was as effective as the long-term one for adolescents with a short duration anorexia nervosa. However, patients with more severe obsessive compulsive thinking, or coming from non-intact families, benefited from the longer treatment.

Strictly speaking, this RCT as such did not provide evidence of benefit from family therapy as there was no alternative form of treatment as a control. Nevertheless the outcomes at the end of 1 year's treatment were highly satisfactory with improvements not reported previously in natural outcome follow-up studies.

(d) Enduring benefits of family therapy

(i) 5-year follow-up with the first Maudsley RCT(110)

Patients who took part in the original Maudsley RCT of family therapy were followed up 5 years after the end of treatment in order to look for evidence of long-term benefit. Follow-up information was obtained on all 57 patients.(110) Apart from three deaths, there was a further overall improvement mainly attributable to the natural outcome of anorexia nervosa.

Within the subgroup of patients with early onset/short history, the mean weight achieved was 103 per cent ABW in patients who had received family therapy. On the Morgan/Russell scale, significantly greater improvement after family therapy was still discernable with a higher proportion of patients achieving a 'good' outcome and a higher average outcome score.

(ii) 5-year follow-up with the Maudsley adolescent RCT(112)

Of the original 40 patients 38 agreed to be reassessed. Compared with the end of treatment there were more patients in the good outcome category and fewer in the poor outcome category, and a further increase in weight. There were no deaths. The main purpose of this study had been to compare CFT and SFT. There was a significant difference between the two groups in the number of patients who resumed normal menstruation, higher in the SFT than in the CFT group. The findings at 1 year in patients from families with raised levels of maternal criticism (high EE) were still evident at 5 years. This group had done less well at the end of treatment in terms of weight and resumption of menstruation if they had been offered CFT.

(iii) 4-year follow-up with the US (Stanford) adolescent RCT(113)

Of the original 86 adolescent patients 71 were followed up. The long-term clinical outcome was good. Again there was little difference between patients treated with short-term or long-term family therapy. The BMI at follow-up for the short-term was 20.6, and the group as a whole showed good psychosocial functioning.

(e) Family therapy conclusions

There is now a strong body of evidence from RCTs that family therapy benefits younger patients with anorexia nervosa. The strength of the evidence in favour of family therapy has grown because of the increasing size of the patient populations tested: 21 in the 1987 Maudsley study, 40 in the 2000 Maudsley study, and 86 in the 2005 Stanford study.

1. From the search for specific components of the family therapy in the Maudsley studies, it can be concluded that the therapy should not be aimed at 'changing the family' but rather at helping them manage a sick family member.
2. Differences in the patients' responses to CFT and SFT were detected when there was a separate analysis for treatment outcome in patients in high and low expressed emotion (EE) families. From this it was concluded that SFT is the more appropriate treatment in families with high expressed emotion.

3 The Stanford study points towards the family therapy of shorter duration (6 months) being acceptable, except in the case of patients with obsessive compulsive thinking or in split families.

4 Finally, it is impressive that the quality of the clinical outcome increases in the long-term follow-ups. The patients in the 1987 Maudsley study showed the best outcome at the end of 5 years. This is not simply due to an expected good natural outcome, as the benefits of family therapy were still evident after 5 years.

Cognitive behavioural therapy

A theory for faulty cognitions maintaining the illness has been put forward by Fairburn *et al.*[(114)] The argument for examining the role of faulty cognitions in anorexia nervosa is inescapable. The original description of perceptual and conceptual disturbances in anorexia nervosa was put forward by Bruch in 1962.[(5)] It was appreciated that faulty attitudes to body size contributed in part to the patient's determination to reduce her food intake and lose weight. These observations led to the development of cognitive behavioural therapy (CBT) for anorexia nervosa. At first the evidence of its benefit relied on clinical impressions and case reports.[(115)] In recent years there have been valiant attempts to assess CBT in adult anorexic patients. It must be said, however, that these studies have met with limited success.

(a) CBT as a post-hospitalization treatment

The most fruitful RCT was conducted at the New York State Psychiatric Institute.[(116)] The design depended on the random allocation to CBT or the control treatment nutritional counselling (NC) of outpatients after discharge from an inpatient programme. Patients were eligible to enter the outpatient trial when they reached at least 90 per cent of ideal body weight. 33 who were eligible were randomly assigned to one or other treatment. The value of each treatment was assessed by its ability to prevent a relapse, defined as a fall in weight below a BMI of 17.5, or the development of medical or psychiatric complications.

Overall treatment failure was counted as the number of patients who had relapsed plus those who had dropped out from the treatment. The main finding is that the CBT group had a lower relapse and dropout rate and a better clinical outcome than the NC group.

(b) Comparison of CBT with a non-specific supportive clinical management (NSCM)

This study was conducted in Christchurch, New Zealand.[(117)] In this randomized controlled trial three therapies were compared:

1 CBT

2 Interpersonal psychotherapy

3 Non-specific supportive clinical management (NSCM).

The hypothesis was that the two specialized psychotherapies would be more effective than NSCM.

56 women were enrolled in the study. In fact the mean weights at baseline were not all that low (mean BMI 17.3). Twenty sessions were provided over a course of 20 weeks. The main assessments were a Global Assessment of Functioning (GAF) scale designed by the authors, body weight and the EDE.

The improvement in the group as a whole was perhaps disappointing with mean weight gains of 2.2 kg for CBT to 4.0 kg for NSCM. The hypothesis was not upheld and the specific therapies were less good than the non-specific supportive clinical management. The main lesson from this study is that good general clinical care combined with supportive psychotherapy can be at least as good as CBT.

(c) Multi-centred US study of CBT on its own or combined with medication[(106)]

An RCT was conducted in three well-established centres in the United States (White Plains New York, Minneapolis, and Stanford). In the original design there were three treatment groups:

1 Medication only

2 CBT only

3 Combined CBT and medication

Altogether 122 patients were randomized to one or other of these treatments. The patients were mainly adult. Their mean BMI (17.7–17.9) suggested the patients were not extremely thin. Intensive treatment was offered for up to 1 year. The patients were withdrawn from the study if they were 'treatment failures'. There were only low rates of completion: 27 per cent of the patients allocated medication, 43 per cent in the CBT group and 41 per cent in the combination group.

The methodological problems prevented an evaluation of the relative effectiveness of the treatments. The overall conclusions were somewhat pessimistic:

> 'It appears premature to conduct randomized controlled trials for *adults with anorexia nervosa* until the reasons for poor acceptance and high dropout rates . . . have been identified, and methods to remedy these serious problems have been devised'.

In fact the investigators were unlucky with the high rate of non-compliance; other studies offering psychotherapy to adult anorexic patients did not encounter such high dropout rates.[(118)]

The specialist eating disorder service

There is evidence that the treatment of anorexia nervosa is superior in specialized eating disorder units (EDUs) to that of general psychiatric units (adult or adolescent) or general medical units. The EDU comprises a team of professionals with training in the treatment of patients with anorexia nervosa and in maintaining the particular therapeutic ethos that is required. An EDU used to provide mainly inpatient care, but in recent years this has been extended to day and outpatient care. The clinical staff consist of a wide range of personnel including a psychiatric leadership and a trained nursing staff. The psychotherapeutic skills may vary but should include family therapy. The ethos of the EDU needs to combine a mix of therapeutic empathy for the patient with the ability to persuade her to return to a normal weight and eating habits. It is essential that the EDU nurse should be able to combine these skills.

This ethos was established in EDUs set-up in London in the 1970s and 1980s, particularly at St George's Hospital, the Royal Free Hospital and the Maudsley Hospital. It is from there that evidence has arisen for the effectiveness of a specialized eating disorder service.

An ambitious study from St George's Hospital, London, initially aimed at evaluating the advantages of three treatment settings.[(96)] Fortunately the study incorporated a control group and the comparison with the active treatment groups yielded the most important results. The four groups were as follows:

1 Inpatient treatment: 4 months on average followed by outpatient psychotherapy.

2 Outpatient treatment combining individual and family therapy.

3 Outpatient group therapy.

4 The control group provided no treatment at the EDU after a 'one-off' evaluation.

90 patients were randomly allocated to one or other of the four options. The study began in the mid-1980s when uncertainty in the subject still warranted from an ethical point of view a random allocation to four groups, including one in which no treatment was provided but the patients returned to the care of their general practitioners. There were methodological difficulties. The patients sometimes dropped out of the treatment when it was not what they wished: out of 30 patients offered inpatient treatment, only 18 accepted it.

At 1 year follow-up there were few clear-cut differences between the patients in the three treatment groups: the inpatients' weights were similar to the outpatients. The clearest finding was that patients allocated to any one of the three treatment groups fared much better than those allocated to the one-off evaluation session only.

The main lesson from this valiant study is that care within an ED service, whether inpatient or outpatient, and irrespective of the specific treatment modality, is superior to treatment received outside an ED service.

(a) Day care and community treatment

There is a paucity of controlled trials of day programmes. An exception is the comparison of inpatient and day treatment carried out in Edinburgh.[119] A traditional inpatient programme, aimed strictly at weight gain, was compared with a more permissive day programme stressing open communication and patient autonomy. The day programme consisted of intensive psychological treatments and was available on 4 days each week. 32 patients who would have merited admission to hospital were randomly allocated to the day programme or the inpatient programme. Although statistically significant differences were not found between the two methods of treatment, the author reported interesting trends in improved outcome using the Morgan/Russell scales. The only advantage conferred by inpatient treatment was a slightly greater weight gain. In contrast, the day programme was more popular with patients who preferred to have a greater say in their rate of weight gain. There was also a greater return of personal autonomy.

(b) Inpatient treatment

Inpatient treatment in recent years has attracted a bad press. It has been argued that there are few RCTs, which have thrown any light on the benefits of inpatient treatments. This is a blinkered approach because RCTs addressed to some of the questions, are either inappropriate or ethically impossible to carry-out. An example of a largely inappropriate question from a clinical point of view is the comparison of inpatient and outpatient treatment in anorexia nervosa because the indications and the patient's suitability for each are very different. It is justified to state this categorically because there now exists solid clinical experience to show what can be achieved by inpatient treatment. The limitations of inpatient treatment are that the benefits may last only a number of months when there is a variable likelihood of relapse. A useful research question would be to identify patients who are most likely to relapse after inpatient treatment. The firm statement made above is warranted because of the valiant study by Crisp and his colleagues[120] previously discussed. Today this study would probably not be possible from an ethical point of view.

The most obvious benefit from inpatient treatment in an EDU is that this is the surest and safest method of improving the patient's nutrition and correcting her weight loss, thereby reversing physical complications, and sometimes saving her life. In various cohort studies the weight gain has varied around 12 kg in 12 weeks.[120–122] There are no comparable rapid improvements with outpatient treatments, not even family therapy in adolescents.

There have been a small number of RCTs in anorexia nervosa in addition to the Crisp *et al* study, and they have addressed narrower questions. For example, a comparison of two different inpatient treatment programmes has yielded the helpful finding that a strict operant conditioning programme offers no advantages over a 'lenient' programme.[123] The value of a specialized eating disorder unit in inducing weight gain was also demonstrated in a cohort of patients admitted to the Maudsley Hospital in 1990. They had previously been admitted to a general psychiatric or medical unit, and information on their previous weights was obtained. In the case of the Maudsley admissions the mean weight rose from 65.8 per cent average body weight (abw) to 90.4 per cent abw; in comparison the admissions elsewhere only led to a mean weight gain from 64.4 to 75 per cent abw.[122]

(c) Compulsory treatments

A study of the use of compulsory treatment in patients admitted to the Eating Disorders Unit at the Maudsley Hospital, comprised 81 patients or16 per cent of admissions. Section 3 of the Mental Health Act, valid for up to 6 months, was the most frequently applied section.[121] The compulsorily admitted patients were compared with a group of voluntary patients. The need for a compulsory admission was found to have two dimensions—the presence of a severe illness and a rejection of treatment. The compulsory patients gained at least as much weight as the voluntary patients but required a longer admission for them to return to a near-normal weight. The compulsory patients represented a selected group by virtue of a more entrenched reluctance to accept treatment. Accordingly it was predicted that in the long term they would fare less well than voluntary patients. The mortality rate of these patients was determined by the National Register, which provided the data at a mean of 5.7 years after the index admission. Ten out of 79 detained patients had died in comparison with two out of 78 voluntary patients, a statistically significant difference. The deaths among the compulsory patients were all due to anorexia nervosa or one of its nutritional complications. Thus the mortality rate among compulsory patients was extremely high at 2.17 per cent per annum, presumably skewed because of the selection factors. Compulsory treatment is an obvious example of the inappropriateness of an RCT.

Treatment: advice on management

It is not possible for the clinician to confine his treatment of anorexia nervosa to those methods that have been subjected to randomized control trials. This does not mean that his treatment is ineffective or unsupported by evidence. The evidence has to be derived from other kinds of studies. They should not be dismissed as mere clinical experience if they can be supported by evidence-based clinical or experimental observations.

The main obstacle to treatment

The avoidance of treatment by the patient is part and parcel of anorexia nervosa and accentuated by her capacity for denial (see p. 783 of this chapter). There have been attempts to predict the likely level of the patient's compliance with treatment. For example, a 'transtheoretical model of change' is aimed at improving the patient's motivation by overcoming ambivalence while at the same time avoiding confrontation.[124] Different stages in the patient's approach to treatment have been recognized: precontemplation, contemplation, preparation, action, maintenance, and relapse prevention. Motivational enhancement therapy is at an early stage of development with only preliminary information on its impact on treatment outcome.

At our present level of knowledge it is simplest to ascertain the patient's attitude to treatment through the mental state examination. At the initial interview she should be asked what weight she would be willing to reach. At this stage it is best to refrain from challenging the patient's weight threshold, even though it will be well below a reasonable therapeutic goal. Having ascertained the limited degree of compliance, the clinician needs to develop a strategy to improve it gradually as treatment proceeds. It is poor clinical practice to place all the onus on the patient herself for accepting or rejecting a package of treatment at the first interview, or even at a later stage. 'Engaging' the patient in treatment is an essential part of most psychotherapeutic methods including CBT.[115] Another tactic for improving the patient's co-operation is to enlist the help of close members of the family. Young patients are likely in any case to require a family treatment.

Inpatient treatment

Although inpatient treatment is less often employed nowadays it will be described first because it is most important in patients who present as emergencies with an urgent need to preserve life and correct serious physical and psychiatric complications.

(a) Indications for admission

- It is tempting to specify a BMI threshold for admission, but it should be remembered that the BMI can only provide a very rough guide with many exceptions. If the BMI is below 14 admission should always be considered, all the more if there has been rapid weight loss during recent weeks. Indeed a BMI of 16 may cause anxiety if it represents a drop in weight from a BMI of 21 in the course of 2 or 3 months. Close attention should be given to the physical manifestations of malnutrition, especially hypoglycaemia and electrolyte disturbances.
- **The BMI may be totally unreliable in patients who have developed oedema as the result of malnutrition, causing a vicarious weight gain, which may deceive the patient and even the clinician into a false sense of security.**
- The BMI is also less reliable in children and adolescents, especially if their growth in height has been retarded thus distorting the calculation for the BMI towards a falsely reassuring value.
- Dangerous or disabling physical complications:
- Emergencies may result from low blood glucose levels, hypokalaemia or hyponatraemia. The electrolyte disturbances are most likely to occur in the presence of self-induced vomiting or laxative abuse. Hyponatraemia may be induced by polydipsia. Signs of proximal myopathy also indicate a need for admission, as do the occurrence of anaemia, low platelet counts (sometimes accompanied by purpura) and impaired liver function tests.
- Severe depression or obsessional behaviour may also arise in part as complications of malnutrition. Suicidal ideas may require admission, but persistent depression of lesser severity may also be an indication, because it renders the patient less amenable to outpatient psychological treatments, as does severe obsessional behaviour affecting the patient's eating pattern.
- Intractable self-induced vomiting or laxative abuse or determined fasting may require a greater supervision than is possible in an outpatient setting. These behaviours are less disconcerting in patients with bulimia and at a reasonable weight, but a severe weight loss makes it probable that vomiting will result in electrolyte disturbances or other physical complications.
- The decision to admit is often determined by the patient not engaging in the recommended outpatient psychological treatment when the malnutrition persists several months to 1 year.
- Young patients with a retarded puberty (premenarchal anorexia nervosa) should elicit an urgent correction of malnutrition, especially if there is evidence of retarded growth and short stature. There is a narrow window of opportunity for regaining stature, which may depend partly on bone age but it is safest to assume that after the age of 16 the probability of resuming growth becomes increasingly limited, especially in girls.

The great advantage of treating a patient in a specialized eating unit is the certainty that considerable benefit will accrue, including a substantial gain in weight, so long as the patient can be persuaded to remain in hospital.[120]

(b) Nursing and dietary care

Inpatient treatment will include a wide range of psychotherapeutic interventions (individual, group, and family) as well as occupational therapy and an educational programme. But the sheet anchor of successful treatment is a well-trained nursing staff working as a team. The role of the medical staff is one of maintaining a high level of expectation that the patient's weight will be restored to a normal (or healthy) level. It is necessary to give the nursing staff moral support so that they can develop their confidence and skills.

There are two main components to the nurses' treatment: their psychotherapeutic input and their supervisory role. The latter should never be draconian. The nursing team establish a relationship of trust with the patient and get to know her personal needs and concerns. The nurses should also be acutely aware of the anorexic patient's tendency to avoid food and exercise excessively. The treatment programme should stress the supportive aspects of the nurse's relationship with her patient rather than the undoubted need for careful supervision. The nurse will come to rely on the daily weight record to monitor the success of her treatment as the weight chart should show a smoothly rising curve. All meals are taken in the ward: thus the anorexic patients constitute a group in which peer interactions take place. The meal is taken in the presence of one or more nurses also seated at the table. The patient learns that she is expected to consume all the food placed before her.

A detailed protocol for the refeeding programme has been produced by Andersen and his group.[120] It is not only the patient who tends to underestimate the food requirements to restore her weight to normal. Metabolic studies have demonstrated that for each kilogram of weight gain a surplus calorie balance of 7500 cal is needed.[111] It is prudent to begin with a modest calorie intake of 1200 to 1500 cal daily during the first 7 days in order to avoid the complications of hypophosphataemia and acute gastric dilation. Thereafter the caloric intake is gradually increased and may rise to 4000 cal. daily. The best diet is that consisting of a wide range of foods including carbohydrate and fat-containing foods. Concentrated foods (e.g. Build-up, Complan, Scandishake, Fortisip, Ensure Plus) may be used to achieve a high caloric intake. The aim is to achieve a positive energy balance of at least 1500 cal daily, leading to a weekly weight gain of 1 to 1.5 kg.

(c) Assessment of progress

Weighing should be a standardized daily procedure before breakfast after the patient has emptied her bladder and while wearing light night clothes. A paradoxical psychological improvement, with a diminution in concern with body size and shape, occurs with weight gain. The improvement is partly through the correction of malnutrition and partly the result of the 'exposure treatment' whereby the patient gradually accepts a higher body weight.

(d) Medication

Exceptionally the patient's tension and depression do not improve and there is a continued resistance to food. It may then be helpful to prescribe moderate doses of olanzapine (not more than 10 mg daily), carefully avoiding a fall in blood pressure, which is a risk in the emaciated patient. In the case of persistent depression, treatment with an antidepressant may be indicated. However, antidepressants are often ineffective in the presence of malnutrition, and by themselves do not assist the patient to gain weight.

(e) General measures

Inevitably the patient will find it irksome to forego home visits during the early period of weight gain. Therefore interesting and therapeutic activities should be provided through group meetings, occupational therapy, and social interactions. Visiting is generally encouraged unless the visiting parents are subjected to emotional appeals to take her home. They may then be asked to postpone their visits or reduce their duration. The monotony can be relieved when the patient's weight gain is on course by providing accompanied outings avoiding mealtimes.

The aim is to restore body weight to a healthy level within 8 to 10 weeks; a further period (usually 2 weeks) in hospital is needed to allow the patient to test her ability to maintain her weight by eating in a general dining room or going on home leave for two or more days at a time. The aim is to effect a smooth transition to day care or outpatient treatment.

Compulsory treatment in anorexia nervosa

The management of patients reluctant to accept essential therapeutic goals requires that they should be gradually engaged in a genuine alliance. However, there remain a minority of patients with whom this strategy fails and whose health and life become endangered. For them, compulsory treatment should be considered.[121] A compulsory admission to hospital is indicated not only when patients threaten suicide or suffer from a life-threatening malnutrition, but also when they fail to respond to simpler measures such as outpatient treatment or day care, or in the event of avoiding treatment altogether. Ill health persisting over the course of several months or the development of serious physical complications (e.g. water and electrolyte imbalance, hypoglycaemia, or myopathy) should also elicit compulsory admission if the patient cannot be persuaded to accept inpatient treatment voluntarily.

The evidence points to the usefulness of a compulsory admission in appropriate circumstances in so far as the patients respond well in the short term. Nevertheless, a patient who has required a compulsory admission carries a higher risk, so that it is essential to safeguard her through a long follow-up.

Day and community treatment

The Edinburgh trial of a day patient programme has already been discussed. At the Toronto Hospital a day hospital programme for eating disorders has been established since 1985.[125] and is now offered on 4 days a week.

The goals are as follows:

1 A normalization of disturbed eating behaviour and weight gain.

2 The identification of psychological and familial processes that serve to perpetuate the eating disorder.

Two meals and a snack are provided during the treatment hours. The staff take turns to supervise the patients during meal times. The psychological treatment consists of intensive group therapy addressing disturbed behaviours around eating and weight, and more general conflicts.

The clinical advantages of day treatment are a reduction in the dependence of patients who need to be able to function outside the hospital. The group treatment provides an atmosphere of mutual support while permitting interventions through group pressures. A wide range of patients can be admitted but those with medical or suicidal risks will elicit inpatient care instead. When patients succeed in reducing their disturbed eating behaviours they may 'act out' by self-harm. The clinical staff may find their skills severely taxed by the continuous staff/patient interaction.

A home oriented service extended to outpatient and day care, has been devised by Robinson (2006) for an area of North London (1.2 million). A wide range of treatments were devised including family interventions and carer support. The educational needs of members of the multi-disciplinary team are well described as are administrative and financial issues. Robinson's book includes an audit on the use of hospital and hostel beds requiring only 4–5 total beds per million population per year.

Outpatient psychotherapies

In the event of a patient's weight loss being less than 20 per cent of her healthy weight, it may be possible to obtain a therapeutic response by outpatient treatment, including attendance at non-specialist general psychiatric clinics or child/adolescent psychiatric services. The feasibility of this approach will depend on the availability of appropriate psychotherapeutic resources. The clinician should guard himself against imaginary conflicts between a psychotherapeutic approach and recording the weight of the patient. It is never justified to accept apparent compliance with psychotherapy if the patient's weight continues to decline.

(a) Family treatments

(i) *Conjoint family therapy*

The frequency of the sessions is determined by clinical need: it averaged 10.5 over the course of 1 year in the Maudsley trial. There are three stages to the therapy:

1 In the first phase the parents are urged to identify their future joint attitude to the feeding pattern that should be adopted by their daughter. With a younger patient the therapist assumes that the parents would initially need to take control of their child's eating.

2 During the second phase the parents are urged to be present together at each meal so that they can reinforce each other's efforts in the practical task of ensuring an improved food intake and a steady weight gain.

3 When the patient's weight is under control, responsibility for continued weight gain is handed back to her. Discussions can then commence on more normal family concerns. With an adolescent patient the main focus is on achieving increased autonomy. The eventual aim is to establish healthy relationships with her parents without the eating disorder as a medium for communication.

(ii) *Separated family therapy*

As in conjoint family therapy the parents are given direct advice on how to manage their daughter's eating problem. The patient herself is provided with individual psychotherapy. The therapist provides counselling about abnormal attitudes to weight and emphasizes the weight issue until steady progress has been made. This method is often preferred by the patient and her parents, largely because it avoids confrontation. It is also easier to gain access to the patient's fears and conflicts.

(b) CBT

CBT has much in common with other methods of treatment including the refeeding programme described under inpatient treatments. It relies on building a positive therapeutic alliance between therapist and patient.

The patient's weight and food intake is monitored at each session and she is told her weight. She is encouraged to think of food as medication and to follow a meal plan. The patient is educated in the disturbances of bodily and psychological function consequent on the state of starvation. The content of the therapy may be divided into two 'tracks'. The first track includes an examination of the behaviours adopted by the patient in order to reduce her weight. The second track is more concerned with psychological themes such as self-esteem, perfectionism, interpersonal functioning, and family conflicts. By asking the patient to give her reasons for specific behaviours, the therapist discovers faulty beliefs and assumptions on her part. For example, the 'anorexic wish' is the patient's wish to recover from her disorder without gaining weight. She is gently persuaded that this is an impossible aim because her real psychological difficulties will remain inaccessible so long as her experiences are clouded by starvation and dieting. The patient also expresses a fear of 'losing control' meaning that she will run the risk of overeating and become fat. It is explained to the patient that her rigid 'control' overeating deprives her completely of choice, and that far from being in control the reality is the converse. It is also useful for the therapist to analyse the pros and cons of maintaining the disorder of anorexia nervosa. The patient often feels more uncomfortable at confronting the hidden rewards of remaining thin.

Having ascertained the particular meanings of attitudes and behaviours for the patient, she is helped to find more adaptive ways of achieving healthier goals, including more relaxed normal eating and weight gain.

(c) Dynamic psychotherapy: therapeutic model

(i) *Crisp's model of anorexia nervosa as a flight from growth*

Crisp has explained how his programme of treatment is based on his model of anorexia nervosa as a refuge from puberty, which the patient has found overwhelming. The youngster reverses her pubertal development by limiting her intake of food.[126] His treatment initially involves an intensive inpatient programme lasting 10 to 12 weeks followed by outpatient treatment for up to 6 years. The advantage of this extensive programme is that it enables the patient to accept gradually an increase in weight while facing up to the feelings of panic and helplessness that originally led her to arrest her puberty through self-starvation. This interpretation is presented to the patient and to her family so that they come to see the psychotherapy as a way of solving the problems.

The model is a useful one even within a more limited outpatient psychotherapeutic setting. Some patients will readily identify their distress when overwhelmed by powerful sexual feelings or when confronted with personal and social responsibilities perceived as the result of growing up. The aims of the psychotherapy are to support the patient while she is beginning to abandon the psychobiological regression of anorexia nervosa. In addition she is encouraged to broaden her perception of herself in ways that are no longer wholly dependent on her physical appearance but include an improved sense of competence and self-esteem. She is helped to tackle personal and social problems from which she had previously escaped so that she can address her own and her parents' concerns about sexuality.

Ethical and medico-legal issues

In the United Kingdom the Mental Health Act Commission[127] has clarified many of the doubts in the minds of clinicians and social workers called upon to consider a compulsory admission under the Mental Health Act 1983. It recognized that anorexia nervosa is a mental disorder within the meaning of the Act and that in some patients their ability to consent may be compromised by fears of obesity or denial of the consequences of their actions. The Mental Health Act Commission concluded that when the patient's health is seriously threatened by food refusal she may be detained in hospital so as to treat the self-imposed starvation. The Commission went as far as to state that nasogastric feeding can be a medical process forming an integral part of the treatment for anorexia nervosa, notwithstanding that nasogastric feeding is seldom required.

Prevention

Preventive measures have been aimed at eating disorders generally rather than just anorexia nervosa. The main approach has been school-based intervention programmes educating adolescent girls into the risks of dieting and other methods of weight control. The commonest outcome has been an increased knowledge about eating disorders without a change in the behaviours, such as dieting, likely to cause them. One controlled study, six weekly sessions were provided by teachers on a wide range of topics covering attitudes and behaviours relevant to eating disorders including a 'non-dieting approach'. Positive changes were detected at a 6-month follow-up but they were modest in size and poorly sustained.[128]

Currently there are active campaigns by the Academy of Eating Disorders and Beat Eating Disorders (UK) to encourage the fashion industry not to employ thin models. Unilever has adopted a policy not to employ models with a BMI less than 18.5. John Lewis requires models to be not less than size 12.

Further information

Robinson, P.H. (2006). *Community treatment of eating disorders.* John Wiley, Chichester.

Russell, G.F.M. (1993). Social psychiatry of eating disorders. In *Principles of social psychiatry* (eds, D. Bhugra and J. Leff). pp. 273–97. Blackwell Science, Oxford.

References

1. Gull, W.W. (1874). Anorexia nervosa (apepsia hysterica, anorexia hysterica). *Transactions of the Clinical Society of London*, **7**, 22–8.
2. Lasègue, C. (1873). De l'anorexie hystérique. *Archives Générales de Médicine*, **21**, 385–403.
3. Brumberg, J.J. (1988). *Fasting girls: the emergence of anorexia nervosa as a modern disease*. Harvard University Press, Cambridge, MA.
4. Bell, R.M. (1985). *Holy anorexia*. University of Chicago Press, Chicago and London.
5. Bruch, H. (1962). Perceptual and conceptual disturbances in anorexia nervosa. *Psychosomatic Medicine*, **24**, 187–94.
6. Russell, G.F.M. (1970). Anorexia nervosa: its identity as an illness and its treatment. In *Modern trends in psychological medicine* (ed. J. Harding Price), pp. 131–64. Butterworths, Norwich.
7. Garner, D.M. and Garfinkel, P.E. (1979). The eating attitudes test: an index of the symptoms of anorexia nervosa. *Psychological Medicine*, **9**, 273–9.
8. Johnson-Sabine, E., Wood, K., Patton, G., *et al.* (1988). Abnormal eating attitudes in London schoolgirls—a prospective epidemiological study: factors associated with abnormal response on screening questionnaires. *Psychological Medicine*, **18**, 615–22.
9. Hoek, H.W. (1991). The incidence and prevalence of anorexia nervosa and bulimia nervosa in primary care. *Psychological Medicine*, **21**, 455–60.
10. van Son, G.E., van Hoeken, D., Bartelds, A.I., *et al.* (2006). Time trends in the incidence of eating disorders: a primary care study in the Netherlands. *The International Journal of Eating Disorders*, **39**, 565–9.
11. Garner, D.M. and Garfinkel, P.E. (1980). Socio-cultural factors in the development of anorexia nervosa. *Psychological Medicine*, **10**, 647–56.
12. Szmukler, G.I., Eisler, I., Gillies, C., *et al.* (1985). The implications of anorexia nervosa in a ballet school. *Journal of Psychiatric Research*, **19**, 177–82.
13. Crisp, A.H., Palmer, R.R.L., *et al.* (1976). How common is anorexia nervosa? A prevalence study. *The British Journal of Psychiatry*, **128**, 549–54.
14. Råstam, M., Gillberg, C., and Garton, M. (1989). Anorexia nervosa in a Swedish urban region. A population based study. *The British Journal of Psychiatry*, **155**, 642–6.
15. Russell, G.F.M. (1993). Social psychiatry of eating disorders. In *Principles of social psychiatry* (eds. D. Bhugra and J. Leff), pp. 273–97. Blackwell Science, Oxford.
16. Milos, G., Spindler, A., Schnyder, U., *et al.* (2004). Incidence of severe anorexia nervosa in Switzerland: 40 years of development. *The International Journal of Eating Disorders*, **35**, 250–61.
17. Lucas, A.R., Beard, C.M., O'Fallen, W.M., *et al.* (1991). 50-year trends in the incidence of anorexia nervosa in Rochester, Minn: a population-based survey. *The American Journal of Psychiatry*, **148**, 917–22.
18. Fosson, A., Knibbs, J., Bryant-Waugh, R., *et al.* (1987). Early onset anorexia nervosa. *Archives of Disease in Childhood*, **62**, 114–18.
19. Favaro, A., Ferrara, S., and Santonastaso, P. (2003). The spectrum of eating disorders in young women: a prevalence study in a general population sample. *Psychosomatic Medicine*, **65**, 701–8.
20. Blake Woodside, D., Garfinkel, P.E., Lin, E., *et al.* (2001). Comparisons of men with full or partial eating disorders, and women with eating disorders in the community. *The American Journal of Psychiatry*, **158**, 570–4.
21. Morgan, H.G. and Russell, G.F.M. (1975). Value of family background and clinical features as predictors of long-term outcome in anorexia nervosa: four-year follow-up study of 41 patients. *Psychological Medicine*, **5**, 355–71.
22. Russell, G.F.M. (1979). Bulimia nervosa: an ominous variant of anorexia nervosa. *Psychological Medicine*, **9**, 429–48.
23. Russell, G.F.M. (1995). Anorexia nervosa through time. In *Handbook of eating disorders: theory, treatment and research* (eds. G. Szmukler, C. Dare, and J. Treasure), pp. 5–17. Wiley, Chichester.
24. Currin, L., Schmidt, U., Treasure, J., *et al.* (2005). Time trends in eating disorder incidence. *The British Journal of Psychiatry*, **186**, 132–5.
25. Campbell, P.G. (1995). What would a causal explanation of the eating disorders look like? In *Handbook of eating disorders: theory, treatment and research* (eds. G. Szmukler, C. Dare, and J. Treasure), pp. 49–64. Wiley, Chichester.
26. Garfinkel, P.E. and Garner, D.M. (1982). *Anorexia nervosa: a multi-dimensional perspective*. Brunner-Mazel, New York.
27. Birnbaum, K. (1923). *Der Aufbau der Psychose*, pp. 6–7. Springer, Berlin.
28. Patton, G.C., Johnson-Sabine, E., Wood, K., *et al.* (1990). Abnormal eating attitudes in London schoolgirls-a prospective epidemiological study: outcome at twelve month follow-up. *Psychological Medicine*, **20**, 383–94.
29. Crisp, A.H. (1970). Premorbid factors in adult disorders of weight, with particular reference to primary anorexia nervosa (weight phobia). A literature review. *Journal of Psychosomatic Research*, **14**, 1–22.
30. Prince, R. (1985). The concept of culture-bound syndromes: anorexia nervosa and brain-fag. *Transcultural Psychiatric Research Review*, **22**, 117–21.
31. DiNicola, V.F. (1990). Anorexia multiforme: self-starvation in historical and cultural context. *Transcultural Psychiatric Research Review*, **27**, 165–96, 245–86.
32. Bryant-Waugh, R. and Lask, B. (1991). Anorexia nervosa in a group of Asian children living in Britain. *The British Journal of Psychiatry*, **158**, 229–33.
33. Mynors-Wallis, L., Treasure, J., and Chee, D. (1992). Life events and anorexia nervosa: differences between early and late onset cases. *The International Journal of Eating Disorders*, **4**, 369–75.
34. Beumont, P.J.V., Abraham, S.F., and Simson, K.G. (1981). The psychosexual histories of adolescent girls and young women with anorexia nervosa. *Psychological Medicine*, **11**, 131–40.
35. Tiller, J. and Treasure, J. (1998). Eating disorders precipitated by pregnancy. *European Eating Disorders Review*, **6**, 178–87.
36. Sloan, G. and Leichner, P. (1986). Is there a relationship between sexual abuse or incest and eating disorders? *Canadian Journal of Psychiatry*, **31**, 656–60.
37. Palmer, R.L., Oppenheimer, R., Dignon, A., *et al.* (1990). Childhood sexual experiences with adults reported by women with eating disorders: an extended series. *The British Journal of Psychiatry*, **156**, 699–703.

38. McClelland, L., Mynors-Wallis, L., Fahy, T., *et al.* (1991). Sexual abuse, disordered personality and eating disorders. *The British Journal of Psychiatry*, **158**(Suppl. 10), 63–8.
39. Wonderlich, S.A., Brewerton, T.D., Jocic, Z., *et al.* (1997). Relationship of childhood sexual abuse and eating disorders. *Journal of the American Academy of Child and Adolescent Psychiatry*, **36**, 1107–15.
40. Minuchin, S., Baker, L., Rosman, B.L., *et al.* (1975). A conceptual model of psychosomatic illness in children: family organization and family therapy. *Archives of General Psychiatry*, **32**, 1031–8.
41. Selvini Palazzoli, M. (1974). *Self-starvation. From the intrapsychic to the transpersonal approach to anorexia nervosa* (trans. A. Pomerans), pp. 202–16. Human Context Books, London.
42. Bruch, H. (1978). *The golden cage: the enigma of anorexia nervosa.* Open Books, London.
43. Dare, C. and Eisler, I. (1997). Family therapy for anorexia nervosa. In *Handbook of treatment for eating disorders* (2nd edn) (eds. D.M. Garner and P.E. Garfinkel), pp. 307–24. Guilford Press, New York.
44. Janet, P. (1903). L'obsession de la honte du corps. In *Les obsessions et la psychasthénie*, Vol. 1, Section 5. Germer Gaillière, Paris.
45. Wonderlich, S.A., Swift, W.H., Slotnick, H.B., *et al.* (1990). DSM-III-R personality disorders in eating disorder subtypes. *The International Journal of Eating Disorders*, **9**, 607–16.
46. Casper, R.C. (1990). Personality features of women with good outcome from restricting anorexia nervosa. *Psychosomatic Medicine*, **52**, 156–70.
47. Simmonds, K. (1916). Über kachexie hypophysaren ursprungs. *Deutsche Medizinische. Wochenschrift*, **42**, 190–1.
48. Russell, G.F.M. (1977). The present status of anorexia nervosa. *Psychological Medicine*, **7**, 363–7.
49. Anand, B.K. and Brobeck, J.R. (1951). Localization of a 'feeding center' in the hypothalamus of the rat. *Proceedings of the Society for Experimental Biology and Medicine*, **77**, 323–4.
50. Schweiger, U., Tuschl, R.J., Laessle, R.G., *et al.* (1989). Consequences of dieting and exercise on menstrual function in normal weight young women. In *The menstrual cycle and its disorders* (eds. K.M. Pirke, W. Wuttke, and U. Schweiger), pp. 142–9. Springer Verlag, Berlin.
51. DeVile, C.H., Sufraz, R., Lask, B., *et al.* (1995). Occult intracranial tumours masquerading as early onset anorexia nervosa. *British Medical Journal*, **311**, 1359–60.
52. Ploog, D.W. and Pirke, K.M. (1987). Psychobiology of anorexia nervosa. *Psychological Medicine*, **17**, 843–59.
53. Lask, B., Gordon, I., Christie, D., *et al.* (2005). Functional neuroimaging in early onset anorexia nervosa. *The International Journal of Eating Disorders*, **37**, S49–51.
54. Strober, M., Lampert, C., Morrell, W., *et al.* (1990). A controlled family study of anorexia nervosa: evidence of familial aggregation and lack of shared transmission with affective disorders. *The International Journal of Eating Disorders*, **9**, 239–53.
55. Bulik, C.M. (2004). Role of genetics in anorexia nervosa, bulimia nervosa and binge eating disorder. In *Clinical handbook of eating disorders* (ed. T.D. Brewerton), pp. 165–82. Marcel Dekker, New York.
56. Holland, A.J., Hall, A., Murray, R., *et al.* (1984). Anorexia nervosa: a study of 34 twin pairs and one set of triplets. *The British Journal of Psychiatry*, **145**, 414–19.
57. Holland, A.J., Sicotte, N., and Treasure, J. (1988). Anorexia nervosa: evidence for a genetic basis. *Journal of Psychosomatic Research*, **32**, 561–71.
58. Blundell, J.E. and Bill, A.J. (1991). Serotonin, eating disorders and the satiety cascade. In *Serotonin-related psychiatric syndromes: clinical and therapeutic links* (eds. G.B. Cassano and H.S. Asikal), pp. 125–9. Royal Society of Medicine Services, London.
59. Szmukler, G.I., Andrewes, D., Kingston, K., *et al.* (1992). Neuropsychological impairment in anorexia nervosa before and after refeeding. *Journal of Clinical and Experimental Neuropsychology*, **14**, 347–52.
60. Kaye, W.H., Gwirtsman, J.E., George, D.T., *et al.* (1988). CSF-5HIAA concentrations in anorexia nervosa: reduced values in underweight subjects normalize after weight gain. *Biological Psychiatry*, **23**, 102–5.
61. Kaye, W.H., Gwirtsman, H.E., George, D.T., *et al.* (1991). Altered serotonin activity in anorexia nervosa after long-term weight restoration: does elevated CSF-5HIAA correlate with rigid and obsessive behavior? *Archives of General Psychiatry*, **48**, 556–62.
62. O'Dwyer, A.-M., Lucey, J.V., and Russell, G.F.M. (1996). Serotonin activity in anorexia nervosa after long-term weight restoration: response to d-fenfluramine challenge. *Psychological Medicine*, **26**, 353–9.
63. Slade, P.D. and Russell, G.F.M. (1973). Awareness of body dimensions in anorexia nervosa: cross-sectional and longitudinal studies. *Psychological Medicine*, **3**, 188–99.
64. Hsu, L.K.G. and Sobkiewicz, T.A. (1989). Body image disturbance: time to abandon the concept for eating disorders? *The International Journal of Eating Disorders*, **10**, 15–30.
65. Hsu, L.K.G. and Lee, S. (1993). Is weight phobia always necessary for a diagnosis of anorexia nervosa? *The American Journal of Psychiatry*, **150**, 1466–71.
66. Blake Woodside, D. and Twose, R. (2004). Diagnostic issues in eating disorders: historical perspectives and thoughts for the future. In *Clinical handbook of eating disorders* (ed. T.D. Brewerton), pp. 1–19. Marcel Dekker, New York.
67. Vandereycken, W. (2007). Denial of illness in anorexia nervosa—a conceptual review: part I diagnostic significance and assessment. *European Eating Disorder Review*, **14**, 352–68.
68. Fichter, M.M. and Pirke, K.M. (1995). Starvation models and eating disorders. In *Handbook of eating disorders: theory, treatment and research* (eds. G. Szmukler, C. Dare, and J. Treasure), pp. 83–107. Wiley, Chichester.
69. Treasure, J.L., Gordon, P.A.L., King, E.A., *et al.* (1985). Cystic ovaries: a phase of anorexia nervosa. *Lancet*, **2**, 1379–82.
70. Treasure, J.L., Wheeler, M., King, E.A., *et al.* (1988). Weight gain and reproductive function: ultrasonographic and endocrine features in anorexia nervosa. *Clinical Endocrinology*, **29**, 607–16.
71. Namir, S., Melman, K.N., and Yager, J. (1986). Pregnancy in restrictor-type anorexia nervosa: a study of six women. *The International Journal of Eating Disorders*, **5**, 837–45.
72. Treasure, J.L. and Russell, G.F.M. (1988). Intrauterine growth and neonatal weight gain in babies of women with anorexia nervosa. *British Medical Journal*, **296**, 1038.
73. Van Wezel-Meijler, G. and Wit, J.M. (1989). The offspring of mothers with anorexia nervosa: a high-risk group for undernutrition and stunting? *European Journal of Pediatrics*, **49**, 130–5.
74. Treasure, J. and Szmukler, G. (1995). Medical complications of chronic anorexia nervosa. In *Handbook of eating disorders: theory, treatment and research* (eds. G. Szmukler, C. Dare, and J. Treasure), pp. 197–220. Wiley, Chichester.
75. Passmore, R. and Eastwood, M.A. (1986). *Human nutrition and dietetics*. Churchill Livingstone, Edinburgh.
76. Handler, C.E. and Pirkin, G.D. (1982). Anorexia nervosa and Wernicke's encephalopathy: an undiagnosed association. *Lancet*, **2**, 771–2.
77. Lask, B. and Bryant-Waugh, R. (1992). Early onset anorexia nervosa and related eating disorders. *Journal of Child Psychology and Psychiatry*, **33**, 281–300.
78. McLoughlin, D.M., Spargo, E., Wassif, W.S., *et al.* (1998). Structural and functional changes in skeletal muscle in anorexia nervosa. *Acta Neuropathologica*, **95**, 632–40.
79. Treasure, J.L., Fogelman, I., Russell, G.F.M., *et al.* (1987). Reversible bone loss in anorexia nervosa. *British Medical Journal*, **295**, 474–5.
80. World Health Organization. (1992). *International statistical classification of diseases and related health problems* (10th revision). WHO, Geneva.

81. Klibanski, A., Biller, B.M.K., Schoenfeld, D.A., *et al.* (1995). The effects of oestrogen administration on trabecular bone loss in young women with anorexia nervosa. *Journal of Clinical Endocrinology and Metabolism*, **80**, 898–904.
82. Serpell, L. and Treasure, J. (1997). Osteoporosis—a serious health risk in chronic anorexia nervosa. *European Eating Disorders Review*, **5**, 149–57.
83. Wakeling, A. and Russell, G.F.M. (1970). Disturbances in the regulation of body temperature in anorexia nervosa. *Psychological Medicine*, **1**, 30–9.
84. Rieger, W., Brady, J.P., and Weisberg, E. (1978). Hematologic changes in anorexia nervosa. *The American Journal of Psychiatry*, **135**, 984–5.
85. Russell, G.F.M. (1966). Acute dilation of the stomach in a patient with anorexia nervosa. *The British Journal of Psychiatry*, **112**, 203–7.
86. Beumont, P.J.V. and Large, M. (1991). Hypophosphataemia, delirium and cardiac arrhythmia in anorexia nervosa. *Medical Journal of Australia*, **155**, 519–22.
87. Russell, G.F.M., Treasure, J., and Eisler, I. (1998). Mothers with anorexia nervosa who underfeed their children: their recognition and management. *Psychological Medicine*, **28**, 93–108.
88. Russell, G.F.M. (1985). Premenarchal anorexia nervosa and its sequelae. *Journal of Psychiatric Research*, **19**, 363–9.
89. Lai, K.Y.C., de Bruyn, R., Lask, B., *et al.* (1994). Use of pelvic ultrasound to monitor ovarian and uterine maturity in childhood onset anorexia nervosa. *Archives of Disease in Childhood*, **71**, 228–31.
90. American Psychiatric Association. (1994). *Diagnostic and statistical manual of mental disorders* (4th edn). American Psychiatric Association, Washington, DC.
91. Beumont, P.J.V., Beardwood, C.J., and Russell, G.F.M. (1972). The occurrence of the syndrome of anorexia nervosa in male subjects. *Psychological Medicine*, **2**, 216–31.
92. Crisp, A.H. and Burns, T. (1990). Primary anorexia nervosa in the male and female: a comparison of clinical features and prognosis. In *Males with eating disorders* (ed. A.E. Andersen), pp. 77–99. Brunner–Mazel, New York.
93. Blake Woodside, D., Garfinkel, P.E., Lin, E., *et al.* (2001). Comparisons of men with full or partial eating disorders, and women with eating disorders in the community. *The American Journal of Psychiatry*, **158**, 570–4.
94. Burns, T. and Crisp, A.H. (1990). Outcome of anorexia nervosa in males. In *Males with eating disorders* (ed. A.E. Andersen), pp. 163–86. Brunner-Mazel, New York.
95. Fichter, M.M. and Daser, C. (1987). Symptomatology, psychosexual development and gender identity in 42 anorexic males. *Psychological Medicine*, **17**, 409–18.
96. Crisp, A.H., Norton, K., Gowers, S., *et al.* (1991). A controlled study of the effect of therapies aimed at adolescent and family psychopathology in anorexia nervosa. *The British Journal of Psychiatry*, **159**, 325–33.
97. Steinhausen, H.-C., Rauss-Mason, C., and Seidel, R. (1991). Follow-up studies of anorexia nervosa. A review of four decades of outcome research. *Psychological Medicine*, **21**, 447–54.
98. Morgan, H.G. and Hayward, A.E. (1988). Clinical assessment of anorexia nervosa. *The British Journal of Psychiatry*, **152**, 367–71.
99. Theander, S. (1985). Outcome and prognosis in anorexia nervosa and bulimia: some results of previous investigations, compared with a Swedish long-term study. *Journal of Psychosomatic Research*, **19**, 493–508.
100. Ratnasuriya, R.H., Eisler, I., Szmukler, G.I., *et al.* (1991). Anorexia nervosa: outcome and prognostic factors after 20 years. *The British Journal of Psychiatry*, **158**, 495–502.
101. Sullivan, P.F. (1995). Mortality in anorexia nervosa. *The American Journal of Psychiatry*, **152**, 1073–4.
102. Steinhausen, H.-C. and Seidel, R. (1993). Outcome in adolescent eating disorders. *The International Journal of Eating Disorders*, **14**, 487–96.
103. Wentz, E., Gillberg, C., Gillberg, I.C., *et al.* (2001). Ten-year follow-up of adolescent-onset anorexia nervosa: psychiatric disorders and overall functioning scales. *Journal of Child Psychology and Psychiatry*, **42**, 613–22.
104. Theander, S. (1992). Chronicity in anorexia nervosa: results from the Swedish long-term study. In *The course of eating disorders* (eds. W. Herzog, H.-C. Deter, and W. Vandereycken), pp. 198–213. Springer-Verlag, Berlin.
105. National Institute of Clinical Excellence. (2004). *Eating disorders: core interventions in the treatment and management of anorexia nervosa, bulimia nervosa and related eating disorders.* Clinical Guideline, 9. National Collaborating Centre for Mental Health, London.
106. Halmi, K.A., Agras, S., Crow, S., *et al.* (2005). Predictors of treatment acceptance and completion in anorexia nervosa: implications for future study designs. *Archives of General Psychiatry*, **62**, 776–81.
107. Russell, G.F.M., Szmukler, G.I., Dare, C., *et al.* (1987). An evaluation of family therapy in anorexia nervosa and bulimia nervosa. *Archives of General Psychiatry*, **44**, 1047–56.
108. Lock, J., Agras, W.S., Bryson, S., *et al.* (2005). A comparison of short—and long-term family therapy for adolescent anorexia nervosa. *Journal of the American Academy of Child and Adolescent Psychiatry*, **44**, 632–9.
109. Eisler, I., Dare, C., Hodes, M., *et al.* (2000). Family therapy for adolescent anorexia nervosa: the results of a controlled comparison of two family interventions. *Journal of Child Psychology and Psychiatry*, **41**, 727–36.
110. Eisler, I., Dare, C., Russell, G.F.M., *et al.* (1997). Family and individual therapy in anorexia nervosa—a 5-year follow-up. *Archives of General Psychiatry*, **54**, 1025–30.
111. Russell, G.F.M. and Mezey, A.G. (1962). An analysis of weight gain in patients with anorexia nervosa treated with high calorie diets. *Clinical Science*, **23**, 449–61.
112. Eisler, I., Simic, M., Russell, G.F.M., *et al.* (2007). A randomized controlled treatment trial of two forms of family therapy in adolescent anorexia nervosa: a five-year follow-up. *Journal of Child Psychology and Psychiatry*.
113. Lock, J., Couturier, J., and Agras, W.S. (2006). Comparison of long-term outcomes in adolescents with anorexia nervosa treated with family therapy. *Journal of the American Academy of Child and Adolescent Psychiatry*, **45**, 666–72.
114. Fairburn, C.G., Shafran, R., and Cooper, Z. (1999). A cognitive-behavioural theory of anorexia nervosa. *Behaviour Research and Therapy*, **37**, 1–13.
115. Garner, D.M., Vitousek, K.M., and Pike, K.M. (1997). Cognitive-behavioural therapy for anorexia nervosa. In *Handbook of treatment for eating disorders* (2nd edn) (eds. D.M. Garner and P.E. Garfinkel), pp. 94–144. Guilford Press, New York.
116. Pike, K.M., Walsh, B.T., Vitousek, K., *et al.* (2003). Cognitive behaviour therapy in the posthospitalisation of anorexia nervosa. *The American Journal of Psychiatry*, **160**, 2046–9.
117. McIntosh, V.V.W., Jordan, J., Carter, F.A., *et al.* (2005). Three psychotherapies for anorexia nervosa: a randomized controlled trial. *The American Journal of Psychiatry*, **162**, 741–7.
118. Dare, C., Eisler, I., Russell, G., *et al.* (2001). Psychological therapies for adults with anorexia nervosa. *The British Journal of Psychiatry*, **178**, 216–21.
119. Freeman, C. (1992). Day patient treatment for anorexia nervosa. *British Review of Bulimia and Anorexia Nervosa*, **6**, 3–9.
120. Andersen, A.E., Bowers, W., and Evans, K. (1997). In-patient treatment of anorexia nervosa. In *Handbook of treatment for eating disorders* (2nd edn) (eds. D.M. Garner and P.E. Garfinkel), pp. 327–53. Guilford Press, New York.

121. Ramsay, R., Ward, A., Treasure, J., *et al.* (1999). Compulsory treatment in anorexia nervosa: short-term benefits and long-term mortality. *The British Journal of Psychiatry*, **175**, 147–53.
122. The Royal College of Psychiatrists. Eating Disorders. (1992). Council Report CR14, p. 13.
123. Touyz, S.O., Beumont, P.J.V., Glaun, D., *et al.* (1984). A comparison of lenient and strict operant conditioning programmes in refeeding patients with anorexia nervosa. *The British Journal of Psychiatry*, **144**, 517–20.
124. Prochaska, J.O. and Di Clemente, C.C. (1992). The transtheoretical approach. In *Handbook of psychotherapy integration* (eds. J.C. Norcross and M.R. Goldfried), pp. 300–34. Basic Books, New York.
125. Kaplan, A.S. and Olmsted, M.P. (1997). Partial hospitalisation. In *Handbook of treatment for eating disorders* (2nd edn) (eds. D.M. Garner and P.E. Garfinkel), pp. 354–60. Guilford Press, New York.
126. Crisp, A.H. (1997). Anorexia nervosa as flight from growth: assessment and treatment based on model. In *Handbook of treatment for eating disorders* (2nd edn) (eds. D.M. Garner and P.E. Garfinkel), pp. 248–77. Guilford Press, New York.
127. Mental Health Act Commission. (1997). *Guidance on the treatment of anorexia nervosa under the Mental Health Act 1983*, pp. 1–6. Mental Health Act Commission, Nottingham.
128. Stewart, D.A., Carter, J.C., Drinkwater, J., *et al.* (2001). Modification of eating attitudes and behaviour in adolescent girls: a controlled study. *The International Journal of Eating Disorders*, **29**, 107–18.

4.10.2 Bulimia nervosa

Christopher G. Fairburn,
Zafra Cooper, and Rebecca Murphy

Introduction

Origins of the concept

The history of the diagnosis bulimia nervosa begins as recently as 1979. It was in this year that Russell published his now seminal paper 'Bulimia nervosa: An ominous variant of anorexia nervosa'[1] in which he described 30 patients (28 women and 2 men), seen between 1972 and 1978, who had three major features in common. First, they had recurrent episodes of uncontrolled overeating; second, they regularly used self-induced vomiting or laxatives as means of weight control; and third, they had a morbid fear of becoming fat. Russell described many other features shared by these patients, including a history of anorexia nervosa (present in 80 per cent), the presence of severe depressive symptoms, and the fact that in most cases their body weight was in the healthy range. He noted that the disorder tended to run a chronic course and that it was 'extremely difficult to treat'. Finally, he suggested that this clinical picture should be viewed as a syndrome, distinct from anorexia nervosa, and he proposed the term 'bulimia nervosa'.

It is difficult to exaggerate the importance of Russell's paper. Its greatest contribution was perhaps its prescience in that it crystallized out from among the range of eating disorders seen in clinical practice a subgroup of patients that was just starting to become more common; it identified its central features; and it gave it an appropriate name.

Events since 1980

Events gathered pace in the 1980s. In 1980 a syndrome termed 'bulimia' was included in DSM-III.[2] This was intended to denote the type of patient that Russell had described, although its diagnostic criteria proved to be overly inclusive. In 1987, the criteria were refined and brought more in line with Russell's original concept. The syndrome was also renamed bulimia nervosa.[3] Also in the early 1980s evidence mounted that bulimia nervosa might be common and this led to a spate of studies of its prevalence. At the same time reports were published describing the successful treatment of these patients, the two most promising approaches being a specific form of cognitive behaviour therapy and the use of antidepressant drugs. By the mid-1980s, both treatments had been tested in the first of what has become a large series of controlled trials.

Now, three decades later, the diagnosis bulimia nervosa is included in both DSM-IV[4] and ICD-10,[5] its prevalence is established, aspects of its aetiology are beginning to be understood, and much has been learned about its treatment.

Classification and diagnosis

The classification of the eating disorders and their principal diagnostic criteria are shown in Table 4.10.2.1. Bulimia nervosa is one of the two main eating disorders recognized in DSM-IV and ICD-10, the other being anorexia nervosa (discussed in Chapter 4.10.1). In addition, in DSM-IV there is a residual category termed 'eating disorder not otherwise specified'. This is reserved for eating disorders of clinical severity that do not meet the diagnostic criteria for anorexia nervosa or bulimia nervosa.[6] In ICD-10, various eating disorder categories other than anorexia nervosa and bulimia nervosa are recognized (for example, atypical anorexia nervosa, atypical bulimia nervosa, overeating associated with other psychological disturbances), although these concepts have never been adequately defined or differentiated.

The relationship between the three DSM-IV diagnoses is represented diagrammatically in Fig. 4.10.2.1. The two overlapping inner circles represent anorexia nervosa (the smaller circle) and bulimia nervosa (the larger circle) respectively, the area of potential overlap being that occupied by those people who would meet the diagnostic criteria for both disorders but for the rule that the diagnosis of anorexia nervosa trumps that of bulimia nervosa (see Table 4.10.2.1). Surrounding these two circles is an outer circle which defines the boundary between having an eating disorder, a state of clinical significance, and having a lesser, non-clinical, eating problem. It is this boundary that demarcates what is, and is not, an eating disorder. Within the outer circle, but outside the two inner circles, lies eating disorder not otherwise specified (eating disorder NOS).

In DSM-IV a new eating disorder diagnosis was proposed termed 'binge eating disorder'. It is designed to denote an eating problem characterized by recurrent binge eating in the absence of the extreme weight-control behaviour seen in bulimia nervosa. Since binge eating disorder is a provisional diagnostic concept, it is currently an example of eating disorder NOS.

The two schemes for classifying eating disorders encourage the view that anorexia nervosa and bulimia nervosa are distinct clinical states. Consideration of their clinical features and course over time does not support this.[7] Binge eating disorder aside, patients with anorexia nervosa, bulimia nervosa, and eating disorder NOS have

Table 4.10.2.1 Classification of eating disorders and their principal diagnostic criteria.

Classification of eating disorders
◆ Anorexia nervosa
◆ Bulimia nervosa
◆ Eating disorder not otherwise specified (eating disorder NOS)
Binge eating disorder (a provisional new diagnosis, currently subsumed under eating disorder NOS)
Principal diagnostic criteria
Anorexia nervosa
1 Over-evaluation of shape and weight (i.e. judging self-worth largely, or exclusively, in terms of shape and weight)
2 Active maintenance of an unduly low body weight (e.g. body mass index < 17.5)
3 Amenorrhoea (in post-menarcheal females who are not taking an oral contraceptive). This criterion is often omitted.
Bulimia nervosa
1 Over-evaluation of shape and weight (i.e. judging self-worth largely, or exclusively, in terms of shape and weight)
2 Recurrent binge eating (i.e. recurrent episodes of uncontrolled overeating)
3 Extreme weight-control behaviour (e.g. strict dieting, frequent self- induced vomiting, or laxative misuse)
4 Diagnostic criteria for anorexia nervosa are not met
Eating disorder not otherwise specified
Eating disorders of clinical severity that do not conform to the diagnostic criteria for anorexia nervosa or bulimia nervosa
Binge eating disorder
Recurrent binge eating in the absence of the extreme weight-control behaviour seen in bulimia nervosa

(Reproduced from Fairburn, C.G. Cognitive Behaviour Therapy and Eating Disorders, copyright 2008, Guildford Press, NY.)

many features in common, most of which are not seen in other psychiatric disorders, and studies of their course indicate that patients migrate between these diagnoses over time: indeed, temporal migration is the norm rather than the exception. This temporal movement, together with the fact that the disorders share the same distinctive psychopathology, has led to the suggestion that the current diagnostic scheme is a poor reflection of clinical reality and that common 'transdiagnostic' mechanisms may be involved in the maintenance of eating disorder psychopathology.[(8)]

Clinical features

The great majority of patients with bulimia nervosa are female and most are in their 20s (although the age range is between 10 and 60 years). In considering the psychopathology of the disorder, a distinction may be drawn between its 'specific' and 'general' features. The former comprises features that are largely peculiar to eating disorders (for example, self-induced vomiting, the over-evaluation of shape and weight), whereas the latter consists of features seen in other psychiatric conditions (for example, depressive symptoms). The clinical features of bulimia nervosa are similar in men and women and in those with and without a history of anorexia nervosa.

Specific psychopathology

(a) Dieting and binge eating

The eating habits of patients with bulimia nervosa are characterized by strict dieting punctuated by repeated episodes of binge eating (see Fig. 4.10.2.2). The dieting is extreme and it is governed by multiple self-imposed dietary rules. These rules tend to be applied to all aspects of eating, including when to eat, what to eat, and how much to eat. As a result, the food eaten (when not binge eating) is restricted in quantity and range.

Recurrent episodes of 'binge eating' interrupt this dieting. (The term binge eating denotes discrete episodes of eating that have two characteristics: first, an unusually large amount of food is eaten,

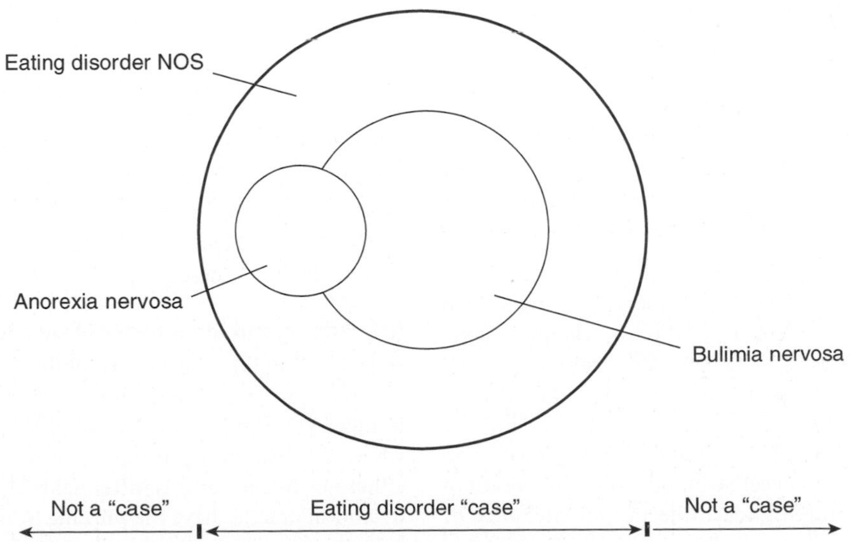

Fig. 4.10.2.1 A schematic representation of the relationship between anorexia nervosa, bulimia nervosa, and eating disorder NOS (Reprinted from Fairburn, C.G. and Bohn, K. Eating disorder NOS (EDNOS): an example of the troublesome "not otherwise specified" (NOS) category in DSM-IV, *Behaviour Research and Therapy*, **43**, 691–701, copyright (2005), with permission from Elsevier).

Day......Thursday.......... Date .....March 21 ....

Time	Food and drink consumed	Place	*	V/L	Context and comments
7.30	Glass water	Kitchen			[8stone 9lbs - really gross] Thirsty after yesterday
8:10	1 bowl muesli with skimmed milk Black coffee	Kitchen	*		Should have had less muesli. Must not binge today.
10:35	Half banana Black coffee	Work - at desk			Better - on track
11:45	Ham and lettuce slimline sandwich Diet coke	In canteen			Usual lunch
6.40 to 7.30	Slice of chocolate cake 1/2 tub ice cream 4 slices of toast with jam Diet coke Another slide of cake 2 slices of toast with jam Diet coke Jam from jar Two kit kats Mars bar Diet coke - large	Kitchen	*	V	Help - I can't stop eating. I'm completely out of control. I hate myself. I am disgusting. Why do I do this? I started as soon as I got in. I've ruined another day.
9:30	Rice cake with fat-free cheese Diet coke	Kitchen			Really lonely. Feel fat and unattractive. Feel like giving up.

Fig. 4.10.2.2 A monitoring record illustrating the eating habits of a patient with bulimia nervosa. Asterisks are used to signify episodes of eating that were viewed by the patient as excessive. The column headed 'V/L' is for recording episodes of self-induced vomiting or laxative misuse.

given the circumstances; and second, there is a sense of loss of control at the time. Some patients with eating disorders have similar episodes of uncontrolled overeating that do not involve the consumption of objectively large amounts of food. These episodes are sometimes referred to as 'subjective binges' although technically speaking they do not meet the definition of a 'binge'.) The frequency and regularity of the binge eating varies. Some patients have episodes almost every day, whereas in others the episodes are intermittent. In DSM-IV, it is specified that the binges should occur on average at least twice a week, but this is an arbitrary figure that has little discriminatory value. Among those patients in whom the binge eating is frequent, the binges have few, if any, obvious triggers, although there may be circumstances under which binge eating is more likely (for example, when alone at home). Among patients in whom the binge eating is less frequent, the binges often have clear precipitants. These tend to be of three overlapping types: first, there is breaking a personal dietary rule (for example, exceeding a daily calorie-limit or eating a banned food); second, there are situations which intensify concerns about shape and weight (for example, receiving an adverse comment about appearance); and third, there is the occurrence of negative moods (often as a result of interpersonal events). All three undermine the maintenance of strict dietary control.

The amount of food eaten during binges varies, both from patient to patient and from episode to episode. Typical episodes involve the consumption of 1000 to 2000 kcal.[(9)] The food eaten generally comprises items that are otherwise being avoided. Thus binges tend to be composed of energy-dense, high-fat items such as chocolate, ice cream, and pastries. Binges come to an end as a result of the combined influence of exhaustion, extreme fullness, a diminution of the drive to eat, and the running out of food supplies. In about three-quarters of patients they are immediately followed by measures designed to counteract the effects of the overeating, the most common being self-induced vomiting and the taking of laxatives or diuretics.

The binges are a source of considerable distress. They magnify these patients' fears of weight gain and fatness, and they may result in shame and self-disgust. For this reason most binges occur in private and are kept secret from others. It is the binge eating that eventually drives these people to seek help.

(b) Purging and other forms of weight control

In DSM-IV bulimia nervosa is subdivided into two types, a purging and non-purging type. In the purging type there is regular self-induced vomiting or the misuse of laxatives or diuretics, or both, whereas in the non-purging type such behaviour ('purging') is either not present or it is infrequent. The majority of patients seen in clinical practice have the purging form of the disorder and it has been the focus of most research.

Self-induced vomiting is the most common form of purging. In most patients it only takes place after binge eating. It is generally achieved by stimulating the gag reflex, using the fingers or some other long object, although in more established cases it can be accomplished with no mechanical aid. The vomiting is repeated until patients think that they have retrieved all the food that they can. Patients get extremely distressed if they are unable to vomit after binge eating: indeed, if they foresee that they may not have the opportunity to vomit, they tend not to binge. A minority of patients also induce vomiting at other times, for example, following smaller episodes of overeating (subjective binges) or ordinary meals or snacks.

The misuse of laxatives or diuretics is somewhat less common than self-induced vomiting. It takes two forms: one is to compensate for specific episodes of binge eating, like self-induced vomiting; and the other is as a general method of weight control (like dieting), in which case it is not tied to particular episodes of overeating. The number of laxatives or diuretics taken varies considerably, sometimes far exceeding the recommended dose.

None of these methods of purging is an effective method of weight control. Self-induced vomiting results in the retrieval of only about half to two-thirds of what has been eaten, the taking of laxatives has a minimal effect on food absorption, and diuretic-taking has none. As a result, a significant proportion of each binge is absorbed.

The weight of most of these patients is in the healthy range (BMI between 20 and 25) due to the effects of the under-eating and over-eating cancelling each other out. As a result they do not experience the secondary psychosocial and physical effects associated with maintaining a very low weight seen in anorexia nervosa.

Other forms of weight-control behaviour are practised by some patients, including over-exercising, the spitting out of food, and the taking of repeated enemas or saunas. Over-exercising is the most common of these, but it is not nearly as prominent or as obviously pathological as in anorexia nervosa. A minority of patients ruminate, that is, repeatedly regurgitate and re-chew food that has been eaten. They may then either re-swallow the food or spit it out. This behaviour is not well-understood.

In the non-purging type of bulimia nervosa there is no vomiting or misuse of laxatives or diuretics, or they occur infrequently. Instead, there is sustained and marked dietary restriction outside the binges. This is both a response to the binge eating and contributor to it, in that this type of eating increases the risk of further episodes. In all other respects the two subtypes of the disorder are similar.

(c) Attitudes to shape and weight

A characteristic set of attitudes to shape and weight is the other distinctive element of the specific psychopathology of bulimia nervosa. Equivalent attitudes are found in anorexia nervosa and most cases of eating disorder NOS. These attitudes are often described as the 'core psychopathology' of eating disorders. They are characterized by an overconcern with shape and weight in which there is a fear of weight gain and fatness that is generally accompanied by a pursuit of weight loss and thinness. Underlying this psychopathology is the tendency to judge self-worth largely, or even exclusively, in terms of shape and weight. Whereas it is usual to evaluate self-worth on the basis of perceived performance in a variety of domains of life (such as interpersonal relationships, work, sport, artistic ability, etc.), people with anorexia nervosa or bulimia nervosa evaluate themselves primarily in terms of their shape and weight. These attitudes and values constitute a good example of an overvalued idea.

Most features of bulimia nervosa can be understood as being secondary to these attitudes to shape and weight. The dieting, purging, and over-exercising are obvious secondary features. In addition, there are direct behavioural expressions of these concerns. For example, many patients repeatedly weigh themselves and scrutinize their appearance in mirrors. Others avoid any knowledge of their weight while being acutely sensitive about their appearance. Some avoid others seeing their body and some even avoid seeing it themselves. This can have a major impact on social and sexual relationships.

The concerns about shape and weight, and eating, have a major effect on others in the patient's immediate environment. Meals are often times of tension and social events which involve eating may be avoided. The feeding of children may be affected[10] and their growth may be impaired[11] (see Chapter 9.3.6).

General psychopathology

General psychiatric symptoms are prominent in bulimia nervosa; more so than in anorexia nervosa. The nature of the comorbid symptoms also differs. Depressive features are particularly striking: indeed, the level of depressive symptoms in bulimia nervosa is equivalent to that seen in major depressive disorder. Anxiety symptoms are also encountered, many of which are directly related to the eating disorder; for example, there is often pronounced anxiety about eating in public. Obsessive-compulsive features are sometimes present, although they are less common than in anorexia nervosa. Similarly, social functioning is less impaired.

The depressive features of bulimia nervosa deserve special mention. In most patients the depressive features can be attributed to the presence of the eating disorder but in a subgroup there appears to be an independent coexisting, but interacting, clinical depression. Features suggestive of such coexisting clinical depressions include the following: recent intensification of depressive features (in the absence of any change in the eating disorder or the patient's circumstances); pervasive and extreme negative thinking (i.e. broader in content than concerns about eating, shape, and weight); hopelessness in general (i.e. seeing the future as totally bleak, seeing no future, resignation); recurrent thoughts about death and dying; suicidal thoughts; guilt over events in the far past; a decrease in involvement with others over and above any impairment that already accompanied the eating disorder (e.g. ceasing to see friends); loss of interest in activities that had been pursued despite the eating disorder (e.g. ceasing to listen to music; ceasing to read newspapers or follow the news); and a decrease in drive and initiative.

These coexisting clinical depressions often go undetected since they are viewed as characteristic of bulimia nervosa. This is unfortunate for two reasons: first, they interfere with the treatment of the eating disorder; and second, they are readily treated with anti-depressant drugs (unlike the secondary depressive features).

A minority of patients with bulimia nervosa have 'impulse-control' problems, such as the overconsumption of alcohol or drugs, or repeated self-harm (e.g. cutting). Some of these patients also meet diagnostic criteria for borderline personality disorder (see Chapter 4.12.2). The prevalence of such features varies according to treatment setting: they are unusual in community samples, whereas they are more frequent among patients seen in specialist treatment centres.

Much more common than frank personality disorders are two traits which are also seen in anorexia nervosa. The first is low self-esteem. This generally antedates the eating disorder, although it is often exaggerated by it. Many patients with bulimia nervosa describe longstanding doubts about their worth and ability, irrespective of their accomplishments. The second is perfectionism, that is, imposing on oneself inordinately high personal standards in a range of domains (for example, work, sport, personal conduct). Since many of these standards are unachievable, it is common for these patients to give long histories of viewing themselves as perpetually failing.

Physical features

There are few physical abnormalities in bulimia nervosa. Body weight is unremarkable in the majority of patients and thus the physical effects of starvation are rarely seen. Nevertheless, menstrual abnormalities or amenorrhoea are present in about a quarter of patients. These are likely to be secondary to the disturbed eating since they generally respond to the successful correction of the eating disorder. On laboratory testing endocrine abnormalities are sometimes encountered and these tend to be mild versions of those found in anorexia nervosa. Fertility appears not to be affected.

Frequent purging, and especially the combination of vomiting and laxative misuse, results in fluid and electrolyte abnormalities in some patients. These abnormalities are varied in nature but most often consist of some combination of hypokalemia, hyponatremia, and hypochloremia. The patients appear to accommodate to these abnormalities since medically serious complications (for example, cardiac arrhythmias) are much less common than might otherwise be expected given the laboratory findings. Some patients experience intermittent oedema particularly if there is a sudden decrease in the extent of their purging.

Localized physical abnormalities include erosion of the dental enamel (especially from the lingual surfaces of the front teeth) among those who have vomited for many years; traumatic calluses on the knuckles of the hand of those who use their fingers to induce the gag reflex (Russell's sign); and enlargement of the salivary glands, especially the parotids, probably as a result of chronic inflammation. A small proportion of patients have raised serum amylase levels usually due to an increase in the salivary isoenzyme.

Relationship to other disorders

Anorexia nervosa and eating disorder NOS

Bulimia nervosa has many features in common with anorexia nervosa and eating disorder NOS, particularly the characteristic attitudes to shape and weight and the behaviour that arises directly as a result.[12] In most cases, bulimia nervosa is preceded either by frank anorexia nervosa (in about a quarter of cases) or an anorexia nervosa-like form of eating disorder NOS. While movement from bulimia nervosa to anorexia nervosa is unusual, progression on to some form of eating disorder NOS is common. Whether it is appropriate to view such patients as having recovered from one psychiatric disorder and developed another is a moot point: rather, it would seem more appropriate to view them as having a single evolving eating disorder.

There is some evidence of co-aggregation between bulimia nervosa, anorexia nervosa, and eating disorder NOS with there being increased rates of all three diagnoses among the relatives of probands with either condition.[13]

Obesity

Few patients with bulimia nervosa are overweight or have obesity. On the other hand there is evidence of raised rates of parental and premorbid obesity.[14] Obesity is an unusual sequel of the disorder although this may be because those at most risk of obesity are less likely to recover and so continue to suppress their weight.

Other psychiatric disorders

As noted above, depressive features are common in bulimia nervosa and they may antedate the eating disorder. The same is true of anxiety and anxiety disorders. Most family studies have found a raised rate of affective disorder among these patients' relatives whereas little is known about the familial relationship between bulimia nervosa and the anxiety disorders.[15] There is a raised rate of alcohol and drug abuse among patients with bulimia nervosa and a raised rate among these patients' relatives.[15] Substance abuse rarely antedates the eating disorder but this is to be expected given the age of onset of substance abuse disorders.

It is hazardous making personality disorder diagnoses among those with eating disorders. This is because eating disorders have their onset in adolescence and they directly affect many of the characteristics upon which personality is judged. Thus there is a risk of overestimating the presence of personality disturbance. Nevertheless, some patients with bulimia nervosa do seem to have a coexisting personality disorder, the most common form being borderline personality disorder. Little is known about the rate of personality disturbance among these patients' relatives although there is evidence of familial co-aggregation of anorexia nervosa and obsessional and perfectionist traits.[15]

Diabetes mellitus

It was thought that eating disorders were over-represented among those with Type I diabetes mellitus. This is now not clear. Controlled studies in which eating disorder features have been assessed by interview rather than self-report questionnaire (the preferred method and one which minimizes the risk of false positive diagnoses) have found little evidence of an elevated rate of anorexia nervosa although the rate of bulimia nervosa may be increased.[16]

Distribution

The fact that it took Russell more than 6 years (1972–1978) to collect 30 cases of bulimia nervosa suggested that the disorder was not common. It is therefore remarkable that within a few years of the publication of Russell's paper it was evident that bulimia nervosa was an important source of psychiatric morbidity among young women.

In the early 1980s large numbers of previously undetected cases were identified using the media.[17,18] These cases were remarkably similar to Russell's, except that almost all were female and a small proportion had a history of anorexia nervosa. Most had kept their eating disorder secret for many years, and because of shame and hopelessness few had sought help. Many thought that they were the only person with this type of eating disorder. Simultaneously however, and doubtless partly as a result of the media attention,

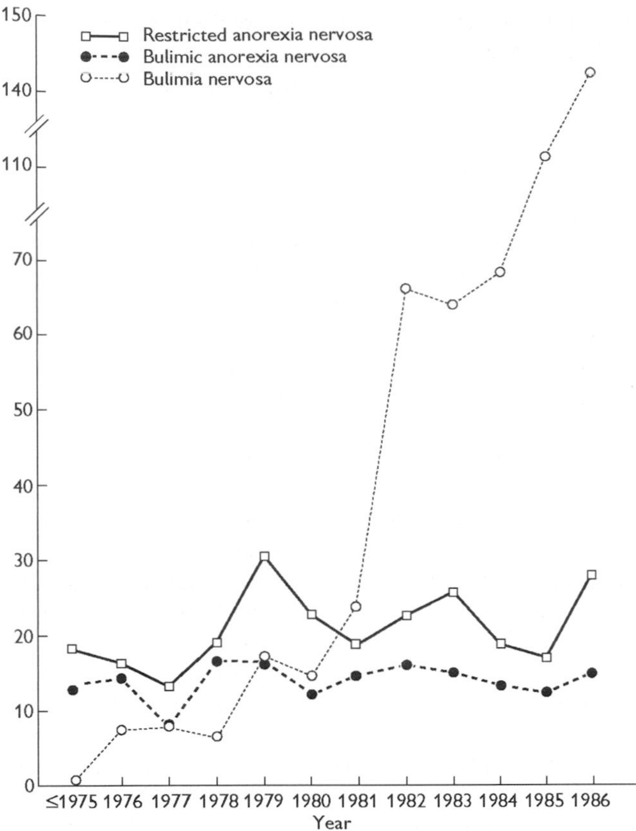

Fig. 4.10.2.3 Rates of referral to a major eating disorder centre in Toronto (1975–1986) (Reproduced from Garner, D.M. and Fairburn, C.G Relationship between anorexia nervosa and bulimia nervosa: diagnostic implications. In *Diagnostic issues in anorexia nervosa and bulimia nervosa* (eds. D.M. Garner and P.E. Garfinkel), copyright 1998, Brunner/Mazel, New York).

there was also a sharp increase in the number of people requesting treatment for bulimia nervosa (see Fig. 4.10.2.3).

The marked increase in the number of patients with bulimia nervosa stimulated interest in the prevalence of the disorder. By 1989 over 50 prevalence studies had been conducted, many of which yielded unrealistically high prevalence figures as a result of using weak assessment and sampling procedures. Gradually methods improved with the result that estimates of the prevalence of bulimia nervosa decreased to more modest and consistent levels with the point prevalence among young adult women (aged 16 to 35 years) being in the region of 1 per cent,[19,20] a similar figure being obtained for lifetime prevalence.[20] The prevalence of bulimia nervosa among men is not known. Among patient samples, male cases are unusual. Bulimia nervosa is thought to be uncommon in non-Western societies although few prevalence studies have been conducted and most have had significant methodological shortcomings.[21]

There have been few estimates of the incidence of bulimia nervosa, and since these have been based upon clinic rather than community samples, they are likely to underestimate the true figures. Even today, many people with bulimia nervosa do not seek help. The lack of reliable community-based incidence figures also makes it impossible to know whether the disorder has become more common since the 1970s or whether the upsurge in cases in the early 1980s was as a result of undetected cases being more likely to seek treatment. Data from the assessment of women in different birth cohorts suggest that the disorder has become much more common[22] although other explanations for the apparent increase cannot be ruled out.

Aetiology

Development of the disorder

As noted in Chapter 4.10.1, anorexia nervosa generally starts in mid-adolescence with a period of voluntary dietary restriction which proceeds to get out of control. As a result body weight falls and a state of starvation develops. Shape and weight concerns may pre-date the onset of the dieting or develop as weight is lost.

Bulimia nervosa starts in a similar way although the age of onset is typically some years later and shape and weight concerns usually antedate the dieting. The dietary restriction resembles that seen in anorexia nervosa and it leads to weight loss sufficient to result in anorexia nervosa in about a quarter of cases. (As a result of referral bias, this proportion is higher in cases seen in specialist centres.) In the remaining cases there is also weight loss but it is less extreme. After a variable length of time (generally within 3 years) dietary control breaks down with the patient's dieting becoming punctuated by episodes of overeating. At first, the episodes of overeating may be modest in size and intermittent, but gradually they become larger and more frequent. As a result, the lost weight is regained and body weight returns to near its original level. By this point the disorder tends to be self-perpetuating. At some stage in this sequence of events, self-induced vomiting and laxative misuse may be adopted to compensate for the overeating. In practice, however, both forms of behaviour have the opposite effect since belief in their effectiveness encourages a relaxation of control over eating. In those who vomit this phenomenon is exaggerated by the discovery that the process is easier after eating large amounts of food.

Predisposing factors and processes

There are many risk factors for the development of bulimia nervosa[14] and these overlap with those for anorexia nervosa[23] (see Table 4.10.2.2).

The risk factors may be usefully divided into a number of categories.

- Demographic factors—these are being female, adolescent and living in a Western society.
- Exposure to an immediate social environment that encourages dieting—this includes being brought up in a family in which there is intense interest in shape, weight, and eating as a result of one or more members either having some degree of eating disorder or having a medical condition that affects eating or weight (such as diabetes mellitus). Extreme occupational or recreational pressures to diet also appear to be associated with increased risk (for example, ballet dancing), although there may also be an element of self-selection. Another important influence is parental and childhood obesity, the rates of which are substa ntially increased in bulimia nervosa. Both are likely to sensitize individuals to their appearance and weight, and thereby make them prone to diet. There is also some evidence that puberty occurs comparatively early which may also magnify concerns about shape.

Table 4.10.2.2 Principal risk factors for anorexia nervosa and bulimia nervosa

General factors
Female
Adolescence and early adulthood
Living in a Western society
Individual-specific factors
Family history
Eating disorder of any type
Depression
Substance abuse, especially alcoholism (bulimia nervosa)
Obesity (bulimia nervosa)
Premorbid experiences
Obstetric complications
Adverse parenting (especially low contact, high expectations, parental discord)
Sexual abuse
Family dieting
Critical comments about eating, shape, or weight from family and others
Occupational and recreational pressure to be slim
Premorbid characteristics
Low self-esteem
Perfectionism (anorexia nervosa and to a lesser extent bulimia nervosa)
Neuroticism
Anxiety and anxiety disorders
Obesity (bulimia nervosa)
Early menarche (bulimia nervosa)
Type I diabetes (bulimia nervosa)

(Reproduced from Fairburn, C.G. Cognitive Behaviour Therapy and Eating Disorders, copyright 2008, Guildford press, NY.)

- Exposure to factors that increase the risk of psychiatric disturbance in general and depression in particular—these include a family history of psychiatric disorder, especially depression, and a range of adverse childhood experiences including parenting deficits and sexual and physical abuse. It was thought that sexual abuse was especially common among those who develop bulimia nervosa, but the balance of evidence suggests that the rate is no higher than that among those who develop other psychiatric disorders.
- Perfectionism and low self-esteem—both traits are common antecedents of anorexia nervosa and bulimia nervosa. Typically they interact resulting in feelings of incompetence and ineffectiveness.
- Family history of substance abuse—there is a raised rate of substance abuse in the families of patients with bulimia nervosa. It is not clear how this increases the risk of bulimia nervosa. Clinical observations suggest that some of those who develop bulimia nervosa learn to modulate their mood by engaging in self-harm (e.g. by cutting themselves) or by consuming large quantities of food, alcohol, or psychoactive drugs.

An important question is how those with anorexia nervosa are able to maintain strict control over their eating whereas this is not true of those with bulimia nervosa. The explanation is unclear but several processes may be of relevance. First, perfectionism is even more pronounced in anorexia nervosa and it may enhance self-control. Second, the vulnerability to obesity found in bulimia nervosa may somehow undermine dietary restraint. Third, the mood lability of bulimia nervosa may also disrupt restraint.

Contribution of genetic factors

The fact that eating disorders run in families suggests that there may be a genetic contribution. In the absence of adoption studies, twin designs have been used to establish its extent.(24) Clinic samples show concordance for anorexia nervosa of around 55 per cent in monozygotic twins and 5 per cent in dizygotic twins, with the corresponding figures for bulimia nervosa being 35 and 30 per cent, respectively.(7,25) These findings suggest a significant heritability to anorexia nervosa but not to bulimia nervosa. Despite this, there is uncertainty as to the size of the genetic contribution to both disorders with there being differing point estimates and wide confidence intervals. The same applies to the contributions of individual-specific and shared (common) environmental factors. A number of issues affect the interpretation of the data. For example, there has been insufficient power to detect shared environmental effects, and established diagnostic criteria have been broadened considerably to increase the number of 'affected' twins available for analysis.

Given the clear and possibly substantial genetic contribution to both disorders, molecular genetic studies have been conducted to identify the underlying loci and genes. Genetic association studies have focussed in particular on polymorphisms in 5-HT (serotonin)-related genes because this neurotransmitter system is important in regulation of eating and mood, but a range of other polymorphisms have also been investigated. Despite this, no associations with eating disorders have been clearly replicated or confirmed in a family study or by meta-analysis. There has been one multi-centre genome-wide linkage study. It found linkage peaks for anorexia nervosa and bulimia nervosa on chromosomes 1, 4, 10, and 14. A further analysis, which covaried for related behavioural traits, identified a different locus on chromosome 1, as well as loci on chromosomes 2 and 13. All these findings await replication.

Neurobiological findings

There has been extensive research into the neurobiology of eating disorders. This has focussed on neuropeptide and monoamine (especially 5-HT) systems thought to be central to the physiology of eating and weight regulation.(26) Of the various central and peripheral abnormalities reported, many are likely to be secondary to the disturbed eating and associated weight loss. However, some aspects of 5-HT function and its receptors remain abnormal after recovery, leading to speculation that there is a trait monoamine abnormality which may predispose to the development of eating disorders or to associated characteristics such as perfectionism. Furthermore, normal dieting in healthy women has been shown to alter central 5-HT function, providing a potential mechanism by which eating disorders might be precipitated in women vulnerable for other reasons.

Brain functional imaging studies have identified altered activity in the frontal, cingulate, temporal, and parietal cortical regions in both anorexia nervosa and bulimia nervosa, and there is some evidence that these alterations persist after recovery.[27] Whether they are a consequence of the eating disorder or have somehow contributed to it is not known.

Maintaining factors and processes

Once established, bulimia nervosa tends to run a chronic course although it commonly evolves into eating disorder NOS. There are a number of processes which account for its self-perpetuating character. These are discussed in Chapter 6.3.2.2 (CBT for eating disorders). They include the ongoing influence of the extreme concerns about shape and weight; the form of these patients' dieting, which encourages binge eating; the mood-modulating effect of binge eating; and the fact that the loss of control overeating perpetuates fears of weight gain.

Assessment

The identification of patients with bulimia nervosa is not difficult so long as the diagnosis is considered. This is important because the shame that characterizes the disorder leads many people to delay seeking help—the average delay between onset and presentation is about 5 years—and when they do present for treatment, some do so indirectly. Thus they may complain of depression, substance abuse, menstrual disturbance, or gastrointestinal symptoms, rather than the eating disorder itself. The best policy is for psychiatrists to always keep in mind the possibility of bulimia nervosa when assessing female patients aged between 16 and 35 years. Negative responses to the following questions should suffice to exclude the disorder:

- 'Do you have any problems with your eating?'
- 'Do you have any problems controlling your eating; that is, problems with binge eating?'
- 'Do you ever make yourself sick or take laxatives to control your weight or shape?'

Patients who present directly complain of having lost control over eating and their assessment is generally straightforward. It should always include an assessment of the extent to which the disorder is interfering with everyday functioning and an evaluation of general psychiatric features and especially those of depression.

The best established measure of eating disorder features is the Eating Disorder Examination.[28] This interview is widely regarded as the 'gold standard' measure of eating disorders, but it is possibly too exhaustive to use on a routine clinical basis. Various self-report questionnaires are available but they provide a more basic level of assessment and they cannot be used to make a clinical diagnosis. The leading self-report measures are the Eating Disorder Inventory[29] and the self-report version of the Eating Disorder Examination.[30]

No assessment is complete without weighing the patient and checking their height. Weighing needs to be done with considerable sensitivity because of these patients' concerns about their weight. A physical examination is not essential unless the patient is underweight (or there are other medical indications), nor are laboratory tests required except in those cases in which there is reason to suspect that there might be fluid or electrolyte disturbance.

Treatment

Given that bulimia nervosa has only recently been described, there has been a remarkable amount of research on its treatment. Over 70 randomized controlled trials have been completed. An authoritative meta-analysis has been conducted by the United Kingdom National Institute for Health and Clinical Excellence or 'NICE'.[31] The majority of the trials have focussed on adults with bulimia nervosa, the treatment of adolescents having received little attention, and almost all these studies have been 'efficacy' rather than 'effectiveness' studies. However, there are reasons to think that their findings are of direct relevance to routine patient care not least because the patients studied have been similar to those seen in clinical practice. Nevertheless, there is a definite need for effectiveness studies particularly now that the main treatment options are clear.

Studies of pharmacological treatment

A variety of drugs have been tested as possible treatments for bulimia nervosa including antidepressants, appetite suppressants, anticonvulsants, and lithium. Only antidepressants have shown promise.

(a) Antidepressant medication

All the major classes of antidepressant drug have been evaluated, including tricyclic antidepressants, monoamine oxidase inhibitors, selective serotonin uptake inhibitors, and atypical antidepressants. The findings have been relatively consistent and may be summarized as follows (adapted from Wilson and Fairburn[32]):

- Antidepressant drugs are more effective than placebo at reducing the frequency of binge eating and purging. On average, among treatment completers there is about a 50 per cent reduction in the frequency of binge eating and a cessation rate of about 20 per cent. The therapeutic effect is more rapid than that seen in depression. There is generally little change in the placebo group. The dropout rate varies but averages about 30 per cent.
- The longer-term effects of antidepressant drugs remain largely untested. Almost all the studies to date have been of their short-term use (16 weeks or less). The findings of the few longer-term studies suggest that outcome is poor and compliance low.[33]
- Few studies have evaluated the effects of antidepressant drugs on features other than binge eating and purging. Mood improves as the frequency of binge eating declines but this effect is common to all treatments for bulimia nervosa. Antidepressant drugs do not appear to modify these patients' extreme dieting which may account for the poor maintenance of change.
- Different antidepressant drugs seem to be equally effective, although there have been no direct comparisons of different drugs.
- With one exception, there have been no systematic dose-response studies. The exception showed that fluoxetine at a dose of 60 mg/day, but not 20 mg/day, was more effective than placebo.[34]
- Patients who fail to respond to one antidepressant drug may respond to another. There have been no drug augmentation studies.
- No consistent predictors of response have been identified. Pretreatment levels of depression appear not to be related to outcome.

- The mechanism(s) whereby antidepressant drugs exert their 'antibulimic' effects is not known. The apparent comparability of different classes of drug implicates a common mechanism but this is unlikely to be their antidepressant action since the response is too rapid and the level of depression does not predict outcome.

Studies of psychological treatment

(a) Cognitive behaviour therapy (CBT)

The most intensively studied psychological treatment is a specific form of CBT.(35,36) This was the first promising treatment described and it remains the leading treatment for the disorder. The treatment and its rationale are described in Chapter 6.3.2.2.

CBT is conducted on an outpatient basis and involves 15 to 20 sessions over about 5 months. It is suitable for all patients bar the small minority (less than 5 per cent) who require hospitalization.

The findings of the studies of CBT (over 20 controlled trials) are summarized below (adapted from Wilson and Fairburn(32)):

- The drop-out rate with CBT (about 20 per cent) is less than that seen with antidepressant drugs. The treatment is also more acceptable to these patients than treatment with medication.
- CBT has a substantial effect on the frequency of binge eating and purging. On average, among treatment completers there is about an 80 per cent reduction in the frequency of binge eating, and a cessation rate of about 60 per cent.
- The effects of CBT appear to be well-maintained. Most of the recent studies have included a 6 to 12-month follow-up period. The relapse rates are low.
- CBT affects most aspects of the psychopathology of bulimia nervosa including the binge eating, purging, dietary restraint, and the over-evaluation of shape and weight. In common with other treatments, the level of depression decreases as the frequency of binge eating declines. Social functioning and self-esteem also improve.
- CBT is more effective than delayed treatment (i.e. a waiting list control group), other psychological treatments (other than possibly interpersonal psychotherapy—see below) and antidepressant drugs at reducing the frequency of binge eating and purging. Among the other psychological treatments studied have been supportive psychotherapy, focal psychotherapy, supportive-expressive psychotherapy, interpersonal psychotherapy, hypnobehavioural treatment, stress management, nutritional counselling, behavioural versions of cognitive behaviour therapy, and exposure with response prevention.
- No consistent predictors of response to CBT have been identified. Severity of symptoms at presentation, a history of anorexia nervosa, low self-esteem, and the presence of borderline personality disorder have been associated with worse outcome in some studies but not others. However, the extent of initial response (over the first 4 weeks of treatment) is a potent and potentially valuable predictor of outcome.(37,38)
- The mechanism(s) of action of CBT have yet to be established although they appear to be mediated at least in part by a reduction in dietary restraint.(39) It also seems that the cognitive procedures are required for progress to be maintained since behavioural versions of the treatment are associated with a greater risk of relapse.(40)
- There is some evidence that the combination of CBT and antidepressant drugs may be more effective than CBT alone in reducing accompanying anxiety and depressive symptoms.
- Simpler forms of CBT may help a small subset of patients although the findings are not consistent. These include brief versions of the treatment and cognitive behavioural self-help in which patients follow a cognitive behavioural self-help programme either on their own (pure self-help) or with the guidance of a therapist (guided self-help). The programme may be delivered via a book, CD-ROM or the internet. This type of treatment is still in its infancy and it has yet to be rigorously evaluated.

(b) Interpersonal psychotherapy (IPT)

IPT is the leading alternative to CBT. This treatment was originally devised by Klerman and colleagues as a treatment for depression (see Chapter 6.3.3).(41) It is a focal psychotherapy, the main emphasis of which is to help patients identify and modify current interpersonal problems. The treatment is both non-directive and non-interpretative and, as adapted for bulimia nervosa,(42) it pays little attention to the patient's eating disorder. It is therefore very different to CBT. There have been two comparisons of CBT and IPT in the treatment of bulimia nervosa and both have found that they are about comparably effective but that IPT takes 4 to 8 months longer to achieve its effects.(40,43) The second of these studies was also designed to identify variables that might allow patients to be matched to CBT or IPT but none emerged.

Management of bulimia nervosa

Given that the leading treatment for bulimia nervosa is CBT, the ideal form of management is the provision of CBT by a therapist trained in its implementation. Unfortunately there is a shortage of the necessary expertise with the consequence that a 'stepped care' approach has been advocated on pragmatic grounds. With such an approach a simple treatment is used first and only if this proves insufficient a more complex and specialized intervention is provided. Three steps may be distinguished.

Step 1—Having established the diagnosis, the first decision is whether the patient may be managed on an outpatient basis. The great majority (over 95 per cent of referrals to non-specialist centres) may be managed this way. Exceptions are patients at significant risk of suicide and the presence of physical complications necessitating inpatient or day patient care. Severe substance abuse requires treatment in its own right, although this can sometimes be integrated with the treatment of the eating disorder. For example, it is possible to adapt CBT for bulimia nervosa so that it addresses the patient's substance abuse at the same time.

Step 2—If the patient is suitable for outpatient-based treatment, guided cognitive behavioural self-help, and/or antidepressant medication is the next step. The former involves following a cognitive behavioural self-help programme under the guidance of a 'facilitator' (a non-specialist therapist). Three cognitive behavioural self-help books are available,(44–46) two of which are direct translations of CBT for bulimia nervosa. There is evidence to support the use of all three and it is a matter of preference which is chosen. Each provides information about bulimia nervosa together with a self-help programme. The role of the facilitator is not to provide treatment as such, as in a conventional 'therapist-led' treatment, but rather to support and encourage the patient to follow the programme. Thus, this is a 'programme-led' form of treatment, and it is this characteristic that makes it suitable for widespread dissemination. Treatment generally takes about 4 months and involves eight to ten meetings with the facilitator, each lasting up to 30 min. It is best if the first few appointments are weekly.

Guided self-help may take place in a variety of settings including primary care. Unfortunately only a small proportion of patients show substantial change and there are no reliable predictors of outcome. Patients who have obtained little benefit after 4 to 6-weeks are unlikely to do so and should be moved on to Step 3.

Antidepressant medication is an alternative to guided self-help. It is important to note that the medication is being used for its antibulimic effect not its antidepressant action. This affects the choice of drug and the dose chosen. The drug of choice is fluoxetine at a dose of 60 mg in the morning. It is usually well tolerated. As with guided self-help, if there has been little benefit after 4 to 6-weeks it is best to move on to Step 3.

A third alternative would be to combine antidepressant medication and guided self-help to see if the two augment each other. This would be a reasonable strategy although there are few data to support it.

Step 3—Patients who do not benefit from cognitive behavioural self-help or antidepressant medication should receive full CBT on a one-to-one basis (see Chapter 6.3.2.2). Ideally this should be delivered by a well-trained therapist who is used to following the protocol.(36)

Step 4—The fourth step is for those who are still symptomatic after having received well-delivered CBT. This step is pragmatic since there are few research findings of relevance. To guide the choice of treatment, the reasons for the poor response need to be carefully considered. Explanations include the presence of an undetected clinical depression; failure of CBT (which itself needs to be explained); poorly delivered CBT; poor patient compliance (which also needs to be explained); and disruption by outside events.

There are a number of different treatment options under these circumstances, the choice depending upon the outcome of the reassessment and the resources available. They include the following:

- Stop treatment and arrange to re-evaluate the patient after an interval of some months. Some patients and therapists 'burn out' after a sustained period of therapeutic work. A break can often be helpful. Deciding to stop treatment should be a joint decision and it is not appropriate with patients who are distressed or with those whose physical or psychological well-being is a cause for concern.
- Embark upon a new psychological treatment. While the obvious choice is IPT, there are no grounds for supposing that patients who fail to respond to CBT will respond to IPT. Indeed, there is evidence that this is not the case.(47) An alternative strategy would be to change the form of the CBT. The re-evaluation of the patient may have resulted in the identification of problems that might be amenable to cognitive behavioural procedures outside the realm of mainstream CBT for bulimia nervosa. Indeed, the fact that this occurs has led to the development of a new 'enhanced' form of CBT for eating disorders that is not only designed to be more potent that the earlier treatment but it also addresses common obstacles to change external to the eating disorder psychopathology (i.e. mood intolerance, clinical perfectionism, low self-esteem, and interpersonal problems).(8,48) It is also of note that this treatment is designed to be suitable for all forms of eating disorder not just bulimia nervosa.
- Arrange for day patient or inpatient treatment. In a small minority of cases outpatient treatment proves not to be sufficient, either because the disorder is resistant to outpatient-based forms of treatment or because the patient's life circumstances are interfering with progress. In such cases day patient or inpatient treatment can be useful. Generally this involves a combination of therapeutic approaches including elements of CBT. It is essential that both day patient treatment and inpatient treatment are followed by outpatient treatment designed to ensure that progress is maintained.

Course and outcome

Much remains to be learned about the course and outcome of bulimia nervosa. It is clear from epidemiological studies that many people do not present for treatment. The course of their disorder is completely unknown. Those who do present tend to do so after a considerable period of time indicating that among this subgroup the disorder has a tendency to run a protracted course. On the other hand, the findings of the treatment studies indicate that the outcome is considerably better than Russell originally suggested, although it must be stressed that even with CBT, the most effective treatment, only about half the patients make a full and lasting recovery.

There have been few studies of long-term course or outcome. A 5-year prospective study of a community sample found that at each assessment point between a half and two-thirds of the cases had an eating disorder of clinical severity, the majority being cases of eating disorder NOS.(49) A 10-year follow-up study found that about 10 per cent met diagnostic criteria for bulimia nervosa and a further 20 per cent had a form of eating disorder NOS.(50) There is no evidence that bulimia nervosa evolves into any other psychiatric disorder, and anorexia nervosa is a very unusual outcome. Body weight changes little over time and, in contrast with anorexia nervosa, the mortality rate appears not to be raised. Robust predictors of long-term course or outcome have been identified.

Acknowledgements

We are grateful to the Wellcome Trust for its support. CGF holds a Principal Research Fellowship (046386). ZC and RM are supported by a programme grant (046386).

Further information

Fairburn, C.G. (ed.). (2008). *Cognitive behavior therapy and eating disorders.* Guilford Press, New York.

International Journal of Eating Disorders.

References

1. Russell, G.F.M. (1979). Bulimia nervosa: an ominous variant of anorexia nervosa. *Psychological Medicine*, **9**, 429–48.

2. American Psychiatric Association. (1980). *DSM-III: diagnostic and statistical manual of mental disorders* (3rd edn). American Psychiatric Association, Washington, DC.
3. American Psychiatric Association. (1987). *DSM-III-R*. American Psychiatric Association, Washington, DC.
4. American Psychiatric Association. (1994). *Diagnostic and statistical manual of mental disorders* (4th edn). American Psychiatric Association, Washington, DC.
5. World Health Organization. (1992). The ICD-10 classification of mental and behavioural disorders. Author, Geneva.
6. Fairburn, C.G. and Bohn, K. (2005). Eating disorder NOS (EDNOS): an example of the troubl esome 'not otherwise specified' (NOS) category in DSM-IV. *Behaviour Research and Therapy*, **43**, 691–701.
7. Fairburn, C.G. and Harrison, P.J. (2003). Eating disorders. *Lancet*, **361**, 407–16.
8. Fairburn, C.G., Cooper, Z., and Shafran, R. (2003). Cognitive behaviour therapy for eating disorders: a 'transdiagnostic' theory and treatment. *Behaviour Research and Therapy*, **41**, 509–28.
9. Walsh, B.T. (1993). Binge eating in bulimia nervosa. In *Binge eating: nature, assessment and treatment* (eds. C.G. Fairburn and G.T. Wilson), pp. 37–49. Guilford Press, New York.
10. Stein, A., Woolley, H., Cooper, S.D., *et al.* (1994). An observational study of mothers with eating disorders and their infants. *Journal of Child Psychology and Psychiatry and Allied Disciplines*, **35**, 733–48.
11. Stein, A., Murray, L., Cooper, P., *et al.* (1996). Infant growth in the context of maternal eating disorders and maternal depression: a comparative study. *Psychological Medicine*, **26**, 569–74.
12. Fairburn, C.G., Cooper, Z., Bohn, K., *et al.* (2007). The severity and status of eating disorder NOS: implications for DSM-V. *Behaviour Research and Therapy*, **45**, 1705–15.
13. Strober, M., Freeman, R., Lampert, C., *et al.* (2000). Controlled family study of anorexia nervosa and bulimia nervosa: evidence of shared liability and transmission of partial syndromes. *American Journal of Psychiatry*, **157**, 393–401.
14. Fairburn, C.G., Welch, S.L., Doll, H.A., *et al.* (1997). Risk factors for bulimia nervosa—a community-based case-control study. *Archives of General Psychiatry*, **54**, 509–17.
15. Lilenfeld, L.R., Kaye, W.H., Greeno, C.G., *et al.* (1998). A controlled family study of anorexia nervosa and bulimia nervosa—psychiatric disorders in first-degree relatives and effects of proband comorbidity. *Archives of General Psychiatry*, **55**, 603–10.
16. Mannucci, E., Rotella, F., Ricca, V., *et al.* (2005). Eating disorders in patients with Type 1 diabetes: a meta-analysis. *Journal of Endocrinological Investigation*, **28**, 417–9.
17. Fairburn, C.G. and Cooper, P.J. (1982). Self-induced vomiting and bulimia nervosa: an undetected problem. *British Medical Journal*, **284**, 1153–5.
18. Fairburn, C.G. and Cooper, P.J. (1984). Binge-eating, self-induced vomiting and laxative misuse—a community study. *Psychological Medicine*, **14**, 401–10.
19. Fairburn, C.G. and Beglin, S.J. (1990). Studies of the epidemiology of bulimia nervosa. *American Journal of Psychiatry*, **147**, 401–8.
20. Hoek, H.W. and van Hoeken, D. (2006). Review of the prevalence and incidence of eating disorders. *International Journal of Eating Disorders*, **34**, 383–96.
21. Keel, P.K. and Klump, K.L. (2003). Are eating disorders culture-bound syndromes? Implications for conceptualizing their etiology. *Psychological Bulletin*, **129**, 747–69.
22. Kendler, K.S., MacLean, C., Neale, M., *et al.* (1991). The genetic epidemiology of bulimia nervosa. *American Journal of Psychiatry*, **148**, 1627–37.
23. Fairburn, C.G., Cooper, Z., Doll, H.A., *et al.* (1999). Risk factors for anorexia nervosa—three integrated case-control comparisons. *Archives of General Psychiatry*, **56**, 468–76.
24. Slof-Op't Landt, M., van Furth, E.F., Meulenbelt, I., *et al.* (2005). Eating disorders: from twin studies to candidate genes and beyond. *Twin Research and Human Genetics*, **8**, 467–82.
25. Bulik, C.M., Sullivan, P.F., Wade, T.D., *et al.* (2000). Twin studies of eating disorders: a review. *The International Journal of Eating Disorders*, **27**, 1–20.
26. Kaye, W.H., Frank, G.K., Bailer, U.F., *et al.* (2005). Serotonin alterations, in anorexia and bulimia nervosa: new insights from imaging studies. *Physiology & Behavior*, **85**, 73–81.
27. Kaye, W.H., Wagner, A., Frank, G., *et al.* (2006). Review of brain imaging in anorexia and bulimia nervosa. In *Annual review of eating disorders Part 2* (eds. S. Wonderlich, J.E. Mitchel, M. de Zwaan, and H. Steiger), pp. 113–29. Radcliffe, Oxford.
28. Fairburn, C.G. and Cooper, Z. (1993). The eating disorder examination (12th edn). In *Binge eating: nature, assessment and treatment* (eds. C.G. Fairburn and G.T. Wilson), pp. 317–60. Guilford Press, New York.
29. Garner, D.M. (1991). *Eating disorder inventory-2*. Psychological Assessment Resources, Odessa, FL.
30. Fairburn, C.G. and Beglin, S.J. (1994). Assessment of eating disorders: interview or self-report questionnaire? *The International Journal of Eating Disorders*, **16**, 363–70.
31. National Collaborating Centre for Mental Health. (2004). Eating disorders: core interventions in the treatment and management of anorexia nervosa, bulimia nervosa and related eating disorders. British Psychological Society and Royal College of Psychiatrists, London.
32. Wilson, G.T. and Fairburn, C.G. (2007). Treatments for eating disorders. In *A guide to treatments that work* (3rd edn) (eds. P.E. Nathan and J.M. Gorman). Oxford University Press, New York.
33. Romano, S.J., Halmi, K.A., Sarkar, N.P., *et al.* (2002). A placebo-controlled study of fluoxetine in continued treatment of bulimia nervosa after successful acute fluoxetine treatment. *American Journal of Psychiatry*, **159**, 96–102.
34. Fluoxetine Bulimia Nervosa Collaborative Study Group. (1992). Fluoxetine in the treatment of bulimia nervosa. A multicenter, placebo-controlled, double blind trial. *Archives of General Psychiatry*, **49**, 139–47.
35. Fairburn, C. (1981). A cognitive behavioural approach to the treatment of bulimia. *Psychological Medicine*, **11**, 707–11.
36. Fairburn, C.G., Marcus, M.D., and Wilson, G.T. (1993). Cognitive-behavioral therapy for binge eating and bulimia nervosa: a comprehensive treatment manual. In *Binge eating: nature, assessment and treatment* (eds. C.G. Fairburn and G.T. Wilson), pp. 361–404. Guilford Press, New York.
37. Agras, W.S., Crow, S.J., Halmi, K.A., *et al.* (2000). Outcome predictors for the cognitive behavior treatment of bulimia nervosa: data from a multisite study. *American Journal of Psychiatry*, **157**, 1302–8.
38. Fairburn, C.G., Agras, W.S., Walsh, B.T., *et al.* (2004). Prediction of outcome in bulimia nervosa by early change in treatment. *American Journal of Psychiatry*, **161**, 2322–4.
39. Wilson, G.T., Fairburn, C.C., Agras, W.S., *et al.* (2002). Cognitive-behavioral therapy for bulimia nervosa: time course and mechanisms of change. *Journal of Consulting and Clinical Psychology*, **70**, 267–74.
40. Fairburn, C.G., Jones, R., Peveler, R.C., *et al.* (1993). Psychotherapy and bulimia nervosa: longer-term effects of interpersonal psychotherapy, behavior therapy, and cognitive-behavior therapy. *Archives of General Psychiatry*, **50**, 419–28.
41. Klerman, G.L., Weissman, M.M., Rounsaville, B.J., *et al.* (1984). *Interpersonal psychotherapy of depression*. Basic Books, New York.
42. Fairburn, C.G. (1997). Interpersonal psychotherapy for bulimia nervosa. In *Handbook of treatment for eating disorders* (eds. D.M. Garner and P.E. Garfinkel), pp. 278–94. Guilford Press, New York.

43. Agras, W.S., Walsh, B.T., Fairburn, C.G., *et al.* (2000). A multicenter comparison of cognitive-behavioral therapy and interpersonal psychotherapy for bulimia nervosa. *Archives of General Psychiatry*, **57**, 459–66.
44. Fairburn, C.G. (1995). *Overcoming binge eating*. Guilford Press, New York.
45. Cooper, P.J. (1995). Bulimia nervosa and binge eating: a guide to recovery. Robinson, London.
46. Schmidt, U.H. and Treasure, J.L. (1993). *Getting better bit(e) by bit(e)*. Erlbaum, London.
47. Mitchell, J.E., Halmi, K., Wilson, G.T., *et al.* (2002). A randomized secondary treatment study of women with bulimia nervosa who fail to respond to CBT. *The International Journal of Eating Disorders*, **32**, 271–81.
48. Fairburn, C.G. (ed.) (2008). *Cognitive behavior therapy and eating disorders*. Guilford Press, New York.
49. Fairburn, C.G., Cooper, Z., Doll, H.A., *et al.* (2000). The natural course of bulimia nervosa and binge eating disorder in young women. *Archives of General Psychiatry*, **57**, 659–65.
50. Keel, P.K., Mitchell, J.E., Miller, K.B., *et al.* (1999). Long-term outcome of bulimia nervosa. *Archives of General Psychiatry*, **56**, 63–9.

4.11

Sexuality, gender identity, and their disorders

Contents

4.11.1 Normal sexual function
Roy J. Levin

4.11.2 The sexual dysfunctions
Cynthia A. Graham and John Bancroft

4.11.3 The paraphilias
J. Paul Fedoroff

4.11.4 Gender identity disorder in adults
Richard Green

4.11.1 Normal sexual function

Roy J. Levin

Introduction

Normal sexual function means different things to different people. It is studied by a variety of disciplines: biology, physiology, psychology, medicine (in the domains of endocrinology, gynaecology, neurology, psychiatry, urology, and venereology), sociology, ethology, culture, philosophy, psychoanalysis, and history. There is often little liaison or cross-fertilization between these disciplines and each has its own literature and terminology. Some are regarded as 'hard science', suggesting hypotheses that can be supported or rejected by experiment, observation, or measurement (evidence-based). Others are looked on as 'soft science', where individual and anecdotal evidence are the norm and are encouraged.

As space is limited, this chapter will characterize 'normal sexual activity' in the Western world mainly from biological, physiological, and psychological aspects but will occasionally utilize other disciplines when they yield insights not available from the 'harder sciences'.

Biological determinants of normal sexual function

Humans are the highest evolved primates. A number of our anatomical/biological features unrelated to reproduction have been described as strongly enhancing our sexual behaviour when compared with other primates,[1] although recent studies have shown that the bonobos (pygmy chimpanzees) also use sex for reasons unconnected with reproduction.[2]

In brief, these features are as follows:

1 The relative hairlessness of our bodies allows well-defined visual displays (see point 6 below) and enhanced tactile skin sensitivity.

2 The clitoris, which is an organ whose sole function is for inducing female sexual arousal/pleasure.

3 Orgasms, in both male and female, provide intense euphoric rewards for undertaking sexual arousal to completion. The female is able to have multiple serial orgasms.

4 The largest penis among primates, whether flaccid or erect, the latter acting as a good sexual stimulator of the female genitalia.

5 Concealed (cryptic) ovulation which could influence males to undertake coitus more frequently to create pregnancy and prevent cuckolding.

6 Well-defined visual sexual displays in the female that are not linked to season or fertility (i.e. breasts, pubic hair, buttocks, and lips). The everted mucous membranes of the lips serve both as a surface display (red, moist, and shiny), and for haptic stimulation during kissing and sucking.

7 Ability of the female to undertake sexual arousal and coitus independent of season, hormonal status, or ovulation. Human females (unlike other primates) can and often do willingly partake of sexual activity and coitus when they are menstruating, pregnant, or menopausal.

8 Development of large mammary glands during puberty which act as visual sexual signals in most cultures.

These biological determinants are augmented by socio-cultural factors:

1 Language, art, and music for erotic stimulation.

2 Facial adornment with make-up to heighten appearance and sex displays (viz., lipstick).

3 Clothing, especially of the female, such as brassières to redefine the shape of breasts, corsets to redefine the shape of the body, and high-heeled shoes to elongate the legs and thrust out the

buttocks. Young adult males use tight trousers to create a genital 'bulge' and to emphasize firm rounded buttocks, the latter being a highly sexually attractive feature to young women.

4 Perfumes and scents to enhance body aroma.

The last three features (2, 3, and 4) use artificial means to enhance normal sexual signals.[1] These biological and socio-cultural factors give human sexual activity an increased appetitiveness and make it more rewarding.

Sexuality as a social construct and the concept of sexual scripting

Laqueur[3] suggests that while the sexual biology remained unchanged, its expression has been influenced over the centuries by culture, social class, ethnic group, and religion. This concept, that human sexuality is a social construct, has been strongly argued by Foucault[4] and promoted by other social constructionist authors.[5] Gagnon and Simon[6] introduced the concept of 'sexual scripting'. Scripts organize and determine the circumstances under which sexual activity occurs, they are involved in 'learning the meaning of internal states, organizing the sequences of specific sexual acts, decoding novel situations, setting limits on sexual responses and linking meanings from non-sexual aspects of life to specifically sexual experience'. Money[7] employed a similar construction in his development of 'love maps' for the individual. While patterns of behaviour are influenced by society and social forces, there is a dearth of evidence to show that sexual identity, orientation, or sexual mechanisms are also influenced.

Modelling normal sexual function—(i) the sex survey

One obvious way of describing normal sexual function is to ask people what they do. Two classic sex surveys were conducted by Kinsey and his coworkers who reported the results of interviews with 12 000 males in 1948[8] and 8000 females in 1953.[9] Their technique of sampling was to interview everyone in specific cooperating groups (clubs, hospital staff, universities, police force, school teachers, etc.). This gave samples of convenience but not a valid statistical sampling of the population. Despite their age and faulty sampling, however, there are still useful data in these surveys. In the sexual climate of the 1950s many of the findings were regarded as highly controversial. Clement[10] has reviewed the subsequent studies of human heterosexual behaviour up to 1990.

Surveys give a selective picture of sexual function. Results depend on the formulation of the questions, they rely on self-reports, and they represent only those prepared to describe their sexual behaviour. It is known, for example, that females tend to under-report their premarital sexual experiences[11] while males tend to over-report their lifetime partners.[11] Berk *et al.*[12] studied the recall by 217 university students of their sexual activity over a 2-week period assessed by questionnaires answered 2 weeks after the recording period, and by daily diaries kept over the same 2 weeks. Subjects reported more sexual activity in the questionnaires than in their diaries. Women reported giving and having more oral sex than the men. Clearly, data from questionnaire surveys should be treated cautiously.

A survey tells only what is frequent and not necessarily what is normal, but the most frequent practices often become identified with normal sexual behaviour. Surveys also vary in the range of behaviours that are asked about, for example coitus without condoms is important in the age of AIDS. Surveys have one great disadvantage, the facts that they produce are often 'perishable'; many aspects of the sex surveys of the pre-pill era, or more recently the pre-AIDS era, are now of use only in a historical or comparative basis.

Two recent well-organized surveys based on samples of the whole population have been undertaken, one in the United States and the other in the United Kingdom. Interestingly, in both surveys, questions about masturbation were disliked by the respondents. In the American survey these questions were asked in a separate self-administered questionnaire, while in the British survey they were abandoned.

The American survey[13] was conducted face to face with 3159 selected individuals who spoke English in representative households by 220 trained interviewers (mainly women). Nearly 80 per cent of the individuals chosen agreed to be interviewed. Men thought about sex often, more than 50 per cent having erotic thoughts several times a day, while females thought about sex from a few times a week to a few times a month. The frequency of partnered sex had little to do with race, religion, or education. Only three factors mattered: age, whether married or cohabiting, and how long the couple had been together. Fourteen per cent of males reported having no sex in the previous year, 16 per cent had sex a few times in the year, 40 per cent a few times a month, 26 per cent two to three times a week, and 8 per cent four times a week. The percentages were similar for women. The youngest and the oldest people had the least sex with a partner; those in their 20s had the most. Of the women aged 18 to 59 years, approximately one in three said they were uninterested in sex, and one woman in five said sex gave her no pleasure. Unlike frequency, reported sexual practices do depend on race and social class. Most practices other than vaginal coitus were not very attractive to the vast majority. In women aged 18 to 44 years of age, 80 per cent rated vaginal coitus as 'very appealing' and an additional 18 per cent rated it as 'somewhat appealing'. Among men 85 per cent regarded vaginal coitus as 'very appealing'. The most appealing activity second after coitus was watching the partner undress, and this was appealing to more men (50 per cent) than women (30 per cent). This reflects the greater voyeuristic nature of men and their willingness to pay to look at women undressing or undressed.

In regard to oral sex, both men and women liked receiving more than giving. This practice varied markedly with race and education, with higher reported rates among better educated white people than among less educated and black people. Some 68 per cent of all women had given oral sex to their partner and 19 per cent experienced active oral sex the last time they had intercourse. Seventy-three per cent of all women had received oral sex from the partner, and 20 per cent had received it the last time they had had intercourse. Corresponding experiences were reported by men.

This survey, unlike many earlier ones, asked about anal sex. Of females aged 18 to 44, 87 per cent thought it not at all appealing, and only 1 to 4 per cent thought it very or somewhat appealing. In males of the same age 73 per cent thought it not at all appealing and rather more than women thought it very or somewhat appealing. Similar reports were obtained from women and men aged 44 to 59.

Regarding masturbation, older people (over 54 years old) had lower rates than at any other age, indicating that they do not use masturbation to compensate for an overall decrease in sexual activity with their partners.

In the United Kingdom survey,[14] 18 876 people were interviewed by 488 interviewers (of whom 421 were women). The sampling used one person per address and the acceptance rate was 71.5 per cent. Questions were asked about the frequency of vaginal coitus, oral sex, and anal sex, but not masturbation. The median number of occasions of sex with a man or woman was five times a month for females aged 20 to 29 and males aged 25 to 34, but declined to a median of two per month for males aged 55 to 59. More than 50 per cent of the females in the 55 to 59 age group reported no sex in the last month, but in this age group females are more likely than men to have no regular partner because they are widowed, separated, or divorced.

Vaginal coitus was reported by nearly all females and males by the age of 25. Fifty-six per cent of males and 57 per cent of females reported vaginal coitus in the previous week, and non-penetrative sex was practiced by 75 per cent men and 82 per cent of women. Twenty-five per cent of males had genital stimulation in the previous 7 days. Cunnilingus and fellatio were common but less practiced than vaginal coitus. Of men and women aged 18 to 44, 60 per cent had oral sex in the previous year but in the 45- to 59-year-old group this fell to 30 per cent for women and 42 per cent for men. This and other sex surveys suggest that the practice of oral sex has increased since the 1950s and 1960s. Anal coitus was infrequent; approximately 14 per cent of the males and 13 per cent of the females had ever undertaken it, and only 7 per cent of males or females had practiced it in the previous year.

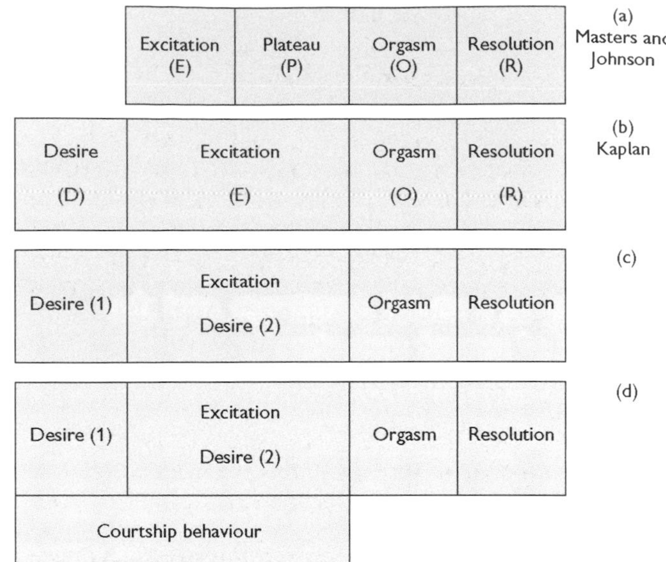

Fig. 4.11.1.1 The development of the human sexual response model from (a) the original **EPOR** model of Masters and Johnson[15] through (b) the desire, excitation, orgasmic, and resolution (**DEOR**) model of Kaplan[17] to (c) the proposed modification with desire phase 1 (before initiation of the excitation phase and desire phase 2 during excitation phase) and finally (d) with added courtship behaviour.

Modelling normal sexual function—(ii) the sexual response cycle

A direct way of investigating normal sexual function is to observe and measure the body changes that take place when men and women become sexually aroused. From these data, models have been constructed of the normal sequence of changes during sexual arousal, coitus, and orgasm. The first models described a simple sequence of increasing arousal and excitement culminating in rapid discharge by orgasm, displayed graphically as an ascent, peak, and then descent. As the investigations became more sophisticated, understanding of the body responses grew and the models became more detailed and complex.[5,15,16]

The EPOR model—a sexual response cycle model

A most successful human sexual response model was that formulated by Masters and Johnson.[15] In the laboratory, they observed the changes that took place in the male and female body and especially the genitals during sexual arousal to orgasm either by masturbation or by natural or artificial coitus with a plastic penis that allowed internal filming of the female genitalia. After studying approximately 7500 female and 2500 male arousals to orgasm in some 382 female and 312 male volunteers over 11 years, they proposed a four-phase, sequential, and incremental model of the human sexual response cycle (Fig. 4.11.1.1). The phases were described as the excitation (**E**) phase (stimuli from somatogenic or psychogenic sources raise sexual tensions), the plateau (**P**) phase (sexual tensions intensified), the orgasmic (**O**) phase (involuntary pleasurable climax), and finally the resolution (**R**) phase (dissipation of sexual tensions). The great success of this **EPOR** model was its wide compass; it could characterize the sexual responses of women and men, both heterosexual and homosexual, ranging from simple petting to vaginal or anal coitus with or without orgasm. However, it had several weaknesses.

Modifying the EPOR model into the DEOR model

The first weakness of the EPOR model is that it was derived from the study of a highly selected group of American men and women volunteers who could arouse themselves to orgasm in a laboratory, on demand, and allow themselves to be watched/filmed or measured for scientific and altruistic (or perhaps exhibitionistic) purposes. The second weakness was the lack of interobserver agreement about the changes observed and of confirmation of their sequential reliability. Robinson[16] examined the **E** phase and **P** phase, and concluded convincingly that the **P** phase was simply the final stage of the **E** phase. Helen Kaplan,[17] a New York sex therapist, proposed that before the **E** phase there should be a 'desire phase' (**D** phase). This proposal came from her work with women who professed to have no desire to be sexually aroused, even by their usual partners. She suggested that the desire must occur before sexual arousal can begin. Kaplan's subjects were attending a clinic and remarkably no studies were ever conducted with a control normal population (either women or men) to investigate whether this 'self-evident' fact was true. Despite this, the **EPOR** model gradually became replaced by the desire, excitation, orgasmic, and resolution phase (**DEOR**) modification. While this is the currently accepted model, the centrality of the desire phase in women remains uncertain (Fig. 4.11.1.1). In a survey of non-clinic sexually experienced women in Denmark, about a third reported that they never experienced spontaneous sexual desire[18] and in an American survey women reported periods of several months when they lacked interest in sex.[13] The other problem with the desire phase is its location in the sequential **DEOR** model.

Sexual desire (D1-proceptive desire) that appears to be spontaneous (but presumably must still be activated by a trigger) should obviously be placed at the beginning of the model (Fig. 4.11.1.1b), while sexual desire (D2-receptive desire) created when the person is sexually aroused by another occurs during the E-phase (Fig. 4.11.1.1c).

It has been proposed[19] that while the DEOR model fits for females in younger couples' relationships for longer maintained ones sexual activity is undertaken often for factors such as intimacy, security, and acceptance and becomes more influenced by cognitive and emotional processes and the possible outcomes of the experience (e.g. mutual pleasure, confirming commitment and trust, enhancing emotional intimacy) rather than proceptive/receptive desires.

Courtship (mating) behaviour—activity initiating normal sexual behaviour

With the possible exception of rape, the pre-initiation of sexual activity normally starts with flirting/courtship behaviours. Sometimes this activity can precede the desire phases; sometimes it occurs during the desire phases, and sometimes in the excitation phase (Fig. 4.11.1.1d).

Evolutionary psychology attempts to explain the strategies of mating.[20] Its message is not always palatable to modern sensitivities about sexual equality. It is argued that women invest more in their offspring than men,[21] that this investment is a scarce resource that men compete for, and that men can enhance their reproductive strategy by mating frequently. Most men are first visually attracted to a possible female sexual partner. They look for youthfulness and physical attractiveness in the form of regular features (symmetry), smooth complexion, optimum stature, and good physique, and they value virginity and chastity. Partner variety is highly desired. Women, however, need to obtain high-quality mates with abundant resources and look for emotional and financial status and security. Clearly the strategies conflict giving rise to different preferences in mate choice and casual sex, and different levels of investment or commitment to relationships.[22]

Once the chosen female (or male) accepts the initiation of flirting/courtship behaviour, the subsequent stages form a stereotyped sequence which is found in many different cultures. The stages are look, approach, talk, touch, synchronize, kiss (caress), sex play, coitus. It is a sequence that the poet Ovid knew in the first century BCE. Morris[1] characterized human courtship behaviour further into 12 basic stages: eye to body, eye to eye, voice to voice, hand to hand, arm to shoulder, arm to waist, mouth to mouth, hand to head, hand to body, mouth to breast, hand to genitals, genitals to genitals. Similar hierarchies have been constructed extending the behaviour to oral-genital contacts.

Although kissing has been described as 'an inhibited rehearsal for intercourse and other sexual practices'[23] and is usually undertaken in the courtship behaviour well before genital activity occurs, it is sometimes thought of as more intimate than coitus. Prostitutes, for example, traditionally do not kiss their clients on the mouth, reserving the activity for their private sexual behaviour. Nicholson[24] has speculated that kissing may be a mechanism by which semiochemicals (similar to pheromones) are exchanged between humans to induce bonding.

Common extragenital changes during sexual arousal

In both males and females, effective sexually arousing stimuli cause a number of physiological changes.[15,25] There is increased respiration, heart rate, and blood pressure, nipple erection, often sweating, and a sex flush (maculopapular skin rash). Muscle tension increases (myotonia) and the pupils dilate. All these changes become more intense as arousal increases. Following orgasm the changes dissipate rapidly (R phase); without orgasm they dissipate more slowly.

The endocrinology of normal sexual function

(a) Peptide hormones and neuropeptides

Prolactin, a peptide hormone, is secreted by cells of the anterior pituitary in both males and females. In females it is a key lactogenic hormone involved in stimulating the manufacture of breast milk but it has no proven physiological reproductive function in males. Pathologically high plasma levels of prolactin (hyperprolactinaemia) are accompanied by disturbances of sexual/reproductive function especially erectile dysfunction in males and inhibition of ovulation in females. The exact causes are unknown. As it is secreted in higher amounts at orgasm in both sexes it has been claimed to be a major factor responsible for 'switching off' sexual arousal but this ignores the fact that women are multiorgasmic while the evidence for this function even in males is unconvincing.[26]

Two neuropeptides, oxytocin and vasopressin (Antidiuretic Hormone, ADH) are hormones and also act as neuropeptide transmitters with distribution in parts of the brain and spinal cord. They are secreted as hormones by the hypothalamus/posterior pituitary with increases at orgasm in both males and females. Oxytocin is often claimed to be responsible for facilitating smooth muscle contractions during ejaculation and uterine contractions during orgasm but the possible role of vasopressin has been ignored. In some animals, oxytocin is involved in pair bonding but the evidence for this in humans is poor.

Males

(a) Androgens

The major steroids influencing normal sexual function in males are the androgens secreted by the testes mainly as testosterone with much smaller quantities of androstenedione and dihydrotestoterone. The adrenal cortex also manufactures and secretes androgens but this amounts only to 2 per cent of the total. Of the total testosterone (260–1000 ng/dl), 95 per cent is bound to plasma proteins; only the unbound fraction (34–194 pg/ml) is an active virilizing hormone.

The development and maintenance of the masculine musculature, bone growth, genitals, and pubic and axillary hair is androgen dependent. The mechanism of the hormonal masculinization of the brain in rodents involves the aromatization of testosterone, but in humans the role of aromatization is still uncertain.

(b) Androgens and male sexual behaviour

The involvement of androgens in adult human male sexual behaviour has been reviewed many times (see Levin[27] for references). Removal of testosterone by castration usually leads to a decrease in sexual activity and drive (libido) in the majority of subjects within

12 months. There is, however, large individual variations, and some castrates retain sexual activity and interest for years.[28] Factors such as adrenal androgens, the availability of sexual partners, and attitude to the operation influence the response. In castrates and in hypogonadal males, replacement of testosterone restores sexual interest and activity.

Females

(a) Oestrogen, progesterone, and androgens

In the female, oestrogen, progesterone, and androgens are involved in differentiating and maintaining genital and breast tissues and in influencing normal sexual function. Female genital development, unlike that of the male, does not appear to need hormonal stimulation as the development of female genital structures are the foetal prototype or default programme.[29] During puberty, ovarian oestrogen and progesterone together with androgens from the adrenal cortex induce growth and functional changes in the internal and external genitalia, breast, and nipples. Oestrogens induce growth in the fallopian tubes, uterus, vagina, and breasts and lay down subcutaneous fat largely in the breast, hip, and thigh regions to create the rounded contours of the female body that are highly attractive to the male. The fat laid down is enough to supply the energy for a pregnancy and the subsequent lactation. Females have a plasma androgen concentration some 10 times less (15–70 ng/dl) than those in the male. Androgens are produced by the ovaries (25 per cent), adrenals (25 per cent) and in peripheral tissues from adrenal-secreted androgen precursors. They are responsible for the development and maintenance of the clitoris, nipples, pubic and axillary hair, and probably the labia, periurethral glans and pelvic-striated musculature. The variation of the androgen levels in the plasma during the menstrual cycle is small and it is the free androgen level (1–21 pg/ml) not the bound that is the active principle.

(b) Role of hormones in female sexuality

While over 60 studies have been undertaken to examine whether the changing hormonal levels of the menstrual cycle influence the sexual arousal of the female,[30] neither oestrogen or progesterone have been found convincingly to play a direct role in influencing the sexual activity of the human female apart from their indirect functions in the maintenance of the structures and functions of the female genitals, especially the vagina.

The role of androgens in female sexuality is not clear-cut.[31] Some propose that, as in the male, it is the major hormonal influence on the female libido. Removal of the adrenals has been shown to reduce desire and ability to reach orgasm. Excess androgens stimulates libido but in pharmacological not physiological doses. Such doses affect the structure and sensitivity of the clitoris (an androgen-sensitive tissue), so the effects on sexuality might not be only brain mediated.

(c) Sexual behaviour during the menstrual cycle

Despite numerous studies it is still uncertain whether female sexual behaviour is influenced by the hormonal changes in the menstrual cycle. Meuwissen and Over[30] surveyed 64 published studies. A significant number showed a premenstrual peak in sexual desire and activity, others a postmenstrual peak, either at menstruation or ovulation but the latter studies often used poor methodology to determine the time of ovulation.

Male genital functions during normal sexual arousal

While the **DEOR** model characterizes the general sexual arousal of humans, a more specific detailed physiological model in males is that of excitation, erection, emission, and ejaculation with orgasm. Each of these is served by separate mechanisms. Although ejaculation and orgasm usually occur temporally together, they also have separate mechanisms.

(a) Excitation

Sexual excitation can occur through any of the five senses by psychogenic or somatogenic stimuli. In special circumstances arousal can become linked to or greatly enhanced by fetishitic association with non-sexual objects such as feminine garments of underwear, rubberware, shoes, furs, etc.

The sexual excitation is manifested in the brain by activation of numerous areas (see section on brain activation during human sexual arousal). Centres in the spinal cord for erection and ejaculation are known from animal studies and it is likely that they also exist in the human cord. They are activated by neural efferent activity from the aroused areas of the brain and initiate erection and ejaculation.

(b) Erection: the conversion of the flaccid urinary penis to the rigid sexual penis

The three longitudinal erectile chambers of the penis are arranged with a side-by-side dorsal pair of corpora cavernosa above the single ventral corpus spongiosum. The corpora cavernosa are covered by the tunica albuginea, a 2-mm thick fibrous membrane which is resistant to stretch. The corpus spongiosum surrounds the length of the penile urethra and is enlarged at its base to form the urethral bulb and distally to create the glans penis. While it becomes engorged with blood during arousal it is not involved in the rigidity of the erection but protects the urethra from closure. The unaroused penis is flaccid because the pudendal arterial blood flow into the erectile tissues is limited by the high sympathetic (adrenergic-mediated) constrictive tone in the smooth muscle of the vessels of corpus cavernosum. On sexual arousal, the sympathetic tone is reduced; the neural innervation of the arteries and cavernosal chambers is activated to release vasoactive intestinal peptide (VIP), a peptidergic vasodilator neurotransmitter that directly relaxes smooth muscle and nitric oxide (NO), the nitrergic neurotransmitter. NO activates the enzyme cyclic guanylase in the smooth muscle cells of the cavernous tissue and blood-vessel endothelium to produce cyclic guanosine monophosphate (cGMP), the second messenger that creates intracellular conditions to relax the muscle. The enzyme phosphodiesterase 5 breaks down the cGMP and inhibitors of this enzyme, which can be taken by mouth, facilitate the attainment of erection even with reduced neural inputs.

The vasodilatation of the arterial supply by VIP together with the relaxation of the vessels of the cavernosal tissue allows them to fill under arterial pressure stretching the chambers until they become stiff against their covering of unyielding tunica albuginea, and the veins (emissary) that pass obliquely through the tunica become occluded greatly reducing penile vascular drainage. The flaccid urinary penis has been converted into the erect rigid sexual penis some 7 to 8 cm longer. The rigidity is essential for successful vaginal penetration and to stimulate its walls (especially the anterior) during penile thrusting. The striated muscles of the pelvic region, namely the ischiocavernosus and bulbocavernosus, are not normally involved in creating penile erection[32] although they can be voluntarily contracted in short bursts to aid its rigidity. The engorged corpus spongiosum is less rigid than the cavernosal chambers making the glans of the penis softer and less damaging to the female labia and vagina.

(c) Internal genitals

The genital fluids of the testes, epididymis, and accessory genital glands of the male are involved in emission. These glands are the bulbo-urethral (Cowper's gland), the prostate (approximately 30 per cent of the total volume of the ejaculate), and the paired seminal vesicles (approximately 60 per cent of the volume of the ejaculate). The fluids from all these together with that of the glands of Littré that line the penile urethra, constitute the ejaculate or semen which has a characteristic odour and rapidly forms a coagulum in contact with air. Subsequently enzymes in the semen break down the coagulum and release the trapped sperm.

(d) Emission

This phase begins with the movement of the various genital fluids into the ducts initiated by the neurally induced contraction of smooth muscles in the capsules of the testes, epididymis, and seminal vesicles. The secretions spurt into the prostatic urethra, and the sphincter of the bladder neck closes to prevent reflux into the bladder. When this happens the male experiences the sensation of 'ejaculatory inevitability' and knows that he will ejaculate within a second or two and that conscious suppression of the ejaculatory reflex is now impossible. The contractions of the smooth muscle of the glandular capsules together with the contraction of the vas deferens and peristalsis in the urethra move the semen along into the penile urethra.

(e) Ejaculation

Within a second or two later the bulbocavernosus muscle of the perineal region contracts clonically, initially at about 1 per 0.8 s, squeezing the urethra and forcing out the ejaculate. As ejaculation proceeds, the interval between each striated muscle contraction gets longer and their force weaker until they gradually die out.[15,32] Their number can vary between 5 and 60. Most of the ejaculate is expressed within the first half dozen contractions. If the striated muscles are paralysed the semen is squeezed out only by the smooth muscle peristaltic contractions which produce a dribbling ejaculate with no projectile force and little pleasurable quality.

(f) Male orgasm

Orgasm, the supreme ecstatic pleasure is experienced just before the striated contractions occur and is then associated, throbbingly, with each subsequent contraction slowly decreasing in intensity and dying away as do the contractions. It is felt as an intense pleasurable throbbing/pumping in the penis and pelvic area and can last from 5 to 60 s. Most males groan with each squirting contraction. Kinsey *et al.*[8] marshalled the evidence showing that orgasm and ejaculation were separate mechanisms. Briefly, orgasm occurs without ejaculation in preadolescent males, in some adult males orgasm does not occur until a few seconds after ejaculation, a few adult males are anatomically incapable of ejaculation but have orgasms, and males who have been prostatectomized cannot have ejaculations but some can have orgasms.

The intensity of orgasm usually varies with the duration of the sexual arousal (the longer it is maintained the greater the subsequent orgasm), the erotic excitement and novelty of the arousing stimuli, and previous ejaculation, especially the interval from the last one (initial ejaculations have usually better orgasms than subsequent ones). Males have a post ejaculation refractory time (PERT) and usually cannot have an erection or another ejaculation until some time has passed. The PERT varies with age and can be anything from minutes, when young, to hours or days when older.[15] It is not known where this inhibitory mechanism resides but animal work suggests that it is in the brain rather than the spinal cord.[33] Some men claim to be able to learn to inhibit ejaculation and yet have repeated serial orgasms.[34]

It has been stated that the larger the ejaculate volume the greater is the orgasmic pleasure,[15] the studies however were flawed because they used men who increased semen volume by abstaining from ejaculation for days. This confounds the effects of semen volume with that of ejaculatory abstinence which itself enhances subsequent sexual pleasure. In fact semen volume does not appear to be the arbiter of pleasure or the trigger for ejaculation.[35] Drugs can induce a 'dry ejaculation' but the pleasure of the orgasm appears unimpaired,[33] and in young boys the pleasure of the early dry orgasm is not noticeably changed when semen becomes added to the ejaculation around puberty.[36]

An ignored feature is whether there is a typology of male orgasms. Most orgasms arise from penile stimulation but they can also be activated by per rectum digital stimulation of the prostate gland. No laboratory study of these orgasms has ever been made but anecdotal reports say that they feel deeper, more widespread and intense and last longer than those from penile stimulation.[37]

Female genital functions during normal sexual arousal

(a) External

(i) Labia

The external female genitalia consist of the outer (majora) and inner (minora) labia containing erectile tissue that surround the vaginal introitus. Normally the outer labia meet and cover the introitus, but in some women the inner labia protrude even when they are sexually unaroused. Sexual arousal creates vasocongestion especially in the labia minora which protrude through the majora adding approximately 1 to 2 cm to the length of the vagina. The labia minora become erotically sensitive to touch and friction when engorged.

(ii) Clitoris

Although the clitoris is the homologue of the penis, its precise anatomical structure is still uncertain. The most recent description by O'Connell *et al.*[38] is of a triplanar complex of erectile tissue with a midline shaft lying in the medial sagittal plane about 2 to 4 cm long and 1 to 2 cm wide, which bifurcates internally into paired curved crura 5 to 9 cm long, and externally is capped with a glans about 20 to 30 mm long with a similar diameter. Two vaginal bulbs of erectile tissue are closely applied on either side of the urethra. The shaft's erectile tissue consists of two corpora cavernosa surrounded by a fibrous sheath (tunica albuginea) and the whole is covered by a clitoral hood formed in part by the fusing of the two labia minora. The uncertainty concerns the location and extent of the female corpus spongiosum. Some describe it as wrapped around the urethra, others state that the vaginal (vestibular) bulbs on either side of the vaginal wall are spongiosus tissue and unite ventrally to the urethral meatus to form a thin strand of erectile tissue ending in the glans. Recent studies by van Turnhout *et al.*[39] have clarified the situation. They confirmed by dissections in fresh cadavers that the bilateral vestibular bulbs terminate into the glans clitoridis.

With sexual arousal, the blood flow to the clitoris is increased probably by a mechanism involving its vipergic (VIP) and nitrinergic (NO) innervation leading to its tumescence (swelling) but, contrary to many inaccurate descriptions, without true erection (i.e. without rigidity). The enhancement of its blood flow is paralleled by an increased sensitivity to touch and friction especially of the glans.

(iii) Periurethral glans

There is a triangular area of mucous membrane that surrounds the urethral meatus, extending from just below the glans of the clitoris to the entrance of the vagina. This area has been called the 'periurethral glans'[25] and is thought to be erotically stimulated, especially during penile thrusting, as it is known that the tissue is pushed and pulled into and out of the vagina by the penile movements.[25] The periurethral glans is actually part of the corpus spongiosum if we accept the anatomical designation of van Turnhout *et al.*[39] which suggest that it is the homologue of the male glans. The extent, mobility, density of innervation, and sensitivity of this erotic site may explain why some women find it easy to reach orgasm during penile thrusting alone.

(b) Internal

(i) Vagina

No single structure can describe the vaginal shape. In sexual quiescence it is a potential space with an H-shaped cross-section and an elongated S-shaped longitudinal section culminating in a cul-de-sac, the anterior wall of which is penetrated by the cervix. The anterior and posterior walls touch but their film of basal vaginal fluid prevents adhesion. This basal fluid is a mixture of fluids from the vagina itself (basal transudate) with uterine and cervical secretions. The squamous epithelial lining of the vagina actively transports sodium ions from the vaginal fluid back into the blood. As fluid follows this ion movement osmotically the vagina is continually producing and reabsorbing its own fluid[25,40] normally lower in sodium and higher in potassium compared to plasma.

Because sexual activity is intermittent, the basal vaginal blood flow is maintained normally at a minimal level by a high adrenergic-mediated vasoconstrictive tone and vasomotion. The latter is the mechanism by which tissue viability is maintained at a basal level by not having all the capillaries open at the same time but rather each one opens and closes randomly to supply by demand its surrounding tissue needs of oxygen and metabolic substrates. On sexual arousal, the blood supply to the vaginal walls is increased by the liberation of VIP from the vipergic neural innervation. This increases the flow through the open capillaries and recruits new ones until all are open and vasomotion disappears,[41] Within seconds this creates blood-vessel engorgement and an increased plasma transudate filters out of the capillaries and percolates between the cells of the epithelium saturating its limited reabsorptive capacity. The newly formed neurogenic vaginal transudate, with its higher sodium ion concentration, creates a lubricating film on the vaginal surface which is essential for painless penile penetration and thrusting. Poor or inadequate lubrication can lead to dyspareunia (painful coitus) and subsequent sexual dysfunction. On cessation of sexual arousal or after orgasm the blood flow returns to the basal level, the fluid is reabsorbed back into the blood following the continuous absorption of sodium ions by the vaginal epithelium and vasomotion is restored.

(ii) Coitus and the vagina

The cul-de-sac of the vagina is expanded during sexual arousal and the uterus with cervix is lifted clear of its posterior wall (vaginal tenting).[15] This vaginal tenting is an important reproductive feature that delays the transport of sperm allowing the ejaculate to decoagulate and initiate motility and pre-capacitation changes that facilitate the process of sperm capacitation (see Levin[40,41] for references). In the ventral–ventral ('missionary') coital position, penile penetration and thrusting stretches and stimulates the structures of the anterior vaginal wall which include the urethra, the 'G spot' (see below), and neural structures in Halban's fascia. All these (the anterior wall erotic complex) are thought to be capable of creating erotic excitement when so stimulated, giving rise to a significant part of the sexual pleasure normally experienced by most women during coitus.

(iii) The erotic structures of the anterior vaginal wall: urethra, 'G spot', and Halban's fascia

The urethra, approximately 4 cm long, is invested with erectile tissue which becomes engorged on sexual arousal. Ultrasound imaging during coitus has shown that the thrusting penis stretches the urethra.[42] There is an area on the anterior vaginal wall a few centimeters from the introitus, at or around the junction of the urethra with the bladder, that becomes swollen and on strong pressure stimulation can induce orgasm. This urethral area was first identified by Grafenberg[43] but the observation was overlooked until its rediscovery by Perry and Whipple[44] who named it the 'G spot' in recognition of the original discoverer. Anatomically, it probably represents the 'paraurethral' or 'periurethral' glands now referred to as the 'female prostate'. In some women these produce at orgasm a small amount of fluid secretion loosely referred to as the 'female ejaculate' (see[25,44] for references). These glands are in the space between the bladder trigone and the neck of the urethra which is filled with fibroelastic mesenchymal lamina rich in vascular lacunae and contains nerve fibres and pseudocorpuscular terminals. This area, known as Halban's fascia[45] when stimulated by pressure (penile or digital) creates intense sexual pleasurable feelings.[44–46] As any pressure stimulus on the anterior vaginal wall will in fact stimulate the G spot, Halban's fascia and the urethra at the same time it makes it difficult to apportion the generation of sexual pleasure to any specific structure.

The involvement of the spinal cord in activating the female erotic structures during sexual arousal has been poorly studied and little is known of possible mechanisms.

(c) Female orgasm

As in the male, the female orgasm creates supreme ecstatic pleasure usually accompanied by throbbing striated muscle contractions, especially of the ischiocavernous and bulbospongiosus muscles, but other pelvic-striated muscles can also be involved.[15,37] Most females groan or moan during these contractions. The induction of orgasm in women by coital stimulation alone is not as frequent as that in the male, about half not achieving orgasm unless clitoral stimulation is also used. The reason for this difference is usually ascribed either to the greater inhibitory education about sexual pleasure experienced by women or the lack of correct genital stimulation. A major difference between males and females is that females can be multiorgasmic because they do not have a PERT after orgasm.(15,23,33) There is mounting evidence that, unlike the unitary concept of the **DEOR** model, the erotic stimulation of different genital sites (especially the anterior vaginal wall compared with the clitoris) induces different types of orgasmic response both subjectively and physiologically.(44,47,48)

Brain activation during human sexual arousal

Before the advent of brain imaging by functional magnetic resonance imaging (fMRI) or positron emission tomography (PET) to identify which areas are activated by and during sexual arousal and orgasm, only limited information was obtained by observing the effects of brain lesions on behaviour, epileptic case studies, electroencephalography (EEG) activity, and rare electrical recordings and stimulations of specific brain areas.(27) Inferences about human sexual arousal mechanisms often had to be made from animal experiments but the problem of species differences always was the spectre in the wings (see comment below).

One type of brain imaging (blood oxygen level dependent [BOLD]) relies on the concept that activation of neurones requires an increased demand for oxygen which normally entails an increase in their blood supply bringing oxygenated blood. The change in the magnetic susceptibilities of the oxygenated and deoxygenated blood is measured and is an index of the increase or decrease in flow to the neuronal area. In the PET technique a short-lived radioactive tracer (often ^{15}O) is injected intravenously and its concentration in the brain area of high blood flow localized by the radioactivity. Both techniques rely heavily on extensive computer programs to correct for a variety of essential artefact corrections one of the most important being corrections for movement. The usual protocol underlying most studies of sexual arousal is to first measure the activity of the brain area under study during a non-sexual basal state (looking at neutral videos) then switching to viewing sexually arousing videos. By subtracting the activity of the neutral from the aroused measurements the remaining activity is assumed to be due the sexual arousal per se. One difficulty is what level (threshold) of activity of a site is to be regarded as physiological. Investigators tend to choose their own criteria making direct comparisons between different studies difficult. Another difficulty is that many areas of the brain are multifunctional (e.g. the amygdala, the periaqueductal grey, the cerebellum) and are thus activated/deactivated by different stimuli (viz., pain, pleasure, fear, anger, emotional processing) the activation/deactivation may be an epiphenomenon of the arousal rather than its cause. Finally, it takes a few seconds to build up a brain scan but neuronal activation takes just hundredths of a second; the image will always lag behind the actual activation so that identifying what is the primary initiator of brain arousal will not be apparent.

Despite all the above caveats about brain imaging one outstanding conclusion is now clear from all the various studies—that there does not appear to be a single site creating arousal or orgasm, multiple site co-activation (also referred to as a neural network) is the rule in both males and females. While a number of the features of brain activation appear common to sexual arousal in the brains of both sexes, the amygdala and hypothalamus are said to be more strongly activated in men when viewing identical sexual stimuli. According to Holstege's group,(47) the first to map brain areas active during ejaculation/orgasm, the strongest activated primary region during male erection/orgasm is the ventral tegmental field region, the midbrain lateral central tegmental field, the zona incerta, the suprafascicular nucleus, the ventroposterior, midline and intralaminar nucleus, and the cerebellum. Decreased activity was seen in the amygdala and adjacent entorhinal cortex. This decrease in the amygdala is said not to occur during women's arousal.(48) Another group.(49) imaging the brain in sexually aroused males reported increased neural activity in areas that included the right frontal cortex, the inferior temporal cortex, the left anterior cingulate cortex, and the right insula. However, only a subset of these areas (anterior cingulate, insula, amygdala, hypothalamus, and secondary somatosensory cortex) were involved in creating a full erection.

Imaging studies undertaken by Komisaruk and Whipple(48) used both women who were paraplegic and some able-bodied women who had the rare ability to create orgasm by mental activity (thoughts) alone. In the former group, where arousal was induced by cervical vibratory stimulation, a large number of sites, including the hypothalamus, were activated by the stimulus used to induce orgasm but in the mental activity group, the only sites activated by thought were regions of the nucleus accumbens, the paraventricular nucleus of the hypothalamus, the hippocampus, and anterior cingulate cortex. The authors suggested that these sites may be specifically related to activate the female orgasm. Interestingly, the amygdala was not activated during these 'thought' induced orgasms. How 'normal' the 'orgasm by thought' group are is yet to be ascertained.

It is unfortunate that while there are now a number of independent studies on brain imaging during sexual arousal the resultant descriptions of the areas claimed to be the activated or deactivated are not in agreement. Part of the problem is that different stimuli, duration of stimuli, data handling, and processing protocols have been used but even these do not explain all the differences. Thus, at present, it is not possible to give a detailed and reliable account of brain activation during sexual arousal.

Summary

Normal human sexual function can be characterized simply by its biological mechanisms which are of obvious importance, not least to reproduction.(41) The mechanisms have changed little over the centuries, but their expression as behaviour, when moulded by historical time, social class, ethnic grouping, religion, and society, creates the changing complex concept of human sexuality. Indeed, it has been said that human sexuality is more about fertilizing relationships than eggs! While we have increased hugely our knowledge about many of the mechanisms involved in human sexuality, the impact of a highly successful oral therapy for erectile dysfunction being an obvious example, those of the brain and spinal cord are practically unexplored. What creates human sexual desire and sexual excitement and what causes them to fade away, where in the brain is the pleasure of orgasms created, why do men have a PERT but not women, are just a few of the fascinating questions that remain to be answered.

Further information

Goldstein, I., Meston, C.M., Davis, S.R., *et al.* (eds.) (2006). *Women's sexual function and dysfunction: study, diagnosis and treatment*. Taylor & Francis, London.

Janssen, E. (ed.) (2007). *The psychophysiology of sex*. Indiana University Press, Bloomington, IN.

Janssen, E., Prause, N., and Geer, J. (2007) The sexual response. In *Handbook of Psychophysiology* (3rd edn) (eds. J.T. Cacioppo, G. Tassinary, and G.G. Bernison), pp. 245–66, Cambridge University Press, New York.

Komisaruk, B.R., Beyer-Flores, C., and Whipple, B. (2006). *The science of orgasm*. The Johns Hopkins University Press, Baltimore, MD.

Lue, T.F., Basson, R., Rosen, R., *et al.* (eds.) (2004). *Sexual medicine- sexual dysfunctions in men and women*. Health Publications, Editions 21, Paris, France.

References

1. Morris, D. (1967). *The naked ape*. Jonathan Cape, London.
2. Heltne, P.G. and Marquardt, L.A. (eds.) (1989). *Understanding chimpanzees*. Harvard University Press, Cambridge, MA.
3. Laqueur, T. (1990). *Making sex: body and gender from the Greeks to Freud*. Harvard University Press, Cambridge, MA.
4. Foucault, M. (1980). *The history of sexuality*. Vintage, New York.
5. Tiefer, L. (1992). Historical, scientific, clinical and feminist criticism of the 'the human sexual response cycle' model. *Annual Review of Sex Research*, **2**, 1–23.
6. Gagnon, J.H. and Simon, W. (1973). *Sexual conduct: the social sources of human sexuality*. Aldine Chicago, IL.
7. Money, J. (1986). *Lovemaps: clinical concepts of sexual/erotic health and pathology, paraphilia, and gender transposition in childhood, adolescence, and maturity*. Irvington, New York.
8. Kinsey, A.C., Pomeroy, W.B., and Martin, C.E. (1948). *Sexual behaviour in the human male*. W.B. Saunders, Philadelphia, PA.
9. Kinsey, A.C., Pomeroy, W.B., Martin, C.E., *et al.* (1953). *Sexual behaviour in the human female*. W.B. Saunders, Philadelphia, PA.
10. Clement, U. (1990). Surveys of heterosexual behaviour. *Annual Review of Sex Research*, **1**, 45–74.
11. Einon, D. (1994). Are men more promiscuous than women? *Ethology and Sociobiology*, **15**, 131–43.
12. Berk, R., Abramson, P.R., and Okami, P. (1995). Sexual activities as told in surveys. In *Sexual nature, sexual culture* (eds. P.R. Abramson and S.D. Pinkerton), pp. 371–86. University of Chicago Press, Chicago, IL.
13. Michael, R.T., Gagnon, J.H., Laumann, E.O., *et al.* (1994). *Sex in America—a definitive survey*. Little, Brown, London.
14. Wellings, K., Field, J., Johnson, A.M., *et al.* (1994). *Sexual behaviour in Britain*. Penguin, Harmondsworth.
15. Masters, W.H. and Johnson, V.E. (1966). *Human sexual response*. Little, Brown, Boston, MA.
16. Robinson, P. (1976). *The modernization of sex*. Cornell University Press, Ithaca, NY.
17. Kaplan, H. (1979). *Disorders of sexual desire*. Simon and Schuster, New York.
18. Garde, K. and Lunde, I. (1980). Female sexual behaviour. A study in a random sample of 40-year-old women. *Maturitas*, **2**, 225–40.
19. Basson, R. (2000). *The female sexual response model revisited. Journal of the Society for Obstetrics and Gynecology of Canada*, **22**, 383–7.
20. Buss, D.M. (1994). *The evolution of desire: strategies of human mating*. Basic Books, New York.
21. Trivers, R.L. (1972). Parental investment and sexual selection. In *Sexual selection and the descent of man 1871–1971* (ed. B. Campbell), pp. 136–79. Aldine, Chicago, IL.
22. Grammar, K. (1989). Human courtship behaviour: biological basis and cognitive processing. In *The sociobiology of sexual and reproductive strategies* (eds. A.E. Rasa, C. Vogel, and E. Voland), pp. 147–69. Chapman & Hall, London.
23. Phillips, A. (1993). *On kissing, tickling and being bored*. Harvard University Press, Cambridge, MA.
24. Nicholson, B. (1984). Does kissing aid human bonding by semio-chemical addiction? *The British Journal* of Dermatology, **111**, 623–7.
25. Levin, R.J. (1992). The mechanisms of human female sexual arousal. *Annual Review of Sex Research*, **3**, 1–48.
26. Levin, R.J. (2007). Sexual activity, health and well being—the beneficial roles of coitus and masturbation. *Sexual and Relationship Therapy*, **22**, 135–48.
27. Levin, R.J. (1994). Human male sexuality: appetite and arousal, desire and drive. In *Appetite: neural and behavioural bases* (eds. C.R. Legg and D. Booth), pp. 127–63. Oxford University Press, Oxford.
28. Bremer, J. (1959). *Asexualisation: a follow up of 244 cases*. Macmillan, New York.
29. Wilson, J. (1978). Sexual differentiation. *Annual Review of Physiology*, **40**, 279–306.
30. Meuwissen, I. and Over, R. (1992). Sexual arousal across phases of the human menstrual cycle. *Archives of Sexual Behaviour*, **21**, 165–73.
31. Hutchinson, K.A. (1995). Androgens and sexuality. *The American Journal of Medicine*, **98**(Suppl. 1A), 111S–15S.
32. Gerstenberg, T.C., Levin, R.J., and Wagner, G. (1990). Erection and ejaculation in man. Assessment of the electromyographic activity of the bulbocavernosus and ischiocavernosus muscle. *British Journal of Urology*, **65**, 395–402.
33. Levin, R.J. (2003). *Is prolactin the biological "off switch" for human sexual arousal? Sexual and* Relationship Therapy, **18**, 239–43.
34. Robbins, M.A. and Jensen, G.D. (1978). Multiple orgasm in males. *Journal of Sex Research*, **14**, 21–6.
35. Levin, R.J. (2005). The mechanisms of human ejaculation—a critical analysis. *Sex & Relationship Therapy*, **20**, 123–31.
36. Langfeldt, T. (1990). Early childhood and juvenile sexuality, development and problems. In *Handbook of sexology*, Vol. 7 (ed. M.E. Perry), pp. 179–200. Elsevier, Amsterdam.
37. Levin, R.J. (2004). An orgasm is . . . who defines what an orgasm is? *Sexual & Relationship Therapy*, **19**, 101–7.
38. O'Connell, H.E., Hutson, J.M., Anderson, C.R., *et al.* (1998). Anatomical relation between urethra and clitoris. *The Journal of Urology*, **159**, 1892–7.
39. van Turnhout, A.A.W.M., Hage, J.J., and van Diest, P.J. (1995). The female corpus spongiosum revisited. *Acta Obstetrica Scandinavica*, **74**, 762–71.
40. Levin, R.J. (1998). Sex and the human female reproductive tract- what really happens during and after coitus. *International Journal of Impotence Research*, **10**(Suppl. 1), S14–21.
41. Levin, R.J. (2005). Sexual arousal—its physiological roles in human reproduction. *Annual Review of Sex Research*, **16**, 154–89.
42. Riley, A.J., Lees, W.R., and Riley, E.J. (1992). An ultrasound study of human coitus. In *Sex matters* (eds. W. Bezemer, P. Cohen-Kettenis, and K. Slob), pp. 29–32. Excerpta Medica, Amsterdam.
43. Grafenberg, E. (1960). The role of urethra in female orgasm. *International Journal of Sexology*, **3**, 145–8.
44. Ladas, A.K., Whipple, B., and Perry, J.D. (2005). *The G spot and other recent discoveries about human sexuality*. Henry Holt & Company Ltd., New York.
45. Minh, H.-N., Smadja, A., and De Sigalony, J.P. (1979). Le fascia de Halban: son role dans la physiologie sexuelle. *Gynaecologie*, **30**, 267–73.
46. Hoch, Z. (1986). Vaginal erotic sensitivity by sexological examination. *Acta Obstetrica et Gynaecologica Scandinavica*, **65**, 767–73.
47. Holstege, G., Geogiadis, J.R., Paans, A.M.J., *et al.* (2005). Brain activation during human male ejaculation. *Journal of Neuroscience*, **23**, 9185–93.
48. Komisaruk, B. and Whipple, B. (2005). Functional MRI of the brain during orgasm in women. *Annual Review of Sex Research*, **16**, 62–86.
49. Ferretti, A., Caulo, M., Del Gratta, C., *et al.* (2005). Dynamics of male sexual arousal: distinct components of brain activiation revealed by fMRI. *NeuroImage*, **26**, 1086–96.

4.11.2 The sexual dysfunctions

Cynthia A. Graham and John Bancroft

Introduction

Sexual relationships are central to the lives of most of us. The sexual component of those relationships can go wrong in various ways. This may be secondary to other difficulties in the relationship, mental health problems, specific sexual vulnerabilities of the individual, or the impact of disease or medication on sexual response. This chapter will describe the more common sexual problems and their prevalence. Evidence related to aetiology of sexual problems and treatment evaluation will be briefly reviewed. In the final section of the chapter, guidelines for the assessment and practical management of sexual problems will be presented.

Historical aspects and some basic concepts

Since 1970, when Masters and Johnson(1) published their groundbreaking book on the treatment of 'human sexual inadequacy', there have been two lines of development in this field, relatively detached from each other until recently: psychological methods of treatment, collectively known as 'sex therapy' and medical interventions, initially focused on erectile problems in men.

The involvement of the medical profession has been substantial, although predominantly involving urologists. Initially there were surgical procedures to implant penile splints or to improve the vascular supply to the penis, and the use of vacuum devices to induce erection mechanically. This was followed by the discovery that injection of smooth muscle relaxants, such as papaverine, phentolamine, or prostaglandin into the erectile tissues of the corpora cavernosa induced erections. Self-injections became widely prescribed. To avoid the need for penile injections, which were not popular among male patients, preparations of prostaglandin for intra-urethral administration became available. This era of medical intervention was characterized by a veritable industry of investigative procedures in attempts to identify local causes for erectile dysfunction (ED). Erectile problems were clearly differentiated into 'organic' and 'psychogenic' subtypes. There was, however, a notable lack of attention to how the brain and psychological processes interacted with these peripheral mechanisms.

Then came the 'Viagra revolution' in the early 1990s. The first oral phosphodiesterase 5 (PDE-5) inhibitor, sildenafil (Viagra®), was found to be effective in enhancing erectile response to sexual stimulation when taken about 1 h before sexual activity. This led to the next phase in the 'medicalization' of male sexual dysfunction, with a shift to the primary care physician as the principle source of treatment and a dramatic reduction in the amount of diagnostic assessment.

The progress of sex therapy has been limited since Masters and Johnson.(1) It has continued to be used, with various adaptations of the original 'sensate focus' approach, incorporating principles of psychoanalytic techniques(2) and cognitive behaviour therapy.(3) The main shortcoming has been inadequate outcome research on the efficacy of these methods.

The next phase in this recent history followed the commercial success of PDE-5 inhibitors for men, with an inevitable quest for a 'Viagra for women'. This has so far proved elusive, but has confronted the 'sexual medicine' community with the complexity of women's sexuality and the need to conceptualize it differently to the sexuality of men.

At the same time, evidence has emerged that treatment of ED with sildenafil and more recent PDE-5 inhibitors, although initially successful in the majority, was being discontinued by a substantial proportion of men.(4) In addition, the female partners of men taking these drugs do not always welcome the associated changes in the sexual relationships.(5) We are now moving into the most recent phase where the 'psychological' and 'organic' approaches, and the professional groups that have been identified with them, have started to interact. There is increasing recognition of the need to integrate psychological and medical methods of treatment,(6,7) but with the important proviso that, at least initially, treatment should focus on the couple and not the individual.

One important aspect of this evolving story is how we define a 'sexual dysfunction', with connotations of abnormal or impaired function, and how it is distinguished from a 'sexual problem' in a more general sense. This issue was epitomized by a publication in the *Journal of the American Medical Association* on the epidemiology of 'sexual dysfunction'.(8) In this widely cited paper, 43 per cent of women and 31 per cent of men were identified as having a 'sexual dysfunction', described as 'a largely uninvestigated yet significant public health problem' (p. 544). The authors commented, 'With the affected population rarely receiving medical therapy for sexual dysfunction, service delivery efforts should be augmented to target high-risk populations'(p. 544).

This dramatic example of 'medicalization', based on extremely limited information from a national survey not designed to assess sexual dysfunction, was effectively challenged by Mercer and colleagues, using data from the UK National Survey of Sexual Attitudes and Lifestyles (NATSAL).(9) This used exactly the same questions as in the Laumann *et al.* study,(8) with the important difference that it was more specific about duration of problems, asking whether particular problems had lasted 'at least 1 month', or 'at least 6 months' during the last year (Laumann *et al.* had asked if symptoms had occurred 'for several months or more' during the last year). Overall, 53.8 per cent of women and 34.8 per cent of men reported at least one sexual problem lasting at least 1 month during the previous year. In contrast, the prevalence of problems lasting 'at least 6 months in the previous year' was 15.6 per cent for women and 6.2 per cent for men. This showed that transient problems were very common, more persistent ones much less so. In both the American and the British study, such problems were related to other problems in the participants' lives, particularly involving impaired mental health (e.g. depression), relationship problems, or significant life stresses.

Relevant to the question of when a sexual problem becomes a 'dysfunction' is a theoretical approach, called the 'Dual Control Model', developed at the Kinsey Institute. This postulates that sexual response results from an interaction between excitation and inhibition, involving relatively discrete neurophysiological systems in the brain.(10) A central assumption of the model is that individuals vary in their propensity for both sexual excitation and sexual inhibition and that 'normal' levels of inhibition are adaptive, reducing sexual responsiveness in circumstances where sexual activity is best avoided. It is predicted that high levels of inhibition may be associated with vulnerability to sexual dysfunction and low levels with an increased likelihood of engaging in high-risk sexual behaviour.[10]

This faces us with the seemingly obvious but fundamental challenge of deciding whether a loss of sexual interest or responsiveness is an understandable or even adaptive reaction to current circumstances, or is a result of 'malfunction' of the sexual response system, which can appropriately be called a 'sexual dysfunction'. This challenge is also central to the relatively new phase of integrated treatment, in which assessment identifies the key factors causing the sexual problem and how they should best be treated. A strategy for carrying out such assessment, which we have called the 'three windows approach', will be outlined below.

Clinical features of sexual problems

Sexual problems in men

The most common problems presented by men are ED and premature ejaculation (PE). Delayed or absent ejaculation is a relatively infrequent complaint. Low sexual desire may be the presenting problem, although in most cases this is combined with ED, and it is not always clear which came first.

(a) Erectile problems

Penile erection is a tangible and fundamental component of a man's experience of sexual arousal and the lack of erection in a sexual situation often has significant negative effects. Irrespective of whether or not there are peripheral explanations for impaired erections (e.g. vascular disease), the reactions of the man and his partner have a major influence on how problematic the erectile difficulty becomes. Erectile difficulties vary in severity; in some men the problem only occurs on a proportion of occasions of sexual activity. The difficulty may be in getting an erection or in maintaining it long enough for satisfactory sexual intercourse.

(b) Low sexual desire

For many men, sexual desire is linked with erectile responsiveness. Many men with low sexual desire also report a reduction in 'spontaneous' erections. However, a man can experience low sexual desire without having any erectile difficulties, although he may require more direct tactile stimulation to achieve erections.

(c) Premature ejaculation (PE)

Ejaculation results from a combination of orgasm and seminal emission, with muscular contractions as part of the orgasmic response resulting in expulsion of the seminal emission. PE is essentially a problem when the man is unable to delay orgasm and ejaculation as he would wish. Not surprisingly, this has led to considerable inconsistencies of definition in the literature. In severe cases, emission occurs before vaginal entry and the orgasmic component may be so reduced that the usual muscle spasms do not occur, resulting in semen seeping out of the urethra rather than being 'ejaculated'.

Premature ejaculation has been categorized as 'primary' (i.e. lifelong) or 'secondary'. Secondary PE is often confounded by erectile problems. If a man is taking a long time to get an erection, he may reach the stimulus intensity required for ejaculation before or soon after erection is achieved.

(d) Delayed ejaculation

Delayed or absent ejaculation occurs in men, although it is much less common than rapid ejaculation. A man might have difficulty ejaculating only during sexual activity with his partner and in some cases only during penetrative intercourse, or the problem may be evident even during masturbation. Delayed or absent ejaculation is a common side effect of selective serotonin re-uptake inhibitor (SSRI) medications, which often prevents orgasm in women as well, suggesting that the primary effect of such drugs is on the triggering of orgasm.

(e) Pain during sexual response

Pain may be associated with prolonged sexual arousal not terminated by ejaculation/orgasm. Such pain is usually experienced in the testes. Pain felt in the urethra may occur during ejaculation. Neither problem is common.

Sexual problems in women

(a) Loss of sexual arousal and/or desire

Most surveys have suggested that low sexual desire is the most common sexual problem reported by women. However, low sexual desire is a heterogeneous problem category and the relationship between sexual arousal and sexual desire in women is particularly complex. Many women do not differentiate between 'arousal' and 'desire'[11] and awareness of 'desire' is usually accompanied by some degree of central arousal, whether or not any genital response is perceived.[12] It has been argued that sexual desire in women is much more likely to be 'receptive' and triggered by a desire for intimacy with one's partner.[13] It is therefore not surprising that there is considerable overlap or comorbidity between problems related to sexual arousal and desire in women.[8]

Although traditionally seen as the counterpart to penile erection in men, vaginal response is not central to the experience of sexual arousal in women. Vaginal dryness may be a problem because of the likelihood of discomfort or pain with intercourse when the vagina is not adequately lubricated, but this symptom does not necessarily indicate lack of arousal. Conversely, a woman may experience lack of sexual arousal and yet have vaginal lubrication. The relevance of vaginal response to sexual arousal in women therefore remains unclear. An increase in vaginal blood flow has been consistently demonstrated in women reacting to sexual stimuli, whether or not they find the sexual stimulus appealing; this led Laan and Everaerd[12] to call this an 'automatic' response. There is no obvious counterpart to this in men. Tumescence of the clitoris, on the other hand, may be more directly comparable to male genital response but this is less easily assessed and less clearly perceived by women, compared with penile erection in men.

Persistent genital arousal disorder (PGAD) is a recently recognized but fairly uncommon sexual problem in women. It is characterized by genital and breast vasocongestion and sensitivity which persists for hours or days and is only temporarily relieved by orgasm; genital sensations are unaccompanied by any subjective sense of sexual desire and excitement but instead are perceived as intrusive. There is no male equivalent to this problem, probably because the post-orgasmic refractory period is more substantial in men.

Much less frequent than loss of sexual arousal or desire is extreme aversion to, and avoidance of all sexual contact with, a sexual partner. This can occur in women and in men.

(b) Problems with orgasm

Difficulty in achieving orgasm is not uncommon in women. Often this is situational in that orgasm is possible with masturbation, but not during sexual interaction with the partner. The capacity to experience orgasm varies considerably across women. Some women reach orgasm easily if sufficient arousal occurs, others may require more specific or more intense stimulation, and an estimated 10–15 per cent are unable to experience orgasm throughout their lives.[14] In identifying a problem as primarily orgasmic, one needs to first establish that appropriate sexual arousal has occurred.

(c) Problems with sexual pain and vaginismus

Pain during attempted or complete vaginal entry (dysparcunia) is a common sexual problem in women with a wide range of possible causes. Sexual pain is also frequently associated with lack of sexual desire and/or arousal. Vaginismus has traditionally been defined as recurrent or persistent involuntary spasm of the musculature of the outer third of the vagina that makes vaginal penetration difficult or impossible. This definition has recently been questioned because of a lack of empirical evidence that vaginal spasms occur in women diagnosed with vaginismus.[15] Vulvar vestibulitis syndrome (VVS) is a condition associated with pain on touching the labia or vaginal introitus. The question of whether these are primarily 'sexual' or pain disorders is currently under debate.[16]

Classification of sexual problems

DSM-IV and ICD classification

The current Diagnostic and Statistical Manual of Mental Disorders (DSM) classification[17] defines sexual dysfunction as characterized by 'disturbance in sexual desire and in the psychophysiological changes that characterize the sexual response cycle and cause marked distress and interpersonal difficulty' (p. 493). There is Hypoactive Sexual Desire Disorder and Sexual Aversion Disorder, defined in the same way for men and women. Female Sexual Arousal Disorder is defined as 'a persistent or recurrent inability to attain, or to maintain until completion of the sexual activity, an adequate lubrication-swelling response of sexual excitement' (p. 502) and, for the male version, erection is the relevant response. Orgasmic Disorder (i.e. delayed or absent orgasm) and Dyspareunia are defined in basically the same way for men and women. Vaginismus is a specifically female diagnosis and Premature Ejaculation an exclusively male disorder.

The International Statistical Classification of Diseases and Related Health Problems[18] covers sexual dysfunctions in one and a half pages, compared with nearly 30 pages in the DSM. The basic categories of dysfunction are similar to those of DSM, but there are few, if any, actual diagnostic criteria given for any of the dysfunctions. ICD-10 also does not require that personal distress or interpersonal problems are present for a diagnosis to be made. Instead, there is the statement 'sexual dysfunction covers the various ways in which an individual is unable to participate in a sexual relationship as he or she would wish' (p. 355).

There has been increasing dissatisfaction with the current classification of sexual dysfunction for women.[19,20]. Major areas of criticism include the high comorbidity between diagnoses of sexual dysfunction and the 'genital' focus of the diagnostic criteria and concomitant neglect of psychological and relationship factors. In response, alternative models of sexual response[13] and women-centred definitions of sexual problems[21] have been proposed.

Epidemiology

There have been at least 12 representative community-based surveys that have assessed the prevalence of sexual problems.[22] Prevalence rates for specific problems vary considerably and whereas several of the studies claim to be reporting prevalence of sexual 'dysfunctions',[8] it is now accepted that the detailed clinical assessment required to identify a sexual dysfunction cannot be undertaken by large-scale surveys.[23] Consequently, more recent surveys have used terms such as 'problems'[9,24] or 'difficulties'.[25] Variability in reported prevalence rates can in part be attributed to variations in how sexual problems are defined, their duration, and how and whether 'distress' about changes in sexual functioning is assessed. In studies of female sexual problems, there has been only limited overlap between what women perceive as problematic and what the researcher or clinician identifies as a problem.[26,27] The variability of prevalence rates is shown in Tables 4.11.2.1 and 4.11.2.2, which compare a number of population-based surveys involving women and men.

There has been more consistency across studies in the associations found between factors of possible aetiological relevance and sexual functioning. In women, sexual problems are more frequent in those with mental health problems and relationship difficulties.[8] In a survey of women aged 20–65 years, all in heterosexual relationships, 24.4 per cent reported marked distress about their sexual relationship and/or their own sexuality.[26] The best predictors of distress were markers of mental health and the quality of the emotional relationship with the partner. Physical aspects of sexual response in women such as arousal and orgasm were poor predictors of distress.

In men, age has a predictable negative effect on erectile function. In one study, complete erectile failure was reported by 5 per cent of men at age 40 and 25 per cent at age 70.[28] A similar age effect is found with loss of sexual desire. In another study, absence of any sexual desire was reported by 2 per cent of men aged 45–59 and 18.2 per cent aged 75+.[29] Contrary to popular belief, PE does not show a clear negative relationship with age.

The association between age and sexual problems in women is more complex. Whereas level of sexual interest typically decreases with age, older women are less likely to regard this as a problem.[26] Older women are much less likely to be in a sexual relationship than older men; the presence or absence of a partner also seems to influence women's sexuality to a greater extent than it does for men.[29] The impact of the menopause is also complex. Although the post-menopausal decline in oestrogens is relevant to vaginal lubrication, other factors such as mental health and the quality of the sexual relationship are more important determinants of sexual well-being.[30]

Aetiology

Before considering the factors that can cause sexual problems, it is worth underlining the important way that sexual function differs from most other physiological response systems. Although involving physiological mechanisms, sexual responses are most often experienced in the context of a relationship. This highlights the

Table 4.11.2.1 Prevalence of specific female problems (%) found in seven community-based surveys

Study	Low sexual interest	Impaired arousal	Impaired lubrication	Impaired orgasm	Pain	Total (one or more problems)
Richters *et al.* (2003)(25)[1]						
At least 1 month	54.8	–	23.9	28.6	20.3	
Mercer *et al.* (2003)(9)[1]						
At least 1 month	40.6	–	9.2	14.4	11.8	53.8
At least 6 months	10.2	–	2.6	3.7	3.4	15.6
Bancroft *et al.* (2003)(26)[3]	7.2	12.2	31.2	9.3	3.3	45
Laumann *et al.* (1999)(8)[1]	31.6	–	20.6	25.7	15.5	43[a]
Fugl-Meyer and Fugl-Meyer (1999)(59)[1]	33.0	–	12.0	22.0	6.0	47
Dunn *et al.* (1999)(24)[2]	–	17.0	28.0	27.0	18.0	41
Osborne *et al.* (1988)(37)[2]	17.0	–	17.0	16.0	8.0	33

[a] Includes additional problem categories not shown in this table.

[1] During last year.

[2] During last 3 months.

[3] During last month.

importance of keeping the interactive relationship components in mind when trying to assess and treat sexual problems. Socio-cultural factors are also crucial to understanding how sexual problems are experienced. Much of the focus in medical treatments of sexual problems has been on the individual patient, with relationship and socio-cultural aspects largely ignored. The more specific aetiological factors can now be considered using the 'three windows approach'.(26)

The first window—the current situation

Through the first window, a variety of factors in the individual's current relationship and situation may be relevant. Relationship problems, particularly resentment and insecurity within a relationship, are of particular importance. For many individuals, feeling secure and being able to 'let go' are necessary for them to enjoy sex. Other factors that may be important include: poor communication between partners about their sexual feelings and needs; misunderstandings and lack of information; unsuitable circumstances and lack of time e.g. fatigue, lack of privacy, and work pressures; concerns about pregnancy or about sexually transmitted diseases; and low self-esteem and poor body image.

Various mechanisms may mediate the effects of the above situational factors on sexual functioning. Reactive inhibition, as postulated by the Dual Control Model,(10) may well be involved in those circumstances associated with a negative emotional response. With stress and fatigue, the mechanisms are less clear, but may entail a transient reduction in the capacity for excitation (i.e. sexual arousability).

Table 4.11.2.2 Prevalence of specific male problems (%) found in five community-based surveys

Study	Low sexual interest	Erectile problem	Premature ejaculation	Delayed ejaculation	Total (one or more problems)
Richters *et al.* (2003)(25)[1]					
At least 1 month	24.9	9.5	23.8	6.3	–
Mercer *et al.* (2003)(9)[1]					
At least 1 month	17.1	5.8	11.7	5.3	34.8
At least 6 months	1.8	0.8	2.9	0.7	6.2
Laumann *et al.* (1999)(8)[1]	14.6	10.2	30.6	7.8	31.0[a]
Fugl-Meyer and Fugl- Meyer (1999)(59)[1]	16.0	5.0	9.0	–	–
Dunn *et al.* (1999)(24)[2]	–	26.0	14.0	–	–

[a] Includes additional problem categories not shown in this table.

[1] During last year.

[2] During last 3 months.

The second window—vulnerability of the individual

Although a wide range of factors can impact on our sexuality, it is also clear that individuals vary substantially in the extent to which they are affected by such factors, particularly in terms of an associated inhibition of sexual response. Such vulnerabilities are likely to have been evident in earlier episodes in the current relationship or in earlier relationships.

(a) Negative attitudes

Long-standing attitudes, usually stemming from childhood, that sex is inherently 'bad' or immoral are likely to interfere with an individual's ability to become involved in and enjoy a sexual relationship.

(b) Need to maintain self-control

In some individuals, a difficulty in 'letting go' sexually reflects a more general need to maintain self-control, particularly in the presence of another person.

(c) Earlier experience of sexual abuse or trauma

There is now an extensive literature on the impact of sexual abuse on subsequent sexual adjustment. Whereas the mediating mechanisms are not well understood and are likely to be complex and varied, a history of such experience should be regarded as potentially relevant to current sexual difficulties.

(d) Propensity to sexual inhibition

The Dual Control Model, discussed earlier, has led to psychometrically validated measures of propensity to sexual excitation and inhibition in men[(31)] and women.[(32)] These are new measures and research exploring their relevance to vulnerability to sexual problems has only recently started. However, using these measures, close to normal distributions of scores for both sexual excitation and inhibition proneness have been reported in men[(31)] and women.[(32)] As predicted, a clear association between low sexual excitation and/or high sexual inhibition propensity and erectile problems in men has been found, but no association with PE.[(33)] One study explored a possible genetic basis for such individual variability in men and found evidence of heritability for propensity to sexual inhibition but not excitation.[(34)] In women, a strong relationship between sexual inhibition scores and reports of sexual problems was found.[(35)] Particularly important was one inhibition subscale (labelled 'arousal contingency') that reflects susceptibility for sexual arousal to be easily affected by situational factors e.g. if the circumstances are not 'just right' or if the woman is distracted. Although further research is needed, these measures of sexual inhibition and excitation may prove valuable in explaining patterns of impaired sexual response and helping in the selection of appropriate treatment. As yet no other personality-related or trait measure has been shown to have clinical value in this respect.

The third window—health-related factors that alter sexual function

The variety of health-related factors are considered under three headings: mental health, physical health, and sexual side effects of medication.

(a) Mental health and sexuality

Psychiatric problems are commonly associated with sexual problems.[(36,37)] Reduction in sexual interest, and to some extent sexual arousability, is generally accepted as a common symptom of depressive illness.[(38)] In contrast, sexual interest tends to be increased in states of elevated mood such as hypomania.[(39)] In a study of men and women with primary loss of sexual interest, the large majority had experienced previous affective disorder, with reduced sexual desire being established during, and persisting after, one of these earlier depressive episodes.[(40)]

We would expect reactive inhibition of sexual interest or response in circumstances eliciting negative mood (i.e. 'reactive depression'). With more endogenous depression, however, reduction of the excitatory component of sexual response is also evident. This is shown clearly in the impairment of nocturnal penile tumescence (NPT) that typically occurs with depressive illness. NPT, while not completely understood, probably results from a 'switching off' of inhibitory tone during REM sleep. This therefore allows expression of 'excitatory tone', presumably impaired in depression with associated metabolic changes.

With anxiety, the clinical evidence is much more limited. Higher rates of sexual dysfunction in patients with anxiety disorders have been reported.[(41)] In the Zurich Cohort Study, a longitudinal study of men and women aged 20–35 years, loss of sexual interest was more prevalent in patients with generalized anxiety disorder, but was not associated with panic disorder, agoraphobia, or social phobia.[(42)] In another study, patients with panic disorder were more likely to report sexual problems, particularly sexual aversion, than social phobics; PE was the most common sexual problem in men with social phobias.[(43)]

Non-clinical, community-based studies have also demonstrated a relationship between mood and sexuality. In the Massachusetts Male Aging Study, an association was reported between ED and depressive symptoms, after controlling for other potential confounding variables such as age and physical health.[(44)] Angst[(42)] found a relationship between depression and loss of sexual interest, particularly marked in women. In a US survey of heterosexual women, scores on a brief measure of mental health were strongly predictive of women's distress about their sexual relationship and their own sexuality.[(26)]

Although most studies have focused on negative effects of mood disorders on sexual interest and response, there is evidence that a minority of individuals experience increased sexual interest during negative mood states. Angst[(42)] reported that among depressed men, 25.7 per cent reported decreased, and 23.3 per cent increased, sexual interest, compared with 11.1 per cent and 6.9 per cent, respectively, of their non-depressed group. In contrast, among depressed women, 35.3 per cent reported decreased sexual interest and only 8.8 per cent reported increased interest (compared with 31.6 per cent and 1.7 per cent, respectively, of their non-depressed group). This paradoxical pattern of increased sexual interest during negative mood states has also been reported in non-clinical samples of men[(45)] and women.[(46)] Although the origins of this pattern are not yet understood, it may well be problematic in various ways; for example, associated with sexual risk-taking or leading to sex being used as a mood regulator.

The impact of schizophrenia on sexuality is complex. Given the importance of dopaminergic neurotransmission to various aspects of sexuality, and the fact that most anti-psychotics are dopamine antagonists, one might expect amplification of sexual interest or response in some form, at least during the more florid type one stage of the illness. Sexual thoughts and behaviours are common in schizophrenia and there may be a relative increase in sexual activity. However, this is typically autoerotic or 'compulsive' without any real 'object-relational' quality.(47) In view of the effects of this illness on interpersonal functioning, this is not surprising. Early studies suggested that loss of sexual interest was less likely in schizophrenia than in other types of psychiatric illness, although female schizophrenics were more likely to report a reduction in sexual interest than males.(47) 'Pre-schizophrenic personality', evident in the history of many cases, may also be associated with an interference with normal sexual development.

(b) Physical health and sexuality

The impact of poor physical health on sexuality may be relatively non-specific. For example, loss of well-being and energy associated with chronic illness is likely to cause reduced sexual interest and arousability. Psychological reactions to the illness or condition (e.g. the effects of breast cancer on a woman's body image and hence her sexual enjoyment) may also be important. In addition there are a variety of ways in which the health problem can directly affect sexual interest and/or response. In most cases we find the evidence much clearer in men than in women.

(i) Damage to the neural control of genital response

This can involve peripheral mechanisms (e.g. autonomic neuropathy and peripheral neuropathy) or disease in the spinal cord (e.g. multiple sclerosis). Injury or surgery causing nerve damage may be involved (e.g. spinal cord injury, prostatectomy, or hysterectomy). The most likely consequences are ED in men and impaired vaginal response in women. There is no clear relationship between neural damage and PE but interference with normal seminal emission can occur, with resulting loss of ejaculation or retrograde ejaculation when, due to nerve damage to the pelvic muscles, the seminal fluid passes backwards into the bladder during ejaculation. Brain abnormalities, such as epilepsy or cerebral tumour, can affect central control of sexual response, the precise effect depending on the site of the abnormality or tumour. In some cases the result is loss of sexual interest and arousability; rarely there is disinhibition of sexual behaviour.

(ii) Impairment of vascular supply of the genitalia

Genital response is dependent on increased arterial inflow as well as alteration in venous outflow. Vascular impairment can result from peripheral vascular disease, affecting the small vessels, or obstruction in a main artery. ED is also common in men who have ischaemic heart disease.

(iii) Alteration of endocrine mechanisms affecting sexual interest, arousal and response

In males any cause of lowered testosterone (T) levels is likely to produce loss of sexual interest and, to a varying extent, impairment of erectile response. Hypogonadism, if severe enough, will also be associated with loss of seminal emission (and usually orgasm).

In women, lack of oestrogen is associated with impaired vaginal lubrication. The effects of sex steroids, either oestrogens or androgens, on sexual interest and arousability, are much less predictable. The evidence is consistent with there being a proportion of women who depend on T for their normal level of sexual interest, but there are many women who can experience substantial reduction in T without obvious adverse sexual effects. The role of oestrogen in the more central aspects of women's sexuality also remains unclear.(48)

Hyperprolactinaemia, usually resulting from pituitary adenomas and hypersecretion of prolactin, may be associated with loss of sexual interest, and in men, with ED. However, this is not always the case. The precise role of prolactin in human sexuality is not understood. Its central control by dopamine and serotonin contributes to the complexity. Adverse effects of hyperprolactinaemia on sexuality are probably more likely in men than women.

(iv) Metabolic disorders

Various forms of metabolic disturbance, such as that associated with hepatic or renal disease, may be associated with adverse effects on sexual interest and response, though the mediating mechanisms are not understood.

Some diseases affect sexuality through more than one of the above mechanisms. Diabetes mellitus is a good example. ED has long been recognized as a complication of diabetes and is more common in Type 1 than Type 2 diabetes. In diabetic men, ED can result from small vessel vascular disease and also autonomic and peripheral neuropathology. Diabetes is associated with hypogonadism in men. Lowered sexual interest and impairment of genital response have also been reported in diabetic women.

(c) Side effects of medication

In considering the complexities of pharmacological effects on sexual function, it is helpful to distinguish between excitatory and inhibitory mechanisms. In the brain, sexual excitation depends to a considerable extent on dopamine (DA) and noradrenaline (NA). DA is involved in the 'incentive motivation system' and is hence relevant to sexual interest. It is the D2 receptor that is most relevant to these sexual effects. It is also involved in the hypothalamic control of genital response. NA, when acting centrally, is involved in central arousal, a key component of sexual arousal though not specific to it. In the periphery, depending on the receptor involved, NA can have inhibitory or enhancing effects on smooth muscle relaxation, a critical aspect of genital response. There are three principal NA receptors of relevance: (i) alpha-1, which is post-synaptic and mediates smooth muscle contractions, inhibiting genital response, (ii) alpha-2 which is principally pre-synaptic, where it increases re-uptake of NA and hence reduces the amount of NA at the synapse, and (iii) beta-2, a peripheral receptor which mediates a relaxing effect of NA on smooth muscle in the urogenital system and elsewhere. Serotonin (5-HT) has a central role in the inhibitory system. The two most relevant receptors are the 5-HT2 receptor, which mediates the inhibitory effects and the 5-HT1A receptor, which is pre-synaptic and, comparable to the alpha-2 receptor, reduces 5-HT transmission. We can now consider the main adverse sexual effects resulting from medication; for a review, see.(49)

(d) Anti-depressants

The clearest examples are the SSRIs which, by inhibiting the 5HT-1A receptor, increase serotonergic transmission. The most predictable effect, in both women and men, is inhibition of orgasm and ejaculation. This effect is being exploited in the treatment of PE, with the development of short-acting SSRIs which can be used as needed prior to sexual activity. Other negative effects include reduced sexual interest and arousability, though they are less predictable and not always easy to distinguish from the sexual effects of the affective disorder being treated. Tricylic anti-depressants also commonly produce sexual side effects. Two anti-depressants which have less sexual side effects are bupropion, which is metabolized into a DA and NA re-uptake inhibitor, and nefadazone, which has a 5-HT2 antagonist effect.

(e) Anti-psychotic medication

These drugs, used for the treatment of schizophrenia and other psychotic disorders, involve a balance of DA antagonist and 5-HT agonist effects. Sexual side effects occur in around 60 per cent of men and 30–90 per cent of women using these drugs. The most common side effects are ED and ejaculatory difficulties in men and orgasmic dysfunction in women. It is not clear to what extent these effects are due to the DA antagonist or 5-HT agonist effects, or a balance of the two.

(f) Anti-hypertensive medication

Many drugs used to treat hypertension interfere with male sexual response. In the case of alpha-1 antagonists (e.g. prazosin), the peripheral effects would be expected to enhance erection, by reducing adrenergic contraction of erectile smooth muscle and indeed priapism is an occasional problem. There is a low incidence of sexual side effects, mainly failure of ejaculation, and central alpha-1 blockade might reduce central arousal. Beta-blockers (e.g. propanalol), by blocking smooth muscle relaxation and leaving the alpha-1 induced contraction unopposed, commonly cause ED. Centrally acting anti-hypertensives (e.g. guanethidine) also interfere with sexual response, impairing erection, and blocking ejaculation. Clonidine, an alpha-2 agonist, causes erectile problems in about 25 per cent of cases. In this case the principal effect is likely to be reduced central arousal. For a review of the effects of anti-hypertensive medication on male sexual response, see.[(50)]

The effects of drugs on women's sexuality have received far less attention. Research has mostly focused on difficulties in achieving orgasm. As orgasm only occurs after sufficient sexual arousal, these effects may reflect impairment of arousal but this has not been adequately assessed. Steroidal contraceptives, although associated with markedly reduced levels of free T, decrease sexual interest only in a minority of women.[(51)] This, again, has been little studied and it remains possible that the adverse effects on sexual interest only occur in those women whose sexuality is 'T dependent'.[(51)]

Management of sexual problems

In this section we will briefly describe the principles of sex therapy and the main forms of pharmacological treatment, followed by an outline of the process of assessment and selection of a suitable treatment plan. The growing awareness of the limitations of pharmacological treatments administered on an individual basis, discussed earlier, has led to recognition that an integration of psychological and pharmacological methods, with emphasis on the couple, may be the most appropriate treatment model in most cases.

Sex therapy

Although the approach first introduced by Masters and Johnson[(1)] has been adapted in various ways, the core treatment techniques remain. Originally developed for helping couples, the techniques can be modified for use with individuals and with same-sex as well as heterosexual couples.

The key elements of the therapeutic process are:

(a) clearly defined tasks are given and the couple asked to attempt them before the next therapy session

(b) those attempts, and any difficulties encountered, are examined in detail

(c) attitudes, feelings, and conflicts that make the tasks difficult to carry out are identified

(d) these are modified or resolved so that subsequent achievement of the tasks becomes possible

(e) the next tasks are set, and so on

The tasks are mostly behavioural in nature. They are chosen to facilitate the identification of relevant issues but in some cases are sufficient in themselves to produce change. The behavioural programme is in three parts. In the first part the couple are asked to avoid any direct genital touching or stimulation and to focus on non-genital contact, alternating who initiates and who does the touching. These first, non-genital steps are effective in identifying important issues in the relationship, such as lack of trust or counter-productive stereotypical attitudes (e.g. once a man is aroused, he can't be expected not to have intercourse). Once this stage can be carried out satisfactorily, and related problematic issues dealt with, the programme moves on to the second part, which allows genital touching to be combined with non-genital touching, with penile–vaginal intercourse still 'out of bounds'. In this second part more intra-personal problems, such as long-standing negative attitudes about sex, or the sequelae of earlier sexual trauma are likely to emerge. In the third part, a gradual approach to vaginal–penile contact and insertion is undertaken. Here the most relevant issues are 'performance anxiety' and fear of pain.

As the behavioural tasks reveal key issues that need to be resolved before moving on to the next stage, a variety of psychotherapeutic approaches, including cognitive behavioural techniques, can be utilized. Although the stage at which particular issues emerge does vary from case to case, there is a tendency for problems identified through the 'first window', particularly those related to lack of trust and unresolved resentment, to appear during the first stage of the programme. Intra-personal issues (e.g. as seen through the 'second window') are more likely to be recognized during the second stage.

The goals of therapy include helping the individual to accept and feel comfortable with his or her sexuality and helping the couple to establish trust and emotional security and to enhance the enjoyment and intimacy of their sexual interaction. An important point is that these goals do not include reversal of specific sexual dysfunctions. There are exceptions; for example, there are specific behavioural techniques to deal with PE and vaginismus (for details of these techniques, see Bancroft.[(52)] However, the overriding principle is that, assuming there is no abnormality of the basic physiological mechanisms involved in sexual response, normal sexual function (in terms of sexual desire, arousal, and genital response) will return once the above goals are achieved. In cases where impairment of physiological mechanisms does exist, the above goals of sex therapy are still helpful and integrate well with the use of pharmacological treatment.

Practical aspects

Although sex therapy varies in duration, 12 sessions over 4 to 5 months is typical. The therapist adjusts to the particular needs of the individual or couple. Treatment begins weekly with the interval between sessions extended once major issues like unexpressed resentment or communication problems have been dealt with. The last two or three sessions are spaced out over a few months so that the couple have an opportunity to consolidate their progress and cope with any setbacks before termination. Open-ended arrangements about length of treatment are best avoided. A specified number of sessions are agreed on at the outset with the proviso that progress will be assessed and a decision made on that basis whether to continue for longer.

A more complete description of the sex therapy process is provided by Bancroft.[52]

Pharmacological treatments for men

(a) Erectile dysfunction. Phosphodiesterase 5 inhibitors

The most important development in this field was the serendipitous discovery that sildenafil (Viagra®), a PDE-5 inhibitor, enhances erectile response. Dose titration is usually required, with available tablets containing 25, 50, or 100 mg. For more severe cases of ED, 100 mg taken about 1 hour before sexual activity is required. The maximal effects last for about 4 h. The most common side effects, that are dose-related, are headache, flushing, and dyspepsia.

Two further PDE-5 inhibitors have been developed and are now in use: tadalafil (Cialis®) and vardenafil (Levitra®). They are both comparable to sildenafil in their efficacy, the main differences being their speed and duration of action. Tadalafil should be taken at least 30 min before sexual activity and has a half-life of 17.5 h; the treatment effect can persist for 24–36 h. Vardenafil is pharmacokinetically similar to sildenafil, but is more potent, with a dose range 5 mg to 20 mg. They are similar in their side effects, though the duration of these relate to the half-life of the drug. For all three drugs, the most important and dangerous drug interaction is with nitrates used for ischaemic heart disease; this is a strong contraindication for the use of PDE-5 inhibitors.

There is now an extensive literature demonstrating the efficacy of sildenafil in the treatment of ED, which has been well reviewed by Rosen and McKenna.[53] Overall, treatment is effective in about 75 per cent of cases. The effectiveness of tadalafil and vardenafil has also been demonstrated.

In spite of their efficacy, the continuing use of PDE-5 inhibitors appears to be limited. In a recent large study done in eight countries, 2912 men identified with ED were followed up; 58 per cent of them had sought medical help for the ED, but only 16 per cent of men maintained their use of PDE-5 inhibitors.[7] Various reasons were given for discontinuation, including lack of appropriate information from the physicians, fear of side effects, partner concerns, and distrust of medications.

(b) Anti-adrenergic drugs

Alpha-2 antagonists may enhance sexual arousal by their central NA effects. One example is yohimbine, which has a modest therapeutic benefit over placebo and is generally well tolerated. Phentolamine is an alpha-1 and alpha-2 antagonist used medically to treat hypertensive crises. It has been used, in combination with papaverine, to induce erection by intra-cavernosal injection, presumably mediated by its alpha-1 antagonist effect. Phentolamine administered systemically can also improve sexual arousal, presumably by blocking both the peripheral alpha-1 receptors and enhancing central arousal by blocking the alpha-2 receptors in the brain. Some evidence of beneficial effects of phentolamine has been reported, although long-term follow-up revealed high attrition.

(c) Dopamine agonists

The main effects of dopamine agonists, such as apomorphine, are to induce genital response, probably via the hypothalamic oxytocinergic system. Early studies with apomorphine in men, while showing positive effects on erection, also demonstrated substantial side effects (mainly nausea and dizziness). Sublingual administration was developed to reduce such side effects and a number of placebo-controlled studies have shown this to improve erectile function[54] but the occurrence of side effects remains a limiting factor.

(d) Melanocortin agonists

A recent development has been bremelanotide (PT-141), a metabolite of melanotan-II, and a melanocortin analogue, which probably works through the same oxytocinergic system as apomorphine. Side effects similar to those with apomorphine occur, and further phase 3 research is required before the clinical value of this compound is established.

(i) Premature ejaculation

The orgasm inhibiting effect of SSRIs (see above) has been exploited in the treatment of PE. Paroxetine, sertraline, and fluoxetine, among others, have all been shown to be effective in this respect. However, continued use is required, and effects may not be apparent during the first week. This raises the issue of side effects and the need to avoid sudden withdrawal.

More recently, PDE-5 inhibitors have been explored as a treatment for PE. However, the benefits are not clear cut and may be restricted to cases of 'secondary' PE. The most likely mechanism of action is reduction of the smooth muscle contraction involved in seminal emission.

(ii) Delayed or absent orgasm/ejaculation

At present there is no accepted pharmacological treatment for delayed or absent ejaculation or orgasm.

(iii) Low sexual desire

The most treatable but relatively infrequent cause of loss of sexual desire in men is hypogonadism. Where androgen deficiency is evident, T replacement is indicated. Currently the most favoured route of administration is transdermal, either using cream or skin patches. One advantage of the transdermal route is that the hormone is absorbed into the skin and then released more gradually into the circulation, maintaining relatively physiological levels. In comparison, intra-muscular injections of T (e.g. T enanthate) produce supraphysiological levels in the circulation, which then steadily decline. Oral routes are complicated by first pass through the liver.

If loss of sexual desire is associated with hyperprolactinaemia, treatment with dopamine agonists, such as bromocriptine, is indicated.

Pharmacological treatments for women

At present pharmacological methods for treating sexual dysfunction in women, although generating much interest and controversy, are very limited. Most attention is currently being paid to the use of T for treating low sexual desire. As considered earlier, the evidence of a role for T in women's sexuality is inconsistent and the likelihood is that it is important for some women and not others.

The most convincing evidence of the benefits of T are in women who have been ovariectomized and have therefore experienced a substantial reduction in their androgen levels. Much of this evidence, however, indicates that supraphysiological levels of T result from treatment; thus, it remains uncertain whether the benefits result from correction of T deficiency or pharmacological effects of high levels of T. For this reason, and because of uncertainty about possible long-term risks, there has been a reluctance to approve such treatments, particularly in women with intact ovaries.(48)

Attempts to treat sexual desire/arousal problems with PDE-5 inhibitors have so far proved unsuccessful, although there may be subgroups of women who benefit. Other pharmacological approaches which are being explored in women include the use of phentolamine, apomorphine, bupropion, and bremelanotide (PT-141). But further research is required before any of these can be recommended for clinical use. For more details of the above treatments, see Bancroft.(52)

Evaluation of treatments

Sex therapy

In a 1997 review, Heiman and Meston(55) concluded that there was evidence for empirically validated treatments for orgasm problems in women and ED in men. There was inadequate support for effective treatments for low sexual desire, sexual aversions, dyspareunia in women and men, and delayed orgasm in men. What is striking is that of the 90 studies involving psychological treatments cited in this review, only two were published since 1990, and 60 of them before 1980.

In the decade since this review, there have been a few controlled trials involving cognitive behaviour therapy (CBT) for women with vaginismus,(56) vulvar vestibulitus,(57) and couples presenting with problems of low sexual desire,(58) all suggesting positive effects. Further outcome studies of psychological therapies that identify predictors of successful outcomes are badly needed.

Combined psychological and medical treatment

There have now been a number of studies in men that have compared combined psychological and pharmacological treatments, with either used separately. These have been reviewed by Althof(6) and include studies combining psychotherapy with sildenafil, and counselling with intra-cavernosal injections or with vacuum devices. In each case, the combination produced significantly better results than the medical treatment alone.

Planning a treatment programme

Assessment

When couples present with sexual difficulties, one of them is usually regarded as having the problem. However, both partners should be carefully assessed whenever possible. There are three stages to assessment; first, to facilitate the decision about whether sex therapy is appropriate; second, to identify issues relevant to the sexual problem that need to be resolved, and third, to determine whether medication or other treatments are required.

Keeping in mind the distinction between a sexual problem that is adaptive or appropriate given an individual's current circumstances and one that is maladaptive (and can perhaps be considered a 'dysfunction'), we can assess each individual's case through the three conceptual 'windows' described earlier. Are there problems in the couple's current relationship or situation, which would make inhibition of sexual responsiveness in either partner understandable or adaptive? Does either individual give a history that suggests vulnerability to sexual problems? Are there are any mental or physical health issues or medication use in either partner that could be having a negative effect on sexual interest or response?

(a) The initial interview

Although not all of the details can be obtained during the initial interview, assessment of the following topics should be carried out: the nature of the problem, including an assessment of level of sexual interest and response in each partner; identification of other assessments that may be needed (e.g. physical examination, blood tests); commitment and motivation of each partner to improving the relationship; and, assessment of the mental state of each partner. If both partners are present, each should be interviewed separately following a conjoint interview. As far as possible, questions should be asked about each individual's sexual history, the nature of the current relationship, contraceptive use and reproductive history, and alcohol or recreational drug use.

At the end of the initial interview, the clinician should provide a preliminary formulation of the nature of the problem and the types of intervention that may be helpful. Whatever treatment methods are used, it is important to continue to see the couple together to monitor progress and provide counselling as needed.

If there is no evidence of causal factors of the kind viewed through the 'first' or 'second' windows (see above), then a trial of pharmacological treatment may be appropriate. In such cases a physical examination and, where relevant, laboratory investigations would normally be arranged before starting treatment. It is important to have a good 'clinical baseline' before embarking on pharmacological interventions.

If there are any indications of problems or issues, particularly of the kind that invoke inhibition of sexual response, which need to be resolved, then pharmacological interventions should not be considered as a first step. In many cases, more assessment is required before such factors can be adequately assessed. There are then two options: (i) further interview(s) to explore such issues or (ii) starting on a programme of sex therapy. The rationale for the second option is as follows. The initial two stages of sex therapy (i.e. involving non-genital and then genital touching with no attempts at vaginal intercourse) are particularly effective at identifying relevant issues underlying the problem. Furthermore, the process involved in those early stages is likely to benefit any sexual relationship, even those without obvious problems. After three or four sex therapy sessions, a re-appraisal would be made and a decision taken whether to continue with sex therapy alone, or to combine it with an appropriate pharmacological method. For example, with a couple where the man has erectile problems, it is easier to assess the indications for the use of a PDE-5 inhibitor after the couple have gone through the first two stages of the programme where there is no 'performance pressure' and no need for an erection to occur. Similarly, it is often informative to see what impact this behavioural programme has on the individual who has complained of reduced sexual desire, before attempting to deal with the problem pharmacologically or hormonally.

Ideally, the use of the pharmacological method should then proceed in combination with the continuation of the sex therapy programme. In that way a gradual transition to a satisfying sexual relationship can be achieved without renewed 'performance pressures'. If, however, progress continues to be made with sex therapy, then the addition of pharmacological interventions may not be necessary. It should be explained to the couple that, whereas pharmacological treatments often have beneficial effects on sexual response, they do not 'cure' the problem, which is likely to recur once the medication is stopped. Furthermore, there are often side effects that have to be dealt with. There is, however, some evidence that when medication is combined with sex therapy, the pharmacological component can be gradually withdrawn, or only used intermittently.

Ethical aspects of clinical management

In assessing individuals or couples with sexual problems it is clearly important to assure them that the information they provide will be treated as highly confidential. It is appropriate to have separate case files for sexual problem clinics, rather than files used in other clinics. In this way the files can be kept secure. Some overview of the information presented to the clinic by the referring clinician should be provided at the start of the assessment. Information to be passed back to the referring clinician by letter or word of mouth should be agreed with the client(s) in advance, particularly if any highly sensitive issue emerged during the assessment. When assessing a couple, and seeing each partner separately, it is important to establish whether each individual agrees to any information not known by the other being shared during the joint sessions (e.g. details of previous sexual relationships). When offering a course of treatment or further assessment, the individual or couple should be fully informed about what is involved before being asked to make their decision.

A more challenging ethical issue relates to cultural values. Much of the process of sex therapy involves the therapist encouraging and 'giving permission' for specific forms of sexual interaction, as well as more general patterns of interaction within the relationship (e.g. 'self asserting' and 'self protecting'). It is important for the therapist to keep in mind that many of these principles are based on western middle class values. When working with a couple from a different culture, or even a different social class to the therapist, there should be awareness, openness, and discussion about contrasting values of cultural or religious origin. In this way differences can be negotiated, rather than have therapist values imposed.

When to seek specialist help

The treatment programme described above can be applied by psychiatrists in practice providing that they (i) are comfortable asking detailed questions about sexual behaviour and response, (ii) have experience working psychotherapeutically with couples, and (iii) are familiar with cognitive behavioural methods of treatment. They have the advantage over many non-medically qualified sex therapists of being able to prescribe medications in combination with a behavioural approach to sex therapy.

Specialist help should be obtained if there is evidence of a physical condition which requires detailed assessment and treatment, or if, after a reasonable trial of integrated psychological and pharmacological treatment, the sexual problem remains unresolved. In some such cases, the specialist help should be from someone with expertise in sexual medicine (e.g. urologist, gynaecologist). In other cases, where the psychological aspects remain unclear or difficult to resolve, referral to an experienced sex therapist is appropriate.

Further information

American Association of Sex Counselors, Educators, and Therapists (AASECT). http://www.aasect.org/.

British Association of Sexual and Relationship Therapists (BASRT) [http://www.basrt.org.uk].

Bancroft, J. *Human sexuality and its problems* (3rd edn). Elsevier, Oxford, in press.

Kingsberg, S., Althof, S.E., and Leiblum, S. (2002). Books helpful to patients with sexual and marital problems. *Journal of Sex & Marital Therapy*, **28**, 219–28.

Leiblum, S.R. (2007). *Principles and practice of sex therapy* (4th edn). Guilford, New York.

References

1. Masters, W.H. and Johnson, V.E. (1970). *Human sexual inadequacy*. Little Brown, Boston.
2. Kaplan, H.S. (1975). *The new sex therapy*. Bailliere Tindall, London.
3. Pridal, C.G. and LoPiccolo, J. (2000). Multielement treatment of desire disorders: integration of cognitive, behavioral, and systemic therapy. In: *Principles and practice of sex therapy* (3rd edn) (eds S.R. Leiblum and R.C. Rosen), pp. 57–81. Guilford Press, New York.
4. Althof, S. (2002). When an erection alone is not enough: biopsychosocial obstacles to lovemaking. *International Journal of Impotence Research*, **14**(Suppl. 1), S99–104.
5. Potts, A., Gavey, N., Grace, V.M., *et al.* (2003). The downside of Viagra: women's experiences and concerns. *Sociology of Health and Illness*, **25**, 697–719.
6. Althof, S. (2006). Sexual therapy in the age of pharmacotherapy. *Annual Review of Sex Research*, **17**, 116–31.
7. Rosen, R.C. (2007). Erectile dysfunction: integration of medical and psychological approaches. In *Principles and practice of sex therapy* (4th edn) (ed. S.R. Leiblum), pp. 277–312. Guilford Press, New York.
8. Laumann, E.O., Paik, A., and Rosen, R.C. (1999). Sexual dysfunction in the United States: prevalence and predictors. *The Journal of the American Medical Association*, **281**, 537–44.
9. Mercer, C.H., Fenton, K.A., Johnson, A.M., *et al.* (2003). Sexual function problems and help seeking behaviour in Britain: national probability sample survey. *British Medical Journal*, **327**, 426–7.
10. Bancroft, J. (1999). Central inhibition of sexual response in the male: a theoretical perspective. *Neuroscience and Biobehavioral Reviews*, **23**, 763–84.
11. Graham, C.A., Sanders, S.A., Milhausen, R.R., *et al.* (2004). Turning on and turning off: a focus group study of the factors that affect women's sexual arousal. *Archives of Sexual Behavior*, **33**, 527–38.
12. Laan, E. and Everaerd, W. (1995). Determinants of sexual arousal: psychophysiological theory and data. *Annual Review of Sex Research*, **6**, 32–76.
13. Basson, R. (2000). The female sexual response: a different model. *Journal of Sex & Marital Therapy*, **26**, 51–64.
14. Kinsey, A.C., Pomeroy, W.B., Martin, C.F., *et al.* (1953). *Sexual behavior in the human female*. Saunders, Philadelphia.
15. Weijmar Schultz, W., Basson, R., Binik, Y., *et al.* (2005). Women's sexual pain and its management. *The Journal of Sexual Medicine*, **2**, 301–16.

16. Binik, Y.M. (2005). Should dyspareunia be retained as a sexual dysfunction in DSM-V? A painful classification decision. *Archives of Sexual Behavior*, **34**, 11–22.
17. American Psychiatric Association. (2000). *Diagnostic and statistical manual of mental disorders* (4th edn, text revision) (DSM-IV). Author, Washington, DC.
18. World Health Organization. (1992). *ICD-10: International statistical classification of diseases and related health problems* (10th edn). Author, Geneva.
19. Bancroft, J., Graham, C.A., and McCord, C. (2001). Conceptualizing sexual problems in women. *Journal of Sex & Marital Therapy*, **27**, 95–103.
20. Tiefer, L. (2001). A new view of women's sexual problems: why new? why now? *The Journal of Sex Research*, **38**, 89–96.
21. The Working Group for a New View of Women's Sexual Problems. (2001). A new view of women's sexual problems. In *A new view of women's sexual problems* (eds E. Kaschak and L. Tiefer), pp. 1–8, The Haworth Press, New York.
22. West, S.L., Vinikoor, L.C., and Zolhoun, D. (2004). A systematic review of the literature on female sexual dysfunction: prevalence and predictors. *Annual Review of Sex Research*, **15**, 40–172.
23. Graham, C.A. and Bancroft, J. (2005). Assessing the prevalence of female sexual dysfunction with surveys: what is feasible? In *Women's sexual function and dysfunction: study, diagnosis and treatment* (eds I. Goldstein, C. Meston, S. Davis, and A. Traish), pp. 52–60. Taylor and Francis, London.
24. Dunn, K.M, Croft, P.R., and Hackett, G.I. (1999). Association of sexual problems with social, psychological, and physical problems in men and women: a cross sectional population survey. *Journal of Epidemiology and Community Health*, **53**, 144–8.
25. Richters, J., Grulich, A.E., de Visser, R.O., *et al.* (2003). Sexual difficulties in a representative sample of adults. *Australian and New Zealand Journal of Public Health*, **27**, 164–70.
26. Bancroft, J., Loftus, J., and Long, J.S. (2003). Distress about sex: a national survey of women in heterosexual relationships. *Archives of Sexual Behavior*, **32**, 193–8.
27. King, M., Holt, V., and Nazareth, I. (2007). Women's views of their sexual difficulties: agreement and disagreement with clinical diagnoses. *Archives of Sexual Behavior*, **36**, 281–8.
28. Feldman, H.A., Goldstein, I., Hatzichristou, D.G., *et al.* (1994). Impotence and its medical and psychosocial correlates: results of the Massachusetts Male Aging Study. *The Journal of Urology*, **161**, 54–61.
29. American Association for Retired Persons (AARP). (1999). *Modern maturity sexuality study*. NFO Research, Inc., Washington, DC.
30. Hayes, R. and Dennerstein, L. (2005). The impact of aging on sexual function and sexual dysfunction in women: a review of population based studies. *The Journal of Sexual Medicine*, **2**, 317–30.
31. Janssen, E., Vorst, H., Finn, P., *et al.* (2002). The Sexual Inhibition (SIS) and Sexual Excitation (SES) Scales: i. Measuring sexual inhibition and excitation proneness in men. *The Journal of Sex Research*, **39**, 114–26.
32. Graham, C.A., Sanders, S.A., and Milhausen, R.R. (2006). The Sexual Excitation/Sexual Inhibition Inventory for Women: psychometric properties. *Archives of Sexual Behavior*, **35**, 397–409.
33. Bancroft, J., Herbenick, D., Barnes, T., *et al.* (2005). The relevance of the dual control model to male sexual dysfunction: the Kinsey Institute/BASRT collaborative project. *Sexual & Relationship Therapy*, **20**, 13–30.
34. Varjonen, M., Santilla, P., Hoglund, M., *et al.* Genetic and environmental effects on sexual excitation and sexual inhibition in men. *The Journal of Sex Research*, **44**, 359–69.
35. Sanders, S.A., Graham, C.A., and Milhausen, R.R. (2008). Predicting sexual problems in women: relevance of sexual inhibition and sexual excitation. *Archives of Sexual Behavior*, **37**(2), 241–51
36. Lindal, E. and Stefansson, J.G. (1993). The lifetime prevalence of psychosexual dysfunction among 55 to 57-year-olds in Iceland. *Social Psychiatry and Psychiatric Epidemiology*, **28**, 91–5.
37. Osborn, M., Hawton, K., and Gath, D. (1988). Sexual dysfunction among middle-aged women in the community. *British Medical Journal*, **296**, 959–62.
38. Beck, A.T. (1967). *Depression: clinical, experimental and theoretical aspects*. Staples Press, London.
39. Segraves, R.T. (1998). Psychiatric illness and sexual function. *International Journal of Impotence Research*, **10**(Suppl. 2), S131–3.
40. Schreiner-Engel, P. and Schiavi, R.C. (1986). Lifetime psychopathology in individuals with low sexual desire. *Journal of Nervous and Mental Disease*, **174**, 646–51.
41. Ware, M.R., Emmanuel, N.P., Johnson, M.R., *et al.* (1996). Self-reported sexual dysfunctions in anxiety disorder patients. *Psychopharmacology Bulletin*, **32**, 530.
42. Angst, J. (1998). Sexual problems in healthy and depressed persons. *International Clinical Psychopharmacology*, **13**(Suppl. 6), S1–4.
43. Figueira, I., Possidente, E., Marques, C., *et al.* (2001). Sexual dysfunction: a neglected complication of panic disorder and social phobia. *Archives of Sexual Behavior*, **30**, 369–77.
44. Araujo, A.B., Durante, R., Feldman, H.A., *et al.* (1998). The relationship between depressive symptoms and male erectile dysfunction: cross-sectional results from the Massachusetts Male Aging Study. *Psychosomatic Medicine*, **60**, 458–65.
45. Bancroft, J., Janssen, E., Strong, D., *et al.* (2003). The relation between mood and sexuality in heterosexual men. *Archives of Sexual Behavior*, **32**, 217–30.
46. Lykins, A., Janssen, E., and Graham, C.A. (2006). The relationship between negative mood and sexuality in heterosexual college women. *The Journal of Sex Research*, **43**, 136–43.
47. Lilleleht, E. and Leiblum, S.R. (1993). Schizophrenia and sexuality: a critical review of the literature. *Annual Review of Sex Research*, **4**, 247–76.
48. Bancroft, J. (2005). The endocrinology of sexual arousal. Starling review. *Journal of Endocrinology*, **186**, 411–27.
49. Mustanski, B. and Bancroft, J. (2006). Sexual dysfunction. In *Psychopharmacogenetics* (eds P. Gorwood and M. Hamon), pp. 479–94. Kluwer Academic Plenum, New York.
50. Bochinski, D. and Brock, G.B. (2001). Medications affecting erectile function. In *Male sexual function: a guide to clinical management* (ed. J.J. Mulcahy), pp. 91–108. Humana, Totowa.
51. Graham, C.A., Bancroft, J., Greco, T., *et al.* (2007). Does oral contraceptive-induced reduction in free testosterone adversely affect the sexuality and mood of women? *Psychoneuroendocrinology*, **32**, 246–55.
52. Bancroft, J. *Human sexuality and its problems* (3rd edn). Elsevier, Oxford, in press.
53. Rosen, R.C. and McKenna, K.E. (2002). PDE-5 inhibition and sexual response: pharmacological and clinical outcomes. *Annual Review of Sex Research*, **13**, 36–88.
54. Von Keitz, A.T., Stroberg, P., Bukofzer, S., *et al.* (2002). A European multicentre study to evaluate the tolerability of apomorphine sublingual administered in a forced dose-escalation regimen in patients with erectile dysfunction. *British Journal of Urology International*, **89**, 409–15.
55. Heiman, J.R. and Meston, C.M. (1997). Empirically validated treatment for sexual dysfunction. *Annual Review of Sex Research*, **7**, 148–94.
56. Van Lankveld, J.D.M., ter Kuile, M.M., de Groot, H.E., *et al.* (2006). Cognitive-behavioral therapy for women with lifelong vaginismus: a randomized waiting-list controlled trial of efficacy. *Journal of Consulting and Clinical Psychology*, **74**, 168–78.
57. Bergeron, S., Binik, Y.M., Khalifé, S., *et al.* (2001). A randomized comparison of group cognitive-behavioral therapy, surface electromyographic biofeedback, and vestibulectomy in the treatment of dyspareunia resulting from vulvar vestibulitis. *Pain*, **91**, 297–306.

58. Trudel, G., Marchand, A., Ravart, M., *et al.* (2001). The effect of a cognitive-behavioral group treatment program on hypoactive sexual desire in women. *Sexual & Relationship Therapy*, **16**, 145–64.
59. Fugl-Meyer, A.R. and Fugl-Meyer, K.S. (1999). Sexual disabilities, problems and satisfaction in 18–74 year old Swedes. *Scandinavian Journal of Sexology*, **2**, 79–105.

4.11.3 The paraphilias

J. Paul Fedoroff

Clinical features

Definition of the condition

The characteristic essential to all paraphilias is the presence of a persistent and/or recurrent, sexually motivated interest that causes harm. This definition has several implications.

Interest versus act

Paraphilias can exist even if they have never been acted upon. By definition, all paraphilias begin with a sexual thought and, like non-paraphilic interests, the majority of sexual fantasies are never fulfilled in reality. Sexual acts are only paraphilic if they are motivated by harmful sexual interests. For example, an individual with paedophilia (sexual interest in children) may act on this interest by masturbating while viewing non-pornographic children's television shows. However, an individual who unintentionally downloads pictures of children from the Internet while meaning to download adult pornography should not be considered paedophilic (even though he or she may still be criminally liable).

Persistent versus opportunistic

Paraphilias are characterized by their persistence. Therefore a single paraphilic thought or activity, especially if it occurs during unusual circumstances, is unlikely to be indicative of a true paraphilia. For example, a woman who while on a vacation and under the influence of alcohol exposes herself once to group of strangers in a bar, would not normally be considered to have exhibitionism (sexual arousal from exposure to strangers). Opportunistic activity that is not sexually motivated, even if it is ongoing, is also exclusionary. A pimp who coerces women to exchange sexual activities for drugs or money, would not meet criteria for sexual sadism even though he repeatedly engages in opportunistic sexual activity with otherwise unwilling participants because, for the pimp, the motivation is financial rather that sexual.

Harm versus happenstance

Many sex acts are intimate. Therefore it should come as no surprise that participants can be harmed. Unfortunately whenever sexual activities are considered, 'harm' tends to be defined somewhat solipsistically. Paraphilias are characterized by sexual interests or behaviours in which harm is more or less inevitable rather than accidental or random. For example, although sexual intercourse may expose the participants to a number of dangers including sexually transmitted diseases, possibly unintended degrees of intimacy, or subsequent events (e.g. pregnancy), by and large, consensual sexual activity between adults does not inevitably lead to disaster.

In contrast, true paraphilic interests are by definition, harmful. For example, a woman who can only become sexually aroused if she is choked to unconsciousness (asphyxophilia), exposes herself to unintended harm including cerebral anoxia and possible death. The paraphilias associated with crime (e.g. voyeurism, exhibitionism, frotteurism, criminal sadism, and paedophilia) involve non-consensual imposition of sexual activity onto others. Other non-criminal paraphilias (e.g. transvestic fetishism) become problematic when they interfere with the ability to maintain a reciprocal emotional relationship. Most men with transvestic fetishism do not seek therapy and there is no indication they should, unless the interest begins to cause harm. Paraphilic transvestites are sufficiently dependent on cross-dressing that it causes distress. Transvestic fetishism is a good example of a paraphilic condition in which the individual symptoms (wearing women's clothing while masturbating or engaging in sexual relations) are not problematic. However, when the sexual interest becomes so pervasive that it interferes with consensual sexual relations, a diagnosis is permissible. Transvestic fetishism is very responsive to treatment with selective serotonergic re-uptake inhibitors prescribed at doses low enough to avoid inhibited orgasm.

Pathologic versus unconventional

While paraphilias are characterized by deviant sexual interests, unconventional interests alone are not sufficient to meet criteria for a true paraphilic condition. This is a persistent source of confusion in two specific situations.

(a) Homosexuality

A primary sexual interest in the same sex (homosexuality) is statistically rare. However, there is nothing about a primary same-sex interest that necessarily leads to harm to anyone. Sexual interest in a woman is no more harmful for a heterosexual man than it is for a lesbian woman. Although homosexuality is statistically and socially unconventional, the absence of inevitable or likely harm excludes same-sexed sexual interest from being paraphilic.

(b) Sadomasochism

Sexual arousal from control (sadism) or from being controlled (masochism) illustrates a second way in which unconventional sexual interests may fail to meet criteria for designation as a paraphilia. While harm is a necessary criterion for paraphilias, it is not sufficient. For example, while many conventional sports involve competition and attempted domination of an opponent, the activity is not primarily sexually motivated. Therefore, although boxing involves the intentional attempt to render an opponent unconscious via infliction of a cerebral concussion (knockout), pugilism is not a paraphilia because it is not primarily sexually motivated.

The converse is also true. Many men and women engage in interactions that are sexually motivated and which involve negotiations about power and control, domination and submission. These themes have become highly organized and regulated within social groups under the general category of 'BDSM' (bondage, domination, submission, sadism, masochism). Publications describing the BDSM 'lifestyle' universally champion the credo: 'safe, sane, and consensual'. Therefore, men and women who engage in 'BDSM' sexual activities, although they may involve statistically and/or socially unconventional activities, do not meet criteria for any paraphilia disorder. In fact, it is arguable that anyone who is sexually aroused by the idea of engaging in 'safe, sane, and consensual' activities is *less* paraphilic than those with conventional sexual interests who are willing to compromise some of these meritorious criteria in pursuit of conventional sexual interactions. For a more complete discussion of sexual violence and sexual sadism.[(1)]

Classification

Table 4.11.3.1 consists of a partial list of the over 100 paraphilic disorders described in the literature. Classification of the paraphilias remains controversial. This is due to two issues. The first is that many paraphilias have been assigned names based on Latin or Greek etymology. For example, retifism refers to a paraphilic interest in shoes more commonly known as a 'shoe fetish' while 'renifleurs' are individuals with sexual arousal from the smell of urine. More complete listings of paraphilic disorders has been

Table 4.11.3.1 Paraphilic sexual disorders

Paraphilia	DSM- IV TR	ICD-10	Essential feature: persistent sexual arousal towards	Comments
Acrotomophilia	302.9	F65.9	Amputees	
Apotemnophilia	302.9	F65.9	Being an amputee	
Asphyxiophilia	302.9	F65.9	Being asphyxiated	Also known as 'autoerotic asphyxia'
Biastophilia	302.9	F65.9	Non-consensual adult intercourse	Also known as paraphilic rapism or raptophilia
Exhibitionism	302.4	F65.2	Exposure to strangers	
Fetishism	302.81	F65.0	Inanimate objects	Not vibrators
Frotteurism	302.89	F65.8	Rubbing groin without consent	ICD has no specific listing
Mysophilia	302.9	F65.9	'Filth'	Typically involving 'soiled' (worn) panties
Necrophilia	302.9	F65.9	Corpses	
Paedophilia	302.2	F65.4	Children	ICD does not differentiate
Attraction				
Males				
Females				
Both				
Exclusivity				
Incest only				
Exclusive				
Non-exclusive				
Polyembolokoilamania	302.9	F65.9	Insertion of objects	Associated with Smith McGinnis syndrome. (Not clearly paraphilic)
Scoptic syndrome	302.9	F65.9	Being castrated	
Scoptophilia	302.9	F65.9	Consensual viewing	Paraphilic only if problematic
Sexual masochism	302.83	F65.5	Loss of control	ICD combines into Sadomasochism
Sexual sadism	302.84	F65.5	Non-consensual control	ICD combines into sadomasochism
Somnophilia	302.9	F65.9	sleeping sexual partner	
Telephone scatalogia	302.9	F65.9	Obscene phone calls	
Transvestic fetishism with gender dysphoria	302.3	F65.1	Wearing clothes of the opposite sex	ICD does not subclassify
Urophilia	302.9	F65.9	Urine	
Voyeurism	302.82	F65.3	Spying	
Paraphilia NOS	302.9	F65.9	Paraphilias not otherwise specified	ICD: Disorder of sexual preference unspecified
Other disorders of sexual preference		F65.8	Other paraphilic disorders	

published (c.f. Love, 1999). In addition, many of the paraphilias involve sexual interest in the characteristics of the sexual partner(s). Often some interest in assuming the same characteristics is evident and receives a unique name. The most obvious example is sadomasochism which the DSM classification divides into sadism and masochism while in the ICD classification the two complimentary conditions are combined.

The second problematic diagnostic issue in the classification of the paraphilias concerns the need to describe both unconventional sexual behaviours and problematic sexual behaviours. For example, while sexual arousal from cross-dressing is unconventional, it technically does not meet criteria for transvestic fetishism unless it causes distress. In the case of paraphilias involving criminal interests (e.g. paedophilia) issues arise if a person reports persistent sexual interest in children but no distress or wish to act on the paedophilic interest. Newer diagnostic criteria likely will address this issue.

Diagnosis and differential diagnosis

Similar to most psychiatric conditions, paraphilic disorders are diagnosed primarily on the basis of self-reported symptoms. Paraphilias differ from most other psychiatric disorders in two ways: (i) many paraphilias involve illegal interests and (ii) objective measures of the primary criteria (in this case sexual interest) are available.

Illegal sexual interests

Paraphilic interests do not necessarily lead to illegal activities, and vice versa. Therefore, 'Not all paedophiles are child molesters and not all child molesters are paedophiles'.

With few exceptions, individuals with paraphilic interests not only know they have abnormal sexual interests but also wish they could replace them with 'normal' ones. Many confuse fantasy with reality, thinking that illegal sexual interests are equivalent to having committed a sex crime. A major issue in the diagnosis of paraphilic disorders is distinguishing between legal and psychiatric concerns (see Management section below for further details).

In addition to legal issues, clinicians should also consider several other diagnostic issues:

(a) False accusations

At one time accusations by children of sexual assault by adults were considered to be almost certainly true since it was assumed that children could not know about sex. A typical assertion would be that a child could not possibly describe acts such as sexual intercourse or ejaculation unless they had been sexually assaulted. Clearly this was before the widespread availability of pornographic videos, DVD's, cable TV networks, and the Internet.

Beginning in the 1990s, adults began to report they had been sexually abused as children but had only recently recovered their memories of the assault. In part this trend seems to have been due to two factors: the decision in the United States to reset the time at which the statute of limitations required a sexual offence to be reported to the time at which the offence was recalled; and the believe that failure to recall sexual abuse was a sign that it had occurred.

(b) False confessions

While less frequent, false reports of paraphilic interests have also been described.(2) The most frequent presentation of false paraphilic symptoms takes the form of a man or woman with depression who reports obsessions involving often exceptionally troubling sex crimes. While a detailed phenomenologic examination of this phenomenon has not been published, several characteristics are typical. The individual often has a history of a mood disorder or is in circumstances in which affective disorders are more likely (e.g. post-partum). The sexual obsession typically involves children to whom the patient has access (it is rare for the patient to report spontaneous fantasies of sexual interactions with unknown children). Most importantly, the fantasies are extremely ego-dystonic. Asked if they ever masturbate to their paraphilic fantasies, they typically respond with horror and, unlike those with true paraphilias, often describe self-loathing indicative of a change in self-esteem due to depression. A danger of false confessions or admission of false paraphilic interests has also been noted in men and women with intellectual disability.

(c) Co-morbid conditions

People rarely seek treatment on their own specifically for paraphilic disorders. This is due to unfortunately widespread false beliefs that (i) there are no effective treatments for paraphilias, (ii) embarrassment about discussing paraphilic symptoms, and (iii) in the case of paedophilia, the mistaken belief that reporting a sexual interest in children necessarily requires that the patient be reported to the police (please see Management below for more comments on this problem). Since paraphilias themselves rarely motivate helpseeking, clinicians should include other conditions in the differential diagnoses both as alternative explanations for the problem and as co-morbid conditions that may be present in addition to the paraphilia. The most frequent of these are mood disorders, substance abuse problems including alcohol, marital disorder, and legal problems.

Less common are organic disorders including brain injuries.(3) Surprisingly, given the importance of sex hormones in the development and expression of sexual characteristics, endocrine disorders affecting the sex hormones are rarely implicated. This may be because testosterone in men with normal or elevated hormone levels are more closely associated with violence and aggression than with alterations in the direction of sexual interest.(1) One exception is hypogonadism associated with Klinefelter's syndrome. In some men with Klinefelter's syndrome, paraphilic problems become apparent when testosterone is prescribed to correct hypogonadism. In those men with Klinefelter's syndrome and paraphilic interests, addition of testosterone appears to unmask rather than cause previously unexpressed paraphilic conditions.

A more controversial question involves a possible association between paraphilias and intellectual disability. Some research has supported the hypothesis that, as a group, men with paedophilia have below average intelligence. However, alternative explanations are possible. For example, most men with paedophilia come to attention when they are arrested. The fact that men with intellectual disability are more likely to be arrested and are over-represented in the criminal justice system may skew the data. Those who live in supervised housing are also more likely to have private activities not only discovered by staff but also labelled by staff as deviant. In addition, men with intellectual disability frequently have impairments in social skills that can certainly contribute to problematic sexual behaviours independent of paraphilic interests. This phenomenon has been described as 'counterfeit deviance'.(4)

One meta-analytic study supporting an association between paedophilia and intellectual disability found the mean I.Q. of sex offenders to be only five I.Q. points below the mean I.Q. of non-sexual offenders.[5] While cognitive ability is important in determining level of risk and in planning treatment (see below) it would be a diagnostic mistake to confirm or refute a diagnosis of paedophilia on the basis of intelligence.

A further area of controversy involves the question of whether having one paraphilia predisposes to having other paraphilias? The answer depends on whether the assessor is a 'lumper' or a 'splitter'. John Money viewed paraphilias as 'vandalized lovemaps' that were unique. He argued that a paedophile might begin by spying on children, then surreptitiously touching them, then engaging in sexual relations. It was his view that it was more accurate to label the disorder as paedophilia (since this explains the motivation behind the varied behaviours) as opposed to making a diagnosis of voyeurism, frotteurism, and paedophilia. Clearly both approaches have strengths and weaknesses. Most important is to be aware of both diagnostic methods when evaluating incidence or prevalence reports.

Epidemiology

Prevalence of paraphilic disorders

Any discussion of the number of people with paraphilic disorders in the population must begin with a series of caveats. The most important is the fact that the majority of the information available is derived from studies of men convicted of sex crimes. This is a significant problem since not all paraphilias are associated with sex crimes. The problem is compounded by the fact that many paraphilic disorders remain undiagnosed either because assessment was never requested, clinicians did not gather sufficient information, or because the person with the paraphilic disorder was unwilling or unable to disclose the symptoms. Further degrees of confusion and subsequent dispute are added by inconsistent application of existing diagnostic criteria (for example confusing child molesters with paedophiles) or by differing opinions about whether or not to subdivide paraphilic disorders (e.g. diagnosing a person who lures children into sexual activity by exposing to them as a paedophile or as both a paedophile and an exhibitionist). To date, insufficient attention has been paid to the importance of precise definitions of what is being measured, the difference between point and period prevalence, and the potentially significant differences attributable to independent characteristics of the populations being studied. For example, a report on the incidence of 'sexual sadism' based on a point prevalence study of sexual assault of women and children in a country in which war is being waged, while important, has little to do with an analysis of the period prevalence of sexual sadism in, for example, North America. There is also an widespread but unwarranted assumption that studies based on criminal populations can be easily generalized to other populations.

Fortunately, with these above caveats in mind, a significant resource to answer epidemiologic questions is now available both in text form and, more importantly, in the form of a constantly updated Internet Web site: http://www.kinseyinstitute.org/ccies/. This Web site, currently under development and hosted on the Kinsey Institute web page, provides free access to reports by noted sexologists on sexual behaviours in 60 countries and six continents. Included in the chapters on most countries are sections dealing with both paraphilic disorders and 'unconventional sexual behaviours'. This is important since different cultures may place different significance on sexual behaviours both in public and private. The fact that each chapter is multi-authored by sexologists who live in the country being described also likely adds to the credibility of the information.

From perusal of the information available several statements about the epidemiology of paraphilic disorders can be made with reasonable confidence.

(a) Men are more likely than women to be arrested for sexually motivated crimes

Most (but not all) illegal activities are non-consensual. Those that are sexually motivated have a high likelihood of being associated with a paraphilia. Data to support this observation is derived primarily from review of the unequal ratio of men and women convicted of sex crimes. While there are increasing numbers of women (especially adolescent females) being convicted of child sexual abuse, men are still the vast majority. From a criminologic perspective men seem more willing to commit crimes of all types, especially those that involve confrontation (verbal, physical, and sexual). This is of significance since two widely employed actuarial risk assessment instruments, the Violence Risk Appraisal Guide (VRAG) and Sex Offender Risk Appraisal Guide (SORAG) rely heavily on the Hare Psychopathy Checklist (HPCL) which itself has been associated with criminal activity independent of sexual interest. This may explain why some researchers believe that a combination of high scores on the HPCL combined with deviant scores on phallometric testing are associated with high risk of re-offence (either violent and sexual) (for more information please see the Hare Web site listed below).

(b) With the exception of internet-related sex crimes, the frequency of sex crimes of all types are on the decline

This welcome finding has been reviewed extensively elsewhere.[6] It is important to note that while this trend of decreasing frequencies of sex crimes excludes countries in the midst of war or major political and social upheaval, the trend is occurring worldwide. Unfortunately the reason for this trend is unknown. One controversial explanation is a wider availability of pornographic materials, beginning with videotapes in the 1980s and now exploding with the Internet. One study noted, during a time of increased availability of pornographic materials, an 85 per cent decrease in numbers of juvenile offenders in Japan from 1803 in 1972 to 264 in 1995.[7] The increase in Internet-related crimes combined with an apparent decrease in other types of sex crimes invites the unproven speculation that one may be substituting for the other.

(c) Paraphilic disorders are not new

A final important point to be made about the epidemiology of paraphilic disorders is that they are not new. Historic texts on the topic clearly describe not only sex crimes but also the same phenomenologic characteristics seen by clinicians today. If there is a change, it is towards increasingly earlier detection of paraphilic behaviours, not only at a younger age,[8] but also before criminal acts have been committed.

Table 4.11.3.2 summarizes generally accepted prevalence estimates for the DSM-IVTR paraphilias.

Table 4.11.3.2 Frequency/prevalance of paraphilias

Paraphilia	Prevalence/frequency	Comments
Exhibitionism	No reliable data	40–60% of females report having been exposed to Evidence suggests a decrease in frequency of exhibitionism after age 40
Fetishism	No reliable data	Depending on population studied, rates range from 0.8% to 18% of men
Frotteurism	No reliable general population data	Only paraphilia claimed to decrease in frequency after age 25 (DSM-IV-TR p. 570)
Paedophilia	Frequency: 300 000 abused children per year in the USA	1988 data; does not account for repeat offences
Sexual sadism	3% to 20% of general population	Data do not distinguish between criminal and non-criminal sexual interests
Sexual masochism	5% to 10% of general population	Data does not distinguish between criminal and non-criminal sexual interests
Transvestic fetishism	1% of men	True prevalence unknown in part due to idiosyncratic diagnostic criteria
Voyeurism	No reliable data	Most studies of voyeurism involve offenders with co-morbid paraphilic interests

Aetiology

Like most psychiatric disorders, the ultimate causes of paraphilic disorders are unknown. Like most groups of psychiatric disorders, they undoubtedly have multiple contributing factors.

Four major explanatory perspectives have been identified: 'disease', 'behavioural', 'dimensional', and 'life story'.[9] Each perspective has had advocates that can be traced to the beginning of the twentieth century.

The disease perspective

The disease perspective is perhaps the most familiar to physicians since it is based upon an attempt to combine signs and symptoms into syndromes or disorders via pathophysiologic mechanisms.

In 1886 Krafft-Ebing published *Psychopathia Sexualis: A Medico-forensic Study* in which he described a large series of patients with a variety of sexual disorders, whom he had examined in his forensic psychiatry practice.[10] Using a disease perspective he advanced the hypothesis that masturbation caused a physiologic imbalance that was a major causal factor in development of sexual deviancy. Krafft-Ebing was widely criticized for his acceptance and perpetuation of the degeneration theory of masturbation (the now discarded theory that masturbation itself could cause progressive degrees of physiologic harm leading to increasingly severe psychopathology), and for his failure to clearly differentiate between extreme and mild forms of sexual deviancy.

While *Psychopathia Sexualis* is now considered a landmark text in human sexuality, its acceptance was limited because it was published at a time when other etiologic explanations for the paraphilias were becoming important. One criticism of Krafft-Ebing's disease perspective was his tendency to focus on illness rather than wellness or normality. In this context, Brautigam's criticism of Krafft-Ebing's *Psychopathia Sexualis* foreshadows current criticisms of etiologic theories of the paraphilias that rely on the disease perspective:

> This first great and distinguished complete presentation and inventory of that field has the character of a large catalogue of perversions. In a picture book-like series are offered the most monstrous cases of his time and history, particularly cases collected by Krafft-Ebing himself as a widely sought medico-legal consultant. The perversions are described in their most extreme forms. This collection of brutal necrophiliacs, anthropophages, sexual murderers,and sodomites, of cunning and cultured sadists, masochists, and transvestites has in its degree of deviation never been surpassed. By this extreme presentation Krafft-Ebing has moved sexual disorders away from general sexuality.[11]

Magnus Hirschfield was a contemporary of Krafft-Ebing who also employed a disease perspective in an attempt to identify abnormal pathophysiology in individuals with identified sexual problems. Although he is best known for his studies of castrated males and for his emphasis on the importance of hormones on sexual behaviour, Hirschfield also drew an important distinction between the simple description of observed behaviours and proof of their aetiology. His argument that describing a behaviour was not sufficient to explain its cause led him to distinguish between homosexuality, transsexualism, and fetishistic transvestism, in which the same behaviour (cross-dressing) could be shown to have different motivations and therefore presumably different causes.[12] His observation that sexual orientation and behaviour may have variable determinants was important since it emphasized the need to look for underlying causes of behaviour from a disease perspective while at the same time opening the door for collaboration with behavioural researchers.

Behavioural perspective

Although Albert Moll felt that sexual disorders could be treated with 'association therapy' (a precursor to modern behaviour modification therapy), he felt learning alone could not account for all sexual deviations:

> Were a single sexual experience, and, indeed, the first sexual experience to induce a lasting association between sex drive and the object of the first sexual experience, then we would have to find sexual perversion everywhere. Where are there to be found people who initially satisfied their sexual impulse in a normal manner?[13]

By extending consideration of sexual development from childhood to adulthood, Moll was able to answer Brautigam's criticism of Krafft-Ebing's research by studying normal as well as abnormal sexuality.

Albert Moll and Alfred Binet, used behavioural perspectives to study sexuality by directing attention to the associations between behaviours and their reinforcers. Binet re-examined the case histories of Krafft-Ebing's patients and argued that sexual deviations which had been presumed to be caused by disease or degeneration could have been caused by learned associations. He noted that many of the reported cases he studied also had 'chance associations' that could explain the development of the sexual deviation. These observations implied that, given a specific set of reinforced experiences, any individual could become paraphilic. The proposition that all people could potentially acquire paraphilias if they were unfortunate enough to have been exposed to the necessary abnormal formative experiences was more fully developed by investigators using a dimensional perspective.

Dimensional perspective

The dimensional perspective is characterized by an avoidance of rigid categorical classifications in favour of continuous descriptors. Variations in sexual interests, including paraphilic interests, are explained as statistical extremes of normal behaviour without necessarily implying that a disease process is present. From a dimensional perspective, paedophilia would be understood as an extreme variation of the widespread tendency to equate youth with sexual attractiveness. The work of Haveloch Ellis is a good example of this approach to sex research. He is most well known for his six volume *Studies in The Psychology of Sex*.[14] A major theme in Ellis' work is the avoidance of a disease perspective as the sole explanation for sexual deviations. Instead of paraphilic disorders, he focused primarily on homosexuality and suggested that homosexuality could be 'latent'. Since degree of 'latency' is a continuous variable it was possible to consider homosexuality as a dimension rather than a disease. This dimensional perspective was later exploited by Kinsey[15] who developed his famous Kinsey scale of sexual orientation that rated men and women on a six point scale. Both Ellis and Kinsey shifted attention from the differences between homosexuals and heterosexuals to their similarities. In this way their work complemented research using disease or behavioural perspectives as well as the work of investigators using a fourth perspective, which focused primarily on the individual's 'life story'.

Life-story perspective

The life-story perspective is characterized by a search for the 'meaning' behind behaviour. This perspective appeals to the self-experienced aspect of life, so life-story perspectives tend to be very compelling and persuasive. For example, in North America, it is rare to find a man with transvestic fetishism that does not recall being dressed as a girl for Halloween. A problem with this approach is that it is often difficult to determine which 'story' is the correct one, or even if a single meaningful connection can be found. For example, there is no evidence that men with transvestic fetishism are more likely to have been dressed as girls when they were children than were other men. Sigmund Freud often used sexual motives to construct a life story that was difficult to disprove. Freud's research method consisted chiefly of interviewing patients and interpreting recurring themes in literature and art. While this approach may seem highly susceptible to bias, it has been surprisingly successful, not only for Freud but for other researchers who have adopted this method of direct interview combined with longitudinal follow-up, to understand the meanings of sexual acts and decisions. The explanations that individuals themselves develop to explain their behaviours are often as important and enlightening therapeutically as their 'true' causes.

Integration of the four perspectives

While each of the four described perspectives provide a unique basis on which to base explanatory theories about the origins of paraphilic disorders, none is mutually exclusive. In the twentieth century, some behaviourists began to acknowledge the importance of non-observable factors such as 'instinct'[16] and later, 'motivation'. Other theorists,[17] while recognizing the importance of behaviourism, emphasized that the 'motivated behaviours' of sleeping, eating, and mating could not reasonably be reduced to simple stimulus response associations. If motivated behaviours could not be fully explained from a single research perspective perhaps an integration of approaches would be more helpful. A good example of an integrated etiologic theory to explain paraphilias is the one advanced by John Money who theorized that all children are born with the potential to develop a full range of sexual interests analogous to the observation that all healthy children at the time of birth are capable of learning to speak any human language. Which language (and by analogy which sexual interests) each child eventually expresses is determined by learning during critical periods of neurologic development.

From extensive research involving patients with genetic and endocrine disorders that interfered with normal anatomic and physiologic sexual development, he theorized that sometime before the onset of puberty, a 'lovemap' was established. He defined lovemap as: 'a developmental representation or template, synchronously functional in the mind and the brain, depicting the idealized lover, the idealized love affair, and the idealized programme of sexuoerotic activity with that lover, projected in imagery and ideation, or in actual performance'.[18] He hypothesized that an individual's lovemap became 'neurologically embedded' or 'imprinted', analogous to the way an individual's native language becomes a 'native tongue'. He believed that each person has a single lovemap (analogous to having a single native language or 'mother tongue') but that each person may never be fully aware of the true nature and details of the lovemap (analogous to not learning the full vocabulary of grammar of a native language). Paraphilias represented what he termed 'vandalized' lovemaps resulting from an abnormal experience during the 'critical period' during which lovemaps are formed.

Course and prognosis

While the incidence of paraphilias (especially those that involve criminal activities) in men is at least 10 times the incidence in women,[19] the majority of both males and females do not develop paraphilias. In addition, unlike sexual orientation, for which there is some evidence of important genetic or at least prenatal influences,[20] and excluding a single retrospective report of possible familial co-morbidity,[21] there is no current evidence of any prenatal factors that cause paraphilic disorders. Similarly the hypothesis that being the victim of sexual abuse predisposes victims to become sex offenders has also been challenged.[22] There is an increasing recognition of the fact that adolescents are capable of committing sex crimes.[8] This edited book concluded that, 'approximately 20 per cent of all rapes and between 30 per cent and 50 per cent of child molestations are perpetrated by adolescent males'. The increasing number of facilities designed to assess and treat juvenile sex offenders, male and female, supports self-report descriptions of paraphilic behaviours beginning in adolescence.

Most crimes (both sexual and non-sexual) are committed by young adult males. One problem in assessing the literature on the frequency of paraphilic behaviours in this age group is the frequent failure to distinguish between current paraphilic acts and those that are recalled. For example, it is not uncommon for a middle-aged man with exhibitionism to recall frequent exhibitionistic activities from his youth[2] but there is no reason to believe that the recollections of the sexual exploits of exhibitionists are any more reliable than the recollections of non-paraphilic men.

To summarize, it is often assumed that anyone who has a paraphilic interest has acted on it. In fact, the DSM-IV diagnostic criteria B requires that the interest has been acted upon or at least caused harm to someone. While cases have been described in which a person engaged in sexual activity without awareness (e.g. engaging in sexual acts while asleep),[23] for the most part, thought precedes action. In fact, it is arguable that a person who fantasizes about paraphilic activities is more paraphilic than one who commits a paraphilic act while fantasizing about a non-paraphilic activity.

Most paraphilic thoughts begin around the time of puberty. If the 'vandalized lovemap' explanation of paraphilias is correct, faulty development of sexual interest likely occurs prior to puberty but is not expressed until there is sufficient increase in sex drive for it to be manifested, first as fantasy and later, by action.

Prognosis is an area of considerable controversy. However, accumulated evidence indicates that the majority of convicted sex offenders do not re-offend (likely fewer that 15 per cent). In addition, evidence indicates that treatments are improving in efficacy (see below).

Evaluation of treatments

In this section 'treatment' refers to intervention with intent to reduce the frequency of unwanted paraphilic symptoms. Studies on the treatment of paraphilic disorders necessarily include participants with diagnosed paraphilias who have not only sought treatment but who have also volunteered for a treatment and have at least started the treatment under study. This represents a group that for obvious reasons may be unrepresentative of the true paraphilic population, the majority of whom likely never seek treatment.

Treatment recommendations should be individualized across paraphilic and co-morbid disorders and to account for individual variation. For example, the treatment approach for an exhibitionist with anti-social personality disorder and heroin dependency will be very different from the treatment of a woman with paedophilia or an adolescent with intellectual disability and transvestic fetishism.

In the past half-century there have been three major innovations in the treatment of paraphilic disorders that have led to significant improvement in prognosis. The first of these was the use of anti-androgen medications.

Interventions to reduce testosterone

Surgical castration has shown a high degree of success, at least in terms of reducing recidivism rates in sex offenders, with reported rates of recidivism after 30 years of follow-up as low as 2.2 per cent for convicted rapists. While this is a remarkable success rate, surgery for this purpose has been criticized on ethical grounds and because reversible interventions, in the form of anti-androgen medications have became available. For a review of the efficacy of castration in the treatment of the sex offender.[24]

Anti-androgens administered either by mouth or by intra-muscular injection were first used in the late 1950s as an alternative to surgical castration. The most common oral anti-androgens prescribed for this purpose are cyproterone acetate (Androcur) (CPA) and medroy-progesterone acetate (Provera) (MPA). Both of these medications are also available in a formulation suitable for intra-muscular injection. Reviews of treatment efficacy of both of these medications are also available.[24]

A review of eight studies involving a total of 452 sex offenders who received treatment with MPA for between 1 and 13 years, recidivism ranged from 1 per cent to 17 per cent.[25] Unfortunately, anti-androgen treatment of sex offenders has been a victim of its own success. Because the success rates were so high in open studies, and because the consequences of recidivism are so great, randomized double-blind treatment studies have been difficult to justify from an ethical perspective. Gonadotropin hormone releasing hormone (GnRH) partial analogs significantly reduce serum testosterone by down-regulating receptors in the anterior pituitary resulting in a decrease in luteinizing hormone which in turn decreases production of testosterone by leydig cells in the testes. Reviews of the apparent impressive efficacy of anti-androgens and GnRH analogs are available.[26]

Selective serotonin re-uptake inhibitors (SSRIs)

Numerous reports have confirmed the apparent efficacy of SSRI and related medications in the treatment of men with paraphilic disorders.[27] Two important prescribing issues are important:

(a) There is no evidence that the efficacy of SSRIs in the treatment of paraphilic disorders is due to suppression of sex drive. Many medications that are more effective in reducing sex drive appear to have little effect on paraphilic interest.

(b) There is no evidence that higher doses of SSRIs are more effective than low doses. In fact, if the prescribed SSRI causes inhibited orgasm, this may be counter-therapeutic since there is a tendency for individuals with paraphilic sexual interests to resort to paraphilic fantasies or acts in order to facilitate orgasm.[28,29]

Psychotherapy

The evidence in support and against various psychotherapeutic interventions has recently been reviewed.[30] Most reviews of psychotherapeutic interventions for paraphilic disorders focus on group therapy (the most common intervention in prisons) or individual psychotherapy (most common in private practices). However, other interventions are also important including marital therapy, family therapy, spousal therapy, occupational therapy, and substance abuse therapy.

Treatment of sex offenders based on psychologic interventions were carefully reviewed by a collaborative group using meta-analytic techniques.[31] A total of 43 published studies involving a total of 9454 sex offenders (5078 treated and 4376 untreated) were analysed. While noting methodologic limitations, there were two important findings: (i) sexual recidivism rates were lower in treated groups (12.3 per cent) than in comparison groups (16.8 per cent) and (ii) efficacy of psychologic treatments appear to have improved since the 1970s. The final results of one important study were not included in the Hanson *et al.* meta-analysis. This was a longitudinal study with stratified randomization into a group that received relapse-prevention group therapy ($n = 167$) or a group that did not ($n = 225$); a third group was matched to the first two groups and consisted of sex offenders who did not volunteer to participate in the study ($n = 220$). Treatment for the first group consisted of 2 years in custody, group relapse-prevention therapy followed by a 1 year mandated programme after release to the community. While results were complicated by a dropout rate in the treatment group of 27 per cent, the third group consisting of 'non-volunteer' controls was found to have the lowest long-term rate of sexual recidivism (19.1 per cent at 12 years follow-up). In comparison, the sub-group that entered therapy but discontinued prematurely had a 35.7 per cent sexual re-offence rate compared to the group that completed the prescribed treatment which had a 21.6 per cent sexual re-offence rate at 12 years follow-up. The final conclusion of this study was that a treatment effect for the cognitive behavioural programme did not produce a significant treatment effect.(32)

The failure to demonstrate the efficacy of 'relapse-prevention' as it was constituted 20 years ago has been regarded by some as a major setback in the field. However, the fact that even in the worst outcome group the majority of sex offenders were not known to have re-offended, the fact that the treatment programme under investigation was 'manualized', and the fact that other important treatment interventions were not employed, makes any conclusion that sex offenders can not be treated unwarranted.

Management

General principles

Summaries of management strategies for individuals with paraphilic disorders and/or sex offence histories are available.(30,33) Specific recommendations for the more commonly encountered paraphilic disorders and for specific paraphilic disorders should also be consulted.(2) An initial approach to the management of paraphilic disorders is summarized in Fig. 4.11.3.1.

Individuals with paraphilic disorders typically are in extreme crisis when they present for treatment. It is important to assist the individual to not only understand that sexual urges are controllable but that sex acts are the person's responsibility. This is often a surprise to people with paraphilias who have lived with the false belief that the difference between themselves and the rest of the world is a lack of will power. It is important to assist in maintaining and establishing a healthy social support system, ideally including family members, spouses, employers, church members, and trusted friends. Group therapy is particularly helpful in assisting to confront cognitive distortions and in demonstrating that others not only do not re-offend but are capable of establishing healthy and fulfilling lives. Medications can be prescribed with the aim of decreasing sexual anxiety and impulsivity (SSRIs), moderating sex drive (anti-androgens), or eliminating sex drive (GNRH

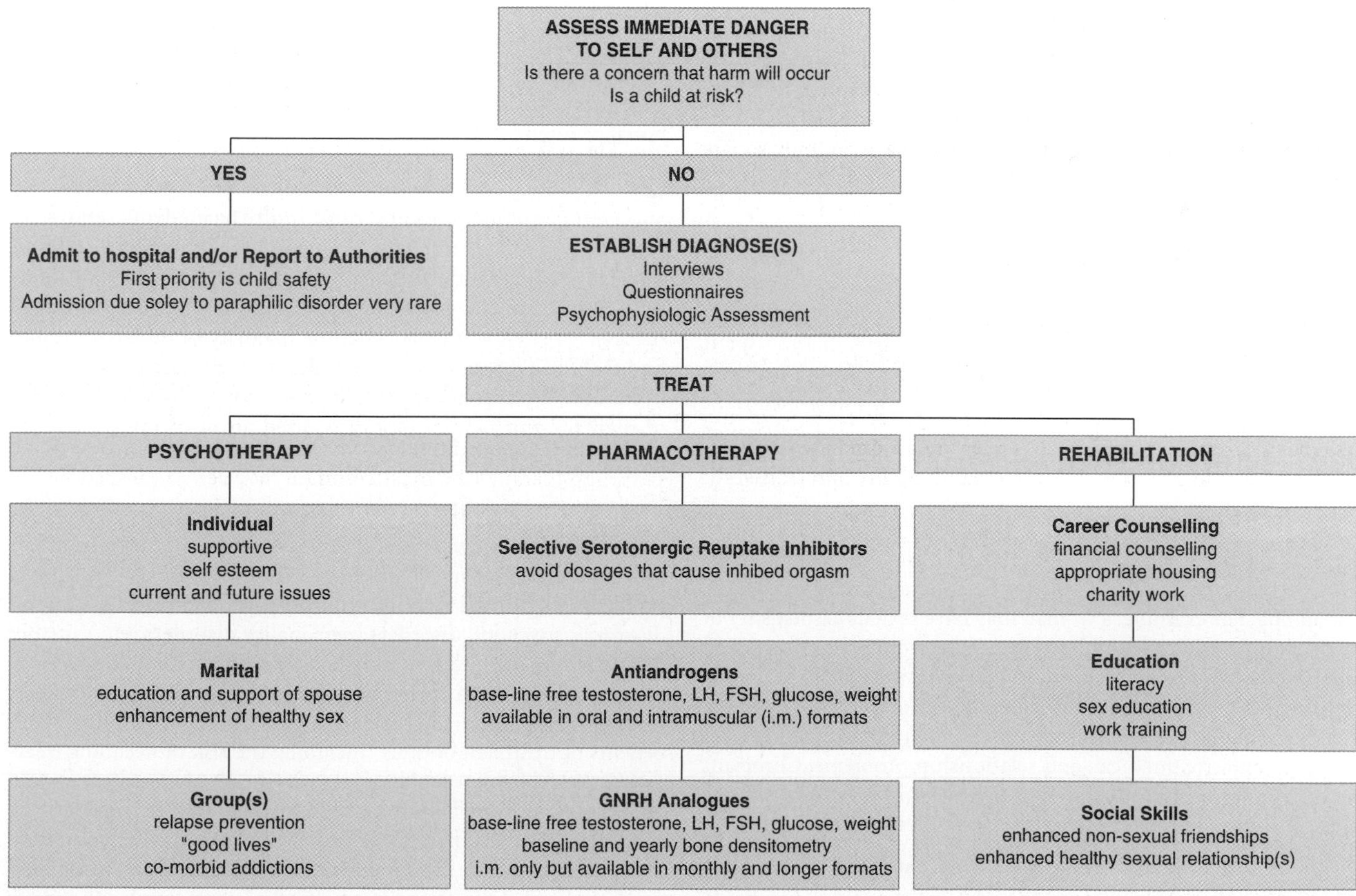

Fig. 4.11.3.1 Management of the paraphilias.

analogues). It is vital, particularly when treating men with paraphilias who have been incarcerated, to assist them in establishing pro-social lifestyles. This includes advice about appropriate work (e.g. avoiding jobs that require contact with children in the case of paedophiles), finding work (some clinics maintain lists of employers willing to hire men they know are in treatment), and ways to spend leisure time in constructive and pro-social ways. A part of the therapy often neglected is the establishment of healthy sexual activities to replace the problematic sexual interests and acts for which therapy was initiated. This frequently involves marital or couple's therapy. Some clinics establish 'spouses' groups to provide independent support, education, and treatment of the spouses of individuals with paraphilias.

In addition, the following general principles are recommended:

(a) Identify for whom you are working

Many paraphilic disorders predispose to unconventional or criminal activities. Most countries now have mandatory reporting requirements for incidents of known or potential sexual abuse of any identifiable child. It is extremely important to establish the limits of confidentiality prior to or at the first meeting. Many clinics post a description of the rules of confidentiality under which they operate. Sometimes it is difficult to be certain for whom one is working. A quick rule of thumb is to ask who is paying for the work and to whom reports will be sent.

(b) Facilitate disclosure

Men and women seeking assessment and treatment for paraphilic disorders almost always think they are the first (and worst) case of their type ever seen. They fear they will be led from the clinic room in handcuffs and be featured on the front page of the following day's newspaper. It is important to dispel these misconceptions not only because it will allow for a more in-depth assessment but also because it is important to dispel a 'me-against-authority' mentality which is common amongst individuals who see themselves as 'outsiders'.

Objective measures of sexual preference (e.g. phallometric testing) are available.(34) Their utility is enhanced if they are used as 'truth facilitators' rather than as 'lie detectors'.(35) While tests based on deception such as surreptitious measurement of time spent viewing pictures are currently widely used, their future utility is questionable since they are valid only if the deception is effective.

Perhaps the greatest truth facilitator is scrupulous adherence to disclosed rules of confidentiality.

(c) Establish what the problem is

Typically, individuals with paraphilic disorders present in crisis. However, the crisis often has only peripheral connection to the paraphilia. For example, a woman may have sexual masochism but seek treatment due to complications arising from major depression or substance abuse. This is true even if she insists that all her problems would end if she could be cured of her masochistic interests. As reviewed above, paraphilic disorders often occur together with other psychiatric, medical, and relationship problems. Clinicians should be wary of limited differential diagnoses, especially those that attribute all problems to a single paraphilia in isolation.

(d) Identify why the patient is seeking treatment now

Most paraphilias begin in childhood or at the time of puberty. However, teenagers rarely self-present for assessment of paraphilic disorders. Therefore, most adults with paraphilic disorders may be assumed to be seeking treatment for a variety of reasons besides having suddenly discovered they have (for example) paedophilia. Frequent motivations include: criminal charges, discovery of problematic behaviours by spouses or family members, and emergence of co-morbid problems such as depression or substance abuse.

For treatment to be successful it is very important to establish what the person seeking treatment thinks is the problem. Failure to do so significantly reduces the likelihood of keeping the person in therapy, establishing a therapeutic relationship, and ultimately the prognosis for a successful outcome.

(e) Avoid one-sided treatment plans

Paraphilic disorders by definition involve an interaction between the most abstract and 'high-level' cognitive processes (sexual fantasies), limbic and sub-cortical neural pathways (sexual arousal patterns), and society. Treatment plans based on single perspectives are unlikely to succeed. Most importantly, it is vital to pay attention to the worldview of the person seeking treatment. While the theory they have may be incorrect, ignoring it is likely to lead to frustration.

(f) Intervene quickly

A common mistake is to assume that because a paraphilia has been present for a long time, that it will take a long time to alleviate the symptoms. Many individuals with paraphilias think they must first review their childhood and all their previous offences before they can think about altering their current problematic behaviours. This is false. On the basis of current evidence, treatment should focus on current and future behaviours with an expectation that sexual behaviours of all types are under voluntary control. Requests to 'taper' problematic sexual behaviours should be dealt with as intentional or unintentional efforts to delay effective intervention.

(g) Be persistent

Successful treatment is not only multi-faceted but above all persistent. A useful strategy is to present treatment as a series of 'experiments' based on feedback about the effectiveness of interventions. Treatment should be presented with the expectation of success. A review of the fact that the majority of outcome studies find that the likelihood of sex offenders to recidivate is less that the likelihood of patients with major depression to have a recurrence of their life-threatening illness, is often an inspiring surprise to people entering therapy.

(h) Be inclusive with treatment

Begin with a thorough assessment and consideration of a complete differential diagnosis. If there are indications of co-morbid problems (e.g. foetal alcohol syndrome, genetic disorders, mood disorders, psychotic disorders, personality disorders, etc.) further investigations and interventions should proceed without delay. Once a diagnosis has been made, all the treatment options should be reviewed with the person seeking treatment (see above). Risks and benefits of treatment options (including the risk of declining treatment) should be thoroughly reviewed. Choice of treatment should be a collaboration between the clinician and person seeking treatment, but ultimately should be informed and voluntary. Typically treatment should include both individual and group psychotherapy. If the person has a sexual partner, couple's therapy is often of assistance. Pharmacologic treatment can include SSRIs (often more effective at doses used for depression as opposed to the higher doses used for obsessive–compulsive disorder), anti-androgens and/or GnRH analogues. Acceptance of treatment with anti-androgens is increased by explaining that treatment effects are reversible. More information about treatment options is available.[2]

(i) Be optimistic

The frequency of sex offences is dropping. The effectiveness of treatment of sex offenders (who are not necessarily paraphilic) is improving. Sex offender re-offence rates are below 15 per cent. New as well as established treatments are available.

Beyond eliminating criminal and harmful sexual behaviours, a key to successful therapy is the establishment of non-criminal and beneficial sexual interests and behaviours. Remarkably, the literature on treatment of paraphilic disorders almost completely ignores the concept of establishing non-paraphilic sexual behaviours as a treatment goal. This is a mistake. Adult men and women rarely want to 'give up' sex. However, if they are provided with the opportunity to improve their sex lives they frequently become enthusiastic (and successful) participants.

Acknowledgements

Dr Fedoroff gratefully acknowledges Drs J. Bancroft, F. Berlin, J. Bradford, E. Coleman, P. Fagin, R. Rosen, and the late J. Money for their significant influences on his thinking about the paraphilias. However, none should be held responsible for any of the opinions expressed in this chapter.

Further information

Web sites

Robert Hare Psychopathy Web site: http://www.hare.org/

Magnus Hirschfeld Archive for Sexology: http://www2.hu-berlin.de/sexology/

Kinsey institute: http://www.indiana.edu/~kinsey/

Useful summaries

Bancroft, J. (in press). *Human sexuality and its problems*. Elsevier Health Sciences In Press.

Love, B. (1999). *Encyclopedia of unusual sex practices*. Greenwich Editions, London.

Money, J. (1986). *Venuses penuses*. Prometheus Books, Buffalo, New York.

Francoeur, R.T. and Noonan, R.J. (eds.) (2004). *The continuum complete international encyclopaedia of sexuality*. Continuum, New York.

Schwartz, B.K. (ed.) (1995–2005). *The sex offender* (Vols. 1–5). Kingston, New Jersey.

References

1. Fedoroff, J.P. (in press). Sadism, sadomasochism, sex and violence. *Canadian Journal of Psychiatry*.
2. Fedoroff, J.P. (2003). Paraphilic worlds. In *Handbook of clinical sexuality for metal health professionals* (ed. S.B. Levine). Brunner/Routeledge, New York.
3. Coleman, E. (2005). Neuroanatomical and neurotransmitter dysfunction and compulsive sexual behavior. In *Biological substrates of human sexuality* (ed. J.S. Hyde), pp. 147–69. American Psychological Association, Washington, DC.
4. Hingsburger, D., Griffiths, D., and Quinsey, V. (1991). Detecting counterfeit deviance: differentiating sexual deviance from sexual inappropriateness. *Habilitative Mental Healthcare Newsletter*, 51–4.
5. Cantor, J.M., Blanchard, R., Robichaud, L.K., *et al.* (2005). Quantitative reanalysis of aggregate data on IQ in sexual offenders. *Psychological Bulletin*, **131**, 555–68.
6. Lalumière, M., Harris, G.T., Quinsey, V., *et al.* (2005). *The causes of rape*. American Psychological Press, Washington, DC.
7. Diamond, M. and Uchiyama, A. (1999). Pornography, rape and sex crimes in Japan. *International Journal of Law and Psychiatry*, **22**, 1–22.
8. Barbaree, H. and Marshall, W.L., (eds.) (2005). *The juvenile sex offender* (2nd edn). Guilford Press, New York.
9. McHugh, P.R. and Slavney, P.R. (1983). *The perspectives of psychiatry*. Johns Hopkins University Press, Baltimore.
10. Krafft-Ebing, R.V. (1906). *Psychopathia sexualis. A medico-forensic study, with especial reference to the antipathic sexual instinct*. Physicians and Surgeons Book Company, New York.
11. Brautigam, W. (1977). Die angliche Beurtelung in Psychopathologie der Sexualitae. In (eds. H. Grese and F. Stutgart).
12. Hirshfield, M. (1910). Die Transvestiten. A. Pulvermacher, Berlin.
13. Moll, A. (1983). Untersuchungen uber die Libido Sexualis. In *Freud, biologist of the mind* (ed. F.J. Sulloway), p. 304. Basic Books, New York.
14. Ellis, H. (1936). *Studies in the psychology of sex*. New York.
15. Kinsey, A.G., Pomeroy, W.B., and Martin, C.E. (1948). *Sexual behavior in the human male*. Saunders, Philadelphia.
16. Darwin, C.R. (1859). *On the origin of species by means of natural selection, or, the preservation of favored races in the struggle for life*. John Murray, London.
17. Lashley, K.S. (1938). The experimental analysis of instinctive behavior. *Psychology Review*, **45**, 445.
18. Money, J. and Lamacz, M. (1989). *Vandalized lovemaps: paraphilic outcome of seven cases in pediatric sexology*. Prometheus Books, Amherst, NY.
19. Fedoroff, J.P., Fischell, A., and Fedoroff, B. (1999). A case series of women evaluated for paraphilic sexual disorders. *The Canadian Journal of Human Sexuality*, **8**, 127–40.
20. Blanchard, R. and Bogaert, A.F. (1996). Homosexuality in men and number of older brothers. *The American Journal of Psychiatry*, **153**, 27–31.
21. Gaffney, G.R., Lurie, S.F., and Berlin, F.S. (1984). Is there familial transmission of pedophilia? *The Journal of Nervous and Mental Disease*, **172**, 546–8.
22. Fedoroff, J.P. and Pinkus, S. (1996). The genesis of pedophilia: testing the abuse to abuser hypothesis. *Journal of Offender Rehabilitation*, **23**, 85–101.
23. Shapiro, C.M., Trajonovic, N.N., and Fedoroff, J.P. (2003). Sexomnia-a new paraphilia? *Canadian Journal of Psychiatry*, **48**, 311–7.
24. Bradford, J. (1987). Medical interventions in sexual deviance. In *Sexual deviance* (eds. D.R. Laws and W. O'Donohue), pp. 449–64. The Guilford Press, New York.
25. Grossman, L.S., Martis, B., and Fichtner, C.G. (1999). Are sex offenders treatable? A research overview. *Psychiatric Services*, **50**, 349–61.
26. Bradford, J.M.W. (2001). The neurobiology, neuropharmacology and pharmacologic treatment of the paraphilias and compulsive sexual behaviour. *Canadian Journal of Psychiatry*, **46**, 26–34.
27. Greenberg, D.M and Bradford, J.M.W. (1997). Treatment of the paraphilic disorders: a review of the role of selective serotonin reuptake inhibitors. *Sexual Abuse: A Journal of Research and Treatment*, **9**, 349–60.
28. Fedoroff, J.P. (1994). Serotonergic drug treatment of deviant sexual interests. *Annals of Sex Research*, **6**, 105–17.
29. Fedoroff, J.P., Peyser, C., Franz, M.L., *et al.* (1994). Sexual disorders in Huntington's disease. *The Journal of Neuropsychiatry and Clinical Neurosciences*, **6**, 147–53.
30. Marshall, W.L., Marshall, L.E., Serran, G.A., *et al.* (2006). *Treating sexual offenders*. Routledge, New York.

31. Hanson, R.K., Gordon, A., Harris, A.J.R., *et al.* (2002). First report of the collaborative outcome data project on the effectiveness of psychological treatment of sex offenders. *Sexual Abuse: A Journal of Research and Treatment*, **27**, 169–95.
32. Marques, J.K., Weideranders, M., Day, *et al.* (2005). Effects of a relapse prevention program on sexual recidivism: final results from California's Sex Offender Treatment and Evaluation Progject (SOTEP). *Sexual Abuse: A Journal of Research and Treatment*, **17**, 79–107.
33. Laws, D.R. and O'Donohue, W. (eds.) (1997). *Sexual deviance: theory, assessment, and treatment*. The Guilford Press, New York.
34. Fedoroff, J.P., Kuban, M., and Bradford, J. (in press). Laboratory measurement of penile response in the assessment of sexual interests. In *Sex offenders: a multi-disciplinary approach to identification, risk assessment, treatment and legal issues* (eds. F. Saleh, J. Bradford, A. Grudzinskas, and D. Brodsky). Oxford Press, New York.
35. Grubin, D. (in press). Using the polygraph to manage risk in sex offenders. In *Assessment and treatment of sexual offenders: a handbook* (eds. A.R. Beech, L.A. Craig, and K.D. Browne). Wiley, London.

4.11.4 **Gender identity disorder in adults**

Richard Green

History

The behavioural phenomenon of transsexualism (now gender identity disorder) is ancient. It has been recorded for centuries and in a broad range of cultures.[1] The historic behavioural picture is comparable to that seen clinically.

In the first half of the twentieth century medical reports of sex reassignment surgery were described in Europe, primarily in Switzerland.[2] In the 1930s a wide-selling biography *Man into Woman* described a Dutch painter who underwent surgical sex reassignment.[3] Contemporary interest in transsexualism surged in 1952 when George Jorgensen, an American, travelled to Denmark and underwent hormonal and surgical treatment to become Christine Jorgensen.[4] The resultant international publicity yielded hundreds of people worldwide applying to the Danish doctors for similar treatment.[5]

By the mid-1960s there were surgeons scattered in several countries performing sex reassignment. Then in the United States at the Johns Hopkins Hospital and the University of Minnesota Hospitals and in the United Kingdom at Charing Cross Hospital, comprehensive sex reassignment programmes commenced. Extensive publicity was given to the Johns Hopkins programme as initially reported in the *New York Times* in 1966. It described the rationale for the programme and in the words of its director, 'if the mind cannot be changed to fit the body, then perhaps we should consider changing the body to fit the mind'.[6]

In 1966 the first professional text on transsexualism was written by Harry Benjamin, widely acknowledged as the 'father of transsexualism'.[7] In 1969 the first multidisciplinary text was edited by the author and John Money.[6] During the past 35 years the recognition of transsexualism, or gender identity disorder, as a treatable condition requiring psychiatric, endocrine, and surgical intervention has been accepted.

Epidemiology

The prevalence of gender identity disorder in adults is estimated from a comprehensive appraisal in the Netherlands at 1 in 10 000 males and 1 in 30 000 females.[8] At nearly all clinical centres the ratio of male-to-female patients ranges from 3:1 to 4:1, in favour of males. In some East European centres the ratio is 1:1 or reversed.[9]

Diagnosis

Diagnostic criteria of gender identity disorder in adults in DSM-IVTR[10] include a stated desire to be the other sex, a desire to live and be treated as the other sex, or the conviction that he or she has the typical feelings and reactions of the other sex. There is a preoccupation for removal of primary and secondary sexual characteristics and for procedures to alter physically the sexual characteristics to simulate the other sex. The condition is not associated with physical intersex. ICD-10 diagnostic criteria are similar but there is no mention of intersex exclusion.[11]

Origins

The search for the origins of transsexualism continues with an increasing bias towards those that are physiological. Some 20 years ago there was a false prophet in the guise of the HY antigen, on the Y chromosome believed to be influential in the development of the testes. A series of male transsexuals were found to be lacking this antigen and the tentative conclusion reached was that its absence resulted in a failure to masculinize the brain in the direction of a male identity.[12] However, the author's collaborative effort to replicate that study was not successful as all the male transsexuals studied appeared to have normal HY antigen.[13]

A more recent finding from the Netherlands implicates the brain region known as the bed nucleus of the stria terminalis. In a series of six male transsexuals studied at post-mortem over a 10-year period the size of the nucleus was comparable to that of typical females and not males.[14] A criticism of this study is that the long-term oestrogen treatment for these males may have altered the size of the nucleus. In response the researchers argue that males treated with anti-male hormone drugs or oestrogen for prostate cancer do not have an alteration in the nucleus size from typical males. However, this treatment may not be comparable to that given to transsexuals. Another criticism is that the sex difference in size of the nucleus does not manifest until early adulthood whereas the symptoms of GID often manifest earlier.

Research with male transsexuals has revealed what might be indirect markers reflecting biological distinctions. In agreement with other researchers' findings that male homosexuals have a greater likelihood of having older brothers,[15] our homosexually oriented male transsexuals also have more older brothers.[16] A theory behind this finding is that there is a progressive immunization with each pregnancy by the pregnant mother against the male foetus reflecting antigenicity of the Y chromosome. This would disrupt typical male development.

A higher ratio of aunts to uncles on the mother's side has also been found in our male transsexuals[17] a finding previously reported by another researcher for male homosexuals.[18] A theory here is that a semilethal factor has been operant in one generation (against uncles) that in the subsequent generation influences brain development resulting in an atypical behavioural pattern (homosexual or transsexual development). The finding is explainable with genomic imprinting where a gene can be dormant in one generation depending on which parent transmitted it.[17]

We also find that both male and female transsexuals are more often non-right-handed.[19] Hand use preference begins in utero and may reflect hormonal levels or cerebral dysfunction.

For female transsexuals, a series of reports indicates a higher rate of polycystic ovarian disease.[20] Although such women secrete higher levels of androgen than typical females in adulthood, prenatal levels are unstudied. However, nearly all patients with polycystic ovarian disease are not transsexual and most female transsexuals do not have polycystic ovarian disease.

Treatment

There have been no randomized controlled trials of treatment and clinical management has evolved from decades of experience.

Prior to recognition of transsexualism as a disorder deserving medical and psychiatric attention many patients self-mutilated or committed suicide[7] Transsexual patients are helped by sympathetic assessment and intervention. However, transsexuals can be difficult patients to treat. It is a rare disorder in which patients make their own diagnosis, 'I am transsexual', and prescribe their own treatment, 'I want sex-change hormones and surgery'. Patients can be demanding and impatient for the therapist's acquiescence. They may be resentful for having to see a psychiatrist, holding the opinion that the desire for hormonal treatment and surgery should be sufficient, and psychiatric agreement should be unnecessary. Some patients will threaten self-mutilation or suicide if their demands and time schedules for demands are not met. Patients need to know that psychological stability is a key ingredient to successful negotiation of the cross-gender living trial period 'Real Life Experience' (see below) and recommendation for surgery, and that suicidal behaviour is a contraindication to going forward.

The general psychiatrist should take a full psychosexual history with emphasis on the onset and development of the gender dysphoria, attempts at treatment, and the patient's long-term goals and appreciation of the obstacles to be confronted. General psychiatric and medical status needs to be understood. A referral is to be made to a specialist centre.

During the past 30 years medical doctors and psychologists specializing in the treatment of transsexualism have worked to develop effective intervention strategies. Early on there was some optimism that extensive, prolonged psychotherapy could modify the patient's gender identity to conform to the patient's birth sex. However, in the vast majority of cases, this was not possible.

During the past 20 years one project undertaken by the Harry Benjamin International Gender Dysphoria Association, the professional body dedicated to the study and treatment of transsexualism, has been setting an extensive series of requirements for evaluation and treatment of gender identity disordered people. This set of guidelines is known as the *Standards of Care*.[21] Their principal purpose is to assure that people presenting with dissatisfaction continuing to live in the sex role to which they were born undergo comprehensive psychiatric and other medical evaluation and enter into an appropriate treatment programme. The programme includes, in addition to ongoing psychiatric or psychological monitoring, possibly endocrine therapy and, depending on the outcome of the graduated trial period of cross-gender living, possibly sex reassignment surgical procedures. The philosophy of treatment is to do reversible procedures before those that are irreversible. Thus, clothing change, name change, and cross-gender role socialization, would precede endocrine treatment with its gradual somatic changes, followed, in carefully selected cases, by surgical treatment.

The screening and evaluation of patients given the opportunity to demonstrate that they will benefit from cross-gender living, perhaps culminating in surgical treatment, is known as the 'Real Life Experience'. This requires that patients live full-time for at least a year and preferably 2 years in that role. The experience includes high doses of cross-sex hormones and full-time employment or full-time student status in the new role for at least a year. If patients can demonstrate to themselves and mental health experts that they have successfully negotiated the 'Real Life Experience' and are adjusting better in this new gender role, they can be referred for surgery.

Hormonal effects

Response to hormonal treatment is variable. This is particularly notable and potentially problematic for males. As with people born female, breast development spans a continuum. Patients may erroneously believe that more oestrogen will result in greater breast development. They neglect the fact that people born female have quite adequate female hormone production but the limiting factor is tissue response. In addition to breast development, male patients report increased hip and buttock fat, skin softening, and loss of sex drive and erection capacity. Vocal retraining is required and perhaps surgical alteration of the larynx to effect a woman's voice. Facial hair removal is required. Some patients opt for major facial contour reconfiguration, performed by a few cosmetic surgeons.

Androgen treatment to the female results in voice deepening, facial hair growth, general body hair growth, menses cessation, clitoral hypertrophy, and increased sex drive. Testosterone effects are very pronounced. The deepening voice and beard growth and perhaps scalp hair loss can metamorphose the female's appearance dramatically.

Surgery

Genital surgical treatment for the male includes penectomy, orchidectomy, and creation of a neovagina. The neovagina may be created from penile skin, perhaps augmented by other skin, or from a portion of large intestine.[22] The cosmetic result is usually very good. The extent of sexual responsivity with the neovagina is mainly anecdotal. Many patients report the subjective experience of orgasm but describe it in a different form from that experienced prior to surgery as a male. Very few physiological measures of the sexual response cycle have been reported with postoperative transsexual patients.[23]

Female transsexuals undergo bilateral mastectomy, and usually hysterectomy and ovariectomy. Genital surgery is an option taken by perhaps half because of the limitations of phalloplasty. Two major approaches are utilized. One is creation of a micropenis from the androgen enlarged clitoris with relocation of the urethra to enable micturition while standing. Prosthetic testes can be incorporated into the labia sutured together. The microphallus will not permit vaginal penetration for intercourse but is erotically sensitive.[24] Alternatively, phalloplasty involves major surgical interventions with scarring at donor sites, particularly the arm.[25] The neophallus is not as close cosmetically to a natural penis as some patients want. It can be made more rigid with an inflatable implant and a conduit for urine may be surgically created. A procedure anastomosing a nerve from the arm to that enervating the clitoris offers promise of erotic sensation along some of the neophallus.

Sex reassignment outcome

Follow-up reports on operated transsexuals are generally quite favourable. An early review of several follow-up studies,[26] reported on 283 male-to-female transsexuals. Results were judged satisfactory for 71 per cent, uncertain for 17 per cent, and unsatisfactory for 12 per cent. For 83 female-to-male transsexuals results were judged satisfactory for 81 per cent, uncertain for 13 per cent, and unsatisfactory for 6 per cent. A more recent report considered reassignment successful in 46 of 50 male-to-female transsexuals and successful in all 61 female-to-male transsexuals.[27] In another study, of 55 male-to-female transsexuals, none regretted surgery and none had significant doubts regarding their reassignment status as women. Of 25 female-to-male transsexuals, at least 90 per cent were judged successful.[28] In a review of the English language literature over a 10-year period for operated transsexuals, 90 per cent of male-to-female transsexuals were judged to be satisfactory and 95 per cent of female-to-male transsexuals were similarly judged successful.[29] The criteria for success in some studies include objective measures of psychological and vocational status, in others the criterion is limited to an absence of regret over the reassignment process.

One study is notable because it effected some randomization of treatment conditions.[30] It was reported on 40 male-to-female transsexuals approved for surgery at Charing Cross Hospital, London. As patients qualified for surgery they were randomly assigned to two groups. Half were operated on in 3 months and the other half were kept on a waiting list for about 2 years. All patients completed a standardized assessment at acceptance for surgery and at the end of 2 years. The group that received the earlier surgery showed significant improvement in a range of psychometric measures and maintained employment. The unoperated group showed no improvement in psychological testing and deteriorated in employment.

Family management

Transsexual patients are often married and have children. When possible, the family should become part of the treatment process. Typically relations are strained with the marital partner of the transsexual and divorce is usual. Particularly when children are involved an effort should be made to deal with the feelings of betrayal or abandonment from the transsexual's spouse that contaminate the continuing relationship between transsexual parent and children. Often there is concern by the parents that the patient's transsexualism will impact adversely on the children. There is concern specifically in areas of gender identity of the children and peer group reactions to the knowledge that one of their age mate's parents is transsexual. However, in the author's research of 34 children of transsexuals who were living with or in regular contact with the transsexual parent, there were no instances of gender identity disorder in the children and no instances of peer group alienation that were especially problematic.[31] Children typically have many questions about the transsexual transformation of that parent that can be answered by the clinician, perhaps with the transsexual present.

The third sex

A recent development in the pattern of patients presenting clinically are those with a transgendered identity, popularly known as 'the third sex'. These males or females do not request 'sex change'. Rather, they want, if male, to be demasculinized and, if female, to be defeminized. Thus males may want castration and penectomy but no oestrogen treatment and no vagina, and females may want mastectomy, perhaps hysterectomy, but no androgen treatment and no phallus.

These patients pose a dilemma for clinicians. The crux of patient management for gender identity disorder is the 'Real Life Experience' (see above), including cross-sex hormonal treatment, the prelude to possible surgical alteration. Reversible procedures precede those that are irreversible in this management strategy. But with third-sex patients, no 'Real Life Experience' is possible. They do not have a trial period. Guidelines for testing the rationality and stability of their requests need to evolve from the body of clinicians currently attempting management of this unique population.

Transsexual patient subgroups

Professionals not experienced in the treatment of large numbers of male-to-female transsexual patients are often unaware that a substantial minority, perhaps a third, are not sexually oriented to male partners. Many of these patients have been married and are fathers, and many will be bisexual or remain sexually attracted to females only after surgery and live as lesbian women. A much smaller number of female-to-male transsexuals are sexually attracted to male partners and live as gay men after reassignment surgery.

In addition to the subtypes of transsexuals based on their sexual orientation, some male transsexual patients evolve through a diagnostic phase more closely fitting fetishistic transvestism. These patients have been more masculine in general lifestyle and appearance than other male transsexuals, cross-dressing has been sexually arousing, and they have usually been heterosexually oriented. However, with the passage of time gender dysphoria increases and fetishistic components of cross-dressing diminish or disappear. Many have been sexually aroused by fantasies of themselves as women.[32] They have been termed 'autogynephiles'. There is some evidence that males evolving through a fetishistic cross-dressing phase, presenting as somewhat older at gender identity clinics, have a poorer prognosis after surgery. However, it is primarily the progression through the 'Real Life Experience' that becomes the critical management guideline for patients, irrespective of their background.

Gender identity as a disorder

A growing movement among transsexual people argues for removal of gender identity disorder from the psychiatric and medical lists of disorders or diseases. These advocates argue that their sexual identity is normal male or female and that surgical correction of their anatomical anomaly is all that is required to allow them to live as normal men or women. Their condition is depicted as distinctive from the recognized traditional forms of mental disorder such as schizophrenia or major depression. Furthermore, carrying a psychiatric diagnosis is stigmatizing. One argument for inclusion of transsexualism in the APA diagnostic manual of disorders is that it follows the criteria of other entries, that is subjective distress and social disadvantage. Another considers third-party payment for treatment. It is unlikely that medical insurance carriers, private or governmental, would fund intervention for a non-medical condition.

Additionally, there is objection by some persons with gender identity disorder to being referred to as transsexual. They prefer the designation 'transwoman' for what has been known as male-to-female transsexualism, and 'transman' for female-to-male transsexualism.

Legal issues

Cultural and legal approaches to transsexualism vary widely across nations and cultures. They are beyond the scope of this chapter. However legal issues in the United States and United Kingdom can be summarized as follows.

Part of the 'Real Life Experience' of cross-gender living includes employment in the desired gender role. However, transsexuals may be the object of employment discrimination based on their transsexualism. In the United States, transsexuals were denied federal protection 20 years ago when the court held that the anti-sex discrimination statute protected men and women, but not transsexuals.(33) Finally, in 2004, another federal court extended employment protection.(34) In the United Kingdom, in 1997, a ruling on an English case before the European Court of Justice held that anti-sex discrimination law, to which all European Union members were subject, did include transsexuals. Thus discrimination in employment was illegal.(35)

Changing sex on one's birth certificate can be an important step in the life of the postoperative transsexual. In its absence, the person's legal sex may remain in the preoperative status, and pose obstacles to a full life. Marriage is a key issue. In the United Kingdom, until recently, postoperative transsexuals could not have a new birth certificate issued and change their legal sex. Thus a male-to-female transsexual could not marry a male and a female-to-male transsexual could not marry a female. This changed in a statute enacted in 2004.(36) In the United States most states permit some birth certificate change. However, that change may not be recognized in another state.

Further information

Barrett, J. (ed.) (2008). *Transsexual and other disorders of gender identity*. Radcliffe Publishing, Oxford.

Ettner, R., Monstrey, S., and Eyler, E. (eds.) (2008). *Principles of transgendered medicine and surgery*. Haworth Press, Binghampton.

References

1. Green, R. (1966). Transsexualism: mythological, historical and cross-cultural aspects. In *Appendix to The transsexual phenomenon* (ed. H. Benjamin). Julian Press, New York.
2. Abraham, F. (1931). Genital alteration in two male transvestites. *Zeitschrift Sexualwissenschaft*, **18**, 223–6.
3. Hoyer, N. (1933). *Man into woman: an authentic record of a change of sex*. E.P. Dutton, New York.
4. Hamburger, C., Sturup, G., and Dahl-Iversen, E. (1953). Transvestism: hormonal, psychiatric and surgical treatment. *The Journal of the American Medical Association*, **12**, 391–6.
5. Hamburger, C. (1953). The desire for change of sex as shown by personal letters from 465 men and women. *Acta Endocrinologica*, **14**, 361–75.
6. Green, R. and Money, J. (eds.) (1969). *Transsexualism and sex reassignment*. Johns Hopkins Press, Baltimore, MD.
7. Benjamin, H. (1966). *The transsexual phenomenon*. Julian Press, New York.
8. Kesteren, P., Gooren, L., and Megens, J. (1996). An epidemiological and demographic study of transsexuals in The Netherlands. *Archives of Sexual Behavior*, **25**, 589–600.
9. Godlewski, J. (1988). Transsexualism and anatomic sex ratio reversal in Poland. *Archives of Sexual Behavior*, **17**, 547–8.
10. American Psychiatric Association. (2000). *Diagnostic and statistical manual of mental disorders* (4th edn, text revision). American Psychiatric Association, Washington, DC.
11. World Health Organization. (1992). *International statistical classification of diseases and related health problems, 10th revision*. WHO, Geneva.
12. Eicher, W., Spoljar, M., Cleve, H., *et al.* (1979). H-Y antigen in transsexuality. *Lancet*, **2**, 1137–8.
13. Wachtel, S., Green, R., Simon, N., *et al.* (1986). On the expression of H-Y antigen in transsexuals. *Archives of Sexual Behavior*, **15**, 49–66.
14. Zhou, J., Hoffman, M., Gooren, L., *et al.* (1995). A sex difference in the human brain and its relation to transsexuality. *Nature*, **378**, 68–70.
15. Blanchard, R. (1997). Birth order and sibling sex ratio in homosexual versus heterosexual males and females. *Annual Review of Sex Research*, **8**, 27–67.
16. Green, R. (2000). Birth order and ratio of brothers to sisters in transsexuals. *Psychological Medicine*, **30**, 789–95.
17. Green, R. and Keverne, E.B. (2000). The disparate maternal aunt–uncle ratio in male transsexuals: an explanation invoking genomic imprinting. *Journal of Theoretical Biology*, **202**, 55–63.
18. Turner, W. (1995). Homosexuality, type 1: an Xq 28 phenomenon. *Archives of Sexual Behavior*, **24**, 109–34.
19. Green, R. and Young, R. (2001). Hand preference, sexual preference, and transsexualism. *Archives of Sexual Behavior*, **30**, 565–74.
20. Futterweit, W., Weiss, R., and Fagerstrom, R. (1986). Endocrine evaluation of 40 female-to-male transsexuals: increased frequency of polycystic ovarian disease in female transsexualism. *Archives of Sexual Behavior*, **15**, 69–78.
21. Harry Benjamin International Gender Dysphoria Association. (1981). *The standards of care for gender identity disorder*. Symposion, Düsseldorf.
22. Schrang, E. (1998). Male-to-female feminizing genital surgery. In *Current concepts in transgender identity* (ed. D. Denny), pp. 315–33. Garland, New York.
23. Green, R. (1998). Sexual functioning in post-operative transsexuals. *International Journal of Impotence Research*, **10**(Suppl. 1), 22–4.
24. Hage, J. and van Turnhout, A. (2006). Long-term outcome of metaidoiplasty in 70 female-to-male transsexuals. *Annals of Plastic Surgery*, **57**, 312–16.

25. Monstrey, S., Hoebeke, P., Dhont, M., *et al.* (2005). Radial forearm phalloplasty, review of 81 cases. *European Journal of Plastic Surgery*, **28**, 206–12.
26. Pauly, I. (1981). Outcome of sex reassignment surgery for transsexuals. *Australian and New Zealand Journal of Psychiatry*, **15**, 45–51.
27. Blanchard, R., Steiner, B., Clemensen, L., *et al.* (1989). Prediction of regrets in postoperative transsexuals. *Canadian Journal of Psychiatry*, **34**, 43–5.
28. Kuiper, B. and Cohen-Kettenis, P. (1988). Sex reassignment surgery. A study of 141 Dutch transsexuals. *Archives of Sexual Behavior*, **17**, 439–57.
29. Green, R. and Fleming, D. (eds.) (1991). Transsexual surgery follow up: status in the 1990s. In *Annual review of sex research* (eds. J. Bancroft, C. Davis, and D. Weinstein). Society for the Scientific Study of Sex, Mount Vernon, IA.
30. Mate-Cole, C., Freschi, M., and Robin, A. (1990). A controlled study of psychological and social change after surgical gender reassignment in selected male transsexuals. *The British Journal of Psychiatry*, **157**, 261–4.
31. Green, R. (1998). Transsexuals' children. *International Journal of Transgenderism*, **2**, 1–7.
32. Blanchard, R. (1989). The classification and labelling of non-homosexual gender dysphorics. *Archives of Sexual Behavior*, **18**, 315–34.
33. Green, R. (1986). Spelling relief for transsexuals: employment discrimination and the criteria of sex. *Yale Law and Policy Review*, **4**, 125–40.
34. Smith,v. City of Salem. (2004). 378 F.3d 566 (6th Cir.)
35. P v. S and Cornwall County Council. (1996). ECRI-2143 C-13/94.
36. Gender Recognition Act. (2004).

4.12

Personality disorders

Contents

4.12.1 Personality disorders: an introductory perspective
Juan J. López-Ibor Jr.

4.12.2 Diagnosis and classification of personality disorders
James Reich and Giovanni de Girolamo

4.12.3 Specific types of personality disorder
José Luis Carrasco and Dusica Lecic-Tosevski

4.12.4 Epidemiology of personality disorders
Francesca Guzzetta and Giovanni de Girolamo

4.12.5 Neuropsychological templates for abnormal personalities: from genes to biodevelopmental pathways
Adolf Tobeña

4.12.6 Psychotherapy for personality disorder
Anthony W. Bateman and Peter Fonagy

4.12.7 Management of personality disorder
Giles Newton-Howes and Kate Davidson

4.12.1 Personality disorders: an introductory perspective

Juan J. López-Ibor Jr.

The goal of psychiatry is the study of mental illnesses. In this chapter we consider the degree to which personality disorders can be considered as mental illnesses.

Basic notions

Personality is the quality that makes each one of us both different from others and consistently recognisable throughout our lives. Hence, there are two approaches to study personality. One is transversal, consisting on description of archetypes of human beings. One of the first to take this approach was Theophrastus (372–287/5 BC) who in his book *The Characters*, portrays thirty-two such prototypes. Some of them can be are easily recognized by present-day psychiatrists, for instance those typified by poor impulse control: The offensive man (*bdeluria*), the unsociable man (*authadeia*), the show-off (*alazoneia*) and the slanderer (*kakologia*); by obsessive traits: the superstitious man (*deisidaimonia*) or by paranoid traits: the suspicious man (*apistia*). The corresponding contemporary approach consists of the isolation of psychological traits or dispositions, to describe permanent inclinations to behave in a preset way.

The longitudinal approach to the study of the personality is based on the notion that there is an initial seed that develops through the lifetime. Sir Francis Galton (1822–1911) was among the first to consider the inheritance of individual differences in humans, although for centuries breeders of dogs, horses or bulls for bullfighting, had been selecting animals for mating on to select desired characteristics whether is be hunting, running or fighting.

Twin and developmental studies have been used. For example, The 'New York Longitudinal Study'[(1)] on infant temperament started in the early 1950s and examined how temperament influences adjustment throughout life. Kagan *et al.*[(2)] followed up a cohort of babies to age 14-17 years and reported that those who were highly reactive when they were babies were more likely to be 'subdued in unfamiliar situations, to report a sour mood and anxiety over the future and to be more religious'.

There are two key features of personality, one of which is temperament and the other character. The two together constitute personality.

Temperament is the innate predisposition to behave in a particular manner. Historically the concept was part of the theory of the four humours, which had corresponding temperaments: *sanguine* (the individual is led by his own pleasure to live), *choleric* (the individual has a feeling of power and shows it), *melancholic* (the individual is dominated by doubts and ruminations) and *phlegmatic* (the individual lacks any links to life, lives without effort nor pleasure). Current research on the biological basis of personality has renewed the interest in temperament.

Character is a configuration of habits, a disposition, consisting in the actualised aspects acquired through learning and shaped by experience.

Psychiatry and abnormal behaviours

Descriptions of individuals with behavioural characteristics of a negative moral or social value exist in every culture and most societies have established institutions in which the marginalized have been confined, as recorded by Foucault.[3] The distinction between immoral behaviour and mental illness was established in France at the end of the eighteenth century, coinciding with the birth of modern psychiatry. The Marquis de Sade was expelled from the Chârenton Hospital because, in words of the director, 'he is not ill, his only madness is vice'.[3] Pinel (1745–1826) considered that, in the case of the young man who in an attack of rage threw a woman into a well, although his ability to judge was clear and intact and although he presented no delusional ideas, his behaviour was characteristic of a mental patient. Consequently, this murderer was diagnosed as suffering from *manie sans délire* and his madness was classified as **reasoning madness** (*folie raisonnante*).[4] This reasoning is similar to that of Cleckley 150 years later who proposed that the social maladaptation of psychopaths is of such high degree that should considered as the result of an underlying psychotic disturbance, being personality disorders are a *mask of sanity*.[5]

Prichard,[6] defined the concept of moral insanity from which, together with the moral degeneration described by Morel (1809–1873),[7] the modern concepts of psychopathy and personality disorders are derived.

Difficulties in the study of personality disorders

Two factors have prevented the development of scientific knowledge in this field: first the negative evaluation of the concept of moral insanity, and second the dualism inherent in psychopathology.

The stigma of personality disorder

The diagnosis of personality disorder generally implies the idea of intractability and frequently leads to a lack of proper medical care. This attitude is the expression of a negative, moralising, and, according to Tyrer *et al.*,[8] delusional attitude of the doctor towards the patient. Cusack and Malaney[9] posed the question as to whether patients with antisocial personality disorders are 'bad' or 'mad'. They attempted to establish differential criteria in order to show that if patients with an antisocial personality disorder are not 'mad', then they must be considered as 'bad' and therefore must be delivered to the judicial system, after diagnosis and treatment of secondary symptoms. In 1999, the UK Government 1999 introduced a new concept: Dangerous and Severe Personality Disorder (DSPD). This subsequently became a treatment and assessment program for individuals who satisfy three requirements: 1) have a severe disorder of personality, 2) present a significant risk of causing serious physical or psychological harm from which the victim would find it difficult or impossible to recover, and 3) the risk of offending should be functionally linked to the personality disorder.[10, 11]

Dualism in psychopathology

Dualism has been present in psychiatry since its origins as specialty. According to Griesinger:[12]

> *It is time that [mental medicine] should be cultivated as a branch of brain pathology and of [the study of] the nervous system in general, and to apply serious diagnostic methods used in all branches of medicine.... Besides this purely medical element, mental medicine has another essential one and which gives a special and proper character to this part of the healing art; it is the psychological study of the aberrations of the intelligence observed in mental illnesses.*

The radical separation between mental-brain illnesses and 'aberrations of intelligence' is fundamental to modern psychopathology. Schneider[13] distinguished between psychoses as pathological conditions of the brain (disease or defective structure) and variations of the psychic way of being. Abnormal personalities, personality disorders, and neurotic disorders belong to the second category.

Schneider[14] defines some **abnormal personalities** in a statistical sense, to describe those individuals whose form of feeling, experience and behaving differs to a certain degree from what is considered to be normal for most individuals in a social group. Some of these are **psychopathic personalities** who, as a result of their abnormality, suffer or make others suffer. It should be stressed that according to Schneider's statistical definition of personality and the dualism of his psychopathological system, the only possible criterion to define a clinical condition in the absence of a brain disease is the suffering, the pathos. Suffering is for Schneider the reason why some people ask for medical care, but not a sufficient criterion for to determine the presence of an illness. Schneider had to add suffering inflicted on others (social suffering) in order to be able to include certain kinds of abnormal personalities characterized by the absence of personal suffering (heartless psychopaths, sociopaths).

It seems acceptable to consider as a patient someone who suffers and asks for clinical care although the criterion for suffering is a weak one when compared with the presence of an illness of an organ. On the contrary, the criterion of induced suffering which characterises some psychopathic personalities, defined following Schneider, is not acceptable in medicine and it is surprising that this has been little criticised. The clue lies in Schneider's definition of personality which *excludes* any biological substrate.[15] The effect of viewing psychopathies as simple variations was to reduce the amount of neurobiological research into the neuroses and personality disorders because they were not considered amenable to natural scientific methods. The study of the personality was left the new psychoanalytical and psychological theories.

Nowadays it is impossible to maintain such a reductionistic perspective, and it is recognised that the morbid nature of personality disorders can be understood through the study of changes in its biological substratum. There are not two kinds of mental disorders, the psychosis which are the consequences of brain illnesses, and the variations of the psychological way of being (neurosis and personality disorders), but two inherent aspects to each disorder. It is essential to consider psychological and psychopathological aspects of psychoses, as well as the brain dysfunction of the variations of the psychic way of being.

Models of personality

The study of personality by the different schools of differential psychology provides a solid background to help to understand the disorders of personality. Unfortunately, these studies have been conducted from different and sometimes contradictory perspectives, which are summarized in the following sections.

Categorical perspective

The categorical perspective is deep rooted in the psychiatric tradition. Categorical models consider discontinuous personality categories. This type of model is used in DSM-IV[16] and ICD-10[17] because of the need for a specific diagnostic, i.e. a categorical approach.

In modern nosology the categorisation of illness is based on the symptoms present and not on their aetiopathology, and says nothing about the nature of the disorders themselves. In the case of personality disorders, the categorisation does not affirm or deny that they are disorders or illnesses, nor does it indicate where the symptoms differ from non-morbid behaviour patterns.

This approach is supported by the notion of ideal types of Weber (1864- 1920), introduced into psychiatry by Jaspers (1883–1969) and more recently by Schwartz and Wiggins.[18] Ideal types are constructs to understand reality: An ideal type is formed by a unilateral accentuation of one or more perspectives and by the synthesis of a great deal of individual phenomena. A type describes the perfect case. Recently Doerr[19] has argued that the ideal types, when well described, become almost real types.

The experimental approach

The experimental approach looks for general laws on personality and establishes causal relations between personality variables. Wundt (1832–1920) studied the effects of modifications of stimuli on the intensity and quality of the subject's experiences introduced them. Pavlov (1849–1936) studied the conditioning of the responses to stimuli and the experimental neurosis. The behavioural approach to the personality was introduced by Watson (1878–1958) who applied objective methods to the study of human behaviour and to the relationship between stimuli and responses. Hull (1884–1952) expanded behaviourism to include learning, feelings, expectations, achievements, goals and motivations. This led to the notion that the stimulus response relationship is influenced by cognitive processes. Perception, memory, language and other functions influence the processing of information of the surrounding world and the information coming from oneself (*self*). Skinner (1904-1990) created a theory of the operating conditioning, result of a non-adaptative learning. From these perspectives, the personality is viewed as a computer which introduces, stores, transforms and produces information, including the contents of the information as well as the process in itself.[20]

The psychoanalytical approach

Freud (1856-1939)[21] proposed in the course of his life three different models of personality: The first was the speculative neuropsychological model of the *Project of a psychology for neuropsychiatrists* (1897) based on the concepts of psychic energy and psychodynamic. The second was the topographic model of the *The Interpretation of Dreams* (1900) where Freud described the conscious, preconscious and unconscious levels. The third is the structural model of *The Ego and the Id* (1923) and of *Inhibition, Symptoms and Anxiety* (1926) where Freud introduced the notions of the Id, the Ego and the Super-Ego. This last model led to a new perspective, the psychology of the Ego and the description of defence mechanisms which have a strong impact on the study of personality in clinical settings. Defence mechanisms distort reality to adapt the subject to it and to reduce anxiety. Some of them are more normal (promote adaptation to the environment), others are pathological (maladjusted or maladaptative).

The correlational approach

The correlation approach explains the individual differences based on personality traits and applying a dimensional model based on statistical correlation. Karl Pearson (1857–1936), the founder of mathematical statistics introduced the correlation coefficient (correlates of cognitive flair with variables like age, gender, weight, height and so on). Charles E. Spearman (1863–1945) applied to research on the traits of personality, a factorial analysis that groups different qualities around a series of correlational factors or dimensions.

Traits are the basic elements of a personality and individual differences are defined and classified along dimensions. The theoretical assumption is that the structure of personality is common to all individuals; it differs in the different combination of traits. Trait is a disposition to respond in a determined way to a determined situation. Traits characterize persons through brief and precise descriptions on stable ways to behave, and as behaviour is consistent, it is possible to predict behaviours. This approach has paved the way to basic dimensions of individual differences.

Dimensional models

Jung (1875-1961) made the first important contribution to the dimensional concept of the personality, based on the concept of trait or disposition.[22] A trait is a permanent inclination towards behaving in a determinant way. Traits are distributed along dimensions which make it possible to classify individuals according to their personality. The different dimensional models are based on the supposition that we all share the same personality structure, differing in the different combination of the mentioned traits. These models have benefited from the innovative statistic techniques, which allows to group different qualities of the individual character around factors of correlation or dimensions.

This dimensional approach raises several questions. How many traits define personality? Are the traits universal? Do traits relate only to manifest behaviours or are they part of feelings, values or thoughts? The problem of the number of dimensions that define personality led to the search for external validators such as biological, cultural and genetic factors. Eysenck[23] identified there are three basic types of personality: extroversion-introversion, neuroticism and psychoticism, each one including multiple levels of traits. For Eysenck and Eysenck,[24] the concept of arousal level is essential. Every individual has an optimal activation level of specific systems of the central nervous system—the better they feel, the better they will perform. This approach has been developed by many authors including Zuckermann,[25] who described sensation-seeking behaviour, Oreland *et al.*,[26] and Siever and Davis,[27] who proposed new traits and dimensions.

Cloninger[28] initially proposed three dimensions: novelty-seeking, harm avoidance, and reward dependence. Latter, he attempted to overcome the dichotomy between dimensional and categorical models by using four temperamental dimensions (novelty-seeking, harm avoidance, reward dependence, and persistence), which are life-long and stable, and three character dimensions (self-direction, co-operation, and self-transcendency) which are variable and susceptible to environmental influences and development.[29]

The five-factor model, based on factorial studies and individual differences[30] has been widely accepted. It comprises the personality dimensions openness, conscientiousness, extraversion, agreeableness, and neuroticism, known by the acronym OCEAN. About 40 per cent of individual personality differences can be explained in terms of heredity.[31] In the five-factor model the same proportion does not apply to each factor; openness to experience appears to have the greatest hereditary input, whereas conscientiousness appears to have the least.

Mathematical tools allow recombining the data in order to find higher order factors of the Big Five. Two of them have appeared in many studies: 1) related to the Big Five trait dimensions Agreeableness, Conscientiousness, and Emotional Stability (meta-trait alpha) and 2) the dimensions Extraversion and Intellect (meta-trait beta).[32] Other have found some extra traits to be added to the Big Five, such as honesty-humility.[33]

An interesting approach is lexicographic, which is based on the examination of relations among personality-descriptive adjectives that are indigenous to various languages. They tend to reveal a structure corresponding closely to the Five-Factor Model, with some differences in the nature of the Agreeableness and Emotionality/Neuroticism factors and also in the existence of a sixth factor, Honesty-Humility.[34] This has been found in different languages such a tagalong with some differences (a Filipino extra factor resembled a Negative Valence or Infrequency dimension).[34] A study with college students yielded seven major dimensions; many of the factors were similar to recognized lexical personality factors. Big Five Conscientiousness and Neuroticism were each strongly associated with a single proverb dimension (interpreted as Restraint and Enjoys Life, respectively). Big Five Agreeableness, Extraversion, and Intellect/Imagination were all associated with several proverb dimensions. Agreeableness was most strongly associated with proverb dimensions representing Machiavellian behaviour and strong Group Ties, and both Extraversion and Intellect showed particularly notable associations with an Achievement Striving dimension. The two remaining proverb dimensions, which represented a belief that Life is Fair and an attitude of Cynicism, could not be accounted for by the Big Five.[35]

Critics of this approach have argued that a) little progress has been made in this area, b) structural models have little direct relevance for psychopathology research, c) the principal methodological tool of structural research–factor analysis–is too subjective to yield psychologically meaningful results and 4), some clinically relevant aspects, such as alexithymia or impulsivity, do not appear in the studies on the structure of personality.

Alexithymia positively correlates with Neuroticism (N) and negatively with Extraversion (E) and Openness (O), whereas no significant relations were found with Agreeableness (A) and Conscientiousness (C).[36] Impulsivity. The term impulsive madness was used in German literature and Jaspers[37] put it in relation to nostalgia and displacement. The balance between social and individual norms is related to the origin of mental disorders. Durkheim[38] introduced the concept of **anomia** when describing a particular form of suicide in individuals who perceive that their own norms and values are no longer relevant and that their relation to the community is weak or non-existent. However, the opposite may also occur. Kraus[39] coined the term **hypernomia** for premorbid personality traits of depressive patients, which consist in an exaggerated form of adaptation to social norms. This personality type is the converse of the impulsive madness that can be characterized as **hyponomic**. We have proposed the term **dysnomic** for obsessive patients[40] who show a distorted adaptation to social norms. For example, patients with obsessions and compulsions related to cleanliness usually appear to be extremely dirty because of their fear of contamination and their unrealistic compulsions, which are based more on 'magic' control than on efficient behaviour oriented towards concrete goals.

The common link in the psychopathology of obsessive-compulsive disorders and the group of impulsive disorders experienced by the **impulsivists**[41] is poor control of the impulses, in the sense that novel interior or exterior experiences are not converted into adequate behavioural patterns. Rather, obsessives abandon actions uncompleted and impulsivists behave in a disorganised manner (acting out). In both cases, 'the irrelevant substitutes the relevant'.[42]

Today, the trend is to look for a classification of personality disorder which will be dimensional, either by selecting one of the existing models by developing a common, integrative representation including the important contributions of each of the models.[43]

Models of personality and personality disorders

The ideal goal of a single structural framework to be applied to normal and abnormal personality is not easy to reach. In a study with the Eysenck Personality Questionnaire-Revised (EPQ-R) the three clusters of personality disorders of DSM found equivocal support. Exploratory principal components analysis and confirmatory factor analysis found four broad factors of personality disorder that overlapped with normal personality traits: an asthenic factor related to neuroticism; an antisocial factor associated with psychoticism; an asocial factor linked to introversion-extraversion; and an anankastic (obsessive-compulsive) factor. In spite of this, there is growing agreement about the number and type of broad personality disorder dimensions; similar dimensions may be found in clinical and non-clinical samples, suggesting that those people with personality disorders differ quantitatively rather than qualitatively from others; and there is substantial overlap between normal and abnormal personality dimensions.[44] For Livesley *et al.*,[45] personality disorders are quantitatively extreme expressions of normal personality functioning developed around four factors: Emotional Dysregulation, Dissocial Behaviour, Inhibitedness and Compulsivity. In the same year, the same group published some different results in another study:[ ] they found 16 basic dispositional traits (anxiousness, affective lability, callousness, cognitive dysregulation, compulsivity, conduct problems, insecure attachment, intimacy avoidance, narcissism, oppositionality, rejection, restricted expression, social avoidance, stimulus seeking, submissiveness, and suspiciousness) and three higher-order patterns (emotional dysregulation, dissocial behaviour, and inhibitedness).[46]

Markon *et al.*[47] have delineated an integrative hierarchical account of the structure of normal and abnormal personality. This hierarchical structure integrates many Big Trait models proposed in the literature. Similarly, O'Connor[48] reanalyzing the published studies found high level of support for both theoretically and empirically based representations of the five-factor model approach to personality disorders. The five-factor model personality dimensions of Neuroticism, Extraversion, and Agreeableness are the most apparent in the DSM-III-R conceptualizations of the personality disorders.[49,50] The five-factor model structure is present although with some variance in the current DSM-IV cluster set.[50]

Mulder and Joyce[51] have attempted to construct a simplified system for the classification of personality disorders related to normally distribute human personality characteristics. A four-factor solution of personality disorder symptoms was obtained and they labelled these factors 'the four As': Antisocial, Asocial, Asthenic and Anankastic. The factors related to the four temperament dimensions of the Tridimensional Personality Questionnaire (TPQ), but less closely to Eysenck Personality Questionnaire (EPQ) dimensions. The four factors were similar to those identified in a number of studies using a variety of assessment methods and this lends some credibility to our findings.

The masking of sanity becomes evident in some dissocial, psychopathic and even criminal behaviours that are the expression of underlying disorders. The issue is very relevant because those can be treated. One example is attention deficit hyperactivity disorder (ADHD) which has important forensic implications. For decades there has been an interest in predicting which children will become psychopaths in order to establish primary prevention interventions. Lynam[52] described the fledgling psychopath, characterized by symptoms of hyperactivity-impulsivity-attention problems and conduct problems are at the greatest risk for becoming chronic offenders. Other authors[53,54] have strongly argued against the clinical-forensic utility of tests designed to assess juvenile psychopathy.

The problems of axis II of the diagnostic and statistical manual

There are several reasons in favour of an independent axis for personality disorders. First it is important not to forget personality in the diagnostic process, especially when using symptomatic classifications (DSM-III / IV and ICD-10). Second, personality may be a predisposing factor, or something essential for the response to treatment and for prognosis.[54] Third personality traits are egosyntonic: they include traits that the subject has accepted as an integrative part of him/herself in a progressive way (when compared to axis I disorders and non-psychiatric illnesses which are something 'that occurs').

Seen from a theoretical perspective, personality disorders may be considered as the expression of the personality's functioning, which is essential for patients, be they psychiatric or not.[45]

But there are also reasons to combine Axis I and Axis II. The better a personality disorder is known and the more biological correlations are found in it, the higher the probabilities it has to be moved to Axis I: Epileptic personality (adhesivity, gliscroidy) became long ago organic disorder of the personality, cyclothymic personality became cyclothymia and depressive personality (at least in part), dysthymia in DSM-III. Schizotypal personality is schizotypal disorder in ICD-10 and several studies emphasise the strong relation of borderline personality disorder and mood (affective) disorders.[55]

Although through most of the 20th century, from K. Schneider to DSM-IV, personality disorders and mental illnesses were studied as separate fields, there has been increasing recognition of the substantial overlap of – and comorbidity between – disorders both within and across axes and interest in the joint study of normal and abnormal personality.[56] In comorbid cases, the personality disorder could be a predisposing factor, a consequence, or an attenuated form of the mental disorder, or it could be independent of the mental disorder. The fact that the association between a mental disorder and a personality disorder is not always fortuitous has been shown by the observation that effective treatment of the former can lead to the disappearance of the latter, as has been demonstrated in the treatment of obsessive-compulsive patients with pharmacotherapy and behavioural therapy.[57]

The main difference between mental and personality disorders may be that the latter are early onset variants with a very chronic course. According to the hypothesis of a spectrum of disorders, personality disorders can often be treated by the same method as those applied to the major psychiatric disorders to which they are related. Patients with anxious or avoidant personality disorder may respond to anxiolytic medication, patients with borderline personality disorder may respond to lithium and antidepressives, patients with schizotypal personality disorder may respond to antipsychotic agents, and patients with disorders characterised by poor impulse control may respond to antidepressives with a selective serotonergic action.

The diathesis-stress model

The diathesis-stress model has been used to explain the relationship between personality and mental disorders. Supposedly broad, innate temperament dimensions, sometimes correlated with somatic characteristics such as body type (Kretschmer [1888–1964]), develop and differentiate themselves through both biologically and environmental events into a hierarchical personality trait structure. At their extremes, are risk factors (diatheses) for psychopathology, especially given adverse life experiences (stress). Rosenthal[58] defined this model as an inherent constitutional predisposition which only becomes apparent under the impact of environmental stress.

The onset early in life, the variability of expression dependent on setting, the greater association with more severe disorders and the acceptance as intrinsic components of functioning by most suffering from personality disorders support the notion that they are diatheses rather than disorders.[59]

Personality disorders have been considered as belonging to the spectrum of major psychiatric disorders. However, it must be remembered that external events, such as brain damage (organic personality disorders), or the psychological impact of a catastrophic event may also lead to personality changes. Severe psychiatric disorders may have a repercussion on the personality of the patient, and other illnesses may also have this effect. For example, chronic pain (of organic nature) can be accompanied by a profound personality change (algogenic psychosyndrome). Hypochondria or dissociative symptoms and traits may become relevant only after the patient has suffered an illness, or a problem related to diagnosis or treatment, or a problem involving the patient–physician relationship.

Recent research has focused on the impact of social conditions in the neuroendocrine regulation of the individual, especially regarding the adaptation to stressful situations. In patients with borderline personality disorder and suicidal impulsive behaviour we have found when compared to the control group, high basal concentrations of cortisol (suggesting a high level of stress) and a very blunted response to the stimulus (suggesting a reduced capacity to respond to external stimulus).[60] A clue to the interpretation of these results lies in the work of Sapolsky,[61] who has studied the adaptation to stress of baboons in the Serengeti savannah in Africa. Males of a lower rank have consistently high concentrations of the stress hormone hydrocortisone in their blood, whereas the concentration is lower in the dominant males. However, in the dominant males hydrocortisone concentrations increase rapidly at times of stress and decrease once the situation is resolved, whereas the lower-order males, who live in a permanent state of stress, are unable to initiate more adaptive resources (increase hydrocortisone secretion) when new stressful events appear. These patterns are the consequence and not the cause of the rank (if the opposite were true, the baboons who were physiologically better able to respond to stressful situations would achieve a higher rank). During periods of revolution, members of the colony hold successively different ranks and, although there is always one dominant animal, the stability of the society is lost and with it the stress-adapted physiology of the dominant males who show prolonged increased hydrocortisone concentrations like the rest of the group. When calm is established again, the normal pattern related to the hierarchical rank of the baboons is restored regardless of what their cortisol secretion pattern was prior to the revolution.

Relational disorders

This model can be applied to the relational disorders or processes. On one side every clinician has the experience of persons whose behavioural problems happen in specific environments (i.e., the family) or in relation to specific persons (i.e., the spouse) while their behaviour is totally normal in the rest of circumstances. Another observation is the case of personality disorders that once beginning to improve after a therapeutic intervention, the whole atmosphere around him or her changes. The patient himself and their relations start to consider that the personality as not a stable and incorrigible set of traits but something that can change for the better. However, it is the influence of child psychiatrists looking for childhood antecedents of mayor psychiatric disorders of adulthood[62] and family therapists that have requested a new diagnostic category to describe these situations.

It has also been claimed that in order to be able to proceed along this line, some problems have to be addressed, although the same may also be present in diagnostic categories accepted in DSM-IV and ICD-10. The main one are: 1) the little consensus on assessment means; 2) the complexity of relational assessment, which results in a lack of well-accepted, evidence-based operational definitions; 3) insufficient empirical testing of relational issues; and 4) the resistance to labeling social difficulties as disorders.[63]

These difficulties can be surmounted if new diagnostic perspectives are implemented. One is the concept of diseases as harmful dysfunctions a view which holds that disorders are harmful failures of biologically selected functions. There are evolutionarily selected functions that depend for their performance on the nature of the interaction between individuals. These relations can fail, even when both individuals are normal, because of mismatches between normal variations. Thus, there are genuine relational dysfunctions that, when harmful, are relational disorders.[64] The Structural Analysis of Social Behavior (SASB) has operationalised interpersonal theory for the research of relational aspects of psychopathology and becoming a useful diagnostic tool.[65]

The research agenda for DSM-V recognizes that the diagnosis of relational disorders is one of the most important gaps in the current DSM-IV.[66] Specific recommendations include developing assessment modules, determining the clinical utility of relational disorders, determining the role of relational disorders in the aetiology and maintenance of individual mental disorders, and considering aspects of relational disorders that might be modulated by individual mental disorders.

Personality disorders vs. personality variants

It is necessary to establish a clear distinction between personality disorders and personality variants, and to view the former as true morbid entities. ICD-10 allows us to differentiate, at least theoretically, personality disorders that appear in the chapter on mental disorders from personalities relevant for medicine in Chapter Z.[67] Personality disorders should be characterised by the presence of symptoms, and relevant personalities by their traits. Symptoms are used as diagnostic criteria in a categorical classification, while psychological traits can be classified according to dimensions.

Personality variants relevant to medicine, although not morbid, play an important role in the aetiopathogenesis of illnesses or are important for prognosis and rehabilitation. The study of the variants of personality also reminds the practitioner of the necessity to identify the uniqueness of the patient's personality.

The frontiers with normal personality are not well explained or justifiable threshold,[68] except for schizotypal disorder and borderline disorder. There are great variations between the different versions of DSM (DSM-III - DSM-III-R) leading in the case of schizotypal disorder to a reduction of prevalence from 11 per cent to 1 per cent.[69]

On the other hand, normal the population also presents maladaptative variants of traits such as: neuroticism, irritability, vulnerability, anxiety, depression, impulsivity, low consciousness, rush, negligence, hedonism, immorality, unreliable, irresponsibility, high antagonism, manipulation, disappointment, exploitation, aggressiveness, cruelty, heartless.

In everyday practice there is a need for categorical approach, essential to define the frontiers of clinical activity, for research, for management and for forensic questions and also of a dimensional approach, to identify functions and its alterations, relevant for interventions with patients. This could be done investigating in new personality models, adopting the multi-axial version of ICD-10[70] (Table 4.12.1.1.), implementing diagnostic system that include a nosographic approach and idiographic perspective[71] or adopting

Table 4.12.1.1 Multiaxial formulation of ICD-10

Axis I	Clinical disorders (DSM-IV axis I, II and III): personality disorders understood as morbid states of the personality
Axis II	Disablement
Axis III	Relevant non morbid circumstances, including variants of the personality (i.e., Type A behaviour) Normal personality traits (i.e.: five factors model)

Table 4.12.1.2 Proposed five axis system (Charney *et al.* 2002)

Axis I: Genotype	Identification of disease-/ symptom-related genes, of resiliency/protective genes and genes related to the therapeutic response and side effects of psychotropic drugs
Axis II: Neurobiological phenotype	Identification of intermediate phenotypes (neuroimaging, cognitive function, emotional regulation) related to genotype and to targeted pharmacotherapy
Axis III: Behavioural phenotype	Range and frequency expressed behaviours associated with genotype, neurobiological phenotype and environment, related to targeted therapies
Axis IV: Environmental modifiers or precipitators	Environmental factors that alter the behavioural and neurobiological phenotype
Axis V: Therapy	Therapeutic options base don the data of axes I to IV

a new multiaxial system[72] (Table 4.12.1.2). Several authors have claimed for a functional psychopathology. Van Praag[73] has recommended a two-tier diagnosis: 1) nosological diagnosis and 2) psychological dysfunctions correlated with biological variables.

The cosmetic of the personality?

Cosmetic or palliative pharmacotherapy is to use a psychotropic agent to make feel better to a person who is not ill. It usually intents to mitigate unwanted or unaccepted personality traits in order to attain a higher order of social normality and acceptability. Kamer[74] has described how a selective serotonin uptake inhibitor used for the treatment of depression and for other psychiatric alterations can remove personality traits in some people. He has considered traits previously considered as an expression of human misery or, in some cases, as the consequence of negative childhood experiences. Kamer even questions whether there could be a 'pandemic' of cosmetic psychopharmacologies which would lead to the disappearance of phenomena such as anguish which are essential for personal realisation in the arts, religion, and creativity. For example, fluoxetine can make non depressed people feel more vital, mentally more alert and become more popular, leading to an increased feeling of wellness. Shyness became a treatable illness when paroxetine was found to improve the symptoms of social phobia and atomoxetine can change the life conditions of adults with a history of ADHD. Most of these cases are probable subthreshold clinical conditions, something which may lead to a change in diagnostic habits, lowering thresholds or modifying criteria. For instance the DSM criteria of suffering or disablement are value loaded, and new values, such as wellbeing may be introduced.

Conclusions

During the last few decades there has been an impressive growth in research and knowledge on personality disorders. There is a strong growing evidence that they are "real" disorders that can be managed in ways similar to the rest of psychiatric disorders. There is also a growing consensus on the need for a new classification able to capture the nuances beyond the rigidity of present nosological systems. There is also a need for a clearer delimitation from normal personality variants something that will have important impacts, for instance in forensic settings or for reimbursement purposes.

Further information

International Society for the Study of Personality Disorders (ISSPD)
isspd@isspd.com info@isspd.com http://www.isspd.com
International Journal of the ISSPD, Guilford Publications, New York
info@guilford.com

References

1. Thomas, A. and Chess, S.1. (1984) Genesis and Evolution of Behavioral Disorders: From Infancy to Early Adult Life. *Am J Psychiatry*, **141**, 1–9.
2. Kagan, J., Snidman, N., Kahn, V., *et al.* (2007) *The preservation of two infant temperaments into adolescence*. Monographs of the Society for Research in Child Development, Serial No. 287, vol. 72, no. 2. Blackwell, Boston.
3. Foucault, M. (1961) *Folie et déraison. Histoire de la folie à l'âge classique*. Plon, Paris.
4. Pinel, P.H. (1809) *Traité médico-philosophique sur l'alienation mentale*. Brosson, Paris.
5. Cleckley, H. (1941) *The mask of sanity*. Henry Kimpton, London.
6. Prichard, J.C. (1835) *A treatise on insanity and other disorders affecting the mind*. Sherwood, Gilbert and Piper, London.
7. Morel, B. (1859) *Traité des dégéneréscences physiques, intellectuelles et morales de l'espèce humaine*. Paris.
8. Tyrer, P., Casey, P., and Ferguson, B. (1991) Personality disorder in perspective. *British Journal of Psychiatry*, **159**, 463–71.
9. Cusack, J.R. and Malaney, K.R. (1992). Patients with antisocial personality disorder. Are they bad or mad? *Postgraduate Medicine*, **91**, 341–4, 349–52, 355.
10. Maden,T. and Tyrer, P. (2003) Dangerous and severe personality disorders: a new personality concept from the United Kingdom. *Journal of Personality Disorders*, **17**, 489–96.
11. Tyrer, P. (2007) An agitation of contrary opinions. *British Journal of Psychiatry*, **190**, (suppl.49), 1–2.
12. Griesinger, W. (1872) *Gesammelte Abhandlungen. Vol. I, Psychiatrische und nervenpathologische Abhandlungen*. Reprinted by Bonset, Amsterdam, 1968.
13. Schneider, K. (1971) *Klinische Psychopathologie* (9th edn). Thieme, Stuttgart.
14. Schneider, K. (1950) *Die psychopathischen Persönlichkeiten* (9th revised edn). Deuticke, Vienna.
15. López Ibor, J.J. (1966) *Las neurosis como enfermedades del ánimo. Gredos, Madrid.*
16. American Psychiatric Association (1994*) Diagnostic and statistical manual of mental disorders* (4th ed.). American Psychiatric Association, Washington, DC.
17. World Health Organization (1992*) The ICD-10 classification of mental and behavioural disorders—clinical descriptions and diagnostic guidelines*. World Health Organization, Geneva.
18. Schwartz, M.A. and Wiggins, O.P. (1987) Diagnosis and ideal types: a contribution to psychiatric classification. *Comprehensive Psychiatry*, **28**, 277-91.
19. Personal communication
20. Pervin, L. (Ed.) (1990) *Handbook of personality: Theory and research*. The Guilford Press. New York.
21. Freud, S., Freud, A., Strachey, J. (1953–1974) *The standard edition of the complete psychological works of Sigmund Freud*. Hogarth Press Richmond UK.
22. Jung, C.J. (1966) *Two essays on analytical psychology*. Princeton University Press, Princeton, NJ.

23. Eysenck, H.J. (1970) *The structure of human personality*. Methuen, London.
24. Eysenck, H.J. and Eysenck, M.W. (1985) *Personality and individual differences: A natural science approach*. Plenum Press, New York.
25. Zuckermann, M. (1979) *Sensation seeking: Beyond the optimal level of arousal*. Erlbaum, Hillsdale, NJ.
26. Oreland, L., Wiberg, A., Åsberg, M., *et al.* (1981) Platelet MAO activity general clinical description of personality disorders and monoamine metabolism in CSF in depressed and suicidal patients and in healthy controls. *Psychiatric Research*, **4**, 21–9.
27. Siever, L.J. and Davis, K.L. (1991) A psychobiological perspective on the personality disorders. *American Journal of Psychiatry*, **148**, 1647–58.
28. Cloninger, C.R. (1987) A systematic method for clinical description and classification of personality variants. *Archives of General Psychiatry*, **44**, 573–88.
29. Cloninger, C.R. (1996) A psychobiological model of temperament and character. Fundamental findings for use in clinical practice. In *New research in psychiatry* (ed. H. Häfner and E.M. Wolpert), pp. 95–112. *Hogrefe and Huber, Göttingen.*
30. McCrae, R.R. and John, O.P. (1992) An introduction to the five-factor model and its applications. *Journal of Personality*, **60**, 175–213.
31. Loehlin, J.C. (1992) *Genes and environment in personality development*. Sage, Newbury Park, CA.
32. Digman, J.M. (1997) Higher-order factors of the Big Five. *Journal Personality and Social Psychology*, **73**, 1246–56.
33. Ashton, M.C. and Lee, K. (2005) Honesty-humility, the big five, and the five-factor model. *Journal of Personality*, **73**, 1321–53.
34. Church, A.T., Reyes, J.A., Katigbak, M.S., *et al.* (1997) Filipino personality structure and the big five model: a lexical approach. *Journal of Personality*, **65**, 477–528.
35. Haas, H.A. (2002) Extending the search for folk personality constructs: the dimensionality of the personality-relevant proverb domain. *Journal of Personality and Social Psychology*, **82**, 594–609.
36. Luminet, O., Bagby, R.M., Wagner, H., *et al.* (1999) Relation between alexithymia and the five-factor model of personality: a facet-level analysis. *Journal of Personality Assessment*, **73**, 345–58.
37. Jaspers, K. (1909) *Heimweh und Verbrechen*. F.C.M. Vogel, Leipzig.
38. Durkheim, E. (1951) *Suicide*. Free Press, Glencoe, IL.
39. Kraus, A. (1977) *Soziales Verhalten und Psychosen manisch-depressiver*. Enke, Stuttgart.
40. López-Ibor, J.J. (1991) Obsessive-compulsive disorder and other disorders. *European Neuropsychopharmacology*, **1**, 275–9.
41. Lacey, J.H. and Evans, C.D.H. (1986). The impulsivist: a multi-impulsive personality disorder. *British Journal of Addiction*, **81**, 641–9.
42. Janet, P. (1903) *Les obsessions et la psychasthenie*. Alcan, Paris.
43. Widiger, TA. (2007) Dimensional models of personality disorder. *World Psychiatry*, **6**, 15–9.
44. Deary, I.J., Peter, A., Austin, E., *et al.* (1998) Personality traits and personality disorders. *British Journal of Psychology*, **89**, 647–61.
45. Livesley, W.J., Jang, K.L., Vernon, P.A. (1998) Phenotypic and genetic structure of traits delineating personality disorder. *Archives of General Psychiatry*, **55**, 941–8.
46. Livesley, W.J. (1998) Suggestions for a framework for an empirically based classification of personality disorder. *Canadian Journal of Psychiatry*, **43**, 137–147.
47. Markon, K.E., Krueger, R.F., Watson, D. (2005) Delineating the structure of normal and abnormal personality: an integrative hierarchical approach. *Journal of Personality and Social Psychology*, **88**, 139–57.
48. O'Connor, B.P. (2002) The search for dimensional structure differences between normality and abnormality.. *Journal of Personality and Social Psychology*, **83**, 962–82.
49. Trull, T.J. (1992) DSM-III-R personality disorders and the five-factor model of personality: An empirical comparison. *Journal of Abnormal Psychology*, **101**, 553–60.
50. Blais, M.A. (1997) Clinician ratings of the five-factor model of personality and the DSM-IV personality disorders. *Journal of Nervous and Mental Diseases*, **185**, 388–93.
51. Parker, G., Hadzi-Pavloic, D., Wilhelm, K. (2000) Modeling and measuring the personality disorders. *Journal of Personality Disorders*, **14**, 189–98.
52. Mulder, R.T., Joyce, P.R. (1997) Temperament and the structure of personality disorder symptoms. *Psychologial Medicine*, **27**, 99–106.
53. Lynam, D.R. (1996) Early identification of chronic offenders: who is the fledgling psychopath? *Psychological Bulletin*, **120**, 209–34.
54. Seagrave, D., Grisso, T. (2002) Adolescent development and the measurement of juvenile psychopathy. *Law and human behavior*, **26**, 219–39.
55. Hart, S.D., Watt, K.A., Vincent, G.M. (2002) Commentary on Seagrave and Grisso: impressions of the state of the art. *Law and human behavior*, **26**, 241–5.
56. Widiger, T.A., Frances, A. (1985) Axis II personality disorders: diagnostic and treatment issues. *Hospital and Community Psychiatry*, **36**, 619–27.
57. Akiskal, H.S., Akiskal, K.K., Perugi, G., *et al.* (2006) Bipolar II and anxious reactive 'comorbidity': Toward better phenotypic characterization suitable for genotyping. *Journal of Affective Disorders*, **96**, 239–47.
58. Clark, L.A. (2005) Temperament as a unifying basis for personality and psychopathology. *Journal of Abnormal Psychology*, **114**, 505–21.
59. Ricciardi, J.N., Baer, L., Jenike, M.A., *et al.* (1992) Changes in DSM-III-R axis II diagnoses following treatment of obsessive-compulsive disorder. *American Journal of Psychiatry*, **149**, 829–31.
60. Rosenthal, D. (1970) *Genetic theory and abnormal behavior*. New York: McGraw Hill.
61. Tyrer, P. (2007) Personality diatheses: a superior explanation than disorder. *Psychological Medicine*, **12**, 1–5.
62. López-Ibor, J.J., Jr, Lana, F., and Sáiz, J. (1991) *Serotonin, impulsiveness and aggression in humans*. In Serotonin related psychiatric syndromes: clinical and therapeutic links (ed. G.B. Cassano and H.S. Akiskal), pp. 35–9. Royal Society of Medicine, London.
63. Sapolsky, R.M. (1990) Adrenocortical function, social rank, and personality among wild baboons. *Biological Psychiatry*, **15**, 862–78.
64. Manzano, J., Zabala, I., Borella, E., *et al.* (1992) Continuity and discontinuity of psychopathology: a study of patients examined as children and as adults. I. Antecedents of adult schizophrenic disorders. *Schweierz Archiv für Neurologie und Psychiatrie,* **143**, 5–25.
65. Lebow, J. and Gordon, K.C. (2006) You cannot choose what is not on the menu—obstacles to and reasons for the inclusion of relational processes in the DSM-V: comment on the special section. *Journal of Family Psychology*, **20**, 432–7.
66. Wakefield, J.C. (2006) Are there relational disorders? A harmful dysfunction perspective: comment on the special section. *Journal of Family Psychology*, **20**, 423–7.
67. Erickson, T.M. and Pincus, A.L. (2005) Using Structural Analysis of Social Behavior (SASB) measures of self- and social perception to give interpersonal meaning to symptoms: anxiety as an exemplar. *Assessment*, **12**, 243–54.
68. Beach, S.R., Wamboldt, M.Z., Kaslow, N.J., *et al.* (Eds.) (2006) *Relational Processes and DSM-V. Neuroscience, Assessment, Prevention, and Treatment*. American Psychiatric Publishing Inc., Washington.
69. World Health Organization (1992) *The ICD-10 International Classification of Mental and Behavioral Disorders. Clinical descriptions and diagnostic guidelines*. Geneva, WHO.
70. Widiger, T.A., Costa, P.T. Jr. (1994) Personality and personality disorders. *Journal of Abnormal Psychology*, **103**, 78–91.

71. Blashfield, R., Blum, N., Pfohl, B. (1992) The effects of changing axis II diagnostic criteria. *Comprehensive Psychiatry*, **33**, 245–5.
72. Janca, A., Kastrup, M., Katschnig, H., *et al.* (1996) The ICD-10 Multiaxial System for Use in Adult Psychiatry: Structure and Applications. *The Journal of Nervous and Mental Diseases*, **184**, 191–192.
73. Mezzich, J.E. (2007) Psychiatry for the Person: articulating medicine's science and humanism. *World Psychiatry*, **6**, 1–3.
74. Charney, D.S., Barlow, D.H., Botteron, K., *et al.* (2002) *Neuroscience research agenda to guide development of a pathophysiologically based classification system. In: A Research Agenda for DSM-V. Kupfer, D., First, M., Regier, D.A. (Eds.), pp:31–83*, American Psychiatric Association, Washington.
75. Van Praag, H.M. (1990). Two-tier diagnosing in psychiatry. *Psychiatry Research*, **34**, 1–11.
76. Kamer, P.D. (1993) *Listening to Prozac*. Viking, New York.

4.12.2 **Diagnosis and classification of personality disorders**

James Reich and Giovanni de Girolamo

Definitions of personality disorders

There has been considerable interest in the study of personality and personality disorder (PD) since early times and in many different cultures. However, as noted by Tyrer *et al.*[(1)] 'The categorization of personality disorder did not receive any firm support until the time of Schneider'. Schneider[(2)] regarded abnormal personalities as 'constitutional variants that are highly influenced by personal experiences' and identified 10 specific types or classes of 'psychopathic personality'. The classification system proposed by Schneider has deeply influenced subsequent classification systems[(1)]: of the 10 types of PD identified by Schneider, eight are closely related to similar types of PD as classified in DSM-III.[(3)] Many of these categories are also represented in DSM-IV[(4)] and ICD-10.[(5)]

Personality is defined in the second edition of the WHO *Lexicon of Psychiatric and Mental Health Terms*[(6)] as 'The ingrained patterns of thought, feeling, and behaviour characterising an individual's unique lifestyle and mode of adaptation, and resulting from constitutional factors, development, and social experience'. Personality disorders, according to the ICD-10 diagnostic guidelines[(5)]:

> . . . comprise deeply ingrained and enduring behaviour patterns, manifesting themselves as inflexible responses to a broad range of personal and social situations. They represent either extreme or significant deviations from the way the average individual in a given culture perceives, thinks, feels, and particularly, relates to others. Such behaviour patterns tend to be stable and to encompass multiple domains of behaviour and psychological functioning. They are frequently, but not always, associated with various degrees of subjective distress and problems in social functioning and performance.

For example, a dependent PD in a favourable environment might not cause dysfunction, but nevertheless might be considered a disorder since it is clinically identical to the same disorder that usually causes dysfunction.

DSM-IV[(4)] defines a PD as 'an enduring pattern of inner experience and behaviour that deviates markedly from the expectations of the individual's culture'. The pattern is manifested in two or more of the following areas: cognition, affectivity, interpersonal functioning, and impulse control. The pattern is inflexible and pervasive across a broad range of situations, has an early onset, is stable and leads to significant distress or impairment.

Personality traits, according to DSM-IV,[(4)] 'are enduring patterns of perceiving, relating to and thinking about the environment and oneself that are exhibited in a wide range of social and personal contexts. Only when personality traits are inflexible and maladaptive and cause significant functional impairment or subjective distress do they constitute PDs.'

ICD and DSM classifications of personality disorders

Table 4.12.2.1 lists the specific PDs as classified in ICD-9,[(7)] ICD-10, DSM-IIIR,[(8)] and DSM-IV.

In the ICD-10 classification, which does not have a multiaxial system for the separate recording of the personality status, PD can be diagnosed together with any other mental disorder, if present. Although a multiaxial system for ICD-10 is being developed, this will not include a separate axis for PDs, as in DSM-IV.

Despite the importance given to behavioural manifestations for the classification and assessment of PDs, personality traits and attitudes are also considered when a diagnosis is made. The ICD-10 diagnostic guidelines subdivide PDs 'according to clusters of traits that correspond to the most frequent or conspicuous behavioural manifestations'. As stressed by Widiger and Frances,[(9)] the reliance on behavioural indicators can improve inter-rater reliability, which reduces the amount of inferential judgement required for the diagnosis, but it does not ensure that the same diagnosis will be made at different times. Moreover, the diagnosis of a PD cannot be based on a single behaviour, as any given behaviour may have multiple causes (e.g. situational and role factors).

There have been four studies that have explored the diagnostic categories for PDs contained in ICD-10 and compared them with the DSM classification. The first[(10)] was carried out among 177 American clinicians who found some degree of overlap between the different categories. When the authors compared the diagnostic categories in ICD-10 with those in DSM-IIIR, they found that only anankastic (ICD) and obsessive–compulsive (DSM) PDs showed a high level of correspondence. The second study[(11)] looked at 52 outpatients and compared DSM-IIIR to ICD-10. It found fair concordance for the diagnosis of 'any PD', but poor agreement for individual PDs; the ICD-10 tended to overdiagnose PDs relative to DSM-IIIR. The third report[(12)] compared ICD-10 and DSM-IV in 58 patients with panic disorder. There was good agreement for the presence of 'any PD', and a reasonable agreement between individual diagnoses (κ ranged from 0.51 to 0.83.), with a tendency for ICD-10 to overdiagnose PDs relative to DSM-IV. In the fourth study,[(13)] ICD-10 criteria were found to have satisfactory inter-rater reliability in a sample of homeless adults.

In the American taxonomic system, a multiaxial classification was first introduced in DSM-III. With the development of DSM-IIIR, more than 100 changes in the classification of PDs were introduced compared with DSM-III.[(14,15)] While the multiaxial and categorical style of classification was maintained, the diagnostic criteria were revised to form a list of symptoms for each PD, of

Table 4.12.2.1 Comparison of different classification systems of personality disorders: ICD-9, ICD-10, DSM-IIIR, and DSM-IV

ICD-9	ICD-10	DSM-III-R	DSM-IV
Paranoid personality disorder	Paranoid personality disorder	Paranoid personality disorder	Paranoid personality disorder
Schizoid personality disorder	Schizoid personality disorder	Schizoid personality disorder	Schizoid personality disorder
Personality disorder with predominantly sociopathic or asocial manifestations	Dissocial personality disorder	Antisocial personality disorder	Antisocial personality disorder
	Emotionally unstable personality disorder:		
Explosive personality disorder	Impulsive type	NA	NA
NA	Borderline type	Borderline personality disorder	Borderline personality disorder
Histrionic personality disorder	Histrionic personality disorder	Histrionic personality disorder	Histrionic personality disorder
Anankastic personality disorder	Anankastic personality disorder	Obsessive-compulsive personality disorder	Obsessive-compulsive personality disorder
NA	Anxious [avoidant] personality disorder	Avoidant personality disorder	Avoidant personality disorder
NA	Dependent personality disorder	Dependent personality disorder	Dependent personality disorder
Affective personality disorder Asthenic personality disorder	Other specific personality disorders	Passive-aggressive personality disorder Schizotypal personality disorder Narcissistic personality disorder Self-defeating personality disorder Sadistic personality disorder	NA Schizotypal personality disorder Narcissistic personality disorder NA NA Personality disorder not otherwise specified

which only a certain number were required for a diagnosis to be reached. In DSM-IIIR, each category of PD comprised 7 to 10 criteria, with the presence of four to six criteria required for diagnosis. DSM-IIIR contained 11 PDs (see Table 4.12.2.1), plus two new disorders (self-defeating PD and sadistic PD) that were not included in DSM-III but were considered as diagnostic categories needing further study. As in DSM-III, the 11 PDs were divided into three clusters:

- cluster A (the 'odd' or 'eccentric' cluster), which included paranoid, schizoid, and schizotypal PD;
- cluster B (the 'dramatic' or 'erratic' cluster), which included histrionic, narcissistic, antisocial, and borderline PDs; and
- cluster C (the 'anxious' cluster), which included avoidant, dependent, obsessive–compulsive, and passive–aggressive PDs.

One study in the United States examined changes in personality diagnoses using DSM-III versus DSM-IIIR.(16) For some categories there was a considerable difference in the frequency of diagnosis: for example, there was an 800 per cent increase in the rate of schizoid PD and a 350 per cent increase in the rate of narcissistic PD diagnosed by the clinicians when DSM-IIIR criteria were applied.

DSM-IV was designed to be a conservative evolution from DSM-IIIR; however, some differences in diagnoses between DSM-IIIR and DSM-IV can be expected.(17) In general, the different DSMs should not be considered interchangeable unless there is specific data supporting agreement of a diagnosis across systems. As shown in Table 4.12.2.1, DSM-IV includes 11 PDs as in the DSM-IIIR classification; slight changes were introduced in the diagnostic criteria, and a new category 'PD not otherwise specified' added. Passive–aggressive, self-defeating, and sadistic PDs (provisionally included in DSM-IIIR) were dropped. The overall effect of these changes will be to increase the concordance between the DSM-IV and the ICD-10 classification systems compared with that between DSM-IIIR and ICD-10. DSM-IV also includes the three clusters present in DSM-IIIR.

Similarities differences between ICD-10 and DSM-IV

Table 4.12.2.1 shows that for seven categories of PD (paranoid, schizoid, dissocial/antisocial, histrionic, anankastic/obsessive–compulsive, anxious/avoidant, and dependent), there is a specific correspondence between ICD-10 and DSM-IV. For three categories, there are differences in nomenclature between the two systems; in particular ICD-10 uses the term 'anankastic' instead of 'obsessive–compulsive', to avoid the erroneous implication of an inevitable link between this type of personality and obsessive–compulsive disorder. ICD-10 also uses the term 'dissocial' instead of 'antisocial', to prevent any possible connotation of stigmatization, and the term 'anxious' instead of 'avoidant'. Moreover, while DSM-IV classifies borderline PD as a specific category, ICD-10 includes it as a subcategory of emotionally unstable PD. Narcissistic and passive–aggressive PDs (present in DSM-IV) are included in ICD-10 under the category of 'other specific PDs'. Finally, while DSM-IV includes schizotypal PD as a PD, ICD-10 classifies it in the overall group of 'Schizophrenia, schizotypal and delusional disorders', to highlight the contiguity between this disorder and the schizophrenia group disorders, as shown by genetic and clinical studies. DSM-IV has the category 'Personality disorders not otherwise specified', while ICD-10 has the category 'Other specific personality disorders'.

Changes in the conceptualization of DSM personality disorders since the last edition of this chapter

Empirical research has advanced in the years following the original chapter in an earlier volume. These changes have impacted our understanding and use of DSM measurement instruments. These changes are that the personality disorders as described by DSM are not as enduring as we once thought. The instruments to measure the DSM PDs have modest agreement at best on the categorical level. Finally these instruments do not seem to adequately fit most of the disorders diagnosed which are diagnosed in the remainder category, 'Personality Disorder NOS'.

1. Research indicating lack of enduring quality of personality disorders.

There has now been considerable research indicating that some aspects of personality are state like. This was a line of research pursued by Reich[18,19] and later confirmed by others.[20] This means that some personality traits may disappear relatively rapidly—the state component. Experienced researchers have also found that even when personality disorders are selected for long-term study by careful methods, significant percentages of these will not be found on retest within a 6 month to several year periods.[21,22]

2. Modest agreement of personality DSM personality disorder instruments.

Research has been fairly consistent from the beginning of DSM instruments that while they may measure aspects of clinical relevance even well-designed instruments of the same design (self-report or semi-structured interview) are compared on categorical diagnoses, the agreements are usually modest at best.[23] (The results improve somewhat when using dimensional measures.) In addition when personality disorders are measured in a clinical population very few fit into the established categories and most wind up in the 'remainder bin' of personality disorder NOS.[24]

3. The problem of chasing changing criteria.

Each time the wording of a questionnaire is changed it can make significant difference in the outcome of the questionnaire or survey even though the changes may seem minor. This means that for every change in a version of the DSM, the DSM personality test developers would theoretically have to do extensive reliability and validity testing all over again. Unfortunately this is a time-consuming and expensive process which is beyond the resources of most DSM test developers. What happens instead is that either they do not update their instrument or update only the questions to conform to the new DSM criteria without doing new validity testing. Although these updated tests may have 'face validity' they (understandably) do not have extensive reliability and validity testing.

4. Conclusions from intervening research on DSM personality instruments.

At the end of the day we are left with the DSM personality measurement instruments being limited by the conceptualizations behind them which may be incorrect. These errors may either by in the enduring nature of the personality disorders and the nature of the proper categories or the nature of the specific criteria for a category. These measures then become good dimensional measures of various aspects of personality pathology and a rough clinical guide for 'disorder'. However, no one should expect that what one of these instruments is measuring is really the same as another. They do, however, conform to the DSM nomenclature.

Categorical versus dimensional styles of classification

In general, researchers involved in the assessment of personality traits tend to use dimensional measures based on normal populations. In contrast, those concerned with personality types and, even more, clinicians concerned with PDs, tend to employ categorical concepts and assessment measures based on these concepts.[15]

Each of the two approaches has specific advantages and disadvantages. The drawbacks of the categorical approach are represented by the difficulty of classifying patients who are at the boundary of different categories or who do not meet the diagnostic criteria for any specific PD, but who still have significant pathology. Other points that should be addressed include the wide variation of symptomatology found within each given category, the need for heterogeneous categories, such as 'mixed' and 'atypical', the need to simplify necessarily complex conditions, the need to define valid cut-off points, and the use of a nominal rather than an ordinal scale.

Those in favour of a dimensional approach argue that PDs differ from normal variations in personality only in terms of degree, and to some extent this is supported by empirical data.[25,26] However, there is evidence that some dimensional models do not account for all of the abnormal personality traits (see discussion on the 'Big five' models below.)

Moreover, it is still unclear whether normal and abnormal personality traits are the same or whether they are qualitatively different. Two main findings seem to support the latter hypothesis: first, normal personality traits are at least moderately heritable, while abnormal personality traits appear less heritable; second, the prevalence rates of PDs found in surveys are much greater than would be expected from the prevalence rates of normal personality traits in the general population. Some researchers[27] have even suggested that an extreme form of a normal personality trait is not necessarily pathological. Although some authors argue that there is no difference between normal and abnormal personality traits,[25] and this is still an area of open inquiry, it does appear more and more likely that there are some abnormal personality traits that differ from normal ones. It is possible that different models may be appropriate in different situations.

1. 'Big Five' personality measures and DSM-IV personality disorders

Since the first edition of this chapter there has been a fair amount of research using the 'big five' personality factors. There is evidence that the big five factors can account for some, but not all of the pathological personality pathology described by the DSM system.[28] However the amount of information also depends on the specific instrument with some with more facets or detail being more able account for aspects of pathological personality. These would be instruments such as the NEO-PI[29] and the five factor model of Cloninger.[30] Also of possible greater utility are dimensional instruments which were designed from the start to measure abnormal as well as normal personality. These include the Schedule for Non-adaptive and Adaptive Personality (SNAP)[31] and Dimensional Assessment of Personality Pathology (DAPP).[32] Also worth noting is a method by Widiger which combines a five factor self-report with a five factor interview in order to obtain more comprehensive personality information.[33]

2. Other non-DSM personality measures from which DSM PD diagnoses can be derived.

There is one measure of DSM-IV personality which is derived from the interpersonal circumplex model. This is the Wisconsin Personality Disorders Inventory (currently in version IV).[34] Although from a fairly different theoretical perspective from the DSM-IV it does have translations to make some DSM-IV diagnoses.[35]

Another unique approach is the Shedler–Westen Assessment Procedure which does not have a patient interview but rather has a clinician who knows the patient do a Q sort procedure. The process is based on distinguishing personality disorders based on prototypes. This procedure can be translated into DSM personality diagnoses. It tends to create fewer diagnoses because the number of descriptors that can be used is limited by the Q sort procedure.[36]

The Millon Clinical MultiAxial Inventory (now in version three) is a very commonly used personality measure. It is now based on evolutionary theory according to its manual. One of the best validated instruments in data-based terms. Unfortunately this data is mostly published in its own manual and not the journal literature. As the population that the instrument was validated on included some fairly severe disorders it is not clear how well the findings would translate into a less severely ill population.[37]

Assessment methods for personality disorders

Table 4.12.2.2 shows the main methods currently available for assessing all PDs. Additional instruments for assessing specified PDs have also been developed—some of the methods listed are

Table 4.12.2.2 Some commonly used assessment methods for all DSM personality disorders

Name of the instrument	Author(s) [(a)]	Method of assessment	Number of Questions	Time required (minutes)
Diagnostic Interview for Personality Disorders (DIPD)	Zanarini	Semistructured interview with patient using DSM-IV criteria	398	60–120
Dimensional Assessment of Personality Disorders (DAPP-BQ)	Livesley & Jackson	Dimensional based of normal and abnormal personality. Has components of DSM-IV PDs	290	45
International Personality Disorder Examination (IPDE)	Loranger *et al.*	Semistructured interview with patient using ICD-10 and DSM-IV criteria	537	150
Millon clinical Multiaxial Inventory (MCMI)	Millon	Self-report by patient using DSM-IV criteria	175	20–30
NEO Personality Inventory-Revised (NEO PI-R)	Costa & McRae	Comprehensive measurement of normal and abnormal personality traits.	240	30–40
Personality Assessment Schedule (PAS)	Tyrer *et al.*	Semistructured interview with informant (s) can derive ICD-10 and DSM-IV diagnoses.	24	60
Personality Diagnostic Questionnaire –Revised (PDQ-4)	Hyler *et al.*	Self-report by patient or informant(s) using DSM-IV criteria	99	30
Personality Disorders Interview-IV	Widiger *et al.*	Semistructured interview with patient using DSM-IV criteria	325	60–120
Schedule for Nonadaptive and Adaptive Personality (SNAP)	Clark	Self report by patient using DSM-IV and dimensional criteria	375	30–60
Shedler-Westen Assessment Procedure	Westen & Shedler	Clinician rated Q sort procedure. Gives abnormal traits, symptoms and defences and can generate DSM-IV diagnoses	200	No interview, based of clinician knowledge of client.
Structured Clinical Interview for DSM-IV Personality Disorders (SCID-II)	First & Gibbon	Semistructured interview with patient using DSM-IV criteria	303	60–90
Structured Interview for DSM Personality Disorders-IV (SIPD)	Pfohl *et al.*	Semistructured interview with patient or informant(s) using DSM-III criteria	337	90
Temperament and Character Inventory (TPQ)	Cloninger *et al.*	Self-report by patient. Temperament and Character dimensions.	240	30–40
Wisconsin Personality Disorders Inventory (WISPI)	Klein *et al.*	Self-report by patient using DSM-III-R criteria. Correlated with interpersonal object relation theory.	214	30

[(a)] For specific references to each instrument please see references.[30, 31, and 33] new, while others have been revised two or three times.[38,39] The following points related to these methods need to be mentioned.

1 The interview measures have generally shown a satisfactory inter-rater reliability, while test–retest reliability has not been well established. However, three methods do show some evidence of good test–retest reliability—the Personality Assessment Schedule (**PAS**),[40] the International Personality Disorder Examination (**IPDE**),[41] and the Structured Clinical Interview for Personality Disorders (**SCID-II**).[42] Many of the methods have been standardized on psychiatric inpatient or outpatient populations; their applicability in epidemiological community studies is largely unknown.[43,44]

2 The various measures tend not to agree with each other on specific diagnoses.[38,39] A measurement on one standardized instrument is not necessarily the same as the measurement on another.

3 Some authors, mostly developers of interview instruments, have in the past stated that self-report measures are not as valid for the measurement and study of personality as interview measures. These arguments tend to be based on the finding that self-report instruments do not agree well with interview instruments, and that a PD diagnosis cannot be made without a clinical interview. The first argument does not hold water, since none of the interview instruments agree well with each other either. Whether self-report instruments can reliably diagnose a PD (as opposed to personality traits) is an open question. However, dimensional interview instruments have high test–retest reliability (some for as long as 30 years) and have been, and will continue to be, a valuable component of personality research, especially where the focus is on dimensions.[45] Self-report instruments measuring DSM disorders tend to disagree with each other in a similar way to the interview instruments. In conclusion, the instrument chosen for any given clinical or research endeavour should reflect the ability of the individual instrument to meet the specific needs of the project. Most researchers now believe that using a self-report, which may be more sensitive but less specific is a good prelude to a semi-structured interview measure.

4 Standardized testing of personality and clinician impression do not tend be in good agreement. This is due both to the tendency of instruments to report more disorders and for clinicians to use idiosyncratic criteria in their diagnoses.[46,47] Standardized measures are a must, however, if the data is to be used for research or public policy purposes.

5 Most personality measurement instruments are affected by the comorbid presence of a non-personality emotional disorder (Axis I disorder in the DSM system). Some structured interviews try to correct for this by asking patients about times when they were not suffering from an Axis I disorder; however, when the Axis I disorder is chronic, this may be difficult to achieve.[41,42] This problem also affects the ability of questionnaires to differentiate between current Axis I disorders and PDs, as this self-judgement of patients who are suffering from a psychiatric condition is frequently impaired.[41] The PDE, PAS, and SCID-II may be less affected by this problem.

6 There is disagreement among experts about the use of informants. Many authors have argued that, besides the patient, a key informant should also be interviewed, given the likelihood that many patients will not reply reliably to questions about their personality and the possibility that informant ratings will differ substantially from patient ones.[41,48] However, even if an informant is interviewed, it is often unclear which source to use to score the test if the interviewee and informant disagree. This tends to reduce their value. More recent research indicates that informants may be of value if their information is in certain areas that are easily observable to then and then are incorporated into the evaluation process in a standardized way.[49]

7 Discriminant validity refers to the ability of a diagnostic system and measurement system to diagnose non-overlapping disorders. Discriminant validity is not high with the ICD-10 and DSM-IV PDs.[50] This means that it is the rule, rather the exception, that multiple personality diagnoses will be made: some studies have provided evidence of this assumption. For instance, in four studies that examined personality comorbidity in a total of 568 patients, the average percentage of multiple diagnoses was 85 per cent.[51] To what extent this reflects the real coexistence of different disorders—with distinct patterns of symptoms, correlates, and course—or if it is simply the effect of an insufficient discriminant validity of current diagnostic systems has still to be clarified.

Further information

Reich, J. (2005). State and trait in personality disorders. In *Personality disorders: current research and treatments* (ed. J. Reich), pp. 3–20. Taylor & Francis, New York.

Reich, J. (2007). State and trait in personality disorders. *Annals of Clinical Psychiatry*, **19**, 37–44.

Widiger, T.A., Costa, P.T., and Samuel, D.B. (2006). Assessment of maladaptive personality traits. In *Differentiating normal and abnormal personality* (2nd edn) (eds. S. Strack and M. Lorr), pp. 311–55. Springer, New York.

References

1. Tyrer, P., Casey, P., and Ferguson, B. (1991). Personality disorder in perspective. *British Journal of Psychiatry*, **159**, 463–71.
2. Schneider, K. (1923). *Die psychopathischen personlichkeiten*. Springer, Berlin.
3. American Psychiatric Association. (1980). *Diagnostic and statistical manual of mental disorders* (3rd edn). American Psychiatric Press, Washington, DC.
4. American Psychiatric Association. (1994). *Diagnostic and statistical manual of mental disorders* (4th edn). American Psychiatric Association, Washington, DC.
5. World Health Organization. (1992). *International statistical classification of diseases and related health problems, 10th revision*. WHO, Geneva.
6. World Health Organization. (1994). *Lexicon of psychiatric and mental health terms* (2nd edn). WHO, Geneva.
7. World Health Organization. (1977). *International classification of diseases, injuries and causes of death, ninth revision*. WHO, Geneva.
8. American Psychiatric Association. (1987). *Diagnostic and statistical manual of mental disorders* (3rd edn, revised). American Psychiatric Press, Washington, DC.
9. Widiger, T.A. and Frances, A. (1985). Axis II personality disorders: diagnostic and treatment issues. *Hospital and Community Psychiatry*, **36**, 619–27.

10. Blashfield, R.K. (1991). An American view of the ICD-10 personality disorders. *Acta Psychiatrica Scandinavica*, **82**, 250–6.
11. Sara, G., Raven, P., and Mann, A. (1996). A comparison of DSM-III-R and ICD-10 personality disorder criteria in an outpatient population. *Psychological Medicine*, **26**, 151–60.
12. Starcevic, V., Bogojevic, G., and Kelin, K. (1997). Diagnostic agreement between the DSM-IV and ICD-10-DCR personality disorders. *Psychopathology*, **30**, 328–34.
13. Merson, S., Tyrer, P., Duke, P., *et al.* (1994). Interrater reliability of ICD-10 guidelines for the diagnosis of personality disorders. *Journal of Personality Disorders*, **8**, 89–95.
14. Gorton, G. and Akhtar, S. (1990). The literature on personality disorders, 1985–1988: trends, issues and controversies. *Hospital and Community Psychiatry*, **41**, 39–51.
15. Widiger, T.A., Frances, A., Spitzer, R.L., *et al.* (1988). DSM-III-R Personality disorders: an overview. *American Journal of Psychiatry*, **145**, 786–95.
16. Morey, L.C. (1988). Personality disorders in DSM-III and DSM-III-R: convergence, coverage and internal consistency. *American Journal of Psychiatry*, **145**, 573–7.
17. Coolidge, F.L. and Segal, D.L. (1998). Evolution of personality disorder diagnosis in the diagnostic and statistical manual of mental disorders. *Clinical Psychology Review*, **19**, 583–99.
18. Reich, J. (2005). State and trait in personality disorders. In *Personality disorders: current research and treatments* (ed. J. Reich), pp. 3–20. Taylor & Francis, New York.
19. Reich, J. (2007). State and trait in personality disorders. *Annals of Clinical Psychiatry*, **19**, 37–44.
20. Clark, L.A. (2005). Stability and change in personality pathology: revelations of three longitudinal studies. *Journal of Personality Disorders*, **19**, 524–32.
21. Zanarini, M.C., Frankenburg, F.R., Hennen, J., *et al.* (2006). Prediction of the 10-year course of borderline personality disorder. *American Journal of Psychiatry*, **163**, 827–32.
22. Skodol, A.E., Gunderson, J.G., Shea, M.T., *et al.* (2005). The collaborative longitudinal personality disorders study (CLPS). *Journal of Personality Disorders*, **19**, 487–504.
23. Widiger, T.A. and Coker, L.A. (2002). Assessing personality disorders. In *Clinical personality assessment. Practical approaches* (2nd edn) (ed. J.N. Butcher), pp. 407–34. Oxford University Press, New York.
24. Verheuk, R. and Widiger, T.A. (2004). A meta-analysis of the prevalence and usage of the personality disorders not otherwise specified (PDNOS) diagnosis. *Journal of Personality Disorders*, **18**, 309–19.
25. Livesley, W.J., Schroeder, M.L., Jackson, D.N., and Jang, K.L. (1994). Categorical distinctions in the study of personality disorders: implications for classification. *Journal of Abnormal Psychology*, **103**, 6–17.
26. Schroeder, M.L. and Livesley, W.J. (1991). An evaluation of DSM-III-R personality disorders. *Acta Psychiatrica Scandinavica*, **84**, 512–59.
27. Birtchnell, J. (1988). Defining dependence. *British Journal of Medical Psychology*, **61**, 111–23.
28. Clark, L.A. and Harrison, J.A. (2001). Assessment instruments. In *Handbook of personality disorders: theory, research and treatment* (ed. W.J. Livesley), pp. 277–306. Guilford Press, New York.
29. Costa, P.T. and McCrae, R.R. (1992). *Revised NEO personality inventory (NEO PI-R) and NEO five-factor inventory (NEO-FFI) professional manual.* Psychological Assessment Resources, Odessa, FL.
30. Cloninger, C.R., Przybeck, T.R., Svrakic, D.M., *et al.* (1994). *The temperament and character inventory (TCI): a guide to its development and use.* Center for Psychobiology of Personality, Washington University, St. Louis, MO.
31. Clark, L.A. (1993). *Schedule for adaptive and nonadaptive personality.* University of Minnesota Press, Minneapolis, MN.
32. Livesley, W.J. and Jackson, D.N. (2006). *Manual for the dimensional assessment of personality pathology.* Sigma, Port Huron, MI.
33. Widiger, T.A., Costa, P.T., and Samuel, D.B. (2006). Assessment of maladaptive personality traits. In *Differentiating normal and abnormal personality* (2nd edn) (eds. S. Strack and M. Lorr), pp. 311–55. Springer, New York.
34. Klein, M.H. and Benjamin, L.S. (1996). *The Wisconsin Personality Inventory-IV.* Wisconsin Psychiatric Institute, Madison, WI.
35. Smith, T.L., Klein, M.H., and Benjamin, L.S. (2003). Validation of the Wisconsin Personality Inventory-IV with the SCID-II. *Journal of Personality Disorders*, **17**, 173–87.
36. Westen, D., Shedler, J., and Bradley, R. (2006). A prototype approach to personality disorder diagnosis, *American Journal of Psychiatry*, **163**, 846–56.
37. Millon, T., Millon, C., Davs R., *et al.* (2006). *MCMI-III manual* (3rd edn). Dicandrien Inc., Minneapolis, MN.
38. de Girolamo, G. and Reich, J.H. (1993). *Personality disorders.* WHO, Geneva.
39. Reich, J.H. (1989). Update on instruments to measure DSM-III and DSM-III-R personality disorders. *Journal of Nervous and Mental Disease*, **177**, 366–70.
40. Tyrer, P., Casey, P., and Gall, J. (1983). Relationship between neurosis and personality disorder. *British Journal of Psychiatry*, **142**, 404–8.
41. Loranger, A.W., Sartorius, N., Andreoli, A., *et al.* (1994). The international personality disorder examination: the World Health Organization/alcohol, drug abuse, and mental health administration international pilot study of personality disorders. *Archives of General Psychiatry*, **51**, 215–24.
42. Ouimette, P.C. and Klein, D.N. (1995). Test-retest stability, mood-state dependence and informant-subject concordance in the SCID-Axis II questionnaire in a non clinical sample. *Journal of Personality Disorders*, **9**, 105–11.
43. Zimmerman, M. (1994). Diagnosing personality disorders. A review of issues and research methods. *Archives of General Psychiatry*, **51**, 225–45.
44. Jackson, H.J., Gazis, J., Rudd, R.P., *et al.* (1991). Concordance between two personality disorder instruments with psychiatric inpatients. *Comprehensive Psychiatry*, **32**, 252–60.
45. Clark, L.A., Livesley, W.J., and Morey, L. (1997). Special feature: personality disorder assessment: the challenge of construct validity. *Journal of Personality Disorders*, **11**, 205–31.
46. Blashfield, R.K. and Herkov, M.J. (1996). Investigating clinician adherence to diagnosis by criteria: a replication of Morey and Ochoa (1989). *Journal of Personality Disorder*, **10**, 219–28.
47. Perry, J.C. (1992). Problems and considerations in the valid assessment of personality disorders. *American Journal of Psychiatry*, **149**, 1645–53.
48. Dodwell, D. (1988). Comparison of self-ratings within informant-ratings of pre-morbid personality on two personality rating scales. *Psychological Medicine*, **18**, 495–502.
49. Ready, R.E., Watson, D., and Clark, L.A. (2002). Psychiatric patient- and informant-reported personality. *Assessment*, **9**, 361–72.
50. Bornstein, R.F. (1998). Reconceptualizing personality disorder diagnosis in the DSM-IV: the discriminant validity challenge. *Clinical Psychology: Science and Practice*, **5**, 333–43.
51. Widiger, T.A. and Rogers, J.H. (1989). Prevalence and comorbidity of personality disorders. *Psychiatric Annals*, **19**, 132–6.

4.12.3 Specific types of personality disorder

José Luis Carrasco and Dusica Lecic-Tosevski

Cluster A personality disorders

Paranoid personality disorder

Pervasive suspiciousness, mistrust, hypersensitivity to criticism, and hostility are the essential features of paranoid personality disorder. These individuals live a restricted emotional and interpersonal life because they fear the malevolent intent of others. As a rule, paranoid people are ready to counter-attack, provoking repeated confrontations. In this way, they induce hostility and resentment in others.

The term paranoia may lead to some confusion if it is not properly delimited. Paranoid had been used as an adjective to label various delusional representations or syndromes. Kraepelin[(1)] differentiated paranoia as a distinct condition characterized by chronic and highly systematized delusional ideas (see Chapter 4.4). Schneider[(2)] described people with this paranoid personality as fanatic psychopaths, stressing their intensity, and rigidity in confrontation with others. He denied any relationship with paranoia. Freud[(3)] and other psychoanalysts construed the paranoid character as a pattern of mistrust and feeling of being attacked, based on distortions and externalization of the person's inner world.

Paranoid personality disorder was included in DSM-III with criteria of suspiciousness, mistrust, hypersensitivity, and restricted affectivity. This last criterion does not appear in DSM-IV and ICD-10, since restricted affectivity is neither necessary nor specific for paranoid personalities. Instead, emphasis is placed on mistrust and sensitivity to setbacks. The DSM-IV criteria for paranoid personality disorder are shown in Table 4.12.3.1.

Table 4.12.3.1 DSM-IV diagnostic criteria for paranoid personality disorder

A. A pervasive distrust and suspiciousness of others such that their motives are interpreted as malevolent, beginning by early adulthood and present in a variety of contexts, as indicated by four (or more) of the following

1. Suspects, without sufficient basis, that others are exploiting, harming, or deceiving him or her
2. Is preoccupied with unjustified doubts about the loyalty or trustworthiness of friends or associates
3. Is reluctant to confide in others because of unwarranted fear that the information will be used maliciously against him or her
4. Reads hidden demeaning or threatening meanings into benign remarks or events
5. Persistently bears grudges, i.e. is unforgiving of insults, injuries, or slights
6. Perceives attacks on his or her character or reputation that are not apparent to others and is quick to react angrily or to counterattack
7. Has recurrent suspicions, without justification, regarding fidelity of spouse or sexual partner

B. Does not occur exclusively during the course of Schizophrenia, a Mood Disorder With Psychotic Features, or another Psychotic Disorder and is not due to the direct physiological effects of a general medical condition.

Note If criteria are met prior to the onset of Schizophrenia, add 'Premorbid', e.g. 'Paranoid Personality Disorder (Premorbid)'

(a) Epidemiology

The prevalence of paranoid personality disorder is estimated at about 0.5 to 1 per cent in the general population and at 10 to 20 per cent among psychiatric patients. The disorder is more commonly diagnosed in males.

(b) Aetiology

This personality disorder has a familial relationship with delusional disorders and with schizophrenia,[(4)] and has been included in the so-called schizophrenic spectrum.[(5)] Deficits in cortical dopamine activity may be associated with a poor conceptual organization that could in turn be responsible for suspiciousness and distorted interpretations.[(6)]

Mistrust and lack of confidence may reflect deficits arising in early developmental stages and resulting in a lack of basic self-confidence.[(7)] Lack of protective care and affective support in childhood could perhaps facilitate the development of paranoid features.

(c) Clinical picture

Paranoid individuals do not often ask for help from psychiatrists. They have no wish to be cured; instead, they believe that they have to be protected from other people's hatred and attacks. Subjects with this personality disorder suspect that others are acting to harm, exploit, or deceive them. These suspections are based not on objective evidence, but on internal conviction and an attempt to find a rational explanation for the supposed wrongs.

Paranoids are reluctant to confide in others; they tend to feel that others are plotting against them, and that the enemy may be found in unexpected places. They do not readily tell others about their suspicions. The disorder may be manifested by irritability, unusual defensive or self-protective behaviours (e.g. locking doors and closing windows and curtains to avoid being spied on, and hiding papers or documents), or emotional detachment.

Paranoid people lack confidence in others. They doubt the loyalty or trustworthiness of friends and partners, and check their behaviour repeatedly for evidence of malevolent intentions. They assume that others are not trustworthy, to the extent that they cannot believe it when friends demonstrate their loyalty. They withhold personal or significant information from friends, fearing that it will be used maliciously against them. They do not form close friendships and are often isolated. When in trouble, paranoids do not expect help from friends or others close to them; instead, they expect to be attacked or ignored.

Many of the suspicious and distrustful attitudes of paranoids are perpetuated by their intense interpersonal sensitivity. They react intensely to any comment or event that may relate to them. Hidden meanings that are demeaning and threatening may be read into benign events or the remarks of others. Unintended errors by colleagues or public servants are taken as deliberate attempts to harm or deceive them. Humorous remarks or jokes may be interpreted as attacks on their character. Paranoids are easily hurt, and their pride is easily damaged by minor critical comments or questioning. They are excessively preoccupied with attacks on their reputation or character, and minor slights may arouse major hostility and a counter-attack. They bear grudges and harbour hostile feelings for a long time, and are unwilling to forgive the insults, injuries, or slights that they think they have received.[8]

Pathological jealousy is a common presentation of paranoid individuals. They have unreasonable doubts about the loyalty and faithfulness of their partners, based on little or no evidence. They may try to gather trivial and circumstantial facts to justify their beliefs. To avoid betrayal they attempt to gain complete control of intimate relationships, continuously questioning, and challenging partners about their whereabouts and intentions.

The interpersonal world of paranoids is a consequence of their suspiciousness and distrust. They have difficulty in relating to others, especially with close relationships. Hostility is always present and can be manifested as excessive argumentativeness, recurrent complaint and confrontation, or hostile aloofness.[8] Although they may appear rational, unemotional, and cold, the affect of paranoids is labile and oversensitive and they may be hostile, stubborn, and sarcastic. This mixture of secretive, cold, hostile, and sarcastic behaviours often elicits a hostile response in others, which confirms the paranoid person's beliefs.

Paranoids blame others for their shortcomings. They are querulous and quick to counter-attack, so that they may become involved in frequent litigation. Since they do not confide in others, paranoids need self-confidence and a sense of autonomy and independence. They need to control people who might be harmful. While they do not accept criticism, they are highly critical.

One group of paranoids are close to Schneider's 'fanatics'.[2] They have hidden grandiose fantasies of power and negative views of other people, especially those belonging to another group who come to be considered as natural enemies. They simplify issues and avoid any ambiguous perspective. Some form cults or other tightly knit groups with people who share their paranoid belief systems.

(d) Course

Paranoid features may be present in childhood and early adolescence in the form of hypersensitivity, social anxiety, poor peer relationships, and eccentricity. These features sometimes elicit teasing from other children, which in turn may aggravate the paranoid attitudes.

In situations of stress, individuals with paranoid personality disorder may respond with brief psychotic episodes. During these episodes, they may have frank delusional ideas or distorted perceptions. Some paranoid personality disorders are the premorbid state for a delusional disorder or even schizophrenia.

Individuals with this personality disorder may be at increased risk for agoraphobia, obsessive–compulsive disorder, and substance abuse or dependence. This personality disorder is often co-diagnosed with schizoid, schizotypal, narcissistic, and avoidant personality disorders.

(e) Differential diagnosis

Paranoid personality disorder should be distinguished from suspicious attitudes towards examination among immigrants, ethnic groups, or political groups. Members of these groups may display defensive and mistrustful behaviours owing to lack of familiarity with the language or the rules of a society, or in response to perceived neglect or rejection. Their behaviour may elicit further rejection from the majority, thus reinforcing the defensive behaviours.

Paranoid personality disorder is distinguished from delusional disorder, paranoid schizophrenia, and depression with psychotic symptoms, all of which are characterized by periods of persistent psychotic symptoms. Paranoid personality disorder present before the occurrence of these syndromes should be diagnosed as 'premorbid'.

People with schizotypal personality disorder are suspicious, have paranoid ideas, and keep their distance from others. However, they also experience perceptual distortions and magical thinking, and are usually odd and eccentric. Schizoid personality disorder is characterized by aloofness, coldness, and eccentricity, but these individuals usually lack prominent suspiciousness or paranoid ideation. Individuals with **avoidant personality disorder** are hypersensitive and do not confide in others. However, their lack of confidence is based on fear of being embarrassed or found inadequate rather than fear of other people's malicious intentions. Some antisocial behaviour by paranoid individuals originates in a wish for revenge or counter-attack, rather a desire for personal gain as in antisocial personality disorder. Paranoid features are often present in narcissistic individuals who fear that their imperfections could be revealed. The differential diagnosis should be based on the predominance of persistent need of praise versus persistent suspiciousness and distrust.

(f) Treatment

Antidepressant and anxiolytic treatment may be useful for anxiety and depression resulting from a paranoid response to stressful situations. Low-dose antipsychotics may be indicated during brief psychotic episodes or when ideas of reference are present.

Psychological treatment is difficult owing to the lack of insight. The approach is to attempt to gain the patient's confidence, avoiding early confrontation of distorted ideas, followed by a slow gentle attempt at cognitive restructuring.

Schizoid personality disorder

Schizoid personality disorder is characterized by a persistent pattern of social withdrawal. Schizoid individuals show discomfort in social interactions and are introverted. They are seen by others as eccentric, isolated, or lonely. DSM-IV diagnostic criteria are shown in Table 4.12.3.2.

This type of personality became recognized in the first two decades of the twentieth century. August Block's description of the shut-in personality and Eugen Bleuler's description of autism distinguished between shy and lonely persons and those who engage in relationships only in fantasy. Psychoanalysts included this term in their writings and developed an approach based on deficient object relations and individuation.[9] Some schizoid personalities have probably been sweet children who were very easy to care for, although giving less joy to their parents and eliciting less stimulation and fewer expressions of emotion than more expressive children.[7]

(a) Epidemiology

The epidemiology of schizoid personality disorder is not clearly established. Recent studies give a median prevalence of 0.5 to 1 per cent (see Chapter 4.12.5).

(b) Aetiology

A familial association may exist between schizotypal personality disorder and schizophrenia.

Table 4.12.3.2 DSM-IV diagnostic criteria for schizoid personality disorder

A. A pervasive pattern of detachment from social relationships and a restricted range of expression of emotions in interpersonal settings, beginning by early adulthood and present in a variety of contexts, as indicated by four (or more) of the following 1 Neither desires nor enjoys close relationships, including being part of a family 2 Almost always chooses solitary activities 3 Has little, if any, interest in having sexual experiences with another person 4 Takes pleasure in few, if any, activities 5 Lacks close friends or confidants other than first-degree relatives 6 Appears indifferent to the praise or criticism of others 7 Shows emotional coldness, detachment, or flattened affectivity
B. Does not occur exclusively during the course of Schizophrenia, a Mood Disorder With Psychotic Features, another Psychotic Disorder, or a Pervasive Developmental Disorder and is not due to the direct physiological effects of a general medical condition

Note If criteria are met prior to the onset of Schizophrenia, add 'Premorbid.' e.g. 'Schizoid Personality Disorder (Premorbid)'.

(c) Clinical picture

People with schizoid personality disorder appear cold, reserved, distant, and unsociable. They lack involvement in everyday events and in the concerns of others. They rarely tolerate eye contact, usually give short answers, and appear uneasy when asked about emotions or feelings. However, they may invest much energy in abstract ideas such as those of mathematics or philosophy.

There is a characteristic lack of emotional expression and low energy. Speech is typically slow and monotonous, and seems to lack associated emotion. Affect is excessively serious or constrained, although some inner fear may be detected by an experienced clinician. If they try to be humorous, they usually give a child-like impression. Psychomotor activity tends to be lethargic, lacking gesture, and rhythmic movement. They may seem absorbed in insignificant matters, keeping quiet and not annoying anybody, as if in their own world. They do not express joy, anger, sadness, or other emotions. Interpersonal communication tends to be formal and impersonal, although not irrational. Threats, real or imagined, are dealt with by fantasized omnipotence or resignation. Aggressive acts are infrequent.

People with schizoid personality disorder characteristically seem to lack interest in the lives and concerns of others. When in a group, they stay unnoticed and detached, seeming indifferent to criticism or praise or to the reactions of others. Schizoids are attracted to solitary hobbies, and may be successful in lonely jobs that others find difficult to tolerate. Many prefer working at night. Usually, they do not seem to suffer because of this detachment and they have no desire for closeness or intimacy. They seldom have close friends or relationships, except with immediate relatives. Their sexual lives may be poor or exist only in fantasy, and some postpone mature sexuality indefinitely. They do not usually marry, although some, especially schizoid women, may passively agree to marriage. However, schizoid individuals may make emotional attachments with animals or inanimate objects.

Schizoid personalities lack insight, and generally have a poorly developed sense of identity and a poor capacity for evaluating interpersonal events. They may appear to be self-absorbed and engage in excessive daydreaming. However, some schizoid individuals have original and creative ideas.

(d) Differential diagnosis

Schizoids have better occupational functioning than patients with **schizophrenia** or **schizotypal personality disorder**, and, although isolated, can have successful careers. Schizophrenic patients exhibit delusional thinking or hallucinations and psychotic episodes. Schizotypal individuals show greater eccentricity and oddness than schizoids, and also have perceptual and thought disturbances including magical thinking.

People with **paranoid personality disorder** may also show social detachment and lack close relationships. However, they show more social engagement than schizoids and may have a history of aggressive behaviour.

Emotional constraint is also present in **obsessive–compulsive personality disorder**, but obsessional patients are more involved in everyday life and concerns, and may be worried by criticism. People with **avoidant personality disorder** are also detached and aloof. However, although they actively avoid interpersonal contact because of fear of rejection or being found inadequate, they have an intense desire for close relationships.

(e) Course

Schizoid personality disorder is usually apparent in early childhood. As with all personality disorders, it is usually long-lasting; however, it is not necessarily lifelong although there is seldom any rapid or profound change. If their deficits are moderate and social circumstances are favourable, some schizoids achieve social and vocational adaptation.

Although this personality disorder is sometimes a precursor of schizophrenia, the number of schizoid patients who go on to develop schizophrenia is unknown.

(f) Treatment

Because they lack insight and have little motivation for change, schizoids seldom seek treatment. Motivation for change may depend on life circumstances and external pressures.

Low-dose antipsychotic medication is useful in some situations. Antidepressants and psychostimulants have also been used with some positive effects.

The psychotherapy of patients with schizoid personality disorder must be based on gaining a therapeutic alliance. Unlike paranoid patients, they may become involved in therapy and reveal fantasies, imaginary friends, and fears of unbearable dependency. Ambivalence may appear because of fear of dependence on the therapist, who must keep the necessary distance to allow a tolerable relationship for the patient.

Social skills training is sometimes useful in improving their awareness of social cues.

Schizotypal personality disorder

Schizotypia is a controversial term in psychiatry. The term was used by Kretschmer[(10)] to denominate the phenotypic characters that antedated the development of schizophrenia. Nevertheless, the term schizotypal personality disorder was not included in psychiatric classifications until the publication of DSM-IIIR in 1987.[(11)] Before

Table 4.12.3.3 DV-IV diagnostic criteria for schizotypal personality disorder

A. A pervasive pattern of social and interpersonal deficits marked by acute discomfort with, and reduced capacity for, close relationships as well as by cognitive or perceptual distortions and eccentricities of behaviour beginning by early adulthood and present in a variety of contexts, as indicated by five (or more) of the following
   1 Ideas of reference (excluding delusions of reference)
   2 Odd beliefs or magical thinking that influences behaviour and is inconsistent with subcultural norms (e.g. superstitiousness, belief in clairvoyance, telepathy, or 'sixth sense'; in children and adolescents, bizarre fantasies or preoccupations)
   3 Unusual perceptual experiences, including bodily illusions
   4 Odd thinking and speech (e.g. vague, circumstantial, metaphorical. overelaborate, or stereotyped)
   5 Suspiciousness or paranoid ideation
   6 Inappropriate or constricted affect
   7 Behaviour or appearance that is odd, eccentric, or peculiar
   8 Lack of close friends or confidants other than first-degree relatives
   9 Excessive social anxiety that does not diminish with familiarity and tends to be associated with paranoid fears rather than negative judgements about self

B. Does not occur exclusively during the course of Schizophrenia, a Mood Disorder With Psychotic Features, another Psychotic Disorder, or a Pervasive Developmental Disorder.

Note If criteria are met prior to the onset of Schizophrenia, add 'Premorbid', e.g. 'Schizotypal Personality Disorder (Premorbid)'.

that date, schizotypal individuals were allocated either with schizoids or with schizophrenics, and were usually labelled as latent schizophrenics or pseudoneurotic schizophrenics. However, the validity of this nosological entity is still controversial and, despite its acceptance in DSM-IV, ICD-10 does not recognize it as a separate personality disorder. Instead, ICD-10 includes the schizotypal syndrome among the psychotic disorders and not as a personality disorder, based on the biological affinities of schizotypal individuals with other schizophrenic patients. DSM-IV diagnostic criteria are shown in Table 4.12.3.3.

(a) Epidemiology

Schizotypal personality disorder is present in 0.5 to 3 per cent of the general population, with no demonstrated differences between sexes. It is more commonly diagnosed in relatives of schizophrenic patients, and the incidence is much higher in monozygotic than in dizygotic twins (33 per cent versus 4 per cent).[4]

(b) Clinical picture

The essential feature of schizotypal individuals is a pattern of peculiarity and oddness in interpersonal relationships with resulting social detachment and lack of close relationships. Because of their distorted reality processing schizotypal individuals feel intensely uncomfortable in the presence of others. Conversely, others feel uneasy in the presence of schizotypals because of their unusual ways of thinking and expressing emotions.

Like schizoids, schizotypals have a decreased desire for intimate contacts, although they may sometimes express unhappiness about their lack of relationships. As a consequence they do not have close friends or confidants other than relatives. They experience intense anxiety in social situations with unfamiliar people. They can interact if necessary, but they prefer to keep aloof because they feel different and are not interested in the concerns of others. Their anxiety in these situations is not based on feelings of inadequacy or fear of humiliation. Rather, it is due to suspicion of the motivation of others, and therefore it is not alleviated as time passes and the situation becomes more familiar. Thus schizotypals feel progressively worse and more reluctant to confide in other people.

Individuals with schizotypal personality disorder often have ideas of reference that is interpretations of casual events as having specific and unusual meanings related to themselves. However, these ideas do not achieve the pathological conviction of delusions. Similarly, these individuals may be preoccupied with superstitions or paranormal phenomena. They may feel that they may read other people's thoughts or influence their behaviour by the power of thought. Their magical thinking is often manifested by ritualized behaviours aimed at avoiding harmful events.

Perceptual disturbances are frequent in schizotypal personality disorder. An experience of a sixth sense is typical, with the 'ability' to notice someone's presence. Distorted perceptions are present in the form of sounds perceived as calling voices or shadows transformed into figures and faces.

Thought processing and speech are characteristically affected. Speech may be constructed in an unusual and idiosyncratic way-generally loose, digressive, or vague, but without actual derailment or incoherence. Responses may be either excessively concrete or far too abstract, and words may be used in unusual ways.

The interpersonal relationships of schizotypal individuals are primarily affected by paranoid and suspicious ideation. They may believe that colleagues at work want to damage their reputation. In addition to the social anxiety of these individuals, this leads to a stiff and constricted contact and affect. They are considered odd and eccentric by others: they have peculiar mannerisms, dress in an unusual and unkempt manner, adopt extravagant postures and clothing combinations, do not obey normal social conventions, and generally avoid eye contact.

(b) Course

Schizotypal features may be present in childhood and adolescence in the form of solitariness, academic underachievement, hypersensitivity, and bizarre fantasies. Schizotypals do not seek treatment because of their personality disorder, but rather because of the presentation of associated depression, dysphoria, and anxiety. In response to stressful situations, these patients may experience transient psychotic episodes lasting from minutes to hours. In some cases, clinical symptoms and duration reach the degree of brief psychotic disorder, schizophreniform disorder, or schizophrenia, with the schizotypal personality disorder as the premorbid state. The prevalence of major depressive episodes is notoriously high, as is co-diagnosis with paranoid, schizoid, avoidant, and borderline personality disorders.

(c) Differential diagnosis

Delusional disorder, **schizophrenia**, and **mood disorder with psychotic symptoms** have to be excluded based on the greater intensity and persistence of psychotic symptoms.

In childhood, it can be difficult to distinguish schizotypal personality disorder from other forms of disorders characterized by odd behaviour, isolation, eccentricity, and peculiarities of language. These include **autistic disorder, Asperger's disorder,** and some **language disorders**. The differentiation with communication disorders is based on the prominence of language symptoms in these children and the compensatory efforts to communicate by gesture and other means. Autism and Asperger's disorder present an even more intense social isolation and indifference, stereotyped behaviours and interests.

Paranoid and **schizoid personality disorders** lack the perceptual and speech impairment of schizotypal personality disorder, as well as the marked eccentricity and oddness. **Avoidant personality disorder**, while including social anxiety and isolation, differs from schizotypal personality disorder in that avoidants have an intense desire for closeness, which is constrained by fear of rejection. Schizotypals do not have a desire for relationships. **Borderline personality disorder** has a high rate of co-occurrence with schizotypal personality disorder and frequently the two disorders cannot be differentiated. Brief psychotic episodes in people with borderline personality disorder are more dissociative-like and generally follow affective shifts in response to stress or frustration. Social isolation in borderline personality patients is generally due to repeated interpersonal failures rather than a persistent lack of desire for relationships and intimacy.

Finally, schizotypal personality disorder must be diagnosed in the cultural context of the patient. It should be noted that some perceptual peculiarities and magical beliefs may be due to culturally determined characteristics. For example, mind reading, voodoo, shamanism, evil eye, and so on should not be considered as personality disorders in some cultural areas.

(d) Treatment

Low-dose antipsychotic medication may be useful for ideas of reference, perceptual disturbances, and other psychotic-like symptoms. Antidepressants are effective when depressive states are associated.

The psychological management of schizotypals should include a prolonged period of gaining the confidence of the patient. However, a particularly careful approach must be adopted owing to the peculiar thought processing of these patients.

Cluster B personality disorders

Antisocial personality disorder

Antisocial personality disorder is characterized by a pattern of disregard for the safety and the rights of others, without feeling remorse. Individuals with this disorder are unreliable, manipulative, incapable of lasting relationships, and unable to conform to social norms. The disorder starts early (before the age of 15), is pervasive, and manifests in variety of contexts. Although social deviance is one of the core features of antisocial personality disorder, it is not synonymous with criminality. Antisocial personality disorder uncomplicated by other disorders is not often met in clinical settings, except forensic psychiatry. However, owing to its impact on family and social environment, it has major public health significance and has been extensively studied in academic psychiatry, psychoanalysis, law, sociology, theology, and literature.

The description of antisocial personality in the last 1970s was mainly based on criminal behaviour[12] and the disorder was conceptualized as synonymous of criminality. Later classifications modified this approach and focused on the personality traits and emotional patterns described in classic descriptions included the classic personality traits leading to the current DSM-IV and ICD-10 classification criteria for antisocial personality disorder. (Tables 4.12.3.4 and 4.12.3.5).

Table 4.12.3.4 SM-IV diagnostic criteria for antisocial personality disorder

A. There is a pervasive pattern of disregard for and violation of the rights of others occurring since age 15 years, as indicated by three (or more) of the following
   1 Failure to conform to social norms with respect to lawful behaviours as indicated by repeatedly performing acts that are ground for arrest
   2 Deceitfulness, as indicated by repeated lying, use of aliases, or conning others for personal profit or pleasure
   3 Impulsivity or failure to plan ahead
   4 Irritability and aggressiveness, as indicated by repeated physical fights or assaults
   5 Reckless disregard for safety of self or others
   6 Consistent irresponsibility, as indicated by repeated failure to sustain consistent work behaviour or honour financial obligations
   7 Lack of remorse, as indicated by being indifferent to or rationalizing having hurt, mistreated, or stolen from another

B. The individual is at least age 18 years

C. There is evidence of conduct disorder with onset before 15 years

D. The occurrence of antisocial behaviour is not exclusively during the course of Schizophrenia or a Manic Episode.

(a) Epidemiology

A prevalence rate of about 3 per cent is consistently found in the general population, and it is more frequent in males than females, with sex ratios ranging from 2:1 to 7:1. It is more common among younger adults, people living in urban areas and lower socio-economic groups.[13]

Table 4.12.3.5 ICD-10 diagnostic criteria for disocial personality disorder

Personality disorder, usually coming to attention because of a gross disparity between behaviour and the prevailing social norms, and characterized by
   (a) callous unconcern for the feelings of others
   (b) gross and persistent attitude of irresponsibility and disregard for social norms, rules and obligations
   (c) incapacity to maintain enduring relationships, though having no difficulty in establishing them
   (d) very low tolerance to frustration and a low threshold for discharge of aggression, including violence
   (e) incapacity to experience guilt and to profit from experience, particularly punishment
   (f) marked proneness to blame others, or to offer plausible rationalizations, for the behaviour that has brought the patient into conflict with society

There may also be persistent irritability as an associated feature. Conduct disorder during childhood and adolescence, though not invariably present, may further support the diagnosis.

Includes: amoral, antisocial, psychopathic, and sociopathic personality (disorder)

Excludes: conduct disorders, emotionally unstable personality disorder

(b) Aetiology

The aetiology of antisocial personality disorder is complex and multifactorial, involving biological, early developmental, and social determinants.

Twin, adoption, and family studies have demonstrated that genetic factors strongly contribute to the development of antisocial personality.[14] Antisocial personality in males is often associated with hysteria in women of the same family which suggests that the two conditions might be alternative expressions of the same genetic endowment, belonging to 'spectrum conditions'.[15] Longitudinal studies of hyperactive children have reported high rates of later (adult) antisocial behaviour, and have suggested a 'developmental' relationship between antisocial behaviour and childhood hyperactivity.

Aggression in antisocial personality disorder is associated with indexes of reduced brain serotonin activity such as low levels of the serotonin metabolite 5-hydroxyindole-acetic acid in the cerebrospinal fluid and[16,17] low platelet monoamine oxidase activity. Reports on minimal brain dysfunctions resulting on frontal-lobe deficiencies and lack of inhibition have also been described.

Parental deprivation, inconsistent maternal care, family violence, and severe childhood physical) abuse have been reported as strong predictors for development of antisocial personality disorders.[12,18]

Social disintegration and chronic criminality can cause episodic antisocial behaviour, reflecting a normal adaptation to an abnormal social environment.[19] However, the multifactorial origin of the antisocial personality disorder and its early onset and manifestations indicate that it cannot be attributed to cultural conflicts and social determinants.

(c) Clinical features and diagnosis

Patients with antisocial personality disorder often appear quite normal, charming, and understanding. However, their history reveals disturbed functioning in the domains of behaviour and self-concept, love and sexuality, interpersonal relations, and cognitive style.[20]

Reckless behaviour unaffected by punishment is typical of antisocial individuals, who are also exploitative, manipulative, demanding, and lacking in a sense of responsibility. An easy-going hedonistic attitude may be interrupted by rage, cruelty, and violence. The absence of internalized moral values is manifested by lying, truancy, running away from home, thefts, fights, substance abuse, and illegal activities may be typical experiences, beginning in early childhood.

An impaired control of impulses and a reduced ability to anticipate the negative consequences of behaviour is typical associated to a marked intolerance to anxiety. Antisocial individuals are egocentric, and unable to feel genuine guilt and remorse. They exhibit intense and persistent anger usually expressed as hostility towards others and they have an incapacity for reflective mourning or sadness. Frequent suicide threats and attempts are also common, as is somatic preoccupation.

Interpersonal relationships of antisocial subjects are characterized by manipulation, exploitation, instability and incapacity for love, and comprehension. Sexual perversions, abuse, and paedophilia are frequent. They display deficient parenting and social dysfunction, and resistance to authorities is pronounced.

The cognitive style of antisocial subjects is characterized by glibness, superficiality of knowledge, and paranoid view of reality.

(d) Comorbidity and differential diagnosis

Antisocial personality disorder is frequently comorbid with **depression**, which usually has atypical features. **Bipolar disorder** (manic phase) and **mental retardation** (learning difficulties) should be excluded. Substance abuse may be comorbid from childhood, and antisocial behaviour may be secondary to premorbid alcoholism type 2. **Atypical schizophrenic disorder** (pseudopsychopathic schizophrenia), **temporal-lobe epilepsy**, or a **limbic-lobe syndrome** should also be excluded.

The presentation of antisocial and criminal behaviour in borderline personality disorder is frequent. However, borderline behaviours are marked by intense affective instability and reactivity and may show some remorse or guilt. Unlike antisocial patients, borderline personality disorders do not lack the capacity for intimacy and emotional investment of others and do not show sadistic behaviours. Self-aggression and suicide attempts are much more prevalent among BPD than in antisocial personality.

Aggressive and defiant behaviours are often present in histrionic personality disorder. Although some aetiologic relationship among both disorders might be possible, as described above, histrionic patients are more impulsive and emotionally driven than antisocial and display intense emotions related with attachments and losses.

(e) Course and prognosis

Antisocial behaviour is most pronounced in early adult years, and gradually decreases with age. Professional motivation and establishing a stable couple or partnership may have beneficial effects. Maturation of the personality might also take with depression or hypochondriasis emerging when rage and aggression are abandoned. Substance abuse and promiscuity are risky behaviours for developing HIV infection.

(f) Treatment

Medication is used to deal with incapacitating symptoms, such as anxiety, rage, depression, and somatic complaints. Selective serotonin reuptake inhibitors, lithium, carbamazepine, clonazepam, and other anticonvulsants have been used to control aggressive behaviour but the effects are much less pronounced than in borderline personality disorder or intermittent explosive disorder. Psychostimulants such as methylphenidate may be useful if there is evidence of attention-deficit hyperactivity disorder. Benzodiazepines are contraindicated since they might cause behavioural disinhibition.

Efficacy of psychotherapy is very little in antisocial patients. Fear of intimacy causes difficulties in establishing a therapeutic alliance, which should be oriented to find alternative defence mechanisms to acting-out and to self-defeating behaviours. Therapeutic communities based on the principles outlined by Maxwell Jones[21] with a general social adjustment as a main task, might give positive results.

Borderline personality disorder

Borderline personality disorder (BPD) is the denomination of a syndromal picture characterized by intense affective instability and impulsivity together with an unstable sense of self-identity. It is often manifested by impulsive self-aggression and suicide attempts, substance abuse, chronic feelings of emptiness, and persistent pattern of severely unstable interpersonal relationships.

The term borderline was first used by Stern[22] in 1938 to denominate a group of syndromes placed in the border between neuroses and psychoses and included also the current label of schizotypal personality disorder and a group of disorders currently classified as psychotic disorders. Only some decades later the term borderline began to be understood as a disorder of character[23] and introduced in DSM-III as a personality disorder, after being separated from schizotypal personality disorder.

Borderline personality disorder derives but is not fully equivalent to the concept of borderline personality organization developed by Kernberg.[24] BPO is a stable permanent state based on three criteria: diffuse identity, primitive defence mechanisms (splitting, denial, and projective identification), and intact reality testing. This personality organization can be found not only in BPD but also in other severe personality disorders and Axis I conditions.

Borderline personality disorder itself can be found in association with so many Axis I and Axis II disorders that its validity as an independent diagnostic category is still weak compared with other personality disorders. Some authors have suggested that borderline personality disorder reflects rather a state of severely impaired personality function than a discrete diagnostic entity.[25] Others have suggested that BPD is an atypical variant of affective disorder and should be included in the affective disorder spectrum.[26] In the ICD-10, this disorder is named as 'emotionally unstable personality disorder', with two subtypes: impulsive and borderline. Borderline subtype is specifically linked to the presence of self-identity weakness and diffusion.

(a) Epidemiology

The number of people suffering from borderline personality disorder ranges from 1.5 to 5 per cent of general population with wide differences between studies because of lack of reliable measures. The prevalence is greater in clinical samples of patients at the outpatient clinics, ranging form 10 to 15 per cent. The disorder is more common in women than in men and is commonly initiated between 18 and 35 years old.[27]

(b) Aetiology

Several factors have been associated with a higher prevalence of borderline personality disorder, including genetic, biological, and developmental findings.[28] Family studies indicate that parents of patients with BPD have a greater incidence of mood disorders but not of schizophrenia. Additionally, there is also high family incidence of antisocial personality disorder and alcoholism.

Among the biochemical findings, those indicating a brain serotonin deficiency are the more consistent. Reduced levels of 5-hydroxyindoleacetic acid in cerebrospinal fluid and blunted prolactin response to serotonin agonists have been demonstrated in association with impulsive aggression, which is a core feature of BPD.[29] Hypothalamic-pituitary—adrenal axis dysfunctions, suggesting increased feedback inhibition, as well as increased sensitivity of some areas of the amigdala, have been reported in samples of BPD patients. Current available data suggest that BPD might be associated with abnormal emotional reactivity in the limbic areas and insufficient regulatory function at the cingulated and prefrontal areas of the brain.[30]

The role of childhood trauma in the development of borderline personality disorder could be crucial. Higher incidence of childhood traumatic experiences, both for sexual/physical abuse or for neglect, has been demonstrated in these patients.[31] Other proposed developmental factors include deficiencies in self and identity development linked to attachment failures with parental figures in the early developmental phases.[32,33]

The onset of BPD needs the interaction of predisposing factors, both biological and developmental, and environmental precipitants. BPD patients seem to be extremely sensitive to frustrations in the intimate relationships, which are commonly detected at the onset of the disorder.

(c) Clinical features and diagnosis

Impulsivity and affective instability, self-aggression, identity disturbance, and unstable/intense interpersonal relationships are the most characteristic manifestations of borderline personality disorder.

Identity weakness and diffusion explain several aspects of borderline personality disorder (Table 4.12.3.6). It is clinically manifested by contradictory character traits and sense of discontinuity of the self and feelings of emptiness.[34] Probably related with this is also the intolerance to be alone and the desperate efforts to avoid abandonment by significant others. The chronic feeling of emptiness is recurrently intensified and unbearable leading to drug abuse and self-defeating behaviours.

The affect of borderline patients is chronically dysphoric and irritated. Their unstable mood is a mixture of depressed affect, anger, loneliness, and emptiness. Impulsive–aggressive behaviour is a core feature of borderline personality disorder and is related with this abnormal affective state.

Cognitive style of borderline patients are easily suggestible and frequently change their decisions. Things and people are seen in black-and-white terms. Transient and brief psychotic episodes are frequent in BPD patients associated with unstructured stressful

Table 4.12.3.6 DSM-IV diagnostic criteria for borderline personality disorder

A pervasive pattern of instability of interpersonal relationships, self-image, and affects and marked impulsivity beginning by early adulthood and present in a variety of contexts, as indicated by five (or more) of the following

1. Frantic efforts to avoid real or imagined abandonment. **Note:** Do not include suicidal or self-mutilating behaviour covered in Criterion 5
2. A pattern of unstable and intense interpersonal relationships characterized by alternating between extremes of idealization and devaluation
3. Identity disturbance: markedly and persistently unstable self-image or sense of self
4. Impulsivity in at least two areas that are potentially self-damaging (e.g spending, sex, substance abuse, reckless driving, binge eating). **Note:** Do not include suicidal or self-mutilating behaviour covered in Criterion 5
5. Recurrent suicidal behaviour, gestures, or threats, or self-mutilating behaviour
6. Affective instability due to a marked reactivity of mood (e.g. intense episodic dysphoria, irritability, or anxiety usually lasting a few hours and only rarely more than a few days)
7. Chronic feelings of emptiness
8. Inappropriate intense anger or difficulty controlling anger (e.g. frequent displays of temper, constant anger, recurrent physical fights)
9. Transient stress-related paranoid ideation or severe dissociative symptoms

situations. Psychotic symptoms may have a typical dissociative-like nature or present as transient self-referential ideation. Rejection sensitivity and suspiciousness usually colours the interpretations of behaviours of others.

Borderline patients are both intensely dependent and hostile towards significant others. Interpersonal relationships are unstable, intense, demanding, clinging, and characterized by alternation between extremes of idealization and devaluation, deriving from the defence mechanism of splitting. Infatuations are followed by devaluation of love objects. There is a tendency towards promiscuity and perversions.

(d) Comorbidity and differential diagnosis

Borderline personality disorder is frequently comorbid with **affective disorders** (major depression, dysthymia, and 'double depression'), **anxiety disorders**, **somatization disorder**, **post-traumatic stress disorder**, and **alcohol abuse**.

Differential diagnosis has to be made with **type II bipolar disorder**. Bipolar patients more often present emotional lability from sadness/apathy to euphoria while BPD patients are characterized by intense and reactive affective instability and shift rather from sadness to tolerable dysphoria. Intermittent explosive disorder also shows impulsive and aggressive behaviours but lacks identity disturbances and affective instability typical of BPD. Mild mental retardation might have intense irritability, lability, and impulsive/aggressive behaviour but lacks chronic feelings of emptiness and self-identity diffusion. Transient psychotic episodes and stress-related referential ideas of BPD should be differentiated from pervasive psychotic-like experiences of schizotypal personality disorder.

Borderline personality disorder has been shown to be associated with most personality disorders, especially with those from the dramatic cluster. The high prevalence of comorbid personality disorders may result from overlapping of diagnostic criteria or reflect the confirmation that there is the underlying borderline personality organization of all severe personality disorders. However, some features like chronic feelings of emptiness, self-mutilation, short-lived psychotic episodes, intense and episodic drug abuse, and intense ambivalent dependency in close relationships suggest a primary diagnosis of BPD.

(e) Course and outcome

Borderline patients often experience profound dysfunction in many important aspects of life including education, jobs, partner relationships, and marriage. Alcohol and psychosexual problems are also frequent. Repeated suicide attempts and premature death from suicide are frequent complications of borderline personality disorder; therefore suicidal gestures and intentions should be always taken seriously. It has been reported that 8 to 10 per cent per cent of all persons with borderline personality disorder commit suicide.[35]

The long-term outcome of borderline patients has not been studied, but the diagnosis is rarely made in patients aged over 40. It is speculated that neural structures and defence mechanisms mature with age and that these changes, together with social learning, reduce symptomatology.

(f) Treatment

Pharmacotherapy is targeted to symptoms such as affective changes (depression, anxiety, rage, dysphoria), cognitive disturbances (brief psychotic episodes or interpretative distortions), and impulsive behavioural dyscontrol.[36] New antidepressants, including SSRIs and venlafaxine, have shown positive effects in treating a broad spectrum of acute symptoms, including depression, hostility, irritability, anxiety, obsessive–compulsive symptoms, suicidal attempts, and impulsivity. Antipsychotics and anticonvulsants may help some patients, even in the absence of EEG or organic changes. There are still no clinical predictors for efficacy, therefore, a pragmatic approach is indicated with patients being treated with two or three drugs in a sequential trial.[36] Suicidal and abusive use of drugs prescribed and non-compliance may be serious problems for treatment of BPD.

Various psychotherapeutical modalities are used, including psychodynamic psychotherapy, supportive psychotherapy, and dialectical–behavioural therapy.

A more structured form of psychoanalytic approach, involving expressive psychotherapy and an active role of psychotherapist have been proposed specifically for BPD. The aims are confrontation of maladaptive defences and interpretation of transference, focusing on the 'here and now', without attempting the achievement of a full genetic reconstruction.[37]

Short-term psychotherapy is useful for managing crises or introducing long-term forms of therapy. Supportive psychotherapy is suggested for more fragile borderline patients, who are prone to serious regression in treatment. In practice, supportive therapy, with a psychoeducational component, has been the most frequently used form of treatment for borderline personality disorder. It is also possible to combine elements of intensive dynamic therapy with supportive therapy, depending on the ego strength of the patients.[38]

Dialectical–behavioural therapy[39] is based on cognitive techniques associated with reality confrontation. The major aim is emotional self-regulation and behavioural self-control and is particularly indicated for control of suicidal and impulsive behaviours and treatment of emotional reactivity.

Histrionic personality disorder

(a) Definition

Histrionic personality disorder derives from the concept of hysterical personality, supported by descriptive literature and clinical tradition but not so much by valid empirical research. It is characterized by excessive emotionality and attention seeking, and by dramatic, colourful, and extroverted behaviour. Egocentric, dependent, and demanding interpersonal relationships are typical of this disorder, which begins in early adulthood and is present in a variety of contexts. The DSM-IV and ICD-10 diagnostic criteria for this disorder are shown in tables 4.12.3.7 and 4.12.3.8.

It was included in scientific medicine by Kraepelin,[40] who described multiple symptoms, including capricious and inconsistent behaviour, histrionic exaggeration, and a life of illness, which captured the core pattern of the illness. Freud[41] recognized the relationship between hysterical neurosis and what he called the 'erotic personality, whose major goal in life is the desire to love or above all to be loved'. Psychoanalytic theorists often distinguish hysterical ('healthier') and histrionic ('sicker') personalities, where the latter has borderline organization and is an exaggeration of the former. Differences between the two concepts are shown in Table 4.12.3.9.

Table 4.12.3.7 DSM-IV diagnostic criteria for histrionic personality disorder

A pervasive pattern of excessive emotionality and attention seeking, beginning by early adulthood and present in a variety of contexts, as indicated by five (or more) of the following

1. Is uncomfortable in situations in which he or she is not the centre of attention
2. Interaction with others is often characterized by inappropriate sexually seductive or provocative behaviour
3. Displays rapidly shifting and shallow expression of emotions
4. Consistently uses physical appearance to draw attention to self
5. Has a style of speech that is excessively impressionistic and lacking in detail
6. Shows self-dramatization, theatricality, and exaggerated expression of emotion
7. Is suggestible, i.e. easily influenced by others or circumstances
8. Considers relationships to be more intimate than they actually are

(b) Epidemiology

The prevalence is found to be 2 to 3 per cent of the general population and 10 to 15 per cent in clinical settings.(42) No significant difference has been found in terms of race and education and is more frequently diagnosed in women than in men. However, some cultural biases associated with sex role stereotypes and emotional expressiveness could lead the lower diagnostic rates in men.(43)

(c) Aetiology

Some studies suggest that histrionic personality runs in families, but evidence for a biological or learning transmission is not yet consistent.(44) Traits such as extraversion, emotional expression, and reward dependence have a strong genetic origin and might be constitutional. Biological findings associated with impulsivity, such as serotonin deficiency, can be found in histrionic patients with marked emotional instability and impulsive behaviours. It has been proposed that histrionic personality in women is genotypically linked to antisocial personality in men.(45)

From a development perspective, histrionic personality is considered to be a result of abnormally intense attachment with parental figures. The erotization component of this attachment in the oedipical phase was classically emphasized in the psychoanalytic research, although recent approaches suggest that there oral/dependent factors, derived from anomalies in earlier phases are of greater importance in the development of the disorder.(46)

Table 4.12.3.8 ICD-10 diagnostic criteria for histrionic personality disorder

Personality disorder characterized by at least three of the following:

(a) self-dramatization, theatricality, exaggerated expression of emotions
(b) suggestibility, easily influenced by others or by circumstances
(c) shallow and labile affectivity
(d) continually seeking for excitement, appreciation by others, and activities in which the patient is the centre of attention
(e) Inappropriate seductiveness in appearance or behaviour
(f) Overconcern with physical attractiveness

Associated features may include egocentricity, self-indulgence, continuous longing for appreciation, feelings that are easily hurt, and persistent manipulative behaviour to achieve own needs

Includes: hysterical and psycho-infantile personality (disorder)

Table 4.12.3.9 Types of histrionism

Hysterical personality	Histrionic personality[a]
Neurotic personality organization	Borderline personality organization
Integrated identity	Diffuse identity
Predominance of repression	Predominance of splitting
Intact reality testing	Intact reality testing (proneness to distortion)
Integrated superego	Marked superego defects
Strongly bonded families	Disturbed, often broken families
Steady educational and vocational careers	Erratic careers
Capable of maintaining long-term friendships	Chaotic interpersonal relationships
Suggestible in triangular relationships	Diffuse suggestibility
Inauthenticity	Multiple identifications
Changing moods	Frequent dysphoria
Sexual inhibition	Promiscuity, perverse tendencies
Competitiveness with the same sex	Less differentiated behaviour toward sexes
Genital traits	Oral/pregenital traits

[a] Includes hysteroid, hysteriform, oral hysteric, and sick hysteric personality disorders. After Akhtar.(31)

(d) Clinical features and diagnosis

Emotionality, dramatization, exhibitionism, egocentricity, and sexual provocativeness are typical of histrionic personalities. However, behavioural expression is not always as manifested and other emotional and cognitive aspects may help for diagnosis.

Histrionic individuals are inappropriately seductive and aggressively demanding. They are self-centred, crave for novelty and excitement, and are prone to temper tantrums. Histrionic subjects are hyperemotional and impulsive, but their emotional enthusiasm is superficial and transient and their mood is labile. They describe their emotions in an inappropriate and exaggerated way in an attempt to obtain attention. Histrionic individuals are suggestible, demanding, accusative, and guilt inducing. In intense stressful situations they can show a dissociative-type of indifference and infantilism.

Histrionic personalities are inclined to sexualize all non-sexual relations, often indiscriminately, not only with a chosen partner but also with a wide variety of persons in various social, occupational, and professional relationships. Pseudosexuality is often accompanied by frigidity. A romantic outlook or a superficially adoring attitude often disguises needs for dependency and emotional attachment to a significant protective figure. Sicker individuals may be promiscuous, and may engage in multiple perverse activities.

Cognitive style is global, impressionistic, and diffuse, and lacks sharpness of detail. Non-verbal communication is better than verbal, speech is inhibited, and education is often superficial. Speech may show malapropisms or slips of the tongue.

The basic belief of histrionic personalities is that others should be impressed, and their basic strategy is dramatization. They blossom when they are the centre of attention and are highly disappointed when they are not, and draw attention to themselves by acting and speaking in a charming flirtatious way. Histrionic individuals quickly respond to others in an intimate way, often treating superficial acquaintances as if they were friends.

(e) Comorbidity and differential diagnosis

There is current evidence that **somatization disorder** (Briquet's syndrome) and **conversion disorder** can occur in conjunction with histrionic personality disorder, as well as **dissociative disorder** and **brief reactive psychosis**.[21] Differential diagnosis should not be difficult, because histrionic personality disorder is a lifelong disturbance with a chronic course, unlike Axis I disorders which are episodic. **Hypomanic and manic states** may be accompanied by seductive behaviour and exaggerated expression of emotions, but can be distinguished from histrionic personality by their episodic nature and the presence of other characteristic symptoms.

A great deal of overlap has been found between histrionic personality disorder and other **Axis II disorders**, defined by DSM-IIIR criteria; of these, the borderline, narcissistic, antisocial, and dependent personality disorders are the most frequent.

Borderline patients have more chaotic interpersonal relationships, make frequent suicide attempts, and are prone to regressive episodes of a psychotic nature. Histrionic individuals share sexual promiscuity, corruptibility, shallow emotions, and a self-centred attitude with antisocial personalities.[47] However, they do not show sustained, calculated, and ruthless disregard of social norms. Narcissists may also seek attention, but they want to be admired for their superiority while histrionic persons are clinging and dependent. Unlike narcissists, histrionic individuals have empathy for other persons. However, the features of the two disorders can be combined.

(f) Course and prognosis

Depressive symptoms, suicide attempts, and frequent use of medical services are common. Histrionic personality may gradually improve with age, as if a maturation of histrionic infantilism occurs over the years.

(g) Treatment

Depressive and anxious symptoms are frequent in histrionic personality disorder and can be alleviated with the use of antidepressants and anxiolytic medications. However, extreme care should be taken for treatment due to the vulnerability of these patients for medication abuse and non-compliance.

Supportive therapy is indicated for acutely distressed histrionic patients, as well as for those at the sicker end of the continuum. Psychoanalytic techniques in histrionic patients[47] are oriented to clarification of the patient's covert inner feelings. Patients are often demanding, want to take a special place in the therapist's life, and act out during therapy sessions, threatening to abandon treatment or undertake dangerous actions. Clear limits should be set and demanding dependent behaviour should not be rewarded.

Narcissistic personality disorder

Narcissistic personality disorder is characterized by an exaggerated sense of self-importance with a lack of sustained positive regard for others. Grandiosity (in fantasy or behaviour) and constant craving for admiration and external gratification are additional features of this disorder. They are present in a variety of contexts and begin by early adulthood.

(a) Historical perspective

The term narcissism originates from the Greek myth of Narcissus who was infatuated with his own reflection in the mirror-lake. Its contemporary usage has many meanings and implications, from its colloquial usage denoting self-centred persons, often with pejorative connotations, to a pathological clinical syndrome. Despite the popularity of the construct, there is still considerable disagreement on the aetiology and phenomenology of narcissistic personality disorder. There is little empirical evidence regarding its description, clinical utility, and validity.

A narcissistic personality has a pathological grandiose self, which hides a diffuse and aimless inner identity. Kernberg argues that self-hatred, rather than self-love, lies at the root of pathological narcissism, and distinguishes between narcissism in the broad sense and the specific pathological structures of the narcissistic personality. According to Kernberg, narcissistic patients function on a borderline level. Malignant narcissism,[37] which develops when primitive aggression infiltrates the pathological grandiose self, lies at the extreme end of a continuum. It is a combination of narcissistic personality disorder, antisocial behaviour, egosyntonic aggression or sadism directed against others, and a strong paranoid orientation (Table 4.12.3.10).

Narcissistic personality disorder was officially accepted in DSM-III. Somewhat refined criteria were adopted in DSM-IV (Table 4.12.3.11), because some studies showed a substantial lack of diagnostic reliability when the DSM-III criteria were used. Narcissistic personality disorder is not included in ICD-10, being mentioned only in the category 'Other specific personality disorders'.

Table 4.12.3.10 Types of narcissism

Normal	Pathological	Malignant
Infantile	Grandiose self-image	Grandiose self-image
Regression or fixation to infantile narcissistic goals in personality disorders (personality traits)	Low self-esteem	Aggression
	Primitive defences	Paranoid traits
	Superego defects	Antisocial behaviour
	Borderline organization	Explosive traits
		Borderline organization
Adult		
Healthy self-esteem regulated by normal self-structure		
Integrated object representations		
Capacity for deep object relations		
Integrated superego		

After Kernberg.[32,37]

Table 4.12.3.11 DSM-IV diagnostic criteria for narcissistic personality disorder

A pervasive pattern of grandiosity (in fantasy or behaviour), need for admiration, and lack of empathy, beginning by early adulthood and present in a variety of contexts, as indicated by five (or more) of the following

1 Has a grandiose sense of self-importance (e.g. exaggerates achievements and talents, expects to be recognized as superior without commensurate achievements)
2 Is preoccupied with fantasies of unlimited success, power, brilliance, beauty, or ideal love
3 Believes that he or she is 'special' and unique and can only be understood by, or should associate with, other special or high-status people (or institutions)
4 Requires excessive admiration
5 Has a sense of entitlement, i.e. unreasonable expectations of especially favourable treatment or automatic compliance with his or her expectations
6 Is interpersonally exploitative, i.e. takes advantage of others to achieve his or her own ends
7 Lacks empathy, i.e. is unwilling to recognize or identify with the feelings and needs of others
8 Is often envious of others or believes that others are envious of him or her
9 Shows arrogant haughty behaviours or attitudes

(b) Epidemiology

The prevalence of narcissistic personality disorder in the community has been found to be around 0.5 per cent.[48] Its prevalence in clinical populations is estimated to range from 1 to 3 per cent, and is more frequently diagnosed among males.

(c) Aetiology

Although no demonstrating evidence is yet available, some aspects of narcissism might be related with inappropriate seeking for excitement and reward and associated to monoamine function abnormalities at the mesolimbic reward systems.

Severe frustration with early objects is considered important in the defensive genesis of narcissistic personality disorder. Behind the compensatory grandiose self, a hungry and inferior real self resides, as the core problem of narcissistic personality disorder. Often, high parental expectations and harsh criticism of the child is present in the family.

(d) Clinical characteristics and diagnosis

Narcissistic patients only seek for help when depressed or involved in interpersonal problems.

An often engaging and attractive appearance masks intense preoccupation with self-regard and an unusual absence of concern for others. Narcissistic individuals may be energetic, capable of consistent work, and socially successful, but this is done in order to obtain admiration. Their successes provide no inner satisfaction and always end with frustration and a feeling of emptiness. Narcissistic grandiosity is often masked by opposing tendencies (false modesty, social aloofness, and a pretended contempt for status). Pathological lying is frequent.

Narcissistic individuals feel bored when the external glitter wears off and there are no new sources to feed their self-esteem, which is extremely fragile. Lacking emotional depth, they do not have genuine feelings of sadness or longing. Anger and resentment laden with vengeful wishes are frequent as a reaction to injured self-esteem. Chronic intense envy is present, as are defences against such envy, particularly devaluation, omnipotent control, and narcissistic withdrawal. They have frequent mood swings, and hypomanic exaltation is often part of the clinical picture.

Narcissistic persons are unable to fall in love, and only have fantasies of ideal love. Sexuality is trivialized, and intercourse is a purely physical pleasure. Promiscuity, perverse fantasies, devaluation of objects, and boredom in relationships are frequent.

Interpersonal relationships are frequently manipulative and exploitative. They idealize people whom they expect to feed their narcissism, but depreciate and treat with contempt others (often former idols) from whom they do not expect to receive anything. They lack empathy and concern for others, who are welcome only as an applauding crowd and as mirrors of success.

Typical defence mechanisms (omnipotence, omniscience, intellectualization, rationalization, idealization, and devaluation) are derived from splitting.

(e) Comorbidity and differential diagnosis

Narcissistic personality disorder is often comorbid with major depression, dysthymic disorder, substance abuse, and anorexia nervosa. Patients meeting criteria for narcissistic disorder have a high overlap with **histrionic, borderline, and antisocial personality disorders**, and also with **schizotypal, paranoid, and passive–aggressive personality disorders**.

Narcissistic personality disorder may display some features of bipolar disorder (manic and hypomanic episodes). However, the mood swings are of limited duration and change rapidly, while insight is maintained and the general integrity of the personality is preserved.

Narcissistic personality disorder is strikingly similar to borderline personality disorder. Phenomenologically, grandiosity is the best discriminator between the two disorders.[49] In narcissistic personality disorder, there is also better impulse control, greater social adjustment and anxiety tolerance, less frequent suicide attempts, and less danger of regressive fragmentation and psychotic episodes.

Narcissistic individuals, especially those manifesting malignant narcissism, may demonstrate antisocial behaviour. However, antisocial individuals are more impulsive and less capable of concentrating on work and career, and they are devoid of guilt feelings. Similarities with histrionic and obsessive–compulsive personalities are superficial, since people with these disorders have a capacity for empathy and a concern and love for others.

(f) Course and prognosis

Patients often become depressed or defensively hypomanic during middle age, when their internal life gradually deteriorates owing to a vicious circle of frustrations and disappointments and diminishing narcissistic supplies. Hypochondriasis and anxiety disorders are frequent complications.

(g) Treatment

Anxiolytic agents and antidepressants may be helpful for alleviating target episodes of mood and anxiety symptoms.

(i) Psychotherapy

Individual psychotherapy is aimed to the analysis of idealizing transference and interpretation of self-grandiosity. However, during the first stages only supportive therapy is recommended with interpretations delayed until confident and integrated attachment with therapist is achieved.

The treatment of narcissistic individuals inevitably arouses serious countertransference problems, because of the emotional detachment, demanding behaviour, and devaluative actions of narcissistic patients. The therapist should have worked through his or her own narcissism and retain an empathic and non-judgemental attitude.

Cluster C personality disorders

Avoidant personality disorder

Avoidant personality disorder was first introduced into psychiatric classification in DSM-III.[11] Before this, such patients were included among the schizoid or dependent patients. The emphasis on avoidant behaviour as a consequence of an intense sensitivity to rejection led to the differentiation of this new personality type.

The characteristic behaviour of the avoidant personality is active isolation from the social environment. Unlike schizoids, who are characterized by passive social isolation, avoidant subjects turn inward to protect themselves because they are extremely sensitive to rejection.[50] They desire interpersonal relationships but they avoid any chance of disapproval. Thus, only relationships that are likely to lead to complete non-critical acceptance are established. The extreme sensitivity to criticism is based on intense feelings of inferiority, poor self-concept and low self-esteem. This disorder is termed anxious personality disorder in ICD-10, since anxiety is considered to be the basic affective feature. The DSM-IV criteria for avoidant personality disorder are shown in Table 4.12.3.12.

(a) Epidemiology

The prevalence of avoidant personality disorder is estimated to be less than 1 per cent in the general population, but almost 10 per cent in clinical populations. No differences between sexes are found.

(b) Aetiology

Some familial transmission is possible, perhaps involving learning and identification, but genetic transmission may also be involved.[51] The biological mechanisms involved in anxiety disorders and social phobia may have a role in the development of this personality disorder. It has been suggested that hypersensitivity of brain areas involved in the separation-anxiety response and overactivity of serotonin limbic neuronal circuits may underlie the avoidant temperament trait.[51]

Psychosocial factors mediate the extent to which biological vulnerability is expressed. Children who are belittled, criticized, and rejected by parents have decreased self-esteem, resulting in social avoidance. These problems are reinforced and perpetuated at school and may generate the expectation of rejection from everyone.[50]

(c) Clinical picture

Avoidant people are characterized by extreme shyness. They appear distant from others and do not express wishes, demands, or opinions. However, this behaviour contrasts with an extreme internal need for warmth and closeness. This contradiction is explained by an exaggerated sensitivity to rejection by others. People with this personality disorder are easily hurt and humiliated by comments from others, which they misinterpret as degrading and disapproving. They tend to be shy, quiet, and inhibited. They say nothing rather than risk being wrong, and they react strongly to any possible indications of mockery or criticism. They usually appear anxious, self-doubting, and insecure when speaking, often use self-defeating expressions, and try to please others. Their tense and fearful demeanour may elicit ridicule from others, which confirms their insecurity. They are concerned with reacting to scrutiny by blushing or crying, which is a cause of further interpersonal avoidance. These patients often choose occupations where no social interaction is needed, and strongly avoid talking in public. The avoidant person lacks intimate relationships with friends or sexual partners unless they anticipate non-critical acceptance.

Patients with avoidant personality disorder perceive themselves as inept and inadequate, and assume that they are unattractive. They tend to see others as negative and potentially harmful. They are inattentive and repeatedly distracted by intrusive thoughts, but they attend intensely to signals of rejection. These people tend to make negative evaluations of situations and exaggerate risk. They have a low tolerance for dysphoric affects, which they avoid by escaping. Escape from reality through fantasy is their usual way of satisfying their needs and relieving frustration.

At interview they may be quite open if they feel accepted. This happens when good rapport is made, which is often easier in clinical than in social situations. However, social limitation outside the office may be intense. Avoidant patients usually feel ashamed about many aspects of their lives and are excessively self-critical, although most of the concerns expressed seem to be trivial.

(d) Course

Avoidant personality disorder may follow childhood fear of strangers and shyness and isolation during school years. However, most shyness in childhood gradually dissipates in adolescence. When it evolves into avoidant personality disorder, the shyness may worsen in adolescence when social and interpersonal relationships become more complex and demanding. The disorder tends to remit or to become less evident in older people.

Avoidant personality disorder is often associated with depressive episodes, dysthymia, and anxiety disorders, particularly social phobia.

Table 4.12.3.12 DSM-IV diagnostic criteria for avoidant personality disorder

A pervasive pattern of social inhibition, feelings of inadequacy, and to negative evaluation, beginning by early adulthood and present in a variety of contexts, as indicated by four (or more) of the following

1. Avoids occupational activities that involve significant interpersonal contact, because of fears of criticism, disapproval, or rejection
2. Is unwilling to get involved with people unless certain of being liked
3. Shows restraint within intimate relationships because of the fear of being shamed or ridiculed
4. Is preoccupied with being criticized or rejected in social situations
5. Is inhibited in new interpersonal situations because of feelings of inadequacy
6. Views self as socially inept, personally unappealing, or inferior to others
7. Is unusually reluctant to take personal risks or to engage in any new activities because they may prove embarrassing

(e) Differential diagnosis

It is often difficult to differentiate avoidant personality disorder and social phobia of the generalized type. Impairment and distress due to the phobic situations is more intense in social phobia, which may have started in middle adulthood rather than adolescence. It is not clear whether the disorders are alternative manifestations of the same condition, or are separate disorders.

Hypersensitivity to rejection and criticism, low self-esteem, and feelings of inadequacy are also features of dependent personality disorder. While the avoidant patient avoids contact, the dependent patient focuses on being cared for. However, the disorders often co-occur and must be diagnosed together.

Schizoid and schizotypal personality disorder are also character ized by social isolation. However, avoidants want to have relationships and suffer for their isolation, while schizoids and schizotypals accept isolation.

People with paranoid personality disorders lack confidence in others. However, avoidants do not confide in others because they fear being found inadequate, whereas paranoids fear malicious intent.

(f) Treatment

Anxiety and hypersensitivity to rejection may improve with anxiolytic medication, β-blockers, monoamine oxidase inhibitors, and antidepressant medication. Medication should be combined with psychological treatment based on reinforcing assertiveness and self-esteem, and restructuring cognitive distortions concerning the self and others. Conscious and unconscious dependency needs should be addressed.

Dependent personality disorder (JLC)

Individuals with this disorder show a persistent and global pattern of behaviours directed at avoidance of the loss of intimate others. To attain this goal, they relinquish their own needs, opinions, expression of feelings, and even their self-identity. In exchange, they get others to take over responsibility for major areas of their lives and to protect them. Their self-concept is characterized by weakness and helplessness, while others are perceived as powerful and protective.

These people were formerly included in different classificatory categories. They belong to the abulic type of Kraepelin and of Schneider[(2)] and were considered as immature personalities.

(a) Aetiology

Classic hypotheses attributing dependent personality to fixation in oral phase of psychosexual development have given way to others indicating that the cause is rather deprivation than overgratification in the oral phase.

Dependent personality was recognized first in DSM-III.[(11)] The description has changed little in DSM-IV (Table 4.12.3.13) and ICD-10.[(52)] The crucial feature in both systems is the urgent need of patients to be cared for by others, with dependence, attachment, and fear of abandonment. Lack of self-confidence was required in DSM-III, but was eliminated from recent classifications because it is not specific to this disorder.

(b) Clinical picture

Dependent patients are passive. They rarely express needs or feelings, especially those that are sexual or aggressive. They tend to avoid responsibilities or decisions in major areas of their lives, such as work and financial or interpersonal relationships. Instead they get others, particularly family or partner, to decide for them or to provide continuous guidance. They depend on others (often one other person, usually the partner or a parent) to decide where they should go, what they should do, and even which clothes they should wear. They manifest self-doubt, pessimism, and a need for affection. They lack aggressiveness and appear helpless. The dependent patient avoids jobs that demand taking responsibility and managing others, and becomes anxious when forced into such situations. These patients seek intensely for companionship and do not tolerate being alone. They may function at an adequate level if in a close and protective relationship, but when left alone they are unable to survive. They believe that they are incapable of functioning independently and require constant assistance. They do not initiate projects, but wait for others who, they believe, will do them better. However, dependent individuals can perform such tasks for other people whom they want to please and to whom they want to attach themselves.

They accept unpleasant tasks, are self-sacrificing, and tolerate verbal, physical, or sexual abuse. Abusive relationships may be accepted as long as the attachment is preserved and is not excessively distorted.

An excessive and unrealistic fear of abandonment is constant in dependent individuals. When an intimate relationship is terminated by separation or death, dependent individuals urgently seek another person who will provide the care and support they seek. Thus they become rapidly and indiscriminately attached to other persons when left alone.

These people are pessimistic, self-doubting, and have low self-esteem. They belittle their capacities and successes and present themselves as inept. They take criticism as a proof of their ineptness and confirmation of their lack of self-confidence.

Table 4.12.3.13 DSM-IV diagnostic criteria for dependent personality disorder

A pervasive and excessive need to be taken care of that leads to submissive and clinging behaviour and fears of separation, beginning by early adulthood and present in a variety of contexts, as indicated by five (or more) of the following

1 Has difficulty making everyday decisions without an excessive amount of advice and reassurance from others
2 Needs others to assume responsibility for most major areas of his or her life
3 Has difficulty expressing disagreement with others because of fear of loss of support or approval. **Note** Do not include realistic fears of retribution
4 Has difficulty initiating projects or doing things on his or her own (because of a lack of self-confidence in judgement or abilities rather than a lack of motivation or energy)
5 Goes to excessive lengths to obtain nurturance and support from others, to the point of volunteering to do things that are unpleasant
6 Feels uncomfortable or helpless when alone because of exaggerated fears of being unable to care for himself or herself
7 Urgently seeks another relationship as a source of care and support when a close relationship ends
8 Is unrealistically preoccupied with fears of being left to take care of himself or herself

(c) Epidemiology

Recent studies have found a median prevalence of 0.7 per cent (see Chapter 4.12.5). Although dependent personality disorder is diagnosed more frequently in women, structured interviews have not shown significant differences between the sexes. Cultural factors may affect the reported prevalence, as passivity, politeness, and submission are normal in some societies.

(d) Course

Dependent personality features present in adolescence may evolve positively in adulthood or lead to a personality disorder. Dependent individuals are at increased risk of depressive, anxiety, and adjustment disorders, particularly in relation to loss of close relationships. Dependent personality disorder may follow separation anxiety in childhood, or chronic physical illnesses in childhood requiring long periods of care and attention.

(e) Differential diagnosis

Dependent personality disorder has some similarities with histrionic personality disorder. Histrionic patients, like dependent patients, adjust their conduct to please other people. Their lives are centred in these others. However, people with histrionic personality disorder obtain attention and care by seductive or manipulative behaviours, whereas people with dependent personality disorder wait passively for others to care for them.[7]

Like people with avoidant personality disorder, dependent individuals may feel devastated by minor criticism or lack of attention from others. However, they lack the sense of embarrassment and social shyness of the avoidant, and fear loneliness or abandonment.

People with dependent and borderline personality disorders share an excessive fear of abandonment. However, borderline individuals react to separation with feelings of emptiness and rage, and are demanding, in contrast with the submissive and appeasing attitude of dependent individuals, which is directed towards finding another person to provide support.

Dependent personality disorder must be differentiated from normal dependent behaviours in specific life situations; for example, elderly people with chronic or debilitating disease may become dependent.

(f) Treatment

Pharmacological treatment is indicated only when depressive or anxiety symptoms are present, especially when associated with separation or loss.

In psychotherapy, the therapist must avoid the development of excessively dependent attachments. Self-confidence and self-esteem should be enhanced and the patient helped to enjoy the feeling of personal autonomy and independence. Cognitive restructuring and social skills training are often useful in bringing these changes about.

Obsessive–compulsive (anankastic) personality disorder

While DSM-IV labels this personality disorder as obsessive–compulsive personality disorder (Table 4.12.3.14), ICD-10 prefers the term anankastic, previously used in European psychiatry to refer to fearful, insecure, and compulsive individuals. The cardinal feature of this disorder is an exaggerated and pervasive attempt to control. Anankastic patients need to control those who are close to them, to control every uncertainty, and to control their own thoughts and emotions. The anankastic lacks an internal sense of security and tries to make the external world totally predictable. The anankastic is afraid of his own internal aggressive drives and avoids free emotional expression. Others perceive this kind of personality as characterized by inflexibility and stubborn inefficiency.

Table 4.12.3.14 DSM-IV diagnostic criteria for obsessive–compulsive personality disorder

A pervasive pattern of preoccupation with orderliness, perfectionism, and mental and interpersonal control, at the expense of flexibility, openness, and effciency, beginning by early adulthood and present in a variety of contexts, as indicated by four (or more) of the following

1 Is preoccupied with details, rules, lists, order, organization, or schedules to the extent that the major point of the activity is lost
2 Shows perfectionism that interferes with task completion (e.g. is unable to complete a project because his or her own overly strict standards are not met)
3 Is excessively devoted to work and productivity to the exclusion of leisure activities and friendships (not accounted for by obvious economic necessity)
4 Is overconscientious, scrupulous, and inflexible about matters of morality, ethics, or values (not accounted for by cultural or religious identification)
5 Is unable to discard worn-out or worthless objects even when they have no sentimental value
6 Is reluctant to delegate tasks or to work with others unless they submit to exactly his or her way of doing things
7 Adopts a miserly spending style toward both self and others; money is viewed as something to be hoarded for future catastrophes
8 Shows rigidity and stubbornness

(a) Epidemiology

The prevalence of obsessive–compulsive personality disorders is about 1 per cent in community samples and up to 10 per cent in psychiatric patients, especially those with depressive and anxiety disorders. It is most frequent among males. Some obsessive–compulsive traits are sanctioned in some cultures, and a personality disorder should not be diagnosed unless the traits are markedly beyond the average for the culture.

(b) Aetiology

Biological factors and learning seem to be involved in the aetiology of obsessive–compulsive personality disorder. The personality may be partly inherited.[53] Early psychodynamic theories linked obsessive personality to the anal phase of psychosexual development between the ages of 2 and 4, when libidinal drives come into conflict with parental attempts to socialize the child, especially in sphincter control and toilet training. Later psychoanalytic theory[54] emphasized earlier manifestations of the child's autonomy versus parental wishes. The expression of drives and emotions, including anger, is shaped by parental responses and may evoke shame and criticism.

This dynamic sequence is reinforced in societies which are strongly influenced by the Protestant work ethic, in families where individual emotions are subordinated to the group, and in societies in which open expression of emotions is discouraged.

(c) Clinical picture

The behaviour of an obsessive–compulsive personality has been consistently described as one of orderliness. The patient is preoccupied with details, and pays attention to rules, procedures, schedules, and punctuality. Patients with obsessional personalities often produce their own detailed lists of symptoms and are annoyed if any item is neglected or misinterpreted. They repeat actions and check for mistakes, despite the inconvenience and annoyance that result from this behaviour. As a consequence, their conduct is frequently inefficient. For example, the combination of unproductive perfectionism and rigidity may lead to difficulty in finishing a written report on time because of excessive correction and rewriting. Since this striving for perfection and order is time consuming, other areas of their lives often appear disorganized. One room or one desk drawer may fall into disarray, or parts of their social or family lives may be disorganized.

People with obsessive–compulsive personality focus on work and productivity. It is difficult for them to take vacations or even to have free time. They do not enjoy leisure activity, which they may consider a waste of time. Often, they need to take work home to alleviate their anxiety. Hobbies and leisure pursuits become formally organized activities. They insist on perfect performance of sports or games and transform them into a serious task requiring careful organization and hard work. Leisure activities may be an unpleasant experience for the others involved, owing to the insistence on rules and standards.

Stubbornness is another characteristic of these people. They need things to be done in their way, and realistic arguments do not usually make them change their insistence. They need others to submit to their way of doing things, and often believe that no one can do the tasks as perfectly as they can. They give detailed instructions, insisting that their way is the only way of doing things, and are irritated if others suggest alternatives. Therefore, they generally insist in doing everything themselves and are unable to delegate, which increases their inefficiency at work. Paradoxically, their stubbornness is associated with doubt. Indecisiveness is a constant characteristic unless they have structured guidelines. They fear making mistakes or misjudgements, and delay repeatedly until they have enough data to take what they consider the only right decision. When rules do not dictate the correct answer to a problem or when procedures for tasks are not laid down, decision-making or task initiation may become a lengthy and painful process.

People with this personality disorder are characterized by excessive conscientiousness and scruples. They are inflexible about matters of morality, ethics, or values. Moral principles and standards of performance have to be followed rigidly, and respect for authority and rules is absolute. Failure to do these things leads to irritation, anger, and self-criticism.

These people are stingy and mean, and often live with standards far below their actual socio-economic status. They dislike spending, believing that money should be saved in case of future difficulties. They have great difficulty in discarding worn-out or worthless objects, believing that they might be useful some day. They may hoard objects such as newspapers or broken appliances, even when they have no sentimental value.

These people are humourless and lack spontaneity of emotional expression. Usually they do not express anger directly. However, they are often angry in situations in which they are unable to control the behaviour of themselves or others. Anger is generally manifested by indirect aggressive acts (such as leaving a small tip or not providing minor help when expected). Their management of anger is closely related to their attitude of dominance–submission towards authority figures. They may be excessively submissive to a person in authority whom they respect, but obstructive with an authority figure whom they do not respect.

The affect of the obsessive person is controlled and stilted. It is not flat or blunted, but constricted. They do not laugh or cry, and feel uncomfortable with people who express their feelings. Their mood is usually serious but may appear anxious or depressed. In a clinical interview they may sit in a stiff unnatural posture, and seldom make spontaneous comments about their emotions. They usually relate their history in a pedantic and circumstantial manner. If interrupted by a question from the doctor, they have to finish their monologue before answering. When asked about feelings, they answer with lists of facts and circumstances. They can label emotions and feelings, but are unable to display them.

In summary, obsessive personalities love order, neatness, and sameness, and hates novelty, spontaneity, and change. They need control, security, and certainty, and avoid creativity, art, and excitement. They mitigate anxiety by following strict rules and repress emotional expression by avoiding spontaneity. They fear their inner fragile and aggressive emotional world.

(d) Course

Like other personality disorders, obsessive–compulsive personality disorder is present in early adulthood and tends to be persistent and constant. However, some adolescents with marked obsessive traits become warm, loving, and tender adults. On the other hand, intense obsessional traits in adolescence are occasionally a premorbid stage of schizophrenia ('pseudoneurotic schizophrenia'). The developmental relationship between obsessive–compulsive personality disorder and obsessive–compulsive disorder is controversial. In the past, it was suggested that most obsessive–compulsive personality disorder evolved to a full obsessive–compulsive disorder, indicating that the two syndromes were expressions of the same basic disorder. More recent investigations[55] indicate that most obsessive–compulsive disorder patients do not have a comorbid obsessive–compulsive personality disorder. A variety of psychiatric disorders may present in a patient with obsessive personality, but depressive and anxiety disorders are the most common, followed by phobic, somatoform, and obsessive–compulsive symptoms. Hypochondriacal syndromes are commonly found in obsessive individuals when they lose control of situations.

Persons with this personality disorder may do well in jobs that demand working with detail, order, and structured procedures, and may adjust to interpersonal relationships with submissive spouses. However, they are particularly vulnerable to unexpected changes in their occupational and social environment. Late-onset depression is a common occurrence in obsessive–compulsive personalities.

(e) Differential diagnosis

The main difficulty in diagnosing obsessive–compulsive personality disorder is to differentiate it from obsessive–compulsive disorder. The latter diagnosis is made when occupational and personal functioning is severely impaired as a consequence of doubt, indecisiveness, hoarding, or any other obsessive behaviour. In many, but not all, cases of obsessive personality, the traits and behaviours are egosyntonic and no resistance is present, in contrast with obsessive–compulsive disorder.

The perfectionism of obsessive personalities may be present in narcissistic personality disorder. However, narcissistic individuals tend to believe that they have achieved perfection, while obsessive individuals tend to be highly critical of their own achievements.

Social detachment and the lack of empathy and warmth may suggest schizoid personality disorder. However, obsessive individuals constrain their emotional expression to keep control of a situation, while schizoids lack the fundamental capacity for affective display or intimacy.

Not all individuals with obsessive traits have obsessive–compulsive personality disorder. Obsessive traits can be adaptive in some situations; it is only when they are maladaptive, inflexible, and persistently cause functional impairment that a personality disorder be diagnosed.

(f) Treatment

Pharmacological treatment may be tried in patients with anxiety and distress due to intense doubts, indecisiveness, and scruples. Benzodiazepines may alleviate tension in these cases. Antidepressants with a serotonergic profile sometimes improve mood and global functioning.

Psychological cognitive treatment, focusing on perfectionism, rigidity, scrupulousness, and intolerance of failure, is the main therapeutic approach. Repressed aggression, guilt, and dependency needs should be addressed using a psychodynamic approach.

Other personality disorders (not included in DSM-IV)

Passive–aggressive (negativistic) personality disorder

(a) Definition

Resistance to demands for adequate social and occupational performance and negativistic attitude are considered to be central features of passive–aggressive personality disorder. A pervasive pattern of argumentativeness, oppositional behaviour, and defeatist attitudes are typical, and are thought to be a covert manifestation of underlying aggression, which is expressed passively and indirectly. Passive–aggressive personalities have interpersonal and cognitive dysfunction and severe impairment in terms of self-image, global mental health, and ability to function at work and in intimate relationships.(56)

Passive–aggressive personality disorder was officially included in DSM-I as the passive–aggressive personality 'trait disturbance' depicted as an immature reaction to military stress by helpless, passive, and obstructive resistant behaviour. However, passive–aggressive disorder was not included in DSM-IV because of the many unsolved problems related to its concept in previous classifications. Instead, it is placed in Appendix B of DSM-IV where it is alternatively called negativistic personality disorder. Research criteria are proposed which are expected to be empirically evaluated and to determine the validity and reliability of this diagnosis (Table 4.12.3.15).

There has been much debate as to whether passive aggression constitutes a personality disorder, a defence mechanism, or a specific maladaptive personality trait (coping style).(57) Surprisingly, empirical literature on the subject is scarce, although passive–aggressive behaviour has been widely recognized by clinicians. An overlap with other personalities has been shown, and it has never been included as a separate category in the *International Classification of Diseases*. The passive–aggressive dimension, as assessed by self-reports, is always high in depressed patients and is state-dependent.(58) Perhaps it would be best to conceptualize passive aggression as a continuum: a passive–aggressive defence mechanism may be normal in some situations, it could be a trait of many personality disorders, and when pronounced and long-lasting it should be designated as passive–aggressive personality disorder.

Table 4.12.3.15 DSM-IV research criteria for passive–aggressive personality disorder

A. A pervasive pattern of negativistic attitude and passive resistance to demands for adequate performance, beginning by early adulthood and present in variety of contexts, as indicated by four (or more) of the following

1 Passively resists fulfilling routine social and occupational tasks
2 Complains of being misunderstood and unappreciated by others
3 Is sullen and argumentative
4 Unreasonably criticizes and scorns authority
5 Expresses envy and resentment toward those apparently more fortunate
6 Voices exaggerated and persistent complaints of personal misfortune
7 Alternates between hostile defiance and contrition

B. Does not occur exclusively during major depressive episodes and is not better accounted for by dysthymic disorder

(b) Epidemiology

The population prevalence ranges from 0.9 to 3 per cent, but in those cases in which a secondary co-occurring diagnosis was assigned, the secondary frequency of passive–aggressive personality disorder was about 10 per cent.(59) Some studies found a higher prevalence in women and others in men.

(c) Aetiology

The cause of the disorder is multidimensional, comprising biological, psychoanalytical, behavioural, interpersonal, and social learning perspectives.

Ambivalence is considered to be a core conflict of passive–aggressive personalities, which originates from fixation to the biting or sucking stages of the oral phase of psychosexual development. Some authors consider masochism to be another precursor of the passive–aggressive personality.

According to the behavioural model, passive–aggressive behaviour is the expression of anger in maladaptive verbal and non-verbal ways that do not lead to rewarding problem-solving Failure to learn appropriate assertive behaviour would be the main aetiological factor.(60)

The primary social factor influencing the development of passive–aggressive patterns would be contradictory parental attitudes in childhood which, being conflicting and incompatible, prevent the child from expressing his feelings directly and thus urge him to develop passive resistance.

(d) Clinical characteristics and diagnosis

Passive–aggressive personalities seek novel and stimulating situations in impulsive ways, while remaining unpredictable.[61] Procrastination and inefficiency are behaviours used to avoid responsibility, which they show by stubborn resistance to the fulfilment of expectations and claiming forgetfulness.

Passive–aggressive individuals easily become irritable and, gloomy and they are resentful and discontent with life. Accumulated anger may be expressed by verbal acting-out, after which passive–aggressive individuals feel guilty and gloomy. Since they have difficulties in expressing emotions directly, they are prone to diffuse somatic complaints, hypochondriasis, and psychosomatic disorders.

Interpersonal ambivalence is a core feature of passive–aggressive personality disorder. Negativism is particularly expressed towards authorities, with whom they are never satisfied and whom they criticize constantly. The argumentative self-detrimental behaviour of passive–aggressive personalities is often experienced by others as punitive and manipulative. Negative verbal comments, which are often caustic, and irritable and moody patterns of communication are typical.

Passive–aggressive individuals are cynical, sceptical, hypercritical, and mistrustful. Disillusioned with life, discouraged, discontented with themselves and with others, they are also pessimistic about the future. They persistently complain and blame others for their own bad luck, feeling themselves to be misunderstood martyrs and victims of destiny.

(e) Comorbidity and differential diagnosis

Passive–aggressive personality disorder is frequently comorbid with major depression, dysthymic disorder, anxiety, panic disorder, and hypochondriasis. Patients with depressive disorders are more aware of their feelings of inferiority and more likely to feel guilty, and their depressed mood is continuous rather than erratically hostile and moody, as in passive–aggressive personality.

Comorbidity with many personality disorders (histrionic, borderline, obsessive–compulsive, dependent, narcissistic) is also frequently observed. People with these personality disorders may use passive aggression as a defence mechanism. Suicide attempts are not as frequent as in histrionic and borderline personality disorders, and features of passive–aggressive personality are less dramatic, affective, openly aggressive, and severe.

(e) Course and prognosis

There are insufficient data on the course and prognosis of passive–aggressive personality disorder. When passive–aggressive people are unable to control their anger, they may experience anxiety, panic states, depressive episodes, chronic depression, and psychosomatic disorders. They are prone to alcohol abuse, and their careers are erratic and stunted despite their abilities (frequent changes of jobs are common). Suicide attempts may complicate this disorder.

(f) Treatment

(i) Pharmacotherapy

Target symptoms, such as depression, anxiety, and somatic complaints, should be treated. Benzodiazepines may be warranted and helpful in the initial period of psychotherapy. The side effects of medication are often the reason for complaints about their psychiatrist's inefficiency. Non-compliance is frequent, reflecting resistance to the therapist. Abuse of medicaments should be controlled and considered seriously.

(ii) Psychotherapy

Psychotherapy is the treatment of choice. Various modes are used, including supportive, psychodynamic, behavioural assertiveness training, and the paradoxical approach in group or individual settings. The goal of treatment should be to help the patient escape from the vicious circle of self-defeating behaviour and develop a mature way of expressing anger and other feelings.

Self-defeating (masochistic) personality disorder

Individuals with masochistic personality disorder persistently seek humiliation and failure, and submit to the will of others.

The term masochism was introduced to psychiatry by Krafft-Ebing in 1882. It is derived from a character in a novel by the German author Leopold von Sacher-Masoch, a man who endured torture, scorn, and humiliation from a woman. Later, Freud conceptualized masochism as the result of aggressive instinct directed towards the self instead of an external object. Reich[62] described the masochistic character as a person who suffered deep frustrations in early developmental stages and needed to express this frustration through suffering inflicted by the love 'objects'. Thus defiance is always present in the masochistic search for love. According to Horney,[63] helplessness and victimization may be a masochistic way of expressing hostility by making others feel shameful. Masochistic suffering may also be used to avoid reproach and responsibility and as a way of restoring a sign of personal value.

(a) Clinical picture

People with self-defeating personality disorder avoid pleasurable experiences and undermine their achievements. They neglect their appearance and live below their means. They accept and endure humiliation, expecting that others will sympathize with them. In this way, they fulfil their expectation that submission will bring love and care. They prefer to relate to people who abuse them and consider those who consistently treat them well to be boring.

These people fail to accomplish tasks of which they are capable and adopt an inferior role. When making appropriate demands, they feel that they are taking advantage of others and adopt an apologetic manner. For them, success is inversely related to inner security. Successful relationships do not make them feel confident, but increase their fears. They tend to believe that all experiences involve future frustration and pain. They may respond to positive personal events with depression and behaviour that negates their accomplishments. They look for people who will respond to their behaviour with disdain, rejection, or cruelty.

People with self-defeating personality disorder do not defend themselves against expressions of disgust and resentment directed towards them and rarely accuse or reproach others. They do not feel confident and are not assertive. They fear that optimism may lead to greater problems.

They are not worried by these attitudes. Rather, masochists believe that by exaggerating their weaknesses and inefficiency they will protect themselves from aggression by others. They feel protected when someone needs something from them, and many non-assertive masochists engage in self-sacrifice for their own protective feelings rather than for the welfare of others. What seems to be a comprehensive and self-sacrificing attitude reflects a lack of confidence and empathy.

The mood of these individuals is usually dysphoric, fluctuating between anxiety and sadness.

(b) Differential diagnosis

Since masochistic personality disorder is not included in DSM-IV, little research has been done on comorbidity or on the validity or specificity of this diagnosis.

Self-defeating attitudes, low self-esteem, and depression may be found in individuals with dependent, borderline, and depressive personality disorders. Some of the characteristics are also found in avoidant personality disorder.

Masochists are prone to mood disorder and dysthymia. Anxiety disorders are frequent. Their fears of abandonment are a persistent source of anxiety. Hypochondriasis and somatization are also common, sometimes as a way of obtaining attention.

(c) Treatment

Antidepressants and anxiolytics may be useful to alleviate a dysphoric state. Psychological treatment should take into account that masochistic patients sometimes induce an aggressive countertransference as a response to their own wish to be hurt. The therapist should gradually clarify the behaviours, which provoke hostile responses and seek to reward adaptive interpersonal behaviours. Training in assertiveness and social skills is sometimes helpful.

Sadistic personality disorder

Sadistic personality disorder is a controversial category, which is not included in either DSM-IV or ICD-10. Some authors, especially those working with perpetrators of abuse, support its inclusion in the diagnostic nomenclature, believing that it is a valid clinical entity, which deserves special treatment. Sadism as a term describing desire to inflict pain upon the sexual object was originally used by Krafft-Ebing.[64] Kernberg[32] connects two dispositions (sadistic and masochistic) into a sadomasochistic character, which includes 'help-rejecting complainers' and often has underlying borderline personality organization.

(a) Aetiology

Subjects with sadistic personality disorder often had a history of significant childhood loss and physical, emotional, or sexual abuse during childhood.[65] Despite their significant psychopathology, sadistic individuals are surprisingly highly functioning, with steady employment and intense long-lasting relationships.

(b) Clinical picture

Sadistic individuals demonstrate a long-standing maladaptive pattern of cruel, demeaning, and aggressive behaviour towards others in order to cause suffering and pain and to establish dominance and control. Sadistic persons are fascinated by violence, weapons, injuries, and torture, and are most frequently encountered in forensic settings among child and partner abusers.

(c) Differential diagnosis

The major distinction for the diagnosis of sadistic personality disorder is from antisocial personality disorder. Sadistic persons may simply represent an aggressive (antagonistic) subtype of psychopathy. Intimidation and sadistic control of others, as well as a fascination with weapons, martial arts, and torture, may be manifested by both antisocial and sadistic individuals. Moreover, both disorders may display 'malignant narcissism',[37] with an admixture of narcissistic, antisocial, sadistic, and paranoid features.

(d) Epidemiology

Existing data[66] suggest that sadistic personality disorder is relatively uncommon, although it may have a higher prevalence in specific forensic populations. Several studies found a high overlap with narcissistic, paranoid, and antisocial personality disorders, which raised the possibility that sadistic personality disorder may not be a distinct entity.

(e) Course

No data are available on the course of this disorder.

(f) Treatment

Sadistic individuals seldom seek treatment, and are usually encountered in forensic settings. No treatment has been successful for this disorder. Since the aetiology is probably multifactorial, there should be multiple approaches to treatment. The primary aim of treatment is control of cruelty and malignant aggression. As with antisocial personalities, selective serotonin reuptake inhibitors and lithium may be beneficial in regulating the serotonergic function that probably underlies the aggressive action, and carbamazepine and clonazepam may act to regulate ictal aggressive outbursts.

Psychotherapy is usually difficult because these individuals lack any desire to change and because there may be serious countertransference problems for the therapists. Small groups may be helpful because there is a dissolution of transference and peer confrontation is accepted more easily.

Depressive personality disorder

This personality disorder is not included in ICD-10 or DSM-IV, although it is considered as a subject for further study in the latter. However, the concept of depressive personality was well recognized in previous decades (e.g. by Kraepelin and Schneider). Depressive personality was seen as a pattern of brooding, pessimism, and low self-confidence,[2] and as a tendency to physical lassitude and suffering. Phenomenological accounts[67] emphasize dependency, orderliness, and adherence to social conventions. The psychoanalytic concept of masochism[47] overlaps to some extent with the classical depressive personality. More recently, Akiskal[68] has discussed the depressive personality as part of a spectrum of affective disorders, reviving Kretschmer's ideas[10] on the role of temperament as the base from where psychiatric disorders develop.

(a) Aetiology

Psychological and biological factors have been suggested as causes of depressive personality disorder. Early losses, inadequate attention from parents, and a punitive superego have been postulated by psychoanalytic authors. Others have suggested that a depressive temperament is genetically related to affective disorder.

(b) Clinical picture

People with depressive personality disorder are submissive, quiet, introverted, and unassertive. Their cognitive style is marked by pessimism, dejection, and self-reproach. They appear gloomy, joyless, cheerless, and unhappy. They are serious and lack a sense of humour. They do not believe that they deserve to be happy. They have a negative view of the past and present and do not expect things to improve. They anticipate failure and dwell on their negative perspective of life. They have a low tolerance to shortcomings and failures, which are seen as confirming their own pessimistic assumptions. They are prone to guilt and judge themselves severely.

Their self-esteem is low and they feel inadequate. They focus on the failings of others and are critical of themselves.

(c) Epidemiology

No data are available on the frequency of this disorder in the population.

(d) Differential diagnosis

Some clinicians doubt whether a distinction can be made between depressive personality disorder and dysthymic disorder. The diagnosis of depressive personality disorder emphasizes cognitive and behavioural aspects rather than the depressed mood. Also, dysthymia, although chronic, has a fluctuating course.

Dysthymic patents generally experience their symptoms as egodystonic, while people with depressive personality disorder think that they have a realistic view of their situation. People with depressive personality disorder may meet the criteria for dependent personality disorder and self-defeating personality disorder, and it is difficult to distinguish between these disorders.

(e) Course

Patients with depressive personality disorder have depressive episodes and dysthymia more frequently than other individuals, and may have difficulties in adapting to stressful or uncertain situations.

(f) Treatment

Antidepressants may be useful when the person is at higher risk for developing a depressive episode. Psychological treatment may be helpful, since these people have a good capacity for introspection and reality testing. Cognitive approaches can help patients to understand their negative views and derogatory attitudes. These patients usually establish a good therapeutic relationship with the clinician.

Personality changes

Enduring personality changes after traumatic experiences

ICD-10 has two categories for personality changes: those occurring after catastrophic situations, and those starting after psychiatric illness. Either diagnosis should be made only when there is evidence of a definite personality change, including cognition, behaviour, and interpersonal relationships. The changes must not be a manifestation of a current mental disorder or the residue of a previous mental disorder. It must not be an exacerbation of a pre-existing personality disorder.

The **aetiology** of the personality change presumably relates to the extreme existential experience of the catastrophic situation or the psychiatric illness.

Examples of catastrophic experiences include life in concentration camps, experiences of disaster, and prolonged exposure to other life-threatening situations. Personality changes following short-term exposure to life-threatening situations, such as a car accident, should not be included in this group, since such changes probably depend on a previous psychological vulnerability. In ICD-10, the symptoms of personality change after catastrophic experiences include hostility and mistrust of the environment, social withdrawal, feelings of emptiness or hopelessness, estrangement, and alertness or feeling on the edge.

When the personality change follows a mental disorder, the cause is related to the stressful experience and the perceived damage to the patient's self-image arising from the disease. Other people's attitudes towards the illness, the subjective emotional experience, and previous psychological adjustment are also important. Features of the personality change after mental disorders include feelings of being stigmatized and consequent withdrawal, passivity, and loss of interests, dependence, excessive demandingness and complaining, and dysphoric–labile mood.

Personality change due to a general medical condition (JLC)

This category, which is included in both ICD-10 and DSM-IV, describes syndromes affecting global features of behaviour, cognition, and emotions, and secondary to the physiological effects of general medical diseases.

The essential feature is a change in personality after a general medical disease. In childhood before a stable pattern of personality has been established, a marked deviation from normal development suggests the diagnosis.

A central feature is loss of control over the expression of emotions and impulses. Affect is commonly labile and shallow, although persistent mild euphoria or apathy may be present, especially when the frontal lobes are affected. The elevated mood of these patients is hollow and silly, unlike that of hypomania. Patients may appear childish, expansive, and disinhibited, but they may admit to not feeling happy. Others are indifferent and apathetic.

Exaggerated expressions of rage and aggression are usually present, often out of proportion to any stressor. Loss of impulse control is also shown in social and sexual disinhibition, inappropriate jokes, and overeating.

(a) Aetiology

In most cases this disorder is associated with structural damage to the brain. Head trauma, cerebral neoplasms, vascular accidents, multiple sclerosis, Huntington's disease, and complex partial epilepsy may all cause personality change, especially when affecting frontal and temporal lobes. Systemic diseases involving the central nervous system, including endocrine disorders, AIDS, lupus erythematosus and chronic metal poisoning, may have the same effect.

Patients with this disorder generally have a clear sensorium but may be inattentive and have some mild cognitive dysfunction. They do not show intellectual deterioration.

(b) Differential diagnosis

In dementia, personality change is accompanied by intellectual deterioration. However, personality change may predate the dementia. Distinction from schizophrenia and other personality disorders is based on the clinical history and the presence of a general medical disease capable of causing personality change.

(c) Treatment

If possible, treatment is directed to the causative condition. Pharmacological treatment of specific symptoms may be useful when depression or inappropriate anger is present.

Further information

Millon, T., and Davis, R. (2000). *Personality disorders in modern life*. John Wiley and sons, Inc., New York.

Schneider, K. (1950). *Psychopathic personalities* (9th edn.). Casell, London. (Original work published in 1923).

Menninger, K. (1940). Character disorders. In *The psychodynamics of abnormal behaviour* (ed. J.F. Brown), pp. 384–403. McGraw-Hill, New York.

Livesley, W.J., Jackson, D.N., and Schroeder, M.L. (1992). Factorial structure of traits delineating personality disorders in clinical and general population samples. *Journal of Abnormal Psychology*, **101**, 432–40.

References

1. Kraepelin, E. (1921). *Manic-depressive insanity and paranoia*. Lingstone, Edinburgh.
2. Schneider, K. (1950). *Psychopathic personalities* (9th edn.). Cassell, London.
3. Freud, S. (1911). Psychoanalytic notes upon an autobiographical account of a case of paranoia. In *Collected papers*, Vol. 3. Hogarth Press, London, 1925.
4. Perry, J.C., and Vaillant, G.E. (1989). Personality disorders. In *Textbook of psychiatry* (eds. H.I. Kaplan and B.J. Sadock), pp. 1352–87. Williams and Wilkins, Baltimore, MD.
5. Kendler, K.S., Masterson, C.C., Ungaro, R., *et al.* (1984). A family history study of schizophrenia related personality disorders. *The American Journal of Psychiatry*, **141**, 424–7.
6. Seiver, L.J. and Davis, K.L. (1991). A psychobiological perspective on the personality disorders. *The American Journal of Psychiatry*, **148**, 1647–58.
7. Millon, T. (1997). *Disorders of personality: DSM-IV and beyond* (2nd edn.). Wiley, New York.
8. American Psychiatric Association. (1994). *Diagnostic and statistical manual of mental disorders* (4th edn.). American Psychiatric Association, Washington, DC.
9. Sullivan, H.S. (1953). *The interpersonal theory of psychiatry*. Norton, New York.
10. Kretschmer, E. (1936). *Physique and character*. Kegan Paul, Trench, Trubner, London.
11. American Psychiatric Association. (1987). *Diagnostic and statistical manual of mental disorders* (3rd edn. revised). American Psychiatric Association, Washington, DC.
12. Robins, L.N. (1966). *Deviant children grown up: a sociological and psychiatric study of sociopathic personality*. Williams and Wilkins, Baltimore, MD.
13. de Girolamo, G. and Reich, J.H. (1993). *Personality disorders*. WHO, Geneva.
14. Crowe, R.R. (1974). An adoption study of antisocial personality. *Archives of General Psychiatry*, **31**, 785–91.
15. Cadoret, R.J. (1978). Psychopathology in adopted-away offspring of biologic parents with antisocial behaviour. *Archives of General Psychiatry*, **35**, 176–84.
16. Coccaro, E.F., Siever, L.J., Klar, H.M., *et al.* (1989). Serotonergic studies in patients with affective and personality disorders. *Archives of General Psychiatry*, **46**, 587–99.
17. Dee Higley, J., Mehlman, P.T., Taub, D.M., *et al.* (1992). Cerebrospinal fluid monoamine and adrenal correlates of aggression in free-ranging rhesus monkeys. *Archives of General Psychiatry*, **49**, 436–41.
18. Glueck, B. and Glueck, E. (1956). *Physique and delinquency*. Harper, New York.
19. Gunderson, J.G. (1984). *Borderline personality disorder*. American Psychiatric Press, Washington, DC.
20. Akhtar, S. (1992). *Broken structure*. Aronson, Northvale, NJ.
21. Jones, M. (1952). *Social psychiatry: a study of therapeutic communities*. Tavistock Publications, London.
22. Stern, A. (1938). Psychoanalytical investigation and therapy in borderline group of neuroses. *Psychoanalytic Quarterly*, **7**, 467–89.
23. Gunderson, J.G. and Kolb, J.E. (1978). Discriminating features of borderline patients. *The American Journal of Psychiatry*, **135**, 792–6.
24. Kernberg, O. (1989). The narcissistic personality disorder and the differential diagnosis of antisocial behaviour. *The Psychiatric Clinics of North America*, **12**, 553–70.
25. Quality Assurance Project. (1991). Treatment outlines for borderlines, narcissistic and histrionic personality disorders. *The Australian and New Zealand Journal of Psychiatry*, **25**, 392–403.
26. Akiskal, H.S. (1981). Subaffective disorders: dysthymic, cyclothymic and bipolar II disorders in the 'borderline realm'. *The Psychiatric Clinics of North America*, **4**, 25–46.
27. Widiger, T.A. and Frances, A. (1989). Epidemiology, diagnosis, and comorbidity of borderline personality disorder. In *American PsychiatricPress review of psychiatry*, Vol. 8 (eds. A. Tasman, R.E. Hales, and A.J. Frances), pp. 8–24. American Psychiatric Press, Washington, DC.
28. Stone, M.H. (1980). *The borderline syndromes. Constitution, personality and adaptation*. McGraw-Hill, New York.
29. Coccaro, E.F., Siever, L.J., Klar, H.M., *et al.* (1989). Sertonergic studies in patients with affective and personality disorders: correlates with suicidal and impulsive aggressive behaviour. *Archives of General Psychiatry*, **46**, 587–99.
30. New, A.S., Hazlett, E.A., Buchsbaum, M.S., *et al.* (2007). Amygdala-prefrontal disconnection in borderline personality disorder. *Neuropsychopharmacology*, **32** (7), 1629–40.
31. Zanarini, M.C., Williams, A.A., Lewis, R.E., *et al.* (1997). Reported pathological childhood experiences associated with the development of borderline personality disorder. *The American Journal of Psychiatry*, **154**, 1101–6.
32. Kernberg, O.F. (1975). *Borderline conditions and pathological narcissism*. Aronson, New York.
33. Gunderson, J.G. (1996). The borderline patient's intolerance of aloneness: insecure attachment and therapist availability. *The American Journal of Psychiatry*, **153**, 752–8.
34. Akhtar, S. (1984). The syndrome of identity diffusion. *The American Journal of Psychiatry*, 141, 1381–5.
35. Gunderson, J.G. and Phillips, K.A. (1995). Personality disorders. In *Comprehensive textbook of psychiatry* (5th edn.) (eds. H.I. Kaplan and B.J. Sadock), pp. 1438–41. Williams and Wilkins, Baltimore, MD.
36. Stein, G. (1992). Drug treatment of personality disorders. *The British Journal of Psychiatry*, **161**, 167–84.
37. Kernberg, O.F. (1984). *Severe personality disorder-psychotherapeutic strategies*. Yale University Press, New Haven, CT.
38. Paris, J. (1994). *Borderline personality disorder-a multidimensional approach*. American Psychiatric Press, Washington, DC.
39. Linehan, M.M., (1987). Dialectical behavior therapy: a cognitive behavioral approach to parasuicide. *Journal of Personality Disorders*, **1**, 328–33.
40. Kraepelin, E. (1913). Hysterical insanity. In *Lectures on clinical psychiatry* (trans. T. Johnstone), pp. 249–58. William Wood, New York.
41. Freud, S. (1931). Libidinal types. In *Standard edition of the complete psychological works of Sigmund Freud*, Vol. 21 (ed. J. Strachey), p. 266. Hogarth Press, London, 1961.
42. Zimmerman, M. and Coryell, W.H. (1990). Diagnosing personality disorders in the community. *Archives of General Psychiatry*, **47**, 527–31.
43. Marmor, J. (1953). Orality in the hysterical personality. *The Journal of the American Psychoanalytic Association*, **1**, 656–71.

44. Torgersen, S. (1980). The oral, obsessive and hysterical personality syndromes. A study of hereditary and environmental factors by means of the twin method. *Archives of General Psychiatry*, **37**, 1272–7.
45. Cadoret, R.J. (1978). Psychopathology in adopted-away offspring of biologic parents with antisocial behaviour. *Archives of General Psychiatry*, **35**, 176–84.
46. Zetzel, E. (1968). The so-called good hysteric. *The International Journal of Psychoanalysis*, **49**, 256–60.
47. Kernberg, O. (1988). Hysterical and histrionic personality disorders. In *The personality disorders and neuroses* (eds. A. Cooper, A. Frances, and M. Sacks), pp. 231–41. J.B. Lippincott, Philadelphia, PA.
48. Zimmerman, M. and Coryell, W.H. (1990). Diagnosing personality disorders in the community. *Archives of General Psychiatry*, **47**, 527–31.
49. Ronningstam, E. and Gunderson, J. (1991). Differentiating borderline personality disorder from narcissistic personality disorder. *Journal of Personality Disorders*, **5**, 225–32.
50. Millon, T. (1981). *Disorders of personality: DSM-III Axis II*. Wiley, New York.
51. Cloninger, C.R. (1986). A unified biosocial theory and its role in the development of anxiety states. *Psychiatric Development*, **3**, 167–226.
52. World Health Organization. (1992). *The ICD-10 classification of mental and behavioural disorders-clinical descriptions and diagnostic guidelines*. World Health Organization, Geneva.
53. Clifford, C.A., Murray, R.M., and Fulker, D.W. (1984). Genetic and environmental influences on obsessional traits and symptoms. *Psychological Medicine*, **14**, 791–800.
54. Erikson, E. (1959). Growth and crises of the healthy personality. In *Psychological issues* (ed. G.S. Klein). International Universities Press, New York.
55. Baer, L. and Jenike, M.A. (1992). Personality disorders in obsessive compulsive disorder. *The Psychiatric Clinics of North America*, **15**, 803–12.
56. Drake, R.E. and Vaillant, G.E. (1985). A validity study of axis II of DSM-III. *The American Journal of Psychiatry*, **142**, 553–8.
57. Perry, J.C. and Flannery, R.B. (1982). Passive-aggressive personality disorder: treatment implications of a clinical typology. *The Journal of Nervous and Mental Disease*, **170**, 164–73.
58. Lecic-Tosevski, D. and Divac-Jovanovic, M. (1996). Effects of dysthymia on personality assessment. *European Personality*, **11**, 244–8.
59. Millon, T. (1993). Negativistic (passive-aggressive) personality disorder. *Journal of Personality Disorders*, **7**, 78–85.
60. Millon, T. (1981). *Disorders of personality. DSM-III: Axis II*. Wiley, New York.
61. Cloninger, C.R. (1987). A systematic method for clinical description and classification of personality variants. *Archives of General Psychiatry*, **44**, 573–88.
62. Reich, W. (1933). *Character analysis* (3rd edn.) (trans. V.R. Carfagno). Farrar, Straus and Giroux, New York.
63. Horney, K. (1945). *Our inner confl icts*. Norton, New York.
64. Krafft-Ebing, R. (1989). *Psychopathia sexualis* (10th edn). Enke, Stuttgart.
65. Gay, M. and Fiester, S. (1991). Sadistic personality disorder. In *Psychiatry* (ed. R. Michaels). J.B. Lippincott, Philadelphia, PA.
66. Fiester, S.J. and Gay, M. (1995). Sadistic personality disorder. In *The DSM-IV personality disorders* (ed. W.J. Livesley), pp. 329–40. Guilford Press, New York.
67. Tellenbach, H. (1980). *Melancholia*. Duquesne University Press, Pittsburgh, PA.
68. Akiskal, H.S. (1989). Validating affective personality types. In *The validity of psychiatric diagnosis* (ed. L. Robins), pp. 217–27. Raven Press, New York.

4.12.4 Epidemiology of personality disorders

Francesca Guzzetta and Giovanni de Girolamo

Introduction

tbegun to be scientifically investigated. This development has taken place because a number of standardized instruments to assess personality and PD in an empirical fashion have been developed, in parallel with the refinement of a valid and reliable diagnostic system based on a categorical approach.

The need for the epidemiological investigation of PDs seems justified for several reasons.

1 As seen in recent epidemiological surveys, PDs are frequent and have been found in different countries and sociocultural settings.

2 PDs can seriously impair the life of the affected individual and can be highly disruptive to societies, communities, and families.

3 Personality status is often a major predictive variable in determining the outcome of Axis I mental disorders and the response to treatment.

In this chapter, we review the epidemiological literature on PDs up to October 2007, focusing on studies carried out since the development of the DSM-III. First, community prevalence studies of PDs are reviewed. We then look at the prevalence of individual PDs in the community. Finally, we consider the prevalence of PDs in clinical populations, and in special settings (e.g. primary care, prisons, etc.).

Community epidemiological studies of unspecified personality disorders

Until the development of the DSM-III diagnostic criteria for PDs and the subsequent availability of standardized assessment instruments, epidemiological studies aimed at assessing the prevalence rate of PDs were hampered by severe methodological limitations, including differences in sampling methods and in diagnostic criteria, the known unreliability of PD diagnoses based on clinical judgement, and the lack of standardized assessment methods. Since 1980, twelve main studies with at least 200 subjects sampled have ascertained the prevalence rate of PDs in different community samples using assessment instruments specific for PD; they are shown in Table 4.12.4.1.

In these studies, the sample sizes ranged between 200 and 2053 subjects, with an average sample of 565.4; all surveyed individuals were evaluated by means of a specific PD assessment instrument, mainly a structured interview. While most studies were carried out in one stage, Lenzenweger *et al.*[(6)] first screened a large sample of university students with a self-administered Axis II inventory, and then interviewed a subgroup of 258 subjects using the International Personality Disorder Examination. The median prevalence rate of any PDs in these eight studies is 12.5 per cent.

Two large community studies[(13,14)] carried out in the USA were not included in Table 4.12.4.1 since PD prevalence rates were based

Table 4.12.4.1 Prevalence rates of personality disorders in epidemiological surveys

Reference	Country	Sample size	Sample features	Diagnostic Criteria	Assessment method	PD prevalence rate (%)
Black *et al.*[1]	USA	247	Relatives of obsessive-compulsive and normal control probands	DSM-III-R	SIPD	**22.3**[a]
Casey & Tyrer[2]	UK	200	Urban and rural residents	ICD-9	PAS	**13.0**
Coid *et al.*[3]	UK	626	Urban and rural residents aged 16–74 and selected in a 2 phase survey (weighted data)	DSM-IV	SCID-II	**4.4**
Crawford *et al.*[4]	USA	644	Individuals re-interviewed from previous surveys, mean age 33.1 years (range 27.7–40.1)	DSM-IV	SCID-II	**15.7**
Klein *et al.*[5]	USA	229	Relatives of normal controls	DSM-III-R	PDE	**14.8**
Lenzenweger *et al.*[6]	USA	258	University students age 18–19 years (two-stage procedure)	DSM-III-R	IPDE	**3.9**[b]
Maier *et al.*[7]	Germany	452	Normal controls, their partners, and relatives	DSM-III-R	SCID-II	**10.0**
Moldin *et al.*[8]	USA	302	Normal controls, parents and their children	DSM-III-R	PDE	**7.3**
Reich *et al.*[9]	USA	235	Urban residents	DSM-III	PDQ	**11.1**
Samuels *et al.*[10]	USA	742	Individuals re-interviewed from previous survey, aged 34–94 years (weighted data)	DSM-IV	IPDE	**9.0**
Torgersen *et al.*[11]	Norway	2,053	Individual from National Register (weighted data)	DSM-III-R	SIPD	**13.4**
Zimmerman & Coryell[12]	USA	797	Relatives of patients and normal controls	DSM-III	SIDP	**14.3**[a]

PAS, Personality Assessment Schedule, IPDE, International Personality Disorder Examination; PDE, Personality Disorder Examination; PDQ, Personality Diagnostic Questionnaire; SCID—II, Structured Clinical Interview for DSM-IV Axis II disorders; SIDP, Structured Interview for DSM-III-R Personality.

[a] Prevalence includes those with 'mixed' and 'not otherwise specified' disorder.

[b] Prevalence was 6.7% 'definite', 11% 'possible', including 'not otherwise specified disorder'.

on screening questions[13] and on a newly developed fully diagnostic structured interview carried out by lay interviewers rather than clinicians, which lacked any accompanying validity data.[14]

In the surveys considered here, the rate of PDs decreases in older age groups; although the sex ratio is different for specific types of PD (e.g. more schizoid, narcissistic, and antisocial PDs among males, more dependent, avoidant, and histrionic PDs among females), the overall rates of PD are about equal for both sexes. Finally, prevalence rates are generally higher in urban populations and lower socio-economic groups.

Community epidemiological studies of specified personality disorders

Table 4.12.4.2 lists the median prevalence rates for specified PDs based on studies that surveyed different types of randomly selected community samples. We will comment on some of the findings. The first column shows the number of studies on which the median prevalence rate is based.

Paranoid personality disorder

The median prevalence rate of paranoid PD is 1.6 per cent. In the study by Baron,[15] paranoid PD was remarkably more common among relatives of schizophrenic probands (7.3 per cent) than among relatives of control probands (2.7 per cent).

Schizoid personality disorder

There have been 13 studies evaluating the prevalence of schizoid PD in the community, with a median prevalence rate of 0.8 per cent. Baron[15] reported a rate of 1.6 per cent of schizoid PD among relatives of schizophrenic probands, but no cases among relatives of control probands.

Table 4.12.4.2 Median prevalence rates of specified personality disorders in epidemiological surveys

PD Category	Number of studies (*N*)	Median prevalence rate (%)
Paranoid	13	1.6
Schizoid	13	0.8
Schizotypal	13	0.7
Antisocial (dissocial)	24	1.5
Borderline	15	1.6
Histrionic	12	1.8
Narcissistic	10	0.2
Obsessive-compulsive	13	2.0
Avoidant (anxious)	13	1.3
Dependent	12	0.9
Passive-aggressive	8	1.7

Schizotypal personality disorder

The median prevalence rate of schizotypal PD is 0.7 per cent. However, in the study by Baron[15] schizotypal PD was remarkably more common among relatives of schizophrenic probands (14.6 per cent) than among relatives of control probands (2.1 per cent). In a similar fashion, Asarnow *et al.*[16] reported significantly higher rates of schizotypal personality disorders in relatives of probands with childhood onset of schizophrenia than in relatives of community controls (4.2 per cent vs. 0 per cent). These results provide additional support for the specific relationship between schizophrenia and schizotypal PD.

Antisocial (dissocial) personality disorder

Antisocial is the most studied PD. Its prevalence has been assessed in 24 epidemiological surveys, with a mean sample size of 2 943 subjects; nine studies used the Diagnostic Interview Schedule as assessment instrument. Antisocial PD seems to have a prevalence of around 1.5 per cent in the general population and to be substantially more frequent among males than females, with sex ratios ranging from 2:1 to 7:1. It is also more common among younger adults, those living in urban areas, and the lower socio-economic classes. People with a diagnosis of antisocial PD are also high users of medical services.

Borderline personality disorder

Borderline PD has been investigated in 15 studies. Swartz *et al.* [17] carried out a study among 1 541 community subjects (between 19 and 55 years of age) at the North Carolina site of the Epidemiologic Catchment Area (ECA) Program, using a diagnostic algorithm derived from the Diagnostic Interview Schedule (**DIS**). They found a rate of 1.8 per cent for borderline PD; the disorder was significantly more common among females, the widowed, and the unmarried. There was a trend towards an increase in the diagnosis in younger, non-white, urban, and poorer respondents. The highest rates were found in the 19 to 34 age range, with the rates declining with age. All borderline respondents had also a DIS DSM-III Axis I lifetime diagnosis.

Although some believe there is a preponderance of females with borderline PD, they do not always take into account that there is also a preponderance of females in the populations studied. There were two studies that did not find a higher female prevalence.[11,18]

Histrionic personality disorder

Histrionic PD has a median prevalence rate of 1.8 per cent, ranging from 0 per cent[3] to 3.2 per cent.[1] A study by Nestadt *et al.*[19] carried out at the Baltimore (Maryland) site of the Epidemiologic Catchment Area Program, ascertained the prevalence of histrionic PD in the community. The authors found a prevalence of 2.1 per cent in the general population, with virtually identical rates in men and women. No significant differences were found in terms of race and education, but the prevalence was significantly higher among separated and divorced persons. It should be noted that the study derived the diagnoses from instruments not originally intended to diagnose PDs; it might be possible that, in some cases, this study has identified personality traits rather than 'true' PDs.

Narcissistic personality disorder

No cases of narcissistic PD were found in five studies. However, Reich *et al.*[9] and Lenzenweger *et al.*[6] found rates of 0.4 per cent and 1.2 per cent respectively, even higher rates were found by Klein *et al.*[5] and Crawford *et al.*[4] who reported prevalence rates of 3.9 and 2.2 per cent respectively.

Obsessive compulsive (anankastic) personality disorder

The median prevalence rate of obsessive compulsive PD, obtained from 13 studies, was found to be 2 per cent, the highest of all PDs. The rate of compulsive PD was especially high in a study in which the Personality Diagnostic Questionnaire was used (6.4 per cent).[6] However, lower rates were reported with structured interviews. A community study, carried out at the Epidemiologic Catchment Area Program Baltimore site, found a prevalence of 1.7 per cent.[20] Males had a rate about five times higher than females. The disorder was also more frequent among white, highly educated, married, and employed subjects, and it was associated with anxiety disorders. However, the study derived the diagnosis from an interview originally not intended to diagnose PDs; this may mean that adaptive obsessive compulsive traits, rather than a 'true' PD, were identified. In the study by Black *et al.* [1] rates of obsessive compulsive PD were higher among relatives of probands with obsessive compulsive disorder compared to relatives of comparison probands (10.8 per cent vs. 7.9 per cent, respectively), however this difference did not reach statistical significance.

Avoidant (anxious) personality disorder

A total of 13 studies have investigated the prevalence of avoidant PD in community samples, with a median prevalence rate of 1.3 per cent. In the study by Asarnow *et al.*[16] avoidant PD occurred more frequently in relatives of schizophrenia probands compared to comparison control probands, also when controlling for schizoid or paranoid PD, and the authors suggest that avoidant PD might be a separate schizophrenia spectrum disorder, and not merely a sub-clinical form of schizoid or paranoid PD.

Dependent personality disorder

In 12 studies in which the frequency of dependent PD was assessed, the median prevalence rate was 0.9 per cent.

Passive-aggressive personality disorder

The median prevalence rate of passive-aggressive PD, obtained from 8 studies, was found to be quite high (1.8 per cent); interestingly, this type of PD has not been included either in DSM-IV or in ICD-10.

Epidemiological studies of personality disorders carried out in psychiatric settings

Table 4.12.4.3 lists the median prevalence rates for any PDs found in 61 studies carried out in inpatient and outpatient psychiatric samples and published between 1981 and October 2007. Only prospective studies that surveyed clinical samples (either inpatients or outpatients) of more than 100 subjects have been considered for

Table 4.12.4.3 Median prevalence rates of PDs among psychiatric patients in prospective studies including more than 100 subjects

Diagnostic category	Number of studies (*N*)	Median sample (*N*)	Median prevalence rates (%)
Alcohol and substance abuse	15	250	57.0
Affective disorder	19	200	49.2
Anxiety disorders	7	200	40.4
Any Axis disorder	20	131	51.0

this analysis. The second column shows the number of studies on which the median prevalence rate is based.

In these studies, subjects have been directly evaluated for the purpose of obtaining PD rates, by means of a standardized assessment instrument specific for PDs. Several other studies, which have evaluated only the prevalence of specified PDs in clinical samples, are not shown here.

In general, the prevalence of PDs among psychiatric outpatients and inpatients is quite high, with a substantial number of studies ($n = 29$) showing a PD prevalence rate equal or higher than 50 per cent of the sample. However, it is difficult to draw more definite conclusions from these studies, because of substantial differences in sampling, diagnostic criteria, timing of the assessment, assessment methods, availability of mental health services, prevalence of Axis disorders, and sociocultural factors.

There are, however, some consistencies across studies that deserve consideration. The most prevalent PD seems to be borderline, both in inpatient and in outpatient settings. The next most common PDs is histrionic, whereas schizoid PD is infrequently diagnosed. Borderline and histrionic PDs are also characterized by the lowest social functioning. They are especially common in inpatient settings, as their symptomatology often results in the patient being admitted to hospital due to their suicidal behaviour, substance abuse, and cognitive-perceptual abnormalities. In outpatient settings, dependent, and passive-aggressive PD are also common.

Especially in inpatient settings, many people who meet the criteria for one PD also meet the criteria for other PDs [21–23]. The highest comorbidity rate appears to occur with borderline PD, with the frequent coexistence of borderline and histrionic PDs, antisocial, schizotypal, and dependent PDs.

With regard to comorbidity between PDs and Axis I disorders, the most common and best-studied patterns are between substance abuse and PDs, affective disorders and PDs, and anxiety disorders and PDs (particularly borderline, antisocial, avoidant, and dependent PDs). Other clinically significant associations have been found between PDs and eating disorders: obsessive-compulsive, avoidant, and dependent PDs are most commonly associated with anorexia nervosa whereas borderline, avoidant, dependent, and paranoid PDs are the most common among individuals with bulimia.[24] High rates of PD (especially borderline and antisocial PDs) have also been detected in patients with selected medical conditions, such as HIV-positive patients.[25,26]

Some studies have assessed the treated prevalence of PD using administrative data (e.g. discharge figures, psychiatric case register data, etc.). In the United States, using data from the 1993 National Hospital Discharge Survey, Olfson and Mechanic[27] found that almost 12 per cent of patients discharged from public general hospitals had a diagnosis of PD, compared with 11 per cent of patients from non-profit hospitals and 5 per cent of patients from proprietary general hospitals.

Some investigations, which compared the hospital admission rates for PD over time, allow us to assess the impact of diagnostic changes. In Denmark, sex- and age-standardized rates of first-admitted borderline patients significantly increased during the 16-year interval between 1970 and 1985, and this might be explained in terms of a change in diagnostic habits.[28] In the United States, comparing the diagnoses given to inpatients in a large university-affiliated mental hospital in the last 5 years of the DSM-II era ($n = 5143$) with those given in the first 5 years of the DSM-III era ($n = 5771$), a marked increase (from 19 per cent to 49 per cent) was found in the diagnosis of PD, together with a decrease in the diagnosis of schizophrenia and a corresponding increase in the diagnosis of affective disorders.[29]

The epidemiological findings in treated samples are especially important if we bear in mind that the presence of a PD among those suffering from other mental disorders can be a major predictor of the natural history and treatment outcome. Therefore, an important clinical implication of these findings is that patients in treatment because of severe Axis I disorders must be carefully assessed with an assessment instrument specific for PDs, because of the high likelihood of diagnosing a PD and the subsequent need to adjust their treatment accordingly.

Epidemiological studies of personality disorders carried out in other settings

A few epidemiological studies on PDs have been carried out among patients attending primary healthcare settings; in these studies between 5 and 8 per cent of patients have been identified as having a primary diagnosis of PD.[21] When the assessment is made independent of the primary diagnosis, however, the average prevalence rate can rise several-fold because of state effects. In a consecutive sample of primary care *attenders*, a PD was diagnosed in 24 per cent of the sample (N=303) and was associated with the presence of common mental disorders and unplanned surgery attendance, indicating that PDs may represent a significant source of burden in primary care.[30]

In other institutional settings, such as prisons, several studies have found very high rates of PDs. In the United Kingdom, two large-scale studies have been completed; in the first, carried out among 750 prisoners representing a 9 per cent cross-sectional sample of the entire male unconvicted population, a PD was diagnosed in 11 per cent of the sample.[31] In the second study, a representative sample of the entire prison population of England and Wales was evaluated; a sub-sample was assessed with the SCID-II administered by a clinician.[32] The prevalence rates for any PD were 78 per cent for male remand prisoners, 64 per cent for male sentenced prisoners, and 50 per cent for female prisoners. In a large meta-analysis by Fazel & Danesh [33] of 28 studies, including a total of 13 844 prisoners, antisocial PD was diagnosed in 47 per cent of subjects. High rates of borderline and antisocial PDs have also been found in a sample ($n = 805$) of women felons entering prison in a North American State.[34]

Conclusions

Up to 30 years ago, the epidemiology of PDs had not received the same amount of attention as that of many other psychiatric disorders. Since then the situation has changed, and we now have data on the prevalence of PD in the community and in psychiatric facilities. Community data come primarily from 12 studies, with a total sample of 6 785 subjects from four countries (Germany, Norway, the United Kingdom, the United States). There are excellent national and cross-national epidemiological data on antisocial personality disorder based on the same diagnostic methods. There are almost no data on other PDs from countries other than the United States, the United Kingdom, Germany and Norway.

One important methodological problem is that some PDs have a very low prevalence rate. Consequently, epidemiological surveys carried out among the general population may require very large samples in order to identify a sufficient number of cases to study demographic correlates and the association of PD with other psychiatric disorders. Future studies should try to address this problem and provide us with more definite epidemiological data. These data will also be invaluable in showing the validity of current classifications and in better delineating the boundaries between different PDs.

Further information

The complete bibliography of studies included in tables 4.12.4.2–4.12.4.3 can be asked from the authors at the e-mail address: f.guzzetta@gmail.com.

Torgersen S. (2005). Epidemiology. In *The American Psychiatric Publishing Textbook of Personality Disorders* (eds. Oldham J.M., Skodol, A.E., Bender, D.S.), pp. 129–41. The American Psychiatric Publishing.

References

1. Black, D.W., Noyes, R., Jr., Pfohl, B., *et al.* (1993). Personality disorder in obsessive-compulsive volunteers, well comparison subjects, and their first-degree relatives. *American Journal of Psychiatry,* **150**(8) 1226–32.
2. Casey, P.R., Tyrer, P.J. (1986). Personality, functioning and symptomatology. *Journal of Psychiatric Research,* **20**(4), 363–74.
3. Coid,J. Yang, M., Tyrer, P. *et al.* (2006). Prevalence and correlates of personality disorder in Great Britain. *British Journal of Psychiatry,* **188**, 423–31.
4. Crawford, T.N., Cohen, P., Johnson, J.G., *et al.* (2005). Self-reported personality disorder in the children in the community sample: convergent and prospective validity in late adolescence and adulthood. *Journal of Personal Disorder,* **19**(1), 30–52.
5. Klein, D.N., Riso, L.P., Donaldson, S.K., *et al.* (1995). Family study of early-onset dysthymia. Mood and personality disorders in relatives of outpatients with dysthymia and episodic major depression and normal controls. *Archives of General Psychiatry,* **52**(6), 487–96.
6. Lenzenweger, M.F., Loranger, A.W., Korfine, L., *et al.* (1997). Detecting personality disorders in a non clinical population. Application of a 2-stage procedure for case identifi cation. *Archive of General Psychiatry,* **54**(4), 345–51.
7. Maier, W. (1992). Prevalence of personality disorders (DSM-III-R) in the community. *Journal of Personal Disorder,* **6**, 186–96.
8. Moldin, S.O., Rice, J.P., Erlenmeyer-Kimling, L. *et al.* (1994). Latent structure of DSM-III-R Axis II psychopathology in a normal sample. *Journal of Abnormal Psychology,* **103**(2), 259–66.
9. Reich, J., Yates, W., Nduaguba, M. (1989). Prevalence of DSM-III personality disorders in the community. *Social Psychiatry Psychiatric Epidemiology,* **24**(1), 12–6.
10. Samuels, J., Eaton, W.W., Bienvenu, O.J., III, *et al.* (2002). Prevalence and correlates of personality disorders in a community sample. *British Journal of Psychiatry,* **180**, 536–42.
11. Torgersen, S., Kringlen, E., Cramer, V. (2001). The prevalence of personality disorders in a community sample. *Archive of General Psychiatry,* **58**(6), 590–6.
12. Zimmerman, M. and Coryell, W. (1989). DSM-III personality disorder diagnoses in a nonpatient sample. Demographic correlates and comorbidity. *Archive of General Psychiatry,* **46**(8), 682–9.
13. Lenzenweger, M.F., Lane, M.C., Loranger, A.W., *et al.* (2007). DSM-IV personality disorders in the National Comorbidity Survey Replication. *Biological Psychiatry,* **62**(6), 553–64.
14. Grant, B.F., Hasin, D.S., Stinson, F.S., *et al.* (2004). Prevalence, correlates, and disability of personality disorders in the United States: results from the national epidemiologic survey on alcohol and related conditions. *Journal of Clinical Psychiatry,* **65**(7), 948–58.
15. Baron, M., Gruen, R., Rainer, J.D., *et al.* (1985). A family study of schizophrenic and normal control probands: implications for the spectrum concept of schizophrenia. *American Journal of Psychiatry,* **142**(4), 447–55.
16. Asarnow, R.F., Nuechterlein, K.H., Fogelson, D., *et al.* (2001). Schizophrenia and schizophrenia-spectrum personality disorders in the fi rst-degree relatives of children with schizophrenia: the UCLA family study. *Archives of General Psychiatry,* **58**(6), 581–8.
17. Swartz, M., Blazer, D., George, L., *et al.* (1990). Estimating the prevalence of borderline personality disorder in the community. *Journal of Personal Disorder,* (4), 257–72.
18. Zimmerman, M. and Coryell, W.H. (1990). Diagnosing personality disorders in the community. A comparison of self-report and interview measures. *Archives of General Psychiatry,* **47**(6), 527–31.
19. Nestadt, G., Romanoski, A.J., Chahal, R., *et al.* (1990). An epidemiological study of histrionic personality disorder. *Psychological Medicine,* **20**(2), 413–22.
20. Nestadt, G., Romanoski, A.J., Brown, C.H., *et al.* (1991). DSM-III compulsive personality disorder: an epidemiological survey. *Psychological Medicine,* **21**(2), 461–71.
21. de Girolamo, G. and Tyrer, P. (1993). *Personality disorders.* Geneva: WHO.
22. Dolan, B., Evans, C., Norton, K. (1995). Multiple axis-II diagnoses of personality disorder. *British Journal of Psychiatry,* **166**(1), 107–12.
23. Zimmerman, M., Rothschild, L. and Chelminski, I. (2005). The prevalence of DSM-IV personality disorders in psychiatric outpatients. *American Journal of Psychiatry,* **162**(10),1911–8.
24. Cassin, S.E. and von Ranson, K.M. (2005). Personality and eating disorders: a decade in review. *Clinical Psychology Review,* **25**(7), 895–916.
25. Erbelding, E.J., Hutton, H.E., Zenilman, J.M., *et al.* (2004). The prevalence of psychiatric disorders in sexually transmitted disease clinic patients and their association with sexually transmitted disease risk. *Sexually Transmitted Diseases,* **31**(1), 8–12.
26. Golding, M. and Pekins, D.O. (1996). Personality disorder in HIV infection. International Review of Psychiatry, (8), 253–8.
27. Olfson, M. and Mechanic, D. (1996). Mental disorders in public, private nonprofit, and proprietary general hospitals. *American Journal of Psychiatry,* **153**(12), 1613–9.
28. Mors O. (1988). Increasing incidence of borderline states in Denmark from 1970–1985. *Acta Psychiatrica Scandinavica,* **77**(5), 575–83.
29. Loranger, A.W. (1990). The impact of DSM-III on diagnostic practice in a university hospital. A comparison of DSM-II and DSM-III in 10,914 patients. *Archives of General Psychiatry,* **47**(7), 672–5.

30. Moran, P., Jenkins, R., Tylee, A., *et al.* (2000). The prevalence of personality disorder among UK primary care attenders. *Acta Psychiatrica Scandinavica*, **102**(1), 52–77.
31. Brooke, D., Taylor, C., Gunn, J., *et al.* (1996). Point prevalence of mental disorder in unconvicted male prisoners in England and Wales. *British Medical Journal*, **313**(7071), 1524–7.
32. Singleton, N., Meltzer, H., Gatward, R., *et al.* (1998). *Psychiatric morbidity among prisoners in England and Wales*. London: Office of National Statistics.
33. Fazel, S. and Danesh, J. (2002). Serious mental disorder in 23 000 prisoners: a systematic review of 62 surveys. *Lancet*, **359**(9306), 545–50.
34. Jordan, B.K., Schlenger, W.E., Fairbank, J.A., *et al.* (1996). Prevalence of psychiatric disorders among incarcerated women. II. Convicted felons entering prison. *Archives of General Psychiatry*, **53**(6), 513–9.

4.12.5 Neuropsychological templates for abnormal personalities: from genes to biodevelopmental pathways

Adolf Tobeña

The scaffolding of personality

Research on human personality has converged upon a 'consensual pathway' indicating that a small number of dimensions can provide the framework for describing the rich variety of human temperaments. These high-level temperamental traits are factorially derived from psychometric measures of individual variation in behaviour, feeling, and thinking,[1,2] and it is assumed that they may reflect the operation of brain systems that are probably multifaceted and multipurpose.[3–5] This global outline of the structure of personality depends on the notion that genetic and developmental dispositions combine with critical nurturing and social conditioning events to form the tapestry of human uniqueness within temperamental clusters. In other words, personality types are expressed through relatively clear-cut and stable phenotypic traits that are accessible to objective measurement at behavioural, emotional, and cognitive levels. These depend, in turn, upon the specific and early organization of particular neurocognitive and neuroendocrine templates.

A handful of 'superfactors' (broad traits or dimensions) apparently capture the essential components of the mosaic of terms and traits used to describe normal personality. These dimensions are *neuroticism*, *extraversion*, *agreeableness/friendliness*, *conscientiousness*, and *intellectual openness*. Neuroticism and extraversion always appear as main stars in these factorial *solutions* whereas the remaining three superfactors—conscientiousness (reliability/persistence), friendliness (as opposed to aggressiveness/hostility) and intellectual curiosity (openness/creativity)—have less regularity on such high-order taxonomies. A five-dimensional structure is advocated by many researchers though dissent is still strong regarding the nature and scope of these superfactors that would define the 'core' of human temperament.[6]

Biological rooting of personality types

Searching for biological substrates of personality dimensions would reinforce their validity as useful constructs but this endeavour was largely neglected by psychometricians devoted to purely descriptive studies and by clinical researchers as well. Some pioneers, like Hans Eysenck at the Institute of Psychiatry, London, tried to root behavioural trait variations within neurobiological concepts[1] following a venerable tradition, which can be traced back as far as Pavlov. These early proposals were rather rudimentary though they served as drivers of subsequent models which focused more tightly on certain brain subsystems as possible sites for the factors underlying normal and abnormal temperaments.[3–5,7–9] Jeffrey Gray, Robert Cloninger, and Larry Siever's ideas were among the more fruitful in an area which has grown steadily and is now an lively field of personality research.[9–11] Progress in basic neuroscience has made it possible to relate a variety of biological measures to paper and pencil or neurocognitive tests distinguishing normal and anomalous temperaments. Biological screening has also increasingly been applied to patients with personality disorders, using the clinical clusters as defined by Diagnostic Systems. Besides these attempts to build psychobiological profiles of normal and abnormal temperaments, converging evidence is used to advocate that categorical and dimensional models for diagnosing personality disorders should be integrated.[12]

To give a broad overview of an area that may be crucial to illuminate the genesis of personality disorders, I shall discuss the studies that, during the last decade, have tried to find genetic traces for personality traits that are both behaviourally consistent and biologically well rooted. Previous work using classical (familial or twin) methods had found substantial heritability estimates for several personality traits.[13] It was thus unsurprising that genetic tracking methods impulsed research aimed at showing that temperamental traits contribute to personality scaffolding via neuroendocrine targets specified by particular genes. I'll be discussing the outcome of some of these efforts and I'll explore afterwards how other basic temperamental traits, rooted within biodevelopmental processes, do mediate enduring neurocognitive organization resulting in long-lasting behavioural styles. Finally I'll outline new avenues for the neuropsychology of personality. My approach is deliberately selective, discussing relevant evidence rather than performing a systematic assessment of the field. For reasons of convenience and possible clinical relevance, I have selected some of the traits heralding sound biological foundations, although they are not necessarily prominent in the state-of-the-art dimensional '*solutions*' for normal and abnormal temperaments.

The genetic saga for novelty-seeking

In 1996 two independent teams reported[14,15] that a particular chromosomal 'locus' was associated with a well-established trait of human temperament—the hunger for novelty and excitement that lies behind sensation-seeking, risk taking, and impulsive behaviours.[5,10] A polymorphism in the sequence of the gene expressing the D4 dopamine receptor (D4DR), located on the short arm of chromosome 11, explained 10 per cent of the genetic variance due to this trait. Individuals with the longer repeat allele at exon III of the *D4DR* gene scored higher in novelty-seeking behaviour (explorers, risk-seekers), whereas those with the shorter allele had lower scores (prudent, cautious). The first of these studies[14] investigated a heterogeneous sample of young Israelis, and showed the association to be independent of ethnicity (Ashkenazim versus Sephardim), sex, or age. The second study, carried out in the United States,[15] used a random sample of people who had initially been recruited in a search for chromosomal regions possibly associated with sexual orientation; this sample mainly comprised white men, although some ethnic minorities were also included. The personality questionnaires were different but very popular in personality research: the Israelis were evaluated using Cloninger's Tridimensional Personality Questionnaire (**TPQ**),[16] which gives direct scores of novelty-seeking, whereas the American study used the Revised NEO Personality Inventory[17] which measures the five superfactors mentioned above, from which scores for novelty-seeking were derived. The results of the two studies were highly concordant.

Despite the modest explanatory power of this reported association, the link between temperamental variability for one trait and a chromosomal polymorphism was the first hint for a direct relationship between a putative 'genetic marker' and a core dimension of normal personality. In this case, the potential genetic marker appeared promising because of the amount of basic and clinical research linking dopaminergic function with the regulation of stimulus-seeking and sensitivity to incentives. In theory, if similar degrees of explained variance were assignable to other sound gene markers associated to *approach/exploring* phenotypes, a substantial part of the heritability of the trait could be explained. Subsequent studies[18,19] failed to replicate these early findings in a consistent way and the optimism receded. The heterogeneity of the samples and the subtleties of the genetics of complex traits were blamed for the disparate results, though the research saga was quite productive: the links between dopamine receptor polymorphisms and novelty-seeking have been intensively searched and the race to find other markers for the same trait was impressive.

Metanalyses suggest that there are subtle connections between dopamine receptor gene variants and *approach/exploring* propensities as measured by personality questionnaires, though the strength of the contribution of every variant is small and hard to establish.[19,20] Moreover, parallel research has established suggestive connections between gene variants regulating other molecular targets (i.e. tryptophan hydroxylase, dopamine transporter, dopamine-beta-hydroxylase, serotonin transporter, MAOA, COMT) that modulate risk-taking behaviours and impulsivity. A handful of genes, thus contribute to differential vulnerabilities for addictive behaviours, a congruent result at the extreme of stimulus-seeking tendencies. Although further and more refined research is required, these data seem to confirm pioneer work, mostly with twins, which had consistently established that novelty-seeking behaviour was moderately heritable (40 to 50 per cent).

Genetics of fearfulness/neuroticism

The aforementioned American team that reported the first associations between novelty-seeking and variants of D4DR gene informed that there was an association between the neuroticism trait and a chromosomal region linked to serotonin neurotransmission involved in modulating anxiety-related traits.[21] The 5-hydroxytryptamine transporter protein (5-HTT) that promotes the reuptake of serotonin into cell membranes is encoded by a gene (*SLC6A4*) located in the q11–q12 segment of chromosome 17. The region governing the transcriptional control of the protein shows a polymorphism that influences its expression and functioning. Individuals carrying the short variant of the polymorphism show a reduced efficiency of serotonin reuptake compared with those possessing the longer variant. The study measured these parameters in the lymphoblasts of two independent samples totalling more than 500 volunteers. Using two different personality questionnaires (NEO and Cattell's 16PF Personality Inventory) and estimated scores on various dimensions of Cloninger's TPQ, the evidence showed that subjects who carried the short variant in the 5-HTT gene polymorphism had higher neuroticism (NEO), anxiety (16PF), and harm-avoidance (TPQ) scores. The results were equally consistent across and within pedigrees. Across the three personality measures, the 5-HTTLPR contributed a modest 3 to 4 per cent of the total variance and 7 to 9 per cent of the genetic variance in anxiety-related traits. It was suggested that, if other genes contributed similar dosage effects to anxiety traits, approximately 10 to 15 genes might be involved in the heritability of neuroticism.

The implication of the serotonin transporter in the potential genetic predisposition towards emotionality traits agrees with many other results. Serotonergic neurotransmission is involved in multiple brain functions with little or no relationship with fear/anxiety regulation, but there is a large body of evidence linking it with the modulation of adaptive responses to serious conflict and emotionally demanding situations.[3] Moreover, many drugs currently used to treat anxious/depressive dysphorias and personality disorders depend on mending serotonergic function. Finally, several studies have shown that variants of the 5-HTTLPR predict differential response on anxious phenotypes: fear-driven amygdala activation[22] and response to pharmacological challenges.[23] Therefore, although the exact role of serotonergic systems in the modulation of emotionality is not fully understood, it is improbable that the neurohormonal adaptations that participate in individual responses to serious emotional conflicts would not include serotonin modulation either through the cell transporter or through the extended family of serotonin receptors and their intracellular targets. Defensive adaptations require however the participation of other central neuromodulators: the CRH-ACTH regulatory cascade, γ-aminobutyric acid, neuropeptide Y, and substance P,[3] are major contenders in this respect and they can be expected to contribute to the genetic mediation of neuroticism.

Polymorphisms in anxious humans versus QTL-genes for fearful rodents

Dozens of studies investigated whether the particular polymorphism in the 5-HTT gene contributes to the tendency for individuals who score higher on neuroticism, in personality tests, to be at higher risk for 'internalizing disorders' (anxiety/depression) and personality disorders (anxiety/affective clusters). The global outcome of that research has been unreliable: though stringent metanalyses confirmed the original association with a modest relevance at explaining the trait variance,[23] subsequent results in large samples of siblings and singletons have been negative.[24] There are other lines of evidence, however, mainly from animal research, that support the claim of a possible genetic basis for fearfulness/emotionality. This evidence is derived from studies of the psychogenetics of emotional susceptibility searching for chromosome loci. In many biological and behavioural tests, comparisons of several reactive and non-reactive strains of mice and rats obtained through artificial selection (forced interbreedings) have narrowed the search for genetic loci thanks to increasingly powerful methods of chromosomal mapping. In a pioneer work with progeny obtained by crossing two strains of mice selected for activity and defecation in an open-field test, three loci (QTLs) which explained most of the genetic variance in emotionality were found on chromosomes 1, 12, and 15 of the murine genome.[25] These data were confirmed and extended by measuring fear responses towards particular cues: the same segment of chromosome 1 was identified as a relevant 'locus' for emotional susceptibility besides other murine chromosomal zones.[9] The importance of the loci at chromosome 1 has been established in studies using heterogeneous and inbred stocks, combining techniques which have permitted to focus the suspicious segment to less than 1 cM and leading to the identification of the first gene linked to murine emotionality: Rgs2, a regulator of G-protein functioning which is highly expressed in the brain.[26] The complexities are nevertheless tremendous because even a QTL like that contains several genes each contributing a very modest part of variation on the phenotype of interest.[9,26]

Several research programmes were concurrently started to determine whether there is also concordance in the chromosomal marking of emotionality in strains of rats differing in fearfulness. The hypoemotional Roman high-avoider (**RHA**) versus the hyperemotional Roman low-avoider (**RLA**) rat lines represented a particularly interesting assay because of the very large body of evidence showing their usefulness as animal models of 'temperamental' styles.[27] Several plausible QTLs were detected but only those located on chromosome 5 and 15 predicted a wide array of anxious/fearful behaviours including spontaneous and learned fears.[28,29] The QTL located at the middle of rat chromosome 5 looks particularly promising because this region is partially syntenic with the human 1p segment where QTLs for neuroticism and liabilities for anxious/depressive dysphorias have been detected.[9,30] The search for plausible genes is, then, much more focused now though they will explain, in all probability, very modest portions of the phenotypic trait variance.[9]

Biodevelopmental mechanisms for affiliative traits

Affiliation (friendliness, sociability, gregariousness, empathy) is another core personality trait that can be measured consistently. Poor or distorted affiliative behaviour is the most predictive marker for a reliable diagnosis of personality disorder.[7,31] Deficits or alterations in affiliative tendencies may show a variety of clinical manifestations: extreme aloofness and detachment, manipulative, non-empathic or exploitative attitudes, and even definite asocial or antisocial tendencies. These behavioural styles appear, in different degrees and combinations, in several clinical categories of abnormal temperament. They could reflect alterations in the functioning of neuroendocrine systems specialized in mediating affective attachments, possibly including subsystems for social reward and social distress.[31] In this respect, an impressive amount of evidence has been gathered (mostly in animals but in humans as well) showing that prosocial behaviours, such as maternal nurturing, friendliness/gregariousness, playful/sexual behaviours, and even cooperativeness in economic interactions, share some neurochemical controls.[31–33]

Central oxytocin and opioid systems are among the more relevant of these modulatory molecules, because several types of attachments (mother–infant bonds, young peer bonds, pair-mating bonds, in-group tendencies) are dramatically altered when the functions of oxytocinergic or opioid systems in the brain are modified. Other centrally acting neuropeptides, such as prolactin and vasopressin, also contribute to particular types of species-specific social bonding. In addition, both the central regulatory monoaminergic systems and the corticotrophin–adrenal cascades that mediate stress adaptations help to organize responses to everyday social challenges.[31] The application of these ideas to personality is still in its infancy and requires the development of consistent scales to be related with sound biological markers.

Neuropeptides, social bonding, and early rearing practices

Theory and research in the psychobiology of social attachments[8,31] has linked the impact of early rearing practices (secure/nurturing mothering versus peer rearing or isolation) with the future organization and functioning of several neuroendocrinological systems. This research has mainly explored the function of the central modulatory monoamines norepinephrine, dopamine, and serotonin, and the hypophyseal–adrenal axis responses to social challenges. The evidence has shown that socially deprived monkeys differ physiologically, behaviourally, and cognitively from mother-reared infants in almost every aspect of what it means to be a social monkey; if the privation extends over the first 6 to 9 months of post-natal life, most effects persist into the adulthood. According to Kraemer[34]: 'The way in which socially deprived individuals orient to and respond physiologically to social stressors is altered and the kind of behavioural differences that seem to be the most important are those usually assigned to the domain of "temperament"'.

With the addition of the central neuropeptide systems that specifically modulate affiliative tendencies, the study of some crucial experiences during early infancy (and probably adolescence) will provide clues to the clarification of the role that developmental processes play in shaping attachment styles. Neural organization depends, to a great extent, on critical environmental inputs to produce enduring behavioural and cognitive adaptation in all domains. Therefore ontogenic factors must be particularly important in modelling social behaviour and in sustaining profiles of affiliative versus non-affiliative temperaments, in the same way as has already been demonstrated for other traits. For instance, in reactive/fearful monkeys, maternal and even grandparental rearing practices can significantly modify future neuroendocrine and behavioural adaptations[35] with parallel data obtained in rats.[36]

Affiliative genes?

These findings do not exclude the participation of genetic dispositions in attachment styles. Some authors have suggested that the operation of 'communicative' or 'affiliative' genes could prime individual tendencies through different sorts of emotional affects.[37] There is a paucity of data on the putative genetic basis of particular attachment styles. When a molecular approach has been used, in rodents, to establish a genetic link between variants of the vasopressin V1a receptor gene with a conspicuous social behaviour such as monogamous pair bonding, the results have been spectacular. After substituting and inserting the V1a receptor gene characteristic of a monogamous species (the prairie voles), both promiscuous mice and meadow voles adopted the pattern of partner preferences and parental behaviours distinctive of the monogamous species. It has been shown, in fact, that socio-behavioural trait differences depend on polymorphisms on the regulatory region of the V1a gene.[38] In rodents and other mammals the neurochemical circuits in the brain regulating attachment/affiliative behaviours are increasingly detailed. In humans the task is just starting and will deeply influence personality research.

Biodevelopmental processes for aggressiveness

Aggressiveness is another temperamental trait that has a very well-founded biodevelopmental basis.[39] Dimensional descriptions of the structure of personality do not always include aggressiveness as a high-level factor, but it is embedded in other traits such as impulsiveness, poor control, or explosive/desinhibited behaviour. However, aggressiveness is a major behavioural trait that has to be taken into account in the routine management of mental disorders, and it is also a prevalent characteristic in personality disorders (generally as an excess, but sometimes because of its absence). In the past, it was extremely difficult to prove that individual variations in aggressive behaviour might be correlated with neurohormonal characteristics. However, this was because of inadequate methods of quantifying biological and behavioural variations.[40]

In humans, the link between lifelong aggressive profiles and familial/subcultural problems is strong indicating that lower socio-economic status, increased rates of abuse, coercive family interactions, and neglect or other adversities contribute to violent behaviour from infancy to adolescence and into adulthood.[39,41] But this cannot obscure the effects of enduring biological dispositions that could, in part, result from the influence of socio-environmental insults to the developing brain. Intensive research in behavioural neuroendocrinology and molecular neuroscience using animal models has shown that aggressive temperaments are associated with both genetic dispositions and critical developmental processes, which affect the function of neuroregulatory controls that either promote or inhibit aggression.

MAO-A functioning and aggression-proneness

It was not surprising, therefore, that an association between a specific gene and an aggressive disorder in humans was early reported[42]: the males of a Dutch family that carried a mutation of the gene for monoaminoxidase A (MAO-A gene situated at chromosome Xp11.23) had a record of severe aggressive incidents in different generations. Subsequent investigations in mice showed that ablating the gene for MAO-A resulted in the 'knockout' mutants being much more aggressive[43] MAO plays an important part in the breakdown of serotonin and other central monoamines, and previous research in humans had found consistent relationships between impulsive or 'poorly controlled' behavioural styles and low-MAO activity, a feature also seen in sensation-seekers. A common polymorphism in the promoter region of the MAO-A gene has been shown to interact with early abuse/neglect in longitudinal studies of large samples of children[44]: only abused kids carrying the genetic variant giving low-MAO-A activity are later at risk of antisocial tendencies or violent/criminal behaviour, during adolescence or young adulthood. Further studies with normative samples differentiated by this polymorphism have permitted to map, through structural and functional neuroimaging, cortico-limbic singularities associated with emotional regulation in the low-MAO-A carriers.[45]

Serotonin/vasopressin ratios

Many other genetically altered animals have been produced that are highly aggressive. Several of them typically show anomalies in serotonin function. Knockout mice that do not express the serotonin 5-HT1B receptors are much quicker to attack intruders[46] an action that can be blocked with targeted serotonergic drugs. All this adds to the evidence obtained from mentally ill patients presenting aggressive outbursts and from chronic offenders in prisons, which shows an inverse relationship between serotonergic function and violent attacks directed towards others or themselves. Taken together, the data appear to suggest that preserved brain serotonin function helps to attenuate aggressive impulses, probably by blocking other neuro-regulatory systems that promote aggression such as sex steroids, insulin, vasopressin, and others. Vasopressin is involved in the establishment of pair bonds and territorial tendencies in mammals, and promotes aggressive behaviour when social/dominance challenges are perceived. There is evidence from adolescent and juvenile hamsters showing that proserotonergic interventions attenuate vasopressin-induced attacks. Patients with personality disorders[47] showed that cerebrospinal fluid levels of vasopressin were positively correlated with a life history of aggression, and with attacks against persons in particular. This was a more poweful relationship than the negative one usually obtained from measurements of serotonergic function and aggression. Other neuromodulators help serotonin to attenuate aggressive outputs: in animals, highly specific genetic techniques of knocking down or targeted regional brain expression of steroid and oxytocin receptors, have been used to identify ensambles of neuromodulators devoted to control aggressiveness, to the point of postulating a landscape of 50 genes to get a sound description to this function.[48]

A prospective landscape including other traits

Temperamental styles in animals show differential clustering of behavioural traits, which correspond to specific (and very complex) neurohormonal profiles. Sometimes, however, a specific genetic modification is sufficient to promote a fully differentiated temperament, as in the case of mice deficient in α-calcium–calmodulin-dependent kinase II (**α-CaMKII**) which show decreased fear responses and increased defensive aggression associated with low-serotonin levels[49] (Table 4.12.5.1).

It is possible that this may also hold for exceptional temperamental combinations in humans. However, we have already established that, when trying to explain the genetic contribution to basic ('universal') personality traits, a multigenic/interactional approach is compulsory to explain just part of the measured variance in each trait (Fig. 4.12.5.1). Nevertheless, this contribution can be very

Table 4.12.5.1 Summary of behavioural phenotypes in α-CaMKII mutant mice

Behavioural phenotype	Heterozygote	Homozygote
Fear-related responses	Decrease	Decrease
Offensive aggression	Normal	Decrease
Defensive aggression	Increase	Decrease
Pain sensitivity	Normal	Increase
Startle response	Normal	Increase
Vigilance	Normal	Increase
Mating	Decrease	Decrease
Maze learning	Normal	Decrease

Reproduced from C. Chen *et al.* Abnormal fear response and aggressive behaviour in mice deficient for alpha-calcium-calmodulin-leinase II. *Science*, **266**, 291–4, copyright 1994, with permission from the American Association for the Advancement of Science.

important, as most of research involving twins has yielded estimates of just over 40 per cent for the genetic input to typical personality traits, with very modest estimations assignable to the so-called shared (familial/cultural) environment. Non-shared environmental influences (from the womb onwards) and genetic–environmental interactions make a well-known contribution to each individual temperament. These complex influences may act first by modelling the development of basic neuroendocrine regulatory systems that cope with natural and social challenges, and second by shaping the neurocognitive architecture that results in an autonomous and particular lifestyle. An interactional approach along these lines is now laying the foundation for a better description of the different factors that contribute to building the typical profiles of normal or abnormal personalities.(50,51)

Such a general scheme must include other traits, in addition to the ones considered so far. For instance, the detection of a substantial genetic contribution to the baseline level of happiness,(52) which all individuals show throughout life independently of the events or episodes that they encounter, must be important for personality diagnoses, because such a 'calibration point' has a direct relationship with the affective tone of optimism or pessimism. Moreover, other traits and measures in the domain of cognitive performance (e.g. attentional spans, perceptual/appraisal reliability, thinking styles, and memory biases) or of character (e.g. religiosity/transcendence, conservatism, altruism, self-directness/self-esteem, and the drive to achieve/enthusiasm) should be incorporated into the whole description of personality structure. This is essential if the aim is to produce a general framework powerful enough to contain the complex categories that clinicians have tried to construct on the basis of systematic observation for more than a century. Cloninger(8,11) and others have advanced proposals along these lines, which have functioned as useful steps to guide empirical work. It must be added that structural and functional neuroimaging techniques have been used to map relations between personality dimensions and brain's regional organization and patterns of activation/deactivation. Although these studies are very preliminary and have been done with convenient samples, they have offered hints of neurocognitive architectures, which tend to confirm, on a broad basis, the neurochemical mechanisms behind the main temperamental traits.(53–55)

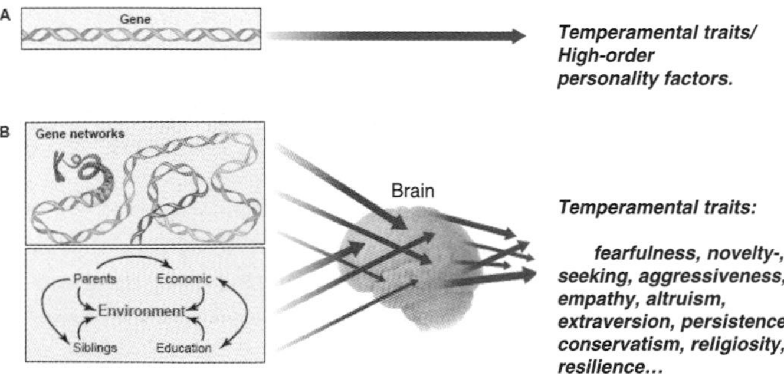

Fig. 4.12.5.1 Two views of the relationships between genes and personality. **A.** Early studies looked for linear relationships between gene markers and temperamental traits or high-order personality factors. **B.** Reality is likely to be far more complex with gene networks interacting with environmental inputs impacting on brain development and leaving enduring neural dispositions that, in turn, influence behavioural, cognitive, and affective styles (temperamental traits). (Reproduced from D. Harner. Rethinking behavior genetics, *Science*, **298**, 71–2, copyright 2004, with permission from the American Association for the Advancement of Science.).

Sophisticating the diagnoses of personality disorders

The evidence discussed so far is starting to have a major impact on the reconceptualizing of the approach that has been applied in psychiatry to the detection and categorization of the elusive profiles of normal and abnormal personalities. It is clear that anchoring some temperamental traits to a sound genetic or biodevelopmental base, and accruing a plausible neurocognitive architecture for it, will not provide a complete solution to the problems encountered in the aetiology and diagnosis of personality disorders. Many additional steps will have to be worked out. But in view of the increasing links that are being established between core personality traits and some genetic/developmental mechanisms, the task of building a solid neuropsychological framework, which would allow improved identification and differentiation of abnormal personalities no longer seems hopeless. In fact, such research is opening up many new avenues for understanding the effects of different factors (innate dispositions, neurodevelopmental organization, neurocognitive architectures, critical social transitions, and repeated stress episodes) on an individual's vulnerability to developing a personality disorder.

Hence, the use of behaviourally well defined and biologically well-established personality measures must be the starting point for achieving the fine-tuned diagnoses increasingly required in modern medicine. Complexity in measurement will increase, but there is no other way of obtaining data that are sufficiently valid to allow understanding of the classical personality disorders. It is hoped that advances in the neuropsychological detection of the more salient 'clinical' profiles within each of the personality subspaces or 'clusters' (at the level of either traits or dimensions), together with a refinement of the neurocognitive and neurohormonal data, will produce much better solutions. Some of the old-established and consistent categories of personality disorders will be confirmed, but it is possible that unexpected 'types' of abnormal personalities, with clinical relevance, will emerge. In this new framework it may be easier perhaps to detect at an early stage those 'exceptional' and 'charismatic', although anomalous, personalities who often impose great social costs and dramatic consequences not only for themselves but also for the group or the society in which they live.[56]

Further information

Archer, J. (2006). Testosterone and human aggression: an evaluation of the challenge hypothesis. *Neuroscience and Biobehavioral Reviews*, **30**, 319–45.

Caspi, A., Roberts, B.W., and Shiner, R.L. (2005). Personality development: stability and change. *Annual Review of Psychology*, **58**, 453–84.

Gosling, S.D. (2001). From mice to men: what can we learn about personality from animal research. *Psychological Bulletin*, **127**, 45–86.

Hariri, A.R. and Holmes, A. (2006). Genetics of emotional regulation: the role of serotonin transporter in neural function. *Trends in Cognitive Sciences*, **10**, 182–91.

Kreek, M.J., Nielsen, D.A., Butelman, E.R., *et al.* (2005). Genetic influences on impulsivity, risk taking, stress responsivity vulnerability to drug abuse and addiction. *Nature Neuroscience*, **8**, 1450–7.

Markon, K.E., Krueger, R.F., Bouchard, T.J. Jr, *et al.* (2002). Normal and abnormal personality traits: evidence for genetic and environmental relationships in the Minnesota study of twins reared apart. *Journal of Personality*, **70**, 660–93.

McGue, M. and Bouchard, T.J. (1998). Genetic and environmental influences on human behavioral differences. *Annual Review of Neuroscience*, **21**, 1–24.

McNaughton, N. and Corr, P..J. (2004). A two-dimensional neuropsychology of defense: fear/anxiety and defensive distance. *Neuroscience and Biobehavioural Reviews*, **28**, 285–305.

Paris, J. (2005). Neurobiological dimensional models of personality: a review of the models of Cloninger, Depue and Siever. *Journal of Personality Research*, **19**, 156–70.

Tobeña, A. (2004). *Deadly martyrs: the biology of lethal altruism*. Bromera Publish.-Valencia University Press, Valencia, Spain.

Young, L.J. and Wang, Z. (2005). The neurobiology of pair bonding. *Nature Neuroscience*, **7**, 1048–54.

References

1. Eysenck, H.J. (1967). *The biological basis of personality*. Charles Thomas, London.
2. McRae, R.R. and Costa, P.T. (1997). Personality trait structure as a human universal. *The American Psychologist*, **52**, 509–16.
3. Gray, J.A. and McNaugthon, N. (2000). *Anxiety: an enquiry into the functions of the septohippocampal system* (2nd edn). Oxford University Press, New York.
4. Cloninger, C.R. (1987). A systematic method for clinical description and classification of personality variants. *Archives of General Psychiatry*, **44**, 573–88.
5. Zuckerman, M. (1994). *Behavioral expressions and biosocial bases of sensation seeking*. Cambridge University Press, New York.
6. Sheller, J. and Westen, D. (2004). Dimensions of personality pathology: an alternative to the five-factor model. *The American Journal of Psychiatry*, **161**, 1743–54.
7. Siever, L.J. and Davis, K.L. (1991). A psychobiological perspective on the personality disorders. *The American Journal of Psychiatry*, **148**, 1647–58.
8. Cloninger, C.R., Svrakic, D.M., and Przybeck, T.R. (1993). A psychobiological model of temperament and character. *Archives of General Psychiatry*, **50**, 975–90.
9. Flint, J. (2004). The genetic basis of neuroticism. *Neuroscience and Biobehavioural Reviews*, **28**, 307–16.
10. Corr, P.J. (2004). Reinforcement sensitivity theory and personality. *Neuroscience and Biobehavioural Reviews*, **28**, 317–32.
11. Sravic, D.M., Draganic, S., Hill, K., *et al.* (2002). Temperament, character and personality disorders: ethiogic, diagnostic, treatment issues. *Acta Psychiatrica Scandinavica*, **106**, 189–95.
12. Widiger, T.A. and Frances, A.J. (2001). Towards a dimensional model for personality disorders. In *Personality disorders and the five-factor model of personality* (2nd edn) (eds. P.T. Costa and T.A. Widiger). American Psychological Association Press, Washington, DC.
13. Markon, K.E., Krueger, R.F., Bouchard, T. J. Jr, *et al.* (2002). Normal and abnormal personality traits: evidence for genetic and environmental relationships in the Minnesota study of twins reared apart. *Journal of Personality*, **70**, 660–93
14. Ebstein, E.P., Novick, O., Umansky, R., *et al.* (1996). Dopamine D4 receptor (D4DR) exon III polymorphism associated with the human personality trait of novelty seeking. *Nature Genetics*, **12**, 78–80.
15. Benjamin, J., Li, L., Greenberg, B.D., *et al.* (1996). Population and familial association between the D4 dopamine receptor gene and measures of novelty seeking. *Nature Genetics*, **12**, 81–4.
16. Cloninger, C.R., Przybeck, T.R., and Svrakic, D.M. (1991). The tridimensional personality questionnaire: US normative data. *Psychological Reports*, **69**, 1047–57.
17. Costa, P.T. and McCrae, R.R. (1992). *Revised NEO personality inventory and NEO five inventory*. Psychological Assessment Resources, Odessa, FL.
18. Lusher, J.M., Chandler, C., and Ball, D. (2001). Dopamine D4 receptor gene (DRD4) is associated with novelty seeking (NS) and substance abuse: the saga continues. *Molecular Psychiatry*, **6**, 497–9.
19. Shinka, J.A., Letsch, E.H., and Crafword, F.C. (2002). DRD4 and novelty seeking: results of a metanalyses. *American Journal of Medical Genetics*, **44**, 643–8.
20. Munafo, M.R., Clark, T.G., Moore, L.R., *et al.* (2003). Genetic polymorphisms and personality in healthy adults: a systematic review and metanalyses. *Molecular Psychiatry*, **8**, 471–84.
21. Lesch, K.P., Bengel, D., Heils, A., *et al.* (1996). Association of anxiety related traits with a polymorphism in the serotonin transporter gene regulatory region. *Science*, **274**, 1527–31.
22. Hariri, A.R., Mattay, V.S., Tessitore, A., *et al.* (2002). Serotonin transporter genetic variation and the response of the human amygdala. *Science*, **297**, 400–03.
23. Smith, G.S., Lothich, F.E., Molhutra, A.K., *et al.* (2004). Effects of serotonin transporter promoter polymorphisms on serotonin function. *Neuropsychopharmacology*, **29**, 2226–34.
24. Willis-Owen, S.A.G., Turri, M.G., Munafò, M.R., *et al.* (2005). The serotonin transporter length polymorphism, neuroticism and depression: a comprehensive assessment of association. *Biological Psychiatry*, **58**, 451–6.
25. Flint, J., Carley, R., DeFries, J.C., *et al.* (1995). A simple genetic basis for a complex psychological trait in laboratory mice. *Science*, **268**, 1432–5.
26. Yakin, B., Willis-Owen, S.A.G., Fullerton, J., *et al.* (2004). Genetic dissection of a behavioral quantitative trait locus shows the Rgs2 modulates anxiety in mice. *Nature Genetics*, **36**, 1197–202.
27. Driscoll, P., Escorihuela, R.M., Fernández-Teruel, A., *et al.* (1998). Genetic selection and differential stress responses: the Roman lines/strains of rats. *Annals of the New York Academy of Sciences*, **851**, 521–30.
28. Fernandez-Teruel, A., Escorihuela, R.M., Gray, J.A., *et al.* (2002). A quantitative trait locus influencing anxiety in the laboratory rat. *Genome Research*, **12**, 618–26.
29. Aguilar, R., Gil, L., Flint, J., *et al.* (2002). Learned fear, emotional reactivity and fear of heights: a factor analytic map from a large F2 intercross of Roman rat strains. *Brain Research Bulletin*, **57**, 17–26.
30. Nash, M.W., Huezo Diaz, P., Williamson, R.J., *et al.* (2004). Genome-wide linkage analyses of a composite index of neuroticism and mood related scales in extreme selected sibships. *Human Molecular Genetics*, **13**, 2173–82.

31. Panksepp, J. (1998). *Affective neuroscience*. Oxford University Press, New York.
32. Insel, T.R., Young, L., and Wang, Z. (1997). Molecular aspects of monogamy. *Annals of the New York Academy of Sciences*, **807**, 302–16.
33. Kosfeld, M., Heinrichs, M., Zak, P.J., *et al.* (2005). Oxytocine increases trust in humans. *Nature*, **435**, 673–6.
34. Kraemer, G.W. (1997). Psychobiology of early social attachment in rhesus monkeys. In *The integrative neurobiology of affiliation* (eds. C.S. Carter, I.I. Lederhendler, and B. Kirpatrick). *Annals of the New York Academy of Sciences*, **807**, 401–18.
35. Suomi, S.J. (1991). Uptight and laid-back monkeys: individual differences in the response to social challenges. In *Plasticity and development* (eds. S.E. Brauth, W.S. Hall, and R.J. Dooling), pp. 27–56. MIT Press, Cambridge, MA.
36. Liu, D., Diorio, J., Tannenbaum, B., *et al.* (1997). Maternal care, hippocampal glucocorticoid receptors and hypothalamic-pituitary-adrenal responses to stress. *Science*, **277**, 1659–62.
37. Buck, R. and Ginsburgh, B. (1997). Communicative genes and the evolution of empathy: selfish and social emotions as voices of selfish and social genes. *Annals of the New York Academy of Sciences*, **807**, 481–3.
38. Hammock, E.A.D. and Young, L.J. (2005). Microsatellite instability generates diversity in brain and sociobehavioral traits. *Science*, **308**, 1630–4.
39. Tremblay, R.E., Hartup, W.W., and Archer, J. (eds.) (2005). *Developmental origins of aggression*, Guilford Books, New York.
40. Adams, D.B. (2006). Brain mechanisms of aggressive behavior: an updated review. *Neuroscience and Biobehavioral Reviews*, **30**, 304–18.
41. Ferris, C.F. and Grisso, T. (eds.) (1996). Understanding aggressive behavior in children. *Annals of the New York Academy of Sciences*, **794**, 98–103.
42. Brunner, H.G., Nelen, M., Breakefiled, X.O., *et al.* (1994). Abnormal behavior associated with a point mutation in the structural gene for monoamine oxidase A. *Science*, **262**, 578–80.
43. Cases, O., Seif, I., Gromsby, J., *et al.* (1995). Aggressive behavior and altered amounts of brain serotonin and noradrenaline in mice lacking MAO-A. *Science*, **268**, 1763–6.
44. Caspi, A., McClay, J., Moffit, T., *et al.* (2002). Role of genotype in the cycle of violence in maltreated children. *Science*, **297**, 851–4.
45. Meyer-Lindenberg, A., Buckholtz, J.W., Kolachana, B., *et al.* (2006). Neural mechanisms of genetic risk for impulsivity and violence in humans. *PNAS*, **103**, 6269–74.
46. Saudou, F., Amarada, G., Dierich, A., *et al.* (1994). Enhanced aggressive behavior in mice lacking 5-HT1b receptor. *Science*, **265**, 1875–8.
47. Coccaro, E.F., Kavoussi, R.J., Hauger, R.L., *et al.* (1998). Cerebrospinal fluid vasopressin levels: correlates with aggression and serotonin function in personality-disordered patients. *Archives of General Psychiatry*, **55**, 708–14.
48. Ogawa, S., Choleris, E., and Pfaff, D. (2004). Genetic influences on aggressive behaviors and arousability in animals. *Annals of the New York Academy of Sciences*, **1036**, 257–66.
49. Chen, C., Rainnie, D.G., Greene, R.W., *et al.* (1994). Abnormal fear response and aggressive behavior in mice deficient for alpha-calcium-calmodulin-kinase II. *Science*, **266**, 291–4.
50. Saudino, K.J. (2005). Behavioral genetics and child temperament. *Journal of Developmental and Behavioral Pediatrics*, **26**, 214–23.
51. Blackburn, R., Logan, C., Renwick, S.D., *et al.* (2005). Higher-order dimensions of personality disorder: hierarchical structure and relationships with the five factor model, the interpersonal cycle and psychopathy. *Journal of Personality Disorders*, **19**, 597–623.
52. Lykken, D.T. and Tellegen, A. (1996). Happiness is a stochastic phenomenon. *Psychological Science*, **7**, 186–9.
53. Pujol, J., Lopez, A., Deus, J., *et al.* (2002). Anatomical variability in the anterior cingulate gyrus and basic dimensions of personality, *Neuroimage*, **15**, 847–55.
54. Kumari, V., Ffytche, D.H., Williams, S.C.R., *et al.* (2004). Personality predicts brain responses to cognitive demands. *The Journal of Neuroscience*, **24**, 10636–41.
55. O'Gorman, R.L., Kumaro, V., Williams, S.C.R., *et al.* (2006). Personality factors correlate with regional cerebral perfusion. *Neuroimage*, **31**, 489–95.
56. Henry, D., Geary, D., and Tyrer, P. (1993). Adolf Hitler: a re-assessment of his personality status. *Irish Journal of Psychological Medicine*, **10**, 148–51.

4.12.6 Psychotherapy for personality disorder

Anthony W. Bateman and Peter Fonagy

Introduction

Psychotherapy has historically been the mainstay of treatment for personality disorder (PD). It remains so. Psychoanalysis was probably the earliest formal treatment for PD, which led to the first clinical descriptions of borderline personality disorder. A parallel but linked development was the application of psychoanalytic ideas in therapeutic communities which have been in existence for over 60 years and remain a treatment context and method for patients with PD. It was only in the 1960s that modified psychotherapeutic treatments were developed. Initially these were based on psychodynamic understanding of PD, but gradually other theoretically and practically driven models have developed, leading to the current situation in which there are behavioural, cognitive, dynamic, and supportive treatments offered in a range of contexts. Some of these methods have more empirical support than others. These methods will be described in this chapter.

Psychological therapies for personality disorders take place against the background of the natural course and outcome of the disorder. Until recently, the natural history of personality disorder had not been systematically studied. Several major cohort follow-along studies have yielded surprising data concerning the rate of symptomatic remissions in a disorder that was assumed to have a lifelong course.[1] For example, over a 10-year follow-along period, 88 per cent of those initially diagnosed with borderline personality disorder appeared to remit in the sense of no longer meeting DIB-R or DSM-III criteria for BPD for 2 years.[2] The symptoms that remit most readily, irrespective of treatment, appear to be the acute ones, such as parasuicide and self-injury, which are the most likely to trigger psychotherapeutic intervention. Temperamental symptoms, such as angry feelings and acts, distrust and suspicion, abandonment concerns, and emotional instability, appear to resolve far more slowly. In the Collaborative Longitudinal Personality Disorder Study (CLPS),[3] when remission was defined as 12 months at two or fewer criteria for PDs, over half of BPD and 85 per cent of major depressive disorder (MDD) patients were reported to remit over a 4-year period. Psychosocial functioning recovered far more slowly than acute symptoms.[1]

There is a considerable body of literature on psychotherapeutic interventions for personality disorders, but significant evidence for effective treatment remains sparse. Much of the literature is dominated by expert opinion, which is not invariably the most helpful guide. In this chapter, we focus on psychological treatments where at least some evidence for treatment effectiveness exists. The evidence is strongest for borderline personality disorder (BPD). Treatment of some other personality disorders, for example schizoid, narcissistic, obsessive–compulsive, dependent, is evidenced mainly by clinical case reports in which theory is combined with clinical description and where, if outcome is measured at all, it is measured for the purpose of illustration and has little probative value.

Assessment of treatment

Any study that seeks to demonstrate the effectiveness of a treatment for PD must fulfil the following requirements:

(a) *Carefully define the target population.* This can be problematic, because the definition of personality disorder (PD) remains controversial, and there is little evidence that the categories of personality disorder have any predictive value in determining response to treatment. Comorbidity must also be considered. Lifetime comorbidity should not be an exclusion criterion for studies, but there is an argument for excluding individuals with current comorbidity. However, in clinical practice, such exclusion is almost impossible.

(b) *Adequately define the treatment and assessment of its specificity.* Personality disorder is a multifaceted condition that is susceptible to a variety of influences, and it justifies the use of complex interventions. These require complex evaluations, which increase the difficulty of interpreting results.

(c) *Establish that treatment is superior to no treatment* since personality disorders show gradual improvement over time.

(d) *Take account of Axis I disorders.* This can be done by excluding patients with Axis I disorders, but PDs are almost always associated with significant Axis I psychopathology. An alternative, which no trial has, to date, attempted, would be to assign patients to treatment group on the basis of matched Axis I disorders. In any case, it must be demonstrated that treatment impacts on personality rather than merely causing a change in mood or psychiatric symptoms.

(e) *Include adequate follow-up*, as some trials report reduced treatment effects during follow-up.

(f) *Address cost-effectiveness* relative to alternative interventions.

(g) *Study treatment effects in standard practice* (pragmatic trials) as well as under strict experimental conditions.

Research trials investigating the effectiveness of treatments for personality disorder have so far singularly failed to meet most of these requirements.

Adverse effects of psychotherapy for personality disorder

It is possible that some psychosocial treatments for personality disorder may have impeded the patient's capacity to recover following the natural course of the disorder and/or prevented them from taking advantage of changes in social circumstances. In Stone's[4] classic follow-up of patients treated nearly 40 years ago, a 66 per cent recovery rate was only achieved in 20 years, about four times longer than reported in the more recent studies. It seems unlikely that the nature of the disorder has changed or that treatments have become markedly more effective rather it is possible that treatments with these adverse effects are being offered less frequently now than in the past, perhaps because of changed patterns of health care, particularly in the United States.

Meta-analyses of psychotherapy and psychosocial treatments

It remains unclear whether the literature is robust enough to withstand the methodology of meta-analysis. The lack of good quality studies, especially randomized trials, the small number of patients in the trials, the heterogeneity of the personality disorders studied, and the variability of outcome measures across studies means that conclusions must remain tentative. One meta-analysis[5] included 15 studies that reported data on pre- to post-treatment effects and/or recovery at follow-up, including three randomized, controlled trials, three randomized comparisons of active treatments, and nine uncontrolled observational studies. They included psychodynamic/interpersonal, cognitive behavioural, mixed, and supportive therapies. All studies reported improvement in personality disorders with treatment. The mean pre–post effect sizes within treatments were 1.11 for self-report measures and 1.29 for observational measures. Among the three randomized, controlled treatment trials, active psychotherapy was more effective than no treatment according to self-report (ES = 0.75), though none of the controls employed an active therapy. Only four studies reported the percentage of cases no longer meeting the criteria for personality disorder. At follow-up (at a mean of 67 weeks), 52 per cent met this criterion. Treatment length was associated with the likelihood of recovery.

A subsequent meta-analysis[6] included psychodynamic therapy and cognitive behaviour therapy (CBT) in the treatment of personality disorders. There were 22 studies of psychodynamic therapy and CBT published between 1974 and 2001 that (1) used standardized methods of diagnosis, (2) applied reliable and valid instruments for the assessment of outcome, and (3) reported data that allowed calculation of within-group effect sizes or included assessment of recovery rates. Because only 11 of the 22 studies were RCTs, ESs were calculated on the basis of pre- to post-therapy change. Fourteen studies included psychodynamic therapy, and 11 studies included CBT. The psychodynamic studies had a mean follow-up of 1.5 years, compared to only 13 weeks for CBT. Psychodynamic therapy yielded an overall effect size of 1.46 ($k = 15$ contrasts), with effect sizes of 1.08 for self-report measures and 1.79 for observer-rated measures. For CBT ($k = 10$ contrasts), the corresponding values were 1.00, 1.20, and 0.87. For more specific measures of personality disorder pathology, a large overall effect size (1.56) for psychodynamic therapy suggested long-term rather than short-term change in personality disorders. For BPD, the ES for psychodynamic therapy was 1.31 ($N = 8$), and for CBT 0.95 ($N = 4$). Treatment length showed a positive but no°nsignificant correlation with outcome in psychodynamic studies ($r = 0.41$); there were too few CBT trials for an equivalent analysis. In the 5 years since 2001, there have been nearly as many new randomized trials of treatments for personality disorder as were included in this meta-analysis, so a further systematic review including only randomized trials is due.

Psychotherapy for borderline personality disorder (BPD)

Several psychosocial treatments for BPD have emerged over the past decade, with one US guideline recommending psychotherapy as the primary treatment for this condition.[7] It is impossible to recommend one specific therapy, because information from research remains inadequate. It has become clear not only that several treatments may be of use, but also that any one treatment by itself, is helpful in only about a half of all cases.[8] Also, there is general consensus that some of the nonspecific elements of psychotherapy may be as important in determining the success of a treatment as the specific techniques. We reviewed treatments shown to be moderately effective and concluded that they share certain common features.[9] They tend to (a) be well-structured, (b) devote considerable effort to enhancing collaboration, (c) have a clear focus, (d) be theoretically highly coherent to both therapist and patient, (e) be relatively long-term, (f) encourage a powerful attachment relationship between therapist and patient, and (g) be well integrated with other services available to the patient. While some of these features may seem to pertain more to a successful research study rather than a successful therapy, the manner in which clinical treatment protocols are constructed and delivered is probably as important in the success of treatment as the intervention itself.

(a) Dynamic psychotherapy

Dynamic psychotherapy has long been recommended for BPD and has now been modified to target the characteristic features of the disorder. Almost all of the first studies examined inpatient treatment using prospective one group pre- to post-test designs.[10] These studies failed to rule out other plausible causes of change, such as passage of time or subsequent outpatient treatment. Stone's[11] report of up to 20 years follow-up of 550 inpatients, most of whom had received some sort of psychosocial intervention, indicated that 66 per cent of patients were functioning well. However, a naturalistic 5-year follow-up of individuals receiving inpatient treatment at the Cassel Hospital in London indicates the need for caution in ascribing benefits to inpatient treatment.[12] Whilst longer term follow-ups are to be applauded, they are hard to interpret, because other therapies are often given subsequent to the original treatment.

Several nonrandomized trials of dynamic psychotherapy have been undertaken by Stevenson, Meares, and colleagues. In an open trial for 48 patients receiving twice-weekly interpersonal-psychodynamic outpatient therapy for 12 months,[13] 30 per cent of the treatment group no longer met DSM-III-R criteria for BPD, while the waiting-list group changed little. Cost–benefit analysis found significant reduction in costs, largely attributable to reduced inpatient stays. A replication study[14] also found significant reduction in symptom severity with the same treatment.

A randomized study of 38 patients with BPD compared an 18-month programme of partial hospitalization using mentalization-based treatment (MBT) with standard psychiatric care.[15] Mentalization entails making sense of the actions of oneself and others on the basis of intentional mental states such as desires, feelings, and beliefs. Outcome measures included frequency of suicide attempts, acts of self-harm, number and duration of inpatient admissions, use of psychotropic medication, and self-report measures including depression, interpersonal function, and social adjustment. After 6 months, patients given MBT showed a statistically significant decrease on all measures in contrast to the control group which showed limited change or deterioration over the same period. This was sustained at the end of the 18 months of treatment and showed further improvement on follow-up after another 18 months. Long-term follow-up 5 years after the initial treatment suggested that the differences between the groups continued, but general social function remained impaired in both groups.[16] The treatment was cost-effective and has been manualized,[17] but as yet the active components remain unclear, and it has not been shown that positive outcomes are correlated with an improvement in mentalizing. (An outpatient version of MBT is currently being evaluated for borderline and antisocial PD in a further randomized controlled trial.) Although promising, this treatment needs further validation by research carried out independently of the originators. Favourable data has recently become available on the effectiveness of a similar programme established in the Netherlands.[18]

Transference-focused psychotherapy (TFP) has also shown good results. In a cohort study,[19] 23 female borderline patients were treated for 12 months. Compared with the year before treatment, the number of patients who made suicide attempts decreased significantly, as did the medical risk and severity of self-injurious behaviour. Also, compared with the previous year, there were significantly fewer hospitalizations and fewer days of psychiatric hospitalization. However, one in five patients dropped out of treatment. A subsequent trial compared TFP, DBT, and supportive therapy.[20] Ninety patients (all but nine of whom were women) were randomized. At the end of 1 year of treatment, the groups did not differ on global assessment of functioning, social adjustment, scores of depression and anxiety, and measures of self-harm. TFP patients improved significantly more than those receiving DBT or supportive therapy on irritability and verbal and direct assault. Patients who received TFP improved most in reflective function, an operationalization of the mentalization construct,[21] but it is not known whether improved reflective function relates to treatment gains at follow-up.

Schema-focused therapy (SFT) has been compared with TFP.[22] Treatment was given by therapists with approved training in the treatment methods administered treatment to 88 patients with borderline personality disorder. In an 'intent to treat' analysis, patients who received TFP showed significantly less improvement than those who received schema-focused CBT over 3 years, and TFP was more expensive. Both groups showed improvement, but changes in the combined measure of outcome in the schema-focused therapy group were greater and more prolonged than in the TFP group. There are several reasons for caution regarding these conclusions. (i) Differences in outcome between the groups can be accounted for almost entirely by the larger dropout early in treatment of patients treated with TFP and disappear when 'completers' are compared. It would be valuable to know why more patients dropped out from TFP at an early stage than from SFT. (ii) Follow-up is required to determine whether treatment gains and group differences are maintained. (iii) In the duration of the treatment period, around 40 per cent of patients could be expected to improve without the treatment.[23] This study also raises the question of how successfully a treatment (TFP) from the US can be transported to a European context.

(b) Group psychotherapy

Noncontrolled studies of day hospital stabilization followed by outpatient dynamic group therapy indicate its utility for BPD.[24] Marziali and Monroe-Blum used group therapy focused on relationship management and without the milieu and social components. A randomized controlled trial found equivalent results between group and individual therapy, suggesting that group therapy is more cost-effective.[25] Further studies are needed to confirm their findings, especially since dropout rates were high.

(c) Cognitive analytical therapy (CAT)

CAT has been manualized for treatment of BPD, and many are enthusiastic about its effectiveness. There are some indications that it may be effective. In a series of 27 patients with borderline personality disorder treated with 24 sessions of CAT, half no longer met diagnostic criteria for personality disorder at 6-month follow-up.[26] More definitive statements about efficacy await results of a randomized trial in progress. Ryle (personal communication) has indicated that patients treated with CAT showed significant improvement on a range of clinical measures but reported no difference between people receiving CAT and those undergoing other psychological treatments. Thus, the effects may be nonspecific. A second randomized trial is in progress comparing CAT with 'best available standard care' for adolescent patients with borderline personality disorder.[27]

(d) Cognitive therapy

Cognitive behavioural formulations of BPD are diverse. In a model derived from 'standard' CBT and modified for personality disorders, Beck and associates[28] define personality in terms of patterns of social, motivational, and cognitive-affective processes, thereby moving away from a primary emphasis on cognitions. However, personality is considered to be determined by 'idiosyncratic structures', known as schemas, whose cognitive content gives meaning to the person, and these schemas are the cornerstone of cognitive formulations of BPD. Young[29] has developed a treatment programme for BPD based on early maladaptive schemas (EMS). These are stable, enduring patterns of thinking and perception that begin early in life and are continually elaborated. EMS are unconditional beliefs linked together to form the core of an individual's self-image. Challenge to these beliefs threatens the core identity which is defended with alacrity, guile, and desperation since activation of the schemas may evoke aversive emotions. The EMS give rise to 'schema coping behaviour', which offers the best adaptation to living that the borderline has found. Schema-focused therapy (SFT) is only just being evaluated, but its adherence to the general requirements of an effective treatment enumerated above suggests that it should be reasonably successful. The recent report comparing SFT with TFP[22] is described above, but SFT has yet to be shown to be more effective than treatment as usual. It is possible that TFP simply induced more negative effects in patients than SFT.

A small ($N = 34$), randomized controlled trial assessed brief cognitive therapy, linked to a manual and incorporating elements of dialectical behaviour therapy, in the treatment of recurrent self-harm in people with cluster B personality difficulties and disorders.[30]

Manual-assisted cognitive treatment (MACT) is a complex six-session treatment based on the theory that deliberate self-harm and suicide attempts stem from distorted cognitive schemas and coping skills deficits.[31] It incorporates elements of bibliotherapy, CBT, and DBT, as well as psychoeducation in relation to self-harm and suicide attempts, and a functional analysis of specific episodes. The treatment also involves strategies to regulate emotion, such as distraction, crisis planning, and problem-solving strategies. Cognitive restructuring strategies and management of negative thinking are incorporated in the second phase of the programme, which includes components for the management of substance abuse and relapse prevention. Its brevity makes MACT a potentially valuable intervention from a public health standpoint. In a clinical trial, 34 self-harm repeaters with a parasuicide attempt in the preceding 12 months were randomly allocated to MACT or treatment as usual (TAU). The rate of suicide acts was lower with MACT, and self-rated depressive symptoms also improved. The mean treatment time was 2.7 sessions, and the average cost of care was 46 per cent less with MACT. A subsequent larger study ($N = 480$) did not find evidence that time to repeat parasuicide was extended following MACT, although there was a decrease in the cost of care.[32] A randomized controlled trial with 104 people with borderline personality disorder with a longer period of treatment (up to 30 sessions) found significant benefit with regard to suicidal behaviour but a nonsignificant increase in emergency presentations in the cognitive behaviour therapy group.[33] The CBT arm used less resources, although no significant cost-effectiveness advantage was demonstrated. Those who received CBT showed less evidence of dysfunctional beliefs, lower state anxiety scores, and less positive symptom distress.

Systems training for emotional predictability and problem solving (STEPPS)[34] is a group treatment offered as an adjunct to other treatments rather than as a sole intervention. It is a 20-week manualized programme of psychoeducation and behavioural management focusing on maladaptive schemas and including both professional and family carers. Subjects are encouraged to continue their usual care, including individual psychotherapy, medication, and case management, and are required to designate a mental health professional who would provide ongoing care and could be reached in a crisis. Data from 52 patients suggests some reduction in impulsive and suicidal behaviour and some improvement on measures of depression, but no follow-up data is yet available. An RCT is currently ongoing. In Holland, a retrospective assessment of the experience of 85 patients enrolled in STEPPS groups[35] reported significant improvement on all subscales of the SCL-90, particularly those assessing anxiety, depression, and interpersonal sensitivity. Patients and therapists reported moderate to high levels of acceptance for the treatment in both studies. As most of the effective programmes for BPD are long-term and expensive, a short-term efficacious treatment will be of great value. However, even if found to be effective in a clinical trial, its effectiveness will depend on the nature of the treatment as usual.

(e) Dialectical behaviour therapy (DBT)

DBT is a special adaptation of CBT, originally used for the treatment of a group of repeatedly parasuicidal female patients with borderline personality disorder. DBT is a manualized therapy[36] which includes techniques at the level of behaviour (functional analysis), cognitions (e.g. skills training), and support (empathy, teaching management of trauma), with a judicious mix of ideas derived from Zen Buddhism. The initial aim of DBT is to control self-harm, but its main aim is to promote change in the emotional dysregulation that is judged to be at the core of the disorder. Thus, the goal of DBT goes far beyond self-harm reduction. The first trial[37] involved 44 females with borderline personality disorder who had made at least two suicide attempts in the previous 5 years, with one in the preceding 8 weeks. Half were assigned to DBT and half to the control condition. Assessments were made during and at the end of therapy and at a 1-year follow-up. Control patients were significantly more likely to attempt suicide spent significantly more time as inpatients over the year of treatment (mean 38.8 and 8.5 days, respectively), and were significantly more likely to drop out of the therapies to which they were assigned (attrition 50 per cent versus 16.7 per cent, respectively).

DBT was less superior at the 1-year follow-up. Follow-up was naturalistic, because the morbidity of the group was thought to preclude termination of therapy at the end of the experimental period. At 6-month follow-up, DBT patients continued to show less parasuicidal behaviour than controls, though there were no between-group differences in days in hospital. At 1 year there were no between-group differences in suicidal behaviour, but DBT patients had had fewer days in hospital. Treatment with DBT for 1 year compared with treatment as usual led to a reduction in the number and severity of suicide attempts and decreased the frequency and length of inpatient admission. However, there were no between-group differences on measures of depression, hopelessness or reasons for living.

The widespread adoption of DBT for BPD and other PDs is a tribute to both the effectiveness of the treatment and its acceptability to patients and families. Several studies have replicated the original Linehan study. Turner observed a decrease in parasuicidal acts and deliberate self-harm at 6 and 12 months in 12 patients treated with DBT compared to 12 treated with client-centred therapy.[38] Koons and colleagues[39] compared DBT with outpatient treatment as usual in 28 participants and found decreases in frequency of parasuicidal acts and self-injury at 3 and 6 months. Bohus and colleagues[40] explored an inpatient adaptation of DBT and found significant improvement in deliberate self-harm but a higher dropout rate. Other studies, however, have shown DBT to be no better than other active treatments such as the 12-step programme for opioid dependence[41] or treatment as usual in a UK context.[42]

Because of severity, symptomatology, and high rates of co-occurring disorders, BPD affects family members, and interventions addressing the needs of family members have been developed using a DBT frame.[43] In a study of a 12-week community-based BPD family education programme, Family Connections (FC),[44] family members showed significant improvements on burden, grief and empowerment, and a reduction in depression. However, the long-term effect of family interventions on the patient's well-being remains to be demonstrated.

It is uncertain which are the active elements of DBT-individual psychotherapy whether skills training, phone consultation, or the consultation team. Two studies examining the process of change in DBT[41,45] had inconclusive results. Nevertheless, adding a DBT skills training group to outpatient individual (non-DBT) psychotherapy does not seem to enhance treatment outcomes. Given that DBT is described as primarily a skills training approach, this finding might indicate that the central skills training component of DBT may not be of primary importance. However, individual DBT focuses on the strengthening of skills learned in the skills groups, and trying to combine a skills training group with an individual therapy that ignores or pays minimal attention to skill strengthening, may invalidate what the patient has learned about utilizing learned skills in an attempt to cope with everyday functioning. Disagreement remains regarding the policy of not admitting patients to hospital, except for a minimum period, since some studies show that the time and structure of an inpatient setting can be used to apparently good effect.[46]

(f) Therapeutic community treatments

A therapeutic community (TC) may be defined as an intensive form of treatment in which the environmental setting provides the core means through which behaviour can be challenged and modified, essentially through group interaction and interpersonal understanding. Therapeutic communities are described in Chapter 6.3.9. Several studies have been completed at the Cassel Hospital, a tertiary referral centre with a psychosocial residential treatment programme which includes daily unit meetings, community meetings, structured activities, co-responsibility planning for the running of the therapeutic community and other structured activities, and formal psychoanalytic psychotherapy (individual and small group). Patients in two different specialist psychosocial programmes (step-down and long-term inpatient) and in general psychiatric treatment as usual (TAU) were assessed at 12 and 24 months. By 24 months, patients in the step-down condition showed significant improvements on all measures.[47] Patients in the long-term residential condition showed significant improvements in symptom severity, social adaptation, and global functioning but no changes in self-harm, attempted suicide, and readmission rates. Over the same period, patients in the TAU group showed no improvement on any variable except self-harm and hospital readmissions. All three groups were followed for 72 months after intake. The specialist step-down condition led to significantly greater change than either the solely inpatient model or TAU in most key dimensions of functioning, even 5 years after the 12 months hospitalization.[48]

While the study appears to show that a step-down programme leads to significant improvement, this conclusion should be qualified by the study's design limitations, including the lack of random assignment to the three conditions and the naturalistic geographical allocation. Overall, these findings are consistent with the general view that extended hospital admission, even to a psychotherapeutically oriented unit, may engender pathological dependency and regression. Against this, a prospective study of 216 patients with severe personality disorder treated at the Menninger Clinic in two psychoanalytically orientated inpatient units[49] found positive change at discharge and 1 year follow-up, with no evidence of deleterious effects due to regression and dependency. As there are now many treatments for personality disorder, therapeutic communities must be evaluated by comparison studies using acceptable experimental designs if they are to be considered a serious treatment approach.

(g) Nidotherapy

Nidotherapy is the name of a new form of systematic management for chronic and persisting mental disorders that concentrates on making environmental changes to bring about a better fit between person and environment.[50] All types of environmental change—physical, social, and personal—are considered relevant.

Nidotherapy is a collaborative treatment 'involving the systematic assessment and modification of the environment to minimize the impact of any form of the disorder on individual or on society'.[50] The word is derived from the Latin nidus or nest, an environment adapted to the object that is occupying it. The therapeutic aim is not to change the person but rather to change the environment so it better fits the person. The therapist should repeatedly question whether interventions given in the course of management incorporate analytic, cognitive, or behavioural psychotherapy—if they do, the intervention is no longer nidotherapy. Nidotherapy involves seeing the world from the patient's standpoint, joint planning of agreed environmental targets, a concentration on finding ways to improve social function, sharing responsibility for the programme so that the patient is the final owner, and the use of independent arbitrators to resolve disagreements about the change that is needed. The programme has several phases: identification of the boundaries of the nidotherapy, full environmental analysis, implementation of agreed environmental change, monitoring progress, and resetting targets. It addresses the patient's physical, social, and personal environments.

This therapy is at its early stages, with little other than anecdotal evidence.[51] Nevertheless, it represents a healthy contrast to the behavioural, cognitive, and analytic approaches which dominate most psychosocial interventions. There is no doubt that a person's environment is an important determinant of their experience and behaviour. This is accepted regardless of theoretical perspective, yet none of these perspectives offers a model of how environments should be modified to be more in line with the capacities of the person who exists within them. Modifying situational constraints may indeed be an independent and effective adjunct to other treatment protocols for personality disorder.

(h) Summary

The findings from the above studies suggest that some of the problems encountered by people with BPD may be amenable to talking/behavioural treatments. Several studies show that the effort by the recipient of care in sticking with the care package is rewarded by a decline in anxiety, depression, self-harm, hospital admission, and use of prescribed medication. A review using Cochrane methodology[52] concluded that the studies are too few and too small to justify full confidence in their results so that current therapies remain experimental. The reviewers suggest that people with BPD, if offered entry into a randomized study of therapies, may wish to consider that outcomes of both experimental and control groups will probably be better than those of standard care outside the trial.

Psychotherapy for avoidant personality disorder

Avoidant PD is the most prevalent personality disorder in the general population.[53] However, avoidant personalities tend to suffer quietly and reject emotional involvement with others. Nevertheless, their distress and functional impairment are probably comparable to those of people with BPD.

Studies of the efficacy of treatment for avoidant PD have been hampered by the close connection of the condition to social phobia. About half of avoidant patients also have a social phobia. There is controversy over the distinction between generalized social phobia and avoidant personality disorder, many authors regarding the latter as an exaggerated type of social phobia.[54] Many studies of social phobia include individuals with avoidant personality disorder. Few trials explicitly focus on this disorder. Most APD patients are treated using behavioural methods including exposure, social skills training, and systematic desensitization. Early studies suggested treatment gains that were maintained for up to 1 year after finishing active treatment.[55]

For phobic anxiety, there is some agreement that the cognitive behavioural strategies involved in traditional treatment tend sometimes to fail with the more severely disturbed patients because of resistance evoked by maladaptive personality traits.[56] Most studies report a pattern of outcome similar to that for generalized social phobia, with similar rate of gains to those without APD but lower end-point functioning,[57] though some report a slower rate of change.[58] Massion *et al.*[59] report a 5-year prospective study examining the impact of personality disorders in 514 patients in the Harvard/Brown anxiety research programme. The presence of a personality disorder reduced the probability of remission in social phobia by 39 per cent. Much of this reduction was explained by the presence of avoidant personality disorder. Alden[60] found that while there were significant improvements on a range of measures, only 9 per cent of patients treated for APD rated themselves as completely improved.

Therapeutic strategies for severe cases of APD should be tailored to the core pathology of the disorder—(1) a despised and unworthy sense of self connected to a punitive and blaming internal other; (2) an avoidant interpersonal style; (3) affect phobia; and (4) pseudomentalization (intellectualization and pretend relations). In achieving somewhat better functioning for avoidant patients, short-term dynamic psychotherapy and cognitive therapy have been shown to have good results.[61] For the more severely disturbed avoidant patients, day treatment programmes are probably more effective[62] than outpatient therapy, where they tend to ossify.[63] An RCT of cognitive behaviour therapy versus psychodynamic therapy for AVPD[64] found greater benefit from cognitive behaviour therapy. Interpersonal therapy and supportive-expressive therapy have also been tried. Patients are often reported to have made substantial gains in all treatment programmes,[65] but many patients who complete treatment still demonstrate a low level of social function.

Psychotherapy for antisocial personality disorder (ASPD)

There are few evaluated therapies for ASPD. The disorder is a common comorbid diagnosis for individuals with substance abuse problems,[66] and a small number of trials have contrasted those with ASPD alone with those with ASPD and depression in the treatment of substance misuse. Outcomes with antisocial personality disorder alone are often poorer than when ASPD is associated with depression. Three studies[67–69] have reported that ASPD alone was an obstacle in the treatment of substance misuse.

Several studies (though few controlled trials) have examined the impact of treatment on individuals within the penal system, at least some of whom, it is likely meet criteria for antisocial personality disorder. Most studies focus on specific categories of offending behaviour (e.g. sexual offences), or on prisoners with problem behaviours, particularly violence.[70] Some studies have focused on individuals who manifest callous-unemotional traits.[71]

There are a few observational studies of individuals detained in high security settings using group CBT,[72] individual and group CBT in the context of a therapeutic milieu,[73] or psychodynamic therapy.[74] While improvements in functioning are noted, there are severe methodological problems such as the absence of control groups and highly reactive measurement of outcome.

Studies reviewed by Warren and colleagues[70] suggest the usefulness of cognitive behavioural or (less frequently) systemic group-based interventions of various kinds for mentally disordered offenders. These include: seven studies of problem-solving skills training, five studies of anger/aggression management, and three studies aimed at social skills problems. Three studies of problem-solving training reported no statistically significant positive effects, while a further three reported some positive results with measures of outcome closely linked to the intervention. Anger management studies were predominantly negative with no statistically significant positive effects reported by the majority of studies and positive results reported only with quite reactive measures or within quasi-experimental studies. Social skills interventions also enjoyed mixed success with either no statistically significant positive effects being reported or positive effects observed only with reactive measures or in uncontrolled studies. While it is not possible to claim that psychotherapy is effective in addressing problems associated with ASPD, there is sufficient preliminary data to justify further inquiry and to counter the therapeutic nihilism that usually pervades this field.

Psychotherapy for other personality disorders

Individuals with **paranoid PD** are highly suspicious of other people, including doctors, and are often unable to acknowledge their own negative feelings towards others. This fact alone means that treatment is problematic, but given that other characteristics include concern that other people have hidden motives, expectation of being exploited by others, inability to collaborate, social isolation, emotional detachment, and overt hostility, treatment becomes nearly impossible. This constellation of characteristics means research on this group of patients is very difficult to conduct, since researchers are inevitably seen as having hidden motives. Whatever treatment method is employed, the first step is the development of a moderately trusting relationship. There is no research specifically investigating the outcome of psychotherapeutic treatment for paranoid personality disorder. However, a number of studies have included patients with paranoid PD in assessment of treatment. In general, the presence of paranoid PD diminishes the effectiveness of psychotherapeutic treatment for other co-occurring personality disorders.

Most of the interest in **schizotypal** personality disorder (STPD) has been in its relationship to schizophrenia, and hence there is little data on outcome of treatment using psychosocial methods. The Chestnut Lodge follow-up study yielded some data suggesting that patients who had schizophrenia plus STPD and had been treated within the psychotherapeutic milieu did slightly better than patients without STPD.[75] This unexpected finding has not been explained.

Winston *et al.*[76] treated 32 patients with a range of personality disorders, predominantly in DSM-III-R cluster C, using two forms of brief psychodynamic therapy (short-term dynamic psychotherapy or brief adaptational therapy) with 40 weekly sessions and waiting-list control. Because of ethical constraints, waiting-list subjects began treatment after 15 weeks. Although both therapies used psychodynamic techniques, brief adaptational therapy employed more cognitive strategies. Contrasted to waiting-list controls, treated patients showed moderate improvements in symptoms and target complaints at post-therapy. Though there were few between-treatment differences, there was more variance in outcome for the patients treated with short-term dynamic therapy, suggesting that for some patients the technique was unhelpful. Gains appeared to be maintained at 18-month follow-up. A larger trial of these therapies with mainly cluster C disorder[77] led to similar findings.

Conclusions

Effectiveness

It is difficult to reach definitive conclusions about the effectiveness of psychotherapy in the treatment of personality disorders, chiefly because RCTs of psychological treatments for PDs are relatively scarce. There is evidence that personality disorders impact negatively on treatments for Axis I presentations. However, the strength and specificity of this evidence varies both across Axis I diagnoses and also across personality disorders.

Historically, studies of psychotherapy for personality disorder have focused on cluster B PDs. Borderline personality disorder is the best studied of the PD diagnoses both from a biological and a psychotherapeutic perspective. The recent growth in the evidence base indicates the feasibility of coherent research programmes with a patient group usually seen as presenting substantial problems of engagement. Evidence from randomized trials suggests that structured treatments employing DBT or a psychodynamic approach are more effective than routine care. Data gathered so far support the use of both behavioural and psychodynamic interventions, while evidence for more short-term cognitive interventions is somewhat equivocal. Since most studies present data from open trials or case-series, only two approaches can be considered 'evidence-based'. The available randomized trials of DBT and psychodynamic treatment are methodologically sound but limited in the latter case by relatively small sample sizes; further, both sets of studies were conducted in the context of clear leadership from the developers. Because, for the most part, contrast was to routine care, it is difficult to ascertain whether outcomes are due to the structured nature of the programmes or their therapeutic orientation.

In relation to antisocial personality disorder, research into treatments has been centred on patients seeking help for substance abuse or individuals seen within the penal system for problems associated with ASPD. There is no clear evidence of treatment efficacy for any one form of intervention. Conclusions in relation to ASPD are limited not only by the small number of trials but also by the methodological limitations of these studies, particularly reactive measures of outcome and complex multifaceted interventions (such as therapeutic communities) where effective transportable components of the treatment package are impossible to disaggregate.

Avoidant personality disorder has received only a modest amount of research attention. Individuals presenting with APD would normally be offered social skills training or cognitive (exposure-based) techniques which are likely to be successful, but the generalization of improvements to other social contexts has not yet been well demonstrated.

Implications for clinical practice

With the exception of cluster B disorders, many individuals with PDs present to services for help with Axis I disorders. Clinicians should be aware that while treatments normally recommended for these problems can still work, they may do so to a lesser extent than would be expected if comorbid PD were not part of the clinical problem. However, they should not assume that this will definitely be the case. The situation is somewhat different in the case of the so-called dramatic PDs. Many of the features of the behaviour of individuals with borderline or antisocial PD create such distress for the people around them that clinicians tend to privilege these features over symptomatic states related to comorbid Axis I disorders when setting goals for treatment.

There is little doubt that psychological therapies have a place in the management of personality disorders, but the methodological shortcomings of the studies so far conducted limit our ability to make practical recommendations. Given the nature of the problem (supposedly enduring problems of character) the fact that few trials conduct follow-up over a longer period or include a contrast or control group over follow-up is a grave limitation of the database. Only two studies (Chiesa's 72 months follow-up and the MBT 5-year follow-up) have demonstrated that post-treatment differences are maintained for extended periods. Clinical experience, somewhat contradicted by recent follow-along data, suggests that many individuals may show periods of complete remission followed by episodes of great severity, and therefore it is crucial to investigate the impact of treatment on this often chronic and cyclic course. DBT has good evidence for its immediate impact on behavioural problems of impulsivity and suicidality, but the evidence for long-term benefit without further treatment is less clear. Psychodynamic approaches aim to change the way the person thinks, and there is some evidence that this approach has some impact on mood states and interpersonal functioning. However, this emphasis on cognitive change requires longer term therapy, with some indication of slower rates of change but perhaps also more sustained gains over follow-up. While shorter interventions are likely to have lower immediate costs, longer ones would be justified if they were more cost-effective in terms of service utilization and other cost-offsets. However, evidence for these kinds of effects is scarce.

Debate about particular forms of therapy may be less relevant than attention to nonspecific factors, especially in the treatment of individuals with cluster B PDs. We have seen that successful approaches usually emphasize the importance of structure, a coherent theoretical base, a higher intensity of treatment than for many Axis I disorders, and especially, attention to the unique set of problems presented by the individual, with a clear psychological formulation guiding treatment. Decisions about which treatment to opt for might be best made with regard to pragmatic considerations rather than argument about which particular course is 'best'. It may even be better to offer patients intensive treatment initially and to follow with short bursts of treatment over a long period of time. The competence and training of senior clinicians who can offer supervision will be especially important, as will the skill mix of staff and the resources (including staffing level) available to the service. These 'nonspecific' issues may be especially pertinent when considering the performance of evidence-based treatments in routine practice. Since systemic factors may be as relevant to success as the type of treatment offered, pragmatic trials would be useful to give an indication of the conditions required to implement evidence-based therapies in routine services.

Further information

Fonagy, P. (ed.) (2007) Special issue on treatment of personality disorder. *Journal of Mental Health*, **16**(1).

Gunderson, J.G. (2001) *Borderline personality disorder: a clinical guide.* American Psychiatric Publishing, Washington, DC.

Lenzenweger, M.F. and Clarkin, J.F. (2004). *Major theories of personality disorder* (2nd edn). Guilford, New York.

Roth, A. and Fonagy, P. (2005). Personality disorders. In *What works for whom? A critical review of psychotherapy research* (2nd edn) (eds. A. Roth and P. Fonagy), pp. 297–319. Guilford, New York.

References

1. Skodol, A.E., Gunderson, J., Shea, M.T., *et al.* (2006). The Collaborative Longitudinal Personality Disorders Study (CLPS): overview and implications. *Journal of Personality Disorders*, **19**(5), 487–504.
2. Zanarini, M.C., Frankenburg, F.R., Hennen, J., *et al.* (2006). The McLean Study of Adult Development (MSAD): overview and implications of the first six years of prospective follow-up. *Journal of Personality Disorders*, **19**(5), 505–23.
3. Grilo, C.M., Sanislow, C.A., Gunderson, J.G., *et al.* (2004). Two-year stability and change of schizotypal, borderline, avoidant, and obsessive-compulsive personality disorders. *Journal of Consulting and Clinical Psychology*, **72**(5), 767–75.
4. Stone, M.H. (1990). *The fate of borderline patients: successful outcome and psychiatric practice.* Guilford Press, New York.
5. Perry, J.C., Banon, E., and Ianni, F. (1999). Effectiveness of psychotherapy for personality disorders. *The American Journal of Psychiatry*, **156**(9), 1312–21.
6. Leichsenring, F. and Leibing, E. (2003). The effectiveness of psychodynamic therapy and cognitive behavior therapy in the treatment of personality disorders: a meta-analysis. *The American Journal of Psychiatry*, **160**(7), 1223–32.
7. Oldham, J.M., Phillips, K.A., and Gabbard, G.O. (2001). Practice guideline for the treatment of patients with borderline personality disorder. *The American Journal of Psychiatry*, **158**(Suppl. 10), 1–52.
8. Roth, A. and Fonagy, P. (2005). *What works for whom? A critical review of psychotherapy research* (2nd edn). Guilford Press, New York.
9. Bateman, A.W. and Fonagy, P. (2000). Effectiveness of psychotherapeutic treatment of personality disorder. *The British Journal of Psychiatry*, **177**, 138–43.
10. McGlashan, T. (1986). The chestnut lodge follow-up study III: long-term outcome of borderline personalities. *Archives of General Psychiatry*, **43**, 20–30.
11. Stone, M. (1993). Long-term outcome in personality disorders. *The British Journal of Psychiatry*, **162**, 299–313.
12. Rosser, R., Birch, S., Bond, H., *et al.* (1987). Five year follow-up of patients treated with in-patient psychotherapy at the Cassel Hospital for nervous diseases. *Journal of the Royal Society of Medicine*, **80**, 549–55.
13. Stevenson, J., Meares, R., and D'Angelo, R. (2005). Five-year outcome of outpatient psychotherapy with borderline patients. *Psychological Medicine*, **35**(1), 79–87.
14. Korner, A., Gerull, F., Meares, R., *et al.* (2006). Borderline personality disorder treated with the conversational model: a replication study. *Comprehensive Psychiatry*, **47**, 406–11.
15. Bateman, A.W. and Fonagy, P. (2001). Treatment of borderline personality disorder with psychoanalytically oriented partial hospitalization: an 18-month follow-up. *The American Journal of Psychiatry*, **158**(1), 36–42.

16. Bateman, A.W. Fonagy P. 8-year follow-up of patients treated for borderline personality disorder—mentalization based treatment versus treatment as usual. *The American Journal of Psychiatry*. submitted.
17. Bateman, A.W. and Fonagy, P. (2004). *Psychotherapy for borderline personality disorder: mentalization based treatment*. Oxford University Press, Oxford.
18. Bales, D., Andrea, H., Smits, M., *et al.* (2007). Mentalization based treatment in the Netherlands: first results. *Biannual meeting of the international society personality disorder*. Den haag, Netherlands.
19. Clarkin, J.F., Foelsch, P.A., Levy, K.N., *et al.* (2001). The development of a psychodynamic treatment for patients with borderline personality disorder: a preliminary study of behavioral change. *Journal of Personality Disorders*, **15**, 487–95.
20. Clarkin, J., Levy, K.N., Lenzenweger, M.F., *et al.* (2007). Evaluating three treatments for borderline personality disorder: a multiwave study. *The American Journal of Psychiatry*, **164**, 922–8.
21. Levy, K.N., Meehan, K.B., Kelly, K.M., *et al.* (2006). Change in attachment patterns and reflective function in a randomized control trial of transference-focused psychotherapy for borderline personality disorder. *Journal of Consulting and Clinical Psychology*, **74**(6), 1027–40.
22. Giesen-Bloo, J., van Dyck, R., Spinhoven, P., *et al.* (2006). Outpatient psychotherapy for borderline personality disorder: randomized trial of schema-focused therapy vs transference-focused psychotherapy. *Archives of General Psychiatry*, **63**(6), 649–58.
23. Zanarini, M.C., Frankenburg, F.R., Hennen, J., *et al.* (2003). The longitudinal course of borderline psychopathology: 6-year prospective follow-up of the phenomenology of borderline personality disorder. *The American Journal of Psychiatry*, **160**(2), 274–83.
24. Wilberg, T., Friis, S., Karterud, S., *et al.* (1998). Outpatient group psychotherapy: a valuable continuation treatment for patients with borderline personality disorder treated in a day hospital? A 3-year follow-up study. *Nordic Journal of Psychiatry*, **52**, 213–22.
25. Marziali, E. and Monroe-Blum, H. (1995). An interpersonal approach to group psychotherapy with borderline personality disorder. *Journal of Personality Disorders*, **9**, 179–89.
26. Ryle, A. and Golynkina, K. (2000). Effectiveness of time-limited cognitive analytic therapy of borderline personality disorder: factors associated with outcome. *British Journal of Medical Psychology*, **73**(Pt 2), 197–210.
27. Ryle, A. (2004). The contribution of cognitive analytic therapy to the treatment of borderline personality disorder. *Journal of Personality Disorders*, **18**(1), 3–35.
28. Alford, B. and Beck, A. (1997). *The integrative power of cognitive therapy*. Guilford, New York.
29. Young, J.E. (1990). *Cognitive therapy for personality disorders: a schema-focused approach*. Professional Resource Exchange, Sarasota, Florida.
30. Evans, K., Tyrer, P., Catalan, J., *et al.* (1999). Manual-assisted cognitive-behaviour therapy (MACT): a randomized controlled trial of a brief intervention with bibliotherapy in the treatment of recurrent deliberate self-harm. *Psychological Medicine*, **29**(1), 19–25.
31. Schmidt, U. and Davidson, K. (2004). *Life after self-harm*. Routledge, London.
32. Byford, S., Knapp, M., Greenshields, J., *et al.* (2003). Cost-effectiveness of brief cognitive behaviour therapy versus treatment as usual in recurrent deliberate self-harm: a decision-making approach. *Psychological Medicine*, **33**(6), 977–86.
33. Davidson, K., Tyrer, P., Gumley, A., *et al.* (2006). A randomized controlled trial of cognitive behavior therapy for borderline personality disorder: rationale for trial, method, and description of sample. *Journal of Personality Disorders*, **20**(5), 431–49.
34. Blum, N., Pfohl, B., John, D.S., *et al.* (2002). STEPPS: a cognitive-behavioral systems-based group treatment for outpatients with borderline personality disorder—a preliminary report. *Comprehensive Psychiatry*, **43**(4), 301–10.
35. Freije, H., Dietz, B., and Appelo, M. (2002). Behandling van de borderline persoonlijk heidsstoornis met de VERS: de Vaardigheidstraining emotionele regulatiestoornis. *Directive Therapies*, **4**, 367–78.
36. Linehan, M.M. (1993). The skills training manual for treating borderline personality disorder. Guilford Press, New York.
37. Linehan, M.M., Heard, H.L., and Armstrong, H.E. (1993). Naturalistic follow-up of a behavioral treatment for chronically parasuicidal borderline patients. *Archives of General Psychiatry*, **50**, 971–4.
38. Turner, R.M. (2000). Naturalistic evaluation of DBT oriented treatment for BPD. *Cognitive Behaviour Practice*, **7**, 413–9.
39. Koons, C.R., Robins, C.J., Tweed, J.L., *et al.* (2001). Efficacy of DBT in women veterans with BPD. *Behavior Therapy*, **32**, 371–90.
40. Bohus, M., Haaf, B., Simms, T., *et al.* (2004). Effectiveness of inpatient dialectical behavioral therapy for borderline personality disorder: a controlled trial. *Behaviour Research and Therapy*, **42**(5), 487–99.
41. Linehan, M.M., Dimeff, L.A., Reynolds, S.K., *et al.* (2002). Dialectical behavior therapy versus comprehensive validation therapy plus 12-step for the treatment of opioid dependent women meeting criteria for borderline personality disorder. *Drug and Alcohol Dependence*, **67**(1), 13–26.
42. Feigenbaum, J.D., Fonagy, P., Pilling, S., *et al.* A pilot randomized control trial of the effectiveness of Dialectical Behavioural Therapy (DBT) for cluster B personality disorder. Submitted.
43. Hoffman, P.D. and Fruzzetti, A.E. (2007). Advances in interventions for families with a relative with a personality disorder diagnosis. *Current Psychiatry Reports*, **9**(1), 68–73.
44. Hoffman, P.D., Fruzzetti, A.E., and Buteau, E. (2007). Understanding and engaging families: an education, skills and support program for relatives impacted by borderline personality disorder. *Journal of Mental Health*, **16**(1), 69–82.
45. Shearin, E. and Linehan, M.M. (1992). Patient-therapist ratings and relationship to progress in dialectical behaviour therapy for borderline personality disorder. *Behavior Therapy*, **23**, 730–41.
46. Bohus, M., Haaf, B., Simms, T., *et al.* (2002). Effectiveness of inpatient dialectical behavioural therapy for borderline personality disorder: a controlled trial. *5th ISSPD European Congress on Personality Disorders—Abstracts*. Munich, Germany: 18.
47. Chiesa, M., Fonagy, P., Holmes, J., *et al.* (2004). Residential versus community treatment of personality disorders: a comparative study of three treatment programs. *The American Journal of Psychiatry*, **161**(8), 1463–70.
48. Chiesa, M., Fonagy, P., and Holmes, J. (2006). Six-year follow-up of three treatment programs to personality disorder. *Journal of Personality Disorders*, **20**(5), 493–509.
49. Gabbard, G.O., Coyne, L., Allen, J.G., *et al.* (2000). Evaluation of intensive inpatient treatment of patients with severe personality disorders. *Psychiatric Services*, **51**(7), 893–8.
50. Tyrer, P., Sensky, T., and Mitchard, S. (2003). Principles of nidotherapy in the treatment of persistent mental and personality disorders. *Psychotherapy and Psychosomatics*, **72**(6), 350–6.
51. Tyrer, P. and Kramo, K. (2007). Nidotherapy in practice. *Journal of Mental Health*, **16**(1), 117–29.
52. Binks, C.A., Fenton, M., McCarthy, L., *et al.* (2006). Pharmacological interventions for people with borderline personality disorder. *Cochrane Database of Systematic Review*, 2006(1), CD005653.
53. Samuels, J., Eaton, W.W., Bienvenu, O.J. III, *et al.* (2002). Prevalence and correlates of personality disorders in a community sample. *The British Journal of Psychiatry*, **180**, 536–42.
54. Rettew, D.C. (2000). Avoidant personality disorder, generalized social phobia, and shyness: putting the personality back into personality disorders. *Harvard Review of Psychiatry*, **8**(6), 283–97.
55. Renneberg, B., Goldstein, A.M., Phillips, D., *et al.* (1990). Intensive behavioral group treatment of avoidant personality disorder. *Behavior Therapy*, **21**, 363–77.

56. Alden, L.E., Taylor, C.T., Laposa, J.M., *et al.* (2006). Impact of social developmental experiences on cognitive-behavioral therapy for generalized social phobia. *Journal of Cognitive Psychotherapy: An International Quarterly*, **20**, 7–16.
57. Scholing, A. and Emmelkamp, P.M. (1999). Prediction of treatment outcome in social phobia: a cross-validation. *Behaviour Research and Therapy*, **37**(7), 659–70.
58. Oosterbaan, D.B., van Balkom, A.J., Spinhoven, P., *et al.* (2002). The influence on treatment gain of comorbid avoidant personality disorder in patients with social phobia. *The Journal of Nervous and Mental Disease*, **190**(1), 41–3.
59. Massion, A.O., Dyck, I.R., Shea, M.T., *et al.* (2002). Personality disorders and time to remission in generalized anxiety disorder, social phobia, and panic disorder. *Archives of General Psychiatry*, **59**(5), 434–40.
60. Alden, L.E. (1989). Short term structured treatment for avoidant personality disorder. *Journal of Consulting and Clinical Psychology*, **56**, 756–64.
61. Svartberg, M., Stiles, T.C., and Seltzer, M.H. (2004). Randomized, controlled trial of the effectiveness of short-term dynamic psychotherapy and cognitive therapy for cluster C personality disorders. *The American Journal of Psychiatry*, **161**, 810–7.
62. Karterud, S., Pedersen, G., Bjordal, E., *et al.* (2003). Day treatment of patients with personality disorders: experiences from a Norwegian treatment research network. *Journal of Personality Disorders*, **17**, 243–62.
63. Wilberg, T., Karterud, S., Pedersen, G., *et al.* (2003). Outpatient group psychotherapy following day treatment of patients with personality disorders. *Journal of Personality Disorders*, **17**, 510–21.
64. Emmelkamp, P., Benner, A., Kuipers, A., *et al.* (2006). Comparison of brief dynamic and cognitive-behavioural therapies in avoidant personality disorder. *The British Journal of Psychiatry*, **189**, 60–4.
65. Barber, J.P., Morse, J.Q., Krakauer, I.D., *et al.* (1997). Change in obsessive-compulsive and avoidant personality disorders following time-limited supportive-expressive therapy. *Psychotherapy*, **34**(2), 133–43.
66. Brooner, R.K., King, V.L., Kidorf, M., *et al.* (1997). Psychiatric and substance use comorbidity among treatment seeking opiate users. *Archives of General Psychiatry*, **54**, 71–80.
67. Woody, G.E., McLellan, T., Luborsky, L., *et al.* (1985). Sociopathy and psychotherapy outcome. *Archives of General Psychiatry*, **179**, 188–93.
68. Alterman, A.I., Rutherford, M.J., Cacciola, J.S., *et al.* (1996). Response to methadone maintenance and counseling in antisocial patients with and without major depression. *The Journal of Nervous and Mental Disease*, **184**(11), 695–702.
69. King, V.L., Kidorf, M.S., Stoller, K.B., *et al.* (2001). Influence of antisocial personality subtypes on drug abuse treatment response. *The Journal of Nervous and Mental Disease*, **189**(9), 593–601.
70. Warren, F., Preedy-Fayers, K., McGauley, G., *et al.* (2003). Review of treatments for severe personality disorder home office online report 30/03 (http://www.homeoffice.gov.uk/rds/pdfs2/rdsolr3003.pdf).
71. Hare, R.D., Hart, S.D., and Harpur, T.J. (1991). Psychopathy and the DSM-IV criteria for antisocial personality disorder. *Journal of Abnormal Psychology*, **100**, 391–8.
72. Quayle, M. and Moore, E. (1998). Evaluating the impact of structured groupwork with men in a high security hospital. *Criminal Behaviour and Mental Health*, **8**, 77–92.
73. Hughes, G., Hogue, T., Hollin, C., *et al.* (1997). First-stage evaluation of a treatment programme for personality disordered offenders. *Journal of Forensic Psychiatry*, **8**, 515–27.
74. Reiss, D., Grubin, D., and Meux, C. (1996). Young psychopaths in special hospital: treatment and outcome. *The British Journal of Psychiatry*, **168**, 99–104.
75. McGlashan, T.H. (1986). Schizotypal personality disorder. Chestnut Lodge follow-up study: VI. Long-term follow-up perspectives. *Archives of General Psychiatry*, **43**(4), 329–34.
76. Winston, A., Pollack, J., McCullough, L., *et al.* (1991). Brief psychotherapy of personality disorders. *Journal of Nervous and Mental Disease*, **179**, 188–93.
77. Winston, A., Laikin, M., Pollack, J., *et al.* (1994). Short-term psychotherapy of personality disorders. *The American Journal of Psychiatry*, **151**, 190–4.

4.12.7 Management of personality disorder

Giles Newton-Howes and Kate Davidson

Introduction

The treatment of personality disorders is a complex but rapidly evolving subject. It is to some extent described elsewhere in Chapters 3.3, 4.12.6, 4.13.1, 5.2.9, 6.3.5, 6.3.9 8.5.6, 9.2.4, 11.3.2, 11.16, and 11.17, and so this chapter excludes a full discussion of psychodynamic interventions, therapeutic communities, interventions for older people and the management of both adolescent and adult offenders.`

Methodological difficulties in evaluating the efficacy of treatment

The requirements for establishing whether a treatment is effective for personality disorders are much more exacting than those for mental state disorders. These can usefully be described under four headings:

- duration of treatment
- comorbidity
- adherence to treatment
- outcome measures.

(a) Duration of treatment

For most mental state disorders it is relatively easy to choose the period over which efficacy has to be demonstrated. In conditions that develop suddenly (e.g. panic), treatment trials could be for a very short time indeed. For others, particularly when maintenance treatment is being evaluated, at least 6 months may be necessary to establish continued efficacy. In the case of personality disorders, it has been thought that efficacy of treatment could not be judged adequately without at least a 2 to 3 year treatment phase. Personality disorder was regarded as being unlikely to change in the short-term. However, these ideas are changing in the light of evidence from longer-term follow-up studies of patients with personality disorder that show that these conditions do change over time in a consistent and predictable manner with substantial numbers of patients achieving full remission in the longer term.[1] If these longer-term follow-up studies are replicated, it would suggest that therapy should aim to accelerate the process of recovery. Determining what constitutes an adequate amount of therapy and over what length of time is an empirical question. More recent studies have offered treatment over 1 year with a 1 year follow-up to examine maintenance of effect[2,3] but other studies have chosen lengthier treatment phases of up to 3 years[4] with some reporting continued therapy in the follow-up phase which does not allow the effect of maintenance of the original effect to be judged.[5] More recent studies, examining the effect of psychological treatments, have included a 1 year follow-up. The purpose of this follow-up period is to determine if treatment effects are maintained following the termination of treatment. Such a requirement is not a purist position; if a treatment for personality disorder appears to be effective over a shorter period, this may be due to change in a concurrent (comorbid) condition. In addition, if a treatment is to be judged efficacious in personality disorder its effects should be lasting beyond the active treatment component.

(b) Comorbidity

Comorbidity has been defined as 'the presence of any distinct clinical entity that has existed or that may occur during the clinical course of a patient who has the index disease under study'.[5] The key word here is 'distinct'. True comorbidity implies the presence of two completely separate disorders in the same person which are not causally related to each other in any way. Co-occurrence ranges from true comorbidity to the presence of the same disorder in two or more different forms.[6]

Comorbidity is the norm for most personality disorders both with other personality disorders or with mental state disorders. Borderline personality disorder is a major offender in this regard. Only about 1 in 20 of such disorders constitutes the pure condition,[7] and multiple comorbidity with four or more disorders is common.

In deciding on the efficacy of any treatment for personality disorder it is impossible to be certain whether observed improvement is in the personality disorder or in a comorbid condition. This problem is made worse because personality assessment is allegedly confounded, or 'contaminated', by the effect of a concurrent mental state disorder. Thus personality status apparently changes during the presence of a mental state disorder such as depression, only to return to the baseline normal subsequently.[8,9] Apparent improvement in a personality disorder following a treatment may be entirely due to improvement in a concurrent mental state disorder. However, this conclusion does not mean that *personality function*, as opposed to *personality disorder*, does not change. The underlying personality may remain stable, but if the setting and circumstances change, and this includes mental state changes, there can be marked changes in adjustment and so the manifestation of disorder will also change.[10]

In view of these problems, a treatment for a personality disorder should ideally be tested in those patients who have that personality disorder only. As these patients are uncommon and atypical, it is difficult to interpret the data from clinical trials.

(c) Adherence to treatment

People with personality disorders do not usually form good relationships with therapists. Although this is in keeping with their problems with relationships elsewhere, it can be a major problem in any form of therapy. The problem is particularly marked with psychotherapy, in which long-held views are challenged by the therapist. The consequence is that many patients dropout of care, and sometimes no amount of therapeutic skill can maintain them in care.[11] The failure to maintain prescribed treatment, in whatever form, is a constant handicap in accumulating an evidence base for interventions in personality disorder. Even within personality disorder there are differences between sub-groups. Most therapeutic trials have been inpatients with borderline personality disorder while those with schizoid, paranoid, histrionic, narcissistic, and antisocial personality disorders appear much less frequently. This is probably related to treatment attitudes. Borderline, anxious, and avoidant personality disorders contain a much higher proportion of treatment seeking (Type S) personality disorders as opposed to treatment resisting (Type R) ones, which are most prominent in those with antisocial, schizoid, and paranoid personalities.[12]

Any study of personality disorder is likely to have a large proportion of dropouts and this complicates the interpretation of the effects of treatment. The exception is when patients are treated in restricted settings such as prisons and other closed facilities,[13] but as these circumstances are abnormal it is difficult to generalize from them.

(d) Outcome measures

The choice of outcome measures is a problem in the assessment of all psychiatric disorders, but difficulty is particularly great in studies of personality disorders. These disorders affect both the individual and society, and a range of outcomes can be measured to cover these possibilities. Forensic psychiatrists and the general public usually consider that the outcome of mentally disordered offenders is best measured by the frequency of reoffending. This is an easily measured and reliable statistic, but it does not necessarily record symptomatic or personality change, and may be distorted by a range of other factors (e.g. patients who spend a long time in hospital or prison are not likely to reoffend). Changes in symptoms also have limited use since they may be a consequence of changes in mental state disorders quite independent of personality. Repeated measures of personality status also have disadvantages since, as noted earlier, they may be affected by changes with concurrent mental state disorder. Personality also changes with ageing irrespective of treatment.[14]

Because of these difficulties, global outcome measures are often used to determine the degree of improvement in personality disorders in long-term follow-up studies, although a battery of measurements is normally used in short-term treatment studies. Unfortunately, there is no standardized set of measures of global outcome. It is reasonable to take into account symptomatic change, social functioning, quality of life, incidents of societal conflict (e.g. police contacts), and reports from informants. Even these may not correctly reflect change in personality status. Thus a person whose personality disorder does not change in any basic way may find an environmental niche in which the personality disturbance does not manifest itself as conflict. Such a person would show improvement on all the items listed above, but the improvement would be a consequence of environmental change, not of personality alteration.

(e) Minimum requirements for establishment of efficacy

The evidence base for effectiveness of treatment in personality disorders is also exacting:

1 The treatment should be effective when used in the pure form of the personality disorder (in an explanatory trial) and subsequently in other forms of the disorder in which comorbidity is more common (pragmatic trial).

2 Efficacy cannot be established satisfactorily unless the treatment is tested in a randomized controlled trial.

3 A suitable control treatment or management needs to be tested against the experimental treatment.

4 Efficacy should only be determined after a period of at least 1 year because of the long duration of personality disorder. More recent randomized controlled trials in borderline personality disorder examining psychological therapies have met these more demanding criteria.[15,16]

Dynamic psychotherapy

This is discussed in chapter 4.12.6.

Cognitive therapies

(a) Cognitive analytical therapy

Cognitive analytical therapy combines cognitive and analytical approaches and has been applied to the treatment of personality disorders, particularly the borderline group.[17] The clinical manifestations of this condition are postulated to be a set of partially dissociated 'self-states' which account for the clinical features of this disorder. Such patients typically describe rapid switching from one state of mind to another, experiencing intense uncontrollable emotions or alternatively feeling muddled, or emotionally cut-off. Such 'dissociative states' (different from the conditions of similar name formerly linked to hysteria) are said to be activated by severe external threats and to be maintained by repetitions of threat and reinforcement by memories or situations which are similar to the original source of threat.

Cognitive analytical therapy is concerned with the identification of these different self-states and helping patients to identify 'reciprocal role procedures', or patterns of relationships which are learned in early childhood and are relatively resistant to change.[18] The patient is taught to observe and try to change damaging patterns of thinking and behaviour which relate to these self-states and to become more self-aware. The therapist's role is to gather information about the patient's experience of relationships and the different states he or she experiences, including interpretation where necessary. Although the standard measure of evidence of effectiveness, the randomized controlled trial, has still not yet been reported for this treatment it has gathered an impressive group of adherents and has become widely used and now has a good theoretical and pragmatic base.[18]

(b) Cognitive behaviour therapy

In its original form, cognitive therapy for depression was used to help the patient to identify and modify dysfunctional thoughts and beliefs through the use of specific cognitive techniques such as Socratic questioning. The focus of therapy was here and now the aim was to return the patient to his or her usual functioning by relieving current symptoms. The cognitive model of personality disorder does emphasize cognitive, emotional, and behavioural factors but the origins of personality problems are regarded as originating in the temperament of the child, childhood development, and experiences. Early infant attachment patterns, the child's internal working model of relationships, self-identity, self-worth, and the emotional availability of the infant's caregivers are central to how the child develops and these shape the adult self-identity, interpersonal relationships in adulthood, and behavioural and emotional coping responses.[19]

One of the first tasks of cognitive therapy in personality disorders is to gain an historical account of the patient's childhood development and background from which the therapist can derive a cognitive formulation linking past difficulties and presenting problems. Through the formulation, and understanding of the patient's view of self and others, unique core beliefs are identified that are linked to affect and to overdeveloped behavioural patterns that prevent the individual from functioning in an adaptive manner, particularly in interpersonal contexts. Therapy focuses on beliefs that concern core concepts about the self and others that have developed from childhood onwards and associated behaviours that have developed as coping strategies. The content and meaning of the beliefs have had an impact on past and present relationships and are likely to impact the therapeutic relationship. These beliefs, formed through negative, possibly abusive and neglectful experiences with others, are likely to have resulted in low self-esteem, hypersensitivity to criticism, and poor relationships with peers, caregivers and others in adolescence. Once a clear understanding of the content of patient's core beliefs and associated overdeveloped or compensatory behavioural patterns has been established, patients are encouraged to test out their beliefs and assumptions about others by learning new, more adaptive strategies for relating to others and to themselves. In borderline personality disorder, typically patients hold beliefs such as 'I am a bad and inadequate person' and 'others will abandon or reject me'. Having formed these beliefs through experiences in childhood, borderline patients, for example, may have learnt to avoid close relationships, are highly sensitized to signs of disapproval in others and have developed a punitive, self-critical style of thinking and behaviour, including self-harm. The emphasis in cognitive therapy is in developing new ways of thinking about self and others and in testing out new ways of behaving that are less self-defeating and more likely to improve the patient's interpersonal skills.[19] In comparison with the treatment of Axis I disorders, cognitive therapy with personality-disordered individuals takes more sessions and spans a longer time because the underlying problems are more pervasive and ingrained. There are other important elements of cognitive and related therapies, of which schema therapy and dialectical behaviour therapy are the most prominent. One of these differences is on the emphasis and attention paid to the therapeutic relationship. In cognitive therapy for personality disorder, more emphasis is placed on establishing and maintaining a therapeutic alliance, as interpersonal difficulties which occur in the patient's life outside therapy are also likely to arise within therapy. This is based on the hypothesis that the patient's core beliefs are consistent across a wide range of settings and therefore are also likely to be manifest in therapeutic relationships. Patients are therefore likely to be highly sensitive to signs of criticism and approval in their therapists. The models of treatment for personality disorder proposed by Beck and Freeman,[20] Davidson,[19] Young,[21] and Linehan[22] have in common an attempt to integrate biological and psychosocial factors. All models of treatment recognize the importance of building a secure therapeutic relationship and transference and countertransference issues in therapy are increasingly recognized as important mediators of the therapeutic process. These therapies utilize cognitive techniques to repair breakdown in communication that can occur during therapy.

Cognitive analytical therapy[18] also gives special attention to this aspect of therapy.

One of the goals of cognitive therapy with personality-disordered patients is to take advantage of these interpersonal difficulties in treatment by identifying and modifying the beliefs underlying them and, by extension, other relationships. Although people with personality disorders can recognize difficulties, they experience the problems as egosyntonic[23] (i.e. accepted as normal because they are an intrinsic part of usual functioning). As a result, alternative and potentially more adaptive beliefs about the self and others need to be identified and evaluated to see if they are indeed more adaptive and embraced as a consequence. These alternative more adaptive beliefs require to be systematically reviewed and reinforced, and new behaviours and ways of relating to others need to be practiced repeatedly if changes are to be consolidated. To achieve these changes, the therapist usually has to adopt a more directive approach than in cognitive therapy for depression and other Axis I disorders, and throughout will be more concerned with identifying and overcoming cognitive, emotional, and behavioural avoidance which maintains core beliefs.

(c) Other related psychological therapies

(i) STEPPS

Systems Training for Emotional Predictability and Problem Solving (STEPPS) is affiliated to the other cognitive psychotherapies. It was developed by Nancee Blum in Iowa and has been extended across several states within the United States and to the Netherlands. It has some of the elements of standard cognitive behaviour therapy and dialectical behaviour therapy and is a manualized programme involving 20 2 h weekly group meetings; with specific goals (or lessons) identified for each session.[24] A randomized controlled trial has just been completed and this shows significant gains in some areas compared with treatment as usual (Black, 2007, APA meeting, San Diego, USA).

(ii) Schema-focused therapy

Schema-focused therapy[21] is now becoming increasingly used in the treatment of borderline and antisocial personality disorders. It is a compendium of cognitive behaviour therapy, object relations theory, and gestalt therapy, and also involving what Young calls 'limited reparenting'. It is given in a relatively intensive form—two to three sessions a week for 1–2 years—but has been shown to be both more effective and cost-effective than transference-focused psychotherapy in a trial of treatments for borderline personality disorder.[28]

(iii) Dialectical behaviour therapy

The era of evidence-based therapy in personality disorder began with a formal trial of dialectical behaviour therapy, a form of cognitive behaviour therapy linked to skills training and detached acceptance (or mindfulness), was compared with treatment as usual in a group of repeatedly self-harming female patients with borderline personality disorder.[28,69] The hypothesis that dialectical behaviour therapy was effective in reducing self-harm was supported. Now several other randomized trials have taken place that show that DBT is particularly effective in reducing self-harm[4,29,30] though in another study, DBT improved hopelessness, depression, anger, and suicidal ideation but showed no difference in suicide attempts.[31]

This treatment has also been used systematically in the treatment of borderline personality disorder and those with comorbid substance abuse.[30] According to Linehan,[22] borderline personality disorder is primarily a dysfunction of emotional regulation which is assumed to have resulted from biological irregularities combined with certain dysfunctional environments. Others in contact with the patient are postulated as reinforcing this dysfunction by discounting or, in Linehan's preferred term, 'invalidating' their emotional experiences. Borderline patients are emotionally vulnerable and have difficulty in regulating patterns of responses associated with emotional states. The maladaptive behaviours which form part of the borderline syndrome can be viewed as either the product of emotional dysregulation or as attempts by the individual at regulating intense emotional states by maladaptive problem-solving strategies. Dialectical behaviour therapy, as its name suggests, contains within it the notion of opposites; common themes that emerge in therapy with borderline patients, such as acceptance of things as they are (so that there is no need for suicidal action), and change (from former maladaptive types of response) may appear incompatible but are synthesized in the therapy.

The essentials of dialectical behaviour therapy[22] are manualized weekly individual psychotherapy, group psychoeducational behavioural skills training, and telephone consultation when considered necessary. Therefore the content comprises a variety of problem-solving techniques including teaching the patient skills to help regulate emotions and tolerate distress, methods for validating the patient's perceptions, and behavioural and psychological versions of meditation skills. Therapists are also trained in case management. 'Core mindfulness skills' are also part of the treatment and involve teaching the patient to observe, describe, and take part in events and responses to events without dissociating from what is happening. The treatment encourages patients to take a non-judgemental approach to events and interactions and to do what is effective in situations rather than what they may feel is the 'right' thing to do.

Summary of cognitive therapies

The collective view of the effectiveness of cognitive and dialectical behaviour therapies is that they are undoubtedly effective Leichsenring and Leibing[32] examined 25 studies (but very few randomized controlled trials) and found cognitive behaviour therapy to be effective (effect size 1.0) but with psychodynamic therapies the effect size was larger (1.46), but the authors emphasized these results were preliminary and need updating. More randomized controlled trials have been carried out into treatments for personality disorder in the last 4 years than in the previous 50 years and further reviews are needed. To date we only have good evidence of effectiveness for borderline personality disorder, but cognitive behaviour therapy has also been shown to be effective in a randomized trial of avoidant personality disorder.[33]

Nidotherapy

Nidotherapy is 'the collaborative systematic assessment and modification of the environment to minimize the impact of any form of mental disorder on the individual or on society'.[25] It was developed specifically for the care of patients with multiple personality and major psychiatric pathology and is particularly focused on Type R (treatment resisting personality disorders). It makes no attempt to treat the patient directly but instead attempts to change the environment so there is a better fit between individual and setting. It is normally carried out individually by a nidotherapist working independently from other clinical services.[26] It has been tested in a randomized trial in which the main gain was in cost savings as patients spent less time in hospital[27] and has also been used for antisocial personality disorder for the reduction of aggression and improvement in social functioning (http://www.controlled-trials.com (ISRCTN96256106)).

Therapeutic community treatments

There has been some confusion regarding the term 'therapeutic community'. It can apply to any form of environment created for a specific treatment but was really introduced and defined in its modern context by Maxwell Jones[34] who created a structure that ran completely counter to that of the traditional (authoritarian) mental hospital. This can be defined as a socially cohesive structure depending on intensive group treatments carried out by its residents. This approach, the democratic therapeutic community, differs from other forms of more coercive communities linked to criminal justice in the United States, often used for substance abusers, which are called concept therapeutic communities.[35,36] Therapeutic communities have very strong advocates and the complexity of the intervention makes it difficult to create a suitable comparison group to act as a control for a randomized trial; to date no such trial has been carried out.

Drug treatment

Drugs are often used for treating personality disorders although it is important to note that none are licensed for the treatment of these conditions. As with other forms of treatment, borderline personality disorder constitutes the largest group in which drug treatment is being used and is therefore worth examining separately. The evidence base for drug treatment is growing and there are now sufficient randomized controlled trials to evaluate and for other studies to be ignored in this review.

Borderline personality disorder

Borderline personality disorder is one of the most heterogeneous of all groups within the personality classification and includes extensive comorbidity with other personality disorders as well as with mental state disorders, particularly mood and stress-related disorders. This hinders the interpretation of Table 4.12.7.1, noting the problems of evaluation referred to at the beginning of this

Table 4.12.7.1 Summary of randomized controlled trials of drugs in the treatment of personality disorder (borderline except where indicated)

Drug group	Individual drug	Size of trial—*n* (ref)	Main outcome measures	Results
Tricyclic antidepressants@	Amitriptyline	61[37]	Depression, aggression, global improvement	Amitriptyline no better than placebo
Selective serotonin reuptake inhibitors (SSRIs)	Fluoxetine	40[38]	Aggression depression,	Fluoxetine superior to placebo
	Fluvoxamine (cross-over study)	38[39]	Mood shifts, aggression, impulsivity	Positive effects of fluvoxamine on mood only
Antipsychotic drugs (both first and second generation)	Haloperidol	61[37] and 108[40]	Depression, hostility, impulsiveness	Haloperidol effective in reducing depression and hostility in first study but not in second
	Olanzapine (wide-dosage range)	40[41]	Aggression, depression, anxiety	Significant improvement in an unrecognized scale (Clinical Global Improvement-BPD) only
	Olanzapine (mean 5.3 mg)	28[42]	'Random effects regression modelling of panel data'	Alleged improvement on composite measure (unsatisfactory)
	Aripiprazole 15 mg/day*	52[43]	Hostility, anger, depression, self-harm	Significant improvement in all measures and reduction in self-harm
Monoamine oxidase inhibitors (MAOIs)	Phenelzine (60 mg/day)	108[40]	Depression, hostility, impulsiveness, anxiety	Phenelzine superior to haloperidol and placebo for anger and hostility
Mood stabilizers and anti-convulsants	Carbamazepine (7 mg/day)†	20[44]	Depression, hostility	
	Sodium valproate (850 mg/day)*	30[45]	Depression, aggression, hostility	
	Sodium valproate*	91[46]	Aggression	
	Lamotrigine*	27[47]	Self-rated anger	
	Topiramate*	56[48]	Anger	

*Patients recruited by advertisement.

†Patients recruited as inpatients.

@A study involving mainly cluster C personality disorders compared the tricyclic antidepressant, dothiepin, with cognitive behaviour therapy and self-help over a 2-year period and showed significantly better response to dothiepin[49] (but study not included as after 2 years there were many deviations from the original protocol.

chapter. The studies are complex, yet the numbers are generally small, the period of treatment variable (8 weeks to 6 months), the dosage of drugs is usually flexible, and the outcomes manifold (and so variable that it is almost impossible to combine the data systematically). Positive publication bias and recruitment of volunteers by advertisement diminish the relationship between this patients group and those in clinical practice.

(i) Antidepressants

Tricyclic antidepressants do not appear to be effective in borderline personality disorder and, interestingly, do not help depressive symptoms preferentially, suggesting that there are subtle differences between the despair and emptiness of the borderline personality disorder and the anhedonia of depressive illnesses. Selective serotonin reuptake inhibitors (SSRIs), have been used in many trials (including some not cited here in which comparisons of inadequately small numbers have been made with psychological treatments) and provide some evidence of a positive effect on aggression and impulsiveness in antisocial personality disorder.[38] Monoamine oxidase inhibitors show reduction of anger and hostility in one trial but conventional risk management uggests that this treatment should only be used in exceptional circumstances.

(ii) Antipsychotic drugs

Although antipsychotic drugs have been tested in the treatment of borderline personality disorder more frequently than any other drug treatment, the results are equivocal. Haloperidol may be effective[37] in the short-term, however continuation studies do not show sustained improvement.[50] Olanzapine has been tested in three trials and, apart from showing consistent weight gain in all of these, has not shown any real evidence of benefit for any of the core symptoms of borderline personality disorder. The only trial showing substantial benefit was carried out with aripiprazole in symptomatic volunteers[43]; as aripiprazole has a complex pharmacological profile with 5-HT and dopamine agonist and antagonist actions this could represent a novel intervention and is worthy of replication.

(iii) Mood stabilizers

Borderline personality disorder is characterized by rapid swings in mood and emotional lability is a core feature. It is therefore not surprising that mood stabilizers have been used in its treatment. Again the results are equivocal and this subject urgently needs the benefit of a large independent trial. The most impressive result has been shown with the anticonvulsant drug, topiramate, which reduces aggression and hostility[48,51] but this finding needs replication. Lithium may also be effective in aggression but a satisfactory level of evidence is lacking.

Critique of drug treatment for borderline personality disorder

The evidence for the value of drug treatment has been influenced greatly by a guideline issued by the American Psychiatric Association in 2001.[49] This was a bold attempt to give clear recommendations to clinicians desperate to find a way through the fog of uncertainty with the abyss of suicide yawning on one side and iatrogenic poly-poly-pharmacy (the patients with this disorder are multiple consumers of prescribed drugs) on the other. There were four recommendations:

1 psychotherapy—both psychoanalytic/psychodynamic therapy, and dialectical behaviour therapy 'have been shown to have efficacy'

2 pharmacotherapy for 'affective dysregulation symptoms' should'be treated initially with a selective serotonin reuptake inhibitor or related antidepressant such as venlafaxine'

3 treatment of 'impulsive-behavioural dyscontrol symptoms' also suggests 'SSRIs are the initial treatment of choice'

4 'low-dose neuroleptics are the treatment of choice for "cognitive-perceptual" symptoms'.

These were criticized heavily at the time for going far beyond the evidence[52–54] and for some treatments, notably cognitive behaviour therapy, neglecting available evidence,[53] and further data accrued over the ensuing years has reinforced these concerns.[15,28,55] The recommendations concerning drug treatments are particularly suspect. There is no evidence worthy of the name that justifies the sub-grouping of borderline personality disorder into 'affective dyscontrol', 'impulsive-behavioural dyscontrol', and 'cognitive-perceptual' categories and these appear to be entities created to justify the use of particular drugs rather than provide a valid subdivision of a complex disorder. The creation of these essentially pseudo-diagnoses allows general conclusions to be made that all the drug treatments are efficacious and that 'taken together, the results of these studies suggest that the choice of medication can be guided as much by tolerability and safety as by symptom presentation'.[56] On the evidence analysed dispassionately this conclusion applies equally well to placebo, whose tolerability and safety are unparalleled.

Flamboyant group (cluster B, not borderline)

The evidence for drug use in other cluster B disorders is very limited. There may be a limited role for the use of mood stabilizers in reducing anger in dissocial personality. Lithium was found to be effective[57] and this action has been found in other settings,[58] but not reproduced in dissocial personality disorder. Carbamazepine has also been found to reduce impulsivity[59] but this result requires replication.

Odd eccentric group (cluster A)

No placebo-controlled, explanatory trials in this group have been conducted and no pragmatic trials provide evidence for drugs that remain in use. A mistrust of treatment given by others limits research and is probably an intrinsic part of the condition.

Anxious fearful group (cluster C)

The diagnostic overlap between cluster C personality disorders and neurotic disorders makes drawing conclusion about drug treatment for this group difficult. No clear explanatory trails have been conducted and the evidence of the effectiveness of antidepressants is confounded by the presence of neurotic disorder.[60,61]

Management

The management of borderline personality disorder can now be directed by a combination of the evidence and clinical judgement. It is clear from the randomized trials of both pharmacological and psychological treatment that an organized plan of care leads to improvement. This includes a consistent approach, a constancy of personnel and adequate access to inpatient care during crisis situations. The cognitively based therapies are effective and pragmatic, providing a higher degree of input to ensure effectiveness. The intermittent addition of low-dose haloperidol or aripiprazole may assist with worsening impulsivity. A trial of topiramate for anger or SSRIs for impulsivity may also be of value. These need to be trialed for a specific period, 4 to 8 weeks, with a clear plan to review or stop if effectiveness is not clear or deteriorates over time. The risks of prescribing need to be carefully weighed against the potential benefits. Polypharmacy increases risk with no evidence of benefit. It is ethically important to ensure all patients have the capacity to consent to treatment, particularly for unlicensed drug use. Because the treatment of personality disorder is among the most complex of complex interventions[(62)] it is likely that several treatments, given in combination in a systematic way, are best suited to many of those who have more severe personality disorders.

The management of other personality disorders remains largely guided by clinical experience. The general principles of service organization remain the same, however decisions regarding psychotherapy and pharmacotherapy need to be tailored to individuals with an expectation of building a body of patient-based evidence, as other evidence is weak. Regular review of a management plan minimizes the likelihood of harm from any one course of action or the neglect of the patient's presentation.

Some management options can now be considered to have a negative risk: benefit ratio. These include behaviour therapy alone, tricyclic antidepressant therapy, and monoamine oxidase therapy.

Organization of services for personality disorder

It is likely that the organization of care for those with personality disorder has a much greater part to play than any specific single treatment in the clinical success of management but it is also fair to add that this conclusion is not based on excellent evidence. What is, however, clear from the randomized trials of both pharmacological and psychological treatment is that an organized plan of care leads to great improvement in those with personality disorder irrespective of the exact nature of the intervention.

Services for the management of personality disorder can include the 'sole practitioner' model (a single therapist seeing the patient), the 'divided function' model (in which part of the patient's care is taken over by specially trained staff whilst others look after other parts), and the 'specialist team' model (in which a specific personality disorder service takes on all aspects of care). The general conclusion is that the 'divided function or specialist team model is probably best for reducing risk and improving outcomes'.[(63)] The general principles of management apply to all personality disorders although the consequences of ignoring them will be greater for the flamboyant cluster of personality disorders than for others.

(a) Consistency

One of the reasons why those with personality disorders create so many problems in therapy is that they are highly sensitive to perceived criticism and are therefore able to detect any inconsistency in their treatment. Sometimes this is a way of deflecting attention away from fundamental problems associated with the personality disorder, but they are nonetheless effective in creating a screen that prevents other issues from being addressed. Clearly the fewer the people involved in care, the less are the chances of creating inconsistency. Keeping the number of main workers to a small number, and maintaining good communication, is a sound goal.

(b) Constancy

It is helpful to avoid changes in staff as far as possible. This is of particular relevance in the treatment of borderline personality disorder in which changes in therapists often re-enact the problems of loss and despair that the patient experiences so commonly in relationships.

(c) Adequate inpatient support

Staff involved in hospital care often believe that people with personality disorders should be kept out of hospital. This belief is based on the observation that such people exploit the opportunities offered by admission and create circumstances whereby it is difficult to discharge them. Much of this is opinion and not founded on evidence. Patients with comorbid mental state and personality disorders actually have better outcomes if they have a hospital-oriented programme of care than treatment in the community, whereas the opposite is true in the absence of personality disorder.[(64)] However, this work was carried out before specific services for personality disorder were set-up in England, the first country in the world to create such services.[(65)] The initial pilot service has just been evaluated and the results are encouraging, but the problem remains that those who wish to seek treatment from these services comprise only a small proportion of the total who suffer.[(72)]

Problems with comorbidity

Perhaps the most important error in management is failure to recognize personality disorder when other psychiatric disorders are more prominent and appear to be the only presenting problem. This is becoming recognized in the development of treatment protocols. This problem is encountered widely in the mental health services among people presenting to emergency psychiatric clinics,[(73)] in services for the homeless mentally ill,[(74)] and among heavy users of psychiatric services[(75)] and those with multiple admissions.[(68)] In all these settings, personality disorder is often not recognized early enough. This is to some extent understandable as the assessment of personality disorder is difficult in, for example, a busy emergency clinic. Nevertheless, failure to achieve a predicted response is often due to an earlier failure to detect the presence of personality disorder.

Conclusions

Some years ago that most sceptical of academic psychiatrists, Michael Shepherd, in referring to the contents of a book entitled *Recent Advances in Psychiatry* commented that the content was more accurately defined as 'recent activities', as 'advances' was too generous a word. Whilst not going quite as far as this in regard to advances in the treatment of personality disorder it is fair to add that the promise of effective therapies across the spectrum of personality dysfunction remains a long way off and we must be very careful not to oversell the evidence. The complexity of personality disorders often requires complex intervention, however, until we are confident that single treatments are effective the arguments for evaluating them in combination have to be very strong on theoretical grounds to justify the cost.

We are still at the stage in which explanatory trials (ones demonstrating efficacy under optimal conditions) are at least as necessary as pragmatic ones (demonstrating benefit in conditions of ordinary practice). These need to be carried out with adequate numbers of patients (at least 50 in each treatment arm rather than an artificially derived sample size to justify a small number) and with good independent assessments carried out by research workers who are masked as much as possible from disclosure of treatment. These requirements are exacting but can be achieved.[67] We also need better pragmatic trials of patients seen in ordinary mental health practice whose treatment and characteristics are both representative and from whom it is possible to generalize findings with confidence. Currently there are very few studies that satisfy this requirement; one recent study combining an educational intervention with problem-solving is an exception.[68]

Despite the caution of these statements these are exciting times in the management of personality disorder. We are no longer listening to the once powerful lobby that claimed that patients with these conditions should not be treated by psychiatric services, or to the pessimists that still regard these conditions as untreatable. We are in the equivalent position as those in the early 1950s who suddenly became aware of the possibility that powerful treatments for severe mental illness were ready and waiting to be used. They do indeed appear to be within reach, but we must use them wisely.

Acknowledgement

The authors would like to thank Professor Peter Tyrer who co-authored the original chapter on which this is based.

Further information

Sampson, M., McCubbin, R., and Tyrer, P. (eds.) (2006). *Personality disorder and community mental health teams, a practitioners guide*. John Wiley & Sons, Ltd., West Sussex. ISBN: 978-0-470-01171-3.

National Institute for Health and Clinical Excellence (UK): http://guidance.nice.org.uk/page.aspx?o=357063&c=91523

References

1. Zanarini, M.C., Krankenburg, F.R., Hennen, J., *et al.* (2003). Longitudinal course of borderline psychopathology: 6 year prospective study. *The American Journal of Psychiatry*, **160**, 274–83.
2. Davidson, K. (2007). *Cognitive therapy for personality disorders: a guide for clinicians* (2nd edn). Routledge, Hove.
3. Verheul, R., van den Bosch, L.M.C., Koeter, W.J., *et al.* (2003). Dialectical behaviour therapy with women with borderline personality disorder. 12-month randomised clinical trial in the Netherlands. *The British Journal of Psychiatry*, **182**, 135–40.
4. Linehan, M.M., Comtois, K.A., Murray, A. M., *et al.* (2006). Two-year randomized controlled trial and follow-up of dialectical behavior therapy vs therapy by experts for suicidal behaviors and borderline personality disorder. *Archives of General Psychiatry*, **63**, 757–66.
5. Feinstein, A. (1970). The pre-therapeutic classification of comorbidity in chronic disease. *Journal of Chronic Diseases*, **23**, 455–62.
6. Tyrer, P. (1996). Comorbidity or consanguinity. *The British Journal of Psychiatry*, **168**, 669–71.
7. Fyer, M.R., Frances, A.J., Sullivan, T., *et al.* (1988). Co-morbidity of borderline personality disorder. *Archives of General Psychiatry*, **45**, 348–52.
8. Coppen, A.L. and Metcalfe, H. (1965). The effect of a depressive illness on MMPI scores. *The British Journal of Psychiatry*, **111**, 236–9.
9. Stuart, S., Simons, A.D., Thase, M.E., *et al.* (1992). Are personality assessments valid in acute major depression? *Journal of Affective Disorders*, **24**, 281–9.
10. Tyrer, P., Coombs, N., Ibrahimi, F., *et al.* (2007). Critical developments in the assessment of personality disorder. *The British Journal of Psychiatry*, **190**(Suppl. 49), s51–9.
11. Adler, G. (1979). The myth of the alliance with borderline patients. *The American Journal of Psychiatry*, **136**, 642–5.
12. Tyrer, P., Mitchard, S., Methuen, C., *et al.* (2003). Treatment-rejecting and treatment-seeking personality disorders: Type R and Type S. *Journal of Personality Disorders*, **17**, 265–70.
13. Soloff, P.H., George, A., Nathan, R.S., *et al.* (1986). Progress in pharmacotherapy of personality disorders: a double blind study of amitriptyline, haloperidol and placebo. *Archives of General Psychiatry*, **43**, 691–7.
14. Seivewright, H., Tyrer, P., and Johnson, T. (2002). Changes in personality status in neurotic disorder. *Lancet*, **359**, 2253–4.
15. Davidson, K., Norrie, J., Tyrer, P., *et al.* (2006). The effectiveness of cognitive behaviour therapy for borderline personality disorder: results from the BOSCOT trial. *Journal of Personality Disorders*, **20**, 450–65.
16. Linehan, M.M., Comtois, K.A., Murray, A.M., *et al.* (2006). Two-year randomized controlled trial and follow-up of dialectical behavior therapy vs therapy by experts for suicidal behaviors and borderline personality disorder. *Archives of General Psychiatry*, **63**, 757–66.
17. Ryle, A. (1997). The structure and development of borderline personality disorder: a proposed model. *The British Journal of Psychiatry*, **170**, 82–7.
18. Ryle, A. and Kerr, I.B. (2002). *Introducing cognitive analytic therapy: principles and practice*. John Wiley, Chichester.
19. Davidson, K. (2007). *Cognitive therapy for personality disorders: a guide for clinicians* (2nd edn). Routledge, London.
20. Beck, A.T. and Freeman, A. (1990). *Cognitive therapy of personality disorders*. Guilford Press, New York.
21. Young, J.E., Klosko, J.S., and Weishaar, M.E. (2003). *Schema therapy: a practitioner's guide*. The Guilford Press, New York.
22. Linehan, M.M. (1992). *Cognitive therapy for borderline personality disorder*. Guilford Press, New York.
23. Alexander, F. (1930). The neurotic character. *International Journal of Psycho-analysis*, **11**, 291–311.
24. Blum, N., Pfohl, B., St. John, D., *et al.* (2002). STEPPS: a cognitive behavioral systems-based group treatment for outpatients with borderline personality disorder-apreliminary report. *Comprehensive Psychiatry*, **43**, 301–10.
25. Tyrer, P., Sensky, T., and Mitchard, S. (2003). The principles of nidotherapy in the treatment of persistent mental and personality disorders. *Psychotherapy and Psychosomatics*, **72**, 350–6.
26. Tyrer, P. and Bajaj, P. (2005). Nidotherapy: making the environment do the therapeutic work. *Advances in Psychiatric Treatment*, **11**, 232–8.
27. Tyrer, P. and Tyrer, S. (2008). Other treatments for persistent disturbances of behaviour. In *Cambridge textbook of effective treatments in psychiatry* (ed. P. Tyrer and K.R. Silk). Cambridge University Press, Cambridge.
28. Giesen-Bloo, J., van Dyck, R., Spinhoven, P., *et al.* (2006). Outpatient psychotherapy for borderline personality disorder: randomized trial of schema-focused therapy vs transference-focused psychotherapy. *Archives of General Psychiatry*, **63**, 649–58.
29. Verheul, R., van den Bosch, L.M.C., Koeter, W.J., *et al.* (2003). Dialectical behaviour therapy with women with borderline personality disorder. 12-month randomised clinical trial in the Netherlands. *The British Journal of Psychiatry*, **182**, 135–40.
30. Linehan, M., Dimeff, L., Reynolds, S., *et al.* (2002). Dialectical behavior therapy versus comprehensive validation therapy plus 12-step for the treatment of opioid dependent women meeting criteria for borderline personality disorder. *Drug and Alcohol Dependence*, **67**, 13–26.

31. Koons, C.R., Robins, C.J., Tweed, J.L., *et al.* (2001). Efficacy of dialectical behavior therapy in women veterans with borderline personality disorder. *Behavior Therapy*, **32**, 371–90.
32. Leichsenring, F. and Leibing, E. (2003). The effectiveness of psychodynamic therapy and cognitive behavior therapy in the treatment of personality disorders: a meta-analysis. *The American Journal of Psychiatry*, **160**, 1223–32.
33. Emmelkamp, P.M.G., Benner, A., Kuipers, A., *et al.* (2006). Comparison of brief dynamic and cognitive-behavioural therapies in avoidant personality disorder. *The British Journal of Psychiatry*, **189**, 60–4.
34. Jones, M. (1953). The therapeutic community: a new treatment method in psychiatry. Basic Books, New York.
35. Campling, P. (2001). Therapeutic communities. *Advances in Psychiatric Treatment*, **7**, 365–72.
36. Rutter, D. and Tyrer, P. (2003). The value of therapeutic communities in the treatment of personality disorder: a suitable place for treatment? *Journal of Psychiatric Practice*, **9**, 291–302.
37. Soloff, P.H., George, A., Nathan, R.S., *et al.* (1986). Progress in pharmacotherapy of personality disorders: a double blind study of amitriptyline, haloperidol and placebo. *Archives of General Psychiatry*, **43**, 691–7.
38. Coccaro, E.F. and Kavoussi, R.J. (1997). Fluoxetine and impulsive-aggressive behaviour in personality disordered subjects. *Archives of General Psychiatry*, **54**, 1081–8.
39. Rinne, T., van den Brink, W., Wouters, L., *et al.* (2002). SSRI treatment of borderline personality disorder: a randomized, placebo-controlled clinical trial for female patients with borderline personality disorder. *The American Journal of Psychiatry*, **159**, 2048–54.
40. Soloff, P.H., George, A., Nathan, S., *et al.* (1993). Efficacy of phenelzine and haloperidol in borderline personality disorder. *Archives of General Psychiatry*, **50**, 377–85.
41. Bogenschutz, M.P. and George Nurnberg, H. (2004). Olanzapine versus placebo in the treatment of borderline personality disorder. *The Journal of Clinical Psychiatry*, **65**, 104–9.
42. Zanarini, M.C. and Frankenburg, F.R. (2001). Olanzapine treatment of female borderline personality disorder patients: a double-blind, placebo-controlled pilot study. *The Journal of Clinical Psychiatry*, **62**, 849–54.
43. Nickel, M.K., Muehlbacher, M., Nickel, C., *et al.* (2006). Aripiprazole in the treatment of patients with borderline personality disorder: a double-blind, placebo-controlled study. *The American Journal of Psychiatry*, **163**, 833–8.
44. De La Fuente, J.M. and Lotstra, F. (1994). A trial of carbamazepine in borderline personality-disorder. *European Neuropsychopharmacology*, **4**, 479–86.
45. Frankenburg, F.R. and Zanarini, M.C. (2002). Divalproex sodium treatment of women with borderline personality disorder and bipolar II disorder: a double-blind placebo-controlled pilot study. *The Journal of Clinical Psychiatry*, **63**, 442–6.
46. Hollander, E., Tracy, K.A., Swann, A.C., *et al.* (2003). Divalproex in the treatment of impulsive aggression: efficacy in cluster B personality disorders. *Neuropsychopharmacology*, **28**, 1186–97.
47. Tritt, K., Nickel, C., Lahmann, C., *et al.* (2005). Lamotrigine treatment of aggression in female borderline-patients: a randomized, double-blind, placebo-controlled study. *Journal of Psychopharmacology*, **19**, 287–91.
48. Nickel, M.K., Nickel, C., Kaplan, P., *et al.* (2005). Treatment of aggression with topiramate in male borderline patients: a double-blind, placebo-controlled study. *Biological Psychiatry*, **57**, 498–9.
49. American Psychiatric Association. (2001). Practice guideline for the treatment of patients with borderline personality disorder. *The American Journal of Psychiatry*, **158**(Suppl.), 1–52.
50. Cornelius, J., Soloff, P., Perel, J., *et al.* (1993). Continuation pharmacotherapy of borderline personality disorder with haloperidol and phenelzine. *The American Journal of Psychiatry*, **150**, 1843–8.
51. Loew, T.H., Nickel, M.K., Muehlbacher, M., *et al.* (2006). Topiramate treatment for women with borderline personality disorder—a double-blind, placebo-controlled study. *Journal of Clinical Psychopharmacology*, **26**, 61–6.
52. McGlashan, T.H. (2002). The borderline personality disorder practice guidelines: the good, the bad, and the realistic. *Journal of Personality Disorders*, **16**, 119–21.
53. Sanderson, C., Swenson, C., and Bohus, M. (2002). A critique of the American Psychiatric Practice Guideline for the treatment of patients with borderline personality disorder. *Journal of Personality Disorders*, **16**, 122–9.
54. Tyrer, P. (2002). Practice guideline for the treatment of personality disorders: a bridge too far. *Journal of Personality Disorders*, **16**, 113–8.
55. Weinberg, I., Gunderson, J.G., Hennen, J., *et al.* (2006). Manual assisted cognitive treatment for deliberate self-harm in borderline personality disorder. *Journal of Personality Disorders*, **20**, 467–82.
56. Zanarini, M.C. (2004). Update on pharmacotherapy of borderline personality disorder. *Current Psychiatry Reports*, **6**, 66–70.
57. Sheard, M.H., Marini, J.L., Bridges, C.I., *et al.* (1976). The effect of lithium on impulsive aggressive behavior in man. *The American Journal of Psychiatry*, **133**, 1409–13.
58. Tyrer, S.P., Walsh, A., Edwards, D.E., *et al.* (1984). Factors associated with a good response to lithium in aggressive mentally handicapped subjects. *Progress in Neuropsychopharmacology & Biological Psychiatry*, **8**, 751–5.
59. Cowdry, R.W. and Gardner, D.L. (1988). Pharmacotherapy of borderline personality disorder: alprazolam, carbamazepine, trifluoperazine and tranylcypromine. *Archives of General Psychiatry*, **45**, 111–9.
60. Deltito, J.A. and Stam, M. (1989). Psychopharmacological treatment of avoidant personality disorder. *Comprehensive Psychiatry*, **30**, 498–504.
61. Ansseau, M., Troisfontaines, B., Papart, P., *et al.* (1991). Compulsive personality as predictor of response to serotonergic antidepressants. *British Medical Journal*, **303**, 760–1.
62. Campbell, M., Fitzpatrick, R., Haines, A., *et al.* (2000). A framework for the design and evaluation of complex interventions to improve health. *British Medical Journal*, **321**, 694–6.
63. Bateman, A.W. and Tyrer, P. (2004). Services for personality disorder: organization for inclusion. *Advances in Psychiatric Treatment*, **10**, 425–33.
64. Tyrer, P., Manley, C., Van Horn, E., *et al.* (2000). Personality abnormality in severe mental illness and its influence on outcome of intensive and standard case management: a randomised controlled trial. *European Psychiatry*, **15**(Suppl. 1), 7–10.
65. National Institute of Mental Health (England). (2003). *Personality disorder: no longer a diagnosis of exclusion*. Department of Health, London.
66. Geller, J.L., Fisher, W.H., McDermeit, M., *et al.* (1998). The effects of public managed care on patterns of intensive use of inpatient psychiatric services. *Psychiatric Services*, **49**, 327–32.
67. Davidson, K.M., Tyrer, P., Gumley, A., *et al.* (2006). Rationale, description, and sample characteristics of a randomised controlled trial of cognitive therapy for borderline personality disorder: the BOSCOT study. *Journal of Personality Disorders*, **20**, 431–49.
68. Huband, N., Duggan, C., McMurran, M., *et al.* Social problem-solving plus psychoeducation for adults with personality disorder: a pragmatic randomised clinical trial. *The British Journal of Psychiatry*, **190**, 307–13.

69. Linehan, M.M., Armstrong, H.E., Suarez, A., *et al.* (1991). Cognitive–behavioral treatment of chronically parasuicidal borderline patients. *Archives of General Psychiatry*, **48**, 1060–4.
70. Zanarini, M.C. and Frankenburg, F.R. (2003). Omega-3 fatty acid treatment of women with borderline personality disorder: a double-blind, placebo-controlled pilot study. *The American Journal of Psychiatry*, **160**, 167–9.
71. Ansseau, M., Troisfontaines, B., Papart, P., *et al.* (1991). Compulsive personality as predictor of response to serotonergic antidepressants. *British Medical Journal*, **303**, 760–1.
72. Crawford, M., Price, K., Weaver, T., *et al.* (2007). Learning the lessons: an evaluation of pilot community services for adults with personality disorder. Department of Health, London.
73. Breslow, R.E., Klinger, B.I., and Erickson, B.J. (1996). Acute intoxication and substance abuse among patients presenting to a psychiatric emergency service. *General Hospital Psychiatry*, **18**, 183–91.
74. North, C.S., Thompson, S.J., Pollio, D.E., *et al.* (1997). *A diagnostic comparison of homeless and nonhomeless patients in an urban mental health clinic. Social Psychiatry and Psychiatric Epidemiology*, **32**, 236–40.
75. Kent, S., Fogarty, M., and Yellowlees, P. (1995). Heavy utilization of inpatient and outpatient services in a public mental health service. *Psychiatric Services*, **46**, 1254–7.

4.13

Habit and impulse control disorder

Contents

4.13.1 Impulse control disorders
Susan L. McElroy and Paul E. Keck Jr.

4.13.2 Special psychiatric problems relating to gambling
Emanuel Moran

4.13.1 Impulse control disorders

Susan L. McElroy and Paul E. Keck, Jr.

This chapter first defines impulse control disorders, and then summarizes available research on the clinical features, epidemiology, psychiatric comorbidity, family studies, psychobiology, and treatment response of the most common of these conditions (except for pathological gambling, which is reviewed in Chapter 4.13.2).

Definitions of impulse control disorders

Historically, impulse control disorders have been broadly defined as harmful behaviours performed in response to irresistible impulses.[1] In DSM-IV, an impulse control disorder is defined as the failure to resist an impulse, drive, or temptation to commit an act that is harmful to the individual or to others.[2] DSM-IV also stipulates that for most impulse control disorders, the individual feels an increasing sense of tension or arousal before committing the act and then experiences pleasure, gratification, or relief at the time of committing the act. In the text describing these disorders, DSM-IV states that after the act, there may or may not be genuine regret, self-reproach, or guilt. In ICD-10,[3] these conditions are classified as habit and impulse disorders and defined as repeated acts that have no clear rational motivation, cannot be controlled, and that generally harm the patient's own interests and those of other people. ICD-10 further states that the behaviour is associated with impulses to action.

In DSM-IV, impulse control disorders are listed in a residual category, 'Impulse control disorders not elsewhere classified', which includes intermittent explosive disorder (IED), kleptomania, pyromania, pathological gambling, trichotill16omania, and impulse control disorders not otherwise specified (NOS). Examples of impulse control disorders NOS are compulsive buying disorder, repetitive self-mutilation, pathological skin picking, and onychophagia (severe nail-biting).[1] In ICD-10, habit and impulse disorders are also listed as a residual category. Similar to DSM-IV, it includes pathological gambling, pathological fire-setting (pyromania), pathological stealing (kleptomania), trichotillomania, other habit and impulse disorders (which includes IED), and habit and impulse disorder, unspecified.

It should be noted that with mounting research, the impulse control disorders are increasingly viewed as complex conditions sharing, in addition to irresistible impulses to perform harmful behaviours, features of trait impulsivity, trait compulsivity, and mood dysregulation, as well as obsessive compulsive mood, and addictive disorders.[1]

Intermittent explosive disorder

Definition and clinical features

Intermittent explosive disorder (IED) is defined in DSM-IV as several discrete episodes of failure to resist aggressive impulses that result in serious assaultive acts or destruction of property (criterion A). Also, the degree of aggression expressed during an episode is grossly out of proportion to any precipitating psychosocial stressors (criterion B) and the explosive episodes are not better accounted for by another mental disorder or due to the direct physiological effects of a substance or a general medical condition (criterion C). Varying definitions of IED based on the DSM-IV criteria have been proposed and used.[4,5] One important set of research criteria for IED, for example, allows for less severe aggressive episodes, such as recurrent verbal outbursts against others without physical aggression, but requires that the aggressive episodes be recurrent and associated with distress or dysfunction.[4] Although ICD-10 lists IED under 'Other habit and impulse disorders', it does not provide specific criteria for its diagnosis.

Regarding phenomenology, persons with IED describe their aggressive episodes as explosive, uncontrollable, unpremeditated, and brief; often provoked by minor stimuli; and associated with various psychological and physical symptoms, especially changes in mood, awareness, and autonomic arousal.[4,6] The frequency of episodes depends in part on how the disorder is defined. In the National Comorbidity Survey Replication (NCS-R), where the DSM-IV A criteria of 'several' episodes was operationalized to be three or more lifetime attacks, persons with IED had a mean of 43 lifetime attacks.

Many persons with IED describe problems with chronic or trait anger and frequent 'subthreshold' aggressive episodes in which they manage to resist enacting aggressive impulses or express them with less destructive behaviours (e.g. screaming rather than assault).[4,6] These subthreshold episodes are similar to the anger attacks (sudden episodes of intense anger with autonomic arousal) often described in patients with mood (bipolar and depressive) disorders.[7]

Of note, the relationship between IED specifically and impulsive aggression in general remains unclear and the two phrases are not necessarily synonymous. In particular, like other impulse control disorders, the aggression of IED usually involves elements of lack of control (e.g. compulsivity) and affect dysregulation (extreme anger, irritability and/or mood instability) as well as impulsivity. Thus, IED may be one form of impulsive aggression.

Epidemiology and course

Once thought to be rare, recent research has shown that IED is common in both clinical and general population samples. In the most rigorous study to date, the NCS-R, lifetime and 12-month prevalence estimates of DSM-IV IED in the general population were 7.3 per cent and 3.9 per cent, respectively.[5] The lifetime and 12-month prevalences of more narrowly defined IED (in which three episodes in the same year were required for diagnosis) were 5.4 per cent and 3.5 per cent, respectively. The disorder is also likely to be common in forensic populations but data are not available.

IED is probably more common in males than females. In the NCS-R, 9.3 per cent of men versus 5.6 per cent of women met lifetime DSM-IV criteria for the disorder. IED begins in childhood or adolescence; follows a chronic or episodic course; and is associated with distress, morbidity (e.g. injuries), and social and occupational impairment.[4-6] For example, in the NCS-R, IED had a mean age of onset of 14 years, was persistent over the life course (with averages of 6.2–11.8 years with attacks), and was associated with substantial role impairment.[5] However, the prevalence of the disorder was significantly lower among persons 60 years and older (2.1 per cent).

Associated psychopathology and comorbidity

IED often co-occurs with other psychiatric disorders.[4–6] In the NCS-R, 81.8 per cent of respondents with lifetime DSM-IV IED met criteria for at least one other lifetime DSM-IV disorder. Specifically, IED was significantly comorbid with all DSM-IV depressive, anxiety, and substance use disorders assessed after controlling for age, sex, and race. It was also significantly comorbid with oppositional defiant disorder, conduct disorder, and attention-deficit/hyperactivity disorder.

Importantly, the boundaries between IED and other conditions characterized by episodic and/or impulsive aggression have not been clearly delineated. Indeed, the comorbidity between IED and both bipolar disorders and Axis II disorders was not assessed in the NCS-R.[5] Comorbidity with Axis II disorders was not determined because the prevalence of these disorders was not evaluated. Comorbidity with bipolar disorders was not assessed because of how IED was defined; cases of IED with lifetime mania or hypomania were excluded from analysis (number not specified) so that the prevalence of IED was not overestimated by cases of bipolar disorder with anger attacks. Of note, although the relationships between IED and both bipolar and cluster B personality disorders remain unclear, clinical studies suggest that patients with IED have high rates of these conditions.[4,6]

Family studies

Family studies suggest that relatives of probands with IED have high rates of impulsive violent behaviour, substance abuse, and possibly mood and other impulse control disorders.[4,6,8,9] In a family history study of patients with temper outbursts meeting the first two DSM-III criteria for IED, non-adopted patients were significantly more likely than adopted patients to have a family history of temper outbursts.[9] Of 25 subjects with DSM-IV IED evaluated via the family history method, 8 (32 per cent) of subjects had a first-degree relative with probable IED, 20 (80 per cent) had at least one first-degree relative with a substance use disorder, 14 (56 per cent) a mood disorder, and 14 (56 per cent) an impulse control disorder.[6] A blinded, controlled family history study using broadly-defined IED criteria found a significantly increased morbid risk of the condition in relatives of affected probands (26 per cent) compared with relatives of control probands (8 per cent).[4]

Psychobiology

Persons with impulsive aggression have been consistently found to have abnormalities in serotonergic function.[4] Although most studies included subjects with impulsive aggression and personality disorders, a few included persons with IED or possible IED. Thus, in a study of 58 violent offenders and impulsive fire-setters, 33 (57 per cent) of whom had DSM-III IED, lower cerebrospinal fluid (CSF) concentrations of 5-hydroxyindoleacetic acid (5-HIAA) were found in the impulsive offenders and fire-setters than in the non-impulsive offenders and normal control subjects.[10]

In a functional magnetic resonance imaging (MRI) study of response to social threat, 10 subjects with IED showed exaggerated amygdala reactivity and diminished orbitofrontal cortex activation to faces expressing anger compared with controls.[11] The authors noted these findings were similar to other disorders characterized by impulsive aggression, including borderline personality and bipolar disorders, and that they supported a link between a dysfunctional frontal-limbic network and aggression.

Treatment response

Clinical experience suggests that IED may be less responsive to insight-oriented and more responsive to cognitive behavioural therapies, particularly those stressing anger management.[4,6,12] Medications reported effective in definite or probable IED, some in controlled trials, include antiepileptics (e.g. phenytoin, carbamazepine, oxcarbazepine), antidepressants (e.g. tricyclics, serotonin reuptake inhibitors), mood stabilizers (e.g. lithium, valproate), β-blockers, psychostimulants, and even antiandrogens. Mood stabilizer monotherapy and antidepressant augmentation of mood stabilizers have both been reported to successfully treat IED and/or anger attacks in patients with bipolar disorders.[6,7] Antidepressants have been reported to be effective in anger attacks associated with major depression.[12] Finally, serotonin reuptake inhibitors, mood stabilizers, antiepileptics, and antipsychotics may be effective for impulsive-aggressive behaviour in personality-disordered patients.[13]

Kleptomania

Definition and clinical features

Kleptomania is defined in DSM-IV as follows:

- recurrent failure to resist impulses to steal objects that are not needed for personal use or for their monetary value (criterion A);
- increasing sense of tension immediately before committing the theft (criterion B);
- pleasure, gratification, or relief at the time of committing the theft (criterion C);
- the stealing is not committed to express anger or vengeance and is not in response to a delusion or a hallucination (criterion D);
- the stealing is not better accounted for by conduct disorder, a manic episode, or antisocial personality disorder (criterion E).

In ICD-10, kleptomania (or pathological stealing) is defined as the repeated failure to resist impulses to steal objects that are not acquired for personal use or monetary gain.

An increasing number of studies have systematically examined the phenomenology of groups of people with DSM-defined kleptomania.[14–17] In these studies, most subjects described irresistible impulses or urges to steal, tension with the impulses, and tension relief either during or shortly after the act of theft (as required by the DSM criteria). Many subjects described the impulses as senseless, intrusive, uncomfortable, and uncontrollable. Many tried to resist the impulses with varying degrees of success. Some reported pleasurable feelings during the act of theft, often described as 'a rush,' 'a high,' or 'a thrill.' Most patients reported instances of impulsive stealing, but some also described premeditated stealing, the aim of which was sometimes to relieve the impulses to steal. Many subjects reported that they had lied to conceal their stealing. Some subjects developed rules for their stealing behaviour—for instance, stealing only from work or from certain types of shops (e.g. drug stores but not department stores), or stealing certain items but not others (e.g. jewellery but not clothing). Many subjects considered their stealing to be wrong, and many, but not all, reported guilt or remorse after stealing. Subjects who had been arrested for shoplifting reported that it had varying effects on their symptoms—some stopped stealing completely, some stopped for a limited amount of time, while others reported that their stealing was unaffected. Some stated they continued to steal once incarcerated.

These studies have also found that some subjects with apparent kleptomania report varying degrees of amnesia surrounding the act of stealing.[17] Many of these subjects deny impulses, tension, or relief with their thefts. Other subjects who are not amnesiac for their stealing episodes may also deny experiencing impulses, tension, relief, and/or pleasure. For these subjects, stealing appears to have become automatic or habit-like.[17]

Epidemiology and course

Kleptomania is presumed to be rare but its prevalence is unknown. Available studies suggest that only a small portion of shoplifters (from none to 8 per cent) represent true cases of kleptomania.[14] However, it has been argued that these rates may be spuriously low because psychiatric evaluations may not have always been sufficiently thorough, operational diagnostic criteria were rarely used, and kleptomania may have been under-represented in the samples due to selection bias (i.e. people with repeated apprehensions were more likely to be legally rather than psychiatrically referred). Also, kleptomania may be relatively common in clinical populations; it was the second most common lifetime impulse control disorder in a group of adult psychiatric inpatients assessed with a structured interview, present in 9.3 per cent of the sample.[18]

Kleptomania is probably more common in women than in men.[14–17] Many cases begin in adolescence or early adulthood, and often follow an episodic or a chronic course.

Associated psychopathology and comorbidity

Clinical studies show that kleptomania often co-occurs with other Axis I psychiatric disorders, including mood, anxiety, substance use, eating, and impulse control disorders.[14–18] In the only controlled study,[16] 10 patients with kleptomania had significantly higher rates of comorbid psychiatric disorders, particularly mood disorders, other impulse control disorders, and substance abuse or dependence (mainly nicotine dependence), than 29 psychiatric comparison patients and 60 patients with alcohol abuse or dependence. Several studies, including the one controlled study, found especially high rates of bipolar disorders.[15–17] Conversely, high rates of kleptomania have been found in women with eating disorders[14] and patients with depressive disorders.[19]

Preliminary data suggest patients with kleptomania may also have high rates of certain Axis II disorders.[17] However, the relationship between kleptomania and antisocial personality disorder is not understood.

Family studies

Uncontrolled studies suggest kleptomania may be associated with increased familial rates of mood, substance use, anxiety, and possibly impulse control disorders.[17] For example, of 103 first-degree relatives of 20 patients with DSM-IIIR-defined kleptomania evaluated blindly by the family history method, 22 (21 per cent) had a major mood disorder, 21 (20 per cent) had a substance use disorder, and 13 (13 per cent) had an anxiety disorder, including seven (7 per cent) with obsessive compulsive disorder[15] Also, two (2 per cent) had apparent kleptomania. However, a controlled family study found similar rates of kleptomania in first-degree relatives of probands with obsessive compulsive disorder and those of control probands.[20]

Psychobiology

Preliminary research suggests kleptomania may be associated with serotonergic and frontal lobe dysfunction. In one study, the number of platelet serotonin transporters, evaluated via [3H] paroxetine binding, was lower in 20 patients with obsessive-compulsive related disorders, including five patients with kleptomania, than in 20 healthy control subjects.[17] In another study, 10 females with DSM-IV kleptomania were more likely than controls to have decreased white matter microstructural integrity in inferior frontal brain regions when evaluated with diffusion tensor imaging.[21]

Treatment response

Although no controlled psychological treatment studies of kleptomania have been published, various types of cognitive behavioural therapy may be effective.[12,17] There are also successful reports of the use of psychodynamic psychotherapies, but there are negative reports as well.[12,15]

Medical treatments with antidepressant, mood-stabilizing, or anxiolytic properties have been reported to be effective in kleptomania, primarily in case reports and case series. These treatments include tricyclics, serotonin reuptake inhibitors, trazodone, lithium, valproate, electroconvulsive therapy, and benzodiazepines.[12,15,17] There are also reports of patients with kleptomania responding to the opioid antagonist naltrexone and the antiglutamatergic agent topiramate.[12,17]

However, in the only controlled pharmacotherapy study of kleptomania published to date, an open-label trial of escitalopram treatment in 24 subjects followed by double-blind discontinuation in 15 of 19 responders, there was no difference in response rate (defined as greater than a 50 per cent decrease in theft episodes per week) between subjects receiving escitalopram (3 [43 per cent]) and those receiving placebo (4 [50 per cent]).[22]

Pyromania

Definition and clinical features

Pyromania is defined in DSM-IV as follows: deliberate and purposeful fire-setting on more than one occasion (criterion A) that is associated with tension or affective arousal before the act (criterion B), fascination with, interest in, curiosity about, or attraction to fire and its situational contexts (criterion C), and pleasure, gratification, or relief when setting fires, or when witnessing or participating in their aftermath (criterion D). Also, the fire-setting is not done for monetary gain, as an expression of sociopolitical ideology, to conceal criminal activity, to express anger or vengeance, to improve one's living circumstances, in response to a delusion or hallucination, or as a result of impaired judgement (criterion E), and is not better accounted for by conduct disorder, a manic episode, or antisocial personality disorder (criterion F). In ICD-10, pyromania (or pathological fire-setting) is defined as multiple acts of, or attempts at, setting fire to property or other objects, without apparent motive, and by a persistent preoccupation with subjects related to fire and burning. The essential features are as follows:

- repeated fire-setting without any obvious motive such as monetary gain, revenge, or political extremism
- an intense interest in watching fires burn
- reported feelings of increasing tension before the act, and intense excitement immediately after it has been carried out.

Although the authors were unable to locate any systematic reports of a group of people with pyromania by either of the above criteria sets, there are numerous case reports and case series of people with repetitive fire-setting behaviour who would probably meet these criteria for pyromania. For example, in what is still probably the largest study of pathological fire-setting, in 1951, Lewis and Yarnell[23] evaluated 1 145 of 2 000 American case records of males 16 years of age and older from the National Board of Fire Underwriters (selection criteria were otherwise not clearly specified). They concluded that 688 of these males were best classified as 'pyromaniacs' as 'they set fires for no practical reason and received no material profit from the act, their only motive being to obtain some sort of sensual satisfaction'. Lewis and Yarnell did not provide quantitative data summarizing these 688 cases, but stated that 50 of the subjects 'approached true pyromania', in that they were able to give a 'classical description of the irresistible impulse'. Specifically, before they set fires, these subjects described 'mounting tension; . . . restlessness; the urge for motion; . . . conversion symptoms such as headaches, palpitations, ringing in the ears, and the gradual merging of their identity into a state of unreality'.

Epidemiology and course

The prevalence of pyromania is unknown.[19] Although there are numerous studies of fire-setting behaviour, few of these studies systematically assessed pyromania in their subjects. Those that did use variable definitions of pyromania and reported widely discrepant rates. For example, in their 1951 study of 1 145 adult males with pathological fire-setting, Lewis and Yarnell[23] reported that 688 (60 per cent) could be classified as having broadly defined pyromania, but only 50 (4 per cent) as having the 'true' disorder.

Pyromania is probably more common in males than females and usually begins in adolescence or early adulthood.[19,23] How often childhood fire-setting represents pyromania is unknown. Clinical descriptions indicate that the course of pyromania may be episodic or chronic, but its course into old age is unknown.

Associated psychopathology and comorbidity

There are no studies of the psychiatric comorbidity of a group of people with well-defined pyromania. However, there are case reports of people with apparent pyromania who have comorbid mood, obsessive compulsive, eating, paraphilic, and possibly psychotic disorders.[23] In addition, impulsive fire-setters have been reported to have high rates of mood, substance use, and cluster B personality disorders, as well as suicide attempts.[10]

Family studies

There are no family history studies of pyromania, but studies of impulsive fire-setters suggest elevated familial rates of substance use disorders.[8]

Biological studies

There are no biological studies of pyromania, but studies of impulsive fire-setters suggest they have abnormalities in central serotonergic neurotransmission.[10]

Treatment response

There are no systematic treatment studies of pyromania.[12,19] There is one case of an 18-year-old male with DSM-IV pyromania and a chief complaint of 'feeling addicted to setting fires' who responded to the combination of topiramate and cognitive behaviour therapy.[24] There is also a case report of two men in both of whom pyromania appeared to be part of a paraphilia and responded to antiandrogen medication.[25]

Clinical reports on the treatment of pathological fire-setting in general stress use of various psychological interventions (e.g. cognitive behavioural, psychoeducational, supportive, and insight-oriented) to address the fire-setting behaviour, and appropriate treatment of any comorbid psychiatric disorders. Preliminary data suggest combined psychosocial treatment approaches may be helpful in reducing further fire-setting behaviour, at least in juveniles.(19)

Trichotillomania

Definition and clinical features

Trichotillomania is defined in DSM-IV as follows:

- recurrent pulling out of one's hair resulting in noticeable hair loss
- an increasing sense of tension immediately before pulling out the hair or when attempting to resist the behaviour
- pleasure, gratification, or relief when pulling out the hair
- the disturbance is not better accounted for by another mental disorder and is not due to a general medical condition (e.g. a dermatological condition)
- the disturbance causes clinically significant distress or impairment in social, occupational, or other important areas of functioning.

In ICD-10, trichotillomania is defined as noticeable hair-loss due to a recurrent failure to resist impulses to pull out hairs. ICD-10 further states the hair-pulling is usually preceded by mounting tension and is followed by a sense of relief or gratification and that the diagnosis should not be made if there is a pre-existing inflammation of the skin, or if the hair pulling is in response to a delusion or a hallucination.

Hair is most often pulled from the scalp but also from the eyelashes, eyebrows, face, axilla, arms, legs, abdomen, and pubis.(26,27) Extracted hair may be chewed or swallowed. Medical complications include trichobezoars (hairballs that form in the stomach) and, uncommonly, obstruction or perforation of the stomach or bowel.

Some authorities have argued that both the DSM-IV and ICD-10 criteria for trichotillomania are too narrow, noting that patients with distressing hair pulling behaviour, especially children, may not always experience impulses and/or tension before hair pulling or relief with or after hair pulling.(26–28) Indeed, for some persons, the hair pulling may be automatic or habit-like and not associated with urges, tension, or relief. In addition, the hair loss may not be noticeable. For this reason and because hair pulling is a self-grooming behaviour, some authorities have argued that trichotillomania should be grouped with other self-grooming behaviours that may become problematic (e.g. skin picking and nail biting, which are discussed later) into a family of grooming disorders or body-focused impulse control disorders.(20,26,27)

Epidemiology and course

The prevalence of DSM-IV or ICD-10 defined trichotillomania is unknown, but survey studies suggest between 0.5 per cent—3.5 per cent of college students report problematic hair pulling.(26,27)

Clinical studies indicate trichotillomania is more common in females than in males; may begin in childhood, adolescence, or adulthood; and may have an episodic or chronic course.(26,27) Spontaneous remissions may occur, particularly in children with recent onset of the disorder.

Associated psychopathology and comorbidity

Trichotillomania often co-occurs with mood, anxiety, eating, substance use, and other impulse control disorders in clinical samples of adults.(26,27) It may also co-occur with various personality disorders, with histrionic, borderline, and obsessive compulsive commonly being cited.(26,27) In paediatric samples, trichotillomania is similarly associated with mood, anxiety, and substance use disorders.(26)

Family Studies

Preliminary family research suggests that trichotillomania may be associated with increased rates of obsessive-compulsive and grooming disorders among first-degree relatives.(26) A controlled family study of 22 probands with compulsive hair pulling, 17 (77 per cent) of whom met DSM-III-R criteria for trichotillomania, found that depression, alcoholism, drug abuse, obsessive compulsive disorder, and antisocial personality disorder were significantly more frequent among the first degree relatives of hair pullers than relatives of control probands.(28) Conversely, another controlled family study found significantly higher rates of grooming disorders (trichotillomania as well as pathological skin picking, pathological nail biting, and impulse control disorder NOS) in first-degree relatives of probands with obsessive compulsive disorder than in first-degree relatives of control probands.(20)

Psychobiology

Neuroimaging studies in subjects with trichotillomania have shown hyperactivity in the cerebellum and right superior parietal lobe as well as possible structural abnormalities of the left putamen, left inferior frontal gyrus, right cuneal cortex, and cerebellum.(26,27,29) Neuropsychological abnormalities found in trichotillomania patients have included increased error rates in spatial processing, divided attention, nonverbal memory, and executive functioning.(26,29)

Genetic studies suggest trichotillomania may be associated with sequence variants in the slit and trk-like 1 (SLITRK1) gene and the T10ZC polymorphism of the serotonin receptor 2A gene.(30,31)

Treatment response

There are a few published reports of the successful treatment of trichotillomania with insight-oriented psychotherapies, but there are many successful reports with various behavioural-based therapies.(12,26,27) Indeed, to date, four randomized, controlled studies supporting the effectiveness of behavioural treatments in adult trichotillomania have been published. In these studies, habit reversal was more effective than negative practice training (N=34); CBT was more effective than clomipramine and placebo (N=16); behaviour therapy was superior to fluoxetine and a wait-list control (N=43); and acceptance and commitment therapy plus habit reversal was superior to wait-list control (N=25).(12,26,27) In addition, one randomized, controlled trial found a cognitive behavioural therapy package of awareness training, stimulus control, and habit-reversal training was superior to minimal attention control in paediatric trichotillomania.(27)

Although many case reports and open trials describe successful treatment of trichotillomania with various serotonin reuptake inhibitors, controlled studies have yielded mixed results.(12,26,27) Two small (N=13 and N=12) double-blind, crossover trials found clomipramine was superior to desipramine and equivalent to fluoxetine (which had beneficial effects), respectively, in reducing hair-pulling symptoms. In contrast, 2 slightly larger (N=21 and N=23) placebo-controlled, double-blind crossover studies of fluoxetine (both up to 80 mg/day) in adult chronic hair pullers found fluoxetine was not superior to placebo in suppressing hair-pulling symptoms.[12,26,27] In addition, as noted earlier, in the two controlled comparisons which found cognitive behaviour therapy or behaviour therapy superior to clomipramine and fluoxetine in 16 and 43 patients with trichotillomania, respectively, neither drug was superior to placebo in reducing trichotillomanic symptoms.[12]

Despite these negative studies, thymoleptics other than serotonin reuptake inhibitors have been reported to be effective for trichotillomania in case reports and case series. These include antidepressants such as imipramine, amitriptyline, isocarboxazid, trazodone, mianserin, and bupropion; the mood stabilizers lithium, olanzapine, and quetiapine; and various antimanic antipsychotics—used as either monotherapy or adjunctively with serotonin reuptake inhibitors.[12,26,27]

Other medications described as being effective for trichotillomania, primarily in case reports or case series, are buspirone, fenfluramine, topiramate, inositol, the progestin levonorgestrel, and naltrexone.[12,26,27,32,33] Naltrexone was reported superior to placebo in one small controlled trial which has only been presented in abstract form.[12] Case reports also describe the successful use of topical steroid ointments in combination with psychotropics when skin is irritated.[12]

Compulsive buying disorder

History and clinical description

Although compulsive buying disorder (also called compulsive shopping, buying mania, and oniomania) is not classified in DSM-IV or ICD-10 as a mental disorder, diagnostic criteria have been proposed.[34,35] These include being frequently preoccupied with buying or subject to irresistible, intrusive, and/or senseless impulses to buy; frequently buying unneeded items or more than can be afforded; shopping for periods longer than intended; and experiencing adverse consequences, such as marked distress, impaired social or occupational functioning, and/or financial problems.[35] Persons with compulsive buying disorder often report irresistible or uncontrollable impulses to buy or shop; mounting tension or anxiety with the impulses; and relief of tension and/or pleasurable feelings (e.g. 'a high', 'a buzz', or 'a rush') with the act of buying or shopping. The disorder is associated with distress, financial and legal difficulties, and impairment in social and vocational functioning.[34,35]

Epidemiology and course

Compulsive buying behaviour is thought to be common, with an estimated lifetime prevalence of 5.8 per cent in the United States general adult population.[36] Indeed, in a recent study of the prevalence of various impulse control disorders in a psychiatric inpatient population, compulsive buying disorder was the most common current (9.3 per cent) and lifetime (9.3 per cent) impulse control disorder diagnosis.[18]

Compulsive buying disorder is probably more common in women than men.[34,35] It may begin in adolescence or adulthood and usually has either an episodic or a chronic course. The course of compulsive buying disorder into old age is unknown.

Associated psychopathology and comorbidity

Compulsive buying disorder often co-occurs with mood, anxiety, substance use, eating, and other impulse control disorders in clinical samples.[34,35] It may also be associated with certain personality disorders, but this comorbidity has received less systematic attention.[34]

Family studies

Preliminary research, including one controlled study, suggests compulsive buying disorder is associated with increased familial rates of mood, substance use, and possibly impulse control disorders.[34,35]

Psychobiology

In a molecular genetic study, no association was found between two serotonin transporter gene polymorphisms and compulsive buying disorder.[34]

Treatment response

Isolated reports of psychoanalytic and insight-oriented psychotherapy in compulsive buying disorder have mostly been unsuccessful. Cognitive behavioural therapy may hold promise. Two patients with compulsive buying disorder each responding to cue exposure plus response prevention after failing clomipramine treatment have been described.[12] In addition, a randomized study found group cognitive behavioural therapy (N=28) superior to wait-list control (N=11) in reducing compulsive buying episodes, time spent buying, and scores on buying symptom measures in 39 patients with compulsive buying disorder.[37] Support groups patterned after Alcoholics Anonymous, such as Debtors Anonymous, self-help books, and financial counselling are available, but their effectiveness has not been formally evaluated.[12,34]

Various antidepressant medications have been reported to be effective for compulsive buying in case reports and open trials, but two randomized, placebo-controlled, double blind studies of fluvoxamine in a total of 54 patients with compulsive buying (N=17 and N=37, respectively) failed to show separation between drug and placebo.[12,34] Both studies, however, were limited by high placebo response rates, possibly due to the use of diaries to record buying behaviour. In a 7-week, open-label trial of citalopram (N=24) followed by a 9-week double-blind, placebo-controlled continuation trial that omitted use of shopping diaries for the 15 subjects who met responder criteria, none of 7 patients randomized to remain on citalopram relapsed as compared with 5 (63 per cent) of 8 patients randomized to receive placebo (P=0.019)[12,34].

Patients with compulsive buying have also been reported to respond to mood stabilizers, naltrexone (at 100 mg/day but not 50 mg/day), and topiramate.[12,34]

Repetitive self-mutilation

Clinical description

Repetitive self-mutilation, also called impulsive deliberate self-harm, parasuicide, or self-injurious behaviour, is the repeated, direct destruction of body tissue without suicidal intent.[38,39] Examples include skin cutting, skin burning, self-hitting, severe skin scratching, and even bone breaking. A wide range of body parts are mutilated, such as arms, legs, abdomen, head, chest, and genitals.

Numerous clinical studies suggest that this syndrome often meets the DSM-IV and ICD-10 definitions of impulse control disorders.[38] Specifically, repetitive self-mutilation is characterized by intrusive, recurrent, and irresistible impulses to harm oneself without suicidal intent that are associated with increasing tension, anxiety, anger, or other dysphoric affective states, along with relief of the uncomfortable affect with or shortly after the act of self-harm. In addition, the act of self-harm is often not associated with pain (i.e. associated with analgesia) and performed privately.[38,39]

Epidemiology and course

The prevalence of narrowly defined repetitive self-mutilation is unknown.[38,39] Clinical studies, however, suggest that the condition is more common in females than males, usually begins early in life (e.g. late childhood, adolescence, and early adulthood), and may persist for 10 to 15 years.[38,39]

Associated psychopathology and comorbidity

Repetitive self-mutilation often co-occurs with other Axis I and II psychiatric disorders.[38,39] These include mood, substance use, eating, psychotic, dissociative, and borderline personality disorders. Repetitive self mutilation may also co-occur with suicide attempts and adverse childhood experiences in patients with certain pathologies, especially borderline personality disorder.[39] Of note, although deliberate self injury is a core feature of borderline personality disorder, not all patients with repetitive self mutilation have borderline personality disorder.[38]

Family history

No family history studies of repetitive self-mutilation have been conducted.

Psychobiology

Although studies have consistently found an association between low central CSF 5-H1AA levels with both impulsive aggression and violent suicide, the results of such studies in patients with repetitive self mutilation have been mixed—with some, but not all, finding similar reductions.[38,39] One study found that broadly-defined self harm was associated with allelic variation in the tryptophan hydroxylase gene (TPH A779C), but not with polymorphisms of five other serotonergic genes.[40]

Studies have found increased pain thresholds in borderline personality patients with repetitive self mutilation who are analgesic to the pain of their self injurious behaviour, suggesting dysfunction the endogenous opioid system.[38,39] In support of this possibility, one study found elevated plasma metenkephalin studies in a small group of analgesic self-injuring persons. Another study, however, found pretreatment with naltrexone did not reduce the anesthesia (as evaluated by the cold pressor test) of a similar group of subjects.[39]

Treatment response

There are no controlled treatment studies of narrowly-defined repetitive self-mutilation. However, two psychological treatments, dialectal behaviour therapy and psychoanalytically-oriented partial hospitalization, have each been shown superior to 'treatment as usual' in decreasing chronic parasuicidal behaviour in women with borderline personality disorder.[39] In addition, a 1998 meta-analysis of 20 treatment trials of broadly-defined deliberate self harm indicated significantly reduced repetition of self harm for problem solving therapy and provision of an emergency contract card in addition to standard care.[41]

Regarding medical treatments, agents with antidepressant, mood-stabilizing, antipsychotic, anticonvulsant, and anti-opiate properties have been reported to be effective in case reports or case series.[12,33,39] In the above noted 1998 meta-analysis, a significantly reduced rate of further self harm was observed for depot flupenthixol versus placebo in the one study of antipsychotic medication that was located and analyzed.[41] The two studies of antidepressants evaluated, however, showed no benefit.

Pathological skin picking

Clinical description

Pathological skin picking (also called neurotic or psychogenic excoriation, compulsive skin picking, dermatotillomania, and *acné excorié*) is excessive scratching, picking, gouging, or squeezing of the skin sometimes in response to an itch or other skin sensation or to remove a lesion on the skin.[42,43] Most patients use fingernails to excoriate the skin, but the teeth and instruments (for example, tweezers, nail files, pins, or knives) are also used. Pathological skin picking causes substantial distress in patients, with most experiencing functional impairment and many reporting medical complications, some severe enough to warrant surgery.

Although not recognized as a distinct DSM-IV or ICD-10 disorder, pathological skin picking resembles an impulse control disorder in that patients sometimes experience an increase in tension prior to picking with transient relief or pleasure with picking or immediately afterwards. Many patients find themselves acting automatically. It also has compulsive features, in that it is repetitive, ritualistic, anxiety reducing, often resisted, and egodystonic. Moreover, some patients describe obsessions about an irregularity on the skin or preoccupations with having smooth skin.

Epidemiology and course

Pathological skin picking may occur in about 2 per cent of dermatology clinic patients, predominately in women, and up to 3.8 per cent of college students.[42,43] The disorder may begin in adolescence or adulthood, and the mean duration of symptoms has ranged from 5 to 18 years, with a better prognosis for patients who have had the symptoms for less than 1 year.[42]

Associated psychopathology and comorbidity

Pathological skin picking often co-occurs with mood, anxiety, and somatoform disorders.[42] It is especially common in body dysmorphic disorder.[43] The comorbidity of pathological skin picking and personality disorders has not been systematically studied.

Family studies

Preliminary family history data suggest first-degree relatives of probands with pathological skin picking may have elevated rates of mood and substance use disorders.[42]

Treatment response

Various behavioural treatments (e.g. habit reversal) may be effective in pathological skin picking.[12] One small placebo-controlled trial (N=21) found that fluoxetine (mean dose of 55 mg/day) may be beneficial[12]. Other serotonin reuptake inhibitors, the tricyclic doxepin (which has been hypothesized to have antipruritic properties due to its antihistaminic effects), inositol, the glutamate-modulating agent riluzole, and certain direct skin treatments (dermatologic and surgical) may also be effective.[12,32,42,44,45]

Onychophagia

Clinical description

Onychophagia is repetitive and excessive nail-biting.[46] The cuticles and skin around the nails are also frequently bitten, picked, or clipped. Onychotillomania, the excessive picking, clipping, or tearing of the nail, may be a variant.

Although not classified as a psychiatric disorder in DSM-IV or ICD-10, onychophagia resembles an impulse control disorder in that the behaviour is often irresistible, automatic, and associated with an increase of tension before and relief or pleasure during or immediately after its enactment.[46] It also has compulsive features in that it is repetitive, resisted, and associated with relief of anxiety.

Epidemiology and course

Nail-biting is more common in children than adults, and may affect 5 to 10 per cent of adults over the age of 30 years.[46] Boys and girls are affected equally until after the age of 10 years, when nail-biting becomes more common in boys.

Associated psychopathology and comorbidity

Onychophagia may be associated with mood, anxiety, and substance use disorders. Of 25 adult subjects who underwent a medication trial for onychophagia, 17 (68 per cent) had a lifetime Axis I psychiatric disorder—despite the exclusion of subjects with obsessive–compulsive disorder, a primary major affective disorder, current substance abuse, or psychosis.[46] Four subjects (16 per cent) had at least one personality disorder.

Family studies

Severe nail biting may be familial.[46,47] Of 112 family members of 25 subjects entering a medication trial for onychophagia, seven (6 per cent) had severe nail-damaging behaviour, four (4 per cent) were severe nail-biters, and three (3 per cent) picked or chewed their hands or feet.[46] In addition, twin studies have found higher concordance rates of nail biting in monozygotic compared with dizygotic twins.[47]

Treatment response

Various cognitive behavioural therapies (especially habit reversal, but also self-monitoring, use of bitter tasting substances, competing responses, and negative practice training) are probably effective in onychophagia.[12] In the only controlled pharmacotherapy study of onychophagia, clomipramine (mean dose 120 mg/day) was superior to desipramine (mean dose 135 mg/day) in eliminating nail-biting, reducing nail-biting severity and impairment, and in improving overall clinical progress.[46]

Conclusion

Growing research shows that the impulse control disorders are much more common than once thought to be. The consistency of the 'structure' of the irresistible impulse (a core disturbance of impulsivity and compulsivity) together with increasing research showing that it responds to certain treatments, especially cognitive-behavioural psychotherapies and medical treatments with thymoleptic or anticraving properties, regardless of its 'content' (the specific impulse experienced), strongly suggest that it is an important psychopathological symptom, and that impulse control disorders are legitimate mental disorders that are in fact likely to be related despite their apparent differences.

Further information

Hollander, E. and Stein, D.J. (eds.) (2006). *Clinical Manual of Impulse-Control Disorders.* American Psychiatric Publishing, Inc., Arlington, VA.

Gabbard, G.O. (ed.) (2007). *Gabbard's Treatments of Psychiatric Disorders* (4th ed.). American Psychiatric Publishing, Inc., Arlington, VA.

References

1. Hollander, E. and Stein, D.J, (eds.) (2006). *Clinical manual of impulse control disorders*. American Psychiatric Publishing, Arlington, VA.
2. American Psychiatric Association. (1994). *Diagnostic and statistical manual of mental disorders* (4th ed.). American Psychiatric Association, Washington, DC.
3. World Health Organization. (1992). *International statistical classifi cation of diseases and related health problems*, 10th revision. WHO, Geneva
4. Coccaro, E.F. and Danehy, M. (2006). Intermittent explosive disorder. In *Clinical manual of impulse control disorders* (eds. E. Hollander and D.J. Stein,), pp. 19–37. American Psychiatric Publishing, Arlington, VA.
5. Kessler, R.C., Coccaro, E.F., Fava, M., *et al.* (2006). The prevalence and correlates of DSM-IV intermittent explosive disorder in the National Comorbidity Survey Replication. *Archives of General Psychiatry*, **63**, 669–78.
6. McElroy, S.L., Soutullo, C.A., Beckman, D.A., *et al.* (1998). DSM-IV intermittent explosive disorder: a report of 27 cases. *Journal of Clinical Psychiatry*, **59**, 203–10.
7. Perlis, R.H., Smoller, J.W., Fava, M., *et al.* (2004). The prevalence and clinical correlates of anger attacks during depressive episodes in bipolar disorder. *Journal of Affective Disorders,* **79**, 291–5.
8. Linnoila, M., DeJong, J. and Virkkunen, M. (1989). Family history of alcoholism in violent offenders and impulsive fire setters. *Archives of General Psychiatry*, **46**, 613–16.
9. Mattes, J.A. and Fink, M. (1990). A controlled family study of adopted patients with temper outbursts. *Journal of Nervous and Mental Disease*, **178**, 138–9.
10. Virkkunen, M., DeJong, J., Bartko, J., *et al.* (1989). Psychobiological concomitants of history of suicide attempts among violent offenders and impulsive fire setters. *Archives of General Psychiatry*, **46**, 604–6.
11. Coccaro, E.F., McCloskey, M.S., Fitzgerald, D.A., *et al.* (2007). Amygdala and orbitofrontal reactivity to social threat in individuals with impulsive aggression. Biological Psychiatry, **62,** 168–71
12. McElroy, S.L. and Keck, P.E. Jr (2007). Impulse control disorders. In *Gabbard's treatments of psychiatric disorders,* (4th edn),(ed. G.O. Gabbard), pp. 877–88. American Psychiatric Publishing, Arlington, VA.
13. Goedhard, L.E., Stolker, J.J., Heerdink, E.R. *et al.* (2006). Pharmacotherapy for the treatment of aggressive behavior in general adult psychiatry: a systematic review. *Journal of Clinical Psychiatry,* **67**, 1013–24.

14. McElroy, S.L., Keck, P.E. Jr, Pope, H.G.J., *et al.* (1991). Kleptomania: clinical characteristics and associated psychopathology. *Psychological Medicine*, **21**, 93–108.
15. McElroy, S.L., Pope, H.G. Jr, Hudson, J.I., *et al.* (1991). Kleptomania: a report of 20 cases. *American Journal of Psychiatry*, **148**, 652–7.
16. Bayle, F.J., Caci, H., Millet, B., *et al.* (2003) Psychopathology and comorbidity of psychiatric disorders in patients with kleptomania. *American Journal of Psychiatry*, **160**, 1509–13.
17. Grant, J.E., (2006). Kleptomania. In *Clinical manual of impulse control disorders* (eds. E. Hollander and D.J. Stein), pp. 175–201. American Psychiatric Publishing, Arlington, VA.
18. Grant, J.E., Levine, L., Kim, D., *et al.* (2005). Impulse control disorders in adult psychiatric inpatients. *American Journal of Psychiatry*, **162**, 2184–8.
19. Lejoyeux, M., McLoughlin, M. and Adès, J. (2006). Pyromania. In *Clinical manual of impulse control disorders* (eds. E. Hollander and D.J. Stein), pp. 229–50. American Psychiatric Publishing, Arlington VA.
20. Bienvenu, O.J., Samuels, J.F., Riddle, M.A., *et al.* (2000). The relationship of obsessive-compulsive disorder to possible spectrum disorders: results from a family study. *Biological Psychiatry*, **15**, 287–93.
21. Grant, J.E., Correia, S. and Brennan-Krohn, T. (2006).White matter integrity in kleptomania: A pilot study. Psychiatry Research, **147**, 233–7.
22. Koran, L.M., Aboujaoude, E.N. and Gamel, N.N. (2007). Escitalopram treatment of kleptomania: an open-label trial followed by double-blind discontinuation. *Journal of Clinical Psychiatry*, **68**, 422–7.
23. Lewis, N.D.C. and Yarnell, H. (1951). Pathological firesetting (pyromania). Nervous and mental disease monograph 82. Coolidge Foundation, New York.
24. Grant, J.E. (2006). SPECT imaging and treatment of pyromania. *Journal of Clinical Psychiatry*, **67**, 998.
25. Bourget, D. and Bradford, J. (1987). Fire fetishism, diagnostic and clinical implications: a review of two cases. *Canadian Journal of Psychiatry*, **32**, 459–62.
26. Franklin, M.E., Tolin, D.F. and Diefenbach, G.J. (2006). Trichotillomania. In *Clinical manual of impulse control disorders* (eds. E. Hollander and D.J. Stein), pp. 1149–73. American Psychiatric Publishing, Arlington, VA.
27. Woods, D.W., Flessner, C., Franklin, M.E., *et al.* (2006). Understanding and treating trichotillomania: what we know and what we don't know. *Psychiatric Clinics of North America*, **29**, 487–501.
28. Schlosser, S., Black, D.W., Blum, N., *et al.* (1994). The demography, phenomenology, and family history of 22 persons with compulsive hair pulling. *Annals of Clinical Psychiatry*, **6**, 147–52.
29. Keuthen, N.J., Makris, N., Schlerf, J.E., *et al.* (2007). Evidence for reduced cerebellar volumes in trichotillomania. *Biological Psychiatry*, **61**, 374–81.
30. Zuchner, S., Cuccaro, M.L., Tran-Viet, K.N., *et al.* (2006). SLITRK1 mutations in trichotillomania. *Molecular Psychiatry*, **11**, 887–9.
31. Hemmings, S.M., Kinnear, C.J., Lochner, C., *et al.* (2006). Genetic correlates in trichotillomania – a case-control association study in the South African Caucasian population. *Israel Journal of Psychiatry and Related Sciences*, **43**, 93–101.
32. Lochner, C., Seedat, S., Niehaus, D.J., *et al.* (2006). Topiramate in the treatment of trichotillomania: an open-label pilot study. *International Clinical Psychopharmacology*, **21**, 255–9.
33. Seedat, S., Stein, D.J. and Harvey, B.H. (2001). Inositol in the treatment of trichotillomania and compulsive skin picking. *Journal of Clinical Psychiatry*, **62**, 60–1.
34. Black, D.W. (2006). Compulsive shopping. In *Clinical manual of impulse control disorders* (eds. E. Hollander and D.J. Stein), pp. 203–28. American Psychiatric Publishing, Arlington, VA.
35. McElroy, S.L., Keck, P.E. Jr., Pope, H.F. Jr., *et al.* (1994). Compulsive buying: a report of 20 cases. *Journal of Clinical Psychiatry*, **55**, 242–8.
36. Koran, L.M., Faber, R.J., Aboujaoude, E., *et al.* (2006). Estimated prevalence of compulsive buying behavior in the United States. *American Journal of Psychiatry*, **163**, 1806 12.
37. Mitchell, J.E., Burgard, M., Faber, R., *et al.* (2006). Cognitive behavioral therapy for compulsive buying disorder. *Behavior Research and Therapy*, **44**, 1859–65.
38. Favazza, A.R. (1998). The coming of age of self mutilation. *Journal of Nervous and Mental Disease*, **186**, 259–68.
39. Simeon, D. (2006). Self-injurious behaviors. In *Clinical manual of impulse control disorders* (eds. E. Hollander and D.J. Stein), pp. 63–81. American Psychiatric Publishing, Arlington, VA.
40. Pooley, E.C., Houston, K., Hawton, K., *et al.* (2003). Deliberate selfharm is associated with allelic variation in the tryptophan hydroxylase gene (TPH A779C), but not with polymorphisms in five other serotonergic genes. *Psychological Medicine*, **33**, 775–83.
41. Hawton, K., Arensman, E, Townsend, E., *et al.* (1998). Deliberate self harm: systematic review of effi cacy of psychosocial and pharmacological treatments in preventing repetition. *British Medical Journal*, **327**, 441–7.
42. Arnold, L.M., Auchenbach, M.B. and McElroy, S.L. (2001). Psychogenic excoriation. Clinical features, proposed diagnostic criteria, epidemiology and approaches to treatment. *CNS Drugs*, **15**, 351–9.
43. Grant, J.E., Menard, W. and Phillips, K.A. (2006). Pathological skin picking in individuals with body dysmorphic disorder. *General Hospital Psychiatry*, **28**, 487–93.
44. Sasso, D.A., Kalanithi, P.S., Trueblood, K.V., *et al.* (2006). Beneficial effects of the glutamate-modulating agent riluzole on disordered eating and pathological skin-picking behaviors. *Journal of Clinical Psychopharmacology*, **26**, 685–7.
45. Bowes, L.E. and Alster, T.S. (2004). Treatment of facial scarring and ulceration resulting from ***acné excorié*** with 585-nm pulsed dye laser irradiation and cognitive psychotherapy. *Dermatologic Surgery*, **30**, 934–8.
46. Leonard, H.L., Lenane, M.C., Swedo, S.E., *et al.* (1991). A double-blind comparison of clomipramine and desipramine treatment of severe onychophagia (nail biting). *Archives of General Psychiatry*, **48**, 821–7.
47. Ooki, S. (2005). Genetic and environmental influences on finger-sucking and nail-biting in Japanese twin children. *Twin Research and Human Genetics*, **8**, 320–7.

4.13.2 Special psychiatric problems relating to gambling

Emanuel Moran

Introduction

Gambling is an activity with the following elements:

- A contract between two or more people, which is based on a forecast of the outcome of an uncertain event involving random processes.
- Property, referred to as the stake, is transferred between those taking part, so that some gain at the expense of others.
- The property transfer depends on the outcome or result of the uncertain event, which has been forecast.
- Participation is voluntary and not necessarily related to gaining the property, but used to obtain an experience.

Clinical features

Gambling misuse is a behavioural disorder that can usually be recognized by the presence of any of the following features:

- Excessive gambling either in terms of the money spent or the time devoted.
- Intermittent or continuous preoccupation with gambling and the development of tolerance and craving for it.
- Loss of control over gambling and 'chasing of losses', despite the realization that damage is resulting.
- Disorder affecting the person who is gambling and the family:
  - financial disturbances, such as debt and shortage;
  - social disturbances, such as loss of employment and friends, running away from home, eviction, marital problems, divorce, behaviour disorders in the children of the family, criminality and imprisonment;
  - psychological disturbances, such as depression and attempted suicide.

Classification

In the past, this syndrome has been referred to as compulsive gambling. However, it is not a true obsessive–compulsive state but a heterogeneous group of conditions, characterized by excessive gambling resulting in disturbance for those involved. The term 'pathological gambling' is more appropriate, since it is not based on any assumptions regarding the underlying processes.(1)

ICD-10(2) describes pathological gambling as a form of behaviour under 'habit and impulse disorders'. On the other hand, DSM-IV(3) implies a homogeneous disease entity and provides criteria for its recognition under 'impulse-control disorders not elsewhere classified'. The ICD-10 approach is preferable since it emphasizes the fact that the condition is a behavioural disorder resulting from faulty habits.

Five varieties of pathological gambling can be recognized(4,5):

- Subcultural gambling arises out of the person's background, which is one of socially accepted heavy gambling.
- Impulsive gambling is characterized by loss of control for varying periods and the tendency to be associated with tolerance, craving, and dependence on the activity.
- Neurotic gambling occurs as a response to an emotional problem, particularly in a disturbed relationship in marriage or during adolescence.
- Symptomatic gambling occurs in mental illness, usually depression, which is the primary disorder.
- Psychopathic gambling is part of the generalized disturbance of behaviour that characterizes antisocial personality disorder.

Diagnosis

For various social reasons, pathological gambling is most easily recognized in men since they tend to patronize those types of gambling that have a high turnover of money so that excess is more likely to become apparent.

Women have tended to gamble on lotteries, bingo, and football pools. These may not involve such large sums of money and excess often presents with disturbances in the social sphere rather than through the accumulation of large debts. However, the greater general acceptance of gambling and the advent of remote gambling via the Internet, television, and mobile devices is changing the situation considerably.

While pathological gambling is seen in all age groups, an increasing number of children and young people are presenting with the condition as a result of gambling on slot/gaming machines. Also, in recent years, remote gambling among children and young people has led to increasing problems. This is in spite of the fact that most jurisdictions treat gambling as an adult activity. Pathological gambling in adulthood frequently has its origins in heavy gambling in childhood and adolescence.

Aetiology and epidemiology

The nature of gambling

The experience of risk provides amusement, thrill, and excitement and is therefore pleasurable. These experiences make gambling attractive and the stake money is used to purchase them, with winnings as an occasional bonus. A few, who gamble professionally, are also able to win money regularly because they have sources of information that reduce the uncertainty, as in betting on horses and dogs. Their gambling is planned and deliberate.

Gambling is usually organized commercially with the odds in favour of the provider. There is therefore an in-built financial disadvantage to those who use the facilities. In slot/gaming machines where the provider is at a distance from the gambling event, this is often not apparent to those who take part.

Commercial gambling involves large sums of money, and has traditionally been confined to licensed premises. Those present have gone there because they have decided to take part in the gambling. However, developments in technology have made it possible to provide gambling facilities on a remote basis via the Internet, television, and mobile devices.

A number of features inherent in the activity of gambling have effects that make it difficult for a person to stop.

Psychological effects

- Underlying all gambling activity is operant conditioning with intermittent variable ratio reinforcement.(6) This is a most effective schedule for habit-formation and produces a stable, persistent response. Consequently, the long-term net gain or loss to those who gamble is almost irrelevant to the continuation of the activity. It is most dramatically seen in slot/gaming machines, which consequently are the main source of profit for the gambling industry.
- Rapid turnover gambling as in casinos restricts the ability of those who gamble to apply any considered judgement. Inevitably, gambling becomes more impulsive, easily leading to excessive participation.
- The assessment of probability of winning (psychological probability) in the gambling situation differs from the mathematical probability. At low probabilities, it is higher than the mathematical probability and at moderate and high probabilities, it is lower. This even occurs in people who are mathematically knowledgeable.

- In a gambling situation involving only random processes, where the outcome of successive events is completely independent, there is usually the irrational belief that a string of losses makes a win more likely. This is the negative recency effect, which is also referred to as the'Monte Carlo Fallacy' since it forms the basis of many spurious gambling systems, especially in roulette. Paradoxically, it is associated with the belief that a string of wins is likely to continue ('a lucky streak'). Also, a 'near win' generally tends to be treated as a prelude to a win. These illogical ways of thinking encourage continuous gambling and are exploited by slot/gaming machines and lottery scratch cards called 'heart stoppers'.
- Large prizes, even at very low probabilities, entice the gambler because of the *possibility* of winning. The stimulant effect of roll-overs in lotteries illustrates this.
- Skill in gambling is usually overrated and often implies an unrealistic ability to control the uncertain event that is the subject of the gamble. Thus, in dog and horse race betting, punters tend to place their bets just before 'the off' in the fantasy that this will affect the result.
- There is a tendency to lose track of time during a gambling session.

These psychological effects have been increased as a result of recent developments in commercial gambling.

- Loyalty cards providing rewards for money spent on gambling in a particular facility.
- Remote gambling on the Internet, television, and mobile devices has resulted in the following:
  - The convenience and anonymity of gambling being available in an isolated domestic setting, without the checks and constraints that can be exercised by the presence of others as in licensed premises.
  - Monetary credit in the form of e-cash systems, reducing the likelihood that those gambling will set a limit on the money staked.
  - Behavioural targeting and messages on some online gambling sites encouraging further gambling when an attempt is made to stop.
  - Difficulty in preventing children and young people from having access, especially since the advent of online social networks.

Physical effects

- A gambling loss in normal subjects immediately results in particular localized activity in the medial frontal cortex of the brain. This is then associated with subsequent *more risky* gambling choices. This is consistent with the negative recency effect.
- Disturbances involving the reward pathways in the brain are significantly associated with excessive gambling.
- There is a great range and strength of emotions during gambling decisions associated with cortical responses in the brain to the expectation of winning money.
- Even normal, social levels of drinking alcohol that alter self-control over decision-making, increase the difficulty in deciding at what point to stop, when losing, in a gambling situation.

Predisposing factors

In the presence of available gambling facilities, certain predispositions may increase the likelihood of pathological gambling.

Morbid risk-taking

Since gambling is a type of risk-taking, it lends itself to be used by those who, for reasons related to their personality, have a high need for risk. They spend large sums of money on the intangible commodity of risk, which may easily pass unnoticed because it is fleeting.

This morbid propensity to take risks shows itself in other ways. Thus, the incidence of attempted suicide is high among those whose gambling is pathological.[5]

Other personality factors

Freud's formulation of gambling was that it resembles masturbation, is a substitute for it, and is resorted to in the context of unresolved Oedipal difficulties.[7] Others have pointed out that pathological gambling may be a manifestation of self-punishment, with an unconscious desire to lose, arising from a psychological mechanism referred to as 'psychic masochism'.[8]

Those whose gambling is pathological appear to have other predisposing personality traits. They view their behaviour as being largely determined by factors outside their personal control. They also tend towards greater impulsivity.[5,9]

Learning processes

Apart from the winnings and losses, the gambling situation itself may affect learning. As far as the random processes inherent in gambling are concerned, all participants, even a total failure, stand on an equal footing. This may be the only circumstance in which some people have this experience. Gambling may therefore provide a means of dealing with morbid anxiety in the presence of feelings of inadequacy, leading to a conditioned avoidance reaction.

Mental disorder

Pathological gambling may occur in any mental disorder. However, it is most commonly associated with depression. More usually, a neurotic type of depression occurs after a bout of heavy gambling with large losses. In symptomatic pathological gambling, the depression is primary and the gambling is a response to the tension and feelings of guilt that occur in depression. This latter situation is similar to alcohol misuse and shoplifting, as part of the depressive syndrome. Pathological gambling may also be a manifestation of antisocial personality disorder.

Misuse of alcohol and pathological gambling can occur together; either may be the primary disorder and either may lead to the other.

Constitutional factors and physical disorder

Twin studies have demonstrated that the likelihood of pathological gambling occurring in a person is influenced, to an important degree, by inherited factors and/or experiences shared during childhood.[10]

There also appears to be a significant association between pathological gambling and genetic abnormalities involving the dopamine reward pathways.[11] Disturbances of serotonergic, noradrenergic, and dopaminergic neurotransmitter systems have all been implicated in the aetiology of pathological gambling. This is particularly so in relation to the arousal, behavioural initiation, behavioural disinhibition, and reward/reinforcement mechanisms that are evident in this condition.(12)

There have been reports of pathological gambling associated with dopamine agonist administration for Parkinsonism.(13)

Course and prognosis

The natural history of pathological gambling is one characterized by exacerbations and remissions, often related to life events. Important elements in this are relationships within the family, especially with the spouse/partner. An example of this is the not infrequent sequence of an exacerbation of heavy gambling in the husband, at the time of the wife's first pregnancy.

The outlook in pathological gambling is usually determined by the integrity of the underlying personality. In those in whom the condition appears as a symptom of a neurotic disorder or depression, the prognosis depends on that of the underlying disorder.

Management and treatment

Pathological gambling involves a whole way of life, which has many ramifications. If its management is to be successful, there need to be major changes in the lifestyle of the person concerned. It is best dealt with by a team approach involving at least a psychiatrist, psychologist, and social worker and must include the spouse/partner. Recently, counselling services have been set up but their efficacy has yet to be established.

Assessment of the problem

The following aspects are important:

- An appraisal of the extent and amount of present gambling.
- A history of the development of the gambling from its early beginnings, which is best done if the person being assessed provides the information by means of a detailed written narrative.
- A discussion of this written narrative.
- An indication of the person's motivation, since many who seek help for pathological gambling readily admit that they enjoy it and only want assistance for the problems that have resulted.
- At least initially, an immediate period of total abstinence from gambling.

Supervision of the finances

Excessive gambling is usually associated with a disturbed appreciation of the value of money. In view of this and the continued temptation to gamble, the family finances should be dealt with as follows:

- All monies should be controlled, at least for some time, by the spouse/partner or some trusted person.
- Regular income from wages/salaries should be paid into a bank account over which the spouse/partner or trusted person has sole control.
- A detailed statement should be drawn up of all the outstanding debts, as well as an inventory of the income and outgoings of the person-seeking help and his or her family.
- The person whose gambling has been pathological should discuss the matter with all creditors and agree a repayment plan. This should be consistent with the person's regular income and circumstances to avoid a situation where there would be the temptation to gamble in order to maintain repayments. Since debts are often considerable, these may have to continue over many years.
- After a period of abstinence from gambling, the person whose gambling has been pathological needs to become gradually involved in working jointly with whoever controls the finances.

Counselling

On the basis of information obtained during the course of the initial assessment, the following aspects need further consideration:

- The features inherent in gambling that affect people so that they find it difficult to stop should be highlighted and discussed.
- Social relationships of the person whose gambling has become pathological and the spouse/partner should be reviewed, especially if there have been serious marital problems predating the pathological gambling.
- The way spare time is spent, what friends are cultivated, and what interests are pursued should be reviewed. Since incitement to gamble will have occurred in the past within specific settings, arrangements need to be made to avoid these or, at least, to be prepared for them.
- A joint contract to be reviewed regularly spelling out in detail those types of behaviour to be avoided as well as those to be encouraged may be found helpful.

Gamblers Anonymous

This form of self-help for pathological gambling is organized in regular local groups. As well as meetings for those who have a gambling disorder, there are also separate ones for their spouses/partners. Quite apart from the valuable work done in the group setting, Gamblers Anonymous provides a useful means of establishing alternative social contacts from those that were associated with gambling. Indeed, for some people, Gamblers Anonymous may be the vehicle through which all the necessary help can be provided. Even if this is not the case, Gamblers Anonymous still provides a valuable form of support for the individual and the family.

Psychological treatments

A variety of psychological treatments have been advocated but, in general, their long-term efficacy has not been established. A good outcome has been reported after a cognitive behavioural approach.(14) Also, controlled gambling, rather than permanent abstinence, has led to a reported successful outcome after behavioural treatment.(15)

Psychiatric treatments

Specialist treatment from a psychiatrist and/or a psychotherapist for a neurotic disorder or severe depression may be required, if these clearly underlie the pathological gambling.

Prevention

In view of the nature of gambling and the importance of the social causation of pathological gambling, it is vital that it should be seen as an activity that requires moderation. Unfortunately, the recent increasing reliance of governments and states on gambling for revenue purposes is resulting in a vast growth in the availability of gambling facilities and the incitements to participate.

This has been associated with public policies that actively promote gambling and also claim to encourage moderation. The inconsistency in trying to do both inevitably has a harmful effect on any educational attempt to provide a sensible attitude to gambling. It also undermines any help for those whose gambling has become excessive.

Further information

Journal of Gambling Studies. Springer. http://www.springer.com/west/home/social+sciences/sociology?SGWID=4-40440-70-35680327-0 Online version available http://www.springerlink.com/content/1050-5350

International Gambling Studies. Routledge. http://www.informaworld.com/smpp/title~content=t713701604~tab=sample?action=view&db=all

References

1. Moran, E. (1970). Gambling as a form of dependence. *British Journal of Addiction*, **64**, 419–27.
2. World Health Organization. (1992). *International statistical classification of diseases and related health problems*, 10th revision. WHO, Geneva.
3. American Psychiatric Association. (1994). *Diagnostic and statistical manual of mental disorders* (4th edn). American Psychiatric Association, Washington, DC.
4. Moran, E. (1970). Varieties of pathological gambling. *The British Journal of Psychiatry*, **116**, 593–7.
5. Moran, E. (1970). Clinical and social aspects of risk-taking. *Proceedings of the Royal Society of Medicine*, **63**, 1273–7.
6. Skinner, B.F. (1966). *Science and human behaviour*. Macmillan, New York.
7. Freud, S. (1961). Dostoevsky and parricide. In *Standard edition of the complete psychological works of Sigmund Freud*, Vol. 21 (ed. J. Strachey), p. 177. Hogarth Press, London.
8. Bergler, E. (1970). *The psychology of gambling*. International Universities Press, New York.
9. Steel, Z. and Blaszczynski, A. (1998). Impulsivity, personality disorders and pathological gambling severity. *Addiction*, **93**, 895–905.
10. Eisen, S.A., Lin, N., Lyons, M.J., *et al.* (1998). Familial influences on gambling behaviour: an analysis of 3359 twin pairs. *Addiction*, **93**, 1375–84.
11. Cummings, D.E. (1998). The molecular genetics of pathological gambling. *CNS Spectrums: International Journal of Neuropsychiatric Medicine*, **3**, 20–37.
12. DeCaria, C.M., Begaz, T., and Hollander, E. (1998). Serotonergenic and noradrenergic function in pathological gambling. *CNS Spectrum: International Journal of Neuropsychiatric Medicine*, **3**, 38–47.
13. O'Sullivan, S.S. and Lees, A.J. (2007). Pathological gambling in Parkinson's disease. *Lancet Neurology*, **6**, 384–6
14. Sylvain, C., Ladouceur, R., and Boisvert, J.M. (1997). Cognitive and behavioural treatment of pathological gambling: a controlled study. *Journal of Consulting and Clinical Psychology*, **65**, 727–32.
15. Blaszczynski, A., McConaghy, N., and Frankova, A. (1991). Control versus abstinence in the treatment of pathological gambling: a two to nine year follow-up. *British Journal of Addiction*, **86**, 299–306.

4.14
Sleep–wake disorders

Contents

4.14.1 Basic aspects of sleep–wake disorders
Gregory Stores

4.14.2 Insomnias
Colin A. Espie and Delwyn J. Bartlett

4.14.3 Excessive sleepiness
Michel Billiard

4.14.4 Parasomnias
Carlos H. Schenck and Mark W. Mahowald

4.14.1 Basic aspects of sleep–wake disorders

Gregory Stores

Introduction

A sound working knowledge of the diagnosis, significance, and treatment of sleep disorders is essential in all branches of clinical psychiatry. Unfortunately, however, psychiatrists and psychologists share with other specialties and disciplines an apparently universal neglect of sleep and its disorders in their training. Surveys in the United States and Europe point to the consistently meagre coverage of these topics in their courses at both undergraduate and postgraduate levels.

The following account is an introductory overview of normal sleep, the effects of sleep disturbance, sleep disorders and the risk of failure to recognize them in psychiatric practice, assessment of sleep disturbance, and the various forms of treatment that are available. The aim is to provide a background for the other chapters in this section.

The close links between the field of sleep disorders and psychiatry which make it essential that psychiatrists are familiar with the field are as follows:

- Sleep disturbance is an almost invariable feature and complication of psychiatric disorders from childhood to old age, with the risk of further reducing the individual's capacity to cope with their difficulties (see Table 4.14.1.3 for further details).
- Sleep disturbance can presage psychiatric disorder.
- Some psychotropic medications produce significant sleep disturbance.
- Of importance to liason psychiatry is the fact that many general medical or paediatric disorders disturb sleep sufficiently to contribute to psychological or psychiatric problems.
- Because of lack of familiarity with sleep disorders and their various manifestations, such disorders may well be misinterpreted as primary psychiatric disorders (or, indeed, other clinical conditions) with the result that effective treatments for the sleep disorder are unwittingly withheld (see later).

Some of these points will be amplified in later sections of this chapter.

Basic features of normal sleep

The scientific study of sleep and its disorders is largely confined to the last several decades. Essentially interdisciplinary advances have displaced earlier speculative accounts including those in psychiatry concerning the significance of dreams, for example. They are well described in recent textbooks of sleep disorders medicine (see recommended sources). Only general points are mentioned here, with special reference to psychiatry where possible.

The nature of sleep

Sleep has characteristic physiological features which distinguish it from other states of relative inactivity. Two distinct sleep states have been defined, that is non-rapid eye movement (**NREM**) sleep and rapid eye movement (**REM**) sleep. The onset of sleep is not simply the shutdown of wakefulness but also the switching between wakefulness, NREM and REM sleep involve complicated active neurochemical mechanisms in different parts of the brain.

The functions of sleep

Debate continues about the various theories concerning sleep, each of which has emphasized physical and psychological restoration and recovery, energy conservation, memory consolidation, discharge of emotions, brain growth and various other biological functions including somatic growth and repair, and maintenance of immune systems. No one theory accounts for all the complexities of sleep and it seems likely that sleep serves multiple purposes.

From the practical point of view, the most obvious observation is that both physical and psychological impairment follows persistent sleep disturbance. Animals totally deprived of sleep for a long periods die with loss of temperature regulation and multiple system failure. As described later, the adverse effects of chronic sleep loss (considered to be common in modern society) on mood, behaviour, and cognitive function can be substantial, with various consequences for personal, social, occupational, educational, and family functioning.

Sleep stages

Conventionally, standard criteria are used to identify different sleep stages according to their characteristic physiological features especially in the electroencephalogram (**EEG**), electrooculogram (**EOG**), and electromyogram (**EMG**).

NREM sleep is divided into four stages of increasing depth. **Stage I** occurs at sleep onset or following arousal from another stage of sleep. This stage represents 4–16 per cent of the main sleep period. **Stage II** contains more slow EEG activity but is still relatively light sleep. It accounts for 45–55 per cent of overnight sleep. **Stage III** (4–6 per cent of total sleep time) contains yet more slow EEG activity. **Stage IV** is characterized by the slowest activity and constitutes 12–15 per cent of sleep. The combination of stages III and IV is called slow wave sleep (**SWS**) or delta sleep and is considered to be the deepest form of sleep from which awakening is particularly difficult. The arousal disorders such as sleepwalking arise from SWS.

REM sleep is physiologically very different. Brain metabolism is highest in this stage of sleep. Spontaneous rapid eye movements are seen and the skeletal musculature is effectively paralysed. Heart rate, blood pressure, and respiration are all variable, body temperature regulation ceases temporarily, and penile and clitoral tumescence occurs. REM sleep usually takes up 20–25 per cent of total sleep time. Most dreams, including nightmares, occur in REM sleep.

Sleep architecture

NREM and REM sleep alternate cyclically throughout the night starting with NREM sleep lasting about 80 min followed by about 10 min of REM sleep. This 90 min sleep cycle is repeated three to six times each night. Each REM period typically ends with a brief arousal or transition into light NREM sleep.

In successive cycles the amount of NREM sleep decreases and the amount of REM sleep increases. SWS is usually confined to the first two sleep cycles. The diagrammatic representation of overnight sleep is known as a **hypnogram**, a simplified form of which is shown in Fig. 4.14.1.1.

In addition to this conventional sleep staging, there has been increasing interest in the microstructural fragmentation of sleep by frequent, brief arousals (seen mainly in the EEG) lasting a matter of seconds without obvious clinical accompaniments. This subtle type of sleep disruption, overlooked by conventional sleep staging, is increasingly associated with impairment of daytime performance, mood, and behaviour.

Circadian sleep–wake rhythms

The timing of sleep (but not its amount) is regulated by a circadian 'clock' in the suprachiasmatic nucleus (**SCN**) of the hypothalamus.

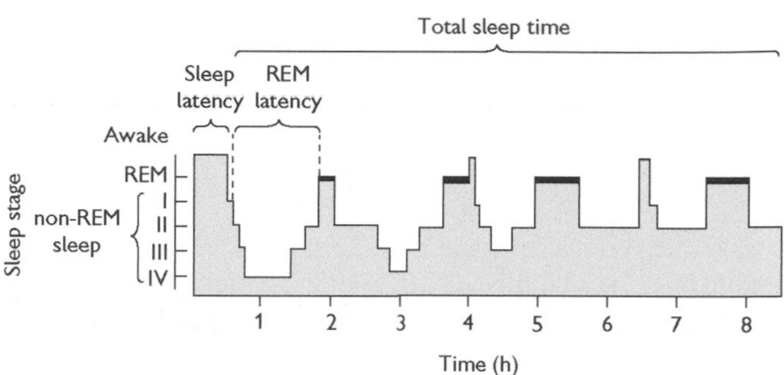

Fig. 4.14.1.1 Diagram of an overnight hypnogram in a young adult.

The intrinsic circadian sleep–wake rhythm is close to 24 h in human adults. Other species are different, an extreme example being dolphins and some other creatures which shut down one cerebral hemisphere at a time ('unihemispheric sleep'), allowing them to be constantly alert. From an early age the individual sleep–wake rhythm has to synchronize with the 24-h day–night rhythm. The main *zeitgeber* by which this is achieved ('entrainment') is sunlight but social cues, such as mealtimes and social activities, are also important.

The SCN also controls other biological rhythms including body temperature and cortisol production with which the sleep–wake rhythm is normally synchronized. In contrast, growth hormone is locked to the sleep–wake cycle and is released with the onset of SWS, whatever its timing.

Melatonin is related to the light–dark cycle rather than the sleep–wake cycle. It is secreted by the pineal gland during darkness and suppressed by exposure to bright light ('the hormone of darkness'). It influences circadian rhythms via the SCN pacemaker which in turn, regulates melatonin secretion by relaying light information to the pineal gland. The widespread popularity of melatonin as a sleep-promoting agent is not justified by what little is known about its action and clinical effectiveness.

Changes with age

Changes in basic aspects of sleep are prominent from birth to old age, although individual differences are seen at all ages. Changes of clinical significance include the following:

- **Total sleep time** decreases with age. Average daily values are as follows: newborns 6–18 h; young children 10 h; adolescents 9 h (although often they obtain significantly less than this); adults 7.5–8 h, including possibly the same in elderly people. The total amount of sleep includes daytime napping in children up to the age of about 3 years.
- **SWS** is particularly prominent in prepubertal children who sleep very soundly. Its decline begins in early adolescence and continues throughout childhood.
- The proportion of **REM sleep** declines from 50 per cent or more of total sleep time in the newborn (more than this in premature babies) to 20–25 per cent by 2 years. This figure remains fairly constant throughout the rest of life. The high level of REM sleep in very early life suggests a role in cerebral maturation but the reason for its persistence throughout life is unclear. Memory processing appears to depend on sleep. However, people deprived

of REM sleep, experimentally or pathologically, can be relatively unaffected either emotionally or cognitively. Deep sleep decreases in the elderly.

- **NREM–REM sleep cycles** occur at intervals of 50–60 min in infants who often enter REM at the start of their sleep period. This interval between sleep cycles remains until adolescence when the periodicity changes to 90–100 min, which persists into adult life. The amounts of NREM and REM in each sleep cycle is about equal in early infancy. Afterwards, NREM sleep (especially SWS) predominates in the earlier cycles and REM sleep in the later cycles.
- **Continuity of sleep** is greatest in pre-pubertal children (as mentioned previously) and least at the extremes of age. Infants are easily awakened and so are the elderly who also wake spontaneously more often. Fragmentation of sleep by brief arousals, or very brief awakenings, is particularly common in old age.
- **Circadian sleep–wake rhythms** change considerably in early development. Full-term neomates show 3–4-h sleep–wake cycles. Sleep periods have largely shifted to the night and wakefulness to daytime by 12 months, except for napping which gradually diminishes and has usually stopped by about 3 years of age. However, a physiological tendency towards an afternoon nap remains throughout the rest of the life. Although repeated brief waking at night is more common in infancy and early childhood than later, it remains a normal occurrence throughout life, increasing in frequency again in old age. The clinical problem arises when there is difficulty returning to sleep after such awakenings.

Psychological effects of sleep disturbance

There is extensive clinical and experimental evidence that sustained sleep disturbance can have serious adverse psychological effects.[1,2] The term sleep disturbance covers the following:

- Loss of sleep (i.e. shortened duration).
- Impaired quality of sleep (repeated disruption of sleep architecture).
- Inappropriate timing of the sleep period in relation to day–night rhythms (as in the various circadian sleep rhythm disorders such as jet lag, shift work, or the more frequently encountered forms seen in clinical practice, as discussed later).

Experimental studies of **total sleep loss** demonstrate a progressive deterioration in cognitive function, mood, and behaviour related to length of sleep loss. However, inter- and also intra-individual differences in susceptibility are seen, reflecting such factors as motivation, personality, and usual sleep requirements. Task characteristics (e.g. brief or prolonged and monotonous tasks), timing of the task in relation to the circadian sleep–wake rhythm, and physical environmental factors such as noise and other distracting stimuli, are also important.

Variations for similar reasons are important in **partial sleep deprivation** experiments which (like those concerning fragmentation of sleep) are much closer to real-life sleep disturbance caused by social activities, job demands, and other aspects of modern lifestyle. These studies raise the issues of how much sleep is needed for optimal daytime functioning and whether these requirements are not being met. It has been argued that there is 'national sleep debt' in the United States and other western countries, and that by sleeping longer than they do habitually, many people would increase their performance and improve their well-being during the day.

The usual subjective effects of sleep disturbance are irritability, fatigue, poor concentration, and depression. More dramatic effects are described with prolonged and severe sleep disturbance, such as disorientation, illusions, hallucinations, persecutory ideas, and inappropriate behaviour with impaired awareness ('automatic behaviour') caused by frequent microsleeps. Psychometric studies have shown that sleep disturbance can produce a range of cognitive impairments, again depending on its duration and individual susceptibility. Sustained attention (vigilance) is particularly vulnerable and possibility abstract thinking and divergent intelligence or creativity.

The experimental findings are in keeping with the results from studies of various occupational groups including junior hospital doctors and drivers of various types of vehicle, in which reduced performance or accidents are associated with sleep disturbance. The common and increasing practice of night-shift work (as part of the '24 h society') is contrary to the fundamental biorhythm of sleeping at night and being awake during the day, and is often accompanied by a reduction in total sleep time and poor quality sleep. It is not surprising that working shifts commonly results in loss of well-being, physical complaints, and impaired productivity and safety, as well as physical disorders. Similarly, the distribution over the 24 h period of road accidents (especially those not involving other vehicles) and other mishaps at work, correspond to that of the levels of sleep tendency assessed objectively. Even industrial and engineering disasters have been attributed to sleep loss and impaired performance on the part of key personnel.

Additional evidence that sleep disturbance affects daytime function comes from neuropsychological studies of certain sleep disorders. Impaired performance on prolonged and complex tasks of subjects with narcolepsy has been shown to be secondary to the effects of their daytime sleepiness rather than an intrinsic neurological deficit. In the many adult patients with obstructive sleep apnoea, attention memory impairment (like depression and irritability commonly reported by these patients) are also largely attributable to daytime sleepiness. There is some evidence that deficits in more complicated 'executive functions' (formulating goals, planning, and carrying out plans effectively) are not necessarily reversed when their sleepiness is relieved by treatment. This might be the result of irreversible anoxic brain changes in the later stages of the condition. Clearly, early detection and treatment of this condition is essential to prevent this happening.

When return to normal sleep is possible, recovery from short periods of sleep disturbance occurs after much less sleep than that originally lost, for example, after one night's sleep following sleep loss over several days and nights. Reversal of the effects of long sleep disturbance in real-life is likely to be complicated, for example by emotional consequences of the disturbance.

Many of the above observations about the psychological effects of sleep disturbance (and their reversibility) have been made on young adult subjects or patients. The area is largely unexplored in other age groups but there is no reason why the general principle should not apply to children and the elderly including demented patients in whom sleep disturbance is particularly prominent.

Another group on whom further research is particularly required are people with learning disabilities (intellectual disability).

The available literature provides good reason to believe that the sleep disorders, especially in the more severely disabled groups, not only affects the majority but also are unusually severe and long-lasting because of lack of appropriate advice and treatment. The sleep disturbance is a problem in its own right and is often associated with various cognitive and behavioural abnormalities which might, at least partly, be the consequence of the sleep disturbance. Sleep disturbance in the duration or the quality of sleep may be one of the few ways of improving to some extent the psychological well-being of people with learning disabilities or dementia (and that of their carers) whose basic condition itself cannot be improved. In the case of the learning disabled, contrary to the common supposition by both professionals and relatives, success can usually be achieved (even in severe and long-standing problems), given an accurate diagnosis of the type of sleep disorder which may be predominantly behavioural or physical in type depending on the cause of the learning disability.

Sleep disturbance in the aetiology of psychiatric illness

Various 'psychotic' and other abnormal psychological phenomena were mentioned earlier resulting from prolonged and severe sleep disturbance, but these are reversed when normal sleep is restored. It remains an open question how often sleep disturbance is a primary cause of psychiatric illness. Evidence is patchy, tentative, and still in need of clarification.

- Over a wide age range, patients with a prior history of insomnia have been found consistently to be at significantly increased risk for severe depression. This could be interpreted in different ways including that sleep disturbance and the depression have a common underlying pathology, or that the sleep problems are an early sign of depression.
- A less fundamental role (but again implying preventative possibilities) is the suggestion that sleep deprivation late in pregnancy and in labour and childbirth at night might trigger post-natal depression.
- Abnormal circadian sleep–wake rhythms have been implicated in various depressive disorders including seasonal affective disorder (SAD). Light therapy has been used to correct the abnormality and relieve the depression and other symptoms.
- Disordered REM sleep mechanisms have (questionably) been considered as fundamental in the development of post-traumatic stress disorder symptoms.
- Some forms of attention-deficit hyperactivity disorder in children are attributed to persistent sleep disturbance.
- In a proportion of patients with schizophrenia, narcolepsy has been reported as the cause of their psychotic symptoms.

Disorders of sleep

Sleep complaints

The starting point for the clinician is the patient's sleep complaint. They are of three basic types:

- Not enough sleep, or unrefreshing sleep (**insomnia**).
- Sleeping too much (**excessive daytime sleepiness** or **hypersomnia**).
- Disturbed episodes during or otherwise related to sleep (**parasomnias**).

The detailed accounts later in this section are organized in relation to these main types of sleep complaint: insomnias (Chapter 4.14.2); excessive daytime sleepiness (Chapter 4.14.3); and parasomnias (Chapter 4.14.4). Sleep problems in childhood and adolescence are discussed in Chapter 9.2.9.

Whatever the clinical setting in which sleep complaints are investigated, the essential aim is to identify the specific sleep disorder from the many other conditions that can give rise to such complaints. Some sleep disorders may cause more than one type of complaint, and a patient may have more than one sleep disorder. The question arises how best to classify the many sleep disorders that have been described.

International classification of sleep disorders—second edition 2005 (ICSD-2)

This system, derived from wide international consultation, is the latest attempt to organize rationally the many ways in which sleep can be disturbed. ICSD-2 replaced the ICSD-Revised scheme outlined in the first edition of this textbook. More than 90 different sleep disorders are grouped as shown in Table 4.14.1.1. The grouping reflects the fact that knowledge about individual sleep disorders is very varied. The basic pathophysiology of some is quite well documented; in others little is known beyond their manifestations, and even they are subject to change as clinical observations improve. As a result, the ICSD-2 groupings are a mixture of those based on a common complaint (e.g. insomnia or hypersomnia), others on presumed aetiology (circadian rhythm sleep–wake disorders), and yet others are grouped according to the organ system from which the problems arise (such as sleep-related breathing disorders). Two additional groups in the system reflect current uncertainty about their status as disorders, or about their true nature.

Each sleep disorder is described in a standardized fashion using a series of sub-headings which include clinical features, demographics, pathology, and differential diagnosis. Treatments are not covered. Some publications are recommended concerning each sleep disorder. An attempt has been made throughout ICSD-2 to highlight aspects of sleep disorders of particular relevance to children.

In all, ICSD-2 provides a concise, easily accessible and up-to-date source of information for consultation by the clinician. Without being over-technical, it is more comprehensive and informative than current ICSD-10 and DSM-IV systems.

Sleep disorders mistaken for primarily psychological or psychiatric conditions

Sleep disorders manifest themselves in many ways. Failure to realize this can result in the misdiagnosis of primary sleep disorders as other types of clinical conditions of psychiatric, neurological, or otherwise medical conditions especially if there is limited familiarity with the sleep disorders field (which, unfortunately, is generally the case). Clearly such mistakes compromise patient care. The following are some of the main examples of this problem. Further details, with examples, are available elsewhere.[(3)]

Table 4.14.1.1 ICSD-2 groups of sleep disorders

I *Insomnias* The many psychological and physical causes of difficulty getting off to sleep, not staying asleep, early morning wakening, and feeling un-refreshed by sleep are included here including stress, poor sleep habits, and various mental and medical conditions.
II *Sleep-related breathing disorders* This group includes the common condition of obstructive sleep apnoea in adults and in children which often causes daytime sleepiness and other serious effects including changes in mood and behaviour. Central apnoea and various types of hypoventilation/hypoxaemic syndromes are also part of this group.
III *Hypersomnias of central origin not due to a circadian rhythm sleep disorder, sleep-related breathing disorder, or other cause of disturbed nocturnal sleep* Included here are narcolepsy and the causes of intermittent or recurrent hypersomnia such as the Kleine–Levin syndrome.
IV *Circadian rhythm sleep disorders* These disorders are characterized by a mistiming (and often disruption) of the sleep period, resulting in insomnia and/or hypersomnia. A prominent example is the delayed sleep phase syndrome common in adolescence. The advanced sleep phase syndrome can be seen in the elderly in which the sleep period begins in the evening with waking early when sleep requirements have been met. Irregular sleep–wake rhythms may be the result of an ill-organized way of life and substance abuse. Jet lag and nightshift work disorder are further examples of sleep problems caused by disturbance of the biological clock controlling the sleep–wake cycle.
V *Parasomnias* These are abnormal behaviours or sensations during or otherwise closely related to sleep. Many can be categorized according to the stage of sleep with which they are usually associated for example NREM sleep (sleepwalking) and REM sleep (nightmares, REM sleep behaviour disorder). Other parasomnias of particular psychiatric interest include sleep-related dissociative disorders and sleep-related eating disorders.
VI *Sleep-related movement disorders* These include the restless leg syndrome and periodic limb movement disorder.
VII *Isolated symptoms, apparently normal variants and unresolved issues*
VIII *Other sleep disorders* The classificatory scheme also includes an appendix on sleep disorders associated with conditions classifiable elsewhere such as sleep-related epilepsy, headaches, gastro-oesophageal reflux. A further appendix is concerned with other psychiatric and behavioural disorders frequently encountered in the differential diagnosis of sleep disorders. This appendix covers mood disorders, anxiety disorders, somatoform disorders, schizophrenia and other psychiatric disorders, personality disorders, and disorders of a psychiatric or behavioural type first diagnosed in infancy, childhood, or adolescence.

- Persistently not obtaining enough sleep, or having poor quality sleep because of interruptions by frequent subclinical arousals (as in obstructive sleep apnoea), is likely to cause tiredness, fatigue, irritability, poor concentration, impaired performance (possibly causing injuries or accidents at work or while driving), or depression. Out of the various possible explanations for such changes of behaviour, sleep disturbance may well be overlooked with failure to appreciate that, with improvement in sleep (which is usually possible with the right advice), such problems can be resolved. Occupational groups at special risk of sleep disturbance and its harmful effects include some clinicians.
- Excessive sleepiness, whatever its cause out of the many possibilities including physical conditions, is often misjudged as laziness, disinterest, daydreaming, lack of motivation, depression, intellectual inadequacy, or a number of other unwelcome states of mind. Sometimes, in very sleepy states, periods of 'automatic behaviour' occur, i.e. prolonged, complex, and possibly inappropriate behaviour with impaired awareness of events and, therefore, amnesia for them. Such episodes, the result of repeated 'microsleeps', can easily be misconstrued as reprehensible or dissociative features, misbehaviour, or prolonged seizure states. The paradoxical effect in young children of sleepiness causing over-activity has sometimes led to a diagnosis of attention-deficit hyperactivity disorder (ADHD) inappropriately treated with stimulant drugs instead of treatment for the sleep disorder.

A number of specific sleep disorders are at particular risk of being misinterpreted.

- In so-called delayed sleep phase syndrome, in which there is difficulty getting to sleep until very late, and problems getting up in the morning because of a shift in this timing of the sleep phase, is considered to be particularly common in adolescents who may be mistakenly thought to be awkward, lazy, irresponsible, or indulging in school refusal of the more usual type. In fact, this sleep disorder at that age is the result of a combination of normal pubertal biological body clock changes and alterations in lifestyle involving staying up late for social reasons or for study.
- It is not generally appreciated that even very complicated behaviour is possible whilst a person is still asleep as in sleepwalking episodes. Those with agitated sleepwalking or sleep terrors may appear to be very fearful and distressed and rush about and cry out as if escaping from danger. Other sleepwalkers develop an eating disorder with excessive weight gain due to the amount of food they consume while they are still asleep at night. Yet others behave in an aggressive or destructive way causing injury to themselves or other people and, at times sexual or other serious offences have been committed during a sleepwalking episode. If it is not known that such complicated actions are compatible with still being asleep, it is likely to be assumed that the person was awake at the time and aware of what he or she was doing, and, therefore, responsible for what had happened.
- Obstructive sleep apnoea is another case in point where this essentially physical disorder may be mistaken for being something very different from its true nature. The impairment of sleep quality, which characterizes this condition, can cause excessive daytime sleepiness, changes of personality, as well as adverse affects on social life and performance at work, as well as intellectual deterioration to the extent that dementia is suspected.
- Narcolepsy/cataplexy is also at serious risk of being misdiagnosed, sometimes for many years. Neurosis or depression is commonly mistaken for the narcolepsy symptoms.
- In REM sleep behaviour disorder there is a pathological retention of muscle tone during REM sleep so that a person can act out their dreams and behave violently if they have violent dreams. The dramatic behaviour that may result, including attacks on the sleeping partner, is easily misconstrued as intentional aggression.

- The complicated behaviour (far removed from that seen in other seizure states) that characterizes nocturnal frontal lobe epilepsy is often mistakenly thought to be evidence of a psychiatric disorder.
- In addition, sleep paralysis may be misconstrued as a psychotic disorder when (not uncommonly) accompanied by hallucinatory experiences.

In addition to sleep disorders being mistaken for psychiatric disorder, the opposite problem arises occasionally, that is some patients simulate excessive daytime sleepiness in order to avoid a psychologically troubling situation. Similarly, apparent parasomnias during sleep have sometimes been shown by polysomnography to occur when the patient is actually awake.

Detection and assessment of sleep disorders

As suggested earlier, evidence of a sleep disturbance should be actively sought in members of the general population and the various groups, including psychiatric patients, who are at special risk of sleep disorders. Otherwise, many instances of even severe sleep disturbance will continue to go unrecognized and untreated.

Sleep history

Routinely, all patients should be asked the following screening questions:

- Do you sleep long enough or well enough?
- Are you very sleepy during the day?
- Do you do unusual things or have strange experiences at night?

Ideally, their partner or other relatives should also be asked the same questions about the patient because the existence or severity of some forms of sleep disturbance are not known to the patient. In the case of children, parents are the main source of information but teachers' observations about daytime sleepiness or disturbance are also important.

If the answer to any of these enquiries is positive, a detailed sleep history is required. As traditional clinical history-taking schedules pay little attention to sleep, additional sleep-related enquiries will need to be made, covering the following points about the sleep problem.

- Precise nature of the sleep complaint, its onset, development, and current patterns.
- Medical or psychological factors at the onset of the sleep problem or which might have maintained it.
- Patterns of occurrence of the symptoms that is factors making them better or worse, weekdays compared to weekends, or work compared with holiday periods.
- Effect on mood, behaviour, work, social life, other family members.
- Past and present treatments for sleep problems and their effects.
- Past and present medication or other treatments for other illness or disorder.

In addition, detailed information is needed concerning the following:

- The patient's typical 24-h sleep–wake schedule. This can usually start with the evening meal, followed by preparation for and timing of bedtime, time and process of getting to sleep, events during the night, time and ease of waking up and getting up, level of alertness, and mental state and behaviour during the day.
- An attempt should be made to establish the duration, continuity, and timing of the patient's overnight sleep as these are the most important aspects of sleep for daytime functioning. It is also important to identify events of particular diagnostic significance, for example loud snoring.
- Sleep hygiene.

Compilation of a sleep history can be aided by the use of a preliminary sleep questionnaire (e.g. ref.[(4)]).

Sleep diary

Systematic recording in a booklet each day over 2 weeks or more, using a standardized format, avoids the bias or distortion of retrospective generalizations.

Other histories

Medical and psychiatric histories should include past and current treatment details (in view of the wide range of illnesses or disorders and their treatment with which sleep disturbance is associated). **Social history** should include occupational, marital, and recreational factors (drinking, smoking, drug use), which may affect sleep. **Family history** may be positive, for example in sleepwalking and associated arousal disorders.

Review of systems

Breathing difficulties and nocturia, for example, are associated with sleep disturbance. Severe obstructive sleep apnoea can cause cardio-respiratory and other cardiovascular complications.

Physical and mental state examination

Particular attention should be paid to the following:

- Evidence of any systemic illness including cardio-respiratory disease or neurological disorder (such as Parkinson's disease or stroke) which may disturb sleep.
- Obesity, oral and pharyngeal abnormalities, retrognathia, or mid-face deformity (predisposing to upper airway obstruction).
- Depression or other psychiatric disorder.
- Intellectual impairment, especially features of intellectual disability or dementia (including specific retardation syndromes) in view of their strong association with sleep disturbance.

Audio–video recording and actigraphy

Audio–video recordings can be very instructive in the parasomnias, sometimes revealing a very different picture than that provided in the clinic. Home video systems can be used where admission to hospital is not feasible. Similarly, monitoring of body movements via means of wrist-watch-like devices (**actigraphy**) can be used at home, if necessary, to quantify basic circadian sleep–wake patterns.

Polysomnography (PSG)

Physiological sleep studies are necessary for diagnosis in only the minority of sleep disorders. Traditionally this has entailed admission to a sleep laboratory. However, especially where such facilities are difficult to obtain, where the laboratory situation is unacceptable to patients (including some children or patients who are psychiatrically disturbed), **home PSG**, using portable systems, is useful, although the procedure has yet to be fully standardized and for some disorders is best seen as only a screening procedure. Recording in the home environment has the further advantage that, if the patient is allowed to adapt to the recording procedure before bedtime, the results from a single night's recording can be representative of the patient's habitual sleep. In contrast 'first night effects' are prominent in laboratory recordings and more than one night of polysomnography is required to allow adaptation to take place.

Basic polysomnography entails the recording of EEG, EOG, and EMG. This allows sleep to be staged and a hypnogram to be compiled as illustrated in Fig. 4.14.1.1. Usually the recording is made overnight but it may be continued during the day if required. Basic measures obtained from this information are as follows: total sleep time, time awake and number of awakenings, amount of REM and NREM sleep and their distribution overnight.

PSG can be extended to additional physiological measures, especially the following:

- Respiratory variables and audio–video recordings for sleep-related breathing problems.
- Additional EEG channels (combined with video) if nocturnal epilepsy is suspected.
- Anterior tibialis EMG for the detection of period limb movements in sleep.

Main indications for PSG are:

- The investigation of excessive daytime sleepiness, including the diagnosis of sleep apnoea, narcolepsy, or PLMS.
- The diagnosis of parasomnias where their nature is unclear from the clinical details, where PSG findings contribute essentially to the diagnosis (e.g. REM sleep behaviour disorder), where the possibility of epilepsy exists, or whether there may be more than one parasomnia present.
- As an objective check on the accuracy of the sleep complaint, or response to treatment.

Other investigations

Further laboratory investigations may be appropriate depending on the nature of the sleep problem and the purpose of the assessment.

- **A multiple sleep latency test (MSLT)**, involving the recording of basic PSG variables, quantifies the degree of daytime sleepiness by measuring the time a patient takes to fall asleep during five opportunities to do so during the day. In adults, a mean sleep latency of 5 min or less indicates pathological sleepiness (usually of organic origin); 5 to 10 min is a grey area which usually includes excessive sleepiness associated with primary psychiatric disorder; while longer than 10 min is normal. These values do not apply in children whose sleep tendency varies with age.
- **HLA typing**, and possibly **CSF hypocretin (orexin) levels** for the investigation of narcolepsy, and **nocturnal penile tumescence monitoring** in the differential diagnosis of organic versus psychogenic impotence, are examples of other specific tests that may be appropriate depending on the clinical problem.

Treatment approaches for sleep disorders

In clinical practice, the pharmacological approach to treatment of sleep problems (especially insomnia) is generally overemphasized, especially in the use of hypnotic-sedative drugs. Table 4.14.1.2 provides some indication of the wide range of available types of treatment, as well as general principles of management, for adults and children. They are roughly arranged in order of the frequency of their use in the comprehensive management of sleep disorders in general. An appropriate choice from this range requires an accurate diagnosis of the underlying sleep disorder. Further details are provided in later contributions to this section on sleep disorders. Claims for the effectiveness of these various measures are based on widespread clinical experience and reports. Few randomized controlled trials have not been published, as yet.

Certain aspects of treatment with special relevance to psychiatric practice are included in Table 4.14.1.3.

Clinical sleep disorders in psychiatric conditions

As mentioned earlier, sleep disturbance is a feature of many psychiatric disorders at all ages. Sometimes a sleep disturbance is profound and constitutes one of the defining characteristics of the psychiatric condition. This aspect of the psychiatric state requires careful definition and quite possibly treatment in its own right, alongside primarily psychiatric help, in order to facilitate recovery.

Table 4.14.1.3 outlines the main types of sleep problem or disorder associated with various psychiatric conditions. Emphasis has been placed on clinical sleep problems rather than PSG abnormalities which are seen in some of the conditions which (although interesting and of potential pathophysiological significance) are

Table 4.14.1.2 Examples of treatment approaches for sleep disorders in adults

General principles
Explain the problem, reassure where appropriate and provide support
Encourage good sleep hygiene (see Chapter 4.14.2)
Where possible treat the underlying cause of the sleep disturbance (e.g. medical or psychiatric disorder)
Take safety or protective measures (e.g. for hazardous parasomnias)
Specific behavioural treatments for insomnia (Chapter 4.14.2)
Chronotherapy (for circadian sleep-wake rhythm disorders)
Sleep phase retiming
Light therapy
Medication
Hypnotics (very selective and short-term)
Stimulants (narcolepsy)
Melatonin (for some circadian sleep–wake rhythm disorders)
Physical measures (e.g. for obstructive sleep apnoea)
Continuous positive airway pressure (CPAP)
Surgery (selected cases)

Table 4.14.1.3 Clinical sleep disturbance in psychiatric disorders

Psychiatric condition	Likely/possible sleep problem/disorder	Possible treatment issues/principles (see also text for general points)
Depression		*General* Emphasis on treatment of depression Possible sleep complications of ADs: drowsiness, insomnia (including SSRIs), RLS, PLMS, RBD
	Insomnia	Early treatment required to prevent worsening of depression Sedating ADs may be helpful
	EDS (minority)	More stimulating ADs may be appropriate Light therapy for SAD
Mania	Profound insomnia	Vigorous treatment required Mood-stimulating drugs may cause arousal disorders
Anxiety disorders	Insomnia and disrupted (poor quality) sleep PTSD nightmares Nocturnal panic attacks	In addition to behavioural treatments; larger dose of antipsychotics at bedtime may be helpful
Eating disorders	Insomnia (especially anorexia nervosa) EDS (especially bulimia nervosa) Sleepwalking with eating behaviours	General principles for insomnia (see Chapter 4.14.2) Possibly SSRIs See Chapter 4.14.4 for management of sleepwalking
Schizophrenia	Insomnia	Most neuroleptics promote sleep As in other psychotic states, behavioural sleep treatments and sleep hygiene are important
Alcohol and other substance abuse (including withdrawal states)	Insomnia including poor qualitysleep Disrupted sleep-wake cycle	Avoid sedative-hypnotic drugs Sleep hygiene principles (Chapter 4.14) and chronotherapy for sleep–wake cycle abnormalities
Alzheimer's disease and other dementing disorders	Progressive insomnia with fragmented sleep and sleep–wake cycle disorders including nocturnal agitated wandering	General principles for insomnia treatments; Sleep problems with some anti-dementia drugs Low-dose antipsychotics, if necessary Promote day–night cues including regular experience of daylight; discourage daytime napping
	RBD	Clonazepam
Child and adult ADHD	Insomnia	Stimulants can add to the sleep problem

KEY:

ADs = Antidepressants

ADHD = Attention-deficit hyperactivity disorder

EDS = Excessive daytime sleepiness

PLMS = Periodic limb movements in sleep

RBD = REM sleep behaviour disorder

RLS = Restless legs syndrome

SAD = Seasonal affective disorder

SSRI = Selective serotonin reuptake inhibitors

not necessarily accompanied by clinical manifestations. A prime example of this is the reduced time between onset of sleep and the start of the first REM sleep period ('REM latency') in certain forms of severe depression. This can be viewed as a type of biological marker which may persist even after the depression itself has lifted, and which may also be seen in relatives of a depressed person with this PSG finding without they themselves suffering from depression. However, the basic significance of reduced REM latency is, as yet, obscure and not helped by the fact that it has also been described in other psychiatric conditions, narcolepsy, following withdrawal from REM sleep-suppressing substances, during recovery from sleep deprivation, and a number of other diverse circumstances.

Another aspect of the pathophysiological relationship between sleep and mood which awaits clarification is a paradox that, while depression is usually associated with sleep disturbance and loss, sleep deprivation is reported to have an antidepressant effect in some patients although the effect does not persist beyond the period of depression.

Clinical sleep disorders associated with neurological and other medical illness

Of obvious relevance to psychiatric practice in general, but liaison psychiatry in particular, is the fact that disturbed sleep (often severe) is associated with many medical conditions. Main examples of this are shown in Table 4.14.1.4 together with mention of treatment issues in relation to each type of illness. Additional general considerations regarding treatment are as follows:

- The main emphasis in the management of sleep disorders in this context should be placed on the treatment of the medical

Table 4.14.1.4 Clinical sleep disturbance in neurological and other medical illness

Medical condition	Likely/possible sleep problem/disorder	Possible treatment issues/principles (see also text for general points)
Parkinson's disease and/or related syndromes	Progressive insomnia including poor quality sleep	Mainly behavioural treatment and sleep hygiene measures as in other insomnias (see Chapter 4.14.2)
	Parasomnias (e.g. nightmares, nocturnal hallucinations)	Consider possible effects of anti-Parkinson's medication on these and other sleep problems
	EDS including sleep attacks	Possibly daytime stimulants
	PLMS	Usual treatments for PLMS, if severe
	RBD	Clonazepam usually effective
Epilepsy	Disrupted sleep depending on type, cause, and severity	Sleep generally improves with seizure control
	EDS	Sedating AEDs can be a factor
Stroke	Insomnia OSA	Usual measures for insomnias
Head injury	Effects depend on type and severity	
	Poor quality sleep	Avoid respiratory depressant substances
	OSA, EDS	Usual measures for OSA (see Chapter 4.14.3)
Neuromuscular disease	OSA, EDS	As above
Tourette syndrome	Disrupted sleep Sleepwalking	Treatment of tic disorder should improve sleep
Cardiovascular disease		
Congestive heart failure	Central sleep apnoea, orthopnoea	Some antihypertensive, hypolipidaemic and antiarrythmic drugs can cause insomnia
Coronary heart disease	Nocturnal angina	Beta blockers can produce insomnia and nightmares
Respiratory disease		
COPD	Nocturnal dyspnoea	Hypnotics contraindicated in respiratory disease
Asthma	Nocturnal awakenings, EDS	Theophylline can cause insomnia
Gastrointestinal disorders (peptic ulcer, reflux oesophagitis)	Nocturnal awakenings	
Rheumatological disorders and other chronic pain conditions (including cancer)	Insomnia, disrupted sleep, EDS	Cortico-steroids and NSAI agents can disturb sleep Major analgesics have sedative effects Various anti-cancer drugs can disrupt sleep
Iron deficiency	PLMS RLS	Treat underlying condition
Endocrine disease		
Diabetes	Awakenings from nocturnia or painful peripheral neuropathy OSA	
Hyperthyroidism	Insomnia	
Myxoedema	OSA	
Chronic renal failure	Sleep disruption EDS OSA RLS and PLMS	Improvement with haemodialysis
ICU patients	Severe sleep disruption and deprivation including sleep–wake cycle disorders causing confusional and psychotic states	Cause of reason for intensive care relevant, plus sleep disrupting effect of ICU environment, procedures and medications
Obesity	OSA	Complications of obesity (e.g. diabetes, joint diseases) affect sleep

KEY

AED = Anti-epileptic drugs
COPD = Chronic obstructive pulmonary disease
EDS = Excessive daytime sleepiness
ICU = Intensive care unit
NSAI = Non-steroidal anti-inflammatory
OSA = Obstructive sleep apnoea
PLMS = Periodic limb movements in sleep
RBD = REM sleep behaviour disorder
RLS = Restless legs syndrome

condition itself, although additional treatment for the sleep disorder may well be required.

- Treatment for other, co-morbid conditions may well be needed, in particular anxiety and depression which will have their own adverse effects on sleep.
- Hypnotic drugs should be used very sparingly (especially in the elderly) because of their potential complications as described in Chapter 6.2.2. In view of their respiratory-depressand effects, benzodiazepines in particular are contraindicated in sleep apnoea and in the presence of other severe respiratory disease.
- The possible effects on sleep of over-the-counter medications also need to be considered. Nasal decongestants and anorectics are stimulants and can cause insomnia. The same is true of caffeine-containing drinks used as 'energy boosters'. Non-prescribed sleeping preparations (which usually contain anti-histamines) may well cause daytime drowsiness.

As mentioned earlier, the link between medical illness and sleep disturbance may operate in the opposite direction. For example, chronic sleep loss or disruption is associated with the development of such chronic health problems as coronary artery disease or diabetes.

Further information

Kryger, M.H., Roth, T., and Dement, W.C. (eds.) (2005). *Principles and practice of sleep medicine* (4th edn). Elsevier Saunders, Philadelphia, PA.

American Academy of Sleep Medicine. (2005). *The international classification of sleep disorders: diagnostic and coding manual* (2nd edn). American Academy of Sleep Medicine, Westchester, IL.

Colton, H.R. and Altevogt, B.M. (eds.) (2006). *Sleep disorders and sleep deprivation: an unmet public health problem*. National Academies Press, Washington, DC. Available from http.//www.nap.edu/catalog/ 11617 html

Shapiro, C. and McCall Smith, A. (eds.) (1997). *Forensic aspects of sleep*. Wiley, Chichester.

References

1. Bonnet, M.H. (2005). Acute sleep deprivation. In *Principles and practice of sleep medicine* (4th edn) (eds. M.H. Kryger, T. Roth, and W.C. Dement), pp. 51–6. Saunders, Philadelphia, PA.
2. Dinges, D.F., Rogers, N.L., and Baynard, M.D. (2005). Chronic sleep deprivation. In *Principles and practice of sleep medicine* (4th edn) (eds. M.H. Kryger, T. Roth, and W.C. Dement), pp. 67–76. W.B. Saunders, Philadelphia, PA.
3. Stores, G. (2007). Clinical diagnosis and misdiagnosis of sleep disorders (Review). *Journal of Neurology, Neurosurgery, and Psychiatry*, **78**, 1293–7.
4. Buysse, D.J., Reynolds, C.F., Monk, T.H., *et al.* (1989) The Pittsburgh sleep quality index: a new instrument for psychiatric practice and research. *Psychiatric Research*, **28**, 193–213.

4.14.2 Insomnias

Colin A. Espie and Delwyn J. Bartlett

Introduction

Most people's experiences of poor sleep are memorable, because sleeplessness and its daytime consequences are unpleasant. There are those, however, for whom insomnia is the norm. Persistent and severe sleep disturbance affects at least one in 10 adults and one in five older adults, thus representing a considerable public health concern. Sleep disruption is central to a number of medical and psychiatric disorders, and insomnia is usually treated by general practitioners. Therefore differential diagnosis is important, and respiratory physicians, neurologists, psychiatrists, and clinical psychologists need to be involved. The purpose of this chapter is to summarize current understanding of the insomnias, their appraisal, and treatment. Particular emphasis will be placed upon evidence-based practical management.

Clinical features

Insomnia often remains unreported, and finally presents when a poor sleep pattern is well established. Alcohol has long been a first-line self-administered sleep aid, and recent years have seen an increasing use of 'over-the-counter' preparations and 'self-help' strategies. The clinical presentation is commonly of a frustrated patient, trapped in a vicious circle of anxiety and poor sleep, who reports having 'tried everything'.[1,2]

There may be concern about the pattern of sleep. This is the most quantifiable aspect of self-report relating to, for example, length of time taken to fall asleep, frequency and duration of wakenings, or total amount of sleep. A poorly established sleep pattern can lead to unpredictability of what sleep will be like on any given night. Patients often report poor quality of sleep, and subjective perceived quality can be a critically important outcome variable. Typical reports relate to light sleep and sleep felt to be unrestorative. Although it may be unclear how such complaints relate to EEG sleep architecture, the clinician should not overlook qualitative report as it may reflect underlying pathophysiology. Concerns are normally expressed also about the daytime effects of poor sleep. These can be cognitive effects, such as fatigue, sleepiness, inattention, and some impairments in performance, or emotional effects, such as irritability and anxiety.[2]

Classification

The *International Classification of Sleep Disorders* (second edition: **ICSD-2**)[3] was published in 2005 and provides the most comprehensive account of sleep disorders, both for descriptive purposes and for differential diagnosis (see Chapter 4.14.1). ICSD-2 describes insomnias as disorders of initiating and maintaining sleep. Patients may have either sleep-onset problems or wakenings from sleep, or both of these. Table 4.14.2.1 summarizes the principal classifications that relate to the insomnias, along with some other sleep disorders where patients commonly present with insomnia symptoms. As can be seen, concomitant symptomatology, potential aetiological factors, and sleeplessness require careful assessment in order to reach a valid diagnosis.

Table 4.14.2.1 The classification and differential diagnosis of the insomnias within ICSD-2

Classification	Sleep disorder	Essential features, complaint of insomnia plus
Insomnias	Psychophysiological insomnia	Learned sleep preventing associations, conditioned arousal, 'racing mind' phenomenon
	Paradoxical insomnia	Complaint of poor sleep disproportionate to sleep pattern and sleep duration
	Idiopathic insomnia	Insomnia typically begins in childhood or from birth
	Insomnia due to a mental disorder	Course of sleep disturbance concurrent with mental disorder
	Inadequate sleep hygiene	Daily living activities inconsistent with maintaining good-quality sleep
	Insomnia due to a medical disorder	Course of sleep disturbance concurrent with mental disorder
	Insomnia due to drug or substance	Sleep disruption caused by prescription medication, recreational drug, caffeine, alcohol or foodstuff
	Adjustment insomnia	Presence of identifiable stressor, insomnia resolves or is expected to resolve when stressor is removed
Sleep-related breathing disorders	Obstructive sleep apnoea syndrome	Excessive sleepiness, obstructed breathing in sleep, associated symptoms include snoring and a dry mouth
	Periodic limb movement disorder	Episodes of repetitive, highly stereotyped limb movements occurring in sleep
	Restless legs syndrome	Strong, nearly irresistible urge to move legs relieved by walking
Circadian rhythm sleep disorders	Delayed sleep phase type	Phase delay of major sleep episode, initial insomnia, excessive sleepiness in morning
	Advanced sleep-phase type	Phase advance of major sleep episode, inability to stay awake in evening, early wakening

Diagnosis and differential diagnosis

Severity of insomnia is judged along dimensions of frequency, intensity, and duration, as well as impact on daytime functioning and quality of life. Generally, the criteria for severe and chronic insomnia are a minimum duration of 6 months with problems presenting three or more nights per week. Restlessness, irritability, anxiety, daytime fatigue, and tiredness commonly accompany such presentations.(2) Mild and moderate insomnia may be diagnosed where problems are less intrusive.

Most patients presenting with insomnia have psychophysiological difficulty initiating and/or maintaining sleep. Usually marked functional effects and somatized tension associated with sleep are evident. The patient reports extreme tiredness while being unable to sleep satisfactorily and appears preoccupied with sleep and its consequences. This contrasts, for example, with the circadian disorders where, in delayed sleep-phase type, the patient may not feel sleepy until late in the normal sleep period, and in advanced sleep-phase type, may waken early and be unable to return to sleep. Taking a history, incorporating screening questions on restlessness, limb movements, and breathing can help to diagnose obstructive sleep apnoea syndrome, periodic limb movement disorder, and restless legs syndrome, although full polysomnographic evaluation may also be required.(4) However, polysomnography is not essential for the diagnosis of insomnia, for which sleep diary monitoring (see Chapter 4.14.1) is usually the most useful form of assessment.(2) Wrist actigraphy is an inexpensive objective evaluation, which estimates sleep/wakefulness based upon body movement.(5) Continuous recordings can be made over 5 to 10 consecutive 24 h periods. It is useful in identifying paradoxical insomnia, and charted data can be inspected for circadian anomalies.

Other causes of insomnia are reported in Table 4.14.2.1 and should not be overlooked. In particular, insomnias due to a drug or substance can include hypnotic-dependent sleep disorder, associated most commonly with benzodiazepine (BZ) drugs where withdrawal leads to exacerbation of the primary problem.(6) This can be mistaken for a severe underlying insomnia and hence reinforce hypnotic dependency. Likewise, a wide range of psychiatric conditions, particularly affective disorders, has associated sleep symptomatology (see Chapter 4.14.1). A primary diagnosis of psychophysiological insomnia cannot be made where diagnostic criteria for DSM-IV Axis I or Axis II disorders are fulfilled. However, it is very important to note that sleep disturbance often precedes depression. The bulk of the psychiatric epidemiological data indicate that insomnia is an independent risk factor for first episode depressive illness, and for recurrence of depression, in adults of all ages.(7,8) Insomnia should not be assumed to be simply a symptom of underlying depression, even when depression is present. Unless the illness courses clearly co-vary it is best to make a diagnosis of co-morbid insomnia. Similar caveats apply to insomnia associated with medical disorders, both in terms of identifying a primary illness, and concluding that insomnia has *the* status of an associated/ co-morbid disorder (see Chapter 4.14.1).

Epidemiology

Insomnia affects one-third of adults occasionally, and 9 to 12 per cent on a chronic basis. It is more common in women, in shift workers, and in patients with medical and psychiatric disorders. Prevalence amongst older adults has been estimated at up to 25 per cent and sleepiness and hypnotic drugs are risk factors for injury and fracture.(9) The decline in prescription of anxiolytics has been greater than the rate of decline for hypnotics [taking BZ and benzodiazepine receptor agonists (BzRAs) together]. Furthermore, there is increasing use of (off-label) sedative antidepressants primarily to treat insomnia.

Aetiology

Many patients report having been marginal light sleepers before developing insomnia.(4) Sleep disturbance often arises during life change or stress, and such adjustment sleep disorder may represent a normal transient disruption of sleep. However, secondary factors, such as anxiety over sleep and faulty sleep–wake conditioning, may exacerbate and maintain the insomnia as a chronic problem when sleep itself becomes a focus for concern. People with insomnia may be hyperaroused relative to normal sleepers, for example having higher levels of cortisol and ACTH, and also find it difficult to 'down-regulate' their arousal at bedtime.[2,10,11]

Course and prognosis

There has been little research on the natural course of insomnia. However, untreated psychophysiological insomnia can last for decades, and may gradually worsen over time. Indeed, there is a developmental trend for sleep pattern to deteriorate, with increasing age. On the other hand, delayed sleep-phase syndrome and insufficient sleep hygiene can be associated with lifestyle problems and may ameliorate as these are resolved. Although certain insomnias *tend* to persist if untreated, prognosis with effective treatment can be very good.

Treatment

A review of the evidence

(a) Drug therapy

Traditionally, insomnia has been treated pharmacologically. Barbiturates were superseded by BZ compounds during the 1960s and 1970s. These drugs were safer in overdose, were thought to have fewer side effects, and to be less *addictive*. Controlled studies have demonstrated that a considerable number of BZ, of short to intermediate half-life, are effective hypnotic agents. However, from the mid-1970s potential problems became apparent, both during administration and withdrawal. Longer-acting hypnotics were prone to carry-over effects of morning lethargy, and shorter-acting drugs to 'rebound insomnia'.[6] Furthermore, tolerance develops, leading either to increased dosing or switching to alternative medication. Although BZs used for short periods/intermittently can maintain effectiveness, these are not the treatment of choice in chronic insomnia,[12] and are contraindicated in older adults and where insomnia may involve sleep-related breathing disorder because of their potentially depressant effects on respiration. A number of BZ compounds have been removed from the market in the United Kingdom, United States, and elsewhere.

Contemporary hypnotic therapy has extended to include BzRAs (often referred to as the 'z' drugs), and more recently melatonin receptor agonists (MeRAs) have been introduced. Whereas the place in therapeutics of MeRAs has yet to become established, the BzRAs are often thought to offer more sustained benefit for insomnia, and to have fewer adverse effects. Nevertheless, there remains uncertainty about the effectiveness of BzRAs in chronic insomnia.[13]

(b) Psychological therapy

Psychological treatment for chronic insomnia, primarily in the form of cognitive behavioural therapy (CBT), has been extensively investigated in over 100 controlled studies during the past 20 years. Five meta-analyses and numerous systematic reviews have demonstrated that CBT is associated with large effect size changes (measured in standardized *z* scores) in the primary symptom measures of sleep latency (difficulty getting to sleep) and wake time after sleep-onset (difficulty remaining asleep).[14,15] Around 70 per cent of patients with persistent sleep problems appear to benefit from CBT and effects are maintained to long-term follow-up. It is thought that CBT achieves these outcomes because it tackles directly the dysfunctional thoughts and maladaptive behaviours that otherwise maintain insomnia. Recent controlled studies have shown that CBT may be effective in general practice settings with nurses delivering the intervention according to a standard protocol.[16,17] Despite the superior efficacy of CBT relative to medication for insomnia, and these recent demonstrations of CBT working in real-world settings, practical problems remain in making CBT widely available.

Within the CBT model, a number of strategies have strong empirical support. Behavioural procedures such as stimulus control and sleep restriction, and cognitive strategies such as paradoxical intention and thought restructuring have been extensively investigated[2,14,15] and are outlined briefly below.

(c) Melatonin, light therapy, and exercise

The pineal hormone melatonin has been the subject of highly publicized claims. However, scientific research has been limited. Several controlled studies support its sleep-promoting effects, but the use of melatonin continues to be controversial. At best it may be useful as a chronobiotic for reducing sleep latency.[18] Several MeRA products are currently under formal evaluation, so more data may be available soon.

Bright light is a potent marker for human circadian rhythms, and has been known for some time to enable the resetting of such rhythms in advanced sleep-phase syndrome and delayed sleep-phase syndrome.[19] The results of studies investigating the efficacy of bright light against psychological treatments for psychophysiological insomnia are awaited. A limiting factor to the value of light therapy is that continued treatment may be required to maintain therapeutic effects.

Athletic people sleep well, although this may be more to do with behavioural patterning than aerobic fitness. Nevertheless, there is evidence that exercise can have positive effects upon sleep quality, particularly if taken late afternoon or early evening, and in otherwise relatively fit individuals.[20] Morning exercise can also be an effective modality to encourage the same waking time and early morning light exposure; which help to reset sleep patterns on a daily basis.

Advice about management

(a) General perspective

Non-pharmacological treatment using CBT procedures should be preferred over pharmacological treatment, in cases of severe persistent insomnia. Hypnotic agents should be recommended mainly for short-term or occasional use, although longer-term trial data are now becoming available. The practitioner should be aware of morning-after effects, and potential problems of withdrawal and dependency, not only with BZs but also possibly with BzRAs. Psychological intervention may also facilitate reduction or discontinuation of medication in hypnotic-dependent person with insomnias.[21] There is limited support for the use of melatonin or exercise as treatments of choice, although light therapy seems effective for circadian disorders.

(b) Using cognitive behavioural therapies

Brief descriptions of effective management strategies are presented in Tables 4.14.2.2 and 4.14.2.3. The following text provides

Table 4.14.2.2 Summary description of sleep hygiene and education components for the treatment of chronic insomnia

Components of sleep education
The need for sleep and its functions
Sleep patterns across the lifespan
Sleep as a process with stages/phases
Factors adversely affecting steep
The effects of sleep loss
The concept of insomnia
Measuring sleep and sleep problems
Components of sleep hygiene treatment
Bedroom comfortable for sleep
Regular exercise, timing, and fitness
Stable and appropriate diet
Undesirable effects of caffeine and other stimulants
Moderation of alcohol consumption
Other common 'self-help' strategies

explanation of underlying psychological models and further information on implementation.

(i) Sleep education and sleep hygiene

The simple provision of information ameliorates the sense of being out of control. Inaccurate attributions are challenged and misunderstandings corrected by understanding what sleep is, how ommon insomnia can be, how sleep changes with age, good sleep hygiene practices, and some facts about sleep loss. Similarly, sleep hygiene provides patients with a starting point for self-management. These techniques are best construed as introductory but they will not of themselves treat insomnia effectively.

Table 4.14.2.3 Summary description of cognitive behavioural components for the treatment of chronic insomnia

Components of stimulus control and sleep restriction treatment
Define individual sleep requirements
Establish parameters for bedtime period (threshold time and rising time)
Eliminate daytime napping
Differentiate rest from sleep
Schedule sleep periods with respect to needs
Establish 7 day per week compliance
Remove incompatible activity from bedroom environment
Rise from bed if wakeful (>20 min)
Avoid recovery sleep as 'compensation'
Establish stability from night to night
Adjust the sleep period as sleep efficiency improves
Components of cognitive intervention
Identify thought patterns and content that intrude
Address (mis)attributions connecting sleep and waking life
Establish rehearsal/planning time in early evening
Relaxation and imagery training
Distraction and thought blocking
Develop accurate beliefs/attributions about sleep and sleep loss
Challenge negative and invalid thoughts
Eliminate 'effort' to control sleep
Motivate to maintain behaviour and cognitive change
Utilize relapse-prevention techniques

(ii) Stimulus control treatment

Stimulus control increases the bedroom's cueing potential for sleep. For good sleepers, the pre-bedtime period and the stimulus environment trigger positive associations of sleepiness and sleep. For the poor sleeper, however, the bedroom triggers associations with restlessness and lengthy night-time wakening via a stimulus-response relationship, thereby continuing to promote wakefulness and arousal. The model is similar to phobic conditions where a conditioned stimulus precipitates an anxiety response.

Treatment involves removing from the bedroom all stimuli which are potentially sleep-incompatible. Reading and watching television, for example, are confined to living rooms. Sleeping is excluded from living areas and from daytime, and wakefulness is excluded from the bedroom. The individual is instructed to get up if not asleep within 15–20 min or if wakeful during the night. Conceptually, stimulus control is a reconditioning treatment which forces discrimination between daytime and sleeping environments.

(iii) Sleep restriction therapy

Sleep restriction restricts sleep to the length of time which the person is likely to sleep. This may be equivalent to promoting 'core sleep' at the expense of 'optional sleep'. Sleep restriction primarily aims to improve sleep efficiency. Since sleep efficiency is the ratio of time asleep to time in bed, it can be improved either by increasing the numerator (time spent asleep) or by reducing the denominator (time spent in bed). People with insomnia generally seek the former, but this may not be necessary, either biologically or psychologically. Sleep restriction first involves recording in a sleep diary and calculating average nightly sleep duration. The aim, then, is to obtain this average each night. This is achieved by setting rising time as an 'anchor' each day and delaying going to bed until a 'threshold time' which permits this designated amount of sleep. Thus, the sleep period is compressed and sleep efficiency is likely to increase. The permitted 'sleep window' can then be titrated week-by-week in 15 increments in response to sleep efficiency improvements.

(iv) Cognitive control

This technique aims to deal with thought material in advance of bedtime and to reduce intrusive bedtime thinking. The person with insomnia is asked to set aside 15 to 20 min in the early evening to rehearse the day and to plan ahead for tomorrow; thus putting the day to rest. It is a technique for dealing with unfinished business and may be most effective for rehearsal, planning, and self-evaluative thoughts which are important to the individual and which, if not dealt with, may intrude during the sleep-onset period.

(v) Thought suppression

Thought-stopping and articulatory suppression attempt to interrupt the flow of thoughts. No attempt is made to deal with thought material *per se* but rather to attenuate thinking. With articulatory suppression the patient is instructed to repeat, subvocally, the word 'the' every 3 s. This procedure is derived from the experimental psychology literature. Articulatory suppression is thought to occupy the short-term memory store used in the processing of information. The type of material most likely to respond is repetitive but non-affect-laden thoughts, not powerful enough to demand attention. Additionally, this technique may be useful during the night to enable rapid return to sleep.

(vi) Imagery and relaxation

There is a wide range of relaxation methods including progressive relaxation, imagery training, biofeedback, meditation, hypnosis, and autogenic training, but little evidence to indicate superiority of any one approach. Furthermore, there is little evidence to support either the presumption that people with insomnia are hyperaroused in physiological terms, or that relaxation has its effect through autonomic change. At the cognitive level, these techniques may act through distraction and the promotion of mastery. During relaxation, the mind focuses upon alternative themes such as visualized images or physiological responses. In meditation the focus is upon a 'mantra' and in self-hypnosis upon positive self-statements. Relaxation may be effective for thought processes that are anxiety-based, confused, and which flit from topic-to-topic.

(vii) Cognitive restructuring

Cognitive restructuring challenges faulty beliefs which maintain wakefulness and the helplessness which many people with insomnia report. It appears to work through appraisal by testing the validity of assumptions against evidence and real-life experience. As an evaluative technique, it may be effective with beliefs that are irrational but compelling. If such thoughts, for example 'I am going to be incapable at work tomorrow', are not challenged, they will create high levels of preoccupation and anxiety and sleep is unlikely to occur. With cognitive restructuring, the person with insomnia learns alternative responses to replace inaccurate thinking.

(viii) Paradoxical intention

Finally, the technique of paradoxical intention is useful in situations where performance anxiety has developed, that is, where the effort to produce a response inhibits that response itself. The paradoxical instruction is to allow sleep to occur naturally through passively attempting to remain quietly wakeful rather than attempting to fall asleep. Paradox may be regarded as a decatastrophizing technique since it appears to act upon the ultimate anxious thought (of remaining awake indefinitely) initially by focusing on and enhancing this thought (a habituation model) and then subjecting it to appraisal through rationalization and experience. By intending to remain awake, and failing to do so, the strength of the sleep drive is re-established, and performance effort is reduced.

Possibilities for prevention

There is insufficient knowledge of the natural course of transient sleep disorders. Mention has been made of adjustment sleep disorder and of the association of life events and stressors with the onset of insomnia. Systematic research is required to establish the 'setting conditions' for the secondary maintenance of insomnia beyond an initial normative reaction to events. Perhaps there is an interaction with a predisposing tendency to light sleep, or with introspection and worry. The instinct to increase opportunity to sleep (spend longer in bed to catch up) when insomnia symptoms develop should probably be resisted. If anything it may be better to advise patients to limit sleep opportunity so that their pattern knits together again more quickly.

The establishment and maintenance of a regular 'tight' routine, both pre-bedtime and in terms of sleep schedule, seem to be important preventive factors. Such chronobehavioural functioning can be at risk of disruption by, for example, jet lag, shift work, weekend patterns differing from weekday, adolescent lifestyle, and retirement. Adherence to, and/or reinstatement of, an adaptive pattern seems crucial.

It is important not to underestimate the importance of attitudes and beliefs in the presentation of insomnia. Exaggerated or emotionally and mentally arousing thoughts should be dealt with promptly. Sleep loss can be distressing, but patients should be reminded that nature seeks to restore equilibrium. What they need to do is to provide the conditions under which sleep can occur rather than attempt directly to control the sleep process. Expectations are important also, since it is the breach of these which generally give rise to anxiety and dysfunctional beliefs about sleep requirements. More often than not sleep-related expectations are unrealistic and require reappraisal, even more so in older adults.

Finally, prevention should be extended to the known extrinsic causes of certain sleep disorders. Where alcohol, stimulants, or proprietary drugs interfere with sleep and the recovery of the normal sleep process, attention should be paid to these factors. Better still, patients should be encouraged to seek advice early rather than go down the path of self-administered treatment. Avoiding the use of hypnotic agents, both in general practice and during acute admissions to hospital, would substantially reduce the number of iatrogenic cases of chronic insomnia.

Further information

Espie, C.A. (2006). *Overcoming insomnia and sleep problems: a self-help guide using cognitive behavioral techniques*. Constable & Robinson Ltd, London [ISBN13: 978-184529-070-2/ ISBN10: 1-84529-070-4].

Perlis, M.L. and Lichstein, K.L. (2003). *Treating sleep disorders: principles and practice of behavioral sleep medicine*. John Wiley & Sons, Inc. Hoboken, NJ [ISBN0-47-44343-3].

Morin, C.M., Bootzin, R.R., Buysse, D.J., *et al.* (2006). Psychological and behavioural treatment of insomnia. Update of the recent evidence (1998–2004) prepared by a Task Force of the American Academy of Sleep Medicine. *Sleep*, **29**, 1398–414.

Morin, C.M. and Espie, C.A. (2003). *Insomnia: a clinical guide to assessment and treatment.* Kluwer Academic/ Plenum Publishers, New York [ISBN 0-306-47750-5].

References

1. Espie, C.A. (1991). *The psychological treatment of insomnia.* Wiley, Chichester.
2. Morin, C.M. and Espie, C.A. (2003). *Insomnia: a clinical guide to assessment and treatment.* Kluwer Academic/Plenum Publishers, New York.
3. American Academy of Sleep Medicine. (2005). *International classification of sleep disorders: diagnostic and coding manual* (2nd edn). AASM, Westchester, IL.
4. Reite, M., Buysse, D., Reynolds, C., *et al.* (1995). The use of polysomnography in the evaluation of insomnia. *Sleep*, **18**, 58–70.
5. Ancoli-Israel, S., Cole, R., Alessi, C., *et al.* (2003). The role of actigraphy in the study of sleep and circadian rhythms. *Sleep*, **26**, 342–92.
6. Kripke, D. (2000). Hypnotic drugs: deadly risks, doubtful benefits. *Sleep Medicine Reviews*, 2000, **4**, 5–20.

7. Cole, M.G. and Dendukuri, N. (2003). Risk factors for depression among elderly community subjects: a systematic review and meta-analysis. *The American Journal of Psychiatry*, **160**, 1147–56.
8. Riemann, D. and Voderholzer, U. (2003). Primary insomnia: a risk factor to develop depression? *Journal of Affective Disorders*, **76**, 255–9.
9. Lichstein, K.L., Durrence, H.H., Reidel, B.W., *et al.* (2004). *The epidemiology of sleep: age, gender and ethnicity*. Lawrence Erlbaum Associates, Mahwah, NJ.
10. Espie, C.A. (2002). Insomnia: conceptual issues in the development, persistence and treatment of sleep disorder in adults. *Annual Review of Psychology*, **53**, 215–43.
11. Perlis, M.L., Pigeon, W., and Smith, M.T. (2005). Etiology and pathophysiology of insomnia. In *The principles and practice of sleep medicine* (4th edn) (eds. M.H. Kryger, T. Roth, and W.C. Dement), pp. 714–25. W.B. Saunders, Philadelphia.
12. NIH. (2005). *State-of-the-science conference statement on manifestations and management of chronic insomnia in adults*. National Institutes of Health, Vol. 22, Number 2. Natcher Conference Center, Bethesda Maryland, USA.
13. NICE. (2004). *Guidance on the use of zaleplon, zolpidem and zopiclone for the short-term management of insomnia*. Technology Appraisal Guidance No.77. National Institute for Clinical Excellence, London.
14. Smith, M.T., Perlis, M.L., Park, A., *et al.* (2002). Behavioral treatment vs pharmacotherapy for insomnia—a comparative meta-analysis. *The American Journal of Psychiatry*, **159**, 5–11.
15. Morin, C.M., Bootzin, R.R., Buysse, D.J., *et al.* (2006). Psychological and behavioural treatment of insomnia. Update of the recent evidence (1998–2004) prepared by a Task Force of the American Academy of Sleep Medicine. *Sleep*, **29**, 1398–414.
16. Espie, C.A., Inglis, S.J., Tessier, S., *et al.* (2001). The clinical effectiveness of cognitive behaviour therapy for chronic insomnia: implementation and evaluation of a Sleep Clinic in general medical practice. *Behaviour Research and Therapy*, **39**, 45–60.
17. Espie, C.A., MacMahon, K.M.A., and Kelly, H.L. (2007). Randomised clinical effectiveness trial of nurse-administered small group CBT for persistent insomnia in general practice. *Sleep*, **30**, 574–84.
18. Mendelson, W.B. (1997). A critical evaluation of the hypnotic efficacy of melatonin. *Sleep*, **20**, 916–19.
19. Czeisler, C.A., Johnson, M.P., Duffy, J.F., *et al.* (1990). Exposure to bright light and darkness to treat physiologic maladaptation to night work. *The New England Journal of Medicine*, **322**, 1253–8.
20. Singh, N.A., Clements, K.M., and Fiatarone, M.A. (1997). A randomized controlled trial of the effect of exercise on sleep. *Sleep*, **20**, 95–101.
21. Morgan, K., Dixon, S., Mathers, M., *et al.* (2003). Psychological treatment for insomnia in the management of long-term hypnotic drug use: a pragmatic randomised controlled trial. *The British Journal of General Practice*, **53**, 923–8.

4.14.3 Excessive sleepiness

Michel Billiard

Introduction

Excessive sleepiness is not an homogeneous concept. It can manifest itself as bouts of sleepiness, irresistible and refreshing sleep episodes, abnormal lengthening of night sleep with a major difficulty waking up in the morning or at the end of a nap or even periods of a week or so of almost continuous sleep recurring at several months' intervals.

According to the recent second edition of the *International Classification of Sleep Disorders* (*ICSD*-2),[1] disorders of excessive sleepiness are distributed within three chapters: sleep-related breathing disorders, hypersomnias of central origin not due to a circadian rhythm sleep disorder, sleep-related breathing disorders, or other cause of disturbed nocturnal sleep, and circadian rhythm sleep disorders.

However in this volume aimed at psychiatrists, the presentation of disorders of excessive sleepiness will obey another logic. Following "Generalities" including epidemiology, morbidity, clinical work-up, and laboratory tests, the various aetiologies will be presented according to the following six subchapters:

- Hypersomnia not due to substance or known physiological condition (non-organic hypersomnia or psychiatric hypersomnia)
- Hypersomnia due to drug or substance
- Behaviourally induced insufficient sleep syndrome
- Hypersomnia in the context of sleep-related breathing disorders
- Hypersomnias of central origin
- And the special case of delayed sleep phase syndrome.

Epidemiology

Contrary to common thinking, excessive sleepiness is neither exceptional nor rare. Epidemiological surveys generally agree on a figure of severe sleepiness (daily and embarrassing) in 5 per cent of the general population and of moderate sleepiness (occasional) in another 15 per cent.[2] Interestingly, only a fraction of these subjects are aware of their condition, due to the fact that they progressively lose reference to a normal state of alertness. As a consequence many subjects will not consult their physician for excessive sleepiness but will be brought to him by the spouse, worried about his or her falling asleep repeatedly in the middle of the day, or even referred by the company's doctor due to unexplained car accidents or poor work efficiency.

Morbidity

Excessive sleepiness has a severe impact on the life of patients. Nearly half of the patients with excessive sleepiness report automobile accidents. Many have lost jobs because of their sleepiness. In addition, sleepiness is disruptive of family life. Cognitive function is also impaired by sleepiness. In children excessive sleepiness has been associated with learning disability and in adults memory problems are frequent.

Clinical work-up and laboratory tests

Whatever the circumstance of the first visit, the patient should be interviewed on the history of excessive sleepiness, the type and severity of it, the associated symptoms, the familial and occupational consequences, the past and current treatments, and the personal and familial medical past-history.

In addition, the subject will complete a self-administered behavioural scale, the Epworth sleepiness scale. This scale asks the subject to rate the probability of dozing from 0 (would never doze) to

3 (high chance of dozing) in eight more or less soporific daily situations. A score of over 10 is taken to indicate abnormal sleepiness.

The subject will then undergo a physical and psychological examination.

Laboratory tests will be chosen according to the clinical impression.

The most frequently used test is the *multiple sleep latency test* (MSLT). The test was developed on the basis of the following principle. The sleepier the subject, the faster he falls asleep. The test is based on 20 min polygraphic recordings (EEG, EOG, EMG) repeated every 2 h (four or five times a day) starting 2 h about after morning awakening. The global sleepiness index is provided by the mean latency to sleep in the four or five tests. A sleep laboratory of less than 5 min indicates pathologic sleepiness, a sleep latency from 10 to 20 min is considerd as normal, and latencies falling between the normal and the pathological values are considered as a diagnostic grey area.

Another test, the *maintenance of wakefulness test* (MWT), is a variant of the MSLT. It was designed to evaluate treatment efficiency in patients with excessive sleepiness. The major difference with the MSLT is in the instruction given to the test subject. The subject being tested is told to attempt to remain awake. The subject is seated in comfortable position in bed, as opposed to lying down in the MSLT, with low lighting behind him (7.5 W at 1 m). Specific recommendations include using a four-trial, 40 min version of the MWT. A mean sleep latency of less than 8 min on the 40 min MWT is abnormal and scores between 8 and 40 min are of uncertain significance.

Prolonged polysomnographic recordings, obtained by either traditional laboratory polysomnographic monitoring or ambulatory recordings, provide a good picture of the actual time asleep within the 24 h period. However, this procedure is neither validated nor standardized.

In addition, whenever there is some doubt about the possibility of hypersomnia associated with a psychiatric disorder, a *psychometric/psychiatric evaluation* will be performed.

Aetiology and treatment

Hypersomnia not due to substance or known physiological condition

It explains about 5 to 7 per cent of cases of hypersomnia seen in sleep disorders centres. Women are more susceptible than men.

Excessive daytime sleepiness is reported. Subjects show an elevated score on the Epworth sleepiness scale. Night sleep is perceived as non-restorative and generally of poor quality. Patients are often intensely focused on their hypersomnia, and psychiatric symptoms typically become apparent only after prolonged interview or psychometric testing. Poor work attendance, abruptly leaving work because of a perceived need to sleep are common. Polysomnography typically shows a prolonged sleep latency, an increased wake time after sleep onset, and a low sleep efficiency. REM latency may be shortened in the case of bipolar disorder. Contrasting with the elevated score on the Epworth sleepiness scale, sleep latency on the MSLT is often within normal limits. A 24 h continuous sleep recording typically shows considerable time spent in bed during day and night, a behaviour referred to as clinophilia, from the Greek κλινη (bed) and φιλεω (love).

Psychiatric interview is essential to diagnose the underlying condition. Causative psychiatric conditions include bipolar type II disorder, dysthymic disorder, undifferentiated somatoform disorder, adjustment disorder, or personality disorder.

Conventional drugs such as antidepressants or anxiolytics are often insufficient. Modafinil, an awakening drug given at a daily dose of 100 to 200 mg, is usually active.

In the group of psychiatric disorders a separate place should be reserved to seasonal affective disorder remarkable for episodes of major depression occurring only during the winter months, associated with fatigue, loss of concentration, increased appetite for carbohydrates, weight gain, and increased sleep duration. Morning bright light treatment (2500 lux for 2 h) is efficient.

Hypersomnia due to drug or substance

A wide spectrum of medications used in psychiatry may be responsible for excessive sleepiness.

(a) Anxiolytics and hypnotics

Benzodiazepines have sedative effects, but these effects vary with dose, administration (single or repeated dose), age, and state of the subject (normal, anxious, or depressed). Non-benzodiazepines usually induce limited sleepiness only.

(b) Antidepressants

Tricyclic antidepressants have sedative properties depending on the molecule, dose, and the subject to whom they are administered. SSRI can also induce sleepiness with high within-patient variability. Venlafaxin, a serotonine, and norepinephrine reuptake blocker may induce excessive sleepiness.

(c) Neuroleptics

The degree of sedation varies widely from subject to subject. Empirically, three-fourth of the patients treated with neuroleptic phenothiazines experience sleepiness in a dependent manner. Among the newer agents clozapine is the most sedating drug, followed by olanzapine and quetiapine. Risperidone and sertindole are less sedating drugs.

Behaviourally induced insufficient sleep syndrome

According to ICSD-2, this syndrome occurs when an individual persistently fails to obtain the amount of sleep required to maintain normal levels of alertness. Behaviourally induced insufficient sleep syndrome is likely the most common cause of daytime sleepiness. In a population-based study conducted in Japan among 3030 subjects aged 20 years and older, 29 per cent slept less than 6 h per night, and 23 per cent reported having insufficient sleep.[(3)] The syndrome is likely to be widespread in truck drivers, working mothers, family doctors, executives, and students. The main symptoms are excessive sleepiness in the afternoon or early evening, decrease of diurnal performances, and, of interest to the psychiatrist, irritability, nervousness, and depression. Diagnosis of the syndrome is relatively easy provided that a thorough interview is conducted. The most rational treatment is an increase of daily total sleep time, either by spending more time in bed at night, or by taking one or two naps per day.

Hypersomnia in the context of sleep-related breathing disorders

The most frequent condition among these disorders is the obstructive sleep apnoea syndrome. This syndrome was first described by

Guilleminault *et al.*[4] It is most frequent in 50-year-old males. According to Young *et al.*[5] the prevalence of obstructive sleep apnoeas accompanied by excessive daytime sleepiness in North America is 4 per cent in men and 2 per cent in women.

Clinical features include night-time and daytime symptoms. Night-time symptoms are represented by loud snoring, apnoeic episodes ending with sonorous breathing resumption, nocturia, severe fatigue upon awakening, and sometimes headache. Daytime symptoms are dominated by excessive sleepiness, which varies in intensity among patients. Other symptoms include irritability, negligence, loss of concentration, loss of libido, impotence, and sometimes depression.

Patients are often obese or mildly obese. High blood pressure is a frequent feature. The ear, nose, and throat examination usually reveals a narrow upper airway due to close-set posterior tonsillar pillars, an abnormally long and hypotonic soft palate, a hypertrophic uvula, or macroglossia.

The positive diagnosis rests on polysomnography allowing the observation of nocturnal disrupted sleep and the identification of apnoeas and of their type (obstructive, central, or mixed) as well as their consequences on heart rate, oxygen desaturation, and degree of somnolence.

Of note, some subjects do not have apnoeas or hypopnoeas but increasing respiratory effort resulting in respiratory effort-related arousals (RERAs) and are believed to be as much at risk for complications. This state is most accurately identified with a quantative measurement of airflow and oesophageal manometry.

Obstructive sleep apnoea patients are at risk for systemic hypertension, occasional arrhythmias and conduction disturbances, cardiac or cerebral ischaemia, functional cognitive impairment, and depression. In a multicentre telephone survey carried-out in 1994–1999 in five European countries, among 18 980 subjects aged 15 to 100 years, 18 per cent of the individuals receiving a diagnosis of major depression also had a sleep-related breathing disorder and 17.6 per cent of the individuals receiving a diagnosis of sleep-related breathing disorder also had a diagnosis of major depression.[6]

There are several possible approaches to treatment:

- Weight loss may be beneficial. Avoidance of alcohol and sedatives should be recommended in all cases.
- Continuous positive airway pressure (CPAP) at night is the most widely used treatment. Good compliance requires proper preparation for the patient and an adaptation period.
- Oral appliances are suitable in mild obstructive sleep apnoea syndrome.
- Surgery consists mainly in nasal reconstruction in case of symptomatic airway blockade caused by bony, cartilaginous, or hypertrophied tissues that interfere with nasal breathing during sleep.

Hypersomnias of central origin

(a) Narcolepsy

First described in 1877[7] and given its name by Gelineau in 1880,[8] narcolepsy is now distinguished into three entities, narcolepsy with cataplexy, narcolepsy without cataplexy, and narcolepsy due to medical condition.

(i) Narcolepsy with cataplexy

Narcolepsy with cataplexy is not an exceptional condition. According to most recent evaluations its prevalence is 0.20 to 0.40 per 1000, i.e. slightly less than the prevalence of multiple sleep sclerosis.

Narcolepsy with cataplexy is characterized by two cardinal symptoms, excessive daytime sleepiness/irresistible sleep episodes and cataplexy, and other clinical features that are not necessarily part of the actual clinical picture.

Excessive sleepiness occurs daily. It comes in waves of varying degree of severity, depending on the individual, building up into irresistible and refreshing episodes of sleep. Excessive sleepiness is brought on by passive situations such as watching TV, being a passenger in a car, or attending a lecture. However it can also awkwardly occur in unexpected situations such as eating, walking, swimming, or driving a car. Excessive sleepiness may lead to automatic behaviour, such as saying totally inappropriate words or sentences, arranging objects in unlikely places, or driving a vehicle to an unintended destination.

Cataplexy is the most specific symptom. It consists of a sudden bilateral loss of voluntary muscle tone with preserved consciousness. It is triggered by environmental factors which are usually positive, such as a fit of laughter, receiving a compliment, humour expressed by the subject himself, the sight of prey for the hunter, the perception of a fish biting at the hook for the angler, a well-caught ball at tennis, or by anger, but almost never by stress or fear. All the striated muscles may be affected except the extra-ocular and respiratory musculature, leading to the progressive slackening of the whole body. More often however the attack is partial, involving certain muscles only, for example the jaw muscles, producing sudden difficulty in articulating words; the facial muscles, responsible for a grimace; or the thigh muscles, causing a brief unlocking of the knees. Consciousness is maintained during the episode. Cataplexy varies in duration from a split second to several minutes. Attack frequency varies from only a few per year, or even less, to several per day. In rare cases, especially after abrupt withdrawal of antidepressant medication, episodes of cataplexy may repeat themselves for minutes or hours, a state referred to as "status cataplecticus".

The other clinical features are deemed accessory to the extent that they are not indispensable for diagnosis.

Hallucinations, whether hypnagogic (at the onset of sleep) or hypnopompic (on awakening), are vivid perceptual experiences, not dreams, either visual, or auditory or kinetic. Patients may perceive someone entering and walking in the room, find themselves flying through the air or falling from a skyscraper. In some cases of unrecognized narcolepsy with daytime hypnagogic/hypnopompic hallucinations, the patient may be mistakenly diagnosed as having a delusional psychosis.

Sleep paralysis is a sudden inability to move during the transition from sleep to wakefulness or vice versa, while the subject is conscious. It is often accompanied by hypnagogic hallucinations. It is very unpleasant. In narcoleptic patients sleep paralysis may last up to 10 min.

Nocturnal sleep disruption occurs in approximately 50 per cent of cases, depending on age and the time elapsed since the onset of condition. The patient typically falls asleep as soon as he gets to bed, but his sleep is disturbed by recurring awakenings. He may complain of disturbing dreams.

REM-sleep behaviour disorder is frequent, either as a mere polysomnographic finding, excess of muscle tone or phasic EMG twitching activity during REM sleep, or as clinically significant complaint manifesting itself as an attempted enactment of distinctly altered, unpleasant, action-filled, and violent dreams in which the individual is being confronted, attacked, or chased by unfamiliar people. Periodic limb movements in sleep are more frequent than in normal subjects.

Physical examination is normal except for a frequently increased body mass index, especially in children at the onset of the condition. Noteworthy is the abolition of deep tendon reflexes during a cataplectic attack.

In a majority of cases, excessive daytime sleepiness is the first symptom to appear. In some patients, cataplexy occurs at the same time as excessive daytime sleepiness, but more often is delayed by one or several years. It is extremely rare for cataplexy to be the first clinical manifestation of narcolepsy with cataplexy.

The clinical diagnosis is based on clinical features. However, additional tests are highly recommended to confirm the diagnosis. The first test is polysomnography followed by an MSLT. At night a sleep onset REM period (SOREMP) is highly specific. It is observed in 25 to 50 per cent of cases. An increase in the amount of stage 1 NREM sleep and repeated awakenings are frequent findings. The MSLT shows a mean sleep latency of less than 8 min and two or more SOREMPs. However, some patients, especially in middle or old age, with clear-cut excessive daytime sleepiness and cataplexy, may have only one SOREMP, or even none during the MSLT procedure.

Today a CSF level of hypocretin-1 below 110 pg/mL is recognized as highly specific and sensitive for narcolepsy with cataplexy. However, up to 10 per cent of narcolepsy with cataplexy patients have normal levels of hypocretin-1.

There is no set pattern of evolution across patients. Excessive daytime sleepiness and irresistible episodes of sleep persist throughout life, but may diminish with age in some subjects. Cataplexy may spontaneously diminish with time or even totally disappear in some patients.

Narcolepsy is a very incapacitating disease. It interferes with every aspect of life. Education, performance at school and workplace, driving capability, recreational activities, interpersonal relationships, sexual life, and self-esteem. Depression is a frequent consequence of narcolepsy.

The mainstay of treatment is pharmacological although taking naps alleviates excessive sleepiness and refraining from emotion may prevent cataplexy.

Modafinil is the first-line treatment of excessive daytime sleepiness and irresistible episodes of sleep. Methylphenidate is less used today. Based on several large randomized controlled trials showing the activity of sodium oxybate on excessive daytime sleepiness and irresistible episodes of sleep, there is a growing practice in the United States to use it for the later indications. However, adverse effects including nausea, nocturnal enuresis, confusional arousals, malaise, and headache are not exceptional. Sodium oxybate is the only registered treatment for cataplexy. Other treatments are antidepressants, including tricyclics, selective serotonion reuptake inhibitors (SSRIS) and more recently new antidepressants such as venlafaxine or atomoxetine, the later being increasingly used despite few or non-randomized placebo-controlled clinical trials. As for disturbed nocturnal sleep the most widely used treatment is still hypnotics. However, the same randomized controlled trials have shown the activity of sodium oxybate against disturbed nocturnal sleep.

(ii) Narcolepsy without cataplexy

Narcolepsy without cataplexy is described as excessive daytime sleepiness and irresistible episodes of sleep unaccompanied by cataplexy. Automatic behaviour may be present as may hypnagogic hallucinations or sleep paralysis. Nocturnal sleep is usually less disturbed than in narcolepsy with cataplexy. When the subject is young, cataplexy may develop later in the course of the disorder.

Given the risk of overdiagnosing, a positive diagnosis of narcolepsy without cataplexy cannot be done without an all-night polysomnography followed by an MSLT documenting a mean sleep latency of less than 8 min and two or more SOREMPs.

(iii) Narcolepsy due to medical condition

As in the two previous categories, the patient has a complaint of excessive daytime sleepiness occurring almost daily for at least 3 months. However, the distinct feature of this subtype of narcolepsy is the existence of a significant underlying medical or neurological disorder accounting for the excessive daytime sleepiness and/or cataplexy.

According to the *ICSD*-2 the diagnosis of narcolepsy due to medical condition can be made only if one of the following is observed:

- a definite history of cataplexy
- a polysomnographic monitoring followed by an MSLT demonstrating a mean sleep latency of less than 8 min with two or more SOREMPs
- hypocretin-1 levels in the CSF lower than 110 pg/ml, provided the patient is not comatose.

In addition, a consistent chronological link with the presumed underlying disease must be established.

Narcolepsy due to a medical condition is extremely rare.

(b) Idiopathic hypersomnia

In comparison with narcolepsy, which is characterized by well-defined clinical, polysomnographic, and biochemical features, idiopathic hypersomnia is not as well delineated.

Its first description dates back to 1976,[(9)] almost a century after that of narcolepsy. According to various sleep disorders centres series populations the ratio of idiopathic hypersomnia to narcolepsy with cataplexy would be around 15 per cent.

Idiopathic hypersomnia includes two forms referred to as idiopathic hypersomnia with long sleep time and idiopathic hypersomnia without long sleep time. The first one is remarkable for three symptoms: a complaint of constant or recurrent excessive sleepiness and unwanted naps, usually longer and less irresitible than in narcolepsy, and non-refreshing irrespective of their duration; night sleep is sound, uninterrupted, and prolonged; morning or nap awakening is laborious. Subjects do not awaken to the ringing of a clock, of a telephone, and often rely on their family members who must use vigorous and repeated procedures to wake them up. Even then patients may remain confused, unable to react adequately to external stimuli, a state referred to as "sleep drunkenness" In contrast, idiopathic hypersomnia without long sleep time stands as isolated excessive daytime sleepiness.

The diagnosis of idiopathic hypersomnia is mainly based on clinical features. However, laboratory tests are necessary to rule out other hypersomniac conditions. Polysomnographic monitoring of nocturnal sleep demonstrates normal sleep, except for its prolonged duration in the case of idiopathic hypersomnia with long sleep time. NREM and REM sleep are in normal proportions. There is no SOREMP. Sleep apnoeas and periodic limb movements should theoretically be absent, but may be acceptable in the case of an early onset of idiopathic hypersomnia and of their late occurrence. The MSLT usually demonstrates a mean sleep latency less than 8 min, but is typically longer than in narcolepsy. Fewer than two SOREMPs are present. In cases with normal MSLT findings, several authors have suggested the use of long-term sleep monitoring to document the excessive amount of sleep.

In contrast with narcolepsy, onset of idiopathic hypersomnia is much more progressive. The disorder is generally stable and long lasting. Complications are mostly social and professional.

Treatment of idiopathic hypersomnia relies mainly on modafinil. However, awakening difficulties are hardly improved by this treatment.

(c) Recurrent hypersomnia

The most classic form of recurrent hypersomnia is the Kleine–Levin syndrome.[10] This is an uncommon disorder with roughly 300 cases published in the world literature. Adolescent males are most commonly affected.

The syndrome is characterized by recurrent episodes of hypersomnia associated with behavioural disorders including binge eating (rapid consumption of a large amount of food on a compulsory manner), oversexuality in the form of sexual advances, shamlessly expressed fantasies or masturbation in public, irritability, odd behaviours (like standing on the head, singing loudly, talking in a childish manner), and cognitive disorders, feeling of unreality, confusion, visual or auditory hallucinations. Simultaneous occurrence of all these symptoms is more the exception than the rule however. During the episode the patient may sleep as long as 14 to 18 h per day, waking or getting up only to eat and void.

Body weight gain of a few kilograms can be observed during the episode.

Amnesia of the episode, transient dysphoria, or elation with insomnia for 1 or 2 days, may follow the episode itself. During asymptomatic intervals patients sleep normally and do not experience behavioural or cognitive disorders.

Diagnosis of the Kleine–Levin syndrome is essentially clinical and laboratory tests merely serve to exclude the possibility of rare recurrent hypersomnias of secondary origin, organic, or psychiatric. Of note due to disordered behavioural features, especially hypersexuality, it is not rare that patients are first hospitalized on psychiatric wards and given antipsychotic drugs.

The course is usually benign with episodes lessening in frequency, duration, and severity. Complications are mainly social and occupational.

Treatment of the Kleine–Levin syndrome is not well codified. The effects of stimulant drugs such as modafinil or methylphenidate on the hypersomniac episodes are difficult to assess given that the methods of evaluation are purely subjective and that the episodes vanish spontaneously within a few days. A prophylactic treatment based on mood stabilizers (carbamazepine, lithium carbonate, and more recently valproic acid) deserves to be prescribed in severe cases. Positive results, that is absence of recurrence of the symptoms throughout the period of administration and recurrence with discontinuation, has been reported.

(d) Hypersomnias associated with various medical disorders

(i) Associated with neurological diseases

Hypersomnia may occur in any intracranial pressure syndrome, but it may also result from tumours affecting the diencephalon, specially the ventro-lateral posterior part of the hypothalamus or the peduncular region, with no associated intracranial hypertension. Cases of narcolepsy secondary to brain tumours affecting the hypothalamus or the midbrain region have been reported.

Uni or bilateral paramedian thalamic infarcts and paramedian pedunculo thalamic infarcts are the most typical causes of hypersomnia of vascular origin.

A non-negligible fraction of patients with Parkinson's disease present excessive sleepiness. This is even more the case of patients with multiple system atrophy.

Normal pressure hydrocephalus, Arnold–Chiari malformation, myotonic dystrophy, may also lead to excessive sleepiness.

(ii) Associated with infectious diseases

Intense fatigue and severe excessive sleepiness may develop in the month following Epstein–Barr disease. The same holds true of atypical viral pneumonia, hepatitis B viral infection and the Guillain–Barré syndrome. Hypersomnia tends to go into gradual remission after several months or years.

Disorders of alertness and/or consciousness are found in virtually all patients affected by viral encephalitis.

Human African Trypanosomiasis (sleeping sickness) is a subacute or chronic parasitic disease caused by the inoculation of a protozoan, *Trypanosoma brucei* transmitted by the tsetse fly. It is endemic to certain regions of tropical Africa. The form found in West and Central Africa is due to *Trypanosoma gambiense*. The invasion of the central nervous system is characterized by meningoencephalitis with abnormal sleepiness, headache, trembling, dyskenesia, choreoathetosis, and mood changes. Polysomnography has shown episodes of sleep occurring randomly day and night and SOREMPs.

(iii) Associated with endocrine diseases

Hypothyroidism and acromegaly are the two main sources of hypersomnia, usually due to obstructive sleep apnoea syndrome.

(iv) Post-traumatic hypersomnia

Excessive daytime sleepiness appearing during the year following a head injury may be considered *a priori* as post-traumatic. This typically presents as extended night sleep and episodes of daytime sleep. Brain imaging may reveal lesions affecting the hypothalamic region or brainstem, midbrain or pontine tegmentum, rarely hydrocephalia, or more often the absence of any significant lesions.

The delayed sleep phase syndrome

The major sleep episode is usually delayed 3 to 6 hours relative to conventional sleep-wake times. Affected individuals complain of great difficulty falling asleep at a socially acceptable time, but once sleep ensues, sleep is reported to be normal. Enforced conventional wake time usually results in morning excessive sleepiness. The disorder has been associated with mental disorders, particularly in adolescents. Schizoid and avoidant personality features are frequently associated with this disorder.

Treatment rests on various approaches including chronotherapy, light exposure, and melatonin therapy.

Conclusion

Hypersomnia deserves to be taken into consideration by the psychiatrist. It may be the consequence of a psychiatric disorder or of its treatment, but it may also be non psychiatric in nature and result in psychiatric symptoms.

Further information

Nofzinger, E.A., Thase, M.E., Reynolds, C.F., *et al.* (1991). Hypersomnia in bipolar depression: a comparison with narcolepsy using the multiple sleep latency test. *The American Journal of Psychiatry*, **148**, 1177–81.

American Academy of Sleep Medicine. (1999). Sleep related breathing disorders in adults: recommendations for syndrome definition and measurement techniques in clinical research. *Sleep*, **22**, 667–89.

Dauvilliers, Y., Arnulf, I., and Mignot, E. (2007). Narcolepsy with cataplexy. *Lancet*, **369**, 499–511.

Billiard, M. and Dauvilliers, Y. (2007). Idiopathic hypersomnia. In *Narcolepsy and hypersomnia* (eds. C.L. Bassetti, M. Billiard, and E. Mignot), pp. 77–87. Informa Healthcare, New York.

Arnulf, I., Zeitzer, J.M., File, J., *et al.* (2005). Kleine-Levin syndrome: a systematic review of 186 cases in the literature. *Brain*, **128**, 2763–76.

Regenstein, Q. and Monk, T. (1995). Delayed sleep phase syndrome: a review of its clinical aspects. *The American Journal of Psychiatry*, **152**, 602–8.

References

1. American Academy of Sleep Medicine. (2005). *International classification of sleep disorders: diagnostic and coding manual* (2nd edn). American Academy of Sleep Medicine, Westchester, IL.
2. Ohayon, M.M., Caulet, M., Philip, P., *et al.* (1997). How sleep and mental disorders are related to complaints of daytime sleepiness. *Archives of Internal Medicine*, **157**, 2645–52.
3. Liu, X., Uchiyama, M., Kim, K., *et al.* (2000). Sleep loss and daytime sleepiness in the general adult population of Japan. *Psychiatric Research*, **93**, 1–11.
4. Guilleminault, C., Tilkian, A., and Dement, W.C. (1976). The sleep apnea syndromes. *Annual Review of Medicine*, **27**, 465–84.
5. Young, T., Palta, M., Dempsey, J., *et al.* (1993). The occurrence of sleep disordered breathing among middle-aged adults. *The New England Journal of Medicine*, **328**, 1230–5.
6. Ohayon, M.M. (2003). The effects of breathing-related sleep disorders on mood disturbances in the general population. *Journal of Clinical Psychiatry*, **64**, 1195–2000.
7. Westphal, C. (1877). Eigentümliche mit Einschlafen verbundene Anfälle. *Archives für Psychiatrie und Nervenkrankheiten*, **7**, 631–5.
8. Gelineau, J. (1880). De la narcolepsie. *Gazette des Hôpitaux* (Paris), **55**, 626–8; 635–7.
9. Roth, B. (1976). Narcolepsy and hypersomnia. *Schweizer Archiv für Neurologie und Psychiatrie*, **119**, 31–41.
10. Critchley, M. (1962). Periodic hypersomnia and megaphagia in adolescent males. *Brain*, **85**, 627–56.

4.14.4 Parasomnias

Carlos H. Schenck, and Mark W. Mahowald

In all of us, even in good men, there is a lawless, wild-beast nature which peers out in sleep. –Plato, *The Republic*

Relevance of parasomnias to psychiatrists

Parasomnias are defined as undesirable physical and/or experiential phenomena accompanying sleep that involve skeletal muscle activity (movements, behaviours), autonomic nervous system changes, and/or emotional-perceptual events.[1] Parasomnias can emerge during entry into sleep, within sleep, or during arousals from any stage of sleep; therefore, all of sleep carries a vulnerability for parasomnias.[1] Parasomnias can be objectively diagnosed by means of polysomnography (i.e. the physiologic monitoring of sleep—figures 4.14.4.1, 4.14.4.2), and can be successfully treated in the majority of cases.[2–5] Understanding of the parasomnias, based on polysomnographic documentation, has expanded greatly over the past two decades, as new disorders have been identified, and as known disorders have been recognized to occur more frequently, across a broader age group, and with more serious consequences than previously understood.[1–10] Parasomnias demonstrate how our instinctual behaviours, such as locomotion, feeding, sex, and aggression, can be released during sleep, itself a basic instinct. There are at least eight reasons why parasomnias should be of interest and importance to psychiatrists:

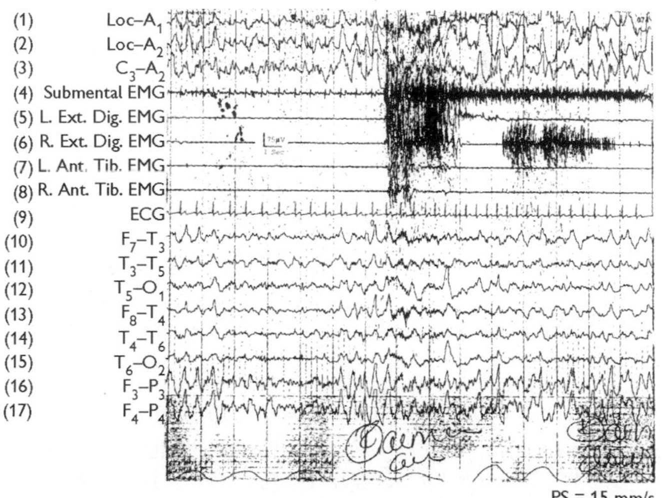

Fig. 4.14.4.1 Polysomnogram of a disordered arousal, with the persistence of sleep, in a 23-year-old man with a history of sleepwalking and sleep terrors. After a behavioural arousal from slow-wave sleep (with arm lifted up and then down), the EEG shows irregular delta and theta activity and superimposed faster frequencies. Immediately preceding the arousal, there is a cluster of three high-amplitude delta waves (channel 3). Electro-occulogram, channels 1. 2; EEG, channels 3, 10–17; EMG, electromyogram. (Reproduced from C.H. Schenck *et al.* Analysis of polysomnographic events surrounding 252 slow-wave sleep arousals in thirty-eight adults with injurious sleepwalking and sleep terrors. *Journal of Clinical Neurophysiology*, **15**, 159–66, copyright 1998, American Clinical Neurophysiology Society)

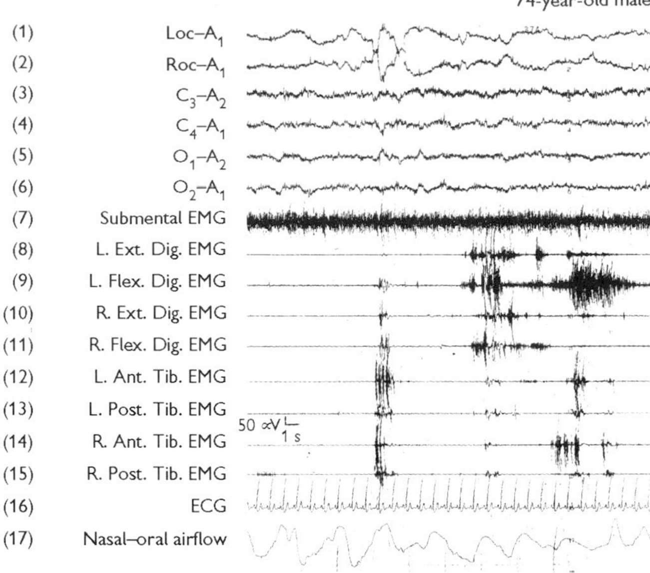

Fig. 4.14.4.2 Polysomnogram of disordered rapid eye movement (REM) sleep in a man with REM sleep behaviour disorder who eventually developed Parkinson's disease. There is complete loss of 'REM-atonia', as the submental electromyogram (EMG) shows continuous muscle tone (channel 7). The appearance of a rapid eye movement (channels 1, 2) signals the onset of excessive muscle twitching in the upper/lower extremity EMGs (channels 8–15). The EEG (channels 3–6) shows the typical low-voltage fast-frequency desynchronized activity of REM sleep. ECG rate (channel 16) remains constant despite generalized muscle twitching, which is a common finding in REM sleep behaviour disorder. Elecro-oculogram: channels 1,2.

1 Parasomnias can be misdiagnosed and inappropriately treated as a psychiatric disorder.

2 Parasomnias can be a direct manifestation of a psychiatric disorder, e.g. dissociative disorder, nocturnal bulimia nervosa.

3 The emergence and/or recurrence of a parasomnia can be triggered by stress.

4 Psychotropic medications can induce the initial emergence of a parasomnia, or aggravate a preexisting parasomnia.

5 Parasomnias can cause psychological distress or can induce or reactivate a psychiatric disorder in the patient or bed partner on account of repeated loss of self-control during sleep and sleep-related injuries.

6 Familiarity with the parasomnias will allow psychiatrists to be more fully aware of the various medical and neurological disorders, and their therapies, that can be associated with disturbed (sleep-related) behaviour and disturbed dreaming.

7 Parasomnias present a special opportunity for interlinking animal basic science research (including parasomnia animal models) with human (sleep) behavioural disorders.

8 Parasomnias carry forensic implications, as exemplified by the newly-recognized entity of 'Parasomnia Pseudo-suicide.' Also, psychiatrists are often asked to render an expert opinion in medicolegal cases pertaining to sleep-related violence.

Classification of parasomnias

Parasomnias can be classified according to whether the signs or symptoms are primary phenomena of sleep itself, or whether they are secondary phenomena derived from various underlying disorders, with sleep facilitating the nocturnal manifestation of these disorders.[6] Table 4.14.4.1 contains such a classification, and provides a context (along with other current sources[1,11]) for the parasomnias to be discussed in this chapter. Parasomnias demonstrate how sleep and wakefulness are not mutually exclusive states. Features of rapid eye movement (REM) sleep, non-REM sleep and wakefulness can occur simultaneously, and with rapid oscillations.[12] Status dissociatus represents the most extreme form of state dissociation.[13]

Clinical evaluation of parasomnias

The evaluation of complex and violent nocturnal behaviours at our centre (Minnesota Regional Sleep Disorders Center) includes the following:[2,14]

1 Clinical sleep-wake interview, with review of medical records, and review of a patient questionnaire that covers sleep-wake, medical, psychiatric and alcohol/chemical use and abuse history, review of systems, family history, and past or current physical, sexual, and emotional abuse.

2 Psychiatric and neurologic interviews and examinations, including psychometric testing.

Table 4.14.4.1 Classification of parasomnias: primary and secondary sleep phenomena

Primary sleep phenomena
Non-REM sleep
Disorders of arousal: sleepwalking/sleep terrors/confusional arousal
REM sleep
REM sleep behaviour disorder (RBD)
Dream anxiety attacks (nightmares)
Miscellaneous (including mixed non-REM/REM sleep)
Parasomnia overlap disorder (sleepwalking/sleep terrors/RBD)
Sleep related eating disorder
Restless legs syndrome/periodic limb movements in sleep
Obstructive sleep apnoea-related parasomnias
Rhythmic movement disorders
Status dissociatus
Bruxism
Secondary sleep phenomena
Central nervous system
Seizures (conventional, unconventional)
Headaches
Psychiatric
Nocturnal dissociative disorders
Nocturnal panic attacks
Nocturnal bulimia nervosa
Post-traumatic stress disorder
Cardiopulmonary (arrhythmias, asthma, etc.)
Gastrointestinal (gastro-oesophageal reflux etc)
Malingering

Modified from Mahowald and Ettinger.[7]

3 Extensive overnight polysomnographic monitoring at a hospital sleep laboratory, with continuous audio-visual recording. Figures 4.14.4.1, 4.14.4.2 depict the polysomnographic montage that includes the electro-oculogram, EEG, chin and four-limb electromyograms, ECG, and nasal-oral airflow (with full respiratory monitoring whenever indicated). Polysomnographic recording speeds of 15 to 30 mm/s are employed in order to detect epileptiform activity. Urine toxicology screening is performed whenever indicated.

4 Daytime multiple sleep latency testing, if there is a complaint or suspicion of excessive daytime sleepiness or fatigue (methods discussed in Narcolepsy chapter).

Causes of sleep related injury

A report on a series of 100 consecutive adults presenting to a multidisciplinary sleep disorders centre on account of sleep-related injury identified five causes:[2]

1 Sleepwalking/sleep terrors (M:F 3:2; mean age of onset, 5 years);

2 REM sleep behaviour disorder (predominantly male; mean age of onset, 57 years)

3 Dissociative disorders (Mostly female mean age of onset, 21 years)

4 Nocturnal seizures (uncommon)

5 Obstructive sleep apnoea/periodic limb movements (uncommon).

The sleep-related injuries included ecchymoses, lacerations, and fractures in 95 per cent, 30 per cent, and 9 per cent of patients respectively.

Non-REM sleep parasomnias: sleepwalking and sleep terrors

The polysomnographic correlates of sleepwalking and sleep terrors were first identified in the 1960s and 1970s by Gastaut and Broughton,[15, 16] Kales *et al.*,[17] and Fisher *et al.*[18] from France, Canada, and the United States. Sleepwalking and sleep terrors are classified as 'disorders of arousal,' and typically arise from delta non-REM (slow wave) sleep and usually affect children, but adults can also be afflicted, and suffer from sleep-related injuries and adverse social consequences.[2,9,10,19–24]

Clinical findings

Sleepwalking (SW) is characterized by complex, automatic behaviours, such as aimlessly wandering about, nonsensically carrying objects from one place to another, rearranging furniture, eating inappropriately, urinating in cupboards, going outdoors, and on rare occasion, driving a car.[1,25,26] The eyes are usually wide open and have a glassy stare, and there may be some mumbling. However, communication with a sleepwalker is usually poor or impossible. Frenzied or aggressive behaviour, the wielding of weapons (knives, guns), or the calm suspension of judgement (e.g. leaving via a bedroom window, wandering far outdoors) can result in inadvertent injury or death to self or others. Homicidal sleepwalking can occur.[25]

Sleepwalking episodes usually emerge 15–120 minutes after sleep onset, but can occur throughout the entire sleep period in adults. The duration of each episode can vary widely. The following is a wife's description.[2]

'He seems to have the strength of 10 men and shoots straight up from bed onto his feet in one motion. He's landed clear across the room on many occasions and has pulled down curtains (bending the rods), upset lamps, and so forth. He's grabbed me and pulled on me, hurting my arms, because he's usually dreaming that he's getting me out of danger . . . He's landed on the floor so hard that he's injured his own body . . . There are low windows right beside our bed and I'm afraid he'll go through them some night.'

Sleep terrors (ST) are characterized by sudden, loud, terrified screaming and prominent autonomic nervous system activation (tachycardia, tachypnea, diaphoresis, mydriasis) that usually appears early in the sleep period, although episodes in adults can occur at any time of the night. The individual may sit up rapidly while screaming, and engage in frenzied activity, such as bolting out of bed, and becoming injured.

Childhood sleepwalking and sleep terrors are characterized by complete amnesia for the events. In adult SW and ST, there can be subsequent recall of the behavioural episode, and also recall of dream-like mentation that usually involves being threatened by imminent danger.[2,27] The distinction between ST and agitated SW in adults is often blurred, with both states being admixed in response to a perceived threat.[24]

The prevalence of SW has been estimated to be as high as 17 per cent in childhood (peaking at age 4–8), and recent data indicate a higher prevalence in adults (4 per cent) than previously recognized.[28–30] The prevalence of ST in children can be greater than 6 per cent and greater than 2 per cent in adults.[1] A familial-genetic basis for SW and ST has been well-established.[30,31] Non-injurious SW does not have a gender preference,[1] although injurious SW appears to be more male-predominant.[2] Sleep terrors do not have a gender preference.[1] 'Confusional arousals' comprise another category of 'disorder of arousal,' and represent partial manifestations of sleepwalking and sleep terrors in which aggression and sexual impulses can be released.[1,10]

Polysomnographic findings

Sleepwalking/sleep terrors episodes arise abruptly during arousals from delta non-REM sleep.[1,15–18] In a systematic study of 38 adults with injurious SW/ST,[24] three postarousal EEG patterns were detected: diffuse, rhythmic delta activity; diffuse delta and theta activity intermixed with alpha and beta activity; and prominent alpha and beta activity. Thus, the postarousal EEG can show the complete persistence of sleep, the admixture of sleep and wakefulness, or complete wakefulness. Figure 4.14.4.1 shows the polysomnogram of a disordered arousal from slow-wave sleep.

Although the sleep architecture (i.e. distribution of sleep stages) is usually normal in SW and ST, the 'micro-structure' of non-REM sleep in adult SW/ST can be perturbed, with increased micro-arousals and increased rate of the 'cyclic alternating EEG pattern'.[1,2, 21,23]

Association with medical and psychiatric risk factors

Sleepwalking and sleep terrors may be triggered by sleep deprivation, febrile illness, alcohol use or abuse, pregnancy, menstruation, obstructive sleep apnea, periodic limb movements, nocturnal seizures, medical and neurological disorders, and psychotropic medications—especially zolpidem, lithium carbonate and anti-cholinergic agents.[1]

A strong association between sleepwalking/sleep terrors and psychopathology in adults was suggested by an early literature, but polysomnograpic monitoring was not conducted, and there were considerable methodological problems. The recent literature reporting PSG-confirmed cases has indicated that most adult cases are not closely associated with a psychiatric disorder, although stress can play a promoting role[2,19,29,22,32]. Genetic-constitutional factors appear to be predominant in adult and childhood sleep-walking/sleep terrors.[1]

Treatment

Treatment (especially in childhood SW/ST) is usually not necessary, other than identifying and minimizing any identified risk factors, and safety measure to avoid accidental injury. In cases involving sleep-related injury, pharmacological treatment is necessary and can be life-saving. A benzodiazepine, such as clonazepam (0.25–1.5 mg) taken 1 hour before sleep onset is usually effective. Alprazolam, diazepam, imipramine, and paroxetine can also be used. Teaching a patient self-hypnosis can be effective in milder cases of either adult or childhood SW/ST.[33] Treatment of any concurrent psychiatric disorder does not usually control sleepwalking/sleep terrors.[2,22] Attempts to waken the patient may cause confusion and distress.

REM sleep behaviour disorder (RBD)

Although various aspects of RBD have been identified by European, Japanese and American investigators since 1966,[34] RBD was not formally recognized and named until 1986–1987,[35,36] and it is incorporated within the international classification of sleep disorders.[1] A typical clinical presentation of RBD is contained in the description of the index case:[35]

> 'A 67-year-old dextral man was referred because of violent behavior during sleep . . . 4 years before referral . . . he experienced the first 'physically moving dream' several hours after sleep onset; he found himself out of bed attempting to carry out a dream. This episode signaled the onset of an increasingly frequent and progressively severe sleep disorder; he would punch and kick his wife, fall out of bed, stagger about the room, crash into objects, and injure himself . . . his wife began to sleep in another room 2 years before referral. They remain happily married, believing that these nocturnal behaviors are out of his control and discordant with his waking personality.'

Mammalian REM sleep, REM atonia, and paradox lost

REM sleep in mammals involves a highly energized state of brain activity, with both tonic (i.e. continuous) and phasic (i.e. intermittent) activations occurring across a spectrum of physiologic parameters.[36] REM sleep has two major synonyms: 'active sleep,' because of the high level of brain activity during REM sleep, and 'paradoxical sleep,' because of the nearly complete suppression of muscle tone despite the high level of brain activity. This generalized skeletal muscle atonia ('REM-atonia') is one of the three defining features of mammalian REM sleep, besides rapid eye movements and a desynchronized EEG. The loss of the customary paradox of REM sleep in RBD bears serious clinical consequences: 'paradox lost' means loss of safe sleep.[9]

Animal model of RBD

In 1965, Jouvet and Delorme reported from France that experimental pontine lesions in cats caused permanent loss of REM-atonia, and the cats displayed attack and exploratory behaviours during REM sleep that resembled dream-enactment (oneirism). This experiment established the first animal model of RBD.[34]

Clinical and polysomnographic findings

Between 1982 and 1991, 96 patients at our centre were diagnosed with chronic RBD. (There is an acute form of RBD that can emerge during withdrawal from ethanol or sedative-hypnotic abuse and with anti-cholinergic and other drug intoxication states.[36] Data on this series[37] are contained in Table 2, and are concordant with the published world literature.[34,36] The older male predominance in RBD is striking, although females and virtually all age groups are represented. Approximately half of RBD cases are closely associated with neurological disorders, predominantly neurodegenerative disorders (especially parkinsonism), narcolepsy and stroke. In fact, RBD may be the first sign of a parkinsonian disorder whose other (classic) manifestations may not emerge until several years or even decades after the onset of RBD.[36,38,39] Thus, routine neurological evaluations are indicated in the long-term management of RBD. The prevalence of RBD is estimated to be from 0.38 per cent to 0.5 per cent.[1] The course is usually progressive; spontaneous

Table 4.14.4.2 Findings in 96 patients with chronic REM sleep behaviour disorder (RBD)

Categories	Percentage (*N*)	Comments
Gender		
Male	87.5 (84)	Mean age of RBD onset (*N* = 90): 52 years (range 9–81)
Female	12.5 (12)	Mean age at polysomnography: 58 years (range 10–83)
Chief complaint		
Sleep injury	79.2 (76)	Ecchymoses (76); lacerations (32); fractures (7)
Sleep disruption	20.8 (20)	
Altered dream process and content	87.5 (84)	More vivid, intense, action filled, violent (reported as severe nightmares)
Dream-enacting behaviours	87.5 (84)	Talking, laughing, yelling, swearing, gesturing, reaching, grabbing, arm flailing, punching, kicking, sitting, jumping out of bed, crawling, running
Clonazepam treatment		
Efficacy (*N* = 67)		
Complete	79.1 (44/67)	Rapid control of problematic sleep behaviours *and* altered dreams, sustained for up to 9 years
Partial	11.9 (8/67)	
Total	91.0 (61/67)	

Modified from Schenck *et al.*[36]

remissions are very rare. Patients with RBD usually have calm and pleasant personalities, and do not display irritability or anger while awake, even though their dreams are highly aggressive.[40] Figure 4.14.4.2 depicts a typical polysomnogram of RBD with attempted dream-enactment.

Association of RBD with psychiatric disorders and Stress

Psychiatric disorders are rarely associated with RBD.[34,41] Fluoxetine treatment of obsessive compulsive disorder,[42] or cessation of use or abuse of REM-suppressing agents (viz. ethanol, amphetamine, cocaine, imipramine) can trigger RBD.[36,43] Tricyclic antidepressants, selective serotonin reuptake inhibitors, venlafaxine, mirtazapine, and monoamine oxidase inhibitors can induce or aggravate RBD. In four cases, major stress involving divorce, automobile accident, sea disaster, or public humiliation triggered RBD.[2,34,43]

Diagnosis of RBD

The diagnostic criteria of RBD are as follows:[1,36]

1 Polysomnographic abnormality during REM sleep: elevated submental electromyographic tone and/or excessive phasic submental and/or limb electromyographic twitching.

2 Documentation of abnormal REM sleep behaviours during polysomnographic studies, or a history of injurious or disruptive sleep behaviours.

3 Absence of EEG epileptiform activity during REM sleep.

Treatment of RBD

Clonazepam is remarkably effective in controlling both the behavioural and the dream-disordered components of RBD, at a usual bedtime dose of 0.5 to 1.0 mg. The long-term efficacy and safety of chronic, nightly clonazepam treatment of RBD has been established.[3] Other treatments include melatonin, pramipexole, etc.[36] Maximizing the safety of the sleeping environment should always be encouraged.

Parasomnia overlap disorder: sleepwalking/sleep terrors/RBD

A group of 33 patients has been reported with polysomnogram-documented sleepwalking, sleep terrors, and RBD.[8] The mean age was 34 years, the mean age of parasomnia onset was 15 years (range: 1–66), and 70 per cent were male. An idiopathic subgroup (N=22) had a significantly earlier mean age of parasomnia onset (9 years) than a symptomatic subgroup (27) whose parasomnia began with either a neurologic disorder (N=6), nocturnal paroxysmal atrial fibrillation (N=1), post-traumatic stress disorder/major depression (N=1), chronic ethanol/amphetamine abuse and withdrawal (N=1), or mixed disorders (schizophrenia; brain trauma; substance abuse [N=2]). The rate of psychiatric disorders was not elevated; group scores on various psychometric tests were not elevated. Forty-five percent (N=15) had previously received psychologic or psychiatric therapy for their parasomnia, without benefit. Treatment, usually with clonazepam, was effective for most patients. The natural history of this disorder is not yet known. Other cases of Parasomnia Overlap Disorder have been reported.[34,36]

Sleep related eating disorder

The 'night-eating syndrome' was first reported in 1955, and featured abnormal eating during full wakefulness in insomniac patients. Over the next 35 years, abnormal nocturnal eating received scant attention in the literature, until a series of 19 cases (expanded to 38 cases) with polysomnographic data was published on the new entity of sleep related eating disorder,[1,4,44] which featured abnormal eating during partial arousals from sleep in patients with other parasomnias or those who were idiopathic. Reports from various countries have now been published.[45–49]

Clinical findings

Pathological sleep-related eating has characteristic features, as identified in two separate series of adult cases.[4,44,48] Neither daytime binge-eating nor obsessive-compulsive disorder was diagnosed in any patient. Sleep-related eating was not associated with either the onset or the course of a psychiatric disorder. Patients do not usually experience hunger or thirst during their 'driven' nocturnal eating and drinking. A typical behavioural sequence consists of 'automatic' arising from bed, and going straight to the kitchen with a compulsive 'out of control' urge to eat. Alcohol is almost never consumed, even in former alcohol abusers. Thick substances, such as milkshakes, peanut butter, and brownies, are preferentially consumed at night. Purging does not take place, either at night or in the morning. Sleep-related eating is usually invariant, and is not influenced by day of the week or sleeping away from home. More than 40 per cent of patients in one series were overweight from the nocturnal eating, according to standardized body mass index criteria.[4]

Sleep related eating is most commonly associated with sleepwalking, but also with restless legs syndrome, obstructive sleep apnoea, narcolepsy, zolpidem/triazolam/midazolam/other psychotropic medication use or abuse, cessation of cigarette smoking, cessation of alcohol, opiate and cocaine abuse; cessation of cigarette smoking; stress (particularly involving separation anxiety), and various medical/neurological disorders (e.g. autoimmune hepatitis, encephalitis, migraines). Rarely, anorexia or bulimia nervosa or a dissociative disorder can be associated with sleep-related eating.[45]

Prescribing a monoamine oxidase inhibitor to a patient with sleep related eating disorder can be hazardous, since indiscriminate food consumption at night could jeopardize the mandatory dietary restrictions of MAOI treatment.

Treatment

Treatment, with one notable exception, is primarily directed at controlling the underlying sleep disorder. For cases associated with restless legs syndrome, therapy with dopaminergics (at times supplemented with an opiate such as codeine) is usually effective; likewise, therapy of obstructive sleep apnoea with nasal continuous positive airway pressure is often effective in controlling the sleep related eating. In contrast, in cases that are idiopathic and in those cases associated with sleepwalking, therapy with the anticonvulsant topiramate (that suppresses overeating urges) was effective in two-thirds of cases in two reported series.[5,50]

Sleep related eating disorder shares many features in common with the 'night eating syndrome' in adults,[49,51] although there are usually major differences in regards to level of consciousness during nocturnal eating, association with other sleep disorders, and response to therapy. It is likely that these two conditions sit at opposite poles of a spectrum of abnormal nocturnal eating.

Sleep related dissociative disorders

A nocturnal dissociative disorder with polysomnographic monitoring was first reported in 1976 by Rice and Fisher in a man with daytime and night-time fugues that began after his father's death.[52] Another polysomnogram-documented case was described in a woman with a history of being physically and sexually assaulted.[1] A series of eight cases was reported from our centre in 1989.[53]

Clinical manifestations

The onset may be sudden or gradual, and the course is chronic. There usually is a history of repeated physical and sexual abuse in childhood and/or adulthood. In a series of eight cases, seven were female who also had daytime states of dissociation with self-mutilating behaviours, such as genital cutting, self-burning, and punching through windows.[53] One male patient had exclusively nocturnal episodes in which he acted like a jungle cat. Patients may report sleep phobia as a consequence of bed-related and sleep-related sexual and physical abuse.

A typical spell during polysomnographic monitoring involves complex and lengthy behaviours that emerge during well-established EEG wakefulness, after a prior episode of sleep.[53] The nocturnal episodes appear to be re-enactments of previous assaults.

Treatment

Treatment involves long-term therapy of the dissociative disorders and of associated psychiatric disorders, usually initiated in a specialized in-patient setting. Bedtime administration of benzodiazepines may aggravate a nocturnal dissociative disorder.

Restless legs syndrome (RLS)

RLS, first described in 1945 by Ekbom from Sweden, is a chronic disorder that often results in severe insomnia, and can be incapacitating.[1,54] It is characterized by unpleasant and at times painful sensations in the lower extremities that emerge during periods of inactivity, particularly during the transition from wakefulness to sleep. These abnormal sensations are relieved by movement or stimulation of the legs, such as walking, stomping the feet, rubbing or squeezing the legs, taking hot showers, or applying hot packs or ointments to the legs.

Both the RLS and the therapeutic interventions just described are incompatible with successful entry into sleep. The more severely affected individuals cannot easily sit still while watching television or a film, or during protracted plane or train journeys. RLS is quite common, affecting up to 10 per cent of the general population, and tends to become more prevalent with increasing age. It affects females more than males. Childhood cases, though rare, at times may masquerade as 'attention deficit disorder with hyperactivity,' or as 'growing pains.'

Most RLS cases are idiopathic with a strong familial basis. Caffeine, fatigue, or stress may worsen the symptoms. There is no evidence that RLS is related to psychiatric disorders, although the symptoms of RLS may suggest a primary anxiety disorder and through impairment of the duration and quality of sleep it can affect daytime mood and behaviour. Also, neuroleptic-induced akathisia can mimic RLS. Secondary RLS can be associated with peripheral neuropathies, renal disease, and psychotropic medications (especially the SSRIs, venlafaxine, and tricyclic antidepressants).

Nearly all patients with RLS have 'periodic limb movements' (PLMs) of non-REM sleep (formerly called 'nocturnal myoclonus'). PLMs are characterized by periodic (every 15–40 sec) movements of the legs, viz. slow dorsi-flexion, which may or may not be associated with arousals. Excessive arousals during sleep from any cause, including PLMs, may result in daytime fatigue or sleepiness.

RLS can usually be diagnosed by history alone, and polysomnographic monitoring is usually not indicated. The syndrome is one of the major organic causes of insomnia, and commonly responds to treatment that includes use of dopaminergics (e.g. pramipexole, ropinerole, levodopa), opiates, and benzodiazepines (e.g. clonazepam). Combinations of these drugs are often necessary. Since RLS is a chronic disorder that often worsens with advancing age, chronic long-term treatment is usually warranted.

Differential diagnosis of dream-enacting behaviours and other parasomnias

A history of dream-enacting behaviours does not automatically implicate RBD. Other diagnoses include sleepwalking/sleep terrors;[2,9] obstructive sleep apnoea, with apnoea-induced arousals from REM sleep being associated with violent behaviours and vivid REM-related dreams;[2,55] nocturnal complex seizures, with the 'dreams' being the seizure equivalents;[34] sleep related dissociative disorders, with the 'dreams' being wakeful memories of past abuse;[53] intoxication states; and malingering.

Other parasomnias of interest to psychiatrists include sexual parasomnias ('sleepsex', 'sexsomnia'),[10] nocturnal panic attacks, which arise from Stages II and III non-REM sleep,[56] sleep related trichotillomania, nocturnal frontal lobe epilepsy,[11] and rhythmic movement disorders of non-REM and REM sleep, including head-banging and body rocking. Finally, expanded knowledge on the parasomnias has allowed for the recognition of a new medical-legal entity called 'parasomnia pseudo-suicide'.[58] This term refers to the unfortunate, but unintentional, fatal consequence of complex, sleep-related behaviours that may be erroneously attributed to suicide.[1]

Forensic guidelines for psychiatrists

The legal implications of automatic behaviour have long been discussed and debated. With regard to sleep-related automatic behaviours, the objective identification of a sleep disorder does not establish causality for any given deed. Guidelines have been developed to assist in determining the role of a sleep disorder in an act of violence.[57]

- There should be reason (by history or by formal sleep laboratory evaluation) to suspect a bona fide sleep disorder. Similar episodes, with benign or morbid outcome, should have occurred previously. (Note that disorders of arousal may begin in adulthood).
- The duration of the action is usually brief (minutes).
- The behaviour is usually abrupt, immediate, impulsive, and senseless—without apparent motivation. Although ostensibly

purposeful, it is completely inappropriate to the total situation, out of (waking) character for the individual, and without evidence of premeditation.

- The victim is someone who merely happened to be present and who may have been the stimulus for the arousal.
- Immediately after return to consciousness, there is perplexity or horror, without an attempt to escape, conceal, or cover up the action. There is evidence of lack of awareness on the part of the individual during the event.
- There is usually some degree of amnesia for the event, however, this amnesia may not be complete.
- In the case of ST or SW or sleep drunkenness, the act may (a) occur on awakening, (rarely immediately upon falling asleep) and usually at least 1 hour after sleep onset; (b) occur on attempts to awaken the subject; and (c) have been potentiated by alcohol ingestion, sedative or hypnotic administration or prior sleep deprivation.

The American Academy of Neurology and other professional organizations have developed guidelines for expert witnesses, with the most stringent being as follows.

- The expert should be willing to submit his or her testimony for peer review.
- The expert must be impartial and be willing to prepare his or her testimony for use by either or both the plaintiff or defendant. Ideally, the expert should assume the role of 'friend of the court.'

Further information

Schenck, C.H., Mahowald, M.W. Parasommias (2008). Associated with sleep-disordered breathing and its therphy, including sexsomnia as a recently recognized parasomnia. *Somnology*, **12**, 38–49.

Howell, M.J., Schenck, C.H., Crow, S.J. (2008). A review of night-time eating disorders. Sleep Medicine Reviews; doi: 10.1016/j.smrv.2008.07.005.

Schenck, C.H. (2005). *Paradox lost: midnight in the battleground of sleep and dreams*. Extreme-Nights, LLC, Minneapolis, Minnesota www.parasomnias-rbd.com

"Sleep Runners: The Stories Behind Everyday Paramnias—Deluxe Academic Edition" (3 DVDs, including 50 minutes of indexed sleep lab parasomnia footage; and CD-ROM), Slow-Wave Films, LLC, St. Paul, Minnesota, 2007. www.sleeprunners.com

www.parasomnias-rbd.com

References

1 American Academy of Sleep Medicine (2005). *International classifi cation of sleep disorders:Diagnostic and coding manual* (2nd edn.). Westchester, Ill:*American Academy of Sleep Medicine.*
2. Schenck, C.H., Milner, D.M., Hurwitz, T.D., *et al.* (1989). A polysomnographic and clinical report on sleep-related injury in 100 adult patients. *American Journal of Psychiatry*, **146**, 1166–73.
3. Schenck, C.H., and Mahowald, M.W. (1996b). Long-term, nightly benzodiazepine treatment of injurious parasomnias and other disorders of disrupted nocturnal sleep in 170 adults. *American Journal of Medicine*, **100**, 548–54.
4. Schenck, C.H., Hurwitz, T.D., O'Connor, K.A., *et al.* (1993). Additional categories of sleep-related eating disorders and the current status of treatment. *Sleep*, **16**, 457–66.
5. Winkelman J.W. (2006). Efficacy and tolerability of open-label topiramate in the treatment of sleep-related eating disorders: an open-label, retrospective case series. *Journal of Clinical Psychiatry*, **67**(11), 1729–34.
6. Mahowald, M.W., and Ettinger, M.G. (1990). Things that go bump in the night: the parasomnias revisited. *Journal of Clinical Neurophysiology*, **7**, 119–43.
7. Ohayon M.M., *et al.* (1997) Violent behavior during sleep. *Journal of Clinical Psychiatry*, **58**, 369–76.
8. Schenck, C.H., Boyd, J.L., and Mahowald, M.W. (1997). A parasomnia overlap disorder involving sleepwalking, sleep terrors, and REM sleep behavior disorder in 33 polysomnographically confirmed cases. *Sleep*, **20**, 972–81.
9. Schenck, C.H. (2005). *Paradox Lost: Midnight In The Battleground Of Sleep And Dreams*. Minneapolis, Minnesota, Extreme-Nights, LLC.
10. Schenck, C.H., Arnulf, I., Mahowald, M.W. (2007). Sleep and sex: what can go wrong? A review of the literature on sleep disorders and abnormal sexual behaviors and experiences. *Sleep*, **30**, 683–702.
11. Kryger, M.H., Roth, T., and Dement, W.C. (2005). *Principles and Practice of Sleep Medicine* (4th edn.). Elsevier: Philadelphia, PA.
12. Mahowald, M.W. and Schenck, C.H. (1992). Dissociated states of wakefulness and sleep. *Neurology*, **42**(Suppl. 6), 44.
13. Mahowald, M.W. and Schenck, C.H. (1992). Status dissociatus—a perspective on states of being. *Sleep*, **14,** 69.
14. Schenck, C.H., Mahowald, M.W. (2005). Rapid Eye Movement Sleep Parasomnias. *Neurologic Clinics*, **23**: 1107–26.
15. Gastaut, H. and Broughton, R. (1965). A clinical and polygraphic study of episodic phenomena during sleep. *Recent Advances in Biological Psychiatry*, **7**, 197–222.
16. Broughton, R. (1968). Disorders of sleep: disorders of arousal? Science, **59**, 1070–8.
17. Kales, A., Jacobson, A., Paulson, J., *et al.* (1966). Somnambulism: psychophysiological correlates. I. All-night EEG studies. *Archives of General Psychiatry*, **14**, 586–94.
18. Fisher, C., Kahn, E., Edwards, A., *et al.* (1973). A psychophysiological study of nightmares and night terrors. I. Physiological aspects of the stage 4 night terror. *Journal of Nervous and Mental Disease*, **157**, 75–98.
19. Kavey, N.B., Whyte, J., Resor, S.R., *et al.* (1990). Somnambulism in adults. *Neurology*, **49**, 749–52.
20. Crisp, A.H., Matthews, B.M., Oakey, M., *et al.* (1990). Sleepwalking, night terrors, and consciousness. *British Medical Journal*, **300**, 360–2.
21. Blatt, I., Peled, R., Gadoth, N., *et al.* (1991). The value of sleep recording in evaluating somnambulism in young adults. *Electroencephalography and Clinical Neurophysiology*, **78**, 407–12.
22. Llorente, M.D., Currier, M.B., Norman, S.E., *et al.* (1992). Night terrors in adults: phenomenology and relationship to psychopathology. *Journal of Clinical Psychiatry*, **53**, 392–4.
23. Zucconi M, *et al.* (1995) Arousal fl uctuations in non-rapid eye movement parasomnias: the role of cyclic alternating pattern as a measure of sleep instability. *Journal of Clinical Neurophysiology*, **12**:147–54.
24. Schenck, C.H., Pareja, J.A., Patterson, A.L., *et al.* (1998). Analysis of polysomnographic events surrounding 252 slow-wave sleep arousals in thirty-eight adults with injurious sleepwalking and sleep terrors. *Journal of Clinical Neurophysiology*, **15**, 159–66.
25. Broughton, R., Billings, R., Cartwright, R., *et al.* (1994). Homicidal somnambulism: a case report. *Sleep*, **17**, 253–64.
26. Schenck, C.H., and Mahowald, M.W. (1995). A polysomnographically documented case of adult somnambulism with long-distance automobile driving and frequent nocturnal violence: parasomnia with continuing danger as a non-insane automatism? *Sleep*, **18**, 765–72.
27. Kavey, N.B. and Whyte, J. (1993). Somnambulism associated with hallucinations.

28. Bixler, E.O., Kales, A., Soldatos, C.R., *et al.* (1979). Prevalence of sleep disorders in the Los Angeles metropolitan area. *American Journal of Psychiatry*, **136**, 1257–62.
29. Klackenberg, G. (1982). Somnambulism in childhood—prevalence, course and behavior correlates. A prospective longitudinal study (6–16 years). *Acta Paediatrica*, **71**, 495–9.
30. Hublin, C., Kaprio, J., Partinen, M., *et al.* (1997). Prevalence and genetics of sleepwalking: a population-based twin study. *Neurology*, **48**, 177–81.
31. Kales, A., Soldatos, C.R., Bixler, E.O., *et al.* (1980). Hereditary factors in sleepwalking and night terrors. *British Journal of Psychiatry*, **137**, 111–18.
32. Crisp. A.H. (1996). The sleepwalking/night terrors syndrome in adults. *Postgraduate Medical Journal*, **72**, 599–604.
33. Hurwitz, T.D., Mahowald, M.W., Schenck, C.H., *et al.* (1991). A retrospective outcome study and review of hypnosis as treatment of adults with sleepwalking and sleep terror. *Journal of Nervous and Mental Disease*, **179**, 228–33.
34. Schenck, C.H., Mahowald, M.W. (2002). REM Sleep Behaviour Disorder: Clinical, Developmental, and Neuroscience Perspectives 16 Years After Its Formal Identification in Sleep, *Sleep*, **25**,120–38.
35. Schenck, C.H., Bundlie, S.R., Ettinger, M.G., *et al.* (1986). Chronic behavioral disorders of human REM sleep: a new category of parasomnia. *Sleep*, **9**, 293–308.
36. Mahowald, M.W., Schenck, C.H. (2005). REM Sleep Parasomnias. In *Principles and Practice of Sleep Medicine* (4th edn.) (eds. M.H. Kryger, T. Roth, W.C. Dement,), pp. 897–916, Elsevier Saunders, Philadelphia, Pennsylvania.
37. Schenck, C.H., Hurwitz, T.D., and Mahowald, M.W. (1993). REM sleep behaviour disorder: an update on a series of 96 patients and a review of the world literature. *Journal of Sleep Research*, **2**, 224.
38. Gagnon J-F, Postuma R.B., Mazza, S., *et al.* (2006). Rapid-eye-movement sleep behavior disorder and neurodegenerative diseases. *Lancet Neurology*, **5**, 424–32.
39. Iranzo, A., Molinuevo, J.L., Santamaria, J., *et al.* (2006) Rapid-eye-movement sleep behavior disorder as an early marker for a neurodegenerative disorder: a descriptive study. *Lancet Neurology*, DOI: 10.1016/S1474-4422(06)70476–8.
40. Fantini, M.L., Corona, A., Clerici, S., *et al.* (2005) Aggressive dream content without daytime aggressiveness in REM sleep behavior disorder. *Neurology*, **65**, 1010-15.
41. Schenck, C.H., and Mahowald, M.W. (1990). A polysomnographic, neurologic, psychiatric and clinical outcome report on 70 consecutive cases with REM sleep behavior disorder (RBD): sustained clonazepam efficacy in 89.5 per cent of 57 treated patients. *Cleveland Clinical Journal of Medical*, **57**(Suppl), 10–24.
42. Schenck, C.H., Mahowald, M.W., Kim, S.W., *et al.* (1992). Prominent eye movements during NREM sleep and REM sleep behavior disorder associated with fl uoxetine treatment of depression and obsessive-compulsive disorder. *Sleep*, **15**:226–35.
43. Schenck, C.H., Hurwitz, T.D., Mahowald M.W. (1988). REM sleep behaviour disorder. *American Journal of Psychiatry*, **145,** 652.
44. Schenck, C.H., Hurwitz, T.D., Bundlie S.R., *et al.* (1991). Sleep-related eating disorders: polysomnographic correlates of a heterogeneous syndrome distinct from daytime eating disorders. *Sleep,* **14**, 419–31.
45. Schenck, C.H., and Mahowald, M.W. (1994). Review of nocturnal sleep-related eating disorders. *International Journal of Eating Disorders*, **15**, 343–56.
46. Spaggiari, M.C., Granella, F., Parrino, L., (1994). Nocturnal eating syndrome in adults. *Sleep*, **17**, 339–44.
47. Manni, R., Ratti, M.T., and Tartara, A. (1997). Nocturnal eating: prevalence and features in 120 insomniac referrals. *Sleep*, **20**, 734–8.
48. Winkelman, J.W. (1998). Clinical and polysomnographic features of sleep-related eating disorder. *Journal of Clinical Psychiatry*, **59**, 14–19.
49. Vetrugno, R., Manconi, M., Ferini-Strambi, L., *et al.* (2006). Nocturnal eating: sleep-related eating disorder or night eating syndrome? A videopolysomnographic study. *Sleep*, **29**: 949–54.
50. Schenck, C.H., and Mahowald, M.W. (2006). Topiramate therapy of sleep related eating disorder. *Sleep*, **29**:A268.
51. Schenck, C.H. (2006). Journal Search And Commentary: A Study of Circadian Eating and Sleeping Patterns In Night Eating Syndrome (NES) Points The Way To Future Studies On NES And Sleep-Related Eating Disorder. *Sleep Medicine*, **7**, 653–6.
52. Rice, E. and Fisher, C. (1976). Fugue states in sleep and wakefulness: a psychophysiological study. *Journal of Nervous and Mental Disease*, **163**, 79–87.
53. Schenck, C.H., Milner, D.M., Hurwitz, T.D., *et al.* (1989b). Dissociative disorders presenting as somnambulism: polysomnographic, video and clinical documentation (8 cases). *Dissociation*, **2**, 194–204.
54. Montplaisir, J., Allen, R.P., Walters, A.S., *et al.* (2005). Restless legs syndrome and periodic limb movements during sleep. In *Principles and Practice of Sleep Medicine* (4th edn.), (eds. M.H. Kryger, T. Roth, W.C. Dement), pp. 839–849. Elsevier Saunders, Philadelphia, Pennsylvania.
55. Iranzo, A. and Santamaria, J. (2005). Severe obstructive sleep apnea/hypopnea mimicking REM sleep behavior disorder. *Sleep*, **28**: 203–06.
56. Shapiro, C.M. and Sloan, E.P. (1998). Nocturnal panic—an underrecognized entity. *Journal of Psychosomatic Research*, **44**, 21–3.
57. Mahowald, M.W. and Schenck, C.H. (1999). Sleep-related violence and forensic medicine issues. In Sleep disorders medicine: basic science, technical considerations, and clinical aspects (2nd edn) (ed. S. Chokroverty), pp. 729–39. Butterworth Heinemann, Boston, MA.
58. Mahowald, M.W., Schenck, C.H., Goldner, M., *et al.* (2003). Parasomnia Pseudo- Suicide. *Journal of Forensic Sciences*, **48**: 1158–62.

4.15

Suicide

Contents

4.15.1 Epidemiology and causes of suicide
Jouko K. Lonnqvist

4.15.2 Deliberate self-harm: epidemiology and risk factors
Ella Arensman and Ad J. F. M. Kerkhof

4.15.3 Biological aspects of suicidal behaviour
J. John Mann and Dianne Currier

4.15.4 Treatment of suicide attempters and prevention of suicide and attempted suicide
Keith Hawton and Tatiana Taylor

4.15.1 Epidemiology and causes of suicide

Jouko K. Lonnqvist

Definition of suicide and the reliability of suicide statistics

Suicidal behaviour or suicidality can be conceptualized as a continuum ranging from suicidal ideation and communications to suicide attempts and completed suicide. A developmental process which leads to suicidal ideation, suicidal communication, self-destructive behaviour, in some cases even to suicide, and its consequences to the survivors is often referred to as a suicidal process. There is no single unanimously accepted definition of suicide, although in most proposed definitions it is considered as a fatal act of self-injury (self-harm) undertaken with more or less conscious self-destructive intent, however vague and ambiguous. Since the deceased cannot testify as to his or her intent, the conclusions about this must be drawn by inference. The evidence required for this inference depends on many factors, for example the mode of death, the use of autopsy, age, gender, social and occupational status, and the social stigma of suicide in the person's culture. The assessment of suicide intent is always based on a balance of probabilities.

Besides the conceptual problems, there are differences in operational definitions of suicidal behaviour which may lead to lack of uniformity of case definition and difficulties in comparing suicide statistics. The reliability of suicide statistics is influenced by whether suicide is ascertained by legal officials as in the United Kingdom and Ireland, or by medical examiners as elsewhere in Europe. In general, suicides tend to be undercounted, whereas non-suicidal deaths are very rarely misidentified as suicides. Most misclassified suicides fall into the category of undetermined deaths and are more like suicides than accidents. Underestimation is reasoned to be less than 10 per cent in the more developed countries, which allows rate comparisons between countries and over time. Despite problems in the recording of suicide, reports on suicide rates among different cultures or people suggest a true variation in suicide mortality.[1,2]

The suicide process and the act of suicide

Suicide is a mode of death usually consequent to a complex and multifaceted behaviour pattern. It is typically seen as the fatal outcome of a long-term process shaped by a number of interacting cultural, social, situational, psychological, and biological factors. Suicide is a rare, shocking, and very individual final act, which often leaves the survivors helpless. The suicide process model is used to organize and clarify the complexity of factors associated with suicide (Fig. 4.15.1.1).

Suicide is usually preceded by years of suicidal behaviour or feelings, and plans and warnings. In about half of all suicides, a previous attempt is found in the person's history, which offers, in theory, an opportunity for suicide intervention wherever suicide attempts occur. Male suicide attempts are more violent and the first attempt more likely to end in death. Successful suicide prevention calls for sensitive understanding of suicidal intent and active early intervention.[3]

Various risk or protective factors underlie suicidal behaviour. An appearance of suicidality means either an intensified effect of risk factors or a weakened effect of protective factors. For example, a separation from someone close may precipitate a suicidal imbalance in a vulnerable person due to the adverse life event as a stressor and the broken social network as a loss of social support.

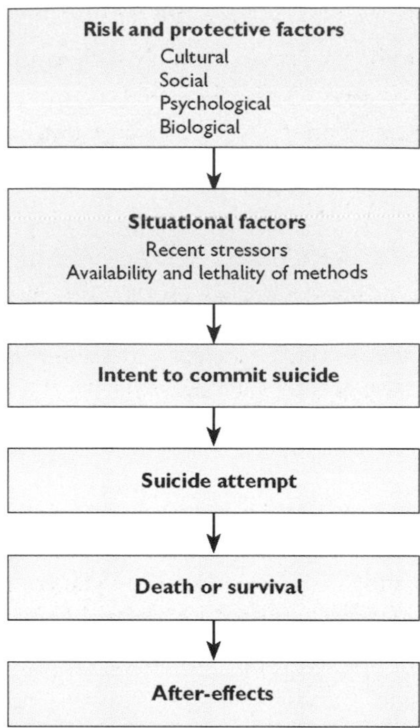

Fig. 4.15.1.1 The suicide process model.

The treating personnel and relatives of the suicide victim tend to overemphasize the meaning of the most recent events in the course of the suicide process. A precipitating factor may well be decisive in explaining the precise timing of suicide in the long course of a person's suicide process. Often, however, it also allows a simple and rational explanation in the face of the complexity of suicide.

The choice of a specific method takes place at the very end of the suicide process and represents the last possibility to intervene. Hanging is universally available and it is the most common suicide method globally. In many countries the ready access to firearms makes them potentially dangerous, especially among male adolescents and young adults. Restricting access to handguns might be expected to reduce the suicide rate of young people. Previously, domestic gas was frequently used as a suicide method, and detoxfication resulted in a significant decrease in suicide rates. Nowadays, the increasing suicide rate in many Asian societies has been largely linked with pesticides and other poisons. Restrictive availability of lethal measures may also be important in the clinical treatment of individual suicidal patients. Restriction in availability of dangerous means is a strategy based on the fact that suicidal crises are often brief, suicidal acts are often impulsive, and the long-term suicide rate of serious suicide attempts is remarkably low.(4–6)

Firearms, carbon monoxide, and hanging are active suicide methods with the highest potential to cause death. Jumping from a height or leaping in the front of a moving vehicle are more passive ways, but are also highly damaging in nature. Poisoning, drowning, or wrist cutting are typically methods which leave more time for help seeking and intervention.

Imitation means learning the use of a specific suicide method from a model which is overtly available in a culture, community, institution, or mass media. Imitation may have a significant effect on the choice of a suicide method, especially at schools, in psychiatric hospital wards, and in the general population of young people. The most famous example of imitation is the effect of Goethe's novel *The Sorrows of Young Werther*, which was widely read in Europe about 200 years ago. The suicide of the hero was imitated to such an extent that authorities in several European countries banned the novel. The 'Werther effect' also appeared after the death of Marilyn Monroe; the suicide rate rose about 10 per cent over the next 10 days. Recommendations for reporting of suicide have encouraged avoidance of repetitive and excessive reports, descriptions of technical details, simplified explanations for suicide, presenting suicide as means of coping with personal problems, or glorifying suicide victims.(7)

Most suicides are solitary and private, but a few result from a pact between people to die together. Suicide pacts are exceptional, accounting for less than 1 per cent of all suicides.

Suicide always has a major impact on the survivors. Suicide is a threatening event not only among close family members, but also in the surrounding population, including treating personnel and the people at the victim's workplace. The major challenges after a suicide, in addition to a normal mourning process, are dealing with shame and guilt feelings, and the crisis of survivors. Sharing of the traumatic experience and social support should be arranged immediately and continued, if necessary, at least some months after the suicide.

Epidemiology and public health aspects of suicide

Every year one million people commit suicide, accounting for 1 to 2 per cent of total global mortality. Suicide is a leading cause of premature death, especially among young adults. It is the fifth highest cause of years of life lost in the developed world. In many westernized countries, suicide is a more frequent cause of death than traffic accidents. According to World Health Organization (**WHO**) statistics, the annual world-wide incidence of completed suicide was 16 per 100 000 persons in 2000. This means that globally one person commits suicide every minute. Suicide is estimated to represent two per cent of the total global burden of disease.

The long-term trend in suicide mortality has been increasing at least during the last 50 years. The rank order of suicide mortality in the European region in 2001 to 2003 shows that most of the countries with high suicide mortality are located in Eastern Europe (Table 4.15.1.1). Outside this region, suicide mortality has been high in Japan and China. Everywhere, the male suicide rate is clearly higher than the female rate; China is the only exception with a very high female suicide rate.

The suicide rate of elderly people has been higher than in the younger age groups almost universally. However, in many Western countries, the suicide rate for people aged 65 years and over has been declining for decades. This change is associated with the growth of the general well being and the better social and health services.

Traditionally the incidence of suicide has been low in the younger age group (15–24), but during the past 40 years the suicide rate has been rising in many Western countries, especially among young males.

Table 4.15.1.1 Suicide rates per 100 000 by country, 2001–2003

European legion	Males	Females
Lithuania	74.3	13.9
Russian Federation	69.3	11.9
Belarus	63.3	10.3
Kazakhstan	50.2	8.8
Estonia	47.7	9.8
Ukraine	46.7	8.4
Latvia	45.0	9.7
Hungary	44.9	12.0
Finland	31.9	9.8
Republic of Moldova	30.6	4.8
Czech Republic	27.5	6.8
Austria	27.1	9.3
France	26.6	9.1
Poland	26.6	5.0
Switzerland	26.5	10.6
Romania	23.9	4.7
Slovakia	23.6	3.6
Ireland	21.4	4.1
Bulgaria	21.0	7.3
Germany	20.4	7.0
Iceland	19.6	5.6
Sweden	18.9	8.1
Portugal	18.9	4.9
Luxembourg	18.5	3.5
Norway	16.1	5.8
Netherlands	12.7	5.9
Spain	12.6	3.9
Italy	11.1	3.3
United Kingdom	10.8	3.1
TFYR Macedonia	9.5	4.0
Uzbekistan	9.3	3.1
Malta	8.6	1.5
Albania	4.7	3.3
Greece	4.7	1.2
Georgia	3.4	1.1
Armenia	3.2	0.5
Azerbaijan	1.8	0.5
Other		
Japan	35.2	12.8
Republic of Korea	24.7	11.2
China (Hong Kong SAR)	20.7	10.2
Australia	20.1	5.3
Canada	18.7	5.2
United States of America	17.6	4.1
Thailand	12.0	3.8
Singapore	11.4	7.6
Kuwait	2.5	1.4

A long list of major public health concerns in the field of suicidology has emerged:

- suicidal ideation and suicide attempts are surprisingly common in the general population
- the high rate of suicides among adolescents and young adults
- unemployment as a major risk factor for suicide
- easy access to lethal suicide methods such as psychotropic or analgesic drugs, guns, and motor vehicles
- high alcohol consumption and increasing substance misuse
- undertreatment of major psychiatric disorders such as depression and schizophrenia
- suicide models projected by the mass media.

These findings indicate that rapid growth and continuous changes in society are simultaneously causing instability and disturbing the development of integration. Some regions and groups of people are inevitably affected negatively by this development, and large numbers of people are thus moving towards a greater risk of suicide.

Determinants of suicide

Usually, suicide has no single cause. It is the endpoint of an individual process, in which several interacting determinants or risk factors can be identified (Tables 4.15.1.2 and 4.15.1.3). Risk factors are by their nature cultural, social, situational, psychological, biological, and even genetic.[8]

(a) Cultural factors in suicide

Culture defines basic attitudes towards life and death, and also towards suicide in society. We still have stigma against suicide. A hundred years ago, suicide was illegal in many European countries. Similarly, most churches overtly opposed suicide and allowed suicide victims to be buried only outside the cemetery. Religion was also a major integrating force between individuals and the community. In a modern secularized society, religion is still a

Table 4.15.1.2 Risk factors for suicide: sociodemographic variables

Gender	Male
Age	Elderly
Social status	Low
Educational status	Low
Marital status	Unmarried, separated, divorced, widowed
Residential status	Living alone
Employment status	Unemployed, retired, insecure employment
Economic status	Weak (males)
Profession	Farmer, female doctor, student, sailor
Special subpopulations	Students, prisoners, immigrants, refugees, religious sects
Special institutions	Hospitals, prisons, army
Region	Uneven distribution locally by urban–rural, residential, or subcultural area
Season and time	Spring and autumn, weekend, evening, anniversary
Life events	Adverse life events such as losses and separations, criminal charges
Social support	Low
Social integration	Lacking

Table 4.15.1.3 Clinical determinants of suicide

Family history	Suicidal behaviour, mental disorders
Mental disorders	Any disorder, depression, substance use disorders, personality disorders, schizophrenia
Contact with psychiatric services	Any contacts, recent contacts, post-discharge period, psychotropic drugs
Psychiatric symptoms	Hopeless, helpless, depressive, psychotic, delirious, anxious, aggressive, introversive
Suicidal behaviour	Previous suicide attempts, suicidal ideations, death wishes, indirect gestures
Physical health	Severe physical illness such as cancer, AIDS, stroke, and epilepsy; permanent sickness
Availability of suicide methods	Easy access to lethal methods

meaningful and protective factor for many individuals in a suicidal crisis. Western culture has had a tendency to emphasize the individuals's free will and the shouldering of responsibility for one's life, while egoistic and anomic trends in society have intensified and altruism has almost disappeared. Such changes may have increased the incidence of suicide in society. The cultural background of suicide is a deep structure inherited over generations. Cultural factors also prevent rapid changes in suicidal behaviour, which is evident among immigrants, whose mode and rate of suicide usually lie somewhere between the original and the host cultures.[(9)]

(b) Sociological theories on suicide

Classic sociology views suicide as a social, not an individual, phenomenon. The suicide victim's moral predisposition to commit suicide, not his or her individual experiences, is felt to be the crucial factor. Moral predisposition means the degree to which the victim is involved in more or less integrated groups and in the values of those groups. Suicides are seen as a disturbance or symptom of a relationship between society and individuals. In 1897, Durkheim published his famous work on suicide and described four basic types. Anomic suicide reflects a situation where an individual is no longer guided by the society due to its weakness, like the suicide of an unemployed and rejected alcoholic without any support from society. Altruistic suicide is illustrated by a society which can exert a strong influence on an individual's decision to sacrifice his or her life, as did the captain of the *Titanic*, for example. Egoistic suicide is an individualistic decision of a person no longer dependent on others' control or opinion such as a person who has arranged an assisted suicide. Fatalistic suicide is seen as a result of strict rules in a society which have proved decisive for the destiny of an individual, for example the suicide of a person held as a slave.[(10)] There are also newer social theories of suicide which stress more the joint effects of social factors. The concept of social isolation has been clinically useful in understanding the socio-ecological and social-psychiatric background of suicide.[(11)] Some sociologists have underlined the individual meanings associated with suicide.

(c) Life events and social support

The life situation preceding suicide is typically characterized by an excess of adverse life events and recent stressors. Usually, the sum effect of events is overwhelming and more important than a single life event. Job problems, family discord, somatic illness, financial trouble, unemployment, separation, and death and illness in the family are the most common life events preceding suicide. Somatic illness and retirement are age-specifically connected with the suicides of elderly men, while separation, financial troubles, job problems, and unemployment are more common among younger men. Severely disabling somatic illness is a very important risk factor for suicide in elderly male patients. In general, suicide among men is more often related to recent stressors than it is among women.

In most cases, life events are not accidental, but are usually also dependent on the individual's own behaviour. Personality features, even mental disorders, often explain the difficulties the victim has had. Among male alcoholics, life stress is connected with family discord and separations in all age groups. Other sources of stress in alcoholic male suicides are unemployment and financial troubles, whereas in depressive non-alcoholic male victims life stress is associated more with somatic illness. Among alcoholic males, adverse life events and living alone clearly have an enhancing effect on suicidality. Among females, life events as psychosocial stress are less strongly connected with suicide. Depression and adverse interpersonal life events are more frequent contributors to female than male suicides.[(12)]

(d) Psychology of suicide

Early psychological theories of suicide focussed on the concept of the self. A classical example is Freud's theory assuming that self-destructive behaviour in depression represents aggression directed against a part of the self that has incorporated a loss or rejection of a love object. In his later theory of suicide, Freud presented the construction of the dual instincts, where Eros is a life-sustaining and life-enhancing drive in constant interaction with Thanatos, the aggressive death instinct.

Later psychodynamic thinking on suicide focussed more on the self in relation to others. Failures in the developmental and adaptational processes are reflected in negative self-images and distorted cognitive schemas, leading to such feelings as depression, hopelessness, rage, shame, guilt, and anxiety. It is widely held that psychological pain is found as a common element at the core of all suicidal behaviours; suicide occurs when the individual can no longer endure the pain. Most recent psychological theories of suicide accept a multifactorial causation of suicide resulting from an interaction of predisposing and precipitating factors.[(13)] A person moves towards a suicidal crisis depending on the stressors and presence or absence of protective factors in his or her life.

(e) Neurobiological determinants of suicide

Suicidal behaviour is highly familial. Relatives of patients who commit suicide are themselves more likely to commit suicide than relatives of patients who do not commit suicide. Liability to suicidal behaviour may be a familially transmitted trait which is partly independent on the specific mental disorders. Since the heritability of liability to suicidal behaviour appears to be on the order of 30–50 per cent, interactions with environmental factors must also be significant.

Results of adoption studies suggest that genetic factors rather than familial environmental factors are the determinants of familial concordance for suicidal behaviour. Among biological relatives of adopted suicide victims there is a higher incidence of suicide than among the relatives of non-suicide controls or among the adoptive relatives of the suicide victims. Also identical twins have a higher concordance for suicide, attempted suicide, and suicide ideation compared with non-identical twins.[14]

The findings that genetic factors contribute to suicidal behaviour has stimulated studies aimed at identifying susceptibility genes. So far molecular genetic studies have focussed on the serontonergic pathway. Two genes have emerged as being involved in the vulnerability to suicidality: the tryptophan hydroxylase 1 (TPH1) gene, as a quantitative risk factor for suicidal behaviour, and serotonin transporter gene (5-HTTLPR), which is consistently associated with impulsive-aggressive personality traits.[15] Patients who have seriously attempted suicide by violent means have low levels of the serotonin metabolite 5-hydroxyindole acetic acid in their cerebrospinal fluid.[16] These and other neurobiological changes are discussed in Chapter 4.15.3.

Basic characteristics of the suicide victim

Persons at greatest risk of suicide are usually middle-aged or older, non-married men with poor social and economic position, and a family history of mental disorders and suicidal behaviour. Usually they are living alone, and often unemployed or with insecure employment. They also typically have marked recent life stress and a weak social network. Most suffer from depression, and feel hopeless and many have a comorbid substance abuse or personality disorder. Almost all elderly victims have comorbid physical illness or are permanently disabled. Most have previously contacted health care, and communicated their suicidal tendencies at least indirectly, although usually without receiving adequate psychiatric treatment. Half of them have previously attempted suicide.

Mental disorders and suicide

Virtually all mental disorders carry an increased risk of suicide.[17] The suicide risk in functional mental disorders is double that in substance use disorders, which in turn carry double the risk of suicide compared to organic disorders. The greatest risk of suicide among all clinical states is in attempted suicide, which carries about 40 times the expected value (Table 4.15.1.4). In anorexia nervosa and major depression, the risk is about 20-fold, and in other mood disorders and psychoses about 10 to 15 times higher than expected. In anxiety, personality, and substance use disorders the suicide risk is at lower levels, but about 5 to 10 times higher than the expected value. In subtance disorders the risk is dependent on the type of disorder, being clearly lowest in alcohol, cannabis, and nicotine abusers.[17]

Psychological autopsy studies have been used to construct an overall view of suicide by collecting all available relevant information on the victim's life preceding his or her death. In psychological autopsy studies, mental disorders of suicide victims have been assessed using DSM-diagnoses and large unselected samples. In two recent meta-analyses[18,19] the victim received at least one diagnosis on Axis I in 87 to 90 per cent of the suicides. In all studies, depressive disorders (43 per cent) and substance use disorders (26 per cent), personality disorders (16 per cent) and psychoses (9 per cent) were frequent and comorbidity was common.

Table 4.15.1.4 Rank order of suicide in mental disorders

Suicide attempt
Anorexia nervosa
Major depression
Mood disorders not otherwise specified
Reactive psychoses
Bipolar disorder
Dysthymia
Schizophrenia
Anxiety disorders
Personality disorders
Substance use disorders

In two European psychological autopsy studies[20,21] from Finland and Northern Ireland, the distribution of the principal diagnoses was similar (Table 4.15.1.5). The most common psychiatric diagnoses in suicide were major depression and alcohol dependence. Major mood disorders together comprised 42 to 36 per cent and substance use disorders, 19 to 30 per cent of all suicides. Comorbidity was a major finding in both samples, most commonly substance use disorder with major depression. A recent European psychological autopsy study gave similar results underlining, however, the role of personality disorders as a risk factor for suicide.[22]

Table 4.15.1.5 Principal diagnoses of suicide victims in Finland and Northern Ireland

Diagnosis	Finland (%) (n = 229)	Northern Ireland (%) (n = 118)
Major depression	30	31
Depressive disorder not otherwise specified	9	—
Dysthymia	—	1
Bipolar disorder	3	4
Alcohol dependence	17	24
Alcohol misuse	2	4
Other substance use disorders	—	2
Schizophrenia	7	6
Schizoaffective disorder	3	1
Other psychoses	3	4
Anxiety disorders	1	5
Adjustment disorder	3	3
Organic mental disorders	2	1
Other Axis I disorders	2	2
Personality disorder	9	3
No diagnosis	2	10
Insufficient information for assessment	7	—

The mortality risk for suicide in major depression is 20 times that expected, and 15-to 20-fold in all affective disorders. Every sixth death among depressive people treated as psychiatric patients is by suicide.[23] The risk of suicide varies across the subclasses of depression, and is related to the selection of suicidal patients for the various types of treatment. The risk is highest for depressive inpatients, even during the postdischarge period, and much lower among psychiatric outpatients, although clearly lowest for those treated for depression in primary care.[24] A meta-analysis found a hierarchy of life-time suicide prevalence: eight per cent in people ever admitted for suicidality, four per cent in patients admitted with affective disorder but not for suicidality, and two per cent in mixed inpatient and outpatient populations.[24]

Depression of suicide victims differ qualitatively from that of living controls; it seems to be more severe and accompanied more often by insomnia, weight or appetite loss, feelings of worthlessness, inappropriate guilt, and thoughts of death or suicidal ideation.[26] In addition, impulsive and aggressive behaviour, alcohol and drug abuse and dependence, and cluster B personality disorders increase the risk of suicide in individuals with major depression.[27] Inadequate and inefficient antidepressant treatment of depressed suicide victims has been a persistent finding in several studies. Less than half of suicide victims with major depression have been in contact with psychiatric care at the time of suicide. However, there is some evidence that good monitoring and maintenance treatment in high-risk groups of patients may be able to decrease their suicide rates.[28]

Alcohol and drugs, often combined, are a major risk or a precipitating factor for suicide. They may intensify the suicidal intent, offer a constantly available suicide method, worsen the somatic status of the victim, and increase the risk of complications after the attempt. Alcohol and drugs impair judgement and lower the threshold to suicide. Alcohol is detected in about every third case at the moment of suicide.[29] The lifetime risk of suicide has been estimated at 7 per cent for alcohol dependence, with only slight variation over the life.[30] The suicide rate in heavy drinking is 3.5 times and in alcohol use disorders ten times higher than that in the general population.[31] In drug dependence or abuse it is 15 times higher than expected.[17,31] The role of substance use disorders varies greatly by country. In a recent study from Estonia, alcohol dependence was found in a half of suicide victims.[32]

The suicide risk in schizophrenia appears to be almost 10 times higher than in the general population.[17] The lifetime risk of suicide in schizophrenia is estimated to be 5 per cent.[30,33] The great majority of schizophrenic patients commit suicide in the active phase of the disorder after having suffered depressive symptoms. Suicide in schizophrenia is thus less of a surprise; it is typically preceded by a previous attempt, and suicidal intent has been communicated at least as often as in non-schizophrenic suicides.[34] Schizophrenic suicide victims differ from other schizophrenic patients by having suicidal thoughts and previous suicide attempts, being more depressive, and having more positive symptoms.[35] Undertreatment, comorbidity, treatment non-compliance, and a high frequency of non-responders are also common problems among schizophrenic suicide victims. Adequacy of comprehensive care is crucial for suicide prevention in schizophrenia, especially among actively psychotic patients with recent suicidal behaviour and depressive symptoms.[36]

Personality disorders are tightly connected with suicide. Most of the suicide victims with personality disorder, especially with borderline and emotionally unstable personality disorder, have also comorbid depressive disorder or substance abuse. They often suffer from impulsive and aggressive behaviour.[20,22,27,38] This kind of comorbidity is very frequent among the young suicide victims.

Mental disorders, particularly depressive disorders, substance abuse, and antisocial behaviour have an important role in the adolescent suicides. The diagnostic distribution of mental disorders among them is surprisingly similar to that of the young and even middle-aged adults.[39]

References

1. Lönnqvist, J. (1977). Suicide in Helsinki: an epidemiological and socialpsychiatric study of suicides in Helsinki in 1960–61 and 1970–71. *Monographs of Psychiatria Fennica*, No. 8.
2. Sainsbury, P. and Jenkins, J.S. (1982). The accuracy of officially reported suicide statistics for purposes of epidemiological research. *Journal of Epidemiology and Community Health*, **36**, 43–8.
3. Isometsä, E.T. and Lönnqvist, J.K. (1998). Suicide attempts preceding completed suicide. *British Journal of Psychiatry*, **173**, 531–6.
4. Ohberg, A., Lonnqvist, J., Sarna, S., *et al.* (1995). Trends and availability of suicide methods in Finland: proposals for restrictive measures. *British Journal of Psychiatry*, **166**, 35–43.
5. Kreitman, N. (1976). The coal gas history: UK suicide rates 1960–1971. *British Journal of Preventive and Social Medicine*, **30**, 83–90..
6. Lewis, G., Hawton, K., and Jones, P. (1997). Strategies for preventing suicide. *British Journal of Psychiatry*, **171**, 351–4.
7. Hawton, K., Fagg, J., Simkin, S., *et al.* (1998). Methods used for suicide by farmers in England and Wales. *British Journal of Psychiatry*, **173**, 320–4.
8. Maris, R.W. (2002). Suicide. *Lancet*, **360**, 319-26.
9. Neeleman, J., Halpern, D., Leon, D., *et al.* (1997). Tolerance of suicide, religion and suicide rates: an ecological and individual study in 19 Western countries. *Psychological Medicine*, **27**, 1165–71.
10. Durkheim, E. (1897). *Le suicide, etude de sociologie*. Alcan, Paris. (English translation: *Suicide*. Routledge and Kegan Paul, London, 1952.)
11. Maris, R.W. (1981). *Pathways to suicide*. John Hopkins Univesrity Press, Baltimore, MD.
12. Heikkinen, M.E., Isometsä, E.T., Marttunen, M.J., *et al.* (1995). Social factors in suicide. *British Journal of Psychiatry*, **167**, 747–53.
13. Farberow, N.L. (1997). The psychology of suicide: past and present. In *Suicide: biopsychosocial approaches* (ed. A.J. Botsis, C.R. Soldatos, and C.N. Stefanis), pp. 147–63. Elsevier, Amsterdam.
14. Brent, D.A., and Mann, J.J. (2005). Family genetic studies, suicide, and suicidal behaviour. *American Journal of Medical Genetics (Semin. Med. Genet.)*, **133**(1), 13–24.
15. Bondy B., Buettner A., and Zill P. (2006). Genetics of suicide. *Molecular Psychiatry*, **11**, 336–351.
16. Mann, J.J. (2003). Neurobiology of suicidal behaviour. *Nature Reviews Neuroscience*, **4**(10), 819–828.
17. Harris, E.C. and Barraclough, B. (1997). Suicide as an outcome for mental disorders. A meta-analysis. *British Journal of Psychiatry*, **170**, 205–28.
18. Cavanagh, J.T.O., Carson, A.J., Sharpe, M. *et al* (2003). Psychological autopsy studies of suicide: a systematic review. *Psychological Medicine*, **33**, 395–405.
19. Arsenault-Lapierre, G., Kim C., and Turecki G. (2004). Psychiatric diagnoses in 3275 suicides: a meta-analysis. *BMC Psychiatry*, **4**, 37.

20. Henriksson, M.H., Aro, H.A., Marttunen, M.J., *et al.* (1993). Mental disorders and comorbidity in suicide. *American Journal of Psychiatry*, **150**, 935–40.
21. Foster, T., Gillespie, K., and McClelland, R. (1997). Mental disorders and suicide in Northern Ireland. *British Journal of Psychiatry*, **170**, 447–52.
22. Schneider, B., Wetterling, T., Sargk, D., *et al.* (2006). Axis I disorders and personality disorders as risk factors for suicide. *European Archives of Psychiatry and Clinical Neuroscience*, **256**, 17–27.
23. Wulsin, L.R., Vaillant, G.E., and Wells, V.E. (1999). A systematic review of the mortality of depression. *Psychosomatic Medicine*, **61**, 6–17.
24. Simon, G.E. and VonKorff, M. (1998). Suicide mortality among patients treated for depression in an insured population. *American Journal of Epidemiology*, **147**, 155–60.
25. Bostwick, J.M. and Pankratz, V.S. (2000). Affective disorders and suicide risk: a reexamination. *American Journal of Psychiatry*, **157**, 1925–32.
26. McGirr, A., Renaud, J., Seguin, M., *et al.* (2007). An examination of DSM-IV depressive symptoms and risk for suicide completion in major depressive disorder: A psychological autopsy study. *Journal of Affective Disorders*, **97**, 203–9.
27. Dumais, A., Lesage, A.D, Alda, M., *et al.* (2005). Risk factors for suicide completion in major depression: a case-control study of impulsive and aggressive behaviors in men. *American Journal of Psychiatry*, **162**, 2116–24.
28. Isometsä, E.T., Henriksson, M.M., Aro, H.M., *et al.* (1994). Suicide in major depression. *American Journal of Psychiatry*, **151**, 530–6.
29. Ohberg, A., Vuori, E., Ojanperä, I., *et al.* (1996). Alcohol and drugs in suicides. *British Journal of Psychiatry*, **169**, 75–80.
30. Inskip, H.M., Harris, E.C., and Barraclough, B. (1998). Lifetime risk of suicide for affective disorder, alcoholism and schizophrenia. *British Journal of Psychiatry*, **172**, 35–7.
31. Willcox, H.C., Conner, K.R., and Caine, E.D. (2004). Association of alcohol and drug use disorders and completed suicide: an empirical review of cohort studies. *Drug and Alcohol Dependence*, **76S**, S11-S19.
32. Kõlves, K., Värnik, A., Tooding, L-M., *et al.* (2006). The role of alcohol in suicide: a case-control psychological autopsy study. *Psychological Medicine*, **36**, 923–930.
33. Palmer, B.A., Pankratz, V.S., and Bostwick, J.M. (2005). The lifetime risk of suicide in schizophrenia. *Archives of General Psychiatry*, **62**, 247–253.
34. Heila, H., Isometsä, E., Henriksson, M.H., *et al.* (1997). Suicide and schizophrenia: a nationwide psychological autopsy study on age- and sex-specific clinical characteristics of 92 suicide victims with schizophrenia. *American Journal of Psychiatry*, **154**, 1235–42.
35. Kelly, D.L., Shim, J-C., Feldman, S.M, *et al.* (2004). Lifetime psychiatric symptoms in persons with schizophrenia who died by suicide compared to other means of death. *Journal of Psychiatric Research*, **38**, 531–6.
36. Heilä, H., Isometsä, E., Henriksson, M.H., *et al.* (1999). Suicide victims with schizophrenia in different treatment phases and adequacy of antipsychotic medication. *Journal of Clinical Psychiatry*, **60**, 200–8.
37. Zouk, H., Tousignant, M., Sequin, M., *et al.* (2006). Characterization of impulsivity in suicide completers: Clinical, behavioral and psychosocial dimensions. *Journal of Affective Disorders*, **92**, 195–204.
38. Brezo, J., Paris, J., and Turecki, G. (2006). Personality traits as correlates of suicidal ideation, suicide attempts, and suicide completions: a systematic review. *Acta Psychiatrica Scandinavica*, **113**, 180–206.
39. Marttunen, M.J., Aro, H.M., Henriksson, M.M., *et al.* (1991). Mental disorders in adolescent suicide: DSM-III-R axes I and II diagnoses in suicides among 13- to 19-year-olds in Finland. *Archives of General Psychiatry*, **48**, 834–9.

4.15.2 Deliberate self-harm: epidemiology and risk factors

Ella Arensman and Ad J. F. M. Kerkhof

Introduction

Deliberate self-harm (DSH) refers to behaviour through which people deliberately inflict acute harm upon themselves, poison themselves, or try do so, with non-fatal outcome. These behaviours are somehow linked to, but do not result in, death. Common to these behaviours is that they occur in conditions of emotional turmoil. In former days these behaviours were often regarded as failed suicides. However, this view did not appear to be correct, and the great majority of patients in fact do not try to kill themselves. Therefore, the term deliberate self-harm was introduced to describe the behaviour without implying any specific motive.[1] But this too has some disadvantages because there is a temporal association between non-fatal and fatal suicidal behaviour; many people who die by suicide have engaged in DSH before. Thus, Kreitman *et al.*[2] introduced the concept of parasuicide to describe behaviour that, mostly without the intention to kill oneself, communicates a degree of suicidal intent. However, both terms, deliberate self-harm and parasuicide, are still somewhat confusing, because in practice they include people who really have the intent of killing themselves but survive the attempt. The difficulty of finding a good terminology for these behaviours is reflected in differences in research populations in empirical studies: some studies are limited to self-poisoning only (overdose), a few studies are restricted to self-injury (wrist cutting) only, some to self-poisoning and self-injury combined, and some studies include behaviours in which, due to last-moment intervention from others, there was no actual self-harm inflicted at all. In recent years the term self-harm is being used in the United Kingdom and North America since the adjective 'deliberate' is not favoured by patients, particularly those who repeatedly engage in acts of self-harm.[3]

In this chapter, we will use the term deliberate self harm interchangeably with attempted suicide to refer to non-fatal suicidal behaviours in which there may have been an intention to die, however ambiguous this intention may have been, and irrespective of other intentions that may have been operating at the same time. It should be stressed that in deliberate self-harm many motives may play a role simultaneously, even contradictory motives such as the hope of being rescued and the wish to continue living. Intentions may vary from attention seeking or communication of despair, appeal for help, to a means for stress reduction. Common to these behaviours is that they are motivated by change: people want to bring about changes in their present situation through the actual or intended harm or unconsciousness inflicted upon the body. Deliberate self-harm may be defined as follows.[4]

> An act with non-fatal outcome, in which an individual deliberately initiates a non-habitual behaviour that, without intervention from others, will cause self-harm, or deliberately ingests a substance in excess of the prescribed or generally recognised therapeutic dosage, and which is aimed at realising changes which the subject desired via the actual or expected physical consequences.

This definition covers deliberate non-fatal suicidal behaviours. Not included are accidental cases of self-poisoning, accidental overdoses of opiates, or self-harmful acts by persons who do not anticipate the consequences of their actions. It does not include automutilation, which is an habitual, often obsessive act of inflicting (minor) self-harm, mostly without a conscious intent of changing the present situation, as with certain persons with learning disability.

Clinical features

Deliberate self-harm can have very different motivations, varying from an intention to die to a cry for help. These behaviours may be well prepared or carried out impulsively, and may have different physical consequences. The degree of lethality and the degree of medical seriousness of the consequences thus depend upon intention, preparation, knowledge and expectations of the method chosen, and sometimes upon coincidental factors such as intervention from others.

It is often difficult to assess the true intent of DSH. Because of fear for consequences, such as admission to a psychiatric hospital, or because of psychological defence mechanisms, people sometimes deny or conceal their intention to die. They also may exaggerate their intention to die in order to receive help. Sometimes people engage in potentially highly lethal self-harming behaviour without any wish to die, for example when they do not have adequate knowledge of the medication used. People who present at a general hospital with minor self-injury or minor self-poisoning may have had strong intentions to die but had insufficient knowledge of the lethality of the method. Therefore, one cannot always reliably infer what the precise meaning of the behaviour was, either from its overt characteristics or from the person's self-report. Among a large sample of adolescents aged 15 and 16 years, Rodham *et al.* found that adolescents who took an overdose more often expressed a wish to die compared to those who engaged in self-cutting.[(5)] Motives associated with self-cutting were self-punishment and interruption, i.e. trying to get relief from a terrible state of mind.

Epidemiology

In the 1960s and 1970s, there was a sharp increase in the number of people treated in hospitals in Europe, the United States and Australia because of intentional overdoses or self-injury. In the 1980s several studies showed a stabilization.[(6,7)] In the early 1990s these numbers increased further in some regions.[(8,9)] The absolute number of persons treated for deliberate self-harm in general hospitals, however, does not adequately reflect the size of the problem. These numbers should be calculated against the size and the characteristics of the population in the areas that are being served by the hospitals. Furthermore, in some countries DSH patients are treated by general practitioners when there is no need for hospital admission. In many instances emergency attendance for overdosing is not even registered. Except for Ireland, where a National Registry of Deliberate Self-Harm has been established,[(10)] there are no national registries that reliably monitor trends in DSH treated in general hospitals. Even though DSH is considered a major problem in the United States, clinical epidemiological research into DSH is uncommon.[(11)] Also, few epidemiological studies on DSH originate from other parts of the world.

Changes over time

In Edinburgh and Oxford, in the United Kingdom, there has been continuous monitoring of deliberate self-harm over a long period of time, where characteristics of persons engaging in DSH have been related to the corresponding population.[(7,12,13)] In these two cities trends in DSH rates have been documented reliably. After a period of stabilization in the 1980s a marked increase was observed. Between 1985 and 1995 the rates of DSH in Oxford increased by 62 per cent in males and 42 per cent in females. The increase in DSH has been most marked among young males. A similar trend has been observed in North Worcestershire where hospital referred cases of DSH were monitored over a period of 20 years (1981–2000).[(14)]

In Canada, the DSH rate was estimated to be around 304 per 100 000.[(15)] In the United States National Institute of Mental Health's Epidemiological Catchment Area study (1980–1985) it was found that 2.9 per cent of the respondents had engaged in DSH at some point of time.[(16)]

So far only one international multicentre study into deliberate self-harm has been conducted taking into consideration the methodological pitfalls outlined above. The World Health Organization (WHO) initiated a collaborative multicentre study in 16 regions in Europe using the same methodology, definition, and case-finding criteria.[(9,17)] The findings were related to the size and characteristics of the corresponding general population in order to investigate rates, trends, risk factors, and social indicators. Most of the epidemiological data presented here have been drawn from that study.[(9,18)]

Differences between countries and regions

There is widespread variation between countries with regard to rates of deliberate self-harm. Based on the latest available data for the years 1995–1999, overall, DSH rates (person-based) were highest in the United Kingdom (Oxford), Belgium (Ghent), Hungary (Pecs) and Finland (Helsinki), with female rates per 100 000 ranging from 83 in Padova (Italy) to 433 in Oxford. Male DSH rates per 100 000 ranged from 53 in Umea (Sweden) to 337 in Oxford.[(9)] Looking at trends over time, an average decrease for male DSH rates of 13 per cent was found comparing average person-based rates for 1989/1993 to the period 1995/1999, with the greatest reduction (70 per cent) in Innsbruck (Austria). For female DSH rates the average decrease in the same period was lower (4 per cent), with the greatest reduction (31 per cent) in Sor-Trondelag (Norway). In addition to medically referred cases of deliberate self-harm, community-based studies show that an even higher proportion of DSH appears to be 'hidden' from health care services.[(19)]

Differences between catchment areas in deliberate self-harm rates in the WHO/EURO study have been studied in relation to socio-economic characteristics of these areas.[(9,20)] No correlations were found with most of the social and economical factors supposedly related to DSH, such as population density, urban–rural distribution, proportion working in agriculture forestry or fishery, sex ratio, percentage aged 40 and over, number of people per household, percentage people living alone, percentage single parent families, per capita income, unemployment rate, life expectancy, mortality rate, infant mortality, crimes per year per 1000, and per capita alcohol consumption. Only two characteristics of the catchment areas seemed to be related to DSH rates: the percentage of divorced people in the area and the percentage receiving social security. Family stability and the percentage of the population relying on welfare both seem to be related to the frequency of DSH, but the interpretation of these findings is difficult because one would expect the other related social indicators of societal cohesion to covary as well.

It is important, however, to realize that the characteristics mentioned above relate to regions or countries, and do not relate to individuals. At individual level, characteristics such as unemployment play an important role, but this does not mean that unemployment rates do explain high DSH rates in a region.[21,22] This relationship holds only for some regions and not for others, as is documented repeatedly.[23] The effect of exposure to risks factors may be due to contextual effects, which arise if individuals' risks of suicidal behaviour depends not only on their personal exposure to risk or protective factors, but also on how these are distributed in their social, cultural or economic environments.[24,25] In a small area study in South East London, Neeleman *et al.* found that the DSH rate of minority groups relative to the white group was low in some areas and high in other areas.

Cultural variation in DSH has been documented from India,[26] Sri Lanka,[27] and Pakistan,[28] and from ethnic groups within Western societies, such as the Inuit in Canada.[29] Neeleman *et al.*[30] studied ethnic differences in DSH in Camberwell, London, and found considerable differences between the DSH rates for white people and for British-born Indian females and African-Caribbeans.[30] Indian females had a particularly high rate, 7.8 times that of white females. Marriage problems seem to be related to DSH in Asian countries such as India, Pakistan, Sri Lanka, and China. Young married women may have serious difficulties after moving in with their husbands' extended families. Dowry problems and problems with in-laws are thought to be precipitants of attempted suicide among young married women. In Asian countries the methods used in DSH reflect differences in accessibility. Self-poisoning with organophosphate pesticides and other household poisons is prevalent. As in the Western world DSH appears to reflect feelings of hopelessness and helplessness in adverse living conditions with no prospect of improvement. Women tend to be more powerless to bring about changes in their living conditions. In Sri Lanka, the continuous warfare, poverty, and the lack of opportunities at home and abroad frustrates the young who are relatively well educated.[27]

Sex and age

In all but one centre (Helsinki) of the WHO Multicentre Study on Suicidal Behaviour the female DSH rates were higher than the male rates. Across the participating regions, on average, the rates for females were 1.5 times higher than those for men. DSH rates were consistently higher among those in the young age groups, with the highest person-based male DSH rates in the age group 25–34 years, whereas for females in most centres the highest rates were found in the age group 15–24 years.[9]

Sociodemographic characteristics

Single and divorced people were over-represented among people who engaged in DSH in the WHO/EURO study.[9,18] Nearly half of the males and 38 per cent of the females were never married. An interaction effect was found for age in that the proportion of single persons among those engaging in deliberate self-harm reduced with increasing age, whereas the proportion of divorced, separated, and widowed people increased with age. Among deliberate self-harm patients who were economically active, a high percentage was unemployed. Based on average DSH rates over the period 1995–1999, 26 per cent of the males and 14 per cent of the females were unemployed.[9]

These findings are consistent with outcomes of earlier research conducted in the United Kingdom, where socio-economic deprivation (low social class and unemployment) repeatedly appear as characteristics of the DSH populations.[22]

These findings indicate that DSH patients disproportionately have had low education, and have high levels of unemployment, poverty, and divorce. The findings may be partly related to underlying common causes, such as the presence of psychiatric disorders, but they also suggest the influence of sociological factors impacting on a relatively economically deprived group in society with a greater share of adversity.[24] Socio-economic deprivation is a well-established determinant of psychiatric morbidity and DSH.[32,33] In contrast with completed suicide, where the presence of psychiatric disorders is well documented (up to 95 per cent of suicides may have suffered from a psychiatric disorder), psychiatric disorders are much less frequent among those who deliberately harm themselves. Among those who engage in DSH for the first time in their lives, the prevalence of psychiatric disorders may be rather low; among repeaters, psychiatric morbidity is considerable.[34,35]

Methods

Methods used in deliberate self-harm are mostly 'non-violent'. In the WHO Multicentre Study, 65 per cent of males and 82 per cent of females took an overdose, based on average DSH rates for the period 1995–1999. Cutting, mostly wrist cutting, was employed in 16 per cent of male cases and 9 per cent of female cases. There are some differences between European countries in the use of particular methods. Based on the years 1995–1999, a relatively high percentage of self-cutting was found in Tallinn (Estonia, 50 per cent), Ljubljana (Slovenia, 30 per cent), and Innsbruck (Austria, 26 per cent). In Szeged (Hungary), 19 per cent of males and 15 per cent of females used poisoning with pesticides, herbicides, or other toxic agricultural chemicals, whereas in other regions this ranged from 0–3 per cent.[9] In Sor-Trondelag, Norway, higher percentages engaged in DSH by deliberate alcohol overdose (6 per cent of males and 5 per cent of females). In general, somewhat older men used the method of jumping or jumping in front of a moving object. In the Oxford studies between 1985 and 1995, 88 per cent of all episodes involved self-poisoning, 8 per cent involved self-injury, and 4 per cent involved both. There was an increase in the use of paracetamol from 31 per cent of poisoning cases in 1985 to 50 per cent in 1995.[6] There was also an increase in antidepressant overdoses and a decrease in overdoses of minor tranquillizers and sedatives. Comparing the early 1990s with the late 1990s, a slight increase was observed in overdose by medication.[9] For all regions the methods used in DSH acts did not covary significantly with age.

The differences in methods between countries may be related to differences in the accessibility of certain methods. Until 1998 paracetamol was available in large quantities in the United Kingdom, unlike other European countries.[36,37] The ingestion of alcohol during or before the act sometimes can be considered to be a part of the actual method of DSH (when used to bring about unconsciousness, or to increase the risk of a fatal outcome), as part of the preparation (to lower the threshold for engaging in an act of DSH, because of disinhibition), or as a long-term risk factor. Hawton *et al.*[38,39] found that 22 to 26 per cent of DSH patients had consumed alcohol at the time of the act (males more frequent than females), and that 44 to 50 per cent had consumed alcohol during the 6 h before the DSH acts, this again being more common in males than in females. About 28 per cent of DSH patients in Oxford appeared to be substance misusers (alcohol and drugs).

General population self-report surveys

General population epidemiological surveys of adolescents indicate that DSH acts occur more frequently than suggested by hospital statistics.[40,41] A number of surveys have been conducted to estimate the prevalence of DSH. Most of these surveys concerned adolescents and were administered anonymously. Most questionnaire studies revealed that between 1 and 20 per cent of respondents had engaged in DSH at some point in time.[41–44] However, the methodology used in the various studies varies considerably and therefore limits comparison of the outcomes. In the study by Hawton *et al.*[41] a minority (12.6 per cent) of adolescents who had engaged in DSH had presented to hospital.

Lifetime prevalence

Based upon the rates from the WHO/EURO study the lifetime prevalence of deliberate self-harm should be around 3 per cent for females and 2 per cent for males, with some variations between countries and regions.[9] DSH acts that did not lead to medical treatment at a hospital or general practitioner's surgery are very difficult to study, because of the limited validity of self-report data. Based on two large community-based surveys, the lifetime prevalence of suicidal ideation varied from 2.6 to 25.4 per cent and for deliberate self-harm this varied from 0.4 to 4.2 per cent.[45,46]

Classification

As previously mentioned, there is a considerable variety of behaviours within the broad category of non-fatal suicidal behaviour. A review of classification studies[34] revealed three types of DSH patients: a 'mild' type, a 'severe' type, and a 'mixed' type in between.

The mild type of DSH encompasses mostly relatively non-violent methods followed by non-serious physical injury. Young age, living together, few precautions to prevent discovery, low level of suicidal preoccupation, low suicidal intent, interpersonal motivation are all characteristics associated with mild forms of attempted suicide/deliberate self-harm. The severe category consists mostly of relatively hard methods followed by serious physical consequences. Older age (over 40), many precautions to prevent discovery, high level of suicidal preoccupation, high suicidal intent, self-directed motivation, often relocated, previous attempted suicides, depression, drug dependence, a high degree of overall dysfunctioning, poor physical health, and previous psychiatric treatment are all characteristics associated with the concept of 'severe' deliberate self-harm. The risk of repetition is greater in the severe type. In between, in the mixed type of DSH, the DSH acts and patients involved show mixed characteristics, which makes this type harder to identify in medical practice.

In order to further refine the classification of deliberate self-harm, Arensman[47] included psychological and personal history variables and these characteristics were studied in relation to recurrent DSH in a follow-up period of 1 year. **The mild DSH type** was validated, approximately 40 per cent of the total sample, as being predominantly younger than 30 years of age, single, living alone or with parents, and having minor injuries because of the index attempt. The mean number of previous DSH acts was 3.7. The repetition rate in the follow-up period for this group was 27 per cent. In the older age group, two groups were distinguished: a moderate group and a group with an extremely high risk for non-fatal repetition were identified. The high-risk group, consisting of approximately 28 per cent of the total sample, suffered more physical injury as a consequence of their deliberate self-harm.

The high-risk group consisted predominantly of females in the age group 30 to 49 years who were divorced or separated, living alone, and who were economically inactive. Most of them had engaged in previous DSH acts (mean number: 5). They had histories of traumatic life events that mostly started early in life. The high-risk group showed the highest scores on depression, hopelessness and expression of state-anger, and two-thirds were diagnosed as having borderline personality disorder. In the follow-up at least 75 per cent engaged in repeated DSH.

The moderate group was characterized by low levels of physical injury following their DSH, they were predominantly aged at least 30 years and married, and scored intermediate on measures of depression, hopelessness, and anger. The mean number of previous attempts was 2.3, and 33 per cent made one or more repeated DSH acts in the follow-up. Surprisingly, this classification into three types of non-fatal suicidal behaviours did not correspond to the levels of reported suicide intent nor to the levels of the different motivations reported (to die, to appeal, to lose consciousness, revenge), underlining the difficulty of classifying DSH according to intentions. Rodham *et al.*[5] found evidence for different subgroups of DSH patients based on DSH methods and motives. For example, they identified a subgroup of female adolescents who engaged in self-cutting and who reported *self-punishment* as the primary motive, followed by *trying to get relief from a terrible state of mind.* Furthermore, *wish to die* as a motive was significantly more often reported by those who took an overdose compared with those who engaged in self-cutting.

Aetiology

The last psychological step towards deliberate self-harm is always set in conditions of emotional turmoil, an emotional crisis. Essential in crisis is the absence of any positive outlook towards the future. People completing suicide do not expect any improvement of their situation in the near or distant future. People who engage in deliberate self-harm indicate that their future is hopeless, but they still seem to have a faint hope, however ambiguous this may be, that the future might improve. In this way deliberate self-harm may be conceived as a self-invented form of crisis intervention. Studies into the cognitive functioning of DSH patients indeed show a global and stable form of negative anticipations and absence of positive anticipations towards the future, probably as a consequence of disturbances in their autobiographical memory, i.e. an overgeneral memory.[48,49] Whenever these anticipations remain overgenerally negative after an act of DSH, it is likely that hopelessness will increase and that this behaviour will occur again.[50]

Precipitants

Difficulties or conflicts that may bring the person to believe that his or her future is without hope can trigger the psychological crisis resulting in deliberate self-harm. DSH is often precipitated by disharmony with key figures, work-related problems, financial difficulties, or physical illnesses. Long-standing relationship problems or feelings of loneliness are especially common. People who engage in DSH have a weak social support system,[48] and they report relational difficulties as major problems in life. They show deficits in interpersonal problem solving, and their future holds no promise. Their emotional status can best be described as a state of learned helplessness, a situation of a blocked escape, in which no solution exists for a perceived insurmountable adversity.[51] This leads to the question as to why these persons have developed such helpless attitudes.

Long-term vulnerability factors

The conflicts experienced by DSH patients in the days before an act of DSH are not different from the same conflicts they have experienced over and over again. Not only recent life events, but also the life events that occurred in their past are important.[47] Many DSH patients, males as well as females, have had traumatic childhood experiences, including physical and emotional neglect, broken homes, other unstable parental conditions, violence, sexual and physical abuse, incest, parents who had psychiatric treatment, who were alcoholics and/or addicted to opiates. Women who have been abused have a much greater probability of becoming a repeater later. In addition they often develop poor relationships, lack self-esteem, and experience overwhelming feelings of helplessness and hopelessness. Any trigger, for example an argument with a friend, may be sufficient to provoke suicidal ideation and behaviour.

DSH patients not only suffer from helplessness with regard to interpersonal conflicts, they also tend to be powerless in other domains of life. The DSH population disproportionately consists of unemployed persons, from low social classes, with low educational levels, economically deprived, divorced, disabled, addicted, incarcerated, and/or lonely. Many have received in- or outpatient psychiatric treatment. These findings are somewhat complicated by the fact that many of these vulnerability factors are strongly interrelated. Unemployment, addiction, and unstable partnership relations all may be caused by psychiatric diseases. For example, unemployment and DSH may both be a consequence of addiction. However, it is not fair to assume that most of the economic deprivation of suicidal patients is explained by their psychiatric condition. The considerable differences between nations in the prevalence of DSH support the importance of socio-economic conditions.

Course and prognosis

Repetition is one of the core characteristics of suicidal behaviour. Among those who die by suicide up to 40 per cent have a history of previous DSH acts.[52] Among DSH patients 'repeaters' are more common than 'first-evers'. Between 30 and 60 per cent of DSH patients engaged in previous acts, and between 15 and 25 per cent did so within the last year.[3,7,53,54]

Risk of suicide after deliberate self-harm

Prospectively, DSH patients have a high risk of dying by suicide. Between 10 and 15 per cent eventually die because of suicide.[11,53] The connection between DSH and suicide lies between 0.5 and 2 per cent after 1 year and above 5 per cent after 9 years.[11] Mortality by suicide is higher among DSH patients who have engaged in previous acts of DSH.[55,56] The risk of suicide after deliberate self-harm for males is nearly twice the female risk, the risk being particularly high in the first year.[57,58] Alcohol and drug abuse and related social deterioration are risk factors for subsequent suicide,[59] as are psychiatric diagnosis (affective disorders, schizophrenia, personality disorders), and a highly lethal non-impulsive index act of DSH. In a large European study focusing on young deliberate self-harm patients, positive correlations were found between rates of DSH and suicide for both males and females, with a statistically significant association among males aged 15–24.[60]

Repetition of deliberate self-harm

Risk of repeated DSH is highest during the first year after an act of DSH, and especially within the first 3 to 6 months.[55,57,61] In the WHO/EURO Multicentre Study on Suicidal Behaviour it was found that at least 54 per cent of DSH patients had engaged in a DSH act before, 30 per cent at least twice. Prospectively, 30 per cent of DSH patients made at least one repeated attempt in a 1-year follow-up.[62,63]

It is hoped for that knowledge of antecedents or risk factors may foster early identification of persons at risk, and improvement of treatment. Many studies have tried to identify risk factors or antecedents and some of these by now are well known. Sociodemographic risk factors associated with repetition are belonging to the age group of 25 to 49 years, being divorced, unemployed, and coming from low social class. Psychosocial characteristics of repeaters are substance abuse, depression, hopelessness, personality disorders, unstable living conditions/living alone, criminal records, previous psychiatric treatment, and a history of stressful traumatic life events, including broken homes and family violence, especially physical and mental maltreatment by partners. Prospectively, a history of previous attempts is one of the most powerful predictors of future non-fatal suicide attempts.[34,51,64,65]

Conclusions

Deliberate self-harm is a major problem in many contemporary societies. DSH seems to reflect the degree of powerlessness and hopelessness of young people with low education, low income, unemployment, and difficulties in coping with life stress. As such, non-fatal suicidal behaviour should be a major concern for politicians. There are substantial differences between communities in the prevalence of deliberate self-harm. This suggests that some communities better meet the needs of their underprivileged youngsters than others do, but we barely understand the differences between communities and nations. Preventive action therefore is difficult to design. There is a need for a better nationwide continuous registration of DSH and related socio-economic conditions. There is also a need for better mental health care management of DSH patients, and for experimental studies on the prevention of repetition. Although we know that persons who engage in DSH are at high risk for future fatal and non-fatal suicidal behaviour, development of effective intervention, and prevention programmes is a key priority.

Further information

Hawton, K. (ed.) (2005). *Prevention and treatment of suicidal behaviour: from science to practice.* Oxford University Press, Oxford.

De Leo, D., Bille-Brahe, U., Kerkhof, A., and Schmidtke, A. (eds.) (2004). *Suicidal behaviour: theories and research findings.* Hogrefe and Huber, Göttingen, Germany.

Van Heeringen, K. (ed.) (2001). *Understanding suicidal behaviour. The suicidal process approach to research, treatment and prevention.* John Wiley & Sons Ltd., Chichester, UK.

Hawton, K. and Van Heeringen, K. (eds.) (2000). *The international handbook of suicide and attempted suicide.* John Wiley & Sons, Chichester, UK.

Website of the International Association for Suicide Prevention (IASP): http://www.med.uio.no/iasp/

References

1. Morgan, H.G., Barton, J., Pottle, S., *et al.* (1976). Deliberate self-harm: a follow-up study of 279 patients. *The British Journal of Psychiatry*, **128**, 361–8.
2. Kreitman, N., Philip, A.E., Greer, S., *et al.* (1969). Parasuicide. *The British Journal of Psychiatry*, **115**, 746–7.
3. Skegg, K. (2005). Self-harm. *Lancet*, **366**, 1471–83.
4. Platt, S., Bille-Brahe, U., Kerkhof, A., *et al.* (1992). Parasuicide in Europe: the WHO/EURO multicentre study on parasuicide. I. Introduction and preliminary analysis for 1989. *Acta Psychiatrica Scandinavica*, **85**, 97–104.
5. Rodham, K., Hawton, K., and Evans, E. (2004). Reasons for deliberate self-harm: comparison of self-poisoners and self-cutters in a community sample of adolescents. *Journal of the American Academy of Child and Adolescent Psychiatry*, **43**, 80–7.
6. Hawton, K. and Fagg, J. (1992). Trends in deliberate self-poisoning and self-injury in Oxford, 1976–1990. *British Medical Journal*, **304**, 1409–11.
7. Platt, S., Hawton, K., Kreitman, N., *et al.* (1988). Recent clinical and epidemiological trends in parasuicide in Edinburgh and Oxford: a tale of two cities. *Psychological Medicine*, **18**, 405–18.
8. Schmidtke, A., Bille Brahe, U., De Leo, D., *et al.* (1996). Attempted suicide in Europe: rates, trends and sociodemographic characteristics of suicide attempters during the period 1989–1992. Results of the WHO/EURO multicentre study on parasuicide. *Acta Psychiatrica Scandinavica*, **93**, 327–38.
9. Schmidtke, A., Bille-Brahe, U., De Leo, D., *et al.* (2004). *Suicidal behaviour in Europe: results from the WHO/EURO multicentre study on suicidal behaviour.* Hogrefe & Huber, Göttingen, Germany.
10. National Suicide Research Foundation. (2007). *National registry of deliberate self harm report—2006.* National Suicide Research Foundation, Cork.
11. Owens, D., Horrocks, J., and House, A. (2002). Fatal and non-fatal repetition of self-harm. Systematic review. *The British Journal of Psychiatry*, **181**, 193–9.
12. Kreitman, N. (1977). *Parasuicide.* Wiley, London.
13. Hawton, K., Fagg, J., Simkin, S., *et al.* (1997). Trends in deliberate self-harm in Oxford, 1985–1995. *The British Journal of Psychiatry*, **171**, 556–60.
14. O'Loughlin, S. and Sherwood, J. (2005). A 20-year review of trends in deliberate self-harm in a British town, 1981–2000. *Social Psychiatr y and Psychiatric Epidemiology*, **40**, 446–53.
15. Sakinofsky, I. (1996). The epidemiology of suicide in Canada. In *Suicide in Canada* (eds. A.A. Leenaars, S. Wenckstern, I. Sakinovsky, D. Dyck, M. Kral, and R. Bland). University of Toronto Press, Toronto.
16. Moscicki, E.K., O'Carroll, P., Rae, D.S., *et al.* (1988). Suicide attempts in the epidemiologic catchment area study. *The Yale Journal of Biology and Medicine*, **61**, 259–68.
17. Kerkhof, A.J.J.M., Schmidtke, A., Bille Brahe, U., *et al.* (1994). *Attempted suicide in Europe.* DSWO-Press/World Health Organization, Leiden and Copenhagen.
18. Schmidtke, A., Bille Brahe, U., De Leo, D., *et al.* (1996). Attempted suicide in Europe: rates, trends and sociodemographic characteristics of suicide attempters during the period 1989–1992. Results of the WHO/EURO multicentre study on parasuicide. *Acta Psychiatrica Scandinavica*, **93**, 327–38.
19. Evans, E., Hawton, K., and Rodham, K. (2004). Factors associated with suicidal phenomena in adolescents: a systematic review of population-based studies. *Clinical Psychology Review*, **24**, 957–79.
20. Bille-Brahe, U., Andersen, K., Wasserman, D., *et al.* (1996). The WHO-EURO multicentre study: risk of parasuicide and the comparability of the areas under study. *Crisis*, **17**, 32–42.
21. Platt, S. (1984). Unemployment and suicidal behaviour: a review of the literature. *Social Science & Medicine*, **19**, 93–115.
22. Platt, S. and Dyer, J. (1987). Psychological correlates of unemployment among male parasuicides in Edinburgh. *The British Journal of Psychiatry*, **151**, 27–32.
23. Adam, K.S. (1990). Environmental, psychosocial, and psychoanalytic aspects of suicidal behavior. In *Suicide over the life cycle* (eds. S.J. Blumenthal and D.J. Kupfer), pp. 39–96. American Psychiatric Press, Washington, DC.
24. Neeleman, J., Wilson-Jones, C., and Wessely, S. (2001). Ethnic density and deliberate self harm: a small area study in south east London. *Journal of Epidemiology and Community Health*, **55**, 85–90.
25. Neeleman, J. (2002). Beyond risk theory: suicidal behaviour in its social and epidemiological context. *Crisis*, **23**, 114–20.
26. Latha, K.S., Bhat, S.M., and D'Souza, P. (1996). Suicide attempters in a general hospital unit in India: their socio-demographic and clinical profile—emphasis on cross-cultural aspects. *Acta Psychiatrica Scandinavica*, **94**, 26–30.
27. Eddleston, M., Rezvi Sheriff, M.H., and Hawton, K. (1998). Deliberate self harm in Sri Lanka: an overlooked tragedy in the developing world. *British Medical Journal*, **317**, 133–5.
28. Khan, M.M., Islam, S., and Kundi, A.K. (1996). Parasuicide in Pakistan: experience at a university hospital. *Acta Psychiatrica Scandinavica*, **94**, 264–7.
29. Kirmayer, L.J., Malus, M., and Boothroyd, L.J. (1996). Suicide attempts among Inuit youth: a community survey of prevalence and risk factors. *Acta Psychiatrica Scandinavica*, **94**, 8–17.
30. Neeleman, J., Jones, P., van Os, J., *et al.* (1996). Parasuicide in Camberwell—ethnic differences. *Social Psychiatry and Psychiatric Epidemiology*, **31**, 284–7.
31. Hawton, K. and Catalan, J. (1982). *Attempted suicide. A practical guide to its nature and management.* Oxford University Press, Oxford.
32. Gunnell, D.J., Peters, T.J., Kammerling, R.M., *et al.* (1995). Relation between parasuicide, suicide, psychiatric admissions, and socioeconomic deprivation. *British Medical Journal*, **311**, 226–30.
33. Congdon, P. (1996). Suicide and parasuicide in London; a small-area study. *Urban Studies*, **1**, 137–58.
34. Arensman, E. and Kerkhof, A.J.F.M. (1996). Classification of attempted suicide: a review of empirical studies, 1963–1993. *Suicide & Life-threatening Behavior*, **26**, 46–67.
35. De Leo, D., Bille-Brahe, U., Kerkhof, A.J.F.M., *et al.* (2004). *Suicidal behaviour: theories and findings.* Hogrefe & Huber, Göttingen, Germany.

36. Hawton, K., Simkin, S., Deeks, J., *et al.* (2004). UK legislation on analgesic packs: before and after study of long-term effect on poisonings. *British Medical Journal*, **329**, 1076.
37. Gunnell, D., Hawton, K., Murray, V., *et al.* (1997). Use of paracetamol for suicide and non-fatal poisoning in the UK and France: are restrictions on availability justified? *Journal of Epidemiology and Community Health*, **51**, 175–9.
38. Hawton, K., Fagg, J., Simkin, S., *et al.* (1997, 1998). *Deliberate self-harm in Oxford, 1996, 1997. Reports from the Oxford monitoring system for attempted suicide.* Warneford Hospital, Oxford.
39. Hawton, K., Simkin, S., and Fagg, J. (1997). Deliberate self-harm in alcohol and drug misusers: patient characteristics and patterns of clinical care. *Drug and Alcohol Review*, **16**, 123–9.
40. Choquet, M. and Ledoux, S. (1994). *Adolescents: enquête nationale.* Inserm, Villejuif Cedex.
41. Hawton, K., Rodham, K., Evans, E., *et al.* (2002). Deliberate self harm in adolescents: self-report survey in schools in England. *British Medical Journal*, **325**, 1207–11.
42. Paykel, E.S., Myers, J.K., Lindentall, J.J., *et al.* (1974). Suicidal feelings in the general population: a prevalence study. *The British Journal of Psychiatry*, **124**, 460–9.
43. Kienhorst, C.W.M., de Wilde, E.J., Diekstra, R.F.W., *et al.* (1991). Construction of an index for predicting suicide attempts in depressed adolescents. *The British Journal of Psychiatry*, **159**, 676–82.
44. Rubinstein, J.L., Heeren, T., Housman, D., *et al.* (1989). Suicidal behavior in 'normal' adolescents: risk and protective factors. *The American Journal of Orthopsychiatry*, **59**, 59–71.
45. Bertelote, J.M, Fleischmann, A., De Leo, D., *et al.* (2005). Suicide attempts, plans, and ideation in culturally diverse sites: the WHO SUPRE-MISS community survey. *Psychological Medicine*, **35**, 1–9.
46. Bernal, M., Haro, J.M., Bernert, S., *et al.* (in press). Risk factors for suicidality in Europe: results from the ESEMED study. *Journal of Affective Disorders*.
47. Arensman, E. (1997). Attempted suicide: epidemiology and classification. Unpublished PhD. Dissertation, University of Leiden, The Netherlands.
48. Williams, J.M.G. (1997). *The cry of pain.* Harmondsworth, Penguin.
49. Sinclair, J.M., Crane, C., Hawton, *et al.* (in press). The role of autobiographical memory specificity in deliberate self-harm: correlates and consequences. *Journal of Affective Disorders*.
50. MacLeod, A.K., Rose, G.S., and Williams, J.M.G. (1993). Components of hopelessness about the future in parasuicide. *Cognitive Therapy and Research*, **17**, 441–55.
51. McAuliffe, C., Corcoran, P., Keeley, H.S., *et al.* (2006). Problem-solving ability and repetition of deliberate self-harm: a multicentre study. *Psychological Medicine*, **36**, 45–55.
52. Maris, R.W. (1992). The relationship of nonfatal suicide attempts to completed suicide. In *Assessment and prediction of suicide* (eds. R.W. Maris, A.L. Berman, J.T. Maltsberger, and R.I. Yufit), pp. 362–80. Guilford Press, New York.
53. Kreitman, N. and Casey, P. (1988). Repetition of parasuicide: an epidemiological and clinical study. *The British Journal of Psychiatry*, **153**, 792–800.
54. Hawton, K. and Fagg, J. (1995). Repetition of attempted suicide: the performance of the Edinburgh predictive scales in patients in Oxford. *Archives of Suicide Research*, **1**, 261–72.
55. Hawton, K. and Catalan, J. (1981). Psychiatric management of attempted suicide patients. *British Journal of Hospital Medicine*, **26**, 365–8.
56. Hawton, K. and Fagg, J. (1988). Suicide and other causes of death, following attempted suicide. *The British Journal of Psychiatry*, **152**, 359–66.
57. Nordstrom, P., Samuelsson, M., and Asberg, M. (1995). Survival analysis of suicide risk after attempted suicide. *Acta Psychiatrica Scandinavica*, **91**, 336–40.
58. Suokas, J. and Lonnqvist, J. (1991). Outcome of attempted suicide and psychiatric consultation: risk factors and suicide mortality during a five year follow-up. *Acta Psychiatrica Scandinavica*, **84**, 545–9.
59. Cullberg, J., Wasserman, D., and Stefansson, C.G. (1988). Who commits suicide after a suicide attempt? An 8 to 10 year follow-up in a suburban catchment area. *Acta Psychiatrica Scandinavica*, **77**, 598–603.
60. Hawton, K., Arensman, E., Wasserman, D., *et al.* (1998). Relation between attempted suicide and suicide rates among young people in Europe. *Journal of Epidemiology and Community Health*, **52**, 191–4.
61. Goldacre, M. and Hawton, K. (1985). Repetition of self-poisoning and subsequent death in adolescents who take overdoses. *The British Journal of Psychiatry*, **146**, 395–8.
62. Kerkhof, A.J.F.M. and Arensman, E. (2004). Repetition of attempted suicide: frequent, but hard to predict. In *Suicidal behaviour: theories and findings* (eds. D. De Leo, U. Bille-Brahe, A.J.F.M. Kerkhof, and A. Schmidtke). Hogrefe and Huber, Göttingen.
63. Arensman, E., Kerkhof, A., Dirkzwager, A., *et al.* (1999). Prevalence and risk factors for repeated suicidal behaviour: results from the WHO/EURO multicentre study on parasuicide, 1989–1992 Report University of Leiden, The Netherlands.
64. Van Egmond, M. and Diekstra, R.F.W. (1989). The predictability of suicidal behaviour: the results of a meta-analysis of published studies. In *Suicide and its prevention* (eds. R.F.W. Diekstra, R. Maris, S. Platt, A. Schmidtke, and G. Sonneck), pp. 37–61. Brill, Leiden.
65. Kreitman, N. and Foster, J. (1991). Construction and selection of predictive scales, with special reference to parasuicide. *The British Journal of Psychiatry*, **159**, 185–92.

4.15.3 **Biological aspects of suicidal behaviour**

J. John Mann and Dianne Currier

Modelling suicidal behaviours

To understand the biological underpinnings of multi-determined behaviours such as suicide and attempted suicide it is necessary to situate them within an explanatory model that can elaborate the causal pathways and interrelations between biological, clinical, genetic, and environmental factors that all play a role in suicidal behaviour. Where possible, such a model should be clinically explanatory, incorporate biological correlates, be testable in both clinical and biological studies, and have some utility in identifying high-risk individuals.

We have proposed a stress–diathesis model of suicidal behaviour wherein exposure to a stressor precipitates a suicidal act in those with the diathesis, or propensity, for suicidal behaviour.[(1)] Stressors are generally state-dependent factors such as an episode of major depression or adverse life event. The diathesis, we have hypothesized, comprises trait characteristics such as impulsive aggression, and pessimism.[(1)] Uncovering the biological mechanisms relevant to the stress and the diathesis dimensions of suicidal behaviour will facilitate the identification of both enduring and proximal markers of risk, as well as potential targets for treatment.

One biological correlate of the diathesis for suicidal behaviour appears to be low serotonergic activity. Abnormal serotonergic function may be the result of numerous factors including genetics, early life experience, chronic medical illness, alcoholism or substance use disorder, many of which have been correlated with increased risk for suicidal behaviour. Moreover, serotonergic dysfunction may underlie recurrent mood disorders or behavioural traits that characterize the diathesis, such as aggression and impulsivity. In terms of stress response, the noradrenergic and HPA axis have been the focus of biological studies in suicidal behaviour. This chapter gives an overview of the major neurobiological findings in suicide and attempted suicide, as well as emerging findings from studies of genes related to those systems.

Serotonergic system

Serotonin is involved in brain development, behavioural regulation, modulation of sleep, mood, anxiety, cognition, and memory and is shown to be disturbed in various psychiatric disorders. Serotonergic function is under genetic control and, moreover, deficits in functioning have been shown to be enduring, marking it as a biological trait. The serotonergic system became a target for investigation in relation to suicide when, more than 30 years ago, Asberg and colleagues observed that depressed individuals who had either attempted suicide by violent means or subsequently died by suicide in the study follow-up period were more likely to have lower CSF 5-HIAA levels.[(2)] Since that time the function of the serotonergic system in suicide and attempted has been examined in many paradigms, and while not all studies agree, there is substantial consensus that individuals who die by suicide, or make serious non-fatal suicide attempts, exhibit a deficiency in CNS serotonin neurotransmission.

Evidence of hypofunction comes from *cerebrospinal fluid* and postmortem studies. 5-hydroxyindoleacetic acid (5-HIAA) is the major metabolite of serotonin and level of CSF 5-HIAA is a guide to serotonin activity in parts of the brain including the prefrontal cortex. There have been over 20 studies of CSF 5-HIAA and suicidal behaviour in mood disorders, and a meta-analysis of prospective studies of 5-HIAA found that in mood disorders lower CSF 5-HIAA increased the chance of death by suicide over fourfold over follow-up periods of 1–14 years.[(3)]

Multiple *postmortem studies* of suicide, report lower brainstem levels of 5-HIAA and serotonin (5-hydroxytryptamine, 5-HT) (see Mann *et al.* for a review[(4)]). These deficits in 5-HT or 5-HIAA are observable across diagnostic groups[(5)] and, despite early reports to the contrary, independent of suicide method. This abnormality appears to be largely specific to the brainstem, and multiple studies have reported no differences between suicides and controls in 5-HT level in other brain regions including the hippocampus, the occipital cortex, the frontal cortex, the temporal cortex, the caudate, the striatum, or the hypothalamus.[(4)] Serotonin neurone cell bodies are in the brainstem raphe nuclei, while their axons innervate most of the brain including the ventral prefrontal cortex. Morphological analysis of stained serotonin neurones in the brainstem of depressed suicides and non-suicides observed greater cell density in the dorsal raphe nucleus in the suicides[(6)] suggesting that reduction in serotonin activity is associated with dysfunctional neurones and not with fewer neurones.

Neuroendocrine challenge studies using fenfluramine provide further evidence of anomalous serotonergic function associated with suicidal behaviour. Fenfluramine is a serotonin-releasing drug and a reuptake inhibitor that may also directly stimulate postsynaptic 5-HT receptors. The release of serotonin by fenfluramine causes a measurable increase in serum prolactin levels that is an indirect index of central serotonergic responsiveness. In depressed patients, those with a history of suicide attempts have a more blunted prolactin response to fenfluramine challenge than non-attempters with some evidence that the effect is more strongly related to seriousness of past attempt.[(7)]

Studies of receptors suggest lower serotonergic transmission in the central nervous system may be accompanied by a compensatory upregulation of some serotonergic postsynaptic receptors such as the 5-HT_{1A} and 5-HT_{2A}, and a decrease in the number of serotonin reuptake sites.[(4)] There is a reported increase in the concentration of the postsynaptic 5-HT_{2A} receptors in the prefrontal cortex of suicides compared with non-suicides.[(8)] This increased binding is reflected in more protein and may be due to elevated gene expression in youth suicide.[(9)] Elevated 5-HT_{2A} binding has also been reported in the amygdala in depressed suicides. In depressed and non-depressed suicides there is evidence that 5-HT_{2A} receptors are upregulated in the dorsal prefrontal cortex but not the rostral prefrontal cortex.[(8)]

Platelet studies examine 5-HT_{2A} in living subjects with respect to non-fatal suicide attempt. 5-HT_{2A} receptors, serotonin reuptake sites, and serotonin second messenger systems are present in blood platelets, and changes in these platelet measurements may reflect similar changes in the CNS. Multiple studies have reported higher platelet 5-HT_{2A} receptor numbers in suicide attempters compared with non-attempters and healthy controls.[(11)]

Studies of second messengers indicate impaired 5-HT_{2A} receptor mediated signal transduction in the prefrontal cortex of suicides, [(12)] and in platelets 5-HT_{2A} receptor responsivity is significantly blunted in patients with major depression who have made high-lethality suicide attempts compared to depressed patients who have made low-lethality suicide attempts.[(13)] The implications of such a defect in signal transduction, if present in the brain, would be that although there may be greater density of 5-HT_{2A} receptors, the signal transduced by 5-HT_{2A} receptor activation may be blunted, which would compound deficient serotonergic input as seen in the lower levels of brainstem serotonin and/or 5-HIAA in suicide victims.

Some *postmortem studies* of the postsynaptic 5-HT_{1A} receptor report higher binding in prefrontal cortex and more rostral segments of raphe nuclei, and lower binding in more caudal raphe nuclei, hippocampus, prefrontal cortex, and temporal cortex.[(7)] Less 5-HT_{1A} autoreceptor gene expression is also reported in the dorsal raphe[(14)] and would favour higher serotonin neurone firing rates.

Postmortem studies of depressed suicides report fewer 5-HT transporters in prefrontal cortex, hypothalamus, occipital cortex, and brainstem.[(15)] Moreover, in suicides this deficit appears localized to the ventromedial prefrontal cortex, whereas depressed individuals who died of other causes had lower binding throughout the prefrontal cortex.[(16)]

The emerging picture from postmortem studies of greater 5-HT_{2A} receptor binding in the frontal cortex of depressed individuals who die by suicide, fewer brainstem 5-HT_{1A} autoreceptors, and fewer serotonin transporters in the cortex, as well as findings of greater tryptophan hydroxylase (the rate-limiting step in serotonin synthesis) immunoreactivity in serotonin nuclei in the brainstem[(17)] all point to homeostatic changes designed to increase deficient serotonergic transmission evidenced by low 5-HIAA in CSF and brain, low 5-HT and 5-HIAA in brainstem, and blunted prolactin response to fenfluramine challenge.

Serotonergic dysfunction and suicide endophenotypes. Increased aggression has been associated with suicide and more highly lethal suicide attempts and impulsivity has shown a stronger relationship to non-fatal suicide attempts.[18] Impulsive aggressive traits are potentially part of the diathesis for suicidal behaviour.[1] Reduced activity of the serotonin system has been implicated in impulsive violence and aggression in studies in a variety of paradigms including: Low CSF 5-HIAA in individuals with a lifetime history of aggressive behaviour with personality and other psychiatric disorders;[19, 20] a blunted prolactin response to serotonin-releasing agent fenfluramine in personality disorder patients,[21, 22] and; greater platelet 5-HT_{2A} binding correlated with aggressive behaviour in personality and other psychiatric disorder patients.[23, 24] In a postmortem study of aggression, suicidal behaviour, and serotonergic function a positive relationship between lifetime history of aggression scores and 5-HT_{2A} binding in several regions of prefrontal cortex of individuals who had died by suicide was found.[25]

Positron emission tomography (PET) studies have shown a deficient response to serotonergic challenge in the orbitofrontal cortex, medial frontal, and cingulate regions in individuals with impulsive aggression compared to controls[26, 27] and lower serotonin transporter binding in the anterior cingulate cortex in impulsive aggressive individuals compared to healthy controls.[28] The prefrontal cortex is important in the inhibitory control of behaviour, including impulsive and aggressive behaviour.[29] Thus aggressive/impulsive traits, related to serotonergic dysfunction, are potentially an aspect of the diathesis for suicidal behaviour, whereby aggressive/suicidal behaviours is manifested in response to stressful circumstances or powerful emotions. This tendency might be conceived of as a diminution in natural inhibitory circuits, or as a volatile cognitive decision style.

Noradrenergic system

Within the stress–diathesis model of suicidal behaviour, it is the confluence of stressful events with the diathesis that is thought to precipitate a suicidal act. Thus, investigating the functioning of stress response systems in suicidal individuals is important for elucidating neurobiological concomitants of suicidal behaviour and identifying targets for preventative intervention. The noradrenergic system and the HPA axis are two key stress response systems.

The majority of norepinephrine neurones in the brain are located in the brainstem locus coeruleus. Postmortem studies of suicides have documented fewer noradrenergic neurones in the locus coeruleus.[30] There are also indications of cortical noradrenergic overactivity including lower alpha and high-affinity $beta_1$-adrenergic receptor binding,[31] and lower β-adrenoceptor density and $alpha_2$–adrenergic binding in the prefrontal cortex in individuals who died by suicide.[23] There is some, but not unanimous, evidence from prospective studies of lower levels of CSF 3-methoxy-4-hydroxphenylglycol (MHPG), a metabolite of noradrenaline, in future suicides,[33] although not in those making non-fatal suicide attempts.[34]

Fewer noradrenergic neurones observed in depressed suicides may indicate a lower functional reserve of the noradrenergic system, which if accompanied by an exaggerated stress response with greater release of noradrenaline may result in norepinephrine depletion leading to depression and hopelessness, both of which are contributory factors to suicidal behaviour.

Noradrenergic and HPA axis responses to stress in adulthood appears to be greater in those reporting an abusive experience in childhood.[35] Such individuals are potentially at greater risk in adulthood for major depression and suicidal behaviour. Childhood abuse may be associated with increased risk for depression and suicidal behaviour because of a dysfunctional stress response both via the noradrenergic system and the HPA axis, and secondary effects of norepinephrine depletion and elevated cortisol levels. There is interaction between the noradrenergic system and the stress response activity of the HPA axis with reciprocal neural connections between corticotropin-releasing hormone neurones in the hypothalamic paraventricular nucleus and noradrenergic neurones in human brainstem and the locus coeruleus.[36]

The hypothalamic-pituitary-adrenal (HPA) axis

The hypothalamic-pituitary-adrenal axis is a major stress response system. Major depression is associated with hyperactivity of the HPA axis,[37] and suicidal patients in diagnostically heterogeneous populations exhibit HPA axis abnormalities, most commonly failure to suppress cortisol normally after dexamethasone.[33] We found most future suicides were dexamethasone suppression test (DST) non-suppressors.[33] In mood disorders, DST non-suppressors had a 4.5-fold greater risk of dying by suicide compared with suppressors.[3] Moreover, non-suppression may be characteristic of more serious attempts that result in greater medical damage[38, 39] or the use of violent method in the suicide attempt.[40] In other indices of HPA axis function suicide attempters had attenuated plasma cortisol responses to fenfluramine although that may indicate less serotonin release and not an HPA abnormality,[41, 42] and lower CSF corticotropin-releasing hormone (CRH) compared to non-attempters,[43] though not all studies agree.

Larger pituitary and larger adrenal gland volumes are reported in depressed suicides,[44, 45] and fewer CRH binding sites in the prefrontal cortex of depressed suicide victims which may mean receptor downregulation due to elevated CRF release.[46]

As with the noradrenergic system, early life adversity appears to have lasting effects on stress response in the HPA axis in adulthood. Abnormalities in HPA axis function have been implicated in poor response to antidepressant treatment, and greater likelihood of relapse in major depression, both of which increase the risk for suicidal acts.[33] Increased anxiety and agitation are another potential pathway whereby abnormal stress response, in both the noradrenergic and HPA axis, contributes to risk for suicidal behaviour.

Other biologic systems

Abnormality in the dopaminergic system has been reported in depressive disorders,[47] however studies of dopaminergic function and suicidal behaviour are relatively few and inconclusive.[48] Low dihydroxyphenylacetic acid levels, indicative of reduced dopamine turnover, in the caudate, putamen, and nucleus accumbens are reported in depressed suicides,[49] although the same group of investigators found no difference in number or affinity of the dopamine transporters.[50] Accordingly, it is unlikely that the reduced dopamine turnover initially observed in depressed suicides is a result of decreased dopaminergic innervation of those regions. Prospective studies disagree as to whether CSF HVA predicts suicidal behaviour.[51–53]

There is a well-documented relationship between thyroid dysfunction and depression[54] and some studies link thyroid function and suicide. Abnormal thyroid-stimulating hormone (TSH) response to thyrotropin-releasing hormone (TRH) has been observed in individuals who died by suicide in a follow-up study. [55] Abnormal TSH response to challenge tests has also been associated with poor response to antidepressant treatment and a higher relapse rate, which may increase risk for suicidal behaviour.[56]

Neurotrophins are involved in brain development and growth, neuronal functioning, and synaptic plasticity. Lower protein levels and gene expression of brain-derived neurotrophic factor (BDNF) in the prefrontal cortex and hippocampus,[57,58] and less mRNA of nerve growth factor, neurotrophin 3 and neurotrophin 4/5 in the hippocampus[59] are reported postmortem in suicides. Lower plasma BDNF has been reported in MDD suicide attempters compared to MDD non-attempters and healthy controls.[60]

Suicide is more common in groups with very low cholesterol levels or after cholesterol lowering by diet (see[61] for a review). This relationship between cholesterol and suicide may be mediated by serotonergic function, as studies of non-human primates on a low-fat diet found lower serotonergic activity and increased aggressive behaviours.[62] Long chain polyunsaturated fatty acids, particularly omega-3, may also be a mediating factor in the relationship between low cholesterol and increased risk for depression and suicide.[63] Lower docosahexaenoic acid percentage of total plasma polyunsaturated fatty acids and a higher omega-6/omega-3 ratio predicted depressed individuals who made a suicide attempt during a 2-year follow-up,[64] and lower eicosapentaenoic acid is found in red blood cells of suicide attempters compared to controls.[65]

Neurobiology, genetics, and suicidal behaviour

Family, twin, and adoption studies support a genetic contribution to suicidal behaviour independent of psychiatric disorder (see Brent and Mann for a review),[66] and genetic studies have sought to determine the responsible genes for suicide and suicide attempt though linkage and SNP association studies. Candidate genes for most studies were selected based on evidence from neurobiological studies in suicide, as a result of which the serotonergic system has been most extensively investigated. A tri-allelic polymorphism in the serotonin transporter promotor has two alleles with lower transcriptional activity and fewer transporters. In varied psychiatric populations, despite some negative findings, the S, or more common lower-expressing allele, has been associated with suicide and with suicide attempts, particularly violent or high-lethality attempts.[67] Functional MRI studies find greater amygdala activation in individuals with the SS genotype when they are exposed to negative stimuli such as angry or fearful faces, negative words, or aversive pictures (see Brown and Hariri 2006 for a review).[68] The amygdala is densely innervated by serotonergic neurones and 5-HT receptors are abundant, and plays a central role in emotional regulation and memory. Excessive responses to emotionally negative events such as abuse, may be over-encoded and contribute to stress-sensitivity in adulthood and thereby to major depression after stress and even suicidal behaviour.

Other genetic studies of the serotonergic system including the 5-HT_{1A}, 5-HT_{2A}, 5-HT_{1B} and other serotonin receptors have largely reported negative results, although there have been some positive findings for the 5-HT_{2A} 102C allele and attempted suicide or suicidal ideation.[67] For tryptophan hydroxylase (TPH1 and TPH2 are two forms of TPH with TPH1 only expressed in the brain during development), associations are reported with suicide and suicide attempt and TPH1 SNPs, however multiple negative findings have also been reported,[67] while haplotype and SNP studies suggest the involvement of the TPH2 gene in suicide and suicide attempt, however again not all studies agree.[67] Monoamine oxidase (MAO-A) plays a key role in metabolism of amines. Low MAO activity results in elevated levels of serotonin, norepinephrine, and dopamine in the brain. The MAO-A gene has functional variable number tandem repeat however no association has been found between this uVNTR and suicidal behaviour, although there is some indication that it may be related to aggression[67] and it is linked to the impact of adversity in childhood on adult antisocial behaviour and trait impulsiveness.[69,70]

Genetic studies in dopaminergic system, noradrenergic system, BDNF, and GABA are few and generally negative,[67] although there are reports of positive association of the catechol-*O*-methyltransferase (COMT), a major catecholamine-catabolic enzyme, gene in Finnish and Caucasian suicide attempters[71] and in Japanese suicides.[72] Inconsistent findings in genetic studies of suicidal behaviour may be due to the complexity of the suicide phenotype, gene–gene interactions, the presence of multiple psychiatric disorders, population racial differences, possible epigenetic effects, and the influence of gene/environment interactions. Nonetheless, new microarray technologies that test expression of thousands of genes simultaneously allowing better gene coverage, and haplotype mapping approaches offer promise for future investigation. Other options include examining more basic endophenotypes such as mood regulation and decision-making.

Genes and environment

Early life stress in conjunction with genetic vulnerability can have enduring effects into adulthood and affect psychopathology and the functioning of biological systems including the serotonergic and stress-response systems (see Mann and Currier 2006).[73] For example monkeys exposed to maternal deprivation in infancy and having the 5-HTTLPR lower expressing S allele in the serotonin transporter gene manifest a lowering of CSF 5-HIAA that persists into adulthood.[74] In 6-month-old macaque monkeys exposed to social stress, those with the S allele had a higher ACTH response, an HPA axis hormone related to stress response, compared with those without that allele and to S allele animals who were maternally reared.[75] Thus the low-expressing S allele not only increased vulnerability to stress in development, but early life stress may further interact with genotype to lower serotonergic function and to increase sensitivity to stressful events later in life, both of which are risk factors for suicidal behaviour.

In human studies, individuals who had experienced childhood maltreatment, those with the low-expressing S allele were at risk for suicidal ideation and suicide attempt,[76] and those with a lower expressing variant of the MAO-A gene were more likely to manifest antisocial behaviour and more impulsivity as adults.[69, 70]

Future directions

There is much still to be learned about the biologic aetiology of suicidal behaviour and the pathways and mechanisms through which biologic dysfunction is involved in suicidal acts. New techniques for imaging the brain, identification of basic intermediate phenotypes and denser gene markers will contribute to elucidating the biological factors and mechanisms involved in suicide and attempted suicide, and identifying potential targets for prevention.

Further information

Mann, J.J. (2003). Neurobiology of suicidal behaviour. *Nature Reviews Neuroscience*, **4**(10), 819–28.

Pandey, G.N. (1997). Altered serotonin function in suicide. Evidence from platelet and neuroendocrine studies. *Annals of the New York Academy of Sciences*, **836**, 182–200.

Mann, J.J. and Currier, D. (2007). A review of prospective studies of biologic predictors of suicidal behavior in mood disorders. *Archives of Suicide Research: Official Journal of the International Academy for Suicide Research*, **11**(1), 3–16.

Bondy, B., Buettner, A., and Zill, P. (2006). Genetics of suicide. *Molecular Psychiatry*, **11**(4), 336–51.

References

1. Mann, J.J., Waternaux, C., Haas, G.L., *et al.* (1999). Toward a clinical model of suicidal behavior in psychiatric patients. *The American Journal of Psychiatry*, **156**(2), 181–9.
2. Åsberg, M., Thorén, P., Träskman, L., Bertilsson, L., and Ringberger, V. (1976). "Serotonin depression"—A biochemical subgroup within the affective disorders? *Science*, **191**, 478–80.
3. Mann, J.J., Currier, D., Stanley, B., *et al.* (2006). Can biological tests assist prediction of suicide in mood disorders? *The International Journal of Neuropsychopharmacology*, **9**(4), 465–74.
4. Mann, J.J., Underwood, M.D., and Arango, V. (1996). Postmortem studies of suicide victims. In *Biology of schizophrenia and affective disease* (ed. S.J. Watson), pp. 197–220. American Psychiatric Press, Washington, DC.
5. Mann, J.J. (1998). The neurobiology of suicide. *Nature Medicine*, **4**(1), 25–30.
6. Arango, V., Underwood, M.D., Gubbi, A.V., *et al.* (1995). Localized alterations in pre- and postsynaptic serotonin binding sites in the ventrolateral prefrontal cortex of suicide victims. *Brain Research*, **688**(1–2), 121–33.
7. Kamali, M., Oquendo, M.A., and Mann, J.J. (2001). Understanding the neurobiology of suicidal behavior. *Depression and Anxiety*, **14**(3), 164–76.
8. Stockmeier, C.A. (2003). Involvement of serotonin in depression: evidence from postmortem and imaging studies of serotonin receptors and the serotonin transporter. *Journal of Psychiatric Research*, **37**(5), 357–73.
9. Pandey, G.N., Dwivedi, Y., Rizavi, H.S., *et al.* (2002). Higher expression of serotonin 5-HT(2A) receptors in the postmortem brains of teenage suicide victims. *The American Journal of Psychiatry*, **159**(3), 419–29.
10. Hrdina, P.D., Demeter, E., Vu, T.B., *et al.* (1993). 5-HT uptake sites and 5-HT_2 receptors in brain of antidepressant-free suicide victims/depressives: increase in 5-HT_2 sites in cortex and amygdala. *Brain Research*, **614**, 37–44.
11. Pandey, G.N. (1997). Altered serotonin function in suicide. Evidence from platelet and neuroendocrine studies. *Annals of the New York Academy of Sciences*, **836**, 182–200.
12. Pandey, G.N., Dwivedi, Y., Pandey, S.C., *et al.* (1999). Low phosphoinositide-specific phospholipase C activity and expression of phospholipase C beta1 protein in the prefrontal cortex of teenage suicide subjects. *The American Journal of Psychiatry*, **156**(12), 1895–901.
13. Malone, K.M., Ellis, S.P., Currier, D., *et al.* (2007). Platelet 5-HT2A receptor subresponsivity and lethality of attempted suicide in depressed in-patients. *The International Journal of Neuropsychopharmacology*, **10**(3): 335–430.
14. Arango, V., Underwood, M.D., Boldrini, M., *et al.* (2001). Serotonin 1A receptors, serotonin transporter binding and serotonin transporter mRNA expression in the brainstem of depressed suicide victims. *Neuropsychopharmacology: Official Publication of the American College of Neuropsychopharmacology*, **25**(6), 892–903.
15. Purselle, D.C. and Nemeroff, C.B. (2003). Serotonin transporter: a potential substrate in the biology of suicide. *Neuropsychopharmacology: Official Publication of the American College of Neuropsychopharmacology*, **28**(4), 613–19.
16. Mann, J.J., Huang, Y.Y., Underwood, M.D., *et al.* (2000). A serotonin transporter gene promoter polymorphism (5-HTTLPR) and prefrontal cortical binding in major depression and suicide. *Archives of General Psychiatry*, **57**(8), 729–38.
17. Boldrini, M., Underwood, M.D., Mann, J.J., *et al.* (2005). More tryptophan hydroxylase in the brainstem dorsal raphe nucleus in depressed suicides. *Brain Research*, **1041**(1), 19–28.
18. Oquendo, M.A., Galfalvy, H., Russo, S., *et al.* (2004). Prospective study of clinical predictors of suicidal acts after a major depressive episode in patients with major depressive disorder or bipolar disorder. *The American Journal of Psychiatry*, **161**(8), 1433–41.
19. Brown, G.L. and Goodwin, F.K. (1986). Cerebrospinal fluid correlates of suicide attempts and aggression. *Annals of the New York Academy of Sciences*, **487**, 175–88.
20. Stanley, B., Molcho, A., Stanley, M., *et al.* (2000). Association of aggressive behavior with altered serotonergic function in patients who are not suicidal. *The American Journal of Psychiatry*, **157**(4), 609–14.
21. Coccaro, E.F., Siever, L.J., Klar, H.M., *et al.* (1989). Serotonergic studies in patients with affective and personality disorders. Correlates with suicidal and impulsive aggressive behavior. *Archives of General Psychiatry*, **46**, 587–99.
22. New, A.S., Trestman, R.F., Mitropoulou, V., *et al.* (2004). Low prolactin response to fenfluramine in impulsive aggression. *Journal of Psychiatric Research*, **38**(3), 223–30.
23. Coccaro, E.F., Kavoussi, R.J., Sheline, Y.I., *et al.* (1997). Impulsive aggression in personality disorder correlates with platelet 5-HT_{2A} receptor binding. *Neuropsychopharmacology: Official Publication of the American College of Neuropsychopharmacology*, **16**(3), 211–16.
24. McBride, P.A., Brown, R.P., DeMeo, M., *et al.* (1994). The relationship of platelet 5-HT_2 receptor indices to major depressive disorder, personality traits, and suicidal behavior. *Biological Psychiatry*, **35**, 295–308.
25. Oquendo, M.A., Russo, S.A., Underwood, M.D., *et al.* (2006). Higher postmortem prefrontal 5-HT2A receptor binding correlates with lifetime aggression in suicide. *Biological Psychiatry*, **59**(3), 235–43.
26. Siever, L.J., Buchsbaum, M.S., New, A.S., *et al.* (1999). D,l-Fenfluramine response in impulsive personality disorder assessed with [^{18}F]fluorodeoxyglucose positron emission tomography. *Neuropsychopharmacology: Official Publication of the American College of Neuropsychopharmacology*, **20**(5), 413–23.
27. New, A.S., Hazlett, E.A., Buchsbaum, M.S., *et al.* (2002). Blunted prefrontal cortical 18fluorodeoxyglucose positron emission tomography response to meta-chlorophenylpiperazine in impulsive aggression. *Archives of General Psychiatry*, **59**(7), 621–9.

28. Frankle, W.G., Lombardo, I., New, A.S., *et al.* (2005). Brain serotonin transporter distribution in subjects with impulsive aggressivity: a positron emission study with [^{11}C]McN 5652. *The American Journal of Psychiatry*, **162**(5), 915–23.
29. de Almeida, R.M., Rosa, M.M., Santos, D.M., *et al.* (2006). 5-HT(1B) receptors, ventral orbitofrontal cortex, and aggressive behavior in mice. *Psychopharmacology*, **185**(4), 441–50.
30. Arango, V., Underwood, M.D., and Mann, J.J. (1996). Fewer pigmented locus coeruleus neurons in suicide victims: preliminary results. *Biological Psychiatry*, **39**, 112–20.
31. Arango, V., Ernsberger, P., Sved, A.F., *et al.* (1993). Quantitative autoradiography of a_1- and a_2-adrenergic receptors in the cerebral cortex of controls and suicide victims. *Brain Research*, **630**, 271–82.
32. De Paermentier, F., Cheetham, S.C., Crompton, M.R., *et al.* (1990). Brain b-adrenoceptor binding sites in antidepressant-free depressed suicide victims. *Brain Research*, **525**, 71–7.
33. Mann, J.J. and Currier, D. (2007). A review of prospective studies of biologic predictors of suicidal behavior in mood disorders. *Archives of Suicide Research: Official Journal of the International Academy for Suicide Research*, **11**(1), 3–16.
34. Lester, D. (1995). The concentration of neurotransmitter metabolites in the cerebrospinal fluid of suicidal individuals: a meta-analysis. *Pharmacopsychiatry*, **28**(2), 45–50.
35. Heim, C. and Nemeroff, C.B. (2001). The role of childhood trauma in the neurobiology of mood and anxiety disorders: preclinical and clinical studies. *Biological Psychiatry*, **49**(12), 1023–39.
36. Austin, M.C., Rice, P.M., Mann, J.J., *et al.* (1995). Localization of corticotropin-releasing hormone in the human locus coeruleus and pedunculopontine tegmental nucleus: an immunocytochemical and in situ hybridization study. *Neuroscience*, **64**(3), 713–27.
37. Carroll, B.J., Feinberg, M., Greden, J.F., *et al.* (1981). A specific laboratory test for the diagnosis of melancholia. Standardization, validation, and clinical utility. *Archives of General Psychiatry*, **38**, 15–22.
38. Norman, W.H., Brown, W.A., Miller, I.W., *et al.* (1990). The dexamethasone suppression test and completed suicide. *Acta Psychiatrica Scandinavica*, **81**(2), 120–5.
39. Coryell, W. (1990). DST abnormality as a predictor of course in major depression. *Journal of Affective Disorders*, **19**(3), 163–9.
40. Roy, A. (1992). Hypothalamic-pituitary-adrenal axis function and suicidal behavior in depression. *Biological Psychiatry*, **32**, 812–16.
41. Duval, F., Mokrani, M.C., Correa, H., *et al.* (2001). Lack of effect of HPA axis hyperactivity on hormonal responses to d- fenfluramine in major depressed patients: implications for pathogenesis of suicidal behaviour. *Psychoneuroendocrinology*, **26**(5), 521–37.
42. Malone, K.M., Corbitt, E.M., Li, S., *et al.* (1996). Prolactin response to fenfluramine and suicide attempt lethality in major depression. *The British Journal of Psychiatry: The Journal of Mental Science*, **168**, 324–9.
43. Brunner, J., Stalla, G.K., Stalla, J., *et al.* (2001). Decreased corticotropin-releasing hormone (CRH) concentrations in the cerebrospinal fluid of eucortisolemic suicide attempters. *Journal of Psychiatric Research*, **35**(1), 1–9.
44. Szigethy, E., Conwell, Y., Forbes, N.T., *et al.* (1994). Adrenal weight and morphology in victims of completed suicide. *Biological Psychiatry*, **36**(6), 374–80.
45. Dumser, T., Barocka, A., and Schubert, E. (1998). Weight of adrenal glands may be increased in persons who commit suicide. *The American Journal of Forensic Medicine and Pathology: Official Publication of the National Association of Medical Examiners*, **19**(1), 72–6.
46. Nemeroff, C.B., Owens, M.J., Bissette, G., *et al.* (1988). Reduced corticotropin releasing factor binding sites in the frontal cortex of suicide victims. *Archives of General Psychiatry*, **45**, 577–9.
47. Dailly, E., Chenu, F., Renard, C.E., *et al.* (2004). Dopamine, depression and antidepressants. *Fundamental and Clinical Pharmacology*, **18**(6), 601–7.
48. Mann, J.J. (2003). Neurobiology of suicidal behaviour. *Nature Reviews Neuroscience*, **4**(10), 819–28.
49. Bowden, C., Cheetham, S.C., Lowther, S., *et al.* (1997). Reduced dopamine turnover in the basal ganglia of depressed suicides. *Brain Research*, **769**(1), 135–40.
50. Bowden, C., Theodorou, A.E., Cheetham, S.C., *et al.* (1997). Dopamine D_1 and D_2 receptor binding sites in brain samples from depressed suicides and controls. *Brain Research*, **752**, 227–33.
51. Roy, A., De Jong, J., and Linnoila, M. (1989). Cerebrospinal fluid monoamine metabolites and suicidal behavior in depressed patients. A 5-year follow-up study. *Archives of General Psychiatry*, **46**, 609–12.
52. Engstrom, G., Alling, C., Blennow, K., *et al.* (1999). Reduced cerebrospinal HVA concentrations and HVA/5-HIAA ratios in suicide attempters. Monoamine metabolites in 120 suicide attempters and 47 controls. *European Neuropsychopharmacology: The Journal of the European College of Neuropsychopharmacology*, **9**(5), 399–405.
53. Placidi, G.P., Oquendo, M.A., Malone, K.M., *et al.* (2001). Aggressivity, suicide attempts, and depression: relationship to cerebrospinal fluid monoamine metabolite levels. *Biological Psychiatry*, **50**(10), 783–91.
54. Jackson, I.M. (1998). The thyroid axis and depression. *Thyroid: Official Journal of the American Thyroid Association*, **8**(10), 951–6.
55. Linkowski, P., Van Wettere. J.P., Kerkhofs, M., *et al.* (1984). Violent suicidal behavior and the thyrotropin-releasing hormone-thyroid-stimulating hormone test: a clinical outcome study. *Neuropsychobiology*, **12**(1), 19–22.
56. Targum, S.D. (1984). Persistent neuroendocrine dysregulation in major depressive disorder: a marker for early relapse. *Biological Psychiatry*, **19**(3), 305–18.
57. Dwivedi, Y., Rizavi, H.S., Conley, R.R., *et al.* (2003). Altered gene expression of brain-derived neurotrophic factor and receptor tyrosine kinase B in postmortem brain of suicide subjects. *Archives of General Psychiatry*, **60**(8), 804–15.
58. Karege, F., Vaudan, G., Schwald, M., *et al.* (2005). Neurotrophin levels in postmortem brains of suicide victims and the effects of antemortem diagnosis and psychotropic drugs. *Brain Research Molecular Brain Research*, **136**(1–2), 29–37.
59. Dwivedi, Y., Mondal, A.C., Rizavi, H.S., *et al.* (2005). Suicide brain is associated with decreased expression of neurotrophins. *Biological Psychiatry*, **58**(4), 315–24.
60. Kim, Y.K., Lee, H.P., Won, S.D., *et al.* (2007). Low plasma BDNF is associated with suicidal behavior in major depression. *Progress in Neuropsychopharmacology and Biological Psychiatry*, **31**(1), 78–85.
61. Golomb, B.A. (1998). Cholesterol and violence: is there a connection? *Annals of Internal Medicine*, **128**, 478–87.
62. Muldoon, M.F., Rossouw, J.E., Manuck, S.B., *et al.* (1993). Low or lowered cholesterol and risk of death from suicide and trauma. *Metabolism: Clinical and Experimental*, **42**(Suppl. 1), 45–56.
63. Brunner, J., Parhofer, K.G., Schwandt, P., *et al.* (2002). Cholesterol, essential fatty acids, and suicide. *Pharmacopsychiatry*, **35**(1), 1–5.
64. Sublette, M.E., Hibbeln, J.R., Galfalvy, H., *et al.* (2006). Omega-3 polyunsaturated essential fatty acid status as a predictor of future suicide risk. *American Journal of Psychiatry*, **163**(6), 1100–2.
65. Huan, M., Hamazaki, K., Sun, Y., *et al.* (2004). Suicide attempt and *n*–3 fatty acid levels in red blood cells: a case control study in China. *Biological Psychiatry*, **56**(7), 490–6.
66. Brent, D.A. and Mann, J.J. (2005). Family genetic studies, suicide, and suicidal behavior. *American Journal of Medical Genetics. Part C, Seminars in Medical Genetics*, **133**(1), 13–24.
67. Bondy, B., Buettner, A., and Zill, P. (2006). Genetics of suicide. *Molecular Psychiatry*, **11**(4), 336–51.

68. Brown, S.M. and Hariri, A.R. (2006). Neuroimaging studies of serotonin gene polymorphisms: exploring the interplay of genes, brain, and behavior. *Cognitive Affective and Behavioral Neuroscience*, **6**(1), 44–52.
69. Caspi, A., McClay, J., Moffitt, T.E., *et al.* (2002). Role of genotype in the cycle of violence in maltreated children. *Science*, **297**(5582), 851–4.
70. Huang, Y.Y., Cate, S.P., Battistuzzi, C., *et al.* (2004). An association between a functional polymorphism in the monoamine oxidase a gene promoter, impulsive traits and early abuse experiences. *Neuropsychopharmacology: Official Publication of the American College of Neuropsychopharmacology*, **29**(8), 1498–505.
71. Nolan, K.A., Volavka, J., Czobor, P., *et al.* (2000). Suicidal behavior in patients with schizophrenia is related to COMT polymorphism. *Psychiatric Genetics*, **10**(3), 117–24.
72. Ono, H., Shirakawa, O., Nushida, H., *et al.* (2004). Association between catechol-O-methyltransferase functional polymorphism and male suicide completers. *Neuropsychopharmacology: Official Publication of the American College of Neuropsychopharmacology*, **29**(7), 1374–7.
73. Mann, J.J. and Currier, D. (2006). Effects of genes and stress on the neurobiology of depression. *International Review of Neurobiology*, **73**, 153–89.
74. Bennett, A.J., Lesch, K.P., Heils, A., *et al.* (2002). Early experience and serotonin transporter gene variation interact to influence primate CNS function. *Molecular Psychiatry*, **7**(1), 118–22.
75. Barr, C.S., Newman, T.K., Shannon, C., *et al.* (2004). Rearing condition and rh5-HTTLPR interact to influence limbic-hypothalamic-pituitary-adrenal axis response to stress in infant macaques. *Biological Psychiatry*, **55**(7), 733–8.
76. Caspi, A., Sugden, K., Moffitt, T.E., *et al.* (2003). Influence of life stress on depression: moderation by a polymorphism in the 5-HTT gene. *Science*, **301**(5631), 386–9.

4.15.4 Treatment of suicide attempters and prevention of suicide and attempted suicide

Keith Hawton and Tatiana Taylor

Introduction

In considering the treatment and prevention of suicidal behaviour account should be taken of recent trends in suicide and attempted suicide, particularly in individual countries. These have been reviewed in other chapters in this section. The term 'attempted suicide' is used in this chapter and includes any act of non-fatal self-poisoning or self-injury, irrespective of motive or intention.

Suicide prevention has been incorporated within the World Health Organization Health for All strategy[1] and has received substantial support from the United Nations.[2] Furthermore, in recent years several countries have developed national suicide prevention programmes. Increased suicide rates in young people have probably acted as a stimulus behind this trend. However, suicide rates in most countries remain higher in older populations and prevention programmes must include this increasingly larger sector of society.

Treatment of suicide attempters

Suicide attempts occur for a wide range of reasons. In many cases the primary aim is not death but some other outcome, such as demonstrating distress to other people, seeking a change in other people's behaviour or temporary escape.[3] This means that a broad range of treatments are required since the needs of individual patients will vary widely (Table 4.15.4.1).

Factors relevant to treatment needs in suicide attempts

(a) Repetition of attempts and risk of suicide

Repetition of attempts is common, with 15 to 25 per cent repeating suicidal acts within a year, and is associated with a greater risk of eventual suicide.[4] The frequency of suicide following attempted suicide varies from country to country,[5] depending on the overall characteristics of the patient population and the rate of suicide in the general population. Prevention of repetition of suicidal behaviour and especially of suicide is a major aim in treating suicide attempters.

(b) Psychiatric and personality disorders

A range of psychiatric disorders are found in suicide attempters.[6] Depression and alcohol abuse are particularly common. In addition, substantial proportions of patients have personality disorders. While treatment directed at the underlying causes of such disorders, where possible, will be important in managing attempted suicide patients, often the disorders themselves will require specific treatment.

(c) Life events and difficulties

Certain problems are particularly common in suicide attempters, including difficulties in interpersonal relationships, especially with partners and with other family members, employment problems, particularly in males, and financial difficulties. Life events, especially disruption in a relationship with a partner, frequently precede suicidal acts.[7]

(d) Poor problem-solving skills

Many suicide attempters have difficulties in problem-solving, particularly in dealing with difficulties in interpersonal relationships.[8] These difficulties are more marked in suicide attempters than in patients with psychiatric disorders who have not carried out a suicidal act.

Table 4.15.4.1 Factors relevant to treatment needs in suicide attempters

Risk of repetition of attempts
Risk of suicide
Psychiatric disorder (especially depression and substance abuse)
Personality disorders
Life events and difficulties
Poor problem-solving skills
Impulsivity and aggression
Hopelessness
Low self-esteem
Motivational problems and poor compliance with treatment

(e) Impulsivity and aggression

There is a strong link between suicidal behaviour and both impulsivity and aggression. There is also accumulating evidence that hypofunction of brain serotonergic systems is linked to aggression (and possibly impulsivity) and also to suicidal behaviour[9] (see Chapter 4.15.3). It is unclear whether this represents a state phenomenon associated with psychiatric disturbance or a trait phenomenon, but current evidence points towards the latter.

(f) Hopelessness and low self-esteem

Hopelessness, or pessimism about the future, which has been shown to be a key factor linking depression with suicidal acts, is an important predictor of repetition of suicidal behaviour, and a risk factor for eventual suicide.[10] Low self-esteem is another important characteristic associated with suicidal behaviour. There is likely to be a link between low self-esteem and a tendency to experience hopelessness when faced by adverse circumstances.

(g) Motivational problems and poor compliance with treatment

Management of suicide attempters is complicated by the fact that some patients appear to be poorly motivated to engage in aftercare. This is also likely to affect compliance with treatments. The style of organization of general hospital psychiatric services (including continuity of care) and the attitudes of clinical staff may be important factors determining whether patients engage in aftercare.

General overview of treatments

Treatments for suicide attempters include both psychosocial and pharmacological approaches. While these are considered separately below, in some patients both will be appropriate. This might be the case, for example, if a patient suffers from depression with biological features in the setting of employment and financial difficulties, when treatment with an antidepressant might be combined with problem-solving therapy.

Psychosocial treatments

A range of psychosocial therapies have been evaluated in suicide attempters in randomized controlled clinical trials. The efficacy of these approaches has been examined in a systematic review of the worldwide literature.[11] The findings from this review and some further studies are summarized below.

(a) Problem-solving

Meta-analysis of the results of trials that have been conducted so far to evaluate the effectiveness of brief problem-solving therapy (see Chapter 6.3.1) compared with treatment as usual indicates a trend towards reduction of repetition of self-harm episodes, but the total numbers of subjects and trials have precluded a definitive result. However, evidence of other positive outcomes, such as reduced levels of depression and hopelessness and improvement in problems, has been convincingly demonstrated in these studies.[12] This approach is useful, either used alone or in the context of other treatment. It is reasonably easily taught and can be used by clinicians from different professional backgrounds.

(b) Psychotherapy

Cognitive behaviour therapy, combined with care management has recently been shown to be effective in reducing frequency of suicide attempts and in producing other positive outcomes.[13] A brief psychological intervention combined with provision of a treatment manual seems to be less effective in the treatment of patients with repeated attempts.[14]

Two trials have been conducted in which an intensive form of psychological treatment known as dialectical behaviour therapy was evaluated.[15,16] Female patients with borderline personality disorders who had a history of repeated self-harm were offered a year of individual and group cognitive behavioural therapy aimed at addressing the patients' problems of motivation and strengthening their behavioural skills, particularly in relation to interpersonal difficulties. Compared with routine care this approach seems to result in a reduction in repetition of self-harm as well as a number of other positive outcomes. Further evaluation of this approach is required to determine if it is effective in male patients and in adolescents, and whether it can be delivered in an abbreviated form. While it is a labour-intensive approach, it appears to be helpful for what is a particularly difficult group of patients.

(c) Outreach

Several trials have been conducted to assess the impact of community outreach, either for all patients or for those that have not attended treatment sessions. Some of these studies have included relatively intensive treatment programmes. Overall these studies indicate that some form of outreach may improve outcome in terms of reducing repetition of attempted suicide. In one study, nurse home visits to encourage non-attending participants to attend outpatient appointments resulted in a significantly greater number of appointments attended as compared to the control group and there was a near significant reduction in the rate of repetition of suicide attempts during the year after study entry.[17] In other studies, telephone contact,[18] and contacting patients regularly by post[19] have also produced promising results. Outreach combined with specific treatment may be useful, perhaps reserved for those who are poorly compliant with aftercare.

(d) Provision of emergency cards

In the United Kingdom there has recently been interest in providing suicide attempters with cards which indicate how they might get emergency help at times of crisis. Two initial, relatively small, studies of this approach, one involving adults and the other young adolescents, produced encouraging results but a larger evaluation did not show the cards to be effective.[20] Provision of emergency cards requires there to be a 24 h service to deal with emergency calls. They might be thought helpful in a minority of cases, but there needs to be careful selection of patients who are offered this facility because of risk of it possibly being abused.

Pharmacological treatments

There have been relatively few treatment trials evaluating the effectiveness of pharmacological agents in suicide attempters. This perhaps reflects the problems of compliance with therapy, which were noted earlier, and risk of overdose.

(a) Antidepressants

A trial in the Netherlands in which paroxetine was compared with placebo in patients who were all repeaters of self-harm but who did not suffer from current depressive disorder showed apparent benefits for a subgroup of patients who received paroxetine, namely those who had a history of between one and four episodes of self-harm. Patients with a history of five or more episodes did not seem to benefit.[21] The findings of this study are clearly of interest (although *post hoc* subgroup analyses of this kind must be treated with caution). Recently there has been much attention to the risk of antidepressants increasing suicidal ideation and acts in adolescents.[22] Also, it has become clear that there is increased risk with all types of antidepressants during the initial period of treatment.[23] These findings have highlighted the need to be cautious in the use of antidepressants, to provide early follow-up after initiating therapy, and to consider combining antidepressant treatment with other therapies, especially for adolescents (in whom only fluoxetine is currently recommended for the treatment of depression).

(b) Neuroleptics

A trial in which the depot neuroleptic flupenthixol was administered monthly in a dose of 20 mg for 6 months to repeaters of self-harm and compared with placebo in similar patients appeared to show that the active drug was effective in reducing the recurrence of self-harm.[24] While this type of study requires replication, perhaps using one of the atypical oral neuroleptics in patients who frequently repeat self-harm may be worth trying.

(c) Lithium

A systematic review of trials of lithium therapy versus a range of other drugs and placebo in patients with affective disorders has shown convincing evidence that lithium may prevent suicide.[25] It is not known if it may be anti-suicidal in other groups of patients.

Management in clinical practice

Before a treatment plan can be formulated a careful assessment must be carried out. In conducting the assessment the clinician needs to try and establish good rapport with the patient and be sensitive to the patient's preferences. The key factors that should be covered during the assessment are listed in Table 4.15.4.2. For the purpose of formulating a management plan it is particularly useful to draw up a problem list which summarizes the patient's current difficulties. This should be done in active collaboration with the patient as far as possible. Qualitative studies have shown that patients appreciate clinicians and other staff keeping them well informed of their mental and physical status and including them in decision-making in regard to their care.[26]

(a) Assessment

During the assessment it is crucial to estimate the risk of suicide or another non-fatal attempt. However, accurate assessment is far from easy. Risk factors for suicide following attempted suicide are shown in Table 4.15.4.3. Because suicide is uncommon, the predictive value of the items is limited. One predictor of suicide risk is the degree of suicidal intent involved in the current attempt (see Table 4.15.4.4). Clinicians should consider the use of the valuable Beck Suicide Intent scale.[27] Factors known to be associated with risk of a further attempt are listed in Table 4.15.4.5. It should be noted that while individuals who score positive on several of these factors will have considerably increased risk of repetition, a substantial proportion of those who repeat will not show these characteristics, i.e. the predictive value of scales to predict repetition is modest.

Table 4.15.4.2 The assessment of attempted-suicide patients

Factors that should be covered
Life events that preceded the attempt
Motives for the act, including suicidal intent and other reasons
Problems faced by the patient
Psychiatric disorder
Personality traits and disorder
Alcohol and drug misuse
Family and personal history
Current circumstances
Social (e.g. extent of social relationships)
Domestic (e.g. living alone or with others)
Occupation (e.g. whether employed)
Psychiatric history, including previous suicide attempts
Assessments that should be made
Risk of a further attempt
Risk of suicide
Coping resources and supports
What treatment is appropriate to the patient's needs
Motivation of patient (and significant others where appropriate, to engage in treatment)

Table 4.15.4.3 Factors associated with risk of suicide after attempted suicide

Older age
Male gender
Unemployed or retired
Separated, divorced or widowed
Living alone
Poor physical health
Psychiatric disorder (particularly depression, alcoholism, schizophrenia, and 'sociopathic' personality disorder)
High suicidal intent in current episode
Violent method involved in current attempt (e.g. attempted hanging, shooting, jumping)
Leaving a note
Previous attempt(s) (including repetitive self-injury)

Table 4.15.4.4 Factors that suggest high suicidal intent

Act carried out in isolation
Act timed so that intervention unlikely
Precautions taken to avoid discovery
Preparations made in anticipation of death (e.g. making will, organizing insurance)
Preparations made for the act (e.g. purchasing means, saving up tablets)
Communicating intent to others beforehand
Extensive premeditation
Leaving a note
Note alerting potential helpers after the act
Subsequent admission of suicidal intent

Table 4.15.4.5 Factors associated with risk of repetition of attempted suicide

Previous attempt(s)
Depression
Personality disorder
Alcohol or drug abuse
Previous psychiatric treatment
Unemployment
Lower socio-economic status
Criminal record
History of violence
Age 25–54 years
Single, divorced, or separated

(b) Treatment

The treatment plan should be drawn up on the basis of the patient's needs and risks. Inpatient psychiatric treatment will usually be indicated for patients with severe psychiatric disorders, especially where immediate risk of suicide appears to be high.

(i) Psychiatric disorders

Major psychiatric disorders should be treated in the usual way, but with particular care about use of medication which might be toxic in overdose. Specific treatment should be provided for alcohol and drug abuse; indeed, a suicide attempt is sometimes the first occasion that abuse may come to clinical attention.

(ii) Community therapy

Most patients can be managed in the community. Brief psychological therapy, with a focus on problem-solving will be appropriate for those patients who have clear problems, such as in interpersonal relationships, employment, or social adjustment. Some form of outreach (e.g. home visiting, telephone contact) may be helpful to increase the proportion of patients who engage in treatment, but is not necessary for most patients. Outreach may be essential in the treatment of patients in remote rural areas in developing countries.

If possible there should be continuity of therapy in terms of the same person who saw the patient in hospital after their attempt providing aftercare as this is likely to result in better compliance with therapy. Longer term cognitive behavioural therapy or dynamic psychotherapy may be required for patients whose attempts are related to traumas, such as sexual abuse, or to personality disorder. People who are repeaters of suicide attempts may also require more intensive treatment, especially those who frequently repeat. If resources permit, the use of a programme based on dialectical behaviour therapy, possibly using a group format for at least part of treatment, might be considered.

(iii) Adolescents

Family therapy may be required for young adolescents, and also for patients with difficulties in relation to children. Group therapy may be helpful for adolescents who are repeaters of self-harm.[28]

Prevention of suicide and attempted suicide

A widely diverse group of individuals are at risk of suicidal behaviour and it occurs in relation to a wide range of problems and situations. For example, suicide may occur in the context of long-term difficulties extending back to childhood, acute severe life events or, and perhaps most importantly, acute or long-term and relapsing mental illness. Because of this the range of potential prevention strategies is also considerable.

Suicide prevention programmes have been established in many countries. This is to be welcomed, not only because of the potential benefits in terms of suicide prevention, but also because of the likely benefits for the broader population of individuals with mental health problems. When considering prevention strategies, it is important to be aware of and sensitive towards issues relating to culture and ethnicity. For example, while suicide rates are generally relatively low in young females in the United Kingdom, this is not the case in young Asian females of the Hindu faith, in which rates appear to be relatively high and greater than those of their male peers.[29] The issues surrounding such deaths are often related to cultural clashes regarding values and expectations between young Asian females and their parents.

While ethical issues in relation to suicide prevention are not dealt with in detail in this chapter, they are none the less highly important.[30] Opinions will vary, for example, about whether suicide should always be prevented. This particularly relates to suicides occurring in the context of terminal and/or painful physical illnesses, and relapsing and debilitating mental illnesses. The ethics of suicide prevention overlap those of assisted suicide and euthanasia. Psychiatrists are increasingly likely to be drawn into debate and controversy about the ethical aspects of these issues, particularly in relation to severe and chronic mental illness, and mental health aspects of assisted suicide and euthanasia in people with severe physical illnesses.

General principles of prevention

Broadly there are two approaches to suicide prevention.[31,32] As described by Rose[33] in the context of prevention of health problems in general, one can distinguish between population approaches, which aim to decrease risk in the population as a whole, and high-risk group strategies, in which specific groups that are at increased risk are targeted. High-risk group strategies often appear more attractive and realistic. However, risk factors for many disorders are widely spread in the population and so the high-risk strategy tends to exclude a large number of people at moderate risk and is often ineffective in reducing the burden of a disease at the population level. Conversely, population strategies may appear more difficult to achieve but are more likely to be effective in reducing population levels of disease (see also Chapter 7.4). The main population and high-risk group strategies in the prevention of suicide and attempted suicide which are considered here are shown in Table 4.15.4.6.

It is unclear if national suicide prevention programmes are effective, although evidence of effectiveness for specific components of such strategies is emerging.[34] The most impressive programme, developed in Finland, was based on information from a detailed national study of all suicides in 1 year and includes a wide range of elements.[35] A decline in the Finnish suicide rate has been attributed to the programme.[36] In England a national suicide prevention strategy with a suicide target was introduced in 2002.[37] Strategies have also been introduced in Scotland[38] and Ireland.[39] While prevention strategies are difficult to evaluate[40] there are indications that programmes for prevention of suicide on a national scale may be effective.

Table 4.15.4.6 Examples of strategies for prevention of suicide and attempted suicide

Population strategies
Reducing availability of means for suicide
Educating primary care physicians
Influencing media portrayal of suicide
Educating the public about mental illness and its treatment
Educational approaches in schools
Befriending agencies and telephone helplines
Addressing the economic factors associated with suicidal behaviour
High-risk strategies
Prevention of suicide in:
Patients with psychiatric disorders
The elderly
Suicide attempters
High-risk occupational groups
Prisoners

Population strategies

(a) Reducing availability of means for suicide

This is the most widely discussed population strategy.[41] It is based on evidence that if the availability and/or danger of a popular method for suicide changes then this tends to have an impact on suicide rates. The general principles of prevention through reducing availability of means are, first, that many suicidal acts occur impulsively and therefore if a dangerous means is available this is more likely to result in death and, secondly, that the eventual suicide rate in survivors of serious attempts is remarkably low. Also the common adage that if people are intent on committing suicide they will find a means is not necessarily correct (see below).

(i) Coal gas

The most cited evidence for the effectiveness of this approach is the reduction in suicides in the United Kingdom which occurred in the 1960s and early 1970s when toxic coal gas supplies were gradually replaced with non-toxic North Sea gas.[42] Prior to this time coal gas poisoning through people placing their head in a gas oven was the most common method of suicide in the United Kingdom. As North Sea gas was gradually introduced the suicide rate dropped steadily, eventually being reduced by approximately a third. It is estimated that as many as 6000 deaths may have been prevented by this change. The effect also illustrates the point that when one method of suicide is no longer available people do not automatically turn to another, or if they do it may be to one that is less likely to cause death. Thus, it was some years before the suicide rate rose again, this being related to an increase in deaths from poisoning with carbon monoxide from car exhausts. Another factor that may have been relevant to the decline in suicides was the reduction in prescribing of barbiturates, these being replaced by far less toxic benzodiazepines.

(ii) Carbon monoxide

Suicide by carbon monoxide poisoning from car exhausts has become less common because cars are now fitted with catalytic converters. This has resulted in a decline in suicide rates in countries where this method of suicide had become more common, particularly in young males.[43]

(iii) Firearms

The widespread availability of guns in certain countries, particularly the United States, has been proposed as an important reason for their relatively high suicide rates. Guns are used in more than half of all suicides in the United States and their use for suicide correlates with the holding of gun licences in households.[44] Some controversy surrounds the question of whether restricting availability of guns leads to a reduction in suicide rates, but the weight of evidence seems to indicate that it does.[45]

(iv) Antidepressants

Given the very strong link between suicide and depression, and the risk of death from overdose of some of the older antidepressants, there has been much debate about whether more extensive use of newer, less toxic antidepressants would prevent suicides. This is not a simple question, as some patients respond better to the older tricyclic antidepressants. Another consideration concerns the cost of the newer antidepressants compared with the older varieties. Also it is very important to remember that most people who are taking antidepressants do not kill themselves with their antidepressants but use other methods. This and the probable selective prescribing of SSRIs to people judged to be at risk may account for the finding that suicide rates were higher in patients taking fluoxetine than patients taking other and in some cases more toxic antidepressants.[46] Nevertheless, common sense dictates that patients known to be at risk, and especially those with a history of suicidal behaviour, should be prescribed the less toxic preparations.

(v) Analgesics

In the United Kingdom and some other countries there has been particular concern about deaths from self-poisoning with paracetamol. Due to evidence that countries which have fewer tablets per pack seem to have a lower rate of mortality from paracetamol self-poisoning and because overdoses of paracetamol are often taken impulsively and involve household supplies, legislation was introduced in the United Kingdom in 1998 to reduce in the number of tablets of paracetamol (and aspirin) available per pack. This resulted in fewer overdoses, decreased cases of hepatotoxicity due to paracetamol toxicity, and a reduced number of deaths from both paracetamol and aspirin.[47]

(vi) Safety measures

Much attention has been paid to improving safety at popular sites for suicide. This includes erecting suicide barriers on bridges, multi-storey car parks, and other sites. If environmental changes are made such that a popular suicide site becomes safer, this does not mean that people at risk automatically move to using another site. For example, erection of barriers on the Clifton Suspension Bridge in Bristol, a popular site for suicide, has resulted in far fewer deaths by jumping.[48]

Clinicians involved in the development of suicide prevention strategies should look very carefully for local patterns which might provide clues about potentially effective measures for reducing access to methods. This could include, for example, ensuring that psychiatric inpatient units are free of hooks, pipes, and other objects or structures from which patients could hang themselves, and that all bed rails are collapsible (compulsory in the United Kingdom), secure fencing of railway lines or waterways close to psychiatric hospitals, and making local popular sites for suicide safer (e.g. suicide barriers on bridges). In addition, attention should be paid to common dangerous methods of self-poisoning. Specific strategies may be required depending on local patterns. For example, the high rates of suicide in rural areas of developing countries due to self-poisoning with pesticides might be reversed with safe-storage programmes.

(b) Education of primary care physicians

Much of the attention regarding improved detection of individuals at risk has concerned the detection and management of depression in general practice. This was stimulated by findings that showed many people who died by suicide or who attempted suicide had seen their general practitioners shortly before these acts. Evidence that an intensive educational programme for general practitioners might be effective in influencing suicide rates comes from a study conducted on the Swedish island of Gotland.[(49)] In the year following this programme the suicide rate dropped significantly, prescribing of antidepressants by general practitioners increased, referrals to psychiatry, especially for depression, decreased, the amount of time lost from work for depression decreased, as did psychiatric admissions. Unfortunately this effect was fairly short-lived in that suicide rates rose again in subsequent years, which the authors attributed to some of the general practitioners having left the island. They also suggested that such programmes need to be repeated.[(50)] It is also important to note that the suicide rate only declined in females. The evidence in this study was based on relatively small numbers, at least with reference to suicide, although the effects on the management and outcome of depression were perhaps more impressive.

While the Gotland study has generated a lot of debate about suicide prevention in primary care, detection of people most at risk in general practice is extremely difficult because a large number of patients share risk factors and because suicide is a rare event. The most pragmatic view is that effective detection and treatment of depression (and other psychiatric disorders) in primary care are extremely important aims in their own rights and that they might also have benefits in terms of preventing some suicides.

Psychiatrists involved in designing suicide prevention strategies might ensure that there are effective local educational programmes for clinicians in primary care and other settings regarding detection and treatment of people with mental disorders.

(c) Influencing media portrayal of suicidal behaviour

Dramatic reporting and portrayal of suicidal behaviour by the media can facilitate suicidal acts in other people. This has been shown in a wide range of studies of both newspaper and television reporting of suicides and fictional presentations of suicidal behaviours in films and television dramas. The impact of media presentations appears to be greatest where the method used in the suicidal act is described in detail, where details of the deceased and/or the site of the act is provided, and for deaths by suicide of celebrities. The largest impact of media influence is on young people, although there is also influence on older people.[(51)]

In each country, consideration should be paid to the development of consensus statements about media policies in relation to reporting and portrayal of suicide,[(52)] which could be produced by joint working parties including representatives of the press, clinical and voluntary agencies, and experts in the field of suicidal behaviour. More difficult is the potentially valuable task of encouraging a policy whereby the media can be used to portray effective coping strategies for people in distress. Such a strategy will need to encompass local cultural factors. Psychiatrists and other professionals developing suicide prevention strategies might examine the practices of their local media with regard to reporting of suicides and, if necessary, hold meetings with media producers to explain the dangers of dramatic and extensive reporting, and also to explore how the media might help in prevention.

Concern is growing about influences on suicidal behaviour through the internet, especially web sites providing instructions on methods of suicide and chat rooms whereby individuals can instruct. Some sites seem to be intended to promote suicide, such as those which initiate meetings between suicidal individuals. Attempts can be made to regulate such sites, but this impossible for sites from other countries. Also, internet providers can be encouraged to ensure that sites offering positive help appear before less desirable sites.

(d) Education of the public about mental illness and its treatment

In view of the very strong link between suicide and mental illness, effective treatment of psychiatric disorders must be a central theme in suicide prevention. However, detection of people with disorders will depend on the awareness that they and those around them have regarding the signs and symptoms of disorder, and their willingness to seek appropriate help.[(53)] These important stages in receiving effective help will depend on the general public's attitudes towards mental illness and knowledge of its nature and the feasibility of treatment. In several countries, programmes to encourage education of the public about psychiatric disorders (especially depression) and to tackle stigmatization of those who are ill have been established. At this stage, evidence is lacking as to whether or not they have been successful. Psychiatrists and their colleagues might consider similar campaigns where these are not already in place, although the method of delivery of messages (e.g. media presentations, leaflets, workshops, articles) will clearly depend on local factors.

(e) Educational approaches in schools

There have been three broad approaches in trying to prevent suicide through school-based programmes.[(54)] The first of these includes teaching about the facts of suicide. Worrying evidence from the United States that such a programme appeared to lead to a small increase in pupils' ratings of the acceptability of suicide as an option compared with the ratings of pupils who did not receive the programme suggests that this is not a wise approach.

Suicidal behaviour in young people often appears to be related to depression, anxiety, low self-esteem, difficulties during upbringing (e.g. abuse, deprivation), life events (especially break-up of relationships, family problems, and bullying), and poor problem-solving skills.[(54)] Also, troubled and suicidal young people most often seek help from their peers. A second school-based strategy has been the development of educational programmes in schools about recognition of psychological distress in individuals and their peers, problem-solving, and peer support. Given the early age at which suicidal behaviour begins, such programmes should probably be targeted at extremely young school children, with later sessions for adolescents.

A third approach is to screen adolescents with questionnaires to detect children and adolescents at risk of psychiatric disorder and possible suicidal behaviour. Pupils that are so detected will then need referral to an appropriate agency for further assessment and possible treatment. While there is some evidence to support such an approach it is not without drawbacks. (Suicide in children and adolescents is considered further in Chapter 9.2.10).

For psychiatrists and others involved in developing local prevention strategies it is important to recognize that school-based approaches to prevention represents is a highly sensitive area and one where the most effective (and least risky) approach is at present unclear. Another important aspect of suicidal behaviour in school pupils is the management of the aftermath of suicides and its impact on other pupils and how to tackle outbreaks of self-harm.[54]

(f) Befriending agencies and telephone helplines

A very important component of suicide prevention policy in many countries is the support provided by largely volunteer staffed befriending agencies and especially telephone helplines. The best known of these is Samaritans. A key principle on which such services are based is that people in distress and at risk of suicide will benefit from being able to discuss their problems with someone entirely confidentially. Recently, more assertive outreach programmes, in which volunteers meet up with distressed individuals such as in prisons and in remote areas, have been added to the traditional telephone service. In the United Kingdom and elsewhere counselling by e-mail and text messaging is being used extensively.

The effectiveness of these approaches is largely unknown. Conducting controlled trials to examine their efficacy is very difficult. Naturalistic studies have produced conflicting evidence about the effectiveness of the Samaritans in the United Kingdom.[55,56] An examination of changes in suicide rates in areas with and without crisis intervention services in the United States suggested that suicide rates in young white females may have been reduced in areas where such services were developed.[57] Given the large numbers of contacts made with Samaritans in the United Kingdom (nearly 5 million in 2005), it appears that the service is valued by people in distress.

Volunteer-run telephone helplines and similar services may benefit greatly from the support and advice of local clinicians, who should regard them as a potentially valuable element in a local suicide prevention strategy.

Addressing the economic factors associated with suicidal behaviour

The association between suicidal behaviour and unemployment and poverty suggests that in order for suicide rates to change markedly these important socio-economic factors must be modified. The big increase in suicide rates during the economic depression of the late 1920s and early 1930s and the statistical association between suicide risk and unemployment would support this. Clearly such factors are increasingly a reflection of the global economic situation, but the strategies of individual governments, particularly in relation to the employment prospects for young people, may be influential. The main role of psychiatrists may be in highlighting these factors. The considerable evidence that changes in the economic environment can exert a powerful influence on suicide rates indicates that governments with serious intentions to reduce suicide rates should address these issues.[32]

Strategies for high-risk groups

There are a wide range of possible prevention strategies which can be targeted at high-risk groups. Here are some of the more important examples of such groups and relevant strategies will be discussed.

(a) Patients with psychiatric disorders

(i) Risk identification

One approach to preventing suicide in people with known psychiatric disorders is to try and use recognized risk factors for suicide in each disorder to identify high-risk patients. The main psychiatric disorders in series of people who have died by suicide are depression (approximately two-thirds), severe alcohol abuse (approximately 15 per cent), and schizophrenia (5–10 per cent).[58] The main suicide risk factors identified in these three disorders include, for example, previous attempts, family history of suicidal behaviour, and living alone. Comorbidity of disorders (e.g. depression and alcohol abuse) and of personality and psychiatric disorders increases risk.

One difficulty in using a risk-identification approach, however, is that the risk factors identified from studies of groups of individuals who have died from suicide are often misleading when applied to individual patients. Also when applying such factors a relatively large number of individuals will appear to be at risk when they may not in fact be so. In clinical practice it is important to be aware of patients who, because of their individual characteristics, are at long-term high risk. Clinicians must also be aware of acute situations which may temporarily increase the risk in patients, be they ones at long-term risk or not.

The most pragmatic approach, therefore, is to ensure that proven effective treatments for patients with these conditions are available and also to be particularly cautious at times of obvious high risk. There are particular periods of risk of suicide for patients with psychiatric disorders. One of these is during the first few weeks after discharge from psychiatric hospital.[59] This emphasizes the necessity for continuity of care at this critical time. Other risk times may be following the break-up of a relationship or other significant loss, during periods of marked hopelessness, shortly after discharge from hospital, and following recent suicidal behaviour by another patient or someone else close to the individual.

(ii) Preventative strategies

Prevention of suicide in patients with psychiatric disorders must be a major element in any suicide prevention strategy.[60] Important strategies in preventing suicide in patients with affective disorders include active treatment of individual episodes of illness, psychological therapy to improve compliance with treatment and assisting individuals to manage their disorder, use of lithium and other mood stabilizers for patients with recurrent bipolar disorders, and use of long-term antidepressants in patients with frequent relapses of depressive disorders. Risk is often greatest during the early stages of a disorder.[53]

The risk factors in schizophrenia indicate that risk tends to be highest between episodes of acute illness when patients may have insight and feel hopeless about their circumstances and prospects. Risk is related more to affective symptoms than core features of the disorders.[61] Continuity of care is likely to be a particularly important factor in preventing suicides in such patients at risk, with care being continued energetically during periods of remission. Community psychiatric nurses have a very important role with such patients. The use of the newer atypical neuroleptics may also be beneficial.[62]

Direct treatment of abuse is likely to be the best preventive strategy for patients with substance abuse disorders, with care taken to manage episodes of depression. The particularly high risk in the weeks following a break-up of a relationship for patients with severe alcohol abuse[63] again points to the need for continuity of support in the community.

The prevention of suicide in patients with comorbid disorders, especially the combination of depression with alcohol abuse and/or personality disorder, is a challenging task, particularly as compliance with treatment is often less good than in patients with single disorders. Effective prevention is likely to depend on close integration of care between different statutory care agencies.

Another important element in prevention in this population is education in suicide risk assessment and management procedures for clinical staff at all levels of seniority. These should be incorporated in educational programmes for risk assessment in general.

(b) Elderly people

In planning suicide prevention in the elderly population, account must be taken of the relative immobility of many older people. In a region of Italy, introduction of a telephone service to provide support and access to emergency help for elderly persons at risk has been associated with an encouraging decline in elderly suicides in the area.[64] This might serve as a model for other countries.

(c) Suicide attempters

In view of the clear association between non-fatal suicidal behaviour and subsequent suicide, establishment of adequate services for suicide attempters, including the provision of careful assessments of patients in the general hospital and offering treatments for which at least some indicators of benefit are available (see above), is an important element in any national suicide prevention strategy. There is good evidence that well-trained, non-medical psychiatric staff can effectively carry out assessments and arrange aftercare. Models for ideal services exist, such as those published by the National Institute for Clinical Excellence[65] in the United Kingdom.

(d) High-risk occupational groups

Certain occupational groups are known to be at relatively high risk of suicide. In the United Kingdom these include farmers, veterinary surgeons, dental practitioners, medical practitioners, pharmacists, and female nurses. It is interesting to note that all these groups have relatively easy access to dangerous methods for suicide. Since prevention through detection of those most at risk encounters the usual difficulties of prevention of relatively rare behaviour using rather crude risk factors, it is probably more important to have general strategies for improving care in individual groups. In doctors, for example, there are some particular difficulties about confidentiality and therefore providing easy means of doctors getting confidential help is important. In farmers, improving the knowledge and attitudes of farming communities towards psychiatric disorder, and removing access to firearms at times of risk, are likely to be important.

(e) Prisoners

There are relatively high suicide rates in prisoners,[66] especially young males held on remand. While one aspect of prevention is through ensuring that prisons and police cells are safe in terms of absence of structures from which inmates can hang themselves, there are a range of other potentially useful and humane strategies. These include careful assessments of new inmates using risk-assessment procedures, training of staff with regard to both assessment skills and attitudes towards mental health problems and suicide prevention, in-reach programmes by befriending organizations such as the Samaritans, and ready access to psychiatric and psychological services. Clinicians involved in local suicide prevention programmes should include prisons in their considerations.

Further information

Hawton, K. (2005). *Prevention and treatment of suicidal behaviour: from science to practice.* Oxford University Press, Oxford.

Hawton, K. and Van Heeringen, K. (2000). *The international handbook of suicide and attempted suicide.* Wiley, Chichester.

National Collaborating Centre for Mental Health. (2004). *Self-harm: the short-term physical and psychological management and secondary prevention of self-harm in primary and secondary care (full guideline) clinical guideline 16.* National Institute for Clinical Excellence, London.

References

1. World Health Organization. (1994). *Ninth general programme of work covering the period 1996–2000.* World Health Organization, Geneva.
2. United Nations. (1996). *Prevention of suicide: guidelines for the formulation and implementation of national strategies.* Department for Policy Coordination and Sustainable Development, New York.
3. Hjelmeland, H., Hawton, K., Nordvik, H., *et al.* (2002). Why people engage in parasuicide: a cross-cultural study of intentions. *Suicide & Life Threatening Behavior*, **32**, 380–93.
4. Zahl, D. and Hawton, K. (2004). Repetition of deliberate self-harm and subsequent suicide risk: long-term follow-up study in 11,583 patients. *The British Journal of Psychiatry*, **185**, 70–5.
5. Owens, D., Horrocks, J., and House, A. (2002). Fatal and non-fatal repetition of self-harm systematic review. *The British Journal of Psychiatry*, **181**, 193–9.
6. Haw, C., Hawton, K., Houston, K., *et al.* (2001). Psychiatric and personality disorders in deliberate self-harm patients. *The British Journal of Psychiatry*, **178**, 48–54.
7. Paykel, E.S., Prusoff, B.A., and Myers, J.K. (1975). Suicide attempts and recent life events: a controlled comparison. *Archives of General Psychiatry*, **32**, 327–33.
8. Williams, J.M.G., Crane, C., Barnhofer, T., *et al.* (2005). Psychology and suicidal behaviour: elaborating the entrapment model. In *Prevention and treatment of suicidal behaviour: from science to practice* (ed. K. Hawton), pp. 71–90. Oxford University Press, Oxford.
9. Mann, J.J. (2003). Neurobiology of suicidal behaviour. *Nature Reviews Neuroscience*, **4**, 819–28.
10. Beck, A.T., Steer, R.A., Kovacs, M., *et al.* (1985). Hopelessness and eventual suicide: a 10 year prospective study of patients hospitalised with suicidal ideation. *The American Journal of Psychiatry*, **145**, 559–63.
11. Hawton, K., Townsend, E., Arensman, E., *et al.* (2005). Psychosocial and pharmacological treatments for deliberate self harm *Cochrane Database of Systematic Reviews*, Issue: 4, Art. No.: CD001764. DOI: 10.1002/14651858.CD001764.

12. Townsend, E., Hawton, K., Altman, D.G., *et al.* (2001). The efficacy of problem-solving treatments after deliberate self-harm: meta-analysis of randomised controlled trials with respect to depression, hopelessness and improvement in problems. *Psychological Medicine*, **31**, 979–88.
13. Brown, G.K., Have, T.T., Henriques, G.R., *et al.* (2005). Cognitive therapy for the prevention of suicide attempts: a randomized controlled trial. *The Journal of the American Medical Association*, **294**, 563–70.
14. Tyrer, P., Thompson, S., Schmidt, U., *et al.* (2003). Randomized controlled trial of brief cognitive behaviour therapy versus treatment as usual in recurrent deliberate self-harm: the POPMACT study. *Psychological Medicine*, **33**, 969–76.
15. Linehan, M.M., Armstrong, H.E., Suarez, A., *et al.* (1991). Cognitive-behavioral treatment of chronically parasuicidal borderline patients. *Archives of General Psychiatry*, **48**, 1060–4.
16. Linehan, M.M., Comtois, K.A., Murray, A.M., *et al.* (2006). Two-year randomized controlled trial and follow-up of dialectical behavior therapy vs therapy by experts for suicidal behaviors and borderline personality disorder. *Archives of General Psychiatry*, **63**, 757–66.
17. Van Heeringen, C., Jannes, S., Buylaert, W., *et al.* (1995). The management of non-compliance with referral to out-patient after-care among attempted suicide patients: a controlled intervention study. *Psychological Medicine*, **25**, 963–70.
18. Vaiva, G., Ducrocq, F., Meyer, P., *et al.* (2006). Effect of telephone contact on further suicide attempts in patients discharged from an emergency department: randomised controlled study. *British Medical Journal*, **332**, 1241–5.
19. Carter, G.L., Clover, K., Whyte, I.M., *et al.* (2005). Postcards from the EDge project: randomised controlled trial of an intervention using postcards to reduce repetition of hospital treated deliberate self poisoning. *British Medical Journal*, **331**, 805–9.
20. Evans, J., Evans, M., Morgan, H.G., *et al.* (2005). Crisis card following self-harm: 12-month follow-up of a randomised controlled trial. *The British Journal of Psychiatry*, **187**, 186–7.
21. Verkes, R.J., Van-der-Mast, R.C., Hengeveld, M.W., *et al.* (1998). Reduction by paroxetine of suicidal behavior in patients with repeated suicide attempts but not major depression. *The American Journal of Psychiatry*, **155**, 543–7.
22. Committee on Safety of Medicines. (2003). Selective serotonin reuptake inhibitors (SSRIs): overview of regulatory status and CSM advice relating to major depressive disorder (MDD) in children and adolescents including a summary of available safety and efficacy data. Medicines and Healthcare products Regulatory Agency, London.
23. Jick, H., Kaye, J.A., and Jick, S.S. (2004). Antidepressants and the risk of suicidal behaviors. *The Journal of the American Medical Association*, **292**, 338–43.
24. Montgomery, S.A., Montgomery, D.B., Jayanthi-Rani, S., *et al.* (1979). Maintenance therapy in repeat suicidal behaviour: a placebo controlled trial. Proceedings of the 10th International Congress for Suicide Prevention & Crisis Intervention. International Association for Suicide Prevention, pp. 227–9. Ottawa, Canada.
25. Cipriani, A., Pretty, H., Hawton, K., *et al.* (2005). Lithium in the prevention of suicidal behaviour and all-cause mortality in patients with mood disorders: a systematic review of randomised trials. *The American Journal of Psychiatry*, **162**, 1805–19.
26. Horrocks, J., Hughes, J., Martin, C., *et al.* (2005). *Patient experiences of hospital care following self-harm—a qualitative study*. Academic Unit of Psychiatry and Behavioural Sciences, Leeds.
27. Beck, A., Schuyler, D., and Herman, J. (1974). Development of suicidal intent scales. In *The prediction of suicide* (eds. A. Beck, H. Resnik, and D.J. Lettieri), pp. 45–56. Charles Press, Maryland.
28. Wood, A., Trainor, G., Rothwell, J., *et al.* (2001). Randomized trial of group therapy for repeated deliberate self-harm in adolescents. *Journal of American Academy of Child and Adolescent Psychiatry*, **40**, 1246–53.
29. Soni Raleigh, V. and Balarajan, R. (1992). Suicide and self-burning among Indians and West Indians in England and Wales. *The British Journal Psychiatry*, **161**, 365–8.
30. Burgess, S. and Hawton, K. (1998). Suicide, euthanasia and the psychiatrist. *Philosophy, Psychiatry and Psychology*, **5**, 113–26.
31. Hawton, K. (2005). *Prevention and treatment of suicidal behaviour: from science to practice*. Oxford University Press, Oxford.
32. Lewis, G., Hawton, K., and Jones, P. (1997). Strategies for preventing suicide. *The British Journal Psychiatry*, **171**, 351–4.
33. Rose, G. (1992). *The strategy of preventive medicine*. Oxford University Press, Oxford.
34. Mann, J.J., Apter, A., Bertolote, J., *et al.* (2005). Suicide prevention strategies. A systematic review. *The Journal of the American Medical Association*, **294**, 2064–74.
35. Upanne, M. (1998). Implementation of the suicide prevention strategy in Finland: first follow-up. In *Suicide prevention: a holistic approach* (eds. D. De Leo, A. Schmidtke, and R.F.W. Diekstra), pp. 219–23. Kluwer Academic Publishers, Dordrecht.
36. Ohberg, A. and Lönnqvist, J. (1997). Suicide trends in Finland 1980–1995. *Psychiatrica Fennica*, **28**, 11–23.
37. Department of Health. (2002). *National suicide prevention strategy for England*. Department of Health, London.
38. Scottish Executive. (2002). Choose life: a national strategy and action plan to prevent suicide in Scotland. The Stationery Office, Edinburgh.
39. Health Service Executive, the National Suicide Review Group, Department of Health and Children. (2005). *Reach out: national strategy for action on suicide prevention 2005–2014*. Health Service Executive, Dublin.
40. Goldney, R.D. (1998). Suicide prevention is possible: a review of recent studies. *Archives of Suicide Research*, **4**, 329–39.
41. Hawton, K. (2005). Restriction of access to methods of suicide as a means of suicide prevention. In *Prevention and treatment of suicidal behaviour: from science to practice* (ed. K. Hawton), pp. 279–91. Oxford University Press, Oxford.
42. Kreitman, N. (1976). The coal gas story: United Kingdom suicide rates 1960–1971. *British Journal of Preventive and Social Medicine*, **30**, 86–93.
43. Amos, T., Appleby, L., and Kiernan, K. (2001). Changes in rates of suicide by car exhaust asphyxiation in England and Wales. *Psychological Medicine*, **31**, 935–9.
44. Kellermann, A.L., Rivara, F.P., Somes, G., *et al.* (1992). Suicide in the home in relation to gun ownership. *New England Journal of Medicine*, **327**, 467–72.
45. Youth Suicide by Firearms Task Force. (1998). Consensus statement on youth suicide by firearms. *Archives of Suicide Research*, **4**, 89–94.
46. Jick, S.S., Dean, A.D., and Jick, H. (1995). Antidepressants and suicide. *British Medical Journal*, **310**, 215–8.
47. Hawton, K., Simkin, S., Deeks, J., *et al.* (2004). UK legislation on analgesic packs: before and after study of long term effect on poisonings. *British Medical Journal*, **329**, 1076–9.
48. Bennewith, O., Nowers, M., and Gunnell, D. (2007). Effect of barriers on the Clifton suspension bridge, England, on local patterns of suicide: implications for prevention. *The British Journal Psychiatry*, **190**, 266–7.
49. Rutz, W., von Knorring, L., and Walinder, J. (1989). Frequency of suicide on Gotland after systematic postgraduate education of general practitioners. *Acta Psychiatrica Scandinavica*, **80**, 151–4.
50. Rutz, W., von Knorring, L., and Walinder, J. (1992). Long-term effects of an educational program for general practitioners given by the Swedish committee for the prevention and treatment of depression. *Acta Psychiatrica Scandinavica*, **85**, 83–8.
51. Hawton, K. and Williams, K. (2005). Media influences on suicidal behaviour: evidence and prevention. In *Prevention and treatment of suicidal behaviour: from science to practice* (ed. K. Hawton), pp. 293–306. Oxford University Press, Oxford.

52. Pirkis, J., Blood, R.W., Beautrais, A., *et al.* (2006). Media guidelines on the reporting of suicide. *Crisis*, **27**, 82–7.
53. Jamison, K.R. and Hawton, K. (2005). The burden of suicide and clinical suggestions for prevention. In *Prevention and treatment of suicidal behaviour: from science to practice* (ed. K. Hawton), pp. 183–96. Oxford University Press, Oxford.
54. Hawton, K. and Rodham, K. (2006). *By their own young hand: deliberate self-harm and suicidal ideas in adolescents*. Jessica Kingsley Publishers, London.
55. Bagley, C.R. (1968). The evaluation of a suicide prevention scheme by an ecological method. *Social Science & Medicine*, **2**, 1–14.
56. Jennings, C., Barraclough, B.M., and Moss, J.R. (1978). Have the Samaritans lowered the suicide rate? A controlled study. *Psychological Medicine*, **8**, 413–22.
57. Lester, D. (1974). Effect of suicide prevention centers on suicide rates in the United States. *Health Service Reports*, **89**, 37–9.
58. Cavanagh, J.T.O., Carson, A.J., Sharpe, M., *et al.* (2003). Psychological autopsy studies of suicide: a systematic review. *Psychological Medicine*, **33**, 395–405.
59. Goldacre, M., Seagroatt, V., and Hawton, K. (1993). Suicide after discharge from psychiatric inpatient care. *Lancet*, **342**, 283–6.
60. University of Manchester. (2006). Avoidable deaths. Five year report of the National Confidential Inquiry into suicide and homicide by people with mental illness. National Confidential Inquiry into Suicide and Homicide by People with Mental Illness, Manchester.
61. Hawton, K., Sutton, L., Haw, C., *et al.* (2005). Schizophrenia and suicide: a systematic review of risk factors. *The British Journal of Psychiatry*, **187**, 9–20.
62. Meltzer, H.Y., Alphs, L., Green, A.I., *et al.* (2003). Clozapine treatment for suicidality in schizophrenia. *Archives of General Psychiatry*, **60**, 82–91.
63. Murphy, G.E., Armstrong, J.W. Jr, Hermele, S.L., *et al.* (1979). Suicide and alcoholism: interpersonal loss confirmed as a predictor. *Archives of General Psychiatry*, **36**, 65–9.
64. De Leo, D., Buono, M.D., and Dwyer, J. (2002). Suicide among the elderly: the long-term impact of a telephone support and assessment intervention in northern Italy. *The British Journal Psychiatry*, **181**, 226–9.
65. National Institute for Clinical Excellence. (2004). Clinical guideline 16. Self-harm: the short-term physical and psychological management and secondary prevention of self-harm in primary and secondary care. National Institute for Clinical Excellence, London.
66. Fazel, S., Benning, R., and Danesh, J. (2005). Suicides in male prisoners in England and Wales, 1978–2003. *Lancet*, **366**, 1301–2.

4.16

Culture-related specific psychiatric syndromes

Wen-Shing Tseng

The concept of culture-related specific (psychiatric) syndromes

In certain ways, all psychiatric disorders are more or less influenced by cultural factors, in addition to biological and psychological factors, for their occurrence and manifestation. 'Major' psychiatric disorders (such as schizophrenia or bipolar disorders) are more determined by biological factors and relatively less by psychological and cultural factors, but 'minor' psychiatric disorders (such as anxiety disorders, conversion disorders, or adjustment disorders) are more subject to psychological causes as well as cultural factors. In addition to this, there are groups of psychiatric disorders that are heavily related to and influenced by cultural factors, and therefore addressed as culture-related specific psychiatric syndromes.

Culture-related specific psychiatric syndromes, also called culture-bound syndromes(1) or culture-specific disorders,(2) refer to mental conditions or psychiatric syndromes whose occurrence or manifestations are closely related to cultural factors and thus warrant understanding and management primarily from a cultural perspective. Because the presentation is usually unique, with special clinical manifestations, the disorder is called a culture-related specific psychiatric syndrome.(3) From a phenomenological point of view, such a condition is not easily categorized according to existing psychiatric classifications, which are based on clinical experiences of commonly observed psychiatric disorders in western societies, without adequate orientation towards less frequently encountered psychiatric conditions and diverse cultures worldwide.

Around the turn of the twentieth century, during a period of colonization by western societies, western ministers, physicians, and others visited faraway countries, where they encountered behaviours and unique psychiatric conditions that they had never experienced at home. Most of these conditions were known to the local people by folk names, such as *latah*, *amok*, *koro*, *susto*, and so on, and were described by westerners as exotic, rare, uncommon, extraordinary mental disorders, mental illnesses peculiar to certain cultures, or culture-bound syndromes. The latter term implies that such syndromes are bound to a particular cultural region.(4)

Recently, however, cultural psychiatrists have realized that such psychiatric manifestations are not necessarily confined to particular ethnic-cultural groups. For instance, epidemic occurrences of *koro* (penis-shrinking panic) occur among Thai or Indian people, not only among the Southern Chinese as originally claimed; and sporadic occurrences of *amok* attacks (mass, indiscriminate homicidal acts) are observed in the Philippines, Thailand, Papua New Guinea, and in epidemic proportions in many places in South Asia,(5) in addition to Malaysia where it was believed to most commonly occur. Terrifying examples of *amok* have recently occurred with frequency on school campuses and in workplaces in the United States.

Therefore, the term culture-bound does not seem to apply, and it has been suggested that culture-related specific psychiatric syndrome would be more accurate to describe a syndrome that is closely **related** to certain *cultural traits* or *cultural features* rather than **bound** specifically to any one *cultural system* or *cultural region*.(4) Accordingly, the definition has been modified to a collection of signs and symptoms that are restricted to a limited number of cultures, primarily by reason of certain of their psychosocial features,(6) even though it is recognized that every psychopathology is influenced by culture to a certain degree.

Subgrouping of culture-related specific syndromes

In order to organize and categorize the various culture-related syndromes, several different subgroup systems have been proposed by different scholars in the past, such as by cardinal symptoms or by 'taxon' (according to a common factor). However, instead of focusing on the clinical manifestation descriptively, it will be more meaningful to subgroup the syndromes according to how they might be affected by cultural factors.

It has been recognized that there are different ways culture contributes to psychopathology. Namely: *pathogenetic effect* (culture has causative effect), *pathoselective effect* (culture selects the nature and type of psychopathology), *pathoplastic effect* (culture contributes to the manifestation of psychopathology), *pathoelaborating effect* (culture elaborates and reinforces certain types of manifestations), *pathofacilitating effect* (culture contributes to the frequent occurrence of particular psychopathologies), or *pathoreactive effect* (culture determines the reaction to psychopathology). Furthermore, culture impacts differently on different types of psychopathology.

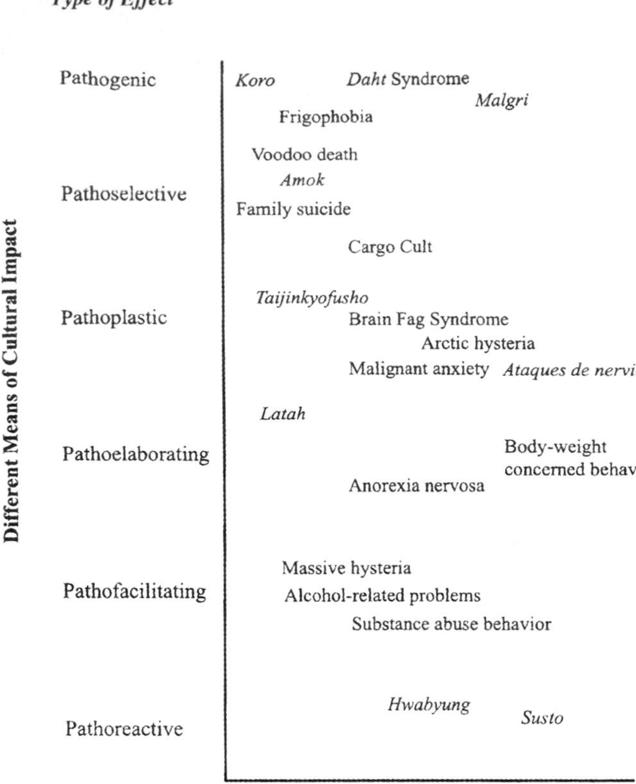

Fig. 4.16.1 Position of culture-related syndromes according to two parameters (This article was published in Handbook of Cultural Psychiatry, Tsend, W.S., copyright Elsevier (2001).)

If the psychopathology is divided into that which is more biologically determined (such as organic mental disorders or major psychiatric disorders), psychologically determined (such as minor psychiatric disorders), or socio-culturally determined (such as culture-related specific syndromes or epidemic mental disorders), it can be said that a pathoreactive effect is observed for all types of psychiatric disorders while a psychogenetic effect is observed mainly for those psychiatric disorders which are more socio-culturally determined, such as culture-related specific syndromes or epidemic mental disorders.

Academically identified culture-related specific syndromes can be compared according to two parameters, namely, the different means of cultural impact and the specificity of the manifestation. It will be useful to determine the basic ways culture contributes to the psychopathology, namely: pathogenic, pathoselective, pathoplastic, pathoelaborating, pathofacilitating, or pathoreactive effects; and to what extent the manifested syndrome is: specific, mixed, or non-specific (Fig. 4.16.1). For example, the primary cultural contribution to *koro* is a pathogenic effect with specific manifestation; to *latah* a pathoelaborating effect with specific manifestation; and to *susto* a pathoreactive effect with non-specific manifestation.

Culture-related beliefs as causes of the occurrence (pathogenetic effects)

(a) Koro (genital-retraction anxiety disorder)

(i) Definition

Koro is a Malay term which means the head of a turtle, symbolizing the male sexual organ which can 'shrink'. Clinically *koro* refers to the psychiatric condition in which the patient is morbidly concerned that his penis is shrinking excessively and subsequently dangerous consequences (such as death) might occur. The manifested symptoms may vary from simple excessive concern to obsessive/hypochondriac concern, intense anxiety, or a panic condition related to the shrinking of the penis. Clinically, this is usually a benign (non-psychotic) condition that occurs in individual, as a sporadic case, but occasionally it may grow to epidemic proportions, so that several hundreds or a thousand people may develop this disorder in a panic manner within a limited time of several weeks or several months. The majority of cases are young males who fear that their penises are shrinking. However, the organ concerned may be any protruding part of the body, such as the nose or ear (particularly when patients are prepuberty children) or the nipples or labia (in females).

Sporadic occurrences of female *koro* cases have never been reported. However, in *koro* epidemics, a small portion of the victims may be female.[7,8] In those cases, the female patients demonstrate slightly different clinical pictures, mainly focusing on the retraction of the nipples and some on the labia. The clinical condition is characterized by a more or less hysterical panic, associated with multiple somatic symptoms, a bewitched feeling, or the misinterpretation or accusation by others of being bewitched.

(ii) Geographic and ethnic group distribution

Cultural psychiatrists originally considered *koro* to be a culture-bound disorder related only to the Chinese. Most Chinese investigators have taken the view that the disorder is related to the Chinese cultural belief in *suoyang*, literally means shrinkage of yang organ due to excess loss of Yang (male) element. It has been speculated further that the occurrence of *koro* among people in South Asian countries, such as Malaysia and Indonesia, was the result of Chinese migrants. However, this cultural-diffusion view is doubted now, since *koro* epidemics have been reported in Thailand and India as well, involving non-Chinese victims.

As a result of the dissemination of knowledge about *koro* as a culture-bound syndrome, there is increased literature reporting so-called *koro* cases from various ethnic groups around the world, such as from the United Kingdom, Canada, and Israel. However, it was pointed out that among the cases reported, all suffered primarily from many psychiatric conditions: affective disorders, schizophrenia and anxiety disorders, drug abuse, or organic brain disorders. Therefore, they were referred as having *koro*-like symptoms, not exactly the same as the *koro* syndrome. It is necessary for clinicians to recognize that *koro* is referred to on different levels as: a symptom, a syndrome, or an epidemic disorder.

(iii) Epidemic of koro

Koro attack may occur occasionally as endemic or epidemic, involving many victims. Epidemic *koro* has been observed in several areas: Guangdong area of China, Singapore, Thailand, and India. As an epidemic, it is manifested as a panic state rather than an anxiety or obsessive state. The epidemic *koro* has tended to occur when there was socio-political stress within the epidemic areas, and an outburst of *koro* by a group of people may be interpreted as a way to deal with the social stress that they encountered.

(iv) Diagnostic issue

Clinicians habitually try to fit pathologies into certain diagnostic categories. Because the patient, based on his misinterpretation, is morbidly preoccupied with the idea that certain ill-effects may occur due to the excessive retraction of his genital organ, the condition may, in a broad sense, be classified as a hypochondriacal disorder as defined in DSM-IV. The condition is also similar to a body dysmorphic disorder, as the patient is preoccupied with a culturally induced, imagined defect in his physical condition. If the focus is on how the patient reacts emotionally, how he responds to the culture-genic stress, with fear, anxiety, or a panic state, anxiety disorder may be considered. However, when we try to categorize culture-related specific syndromes according to the existing nosologically oriented classification system, their meaning and purpose are lost.

(v) Therapy

As for therapy of sporadic individual cases, assurance may be provided or medical knowledge offered in the form of educational counselling to eliminate the patient's concern about impending death. This supportive therapy may work in many cases, but, for someone who firmly believes the *koro* concept, it may not. In general, a young, unmarried male, who lacks adequate psychosexual knowledge and experience, will respond favourably to therapy. If necessary, it is desirable to work on issues such as the patient's self-image, self-confidence, or his masculinity.

(b) Dhat syndrome (semen-loss anxiety)

Very closely related to the genital-retraction anxiety disorder (*koro*) is the semen-loss or semen-leaking anxiety disorder, or spermatorrhea, also known by its Indian folk name, *dhat* syndrome. The *dhat* syndrome refers to the clinical condition in which the patient is morbidly preoccupied with the excessive loss of semen from an improper form of leaking, such as nocturnal emissions, masturbation, or urination. The underlying anxiety is based on the cultural belief that excessive semen loss will result in illness. Therefore, it is a pathogenically induced psychological disorder.[9,10] The medical term spermatorrhea is a misnomer, as there is no actual problem of sperm leakage from a urological point of view.

From a clinical point of view, the patients are predominantly young males who present vague, multiple somatic symptoms such as fatigue, weakness, anxiety, loss of appetite, and feelings of guilt (about having indulged in sexual acts such as masturbation or having sex with prostitutes). Some also complain of sexual dysfunction (impotence or premature ejaculation). The chief complaint is often that the urine is opaque, which is attributed to the presence of semen. The patient attributes the passing of semen in the urine to his excessive indulgence in masturbation or other socially defined sexual improprieties.[11] The syndrome is also widespread in Nepal, Sri Lanka (where it is referred to as *prameha* disease), Bangladesh, and Pakistan.

(c) Sorcery fear and voodoo death (magic-fear-induced death)

The peculiar phenomenon of voodoo death refers to the sudden occurrence of death associated with taboo-breaking or curse fear. It is based on the belief in witchcraft, the putative power to bring about misfortune, disability, and even death through spiritual mechanisms.[12] A severe fear reaction may result from such beliefs, which may actually end in death. From a psychosomatic point of view, it would be psychogenically induced death. From a cultural psychiatric perspective, it is another example of culture-induced morbid fear reaction.

Medically it has been recognized that sudden death was related to psychological stress occurring during experiences of acute grief, the threat of the loss of a close person, personal danger, or other stressful situations. It has been speculated that the cause of death was possibly from natural causes; the possible use of poisons due to sorcery or witchcraft; excessive fear reaction; or death from dehydration or existing physical illness due to old age.

Culture-patterned specific coping reactions (pathoselective effect)

(a) Amok (indiscriminate mass homicide attacks)

(i) The nature of the behaviour

Amok is a Malay term that means to engage furiously in battle. Clinically *amok* refer to an acute outburst of unrestrained violence associated with (indiscriminate) homicidal attacks, preceded by a period of brooding and ending with exhaustion and amnesia.[13] *Amok* homicides are distinct from other murders: the killer chooses an extremely destructive weapon, a crowded location, and insanely and indiscriminately kills a large number of people.[14]

There has been much speculation as to why *amok* behaviour tends to occur in Malay society. One explanation is its connection to the religious background of the people. Muslims are not permitted to commit suicide, which is considered a most heinous act in the Mohammedan religion. In the past, aggressive-homicidal behaviour influenced by infectious diseases has been considered, along with malaria, dengue, neurosyphilis, epilepsy, and so on, as biological in some cases. From a psychological point of view, an extraordinary sensitivity to hurt and the tendency to blame others for one's own difficulties are considered possible causes for the phenomenon. Loss of social standing, by way of insult, loss of employment, or financial loss, has been posited as a precipitating event for *amok*.

(ii) Amok behaviour in other areas

The outburst of aggressive (mass) homicidal behaviour is not necessarily confined to one cultural area, but can potentially be observed elsewhere, such as the territory of Papua and New Guinea, or many areas in South Asia, such as Thailand, the Philippines, Lao, and Indonesia.[5] It has challenged the previous view that *amok* occurs endemically within a particular society. It has been indicated that *amok* could happen in a fashion by communicability and through transmission from one population to another.[5] During the past decade in the United States, there have been increasing episodes of massive (and aimless) killing of people in neighbourhoods, workplaces, and of teachers/students in schools by deadly military weapons. These are American versions of *amok* attacks.

(b) Family suicide

When adults encounter severe difficulties (such as financial debt or a disgraceful event), there are many ways to deal with such problems. As one of the ways to cope with the difficult situation, Japanese parents, may decide to commit suicide together with their young children. This stress-coping method is based on the cultural belief that it would be disgraceful to live after a shameful thing had happened, and that the shame would be relieved by ending one's life. This is coupled with the belief that the children, if left as orphans (after parents' committing husband–wife double suicide), would be mistreated by others. 'Blood is thicker than water' is the common saying reflecting the emphasis of blood-related family tie. Therefore, it would be better for them to die with their parents. This unique way of solving problems was often observed in Japan in the past. It is declining now but still observed some times.

(c) Cargo-cult syndromes (millenniary delusions)

Numerous social and behaviour scientists have noted that, historically, there have been occurrences of crisis cults in many different countries. The Taiping (Great Peace) Rebellion in China, Kikuyu maumau in Kenya, and the Ghost Dance of the Plains Indians of North America are some examples. Central to all these cultures are marked feelings of inferiority, conflict, and anxiety among the member-participants after being exposed to other, superior cultures and an attempt to renovate their self-images. Underlying these non-logical, magic-religious endeavours is a strong wish for resolution of their social, economic, and political problems and for a new and better way of life, such as that of the invading, superior cultures.

One kind of crisis cult is the cargo cult that has repeatedly arisen in Melanesia over the past century as a means of obtaining the manufactured articles possessed by European invaders.[15] Cargo is a neo-Melanesian or pidgin word that designates all of the manufactured goods, including canned foods and weapons, possessed by the Europeans, which are greatly desired by the indigenous people. Without knowing how the cargo was manufactured in the home countries of Europe, based on their own folk beliefs, the local people thought that it was given to the white people by their powerful ancestors through the performance of proper rituals. Accordingly, the local people tried to perform the white people's rituals, in the hopes that their ancestors would send them a lot of cargo and their lives would eventually be full of wealth. This behaviour might be individual, or it might involve a group of followers that gave up their normal lives to perform religious rituals, waiting for the arrival of the cargo, not only for several months, but for many years. They would become collectively deluded and led by a cult leader. As a culture-related specific syndrome, it may be understood that culture contributed to the stress that was encountered and also shaped the unique, pathological pattern of coping with it, a combination of pathogenic and pathoselective effects.

Culture-shaped variations of psychopathology (pathoplastic effect)

This category includes a group of disorders that manifests a clinical picture that is considerably different from the ordinal symptomatology of identified disorders described in current psychiatric classifications (of Euro-American origin). It is considered that the uniqueness of the symptomatology may be culturally attributed, i.e. due to cultural pathoplastic effects. Culture affects not only the content of symptoms, but, even more, the total clinical picture by the absence, addition, or variation of symptoms, resulting in considerable change in the manifestations of variations or subtypes of universally recognized psychiatric disorders.

(a) Anthropophobia (interpersonal relation phobia)

(i) Definition and nature of the disorder

Anthropophobia is the English translation for the Japanese term *taijin-kyofu-shio*. In Japanese, *taijin* means interpersonal, *kyofu* means phobic, and *shio* means syndrome or disorder. Therefore, *taijin-kyofu-shio* literally means the disorder with fear of interpersonal relation.[16] *Taijinkyofushio* is said to be prevalent among Japanese and is considered a culture-related psychiatric disorder. According to the clinical study, the onset of illness was as early mostly between 15 and 25 years, more prevalent among males than female. The cardinal symptoms manifested by the patients are: fear of one's bodily odours, fear of flushing, fear of showing odd attitudes towards others, fear of eye contact with others, concern about others' attitudes towards oneself, and fear of body dysmorphia.

(ii) Dynamic interpretation and culture formulation

The characteristic of *taijinkyofushio* is that the fear is induced in the presence of classmates, colleagues, or friends, those who are neither particularly close (such as family members) nor totally strange (such as people in the street). In other words, subjects are concerned with how to relate to people of intermediate familiarity. It is towards these people that a person must exercise delicate social etiquette. This is different from social phobia described in western societies, where patients have fear of socializing with strangers.

Culturally it has been explained that Japan is a situation-oriented society, very much concerned with how others see one's behaviour. It is considered that the act of staring at the person to whom one is talking is quite extraordinary and considered to be rude. Thus, there are cultural characteristics that cause Japanese to be hypersensitive about looking at and being looked at.

Taijinkyofushio is a psychological disorder of the adolescent. It is closely related to the problems associated with psychological development in the area of socialization. The Japanese child is raised in an atmosphere of indulgence and trust. However, when this protected child enters the wider world of junior high school, he or she faces multiple tasks: coping with conflict between biological needs and social restrictions, personal identity problems, and an increasing need for acceptance and love by others in social settings. This intensifies a feeling of unworthiness, making him or her more concerned about others' sensibilities and reactions.

(b) Brain fag syndrome

This syndrome was described originally as a very common minor psychiatric disorder occurring among the students of Southern Nigeria. Clinically, it is characterized by subjective complaints of intellectual impairment, (visual) sensory impairment, and somatic complaints, mostly of pain or a burning sensation in the head and neck. The student-patients often used the term brain fag to complain that they were no longer able to read, grasp what they were reading, or recall what they had just read, basically stressing their difficulty in mental function. Therefore, the term brain fag syndrome was suggested for this distinct clinical mental condition.[17]

In Nigeria, education was often a family affair, in which one of the brighter children was supported financially by family members; the educated member in turn was expected to be responsible for other family members when the need arose. Because of this family aspect of education, the student was burdened by the responsibility of maintaining the family's prestige. Thus, his or her academic success or failure was associated with great stress. Therefore, it can be said that this syndrome is adjustment disorder with somatic feature and its symptomatology is shaped by culture.

(c) Arctic hysteria (pibloktoq)

Arctic (or polar) hysteria, also known by the local name *pibloktoq*, refers to a unique hysterical attack observed among the polar Eskimo people living in Arctic areas. The clinical condition is characterized by the sudden onset of loss or disturbance of consciousness. During the attack, as the patient may show various abnormal behaviours, such as tearing off his or her clothing, glossolalia, fleeing (nude or clothed), rolling in the snow, throwing anything handy around, performing mimetic acts, convulsion, or other bizarre behaviour. This emotional outburst occurs predominantly in women, but occasionally among men.[(18)]

No specific precipitating causes are noted. It has been speculated that the reaction is a manifestation of the basic Eskimo personality. Because the reaction is prevalent in winter, it is also thought that it may be related to increased threats of starvation or higher accident rates. Generally, it is suspected that the disorder is due to some basic, underlying anxiety, triggered by severe, culturally typical stresses: fear of certain impending situations, fear of loss, or fear of losing emotional support, including the sense of being on safe, solid, familiar ground.

(d) Malignant anxiety

A special, intensified form of anxiety disorder, termed as malignant anxiety, was reported to occur in Africa.[(19)] The condition was characterized by intense anxiety, extreme irritability, restlessness, and intense fear, and, therefore, named it malignant anxiety. It was referred to as frenzied anxiety as well. Often, the patient claimed that there was a change in his sense of self and reality, but there was no sign of personality deterioration or disintegration and no latent or overt psychotic symptoms. However, patients often suffered from intense feelings of anger that led to homicidal behaviour. The condition usually occurred in sporadic cases, but occasionally as an endemic. The disorder was thought to be situation related, associated with problems of adaptation to new and stressful life situations. Very often the patients were culturally marginal persons, who were in the process of renouncing their age-old cultures, but had failed to assimilate the new.

Culturally elaborated unique behaviour (pathoelaborating effect)

(a) Latah (startle-induced dissociative reaction)

(i) Defining the condition

Latah is a Malay word referring to the condition in which a person, after being startled by external stimuli, such as being tickled, suddenly experiences an altered consciousness and falls into a transient, dissociated state, exhibiting unusual behaviour (such as echolalia, echopraxia, or command automatism), including explosive verbal outbursts, usually of erotic words that are not ordinarily acceptable.[(20)] Beside Malaysia, the phenomenon has been observed in other places around the world and has been given various folk names: in Burma (where it is called *yaun*), Indonesia, Thailand (*bah-tsche*), the Philippines (*mali-mali*), indigenous tribes in Siberia, Russia (*myriachit*), and among the Ainu in Japan (who call it *imu*).

The *latah* reaction is found predominantly among women, although men may occasionally be involved. It was found that *latah* tends to run in families. In the past, it was primarily young women who were involved in *latah*. Most of the subjects found now are beyond middle age. Most cases are found in rural areas. Some develop *latah* reactions insidiously, without any precipitating events, whereas others symptoms occur after they endure psychologically stressful events. The loss of a significant person usually occurs shortly before the first experience of *latah* reaction. Once the reaction is experienced, it becomes habitual, and, thereafter, any sudden stimulation may provoke it. Hearing a sudden noise or being suddenly touched or poked by others may cause *latah*. Throwing a rope or other snake-like object in front of the person or simply shouting snake! will sufficiently startle the person to start a *latah* reaction.

The condition may last for several minutes or several hours if the person is continuously provoked. After the dissociative reaction is over, the subject usually claims amnesia and is puzzled about what had happened. Often, the subject is very apologetic and embarrassed for the (socially) inappropriate things he or she may have said (sexually coloured, dirty words) or done (such as touching men) during the attack.

(ii) Aetiological speculations

Anthropologists have tried to understand the *latah* condition from a cultural point of view. It has been pointed out that the *latah* reaction is remarkably congruent with the cultural themes emphasized, but in a paradoxical way. It is a peculiarly appropriate means of communicating marginality to others. The *latah* subjects are engaging in a performance, a role, and theatre, a culture-specific idiom expressing marginality while simultaneously reaffirming normative boundaries. The traditional polygamous Malay extended family structure is male dominated. Within this cultural system, *latah* is socially accepted as a female attention-seeking response, one of the few permissible overt, excitable, aggressive, and/or sexual demonstrations. In other words, *latah* is a culturally sanctioned emotional outlet for females. It is also a culturally elaborated unique behaviour.[(21)]

Cultural influence of prevalent occurrence of disorders (pathofacilitating effects)

This category includes several conditions that are commonly known as psychiatric disorders. There is nothing particular about them in terms of clinical manifestation (thus, they are not *specific* or *unique* disorders). However, their prevalence is influenced strongly enough by cultural factors that they may be viewed as heavily culture-related syndromes, rather than merely *ordinary* psychiatric disorders. Among this group of disorders, massive hysteria, group suicide, alcohol-related problems, or substance abuse are some of the examples.

Cultural interpretation of certain mental conditions (pathoreactive effect)

(a) Ataques de nervios (attack of nerves)

The folk name, *ataques de nervios*, literally meaning attack of nerves, refers to a stress-induced, culturally shaped unique emotional reaction with mixed anxiety-hysterical features.[(22)] This is an illness category used frequently by Hispanic people.

Initially observed among Puerto Rican army recruits, it was also labelled Puerto Rican syndrome. This condition typically occurs at funerals, in accidents, or in family conflicts, and calls forth family or other social supports. Commonly experienced symptoms include shaking, palpitations, a sense of heat rising to the head, and numbness, symptoms resembling a panic attack. The individual may shout, swear, and strike out at others, and finally fall to the ground, manifesting convulsion-like movements.

Based on clinical study, it has been reported that most of the patients (about 80 per cent) were female. From a clinical, diagnostic point of view, according to DSM-III-R criteria, the condition belongs to many subtypes of disorders, including panic disorder, recurrent major depression, generalized anxiety disorder, non-specific anxiety disorder, and others. Because the clinical picture is of a mixed, rather than a specific, nature, it may be interpreted simply as a folk label for an emotional reaction based on psychoreactive effect. It may be understood as an acute episode of social and psychological distress related to upsetting or frightening events in the family sphere. Focusing on symptoms alone misses what is most salient and meaningful about illness categories.

(b) Hwabyung (fire sickness)

Hwa-byung in the Korean language literally means fire (*hwa*) sickness (*byung*). Based on a traditional Chinese medical concept that is still prevalent in Korea, that an imbalance among the five elements within the body (metal, wood, water, fire, and earth) may cause physical disorders, laypeople in Korea use the folk term fire sickness to describe ill conditions. This is a folk idiom of distress characterized by a wide range of somatic and emotional symptoms. About three-fourths of the patients that complained of *hwabyung* were women, who linked their conditions to anger provoked by domestic problems, such as their husbands' extramarital affairs and strained in-law relationships. Culturally, it has been explained that male chauvinism has always been dominant in Korean society, and women tend to suffer from their vulnerable status. When a housewife is mistreated by her husband or is having troubles with her in-laws, she has to suppress her emotional reactions so that there will be no disturbance in the stability of the family. As a woman, she is taught to accept defeat, bear frustration, and suppress her hatred. As a result, accumulated resentment (*hahn* in Korean) becomes a major issue for some women. This is the core dynamic for understanding *hwabyung*.(23)

Cultural factors may indirectly contribute to the occurrence of particular psychological problems that are encountered by Korean women, but through pathoreactive effect, emotional reaction was labelled by laymen as an indication of fire sickness (*hwabyung*).

(c) Susto (soul loss)

Susto is a Spanish word that literally means fright. The term is widely used by people in Latin America to refer to the condition of loss of soul.(24) It is based on the folk belief that every individual possesses a soul, but, through certain experiences, such as being frightened or startled, a person's soul may depart from the body. As a result, the soul-lost person will manifest certain morbid mental conditions and illness behaviour. The remedy for such a condition is to recapture the soul through certain rituals. The concept of loss of soul as a cause for sickness is prevalent around the world, and that terms similar, or equivalent, to *susto* are found widely distributed across many different cultural groups, such as *el miedo* (fright) in Bolivia, *lanti* in the Philippines, or *mogo laya* in Papua New Guinea.

It should be pointed out that, although the cause is attributed to spiritual-psychological reasons relating mostly to a frightening experience or misfortune, from a clinical point of view, the manifested syndrome is quite heterogeneous, without a commonly shared syndrome. The victim may manifest loss of appetite, sleep disturbance, reduced strength, absentmindedness, headache, dizziness, or other somatic symptoms, as well as emotional symptoms of depression, anxiety, or irritability. Therefore, strictly speaking, it is not a culture-related specific syndrome derived from psychogenic or psychoplastic effects. It is culture-related *only* in the sense that the morbid condition is interpreted after the fact according to folk concepts of aetiology and certain ways of regaining the lost soul, such as rituals, are offered. Therefore, the role of culture is interpretation of and reaction to the illness.

Final comments

Diagnosis and classification issues

Associated with the increased awareness of the impact of culture on psychiatric classifications, there is controversy regarding how to deal with culture-related specific syndromes from a diagnostic point of view.(12) Some clinicians feel strongly that various known culture-bound syndromes (such as *koro* or *hwabyung*) should be officially recognized and included in the present classification system.

However, it needs to be pointed out that the present DSM classification system is based on the descriptive approach, categorizing psychiatric disorders by certain sets of manifested symptomatology. If we try to fit culture-related specific syndromes into the categories of the existing classification system or try to create new categories of disorders, they will be classified as NOS (not otherwise specified) or, at best, as variations of presently recognized disorders. Most importantly, by squeezing the culture-related specific syndromes into the descriptive-oriented classification system, we will lose the unique meaning of the syndromes from a cultural perspective.(25)

Culture-related specific syndromes in western societies

Another point that must be made is that, by definition, culture-related specific syndromes should be able to be discovered everywhere, as every society, no matter East or West, has its own culture. However, the trend has been to consider that most culture-related specific syndromes (such as *koro*, *amok*, or *dhat* syndromes) occur in non-western societies. This is because they were considered peculiar phenomena observed in areas previously colonized by western people and they simply did not fit the classification system developed for Euro-American populations. This trend is now changing. There is an increased interest in recognizing syndromes in our own western cultures that are heavily culture-related.(26) Several psychiatric disorders have been suggested by various scholars for consideration as western culture-related syndromes. These include: anorexia nervosa, obesity, drug-induced dissociated states, and multiple personality, disorders that are seldom observed or concerned in non-western societies. Because these conditions are already recognized in the existing western nosological system, they are, in a sense, not viewed as specific syndromes. However, they can be viewed as culture-related psychiatric conditions that are influenced by the pathoelaborative, pathofacilitative, or pathoplastic effects of western culture.

Clinical implications for general psychiatry

Even though the encounter of culture-related specific psychiatric disorder in our daily psychiatric practice is relatively rare, the purpose of examining such specific syndromes has its significant purpose and implications. Through such unique examples, it helps us to appreciate the cultural attribution to the stress formation, reaction pattern, symptom manifestation, occurrence of frequency of disorders, and reaction to the disorders. It also concerns how to work on therapy for the disorder by complying patient's cultural background.

Further information

Tseng, W.S. (2001). D: 13. Culture-related specific syndromes. In *Handbook of cultural psychiatry* (ed. W.S. Tseng), pp. 211–63. Academic Press, San Diego.

References

1. Yap, P.M. (1967). Classification of the culture-bound reactive syndromes. *The Australian and New Zealand Journal of Psychiatry*, **1**, 172–9.
2. Jilek, W.G. and Jilek-Aall, L. (2001). Culture-specific mental disorders. In *Contemporary psychiatry. Psychiatry in special situations*, Vol. 2 (eds. F. Henn, N. Sartorius, H. Helmchen, *et al.*), pp. 219–45. Springer, Berlin.
3. Tseng, W.S. (2001). *Handbook of cultural psychiatry*. Academic Press, San Diego.
4. Tseng, W.S. (2006). From peculiar psychiatric disorders through culture-bound syndromes to culture-related specific syndromes. *Transcultural Psychiatry*, **43**, 554–76.
5. Westermeyer, J. (1973). On the epidemicy of *amok* violence. *Archives of General Psychiatry*, **28**, 873–6.
6. Prince, R. and Tcheng-Laroche, F. (1987). Culture-bound syndromes and international disease classifications. *Culture, Medicine and Psychiatry*, **11**, 3–19.
7. Chowdhury, A.N. (1994). Koro in females: an analysis of 48 cases. *Transcultural Psychiatric Research Review*, **31**, 369–80.
8. Tseng, W.S., Mo, G.M., Hsu, J., *et al.* (1988). A sociocultural study of koro epidemics in Guandong, China. *The American Journal of Psychiatry*, **145**, 1538–43.
9. Malhotra, H.K. and Wig, N.N. (1975). Dhat syndrome: a culture-bound sex neurosis of the orient. *Archives of Sexual Behavior*, **4**, 519–28.
10. Neki, J.S. (1973). Psychiatry in south-east Asia. *The British Journal of Psychiatry*, **123**, 256–69.
11. Bhatia, M.S. and Malik, S.C. (1991). Dhat syndrome—a useful diagnostic entity in Indian culture. *The British Journal of Psychiatry*, **159**, 691–5.
12. Hughes, C.C. (1996). The culture-bound syndromes and psychiatric diagnosis. In *Culture and psychiatric diagnosis: a DSM-IV perspective* (eds. J.E. Mezzich, A. Kleinman, H. Fabrega, Jr, *et al.*), pp. 289–307. American Psychiatric Press, Washington, DC.
13. Yap, P.M. (1951). Mental diseases peculiar to certain cultures: a survey of comparative psychiatry. *The Journal of Mental Science*, **97**, 313–27.
14. Westermeyer, J. (1972). A comparison of *amok* and other homicide in Laos. *The American Journal of Psychiatry*, **129**, 703–9.
15. Burton-Bradley, B.G. (1975). Cargo cult. In *Stone age crisis: a psychiatric appraisal* (ed. B.G. Burton-Bradley), pp. 10–31. Vanderbilt University Press, Nashville, TN.
16. Kitanishi, K. and Mori, A. (1995). Morita therapy: 1919 to 1995. *Psychiatry and Clinical Neurosciences*, **13**, 31–7.
17. Prince, R. (1960). The brain fag syndrome in Nigerian students. *The Journal of Mental Science*, **104**, 559–70.
18. Foulks, E.F. (1972). The Arctic hysterias of the North Alaskan Eskimo. In *Anthropological studies* (No. 10) (ed. D.H. Maybury Lewis). American Anthropological Association, Washington, DC.
19. Lambo, T.A. (1962). Malignant anxiety: a syndrome associated with criminal conduct in Africans. *The Journal of Mental Science*, **108**, 256–64.
20. Simons, R.C. (1980). The resolution of the latah paradox. *The Journal of Nervous and Mental Disease*, **168**, 195–206.
21. Simons, R.C. (1996). *Boo!—culture, experience, and the startle reflex*. Oxford University Press, New York.
22. Guarnaccia, P.J. (1993). Ataques de nervios in Puerto Rico: culture-bound syndrome or popular illness? *Medical Anthropology*, **15**, 157–70.
23. Min, S.W.K. (2006). Hwabyung: a culture-related chronic anger syndrome of Korea. The First World Congress of Cultural Psychiatry Proceeding. (S-III-23).
24. Rubel, A.J. (1964). The epidemiology of a folk illness: *Susto* in Hispanic America. *Ethology*, **3**, 268–83.
25. Pfeiffer, W.M. (1982). Culture-bound syndromes. In *Culture and psychopathology* (ed. I. Al-Issa). University Park Press, Baltimore.
26. Littlewood, R. and Lipsedge, M. (1986). The culture-bound syndromes of the dominant culture: culture, psychopathology and biomedicine. In *Transcultural psychiatry* (ed. J.L. Cox), pp. 253–73. Croom Helm, London.

Index

Note: Page numbers in **bold** refer to main entries. Those in *italic* refer to figures and / or tables. Alphabetical order is word-by-word.

AA (Alcoholics Anonymous) 451–2, 459, 1279, 1352
AACD (age-associated cognitive decline) 1535
AAI (Adult Attachment Interview) 309–10
AAMI (age-associated memory impairment) 1534–5, 1535–6
Abbreviated Injury Scale 1105
ABC analysis 96, 413–14
ABC medical assessment 1106
ABC transporters and complementary medicines 1249–50, *1250*
Abel Screen 1962
Aberrant Behavior Checklist 94, 1823
ability, general, assessment of 87, *88*
ablative neurosurgery *see* neurosurgery for mental disorder
abortion 1119, 1883
  late 1119
  self-induced 1117
Abraham, Karl 306
abridged somatization index 1000
absolute risk reduction 128
abstinence
  from alcohol 450
  in psychoanalysis 1339
abulia 379
acamprosate 454, **1246**, 1542
'accident neurosis' 1055
accidents **1105–13**
  classification of physical injury 1105
  compensation claims 1111–12
  epidemiology 1105
  litigation following 1111–12
  needs of significant others 1108
  and psychiatric disorder 1105
  psychological trauma 1105–6
    assessment at accident scene 1106–7
    long-term assessment and treatment 1110–11
    responses seen in emergency room 1107–8
    treatment during hospital stay 1108–10, *1109*
  and sleep disturbance 926, 1108
acetylcholine 429
  and the basal forebrain 150
  identification 168
  and memory 253
  receptors *173*, 206, 1171
  role in neurodevelopment 159
  in substance use disorders *429*
acetylcholinesterase 155
aciclovir *1091*
acné excorié 618, 917–18, 1044
acromegaly and hypersomnia 942
acrotomophilia *833*
ACSeSS (Admission Criteria to Secure Services Schedule) 2018
ACT *see* assertive community treatment
ACTH 170
  in depression 661
  and insomnia 935
  release in response to stress 1135
  tumours producing 1101
actigraphy 934, 1697
acting out 299, 300
Action Program Test *90*
action-taking, legal aspects 1895–900
Active Life Expectancy 1509–10
activities of daily living (ADL)
  in Alzheimer's disease 335
  instrumental 337
  in mild cognitive impairment 1535
activity scheduling in body dysmorphic disorder 1047
acute and transient psychotic disorders **602–8**
acute intermittent porphyria 212
acute polymorphic disorder with symptoms of schizophrenia 605, 1124
acute polymorphic psychotic disorder without symptoms of schizophrenia 604–5
acute renal failure 1087
acute schizophrenia-like psychotic disorder 536, 603, 605
Acute Stress Disorder Interview 695
Acute Stress Disorder Scale 695
acute stress reactions **693–9**, 716
  aetiology 696
  assessment 695
  childhood and adolescence 1729
  classification 693, 694
  clinical features 693–4
  comorbidity 696
  course and prognosis 696–7
  diagnosis 694–5, *694*
  differential diagnosis 695
  epidemiology 695–6
  following an accident 1107, 1108
  in HIV/AIDS 1091
  and offending 1923
  predictors of 697
  prevention 698
  treatment and management 697–8
  victims of criminal activity 1984–5
AD *see* Alzheimer's disease
Adaptive Behaviour Scales 1821
ADARDS unit 1583
ADAS-Cog (Alzheimer's Disease Assessment Scale-Cognition) 1240
addiction
  'primary addiction' theory 434
  role of personality 428–9
  routes and risks of 430–1, *431*
  self-medication hypothesis 434
  use of term 427
Addiction Severity Index 1164
Addison's disease 1086
adenine 223
adenosine receptors *173*
  adenylate cyclase 174, 176, 473, 1201
ADH *see* alcohol dehydrogenase; vasopressin
ADHD *see* attention-deficit hyperactivity disorder
adjustment disorders **716–24**, **1066–9**
  acute 717
  aetiology 720, 1067–8
  and age 719, 721–3
  associated features 719
  childhood and adolescence 721–3
    after diagnosis of physical illness 1741, 1742
    diagnostic criteria 1669–70, *1671*
  chronic 717
  classification 106, 1066–7
  clinical features 720
  comorbidity 719
  course and prognosis 1068
  definitions 716–19, *716*, *717*, 1066–7
  and deliberate self-harm/suicide 718, 722
  diagnosis 1067, 1669–70, *1671*
  differential diagnosis 695, 1067, 1657
  elderly people 1552

adjustment disorders (*cont.*)
  epidemiology 719, 1067
  and offending 1923
  postoperative 1099–100
  stressors 718, 720
  subtypes *717*, 720
  symptom profile 717–18
  in terminal illness 1069–70
  treatment and management 720–3, 1068–9, *1069*, 1278
ADL *see* activities of daily living
Admission Criteria to Secure Services Schedule 2018
ADMP 73
adolescence *see* childhood and adolescence
Adolescent Transitions Program 1790
adoption 1120
  effects on child and adult mental health **1747–52**
  history-taking 1601
  open 1747
  total severance model 1747
adoption studies **216**
  anxiety disorders 1667
  attention-deficit hyperactivity disorder 1646
  conduct disorder 1659
  in gene–environment interaction 217–18
  mood disorders 651
  offending behaviour 1918
  schizophrenia 548–9, 553–4
adrenaline 150
  in conduct disorder 1658
  functions 161
adrenergic receptors 1171
  antidepressant actions at 1172, 1187
  antipsychotic actions at 1209, *1211*
  and depression 1185, *1185*
  in generalized anxiety disorder 732
  and post-traumatic stress disorder 706
  and suicidal behaviour 965
adrenocorticotropic hormone *see* ACTH
Adult Attachment Interview 309–10
Adult Memory and Information Processing Battery 88
advance directives 30, 1577, 1899
advanced glycosylation end products 1509
advanced sleep phase syndrome 1261, 1699
aetiology
  contribution of epidemiology **280–9**
  contribution of genetics **212–22, 222–33**
  contribution of social sciences **268–75, 275–9**
Afa 1420
affective blunting in schizophrenia 529
affective psychosis and Prader Willi syndrome 1826
affects
  Freudian theories of 295
  and object-relations theory 302, 303
affiliative traits 886, 888
Africa
  attitudes to psychiatric disorder 6
  psychiatric nurses in 1406–7
age-associated cognitive decline 1535
age-associated memory impairment 1534–5, 1535–6
age of consent 1899–900
age of criminal responsibility 1945, 1954
AGE products 1509
ageing
  as an energy crisis 1509
  biology of **1507–11**
  and circadian rhythms 1572
  and culture 1512–13
  and dementia 1520
  dietary modification 1509
  disengagement theory of 1512
  genomic theories 1507–8
  and life expectancy 1507, 1509–10
  and mitochondria 223
  and modernization 1512
  and narrative gerontology 1514–15
  population 1579
  and schizophrenia 544–5
  and sexual function 1569, *1569*
  and sleep 925–6, 1571–2
  social constructionist approach 1515
  sociology of **1512–16**
  stochastic theories 1508–9
  successful 1512
  and transitions 1513–14
  see also elderly people
aggression
  adolescent *see* antisocial behaviour, adolescent
  in antisocial personality disorder 866
  biodevelopmental processes 889
  and body dysmorphic disorder 1044
  in conduct disorder 1656
  in dementia 336, 1920–1, 1928–9
  as a diagnostic feature 1928–9
  and epilepsy 1078, 1864, 1929, 1929–30
  following an accident 1107, 1108, 1920
  following head injury 393, 396, 1929
  and Huntington's disease 1929
  ictal 1930
  impulsive/episodic 912
  information-processing model 1658
  and intellectual disability 1855–6, 1929
  neurobiological determinants 1917–18
  passive 876
  in physical illness 1132–3
  severe maladaptive in childhood and adolescence 1798
  and substance use disorders 1926
  and suicide 970
  and Wernicke–Korsakoff syndrome 1929
  see also violence
aggressive drive 294, 295, 302
agitation
  in dementia 413–15
  in elderly people 1527
  following head injury 393, 396
  in physical illness 1132–3
  postoperative 1098–9
  in schizophrenia 529
agnosia in Alzheimer's disease 334
agomelatine 671
agonists 1171
agoraphobia 52, 750, 752
  elderly people 1559
  with panic disorder 740–1, 750–64
agranulocytosis, drug-induced 1223
agraphia, pure 54
agreeableness 850, 886, 888
AIDS *see* HIV/AIDS
AIS (Abbreviated Injury Scale) 1105
akathisia *58*, *730*, 1222
akinesia 58, *58*
Alanon 1352
alarm clock, dawn-simulating 1261
alcohol
  abstinence vs. controlled drinking 450
  addictiveness *431*
  advertising/promotion restrictions 470
  age limits on drinking 469–70
  as anxiolytic 1178
  awareness of compulsion to drink 439
  binge drinking 646
  control of availability and conditions of use 469–70
  drink-seeking behaviour 438
  drinking repertoire 438
  drug interactions 1175
  education about 468
  effects on sleep 1572
  'expectancies' 434
  'harmful use' 440
  integrated societal policy 471
  intoxication 442–3
    as a legal defence 1901
    and offending 1926, 1927–8
  legal prohibitions on 468
  paradoxical reactions with 1180
  'pathological intoxication' 442, 1926
  rationing sales 470
  reinstatement of drinking after abstinence 439
  relationship between consumption and violence 1926
  sensitivity to 435
  taxes on 470
  temperance movement 470
  tolerance to 438
alcohol abuse, terminology 439–40
alcohol dehydrogenase 435
alcohol dependence syndrome **437–42**
  and classification 439
  clinical features 438, *438*
  elements of 438–9
  validity of 438
alcohol-induced amnesia 404, 443
alcohol-induced dementia 182–3, **399–402**, 444, 1541
alcohol-related brain damage 182–3, **399–402**, 444, 1541
alcohol-related neurodevelopmental disorder 1615, 1841
alcohol-related problems 438, **440–1**
Alcohol Stroop Test 265
alcohol use
  assessment 442, 448
  guidelines for safety 432
  and health 1136
  recommended intake for elderly people 1540
alcohol use disorders (AUDs)
  and accidents 1110
  aetiology **432–7**
    biopsychosocial model *433*
    genetic factors 434–6
    psychological factors 433–4
    sociocultural factors 433
  and anxiety 427
  assessment 448
    instruments 1484, 1542
  in childhood and adolescence 456, 464
  as a chronic relapsing disorder 447–8
  classification 437
  cognitive assessment 92
  comorbidity 427, 434, 443–4

benzodiazepine misuse 492
bipolar disorder 646
bulimia nervosa 804, 806
cyclothymia/cyclothymic disorder 687
depression 649
panic disorder 455, 752
services for 465
sleep-wake disorders *931*
treatment 455–6
and dopamine receptors 229
effects on family and carers 452–3, 465
elderly people 1519, *1540*, **1540–2**, *1541*
and employment 456
ethnic minorities 464
family history positive 434, *434*
global disease burden 10, 467
and head injury 393–4
in health care workers 457
and homelessness 456, 464
informants 448
inpatient care 1453
and intoxication 442–3
and jealousy 620
late-onset 1540
legal issues 1927–8
levels of severity *1541*
and liver transplantation 456
memory impairment in 404
mental health services **459–67**
neuropathology 182–3, *183*
parental, effects on child development 1754
and personality 434
physical disorders associated 444–5
in pregnancy 1117, 1448, 1614–15, 1754, 1826, 1841
prevalence *285*
prevention **467–72**, 1448–9
deterrence 468
education/persuasion 468
harm reduction strategies 469
providing/encouraging alternative activities 468–9
regulating availability and conditions of use 469–70
social, religious and community movements 470
preventive/prevention paradox 460, 467
in primary care, detection 1484
reasons for 427
relapse prevention 450–2, *450*, *451*
spectrum of 459–60, *460*
and suicide 427, 444, 955, 956
terminology 437
treatment **5521–33**, 428
Alcoholics Anonymous 451–2, 459, 1279, 1352
brief interventions 460–1, 463
community-based 461–2
coping skills therapies 451
cost-effectiveness 462–3
counselling 1279
cue exposure 451
deterrent medication 453–4, 1542
effectiveness 470–1
follow-up 457
inpatient 449, 455–6, 461
matching of patients to 452, 455, 456, 462
motivational interviewing 451
pharmacotherapy 1246
spectrum of 459–60, *460*
starting 448
stepped care 462
treatment gap *13*
type I/type II 429
in women 454–5, 464
see also alcohol dependence syndrome
Alcohol Use Disorders Identification Test 284, 460, 1542
alcohol withdrawal 443
alleviation by further drinking 439
complementary medicines 1249
explanation of symptoms 448
inpatient 449, 461
medical assistance 448–9, *449*, 1542
outpatient 448, 461–2
with perceptual disturbance 443
psychosis in 58, 443, 449–50, 538
with seizures 443, 449
symptoms 438–9
tachycardia in 448
and violence 1926
alcoholic blackouts 404, 443
alcoholic hallucinosis 443, 538
Alcoholics Anonymous 451–2, 459, 1279, 1352
alcoholism 437
see also alcohol use disorders
aldehyde dehydrogenase (ALDH) 435
ALE (Active Life Expectancy) 1509–10
alexia 54
alexithymia 850, 1005
algogenic psychosyndrome 851
ALI hierarchy 1372, *1372*
alleles 212–13, 226
association studies 220–1, *220*
allocortex 148, *149*
allostatic load and ageing 1507
alogia 53
1-α-acetylmethadol hydrochloride 1243–4
α-calcium calmodulin-dependent kinase II (α -CaMKII) 889, *890*
α-crystalin 362
α-melanocyte stimulating hormone (α -MSH) 170
α-secretase 338
alpha-synuclein protein/gene 362, 365, 369
α2-agonists in opioid detoxification 477
alprazolam
antipanic actions 1180
in cancer *1102*
in delirium 1533
in panic disorder 756–7, *756*
pharmacokinetics *1172*, 1179
potential for misuse 491
in social anxiety disorder 743
alternative medicine *see* complementary medicines
Alzheimer's disease (AD) **333–43**
aetiology and molecular neurobiology 337–9
and ageing 1520
assessment 92, 265–6, 337, 1240
behavioural and psychological symptoms *413*
biomarkers 341
carers 340
classification 336
clinical features 334–6
cognitive impairment in 334–5
delaying onset/disease modification 341, 1538
and delirium 1532
and depression 335
diagnosis 336–7
differential diagnosis 347, 364, 373, 380
and Down syndrome 1584, 1827, 1839, 1865, 1880
early detection 265–6, 1519–20
epidemiology **1519–22**
functional impairment in 335
genetic counselling 340
genetics 227, 339, 1521
history of disorder 334
history-taking 336–7
impact 1522
incidence and risk factors 1520–2, *1520*, *1522*
Lewy body variant 362
and mild cognitive impairment 1534, *1534*, 1535–6, 1538
neurofibrillary tangles 337–8, 339
neuropathology 337–9
amyloid cascade hypothesis 338
cholinergic hypothesis 338, 1240–1
presenilin genes 339
personality change in 335–6
prevention 341
psychoses in 335
risk reduction/protective factors 1521–2, *1522*, 1538
and sleep-wake disorders *931*
sporadic/familial 339
translational research 341
treatment and management 339–41, 1240–1
Alzheimer's Disease Assessment Scale-Cognition 1240
amantadine 374, 1226, 1876
ambitendency 58
aMCI (amnestic mild cognitive impairment) 1520, 1535
amenorrhoea in anorexia nervosa 782, 783, 787
AMHPs (approved mental health practitioners) 1410
amimia 346
amines *168*
amino acids *168*
amisulpride 1209
administration 1220
adverse effects *1212*
pharmacodynamics 1210
pharmacokinetics 1222
amitriptyline *670*
adverse effects *1191*
in anxiety disorders 1182
in cancer *1103*
dosage *1196*
drug interactions 1175, 1233
in personality disorders *905*
pharmacodynamics *1173*, *1187*
pharmacokinetics *1172*, *1189*
amnesia 59
alcohol-induced 404, 443
in Alzheimer's disease 334
anterograde 59, 92, 252, 391
assessment of awareness of 420–1
assessment of functional consequences 420
assessment of memory 89, *89*, 253, 254, 255–6, 264, 420–1, *420*
in brain tumour 1075
and cerebrovascular disease 407
for criminal offences 405, 1927
in dementia 59
dissociative 714, 715, 1012
following ECT 404, 1257
following hypoxia 406–7

amnesia (*cont.*)
in fugue states 404–5
global 59
in herpes encephalitis 406
malingered 1055–6
memory remediation and rehabilitation 421–4, *422*
partial 59
persistent 405–8
post-traumatic 388, 390–1, 404, 407
in post-traumatic stress disorder 404, 714
psychogenic 59
psychogenic focal retrograde 405
retrograde 59, 252, 408
following head injury 388, *388*, 391
selective 57
transient 403–5
transient epileptic 403
transient global 59, 403
use of memory aids and strategies 420, *421*
in vascular dementia 379
in Wernicke–Korsakoff syndrome 92, 405–6
see also memory impairment
amnesic syndromes **403–11**
associated with alcohol use 1541
elderly people 1531
amnestic mild cognitive impairment 1520, 1535
amok 606, 979, **981**
amotivational syndrome, cannabis-associated 508
amoxapine 669
adverse effects 1190, *1191*
dosage *1196*
pharmacodynamics *1187*
pharmacokinetics *1189*
AMPA receptors 172, *173*, 174, 1171
AMPAkines 174
amphetamine **482–6**
addictiveness *431*, 483
in attention-deficit hyperactivity disorder 1241, 1876
effects of 483, *483*
in intellectual disability 1876
misuse
aetiology 484
complications associated 484–5
course and prognosis 484–5
diagnosis 483–4
epidemiology 484
prevention 485
treatment and management 485
pharmacodynamics 1172
preparations 482–3
psychosis due to 485
withdrawal 483, *483*
amphotericin B *1091*
ampicillin 1532
amygdala 152, 152–3, 158, 201
and associative learning 258
and emotion 258, 259, 264
and fear/anxiety 1666, *1667*, 1668
in generalized anxiety disorder 732–3
and memory 251, 253, 259, 264
and orbitofrontal cortical development 1919
amygdalotomy 1267
amylase serum levels in bulimia nervosa 804
amyloid 338
amyloid precursor protein 338
anabolic steroid abuse 1045
anaclitic type 316
anaemia 785, 1087–8
anaesthesia, glove and stocking 57
anaesthetics, adverse effects *730*
anal phase of development 294, 295
analgesics
combination formulations 1169
in somatization disorder 1009
suicide risk 973
analysis of variance 138
analytical behaviourism 133–4
analytical functionalism 134–5
anandamide 172, 429, *429*, 507
anankastic personality disorder *see* obsessive–compulsive disorder
anankastic phenomena 52
androgen therapy in gender identity disorder 843
androgens 815–16, 816, 826
androstenedione 815
anencephaly 156
aneuploidy 228
aneusomy 228
angel dust *see* phencyclidine
Angelman syndrome
behavioural and psychiatric aspects 1841–2
and epilepsy 1864, 1865
genetics 213, 224, 229, 1841, 1865, *1866*
physical characteristics 1841
prevalence 1841
Anger Coping and Coping Power Programme 1662, 1782
anger management
in adjustment disorders *1069*
in antisocial personality disorder 898
in anxiety disorders 1295–6
in conduct disorder 1662, 1782
in intellectual disability 1874
aniracetam 1240
Anna O 1338
anomia 253, 850, 1449
anorexia nervosa **777–800**
and adverse life events 779–80
aetiology 778–82
biomedical factors 781–2
family factors 780
multidimensional approach 778–9, *779*
sociocultural factors 779
age at onset 778
assessment instruments 777
and body image 57
and child sexual abuse 780
childhood and adolescence 1784
classical post-pubertal 782–6
classification and diagnosis 787–8, 800–1, *801*
course and prognosis 788–9
as culture-bound syndrome 779
and depression 783, 787
differential diagnosis 784, 787
early onset/premenarchal 786–7, 788–9
epidemiology 777–8
ethical issues 796
and gender 778
genetics 781–2, 806
history of concept 777
hypothalamic model 781
incidence 778
maintenance 1299
in males 788
malnutrition in 784–6
medico-legal issues 796
mortality 788–9
myopathy in 785
and obsessive–compulsive disorder 783
osteoporosis in 785
overlap with bulimia nervosa 800, *801*
and parenthood 786
and personality disorders 780–1, 884
and postnatal depression 780
and pregnancy 780, 784, 1118
prevalence 778
prevention 796–7
psychopathology 779, 783, 786–7
relationship with other eating disorders 804
risk factors *806*
and socio-economic status 778
and suicide 955
temperature regulation in 785
treatment 789–96
antidepressants 795, 1193
cognitive-behaviour therapy 792, 796, **1298–303**
compliance 794
complications 786
compulsory 793, 795
day care/community 793, 795
dietary care 794–5
dynamic psychotherapy 796
eating disorder units 792–3
family therapy 790–2, *790*, 796
inpatient 792–3, 793, 794–5
interpersonal psychotherapy 792
nursing 794–5
ANOVA 138
Antabuse® **453**, *730*, **1246**, 1542
antagonists 1171–2
anterior capsulotomy 1267, *1269*, Plate 15
anterior cingulate cortex 245
anterior cingulotomy 1267, *1270*, Plate 16
anterior commissure 151, 157
anthropology *see* social and cultural anthropology
anthropophobia 982
anti-androgens in the paraphilias 838
anticholinergics
adverse effects 365, 487, 1225
anxiety *730*
delirium 331, 1532
memory loss 404
parasomnias 946
in management of antipsychotic adverse effects 1225
anticipation 213, 228, 652
antidepressants 669–71, *670*, **1185–98**
in adjustment disorders 721, 1068
administration and dosage 1195, *1196*
adverse effects 674, 1190–3, *1191*, *1192*
anxiety *730*
cardiotoxicity 1794–5
epileptogenicity 1078
sexual dysfunction 826–7
suicide risk 971, 973, 1192, 1668, 1707–8, 1796, 1923
in alcohol use disorders 455
in anorexia nervosa 795, 1193–4
in anxiety disorders 1182, 1193
and attempted suicide 670, 674
in attempted suicide 970–1, 1192
in bipolar disorder 671–2
in bulimia nervosa 807–8, 809, 1193–4
in cancer 1102, *1103*

in childhood and adolescence 674–5, 1676, 1794–5, 1796
choice of 674
classes of 1186–8, *1187*
complementary medicines 1248
contraindications 1194
delayed onset of effects 176, *176*
in dementia 416
dosage 674–5
drug interactions 1194–5, *1195*
in dysthymia/dysthymic disorder 684–5
in elderly people 674, 1554–5, *1554*
in generalized anxiety disorder 735
history of 1185–6, *1185*
in HIV/AIDS 386, 1092
indications 674, 1193–4, *1193*
in intellectual disability 1875–6
in obsessive–compulsive disorder 768–9, 770, 1193, 1687–8, *1687*
overdose 1192
in persistent somatoform pain disorder 1033–4
in personality disorders *905*, 906
pharmacodynamics 1172–3, *1173*, 1186–8, *1187*
pharmacokinetics *1172*, 1188–9, *1189*
in post-traumatic stress disorder 709
precautions with 1796
in pregnancy 675, 677, 761–2, 1117, 1192
prescription in physical illness 674, 1132
and surgery 1097–8
switching between 674
in terminal illness 1070
theories regarding actions of 1185–6, *1185*
withdrawal 1195
see also specific drugs and types of drugs
antiemetics
adverse effects 1101
in chemotherapy 1101
antiepileptic drugs **1231–40**
adverse effects
anxiety *730*
behavioural disorders 1867–8
on cognitive function 92
teratogenicity 1169
in anxiety disorders 1182
in bipolar disorder 671, 672, 1556
in childhood and adolescence 1798
with psychiatric/behaviour disorder and intellectual disability 1852
choice of 1866–7
drug interactions 1866
in elderly people 1556
in epilepsy 1080
with intellectual disability 1866–7, *1867*
in intellectual disability 1852, 1866–7, *1867*, 1876
in Landau–Kleffner syndrome 1627
in personality disorders *905*, 906
pharmacokinetics *1867*
structures *1232*
withdrawal 1867
see also specific drugs
antihistamines
in anxiety disorders 1182
in management of antipsychotic adverse effects 1225
antihypertensives, adverse effects 827
antilibidinal drugs in intellectual disability 1876
antilibidinal object 308
antioxidants
and longevity 1509
in tardive dyskinesia 1249
anti-PrP antibodies 359
anti-psychiatrist movement 28
antipsychotics **1208–31**
in acute and transient psychotic disorders 606
administration 1213–22, *1214*
adverse effects 58–9, *1212*, 1222–5
acute sensitivity reactions in dementia with Lewy bodies 361–2, 365
akathisia *730*, 1222
anxiety 1101
in childhood and adolescence 1677, 1797–8
cognitive impairment 580
diabetes 1085
dystonia 1222
in elderly people 1548
epileptogenicity 1078, 1223
hyperprolactinaemia 1086, 1217, 1223
hypersomnia 939
hypotension 1223, 1529
management 1225
'neuroleptic toxicity' 588
parkinsonism 580, 1222–3
sexual dysfunction 827
tardive dyskinesia 1223
see also neuroleptic malignant syndrome
in alcohol withdrawal 449–50
antidepressant actions 581
in anxiety disorders 1182
in attempted suicide 971
in attention-deficit hyperactivity disorder 1652
atypical 1172, 1209, *1209*
in autism and other pervasive developmental disorders 1640
in bipolar disorder 677
in cancer *1104*
in childhood and adolescence 1677, 1796–8, 1852
classification 1209–10, *1209*
complementary medicines 1249
in delirium 331
in dementia 414–15
in dementia with Lewy bodies 367
depot formulations 581–2
drug interactions 1221–2
high-potency 1209
in HIV/AIDS 386, 1092
in Huntington's disease 374
indications and contraindications 1225
in intellectual disability 1875
low-potency 1209
mid-potency 1209
in personality disorders 600, *905*, 906
PET/SPET imaging studies 189–90
pharmacodynamics 1172, 1210, *1211*, 1212–13, *1212*
pharmacokinetics *1172*, 1221–2
polypharmacy 587–8
in pregnancy 677, 1118
resistance to 582, 590, 1213
risk: benefit appraisal 585, *586*
in schizoaffective disorder 598
in schizophrenia 579–82, *579*, 585, 586–8, *586*, 1213, *1215*, 1548
and surgery 1098
in tic disorders 1073, 1688
typical (first generation) 1209, *1209*
antisocial behaviour, adolescent 1654, **1945–59**
assessment 1947–8, *1949*
and attention-deficit hyperactivity disorder 1948–9
and autism spectrum disorders 1950
and capacity 1954–5
and conduct disorder 1946, 1948–9
and depression 1949
and early-onset psychosis 1950
epidemiology 1945
girls 1955–6
interventions 1950–7, *1951*
justice system 1945, 1947
legal issues 1954–5
and mental disorder 1946–7, 1948–50, 1951–2
pathways of care 1947
pathways to *1946*
and post-traumatic stress disorder 1949–50
protective factors 1947, *1947*
risk factors *1946*, 1947
antisocial behaviour, adult *see* offending
antisocial personality disorder **865–6**
aetiology 866
classification 851, *856*, *865*
clinical features 866
comorbidity 866
course and prognosis 866
and deception 1049
diagnosis 866
differential diagnosis 866, 1657
in elderly people 1561, *1562*, 1563
epidemiology 865, *882*, 883
following head injury 391
and genetic–environmental interactions 315
offenders 1921
prisoners *1933*
relationship with attention-deficit hyperactivity disorder 1931
terminology 856
treatment 866, 898, 898–9, 904
anxiety
as an alarm signal 295
anticipatory 751
and arousal 55
assessment instruments 1164
in bulimia nervosa 803
in cancer 1101–2, *1101*
in childhood and adolescence
assessment 1665
with intellectual disability 1851–2
with physical illness 1742–3
and conversion disorder 1014–15, 1015
counselling in 1278
definition 1664
in depression 634
'depressive' 307
and diabetes mellitus 1085
drug-induced symptoms resembling *730*
elderly people 1558–61
and epilepsy 1080
following an accident 1106, 1108–9
and functional symptoms 993
and hyperthyroidism 1085
malignant 983
pathophysiology 1666–8, *1667*
in physical illness 1131–2, 1742–3
in pregnancy 1117
preoperative 1097

anxiety (*cont.*)
  and sexuality 825
  in Tourette syndrome 1073
  trait 1137
  in vascular dementia 379
  and ventricular dysrhythmias 1081
anxiety disorders
  acute-on-chronic 1180
  alcohol-induced 427, 434, 444, 455
  assessment 1289, *1289*
  with attention-deficit hyperactivity disorder 1650
  and bipolar disorder 646
  childhood and adolescence **1664–9**
    assessment 1665
    clinical course and outcome 1666
    clinical presentation 1665–6
    comorbidity 1666, 1673
    differential diagnosis 1671
    epidemiology 1665–6
    pathophysiology 1666–8, *1667*
    treatment 1668, 1779–80
  chronic 1180
  and chronic fatigue syndrome 1037
  classification 105
  cognitive content 1286–7
  cognitive model of 1289–90, *1290*
  definition 1664
  and depression 649
  elderly people 1531, 1579
  following head injury 393
  following stroke 1071–2
  genetics 1667
  and hypochondriasis 997, 1024, 1027
  and intellectual disability 1855
  and kleptomania 1943
  and pain 1030
  parental, effects on child development 1754
  and persistent somatoform pain disorder 997, 1032
  postpartum 1121–2
  prevalence *285*
  and sleep-wake disorders *931*
  and somatization disorders 996
  and stress 1667–8
  and suicide 955
  treatment
    antidepressants 1182, 1193
    cognitive-behaviour therapy **1285–98**, 1668, 1779–80
    interpersonal psychotherapy 1324
    neurosurgery 1267
    see also anxiolytics
  vulnerability to 732, 734–5
  see also generalized anxiety disorder
anxiety management
  in depression in elderly people 1555
  in obsessive–compulsive disorder 1685
'anxiety neurosis'/'anxiety state' 729
anxiety programme 1285
anxiolytics 1178–9
  in cancer 1101–2, *1102*
  clinical effects 1179–81
  complementary medicines as 1248
  intravenous, in conversion disorder 1019
  in obsessive–compulsive disorder 769
  in pregnancy 1117
  withdrawal from *730*
anxious personality disorder *see* avoidant personality disorder
AO (assertive outreach) teams 1455, 1457–8, *1457*
apathy
  in dementia 416
  following an accident 1106
  following head injury 391, 392, 396
  following neurosurgery for mental disorder 1269
aphasia 53
  acquired childhood 1712
  acquired epileptic 1626–7, 1639, 1864
  in Alzheimer's disease 334
  assessment 89
  jargon 54
  progressive non-fluent 344
aphonia 53
Aplysia 315
APOE gene/apoE protein and Alzheimer's disease 339, 1521
apotemnophilia *833*
APP gene/APP protein 338, 339
applied tension in specific phobia 746
appraisal delay 1137
approved mental health practitioners 1410
'approximate answers' 54, 1055
apraxia in Alzheimer's disease 334
archicortex 158
Arctic hysteria 983
Argentina, attitudes to psychiatric disorder 6
aripiprazole 1209, *1209*
  administration *1214*, 1219–20
  adverse effects *1212*, 1225
  in bipolar disorder in elderly people 1556
  in childhood and adolescence 1797
  in personality disorders *905*, 906
  pharmacodynamics 1210, *1211*
  pharmacokinetics 1222
  pharmacology 1210
Aristotle 133
arithmetical skills, specific disorders of 1629–30
ARND (alcohol-related neurodevelopmental disorder) 1615, 1841
aromatherapy in dementia *414*
arousal and anxiety 55
array CGH 1831
arson 1924, **1965–9**
  by children/adolescents 1954
  characteristics of fire-raisers 1966
  classification 1966, *1966*
  historical context 1965
  legal aspects 1966
  management 1967–8
  motivation *1966*, 1967
  prevalence 1965–6, *1965*
art therapy 1352, **1413–17**
  with children 1414
  contextual issues 1415–16
  definitions 1413
  with elderly people 1415
  historical development 1414
  with offenders 1415
  people with intellectual disability 1414–15
  in physical illness 1415
  in psychotic illness 1415
  research 1416
  in selective mutism 1714
artefactual illness 57
articulatory suppression in insomnia 936–7
artificial insemination 1114–15
ascending reticular activating system in Alzheimer's disease 1240
ascertainment
  in family studies 215
  in twin studies 216
aschemazia 57
asenapine 1209, 1210, 1220–1
aspartylglucosaminuria 1865
Asperger's syndrome **1638–9**
  aetiology 1639
  clinical features 1638
  course 1639
  definition 1638, *1638*
  demographics 1639
  differential diagnosis 865
  epidemiology 1639
  and juvenile delinquency 1950
  management 1640
  and offending 1921
  prognosis 1639
asphyxiophilia 832, *833*
aspirin, drug interactions 1232
assertive community treatment (ACT) 1402
  in alcohol use disorders 462
  in schizophrenia 584
assertive outreach teams 1455, 1457–8, *1457*
assessment
  acute stress reactions 695
  adolescent antisocial behaviour 1947–8, *1949*
  alcohol use 442, 448
  alcohol use disorders 448
  Alzheimer's disease 92, 265–6, 337, 1240
  anxiety, in childhood and adolescence 1665
  anxiety disorders 1289, *1289*, 1665
  attention 60, 88–9, 264–5
  attention-deficit hyperactivity disorder 1645, 1782–3
  behavioural methods 94, 96–7, *96*
  benzodiazepine misuse/dependence 492
  bereavement 726–7
  bulimia nervosa 807
  by community mental health teams 1455
  and categories of information 63
  character 80–1, *80*, 82–3
  in childhood and adolescence 90, **1600–6**
    content of the clinical interview 1600–1, *1602*
    developmentally sensitive techniques 1601, 1604–5
    laboratory tests 1605–6, *1605*
    mood disorders 1675
    need for multiple informants 1600
    structure of the clinical interview 1601, 1603–4, *1603*
  concentration 60, 88–9
  and concepts of disablement 65
  and the concepts of disease, illness and sickness 63–4
  concepts underlying procedures 63–7
  condensation and recording of information 73–4
  conduct disorder 1657, 1781–2
  and confidentiality 67
  in consultation-liaison psychiatry 1146
  contextual influences 67
  and culture 67
  depression 660
  and diagnoses 74
  and the diagnostic process 64–5

distinction between form and content of symptoms 63
elderly people **1524–9**
after treatment 1528–9
history-taking 1526
mental state examination 1526–7, *1528*
physical 1527–9
setting for 1525–7
formulation 73–4
from complaint to formulation 66, *66*
general ability 87, *88*
instruments *see* assessment instruments
intellectual disability 1821–3
intelligence 22, 54, 87, *88*, 263–4
and life events 66–7
mania 1675
memory 89, *89*, 253, 254, 255–6, 264, 420–1, *420*
mental health services **1463–72**
mild cognitive impairment 1536
as a multi-disciplinary activity 62, 68
obsessive–compulsive disorder 1783
offenders with mental disorder 2011–12, 2018
personality 72–3, **78–85**, 286, 1164–5
personality disorders 858–9, *858*
principles in general psychiatry **62–78**
privacy of interviewing 67
and prognosis 74
and psychodynamics 67
psychometric 85–7
psychophysiological methods 97
refugees 1496–7
and reviews 74
sequence of 66
sleep-wake disorders 929–30
in childhood and adolescence 1696–7, *1696*
somatization disorder 1005–6, *1005*
summary 73–4
temperament 79–80, *80*
urgent 68
use of interpreters 67
and written reports 74–6
see also cognitive assessment; needs, assessment; neuropsychological assessment
Assessment and Reduction of Psychiatric Disability 572
assessment instruments **69–73**
acute stress reactions 695
administration 95–6
alcohol use disorders 1484, 1542
anorexia nervosa 777
anxiety 1164
behavioural 94, 96–7, *96*
behavioural and psychological symptoms in dementia 413
'bottom-up' organization 71
in childhood and adolescence 1591
with intellectual disability 1860
cognitive and neuropsychological functioning 87–9, *88*, *89*, *90*, 263–7
comprehensive 73
computer-based 70, 263
content and format 95, *95*
contents of a good test manual *87*
and context 268
creation 96
delirium 328
depression 69, 70, 1163–4, 1306, 1484, 1551, *1552*
developments since the 1950s 70–2
disablement 284
in epidemiology 284–6
evaluation criteria 95
in evaluation of psychotherapy 1163–5
of functioning 1165
information regarding 89
investigator-based 269
mental state and behaviour 69–70
multiaxial descriptive systems 73
multiple measures 96
needs 73, 94, 1433–4
in needs assessment 73, 1433
for negative symptoms 72
numeric analogue scales 1032
for personality 72–3, 81–2, *81*
personality disorders 858–9, *858*
post-traumatic stress disorder 703
psychometric adequacy 95
psychopathology 1164
psychoses 1164
purpose of 94
quality of life 73, 1165
for quantification of clinical outcome 73
questionnaires **94–8**
rating scales **94–8**
reasons for development of structured interviewing and rating scales 69
response coding 97
for risk 1994, 1996–7
screening 69
self-esteem 1164
sensitivity and specificity 140–1, 284
service utilization 1165
standard vs. individualized 97
standardized interview schedules 14, 284
substance use disorders 1164
'top-down' organization 71
understanding and choice of 89–90
usefulness 1595
validity 140–1, 284
verbal descriptor scales 1033
visual analogue scales 1032
see also specific instruments
assisted reproduction 1114–15
association therapy 836–7
associative learning 258, 696
asthma 1082
brittle 1050
and sleep-wake disorders *932*
astroglia 157
astrology 1420
Asylum Act 1828 19
asylums 17–18, 18–19, 22, 24
ataques de nervios 983–4
ataxia
cerebellar, in alcohol use disorders 445
in HIV-associated dementia 384
atmosphere, delusional 51
atomoxetine 1688, 1795–6
adverse effects 1795
in attention-deficit hyperactivity disorder 1241, 1648, 1650
and epilepsy 1650
precautions with 1795
suicidal risk 1796
ATP (Adolescent Transitions Program) 1790
ATP receptors *173*
attachment theory 242–3, *242*, 285, **309–10**, 1725
and child abuse 1735
and child neglect 1736
and conduct disorder 1659
and generalized anxiety disorder 734
internal working model (IWM) 243
and mentalization 1948
mother–infant 1123–4
and neuropeptides 888
and offending 1910
prenatal 1116–17
and psychopathology 243
secure/insecure attachment 242, *242*, 309–10, 1725
and separation 1758
and stalking 1972
and transference 1342–3
attention **245–9**
assessment 60, 88–9, 264–5
in attention-deficit hyperactivity disorder 1643
brain regions involved *246*
deficit 60
and delirium 325, 326
and depression 92
disorders of 60
divided 247–8
effects of disturbed sleep 926
and emotion 259
executive control 248–9, *248*
following head injury 390
phasic 247
selective 60, 245–7, 264, 1288
shared 60
in somatization disorder 1005
sustained 247, 264
vigilant 59, 247, 264
attention-deficit hyperactivity disorder (ADHD) 60, 1613, **1643–54**
in adult life 1647–8, 1652
aetiology 1646–7
assessment 1645, 1782–3
classification 1643
clinical features 1643
comorbidity 427, 646, 1073, 1644, 1650, 1673, 1682, 1931
course and prognosis 1647–8
diagnosis 1643–5, 1849
differential diagnosis 1644–5, 1657, 1671
epidemiology 1645–6
and gender 1646, 1828
genetics 1590, 1646
hyperactive/impulsive subtype 266
and intellectual disability 1850–1, 1876
and juvenile delinquency 1948–9
legitimacy of diagnosis 28
neuropsychological assessment 266
and offending 1931
pathogenesis 1647
prisoners 1931
refractory 1651–2
relationship with antisocial personality disorder 1931
and sleep-wake disorders 927, *931*, 1695, 1697
and speech and language disorder/difficulty 1714
and stigma 1651
treatment and management 1241–2, 1648–52, 1782–3, 1876
attentional blink paradigm 247
attributional style 653

atypical schizophrenic disorder 866
AUDIT (Alcohol Use Disorders Identification Test) 284, 460, 1542
audit of consultation-liaison psychiatric services 1147
AUDs *see* alcohol use disorders
aura 60, 1077
Australia, neurasthenia as diagnostic entity 1061
autism **1633–6**
  aetiology 227, 1635–6
  atypical 1639
  classification 1623
  clinical features 1633
  comorbidity 1852
  course 1635
  definition 1633–4, *1634*
  demographics 1634–5
  differential diagnosis 865, 1639, 1644–5, 1657
  and Down syndrome 1839
  epidemiology 1634–5
  and epilepsy 1852
  and fragile-X syndrome 1635
  and gender 1828
  genetics 1635–6
  and intellectual disability 1852, 1855
  and juvenile delinquency 1950
  and offending 1921
  and parental psychiatric disorder 1885
  prevention 1640
  prognosis 1635
  and sleep disorder 1697
  and specific language impairment 1713
  treatment and management 1639–40, 1875
  and tuberous sclerosis 1075, 1635
Autobiographical Memory Interview 89
autoerotic asphyxia 1703
autogynephiles 844
automatic behaviour in sleep-wake disorders 926, 928, 940, 945
  legal issues 948–9
automatic obedience 58
automatic thoughts *see* negative automatic thoughts
Automatic Thoughts Questionnaire 1165
automatism
  and epilepsy 403, 1077
  'insane' 405, 1901
  'sane' 405
  violent 1930
autonomic failure with syncope and orthostatic hypotension 361
autonomy, legal aspects 1895–900
autoprosopagnosia in Alzheimer's disease 334
autoscopy 56
autosomal dominant disorders 212, 1831
autosomal recessive disorders 212, 1831
Avena sativa 1248
avoidance 1287–8
  in chronic fatigue syndrome 1039
  following an accident 1107
  and hypothalamic–pituitary–adrenal axis 658
  in obsessive–compulsive disorder 768
  and pain-related fears 1033
  in panic disorder 751
  and phobias 745
avoidant personality disorder **872–3**
  aetiology 872
  classification *856*, 872, *872*
  clinical features 872
  course 872
  differential diagnosis 862, 863, 865, 873
  in elderly people 1562, *1562*
  epidemiology 872, *882*, 883
  and social anxiety disorder 740, 897
  terminology 856
  treatment 873, 897, 898
AVON Mental Health Measure 1434
awareness of activity, disorder of 56
awareness of singleness, disorder of 56
ayahuasca 488, 501
azapirones 735
azoospermia 1114
azotaemia 1087

Babinski reflex 158
Baby X experiments 1719
BAC (blood alcohol concentration) 442, 448
bah-tsche 983
Bali, attitudes to psychiatric disorder 7
Balint, Michael 308–9, 313
Banisteriopsis (ayahuasca) 488, 501
barbiturates 1178
  addictiveness *431*
  duration of action 1178
  history of 1178
  see also specific drugs
basal ganglia 154–5, *154*
  in alcohol use disorders *183*
  and memory 254
  in obsessive–compulsive disorder 1684
  in schizophrenia *178*
  in tic disorders 1684
basic assumption theory 1353, 1356
'battered child syndrome' 1734–5
Bayley Developmental Scale 1821
BDD *see* body dysmorphic disorder
BDI (Beck Depression Inventory) 719, 1163–4, 1306, 1486, 1675
BDNF (brain-derived neurotrophic factor) *160*, 171, 225, 652, 966, 1199, 1201, 1674, 1684
BDQ (Brief Disability Questionnaire) 284
'BDSM' sexual activities 832–3
BDT (brief dynamic therapy) 720
'Beating the Blues' 1485
Bech-Rafaelsen Mania Scale 1164
Beck, A.T. 1304
Beck Anxiety Inventory 1164
Beck Depression Inventory 719, 1163–4, 1306, 1486, 1675
Beck Self-Concept Test 1164
Bedford College Life Events and Difficulties Schedule 1065
Beers, Clifford 22
behaviour
  assessment instruments 69–70
  and the unconscious 313
behaviour modification
  in attention-deficit hyperactivity disorder 1649
  in autism and other pervasive developmental disorders 1640
  in children and adolescents with psychiatric/behaviour disorder and intellectual disability 1852
behaviour therapy
  in agitation and challenging behaviour in dementia 413–14
  attention-deficit hyperactivity disorder 1648
  in children and adolescents with intellectual disability and psychiatric/behavioural disorder 1852
  depression 15
  history of 23
  nicotine dependence 512
  obsessive–compulsive disorder 770
  panic disorder 758
  with sex offenders 1963
  trichotillomania 915
  see also cognitive-behaviour therapy; exposure
behavioural activation in depression in elderly people 1555
behavioural and psychological symptoms in dementia 412–17, *413*, *414*
Behavioural Assessment of the Dysexecutive Syndrome 93
behavioural experiments in anxiety disorders *1294*, 1295
behavioural factors influencing health 1135–7
behavioural inhibition 1667
  and generalized anxiety disorder 733, *733*
  and panic disorder 754, 762
Behavioural Pathology in Alzheimer's Disease 413
behavioural phenotypes 1592, 1838, 1850, *1851*, 1858
  foetal alcohol syndrome 1614–15
  neurogenetic syndromes 1613–14
behavioural programmes in intellectual disability 1874
behaviourally-induced insufficient sleep syndrome 939
behaviourism 133–4
  and personality 849
Benedict, Ruth 276
benefit-finding 1066
benefits,measurement of 1475
benzhexol 1532
benzodiazepine receptor agonists (BzRAs) 934
  in insomnia 935
  partial 1181–2
benzodiazepine receptors 1171, 1179
  in generalized anxiety disorder 733, *734*
benzodiazepines
  in acute and transient psychotic disorders 607
  addictiveness *431*
  adverse effects 934, 939, 1180, 1183
  in alcohol withdrawal 449, *449*, 1542
  antiepileptic properties 1080, 1231
  as anxiolytics 1178, 1179–80
  in bipolar disorder 677
  in breastfeeding 1121, 1180
  in cancer 1101–2, *1102*, *1104*
  cross-tolerance 491
  in delirium 331, 1533
  in dementia 415
  development 1178
  effects on memory 409, 1179
  in generalized anxiety disorder 735
  in Huntington's disease 374
  as hypnotics 1179, 1182–3
  indications 1179–80
  in insomnia 934
  long-term use 1179
  in management of antipsychotic adverse effects 1226
  management of withdrawal 1181, *1181*
  misuse/dependence **490–3**, 1182
    with alcohol dependence 492
    assessment 492
    by injection 491

cross-dependence 491
dependence at therapeutic doses 491, 1180–1, 1183
and drug formulation 430
elderly people 1543
epidemiology 490–1
management 491–2
with opiate abuse 492–3
patterns of use 490–1
potential for 491
overdose 1180
in panic disorder 756–7, *756*
pharmacodynamics 1171
pharmacokinetics *1172*, 1178–9
pharmacology 1179
in postoperative delirium 1099
in post-traumatic stress disorder 710
in pregnancy 762, 1117, 1180
preoperative 1097
prescriptions 492
in schizophrenia 591–2
in social anxiety disorder 743, 744
in specific phobia 746
in status epilepticus 1867
in terminal illness 1070
tolerance to 1179, 1180–1
benztropine 1225
bereavement **724–8**
after infant loss 725, 1120
assessment 726–7
in childhood and adolescence 235, **1758–60**
and depression 725
factors affecting course and outcome 725–6
in intellectual disability 1881
management 726–7
neurobiology 725
phenomenology of 'normal grief' 725
physical and mental health consequences 726
violent traumatic 1985
see also grief
Bergmann glia 158
beri-beri in anorexia nervosa 785
β-adrenergic stimulants *730*
β-amyloid protein
in Alzheimer's disease 338
in dementia with Lewy bodies 362
in mild cognitive impairment 1537
β-arrestins 175
β-blockers
adverse effects 827
in anxiety disorders 1182
in children and adolescents with psychiatric/behaviour disorder and intellectual disability 1852
in intellectual disability 1876
in management of antipsychotic adverse effects 1226
in social anxiety disorder 743
in specific phobia 746
β-crystalin 362
β-endorphin 170, *171*
β-secretase 338
Better Services for the Mentally Ill 24
biastophilia *833*
bifeprunox 1209
bilateral frontal lobotomy 1267
Binet–Simon scale 22
binge eating disorder 800, *801*, 1299
Binswanger's disease 377
bioavailability 1170
biofeedback in persistent somatoform pain disorder 1034
biomarkers in Alzheimer's disease 341
Bion, Wilfred 308, 1353, 1355
biopsychosocial model 64, 207, *208*, *433*, 990, *991*
biperiden 1225
bipolar disorder
age of onset 665
anticipation in 652
biphasic episodes 665
childhood and adolescence
aetiology 1674
assessment and monitoring 1675
course 1673–4
diagnostic criteria 1671, *1672*
differential diagnosis 1645, 1657, 1671–3
environmental risk factors 1675
epidemiology 1673–4
neurocognitive factors 1675
treatment and prevention 1676–7
classification 639–40, 643, *643*
comorbidity 645, 646
course 665–6
and cyclothymia/cyclothymic disorder 688
definition of bipolar 638
diagnosis 645–6
differential diagnosis 866, 868, 871
duration of episodes 665
elderly people 1556–7
epidemiology 645–7, 650–1
genetics **650–8**
global disease burden 645
history of concept 631
hyperthymic 638
and intellectual disability 1827, 1854–5
late-onset 665
mixed states 636, 638
mortality associated 666
outcome 666
overlap with other disorders 645
overlap with schizophrenia for susceptibility 652
patient state fluctuations within 632–3, *632*, *633*
pharmacogenetics 653
in pregnancy 677
prevalence 646
prisoners *1934*
psychosocial factors 653
psychotic 665
rapid cycling 636, 668, 677
recurrence 665–6
risk factors 646, 1675
social functioning in 653
subtypes 631, 638, 643, 665
and suicide 1704
and surgery 1098
treatment
acute 671
continuation 677
and course 667
electroconvulsive therapy 1253–4
interpersonal and social rhythm therapy 1323
long-term 678
maintenance 671–2, 677
management of 677–8
neurosurgery 1268
psychotherapy 673
treatment gap *13*
and use of mental health services 646
bipolar spectrum 680
birth certificate, change of sex on 845
birth season and schizophrenia 547, 556
birth weight
and HPA function 659
and schizophrenia 548
blackouts, alcoholic 404, 443
Bleuler, Eugen 522, 531, 603, 631, 1546–7
blindness, hysterical 1017
blood alcohol concentration 442, 448
blood transfusion and Creutzfeldt–Jakob disease transmission 355, 356, 358
BMI *see* body mass index
BMP (bone morphogenetic protein) 156
bodily distress disorder 1000, *1000*, 1003
epidemiology 1003, 1004
bodily preoccupation
in body dysmorphic disorder 1043–4
in hypochondriasis 1022
body, dislike of 57
body awareness disorders 57
body dysmorphic disorder (BDD) 57, **1043–9**
association with aggression and violence 1044
childhood and adolescence 1045
classification 1022, 1045
clinical features 1043–5
comorbidity 1044–5
course 1046
cross-cultural aspects 1045
delusional 618, 1044, 1045
diagnosis 1045–6, *1045*
epidemiology 1046
and gender 1045
and hypochondriasis 1045
non-delusional 1045
and obsessive–compulsive disorder 1044, 1045
pathogenesis 1046
and pregnancy 1116
prevalence 997–8, *998*
prevention 1048
prognosis 1046
puerperal 1120
and requests for cosmetic treatment 1046, 1096
and suicidality 1044
treatment and management 1046–8
body image
distortion 57
disturbance 783
and eating disorder 57
organic changes in 57
body mass index (BMI) 784
in anorexia nervosa 784, 794
and depression 1674
body weight
in anorexia nervosa 782, 784
in bulimia nervosa 803, 804
Bolam test 1902, 1905
bone morphogenetic protein 156
bonobo 812
Borago officinalis (borage) 1248
borderline personality disorder **866–8**
aetiology 867
and bulimia nervosa 803, 804
childhood and adolescence 1673
classification *856*, 867, *867*

borderline personality disorder (*cont.*)
clinical features 867–8
comorbidity 868, 884, 902
course and outcome 868, 892
and deception 1049
diagnosis 867–8
differential diagnosis 682, 865, 866, 868, 871, 874
elderly people *1562*, 1563
epidemiology 867, *882*, 883
following head injury 391
treatment 318–19, 868, 894–7, 898, 902, 903, 904, 905–6, *905*, 1364–5
borderline personality organization 867
boredom and substance use disorders 427
Borrelia burgdorferi 1094–5
Boston Diagnostic Aphasia Examination 89
Boston Naming Test 89
Botswana, life expectancy 1507
bouffée délirante 603, 604, 606
with symptoms of schizophrenia 605
boundaries of self, awareness of 56
boundary violation 1338
bovine spongiform encephalopathy 351, 352, 355
Bowlby, John 242, 309–10, 1725
boxing 395
BPSDs (behavioural and psychological symptoms in dementia) 412–17, *413*, *414*
Brachman-de Lange syndrome *see* de Lange syndrome
brachycephaly 1839
bradyphasia 53
bradyphrenia in brain tumour 1075
brain
activation during sexual arousal 819
alcohol-related damage 182–3, **399–402**, 444, 1541
anatomy **144–56**
in anorexia nervosa 781
anoxia 1091
applications of PET 187–8
in autism 1636
congenital anomalies 538
in delusional disorder 614
in delusional misidentification syndrome 623–4
development 156–7, *157*
effects of substance use disorders 429–30, *429*
fear and anxiety circuit 754–5
glucose metabolism 187–8
hemispheric shape and formation of gyri 159
histogenesis 158–9
hypoperfusion in depression 660
injury *see* head injury
ischaemia 387
magnetization 191
mapping 187–8
and mind **133–6**
and psychodynamic psychiatry 315–16
neural induction 156
neuronal death 387
neuronal networks 201–5
in obsessive–compulsive disorder 768
oedema 387, 1084–5
pathology *see* neuropathology
regional blood flow 187–8
in chronic fatigue syndrome 1039
in frontotemporal dementia 347, Plate 12
and neural activity 197
regions involved in attention *246*
reward circuit 430
in schizophrenia 562–4, *563*
tumours 407, 942, 1075, 1929
in vascular dementia 376
visual areas *147*, 152
see also specific areas
brain-derived neurotrophic factor *160*, 171, 225, 652, 966, 1199, 1201, 1674, 1684
brain fag syndrome 982–3
brain slices 202–3
brainstem 150–1
in alcohol use disorders *183*
histogenesis 158
in mood disorders *182*
in schizophrenia *178*
Brazil, attitudes to psychiatric disorder 6
breastfeeding 1120
and opioid use 480
pharmacotherapy 1123
antidepressants 675
benzodiazepines 1121, 1170
dosage regimens 1169–70
breathing retraining in panic disorder 761
breeder effect 549
bremelanotide in sexual dysfunction 828
Brief Cognitive Rating Scale 1240
Brief Disability Questionnaire 284
brief dynamic therapy 720
brief focal psychotherapy 1327, 1330–1, *1331*
Brief Psychiatric Rating Scale 70, 524, 1164
brief psychodynamic psychotherapy *see* psychodynamic psychotherapy, brief (short-term)
brief psychotic disorder 606, 695
brief reactive psychosis 870
brief solution-focused therapy 1276
brief supportive therapy 720
Brief Symptom Inventory 1164
bright light therapy in dementia *414*
Briquet's syndrome 999
British Crime Survey 1984
Brixton Test *90*
broad-focus short-term dynamic psychotherapy 1333
Broca's area 144, 146, 153, *153*
Broca's dysphasia 1527
brofaromine
adverse effects *1191*
dosage *1196*
pharmacodynamics *1187*, 1188
pharmacokinetics *1189*
in social anxiety disorder 743
bromides 1178
4-bromo-2,5-dimethoxyphenethylamine 501
bronchodilators *730*, 1101
brucellosis 1095
BSE (bovine spongiform encephalopathy) 351, 352, 355
BST (brief supportive therapy) 720
Building Bridges project 1411
bulbo-urethral gland 817
bulimia nervosa **800–11**
aetiology 805–7
anxiety in 803
assessment 807
attitudes to shape and weight 803
binge eating in 801–2
and child sexual abuse 780
childhood and adolescence 1784
classification and diagnosis 800–1, *801*
clinical features 801–4
course and outcome 809
depression in 803, 804
development 805
and diabetes mellitus 804
dieting in 801–2
epidemiology 804–5, *805*
general psychopathology 803 4
genetics 806
impulse control problems in 803
maintaining factors 807, 1299
neurobiology 806–7
and obesity 804
origins of the concept 800
overlap with anorexia nervosa 800, *801*
perfectionism in 804, 806
and personality disorder 803, 884
physical features 804
and pregnancy 1118
purging/non-purging 802–3
relationship with other eating disorders 804
risk factors 805–6, *806*
self-esteem in 804, 806
and substance use disorders 804, 806
treatment and management 807–9, 1193–4, 1298–303, 1323–4, 1784
weight control methods 802–3
buprenorphine 475, **1244**
detoxification 476–7
maintenance treatment 476, 479
metabolism 473
in pregnancy 1118
prescription 479
in substance use disorders 429–30
bupropion *670*, 671
adverse effects 1190–1, *1191*
in body dysmorphic disorder 1047
in cancer *1103*
in childhood and adolescence 1676
dosage 1195, *1196*
in panic disorder 757
pharmacodynamics *1187*, 1188
pharmacokinetics 1189, *1189*
in smoking cessation 512
burglary, victims of 1986
burns *see* accidents
Burton, Richard, *Anatomy of Melancholy* 629–30, *630*
buspirone 1178, 1181, 1212
in body dysmorphic disorder 1047
in children and adolescents with psychiatric/behaviour disorder and intellectual disability 1852
in generalized anxiety disorder 735, 737
in panic disorder 757
pharmacodynamics 1172
in social anxiety disorder 743
Butler Report 2015
butobarbitone 1178
butyrophenones in pregnancy 1118
BzRAs *see* benzodiazepine receptor agonists
2C-B 501
2C-T2 501

CACE estimation 142
caffeine, addictiveness *431*
CAGE 1519, 1542
Cajal–Retzius cells *148*, 158
calcitonin gene-related peptide 206

calcium carbimide 453
calcium-channel blockers, L-type 1200–1, 1201, 1203, *1203*
see also nimodipine
California Verbal Learning Test 253, 264
calorie restriction and modification of ageing 1509
CAM (Confusion Assessment Method) 328, 1531
Camberwell Assessment of Need 94, 1434
Camberwell Family Interview 268
Cambridge Mental Disorders of the Elderly Examination 336
Cambridge Neuropsychological Test Automated Battery 255, 263
Cambridge–Somerville Study 1910
Cambridge Study in Delinquent Development 1908, 1909, 1910, 1911, 1912, 1912–13
CAMDEX 336
CAMHS *see* mental health services, child and adolescent
cAMP (cyclic adenosine monophosphate) 175
Camphill communities 1392
CAN (Camberwell Assessment of Need) 94, 1434
Canada, attitudes to psychiatric disorder 6
cancer **1100–5**
and alcohol consumption 446
and anxiety 1101–2, *1101*
childhood and adolescence 1743
delirium in 1103–4, *1104*
fatigue in 209, *210*
and mood disorders 649, 1102, *1102*, *1103*
parental, effects on child development 1754–5
and suicide 1102–3
candidiasis, systemic 997
cannabinoids
addictiveness *431*
endogenous 429
receptors *173*, 1171
cannabis **507–10**, 515
acute psychological effects 507
amotivational syndrome associated 508
behavioural effects in adolescence 508
chronic psychological effects 507
cognitive effects 92, 507–8
dependence 507
and flashbacks 508
patterns of use 507
in pregnancy 1117
psychosis 507, 538
and schizophrenia 507, 546
cannibalism 351, 354
CANTAB (Cambridge Neuropsychological Test Automated Battery) 255, 263
CANTAB Paired Associate Learning test 264, 266
CANTOUs 1583
capacity
and cognitive assessment 90–1
and consent to surgery 1096–7
Council of Europe Principles Concerning the Legal Protection of Incapable Adults 1896
elderly people 1577
following head injury 397
independent advocate 1898
and juvenile delinquency 1954–5
lack of 1898–9
legal aspects 1895–900
tests of 1897
Capgras syndrome 335, 392, 610, 623
CAPS (Clinician Administered PTSD Scale) 703
Caracas Declaration 1427
carbamazepine 1198, 1200, **1233–5**
adverse effects *1200*, 1204, 1233–4, 1867–8
in bipolar disorder 671, 672
in childhood and adolescence 1677
choice of 1866
in dementia 415
dosage and administration *1233*, 1234–5
drug interactions 1175, 1205–6, 1232, 1234, *1234*, 1866
indications and contraindications 1234
mechanism of action *1200*
monitoring therapy 1176
overdose 1234
in personality disorders *905*
pharmacokinetics 1203, 1233, *1867*
pharmacology 1201, *1202*, *1203*, 1233
in pregnancy 1118, 1234
response correlates *1199*
in schizophrenia 591
structure *1232*
therapeutic profile *1199*
withdrawal 1206–7, 1234
carbon monoxide poisoning 406–7, 973
carcinoid tumours 1101
card-sorting games 1778
'cardiac invalidism'/'cardiac neurosis' 1025, 1138, 1559
cardiac myopathy in alcohol use disorders 446
Cardinal Needs Schedule 1434
cardiovascular disease 1081–2
in alcohol use disorders 446
and sleep-wake disorders *932*
cardiovascular system, in chronic fatigue syndrome 1038
care management, in mental health social work 1410–11
care programme approach (CPA)
in community mental health services 1455, *1456*, *1457*
to manage risk of homicide 1939
in services for people with intellectual disability 1888
caregiver-mediated interventions **1787–93**
adolescents 1790
background 1787
mediators of efficacy 1790–1
pre-natal and early childhood 1787–8
preschool years 1788–9
school-aged children 1789–90
carers
in Alzheimer's disease 339
burdens on 1401
in dementia 417–18
effects of personality change following head injury 391
of elderly people with intellectual disability 1880–1
impact of caring on 1465
of people with alcohol use disorders 452–3, 465
role in treatment of intellectual disability 1873
Carers and Users Experience of Services 1434
cargo-cult syndrome 982
CARITAS principles 1580
Cartesian dualism 133, 989
CAS (childhood apraxia of speech) 1712
case ascertainment 283
case-control studies 282
case-finding 541
case management 584, 1402, 1455
castration
chemical 838
and libido 815–16
surgical 838
castration anxiety 294
CAT *see* cognitive analytical therapy
CAT (community alcohol team) model 461
catalepsy 58, *58*
cataplexy
misdiagnosis 928
with narcolepsy 940–1
catastrophizing 1137–8
catatonia 58
elderly people 1531
excited 529
malignant 529, 1254
retarded 529
in schizophrenia 529
treatment 1254
catecholamines
in cocaine use 485
and depression 1185, *1185*
effects on memory 409
in methamphetamine use 497
in post-traumatic stress disorder 706
category fallacy 276
Catherine of Siena, St 777
caudate nucleus 154, 159, 1684
CBD *see* corticobasal degeneration
CBGT (cognitive-behavioural group therapy) 742, 744
CBT *see* cognitive-behaviour therapy
CD *see* conversion disorder
CDCS *see* cri-du-chat syndrome
CDR (Clinical Dementia Rating) scale 1535
CDRPs (Crime and Disorder Reduction Partnerships) 515
CDRS-R (Children's Depression Rating Scale, Revised) 1675
CEA *see* cost-effectiveness analysis
CEACs (cost-effectiveness acceptability curves) 1475, *1475*
Center for Epidemiologic Studies Depression Scale 284, 1675
central nervous system
malformations leading to intellectual disability 1832
neural induction 156
organogenesis 156–7, *157*
central pontine myelinolysis 445
central sleep apnoea 1083
central state materialism 134
central sulcus 144–5
centromeres 223
cephalic flexure 156
CER *see* control event rate; cost-effectiveness ratio
CERAD (Consortium to Establish a Registry for AD) 336
cerebellum 155
in alcohol use disorders *183*
development 157, *157*
effects of alcohol use disorders 445
histogenesis 158

cerebellum (*cont.*)
  and memory 254
  in mood disorders *182*
  in schizophrenia *178*
cerebral contusions 387, *388*, 389
cerebral cortex
  association pathways for hearing *147*, 152
  association pathways for somatic sensation *146*, 152
  association pathways for vision *147*, 152
  commissural connections 151
  effects of alcohol use disorders 444
  general connectivity pattern 149–50, *149*
  histogenesis 158–9, *159*
  olfactory pathways to *147*, 152
  speech areas 153, *153*
  structure and organization 144–8, *145*, *146*, *147*
  subcortical afferents to 150–3, *153*, Plate 2
  subcortical efferent pathways 154–6, *154*
cerebral palsy 1740
cerebrasthenia 1060
cerebrospinal fluid 157
  in anorexia nervosa 782
  in frontotemporal dementias 347
  in HIV-associated dementia 385
  in mild cognitive impairment 1538
cerebrovascular disease
  and amnesia 407
  and vascular dementia 366, 378, *378*
cervical flexure 156
CES-D (Center for Epidemiologic Studies Depression Scale) 284, 1675
CFS *see* chronic fatigue syndrome
CGA (common geriatric assessment) 1581
CGRP (calcitonin gene-related peptide) 206
challenging behaviour in dementia 413–15
Change for Children Programme 1946
character 79
  analysis 299–300
  assessment 80–1, *80*, 82–3
  definition 847
  development *84*
  dimensions 80–1, *80*, 316
  and personality 316–17
  psychoanalytic approaches 295–6
Charcot, Jean-Martin 20–1
Charles Bonnet syndrome 1531
'chasing the dragon' 473
chemokines *168*, 171
chemotherapy, anticipatory disorders 1101
chien 1420
child abuse and neglect **1731–9**
  and adoption outcome 1750
  characteristics of abused child 1734, 1736
  characteristics of abusers 1734–5, 1736, 1736–7
  and chronic pain 1033
  and conduct disorder 1660
  emergency presentation 1810
  epidemiology 1732
  and factitious disorder 1051
  false and recovered memories 713–15
  and filicide 1125
  and hypochondriasis 1025
  induced factitious disorder 1054, 1697, 1737, 1923–4
  and mental health social work 1409
  and mood disorders 1675
  neglect 1735–6
  and offending 1910
  physical abuse 1734–5
  prevention 1737–8, 1788
  psychodynamic theories 316
  psychological maltreatment (emotional abuse) 1736–7
  role in aetiology of psychiatric disorder 286
  treatment and management 1738
child and adolescent mental health services *see* mental health services, child and adolescent
Child Behaviour Checklist 1718
child-care 1727
child guidance movement 1381
child molesting (paedophilia) 832, *833*, *836*, 1960–1, 1962
child pornography 1961
child protection
  and psychiatric reports 75
  role of school 1814
Child PTSD Symptom scale 1730
child sexual abuse
  aetiological factors 1733
  characteristics of abused child 1733
  characteristics of abusers 1733
  clinical features 1732
  course and prognosis 1733, *1734*
  definition 1732
  diagnosis 1732–3
  and eating disorders 780
  false accusations 834
  false and recovered memories 713–14, 834
  prevalence 1960
  and sexual dysfunction 825
  within-family 1733
childbirth 1118–20
  post-traumatic stress disorder following 1121
  querulant reactions to 1121
childhood and adolescence
  acute behavioural disturbance 1810
  acute stress disorder 1729
  adjustment disorders 721–3
    after diagnosis of physical illness 1741, 1742
    diagnostic criteria 1669–71, *1671*
  adolescents 1945
    interviewing 1601
  adverse experiences 271–2, 1724
    and borderline personality disorder 867
    and mood disorders 648, 658–9
    and panic disorder 754, 762
  aggression, severe maladaptive 1798
  alcohol use disorders 456, 464
  antisocial behaviour 1654, **1945–59**
  anxiety
    assessment 1665
    with intellectual disability 1851–2
    with physical illness 1742–3
  anxiety disorders **1664–9**
    assessment 1665
    clinical course 1666
    clinical presentation 1665–6
    comorbidity 1666, 1673
    differential diagnosis 1671
    epidemiology 1665–6
    pathophysiology 1666–8, *1667*
    treatment 1668, 1779–80
  art therapy 1414
  assessment 90, **1600–6**
    content of the clinical interview 1600–1, *1602*
    developmentally sensitive techniques 1601, 1604–5
    laboratory tests 1605–6, *1605*
    mood disorders 1675
    need for multiple informants 1600
    structure of the clinical interview 1601, 1603–4, *1603*
  'at risk' children 1803
  behavioural effects of cannabis in adolescence 508
  bereavement 235, **1758–60**
  bipolar disorder
    aetiology 1674
    assessment and monitoring 1675
    course 1673–4
    diagnostic criteria 1671, *1672*
    differential diagnosis 1645, 1657
    environmental risk factors 1675
    epidemiology 1673–4
    neurocognitive factors 1675
    treatment and prevention 1676–7
  body dysmorphic disorder 1045
  borderline personality disorder 1673
  cancer 1743
  caregiver-mediated interventions **1787–93**
  cerebral palsy 1740
  chronic fatigue syndrome 1745–6, 1784
  chronic renal failure 1741, 1743
  classification 104, **1589–94**
  cognitive assessment 90
  cognitive-behaviour therapy 1767, **1777–86**
    anxiety disorders 1668, 1779–80
    attention-deficit hyperactivity disorder 1782–3
    chronic fatigue syndrome 1784
    conduct disorder 1781–2
    depression 1675–6, 1780–1
    eating disorders 1784
    failure to engage/respond 1779
    following attempted suicide 1707
    inclusion of cognitive component 1778–9
    non-organic pain 1784
    obsessive–compulsive disorder 1686–7, *1686*, 1783–4
    post-traumatic stress disorder 1784
    psychiatric/behaviour disorder with intellectual disability 1852
    substance abuse 1784
    technique and management 1778
    working with parents 1778–9
  cognitive therapy 1610, 1767, 1783
  comorbidity in 1591, 1600
  confusional state 1742
  conversion disorder 1745
  counselling **1764–9**
    approaches to 1766–8
    measures of effectiveness and outcome 1769
    practical issues 1768
    in psychiatric/behaviour disorder and intellectual disability 1852
    supportive 1767
    training and supervision 1768–9
    treatment setting and process 1766
  cross-gender behaviour 1718–19
  cyclothymic disorder 1671, *1672*
  cystic fibrosis 1743
  definitions and terminology 1764–5
  deliberate self-harm 972, 1601, 1703

depression
  acute management 1677
  aetiology 1674
  assessment and monitoring 1675, 1780–1
  course 1673
  diagnostic criteria 1669, *1670*
  differential diagnosis 1657, 1671–3
  double 1673
  environmental risk factors 1675
  epidemiology 1673–4
  minor 1669
  neurocognitive factors 1674–5
  neuroendocrine studies 1675
  sequelae 1674
  treatment and prevention 674–5, 1322, 1668, 1675–6, 1780–1, 1794–5, 1796
developmental disorders 1591, *1591*
  see also specific developmental disorders
developmental history 1600–1, 1822
diabetes mellitus 1741
disruptive (externalizing) disorders 1591, *1591*, 1654
dysthymia/dysthymic disorder 683, 1669, *1670*, 1673
eating disorder
  atypical 787
  differential diagnosis 1672
  treatment 1784
  see also specific eating disorders
effects of parental mental/physical illness on development **1752–8**
electroconvulsive therapy 1256
emergencies in **1807–11**
emotional (internalizing) disorders 1591, *1591*, 1654
environmental factors affecting mental health **1724–8**
  child care 1727
  family 1725–7
  peers 1727
  schooling 1727
  social 1727–8
epidemiology of psychiatric disorders **1594–9**
epilepsy
  aetiology 1619–20
  classification 1619
  clinical features 1618–19
  course and prognosis 1618–19, 1620
  diagnosis 1619
  differential diagnosis 1619
  epidemiology 1619
  with intellectual disability *1861*, *1863*, 1864
  management 1620
  prevention 1620
  psychiatric disorder associated 1740
  salient non-epileptic episodes *1861*
estimating the burden of psychiatric disorders 1595–6
factitious disorder in 1050
factors related to development of chronic pain 1033
factors related to development of hypochondriasis 1025
gender identity disorder **1718–23**
  aetiology 1719–20
  assessment 1721
  clinical features 1718–19
  epidemiology 1718
  longitudinal studies 1720–1
  and mental disorder 1721
  treatment 1721–2
group therapy 1768
head injury 394–5, 1616–18
headache 1745
health promotion in 1610
Huntington's disease in 372–3
hypersexuality 1671
intellectual disability
  and antisocial behaviour 1946
  and anxiety 1851–2
  and bereavement 1759
  and depression 1852
  effects on family 1883–4
  prevalence 1878
  psychiatric and behaviour disorders associated **1849–53**, 1879
  special needs of adolescents 1878–80
  transition to adulthood 1878–9
interests/hobbies/talents 1601
juvenile delinquency *see* juvenile delinquency
and life events 1601
looked after children **1799–802**
mania 1670–1, 1675, 1677
media exposure 1601
medical history 1601
mental health services *see* mental health services, child and adolescent (CAMHS)
mental status examination 1601, *1602*
mood disorders **1669–80**
  aetiology 1674
  clinical picture 1669–71, *1670*, *1672*
  comorbidity 1673
  course 1673–4
  differential diagnosis 1657, 1671–3
  epidemiology 1673–4
  with intellectual disability 1852
  neurocognitive factors 1675
  sequelae 1674
  treatment and prevention 1675–7
natural emotional healing 1765–6
neuropsychiatric disorders **1612–22**
neuropsychological assessment 1590–1, 1605
obsessive–compulsive disorder 1613, **1680–93**
  aetiology 1683–5
  age of onset 1681
  classification 1682
  clinical features 1680–1
  comorbidity 1681–2
  course and prognosis 1685
  diagnosis 1682–3
  differential diagnosis 1682–3
  epidemiology 1683
  and gender 1681
  with intellectual disability 1852
  prevention 1690
  refractory 1688
  treatment 1685–90, *1686*, *1687*, 1783–4
opioid dependence 480
pain in 1744–5
persistent somatoform pain disorder 1745
pharmacotherapy **1793–9**
  antidepressants 674–5, 1668, 1676, 1794–5, 1796
  antipsychotics 1677, 1796–8, 1852
  atomoxetine 1795–6
  developmental issues 1794
  dosage regimens 1169
  mood stabilizers 1798, 1852
  as part of multimodal treatment 1793–4
  with psychiatric/behaviour disorder and/or intellectual disability 1798, 1852
  rapid tranquillization 1798
  stimulants 1795
  symptom-based approach 1794
physical illness
  effects of psychiatric disorder on course and outcome 1744
  psychiatric disorder associated 1740–3
post-traumatic stress disorder 237–8, **1728–31**, 1741, 1744, 1759, 1784, 1851–2
prevention in 1606, 1609–11
psychodynamic psychotherapy **1769–77**
  background 1770
  classical technique 1770–1
  definition 1764
  efficacy 1773–4
  indications and contraindications 1772
  limitations 1774
  managing treatment 1772–3
  procedure selection 1772
  psychodynamic technique 1771–2
psychopathic personality 1950
psychoses
  differential diagnosis 1673
  and juvenile delinquency 1950
psychotherapy **1764–9**, **1769–77**
  approaches to 1766–8
  confidentiality 1768
  consent for 1765
  and culture 1768
  differences from adult psychotherapy 1765, *1765*
  ending 1768
  failure to attend 1768
  focus on past vs. focus on present 1767
  individual vs. group therapy 1768
  involvement of parents and school 1768
  limit-setting vs. free expression 1767
  measures of effectiveness and outcome 1769
  record-keeping 1768
  training and supervision 1768–9
  treatment setting 1766
rapid tranquillization 1798
reaction to death of a parent 1758–60
relationship between physical and mental health **1739–47**
residential care **1799–802**
role of child psychiatrist in schools and colleges **1811–16**
schizophrenia 1613
  differential diagnosis 1673
  risk factors for development 556–7
sleep disorders **1693–702**
  assessment 1696–7, *1696*
  developmental effects 1695
  effects on parenting and the family 1694–5
  excessive daytime sleepiness 1699–701, *1700*
  manifestations 1695
  misinterpretation 1695
  parasomnias 1701–2
  parental influences 1694
  patterns of occurrence 1695
  risk factors 1697–8
  sleeplessness 1698–9
  treatment and prognosis 1695–6
sleep physiology 1693–4

childhood and adolescence (*cont.*)
social anxiety disorder 740, 1664, 1666
social functioning 1593
somatization and somatization disorder 1744, *1744*
special educational needs 1815
specific phobia 1664, 1665, 1666, 1741, 1742
speech and language disorder **1710–17**
substance use disorders 1600, 1604
comorbidity 1673
differential diagnosis 1672
treatment 1784
suicide and attempted suicide 1674, **1702–10**
aetiology 1705–6, *1705*, *1706*
assessment 1703–4
associated diagnoses 1704
clinical features 1703
course and prognosis 1706
epidemiology 1704–5
prevention 1708–9
treatment 1706–8
temperament 235, 238, *238*, 1601, 1665, 1667
in intellectual disability 1850
terminal illness 1743–4
therapeutic communities 1397
tic disorders 1073, **1680–93**
aetiology 1683–5
age of onset 1681
classification 1682
clinical features 1681
comorbidity 1681–2
course and prognosis 1685
diagnosis 1682–3
differential diagnosis 1682–3
epidemiology 1683
and gender 1681
prevention 1690
treatment 1685–90
Tourette syndrome 1613, 1680–93
trauma in 1601, 1697, **1728–31**, 1744, 1762
victims of criminal activity 1986–7
wish for behavioural change in 1600
witnesses, children as **1761–3**
childhood apraxia of speech 1712
childhood disintegrative disorder **1637**
Children Act 1989 1732
Children's Depression Inventory 1675, 1780
Children's Depression Rating Scale, Revised 1675
Children's Global Assessment scale 1593
Children's Memory Scale 89, *89*
Children's PTSD Inventory 1730
Children's Revised Impact of Events scale 1730
Children's Yale-Brown Obsessive-Compulsive Scale 1681
China
attitudes to psychiatric disorder 6
neurasthenia as diagnostic entity 1061, 1062
and Pavlovian theory 1061
psychiatric nurses in 1407
Chinese Classification of Mental Disorders 1062
Chinese traditional medicine 1249
chloral 1178
chloramphenicol 1091
chlordiazepoxide 1178
in alcohol withdrawal 449, *449*
pharmacokinetics *1172*
chlormethiazole *see* clomethiazole
chlorpromazine 1209, *1209*, 1262
administration 1213–14, *1214*
adverse effects *1212*, 1222
in anxiety disorders 1182
in cancer *1104*
development 1208–9
pharmacodynamics *1211*
pharmacokinetics *1172*
cholecystokinins 171, *171*
in generalized anxiety disorder 734
in panic disorder 754
cholesterol and suicide 966
cholinergic anti-inflammatory pathway 206
cholinergic system
and alcohol-related brain damage 400
in Alzheimer's disease 338, 1240–1
anticholinergic action at 1225
antipsychotic actions on 1210, *1211*
and cortical function 150, 151
and delirium 330, 1532
in depression 660
effects of PCP on receptors 487
in head injury 388
and memory 253
and neurotrophic factors *160*
in schizophrenia 180
cholinesterase inhibitors
in Alzheimer's disease 1240–1, 1538
in dementia 415
in dementia with Lewy bodies 366–7
effects on memory 409
in mild cognitive impairment 1538
in vascular dementia 381
cholinomimetics in Alzheimer's disease 1241
chorea 371
chorea acanthocytosis 373
Christian religious healing 1420
chromatids 223
chromatin remodelling 225
chromosomes 218, 223
anomalies 1831
autosomal 218, 223
rearrangements 228–9, 1831
recombination 223, 226
sex *see* sex chromosomes
telomere loss 1508
chronic benign pain syndrome 1003
chronic cutaneous dysaesthesia 618
chronic fatigue syndrome (CFS) **1035–43**
aetiology 1038–40, *1040*
assessment 1040–1
attribution to organic disease 1039
case formulation 1041
childhood and adolescence 1745–6, 1784
classification 1003, 1036–8
clinical features 1036, *1036*
controversial aspects 990
coping strategies 1039
course 1040
diagnosis 1036–8, 1041
differential diagnosis *1041*
epidemics 1038
epidemiology 997, 1038
genetics 1038
international consensus definition *1037*
overlap with psychiatric syndromes 1037–8
pathophysiology 1038–9
and personality 1039
prevalence 1038
prevention 1042
prognosis 1040
psychopathology 1039–40
and sleep disorder 1697
and somatization 1039
and stigma 1039–40
treatment and management 1034, 1040–2, *1041*, 1784
chronic obstructive pulmonary disease *932*, 1082
chronic renal failure 1087
childhood and adolescence 1741, 1743
and sleep-wake disorders *932*
chronic stress reaction and post-traumatic stress disorder 706
CI (confidence interval) 126, 128
CIDI (Composite International Diagnostic Interview) 69, 70, 72, 284, 542, 1023, 1438
cimetidine 1532
CIND *see* cognitive impairment, non-dementia
cinnarizine 1240
circadian rhythms 1260
and bipolar disorder 647
disorders 1261
effects of ageing 1572
sleep–wake 925, 926
circle time 1814
circular causality 1371
circular questioning 1387
circular sulcus 145
circumstantiality 53
citalopram *670*
adverse effects *1191*
in body dysmorphic disorder 1046
in cancer *1102*, *1103*
in childhood and adolescence 1676
in dementia 415
in depression in elderly people 1554, *1554*
dosage *1196*
in obsessive–compulsive disorder *1687*
in panic disorder *756*
pharmacodynamics 1186, *1187*
pharmacokinetics 1188–9, *1189*
CIWA-Ar (Clinical Institute Withdrawal Assessment for Alcohol-Revised Version) *1542*
CJD *see* Creutzfeldt–Jakob disease
CJITS (Criminal Justice Integrated Teams) 515
CL psychiatry *see* consultation-liaison (CL) psychiatry
Clarke Sex History Questionnaire for Males 1962
classification **99–121**
in childhood and adolescence **1589–94**
conceptual issues 99–100
definition 99
development of systems 100–2
and diagnostic instruments 64
and epidemiology 1607
goals 99
history of 631
in primary care 1483–4
Classification of Violence Risk 1996, 1998
claustrophobia 52
claustrum 151
Claviceps purpurea 487
see also hydergine
cleft lip/palate 1711, 1712
Client Service Receipt Inventory 1474
clinical assessment *see* assessment
Clinical Dementia Rating scale 1535
Clinical Institute Withdrawal Assessment for Alcohol-Revised Version *1542*

clinical neuropsychology 262
clinical practice guidelines 123, 124
Clinician Administered PTSD Scale 703
Clinician Assessment of Fluctuation Scale 363
clinophilia 939
clitoris 812, 817–18, 822
clobazam 1080, *1172*
clomethiazole **1246–7**
  pharmacodynamics 1171
  pharmacokinetics 1170
clomipramine *670*
  adverse effects *1191*, 1687
  in body dysmorphic disorder 1046, 1047
  in childhood and adolescence 1676
  in depersonalization disorder 775
  dosage *1196*
  in intellectual disability 1875
  in obsessive–compulsive disorder 768–9, 769–70, 1193, 1687, *1687*
  in panic disorder 756, *756*
  pharmacodynamics *1173*, 1186, *1187*
  pharmacokinetics *1172*, *1189*
clonazepam 1080
  in cancer *1102*
  in obsessive–compulsive disorder 769
  in panic disorder *756*, 757
  pharmacokinetics *1867*
  potential for misuse 491
  in REM sleep behaviour disorder 947
  in social anxiety disorder 743
clonidine **1245**
  in attention-deficit hyperactivity disorder 1651
  in intellectual disability 1876
  in opioid detoxification 477
  in smoking cessation 512
  in tic disorders 1073, 1688
'closed-loop' tasks 254
clozapine 1209
  administration *1214*, 1215–16
  adverse effects *1212*, 1223–4
  in childhood and adolescence 1797
  in intellectual disability 1875
  pharmacodynamics 1172, *1211*, 1213
  pharmacokinetics *1172*, 1221
  in schizophrenia 580, 582, 592
'Club House' 1453
CMHCs (community mental health centres) 1454
CMHTs *see* community mental health teams
CNS (Cardinal Needs Schedule) 1434
cobalamin deficiency 1087–8
cocaine **482–6**
  addictiveness *431*, 483
  aetiology of use 484
  classification of disorders relating to 483, *484*
  cognitive effects 92
  complications associated 484–5
  course and prognosis of use 484–5
  diagnosis of use 483–4
  effects of 483, *483*
  epidemiology of use 484
  in pregnancy 1118, 1615–16
  prevention of misuse 485
  psychosis due to 485, 538
  routes of use and risk associated 430, 483
  treatment and management of use 485
  withdrawal 483, *483*
Cochrane Collaboration 123–4, 578
Cochrane Database of Systematic Reviews 1156–7
Cochrane Library 1156–7
codeine 430
  metabolism 473–4
  in opiate abuse 1244
coenaesthesia 50
coenestopathic states 1030
Coffin–Lowry syndrome 1839
  behavioural and psychiatric aspects 1842
  genetics 1842
  physical characteristics 1842
  prevalence 1842
COGA (Collaborative Study on the Genetics of Alcoholism) 435
cognitive analytical therapy (CAT) 903–4, 1278
  borderline personality disorder 895
cognitive assessment **85–94**
  in alcohol abuse and dependence 92
  attention 60, 88–9
  and capacity 90–1
  childhood and adolescence 90
    with intellectual disability 1850
  concentration 60, 88–9
  in dementia 92
  in depression 92
  in drug abuse 92–3
  ecological validity 92, *92*
  elderly people 1527
  in epilepsy 92
  estimating premorbid ability 90, *90*
  frontal and executive functions 89, *90*
  general ability 87, *88*
  generalizability theory 92
  intelligence 87, *88*
  language 89
  and malingering 91
  memory 89, *89*, 253, 254, 255–6, 264, 420–1, *420*
  in parkinsonism 92
  principles 85–7, *85*, *86*
  protocol 91, *91*
  in schizophrenia 93, 265, 531–4
  sources of tests and test data 89
  speed of processing 87–8, *88*
  understanding and choice of tests 89–90
  see also neuropsychological assessment
cognitive-behaviour therapy (CBT)
  acute stress reactions 697
  adjustment disorders 720, 1068
  anxiety disorders **1285–98**
    in childhood and adolescence 1668, 1779–80
  attempted suicide 970
  for auditory hallucinations 1314, 1317
  bipolar disorder 673
  body dysmorphic disorder 1047
  childhood and adolescence 1767, **1777–86**
    anxiety disorders 1668, 1779–80
    attention-deficit hyperactivity disorder 1782–3
    chronic fatigue syndrome 1784
    conduct disorder 1781–2
    depression 1675–6, 1780–1
    eating disorders 1784
    failure to engage/respond 1779
    following attempted suicide 1707
    inclusion of cognitive component 1778–9
    non-organic pain 1784
    obsessive–compulsive disorder 1686–7, *1686*, 1783–4
    post-traumatic stress disorder 1784
    psychiatric/behaviour disorder with intellectual disability 1852
    substance abuse 1784
    technique and management 1778
    working with parents 1778–9
  in chronic fatigue syndrome 1030, 1042
  comparison with other psychotherapies 1321, 1333–4, *1333*
  compulsive buying/shopping disorder 916
  computerized 1406
  conversion disorder 1019
  and counselling 1277
  delusions/delusional disorder 1314, 1315–17, *1315*, 1920
  depersonalization disorder 775
  depression 672–3, 676, **1304–13**
    advantages of 1304
    background 1304
    childhood and adolescence 1675–6, 1780–1
    demands of 1304
    in elderly people 1555
    ending treatment 1310–12
    indications and contraindications 1305–6
    management of treatment 1307–12, *1308*, *1309*
    selection for 1306–7
    technique 1304–5
  eating disorders 792, 796, 808, 808–9, **1298–303**, 1784
  following attempted suicide 1707
  in generalized anxiety disorder 735–6
  guided self-help 808–9
  historical development 1286
  in HIV/AIDS 1092
  hypochondriasis 1026–7
  insomnia 935–6, *936*
  in intellectual disability 1874
  obsessive–compulsive disorder 770, 1686–7, *1686*, 1783–4
  panic disorder 758, 761
  persistent somatoform pain disorder 1034
  personality disorders 903–4
    antisocial 898
    avoidant 897
    borderline 895
  post-concussion syndrome 396
  provision by psychiatric nurses 1406
  for refugees 1497
  schizophrenia 582–3, **1313–18**
  sex offenders 1963
    juvenile 1953
  social anxiety disorder 741–2, 742, 744
  somatization disorder 1008–9, *1009*
  substance use disorders 428, 1784
  therapeutic alliance in 903, 1307
  tic disorders 1686–7
  training 1297, 1312
  trauma-focused 708–9, 1109, 1111, 1730
  with victims of criminal activity 1988
cognitive-behavioural group therapy 742, 744
cognitive control in insomnia 936
cognitive deficits and distortions
  in childhood and adolescence
    in anxiety disorders 1779
    attention-deficit hyperactivity disorder 1782
    in conduct disorder 1781
    in depressive disorders 1780–1
    in obsessive–compulsive disorder 1783
  malingered 1055–6

cognitive development 1777–8
  and developmental psychology 238–40, *239*
  history-taking 1600
cognitive dissonance and the placebo response 1142
cognitive dysmetria 563
Cognitive Estimates Test *90*
cognitive impairment
  in Alzheimer's disease 334–5
  in autism 1633
  cannabis-associated 92, 507–8
  due to disturbed sleep 926
  following head injury 390–1, *395*
  following stroke 1071
  in frontotemporal dementias 347
  mild *see* mild cognitive impairment
  in multiple sclerosis 1074
  non-dementia 1519, 1520, *1521*, 1535, *1535*, 1536, 1537
    vascular 378–9
  in Parkinson's disease 368
  postoperative 1099
  prior to surgery 1098
  in schizophrenia 93, 265, 528, **531–4**, 580
  in schizotypal personality disorder 533
  vascular 378–9
cognitive models of illness 1138
cognitive neuropsychology 262
cognitive neuroscience 262
cognitive reactivity 1304
cognitive restructuring
  in anxiety disorders 1293, *1293*
  in body dysmorphic disorder 1047
  in generalized anxiety disorder 736
  in panic disorder 761
  in sleep disorders 937, 1572
  in social anxiety disorder 742
  social anxiety disorder 742
  in specific phobia 746
cognitive schemas 52, 1778
  maladaptive 1778
    early 895
  negative 1304
  and reporting of physical symptoms 1137
cognitive stimulation in dementia *414*
Cognitive Test for Delirium 326
cognitive theory
  and hypochondriasis 1025
  and somatization disorder 1005
cognitive therapy 310, 311, 1940
  attention-deficit hyperactivity disorder 1648
  childhood and adolescence 1610, 1767, 1783
  and concept of depression 15
  and counselling 1277
  for delusions 1980
  family-based 1707
  group setting 1351
  history of 23
  in morbid jealousy 1920
  personality disorder 903–4
    borderline 895
  post-traumatic stress disorder 708–9
  schizophrenia 1315–17, *1315*, 1317
  substance use disorders 428
  see also cognitive-behaviour therapy
Cognitive Therapy Scale 1311
Cohen–Mansfield Agitation Inventory 413
cohort 1513
cohort studies 282, 283, 541, 557, 568
collaborative care 1483, 1486, 1487
  in adjustment disorders 1068
Collaborative Study on the Genetics of Alcoholism 435
collagen, cross-linkage 1508
colleges
  psychiatrist as advisor 1815
  see also schools
coma 59
  following head injury 388
  Glasgow Coma Scale 388, *388*
commissural plate 157
commissure of the fornix 151
common geriatric assessment 1581
communication
  doctor–patient 1138–9
  in intellectual disability 1873
  skills training 1139, 1375–6
communication disorders *see* specific developmental disorders, of speech and language
community, prevalence of mental disorders *1480*
community alcohol team model 461
community care 584
  global survey 11
  history of 24
  and rehabilitation 1400
community diagnosis 280
community mental health centres 1454
Community Mental Health in ID Service 1888–9
community mental health teams (CMHTs) 584, 1454–5, *1456*, *1457*, 1458
  services for people with intellectual disability 1888–9
  see also mental health services, community
community outreach in attempted suicide 970, 972
community psychiatric nurses (CPNs) 1404–5
  in treatment of alcohol use disorders 462
  see also psychiatric nurses
community reinforcement 456, 462
community substance misuse teams 479
community treatment orders 1411, 1458
comorbidity 278, 990
  in childhood and adolescence 1591, 1600
  in primary care 1483
  see also under specific disorders
compartmentalization phenomena 1012, *1012*
compensation claims
  and conversion disorder 1016
  and persistent somatoform pain disorder 1034
'compensation neurosis' 700
competence 29
  abilities involved 1897
  best interest approach 1899
  functional approach 1898
  and juvenile delinquency 1954–5
  lack of 1898–9
  legal aspects 1895–900
  outcome approach 1897–8
  status approach 1897, 1899–900
  tests of 1897
complementary medicines 15, **1247–51**
  antipsychotics 1249
  anxiolytics and sedatives 1248
  in chronic fatigue syndrome 1042
  in chronic somatic conditions 1249
  cognitive enhancers 1247–8
  determinants of pharmacological properties *1248*
  and diagnosis 65
  drug interactions 1249–50, *1250*
  mood disorders 1248
  in movement disorders 1249
  in neurasthenia 1063
  psychoses 1249
  for refugees 1497
  smoking cessation 512
  in substance use disorders 1249
'complex medically ill' 1144
complex regional pain syndrome, type 1 1015, 1050
Complexity Prediction Instrument 1145
Complier-Average Causal Effect of Treatment 142
Composite Disability Malingering Index 1054–5
Composite International Diagnostic Interview 69, 70, 72, 284, 542, 1023, 1438
Comprehensive Psychopathological Rating Scale 70
COMPRI (Complexity Prediction Instrument) 1145
compulsions 52, 53, 1680
  in body dysmorphic disorder 1044, *1044*
  in obsessive–compulsive disorder 765–6
compulsive buying/shopping disorder **916**
computed tomography (CT)
  alcohol-related dementia 400
  anorexia nervosa 781
  epilepsy 1619
  frontotemporal dementias 347
  head injury 389
  HIV-associated dementia 385
  obsessive–compulsive disorder 768
  schizophrenia 563–4
  vascular dementia 376
  Wernicke–Korsakoff syndrome 400, 406
COMT gene 255, 256, 555, 559, 1646
concealment of treatment allocation 127
concentration
  assessment 60, 88–9
  disorders of 60
  following head injury 390
concentration camp survivors 1494
conditioning 250, 254, 258
  in acute stress reactions 696
  in obsessive–compulsive disorder 768
  and phobias 745
  and post-traumatic stress disorder 705
  and substance use disorders 428, 434
conduct disorder **1654–64**
  adolescent onset 1655, 1658
  adult outcome 1660–1, *1660*
  aetiology 1658–60
  and age 1655
  assessment 1657, 1781–2
  and bipolar disorder 646
  classification 1656–7
  clinical features 1655–6
  comorbidity 1644, 1657
  confined to the family context 1656
  course 1660–1
  depressive 1657
  differential diagnosis 1657, 1671
  early-onset 1655, 1656, 1658, 1788
    and outcome 1660, *1660*
  epidemiology 1658
  and gender 1655, 1658
  genetics 1658
  hyperkinetic 1644, 1657

and intellectual disability 1657, 1851
and juvenile delinquency 1946
life-course persistent 1658
pattern and setting of behaviour 1655
and perinatal complications 1658
prevention 1663, 1788
prognosis 1660–1
protective factors 1660
and pulse rate 1658
relation to other disorders 1654
risk factors 1658–60
role of neurotransmitters 1658
as a social problem 1654–5
socialized 1656
and suicide 1704
treatment and management 1661–3, 1781–2
unsocialized 1656
verbal deficits in 1658
wider impact of 1655–6
conduction dysphasia 54
confabulation 59, 403, **408**, 1049
following head injury 392
momentary/provoked 408
in post-traumatic stress disorder 404
spontaneous 408
in Wernicke–Korsakoff syndrome 405
confidence interval 126, 128
confidentiality
in childhood and adolescence
assessment 1605
psychiatric emergencies 1811
psychotherapy 1768
and clinical assessment 67
and domestic violence 1982
and expert witnesses 2006–7
in factitious disorder 1053
in higher/further education 1815
in the paraphilias 840
and reports 75
in schools liaison service 1813
confounding factors 285
confrontation in factitious disorder
1052–3, *1053*
Confusion Assessment Method 328, 1531
confusional state 59
in brain tumour 1075
in childhood and adolescence 1742
following an accident 1110
following neurosurgery for mental
disorder 1268
post-ictal 403
see also delirium
congenital rubella syndrome 548, 1635, 1850,
1852, 1863
congestive heart failure in anorexia nervosa 785
congophilic angiopathy 338
Conners' Parent Rating Scale 1241, 1645
Conners' Teacher Rating Scale 1241, 1645, 1813
connexions advisors 1812
conscientiousness 850, 886
conscious mental states 135
conscious thinking 294
consciousness
clouding of 59, *59*, 60
concept of 59
disorders of 59–60
heightened 59
loss of following head injury 388
narrowing of 60
consent *see* informed consent
Consortium to Establish a Registry for AD 336
constipation and depression 641
consultation
communication in 1138–9
in consultation-liaison psychiatry 1145
patient-centred/doctor-centred 1139
consultation-liaison (CL) psychiatry 990, 1135,
1144–8, 1487
audit 1147
current levels of service delivery 1144
for elderly people 1583
Psych-Med unit 1145
screening in 1145–6, *1146*
service organization 1146–7, *1147*
staffing 1146
training 1147
types of service delivery 1145–6, *1145*, *1146*
container-contained theory 308
contiguous gene syndromes 228
contingency management in opioid
dependence 477
continuous performance tests 247
contracts in psychoanalysis 1341
control
delusions of 51, 56
perceived lack of in generalized anxiety
disorder 734
control event rate 128
contusions, cerebral 387, *387*, 389
conversion 1012
pain as form of 1031–2
conversion disorder (CD) 57, **1011–21**
childhood and adolescence 1745
chronic 1017
classification 106, *993*, 994
clinical features 1014–17
comorbidity 870, 1015
and culture 14–15
definitions 1012, *1012*
differential diagnosis 695, 1003, 1012, *1012*
epidemiology 998, 1014
examination 1015–16
mimicking surgical conditions 1096
and pain 1031–2
pathophysiology 1013–14, *1013*, *1014*
prognosis 1017–18
role of volition 1012
sleep-related 948
treatment and management 1018–20, *1019*
conversion symptoms 57
Cool Kids programme 1779
cooperativeness 80, *80*, 83, 316, 850
cooperatives 1401
Coordinators of Services for the Elderly
project 1584
COPD (chronic obstructive pulmonary
disease) *932*, 1082
COPE programme 1779
coping
active/engaged/approach 1066
behavioural 1066
in chronic fatigue syndrome 1039
with depression 1306
emotion focused 1066
failure 1067
with illness 1065–71
and immune function 207
passive/disengaged/avoid 1066
problem focused 1066
with schizophrenia 1313–14, 1315
social 1066
in social anxiety disorder 744
and somatization disorder 1009
styles 1066
techniques 1066
with terminal illness 1069–70
Coping Power Programme 1662, 1782
coping strategy enhancement 451, 1313–14,
1315, 1662, 1782
coprolalia 1073, 1681
copropraxia 1073
Cornell scale for depression in dementia 413
coronary heart disease
and alcohol consumption 446
and sleep-wake disorders *932*
and type A personality 1136
and type D personality 1136
corpus callosum 151, 157, 180
corpus striatum 158, 159
correlation coefficient 849
Corsi blocks 255
cortical dysplasia 159, 1863
cortical plate 158
corticobasal degeneration (CBD) 344
aetiology 348
differential diagnosis 347–8
neuropathology 345
corticobulbar pathway 156
corticopontine pathway 155
corticospinal tract 156, 158
corticosteroids
adverse effects
anxiety 1101
in childhood and adolescence 1673
psychosis 539
in Landau–Kleffner syndrome 1627
release in response to stress 1135
corticostriate pathway 154–5, *154*
corticotrophin-releasing hormone (CRH)
163, *171*
and depression 163–4, 166, 659, 661
functions 161
and immune function 206
in post-traumatic stress disorder 706
and suicide 965
cortisol
and aggressive/antisocial behaviour 1918
and chronic fatigue syndrome 1039
and depression 660–1, 1675
and fibromyalgia 1039
in generalized anxiety disorder 732
hypersecretion 1086
and insomnia 935
and the sleep–wake cycle 925
COSE project 1584
cosmetic psychopharmacology 28–9
cosmetic treatment in body dysmorphic
disorder 1046, 1096
cost-benefit analysis 1474, 1475
cost-consequence analysis 1475
cost-effectiveness acceptability curves
1475, *1475*
cost-effectiveness analysis (CEA)
1463, 1474, 1475
alcohol use disorders services 462–3
child and adolescent mental health
services 1476–7
mental health interventions in developing
countries 1477, *1478*
research study design 1475–6

cost-effectiveness ratio, incremental
124, 1475, *1475*
cost-per-QALY approach 1475, 1476
cost-utility analysis (CUA) 1474, 1475
of depression treatment in primary care 1476
costs, measurement of 1474–5
Cotard's syndrome 56
Council of Europe, Principles Concerning the Legal Protection of Incapable Adults 1896
counselling **1272–85**
adjustment disorders 721, 1278
alcohol use disorders 1279
anxiety 1278
applications 1278–80
bereavement 726–7, 1279
childhood and adolescence **1764–9**
approaches to 1766–8
measures of effectiveness and outcome 1769
practical issues 1768
with psychiatric/behaviour disorder and intellectual disability 1852
supportive 1767
training and supervision 1768–9
treatment setting and process 1766
cognitive–behavioural models 1275, 1277
cognitive models 1275
core conditions 1274–5
couple 1370
definitions 1273
depression 672, 676, 1278
eclectic-integrative approaches 1278
in educational settings 1281
effectiveness 1274
electronic delivery 1282
existential approaches 1277
following abortion 1119
genetic *see* genetic counselling
grief 726–7, 1279
in HIV/AIDS 1280–1
in hospitals and clinics 1280–1
humanistic–existential models 1275, 1276–7
information-giving in 1275–6
key elements and goals *1273*
methods and techniques 1275–8
mothers giving up children for adoption 1120
pathological gambling 922
person-centred (client-centred) 1275, 1276–7
postnatal depression 1280
practice 1274
in primary care 1280, 1485–6
psychodynamic models 1275, 1277–8
and psychotherapy 1273–4, 1765
rape victims 1986
in relationship problems 1278–9
schools of 1275, *1275*
settings 1280–2, 1485–6
skills 1274
smoking cessation 511–12
stress disorders 1278
substance use disorders 1279
telephone helplines 1282
theoretical approaches to 1275, *1275*
therapeutic alliance in 1275
training, accreditation and registration 1282–3
trauma 1279–80
in the voluntary sector 1279, 1281
in the workplace 1281–2
counselling psychology 1274
counterfeit deviance 834–5
countertransference
in brief psychodynamic psychotherapy 1329, 1330
broad/totalistic view 314, *315*
complementary 1343
concordant 1343
joint creation 314, *315*
narrow view 314, *315*
and non-compliance 317
object-relations theory model 298–9
in physician-assisted suicide 318
and projective identification 308
in psychoanalysis 1343–4
and psychodynamic psychiatry 314, *315*, 318
Countertransference Questionnaire 1344
couple counselling 1370
couple therapy 1365–6, **1369–80**
adjustment disorders *1069*
alcohol use disorders 452–3
assessment and selection 1373
behavioural 452–3, 1371
behavioural–systems 1372–8
cognitive-behavioural 1371
and culture 1377–8
depression 15, 672
distinction from couple counselling 1370
efficacy 1378–9
indications and contraindications 1373
intersystem model 1372
mixed/eclectic approach 1371–2
paraphilias 838, 840
process 1373–5
psychoanalytic/psychodynamic 1370–1
psychodynamic–behavioural 1372
rational–emotive 1371
substance use disorders 516
systems approach 1371
techniques 1375–7
training in 1379
Court of Protection 1898–9
Court reports 1928, *2004*, **2005–6**
courtship behaviour 815
COVR (Classification of Violence Risk) 1996, 1998
Cowper's gland 817
CPA *see* care programme approach
CPNs *see* community psychiatric nurses
CPSS (Child PTSD Symptom scale) 1730
CR (calorie restriction) and modification of ageing 1509
CR/HT (crisis resolution/home treatment) teams 1458, *1458*
crack 430, *431*, 483
see also cocaine
cranial nerve development 157
'crashing' 497
craving 427, 428, 483
cre recombinase 230
creatinine 1204
creative thought 308
Creutzfeldt–Jakob disease (CJD) 351, 1903
aetiology 351–2
amyotrophic 354
ataxic 354
atypical 354
Heidenhain's variant 354
iatrogenic *353*, 355
panencephalopathic 354
prevention 358–9
sporadic/classical 352, 353–4, *353*
variant 351, *353*, 355–6
aetiology 351–2
secondary (iatrogenic) *353*, 356
CRH *see* corticotrophin-releasing hormone
cri-du-chat syndrome (CDCS)
behavioural and psychiatric aspects 1842
genetics 1842
physical characteristics 1842
prevalence 1842
crime analysis 1914
Crime and Disorder Act 1998 1982, 1987–8
Crime and Disorder Reduction Partnerships 515
criminal activity *see* offending
Criminal Damage Act 1971 1966
Criminal Justice Integrated Teams 515
criminal liability 1900–1
Criminal Procedure (Insanity and Fitness to Plead) Act 1991 1901
criminal victimization **1984–90**
criminogenic factors 1911, 1917, 1918, 2011, 2012
crisis cults 982
crisis houses 1458
crisis resolution/home treatment teams 1458, *1458*
criterion variance 284
Crohn's disease 1083–4
cross-cultural comparisons 276, *277*
cross-fostering study 216
cross-sectional studies 282
crowding of thoughts 53
CRPS I (complex regional pain syndrome type I) 1015, 1050
cryptographia 54
cryptolalia 54
crystal/crystalline methamphetamine hydrochloride **497–8**
CT *see* computed tomography
CTOs (community treatment orders) 1411, 1458
CUA *see* cost-utility analysis
cue exposure in alcohol use disorders 451
CUES (Carers and Users Experience of Services) 1434
'cult of thinness' 779
cultural competence 1502–4, *1503*
culture
in acute and transient psychotic disorders 606
and ageing 1512–13
and body dysmorphic disorder 1045
and care pathways **1438–45**
in child and adolescent psychotherapy 1768
and clinical assessment 67
and the concept of depression 15
and conversion hysteria 14–15
and couple therapy 1377–8
cultural critique of biomedicine 276–7
cultural formulations 278
and deliberate self-harm 958–9
and depression 14, 1496
and help-seeking behaviour 15, 1441–2
and hypochondriasis 1025–6
and indigenous folk healing practices 1418
and intellectual disability 1879–80, 1881
and mania 14
and marriage 1370
and mental health services for ethnic minorities **1502–4**

and neurasthenia 1060–1
and neuroses 14
and normal sexual function 812–13
and the phenomena of psychiatric disorder 47
and provision of services 277–8
and reaction to loss of a parent 1758
and refugee assessment, diagnosis and treatment 1496, *1496*, 1498
role in caregiver-mediated interventions 1791
and schizophrenia 14, 546, 557, 571–3, *572*
and social and cultural anthropology 275–9
and somatization disorders 996
and stigma 6–7
and suicide 953–4, 1704
transcultural psychiatry **13–16**
and treatment 1442–3
culture of blame 1991–2
culture-related specific psychiatric syndromes 14, **979–85**, 1439
acute and transient psychotic disorders 606
anorexia nervosa as 779
concept of 979
subgroups 979–80, *980*
in western societies 984–5
current awareness 124–5, *125*
Cushing's syndrome 1086
CVLT (California Verbal Learning Test) 253, 264
CY-BOCS (Children's Yale-Brown Obsessive-Compulsive Scale) 1681
cyberstalking 1970
'cyber suicide' 1706
cyclic adenosine monophosphate 175
d-cycloserine
adverse effects *1091*
in social anxiety disorder 743
in specific phobia 746
cyclothymia/cyclothymic disorder 632, **686–9**
aetiology 688–9
childhood and adolescence 1671, *1672*
clinical features 687–8
course 687–8
diagnosis 687–8
epidemiology 688, *689*
historical perspective 686
management 689
prevention 689
relationship to bipolar disorder 688
CYP system
and antidepressants 1188
and antipsychotics 1221, 1222
and complementary medicines 1249, *1250*
inhibitors 1795
and opioid metabolism 473–4
and pharmacokinetics 1170, *1172*
cyproterone acetate 838, 1963–4
cystic fibrosis 1743
cytokines *168*, 171, 209
cytomegalic inclusion disease 1863
cytosine 223

Da Costa syndrome 751
DAG (diacyl glycerol) 174, 175
DALE (Disability-Adjusted Life Expectancy) 1510
DALYs (Disability-Adjusted Life Years) 10, 645, 1477, 1510
dangerous and severe personality disorders 848, 2015, 2018
DAPA-PC (Drug Abuse Problem Assessment for Primary Care) 1484
DAPP-BQ (Dimensional Assessment of Personality Disorders) 858, *858*
DARE database 1156
DAS (Disability Assessment Schedule) 284
'date rape' 409, 491
DATs (Drug Action Teams) 515–16
DAWBA (Development and Well-Being Assessment) 1595–6
dawn-simulating alarm clock 1261
day hospitals
acute 1453
in Alzheimer's disease 340
in anorexia nervosa 793, 795
in community mental health services 1453
for elderly people 1583
daydreaming 294, 1941
DBS (deep brain stimulation) 671, 769, 1073–4, 1258, **1269–70**
DBT *see* dialectical behaviour therapy
DC-LD (Diagnostic Criteria for Psychiatric Disorders for Use with Adults with Learning Disabilities/Mental Retardation) 1826–7, 1850
de Lange syndrome
behavioural and psychiatric aspects 1842
genetics 1842
physical characteristics 1842
prevalence 1842
de-affectualization 774
debriefing
critical incident stress 697
emergency workers 1110
trauma story 1497
deceitfulness in conduct disorder 1656
decentring technique 1374
deception 1941
decision-making
and emotion 260–1
legal aspects 1895–900
deep brain stimulation 671, 769, 1073–4, 1258, **1269–70**
deep lateral sulcus 144, 145
de-escalation techniques 1404
defence mechanisms 310, 849
avoidant 1339–40
in brief psychodynamic psychotherapy 1328–9
classification 1339–40
in obsessive–compulsive disorder 768
and personality development 316–17
primitive/mature 1339
and psychoanalysis 293–4, 1339–40
and resistance 315, 317
defensive organizations 1339
dehydration and ecstasy use 495
de-ideation 774
deinstitutionalization
and burden of care 1401
and intellectual disability 1881, 1887, 1890
and mental health social work 1408, 1411
and prevalence of mental disorder among prisoners 1934
and psychiatric nursing 1403
déjà vu 59, 250
delay aversion in attention-deficit hyperactivity disorder 1647
delayed sleep phase syndrome 928, 942–3, 1261, 1695, 1700
deliberate self-harm (DSH) 955, **957–63**
and adjustment disorders 718, 722
aetiology 960–1
and age 1704
in anorexia nervosa 782–3
assessment 971, *971*
in childhood and adolescence 972, 1601, 1703
choice of method 959–60
classification 960
clinical features 958
course and prognosis 961
definition 957–8
elderly people 1551, **1564–7**
epidemiology 958–60
high-risk 960
impulsive 916–17
and intellectual disability 1856
and liability of mental health service providers 1905
lifetime prevalence 960
mild 960
moderate 960
in physical illness 1133
precipitants 961
prevention **972–6**
repetition 961, 969, 971, *972*
and risk of suicide 961, 971, *971*, *972*
self-report surveys 960
sociodemographic characteristics 959
in Tourette syndrome 1073
treatment **969–72**
vulnerability factors 961
delineation of syndromes 281
délire d'emblée 603, 604
delirium 49, **325–33**
aetiology 330, *330*
at childbirth 1118
in cancer 1103–4, *1104*
and cholinergic system 330, 1532
classification 105, 327, 1531
clinical features 326–7, *326*
comorbidity 327
and consciousness 59
and dementia 327, 329, 332, 1532
diagnosis 327–8
differential diagnosis 327–8, *328*, 364
drug-induced 1532
elderly people 1529, **1530–4**
aetiology 1532, *1532*
classification 1531
clinical features 1530–1
complications 1533
course and prognosis 1532
diagnosis 1531
differential diagnosis 1531, 1559
epidemiology 1531–2
prevention 1533
treatment and management 1532–3
epidemiology 328–9
in HIV/AIDS 1092–3, *1093*
hyperactive 327, 1531, 1532, 1533
hypoactive 327, 1530–1, 1532, 1533
investigation 330, *330*
mixed 327
mortality risk 329
neuropathogenesis 330–1, *330*
outcome 328–9
phencyclidine-induced 486–7
in pneumonia 1091
postoperative 1098–9
post-seizure 1257

delirium (*cont.*)
prevention 331, 1533
psychosis in 327
risk factors 329, *329*
subsyndromal 325, 328, 1531
treatment and management 331–2, *1104*, 1255
tremor in 58
Delirium Rating Scale 1531
Delirium Rating Scale-Revised-98 328
Delirium Symptom Interview 1531
delirium tremens 58, 327, 443
prevention 450
treatment 449–50
delusional atmosphere 51
delusional disorder **609–28**
aetiology 613–14
clinical features 613–15
diagnostic criteria 103–4, 613, *613*
differential diagnosis 864
elderly people 1552
erotomanic 621–2
features of delusions in 612
genetics 614
grandiose 622
and homicide 1920
induced 610, 624–5
jealous 51, 619–21, 1920, 1967
litigious 616, 1977–80
mixed/unspecified 623
and mood disorders 614
nomenclature 610–11
and offending 1920
persecutory 616
somatic 617–19, 1024
and stalking 1920
subtypes 613, *613*, 615–23
treatment 625–7, 1920
and violence 1920
delusional disorientation 392
delusional intuition 51
delusional misidentification syndrome 51, 392, 609–10, 611, 622, **623–4**
delusional perception 51, 527–8
delusional states, systematized 1030
delusions 49
in acute and transient psychotic disorders 602–8
in Alzheimer's disease 335
autistic 51
autochthonous 51
in body dysmorphic disorder 618, 1044, 1045
clinical aspects 611–12
cognitive-behaviour therapy 1314, 1315–17, *1315*
content of 51
of control 51, 56
definition 50–1, 611
in delirium 327
in delusional disorder 612
in dementia with Lewy bodies 361
dental 619
and depression 51, 639, 641, 674, 1253
differential diagnosis of cause 537
of disease transmission 619
following head injury 392
in frontotemporal dementias 346
genesis 51
grandiose 51
of guilt 51
of halitosis 618–19
hypochondriacal 51
and jealousy 51, 619–21, 1920, 1967
of love 51
memory 51, 59
millenniary 982
and misidentification 51, 392, 609–10, 611, 622, **623–4**
mood-congruent/-incongruent 537, 641
in multiple sclerosis 1074
nihilistic 56
and pain 1030
as paranoid defence 1314
of parasitosis/infestation 50, 51, 618
in Parkinson's disease 1072
of persecution 51
polarized 51
of pregnancy 1115
primary 51, 611
religious 51
in schizophrenia 526–7
secondary 51, 611
of sexually transmitted disease 619
of smell 618–19
structure of 51
and violence 1929
dementia 54
and ageing 1520
and aggression 336, 1920–1, 1928–9
agitation in 413–15
alcohol-related/alcohol-induced **399–402**, 1541
apathy in 416
behavioural and psychological symptoms 412–17, *413*, *414*
carers 417–18
challenging behaviour in 413–15
cholinergic hypothesis 338, 1240–1
classification 105
cognitive assessment 92
definitions 411
delaying onset 1538
and delirium 327, 329, 332, 1532
depression in 416
differential diagnosis 1531
distinction from delirium 327, *328*
distinction from depression 1551, *1551*
disclosure of diagnosis 411
and Down syndrome 1584, 1827, 1839, 1865, 1880
and driving 412
early-onset 411–12, 1584
elderly people
differential diagnosis 1558–9
early detection 1519–20
epidemiology **1519–22**, 1579–80
impact 1522
incidence and risk factors 1520–2, *1520*, *1522*
presentation in primary care 1483
end-stage management 418
epidemiology 1579–80
frontotemporal (FTD) 258–9, **344–50**, 1519
aetiology and pathogenesis 348
and aggression 1928–9
behavioural and psychological symptoms *413*
classification *344*, 347
clinical features 345–6
differential diagnosis 347–8, *347*, 373
epidemiology 345
genetics 348
investigations 347, Plate 12
Lund–Manchester consensus on clinical criteria 345, *345*, 347
neuropathology 344–5
with parkinsonism 344–5, 346, 348
physical signs 346
treatment and care 348–9
genetic counselling and testing 411, *412*
HIV/AIDS **384–6**, 1091
classification 384
clinical features 384
course and prognosis 385
diagnosis 384–5
differential diagnosis 384–5
epidemiology 385
pathogenesis 385
severity levels 384
treatment and management 385–6
in Huntington's disease **371–5**
and intellectual disability 1827, 1828, 1855
with Lewy bodies (DLB) **361–8**
behavioural and psychological symptoms *413*
clinical diagnosis 363–4, *363*
clinical features 335, 361–2
course and prognosis 365
diagnosis 336
differential diagnosis 364, *364*, 369
epidemiology 364–5
genetics 365
investigations 364
management 365–7, *366*
pathological classification 362
pathological criteria *362*
relationship with dementia in Parkinson's disease 362–3
management **411–19**
mania in 416
memory impairment 59
and mild cognitive impairment 1534, *1534*, 1535–6, 1538
mixed pathologies 336
in motor neurone disease 344, 345, 347, 348
and offending 1920–1
pain in 418
in Parkinson's disease 92, 362–3, **368–71**, *370*
psychomotor disturbance in 59
psychosis in 416
risk assessment and management 417, *417*
risk reduction/protective factors 1521–2, *1522*
semantic 344, 346
severity stages 1535
sexual behaviour disorders 416
and sexuality 1568
and sleep-wake disorders 416–17, *931*, 1572, 1573
structural MRI 195
subcortical 368–9
treatment
complementary medicines 1247–8
pharmacotherapy 1240–1
urinary incontinence in 417
vascular (VaD) **375–84**, 1519
acute onset *378*
aetiology 376
behavioural and psychological symptoms *413*
classification 377
clinical criteria 377–8, *377*, *378*

clinical features 379
cortical (multi-infarct) 375, 377, *378*
course and prognosis 379
diagnosis 379–80
differential diagnosis 348, 364, 380
epidemiology 380–1
incidence 1520
mixed cortical and subcortical *378*
NINDS-AIREN criteria 377, 378, *378*
pathophysiology 376
prevention 381, 1447
risk factors 376
subcortical (small-vessel) 377, *378*
treatment 381
wandering in 415
see also Alzheimer's disease
dementia infantilis **1637**
dementia paralytica 1093
dementia praecox 522, 540, 568, 603, 631, 1547
see also schizophrenia
DemTect 1536
denial 298
in anorexia nervosa 783
as coping behaviour 1066
dental enamel erosion in bulimia nervosa 804
dentate gyrus 148
dentatorubropallidoluysian atrophy *228*, 373
deoxyhaemoglobin 197
deoxyribonucleic acid *see* DNA
dependence
distinction between physical and psychological 427–8
spectrum of 427–8
use of term 427
dependent personality disorder **873–4**
aetiology 873
classification *856*, 873, *873*
clinical features 873
course 874
differential diagnosis 874
elderly people *1562*
epidemiology 874, *882*, 883
treatment 874
depersonalization 55, 56, 1012
definition 774
in delirium 327
distinction between primary and secondary 775
epidemiology 775
following an accident 1107
following head injury 392
in neurological disorders 775
victims of criminal activity 1984
depersonalization disorder **774–6**
aetiology 775
classification 774
clinical features 774
course and prognosis 775
diagnosis and differential diagnosis 774–5
epidemiology 775
treatment and management 775–6
deprenyl 385
depression
aetiology
genetic 648, **650–8**
integrated model 649
neurobiological **658–65**
age of onset 667
and alcohol use disorders 649
and anorexia nervosa 783, 787
anticipation in 652
and antisocial personality disorder 866
and anxiety disorder 649
anxious 641–2, 642
assessment 660
assessment instruments 69, 70, 1163–4, 1306, 1484, 1551, *1552*
atypical 635
and bereavement 725
binary model 638
and body mass index 1674
in bulimia nervosa 803, 804
childhood and adolescence
acute management 1677
aetiology 1674
assessment and monitoring 1617–16, 1780–1
course 1673
diagnostic criteria 1669, *1670*
differential diagnosis 1657, 1671–3
double 1673
environmental risk factors 1675
epidemiology 1673–4
minor 1669
neurocognitive factors 1674–5
neuroendocrine studies 1675
sequelae 1674
treatment and prevention 674–5, 1322, 1668, 1675–6, 1780–1, 1794–5, 1796
and childhood adverse experiences 648, 658–9
chronic 667
and chronic fatigue syndrome 1037
classification 638–9, 640–2
clinical features 633–5, *633*, 640–1
cognitive assessment 92
cognitive model 1304–5, *1305*, 1307
cognitive vulnerability to 1304
concept of 15
and conversion disorder 1015
coping strategies 1306
and corticotrophin-releasing hormone 163–4, 166, 659, 661
and cortisol 660–1, 1675
course 271, 667
and culture 14, 1496
definition 637
in dementia 416
in dementia with Lewy bodies 361, 367
diagnosis 647, 1306
differential diagnosis 327, *328*, 643–4, 741, 766, 1004, 1024, 1531
distinction from dementia 1551, *1551*
double 681, 683, 1673
drug-induced 1551, *1552*
duration and severity of episodes 633–4, 667
dysfunctional cognition in 653
elderly people **1550–6**
aetiology *1552*, 1553
assessment 1527, 1551–2
clinical features 1551
in the community 1517
course and prognosis 1553
diagnosis 1551–2
differential diagnosis 373, 1552, 1558
epidemiology 1517–18, 1552–3, 1579
factors influencing presentation *1551*
in hostels and nursing homes 1518
investigations 1551–2, *1553*
mortality associated 1553
prevention 1555–6
in primary care 1482–3, 1518
resistant 1555
treatment and management 674, 1554–5
endogenous/melancholic 630, 631, 638, 640–1
epidemiology **647–9**, 650–1
following abortion 1119
following an accident 1109–10
following ecstasy use 495
following head injury 393, 396
following miscarriage 1119
functional anatomy 189, 660
and functional symptoms 993
and gender 271, 648, 653–4
and generalized anxiety disorder 731
global disease burden 645, 1185
history of 629–30
hostile 641–2, 642
and hypochondriasis 997, 1024, 1027
and immune function 207
and intellectual disability 1827, 1852, 1854–5
and juvenile delinquency 1949
and kleptomania 1943
and life events 269–73, *270*, *271*, 648, 659
lifespan perspective 271–2
maintaining factors 659–63
major
classification 639
diagnosis 647
with psychotic features 634, 639
recurrent 634
stages leading to *634*
with/without melancholia 634
and marital conflict 1753
and marital status 648
masked 1030, 1527
melancholic 270
minor 668
models 638–9
monoamine theory 662
mortality associated 667–8
and neurasthenia 1063
neuroendocrine challenge tests 660
neurotic 270, 638, 641
offenders 1923, *1933*
outcome 667
and pain 1029, 1030
and panic disorder 752
parental, effects on child development 1752–3
and patient state fluctuations within mood disorders 632–3, *632*, *633*
and persistent somatoform pain disorder 997
and personality 648
and personality disorders 649
pharmacogenetics 653
in physical illness 648–9, 1132
Alzheimer's disease 335
cancer 649, 1102, *1102*, *1103*
COPD 1082
Cushing's syndrome 1086
diabetes mellitus 649, 1085
epilepsy 1080
HIV/AIDS 1092
Huntington's disease 371
hyperthyroidism 1085
hypothyroidism 1085
infection 1091
multiple sclerosis 1074

depression (*cont.*)
in physical illness (*cont.*)
myocardial infarction 649, 1082
Parkinson's disease 648–9, 1072
population perspective 272–3, *272*
post-hysterectomy 1116
post-psychotic 589, 626
post-stroke 1071, 1555
precipitating factors 659
in pregnancy 653, 1117, 1322
prevalence 647–8
primary 637
in primary care
detection and assessment 1476
elderly people 1518
treatment 1322, 1476
prisoners 1923, *1933*
psychosocial factors 271, 653
psychotic/delusional 51, 639, 641, 674, 1253
reactive 630, 631, 638, 641
recurrence 634–5, 667, 671
in refugees 1495
relapse 671
remission 271
resistant 675, Plate 14
risk factors 648–9, 658–9, 1675
in schizophrenia 529, 573
seasonal 635
secondary 637
and sexuality 825
and shoplifting 1943
situational 642
and sleep-wake disorders 634, 661–2, 927, 931, *931*, 934, 1697
social functioning in 653
and somatization disorders 996
spectrum model 642
and substance use disorders 649
subsyndromal symptomatic (SSD) 719
subtypes 630, 631, 638, 640–2, *640*, 647
and suicide 634, 955, 1704
and temperament 654, 658
in terminal illness 1070
thyroid abnormalities in 661
in Tourette syndrome 1073
treatment **669–77**
cognitive-behaviour therapy 672–3, 676, **1304–13**, 1555, 1675–6, 1780–1
combined psychotherapy and pharmacotherapy 672–3
complementary medicines 1248
continuation 671, 675, 677
counselling 672, 676, 1278
deep brain stimulation 671, 1270
electroconvulsive therapy 671, 1252–3
in HIV/AIDS 1092
interpersonal psychotherapy 672–3, 676, 1322–3, 1555, 1676
maintenance 671, 675–6, 677
management 673–7
marital therapy 672
neurosurgery 1267, 1268
in primary care 1476
in resistant depression 675
setting 673
transcranial magnetic stimulation 671, 1264
vagus nerve stimulation 671, 1269
see also antidepressants *and specific drugs*
treatment gap *13*
tryptophan depletion 662
unipolar
definition 638
history of concept 631
as unitary disorder 638
and use of mental health services 649
vascular, elderly people 1551, 1553
in vascular dementia 379
and ventricular dysrhythmias 1081
depressive condition, definition 637
depressive episode disorder 633
depressive equivalent 1030
depressive personality disorder 878–9
depressive position 307
deprivation and psychiatric disorder in intellectual disability 1828
derailment 53
derealization 56, 774, 1012
following an accident 1107
following head injury 392
victims of criminal activity 1984
dermatotillomania (pathological skin picking) 618, **917–18**, 1044
Descartes, René 133, 989
description, personal and subpersonal levels 135
descriptive phenomenology **47–61**
definition 47
disorders of attention and concentration 60
disorders of consciousness 59–60
disorders of intellectual performance 54
disorders of memory 59
disorders of mood 54–5
disorders of perception 48–50
disorders of personality 60
disorders of self and body image 56–7
disorders of thinking 50–4
language and speech disorder 53–4
motor symptoms and signs 58–9
principles 47–8
theoretical bases 48
desensitization
in obsessive–compulsive disorder 770
systematic 1097
designer drugs 494
desipramine *670*, 1185
adverse effects *1191*, 1193
in body dysmorphic disorder 1046
in cancer *1103*
dosage *1196*
pharmacodynamics *1173*, *1187*
pharmacokinetics *1172*, 1188, *1189*
desomatization 774
detachment phenomena 1012
Determinants of the Outcome of Severe Mental Disorders 14, 572, *572*
devaluation 298
developing countries
cost-effectiveness analysis of mental health interventions 1477, *1478*
prevalence of intellectual disability 1825
psychiatric nurses in 1406–7
Development and Well-Being Assessment 1595–6
Developmental Behaviour Checklist 1850
Developmental Behaviour Checklist for Adults 1828
developmental disorders 1591, *1591*
and schizophrenia 548
see also pervasive developmental disorders; specific developmental disorders
developmental history 1600–1, 1822
developmental neuropsychiatry **1612–22**
developmental perspective
environmental risks 1724–8
pharmacotherapy 1794
in psychodynamic psychiatry 314
reasons for taking 234–5
developmental psychology **234–45**
cognitive development 238–40, *239*, 1777–8
critical issues 235–7
and effects of parental mental/physical illness **1752–8**
and individual differences 238
language development 240–1, *241*, 1623, 1710–11
memory development 241–2, *241–2*
models and theories 234–5
neonatal/early infancy stage 238–9
social and emotional development 242–3, *242*
stage theories 234–5, 239–40, *239*
developmental psychopathology 237–8, 1612–13
and attachment 243
and classification in childhood and adolescence **1589–94**
and epidemiology 1608
and individual differences 238
in infancy 238–9
linking to developing children 238–42
Piaget's work 239–40, *239*
developmental scales 1821
developmental stages 1764, 1777
developmental toxicology 1614
deviance, subcultural 1657
dexamethasone, in generalized anxiety disorder 732
dexamethasone–CRF test 164, 1252
Dexamethasone Suppression Test (DST)
in depression 661, 1252
in elderly people 1552
in obsessive–compulsive disorder 768
and suicide 965
dextroamphetamine
in attention-deficit hyperactivity disorder 1648
in cancer *1103*
in terminal illness 1070
dhat 606, **981**
diabetes insipidus, lithium-induced 1204
diabetes mellitus 1085
brittle 1050
and bulimia nervosa 804
in childhood and adolescence 1741
depression in 649, 1085
and schizophrenia 546
sexual dysfunction in 826
and sleep-wake disorders *932*
diacetylmorphine *see* heroin
diacyl glycerol 174, 175
diagnosis **99–121**
additional/subsidiary 74
alternative 74
and clinical assessment 64–5, 74
and complementary medicine 65
cultural critique 276–7
definition 99
differential 74

and disorder 64–5
division between medical and psychiatric 989–90, 992
ethical issues 28–9
main 74
multiaxial systems 73, 100–1, 990, *990*
provisional 74
role of value judgement 29
and social control 29
diagnosis related groups 1430
Diagnostic and Statistical Manual of Mental Disorders, development 100–2
Diagnostic and Statistical Manual of Mental Disorders, DSM-II
hypochondriasis 1022
neurasthenia 1060
Diagnostic and Statistical Manual of Mental Disorders, DSM-III 26, 631
alcohol dependence and alcohol abuse 437
autism 1633
bulimia 800
depression 638–9
development 100–1
dysthymic disorder 1060
generalized anxiety disorder 729–30
multiaxial descriptive systems 100–1
panic disorder 751
post-traumatic stress disorder 693
schizophrenia 1547
sexism in 28
somatoform disorders 105, 993–4, 999, 1022
Diagnostic and Statistical Manual of Mental Disorders, DSM-III-R 101
alcohol dependence syndrome 437
depression 639
panic disorder 751, 752
personality disorders 855–6, *856*
post-traumatic stress disorder 693
schizophrenia 1547
Diagnostic and Statistical Manual of Mental Disorders, DSM-IV **113–20**
acute PCP intoxication 486
acute stress disorder 693, 694, *694*
adjustment disorders 106, *716*, 717–19, *717*, 1067
alcohol use disorders 439, *440*
Alzheimer's disease 336
attention deficit-hyperactivity disorder 1643
bipolar disorder 639
body dysmorphic disorder 1045–6
categorical approach 849
as classification of disorders 64
communication disorders 1623, *1623*
comparison with ICD-10 102–4
cultural critique 276
and cultural formulation 278
cyclothymic disorder 686
delirium 327, 1531
delusional disorder 609, 613, *613*
delusions 611
depersonalization disorder 774
depression 633, *633*, 639, 640
development 101–2
disorders relating to cocaine 483, *484*
dysthymic disorder 681
eating disorder 106, 787–8, 800–1, *801*
ethical issues in diagnosis using 28
factitious disorder 106, 1049, 1050
frontotemporal dementias 348
generalized anxiety disorder 730, *730*
impulse control disorders 911
intellectual handicap 1820, *1820*
learning disorders 1623, *1623*
malingering 1054
mania 635, *635*
mental retardation (intellectual handicap) 1820, *1820*
motor skills disorder 1623, *1623*
multiaxial descriptive systems 73
obsessive–compulsive disorder 765, 1682
panic disorder 750–1, 751, 752
pathological gambling 920
personality disorders 106, 851, 855–8, *856*
antisocial personality disorder *865*
avoidant personality disorder *872*
borderline personality disorder *867*
dependent personality disorder *873*
histrionic personality disorder *869*
narcissistic personality disorder *871*
obsessive–compulsive personality disorder 874, *874*
paranoid personality disorder 861, *861*
passive–aggressive personality disorder 876, *876*
schizoid personality disorder 863, *863*
schizotypal personality disorder 864, *864*
pervasive developmental disorders 1633, 1639
post-traumatic stress disorder 701, *702–3*, 703
in primary care 1483–4
relational problems 1382
schizoaffective disorder 597–8
schizophrenia 105, 534, *534*, *536*, 541, 568–9, 571
sexual dysfunction 823
social anxiety disorder 740
somatoform disorders 993–4, *993*, 1003, 1062
body dysmorphic disorder 1045–6
conversion disorder 106, 1012
hypochondriasis 996–7, 1022–3, *1022*
persistent somatoform pain disorder 993–4, 1029–30
somatization disorder 996, 999–1000, 1003
specific phobia 745
substance-induced persisting dementia 399, *399*
substance use disorders 439, *440*
tic disorders 1682
use in epidemiology 283
vascular dementia 377, *377*
Diagnostic and Statistical Manual of Mental Disorders, DSM-IV-PC 1483–4
Diagnostic and Statistical Manual of Mental Disorders, DSM-IV-TR 102
bereavement 1758
in childhood and adolescence 104, 1592–3
conduct disorder 1657
and epidemiology 1607
intellectual disability 1825
intellectual disability with psychiatric disorder 1826, 1849, 1850
schizophrenia 1547
and stressors 718
structure 104–6
Diagnostic and Statistical Manual of Mental Disorders, DSM-V, research planning for 106–8, 852
Diagnostic Criteria for Psychiatric Disorders for Use with Adults with Learning Disabilities/ Mental Retardation 1826–7, 1850
Diagnostic Criteria for Research 71
Diagnostic Interview for Personality Disorders *858*
Diagnostic Interview Schedule 71–2, 542, 765
dialectical behaviour therapy (DBT) 304
attempted suicide 970, 1707
personality disorders 318–19, 868, 895–6, 904, 1563
diazepam 1178
in alcohol withdrawal 449
in cancer *1102*
in delirium 1533
dosage 1180
drug interactions 1232
as a hypnotic 1182
in panic disorder *756*, 757
pharmacokinetics *1172*, 1178
potential for misuse 491
rebound and withdrawal symptoms 1180–1
in status epilepticus 1867
didanosine *1091*, 1092
diencephalon 156
diet
and attention-deficit hyperactivity disorder 1646–7, 1648
elderly people 1529
elimination 1648
and modification of ageing 1509
and monoamine oxidase inhibitors 1187–8, 1192, *1192*
difference scores 87
abnormality 87
reliability 87
differential reinforcement of other behaviour 414
diffuse axonal injury 387
digit span 89, 255, 264
digoxin 1532
dihydrocodeine 474, 1244
dihydroergotoxin 1240
dihydrotestosterone 815
diltiazem 1201, 1206
Dimensional Assessment of Personality Disorders 858, *858*
2,5-dimethoxy-4-ethylthio-β-phenethylamine 501
dimethyltryptamine 488, 489, 501
diminished responsibility defence 1901, 1922, 1923, 1928, 1937, 1939, 1940
Dioscorea alata 1249
DIPD (Diagnostic Interview for Personality Disorders) *858*
diphenhydramine 1226
direct questioning in child and adolescent assessment 1604–5
DIS (Diagnostic Interview Schedule) 71–2, 542, 765
disability
definition 389
measurement of 1465
Disability-Adjusted Life Expectancy 1510
Disability-Adjusted Life Years 10, 645, 1477, 1510
Disability Assessment Schedule 284
disablement 283
concepts of 65, *66*
measurement of 284
disasters 1108
DISC1 gene 229, 555
discrimination 11
and stigma 5, 6, 7

disease, concept of 62, 63–4, 277–8
disinhibition
in Alzheimer's disease 335
in attention-deficit hyperactivity disorder 1647
and hallucinations 50
disintegrative psychosis **1637**
disorientation 59
delusional 392
disposable soma theory 1509
dissocial personality disorder *see* antisocial personality disorder
dissociation 1012, *1013*
in acute stress reactions 693, 694, 696
following an accident 1106–7
victims of criminal activity 1984
dissociative disorder *see* conversion disorder
dissolution du langage 346
disulfiram **453**, *730*, **1246**, 1542
diuretic abuse
in anorexia nervosa 784
in bulimia nervosa 802, 803
diurnal rhythm disturbances 55
divalproex 1677
divination 1420
divorce 1369–70, 1601, 1726
counselling 1278–9
DLB *see* dementia, with Lewy bodies
DMIS (delusional misidentification syndrome) 51, 392, 609–10, 611, 622, **623–4**
DNA
cloned 231
cross-linkage 1508
deletions/insertions 227
free radical damage 1509
hybridization 226
methylation 224, 1508
microsatellites 226
mitochondrial (mtDNA) 223, 1832
age-related defects 1508
free radical damage 1509
non-coding sequences 218
nuclear (nDNA) 223
accumulated somatic mutations 1508
pooling 221
replication 223
short tandem repeats (STRs) 226
single nucleotide polymorphisms (SNPs) 218, 226, 227
structure and function 223
transcription 223–4, *224*
effects of ageing on 1507
DNA microarray studies 1509, 1510
DNA repair genes 1508
doctor–patient communication 1138–9
domestic violence 1449, **1981–3**
and conduct disorder 1659–60
during pregnancy 1117
Dominica, attitudes to psychiatric disorder 6
dommage par ricochet 1902
Domus units 1583
donepezil
in Alzheimer's disease 409, 1241, 1538
in dementia 415
in mild cognitive impairment 1538
in Parkinson's disease 370–1
in vascular dementia 381
donor insemination 1114–15
Doose syndrome 1863–4
dopamine agonists
adverse effects 539
in sexual dysfunction 828
dopamine dysregulation syndrome 1073
dopaminergic system and dopamine receptors *173*, 511, 1171
and alcohol use disorders 229
antipsychotic actions at 1171–2, 1209, 1210, *1211*
and attention-deficit hyperactivity disorder 1646
in autism 1636
and cortical function 151
in delirium 330
dopamine transporters 169, *170*
effects of amphetamines/cocaine on 482, 1172
effects of nicotine 510
effects of transcranial magnetic stimulation 1263
and neurotrophic factors *160*
and novelty-seeking 886–7
in obsessive–compulsive disorder 767
PET/SPET imaging *186*, 187, 188, 189–90
and schizophrenia 180, 188, 561–2
and sexual function 826
in social anxiety disorder 741
and substance use disorders 429
in substance use disorders 429, *429*, 436
and suicide 965–6
and Tourette syndrome 1073, 1684
Doppelgänger 623
dorsal horn 157
dorsal parieto-frontal network 245
dorsal roots 158
dosulepin (dothiepin) 670
'double-bind' 1053, 1381
double orientation 392
double phenomenon 56
Doublecortin 158
Down syndrome
and autism 1839
behavioural phenotype 1613, 1839, *1851*, 1858
and dementia 1584, 1827, 1839, 1865, 1880
effects on the family 1883–4
and epilepsy 1864, 1865
genetics 228, 1831, 1838–9
infantile spasms in 1863
and intellectual disability 1839
and mania 1826
and parental psychiatric disorder 1885
physical characteristics 1839, 1850
prevalence 1825, 1838–9
prevention 1448
downward comparison 1066
doxepin *670*
adverse effects *1191*
in anxiety disorders 1182
dosage *1196*
pharmacodynamics *1187*
pharmacokinetics *1189*
drawings in child and adolescent assessment 1604
dreams
analysis 299, 306
and the unconscious 313
dressing dyspraxia 1527
DRGs (diagnosis related groups) 1430
drift effect 549
drive-defence model 313
drive theory 294, 295, 302, 306
driving
and dementia 412
elderly people 1577–8
legislation regarding alcohol consumption 468, 469
measures to reduce casualties 468, 469
DRO (differential reinforcement of other behaviour) 414
droperidol *1209*
pharmacodynamics *1211*
pharmacokinetics *1172*
DRPLA (dentatorubropallidoluysian atrophy) *228*, 373
DRS-R98 (Delirium Rating Scale-Revised-98) 328
Drug Abuse Problem Assessment for Primary Care 1484
Drug Action Teams 515–16
drug therapy *see* pharmacotherapy
DSH *see* deliberate self-harm
DSM *see entries under* Diagnostic and Statistical Manual of Mental Disorders
DSPD 848, 2015, 2018
DST *see* Dexamethasone Suppression Test
dual instinct/drive theory 294, 295, 302, 306
dualism 133, 989–91
in psychopathology 848
Duchenne muscular dystrophy
behavioural and psychiatric aspects 1843
genetics 1843
physical characteristics 1843
prevalence 1843
duloxetine 670, *670*
adverse effects *1191*, 1555
in cancer 1102
in depression in elderly people 1554, *1554*
dosage *1196*
pharmacodynamics 1186, *1187*
pharmacokinetics 1189, *1189*
duration of untreated psychosis (DUP) 536, 590
and prognosis 1459
and response to treatment 573
Dyadic Adjustment Scale 1165
dynamic child psychotherapy *see* psychodynamic psychotherapy, childhood and adolescence
dynorphin 171, *171*
dysaesthesia, chronic cutaneous 618
dysarthria 53, 1711, 1712
in HIV-associated dementia 384
dysbindin gene 179, 230, 555
dyscalculia 1629–30
Dysexecutive Questionnaire *90*
dysexecutive syndrome
assessment 89, *90*
features *90*
following head injury 390
in parkinsonism 92
in schizophrenia 93
in vascular dementia 379
dysfunctional assumptions 1286
Dysfunctional Attitudes Scale 1165
Dysfunctional Thoughts Record 1309–10, *1309*, 1311
dyskinesias in Huntington's disease 371
dyslexia 1627–9
surface 406
dysmorphophobia *see* body dysmorphic disorder
dysnomia 850
dyspareunia 823

dysphasia 53
  Broca's 1527
  conduction 54
  and delirium 326
  elderly people 1527
  following head injury 391
  nominal 54, 334
  primary motor 54
  primary sensory 54
  Wernicke's 1527
dysphonia 53
dyspraxia
  in Alzheimer's disease 334
  dressing 1527
dysprosody following head injury 391
dysthymia/dysthymic disorder **680–6**, 1060
  aetiology 683–4
  childhood and adolescence 683, 1669, *1670*, 1673
  classification 681
  clinical features 681–2, *682*
  concept of 680
  course and outcome 668, 682–3, *683*
  diagnosis 681–2
  elderly people 1552
  epidemiology 683
  historical perspective 680–1
  and intellectual disability 1855
  interpersonal psychotherapy 1323
  prevention 686
  relationship with major depressive disorder 684, *684*
  treatment 684–6
dystonia
  drug-induced 1222
  psychogenic 1016
dystrobrevin-binding protein-1 555

EAPs (employee assistance programmes) 1281–2
early infantile epileptic encephalopathy 1862
early intervention teams 1459, *1459*
early morning wakening in depression 634, 661–2
early myoclonic epileptic encephalopathy 1862
Eating Attitudes Test (EAT) 777
eating disorder
  atypical 787
  and body image 57
  childhood and adolescence
    atypical 787
    differential diagnosis 1672
    treatment 1784
  classification and diagnosis 106, 800–1, *801*
  cognitive-behaviour therapy 792, 796, 808, 808–9, **1298–303**, 1784
  maintenance 1299
  'not otherwise specified' 800, *801*, 804
  parental, effects on child development 1753–4
  and pregnancy 780, 784, 1118
  relationships between 804
  sleep-related *931*, 947–8
  temporal migration between disorders 801
  see also anorexia nervosa; bulimia nervosa
Eating Disorder Examination 807, 1163
Eating Disorder Inventory 807
eating disorder units 792–3
Ebstein's anomaly 1118, 1169
Echinacea purpurea (echinacea) 1249, *1250*
echo de la pensée 49
echo phenomena 54, 58, *58*
echolalia 54, 58, *58*, 1681, 1713
  in Alzheimer's disease 334
  in autism 1633
  in frontotemporal dementias 346
  in Tourette syndrome 1073
echopraxia 58, *58*
  in Tourette syndrome 1073
eclectic therapy 1278
ECLW Collaborative Study 1144, 1146
ecstasy **494–7**
  addictiveness *431*
  effects on memory 409
  neuropsychological impairment due to 496
  neurotoxicity 496, *496*
  physical effects and complications 495, *495*
  pill testing 494
  preparations and purity 494
  prevalence and patterns of use 494–5
  psychological effects and complications 495–7, *495*, 538
  routes of use 494
ECT *see* electroconvulsive therapy
ectoderm 156
ED *see* erectile dysfunction
Edinburgh Postnatal Depression Scale 1122
education
  higher/further 1815
  and intellectual disability 1873, 1884
  role of the child psychiatrist **1811–16**
  school liaison service 1812–13
  see also schools
education welfare officer 1812
educational psychologist 1812
EDUs (eating disorder units) 792–3
EEG *see* electroencephalography
EER (experimental event rate) 128
efavirenz *1091*
Effective Black Parenting Program 1791
effectiveness 1609
  measurement of 1475
efficacy 1609
effort testing 1055, 1056
ego 294, 306, 313, 849
  defences 297, 310
  structure and functions 295–6, 316
ego ideal 296
ego identity 295
ego psychology 295, 313, 1339
  and mental health social work 1408–9
egocentricity 1777
eicosapentaenoic acid 1248
EIS (early intervention teams) 1459, *1459*
ejaculation 817
  delayed 822
  premature 822, 828
el miedo 984
elation in Alzheimer's disease 335
elderly people
  abuse of 1575–6, *1575*
  adjustment disorders 1552
  agoraphobia 1559
  alcohol intake recommendations 1540
  alcohol use disorders 1519, *1540*, **1540–2**, *1541*
  anxiety 1558–61
  anxiety disorders 1531, 1579
  art therapy 1415
  assessment **1524–9**
    after treatment 1528–9
    common geriatric assessment 1581
    history-taking 1526
    mental state examination 1526–7, *1528*
    physical 1527–9
    setting for 1525–7
  bipolar disorder 1556–7
  boundaries of normality 1574–5
  capacity 1577
  cognitive assessment 1527
  definitions 1579
  deliberate self-harm 1551, **1564–7**
  delirium 1529, **1530–4**
    aetiology 1532, *1532*
    classification 1531
    clinical features 1530–1
    complications 1533
    course and prognosis 1532
    diagnosis 1531
    differential diagnosis 1531, 1559
    epidemiology 1531–2
    prevention 1533
    treatment and management 1532–3
  delusional disorder 1552
  dementia
    differential diagnosis 1558–9
    early detection 1519–20
    epidemiology **1519–22**, 1579–80
    impact 1522
    incidence and risk factors 1520–2, *1520*, *1522*
    presentation in primary care 1483
    see also Alzheimer's disease
  demography 333–4, 1517, *1517*
  dependence 1575–8
  depression **1550–6**
    aetiology *1552*, 1553
    assessment 1527, 1551–2
    clinical features 1551
    in the community 1517
    course and prognosis 1553
    diagnosis 1551–2
    differential diagnosis 373, 1552, 1558
    epidemiology 1517–18, 1552–3, 1579
    factors influencing presentation *1551*
    in hostels and nursing homes 1518
    investigations 1551–2, *1553*
    mortality associated 1553
    prevention 1555–6
    in primary care 1482–3, 1518
    resistant 1555
    treatment and management 674, 1554–5
  driving 1577–8
  dysphasia 1527
  dysthymic disorder 1552
  epilepsy with intellectual disability 1864
  ethical issues 1576–7
  ethnic minorities 1585
  falls 1528–9
  group therapy 1366
  homicide by 1938
  hypomania 1527
  illicit drug use 1544
  indirect self-destructive behaviour 1565
  intellectual disability 1584, 1864
    carers 1880–1
    health needs 1880
    life expectancy 1880
    with psychiatric/behavioural disorders 1858–9

elderly people (*cont.*)
legal issues 1577–8
life events 1559–60
loss of capacity 1575–8
mania 1527, 1556–7
medication use disorders **1543–5**, *1544*
mental health services 1574–5, *1575*, **1579–86**
academic units 1584
CARITAS principles 1580
community services 1582
comprehensive 1581
consultation-liaison services 1583
core business 1581
core components 1581–4, *1582*
day hospitals 1583
inpatient units 1582–3
integrated 1581
long-term care 1583
need for 1579–80
patient-centred 1580–1
planning to commissioning 1584–5
primary care collaborations 1583–4
principles of good service delivery 1580–1
residential care 1583
respite care 1583
special components 1584
mood disorders **1550–8**
neurotic (stress-related) disorder **1558–61**
aetiology 1559–60
clinical features 1558
course and prognosis 1560
diagnosis and differential diagnosis 1558–9
epidemiology 1559
treatment 1560
nicotine use 1544
nutrition 1529
obsessive–compulsive disorder 1558
paranoia **1546–50**, 1559
parasomnias 1572
personality disorders **1561–4**
aetiology 1562–3
clinical features 1561–2
course and prognosis 1563
diagnosis 1562
epidemiology 1518, 1562–3, *1562*
treatment and management 1563–4
pharmacotherapy 1573
dosage regimens 1169
physical illness 1559
in primary care 1482–3, 1518, 1584
prisoners 1584
psychological treatments 1574
psychoses 1518–19
referral process 1524
residential services 1518, 1583
schizoaffective disorder 1552
schizophrenia **1546–50**, 1552
aetiology 1548
classification 1546–7
clinical features 1546
course and prognosis 1548
diagnosis 1547
differential diagnosis 1547, 1559
epidemiology 1547
treatment and management 1548–9
self-esteem 1559
sexuality **1567–70**
sleep disorders 1571–3
substance use disorders 1519, **1540–6**
suicide 976, 1518, 1527, 1551, **1564–7**
thought content 1527
treatment, special features **1571–8**
electrical allergy 997
electroconvulsive therapy (ECT) **1251–60**
body dysmorphic disorder 1047
in childhood and adolescence 1256
choice of 675
in combination with drug therapy 1257
comparison with transcranial magnetic stimulation 1264–5
continuation 1257
contraindications 1252, *1252*, 1257
in elderly people 1555, 1556
future of 1258
indications 1252–5, *1252*
mechanism of action 1257–8
mood disorders 671, 1252–4
origins 1251–2
in pregnancy 1117
risks 404, 1257
schizoaffective disorder 598
schizophrenia 592
stigma attached 1251, 1258
suggested replacements for 1258
treatment
principles 1256–7
process 1256–7
electroencephalography (EEG)
Alzheimer's disease 337
in antisocial behaviour 1918
Creutzfeldt–Jakob disease 353
delirium 328
dementia with Lewy bodies 364
early infantile epileptic encephalopathy 1862
in electroconvulsive therapy 1257
epilepsy 1078, 1862
frontotemporal dementias 347
head injury 389
infantile spasms 1862–3
Lennox–Gastaut syndrome 1863
psychogenic seizures 1864
schizophrenia 563
sleep stages 925
vascular dementia 380
electromyography, sleep stages 925
electro-oculography, sleep stages 925
EMDR *see* eye movement desensitization and reprocessing
emergencies
assessment 68
in childhood and adolescence **1807–11**
emergency cards in attempted suicide 970
emergency workers, debriefing 1110
emics 276
emission 817, 822
emotion
anatomy of **257–62**
and decision-making 260–1
immune modulation 209
and memory 259
and perception 259–60
role of the amygdala 258, 259
emotional development 242–3, *242*
history-taking 1601
emotional lability
following stroke 1071
in multiple sclerosis 1074
in vascular dementia 379
emotional learning 258–9
emotional memory 264
emotional reasoning 1288
emotional stability 850
emotional withdrawal in depression 634
empathogens 495
empathy 47
employee assistance programmes 1281–2
employment
and alcohol use disorders 456
employee assistance programmes 1281–2
supported 1401
empty nest syndrome 1513
encephalitis 1095
herpes 406, 1095
motor sequelae 59
encephalitis lethargica 59
encephalopathy
chronic traumatic 395
early infantile epileptic 1862
early myoclonic epileptic 1862
hepatic 445, 1084–5
mitochondrial 1864, 1865, *1866*
ENCODE project 224
end-stage renal disease 1087
Endicott Work Productivity Scale 1165
endocannabinoids *168*, 172, 429, *429*, 507
endophenotypes 266, 652, 1667
endorphins 170, 429, *429*
engagement techniques in child and adolescent assessment 1604
engrams 250, 253
enkephalins 429, *429*
enmeshment 1371
entactogens 495
entorhinal cortex 146, 152, 180, 251–2, 564, 1537–8
entrainment test in psychogenic tremor 1016
enuresis, nocturnal 1702
environment
factors in attention-deficit hyperactivity disorder 1646
factors in bipolar disorder 1675
factors in child development 1724–8
factors in conduct disorder 1658–9
factors in depression 1675
factors in offending 1913–14
factors in schizophrenia 555–8
host–agent–environment model 1608
interactions with genetic factors 214–18, 221, 229, 315, 558–9, 1608, 1725
envy 307
ependymal cells 157
Epidemiological Catchment Area study 72, 541, 645, 1926, 1937
epidemiology
in childhood and adolescence 1594–9
and classification 1607
contribution to aetiology **280–9**
developmental 1607
and ethnicity 277
genetic 286, 650–1, 1597–8
Goldberg–Huxley model 1480, *1481*
intergenerational 1598
life course 1598
matrix for studies *287*, 288
measurement of symptoms 284–6
and prevention science 1598
in primary care 1480–2, *1481*, *1482*
in public health 1607–8

sampling principles 282–3
specifying disorders 283–4
strategies 286, *287*, 288
study design 282
and transcultural psychiatry 14
uses of 280–1
epigenetics 218, 225
epilepsia partialis continua 1531
epilepsia partialis Kojewnikow 1864, 1867
epilepsy **1076–81**
absence 204, 1077
aetiology 1078, 1619–20
and aggression 1078, 1864, 1929, 1929–30
and Angelman syndrome 1864, 1865
and anxiety 1080
with attention-deficit hyperactivity disorder 1650
aura 60, 1077
and autism 1852
automatism 403, 1077
benign focal 1618
in childhood and adolescence
aetiology 1619–20
classification 1619
clinical features 1618–19
course and prognosis 1618–19, 1620
diagnosis 1619
differential diagnosis 1619
epidemiology 1619
with intellectual disability *1861*, *1863*, 1864
management 1620
prevention 1620
psychiatric disorder associated 1740
salient non-epileptic episodes *1861*
classification 1076–7, 1619, 1862–4, *1863*
cognitive assessment 92
and conversion disorder 1015
and crime 1079–80
definition 1860–1
and depersonalization 775
and depression 1080
diagnosis 1078, 1619, 1861–2
differential diagnosis 538, 1078, 1619, 1861–2, *1862*
and Down syndrome 1864, 1865
elderly people with intellectual disability 1864
epidemiology 1078, 1619
experimental
kindling 204
tetanus toxin model 204
and fragile-X syndrome 1864, 1865
frontal-lobe
behavioural abnormalities associated 1864
in childhood and adolescence 1618
and gamma rhythms 203
generalized 1077
genetics 159, 1620
ictus 1077
imaging 1078, 1862, 1930
in infancy 1861
and intellectual disability 92, 1828
in adults and elderly people 1864
aetiology and pathogenesis 1865–6, *1865*, *1866*
behavioural disorders 1864
in childhood and adolescence *1863*, 1864
diagnosis 1861–2
differential diagnosis 1861–2, *1863*
epidemiology 1864–5
in infancy 1861, 1862–4, *1863*
prognosis 1868
treatment 1866–8, *1867*
and memory 92
myoclonic
in childhood and adolescence 1864
in infancy 1863
with ragged red fibres 1865, *1866*
myoclonic–astatic 1863–4
and neuronal networks 201, 203–4
nocturnal seizures 1702
Northern 1864, *1866*
and offending 1079–80, 1920, 1929–31
partial 1077
and personality disorder 1079
pharmacotherapy **1231–40**
in intellectual disability 1866–7, *1867*
post-traumatic 394
prevention 1620
prodrome 1077
progressive myoclonus 1864
progressive partial 1864
psychiatric consequences 1078–80
psychosis
chronic interictal 1079
postictal 1079
and Rett's syndrome 1864, 1864–5
and schizophrenia 1079
and sexual function 1079
and sleep-wake disorders *932*
and social development 1079
and suicide 1080
syndromes 1077–8, 1861
temporal lobe (limbic) 59, 201, 1077
behavioural abnormalities associated 1864
in childhood and adolescence 1618
differential diagnosis 866
effects on learning and memory 204
and personality traits 1930
and transient global amnesia 403
treatment and management 1080, 1620
in tuberous sclerosis 1075
epistasis 229
EPQ-R (Eysenck Personality Questionnaire) 81, *81*, 286, 850
Epstein–Barr virus
and chronic fatigue syndrome 1038
and hypersomnia 942
and infectious mononucleosis 1095
Epworth sleepiness scale 938–9
erectile dysfunction (ED) 822
in dementia 416
in elderly people 1569
medical intervention 821
pharmacotherapy 821, 828
in physical illness 826
see also sexual dysfunction
ergot 487
Eriksen Flanker paradigm 265
erotomania 621–2, 1920
error (*e*) 85
error catastrophe 1507
errorless learning 423–4
escitalopram *670*
adverse effects *1191*
in body dysmorphic disorder 1046
in cancer *1102*, *1103*
in depression in elderly people 1554, *1554*
dosage *1196*
in obsessive–compulsive disorder *1687*
in panic disorder *756*
pharmacodynamics 1186, *1187*
pharmacokinetics 1188–9, *1189*
in social anxiety disorder 743
ESEMed Study 1433
Esquirol, Jean-Etienne Dominique 18
estavudine 1092
eszopiclone *1102*, 1179, 1182–3
ethambutol 1094
ether 503
ethics and ethical issues **28–32**
anorexia nervosa 796
care ethics 31
codes of 30–1
in cognitive-behaviour therapy in childhood and adolescence 1778–9
in community mental health services 1457–8
and diagnosis 28–9
expert witnesses 2004–5, *2005*
factitious disorder 1053–4
malingering 1058
in management 40–1
in management of sexual dysfunction 830
and neurosurgery for mental disorder 1267–8
old age psychiatry 1576–7
in prevention of intellectual disability 1835
principle-based 31
sexual offences 1964
and treatment 29–30
and values 32–3
Ethiopia, attitudes to psychiatric disorder 6
ethnic cleansing 1495
ethnic conflict 1494
see also refugees
ethnic minorities
adoption outcomes 1750–1
alcohol use disorders 464
care pathways 1439, 1440–1
caregiver-mediated interventions 1791
criminal victimization 1987
culturally informed services for 277
effects of a child with intellectual disability 1884
elderly people 1585
intellectual disability 1879–80, 1881
mental health services 277, **1502–4**
schizophrenia 549, 557–8
voluntary organizations supporting 1491–2
ethnographic database *277*
ethnography 275–6, *277*
ethosuxumide *1867*
etifoxine in adjustment disorders 721
euphoria 55
in multiple sclerosis 1074
European Consultation-Liaison Workgroup Collaborative Study 1144, 1146
European Convention on Human Rights 1899, 1900, 1904, 2015
European Declaration for Mental Health 1427
evening primrose oil 1249, *1250*
event rate 128
event sampling 97
evidence-based medicine **122–8**, 578
appraisal of evidence 126, *126*, *127*
and clinical practice guidelines 123, 124
and current awareness 124–5, *125*
evidence hierarchy 123, *1465*
finding evidence 123–6, *125*

evidence-based medicine (*cont.*)
formulating a structured clinical question 122–3
stages *122*
and study design *123*
and systematic reviews 123–4
types of clinical question *123*
use of electronic communication and the Internet 124
using research findings with individual patients 126–8
and values-based practice 33
Evidence-Based Mental Health 125, *125*
evoked potentials in schizophrenia 563
EWO (education welfare officer) 1812
exaggeration *see* malingering
exalted stage 58
excellence, concepts of 43–4, *44*
exclusion criteria 100
excoriation, neurotic/psychogenic 618, **917–18**, 1044
executive control systems 248–9, *248*
executive function 262
assessment 89, *90*, 265
and attention-deficit hyperactivity disorder 1647
exercise
and anorexia nervosa 782
in chronic fatigue syndrome 1040, 1042
in dementia *414*
in depression in elderly people 1555
excessive, in bulimia nervosa 803
and health 1136
in insomnia 935
in persistent somatoform pain disorder 1034
exhibitionism 832, *833*, *836*, 1960, 1961
exons 224
expanded trinucleotide repeat sequences 652
experimental event rate 128
expert opinion 75
expert witness 1112, 1901, **2003–8**
accreditation 2004
common knowledge rule 2003
and confidentiality 2006–7
Court appearance 2007
dual role 2004–5, *2005*
ethical issues 2004–5, *2005*
immunity from suit 2003
regulatory rules 2004, *2004*
reliability 2004
reports 1928, *2004*, **2005–6**
and risk assessment 2005
explanation, personal and subpersonal levels 135
explanatory gap 135, 278
explanatory models 278
explanatory therapy in hypochondriasis 1026
exposure 55, 1668
in anxiety disorders 1294–5
in body dysmorphic disorder 1047
graded 1779
imaginal 742, 746, 1295
in vivo 742, 746
interoceptive 761
in panic disorder 758, 760–1
in post-traumatic stress disorder 708, 1295
social anxiety disorder 742
in specific phobia 746
virtual reality 746
exposure and response prevention in tic disorders 1687
expressed emotion and schizophrenia 575, 583
expression 213
expressive/exploratory psychotherapy *see* psychoanalytic psychotherapy
expressive language disorder 1625–6
extinction 250, 254, 1668
extradural haemorrhage 387
extraversion 81, *81*, 632, 633, 654, 850, 886
eye, development 157
eye movement abnormalities in schizophrenia 563
eye movement desensitization and reprocessing (EMDR) 1497
adjustment disorders 720
in childhood trauma 1730
delusional disorder 1920
following accidents 1109, 1111
post-traumatic stress disorder 709
Eysenck, Hans 1158
Eysenck Personality Questionnaire 81, *81*, 286, 850

fabricated or induced illness 1054, 1697, 1737, 1923–4
facial erythema in alcohol use disorders 446
factitious disorder 994, **1049–54**, 1941
aetiology 1051
classification 106, 1050
clinical features 1049–50
cognitive-behavioural conceptualization 1051, *1052*
course 1051
diagnosis 1050
diagnostic criteria 1049
diagnostic problems 1049
differential diagnosis 1003, 1012, *1012*, 1050–1
electronic 1050
epidemiology 998, 1051
ethical and legal issues 1053–4
in health care workers 1054
induced 1054, 1697, 1737, 1923–4
obstetric 1050, 1118
and pathological lying 1049
prognosis 1051
subtypes 1050
and surgery 1096
treatment and management 1052–4
Fahr's syndrome 373
fail, right to 1408
Fairbairn, W.R.D. 308
Faith Links project 1411
falls, elderly people 1528–9
false attribution 1054
false memories 59, 250, 403, 408, **713–16**
false-self–real-self distinction 309
familial schizotypal disorder 599
familicide 1923
Families and Schools Together Track programme 1663, 1789
family
assessment 1382–3, 1384–6
and borderline personality disorder 896
burdens on 1401
caregiver-mediated interventions **1787–93**
changes in patterns of 1726–7
and child neglect 1736
and child physical abuse 1735
and child sexual abuse 1733
and conduct disorder
factors in 1659–60
impact of disorder 1655–6
involvement in management 1663
criminal activity by 1659, 1911–12
and cultural variation in care pathways 1439
as decision-makers 1895
disruption 1910–11
effects of alcohol use disorders 452–3, 465
effects of child with intellectual disability **1883–6**
effects of child with physical illness 1742
effects of childhood and adolescent sleep disorders 1694–5
effects of dementia 417–18
effects of Huntington's disease 374
effects of personality change following head injury 391
factors affecting child mental health 1725–7
factors in anorexia nervosa 780
factors in offending 1910–12
factors in schizophrenia 536, 548–9, 553–5
in gender identity disorder 844
history 215, 1601
impact of caring on 1465
involvement in management of somatization disorder 1009
involvement in rehabilitation of delirium 1533
large 1912
nontraditional configurations 1787
reaction to illness 1066
of refugees 1497
role in treatment of intellectual disability 1873
single-parent 1369–70, 1601, 1726–7, 1910, 1911
step-families 1370, 1726–7
suicide 981–2
Family-Check-Up 1790
family crisis intervention 1382
family focused treatment 1677
family intervention 1401
family interview 1386
family life cycle 1373–4
family-mediated interventions *see* caregiver-mediated interventions
family myths 1066
family studies **215**
anxiety disorders 1667
intermittent explosive disorder 912
kleptomania 913
mood disorders 651
trichotillomania 915
family support teams 1411
family therapy **1380–91**
adjustment disorders *1069*
anorexia nervosa 790–2, *790*, 796
assessment in 1384–6
in attempted suicide 1707
bipolar disorder 673
in childhood trauma 1730
conduct disorder 1661–2, 1782
conjoint 790–1
contraindications 1383
course 1386
elderly people 1574
historical context 1380–1
indications 1382–3
Milan approach 1381, 1387
persistent somatoform pain disorder 1034

family therapy (*cont.*)
  post-modern developments 1381–2
  problems encountered in 1388
  psychoanalytic and related approaches 1381
  psycho-educational approach 1382
  research 1388–9
  role of the therapist 1386–7
  schizophrenia 583–4
  separated 790–1
  systems-oriented 1381, 1381–2
  termination 1387–8
  training in 1389–90
  transgenerational 1381
family tree 1381, 1384, *1384*
famine oedema 785
fantasy (gamma hydroxy butyrate) 409, **498–9**
fantasy thinking 50
FAS *see* foetal alcohol syndrome
FASD (foetal alcohol spectrum disorder) 1614–15, 1841
FAST (Functional Assessment Staging) scale 335, 337
'Fast Track' programme 1598, 1663, 1789
fatigue
  differentiation from chronic fatigue syndrome 1037
  in physical illness 209, *210*
  as a symptom 1035–6
  see also chronic fatigue syndrome
FCU (Family-Check-Up) 1790
fear
  definition 1664
  pathophysiology 1666–7, *1667*
  pathways *732*
fear conditioning paradigm 1666
'fear of fatness' 783
FEAR plan 1779
feeling states, neurobiology of 260–1
feelings, definition 260
Feighner criteria 100
Ferenczi, Sandór 1338
fertility and schizophrenia 545
fetishism *833*, *836*
FFT (family focused treatment) 1677
fibroblast growth factor (FGF) 156
fibromyalgia 990, 997, 1003, 1037
  and cortisol 1039
  treatment and management 1034
fight response following an accident 1107
FII (induced factitious disorder) 1054, 1697, 1737, 1923–4
filicide 1125, 1923
Finnish disease heritage 1831
fire-raising/fire-setting *see* arson; pyromania
fire sickness (*hwabyung*) 984
5p-syndrome *see* cri-du-chat syndrome
fixations 297
flashbacks
  cannabis 508
  in hallucinogen persisting perception disorder 488
  in post-traumatic stress disorder 404, 701
FLD *see* frontal lobe degeneration of non-Alzheimer type
flesinoxan 735
flexibilitas cerea 58, *58*
flight of ideas 53
  slow 1527
flight response following an accident 1106
flooding in panic disorder 761
floppy infant syndrome 1117
fluency disorders 53, 1623, 1712
flumazenil 1172, 1176, 1180
flunarizine 1201
flunitrazepam 409, 491, 1178, 1183
fluoxetine
  adverse effects 1173, *1191*
  in body dysmorphic disorder 1046
  in bulimia nervosa 807
  in cancer *1102*, *1103*
  in childhood and adolescence 1676
  and cosmetic psychopharmacology 29
  delayed onset of effects 176
  in depression *670*
    continuation treatment 671
    in elderly people 1554, *1554*
  dosage 674, *1196*
  drug interactions 1233
  in intellectual disability 1875
  in obsessive–compulsive disorder 769, *1687*
  in panic disorder *756*
  in personality disorders *905*
  pharmacodynamics *1173*, *1187*
  pharmacokinetics *1172*, 1188, *1189*
  in pregnancy 1117
  in selective mutism 1714
  in social anxiety disorder 743
flupenthixol
  in attempted suicide 971
  pharmacokinetics *1172*
fluphenazine *1209*
  administration *1214*
  adverse effects *1212*, 1222
  in intellectual disability 1875
  pharmacodynamics *1211*
flurazepam *1172*, 1179
fluvoxamine *670*
  adverse effects *1191*
  in body dysmorphic disorder 1046
  in depression in elderly people *1554*
  dosage *1196*
  drug interactions 1175
  in intellectual disability 1875
  in obsessive–compulsive disorder 769, *1687*
  in panic disorder *756*
  in personality disorders *905*
  pharmacodynamics *1173*, *1187*
  pharmacokinetics *1172*, 1189, *1189*
  in social anxiety disorder 743
  in Wernicke–Korsakoff syndrome 409
fMRI *see* functional magnetic resonance imaging
focal conflict theory 1357
focal psychotherapy 1327, 1330–1, *1331*
foetal alcohol spectrum disorder 1614–15, 1841
foetal alcohol syndrome (FAS) 445, 1117, 1754
  aetiology 1615
  behavioural phenotype 1615
  classification 1841
  clinical features 1614–15, 1646, 1841
  epidemiology 1615
  natural history 1615
  neurological and behavioural aspects 1841
  prevalence 1826, 1841
  prevention 1448
  treatment and management 1615
foetal valproate syndrome 1118
foetus
  abuse of 1117
  adverse environment 659, 1725
  death *in utero* 1119
  effects of maternal alcohol use *see* foetal alcohol syndrome
  effects of maternal substance use 480, *480*, 1117–18, 1614, 1615–16
  mother–foetus relationship 1117
  prenatal diagnosis of intellectual disability 1833–4
folic acid deficiency 1087–8
folie à deux 610, **624–5**
folk healing practices **1418–22**
follicle-stimulating hormone in anorexia nervosa 783
follow-back studies 556–7, 568
food avoidance emotional disorder 787
food diary *802*
food fads 787
food intake history in anorexia nervosa 782
food refusal 787
forced choice testing 94, 1057
forebrain 156–7
forensic mental health services 2013, **2015–21**
  capacity planning 2017–18
  community 1459
  international context 2016
  philosophy and theoretical models 2015–16
  private 2017
  pyramid planning 2017
  security 2015, 2016–17
  service structure 2017–18
  service users 2018–20
  super-specialist 2017
foresight 80, *80*, 82, 83
formal thought disorder 52
formulation 68, 73–4
  cultural 278
  in psychoanalysis 1341–2
fornix 155–6
fortune-telling 1420
foscarnet *1091*
fosphenytoin in status epilepticus 1867
foster care 1787, 1790, 1800, 1801
  effects on child and adult mental health **1747–52**
  forensic/multidimensional treatment 1790, 1953
  long-term 1749–50
  short-term 1748–9
  treatment 1662
Foulkes, S.H. 1353, 1357
14-3-3 protein 353
fourth ventricle 157
fragile X-associated tremor ataxia syndrome *228*
fragile-X syndrome
  and autism 1635
  behavioural phenotype 1613, 1614, 1840, *1851*, 1858
  effects on the family 1884
  and epilepsy 1864, 1865
  genetics 212, 213, 228, *228*, 1832, 1839–40, 1865, *1866*
  physical characteristics 1840
  prevalence 1839–40
  psychiatric aspects 1840
fragile-XE syndrome *228*
FRAMES 450, *450*
framing effect 261

France
CANTOUs 1583
community mental health teams 1454
and dual-drive theory 302
history of psychiatry 17, 19, 20, 22, 23, 24, 26, 603, 630, 848
involuntary admission in 1440
legal aspects 1901, 1902
prion disease 355, 357
fraud 1941
free association 293–4, 297, 1328, 1770
free-floating discussion 1357, 1360, 1363
free radicals, role in ageing 1509
freeze response following an accident 1106
Frégoli syndrome 623
Freud, Anna 310, 1683, 1770
Freud, Sigmund 20–1, 293, 1337, 1770
dual-drive theory 294, 295, 302, 306
models of personality 849
and neurasthenia 1060
and obsessional neurosis 768
and obsessive–compulsive phenomena 1683
and panic disorder 751
and psychodynamic psychiatry 313
and psychosexual development 235
structural theory 294–6
theories on suicide 954
theory of the mental apparatus 293–4
therapeutic technique 1338
topographic theory 294
Freudian slips 313
Friedrich ataxia *228*
friendliness 886, 888
FRIENDS programme 1780
Fromm, Eric 311
Fromm-Reichmann, Freida 310
frontal eye field 245
frontal leucotomy 1267
frontal lobe degeneration of non-Alzheimer type (FLD) 344
aetiology 348
age at onset 345
clinical features 345–6
investigations 347
frontal-lobe syndrome 89
frontal lobes
and aggressive/antisocial behaviour 1917–18
in alcohol use disorders *183*
anatomy 145–6, *145*
association connections *145*, 153
lesions 265, 1917–18
in schizophrenia *178*
frontotemporal lobar degeneration (FTLD) 344, *344*
classification 344, *344*
epidemiology 345
physical signs 346
ubiquitinated 344
frotteurism 832, *833*, *836*
FTD *see* dementia, frontotemporal
FTDP-17 344–5, 346, 348
FTLD *see* frontotemporal lobar degeneration
fugue states 57, 404–5
functional analysis 96
Functional Assessment Staging scale 335, 337
functional disorders 990
functional family therapy 1661, 1782
functional magnetic resonance imaging (fMRI) **196–201**
alcohol-related dementia 401
Alzheimer's disease 337
anxiety disorders in childhood and adolescence 1668
artefacts 197–8
cerebral activation and blood-flow changes 197
comparison with PET and SPET 186–7, 196–7
data analysis 199–201
activation mapping 200, Plate 10
movement estimation and correction 199
multivariate approaches 200
statistical models for the neurovascular response 199–200
visualization 201, Plate 11
within- and between-group 200–1
depression 660
and emotions 257–8
endogenous contrast agents 197
epilepsy 1862
experimental design 198–9
blocked periodic design 198, *199*
event-related design 199
parametric design 199
hardware 198
imaging sequences 197
echoplanar imaging 197
gradient echo sequence 197
intermittent explosive disorder 912
in pathological lying 1049, 1051
schizophrenia 562–3
functional neuroimaging
and aggressive/antisocial behaviour 1918
alcohol-related brain damage 401
anorexia nervosa 781
attention-deficit hyperactivity disorder 1647
conversion disorder 1013
and emotion 257–8, 260, 261
epilepsy 1078, 1079
post-traumatic stress disorder 706–7
schizophrenia 562–3
with violence 1919
see also specific techniques
functionalism 134
challenges to 134–5
fusion of thought 53

G (gamma hydroxy butyrate) 409, **498–9**
G protein-coupled receptors 172, *173*, 174, *175*, 202, 1171
regulation 175
G-proteins 174–5, 473, 1201
'G spot' 818
G72 gene 555
GABA 148, 155, 429
and body dysmorphic disorder 1046
effects of valproate on 1231
and epilepsy 1619, 1865
hippocampus 202
in opioid neurobiology 473
in panic disorder 754
role in neurodevelopment 159
and schizophrenia 562
in substance use disorders *429*
transporters 169, *170*
GABA receptors 1171
action of benzodiazepines at 1171, 1179
in generalized anxiety disorder 733, *734*
hippocampal 202
ligand-gated ion channels *173*, 174
gabapentin 1237
drug interactions 1866
pharmacokinetics *1867*
in social anxiety disorder 743
Gabitril (tiagabine) 1237, *1867*
gaboxadol 1183
GAD *see* generalized anxiety disorder
GAF (Global Assessment of Functioning scale) 73, 1165, 1593
gait abnormalities 57
galanin 171, *171*
receptors *173*
galantamine
in Alzheimer's disease 409, 1241
in vascular dementia 381
Gamblers Anonymous 922, 1352
gambling, pathological **919–23**
addictiveness *431*
aetiology 920–1
classification 920
clinical features 920
course and prognosis 922
diagnosis 920
epidemiology 920–1
impulsive 920
neurotic 920
predisposing factors 921–2
prevention 923
psychopathic 920
subcultural 920
symptomatic 920
treatment and management 922
γ-aminobutyric acid *see* GABA
gamma butyl-lactone 498
gamma hydroxy butyrate 409, **498–9**
γ-linolenic acid 1248, 1249
gamma rhythms 203
ganciclovir 1092
ganoderic acid 1063
Ganoderma lucidum 1063
Ganser syndrome 1049, 1055
Gastaut–Geschwind syndrome 1930
gastroesophageal reflux *932*, 1084
gastrointestinal disorders 1083–4
in rapid refeeding 786
and sleep-wake disorders *932*
Gaucher disease type 3 1865
GBH (gamma hydroxy butyrate) 409, **498–9**
GBL (gamma butyl-lactone) 498
GDS *see* Geriatric Depression Scale; Global Deterioration Scale
Gedankenlautwerden 49
gender
and anorexia nervosa 778
and anxiety disorders 1666
and attention-deficit hyperactivity disorder 1646, 1828
and autism 1828
and body dysmorphic disorder 1045
and childhood OCD and tics 1681
and conduct disorder 1655, 1658
and deliberate self-harm 959
by elderly people 1565
and hypochondriasis 997
and mood disorders 271, 648, 653–4
and offending 1909
and prevalence of somatization disorders 996
and psychiatric disorder in intellectual disability 1828

and schizophrenia 544–5
and social anxiety disorder 741
and specific phobia 745
and suicide 1704
gender identity 57
gender identity disorder 57, 106, **842–6**
childhood and adolescence **1718–23**
aetiology 1719–20
assessment 1721
clinical features 1718–19
epidemiology 1718
longitudinal studies 1720–1
and mental disorder 1721
treatment 1721–2
diagnosis 842
epidemiology 842
and homosexuality 1720
legal issues 845
origins 842–3
patient subgroups 844
Real Life Experience 843, 844
treatment and management 843–4
validity 845
General Health Questionnaire 69, 283, 284
general hospitals
liaison visits to 1525
organization of psychiatric services **1144–8**
'general neurotic syndrome' 682
general paresis (of the insane) 1093
general practitioners (GPs)
ability to detect psychiatric morbidity 1482
education regarding suicide risks 974
expectations of psychiatrists 1486–7
training in psychiatry 1487–8
generalizability theory 92
generalized anxiety disorder (GAD) **729–39**
aetiology 732–5, *732*, *733*, *734*
in childhood and adolescence 1664
clinical presentation 1665
outcome 1666
prevalence 1666
clinical features 729
cognitive content 1286–7
comorbidity 731, *731*, 736
course and prognosis 735
and depression 731
diagnosis 729–30, *730*
differential diagnosis 730–1, *730*, 741, 752, 1004, 1024
epidemiology 731
following stroke 1071
genetics 732
and life events 735
and neurasthenia 1063
treatment and management 735–7
validity of disorder 731
vulnerability to 734–5
generation 1513
genetic counselling 1281
Alzheimer's disease 340
dementia 411
Huntington's disease 374–5
in intellectual disability 1825, 1884
genetic epidemiology 286, 650–1, 1597–8
genetic tagging 231
genetic testing
dementia 411, *412*
Huntington's disease 374–5
genetics
and ageing 1507–8
analysis methods 216–17
candidate genes 220–1, 651
components of phenotypic variation 214
continuous traits 213, *213*
and epidemiology 286, 650–1, 1597–8
functional analysis 230–2
gene association studies 220–1, *220*, 226–7, 230, 651
gene copy-number variants 230
gene–environment correlation 214
gene–environment interactions (GXE) 214–18, 221, 229, 315, 558–9, 1608, 1725
gene expression control errors 1508
gene expression regulation 218, 223–6, *224*
gene interactions (epistasis) 229
gene mapping 218, 226–7
gene mutations 1508, 1831–2
Mendelian 227–9
mis-sense 227
non-sense 227
point 227–8
and psychiatric disorders 227–9, *228*
triplet repeats 228, *228*
genome organization 223
genotyping 226
and intellectual disability 1831–2, *1831*, 1838
with behavioural/psychiatric disorder 1858
and life expectancy 1507
linkage analysis 218–20, *218*, 227, 230, 651
markers 218, 226
Mendel's laws 212
model fitting 217
molecular **222–33**, 286
multiple regression analysis 217
neurodevelopmental disorders 159
neurogenetic syndromes 1613–14
non-additive genetic effects 214
nucleic acid structure and function 223
path analysis 217, *217*
patterns of inheritance 212–13, *213*
and personality traits 886–8, 888–9, *890*
polymorphism 218
psychiatric–behavioural 1597–8
psychiatric disorders
in childhood and adolescence 1590
complex 229–30
Mendelian/single-gene 212–13, 213, 227–9, *228*
quantitative **212–22**
research methods 215–16
whole genome association (WGA) studies 221, 229–30
specific disorders
alcohol use disorders 434–6
Alzheimer's disease 227, 339, 1521
Angelman syndrome 213, 224, 229, 1841, 1865, *1866*
anxiety disorders 1667
attention-deficit hyperactivity disorder 1590, 1646
autism 1635–6
body dysmorphic disorder 1046
chronic fatigue syndrome 1038
Coffin–Lowry syndrome 1842
conduct disorder 1658
cri-du-chat syndrome 1842
de Lange syndrome 1842
delusional disorder 614
dementia with Lewy bodies 365
Down syndrome 228, 1831, 1838–9
Duchenne muscular dystrophy 1843
eating disorders 781–2, 806
epilepsy 159, 1620
fragile-X syndrome 212, 213, 228, *228*, 1832, 1839–40, 1865, *1866*
frontotemporal dementias 348
generalized anxiety disorder 732
Huntington's disease 372
hypochondriasis 1024
Klinefelter syndrome 1840
Lesch–Nyhan syndrome 1843
mood disorders 648, **650–8**, 658
mucopolysaccharidoses 1843
neurofibromatosis type 1 1843, *1866*
obsessive–compulsive disorder 768, 1684
offending 1918
panic disorder 753–4
phenylketonuria 212, 214, 1844
post-traumatic stress disorder 707
Prader–Willi syndrome 213, 224, 229, 1844
Rett's syndrome 224, 229, 1637, 1844, *1866*
Rubinstein–Taybi syndrome 1845
schizophrenia 547, 548–9, 553–5, 565–6, *565*
Smith–Lemli–Opitz syndrome 1845
Smith–Magenis syndrome 1845
smoking addiction/nicotine dependence 510–11
substance use disorders 428–9
suicide 954–5, 966–7
tic disorders 229, 1073, 1684
tuberous sclerosis 1075, 1845, *1866*
Turner syndrome 224, 1840
velo-cardio-facial syndrome 1846
Williams syndrome 1846
X-linked intellectual disability 1839
XXX syndrome 1841
XYY syndrome 1841
genital herpes 1094
genital-retraction anxiety disorder (*koro*) 606, 779, 979, **980–1**
genogram 1381, 1384, *1384*
genome organization 223
genotype 212, 226
genotyping 226
gentamicin *1091*
geophagia 1116
gepirone 735
Geriatric Depression Scale 719, 1551, *1552*
German chamomile 1248
Gerstmann–Straussler(–Scheinker) syndrome 351, 356–7
Gestalt therapy 1277
gestational substance use 480, *480*, 1117–18, 1614, 1615–16, 1754
GHB (gamma hydroxy butyrate) 409, **498–9**
GHQ (General Health Questionnaire) 69, 283, 284
GHQ-12 284
GHRF (growth hormone-releasing factor) 165, *171*
Gillick Rules 1899
Ginkgo biloba
adverse effects 1248
as cognitive enhancer 1247–8
drug interactions *1250*
in neurasthenia 1063
ginseng see Panax ginseng
GIPs (GPCR-interacting proteins) 175
give way weakness in conversion disorder 1016

Glasgow Coma Scale 388, *388*
glioblasts 157
gliosis in schizophrenia 180–1, *180*, *181*
Global Assessment of Functioning scale 73, 1165, 1593
global burden of disease 645
alcohol use disorders 10, 467
mental disorder 10–11, 1428, 1606
in childhood and adolescence 1595–6
mood disorders 645, 1185
smoking 510
Global Deterioration Scale 1535
globus pallidus 154, 155, 1684
glove and stocking anaesthesia 57
glutamate 429
and epilepsy 1619, 1865
hippocampus 202
ligand-gated ion channels 172, *173*, 174
in obsessive–compulsive disorder 1684
in opioid neurobiology 473
role in neurodevelopment 159
and schizophrenia 562
in substance use disorders *429*
transporters 170, *170*
glutamate receptors, hippocampal 202
Glyccirhiza glabra 1249
Glycine max 1249
glycine receptors 1171
glycine transporters 169–70, *170*
glycosylation (glycation) of proteins 1508–9
GNP and population mental well-being 1428
GnRH (gonadotrophin-releasing hormone) 162, 165
GnRH analogs in the paraphilias 838
Go-No-Go tasks 266
Goldberg–Huxley model 1480, *1481*
gonadotrophin-releasing hormone 162, 165
good-enough mother 309
goserelin 1964
GPCR-interacting proteins 175
GPCR kinases 175
GPs *see* general practitioners
graded activity in adjustment disorders *1069*
Graded Naming Test 89, 266
graduate mental health workers 1485
grandiose delusions 51
grandparenting
effects of a grandchild with intellectual disability 1884
roles 1514
transition to 1513–14
green (ketamine) 489, **499–500**, 1186
grief
after diagnosis of intellectual disability in a child 1883
after infant loss 725, 1119–20
assessment and management 726–7
counselling in 726–7, 1279
normal 725
traumatic 725, 1985
see also bereavement
Griffiths Developmental Scale 1821
grimacing *58*
grooming 1961, 1962
gross national product and population mental well-being 1428
group-analytic group therapy 1351, 1353, 1355, 1357–8, *1357*, *1358*
group-as-a-whole 1353
group homes 1454
group matching 1468
group therapy **1350–69**
activity 1351–2
antisocial personality disorder 898
basic methods 1351–3
bipolar disorder 673
borderline personality disorder 895, 1364–5
boundary events 1363
brief 1366
childhood and adolescence 1768
chronic mental disorder 1364
cognitive-behavioural 742, 744
curative factors 1355, *1356*
domestic violence perpetrators 1982–3
elderly people 1366
fostering therapeutic norms 1363
group-analytic 1351, 1353, 1355, 1357–8, *1357*, *1358*
group development theory 1358–60
historical aspects 1353–4
homogeneous/heterogeneous groups 1362
hypochondriasis 1027
interpersonal 1351, 1355, *1356*
intervention guidelines 1363, **1363**
language of the group 1360
leadership 1350–1, 1360–2
multiple family 1382, 1389
with offenders/prisoners 1365
optimal/sub-optimal size 1363
organizing principles *1353*
outpatient 1364, **1365**
in the paraphilias 838, 839
in physical illness 1364
problem-solving 1351, 1352
psychoanalytic 1351
psychodynamic 1352–3, 1354–8
psychoeducational 1351, 1352, 1364
research and evaluation 1366
schizophrenia 1364
selection and composition 1362, *1362*
service planning 1366–7
setting 1364
short-term dynamic 1351
smoking cessation 512
supportive 1352
systems-centred 1351
Tavistock 1351, 1355–7, *1356*
therapeutic goals 1350, *1351*
therapist 1354, *1354*
with trauma victims 1365
'growing pains' 1695
growth
arrested in anorexia nervosa 787
drug-induced retardation 1795
growth hormone 164–5
and immune function 206
and sleep 1695
and the sleep–wake cycle 925
growth hormone-inhibiting hormone 165
growth hormone-releasing factor 165, *171*
GSS (Gerstmann–Straussler–Scheinker syndrome) 351, 356–7
guanfacine 1651, 1688
guanine 223
guanylate cyclase 176
guardianship 29–30, 1895, 1898
guided imagery and recovered memories 715
Guillain–Barré syndrome 942
guilt
delusions of 51
and depression 634
unconscious 294
gynaecological conditions **1114–16**

HAART in HIV-associated dementia 385
habit reversal
in body dysmorphic disorder 1047
in tic disorders 1687
Hachinski Ischaemia Score 379, *379*
HADS (Hospital Anxiety and Depression Scale) 1486
haematological disorders 1087–8
haemodialysis 1087, 1139
haemoglobin 197
Halban's fascia 818
halitosis, delusions of 618–19
Hallowell, Irving 276
hallucinations 49
aetiological theories 50
after infant loss 1120
in alcohol withdrawal 443, 538
in Alzheimer's disease 335
associated with simple partial seizures 1864
auditory 49
cognitive-behaviour therapy 1314, 1317
transcranial magnetic stimulation therapy 1265
bodily/tactile/coenaesthetic 50
in delirium 327
in delusional disorder 609, 610, 613, 615
in dementia with Lewy bodies 335, 361
and depression 641
differential diagnosis of cause 537
and disinhibition 50
following head injury 392
in frontotemporal dementias 346
gustatory 50
hypnagogic 50, 940, 1702
hypnopompic 940, 1702
mood-congruent/-incongruent 537, 641
olfactory 50
and overstimulation 50
in Parkinson's disease 1072
phencyclidine-induced 487
and psychodynamic psychiatry 315–16
in schizophrenia 527, 573–4
somatic 1030
visual 49–50
hallucinogen persisting perception disorder 488–9
hallucinogenic mushrooms 488
hallucinogens **487–9**
acute effects 488
addictiveness *431*
adverse effects 488–9
botanical 488
epidemiology of abuse 488
human experimentation with 489
preparations 488
hallucinosis, alcoholic 443, 538
haloperidol 1209, *1209*
administration 1213, *1214*
adverse effects *1212*, 1222
in alcohol withdrawal 449–50
in autism 1875
in cancer *1104*
in children and adolescents with psychiatric/behaviour disorder and intellectual disability 1852
in delirium 331, 1533

in dementia 414
in elderly people 1556
in Huntington's disease 374
in personality disorders 600, *905*, 906
pharmacodynamics *1211*, 1212
pharmacokinetics *1172*
in postoperative delirium 1099
in schizophrenia 586
in tic disorders 1073, 1688
Hamilton Anxiety Rating Scale 1164
Hamilton's Rating Scale for Depression 69, 70, 634, 1163, 1164
hand use preference and gender identity disorder 843
handicap
adjustment to **1065–71**
definition 389
HapMap (International Haplotype Map) 222, 227
'happy puppet' syndrome *see* Angelman syndrome
Hardy–Weinberg equilibrium 213, 226
Hare Psychopathy Checklist 835
harm-avoidance 79–80, *80*, 316, *316*, 849
'harmful dysfunction' concept 28
harmine 501
Harvard Trauma Questionnaire 1497
hashish *see* cannabis
hate crimes 1987
Hayling Test *90*
HCR-20 (Historical Clinical Risk-20) 1927, 1994, 1997, 1998, 2018
head-banging 1601
head injury **387–99**
agitation and aggression following 393, 396, 1929
and alcohol use disorders 393–4
amnesia following 404, 407
and attention-deficit hyperactivity disorder 1646
and boxing 395
and capacity 397
in childhood and adolescence 394–5, 1616–18
closed 387–8, 394, 1617
cognitive impairment following 390–1, *395*
and delusional disorder 614
and depression 92
differential diagnosis 695
early symptoms 392
epidemiology 388–9
epilepsy following 394
as form of torture 1495
function and health 389
immediate response to 1107
and insight 397
investigations 389
late effects 388
long-term outcome 389–90
loss of consciousness 388
malingering following 1055
management of sequelae 395–7
mood disorders following 393, 396
neuropathology 387–8, *387*
and offending 1920
open 387, 394, 1617
personality change following 391
post-concussion syndrome 394, 395–6, 1929
psychological sequelae 390
psychosis following 392–3
recovery from 389–90
refugees 1495
severity 388, *388*
and sleep-wake disorders *932*, 942, 1698
Head Start programme 1788
headache
in childhood and adolescence 1745
following neurosurgery for mental disorder 1268
induction by transcranial magnetic stimulation 1263
health
behavioural factors influencing 1135–7
beliefs 1136–7
definition 1606
and lifestyle 1136
and personality 1136
and stress 1135–6
Health and Education for Life Project 1814–15
Health Anxiety Inventory 1023
Health Belief Model 1137, 1140
health care behaviour 1138–40
health care services
high users 1137–8
types 44–5
health care workers
alcohol use disorders 457
assaults on 1986
factitious disorder 1054
Health Maintenance Organization 45
Health of the Nation Outcome Scale 70, 73
health promotion
in childhood and adolescence 1610
comparison with prevention 1609
see also prevention, primary
health psychology **1135–43**
behavioural factors influencing health 1135–7
health care behaviour 1138–40
symptoms and illness behaviour 1137–8
treatment behaviour 1140–2
health-related behaviour 1136–7
health-risk behaviours 1136
Health Technology Appraisals 124
health visitors 1486
Healthy Start programme 1788
hearing, cortical association pathways *147*, 152
heavy metal exposure 1825
Helicobacter pylori 1084
Heller's syndrome **1637**
HELP (Health and Education for Life Project) 1814–15
help-seeking behaviour
and culture 15, 1441–2
delay in 1137
hemisensory syndrome 1017
hemispherectomy 1867
hepatic encephalopathy 445, 1084–5
hepatitis B infection
and hypersomnia 942
and opioid use 475
and substance use disorders 430
hepatitis C infection
and opioid use 475
and substance use disorders 430
hepatocerebral degeneration 445
hepatolenticular degeneration 537, 1084
heritability 214
broad-sense 214
narrow-sense 214
heroin 430, 473, 515
action at opioid receptors 473
administration routes 473
brown 473
complications of use 474–5, *475*
dependence 474
assessment 478
in childhood and adolescence 480
confirmation of 478
management 477–9
outcome 481
treatment 475, 476–8, 479, 1242–7
detection 473
epidemiology of use 474
metabolism 473–4, *474*
overdose 474–5, 479, *480*
in pregnancy and breastfeeding 480, *480*, 1615–16
prescription 476
tolerance 473, 474, 478
withdrawal 474
measurement 478, *478*
see also opioids; substance use disorders
herpes
encephalitis 406, 1095
genital 1094
heterozygosity 212, 226
5-HIAA *see* 5-hydroxyindoleacetic acid
hierarchy of evidence 123, *1465*
highly active antiretroviral therapy in HIV-associated dementia 385
hindbrain 156, 157
hippocampal formation 148, *149*, 182, 202, 251–2, *252*, 733
hippocampus 158, 159, 251
anatomy of neuronal network 202–3, *202*
cortical projections to 155–6
emergent properties of networks 203
in epilepsy 203–4
evoked responses 202
and fear/anxiety 1666–7, *1667*
lesions 252, *252*
local circuits 202
and long-term potentiation 251, *251*
and memory 204, 251–3, *251*, 259
rhythms 203
in schizophrenia 179–80, *179*
structure and organization 146, 148, *149*
HIS syndrome 1909
histaminergic system 151, 1210, *1211*
histones 223, 225
historical background
Alzheimer's disease 334
anorexia nervosa 777
art therapy 1414
barbiturates 1178
biological and psychological model of mental disorder 19–20
bipolar disorder 631
community care 24
depression 629–31
diagnostic systems 631
family therapy 1380–1
hypochondriasis 1021–2
mental health social work 1408
mood disorders **629–31**
neuropsychiatry 20
neuroses 20–1
neurosurgery for mental disorder 1266–7
pharmacotherapy 25
psychiatry as a medical specialty **17–27**

historical background (*cont.*)
psychiatry as profession 18
psychoanalysis 23, 1338–9
psychodynamic psychiatry 23
psychotherapies 20–1
schizophrenia **521–6**
sexual dysfunction 821–2
social aspects of psychiatry 18–19
Historical Clinical Risk-20 1927, 1994, 1997, 1998, 2018
histrionic personality disorder **868–70**
aetiology 869
classification *856*, *869*
clinical features 869–70
comorbidity 870, 884
course and prognosis 870
and deception 1049
diagnosis 869–70
differential diagnosis 866, 870, 874
in elderly people 1562, *1562*, 1563
epidemiology 869, *882*, 883
treatment 870
HIV/AIDS **1091–3**
acute stress reaction in 1091
counselling in 1280–1
delirium in 1092–3, *1093*
delusions of 619
dementia in **384–6**, 1091
depression in 1092
effects on family members 1742
interpersonal psychotherapy (IPT-HIV) 1092, 1322
mania in 1092
nature of neuropsychiatric disorders in 1091
and opioid use 475
opportunistic CNS infections 1093
parental, effects on child development 1755
prevention 1447
psychosis in 1092
and stigma 1091
and substance use disorders 430
and syphilis 1093
HLA typing in sleep-wake disorders 930
HMO (Health Maintenance Organization) 45
home treatment programmes for schizophrenia 584
home visitation programme 1788, 1789
homelessness **1500–2**
and alcohol use disorders 456, 464
barriers to care 1500–1
definition 1500
demography 1500
and psychiatric disorder 1500
service organization and delivery 1501
homicide **1937–40**
altruistic 1923
by children/adolescents 1952–3
by elderly people 1938
by spouse/partner 1981
and delusional disorders 1920
female perpetrators 1938
general population 1937
infant 1119, 1125, 1937–8
longitudinal trends 1939–40
mass 606, 979, 981, 1938
methods 1937
multiple 1938
perpetrators with mental health service contact 1938–9
perpetrators with schizophrenia 1939, 1995
and personality disorder 1921
risk assessment 1939–40
secondary victims 1985
serial 1938
'stranger' 1937
and substance use disorders 1926
suicide following 1923, 1938
Homicide Act 1957 1901
homosexuality 832
and gender identity disorder 1720
and hate crimes 1987
homozygosity 212, 226
honesty-humility 850
Hong Kong
attitudes to psychiatric disorder 6
neurasthenia 1061
HONOS (Health of the Nation Outcome Scale) 73
Hoover's sign 1016
Hopelessness Scale 1165
Hopkins Symptom Checklist 284, 1497
Hopkins Verbal Learning Test 253
hops 1248
Horney, Karen 310–11
Hospital Anxiety and Depression Scale 1486
hospitals
counselling in 1280–1
schools 1815
see also day hospitals; general hospitals; secure hospitals
host–agent–environment model 1608
hostels 1454
housing, supported 1400
HOX genes 1614
HPA axis *see* hypothalamic–pituitary–adrenal (HPA) axis
HPCL (Hare Psychopathy Checklist) 835
HPPD (hallucinogen persisting perception disorder) 488–9
5-HT and 5-HT receptors *see* serotonergic system and serotonin receptors
5-HT_{1A} partial agonists 1181
see also buspirone
HTAs (Health Technology Appraisals) 124
Hughlings-Jackson, J. 523
Human Genome Project 218, 222, 1510
human rights
European Convention on Human Rights 1899, 1900, 1904, 2015
Human Rights Act 1998 2015
and mental health public policy 1427
and refugees 1493
UN Declaration of Human Rights 1427, 1494
violations of 11
Humulus lupulus 1248
Hunter syndrome 1843
huntingtin gene 372
Huntington disease-like 2 228, 373
Huntington's disease 212, 213, 228, 228, **371–5**
and aggression 1929
in childhood and adolescence 372–3
clinical features and course 371–2
diagnosis 372–3
differential diagnosis 348, 373–4
genetics 372
pathology 372
risk of 374–5
subcortical triad of symptoms 369
treatment and management 374
Hurler syndrome 1843
hwabyung 984
HY antigen 842
hydergine
adverse effects 1248
as cognitive enhancer 1248
drug interactions *1250*
hydrocephalus following head injury 388
hydrocortisol in acute stress reactions 697
5-hydroxyindoleacetic acid (5-HIAA)
in anorexia nervosa 782
in borderline personality disorder 867
and intermittent explosive disorder 912
and repetitive self-mutilation 917
and suicide 964, 965
hyperactivity
and offending 1909
see also attention-deficit hyperactivity disorder
hyperactivity–impulsivity–attention deficit syndrome 1909
hyperarousal following an accident 1107
hypercalcaemia 1085–6
hypercarotenaemia in anorexia nervosa 785
hypercortisolaemia in depression 660–1, 1252, 1258
hyperdopaminergia 562
hyperemesis gravidarum 1116
hyperforin 1249
hyperglycinaemia 1863
hypergraphia 1079
Hypericum perforatum (St John's wort) 386, 686, 1248, *1250*, 1262
hyperkinetic disorder *see* attention-deficit hyperactivity disorder
hyperkinetic stereotyped movement disorder 1633
hyperkinetic syndrome 1654, 1657
see also attention-deficit hyperactivity disorder
hypernomia 850
hyperparathyroidism 1085–6
hyperphagia with seasonal affective disorder 1260
hyperprolactinaemia 815, 826, 1086, 1217, 1223
hyperreflexia in HIV-associated dementia 384
hypersalivation, drug-induced 1223
hyperschemazia 57
hypersexuality
in childhood and adolescence 1671
in Huntington's disease 373
hypersomnia 927, *928*, **938–43**, 1083, 1699–701, *1700*
aetiology 939–43
assessment 938–9
of central origin 940–2
epidemiology 938
idiopathic 941–2
misdiagnosis 928
morbidity 938
with physical illness 942
post-traumatic 942
recurrent 942
with seasonal affective disorder 1260
with sleep-related breathing disorder 939–40
substance-induced 939
treatment 939–43
hypertension 1081
and alcohol consumption 446
hyperthermia and ecstasy 495
hyperthymia **690–1**

hyperthyroidism 1085
  panic-like symptoms 752
  and sleep-wake disorders *932*
hyperventilation
  in chronic fatigue syndrome 1038
  following an accident 1106
hypnogram 925, *925*, 930
hypnosis
  in conversion disorder 1019
  in persistent somatoform pain disorder 1034
  in post-traumatic stress disorder 709
  and recovered memories 715
hypnotics 1178, 1179
  abuse 1183
  adverse effects 1183
  in cancer 1101–2, *1102*
  clinical effects 1182–3
  dependence 1183
  half-lives *1183*
  rebound 1183
  residual effects 1183
hypocalcaemia 1085
hypochloraemia in bulimia nervosa 804
hypochondriacal delusions 51
hypochondriasis 57, **1021–9**
  aetiology and pathogenesis 1025–6
  assessment instruments 1023, *1023*
  and body dysmorphic disorder 1045
  and chronic fatigue syndrome 1037
  classification 993–4, *993*, 994, 1022–3, *1022*
  clinical features 1022, *1022*
  cognitive and perceptual factors 1025
  comorbidity 1024, 1027
  complications 1026
  conceptualizations 1022
  controversial aspects 997
  correlates and risk factors 997, 1024
  course 1026
  definitions 996
  developmental factors 1025
  differential diagnosis 1003, 1023
  epidemiology 996–7, *998*, 1024–5
  family studies 1024
  and functional symptoms 992
  history of disorder 1021–2
  interpersonal factors 1025
  and life events 1025
  monosymptomatic 997–8
  morbidity 1024–5
  and pain 1031
  and personality 1025
  phenomenology 996
  prevalence 996–7, *998*, 1024
  prognosis 1026
  and service utilization 1024–5
  and sexually transmitted diseases 1094
  social and cultural factors 1025–6
  and somatic delusional disorder 617–18
  subtypes 1022
  treatment and management 1026–8, *1027*, 1034
  twin studies 1024
  validity of diagnosis 1023
hypocretin 930, 941
hypofrontality in schizophrenia 188–9, 562
hypoglycaemia in anorexia nervosa 785
hypogonadism 826, 828, 834
hypokalaemia in bulimia nervosa 804
hypomania 631
  in Alzheimer's disease 335
  and attempted suicide 1704
  clinical features 635, *635*
  definition 638
  differential diagnosis 644, 870
  duration 646
  elderly people 1527
  see also cyclothymia/cyclothymic disorder
Hypomania Checklist 635
hypomobility 58
hyponatraemia
  in anorexia nervosa 794
  in bulimia nervosa 804
hyponomia 850
hypoparathyroidism 1085
hypophosphataemia in rapid refeeding 786
hypopituitarism 781, 1086
hyposchemazia 57
hypotension
  and chronic fatigue syndrome 1038
  drug-induced 1190, 1223, 1529
  in frontotemporal dementias 346
hypothalamic–growth hormone axis 164–5
hypothalamic–pituitary–adrenal (HPA) axis **164–5**
  in anorexia nervosa 784
  and avoidance response 658
  and birth weight 659
  in borderline personality disorder 867
  effects of stress on 206–7
  in generalized anxiety disorder 732
  in post-traumatic stress disorder 706
  and suicide 965
hypothalamic–pituitary–gonadal axis **165**
  in anorexia nervosa 781, 783–4
hypothalamic–pituitary–thyroid axis **163**
  in anorexia nervosa 784
  in post-traumatic stress disorder 706
hypothalamic–prolactin axis 165–6
hypothalamotomy 1267
hypothalamus
  and circadian rhythms 1260
  components of the hypothalamic–pituitary–end-organ axes 162–3, *162*
  feeding centre 781
hypothermia in anorexia nervosa 785
hypothyroidism 163, 1085
  congenital 1616
    physical and cognitive characteristics 1842
    prevalence 1825–6, 1842
  in depression 661
  in Down syndrome 1839
  and hypersomnia 942
hypoxia, amnesia following 406–7
hysterectomy 1116
hysteria 57, 1021
  see also conversion disorder
hysterical blindness 1017

ibogaine 488, 1249, *1250*
IBS (irritable bowel syndrome) 997, 1003, 1037, 1083
ICD *see entries under*International Classification of Diseases
ice (methamphetamine) **497–8**
'ice-pick' lobotomy 1267
ICER (incremental cost-effectiveness ratio) 124, 1475, *1475*
ICESCR (International Covenant on Economic Social and Cultural Rights) 1427
ICF (*International Classification of Functioning, Disability and Health*) 65, 389, 1399, 1820–1, *1821*
ICIDH (*International Classification of Impairments, Disabilities and Handicaps*) 65, 389, 1399, 1820
ICM (intensive case management) 1402
ICPC-2-R (International Classification for Primary Care) 1484
ICSD-2 (International Classification of Sleep Disorders) 927, *928*, 933, *934*, 938, 1695, 1698
ICU (intensive care units) 1139
id 294–5, 306, 313, 849
id resistances 297
ideal object 308
ideal types 849
idebenone 1240
identity, disorder of awareness of 56
identity theft 1970
identity theory 134
idiopathic CNS hypersomnia 1701
idiopathic infantile hypercalcaemia *see* Williams syndrome
IDO (indoleamine 2,3 dioxygenase) 209
IED (intermittent explosive disorder) 911–13
Ifa 1420
IGFs (insulin-growth factors) 206
IL-1 (interleukin-1) 209
illness
  cognitive models 1138
  concept of 62, 63–4, 277–8
  coping with 1066
  definition 989
  as a demand/threat 1066
  division into 'medical' and 'psychiatric' 989
  interpersonal basis of experience 277
  perceptions 1138
  phobia of 52, 1022, 1023
  resources for response to 1066
  self-regulatory model 1138
  as a stress 1065
  see also mental disorder; physical illness; terminal illness
Illness Attitude Scales 1023
illness behaviour and somatization disorder 1003, 1009
illness deception model *1051*
illness delay 1137
illness self-management in schizophrenia 583
illusions 49, 1030
  in delirium 327
  iloperidone 1209
  administration 1220–1
  pharmacodynamics 1210
  pharmacokinetics 1222
ILPs (independent learning plans) 1716
imagery 49, 1779
  in insomnia 937
imagery modification 1292–3
images, negative 1288
imipramine *670*, 1185
  adverse effects *1191*
  delayed onset of effects 176
  dosage *1196*
  in generalized anxiety disorder 735
  in panic disorder 756, *756*
  pharmacodynamics *1173*, *1187*
  pharmacokinetics *1172*

immune system **205–11**
in chronic fatigue syndrome 1039
effects of echinacea 1249
effects of stress 205, 207, 1135–6
modulation of emotion and mood 209
neural influences 206–7
receptors 206
as sensory organ 207, 209
Impact of Event scale 703
impact rule 1902
impairment 389
imprinting 213, 224–5
defects 229
Improvement Foundation 1488
impulse control disorders **911–19**
in bulimia nervosa 803
definitions 911
and offending 1924
impulse control enhancement 1771–2
impulsivity 850
in attention-deficit hyperactivity disorder 1643
and offending 1909
and suicide 970
imu 983
in vitro fertilization (IVF) 1115
and intellectual disability 1883
inappropriate affect in schizophrenia 529
incidence 281, 1607
secular changes in 280–1
inclusion criteria 100
Incredible Years, The 1788
incremental cost-effectiveness ratio 124, 1475, *1475*
indeloxazine 1240
independent learning plans 1716
India
Action for Mental Illness 1491
attitudes to psychiatric disorder 6
cost of psychiatric disorder 11
psychiatric nurses in 1407
traditional medicine 1061
indigenous folk healing practices **1418–22**
indoleamine 2,3 dioxygenase 209
infancy
caregiver-mediated interventions 1787–8
death in 1119
epilepsy with intellectual disability 1861, 1862–4, *1863*
maternal anxieties about infant health and survival 1121–2
mother–infant relationship disorders 1123–4
psychoanalytic theories of sexuality 294–5
relinquishment in 1120
sleeplessness in 1698
see also childhood and adolescence
infanticide 1119, 1125, 1937–8
infantile spasms 1618, 1862–3, 1867
infection **1090–5**
and chronic fatigue syndrome 1038–9
and hypersomnia 942
and obsessive–compulsive disorder 1685
opportunistic in HIV/AIDS 1093
pharmacotherapy 1091, *1091*
prenatal exposure to, and schizophrenia 547–8, 556
and tic disorders 1073, 1685
see also specific infections
infectious mononucleosis 1095
inferior frontal gyrus 245
inferior parietal lobe 245
inferior temporal sulcus 146
inferotemporal cortex 146, 148
infertility 1114–15
see also fertility
inflammatory bowel disease 1083–4
influenza, prenatal exposure to 547–8
information
analysis and integration *65*
categories 63
condensation and recording 73–4
effects on stigma 5–6
keeping up to date with **122–9**
objective 63
scientific 63
subjective 63
information-giving in counselling 1275–6
information variance 284
informed consent 29, 1895
for neurosurgery for mental disorder 1267–8
in psychiatric emergencies in childhood and adolescence 1811
for psychotherapy in childhood and adolescence 1765
for surgical procedures 1096–7
inhalant abuse *see* volatile substance abuse
inheritance
multifactorial 213
patterns of 212–14, *213*
polygenic 213
inhibition, sexual 825
injury *see* accidents; head injury; sleep-related injury
Injury Severity Score 1105
inositol 176
inositol triphosphate 174, 176
inpatient care
in alcohol use disorders 449, 455–6, 461
anorexia nervosa 792–3, 793, 794–5
in community mental health services 1452–3
containment of violent behaviour 1404
diagnosis-specific 1453
for elderly people 1582–3
global survey 12, *12*
health psychology of 1139–40
and psychiatric nursing 1404
stress associated 1139–40
and suicide 1404
insanity defence 1900–1, 1922–3, 1923, 1928
insight 56, 80, *80*, 83
in body dysmorphic disorder 1044
following head injury 397
measurement 56
in psychoanalysis 1340
in schizophrenia 528
insistence on sameness in autism 1633
insomnia 927, *928*, **933–8**, 1182
aetiology 934–5
childhood-onset/idiopathic 1699
classification 933
clinical features 933
course and prognosis 935
and depression 934
diagnosis 934
differential diagnosis 934
epidemiology 934
fatal familial 352
prevention 937
rebound 935
treatment and management 935–7
institutional racism 276
institutionalization 236–7, 1393, 1396
insula 145, 148, 152, 260
insulin-growth factors 206
insulinoma 1101
integration 1278
intellect/imagination 850
intellectual disability 1861
in adults 1884
aetiology 1821–2, **1830–7**
assessment 1833–4, *1833*
central nervous system malformations 1832
classification of causes 1830, *1831*
complexity of causes 1830
external prenatal factors 1832
genetic factors 1831–2, *1831*, 1838
importance of confirmation of 1834
paranatally-acquired disorders 1832
postnatally-acquired disorders 1833
untraceable/unclassified 1833
and aggression 1855–6, 1929
anger management 1874
and anxiety 1851–2
and anxiety disorders 1855
and art therapy 1414–15
assessment 1821–3
and attention-deficit hyperactivity disorder 1850–1, 1876
and autism 1852, 1855
behavioural programmes 1874
and bereavement 1881
and bipolar disorder 1827, 1854–5
characterization 1821–2
childhood and adolescence
and antisocial behaviour 1946
and anxiety 1851–2
and bereavement 1759
and depression 1852
effects on family 1883–4
prevalence 1878
psychiatric and behaviour disorders associated **1849–53**, 1879
special needs of adolescents 1878–80
transition to adulthood 1878–9
classification 54, *86*, 1592, *1593*, 1819–21, *1820*, *1821*
cognitive-behaviour therapy 1874
communication skills 1873
and conduct disorder 1657, 1851
and consent to sexual activity 1900
and culture 1879–80, 1881
definitions 1825
and deinstitutionalization 1881, 1887, 1890
and deliberate self-harm 1856
and dementia 1827, 1828, 1855
and depression 1827, 1852, 1854–5
diagnosis 1833–4, *1833*
multiaxial 1871–2
differential diagnosis
antisocial personality disorder 866
pervasive developmental disorders 1639
specific developmental disorders 1623
and dysthymia/dysthymic disorder 1855
and education 1873, 1884
effects on the family **1883–6**
elderly people 1584, 1864
carers 1880–1
health needs 1880
life expectancy 1880

with psychiatric/behavioural disorders 1858–9
and epilepsy 92, 1828
in adults and elderly people 1864
aetiology and pathogenesis 1865–6, *1865*, *1866*
behavioural disorders 1864
in childhood and adolescence *1863*, 1864
diagnosis 1861–2
differential diagnosis 1861–2, *1863*
epidemiology 1864–5
in infancy 1861–2, 1862–4, *1863*
prognosis 1868
treatment 1866–8, *1867*
ethnic minorities 1879–80, 1881
health inequalities 1819
and IQ 1820, 1825
mental state examination 1823
needs assessment 1823–4
normalization 1872
and offending 1856
and oppositional-defiant disorder 1851
and paraphilias 834
and parenthood 1885
and personality disorders 1856
pharmacotherapy 1875–6
prevalence 1825–6
prevention 1447–8, *1448*
coordinated 1835
ethical issues 1835
primary 1834
secondary 1834–5
tertiary 1835
psychiatric and behaviour disorders in adults **1854–60**
aetiology 1857–8
assessment 1822–3, 1856
and baseline exaggeration 1854
classification 1857
clinical features 1854–6
and cognitive disintegration 1854
and deprivation 1828
diagnosis 1822–3, 1856–7
in elderly people 1858–9
epidemiology 1826–7, *1827*, 1857
and intellectual distortion 1854
and levels of support 1828
and life events 1828
mental health service planning and provision 1887–92
outcome measurement 1889
and physical illness 1828
protective and vulnerability factors 1827–8
and psychological masking 1854
residential programmes 1889
and smoking 1828
staffing and training 1889–90
vocational programmes 1889
psychiatric and behaviour disorders in childhood and adolescence **1849–53**
assessment 1822–3
classification 1849–50
diagnosis 1822–3, 1849–50
management principles 1852–3
and physical illness 1850
social and family influences 1850
psychodynamic psychotherapy 1874–5
and psychoses 1826, 1827, 1854
rational emotive therapy 1874
and schizophrenia 1827, 1854
self-help skills 1873
and sexual relationships 1873, 1879
and sleep-wake disorders 926–7, 1694, 1697–8
and social inclusion 1819
and social relationships 1873
social role valorization (SRV) approach 1409–10
spectrum of 1819
and speech and language disorder/difficulty 1712
and stereotypic movement disorder 1683, 1851
and sterilization 1116
syndromes **1838–48**
therapeutic communities 1397
and tic disorders 1851
treatment **1871–7**
methods 1873–6
therapeutic environment 1872–3
in tuberous sclerosis 1075
United Nations Declaration on the Rights of Mentally Retarded Persons 1895–6
X-linked 1831–2, 1839–40, 1842
see also specific disorders and syndromes
intellectual openness 886
intellectual performance disorders 54
intellectualization 294
intelligence
assessment and measurement 22, 54, 87, *88*, 263–4
conceptualization 54, 263–4
and offending 1909–10
premorbid 90, *90*, 264, 548
intelligence quotient *see* IQ
intensive care units 1139
intensive case management 1402
intention-to-treat analysis 128, 142, 1155
intentional communities 1392
interactive techniques in child and adolescent assessment 1605
interferon *1091*
interleukin-1 209
INTERMED-method 1145, *1146*
intermetamorphosis 623
intermittent explosive disorder 911–13
internal consistency of a test *85*
international agencies and mental health public policy 1427
International Bill of Rights 1427
International Classification of Diseases, development and early editions 100–2
International Classification of Diseases, ICD-9 100, 631
alcohol dependence syndrome 437
autism 1633
neurasthenia 1060
personality disorders *856*
International Classification of Diseases, ICD-10 **108–13**, 631
acute stress reactions 693, 694, *694*
adjustment disorders *717*, 1066–7
alcohol use disorders 439, *440*
Alzheimer's disease 336
Asperger's syndrome 1638, *1638*
autism 1633–4, *1634*
bipolar disorder 639
categorical approach 849
in childhood and adolescence 1592–3
childhood disintegrative disorder *1637*
as classification of disorders 64
Clinical Descriptions and Diagnostic Guidelines (Blue Book) 103
comparison with DSM-IV 102–4
conduct disorder 1656, 1657
cultural critique 276
cyclothymic disorder 686
delirium 327, 1531
delusional disorder 103–4, 609, 613, *613*
depersonalization disorder 774
depression 633, *633*, 639
development 100–2
Diagnostic Criteria for Research (Green Book) 103
disorders relating to cocaine 483, *484*
dysthymic disorder 681
eating disorder 787, 800–1
and epidemiology 1607
ethical issues in diagnosis using 28
frontotemporal dementias 348
generalized anxiety disorder 730, *730*
hyperkinetic disorder 1643
impulse control disorders 911
intellectual disability 1825
with psychiatric disorder 1826, 1849–50
malingering 1054
mania 635, *635*
multiaxial version 73, 103
neurasthenia 1062
obsessive–compulsive disorder 1682
panic disorder 751–2
pathological gambling 920
personality disorders 852, *852*, 855–7, *856*
antisocial personality disorder *865*
dependent personality disorder 873
histrionic personality disorder *869*
obsessive–compulsive personality disorder 874
paranoid personality disorder 861
pervasive developmental disorders 1623, 1633, 1639
post-traumatic stress disorder 701, *702–3*, 703
in primary care 1483–4
Primary Health Care version (PHC) 103
Rett's syndrome 1636, *1636*
schizoaffective disorder 598
schizophrenia 103–4, 534, *534*, *536*, 541, 569, 571, 1547
sexual dysfunction 823
Short Glossary of ICD-10 103
social anxiety disorder 740
somatoform disorders 104, *993*, 994, 1003
body dysmorphic disorder 1045–6
conversion disorder 1012
hypochondriasis 997, 1022–3
persistent somatoform pain disorder 997, 1029–30
somatization disorder 996, 999–1000, 1003
specific developmental disorders 1623, *1623*, 1627
specific phobia 745
structure 102–4
substance use disorders 439, *440*
tic disorders 1682
use in epidemiology 283
vascular dementia 377–8, *377*
International Classification of Diseases, ICD-10-PHC 1483–4

International Classification of Diseases, ICD-11, research planning for 106–8
International Classification of Functioning, Disability and Health 65, 389, 1399, 1820–1, *1821*
International Classification of Impairments, Disabilities and Handicaps 65, 389, 1399, 1820
International Classification for Primary Care 1484
International Classification of Sleep Disorders 927, *928*, 933, *934*, 938, 1695, 1698
International Covenant on Economic, Social and Cultural Rights 1427
International Covenant on Political and Civil Rights 1427
International Haplotype Map 222, 227
International Initiative for Mental Health Leaders 1488
International Personality Disorder Examination 72, *858*, 859
International Pilot Study of Schizophrenia 14, 71, 523, 527, 528, 540–1, 541, 572, 574
International Study of Schizophrenia 572–3, *572*, 574
Internet
 counselling services based on 109, 1814–15
 and suicide pacts 1706
 use in evidence-based medicine 124
interneuronal network gamma 203
interpersonal and social rhythm therapy 647, 673, 1319, 1323
interpersonal counselling 1324
interpersonal development 1600–1
interpersonal group therapy 1351, 1355, *1356*
interpersonal inventory 1320
interpersonal psychoanalysis 310
interpersonal psychotherapy (IPT) 1278, **1318–26**
 adjustment disorders 1068, *1069*
 anorexia nervosa 792
 anxiety disorders 1324
 avoidant personality disorder 897
 background 1319
 bipolar disorder 1323
 bulimia nervosa 808, 809, 1323–4
 by telephone 1324
 comparison with other psychotherapies 1321, 1333–4, *1333*
 contraindications 1319
 conversion disorder 1019
 depression 672–3, 676, 1322–3
  in childhood and adolescence 1322, 1676
  in elderly people 1555
  maintenance treatment 1322–3
  and marital conflict 1322
  peripartum 1322
  in primary care 1322
 dysthymia/dysthymic disorder 686, 1323
 in HIV/AIDS 1092, 1322
 indications 1319
 phases of treatment 1319–20
 predictors of response to 1324
 for refugees 1497
 research 1324
 substance use disorders 1324
 techniques 1320–1
 training in 1325
interpersonal relation phobia 982
interpersonal skills training in conduct disorder 1662
interpretationism 134–5
interpreters
 mental health professionals as 67
 use in assessment 67
interval scales 86
interventricular foramen 157
interviewing, privacy of 67
intracerebral haemorrhage 387
introjection 294
introjective type 316
introns 224
introversion 81, 632, 633, 635, 654, 850, 862, 878
intrusion following an accident 1107
intuition, delusional 51
invasion of privacy in diagnosis of factitious disorder 1053
Inventory of Depressive Symptomatology 1163
Inventory of Interpersonal Problems 1165
iodine deficiency 1448, 1825
Iowa Gambling Task 265
Iowa Strengthening Families program 1790
IP_3 (inositol triphosphate) 174
IPC (interpersonal counselling) 1324
IPDE (International Personality Disorder Examination) 72, *858*, 859
iproniazid 1185, 1190
ipsapirone in generalized anxiety disorder 735
IPSRT (interpersonal and social rhythm therapy) 647, 673, 1319, 1323
IPT *see* interpersonal psychotherapy
IPT-HIV 1092, 1322
IQ 54, 263–4
 classification *86*
 difference scores 86, *86*
 and intellectual disability 1820, 1825
 and offending 1909–10
 population distribution 1825
 premorbid, strategies for estimation 90, *90*
 scores 86
 tests 67, *88*
 z-scores and percentiles *86*
Irish Affected Sib Pair Study 435
iron deficiency *932*, 1088
irresponsibility in elderly people 1561
irritable bowel syndrome 997, 1003, 1037, 1083
irritable heart syndrome 751
Islamic communities, attitudes to psychiatric disorder 7
isocarboxazid 670, *670*
 adverse effects 1190, *1191*, 1193
 dosage *1196*
 limitations on use 1187
 pharmacodynamics *1187*
 pharmacokinetics *1189*
isolation 294
isoniazid
 adverse effects *1091*
 in tuberculosis 1094
isoproterenol 754
isoxsuprine 1240
ISS (Injury Severity Score) 1105
ITT (intention-to-treat analysis) 128, 142, 1155
IVF *see in vitro* fertilization

Janet, Pierre 20, 21
Japan
 attitudes to psychiatric disorder 7
 life expectancy 1507
 neurasthenia 1061
jargon aphasia 54
Jaspers, Karl 523
jealousy 619–20
 cognitive therapy 1920
 delusional 51, 619–21, 1920, 1967
 pathological 51, 620–1, 862, 1920, 1998
jet (ketamine) 489, **499–500**, 1186
jet lag 1261
journals
 current awareness 124–5, *125*
 systematic reviews in 1156
judgement 80, *80*, 83
'Just Say No' campaign 1598
juvenile delinquency 1654, **1945–59**
 assessment 1947–8, *1949*
 and attention-deficit hyperactivity disorder 1948–9
 and autism spectrum disorders 1950
 and capacity 1954–5
 and conduct disorder 1946, 1948–9
 and depression 1949
 and early-onset psychosis 1950
 epidemiology 1945
 girls 1955–6
 interventions 1950–7, *1951*
 justice system 1945, 1947
 legal issues 1954–5
 and mental disorder 1946–7, 1948–50, 1951–2
 pathways of care 1947
 pathways to *1946*
 and post-traumatic stress disorder 1949–50
 protective factors 1947, *1947*
 risk factors *1946*, 1947

K (ketamine) 489, **499–500**, 1186
Kahlbaum, Karl 521
kainate receptors 172, *173*, 1171
kava 1248, *1250*
Kendra's Law 2015
Keppra *see* levetiracetam
Kernberg, Otto 311
ketamine 489, **499–500**, 1186
ketoconazole *1091*
kidney, transplantation 1087
kindling 204
kissing 815
Klein, Melanie 306–7, 308, 1770
Kleine–Levin syndrome 942, 1701
kleptomania **913–14**, 1924, 1942–3
Klinefelter syndrome 834
 behavioural and psychiatric aspects 1840
 genetics 1840
 physical characteristics 1840
 prevalence 1840
Klüver-Bucy syndrome 258–9, 346
knockout/knock-in technology 230, 231
Kohlberg, Lawrence 235
Kohut, Heinz 311
koro 606, 779, 979, **980–1**
Korsakoff syndrome *see* Wernicke–Korsakoff syndrome
Kraepelin, Emil 522, 531, 540, 568, 603, 609, 610, 630, 681
kudzu 1249
kujibiki 1420
kuru 351, 354–5
'la belle indifference' 1016

LAAM 1243–4
labelling 5
labia 817
lacunar state 377
Lafora disease 1864, *1866*
Laing, R.D. 24, 309
lamina terminalis 157
lamotrigine 1198, 1200, **1235**
adverse effects *1200*, 1204, 1235
in bipolar disorder 671, 677
in childhood and adolescence 1798
in cyclothymia/cyclothymic disorder 689
in depersonalization disorder 775
dosage and administration *1233*, 1235, *1236*
drug interactions 1206, 1232, 1235, 1866
in epilepsy 1080
indications and contraindications 1235
mechanism of action *1200*
overdose 1235
in personality disorders *905*
pharmacokinetics 1203, 1235, *1867*
pharmacology 1235
in pregnancy 1235
response correlates *1199*
in schizophrenia 591
structure *1232*
therapeutic profile *1199*
withdrawal 1206–7, 1235
Landau–Kleffner syndrome 1618, 1626–7, 1640, 1712, 1864
language *see* speech and language development; speech and language disorder/difficulty
lanti 984
lasting power of attorney 1577
latah 606, **983**
late paraphrenia 1547
lateral horn 157
lateral ventricles 157, 159
laurasidone 1209
Lavandula angustifolia (lavender) 1248
law and psychiatry *see* legal issues
laxative abuse
in anorexia nervosa 783, 784, 794
in bulimia nervosa 803
learned helplessness 684, 1982
learning, in epilepsy 204
learning disability *see* intellectual disability
learning disorders 1623, *1623*, 1627–31
learning mentors 1812
legal issues
action-taking 1895–900
anorexia nervosa 796
arson 1966
decision-making 1895–900
factitious disorder 1053–4
gender identity disorder 845
juvenile delinquency 1954–5
law relating to people with mental disorder **1895–907**
malingering 1058
old age psychiatry 1577–8
paraphilias 834
responsibility 1900–5
sleep–wake disorders 948–9
substance use disorders 1927–8
Leibniz, Gottfried 133
lemon balm 1248
Lennox–Gastaut syndrome 1618, 1862, 1863
Lesch–Nyhan syndrome
behavioural and psychiatric aspects 1838, 1843
behavioural phenotype 1613, 1614
genetics 1843
physical characteristics 1843
prevalence 1843
Letter–Number Span 255
leuprolide acetate 1964
Level of Service Inventory, Revised 2011
levetiracetam 1237
drug interactions 1866
in epilepsy 1080
pharmacokinetics *1867*
levodopa
adverse effects *730*
in dementia with Lewy bodies 366
Lewis, David 134
Lewy bodies 361
composition 362
cortical 362
in Parkinson's disease 361, 369
sites 362
subcortical 362
Lewy body disease *see* dementia, with Lewy bodies
Lewy neurites 362
in Parkinson's disease 369
lexipafant 386
liability
for clinical negligence 1902
criminal 1900–1
of mentally ill people in negligence 1903–4
to mentally ill people who self-harm 1905
of providers of mental health services 1904–5
for psychiatric injury 1902–3
to third parties for acts by mentally ill people 1904
tortious 1901–5
vicarious 1904–5
liaison, in consultation-liaison psychiatry 1145
libidinal object 308
libido 294, 295
and castration 815–16
in epilepsy 1079
postnatal loss 1121
reduced/low 822
in dementia 416
management 828
LIFE (Longitudinal Interval Follow-up Evaluation) 1165
life course 1512
perspective 1513–14
structuring through age 1512–13
life events
and aetiological models 269–71
and anorexia nervosa 779–80
in clinical assessment 66–7
and conversion disorder 1014
and depression 269–73, *270*, *271*, 648, 659
effects on children and adolescents 1601
elderly people 1559–60
and exposure to adversity 286
and generalized anxiety disorder 735
and hypochondriasis 1025
and immune function 207
involving danger 270
involving entrapment 270
involving humiliation 270
involving loss 270
and mania 647
and mood disorders 269–73, *270*, *271*, 659
and psychiatric disorder in intellectual disability 1828
and schizophrenia 558, 575
and suicide 954, 969, 1705
Life Events and Difficulties Schedule 67, 269–71
life expectancy
and ageing 1507, 1509–10
healthy 1509–10
and population ageing 1579
life skills training *see* social skills training
life stories 1514–15
life table analysis 215
life transitions 1513–14
lifechart 67, 73
lifestyle
and ageing 1507
and health 1136
LIFT (Linking the Interests of Families and Teachers) programme 1789
ligand-gated ion channels 172, *173*, 174
light box 1261
light visors 1261
limbic cortex 150, 152–3, 1267
limbic leucotomy 1267
limbic-lobe syndrome 866
lingzhi 1063
linkage disequilibrium 220, 221, 651
Linking the Interests of Families and Teachers programme 1789
lipid metabolism disorders 1084
lipofuscin 1508
liquid ecstasy (gamma hydroxy butyrate) 409, **498–9**
liquorice 1249
LIS1 protein 158
literature searches 123
lithium 1198, **1198–208**
adverse effects *1200*, 1204
in childhood and adolescence 1677
hypothyroidism 1085
risk factors 1175
teratogenicity 1169–70
in attempted suicide 971, 1707
in autism and other pervasive developmental disorders 1640
in bipolar disorder 671, 677
in body dysmorphic disorder 1047
and breast-feeding 1169–70
in childhood and adolescence
depression 1677
psychiatric/behaviour disorder and intellectual disability 1852
comparison of immediate-release and modified-release 1169, *1169*
continuation treatment 671
in cyclothymia/cyclothymic disorder 689
drug interactions 1175, 1205
in elderly people 1556
historical perspective 1200
in HIV/AIDS 1092
in Huntington's disease 374
indications and contraindications 1205
in intellectual disability 1875
maintenance treatment 671
mechanism of action *1200*
monitoring therapy 1176
in personality disorders 906

lithium (*cont.*)
pharmacodynamics 1172
pharmacokinetics 1170, *1172*, 1202–3
pharmacology 1201, *1202*, *1203*
in pregnancy 677, 1118, 1205
psychoprophylactic use 1448
in resistant depression 675
response correlates *1199*
in schizophrenia 591
and surgery 1097
therapeutic profile *1199*
withdrawal 1206
litigation
and conversion disorder 1016
following accidents 1111–12
and malingering 1057
and persistent somatoform pain disorder 1034
vexatious *see* querulous behaviour
liver
effects of alcohol use disorders 445, 446, 456
transplantation 456
local worlds 277
locus coeruleus 151
LOD score 219, 222
lofepramine *670*
lofexidine 477, **1245**
Logical Memory test 264
logistic regression 141
logoclonia 53
logorrhoea 53
long-term plasticity 251
long-term potentiation 202, 231, 251, *251*
longevity
and need for mental health services 1579–80
and rate of living 1508
variance in 1507
Longitudinal Interval Follow-up Evaluation 1165
loosening of association 53, 528
Lophophora williamsii 488
loprazolam 1179
lorazepam 1178
in adjustment disorders 721
adverse effects 1180
in alcohol withdrawal 1542
in cancer *1102*, *1104*
in delirium 1533
in dementia 415
dosage 1180
indications 1178
in panic disorder *756*, 757
pharmacokinetics *1172*, 1178
potential for misuse 491
in status epilepticus 1867
in terminal illness 1070
love, delusions of 51
love maps 813, 837
loxapine *1209*
administration *1214*
adverse effects *1212*
pharmacodynamics *1211*
LSD 487
acute effects 488
adverse effects 488–9
differential diagnosis of intoxication 487
epidemiology of use 488
preparations 488
psychosis induced by 489, 538
use in pregnancy 1117
LSI-R (Level of Service Inventory, Revised) 2011
LTP (long-term potentiation) 202, 231, 251, *251*
LTPP (long-term psychodynamic psychotherapy) 318–19, 1327, 1329, 1338, 1345
Lunacy Act 1845 19
luteinizing hormone in anorexia nervosa 783
lying 1941
pathological 54, 871, 1049, 1051, 1941
Lyme disease 1094–5
Lyrica (pregabalin) 743, 1182, 1237
lysergic acid diethylamide *see* LSD

MacArthur Risk Assessment Study 1937
machine functionalism 134
McNaghten rules 1900–1, 1928
MACT (manual-assisted cognitive treatment) 895
made acts 527
Madrid Declaration 40, 40–1
magersucht 783
magic-fear-induced death 981
magnetic resonance imaging see functional magnetic resonance imaging; structural magnetic resonance imaging
magnetic resonance spectroscopy 186
alcohol-related brain damage 401
epilepsy 1862
lithium therapy 1202
mood disorders in childhood and adolescence 1674
magnetization 191, *192*
magnetoencephalography in epilepsy 1862
maintenance of wakefulness test 939
make-belief 1941
Malan, David 310
malaria 1447
malarial fever therapy 1251
mali-mali 983
malingering 57, 994, 1049, **1054–8**, 1096, 1941
aetiology 1057
assessment instruments 1057
classification 1056
clinical features 1055–6
and cognitive assessment 91
and cognitive deficit 1055–6
course 1057
definition 1054
diagnosis 1056
differential diagnosis 1003, 1012, *1012*, 1051, 1056
epidemiology 1054–5
ethical and legal issues 1058
following accidents 1111
partial 1054
and physical disease 1056
and post-traumatic stress disorder 1055
prevention 1058
prognosis 1057
and psychoses 1055
pure 1054
symptom validity tests 1057
treatment and management 1057–8
malnutrition
in alcohol use disorders 445
in anorexia nervosa 784–6
managed care 45
management **39–46**
activities 41
basic concepts 40
categories 41
definition 40
ethical aspects 40–1
functions 40
information systems 42
levels and styles 42
quality 43–4, *44*
risk 44
roles and responsibility of managers of clinical units 42
and strategic planning 43
management by objectives 43
management science 42
mania
assessment 1675
childhood and adolescence 1670–1, 1675, 1677
clinical features 635–6, *635*
cultural influences 14
and Cushing's syndrome 1086
definition 638
in dementia 416
differential diagnosis 644, 870, 1531
and Down syndrome 1826
duration and severity of episodes 635–6
elderly people 1527, 1556–7
endophenotype 266
following head injury 393
in HIV/AIDS 1092
and life events 647
and offending 1923
and patient state fluctuations within mood disorders 632–3, *632*, *633*
and physical illness 1132
postpartum 647
with psychotic features 636
risk factors 646–7
and sleep-wake disorders *931*
stages of *636*
treatment 677–8, 1253–4
unipolar 633
without psychotic features 635–6
mania à potu 60
Mania Rating Scale 1675
manic episode disorder 633
mannerisms 58, 58
manual-assisted cognitive treatment 895
MAO-A see monoamine oxidase-A
MAOIs see monoamine oxidase inhibitors
Map Search 88, 89
maple syrup urine disease 1863
maprotiline 669
adverse effects *1191*
dosage *1196*
pharmacodynamics *1173*, *1187*
pharmacokinetics *1172*, *1189*
Marchiafava–Bignami syndrome 445
marijuana *see* cannabis
marital conflict
and conduct disorder 1659–60
and depression 1753
effects on child mental health 1726
interpersonal psychotherapy (IPT-CM) 1322
and mood disorders 653
and offending 1910–11
marital status, and depression 648
marital therapy *see* couple therapy
Maroteaux-Lamy syndrome 1843
marriage 1369–70
consanguineous 1825
counselling 1278–9

and culture 1370
masochism 832–3, *833*, *836*, 877, 878
masochistic personality disorder 877–8
massacre, autogenic (self-generated) 1938
MAST-G 1519
masturbation
degeneration theory 836
surveys of 813–14
'matchbox' sign 618
matching 1468
maternal deprivation 285
maternity blues 1121
mathematics disorder 1630
mating behaviour 815
Matricaria recutita 1248
MATRICS battery 263, 265
Matrix Model 1463, *1464*, 1889
Mayo Fluctuations Composite Scale 363
MBDB (*N*-methyl-1-(1,3-benzodioxol-5-yl)-2-butanamine) 494
MBO (management by objectives) 43
MBT (mentalization-based therapy) 304, 894, 1341
MCI *see* mild cognitive impairment
MCMI (Millon Clinical Multiaxial Inventory) 858, *858*, 1962
MDA (methylenedioxyamphetamine) 494
MDAS (Memorial Delirium Rating Scale) 328
MDEA (methylenedioxyethylamphetamine) 494
MDMA *see* ecstasy
MDT (mode deactivation therapy) 1953
ME *see* chronic fatigue syndrome
Mead, Margaret 276
mean 86
mean green (ketamine) 489, **499–500**, 1186
Measure of Parenting Style 286
measurement scales 85–6
MECA (Methods for the Epidemiology of Child and Adolescent Mental Disorders) study 1594
media, exposure to in childhood and adolescence 1601
medial temporal lobe
and declarative/episodic memory 251–3, *252*
in mild cognitive impairment 1537–8
median 86
medical anthropology 276
medical practice models 64
medical pupil referral units 1815
Medical Research Council *see* MRC
medical sociology **268–75**
context and measurement 268
life events and building aetiological models 269–73
methodological considerations 269
medical students' disease 1137
Medical Symptom Validity Test 1057
medication use disorders in elderly people **1543–5**, *1544*
meditation 1418
medroxyprogesterone acetate 838, 1964
meiosis 223
melancholia 681, 1021
features 640–1
treatment 1252–3
melanocortin agonists in sexual dysfunction 828
MELAS (mitochondrial encephalopathy with lactic acidosis and strokes) 1865, *1866*
melatonin 925, 935, 1183, 1248, *1250*, 1262
melatonin receptor agonists in insomnia 935
Melissa officinalis 1248
memantine
in Alzheimer's disease 1241
in dementia 415
in HIV-associated dementia 385
in vascular dementia 381
Memorial Delirium Rating Scale 328
memory
in acute stress reactions 696
in anxiety disorders 1288
assessment 89, *89*, 253, 254, 255–6, 264, 420–1, *420*
biographical 59
cellular and molecular mechanisms 251, *251*
classification 250–1, *250*
declarative (explicit) 59, 250, 313
assessment and neuropsychology 253
neural system 251–3, *252*
delusional 51, 59, 611
and depression 92
development 241–2, *241–2*
distortion following head injury 392
effects of benzodiazepines 1179
emotional 264
encoding 264
enhancement 396–7
and epilepsy 92, 204
episodic *241*, 250, 264, 407, 1179, 1761
assessment and neuropsychology 253
and emotions 259
neural system 251–3, *252*, 259
eye witness *241–2*
false 59, 250, 403, 408, **713–16**
immaturity in childhood 1761
long-term (remote/secondary) 59, 250, 407
remediation 421–4, *422*
and mood disorders 59
non-declarative (implicit) *241*, 250, 313, 407
assessment and neuropsychology 254
neural systems 254
preverbal (eidetic) 1761
procedural 59, 250, 254, 313–14
prospective 407
in psychiatric practice 249–50
psychology and biology **249–57**
rate of forgetting 253
recognition *241*, 264
recovered 714–15, 834
remediation and rehabilitation 421–4, *422*
repression 293–4, 314
retrieval 264
role of amygdala 264
semantic 250, 264, 406, 407
short-term/recent 59, 250, 264, 407
visual 247–8
situationally accessible 696
ultrashort-term (sensoric/echoic/iconic) 59, 250
verbally accessible 696
working/primary *242*, 250, 264, 407
assessment and neuropsychology 255–6
neural systems 254–5
remediation 421
and schizophrenia 255
memory aids
assessment of use 420, *421*
electronic 423
memory clinics 1584
memory impairment, age-associated (AAMI) 1535, 1535–6
see also amnesia
memory strategy training 423
Mendel, Gregor 212
meningitis
and chronic fatigue syndrome 1038
cryptococcal 1093
prevention 1447
tuberculous 1094
menopause 823
menstrual cycle and sexual behaviour 816
menstruation 1114
and anorexia nervosa 782, 783, 787
Mental Capacity Act 2005 1897, 1898–9
mental causation 134
Mental Deficiency Act 1913 1819
mental disorder
disease burden 10–11, 467, 1428, 1606
in childhood and adolescence 1595–6
and juvenile delinquency 1946–7, 1948–50
interventions 1951–2
myth of 28
and offending **1917–26**, 2009–10
parental, effects on child development 1752–4, 1755–6
phenomena of 47
prevalence in the community *1480*
prevalence in general hospital population 1144
prevalence in primary care 1480–2, *1481*, *1482*
prisoners **1933–6**
scope of term 1933
and violence 1937
as worldwide public health issue **10–13**
mental health, definition 1606–7
Mental Health Act 1930 22
Mental Health Act 1959 1898
Mental Health Act 1983 1491, 1905
Mental Health Alliance 1491
mental health budgets, global survey 11, *11*
mental health legislation, global surveys 11, *11*
mental health literacy 5
mental health nurses *see* psychiatric nurses
mental health professionals
burnout 1449, *1449*
in consultation-liaison psychiatry 1146
engagement in risk assessment 1993–4
global survey *11*, 12
as interpreters 67
perceptions of need 1433
in primary care 1485–6
recruitment 1429
role in primary prevention 1449–50, *1450*
stalking of 1972
working with people with intellectual disability and psychiatric disorder 1889–90
see also specific professions
mental health public policy **1425–31**
comparative 1426–7
definitions 1425
and economic impact of disease burden 1428
and equitable resource allocation 1430
function 1426
and funding 1429–30
global surveys 11, *11*
and human resources 1429
and human rights 1427

mental health public policy (*cont.*)
implementation 1428–9
and international agencies 1427
need for 1427–8
positive and negative drivers 1425–6
scope of development 1428
mental health resources
allocation 1473
equitable allocation and mental health public policy 1430
global 11–12
insufficiency 1473–4
mental health services
for adults with intellectual disability **1887–92**
for alcohol use disorders **459–67**
assessment of utilization 1165
for bipolar disorder 646
child and adolescent (CAMHS) **1802–7**, 1946
accessibility 1805–6
client groups 1803
cost-effectiveness analysis 1476–7
evidence-based development 1804
inclusion of schools 1811–12
inclusion of speech and language therapists 1716
multi-disciplinary teams 1812
prioritizing need 1803–4
provision of interventions 1804–5
quality 1806
referrals to 1811
role in medico-legal assessment 1954–5
role in special education 1815
school liaison service 1812–13
service structure 1805
staffing 1805
community **1452–62**
acute beds 1452–3
assertive outreach teams 1455, 1457–8, *1457*
community mental health centres 1454
community mental health teams 584, 1454–5, *1456*, *1457*, 1458, 1888–9
community substance misuse teams 479
crisis teams 1458, *1458*
day care 1453
development principles *1461*
diagnosis-specific teams 1459
early intervention teams 1459, *1459*
for elderly people 1582
ethical aspects 1457–8
forensic teams 1459
inpatient beds 1452–3
monitoring and review 1460
and needs of offenders/prisoners 1934
office-based care 1454
outpatient clinics 1454
planning 1459–60
rehabilitation in 389–90, 1459
residential care 1453–4
supported accommodation 1453–4
culturally competent 1502–4, *1503*
dangerous and severe personality disorder (DSPD) services 2015, 2018
and depression 649
economic analysis **1473–9**
examples 1476–7, *1478*
macro-level 1473–4, *1473*
micro-level 1474–6
for elderly people 1574–5, *1575*, **1579–86**
academic units 1584
CARITAS principles 1580
community services 1582
comprehensive 1581
consultation-liaison services 1583
core business 1581
core components 1581–4, *1582*
day hospitals 1583
inpatient units 1583
integrated 1581
long-term care 1583
need for 1579–80
patient-centred 1580–1
planning to commissioning 1584–5
primary care collaborations 1583–4
principles of good service delivery 1580–1
residential care 1583
respite care 1583
special components 1584
for ethnic minorities 277, **1502–4**
evaluation **1463–72**
definitions and conceptual framework 1463
key challenges *1470*
Matrix model 1463, *1464*
outcome measures 1464–5, *1464*
purpose of 1463, *1464*
research design 1465–9, *1465*, *1466*, *1467*, *1468*, *1469*
financing 11, *11*
forensic 2013, **2015–21**
capacity planning 2017–18
community 1459
international context 2016
philosophy and theoretical models 2015–16
private 2017
pyramid planning 2017
security 2015, 2016–17
service structure 2017–18
service users 2018–20
super-specialist 2017
global improvement 12–13
for homeless people 1501, *1501*
integrated 990, 1460
liability of providers 1904–5
for mothers 1124–5
needs *see* needs
for offenders 1934–5
forensic 1459, 2013, **2015–21**
general psychiatric services **2009–14**
needs 1934–5
provision in prisons 1934–5
organization in general hospital departments **1144–8**
for personality disorder 907
primary care 1486
research on 281, 1452
for schizophrenia 584–5
for substance use disorders **515–20**
see also consultation-liaison (CL) psychiatry
mental health social work **1408–13**
behavioural 1409
care management 1410–11
crisis approach 1409
historical development 1408
innovative practice 1411
legal and policy framework 1410–11
problem-solving approach 1409
psychodynamic approaches 1408–9
social dimension 1409
social role valorization (SRV) approach 1409–10
strengths model 1410
task-centred 1409
values underpinning 1408
mental hygiene 22
mental retardation *see* intellectual disability
mental status examination (MSE)
assessment instruments 69–70
in childhood and adolescence 1601, *1602*
in intellectual disability 1823
see also Mini-Mental State Examination
Mental Status Schedule 71
mentalization 1948
mentalization-based therapy 304, 894, 1341
meprobamate 1178
MeRAs (melatonin receptor agonists) in insomnia 935
mescaline 488
mesencephalon 156, 157
mesoridazine *1209*
administration *1214*
adverse effects *1212*
meta-analysis 229, 1155, 1465–6, *1466*
metabolic disorders 1084–5
metabolic enhancers 1240
metachromatic leukodystrophy 537
meta-communications 1381
metencephalon 157
meth (methamphetamine) **497–8**
methadone 475, **1243**
action at opioid receptors 473
detoxification 477
injectable 476
maintenance treatment 476, 479
metabolism 473
in pregnancy 1118, 1615–16
prescription 479
methamphetamine **497–8**
Methods for the Epidemiology of Child and Adolescent Mental Disorders study 1594
methohexitone 1178
18-methoxycoronaridine 1249
N-methyl-1-(1,3-benzodioxol-5-yl)-2-butanamine 494
methylenedioxyamphetamine 494
methylenedioxyethylamphetamine 494
3,4-methylenedioxymethamphetamine *see* ecstasy
methylphenidate 1795
abuse potential 1795
adverse effects 1650, 1795
in attention-deficit hyperactivity disorder 1241, 1648, 1650, 1876
in cancer *1103*
and epilepsy 1650
in HIV-associated dementia 386
in intellectual disability 1876
in narcolepsy with cataplexy 941
precautions with 1795
rebound effects 1795
in terminal illness 1070
metoclopramide 1101
Mexico, attitudes to psychiatric disorder 6
Meyer, Adolf 22
MFQ (Mood and Feelings Questionnaire) 1675, 1780
MFTG (multiple family group therapy) 1382, 1389

mianserin *670*, 671
adverse effects 1191, *1191*
in depression in elderly people 1554, *1554*
dosage *1196*
pharmacodynamics *1173*, *1187*, 1188
pharmacokinetics *1172*, *1189*
midazolam *1104*
midbrain 156, 157
'midweek blues' 495
migraine
and depersonalization 775
and transient global amnesia 403
migration and schizophrenia 286, 549, 557–8
mild cognitive disorder 1534
mild cognitive impairment (MCI) 266, 1519, **1534–9**, 1574
aetiology 1537, *1537*
amnestic 1520, 1535
assessment 1536
biomarkers 1537–8
clinical staging scales 1535
cognitive assessment 1536
definition 1520, 1534
diagnosis 1536–8, *1537*
diagnostic criteria 1535
epidemiology 1535–6, *1536*
mortality risk 1536
neuroimaging 1537–8
neuropsychiatric symptoms 1537
nosology 1534–5, *1534*
progression to dementia 1535–6
reversion to normal 1536
treatment and management 1538
vascular 407
mild neurocognitive disorder 1534
millenniary delusions 982
Millon Clinical Multiaxial Inventory 858, *858*, 1962
milnacipran
adverse effects *1191*
dosage *1196*
pharmacodynamics 1186, *1187*
pharmacokinetics 1188, *1189*
mind–body dualism 133, 989–91
mind–body literature 205
mind–brain relation **133–6**
and psychodynamic psychiatry 315–16
mindfulness-based cognitive therapy 1310
mindfulness skills in body dysmorphic disorder 1047
mini-ethnography 278
'minimal brain dysfunction' 1631, 1643
Mini-Mental State Examination (MMSE) 87, 284
in Alzheimer's disease 337, 1240
in delirium in elderly people 1531
with elderly people 1527, *1528*
extended 1527, *1528*
in Huntington's disease 373
in mild cognitive impairment 1536
sensitivity to education 284
in vascular dementia 380
Minnesota Multiphasic Personality Index
use in malingering 1057
use with sex offenders 1962
'miracle question' 1276
mirror retraining in body dysmorphic disorder 1047
mirror sign 334
mirror therapy in adjustment disorders 720
mirroring 311, 1357
mirtazapine *670*, 671
adverse effects 1191, *1191*, 1555
in cancer *1103*
in depression in elderly people 1554, *1554*
dosage *1196*
in panic disorder 757
pharmacodynamics *1187*, 1188
pharmacokinetics *1189*
miscarriage 1119
misidentification, delusional 51, 392, 609–10, 611, 622, **623–4**
misidentification syndromes
in Alzheimer's disease 335
delusional 51, 392, 609–10, 611, 622, **623–4**
and risk of violence 1998
mission statement 43
Misuse of Drugs Act 1971 1927
Mitchell, Stephen 311
mitochondria 223
and ageing 1508
mitochondrial disorders 1832
mitochondrial encephalopathy with lactic acidosis and strokes 1865, *1866*
mitochondrial encephalopathy with ragged red fibres 1864
mitral valve prolapse 752
mixed anxiety-depressive disorder 718–19
MMSE *see* Mini-Mental State Examination
mobile phones, counselling services using 1814–15
MoCA (Montreal Cognitive Assessment) 1536
moclobemide 670, *670*
adverse effects *1191*, 1555
in depression in elderly people *1554*
dosage 674, *1196*
pharmacodynamics 1172, *1187*, 1188
pharmacokinetics *1172*, *1189*
in social anxiety disorder 743
modafinil
in attention-deficit hyperactivity disorder 1241, 1651
in cancer *1103*
in hypersomnia 939
in narcolepsy with cataplexy 941
mode 86
mode deactivation therapy 1953
model fitting 217
models of medical practice 64
Modified Card Sorting Test *90*
Modified Six Elements Test *90*
Modified Social Stress Model 505
mogo laya 984
molecular genetics 1598
gene–environment interactions 214–18, 221, 229, 315, 558–9, 1608, 1725
intermediate phenotypes 221
molindone *1209*
administration *1214*
adverse effects *1212*
pharmacodynamics *1211*
Mongolia, attitudes to psychiatric disorder 6
monoamine oxidase-A (MAO-A)
and aggression 889, 1918
and antisocial personality disorder 315, 1918
and conduct disorder 1658
monoamine oxidase inhibitors (MAOIs)
adverse effects 674, 1187–8, 1190, *1191*, 1192, *1192*
in anxiety disorders 1182
in attention-deficit hyperactivity disorder 1651
in body dysmorphic disorder 1047
choice of 674
dietary interactions 1187–8, 1192, *1192*
dosage *1196*
drug interactions 1175, 1194–5, *1195*
in HIV-associated dementia 385
introduction 1185, *1185*
irreversible 670, *670*, 1187
in panic disorder *756*, 757
in personality disorders *905*, 906
pharmacodynamics 1173, 1186–7, 1186–8, *1187*
pharmacokinetics *1172*, 1189, *1189*
in post-traumatic stress disorder 709
reversible 1187
in social anxiety disorder 743
and surgery 1097–8
monoamines
and depression 662
inhibition of reuptake 1172, *1173*
and phototherapy 1260
monosomy 228
Montreal Cognitive Assessment 1536
mood
in alcohol withdrawal 439
definition 54, 629
delusional 51, 611
depressed 637
immune modulation 209
Mood and Feelings Questionnaire 1675, 1780
Mood Disorder Questionnaire 635
mood disorders 54–5
aetiology
genetic **650–8**
neurobiological **658–65**
alcohol-induced 427, 434, 444, 455
anticipation in 652
in cancer 1102, *1102*, *1103*
childhood and adolescence **1669–80**
aetiology 1674
clinical picture 1669–71, *1670*, *1672*
comorbidity 1673
course 1673–4
differential diagnosis 1657, 1671–3
epidemiology 1673–4
with intellectual disability 1852
neurocognitive factors 1674–5
sequelae 1674
treatment and prevention 1675–7
classification 104, 105, 631, **638–43**, 665
clinical features **632–7**
concept of unipolar and bipolar disorders 631
course and prognosis **665–9**
definitions 637–8
and delusional disorder 614
diagnosis **637–45**
stability of 665
differential diagnosis 643–4
elderly people **1550–8**
epidemiology **645–50**, 650–1
following head injury 393, 396
and gender 271, 648, 653–4
genetics 658
history of **629–31**
and life events 269–73, *270*, *271*, 659
maintaining factors 659–63
and memory 59

mood disorders (*cont.*)
mixed states 636, 638
neurobiology **658–65**
neuropathology 181–2, *182*
and neuroticism 658
and offending 1923
organic 1552
and pain 1030
patient state fluctuations within 632–3, *632*, *633*
and persistent somatoform pain disorder 1032
pharmacogenetics 653
and physical illness *1128*
precipitating factors 659
prevalence *285*
prevention 1448, 1675–7
psychosocial factors 653
with psychotic symptoms 864
rapid cycling 636, 668
risk factors 658–9
and sexuality 825
social functioning in 653
and socio-economic status 654
subthreshold **680–92**
and surgery 1097–8
and temperament 654, 658, 680
thinking in 52
treatment **669–80**, 1252–4
complementary medicines 1248
phototherapy 1261
see also specific disorders
mood stabilizers **1198–208**
in childhood and adolescence 1798, 1852
see also specific drugs
Moodgym 1406
MOPS (Measure of Parenting Style) 286
moral development, history-taking 1601
moral judgement 235
'moral treatment' 17, 1392
morality, conventional/pre-conventional 1762
morbid risk 215
morbidity
continuous measures 283
hidden and conspicuous in primary care 1482
and poverty 278
Morel, Bénédict-Auguste 521
Moreno, Jacob 1353
morphine 430
detection 473
metabolism 473, *474*
morphometry 195, Plate 9
Morquio syndrome 1843
mosaicism in Down syndrome 1839
mother–foetus relationship 1117
mother–infant relationship disorders 1123–4
motility disorder 58, *58*
motivated sleep phase syndrome 1700
Motivational Assessment Scale 1823
motivational enhancement therapy 451, 794
motivational interviewing
in adjustment disorders *1069*
in alcohol use disorders 451
in body dysmorphic disorder 1047
in cognitive-behaviour therapy in childhood and adolescence 1779
in opioid dependence 477, *477*, 479
in rehabilitation 1400
in substance use disorders 428
motor co-ordination in schizophrenia 529
motor neurone disease 348
with dementia 344, 345, 347, 348
motor skills disorder 1623, *1623*, 1631
motor symptoms and signs, descriptive phenomenology 58–9
mourning 724
pathological 296
religious ceremony 1419
see also bereavement
movement disorders
complementary medicines 1249
in conversion disorder 1016, *1016*, 1017
differential diagnosis 373
MR (morbid risk) 215
MRC
framework for evaluation of complex intervention 1465, *1466*
Needs for Care Assessment 73, 1433–4
MRI *see* structural magnetic resonance imaging
MSE *see* mental status examination
MSI-II (Multiphasic Sex Inventory II) 1962
MSLT *see* multiple sleep latency test
mtDNA *see* DNA, mitochondrial
MTFC (Multidimensional Treatment Foster Care) 1790, 1953
mucopolysaccharidoses
behavioural and psychiatric aspects 1843
classification 1843
genetics 1843
physical characteristics 1843
prevalence 1843
muddling 53
MUDs (medication use disorders) in elderly people **1543–5**, *1544*
multiaxial descriptive systems 73, 990, *990*
in childhood and adolescence 1592–3
Multidimensional Treatment Foster Care 1790, 1953
multi-disciplinary practice 68
multi-disciplinary team
agreement on terminology used 64
in Alzheimer's disease 341
care planning 68–9
in child and adolescent mental health services 1812
and clinical assessment 62, 68
community mental health teams 584, 1454–5, *1456*, *1457*, 1458, 1888–9
community old age mental health services 1582
in consultation-liaison psychiatry 1146
key worker/case manager 68–9
leadership 68
membership 68–9
for people with intellectual disability 1888
values in 33–5, *34*
values-based practice *34*, 35, *36*
multi-disciplinary teamwork 68
Multiphasic Sex Inventory II 1962
multiple causation 314
multiple chemical sensitivity 997, 1002
multiple family group therapy 1382, 1389
multiple personality disorder 56, 1923
multiple regression analysis 217
multiple sclerosis **1074**
cognitive impairment in 1074
depression in 1074
emotional lability in 1074
euphoria in 1074
psychotic symptoms 1074
multiple sleep latency test (MSLT) 930, 939, 945
in childhood and adolescence 1697
multi-sensory therapy *414*
multisomatoform disorder *998*, 1000
multi-system atrophy 364, 942
multisystemic therapy 1598, 1661–2, 1782
Munchausen syndrome *see* factitious disorder
Munchausen syndrome by proxy 1054, 1697, 1737, 1923–4
muscarinic agonists in Alzheimer's disease 1241
muscle dysmorphia 1044–5
mushrooms, hallucinogenic 488
music therapy *414*, 1352
mutism 54, 58, *58*
in frontotemporal dementias 346
selective 1639, 1714
MWT (maintenance of wakefulness test) 939
myalgic encephalomyelitis *see* chronic fatigue syndrome
myelasthenia 1060
myelencephalon 157
myocardial infarction 649, 1081–2
myocardial ischaemia 1081–2
myopathy
in alcohol use disorders 446
in anorexia nervosa 785
myotonic dystrophy *228*
myriachit 983
mysophilia *833*
mythomania 54
myxoedema and sleep-wake disorders *932*
nadolol 1876
Nagel, Thomas 135
nail-biting 918
nalmefene 454
naloxone 473, 475, 479, 1232, **1245**
in children and adolescents with psychiatric/behaviour disorder and intellectual disability 1852
in depersonalization disorder 775
in pregnancy 1118
naltrexone
in alcohol use disorders 454, 1542
in children and adolescents with psychiatric/behaviour disorder and intellectual disability 1852
in intellectual disability 1876
in opioid use 477, 1245
naratriptan 1171
narcissism 57, 296
healthy 311
history of concept 870
malignant 870, 871
types *870*
narcissistic loss 1106
narcissistic personality disorder 296, **870–2**
aetiology 871
classification *856*, 871, *871*
clinical features 871
comorbidity 857–71
course and prognosis 872
and deception 1049
diagnosis 871
differential diagnosis 871, 876
in elderly people *1562*
epidemiology 871, *882*, 883
historical perspective 870
treatment 871–2

narcolepsy **940–1**, 1695, 1701
with cataplexy 940–1
misdiagnosis 928
in physical illness 941
and schizophrenia 927
without cataplexy 941
Narcotics Anonymous 477, *477*, 1279
NARIs (noradrenaline reuptake inhibitors) 670, *670*
narrative gerontology 1514–15
National Adult Reading Test (NART) 264, 389
National Comorbidity Survey 541, 645
National Comorbidity Survey Replication 1595, 1596
National Confidential Inquiry into Suicide and Homicide by People with Mental Illness 1937, 1938, 1939
National Drug and Alcohol Treatment Utilization Survey 463–4
National Drug Treatment Monitoring System 515
National Health Service and Community Care Act 1432
National Healthy School Standard 1814
National Institute for Health and Clinical Excellence (NICE) 789
clinical practice guidelines 124
National Institute of Neurological and Communicative Disorders and Stroke–AD and Related Disorders Association 336, 348
National Institutes of Mental Health 23
National Psychiatric Morbidity Survey 645, 647
National Schizophrenia Fellowship 1490–1
National Service Framework for Children, Young People and Maternity Services 1946
National Survey of Health and Development 1911, 1912
National Survey of Sexual Attitudes and Lifestyles 821
National Trailblazer network 1487–8
National Treatment Agency for Substance Misuse 515–16
National Treatment Outcome Research Study 1927
NATSAL (National Survey of Sexual Attitudes and Lifestyles) 821
nausea in alcohol withdrawal 439
NDATUS (National Drug and Alcohol Treatment Utilization Survey) 463–4
nDNA *see* DNA, nuclear
necrophilia *833*
needs **1432–7**
for action 1433
assessment 73, 94, 1433–5, *1435*, 1823–4
population-level 1434–5, *1435*, 1459
definitions 1432–3
in evaluation of mental health services 1465
of families with a member with intellectual disability 1885–6
hierarchy of 1432
for improved health 1432
needs-led care planning 1432
patient and staff perceptions 1433
relationship between individual and population 1435
for services 1433
Needs for Care Assessment 73
nefazodone
adverse effects 1190, *1191*
dosage *1196*
pharmacodynamics *1187*, 1188
pharmacokinetics 1189, *1189*
negation 294
negative automatic thoughts 761, 1165, 1286, 1287–9, *1287*, 1291–2, 1304–5, 1306, *1306*, 1307, 1308–10, *1309*
negative emotionality
and health 1136
and hypochondriasis 1025
negative images 1288
negativism 58
negativistic personality disorder *see* passive–aggressive personality disorder
negligence 1901–2
clinical 1902
difference between acts and omissions 1905
liability of mentally ill people 1903–4
liability to mentally ill people who self-harm 1905
liability of providers of mental health services 1904–5
liability for psychiatric injury 1902–3
liability to third parties for acts by mentally ill people 1901–5
NEO Personality Inventory-Revised (NEO PI-R) 81, *81*, 654, 847–58, *858*, 887, 1164
neo-behaviourism 134–5
neocortex 202
in absence epilepsy 204
connection 149, Plate 1
development 158–9, *159*
in epilepsy 203
and memory 253
and priming 254
structure 147, *148*, Plate 1
neologisms 54
neonates
abilities 238
cocaine withdrawal syndrome 1118
death of 1119
mother–infant relationship disorders 1123–4
narcotics withdrawal syndrome 1118
neonaticide 1118–19, 1125
nerve gas 1241
nerve growth factor *160*, 966
nesting behaviour 1117
neural crest 156
neural groove 156
neural induction 156
neural plasticity 251
neural plate 156
neural tube 156, 157
neurasthenia *993*, 994, 1003, 1035, **1059–64**
aetiology 1062–3
and chronic fatigue syndrome 1037
classification 1062
comorbidity 1063
concept of 1059–60
course and prognosis 1063
and culture 1060–1
current usage 1062
definition 1060
as diagnostic entity 1059–60
differential diagnosis 1062
epidemiology 1062, *1062*
and stigma 1040
treatment 1063
neuregulin 1 (NRG1) gene 179, 230, 555, 565
neuroanatomy **144–56**
neurobehavioural teratology 1614
neuroblasts 157
neurocirculatory asthenia 751
neurodevelopment **156–60**
brainstem histogenesis 158–9
cerebellum histogenesis 158
cerebral cortex histogenesis 158–9, *159*
CNS organogenesis 156–7, *157*
environmental risks 1724
genetic factors 159
hemispheric shape and formation of gyri 159, *159*
neural induction 156
spinal cord histogenesis 157–8
neurodevelopmental disorders 1613
alcohol-related 1615, 1841
genetics 159
see also specific disorders
neuroectoderm 156
neuroendocrine 'window' strategy 161
neuroendocrinology **160–7**, 205, 781, 889
neurofibrillary tangles in Alzheimer's disease 337–8, 339
neurofibromatosis type 1
behavioural and psychiatric aspects 1075, 1844
expression 213
genetics 1843, *1866*
physical characteristics 1843–4
prevalence 1843
neurofibromatosis type 2, psychiatric aspects 1075
neurogenetic syndromes 1613–14
neurokinins *171*
neuroleptic malignant syndrome 1223, 1531
in HIV/AIDS 386, 1092
and malignant catatonia 529
treatment 1254
neuroleptics *see* antipsychotics
neuroligins 227
neurological disorders **1071–6**
see also specific disorders
neuromodulators 168
neuronal ceroid lipofuscinoses 1865, *1866*
neuronal networks **201–5**
and gamma rhythms 203
hippocampal 202–3, *202*
realistic computer simulations 203
neuronal specific enolase 353
neurones
death from traumatic brain injury 387
development 157
endocrine functions **160–7**
neocortical 148, *148*
in schizophrenia *178*, 180
NeuroPage 423
neuropathology **177–85**
alcohol use disorders 182–3, *183*
Alzheimer's disease 337–9
corticobasal degeneration 345
delirium 330–1, *330*
frontotemporal dementia 344–5
head injury 387–8, *387*
Huntington's disease 372
mood disorders 181–2, *182*
Pick's disease 344
progressive supranuclear palsy 345
schizophrenia and psychoses 178–81, *178*, *179*, *180*, *181*
neuropeptides *168*, 170–1, *171*, 206
neuropores 156

neuropsychiatry
  developmental **1612–22**
  history of 20
neuropsychological assessment **262–7**
  in Alzheimer's disease 265–6
  in anorexia nervosa 783
  in attention deficit hyperactivity disorder 266
  in childhood and adolescence 1590–1, 1605
  in depression 660
  domains 263–6
  functions 263
  head injury 389
  in HIV-associated dementia 384–5
  in mild cognitive impairment 1536
  in obsessive–compulsive disorder 266
  principles 263
  in schizophrenia 93, 265, 531–4
  in transient global amnesia 403
neuroses
  cultural influences 14
  historical background 20–1
neurosurgery for mental disorder (NMD) 769, **1266–9**
  adverse effects 1268–9
  definition 1266
  ethical considerations 1267–8
  historical overview 1266–7
  inclusion and exclusion criteria *1268*
  indications 1267
  mechanism of action 1268
  outcomes 1268
  procedures 1267, *1269*, *1270*
  stereotactic procedures 1267
neurosyphilis 537, 1093
neurotic (stress-related) disorder, elderly people **1558–61**
  aetiology 1559–60
  clinical features 1558
  course and prognosis 1560
  diagnosis and differential diagnosis 1558–9
  epidemiology 1559
  treatment 1560
neuroticism 81, *81*, 850, 886
  and body dysmorphic disorder 1046
  and high health service use 1137
  and hypochondriasis 1025
  and mood disorders 658
  and serotonergic system 887–8
  and subthreshold mood disorders 680
  subtypes 632
neurotransmitter receptors 172
  drug actions at 1171
    agonist 1171
    antagonist 1171–2
    partial agonist 1172
  ionotropic 1171
  metabotropic 1171
neurotransmitters **168–77**
  in anorexia nervosa 782
  in autism 1636
  chemokines and cytokines as 171
  and chronic fatigue syndrome 1039
  co-localization with neuropeptides 171
  in conduct disorder 1658
  definition 168
  and drug pharmacodynamics 1173
  hippocampus 202
  as hormones 161
  neuropeptides 170–1, *171*
  and phototherapy 1260
  primary 429
  principles of transmission 168, *169*
  retrograde messengers 171–2
  role in neurodevelopment 159
  secondary 429
  small molecule 168
  in substance use disorders 429, *429*, 435–6
  transporters 168–70, *170*
    plasma membrane 169–70, *170*
    vesicular 170, *170*
  see also specific substances
neurotrophic factors 159, *160*, *168*, 171, 1186
  see also specific factors
neurotrophin receptors 158
neurovascular coupling 197
neutralizing activities in obsessive-compulsive disorder 1783
New Zealand, Mental Health Foundation 1491
Newcastle Thousand-Family Study 1910
Newton, Isaac 133
NGF (nerve growth factor) *160*, 966
NGOs (non-governmental organizations) 1491
Nicaragua, attitudes to psychiatric disorder 6
NICE *see* National Institute for Health and Clinical Excellence
nicotine replacement therapy 512
nicotine use *see* smoking
nidotherapy 896–7, 904–5
nifedipine 1201
night-eating syndrome *931*, 947–8
night-time fears 1698–9
nightmares 1108, 1702
  in post-traumatic stress disorder 701
nihilistic delusions 56
nimodipine 1198, 1201, 1203
  adverse effects *1200*, 1204–5
  drug interactions 1206
  in HIV-associated dementia 385
  indications and contraindications 1205
  mechanism of action *1200*
  pharmacokinetics 1201
  response correlates *1199*
  therapeutic profile *1199*
  in vascular dementia 381
  withdrawal 1207
NINCDS–ADRDA 336, 348
Nisonger Child Behaviour Rating form 1850
nitrazepam *1172*, 1179
nitric oxide, as retrograde messenger 172
nitroglycerin in HIV-associated dementia 385
nitrous oxide 503
NMD *see* neurosurgery for mental disorder
NMDA receptors 172, *173*, 231, 1171
  action of lithium at 1201
  in alcohol withdrawal 443
  antibodies against 1086
  and depression 1186
  and long-term plasticity 251
  and long-term potentiation 251
  and schizophrenia 562
NMR (nuclear magnetic resonance) 191–2
NNT (number needed to treat) 127, 128, *128*
NO as retrograde messenger 172
'no-suicide' contracts 1707
nocebo effects 1141
nociception 473
nocturnal enuresis 1702
nocturnal penile tumescence 825, 930
nominal scales 85–6
non-compliance *see* treatment, non-compliance
non-experimental descriptive studies 1468–9
non-governmental organizations 1491
nootropic agents 1240
noradrenaline reuptake inhibitors 670, *670*
noradrenergic storm 473, 476
noradrenergic system and noradrenaline receptors *173*, 482, 1171, 1172
  and depression in childhood and adolescence 1675
  in generalized anxiety disorder 732
  noradrenaline transporters 169, *170*
  in panic disorder 754
  in post-traumatic stress disorder 706
  and sexual function 826
  and substance use disorders 429
  and suicide 965
nordiazepam 1178
norepinephrine *see* noradrenergic system and noradrenaline receptors
Northfield Hospital 1353
nortriptyline *670*
  adverse effects *1191*
  in cancer *1103*
  dosage 1195, *1196*
  pharmacodynamics *1173*, *1187*
  pharmacokinetics *1172*, 1188, *1189*
  in smoking cessation 512
Notch protein 339
notochord 156
novelty-seeking 80, *80*, 316, *316*, 654, 849, 886–7
NRT (nicotine replacement therapy) 512
NSE (neuronal specific enolase) 353
NT-3 *160*
NTA (National Treatment Agency for Substance Misuse) 515–16
nuclear magnetic resonance 191–2
nucleosomes 223, 225
nucleus accumbens 154
  in substance use disorders 430
nucleus basalis of Meynert, in Alzheimer's disease 1240
number needed to treat 127, 128, *128*
Nuremberg Statement 30

oats 1248
obesity
  and body image 57
  and bulimia nervosa 804
  psychiatric disorders associated 1084
  and schizophrenia 546
  and sleep-wake disorders *932*
object relations 295, **306–12**, 313, 1337
  Balint's work 308–9
  Bion's work 307–8
  Bowlby's work 309–10
  and character 316
  conflictual model 308
  and countertransference 298–9
  deficit model 308
  development from drive theory 306
  Fairbairn's work 308
  internalization 301–2
  Klein's work 306–7, 308
  overview and critique of psychoanalytic theories 301–3
  and personality development 316
  and psychoanalytic treatment 297
  and transference 298–9
  unconscious internal 297, 314

Winnicott's work 309
object representation 298, 302–3
Objective Opiate Withdrawal Scale 478, *478*
observed score (*x*) 85
obsessions 52, 53, 1680
as conditioned stimuli 768
in obsessive–compulsive disorder 765–6
and querulous behaviour 1979
obsessive–compulsive disorder (OCD) **765–73**
aetiology 767–8, 1683–5
and anorexia nervosa 783
assessment 1783
and body dysmorphic disorder 1044, 1045
in cancer 1101
childhood and adolescence 1613, **1680–93**
aetiology 1683–5
age of onset 1681
classification 1682
clinical features 1680–1
comorbidity 1681–2
course and prognosis 1685
diagnosis 1682–3
differential diagnosis 1682–3
epidemiology 1683
and gender 1681
with intellectual disability 1852
prevention 1690
refractory 1688
treatment 1685–90, *1686*, *1687*, 1783–4
classification *856*, 1682
clinical features 765–6, 1680–1
cognitive content 1287
comorbidity 765, 1681–2
course and prognosis 766–7, 1685
diagnosis 765–6, 1682–3
differential diagnosis 766, 863, 875–6, 1004, 1023–4, 1639, 1682–3
elderly people 1558
epidemiology 765, 1683
genetics 768, 1684
neuropsychological assessment 266
and offending 1923
prisoners *1934*
puerperal 1121–2
and schizophrenia 766
and sleep disorder 1697
stalking as 1972
terminology 856
and tic disorders 765, 1073, 1681
treatment
in childhood and adolescence 1685–90, *1686*, *1687*, 1783–4
cognitive-behaviour therapy 770, 1686–7, *1686*, 1783–4
deep brain stimulation 769, 1270
long-term 769
neurosurgery 769, 1267, 1268
pharmacotherapy 768–70, 1193, *1686*, 1687–8, *1687*
psychological therapies 770, 1783–4
transcranial magnetic stimulation 1265
treatment gap *13*
obsessive–compulsive personality disorder 765, **874–6**
aetiology 874
classification 874, *874*
clinical features 875
course and prognosis 875
defence mechanisms 317
differential diagnosis 875–6
in elderly people 1562, *1562*
epidemiology 874, *882*, 883
treatment 876
obstetric complications
and conduct disorder 1658
and schizophrenia 548, 555–6
obstetric liaison services 1118, 1124
obstructive sleep apnoea (OSA) 928, 1083
early-onset 1695, 1700
in elderly people 1572
hypersomnia in 939–40
occipital lobe 146, *147*
in alcohol use disorders *183*
in schizophrenia *178*
occupation, and risk of suicide 976
occupational therapy 1034, 1351–2, 1400–1
OCD *see* obsessive–compulsive disorder
OCEAN 850
odds ratios 126, *127*, 128, 141, 282
oedema, famine 785
Oedipus complex 307
negative 294
positive 294–5
and the superego 296
Oenothera biennis oil 1249, 1250
oesophageal dysmotility 1083
oestrogens 816, 826
therapy
in gender identity disorder 843
sex offenders 1963–4
off time 1515
offenders
amnesia for crimes 405, 1927
art therapy 1415
assessment 2011–12, 2018
depression 1923
group therapy 1365
mental health services for
development 1934–5
forensic 1459, 2013, **2015–21**
general psychiatric services **2009–14**
needs 1934–5
provision in prisons 1934–5
need for psychiatric assessment and treatment 1918
outcome assessment 2020
sexual *see* sex offenders
therapeutic communities 1396
treatment 2012–13, 2018–20, *2019*
versatility 1909
see also prisoners
offending
acquisitive 1927
in adolescence *see* juvenile delinquency
amnesia for 405, 1927
and attention-deficit hyperactivity disorder 1931
and autism 1921
and child abuse and neglect 1910
and child-rearing practices 1910
and cognitive disorder **1928–32**
and community influences 1913–14
concentration in families 1659, 1911–12
criminogenic factors 1911, 1917, 1918, 2011, 2012
and delusional disorder 1920
and dementia 1920–1
epidemiology 1908–9
and epilepsy 1079–80, 1920, 1929–31
and gender 1909
genetic factors 1918
and head injury 1920
and hyperactivity and impulsivity 1909
impact of criminal victimization **1984–90**
and impulse control disorders 1924
and intellectual disability 1856
and intelligence 1909–10
and marital conflict 1911
measurement 1908–9
and mental disorder **1917–26**, 2009–10
and mood disorders 1923
neurobiological determinants of 1917–18
and neurotic disorders 1923
and opioid use 474, 480
and peer influences 1912–13
and personality disorder 865, 866, 1921–3
protective factors 1909
psychosocial causes **1908–16**
risk factors 1909
family 1910–12
individual 1909–10
social 1912–14
and schizophrenia 1918–20
and school influences 1913
self-reported 1908
and situational influences 1914
and socio-economic status 1912
and substance use disorders **1926–8**
and violence 1918, 2010–11
Ohtahara syndrome 1862
olanzapine 1209, *1209*
administration *1214*, 1217–18
adverse effects *1212*, 1224
in bipolar disorder 672
in elderly people 1556
in cancer *1104*
in childhood and adolescence 1677, 1797
in delirium 331
in dementia 415
and diabetes mellitus 1085
in personality disorders *905*, 906
pharmacodynamics 1210, *1211*, 1213
pharmacokinetics 1221
old age/older people *see* elderly people
olfactory pathways to the cerebral cortex *147*, 152
olfactory reference syndrome 618
olfactory tubercle 154
omega-3 fatty acids 1248, *1250*, 1676
omnipotence 298
omnipotent control 298
on time 1515
One Day Fluctuation Assessment Scale 363
oneiroid state 60, 392, 603, 605
onychophagia 918
onychotillomania 618, 918
'open-loop' tasks 254
openness 850
opiate neurotransmitter pathway, in substance use disorders 429
opioid antagonists *see* naloxone; naltrexone
opioid receptors *173*, 473, 1171
opioid substitution/maintenance treatment 475, 476, 479, 1243–4
opioids **473–82**
addictiveness *431*
as anxiolytics 1178
cognitive effects 92
complications of use 474–5, *475*
definition 473

opioids (*cont.*)
dependence 473, 474
assessment 478
in childhood and adolescence 480
confirmation of 478
management 477–9
outcome 481
psychiatric comorbidity 475, 492–3
relapse prevention 477
treatment 475, 476–8, 479, 1242–7
detoxification 476–7
effects *474*
epidemiology of use 474
metabolism 473–4, *474*
neurobiology 473
and offending 474, 480
overdose 474–5, 479, *480*
in pregnancy and breastfeeding 480, *480*, 1117–18, 1615–16, 1754
routes of use and risk associated 430, 473
in terminal illness 1070
tolerance 473, 474
assessment of 478
use by elderly people 1543
withdrawal 473, 474
measurement 478, *478*
opioids, endogenous 170, *171*, 429
in autism 1636
in post-traumatic stress disorder 706
in substance use disorders *429*
opium 473
opportunity costs in service planning 1459
oppositional defiant disorder
comorbidity 1682
diagnosis 1656
differential diagnosis 1671
with intellectual disability 1851
treatment 1781–2
optic nerve development 157
optical distortions 49
optimism
and health 1136
and immune function 207
OQ-45 1165
oral contraceptives, drug interactions 1174
oral phase of development 294, 295
orbitofrontal cortex 146, 1919
ordinal scales 86, 95
orexin (hypocretin) 930, 941
orgasm 812
female 818–19
problems 823
male 817
delayed/absent 828
ORLAAM® 1243–4
OSA *see* obstructive sleep apnoea
osteoporosis in anorexia nervosa 785
Othello-type syndrome 1967
out-of-body experiences 1012
outcome measures 73
in evaluation of mental health services 1464–5, *1464*
psychometric properties 1465
outpatient care in community mental health services 1454
ovaries, in anorexia nervosa 784, 787
overactivity in attention-deficit hyperactivity disorder 1643
overdetermination 314
oversedation 1178, 1180
overstimulation and hallucinations 50
overvalued ideas 52, 57, 611, 803
oxazepam
in dementia 415
pharmacokinetics *1172*, 1178
in terminal illness 1070
oxcarbazepine 1198, 1237
adverse effects 1204
in childhood and adolescence 1677
dosage and administration *1233*
pharmacokinetics *1867*
structure *1232*
oxiracetam 1240
oxytocin 815, 888

P-glycoprotein 1170, 1249–50, *1250*
p11 175
p73 protein 158
P300 event-related brain potential 435
Paced Auditory Serial Addition Test 87–8, *88*
paediatric autoimmune neuropsychiatric disorder associated with streptococcal infection 1073, 1685
paedophilia 832, *833*, *836*, 1960–1, 1962
pain
acute 1029, 1033
affective dimension 1033
assessment 1032–3
assessment instruments 1032–3
behaviours 1032, 1033
beliefs 1032, 1033
in cancer 1103
in childhood and adolescence 1744–5
chronic 1029, 1030, 1033
neuropathic 1265
and sleep-wake disorders *932*
chronic benign pain syndrome 1003
clinics/treatment centres 1034
definition 1029
and delusions 1030
in dementia 418
and depression 1029, 1030
during sexual arousal 822
following an accident 1107, 1110
history 1032
low threshold 1096
in mood-/anxiety-related disorders 1030
non-operant 1033
non-organic 1784
operant 1033
in organic disorders 1030
postoperative management 1099
and post-traumatic stress disorder 1030–1
and the psychiatrist 1029
psychogenic 57
as a psychopathological entity 57
and psychoses 1030
psychosocial contributions to development 1033
sensory dimension 1033
and somatization 1030, 1031–2
and somatoform disorders 1031–2
and substance use disorders 427
syndromes of uncertain origin 1030
topographical distribution 1033
treatment and management 1033–4
pain disorder *see* persistent somatoform pain disorder
paired matching 1468
PAL (CANTAB Paired Associate Learning test) 264, 266
palaeocortex 158
palilalia 346, 1681
palimpsest 59
paliperidone 1209, *1209*
administration *1214*, 1220
adverse effects 1225
pharmacodynamics 1210
pharmacokinetics 1221
palliative care in dementia 418
palm sign 487
palmar erythema in alcohol use disorders 446
Panax ginseng
adverse effects 1248
as cognitive enhancer 1247–8
drug interactions *1250*
in neurasthenia 1063
pancreas, effects of alcohol use disorders 446
PANDAS 1073, 1685
panic attack/panic disorder **750–64**
aetiology 753–5
with agoraphobia 740–1, 750–64
and alcohol use disorders 455, 752
biological models 754–5
in cancer 1101
in childhood and adolescence 1664
clinical presentation 1665
prevalence 1666
classification 751
clinical features 750–1
cognitive content 1286
comorbidity 752, 761
and COPD 1082
course and prognosis 755
and depression 752
diagnosis 752–3
differential diagnosis 752, *753*, 1004, 1023, 1078, 1864
epidemiology 753
following an accident 1106
genetics 753–4
hallucinogen-induced 488
in HIV/AIDS 1091
and hypochondriasis 997
limited symptom attacks 751
and neurasthenia 1063
nocturnal attacks 751
in physical illness 1131
and pregnancy 761–2
prevention 762
prevention of recurrence 759
in primary care setting 753
puerperal 1121
risk factors 753
and separation anxiety disorder 1665
situational attacks 750
situationally predisposed 750
and sleep disorders 1697
with social phobia 750
and suicide 1704
treatment and management 755–62, 1180
cognitive-behaviour therapy 758, 761
continuation/maintenance 758
discontinuation 760
ethical issues 762
exposure treatments 758, 760–1
hyperstimulation reaction 756, 759–60
pharmacotherapy 755–7, *756*
psychodynamic psychotherapy 758

resistance to 761
treatment gap *13*
Panic Disorder Severity Sale 760
Papaver somniferum 473
papaverine 1240
Papez circuit 733
para-aminosalicylate *1091*
paracetamol poisoning 973
paradoxical intention in insomnia 937
paradoxical interventions 1377
paragrammatism 54
parahippocampal gyrus 146, 153
paraldehyde 1178, 1867
paralysis 57
in conversion disorder 1016
paramnesia 59
paraneoplastic syndromes 1101
paranoia
definition 861
elderly people **1546–50**, 1559
querulous *see* delusional disorder, litigious
see also delusional disorder
paranoia acuta 603, 605
paranoid personality disorder **861–2**
aetiology 861
classification *856*, 861, *861*
clinical features 861–2
course 862
defence mechanisms 317
differential diagnosis 862, 863, 865
in elderly people 1562, *1562*
epidemiology 861, 882, *882*
nomenclature 610
treatment 862, 898
paranoid psychoses following head injury 392–3
paranoid–schizoid position 307
'paranoid spectrum' 609, 610–11
paraphasia 54
paraphilias **832–42**, 1961
aetiology 836–7
assessment 1962
classification 833–4, *833*
clinical features 832–3
co-occurrence 1962
comorbidity 834–5
course and prognosis 837–8
diagnosis 834–5
differential diagnosis 834–5
epidemiology 835, *836*
false accusations 834
false confessions 834
in Huntington's disease 373
and intellectual disability 834
legal issues 834
overlap with sexual offences 1960
treatment and management 838–41, *839*, 1963–4
paraphrenia 609, 610, 623
late 1547
paraplegia, in conversion disorder 1016
parapraxes 313
paraschemazia 57
parasitosis, delusion of 50, 51, 618
parasomnia pseudo-suicide 948
parasomnias 927, *928*, **943–50**, 1695
in childhood and adolescence 1701–2
classification 944, *944*
clinical evaluation *943*, 944–5, *945*
definition 943
differential diagnosis 948
in elderly people 1572
overlap disorder 947
relevance to psychiatrists 943–4
parasuicide 916–17, 957, 1703
parasympathetic nervous system 156
parasyntax 54
parathyroid adenoma 1101
Parent–Child Interaction Training 1788–9
Parental Bonding Instrument 286, 648
parenting
and attachment 309
and conduct disorder 1659–60, 1661, 1662
factors affecting child mental health 1725–7
and gender identity disorder in childhood and adolescence 1719–20
and generalized anxiety disorder 734
and mood disorders 653
negative 1788, 1789
and offending 1910
positive 1788, 1789
style 286
parents
abusive 1734
and assessment in childhood and adolescence 1600, 1602, *1603*, 1605
in child and adolescent psychiatric emergencies 1808, 1809
child's reaction to death of 1758–60
conflict between
and conduct disorder 1659–60
and depression 1753
effects on child mental health 1726
interpersonal psychotherapy (IPT-CM) 1322
and mood disorders 653
and offending 1911
criminal activity by 1659, 1911–12
effects of child with intellectual disability 1884, 1885
effects of child with physical illness 1742
effects of childhood and adolescent sleep disorders 1694–5
factors affecting child mental health 1726–7
good-enough mother 309
influence on childhood and adolescent sleep disorders 1694
interviewing 1601, *1603*
involvement in cognitive-behaviour therapy 1778–9, 1780
involvement in pharmacotherapy 1794
involvement in psychotherapy 1768, 1771
late-life 1514
mental disorder
alcohol use disorders 1754
anxiety disorders 1754
depression 1752–3
eating disorders 1753–4
effects on child development 1752–4, 1755–6
schizophrenia 1753
substance use disorders 1754
neglectful 1736
people with intellectual disability as 1885
physical illness
cancer 1754–5
effects on child development 1754–6
HIV/AIDS 1755
single 1369–70, 1601, 1726–7, 1910, 1911
training programmes 1661, 1787–93
in attention-deficit hyperactivity disorder 1648
in conduct disorder 1782
young 1910
parietal lobe 146, *146*
in alcohol use disorders *183*
in schizophrenia *178*
parieto-occipital sulcus 145
parkinsonism
in dementia with Lewy bodies 361
drug-related 580, 1222–3
with frontotemporal dementia 344–5, 346, 348
treatment 1255
Parkinson's disease **1072–3**
cognitive assessment 92
dementia in 92, 362–3, **368–71**, *370*
depression in 648–9, 1072
diagnosis 369
differential diagnosis 373
dopamine dysregulation syndrome 1073
hypersomnia in 942
Lewy bodies in 361, 369
mortality in 370
psychotic symptoms in 1072
sleep-wake disorders *932*, 1072
transcranial magnetic stimulation 1265
paroxetine *670*
adverse effects *1191*
in attempted suicide 970–1
in cancer *1102*, *1103*
in depression in elderly people *1554*
dosage *1196*
in generalized anxiety disorder 735
in obsessive–compulsive disorder 769, *1687*
in panic disorder *756*
pharmacodynamics *1173*, *1187*
pharmacokinetics *1172*, 1189, *1189*
in post-traumatic stress disorder 709
in pregnancy 1117
in social anxiety disorder 743
partial arousal disorder 1702
partnerships 40
parturition *see* childbirth
PAS (Personality Assessment Schedule) *858*, 859
PASAT (Paced Auditory Serial Addition Test) 87–8, *88*
Passiflora incarnata (passion flower) 1248, 1249, *1250*
passive–aggressive personality disorder *876*, **876–7**, *1562*
epidemiology *882*, 883
passivity experience 56
passivity of thought 53
path analysis 217, *217*
pathological jealousy 51, 620–1, 862, 1998
pathological lying 54, 871, 1049, 1051, 1941
pathways to care 281, *281*
and culture **1438–45**
filters on 1440–2, *1441*
international comparisons 1438–9, *1439*
pathways out of care 1443
patient delay 1137
patient expected event rate 128
Patient Health Questionnaire 1145
Patient Health Questionnaire-9 1484, 1486
patient-intervention studies 1139

patients
  doctor–patient communication 1138–9
  education 4, 1198
  expectations, and the placebo response 1142
  information for 1140
  perceptions of need 1433
  perspective on services **3–4**
  protection, and psychiatric reports 75
  satisfaction 1138–9, 1465
Pavlovian theory 1061
PBI (Parental Bonding Instrument) 286, 648
PCIT (Parent–Child Interaction Training) 1788–9
PCL-R (Psychopathy Check List-Revised) 1921, 2011
PCMHWs (primary care mental health workers) 1485
PCP *see* phencyclidine
PCR (polymerase chain reaction) 223, 226
PD *see* personality disorders
PDA (panic disorder with agoraphobia) 740–1, 750–64
PDDs *see* pervasive developmental disorders
PDEs (phosphodiesterases) 176
PDQ-4 (Personality Diagnostic Questionnaire-Revised) *858*
PDS (Post-traumatic Stress Diagnostic scale) 703
PDSS (Panic Disorder Severity Sale) 760
PEA (prenatal exposure to alcohol) 1841
PEER (patient expected event rate) 128
peer pressure, and substance use disorders 427
peer relationships, and conduct disorder 1659
pellagra 1447
pemoline 1648, 1652
penetrance 213
penicillin
  adverse effects *1091*
  in syphilis 1094
penile plethysmography 840, 1962, 1964
penis
  erection 816–17
  nocturnal penile tumescence 825, 930
Penn State Worry Questionnaire 1163
pentagastrin in panic disorder 754
pentosan polyphosphate 359
pentoxifylline in HIV-associated dementia 385–6
peptic ulcer disease *932*, 1084
peptide T in HIV-associated dementia 385
percentile 86, *86*
perception
  and consciousness 59
  delusional 51, 527–8
  disorders of 48–50
  disturbance in schizotypal personality disorder 864
  and emotion 259–60
perceptual priming 696
perfectionism
  in bulimia nervosa 804, 806
  and chronic fatigue syndrome 1036
  and psychoanalysis 1341
  and somatization disorder 1002
periodic limb movements in sleep 948, 1572, 1695, 1700
peripheral nervous system, in mood disorders *182*
peripheral neuropathy
  in alcohol use disorders 446
  disulfiram-induced 453
peripheral oedema in anorexia nervosa 784
perirhinal cortex 146, 152–3, 153, 252, 406
periurethral glans 818
perphenazine *1209*
  administration *1214*
  adverse effects *1212*
  pharmacodynamics *1211*
persecution, delusion of 51
perseveration 53
  in Alzheimer's disease 334
  in frontotemporal dementias 346
persistence 80, *80*, 316, *316*, 849
persistent genital arousal disorder 822
persistent somatoform pain disorder 57, *993*, 1003, **1029–35**
  assessment 1032–3
  assessment instruments 1032–3
  childhood and adolescence 1745
  classification 997, 1029–30
  comorbidity *1031*, 1032
  correlates 997
  diagnostic and clinical features 1029–30
  differential diagnosis 1003, 1029, 1030–2, *1031*
  epidemiology 997, *998*, 1032
  phenomenology 997
  prevalence 997, *998*
  prognosis 1034
  and psychosocial contributions to development of pain 1033
  treatment and management 1033–4
persistent vegetative state in Huntington's disease 373
Personal, Health and Social Education 1814
personality
  abnormality 60
  accentuated type 73
  and addiction 428–9
  and alcohol use disorders 434
  in Alzheimer's disease 335–6
  assessment 72–3, **78–85**, 286, 1164–5
  change
    due to a general medical condition 879, 1929
    following head injury 391
    following traumatic experiences 879, 1110–11
  and character 316–17
  and chronic fatigue syndrome 1039
  definition 60, 79, 855
  and depression 648
  development *316*
    psychodynamic approaches 316–17
  domestic violence perpetrators 1982
  effects of neurosurgery for mental disorder 1269
  and health 1136
  histrionic 868, *869*
  and hypochondriasis 1025
  hysterical 868, *869*
  models 848–50
    categorical 849
    correlational 849
    dimensional 849–50
    experimental 849
    Five-Factor 238, 850, 857–8, 1164
    and personality disorders 850–1
    psychoanalytical 849
    psychobiological 316
  neuropsychology **886–92**
  premorbid 1526
  quantitative description of 79–81, *80*
  and somatization disorder 1002
  studies 848
  and subthreshold mood disorders 680
  and temperament 316, *316*
  traits 79–81, *80*, 286, 849–50, 855, 857, 886
    biological factors 886–92
    and genetics 886–8, 888–9, *890*
    and head injury 390
    normal/abnormal 857
    psychometric testing 81–2, *81*
  type A 1082, 1136
  type B 1136
  type D 1082, 1136
  typology 60
  variants 852–3, *852*
Personality Assessment Inventory 1962
Personality Assessment Schedule *858*, 859
Personality Diagnostic Questionnaire 1562
Personality Diagnostic Questionnaire-Revised *858*
Personality Disorder Questionnaire 1164
personality disorders (PD) **847–55**
  assessment 858–9, *858*
  changes in conceptualization 857
  and character dimensions 316
  classification 106, 850–1, 851, 852, *852*, *853*, 855–8, *856*
  cluster A 856, **861–5**
    drug treatment 906
    and reward-dependence 316
  cluster B 856, **865–72**
    and attempted suicide 1704
    drug treatment 906
    and novelty-seeking 316
  cluster C 856, **872–6**
    drug treatment 906
    and harm-avoidance 316
    long-term psychodynamic psychotherapy 318
  comorbidity 780–1, 803, 884, 893, 902, 907
  course 892–3
  dangerous and severe 848, 2015, 2018
  definitions 60, 855, 893
  and depression 649
  diagnosis **855–60**, 890–1
  distinction from personality variants 852–3, *852*
  elderly people **1561–4**
    aetiology 1562–3
    clinical features 1561–2
    course and prognosis 1563
    diagnosis 1562
    epidemiology 1518, 1562–3, *1562*
    treatment and management 1563–4
  epidemiology **881–6**
    community studies 882–3, *882*
    studies in a psychiatric setting 883–4
  and epilepsy 1079
  features *82*
  history of concept 847–8
  and homicide 1921
  and intellectual disability 1856
  and kleptomania 1943
  and models of personality 850–1
  and offending 865, 866, 1921–3
  and persistent somatoform pain disorder 1032

and physical illness 1132
prisoners 1921, 1933, *1933*
psychoanalytic approach 294, 296
qualitative clusters and subtypes *83*
and stigma 848
stress–diathesis model 851–2
and suicide 955, 956, 969
and surgery 1098
and temperament dimensions 316
in Tourette syndrome 1073
treatment **901–10**
adherence to 902
cognitive 895, 903–4
drug treatment 600, 905–6, *905*
duration 901–2
evaluation of efficacy 901–3
nidotherapy 896–7, 904–5
outcome measures 902
psychotherapy **892–901**, 1395–6
service organization 907
therapeutic communities 892, 896, 905, 1395–6
type R (treatment resisting) 902
type S (treatment seeking) 902
see also specific personality disorders
Personality Disorders Interview-IV *858*
PERT (post ejaculation refractory time) 817, 822
pervasive developmental disorders (PDDs) 1613, **1633–42**
with attention-deficit hyperactivity disorder 1650
classification 1623
differential diagnosis 1639
prevention 1640
and social phobia 1665
treatment and management 1639–40
see also specific disorders
pervasive refusal syndrome 787
PET *see* positron emission tomography
pet therapy in dementia *414*
peyote 489
PFAE (possible foetal alcohol effects) 1841
PGAD (persistent genital arousal disorder) 822
phaeochromocytoma 1101
phallometry 840, 1962, 1964
phantasy, unconscious 307
phantom bite syndrome 619
pharmacodynamics 1168, **1171–3**
in childhood and adolescence 1794
pharmacogenetics 221
mood disorders 653
pharmacokinetics 1168, **1170–1**, *1172*
bioavailability 1170
in childhood and adolescence 1794
clearance 1170–1
half-life 1170–1
protein binding 1170
pharmacotherapy **1168–77**
acute stress reactions 697
adjustment disorders 721, 1068
adverse effects *427*, **1173–5**
anxiety *730*
collateral 1173
dose-related 1173
DoTS classification 1173, *1174*
hypersusceptibility 1173
risk factors 1174–5
sexual dysfunction 826–7
susceptibility factors 1174–5, *1175*
time-related 1173–4, *1174*
toxic 1173
withdrawal syndromes 1175
alcohol use disorders 1246
Alzheimer's disease 1240–1
attempted suicide 970–1
attention-deficit hyperactivity disorder 1174–2, 1648, 1650, 1876
beliefs about 1141
body dysmorphic disorder 1046–7, 1047–8
in breastfeeding 1121, 1123, 1169–70, 1180
with brief psychodynamic psychotherapy 1329
bulimia nervosa 807–8
childhood and adolescence **1793–9**
antidepressants 674–5, 1668, 1676, 1794–5, 1796
antipsychotics 1677, 1796–8, 1852
atomoxetine 1795–6
developmental issues 1794
dosage regimens 1169
mood stabilizers 1798, 1852
as part of multimodal treatment 1793–4
with psychiatric/behaviour disorder and/or intellectual disability 1798, 1852
rapid tranquillization 1798
stimulants 1795
symptom-based approach 1794
chronic fatigue syndrome 1040, 1042
in combination with electroconvulsive therapy 1257
comparisons with psychotherapy 1162
conversion disorder 1019–20
cosmetic/palliative 853
delirium 331–2
in cancer patients *1104*
dementia with Lewy bodies 365–7
depersonalization disorder 775
dosage regimens 1168–70
in childhood and adolescence 1169
combination formulations 1169
elderly people 1169
maintenance dose 1171, *1171*
modified-release (depot) 1169, *1169*, 1171, 1486
parenteral 1169
in pregnancy and breast feeding 1169–70
drug interactions 1175–6
dynamic 317
dysthymia/dysthymic disorder 684–5
elderly people 1573
dosage regimens 1169
epilepsy **1231–40**
with intellectual disability 1866–7, *1867*
erectile dysfunction 821, 828
following head injury 396–7, *396*
generalized anxiety disorder 735, 736, 737
history of 25
hypochondriasis 1027
in infectious disease 1091, *1091*
in intellectual disability 1875–6
mild cognitive impairment 1538
minimum effective dose (MED) 1794
monitoring 1176
obsessive–compulsive disorder 768–70, *1686*, 1687–8, *1687*
panic disorder 755–7, *756*
personality disorders 600, 905–6, *905*
pharmacodynamics *see* pharmacodynamics
pharmacokinetics *see* pharmacokinetics
in physical illness with psychiatric disorder 1130–1
post-traumatic stress disorder 709–10
prescribing and management by psychiatric nurses 1405–6
in rehabilitation 1400
schizophrenia 579–82, *579*, 585, 586–8, *586*
social anxiety disorder 742–4
somatization disorder 1009
specific phobia 746
substance use disorders **1242–7**
and surgery 1097–8
in terminal illness 1070
tic disorders 1687–8
vascular dementia 381
see also specific drugs and types of drugs
phasic alertness 247
phencyclidine (PCP) **486–7**
acute physiological effects 486
adverse effects 486
delirium due to 486–7
dependence 487
epidemiology of abuse 486
psychosis due to 487, 538
use in pregnancy 1117
phenelzine 670, *670*
adverse effects *1191*, 1193
dosage *1196*
limitations on use 1187
in panic disorder *756*
in personality disorders *905*
pharmacodynamics *1187*
pharmacokinetics *1172*, *1189*
in post-traumatic stress disorder 709
in social anxiety disorder 743
phenobarbitone 1178
adverse effects 1673
choice of 1866–7
drug interactions 1866
in epilepsy 1080
pharmacokinetics *1867*
phenomenology
definition 47
descriptive **47–61**
phenothiazines in pregnancy 1117, 1118
phenotype 212
components of variation 214
intermediate 221
phentolamine 828
phenylketonuria
behavioural and psychiatric aspects 1844, 1852
genetics 212, 214, 1844
infantile spasms in 1863
physical characteristics 1844
prevalence 1825–6, 1844
prevention 1448
phenytoin 1231
adverse effects 1868
in alcohol withdrawal 449
choice of 1866–7
drug interactions 1175, 1232, 1866
in epilepsy 1080
pharmacokinetics 1170, *1170*, *1867*
in status epilepticus 1867
phobias *see* specific phobia *and other phobias*
phobic–anankastic syndromes 52
phonological speech disorder 1624–5, 1711, 1712
phosphodiesterases 176

phototherapy 670, 927, **1260–2**
administration 1262
adverse effects 1261–2
drug interactions 1262
forms 1261
indications and contraindications 1261
in insomnia 935
mechanism of action 1260
withdrawal 1262
PHQ (Patient Health Questionnaire) 1145
PHQ-9 (Patient Health Questionnaire-9) 1484, 1486
PHSE (Personal, Health and Social Education) 1814
physical illness
adjustment to **1065–71**, 1741, 1742
antidepressant therapy in 674, 1132
art therapy 1415
differentiation from mental disorder 989
differentiation from panic disorder 752, *753*
effects on family 1742
elderly people 1559
group therapy 1364
immune system involvement 209, *210*
and intellectual disability 1828, 1850
parental, effects on child development 1754–6
personality change due to 879
with psychiatric disorder 546, **1081–90**
in childhood and adolescence **1739–47**
course and prognosis 1129–30
depression 335, 371, 648–9, 1072, 1074, 1080, 1082, 1085, 1086, 1091, 1092, 1102, 1132
diagnosis and differential diagnosis 1129, *1129*
epidemiology 1128, *1128*
management **1128–34**
of refugees 1495
sexual dysfunction in 826
with sleep-wake disorders 931, *932*, 933, 941, 942
see also illness *and specific illnesses*
physicalism, *a priori* 134
physiognomy 1420
physiological deconditioning 1036
physiotherapy in persistent somatoform pain disorder 1034
physostigmine 331–2, 1241
phytoestrogens 1249
Piaget, Jean 235, 239–40, *239*, 1777
pibloktoq 983
pica 1116
Pick bodies 344
Pick cells 344
Pick's disease 228, 344
age at onset 345
clinical features 345–6, 346
epidemiology 345
investigations 347
neuropathology 344
Picture Vocabulary Test 239
'pill bottle' sign 618
pimozide *1209*
in body dysmorphic disorder 1047
pharmacodynamics *1211*
in tic disorders 1073, 1688
pindolol 1172
Pinel, Philippe 17–18
Piper methysticum (kava) 1248, *1250*
piracetam 1240
Pittsburgh Youth Study 1908, 1910, 1912, 1913
pituitary
components of the hypothalamic–pituitary–end-organ axes 162–3, *162*
see also specific axes
Place, U.T. 134
placebo response 1141–2, 1794
plaques
in Alzheimer's disease 338
in dementia with Lewy bodies 362
plate 12
play
development of *1766*
enhancement of capacity for 1772
play therapy 306–7, 1765, 1766, 1770
in selective mutism 1714
pleasure principle 294, 295
pleasure-seeking behaviour and substance use 426
pleiotropy 224
PLMS (periodic limb movements in sleep) 948, 1572, 1695, 1700
PMR (progressive muscle relaxation), in generalized anxiety disorder 736
pneumonia and delirium 1091
Point of Service 45
polar hysteria 983
polyclinics 1454
polycystic ovarian disease and gender identity disorder 843
polyembolokoilamania *833*
polygraphy, use with sex offenders 1962, 1964
polymerase chain reaction 223, 226
polysomnography 930
in childhood and adolescence 1695, 1696, 1699
in hypersomnia 939
in insomnia 934
in parasomnias 943–4, *943*, *944*
REM sleep behaviour disorder 946–7
sleepwalking/sleep terrors 945
POMC (proopiomelanocortin) 170
pooled odds ratio 126
population stratification 651
poriomania 1930
pornography 1961
porphyria, acute intermittent 212
Portland Digit Recognition Test 1057
POS (Point of Service) 45
positron emission tomography (PET) **185–91**, Plates 3–6
alcohol-related dementia 401
comparison with functional magnetic resonance imaging 186–7, 196–7
comparison with SPET 185
data collection and analysis 186
depression 189, 660
during antipsychotic use 189–90
during heroin use 428, Plate 13
and emotions 257–8
epilepsy 1619, 1862
frontotemporal dementias 347
head injury 389
imaging strategies 187, *187*
isotopes *186*
production 185
limitations 186–7
methodology 185
mild cognitive impairment 1538
obsessive–compulsive disorder 768
schizophrenia 188–9, 562–3
of transcranial magnetic stimulation 1263
vascular dementia 380
Wernicke–Korsakoff syndrome 406
Posner covert spatial attentional task 265
possession disorder 56
possession states 276
possible foetal alcohol effects 1841
postcentral gyrus 146
postcentral sulcus 146
post-concussion syndrome 394, 395–6, 1929
post-ejaculation refractory time 817, 822
postnatal depression 1122, 1486
and anorexia nervosa 780
counselling in 1280
effects on child development 1753
interpersonal psychotherapy 1322
and sleep deprivation in pregnancy 927
postpartum psychiatry 647, 653, 1121–5
Post-traumatic Stress Diagnostic scale 703
post-traumatic stress disorder (PTSD) **700–13**
and acute stress reactions 693, 696
aetiology 696, 705–7, *707*
amnesia in 404, 714
animal models 707
assessment instruments 703
behaviours that maintain the symptoms 706
biological factors 706–7
childhood and adolescence 237–8, **1728–31**, 1741, 1744, 1759, 1784, 1851–2
classification 693, 701, *702–3*
clinical features 701
cognitive content 1287
comorbidity 704–5
course and prognosis 707–8
diagnosis 701, *702–3*, 703
differential diagnosis 695, 701, *702–3*, 703
epidemiology 703–5
flashbacks in 404
following accidents 1109, 1110–11
following childbirth 1121
following surgery 1099
genetics 707
and intellectual disability 1851–2
and juvenile delinquency 1949–50
malingered 1055
and offending 1923
and pain 1030–1
partial 704
and physical illness 1131
prevalence 704
prevention 697, 698, 1109, 1279–80
prisoners *1934*
in refugees 1495, 1497
risk factors *707*
and sleep-wake disorders 927
subsyndromal 1110
treatment and management 708–10, 1295, 1497, 1784
victims of burglary/robbery 1986
victims of criminal activity 1984, 1985
victims of rape/sexual assault 1986
victims of terrorism 1987
postural hypotension
and chronic fatigue syndrome 1038
drug-induced 1190, 1223, 1529
posturing 58, *58*
poverty
and child mental health 1727–8

  and conduct disorder 1659
  and homelessness 1500
  relationship with morbidity and mortality 278
PPG (penile plethysmography) 840, 1962, 1964
PPO (Preferred Provider Organization) 45
practice nurses 1486
Prader–Willi syndrome 1841
  and affective psychosis 1826
  behavioural phenotype 1613, 1614, 1838, 1844, *1851*, 1858
  cognitive and psychiatric aspects 1838, 1844
  genetics 213, 224, 229, 1844
  physical characteristics 1844
  prevalence 1844
Pragmatic Language Impairment 1713
pragmatics, difficulties with 1711, 1713
prameha 981
Precaution Adoption model 1137
precentral gyrus 145
precentral sulcus 145
preconscious 294, 295
prediction errors 259
predictive learning 258–9
prednisolone 1532
Preferred Provider Organization 45
prefrontal cortex
  in conversion disorder 1013, *1013*, *1014*
  and declarative memory 253
  dorsolateral
    transcranial magnetic stimulation 1264
    and working memory 254–5
  and fear/anxiety 1667, *1667*
  lateral 146
  medial 146
  ventral, in obsessive–compulsive disorder 1684
pregabalin 743, 1182, 1237
pregnancy
  adjustment to 1116
  alcohol use disorders in 1117, 1448, 1614–15, 1754, 1826, 1841
  anxiety in 1117
  and attachment 1117
  bipolar disorder in 677
  and body dysmorphic disorder 1116
  delusions of 1115
  denial of 1116
  depression in 653, 1117, 1322
  domestic violence during 1117
  early, and offending 1910
  and eating disorders 780, 784, 1118
  ectopic 1119
  electroconvulsive therapy in 1117
  factitious disorder in 1050, 1118
  foetal abuse in 1117
  and panic disorder 761–2
  pharmacotherapy in
    antidepressants 675, 677, 761–2, 1117, 1192
    antiepileptic drugs 677
    antipsychotics 677, 1118
    anxiolytics 1117
    benzodiazepines 762, 1117, 1180
    butyrophenones 1118
    carbamazepine 1118, 1234
    dosage regimens 1169–70
    lamotrigine 1235
    lithium 677, 1118, 1205
    phenothiazines 1117, 1118
    propranolol 1117
    topiramate 1236
    valproate 1118, 1169, 1232
  premarital 272
  psychosis in 1118
  and schizophrenia 548
  sleep deprivation in 927
  smoking in 1646
  substance use disorders in 480, *480*, 1117–18, 1614, 1615–16, 1754
  and suicide 1116, 1119
  surrogate 1115
  termination *see* abortion
  volatile substance abuse in 504
  see also obstetric complications
prejudice and stigma 6
premenstrual tension/syndrome 1114
premotor cortex 145
prenatal exposure to alcohol 1841
pre-occipital sulcus 145
preparedness theory and phobias 745
Preparing for the Drug Free Years programme 1790
presenilins 227, 339
Present State Examination 71, 269, 272, 523, 534, 542
pre-speech 240
pre-supplementary area 245
prevalence 281, 1607
  estimation 138–41
  lifetime 215, 542
  point 215, 542
  typical estimates 285, *285*
prevention
  alcohol use disorders **467–72**, 1448–9
  Alzheimer's disease 341
  anorexia nervosa 796–7
  autism 1640
  body dysmorphic disorder 1048
  child abuse and neglect 1737–8, 1788
  in childhood and adolescence 1606, 1609–11
  chronic fatigue syndrome 1042
  comparison with health promotion 1609
  conduct disorder 1663, 1788
  Creutzfeldt–Jakob disease 358–9
  cyclothymia/cyclothymic disorder 689
  deliberate self-harm **972–6**
  delirium 331, 1533
  Down syndrome 1448
  dysthymic disorder 686
  epilepsy 1620
  evidence-based 1608–9
  foetal alcohol syndrome 1448
  HIV/AIDS 1447
  indicated 1609, 1610
  infectious diseases 1447
  intellectual disability 1447–8, *1448*, 1834–5
  iodine deficiency 1448
  malingering 1058
  mood disorders 1448, 1555–6, 1675–7
  panic disorder 762
  pervasive developmental disorders 1640
  phenylketonuria 1448
  post-traumatic stress disorder 697, 698, 1109, 1279–80
  primary **1446–51**, 1598, 1609
    responsibility for 1449–50, *1450*
  and public health 1606–7
  relapse 1448
  research cycle 1608–9
  role of epidemiology 281
  schizophrenia 550, 589, 1448
  schizotypal personality disorder 601
  secondary 1446, 1598, 1609
  selected 1609, 1610
  social anxiety disorder 744
  specific phobia 746
  staff burnout 1449, *1449*
  suicide **969–78**, 1449, 1708–9, 1992
  tertiary 1446, 1598, 1609
  theoretical models 1608
  three-level concept 1446
  universal 1609, 1610
  vascular dementia 381, 1447
  violent behaviour 1449
  volatile substance abuse 505
  Wernicke–Korsakoff syndrome 450, 1542
'primary addiction' theory 434
primary auditory cortex 146
primary care **1480–9**
  alcohol use disorder detection 1484
  assessment in 67
  classification in 1483–4
  clinical presentation in 1482–3
  counselling in 1280, 1485–6
  depression
    detection and assessment 1476
    elderly people 1518
    treatment 1322, 1476
  elderly people 1482–3, 1518, 1584
  epidemiology 1480–2, *1481*, *1482*
  hidden vs. conspicuous morbidity 1482
  interface with secondary care 1486–7
  management of psychiatric disorder 1485–6, *1485*
  mental health professionals 1485–6
  mental health services 1486
  panic disorder 753
  prevalence of personality disorders 884
  prevalence of psychiatric disorder 1480–2, *1480*, *1481*, *1482*
  psychiatric nurses in 1406
  refugee clinics 1496
  social worker attachment 1411
  somatization in 1482
  training in mental health 1487–8
primary care mental health workers 1485
primary child mental health workers 1812
primary identification 1344
primary motor cortex 145
primary somatic sensory cortex 146
primary visual cortex 152
primidone
  choice of 1866–7
  pharmacokinetics *1867*
priming 250, 254
primitive defensive operations 298–9
primitive idealization 298
principlism 31
prion disease **351–61**
  acquired 352, 354–6
  aetiology 351–2
  clinical features 352–3
  diagnosis 352–3, *353*
  inherited 352, *353*, 356–8
  pre-symptomatic and antenatal testing 358
  prevention 358–9
  prognosis and treatment 359
  species barrier/transmission barrier 352
  sporadic 352, *353*
  subclinical infection 352

prion protein 351, 353–4
prisoners
attention-deficit hyperactivity disorder 1931
bipolar disorder *1934*
depression 1923, *1933*
elderly 1584
female 1934, 1935
group therapy 1365
Integrated Drug Treatment System 515
mental disorder **1933–6**
prevalence 1933–4, *1934*
mental health services for 1934–5
obsessive–compulsive disorder *1934*
personality disorder 1921, 1933, *1933*
post-traumatic stress disorder *1934*
prevalence of personality disorders 884–5
psychopathy 1921
psychoses 1933, *1933*
risk of suicide 976
schizophrenia 1934, *1934*
substance use disorders 480, *1934*
see also offenders
prisons, psychiatric nursing in 1404
Pritchard, J.C. 18–19
private symbolism 54
PRNP gene 351, 352–3, 357
mutations 357–8, *357*
probability 1997
problem list 73, 74
problem-solving therapy 1276
adjustment disorders 1068
antisocial personality disorder 898
attempted suicide 970
conduct disorder 1781–2
depression 1555
elderly people 1555, 1574
group setting 1351, 1352
procarbazine 1092
processing speed, assessment of 87–8, *88*
prochlorperazine 1101
procyclidine 1225
Profile of Mood States 717
progesterone 816
progranulin gene/protein 348
progressive multifocal leucoencephalopathy in HIV/AIDS 1093
progressive muscle relaxation in generalized anxiety disorder 736
progressive subcortical gliosis 348
progressive supranuclear palsy 344
differential diagnosis 348, 364
neuropathology 345
Project Atlas 11
Project MATCH 452, 455, 456, 462
projection 294, 299, 307, 1339
projective identification 298–9, 307–8, 316, 1339, 1340, 1344, 1770
projective techniques in child and adolescent assessment 1604
prolactin 165–6, 815
in electroconvulsive therapy 1257
hyperprolactinaemia 815, 826, 1086, 1217, 1223
and seizures 1078
and social bonding 888
prolonged grief disorder 726
promazine *1209*
proneurones 157, 158
proopiomelanocortin 170
propentofylline in vascular dementia 381
property destruction in conduct disorder 1656
propofol
in cancer *1104*
in conversion disorder 999
propranolol
in acute stress reactions 697
in dementia 415
in intellectual disability 1876
in panic disorder 757
in pregnancy 1117
Prospective and Retrospective Memory Questionnaire 420
prospective longitudinal (cohort) studies 282, 283, 541, 557, 568
prostate 817
Protection-Motivation Theory 1137
protective factors 1607
protein kinase C 1201
proteins
glycosylation (glycation) 1508–9
post-synthetic modification 1508–9
proton magnetic resonance spectroscopy *see* magnetic resonance spectroscopy
protryptylene *670, 1187, 1189, 1191, 1196*
PrP (prion protein) 351, 353–4
PSE (Present State Examination) 71, 269, 272, 523, 534, 542
pseudocorrelation 1608
pseudocyesis 1115
pseudodementia 335, 1551, *1551*
in HIV/AIDS 385
treatment 1253
pseudohallucination 49
pseudologia fantastica (pathological lying) 54, 871, 1049, 1051, 1941
pseudoneurasthenias 1060
pseudoseizures 1078, 1619, 1861
pseudosexuality 869
pseudo-status 1050
psilocin 488
psilocybin 488, 489
psoriasis in alcohol use disorders 446
Psychiatric Assessment Schedule for Adults with Developmental Disorders 1823
psychiatric disorder/psychiatric illness *see* mental disorder
psychiatric injury 1902–3
psychiatric nurses **1403–7**
community 462, 1404–5
in consultation-liaison psychiatry 1146
in the developing world 1406–7
global survey 12, *12*
in inpatient settings 1404
prescribing and medication management 1405–6
in primary care 1406
in prison settings 1404
provision of cognitive-behaviour therapy 1406
psychosocial interventions in the community 1404–5
psychiatric services *see* mental health services
Psychiatric Status Schedule 71
psychiatrists
cooperation with GPs 67
global survey 12, *12*
GPs' expectations of 1486–7
as managers **39–46**
in the multi-disciplinary team 68
role in rehabilitation 1400
psychic determinism 314
psychic retreat 308
PSYCHLOPS 1274
Psych-Med unit 1145
psychoanalysis **293–305**, 1327, **1337–50**
abstinence in 1339
aspects of 293
constructivist 299
contemporary techniques 299–300, 1339–40
defence mechanisms 293–4, 1339–40
definitions 293, 297
derived treatment modalities 300–1
efficacy 1345–6
ending treatment 1345
formulation 1341–2
history of therapeutic approach 23, 1338–9
indications and contraindications 301, 1341
interpersonal 310
interpretation in 1344–5
modes of therapeutic action 1340–1
and object-relations theory 297, 301–3, 306–12
objectivist 299
outcome research 303–4
and personality 849
personality disorders 892
principal features of techniques 1339–41
and psychopathology 296–7
and regression in 297, 1342
relational 1337, 1340
resistance to 1342
selection procedures 1341
starting treatment 1341–2
structural theory 294–6
supportive and directive interventions 1342
theories 293–6, 1337–8
therapist neutrality 1339, 1340
training in 1346
treatment duration 1327, 1341
treatment formulation 297
treatment management 1341–5
treatment process 297–8
see also psychodynamic psychiatry
psychoanalytic psychotherapy 300
indications and contraindications 301
outcome research 303–4
psychodrama groups 1351, 1353
psychodynamic counselling 1275, 1277–8
psychodynamic psychiatry **313–20**
basic principles 313–15, *313*
and clinical assessment 67
and conversion disorder 1011
and countertransference 314, *315*, 317–18
definition 313
developmental orientation 314
future directions 319
history of 23
and mental health social work 1408–9
and the mind–brain interface 315–16
multiple-treater settings 317
and personality development 316–17
and pharmacotherapy 317
and psychic determinism 314
and resistance 315, 317
and somatization disorder 1004
and transference 314
two-person concept 317–18
and the unconscious 313–14
and the uniqueness of the individual 314

psychodynamic psychotherapy 313, 1327, 1337
anorexia nervosa 796
avoidant personality disorder 897
borderline personality disorder 318–19, 894
brief (short-term) 318, **1327–37**
adjustment disorders 1068
background 1327
comparison with interpersonal psychotherapy and cognitive-behaviour therapy 1333–4, *1333*
comparison of therapies 1329–33
in conjunction with pharmacotherapy 1329
duration of treatment 1330
efficacy 1334–5
evaluation and setting 1327–8
focus of 1329
practical problems in 1334, *1334*
research 1334–5
schizotypal personality disorder 898
technique 1328–9
childhood and adolescence **1769–77**
background 1770
classical technique 1770–1
definition 1764
efficacy 1773–4
indications and contraindications 1772
limitations 1774
managing treatment 1772–3
procedure selection 1772
psychodynamic technique 1771–2
trauma 1730
definition 318
in depression in elderly people 1555
expressive–supportive continuum *318*, 1327
in intellectual disability 1874–5
long-term 318–19, 1327, 1329, 1338, 1345
see also psychoanalysis
panic disorder 758
post-traumatic stress disorder 709
schizophrenia 583
in sexual abuse by children/adolescents 1953
psychoeducation 1276
in anxiety disorders 735–6
in attention-deficit hyperactivity disorder 1648–9
in bereavement 726
in body dysmorphic disorder 1047
in borderline personality disorder 868
in cyclothymia 689
in dementia 386, 411, *414*, 418
in family therapy 1382
group setting 1351, 1352, 1364
in hyperthymia 691
in interpersonal psychotherapy 1321
in manual-assisted cognitive treatment 895
in mood disorder 676, 677, 1554
in childhood and adolescence 1676, 1677
in psychodynamic child psychotherapy 1771, 1773
in schizophrenia 583, 1448
in somatization disorder 1008
in systems training for emotional predictability and problem solving 895
use by psychiatric nurses 1405, 1406
psychogeriatric services *see* mental health services, for elderly people
psychological anthropology 276
psychological first aid 726
Psychological Impairments Rating Scale 72
psychological pillow 58
psychological refractory period 248
psychologists, global survey 12, *12*
Psychology of Criminal Conduct 2011
psychometric tests 81–2, *81*, 85–7
clinical value 84
in hypersomnia 939
sex offenders 1962
psychomotor acceleration 55
psychomotor agitation *58*
psychomotor development, history-taking 1600
psychomotor retardation 55, *58*
in vascular dementia 379
psychoneuroendocrinology 161
psychoneuroimmunology **205–11**, 1039, 1249
early investigations 205–6
effects of stress on immune system 205, 207, 1135–6
immune modulation of emotion and mood 209
immune system as sensory organ 207, 209
neural influences on immune system 206–7
receptors in the immune system 206
psycho-oncology **1100–5**
Psychopathia Sexualis (Krafft-Ebing) 836
psychopathology
assessment instruments 1164
and attachment theory 243
culture-related variations 982–3
definition 47
descriptive 47
distinction between form and content 48, 63
distinction between process and development 48
dualism in 848
explanatory 47
phenomenological 47–61
and psychiatric diagnosis 989
and psychoanalysis 296–7
psychopathy
in childhood and adolescence 1950
diagnosis 1921
in offenders/prisoners 1921–2
prediction of 851
Psychopathy Check List-Revised 1921, 2011
psychopharmacology, cosmetic 28–9
psychoprophylactics 1448
psychoses
acute and transient disorders **602–8**
in alcohol withdrawal 58, 443, 449–50, 538
in Alzheimer's disease 335
art therapy 1415
assessment instruments 1164
childhood and adolescence
differential diagnosis 1673
and juvenile delinquency 1950
cognitive model 1314
complementary medicines 1249
cultural influences 14
cycloid 574, 603, 605, 1124
and delirium 327
in dementia 416
differential diagnosis 536–9, 1004
drug-induced
cannabis 507, 538
differential diagnosis 538–9
hallucinogens 489
phencyclidine 487
prescribed medication 539
stimulants 485, 498
elderly people 1518–19
and epilepsy
chronic interictal 1079
postictal 1079
factitious 1055
and filicide 1125
first episode 573, 1396
following an accident 1110
following head injury 392–3
in HIV/AIDS 1092
and intellectual disability 1826, 1827, 1854
malingered 1055
menstrual 1114
monosymptomatic hypochondriacal 617–19
in multiple sclerosis 1074
and pain 1030
paranoid 392–3, 485
in Parkinson's disease 1072
and physical illness 546, 1132
postabortion 1119
postpartum 647, 1124
in pregnancy 1118
prisoners 1933, *1933*
psychogenic 603
puerperal 1114
reactive 574
schizophreniform 536, 603, 605
secondary to organic disorder 537–8
and surgery 1098
treatment 1254–5
very-late-onset schizophrenia-like 1518–19
psychosexual development 235
hormonal influences 1720
variation in 1718–19
psychosocial functioning
assessment 73, 1164, 1593
in body dysmorphic disorder 1044
psychosocial interventions in dementia 414, *414*
psychosocial vulnerability and depression 271
psychostimulants
in cancer 1102, *1103*
in terminal illness 1070
psychosurgery *see* neurosurgery for mental disorder
psychotherapy
in autism and other pervasive developmental disorders 1640
childhood and adolescence **1764–9, 1769–77**
approaches to 1766–8
confidentiality 1768
consent for 1765
and culture 1768
differences from adult psychotherapy 1765, *1765*
ending 1768
failure to attend 1768
focus on past vs. focus on present 1767
individual vs. group therapy 1768
involvement of parents and school 1768
limit-setting vs. free expression 1767
measures of effectiveness and outcome 1769
record-keeping 1768
training and supervision 1768–9
treatment setting 1766
comparisons with pharmacotherapy 1162
and counselling 1273–4, 1765
definition 1764
empirically supported 672

psychotherapy (*cont.*)
evaluation **1158–67**
internal vs. external validity 1159
measurement of therapeutic change 1163–4
outcome assessment strategies 1163
patient selection 1163
research design 1161–5
research planning 1159, *1160*
selection criteria for outcome studies 1159, 1161
treatment standardization 1161, *1161*
historical background 20–1
hypochondriasis 1026–7
in the paraphilias 838–9
personality disorders **892–901**
process-orientated/outcome-orientated 672
treatment manuals 1161
see also specific therapies
psychoticism 81, *81*
PTSD *see* post-traumatic stress disorder
PTSD Checklist 703
puberty, delayed/arrested in anorexia nervosa 787, 794
public attitudes and stigma **5–9**
public health
epidemiology 1607–8
and prevention 1606–7
psychiatric disorder as worldwide issue **10–13**
public policy
influence on mental health 1426, *1426*
see also mental health public policy
publication bias 229
Pueraria lobata 1249
puerarin 1249
puerperal psychosis 1124
puerperium
anxiety disorders in 1121
depression in 1122, 1280, 1322, 1486
normal 1120–1
obsessive–compulsive disorder in 1121–2
Puerto Rican syndrome 983–4
pulmonary embolism 1082–3
pulmonary oedema in anorexia nervosa 785
pulse rate and conduct disorder 1658
pulvinar sign 356
punch-drunk syndrome 395
puppets 1778
pure agraphia 54
purines *168*
Purkinje cells 158
putamen 154, 159, 1684
Putnam, Hilary 134
pyramidal cells 148
pyramidal tract 156, 158
pyrazinamide 1094
pyromania **914–15**, 1924, 1965, 1967, 1968

Q fever 1038
QALYs (Quality-Adjusted Life Years) 124, 1475, 1510
quality of life
in alcohol use disorders 463
in Alzheimer's disease 339
assessment instruments 73, 1165
in body dysmorphic disorder 1044
in evaluation of mental health services 1465
quality management 43–4, *44*
quasi-experimental studies 1468
querulant reactions to childbirth 1121
querulous behaviour 616, **1977–80**
assessment 1978–9, *1979*
clinical features 1977–8
management 1979–80
questionable dementia *see* mild cognitive impairment
questionnaires 62, **94–8**
administration methods 95–6
in childhood and adolescence 1591
content and format 95, *95*
creation 96
in epidemiology 284
evaluation criteria 95
forced-choice questions 94
multiple measures 96
psychometric adequacy 95
purpose of 94
reasons for development 69
self-report measures 94
standard vs. individualized 97
see also assessment instruments
quetiapine 1199, 1209, *1209*
administration *1214*, 1218
adverse effects *1212*, 1224
in bipolar disorder in elderly people 1556
in cancer *1104*
in childhood and adolescence 1677, 1797
pharmacodynamics 1210, *1211*, 1213
pharmacokinetics 1221–2
quinacrine 359
quinalbarbitone 1178

rachischisis 156
racism, institutional 276
RAD (reactive attachment disorder) 243, 1590, 1639, 1645
'railway spine syndrome' 700, 1902
random sampling 139
randomized controlled trials (RCTs) 123, 1158, 1466–8, 1608
advantages 1151–2, *1467*
appraisal 126, 127–8
biases 1151–2
blinding 127
cluster 1470
comparative designs 1162
concealment of treatment allocation 127
control groups 1162
criteria for quality evaluation *1467*
design and analysis 141–2
differential drop-out 128
dismantling designs 1162
effectiveness 1466–8, *1468*, 1469–70, *1469*
efficacy 1466–8, *1468*
generalizability 1152
inapplicable situations *1467*
inclusion and exclusion criteria 128
intention-to-treat analysis 128
limitations/disadvantages 1151–2, *1467*
meta-analysis 229, 1155, 1465–6, *1466*
power calculation 1151
preference 1470
psychotherapy 1162–3
rogue results 1152
systematic reviews *see* systematic reviews
validity 127–8
rape 1498
crisis centres 1988
date 409, 491
definition 1985
offenders 1961
victims 1985–6
raphe nuclei 150–1
Rapid Risk Assessment of Sex Offender Recidivism 1963
rapid tranquillization 1404
in childhood and adolescence 1798
rapists, personality disorder 1921
Ras proteins 175
Rasmussen syndrome type 2 1864, 1867
Rat Man 1683
rate of living and longevity 1508
rating scales/schedules 62, **94–8**
content and format 95, *95*
creation 96
evaluation criteria 95
multiple measures 96
psychometric adequacy 95
purpose of 94
reasons for development 69
standard vs. individualized 97
see also assessment instruments
rational emotive therapy in intellectual disability 1874
rationalization 294
Rauvolfia serpentina (rauwolfia) 1249, *1250*
Raven's Progressive Matrices Test 87, 264, 1909
RBD *see* REM sleep behaviour disorder
RC (residential continuum) 1400
RCTs *see* randomized controlled trials
RDC (Research Diagnostic Criteria) 100, 523, 534, 751
reaction formation 294
reactive attachment disorder 243, 1590, 1639, 1645
reactive oxygen species, role in ageing 1509
reactivity 95
Read codes 1484
reading disorder 1627–9
reality orientation in dementia *414*
reality principle 294, 295
reassurance, in medical consultations 1138
reassurance-seeking, in hypochondriasis 1022
re-bonding 1514
reboxetine 670, *670*
adverse effects 1190, *1191*
dosage *1196*
in panic disorder 757
pharmacodynamics *1187*
pharmacokinetics *1189*
receptive language disorder 1626
reciprocity negotiation 1375
Recognition Memory Test 89
recovered memories 714–15, 834
recovery model 1491
recreational drugs
classification 1927
use by elderly people 1544
see also substance use disorders *and specific drugs*
reductionism 134
reduplicative paramnesia 392
Reelin 158
refeeding 795
complications 786
referential thinking in body dysmorphic disorder 1044
reflective awareness 308
reflex sympathetic dystrophy 1015, 1050
reflexive function 310

refugees **1493–500**
assessment 1496–7
conceptual outcome models 1494–5, *1495*
cultural factors 1496, *1496*, 1498
definition 1493–4, *1493*
depression 1495
families 1497
head injury 1495
health status and physical illness 1495
internally displaced 1493
long-term functional impairment and disability 1495–6
post-traumatic stress disorder 1495, 1497
principle of *non-refoulement 1493*, 1494
protection of 1493–4
psychiatric symptoms and illness 1495–6
risk and resiliency factors 1498
screening 1496–7
somatic complaints 1497
torture 1494, 1495
trauma 1494–6, *1495*, 1496–7, 1497
treatment 1497–8
Regional Care Services Improvement Partnership Development Centres 1488
regression
as coping strategy 1066
in psychoanalysis 297, 1342
regressive transference neurosis 297–8
rehabilitation 1352, **1399–403**
in community mental health services 389–90, 1459
core elements *1402*
current approaches 1400–2
development of environmental resources 1402
and family intervention 1401
and participation in the community 1402
role of psychiatrist 1400
social skills training 583, 898, 1401, 1968
target population 1399–400
vocational 583, 1400–1, 1889
reinforcer devaluation 258
Relate 1370
relationship counselling 1278–9
relative risk 126, 128, 282
relaxation techniques
applied relaxation 746
in insomnia 937
in persistent somatoform pain disorder 1034
progressive muscle relaxation 736
in sleep disorders 1572
in specific phobia 746
reliability 85, 92, 95, 137–8
in classification in childhood and adolescence 1591
inter-rater/inter-observer *85*, 95, 263, 1465
models and definitions 137–8
of outcome measures 1465
parallel-form *85*, 1465
split-half *85*, 1465
test–retest *85*, 263, 1465
types *85*
religious delusions 51
religious healing ceremonies 1419–20
REM-atonia 946
REM latency 684, 931
REM sleep behaviour disorder (RBD) 928, **946–7**, 1695
association with psychiatric disorders and stress 947
clinical and polysomnographic findings 946–7
in dementia 416–17
diagnosis 947
in elderly people 1572
in narcolepsy with cataplexy 941
overlap with other parasomnias 947
treatment 947
reminiscence therapy *414*, 1574
remoxipride 1209–10
repetition compulsion 299
repetitive self-mutilation 916–17
repetitive transcranial magnetic stimulation *see* transcranial magnetic stimulation
reports 74–6
and confidentiality 75
expert witness 1928, *2004*, **2005–6**
partiality 75
principles 75
purposes 75
structure 75–6
repression 294
RERAs (respiratory effort-related arousals) 940
Rescorla–Wagner learning rule 259
rescue workers, debriefing 1110
research
on aetiology 281–6
on art therapy 1416
in epidemiology of child and adolescent psychiatric disorder 1597–8
in evaluation of mental health services 1465–9, *1465*, *1466*, *1467*, *1468*, *1469*
and evidence-based medicine 122–8
longitudinal 1597
on mental health services 281, 1452
patient selection 1163
study design 282, 1161–3, 1465–9, *1465*, *1466*, *1467*, *1468*, *1469*, 1475–6
using with individual patients 126–8
Research Diagnostic Criteria 100, 523, 534, 751
reserpine 1172, 1249
residential continuum 1400
residential services
in childhood and adolescence **1799–802**
in community mental health services 1453–4
for elderly people 1518, 1583
for people with intellectual disability and psychiatric disorder 1889
resilience 1607
and adoption/foster care 1748
in childhood 1660, 1803
of refugees 1498
resistance
in adolescence 1603–4
and non-compliance 317
to psychoanalysis 1342
in psychodynamic psychiatry 297, 315, 317
repression 1342
transference 1342
resistance to change in autism 1633
respiratory effort-related arousals 940
respiratory perturbation and anxiety disorders 1667
respiratory system
in anorexia nervosa 785
in chronic fatigue syndrome 1038
disorders *932*, 1082–3
respite care
in community mental health services 1458
for elderly people 1583
response inhibition/prevention 249, 1047
responsibility
criminal 1945, 1954
diminished 1901, 1922, 1923, 1928, 1937, 1939, 1940
legal aspects 1900–5
in obsessive–compulsive disorder 1783
see also diminished responsibility defence
restless legs syndrome **948**, 1572, 1695
restraint 1133, 1404
restriction fragment length polymorphisms 218
Rethink 1490–1
reticular nucleus 150
retifism 833
retinal development 157
retirement 1514
Retreat, York 17–18
retrograde messengers 171–2
Rett's syndrome 1614, **1636–7**, 1698
aetiology 1637
behavioural and psychiatric aspects 1845
clinical features 1636
course 1637–8
definition 1636, *1636*
demographics 1636
epidemiology 1636
and epilepsy 1864, 1864–5
genetics 224, 229, 1637, 1844, *1866*
management 1640
physical characteristics 1845
prevalence 1844
prognosis 1637–8
revenge and fire-raising 1967
reverse bonding 1514
reversed role play 1376
reversible inhibitors of monoamine oxidase (RIMAs) 670, *670*
pharmacodynamics 1173
in social anxiety disorder 743
reviews 1152
and clinical assessment 74
'reward deficiency syndrome' hypothesis 434
reward-dependence 80, *80*, 316, *316*, 849
Rey 15-item test 1057
Rey Auditory-Verbal Learning Test 89, 264
Rey–Osterrieth Complex Figure Test 89
Reynolds Adolescent Depression Scale 1675
rhombencephalon 156, 157
rhombomeres 157
rhythmic movement disorder, sleep-related *928*, 1702
ribonucleic acid *see* RNA
rifampicin
adverse effects *1091*
in tuberculosis 1094
RIMAs *see* reversible inhibitors of monoamine oxidase
rimonabant 513
risk 1991–2
individual, application of population data 281
modelling patterns of 141
risk analysis 44
risk assessment 1991–2
contemporary approaches 1992–3
and contingency plan 1455, *1457*
and culture of blame 1991–2
in dementia 417, *417*
and expert witnesses 2005
limits of mental health professionals' engagement 1993–4

risk assessment (*cont.*)
offenders using drugs/alcohol 1927
violence **1991–2002**
approaches 1994–5
by stalkers 1972–4, *1973*
evaluating levels of risk 1998–9
instruments 1994, 1996–7
practicalities 1997–2000
utility 1995–6
risk difference 128
risk factors 1607–8
Alzheimer's disease 1520–2, *1520*, *1522*
anorexia nervosa *806*
antisocial behaviour by adolescents *1946*, 1947
bipolar disorder 646–7, 1675
bulimia nervosa 805–6, *806*
causative 1607
in child and adolescent psychiatric disorders 556, 1590, 1675
conduct disorder 1658–60
delirium 329, *329*
dementia 376, 1520–2, *1520*, *1522*
depression 648–9, 658–9, 1675
fixed 1607
hypochondriasis 997, 1024
independent 1608
malleable 1607
mania 646–7
mediating 1608
moderating 1608
offending 1909–14
overlapping 1608
panic disorder 753
post-traumatic stress disorder *707*
proxy 1608
and refugee vulnerability 1498
schizophrenia 547–9, **553–61**
sleep-wake disorders 1696–7
suicide 951–2, *953*, 971, *971*, *972*, 1449
Risk for Sexual Violence Protocol 1998
risk management 44
offenders using drugs/alcohol 1927
of violence towards others 1997–8, 1999–2000, *1999*
risk-taking, morbid 921
risperidone 1209, *1209*
administration *1214*, 1216–17
adverse effects *1212*, 1224
in attention-deficit hyperactivity disorder 1652
in bipolar disorder, in elderly people 1556
in cancer *1104*
in childhood and adolescence 1797
mania 1677
with psychiatric/behaviour disorder and intellectual disability 1852
in delirium 331
in dementia 415
in HIV/AIDS 1092
in intellectual disability 1875
long-acting injectable 581
pharmacodynamics 1172, 1210, *1211*, 1213
pharmacokinetics *1172*, 1221
in schizotypal personality disorder 600
in tic disorders 1688
Ritalin® *see* methylphenidate
rivastigmine
in Alzheimer's disease 409, 1241, 1538
in dementia 415
in Parkinson's disease 370–1
in vascular dementia 381
Rivermead Behavioural Memory Test 89
Rivers, W.H.R. 276
RLS (restless leg syndrome) **948**, 1572, 1695
RNA
cross-linkage 1508
double-stranded (dsRNA) 225
messenger (mRNA) 224–5, *224*
micro (miRNA) 225
non-coding 229
small interfering (siRNA) 225
structure and function 223
road traffic accidents *see* accidents
robbery, victims 1986
ROC curve 140, 1995
Rochester Youth Development Study 1910, 1913
rofecoxib in Alzheimer's disease 1538
Rogers, Carl 1273, 1274, 1276
Rohypnol (flunitrazepam) 409, 491, 1183, 1188
ROI morphometry 195
role play, reversed 1376
role reversal 308
role theory and transitions 1514
rolipram 176
ROM (routine outcome measures) 1460
ROS (reactive oxygen species), role in ageing 1509
Rosenberg Self-Esteem Scale 1164
Rough Sleepers Initiative 1501
routine outcome measures 1460
RRASOR (Rapid Risk Assessment of Sex Offender Recidivism) 1963
RSVP (Risk for Sexual Violence Protocol) 1998
rTMS *see* transcranial magnetic stimulation
Rubinstein–Taybi syndrome
behavioural and psychiatric aspects 1845
genetics 1845
physical characteristics 1845
prevalence 1845
Rule Shift Cards Test *90*
rule violation in conduct disorder 1656
'rum fits' 443
rumination
in anxiety disorders 1288–9
in bulimia nervosa 803
Russell's sign 804
Russia, neurasthenia as diagnostic entity 1061
Ryle, Gilbert 133

S-100b 353
S-adenosylmethionine 1248
sacrificial ritual 1419
SAD *see* seasonal affective disorder; separation anxiety disorder
sadism 832–3, *833*
criminal 832
sexual 832, *836*
sadistic personality disorder 878, 1921
sadomasochism 832–3, 878
SAFE Children (Schools and Families Educating Children) programme 1789
safety behaviours
in anxiety disorders 1287–8, *1288*, 1290
in body dysmorphic disorder 1044, *1044*
sage 1248
St John's wort 386, 686, 1248, *1250*, 1262
salivary gland enlargement in bulimia nervosa 804
Salpêtrière asylum 17, 18
Salvia divinorum 488
Salvia officinalis 1248
SAMe (*S*-adenosylmethionine) 1248
sample bias 282–3
sampling 96–7, 138–9, 1595
principles 282–3
structural MRI studies 194
Sanfillipo syndrome 1843
SARA (Spousal Assault Risk Assessment) 1998
SARCs (Sexual Assault Referral Centres) 1986
SASB (Structural Analysis of Social Behavior) 852
satiety cascade 782
SATs (Standard Assessment Tests) 1715
Scale for the Assessment of Negative Symptoms 69, 72, 524
Scale for the Assessment of Positive Symptoms 524
SCAN (Schedules for Clinical Assessment in Neuropsychiatry) 70, 71, 72, 284, 542, 719
scapegoating 317
Schedule for Affective Disorders and Schizophrenia 70, 71, 523
Schedule for Nonadaptive and Adaptive Personality 858, *858*
Schedules for Clinical Assessment in Neuropsychiatry 70, 71, 72, 284, 542, 719
schema-coping behaviour 895
schema-focused therapy 894, 895, 904, 1778
Schie syndrome 1843
schizoaffective disorder **595–602**
classification 596–7
clinical features 595–6
course and outcome 574, 596–7
diagnosis 597–8
differential diagnosis 537, 597–8
elderly people 1552
epidemiology 598
family studies 596
management 598–9
premorbid function 595
subtypes 597
schizoid personality disorder **862–3**
aetiology 862
classification *856*, 863, *863*
clinical features 863
course 863
differential diagnosis 862, 863, 865, 876
in elderly people 1562, *1562*
epidemiology 862, 882, *882*
treatment 863
schizoid thought 308
schizophrenia
admission policies *585*
and age 544–5
age of onset 558, 1547
atypical/unsystematic 574
catatonic *535*
cerebral atrophy in 536
childhood and adolescence 1613
differential diagnosis 1673
risk factors for development 556–7
classification **535–6**, 1546–7
clinical features **526–31**
anxiety and somatoform disorders 530
emotional disorders 529
motor disorders 529
thought and perception disorders 526–8
volition disorders 529–30
cognitive impairment 93, 265, 528, **531–4**, 580

comorbidity
physical disease 546
substance use disorders 427, 507, 546, 558, 1919
coping strategies 1313–14
course and outcome *536*, **568–78**
definitions and assessment of variables 569
elderly people 1548
methodological factors 568–74
patterns and stages 571
predictors 574–6, *575*
and risk factors 558
study results 569, *570*
cultural and geographic variations 14, 546, 557, 571–3, *572*
delusions 526–7
depression in 529, 573
developmental antecedents 548
and diabetes mellitus 1085
diagnosis and diagnostic criteria 103–4, 105, 522–3, **534–6**, *535*, 1547
diagnostic process 539
early diagnosis 536
and epidemiology 541
influence on outcome studies 568–9
differential diagnosis 327, *328*, 536–9, 863, 864, 1547
dimensions of psychopathology 530, *530*
disease and disability burden 546–7
disease expectancy/morbid risk 544
as a disorder of brain maturation 180–1, *180*, *181*
elderly people **1546–50**, 1552
aetiology 1548
classification 1546–7
clinical features 1546
course and prognosis 1548
diagnosis 1547
differential diagnosis 1547, 1559
epidemiology 1547
treatment and management 1548–9
emergencies 590
epidemiology **540–53**
case finding 541
descriptive 542–7
in elderly people 1547
future issues 549–50
historical landmarks *540*
incidence 542–4, *544*, *545*
methods and instruments 541–2
prevalence 542, *543*
and epilepsy 1079
ethnic minorities 549, 557–8
and expressed emotion 575, 583
family factors 536, 548–9, 553–5
and fertility 545
and fire-raising 1967
first-rank (Schneiderian) symptoms 523, 526, 527–8, *527*, 535–6, 573–4
following head injury 392
and gender 544–5
genetics 547, 548–9, 553–5, 565–6, *565*
hallucinations 527, 573–4
hebephrenic (disorganized) *535*, 574
history of concept **521–6**
homicide by people with 1939, 1995
insight in 528
and intellectual disability 1827, 1854
and juvenile delinquency 1950
late-onset 1547
markers 536
mental health services 584–5
models
genetic 554
gene–environment interaction 558–9
stress–diathesis 507, 558–9, 1313
mortality associated 545–6
name change in Japan 7
and narcolepsy 927
natural history 569–70
negative symptoms 535
concept of 522, 523–5
dimensions 530
treatment 580, *589*, 1265, 1548
neurobiology **561–8**
functional 561–3
structural 563–4
theories based on 564–6, *565*, *566*
neuropathology 178–81, *178*, *179*, *180*, *181*
neuropsychological assessment 93, 265, 528, **531–4**
and obsessive–compulsive disorder 766
and offending 1918–20
and optical distortions 49
overlap with bipolar disorder for susceptibility 652
paranoid *535*, 574, 609, 610
parental, effects on child development 1753
PET/SPET imaging 188–9, 562–3
positive symptoms 523
concept of 523–5
dimensions 530
drug therapy 579–80
and pregnancy/birth complications 548
premorbid intelligence 548
premorbid personality 536
premorbid social impairment 548
prevention 550, 589, 1448
prisoners 1934, *1934*
prodrome 573, 589–90
pseudoneurotic 875
pseudopsychopathic 866
and pulmonary embolism 1083
recovery 576
relapse 581
remission 589
residual *535*
risk factors 547–9, **553–61**
and age of onset 558
birth season 547, 556
childhood 556–7
environmental 555–8
familial/genetic 547, 548–9, 553–5, 565–6, *565*
life events 558, 575
migration 286, 549, 557–8
model based on 558–9
obstetric complications 548, 555–6
and outcome 558
paternal age 555
prenatal exposure to infection 547–8, 556
social and geographic 557–8
and sexuality 825–6
simple *535*, 574
and sleep-wake disorders *931*
and social class 549
and stigma 5, 6–7, 539
subtypes 534, *535*, 549
prognosis 574
and suicide 545–6, 956
and surgery 1098
syndromes of symptoms 530, *530*
systematic 574
treatment and management **578–95**
acute phase 586–8
adjunctive medication 591–2
cognitive-behaviour therapy 582–3, 1313–18
of cognitive impairment 533
drug therapy 579–82, *579*, 585, 586–8, *586*, 1213, *1215*, 1548
elderly people 1548–9
electroconvulsive therapy 1255
in emergencies 590
family therapy 583–4
group therapy 1364
maintenance 581–2, 589
outline plan *587*
poor response to 590–2
post-acute phase 588
principles 585, *586*
psychodynamic psychotherapy 583
psychoeducation 583
research 592
resistance to 582, 590–2
social skills training 583
transcranial magnetic stimulation 1265
treatment gap *13*
type I 524, 535–6
type II 524, 535–6
undifferentiated 535, 574
and violence 1919, *1999*
risk assessment 1995
and working memory 255
schizophreniform psychosis 536, 603, 605
schizotaxia 599
schizotypal personality disorder **599–601**, **863–5**
classification 103–4, 599–600, *856*, 864, *864*
clinical features 599, 864
cognitive impairment in 533
course 864
diagnosis 600
differential diagnosis 600, 862, 863, 864–5
in elderly people *1562*, 1563
epidemiology 600, 864, *882*, 883
prevention 601
terminology 856–7
treatment and management 600–1, 865, 898
schnauzkrampf 58
Schneider, Kurt 522–3, 526, 681, 682, 686
school nurse 1812
'school phobia' 1665
schools
child psychiatrist as consultant to **1811–16**
establishing a school liaison service 1812–13
factors in offending 1913
in hospital 1815
intervention strategies based in 1814–15
involvement in psychotherapy 1768
problems associated with conduct disorder 1656, 1662
role in child mental health 1727
role in child protection 1814
special 1815
see also education
Schools and Families Educating Children programme 1789
Schwartz, Emanuel 1354

SCID-II (Structured Clinical Interview for DSM-IV Personality Disorders) *858*, 859
SCL-90-R 1164
scopolamine, effects on memory 409
scoptic syndrome *833*
scoptophilia *833*
scrapie 351
screening
  for alcohol use disorders in elderly people 1542
  in consultation-liaison psychiatry 1145–6, *1146*
  for domestic violence 1982
  instruments 69
  refugees 1496–7
sculpting 1376
SCUs (specialized care units) 1583
SD (standard deviation) 86
SEAL (Social and Emotional Aspects of Learning) 1814
Searles, Harold 310
season
  and bipolar disorder 646–7
  and depression 635
  seasonal affective disorder (SAD) 927, 939, 1260, 1261, 1262
  course and outcome 668
  treatment 671
seasonal rhythms 1260
Seattle Social Development Project 1912–13
second messengers 175–6, *175*, 1172
  downstream signalling cascades 176
second somatic sensory cortex 146
Secure Children's Homes 1945
secure hospitals 2015, 2016–17
  admission criteria 2018
Secure Needs Assessment Profile 2018
Secure Training Centres 1945
security 2015, 2016–17
  levels 2017
  physical 2016
  procedural 2016
  relational 2016–17
  treatment as 2017
sedatives *see* anxiolytics
segmental aneusomy syndromes 228
seizures
  absence 204, 1077
  in alcohol withdrawal 443, 449
  classification 1076–7, *1077*, 1862, *1863*
  definition 1076
  differential diagnosis of epileptic and psychogenic 1861, *1862*
  drug-induced 1223, 1795, 1795–6
  exercise-induced 1861
  factors provoking 1861
  focal 1862, *1863*
  following neurosurgery for mental disorder 1269
  in frontotemporal dementias 346
  generalized 1077, 1619, *1863*
    secondary 1862, *1863*
  iatrogenic 1078
  induction by transcranial magnetic stimulation 1263
  myoclonic 1077
  nocturnal 1702
  partial 1077, 1619
    complex 201, 1077, 1619, *1863*, 1864
    simple 1861, *1863*, 1864
  primary generalized 1862, *1863*
  provoked 1078
  psychogenic 1016–17, 1080, 1861, *1862*, *1863*, 1864
  threshold 204
  tonic–clonic 1077, *1863*
  treatment 1080
  withdrawal 1861
  see also epilepsy
selective eating 787
selective mutism 1639, 1714
Selective Reminding Test 253
selective serotonin reuptake inhibitors *see* SSRIs
selegiline
  adverse effects *1191*
  dosage *1196*
  pharmacodynamics *1187*, 1188
  pharmacokinetics *1189*
selenium 1248
self
  disorders of 56
  and the ego 295
self-actualization 1276
self-awareness 82, *83*
self-deception 1941
self-defeating personality disorder 877–8
self-directedness 80–1, *80*, 83, 316, 849–50
self-esteem 311
  assessment instruments 1164
  in bulimia nervosa 804, 806
  and chronic fatigue syndrome 1036
  and defence mechanisms 317
  and domestic violence 1982
  and the ego ideal 296
  elderly people 1559
  in hypochondriasis 1022
  and suicide 970
  and vocational rehabilitation 1401
self-harm *see* deliberate self-harm
self-help groups 1449
self-help skills, in intellectual disability 1873
self-image, in adolescence 1604
self-mutilation, repetitive 916–17
self-objects 311
self-psychology 313
  and somatization disorder 1004–5
Self-Regulatory Model 1138, 1140–1
self-report scales 4, 94
self-representation 298, 302–3
self-soothing 1694, 1698
self-states 903
self-structures 316
self-transcendence 80, *80*, 83, 316, 850
Selves Questionnaire 1164
SEM (standard error of measurement) 85
semantic–pragmatic disorder 1713
semen 817
semen-loss anxiety 606, **981**
seminal vesicles 817
SENCO (special educational needs coordinator) 1812
sensate focus exercise 1569
sensory dysfunction in conversion disorder 1017
sensory-specific satiety 258
separating 5
separation anxiety
  and intellectual disability 1851
  and panic disorder 754
separation anxiety disorder (SAD)
  clinical presentation 1665
  outcome 1666
  prevalence 1666
septohippocampal system, in generalized anxiety disorder 733, *733*
serotonergic system and serotonin receptors *173*, 174, 1171
  action of antipsychotics on 1170, 1209, 1210, *1211*
  action of anxiolytics on 1178
  and aggressive/antisocial behaviour 889, 1918
  and attention-deficit hyperactivity disorder 1646
  in autism 1636
  and chronic fatigue syndrome 1039
  and cortical function 151
  in depression 189, 660, 662, 1185, 1186
    in childhood and adolescence 1675
    genetics 652
  and eating disorders 782, 806
  effects of ecstasy 496
  in generalized anxiety disorder 733–4
  knockout studies 231
  and memory impairment 409
  and neuroticism 887–8
  in obsessive–compulsive disorder 767, 1683–4, 1684
  in panic disorder 754
  PET/SPET imaging *186*, 187, 189
  in post-traumatic stress disorder 706
  and schizophrenia 562
  serotonin transporter 169, *170*, 189, 221, 273, 286, 658, 887, 1674
  and sexual function 826
  in social anxiety disorder 741
  and substance use disorders 429
  in substance use disorders *429*, 436
  and suicide 955, 964–5, 970, 1705
  and Tourette syndrome 1073
serotonin and noradrenaline reuptake inhibitors *see* SNRIs
serotonin supplementation 1248
serotonin syndrome 1173, 1176, 1192, 1194, 1254
sertindole 1209
sertraline *670*
  adverse effects *1191*
  in cancer *1102*, *1103*
  in childhood and adolescence 1676
  in depression in elderly people 1554, *1554*
  dosage *1196*
  in obsessive–compulsive disorder 1687, *1687*
  in panic disorder *756*
  pharmacodynamics *1173*, *1187*
  pharmacokinetics *1172*, 1188, *1189*
  in social anxiety disorder 743, 744
SES *see* socio-economic status
Settlement Movement 1408
sex chromosomes 218, 223, 225
  abnormalities 1840–1
sex-linked disorders 212
Sex Offender Risk Appraisal Guide 835, 1963
sex offenders **1960–4**
  assessment 1961–2
  classification 1960–1
  definitions 1960
  ethical issues 1964
  and the general psychiatrist 1960
  juvenile 1953–4

mood disorders 1923
personality disorder 1921
risk assessment 1963, *1963*
treatment 1963–4
sex reassignment surgery 842, 843–4
sex therapy 821, **827–8**, 829
sexual arousal
brain activation during 819
extragenital changes 815
female 816, 817–19
loss of 822
male 816–17
pain during 822
Sexual Assault Referral Centres 1986
sexual disinhibition in dementia 416
sexual dysfunction **821–32**
aetiology 823–7
assessment 829–30
classification 823
clinical features 822–3
definitions and terminology 821–2
in dementia 416
drug-induced 826–7, 1190
Dual Control Model 821, 824
in elderly people 1569, *1570*
in end-stage renal disease 1087
epidemiology 823, *824*
historical aspects 821–2
and mental health 825–6
in physical illness 826
treatment and management 827–30, 1569–70
sexual function
and epilepsy 1079
and mental health 825–6
normal **812–20**
biological determinants 812–13
DEOR model 814–15, *814*
in elderly people 1569, *1569*
endocrinology 815–16
EPOR model 814–15, *814*
initiating activity 815
modelling 813–15
surveys 813–14, 821–2
sexual inhibition 825
Sexual Offences Act 1956 1899–900
Sexual Offences Act 2003 1900, 1985
sexual orientation, of elderly people 1568
sexual orientation disturbance, legitimacy of diagnosis 28
sexual scripting 813
Sexual Violence Risk-20 1998
sexuality
assessment in childhood and adolescence 1604
and dementia 1568
in elderly people 1567–70
and fire-raising 1967
in Huntington's disease 373
and intellectual handicap 1873, 1879
psychoanalytic theories 294–5
as a social construct 813–15
sexually transmitted disease (STD) 1094
delusions concerning 619
and stigma 1091
see also specific diseases
SF-12 284
SF-36 284
shabu (methamphetamine) **497–8**
shamanism 1419
shared care plans 1487
shared care register 1487
shared psychotic disorder 610, **624–5**
Shedler-Westen Assessment Procedure 858, *858*
'shell shock' 700
shenjing shuairuo 1061
shift work and sleep disturbance 926
shin-byung 606
shinkeishitsu 1061
shoplifting 1923, 1924, 1943
short-term anxiety-provoking psychotherapy 1327, 1331–2
SIADH and ecstasy 495
sialidosis 1864, 1865
Siberia, attitudes to psychiatric disorder 6
siblings
effects of loss of sibling 1120, 1759
effects of sibling with intellectual disability 1884–5
effects of sibling with physical illness 1742
sick role 1320, 1321
sickness, concept of 62, 63–4
SIDS (sudden infant death syndrome) 1119, 1698
siege experience 49–50
sign language
in autism 1639
in expressive language disorder 1626
in receptive language disorder 1626
signs, definition 47
sildenafil 821, 828
Silence of the Mind meditation 82
simple phobia *see* specific phobia
simulated presence, in dementia *414*
single-case studies 1161
single nucleotide polymorphisms 218, 226, 227
single-photon emission tomography (SPET/SPECT) 185
Alzheimer's disease 337
comparison with functional magnetic resonance imaging 186–7, 196–7
comparison with PET 185
data collection and analysis 186
dementia with Lewy bodies 364
depression 189, 660
during antipsychotic use 189–90
in epilepsy 1862
frontotemporal dementias 347, Plate 12
head injury 389
imaging strategies 187, *187*
isotopes *186*
limitations 186–7
methodology 185
schizophrenia 188–9
vascular dementia 380
Six Elements Test 265
skin
delusions concerning 50, 51, 618
effects of alcohol use disorders 446
skin picking, pathological/compulsive 618, **917–18**, 1044
Slavson, S.R. 1353
sleep **924–6**
active 946
architecture 925
changes with age 925–6, 1571–2
and chronic fatigue syndrome 1036, 1039
circadian rhythms 925, 926
and depression, in childhood and adolescence 1675
deprivation, in the puerperium 1120
functions 924–5
insufficient 1700
nature of 924
non-rapid eye movement (NREM) 924, 925
paradoxical 946
physiology, in childhood and adolescence 1692–3
rapid eye movement (REM) 924, 925, 946, 1694
REM latency 684, 931
requirements *1694*
slow wave (SWS) 925, 1694
stages 925
unihemispheric 925
sleep debt 1700
sleep diary 929, 934, 1696
sleep drunkenness 941
sleep education 936, *936*
sleep efficiency 936
sleep history 929, 1696
sleep hygiene 936, *936*
sleep onset REM period 941
sleep paralysis 929, 940
sleep questionnaire 1696
sleep-related dissociative disorder 948
sleep-related eating disorder *931*, 947–8
sleep-related injury 945
sleep-related rhythmic movement disorder *928*, 1702
sleep restriction therapy 936
sleep terrors 928, **945–6**, 1702
sleep-wake cycle, in delirium 326–7
sleep-wake disorders **924–33**
in aetiology of psychiatric illness 927
and alcohol use disorders *931*
and anxiety disorders *931*
assessment 929–30
and attention-deficit hyperactivity disorder 927, *931*, 1695, 1697
audio–video recordings 929
and autism 1697
and cardiovascular disease *932*
childhood and adolescence **1693–702**
assessment 1696–7, *1696*
developmental effects 1695
effects on parenting and the family 1694–5
excessive daytime sleepiness 1699–701, *1700*
manifestations 1695
misinterpretation 1695
parasomnias 1701–2
parental influences 1694
patterns of occurrence 1695
risk factors 1697–8
sleeplessness 1698–9
treatment and prognosis 1695–6
and chronic fatigue syndrome 1697
and chronic pain *932*
and chronic renal failure *932*
circadian rhythm *928*
classification 927, *928*
delayed sleep phase syndrome 928, 942–3, 1261, 1695, 1700
and dementia 416–17, *931*, 1572, 1573
in dementia with Lewy bodies 362
and depression 634, 661–2, 927, 931, *931*, 1697
detection 929–30
and eating disorder *931*

sleep-wake disorders (*cont.*)
elderly people 1571–3
and endocrine disease *932*
and epilepsy *932*
following stroke *932*
and gastrointestinal disorders *932*
and head injury *932*, 942, 1698
hypersomnia *see* hypersomnia
hypnotic-dependent 934
insomnia *see* insomnia
and intellectual disability 926–7, 1694, 1697–8
in intensive care patients *932*
and iron deficiency *932*
legal issues 948–9
and mania *931*
mistaken for primarily psychological/psychiatric conditions 927–9
in neurological and physical illness 931, *932*, 933, 941, 942
and obesity *932*
and obsessive–compulsive disorder 1697
and panic disorder 1697
parasomnias *see* parasomnias
in Parkinson's disease *932*, 1072
phototherapy 1261
postoperative 1099
and post-traumatic stress disorder 927
in psychiatric conditions 930–1, *931*
psychological effects of sleep disturbance 926–7
REM sleep behaviour disorder 928, 1572, 1695
and respiratory disease *932*
and schizophrenia *931*
sleep-related breathing disorders *928*
sleep-related movement disorders *928*, 1702
and substance use disorders *931*
and tic disorders 1697
and Tourette syndrome *932*, 1697
treatment approaches 930, *930*
sleepiness, excessive daytime *see* hypersomnia
sleeplessness
in childhood and adolescence 1698–9
partial 926
total 926
sleepwalking 928, **945–6**, 1702, 1930
SLI (Specific Language Impairment) 1710, **1713–15**
SLITRK1 gene 229
SLT *see* speech and language therapy
Sly syndrome 1843
small G proteins 175
Smart, J.J.C. 134
smell, delusions of 618–19
Smith–Lemli–Opitz syndrome
behavioural phenotype 1845, *1851*
genetics 1845
physical characteristics 1845
prevalence 1845
psychiatric aspects 1845
Smith–Magenis syndrome
behavioural and psychiatric aspects 1845
genetics 1845
physical characteristics 1845
prevalence 1845
smoking
addictiveness *431*
by elderly people 1544
by psychiatric patients 511
cessation treatments 511–13
disease burden 510
genetic factors 510–11
and health 1136
mortality associated 510
and nicotine dependence **510–15**
in pregnancy 1646
prevalence 510
and psychiatric disorder in intellectual disability 1828
and schizophrenia 546
withdrawal symptoms 511
snake-handling cult 1419–20
SNAP *see* Schedule for Nonadaptive and Adaptive Personality; Secure Needs Assessment Profile
snoezelen therapy *414*
snow (cocaine) 430
SNPs (single nucleotide polymorphisms) 218, 226, 227
SNRIs 670, *670*
adverse effects 674
in childhood and adolescence 1796
in generalized anxiety disorder 735
in panic disorder 756, *756*
in persistent somatoform pain disorder 1034
pharmacodynamics *1173*, 1186, *1187*
in somatization disorder 1009
Social Adjustment Scale 1165
social and cultural anthropology 14, 15, **275–9**
Social and Emotional Aspects of Learning 1814
social anxiety disorder **739–44**, 1639
aetiology 741
and avoidant personality disorder 740, 897
and body dysmorphic disorder 1044
childhood and adolescence 740, 1665, 1666
classification 740–1
clinical presentation 740
cognitive content 1286
comorbidity 740, 744
course 741
differential diagnosis 740–1, 752, 873
epidemiology 741
functional impairment in 740
generalized/non-generalized 740
and offending 1923
with panic disorder 750
prevention 744
secondary to physical disorder 740
and substance use disorders 427
treatment and management 741–4
social bonding 888–9
social capital 1610
social cognition models 1136–7, 1140–1
social communication, problems with 1711, 1713
social constructionism and ageing 1515
social development 242–3, *242*
social drift 557
social inclusion 1819
social learning theory
and alcohol use disorders 434
and offending 1910
social phobia *see* social anxiety disorder
Social Readjustment Rating Scale 1065
social role valorization 1409–10
social skills training 1401
antisocial personality disorder 898
fire-raising 1968
schizophrenia 583
social stress theory, and transitions 1514
social suffering 848
social support
in bereavement 726
and group therapy 1352
in mood disorders 653
and psychiatric disorder in intellectual disability 1828
and response to illness 1066
and suicide 954
social theory *277*
social withdrawal in depression 634
social work *see* mental health social work
social workers
approved 1410
attachment to primary care 1411
global survey 12, *12*
socio-economic status (SES)
and anorexia nervosa 778
and anxiety disorders 1666
and child mental health 1727–8
and deliberate self-harm 959
and mood disorders 654
and offending 1912
and schizophrenia 549, 557
sociology of ageing **1512–16**
sociometry 1353
sociosomatic processes 278
sodium oxybate 941
sodium valproate *see* valproate
Solution Oriented Schools 1814
solvent abuse *see* volatile substance abuse
somatic sensation, cortical association pathways *146*, 152
somatization 57, 278, 989–90
by refugees 1497
in childhood and adolescence 1744, *1744*
and chronic fatigue syndrome 1039
cultural influences 15
definitions 996
and pain 1030, 1031
presentation in primary care 1482
subthreshold 996, *998*
and surgery 1096
somatization disorder **999–1011**
abrupt onset 1002
aetiology 1004–5
assessment 1005–6, *1005–6*
in childhood and adolescence 1744
and chronic fatigue syndrome 1037
classification *993*, 994, 999–1000, 1003
clinical features 1000–2
physical symptoms 1000–2, *1001*
psychological symptoms 1002
comorbidity 57, 870, 1002, 1004
controversial aspects 996
and conversion disorder 1015
correlates 996
course 1005
diagnosis 1003
differential diagnosis 1003–4, 1023–4
dystonia in 1016
epidemiology 996, 1004
examination 1005–6
family transmission 1004
and illness behaviour 1002
mimicking surgical conditions 1096
and pain 1031
phenomenology 996
prevalence 996, *998*, 1004
prognosis 1005
TERM model 1005, 1008, *1008*

treatment and management 1006–10, *1008*, *1009*, 1034
somatoform autonomic dysfunction *993*, 994, 1003, 1003–4
differential diagnosis 1030
and pain 1031
somatoform disorders 57, 989–90
acute/chronic 1003
assessment 994–5, *995*
and chronic fatigue syndrome 1037
classification 104, 105, 993–4, *993*, 999–1000, 1003, 1023
comorbidity 57, 994, 1002, 1004
differential diagnosis 1050–1
epidemiology **995–9**
mimicking surgical conditions 1096
multisymptomatic 1003
and pain 1031–2
problems in definition 994
treatment 994–5, *995*
undifferentiated/not otherwise specified *993*, 994, 1000, 1003, 1036, 1062
see also specific disorders
somatomedin C 165
somatosensory amplification 1025
somatostatin 165, *171*
somnophilia *833*
SORAG (Sex Offender Risk Appraisal Guide) 835, 1963
sorcery, fear of 981
SOREMP (sleep onset REM period) 941
SOS (Solution Oriented Schools) 1814
Soteria model 1393, 1396
South Africa, attitudes to psychiatric disorder 6
South Verona Outcome Study 1468–9
soy 1249
spasm, in conversion disorder 1016
spatial cueing task 246
special educational needs, meeting 1815
special educational needs coordinator 1812
Special K (ketamine) 489, **499–500**, 1186
specialized care units 1583
specific developmental disorders **1622–32**
classification 1623
diagnosis *1623*
differential diagnosis *1623*, 1639
mixed *1623*
of motor function 1623, *1623*, 1631
of scholastic skills 1623, *1623*, 1627–31
of speech and language 1622–7, *1623*
Specific Language Impairment 1710, **1713–15**
specific phobia 52, **744–50**
aetiology 745
age at onset/seeking treatment 745
in cancer 1101
childhood and adolescence 1664, 1665, 1666, 1741, 1742
classification 745
clinical features 744–5
comorbidity 745
course 745–6
differential diagnosis 766
epidemiology 745
functional impairment in 744–5
and gender 745
of illness 52, 1022, 1023
prevention 746
subtypes 745
and surgical procedures 1097
treatment and management 746
specific reading disorder 1627–9
specific speech articulation disorder 1624–5
specific spelling disorder 1629
speech and language development 240–1, *241*, 1623, 1710–11
speech and language disorder/difficulty
assessment 89
and attention-deficit hyperactivity disorder 1714
in autism 1633
in childhood and adolescence **1710–17**
classification 1711
and conduct disorder 1658
course and prognosis 1715
definitions 53
diagnosis and differential diagnosis 1712
disturbance in generation and articulation of words 53
disturbance in talking 53–4
due to sensory or CNS impairment 1623–4
expressive 1625–6
features of difficulties 1711
in frontotemporal dementias 346
identification 1715
and intellectual disability 1712
management 1715–16
and motility disorder 58
organic language disorders 54
receptive 1626
in schizotypal personality disorder 864
specific developmental disorders **1622–7**, *1624*
speech and language therapy (SLT) 1714, 1716
expressive language disorder 1625–6
selective mutism 1714
speech articulation disorder 1624–5
speed *see* amphetamine
Speed of Comprehension Test 88
spelling disorder 1629
SPET *see* single-photon emission tomography
spider naevi in alcohol use disorders 446
spina bifida occulta 156
spinal cord
histogenesis 157–8
neural induction 156
spinobulbar muscular atrophy *228*
spinocerebellar ataxia *228*
spinocerebellar degeneration 373
spiny stellate cells 148
spirit dancing ceremony 1419
spirit mediumship 1418–19
splitting 295, 297, 298, 307, 317, 1339
Spousal Assault Risk Assessment 1998
Sprachverödung 346
SPT *see* supportive psychotherapy
SRM (Self-Regulatory Model) 1138, 1140–1
SRV (social role valorization) 1409–10
SSD 719
SSP (Strange Situation Procedure) 242
SSRIs 670, *670*, 1178
in adjustment disorders 721, 1068
adverse effects 674, 1190, *1191*, 1687–8
aggression 1923
in elderly people 1555
sexual dysfunction 826
sleep disorders 1572
suicidal ideation/behaviour 1668, 1707–8, 1923
in anxiety disorders 1182
in childhood and adolescence 1668
in attempted suicide 1707–8
in autism and other pervasive developmental disorders 1640
in body dysmorphic disorder 1046, 1047–8
in cancer 1101–2, 1102, *1102*, *1103*
in childhood and adolescence 1668, 1676, 1796
choice of 674
in chronic fatigue syndrome 1040
in conversion disorder 1019–20
in dementia 416
in depression
in childhood and adolescence 1676
in elderly people 1554, *1554*
dosage *1196*
drug interactions 1175–6
in dysthymia/dysthymic disorder 685
in generalized anxiety disorder 735
in HIV/AIDS 386, 1092
in Huntington's disease 374
in hypochondriasis 1027
in intellectual disability 1875
in obsessive–compulsive disorder 769–70, 1687–8, 1688–9
in panic disorder 756, *756*, 759
in the paraphilias 838
in persistent somatoform pain disorder 1034
in personality disorders *905*, 906
pharmacodynamics *1173*, *1187*, 1188
pharmacokinetics *1172*, 1188–9, *1189*
in post-traumatic stress disorder 709
in premature ejaculation 828
in smoking cessation 513
in social anxiety disorder 743, 744
in somatization disorder 1009
and suicide risk 674
and surgery 1097–8
SSRT (stop signal reaction time task) 266
staff burnout, prevention 1449, *1449*
staff counselling services 1281–2
stages of change model 428
stalking 1917, **1970–6**
assessment 1974
and attachment 1972
classification and typology of stalkers 1971
definition 1970
and delusional disorders 1920
duration 1972
epidemiology 1970
of health professionals 1972
impact on victims 1970–1
management 1974
as obsessive–compulsive disorder 1972
psychopathology 1971–2
reduction of impact on victim 1974
risk assessment and management 1972–4, *1973*
risk of violence 1973–4, 1998
stammering 53
Standard Assessment Tests 1715
standard deviation 86
standard error of measurement 85
standard score (z) 86, *86*
standardized interview schedules 14, 284
Stanford Acute Stress Reaction Questionnaire 695
starflower 1248
startle-induced dissociative reaction 606, **983**
startle response 732, 1667
STATIC-99 1963, 1994, 1996, 1997, 1998

statistics **137–43**
- evaluating treatment effects 141–2
- modelling patterns of risk 141
- prevalence estimation 138–41
- reliability of instruments 137–8
- structural MRI studies 194–5, 196
- systematic reviews 1155–6

status cataplecticus 940
status dissociatus 944
status epilepticus 1077
- absence 1864
- complex partial 1077
- electrical 1864
- in intellectual disability 1867
- treatment 1255, 1867

status loss 5
STD *see* sexually transmitted disease
stealing, pathological **913–14**, 1924, 1942–3
stem cells
- adult, and study of ageing 1510
- embryonic, recombination studies 230

step-families 1726–7
stepped-care model 1006–7
- in adjustment disorders 1068, *1068*
- in anorexia nervosa 789
- in primary care 1484, *1485*

STEPPS (systems training for emotional predictability and problem solving) 895, 904
stereotyped behaviour in frontotemporal dementias 346
stereotypic movement disorder with intellectual disability 1683, 1851
stereotypy 5, 58, *58*
sterilization 1115–16
stigma **5–9**, 11, 1585
- and attention-deficit hyperactivity disorder 1651
- and chronic fatigue syndrome 1039–40
- combating 1408
- component processes 5
- definition 5
- and dementia 411
- and electroconvulsive therapy 1251, 1258
- global patterns of 6–7
- limitations of work on 5–6
- and neurasthenia 1040
- and personality disorder 848
- and rehabilitation 1402
- and schizophrenia 5, 6–7, 539
- in sexually transmitted disease 1091
- and suicide 953

still face paradigm 240
stillbirth 1119
stimulants *see specific drugs*
stimulus-bound behaviour 58
stimulus control in sleep disorders 936, 1572
stimulus entrapment 1005
stop signal reaction time task 266
story telling 1778
STPP *see* psychodynamic psychotherapy, brief (short-term)
Strange Situation Procedure 242
strategic therapy 1381
stratum pyramidale 148
Strengths and Difficulties questionnaires 1813
streptococcal infection
- and obsessive–compulsive disorder 1616–85
- and tic disorders 1073, 1685

streptomycin
- adverse effects *1091*
- in tuberculosis 1094

stress
- acute/chronic 720
- and adjustment disorders 720
- and ageing 1507, 1508
- and anxiety disorders 1667–8
- associated with inpatient care 1139–40
- and counselling 1278
- definitions 1065
- disorders induced by/related to 716
  - *see also specific disorders*
- effects on immune system 205, 207, 1135–6
- and health 1135–6
- illness as 1065
- and inflammatory bowel disease 1083–4
- and irritable bowel syndrome 1083
- modifiers 720
- and myocardial ischaemia 1081–2
- and REM sleep behaviour disorder 947
- and somatization disorder 1009
- transactional model 1065
- and transient global amnesia 403
- and ventricular dysrhythmias 1081
- *see also* acute stress reactions

stress–diathesis model
- personality disorders 851–2
- schizophrenia 507, 558–9, 1313
- suicide 963–4, 965

stress management (stress inoculation), in post-traumatic stress disorder 709
'stress response syndromes' 717
stressors
- in acute stress reactions 694
- traumatic 701

stria of Gennari 146
stria terminalis, bed nucleus
- in gender identity disorder 842
- in generalized anxiety disorder 733

striate cortex 146
striatum 154–5, 1684
stroke **1071–2**
- anxiety following 1071–2
- depression following 1071, 1555
- emotionalism following 1071
- sleep-wake disorders following *932*

Stroop Test *90*, *248*, 249, 255, 265
Structural Analysis of Social Behavior 852
structural magnetic resonance imaging (MRI) **191–6**
- alcohol-related dementia 400–1
- Alzheimer's disease 337
- artefacts 193–4, Plate 7
- in chronic fatigue syndrome 1039
- clinical data analysis 195
- in conjunction with PET 187
- Creutzfeldt–Jakob disease
  - sporadic/classical 353
  - variant 356
- dementia with Lewy bodies 364
- diffusion-weighted imaging 193, Plate 8
- epilepsy 1078, 1619, 1862, 1930
- frontotemporal dementias 347
- hardware 194
- head injury 389
- HIV-associated dementia 385
- Huntington's disease 372
- Korsakoff syndrome 406
- mild cognitive impairment 1537–8
- morphometry 195, Plate 9
- obsessive–compulsive disorder 768
- post-traumatic stress disorder 706
- quantitative data analysis 195–6, Plate 9
- safety 193
- scanner suite 194
- schizophrenia 179–80, *179*, 563–4
- spin echo sequence 192, *192*
- structural imaging sequences 193
- studies 194–5
- tissue contrast 192–3, *193*, Plate 7
- vascular dementia 377, 380

structural theory 294–6
Structured Clinical Interview for DSM-III and DSM-IV 70, 71, 695, 703, 1023, 1164
Structured Clinical Interview for DSM-IV Personality Disorders *858*, 859
Structured Interview of the Five-Factor Model of Personality 1164
structured interviewing *see* questionnaires
Structured Inventory of Malingered Symptoms 1057
student counselling services 1281
stupor 58, *58*
Sturge–Weber syndrome 1867
stuttering 53, 1623, 1712
subacute spongiform encephalopathies *see* prion disease
subarachnoid haemorrhage 407
subcaudate tractotomy 1267
subcultural deviance 1657
subdural haemorrhage 387
subiculum 148
subjective experience, categorization of 48
sublimation 297
subsidiarity 1896
substance P 155, 170, *171*, *173*, 206
substance use disorders
- and accidents 1110
- amphetamine **482–6**
- assessment instruments 1164
- childhood and adolescence 1600, 1604
  - comorbidity 1673
  - differential diagnosis 1672
  - treatment 1784
- classification 105
- cocaine **482–6**
- comorbidity
  - attention-deficit hyperactivity disorder 427, 1650
  - bipolar disorder 646
  - body dysmorphic disorder 1044
  - bulimia nervosa 804, 806
  - in childhood and adolescence 1673
  - cyclothymia/cyclothymic disorder 687
  - depression 649
  - persistent somatoform pain disorder 1032
  - schizophrenia 427, 507, 546, 558, 1919
  - social anxiety disorder 427
  - somatization disorder 1002
- and conditioning 428, 434
- effects on the brain 429–30, *429*
- elderly people 1519, **1540–6**
- genetics 428–9
- global disease burden 10
- hallucinogens 487–9
- and homicide 1926
- and infection 430
- inpatient care 1453
- legal issues 1927–8

motivation for 426–7
and offending **1926–8**
opioids **473–82**
and pain 427
parental, effects on child development 1754
PCP **486–7**
pharmacological aspects **426–32**
in pregnancy 480, *480*, 1117–18, 1614, 1615–16, 1754
prevalence *285*
prisoners 480, *1934*
psychological aspects **426–32**
relapse prevention 428
routes and risks of addiction 430–1, *431*
services **515–20**
commissioning 517–19
levels 516–17
local coordination 515–16
needs assessment 517, 518–19
performance analysis 519–20
target groups 517–18
and sleep-wake disorders *931*
and suicide 955, 956, 1704
and surgery 1098
terminology 427–8
treatment
cognitive-behaviour therapy 428, 1784
complementary medicines 1249
counselling 1279
interpersonal psychotherapy 1324
motivational interviewing 428
outcome 519, *519*
pharmacotherapy **1242–7**
and stages off change model 428
therapeutic communities 1396
tiered 516–17
and violence 1449, 1926
risk management 1999
see also specific substances
substantia nigra 154
subthalamic nucleus 154
subthreshold disorders **680–92**, 716, 718–19, 722
see also specific disorders
sucralfate 1175
sudden infant death syndrome 1119, 1698
suffering 848
suicidal ideation 951, 952, 955
and antidepressants 971, 973, 1192, 1668, 1707–8, 1796, 1923
in childhood and adolescence 1703
in parents 1923
prevalence 960
provoking factors 961
see also suicide
suicide
and adjustment disorders 718, 722
and aggression 970
and alcohol use disorders 427, 444, 955, 956
altruistic 954
anomic 954
and anorexia nervosa 955
and anxiety disorders 955
attempted *see* deliberate self-harm
biological aspects **963–9**
and bipolar disorder 1704
and body dysmorphic disorder 1044
by imitation (Werther effect) 952, 1706
by inpatients 1404
and cancer 1102–3
childhood and adolescence 1674, **1702–10**
and choice of antidepressants 670, 674, 970–1, 1192
choice of method 952, 973
and conduct disorder 1704
cultural factors 953–4, 1704
definition 951
and depression 634, 955, 1704
determinants 953–5, *954*
education regarding 974
egoistic 954
elderly people 976, 1518, 1527, 1551, **1564–7**
and electroconvulsive therapy 1255
epidemiology **951–7**
and epilepsy 1080
ethical issues 30
extended 1923
family 981–2
fatalistic 954
following head injury 393
following homicide 1923, 1938
and gender 1704
genetics 954–5, 966–7
global statistics 10
and hypochondriasis 1026
and hypothalamic–pituitary–adrenal axis 965
and impulsivity 970
indirect 1565
and life events 954, 969, 1705
media portrayal of behaviour 974
and mental disorders 955–6, *955*
modelling behaviour 963–4
neurobiology 954–5, 966–7
'no-suicide' contracts 1707
and noradrenergic system 965
pacts 952, 1706
and panic disorder 1704
and personality disorders 955, 956, 969
in physical illness 1133
physician-assisted 318
and pregnancy 1116, 1119
prevention **969–78**, 1449, 1708–9, 1992
and problem-solving 969
process 951–2, *952*
protective factors 951–2
psychology of 954
public health aspects 952–5
rates 952–3, *953*
rational 30, 1565
reliability of statistics 951
risk after deliberate self-harm 961
risk behaviours in childhood and adolescence 1605
risk factors 951–2, *953*, 971, *971*, *972*, 1449
role of internet 1706
and schizophrenia 545–6, 956
and self-esteem 970
and serotonergic system 955, 964–5, 970, 1705
and social support 954
sociological theories 954
and somatization disorder 1002
stigma of 953
stress–diathesis model 963–4, 965
and substance use disorders 955, 956, 1704
and terminal illness 1070
victim characteristics 955
Sullivan, Harry Stack 310
sulphonamide *1091*
sulpiride in tic disorders 1073, 1688
sumatriptan 1171
sundowning 336
suoyang 980
super K (ketamine) 489, **499–500**, 1186
superego 294, 296, 306, 313, 849
superego defences 297
superior parietal lobe 245
superior temporal sulcus 146
supervisory attention system 249
supported employment 1401
supported housing 1400
supportive-expressive therapy, avoidant personality disorder 897
supportive psychotherapy (SPT) 300–1
borderline personality disorder 868
elderly people 1574
indications and contraindications 301
outcome research 303–4
personality disorders 318–19
post-traumatic stress disorder 709
suprachiasmatic nucleus, and circadian rhythms 925, 1260
SureStart programme 1663
surgery **1096–100**
assessment of response to 1097
capacity to consent to 1096–7
postoperative complications and interventions 1098–100
preoperative assessment and intervention 1096–8
transplantation 456, 1087, 1097
see also neurosurgery for mental disorder
surrogate motherhood 1115
surveys
in case-finding 541
design 139, 541
results analysis 139–40
survivor guilt 1106
susto 984
SVR-20 (Sexual Violence Risk-20) 1998
SWAN scale 1645
SWAP-200 1164
sweating in alcohol withdrawal 439
Sydenham's chorea 767, 1685
Sylvian fissure 144
sympathetic nervous system 156, 206
symptom validity tests in malingering 1057
symptoms
conversion 57, 1012–13
definition 47
developmental differences in expression 1600
dissociative 1012–13
distinction between form and content 48, 63
effects on function 63
elaboration 57
feigning 57
functional (without organic pathology/ medically unexplained) 989–90, 992, 999
aetiology 992–3
assessment and treatment principles 994–5, *995*
atypical nature 1001
classification 993–4
descriptions 1001, *1001*
epidemiology 995–9
and psychiatric disorder 993
terminology 992
measures of severity 1465
negative, assessment instruments 72
prodromal/subthreshold 1607

symptoms (*cont.*)
psychology of 1137
subjective 1000
understanding of 47–8
syndrome of subjective doubles 623
syntax, problems with 1711
syphilis **1093–4**
meningovascular 1093
systematic lupus erythematosus 1086–7
systematic reviews 123–4, *126*, 1152–3, 1466, *1466*
advantages 1153
limitations 1153–4
methods 1154–6
sources 1156–7
systems theory in family therapy 1381–2
systems training for emotional predictability and problem solving 895, 904

T helper cells and immune function 206
T3 (triiodothyronine) 163, 675, 784
T4 (thyroxine) 163, 1101
TA (transactional analysis) 1277
Tabernanthe iboga 488, 1249, *1250*
tabes dorsalis 1093–4
tachycardia in alcohol withdrawal 448
tachykinin receptors *173*
tachykinins 171, *171*
tachyphasia 53
tacrine 1241
tadalafil 828
taijinkyofushio 982
Taiwan, neurasthenia 1061
tandospirone 735, 1212
tangentiality 53
tanning, compulsive 1044
tardive dyskinesia 59
complementary medicines 1249
differential diagnosis 373
drug-induced 1223
tau protein 228
in Alzheimer's disease 338, 339
in dementia with Lewy bodies 362
in frontotemporal dementias 344, 347
in mild cognitive impairment 1537
tauopathies 338
Tavistock Clinic 1353, 1408
Tay-Sachs disease 1825, 1865
TDP-43 protein 348
TEACH (Tests of Everyday Attention for Children) 89
teachers
and schools liaison service 1813
training in mental health 1812
technical eclecticism 1278
teeth, enamel erosion in bulimia nervosa 804
Tegretol *see* carbamazepine
telencephalon 156–7
telephone helplines 975, 1282, 1708, 1805–6
telephone scatalogia *833*, 1961
Telephone Search 88, 89
telomerase 1508
telomeres 223
loss with age 1508
temazepam 1179
in cancer *1102*
as a hypnotic 1183
misuse 430, 491, 1179, 1183
pharmacokinetics *1172*, 1178
temperament 79
assessment 79–80, *80*, 680
clinical 82–3
in childhood and adolescence 235, 238, *238*, 1601, 1665, 1667
with intellectual disability 1850
definition 847
dimensions 79–80, *80*, 316, *316*
hyperthymic **690–1**
and mood disorders 654, 658, 680
and personality 316, *316*
Temperament and Character Inventory 79, *80*, 81, *81*, *858*
temperature regulation, in anorexia nervosa 785
temporal difference learning 259
Temporal Judgement Test *90*
temporal lobes
in alcohol use disorders *183*
anatomy 146, *147*, 148
in mood disorders *182*
in schizophrenia *178*
temporoparietal junction 245
TEMPS-A 680
Tenancy Sustainment Programme 1501
teratology, neurobehavioural 1614
TERM model 1005, 1008, *1008*
terminal illness
adjustment to 1069–70
art therapy 1415
in childhood and adolescence 1743–4
terrorism 1987
Test of Everyday Attention 89
Test of Malingered Memory *see* ToMM
testosterone 815, 834
interventions to reduce levels 838
reduced levels 826
replacement therapy 828
therapy in gender identity disorder 843
testosterone antagonists in adolescents with intellectual disability 1852
Tests of Everyday Attention for Children 1647
tetrabenazine in Huntington's disease 374
tetracyclic antidepressants
pharmacodynamics *1173*
pharmacokinetics *1172*
tetracycline transactivator system 230, 231
δ-9-tetrahydrocannabinol 172, 507
TF-CBT (trauma-focused cognitive-behaviour therapy) 708, 1109, 1111, 1730
TFP (transference-focused psychotherapy) 304, 318–19, 894, 895, 904
TGA (transient global amnesia) 59, 403
thalamus
in absence epilepsy 204
in alcohol use disorders *183*, 400, 406
cortical projections 150, Plate 2
development 158
infarction 407
and memory 254
in neurofibromatosis 1844
in obsessive–compulsive disorder 1684
in schizophrenia *178*, 180
THC (δ-9-tetrahydrocannabinol) 172, 507
theft **1941–3**
in conduct disorder 1656
management 1942
motivational classification 1941–2
prevalence 1941
shoplifting 1943
types of 1941
see also kleptomania
Theory of Reasoned Action/Theory of Planned Behaviour 1137, 1140
therapeutic alliance 299
in brief psychodynamic psychotherapy 1328
in cognitive-behaviour therapy 903, 1307
in counselling 1275
importance of 317
in rehabilitation 1400
therapeutic communities **1391–8**
addiction 1391
background 1392–3
in childhood and adolescence 1397
core standards 1392, *1392*
culture of enquiry 1393
definitions 1392
in first episode psychosis 1396
indications and contraindications 1394, *1395*
in intellectual disability 1397
living–learning situation 1393
for offenders 1396
pathways and process 1394–5
in personality disorders 892, 896, 905, 1395–6
principles (themes) 1392
research evidence 1395–7
in severe and enduring mental disorder 1396–7
staff and client roles *1394*
staff training 1393–4
in substance use disorders 1396
technique 1393
therapeutic index 431
therapist
in family therapy 1386–7
in group therapy 1354, *1354*
neutrality 1339, 1340
theta rhythm 203
thiamine
deficiency
in alcohol use disorders 405, 408–9, 444–5
in anorexia nervosa 785
supplementation in alcohol withdrawal 450
thinking
abstract 53
acceleration of 53
concrete 53
control of 53
disorders of 50–4
fantasy/dereistic/autistic 50
flow of 52–3
imaginative 50
incoherent 53
in mood disorders 52
negative 52
overinclusive 53
rational/conceptual 50
retardation of 53
types of 50
thiopentone 1178
thioridazine *1209*
administration *1214*
adverse effects *1212*, 1222, 1532
pharmacodynamics *1211*
pharmacokinetics *1172*
pharmacology 1210
thiothixene *1209*
administration *1214*
adverse effects *1212*
pharmacodynamics *1211*
third sector *see* voluntary organizations

third sex 844
Thorn Initiative 1405
thought-action fusion in obsessive–compulsive disorder 1783
thought blocking 53
thought broadcast 527
thought content, elderly people 1527
Thought Disorder Index 528
thought disorders
  differential diagnosis 538
  in schizophrenia 527, 573
thought insertion 527
Thought, Language and Communication Scale 528
thought process abnormalities in delirium 326
thought stopping
  in insomnia 936–7
  in obsessive–compulsive disorder 770
thought withdrawal 527
threat-control override 1919
thymine 223
thyroid
  function
    in depression 661
    and suicide 966
  tumours 1101
thyroid-stimulating hormone 163, 966, 1204
thyrotrophin, in depression 661
thyrotrophin-releasing hormone 163, *171*, 706, 966
thyroxine 163, 1101
tiagabine 1237, *1867*
tianeptine 1186
tiapride 1688
tic disorders
  childhood and adolescence 1073, **1680–93**
    aetiology 1683–5
    age of onset 1681
    classification 1682
    clinical features 1681
    comorbidity 1681–2
    course and prognosis 1685
    diagnosis 1682–3
    differential diagnosis 1682–3
    epidemiology 1683
    and gender 1681
    prevention 1690
    treatment 1685–90
  chronic motor 1682
  chronic vocal 1682
  genetics 229, 1073, 1684
  and intellectual disability 1851
  and obsessive–compulsive disorder 765, 1073, 1681
  secondary 1073
  transient 1073, 1682
  see also Tourette syndrome
tics 58, *58*, 1681
  complex motor 1681
  complex verbal 1681
  motor 1073, 1681
  phonic 1073
  secondary 1683
  stimulant-induced 1651
  vocal 1681
time-limited psychotherapy 1327, 1332–3
time out on the spot 414
time sampling 97
timetabled tasks 1376–7
tina (methamphetamine) **497–8**
tinnitus, chronic 1265
TMS *see* transcranial magnetic stimulation
TNF- α (tumour necrosis factor- α) 209
tobacco *see* smoking
tocophobia 1117, 1121
Token Test 89
tolerance 427, 428
'tomboyism' 1719
ToMM 1057
TOOTS (time out on the spot) 414
topiramate (Topamax) **1236–7**
  adverse effects 1236
  dosage and administration 1237
  drug interactions 1236–7
  in epilepsy 1080
  indications and contraindications 1236
  overdose 1236
  in personality disorders *905*, 906
  pharmacokinetics 1236, *1867*
  pharmacology 1236
  in pregnancy 1236
  structure *1232*
  withdrawal 1237
topographic theory 294
torture
  of refugees 1494, 1495
  of women 1498
torulosis 1093
Tourette syndrome **1073–4**
  aetiology 1073
  childhood and adolescence 1613, 1680–93
  differential diagnosis 1644
  epidemiology 1073
  genetics 229, 1073, 1684
  with intellectual disability 1851
  and obsessive–compulsive disorder 765, 1073
  psychiatric comorbidity 1073
  and sleep-wake disorders *932*, 1697
  treatment and management 1073–4
  see also tic disorders
Tower of London task 255, 265
toxoplasmosis 1863
  in HIV/AIDS 1093
  maternal, and schizophrenia 548
toys, in child and adolescent assessment 1604
TPQ *see* Temperament and Character Inventory; Tridimensional Personality Questionnaire
traditional healers 15
  and diagnosis 65
  use by refugees 1497
Trail Making Test *90*, 326
Trailblazers 1487–8
training
  approved social workers 1410
  in child and adolescent psychotherapy/counselling 1768–9
  in cognitive-behaviour therapy 1312
  community psychiatric nurses 1405
  in consultation-liaison psychiatry 1147
  in counselling 1282–3
  in couple therapy 1379
  in family therapy 1389–90
  in interpersonal psychotherapy 1325
  primary care workers 1487–8
  in psychoanalysis 1346
  staff in therapeutic communities 1393–4
  staff working with adults with psychiatric disorder and intellectual disability 1889–90
trance 276
  and filicide 1125
trance-based healing systems 1418–19
tranquillizers *see* anxiolytics
transactional analysis 1277
transcranial magnetic stimulation (TMS/rTMS) 671, 1258, **1263–6**
  adverse effects 1263
  in chronic neuropathic pain 1265
  in chronic tinnitus 1265
  comparison with ECT 1264–5
  in depression 1264
  mechanism of action 1263
  in obsessive–compulsive disorder 1265
  in Parkinson's disease 1265
  in post-stroke depression 1555
  in schizophrenia 1265
  sham treatment 1264
  technique 1263–4
transcription factors 224
transcultural psychiatry **13–16**
  clinical relevance 13–14
  and epidemiology 14
  and social anthropology 15
transference 297–8, 298–9, 300, 1338, 1342–3
  bidimensional quality 314
  in brief psychodynamic psychotherapy 1328–9, 1330
  in childhood psychodynamic psychotherapy 1765, 1772
  dimensions 1343
  eroticized 1343
  idealizing 1343
  mirroring 1343
  and non-compliance 317
  object-relations theory model 298–9
  and play 1770
  and psychodynamic psychiatry 314
  and resistance 315
  reverse 1343
transference-focused psychotherapy 304, 318–19, 894, 895, 904
transformation 294
transgenic animals 230
transient global amnesia 59, 403
transient ischaemic attacks 364, 403
transitional objects 309, 1603, 1694
  in pharmacotherapy 317
transitional space 1770
transketolase 408
transmission disequilibrium test 220, *220*
transorbital lobotomy 1267
transplantation surgery 456, 1087, 1097
transsexualism *see* gender identity disorder
transtheoretical model 1137
transvestic fetishism 832, *833*, 834, *836*, 837, 844
tranylcypromine 670, *670*
  adverse effects *1191*
  dosage *1196*
  drug interactions 1175
  limitations on use 1188
  in panic disorder *756*
  pharmacodynamics *1187*
  pharmacokinetics *1172*, *1189*
trauma
  assessment 1496–7
  associated with post-traumatic stress disorder 704
  in childhood and adolescence 1601, 1697, **1728–31**, 1744, 1762

trauma (*cont.*)
counselling following 1279–80
creeping 1903
debriefing 1497
group therapy with victims 1365
nature of memories of 705–6
personal meanings of events 705
prevalence 704
to refugees 1494–6, *1495*, 1496–7, 1497
story 1497
see also accidents
trauma-focused cognitive-behaviour therapy 708, 1109, 1111, 1730
traumatic bonding 1982
trazodone *670*, 671
adverse effects 1190, *1191*
in anxiety disorders 1182
in cancer *1103*
in dementia 415
dosage *1196*
in elderly people 1554, *1554*
in generalized anxiety disorder 735
pharmacodynamics *1173*, *1187*, 1188
pharmacokinetics *1172*, 1189, *1189*
as sedative 1194
treatment
adherence to 1140
behaviour 1140–2
cultural variations in 1442–3
ethical issues 29–30
evaluation 141–2
physical treatment **1151–8**
psychotherapy **1158–67**
involuntary/compulsory 30, 1053–4
manuals 1161
non-compliance
determinants 1140–1
and estimation of efficacy 142
incidence 1140
intentional/unintentional 1140
psychodynamic approaches to 317
refusal
advance directives 1577
in physical illness 1133
right to 29–30, 1565
in surgery 1096–7
right to effective 29
right to 29
as security 2017
treatment foster care, in conduct disorder 1662
treatment gap 12, *13*
Treatment Outcomes Profile 519, *519*
Treatment Services Review 1165
tremor
in alcohol withdrawal 438–9
in HIV-associated dementia 384
lithium-induced 1204
psychogenic 1016
Treponema pallidum 1447
TRH (thyrotrophin-releasing hormone) 163, 171, 706, 966
triangular model 310
triazolam 1169
adverse effects 1183
potential for misuse 491
trichobezoars 915
trichotillomania 618, **915–16**
tricyclic antidepressants 669–70, *670*
in adjustment disorders 1068
adverse effects 674, 1188, *1191*
delirium 1532
in elderly people 1555
hypersomnia 939
postural hypotension 1529
sexual dysfunction 826–7
in attention-deficit hyperactivity disorder 1651
in cancer 1102, *1103*
in childhood and adolescence 1676, 1796
in conversion disorder 1019–20
drug interactions 1194
in elderly people 1554, *1554*
in HIV/AIDS 386, 1092
in panic disorder 756, *756*
in persistent somatoform pain disorder 1034
in personality disorders *905*, 906
pharmacodynamics *1173*, 1186, *1187*
pharmacokinetics *1172*, 1188, *1189*
in post-traumatic stress disorder 709
slow metabolisers/slow hydroxylation 1188
in somatization disorder 1009
suicide risk 674, 1707
Tridimensional Personality Questionnaire 654, 851, 887
trifluoperazine *1209*
administration *1214*
adverse effects *1212*
in anxiety disorders 1182
pharmacodynamics *1211*
pharmacokinetics 50
trihexylphenidyl 1225
triiodothyronine 163, 675, 784
Trileptal *see* oxcarbazepine
trimethoprim-sulphamethoxazole *1091*
trimipramine *670*, *1187*, *1189*, *1191*, *1196*
Triple P programme 1791
trisomy 228
trisomy 21 *see* Down syndrome
Trk (tyrosine kinase) receptors 159
true score (*t*) 85, 92
trypanosomiasis 942
tryptamine 500–1
tryptophan 662, 1248
tryptophan hydroxylase (TPH1) gene 652
TSH (thyroid-stimulating hormone) 163, 966, 1204
tTA system (tetracycline transactivator system) 230, 231
tuberculosis **1094**
tuberous sclerosis
and autism 1075, 1635
behavioural and psychiatric aspects 1075, 1846, 1852
effects on the family 1884
genetics 1075, 1845, *1866*
infantile spasms in 1863
physical characteristics 1846, 1850
prevalence 1845
'Tuesday blues' 496
Tuke, William 17
tumour necrosis factor-α 209
Turkey, attitudes to psychiatric disorder 6
Turner syndrome
behavioural and psychiatric aspects 1840–1
genetics 224, 1840
mouse model 225
physical characteristics 1840
prevalence 1840
12-step programmes 451–2, *452*, 477, *477*
twilight states 60, 1531
twin similarity questionnaire 216
twin studies **215–16**
anxiety disorders 1667
attention-deficit hyperactivity disorder 1646
autism 1635–6
chronic fatigue syndrome 1039
conduct disorder 1659
depression 649
eating disorders 781–2, 806
in gene–environment interaction 217–18
hypochondriasis 1024
longevity 1507
mood disorders 651
obsessive–compulsive disorder 768
post-traumatic stress disorder 707
schizophrenia 554
social anxiety disorder 741
specific phobia 745
two-by-two table 280, *280*
tyrosine kinase receptors 159

ubiquitin
in frontotemporal dementias 344
in Lewy bodies 362, 369
ulcerative colitis 1083–4
unconscious
dynamic 294
and the ego 295
Freudian theory of 293–4
and the id 294–5
in psychodynamic psychiatry 313–14
unconscious phantasy 307
uncus 146
UNHCR (United Nations High Commission for Refugees) 1493
Unified PD Rating Scale 363
United Kingdom
cost of psychiatric disorder 11
national prevalence study of psychiatric disorder in childhood and adolescence 1595–6
neurasthenia as diagnostic entity 1061
United Nations
Convention against Torture and Other Cruel Inhuman or Degrading Treatment or Punishment 1494
Convention on the Rights of the Child 1731
Convention on the Rights of Persons with Disabilities 1896–7
Declaration of Human Rights 1427, 1494
Declaration on the Rights of Mentally Retarded Persons 1819, 1895–6
High Commission for Refugees 1493
MI principles 1427
United States
art therapy 1414
attitudes to psychiatric disorder 6
child abuse legislation 1732
cost of psychiatric disorder 11
group therapy 1353–4
neurasthenia as diagnostic entity 1060, 1061
United States–United Kingdom Diagnostic Project 71
universe score 92
Unverricht–Lundborg disease 1864, *1866*, 1868
uracil 223
urbanization 1728
urinary incontinence
in dementia 417

following neurosurgery for mental disorder 1268
urocortin 661
urophilia *833*
utility, measurement of 1475
utilization behaviour in frontotemporal dementias 346
utilization delay 1137

VaD *see* dementia, vascular
vagina 818, 822
vaginismus 823
vagus nerve stimulation 671, 1258, **1269**
Valeriana officinalis (valerian) 1248, 1249, *1250*
validation therapy in dementia *414*
validity 85, 92, 95
of assessment instruments 140–1, 284
in classification in childhood and adolescence 1590–1
concurrent *86*
construct *86*
content *86*
discriminant 859
face *86*
factorial *86*
incremental *86*
internal vs. external 1159
of outcome measures 1465
predictive *86*
of randomized controlled trials 127–8
of systematic reviews *126*
types *86*
valproate 1198, 1200, **1231–3**
adverse effects 1169, *1200*, 1204, 1232
in bipolar disorder 671, 672, 677, 1556
in childhood and adolescence 1798
choice of 1866
in cyclothymia/cyclothymic disorder 689
in dementia 415
dosage and administration 1233, *1233*
drug interactions 1175, 1205, 1232–3, 1866
indications and contraindications 1232
mechanism of action *1200*
monitoring therapy 1176
overdose 1232
in personality disorders *905*
pharmacodynamics 1173
pharmacokinetics 1203, 1232, *1867*
pharmacology 1201, *1202*, *1203*, 1231–2
in pregnancy and breast feeding 1118, 1169, 1232
response correlates *1199*
in schizophrenia 591
structure *1232*
therapeutic profile *1199*
withdrawal 1206–7, 1233
valpromide 1231
value learning 259
values **32–8**
ethical 32–3
in the multi-disciplinary team 33–5, *34*
values-based practice **32–8**
and evidence-based medicine 33
key points *37*
key skills areas *33*
in the multi-disciplinary team *34*, 35, *36*
values statement 43
Valuing People 1819, 1878, 1879
vardenafil 828
varenicline 513
vasopressin 815
and aggressiveness 889
and social bonding 888
vCJD *see* Creutzfeldt–Jakob disease, variant
velo-cardio-facial syndrome
behavioural and psychiatric aspects 1826, 1846
genetics 1846
physical characteristics 1846
prevalence 1846
veneroneurosis 1094
venlafaxine 670, *670*
adverse effects *1191*
in body dysmorphic disorder 1047
in cancer *1103*
in childhood and adolescence 1676
dosage *1196*
drug interactions 1176
in elderly people 1554, *1554*
in generalized anxiety disorder 735
in panic disorder 756, *756*
pharmacodynamics *1173*, 1186, *1187*
pharmacokinetics 1188, *1189*
in social anxiety disorder 743, 744
ventilators, weaning from 1099
ventral anterior nucleus 150
ventral horn 157
ventral lateral nucleus 150
ventral parieto-frontal network 245
ventral root 157
ventricular dysrhythmias 1081
ventricular zone 157
ventriculomegaly 388
verapamil 1200–1, 1201, 1205, 1206
verbal fluency tests 264
verbal recall 264
verbigeration 54, 58, *58*
very-late-onset schizophrenia-like psychosis 1518–19
vesicular monoamine transporters 170, *170*
Viagra® (sildenafil) 821, 828
victims
of burglary/robbery 1986
in childhood and adolescence 1986–7
empathy with 2000
of hate crimes 1987
impact of criminal victimization **1984–90**
immediate and short-term effects 1984–5
long-term effects 1985
primary 1902
of rape/sexual assault 1985–6
secondary 1902–3, 1985
support groups 1986, 1987, 1988
of terrorism 1987
treatment 1987–8
of workplace violence 1986
video replay techniques, psychological 1109
video-telemetry, in epilepsy 1078
vigabatrin
adverse effects 1079
in epilepsy 1080
pharmacokinetics *1867*
vigilance 59, 247, 264
Vineland Adaptive Behaviour Scales 1821
violence
adolescent *see* antisocial behaviour, adolescent
and alcohol consumption 1926
in alcohol use disorders 453
and body dysmorphic disorder 1044
and delusional disorder/delusions 1920, 1929
domestic 1449, **1981–3**
and conduct disorder 1659–60
during pregnancy 1117
gender-based 1495, 1498
homophobic 1987
in inpatient settings 1404
and mental disorder 1937
and offending 1918, 2010–11
prevention 1449
racially-motivated 1987
to refugees 1494–6, *1495*
risk assessment and management **1991–2002**
and schizophrenia 1919, 1995, *1999*
situational factors 1914
and stalking 1973–4, 1998
and substance use disorders 1449, 1926, 1999
in the workplace 1986
see also aggression
Violence Risk Appraisal Guide 835, 1994, 1996, 1997, 1998
viral infection
and chronic fatigue syndrome 1038–9
and hypersomnia 942
risk of in opioid use 475
Virchow, Rudolph 276
vision
cortical association pathways *147*, 152
dysfunction in conversion disorder 1017
impairment following head injury 391
vision statement 43
visual backward masking paradigm 259
Visual Object and Space Perception Battery 264
visual search paradigm 246–7
vitamin A, teratogenic effects 1614
vitamin B1 deficiency
in alcohol use disorders 405, 408–9, 444–5
in anorexia nervosa 785
vitamin B12 deficiency 1087–8
vitamin E
as cognitive enhancer 1248
drug interactions *1250*
in tardive dyskinesia 1249
'vitamin K' (ketamine) 489, **499–500**, 1186
VMAT (vesicular monoamine transporters) 170, *170*
VNS (vagus nerve stimulation) 671, 1258, **1269**
vocabulary, problems with 1711
vocational training/rehabilitation 1400–1
for people with intellectual disability and psychiatric disorder 1889
in schizophrenia 583
volatile substance abuse (VSA) **502–6**
cognitive effects 92–3
health issues 504
mortality associated 503–4, *504*
in pregnancy 504
prevalence 503
prevention 505–6
product range *503*
treatment 504–5
volition 1012
disorders in schizophrenia 530
voluntarism 29
voluntary organizations
and community mental health services 1460
counselling by 1279, 1281
role of **1490–2**

vomiting
in alcohol withdrawal 449
in anorexia nervosa 782–3, 784, 794
in bulimia nervosa 802–3
voodoo death 981
voyeurism 832, *833*, *836*, 1960, 1961
VRAG (Violence Risk Appraisal Guide) 835, 1994, 1996, 1997, 1998
VRE (virtual reality exposure) 746
VSA *see* volatile substance abuse
vulvar vestibulitis syndrome (VVS) 823

WAIS-III^UK (Wechsler Adult Intelligence Scale-Third Edition UK Version) 87, *88*, 89, 264
wandering in dementia 415
warfarin
adverse effects 1532
drug interactions 1174, 1233
waxy flexibility 58, *58*
Wechsler Adult Intelligence Scale - Third Edition UK Version 87, *88*, 89, 264
Wechsler Intelligence Scale for Children - IV UK Version 87, *88*
Wechsler Memory Scale - Third Edition 89, *89*, 253, 255, 264
Wechsler Objective Reading Dimensions Test 89
Wechsler Preschool and Primary Scale of Intelligence - Revised 87
Wechsler Scale for IQ 1821
Wechsler Test of Adult Reading 264
Weekly Activity Schedule 1307–8, *1308*
weight gain
in antipsychotic therapy 1223
following neurosurgery for mental disorder 1269
following weight loss 1084
weight loss 1084
Wernicke–Korsakoff syndrome 59, 92, **399–402**, 405–6, 408–9, 444–5, 785
and aggression 1929
memory impairment 252
neuropathology 182–3
prevention 450, 1542
Wernicke's area 153, *153*
Wernicke's dysphasia 1527
West syndrome 1862, 1863
Western Aphasia Battery 89
WFSAD (World Fellowship for Schizophrenia and Applied Disorders) 1491
'what if' syndrome 751
wheel of change *451*
whiplash injury and whiplash-associated disorder 1002, 1056, 1108
Whiteley Index 1023
whizz *see* amphetamine
WHO *see* World Health Organization
WHO/PIRS (Psychological Impairments Rating Scale) 72
whole-person medicine 66
widowhood 1513
wild yam 1249
Williams syndrome
behavioural phenotype 1613, 1614, 1846, *1851*, 1858
genetics 1846
physical characteristics 1846
prevalence 1846
psychiatric aspects 1846
Willis, Thomas 630, *631*
Wilson's disease 537, 1084
Winnicott, Donald 309, 313, 1770
WISC-IV^UK (Wechsler Intelligence Scale for Children - IV UK Version) 87, *88*
Wisconsin Card Sort test *248*, 249, 255, 265, 266, 563
Wisconsin Personality Disorders Inventory (WISPI) 858, *858*
withdrawal 427
schizoid 308
witnesses
children as **1761–3**
expert *see* expert witness
WMT (Word Memory Test) 1057
Wnt (wingless) gene 156
Wolf, Alexander 1354
women
alcohol use disorders 454–5, 464
homicide by 1938
torture 1498
word-blindness, pure 54
word-deafness, pure 54
word-dumbness, pure 54
Word Memory Test 1057
word salad 54
working through 299, 1340
workplace
counselling services 1281–2
violence 1986
World Development Report: investing in health 10
World Fellowship for Schizophrenia and Applied Disorders 1491
World Health Organization (WHO)
CHOICE project 1477
Division (Section) of Mental Health 23
Health for All 969
and mental health public policy 1427
Project Atlas 11
World Health Report 2001 10, 12, 1427, 1606
World Mental Health Survey 645
World Psychiatric Association 23
WPPSI-III (Wechsler Preschool and Primary Scale of Intelligence - Revised) 87
wrist actigraphy 934, 1697
WTAR (Wechsler Test of Adult Reading) 264
X chromosome 223
females with single 225
inactivation 224
X-linked intellectual disability (X-linked mental retardation) 1831–2, 1839–40, 1842
xanomeline 1241
XXX syndrome
behavioural and psychiatric aspects 1841
genetics 1841
physical characteristics 1841
prevalence 1841
XYY syndrome
behavioural and psychiatric aspects 1841
genetics 1841
physical characteristics 1841
prevalence 1841

yaba (methamphetamine) **497–8**
Yale-Brown Obsessive-Compulsive Scale 1163
Yalom, Irving 1354, 1355
yaun 983
yearning 725
Yi-Jing 1420
yohimbine 706, 754, 828
Young Mania Rating Scale 1164, 1675
Young Offenders Institutions 1945
Youth Justice System 1945, 1947
Youth Offending Teams 1945

zalcitabine *1091*
zaleplon *1102*, 1178, 1179, 1183
zar ceremonies 1419
zeitgebers 1260, 1261
zidovudine *1091*, 1092
zimelidine 409
ziprasidone 1199, 1209, *1209*, 1797
administration *1214*, 1218–19
adverse effects *1212*, 1224
pharmacodynamics 1210, *1211*
pharmacokinetics 1222
ZKPQ (Zuckerman–Kuhlman Personality Questionnaire) 81, *81*
zolmitriptan 1171
zolpidem 1178, 1179, 1182–3
in cancer *1102*
pharmacodynamics 1171
zonisamide (Zonegran) 1198, 1237
Zoo Map Test *90*
zopiclone 1171, 1178, 1179, 1182–3
zotepine 1209
Zuckerman–Kuhlman Personality Questionnaire 81, *81*
zuclopenthixol *1172*
Zung's Self-Rating Anxiety Scale 717
Zung's Self-Rating Depression Scale 717